LNMP	last normal menstrual period
LP	lumbar puncture
LUL	left upper lobe
MAR	medication administration record
MDI	metred-dose inhaler
mEq	milliequivalents
mm Hg	millimetres of mercury (measure of BP)
MRI	magnetic resonance imagery
MRSA	methicillin-resistant *Staphylococcus aureus*
MS	multiple sclerosis
NANDA	North American Nursing Diagnosis Association
NG	nasogastric
NPO	nil per os (L.); nothing by mouth
NS	normal saline (solution)
nsg	nursing
NVS	neurological vital signs
o.d.	once daily
OT	occupational therapy; occupational therapist
OTC	over-the-counter (drugs)
ORIF	open reduction and internal fixation
p	post (L.); after
PC	potential complication
PCA	patient-controlled analgesia
pCO_2	carbon dioxide partial pressure (tension)
PCP	*Pneumocystis carinii* pneumonia
PEFR	peak expiratory flow rate
PEG Tube	percutaneous endoscopic gastrostomy
pO_2	oxygen partial pressure (tension)
PHC	primary health care
PICC	peripherally inserted central catheter
PID	pelvic inflammatory disease
PLISSIT	permission, limited information, specific suggestions, intensive therapy (model)
PM	postmortem
PMI	point of maximal impulse
PPN	peripheral parenteral nutrition
PO	per os (L.); by mouth
prn	pro re nata (L.); as necessary
pt	patient
PT	physiotherapy; physiotherapist/ prothrombin time
PTT	partial thromboplastin time
PVR	postvoid residual
q	every
qh	every hour
q.i.d.	four times daily
q2h	every two hours
R	right
RBC	red blood cell
RDS	respiratory distress syndrome
REM	rapid eye movement (sleep)
RLL	right lower lobe
RML	right middle lobe
RN	registered nurse
ROM	range of motion
RSV	respiratory syncytial virus
RUL	right upper lobe
r/t	related to
$\bar{s}$	sine (L.); without
SA	surface area
SaO_2	oxygen saturation (of hemoglobin)
STAT	immediately
STD	sexually transmitted disease
SW	social work; social worker
T&A	tonsillectomy and adenoidectomy
TAH	total abdominal hysterectomy
TB	tuberculosis
TENS	transcutaneous electrical nerve stimulation
TIA	transient ischemic attack
t.i.d.	three times daily
TKVO	to keep vein open
TLC	total lymphocyte count
TO	telephone order
TPA	transluminal percutaneous angioplasty
TPN	total parenteral nutrition
TSE	testicular self-examination
U/A	urinalysis
US	ultrasound; ultrasonic
UTI	urinary tract infection
VO	verbal order
VRE	vancomycin-resistant enterococci
VS	vital signs
WBC	white blood cell count
WHO	World Health Organization
WNL	within normal limits

NURSING FOUNDATIONS

A Canadian Perspective

Second Edition

NURSING FOUNDATIONS

A Canadian Perspective

2nd Edition

BEVERLY WITTER DU GAS
Adjunct Professor
School of Nursing
University of British Columbia
Vancouver, British Columbia

LYNNE ESSON
Clinical Associate
Undergraduate Program Advisor
School Of Nursing
University of British Columbia
Vancouver, British Columbia

SHARON E. RONALDSON
Instructor
Faculty of Nursing Department
Langara College
Vancouver, British Columbia

Prentice Hall Canada Inc. Scarborough, Ontario

Canadian Cataloguing in Publication Data

Du Gas, Beverly Witter, 1923–
Nursing Foundations

2nd ed.
Includes index.
ISBN 0-13-899527-3

1. Nursing. 2. Nursing–Canada. I. Esson, Lynne.
II. Ronaldson, Sharon E. III. Title.

RT41.D84 1999 610.73 C98-932579-2

Prentice-Hall, Inc., Upper Saddle River, New Jersey
Prentice-Hall International (UK) Limited, London
Prentice-Hall of Australia, Pty. Limited, Sydney
Prentice-Hall Hispanoamericana, S.A., Mexico City
Prentice-Hall of India Private Limited, New Delhi
Prentice-Hall of Japan, Inc., Tokyo
Simon & Schuster Southeast Asia Private Limited, Singapore
Editora Prentice-Hall do Brasil, Ltda., Rio de Janeiro

ISBN 0-13-899527-3

Acquisitions Editor: Linda Bain
Developmental Editor: Maurice Esses
Production Editor: Kelly Dickson
Copy Editor: Francine Geraci
Production Coordinator: Deborah Starks
Permissions/Photo Research: Susan Wallace-Cox, Michaele Sinko
Art Direction: Julia M. Hall
Cover and Interior Design: Lisa LaPointe
Cover Image: Ron Chapple/Masterfile
Page Layout: Debbie Kumpf
Medical Illustrations: Dave Mazierski, Lianne Friesen, Stephen Mader

3 4 5 03 02 01

Printed and bound in the USA.

Statistics Canada information is used with the permission of the Minister of Industry, as Minister responsible for Statistics Canada. Information on the availabilty of the wide range of data from Statistics Canada can be obtained form Statistics Canada's Regional Offices, its World Wide Web site at http://www.statcan.ca, and its toll-free access number 1-800-263-1136.

Page 1258, The Bill of Rights, was created at a workshop on "The Terminally Ill Patient and Helping Person," in Lansing, Mich., sponsored by the Southwestern Michigan Inservice Education Council and conducted by Amelia J. Barbus, Associate Professor of Nursing, Wayne State University, Detroit.

Contributors

Melanie Basso, RN, MSN
Instructor
Nursing Faculty
Langara College
Vancouver, British Columbia

Sandra L. Beard, RN, BSN, MSN(c)
Nurse Educator, Emergency
The Richmond Hospital
Richmond, British Columbia

Joan Bottorff, RN, PhD
Associate Professor
Associate Director Research
School of Nursing
The University of British Columbia
Vancouver, British Columbia

Frances Fothergill-Bourbonnais, RN, PhD
Professor
School of Nursing
University of Ottawa;
and Institute of Palliative Care
Ottawa Hospital, Alta Vista Site
Ottawa, Ontario

Elaine Carty, RN, MSN
Professor
School of Nursing
The University of British Columbia
Vancouver, British Columbia

Anne Compton, BA, RN
Clinical Nurse Leader
Canuck Place
Vancouver, British Columbia

Susan Cush, RN, BSN
Nurse Clinician/Educator
General Surgery
St. Paul's Hospital
Vancouver, British Columbia

Betty Davies, RN, PhD
Professor
School of Nursing
The University of British Columbia
Vancouver, British Columbia

Kathleen (Amy) Doi, RN BHSN, MAdEd
Nursing Resource Coordinator
University College of the Cariboo
Kamloops, British Columbia

Lenore Du Gas, RN, ET, BSN
Enterostomy Therapist
Prince George Regional Hospital
Prince George, British Columbia

Mary Jane Duke, RN MSN
Lecturer
School of Nursing
The University of British Columbia
Vancouver, British Columbia

Wendy Dickson Fallis, RN, BSN, MN, Dipl.PHNrsg
Director
Department Of Research and Evaluation
Victoria General Hospital
Winnipeg, Manitoba

Linda Gomez, RN MSN
Selkirk College (Castlegar Campus)
Castlegar, British Columbia

J. Kirstine Griffith, BASc, MA
Nurse Educator, Author
Vancouver, British Columbia

Susan E. Hicks, RN, MSN
Nursing Policy Consultant
Canadian Nurses Association
Ottawa, Ontario

Lisa R. Jarvis, RDN, BHE, MEd
Nutrition Support Dietician
St. Paul's Hospital (Vancouver, British Columbia)

Emily R. Knor, RN, BSN, MA(Educ)
Coordinator, Flexible Assessment and Instructor
Nursing Faculty
Langara College
Vancouver, British Columbia

Frank J. Knor, BEd, BLS, MLS
Library Systems Coordinator
British Columbia Institute of Technology
Vancouver, British Columbia

Faye S. Lapka, RN, BA, BSc, MCS, CHN
Vancouver Richmond Health Board
Vancouver, British Columbia

Kathleen de Leon-Demaré, MN, RN, FNP
Assistant Professor
Faculty of Nursing
University of Manitoba
Winnipeg, Manitoba

Elizabeth Lindsey, RN, PhD
Associate Professor
School of Nursing
University of Victoria
Victoria, British Columbia

Tina Lobin
Statistical Clerk
Canadian Nurses Association
Ottawa, Ontario

Colleen McEwan, RN, BSN, MA
Practice Improvement Leader
The Richmond Hospital
Richmond, British Columbia

Marian MacKinnon, RN, MN
Assistant Professor
School of Nursing
University of Prince Edward Island
Charlottetown, Prince Edward Island

Connie D. Magnusson, RN, BSN, MEd
Project Director
Patient Care Management System
Simon Fraser Health Region
New Westminster, British Columbia

Karen Malfesi-Merrit, RN, BSN
Nurse Clinician
St. Paul's Hospital
Vancouver, British Columbia

Tiina K. Mettala, RN
Trauma Nurse
Vancouver General Hospital and Health Sciences Centre
Vancouver, British Columbia

Heather S. Millar, RN, BSN
Vice President, Research and Technology
Nico-Environmental Health Strategies
Vancouver, British Columbia

Cherry Nettleton, RN, BSN
Instructor
Nursing Faculty
Kwantlen University College
Surrey, British Columbia

Connie K. Ordish, RN, BSN, MSN
Instructor
Nursing Faculty
Kwantlen University College
Surrey, British Columbia

Wendy Otsu, RN, BSN, CNA
Patient Educator
St. Paul's Hospital
Vancouver, British Columbia

Lynda Kushnir Perkul, RN, BSN, MScAdmin
Supervisor, Employee Health Centre
Crown Life Insurance Company;
Regina, Saskatchewan
and President
Canadian Nurses Association (1998-2000 Biennium)

Patricia (Paddy) Rodney, RN, MSN, PhD
Assistant Professor
School of Nursing
University of Victoria;
and Research Associate
Centre for Applied Ethics
The University of British Columbia
Victoria, British Columbia

Kelli I. Stajduhar, RN, MSN
Doctoral Student, The University of British Columbia;
and Clinical Nurse Specialist
Palliative Care
Capital Health Region
Victoria, British Columbia

Charlotte Thompson, RN, CNM, BSN, MSN
Regional Nursing Consultant
Health Canada, Medical Services, Pacific Region
Vancouver, British Columbia

Moira M. Walker, RN, CIC
Senior Infection Control Nurse
Vancouver General Hospital and Health Sciences Centre
Vancouver, British Columbia

Jackie Wells
Physiotherapist
Richmond, British Columbia

Bow Wong, RN, BSN, MEd
Instructor
Nursing Faculty
Langara College
Vancouver, British Columbia

Glennis Zilm
Writer and Editor in the nursing field
White Rock, British Columbia

Brief Table of Contents

Detailed Table of Contents

Chapter 5

Chapter 6

Chapter 25

Chapter 26

Unit 6

Protection and Safety Needs 943

Chapter 30

Chapter 31

Chapter 32

Preface

We have written this book to provide a basic nursing text for students and their teachers that reflects current trends in health care in Canada and around the world. The main orientation of this second edition of *Nursing Foundations* is one of health promotion based on health rather than illness, with an emphasis on the socioeconomic and environmental determinants of health and well-being that go beyond the lifestyle model. As so beautifully and succinctly stated by Sister Simone Roach, nursing is the professionalization of caring. This philosophy is evidenced in a holistic approach to the care of individuals, families, and communities.

We believe that beginning nursing students should have an understanding of the health care system in which they will practise as graduates; the philosophy on which the system is based; and their role in providing nursing services to individuals, families, and communities. We also believe that in introductory courses in nursing, students should gain a solid foundation of knowledge and skills on which to build in more senior courses.

Throughout this text, we have chosen to use the term "patient" rather than "client" to refer to the recipient of nursing care. We do so because "client" is a generic term that can refer to anyone who seeks help from a professional practitioner, regardless of the nature of that person's practice. That is to say, a person becomes a "client" when seeking the services of a lawyer, an engineer, an accountant, or any other individual who has special qualifications for practice in his or her field. By contrast, the term "patient" refers specifically to an individual who has sought the help of a health professional. In this sense, although both "client" and "patient" are correct, the term "patient" is more specific.

Content and Organization

The book is divided into 37 chapters, organized into 7 units. In Unit 1 (Health Care and the Practice of Nursing), we introduce students to the role of the nurse in today's health services in hospitals and in the community at large. Writing from a Canadian perspective, we first discuss the changing views on health and its determinants as they have evolved over the years. We then describe the development and present structure of Canada's health care system and the services provided for people under our national health insurance program—services that are increasingly based on a primary health care philosophy that emphasizes health promotion throughout the life cycle. In the remaining chapters of this unit, we outline nursing practice and nursing education in Canada, the legal and ethical aspects of practice, and the role of research in nursing practice.

In Unit 2 (Dimensions of Health), we focus on health as it relates to basic human needs of the individual, the family, and the community. And we have devoted Chapter 12 to meeting the health needs of people of different cultural, spiritual, and ethnic backgrounds, including the people of Canada's First Nations.

In Unit 3 (Skills Basic to Nursing Practice), we introduce students to the theoretical basis of nursing and the critical thinking skills that they need to develop. We also discuss the methodology of nursing practice, giving both a conceptual framework and the tools required to begin clinical practice.

In the second half of the book, we introduce students to the care of people who need help in meeting their basic needs, regardless of their medical diagnosis. We address physiological needs (Unit 4), activity needs (Unit 5), protection and safety needs (Unit 6), and psychosocial needs (Unit 7). In each of these units, we consider needs throughout the life cycle. We place particular emphasis on the nurse's role in promoting optimal health by helping people to make decisions and take control of their own health and by providing supportive assistance as needed. We use the nursing process as an organizing framework by covering the assessment, diagnostic reasoning, planning, implementation, and evaluation of nursing care related to each basic need. Throughout these units, we highlight key principles, guides for taking a patient's history, strategies for health promotion, practices of community health care, and gerontological considerations by means of special Boxes (as described below under Features). And we clearly explain specific Procedures, giving the rationale for each step.

New to this Edition

To reflect advances in nursing and recent changes in the health-care environment in Canada, we have thoroughly updated all the material. And to better suit the users of this book, we have made the following important changes to the content and organization of the book:

An entirely new chapter devoted to **Critical Thinking** has been added as Chapter 14.

An entirely new section devoted to **Spirituality** has been incorporated in Chapter 12 (Ethnicity, Spirituality, and Health).

More material on **Cultural Diversity** has been added throughout the book.

More material on **Community Health Care** has been added in the body of the text and in the form of new Community Health Promotion Boxes.

More material on **Gerontology** has been added in the body of the text and in the form of new Gerontology Boxes.

The **In Review** summaries near the ends of chapters have been reorganized in point form.

The Learning Activities at the ends of the chapters have been changed to **Critical Thinking Exercises**.

The references listed at the ends of the chapters have been divided into **References** and **Additional Readings**.

The full **Code of Ethics for Registered Nurses** (March 97) is reprinted near the end of the book as the new Appendix A.

Information about **CNA Nurse Registration/Licensure Examinations** has been updated as the new Appendix B.

The Internet, Nursing Research and Continuing Education are discussed as the new Appendix C. In addition to presenting an overview of the Internet and tips for searching, it provides an annotated list of Internet sites for each of the following:

- Indexes and Databases for Nursing and Medical Research
- Canadian and International Health Resource Associations and Organizations
- Employment, Career, and Job Search Links
- General Health, Nursing, and Medicine References
- General Science References

Finally, in response to requests and suggestions by instructors and students alike, we have strengthened the pedagogical features of the book by adding important new elements (as described below).

Features

We have enhanced the features for this edition to facilitate learning and highlight applications. A complete listing of all the Procedures and of each type of Box described below is given on the back endpapers.

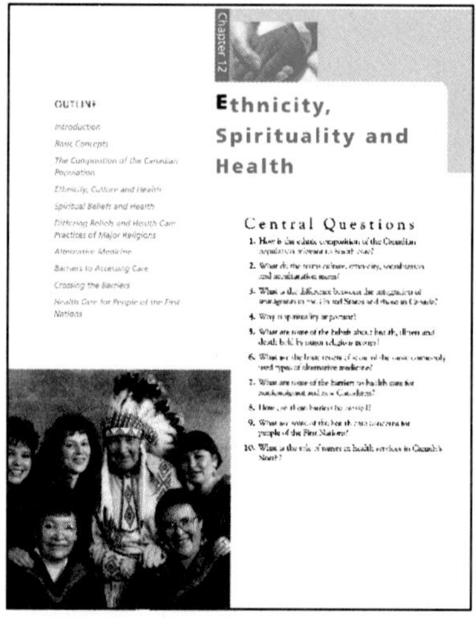

- An **Outline** and a set of **Central Questions** open each chapter.

- **Key terms** are boldfaced where they are defined in the text. They are also listed in chronological order, with page references, near the end of each chapter. For easy reference, all the key terms and their definitions are collated in a Glossary near the end of the book.

PROCEDURE 16.4 Measuring Blood Pressure

- **Procedures** in Units 3, 4, 5, 6, and 7 provide step by step actions, along with their rationales, for performing particular procedures.

HEALTH history guide Pain Experience

- **Health History Guide Boxes** in Units 4, 5, 6, and 7 present the important questions to ask when taking a patient's history to assess a particular problem.

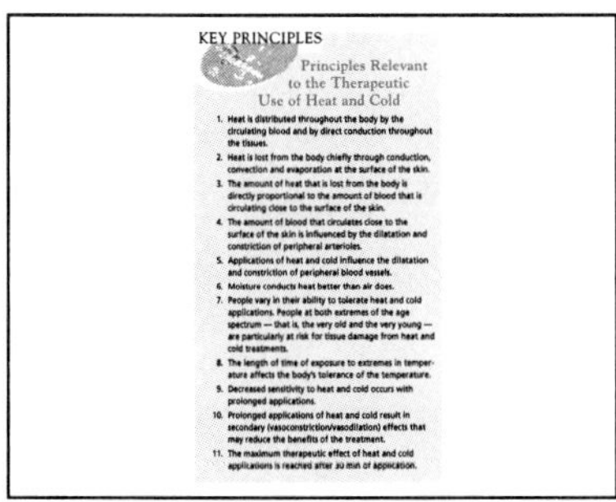

- **Key Principles Boxes** in Units 4, 5, 6, and 7 highlight important physiological principles that help to determine effective care treatment.

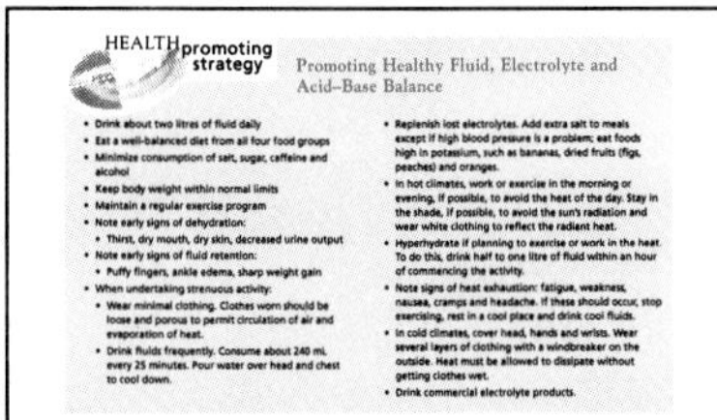

- **Health Promoting Strategy Boxes** in Units 4, 5, 6, and 7 summarize important strategies for maintaining wellness.

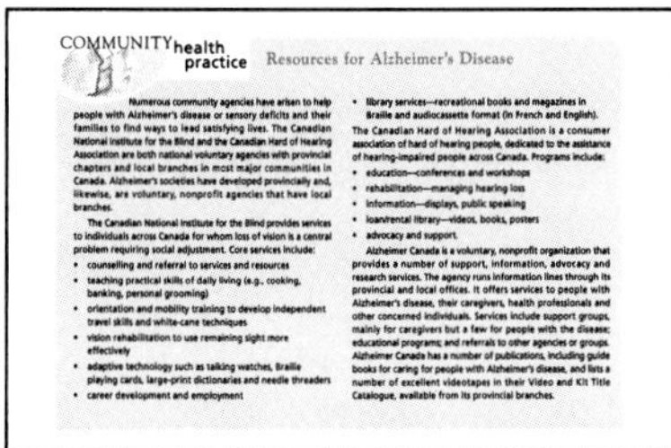

- **Community Health Practice Boxes** in Units 2, 3, 4, 5, 6, and 7 highlight practices of health care in our communities in settings other than hospitals.

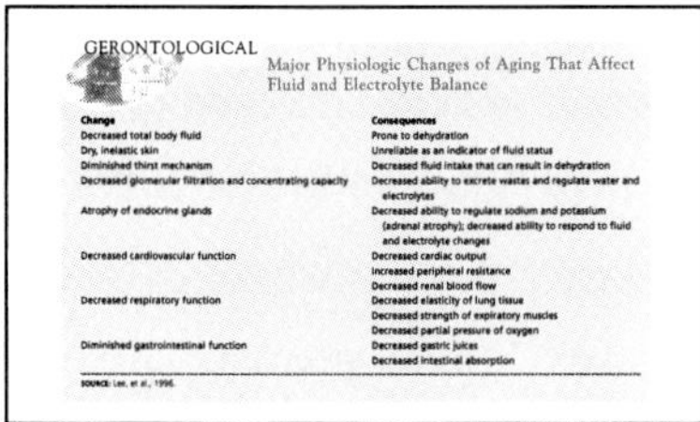

- **Gerontological Boxes** in Units 4, 5, 6, and 7 focus on health concerns that become more prominent in the elderly.

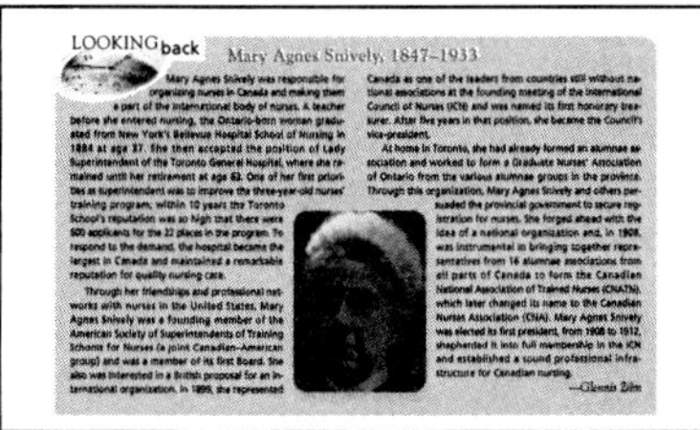

- **Looking Back Boxes** in Units 1 and 2 provide historical vignettes of prominent women who have helped shape the development of nursing in Canada.

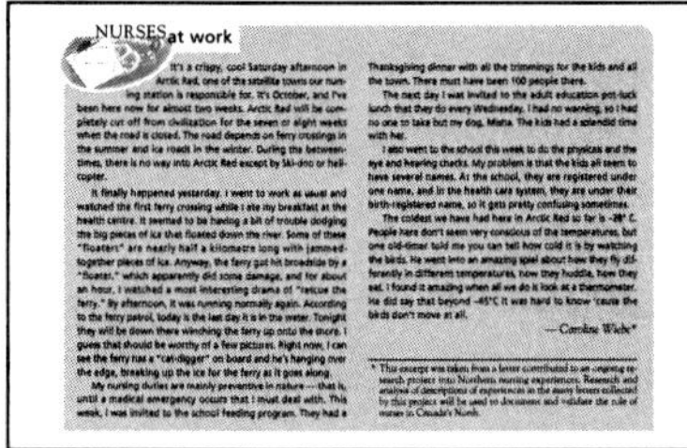

- **Nurses at Work Boxes** in Units 2, 3, and 6 provide modern vignettes of nurses at work to show the diversity of current nursing practice in Canada.

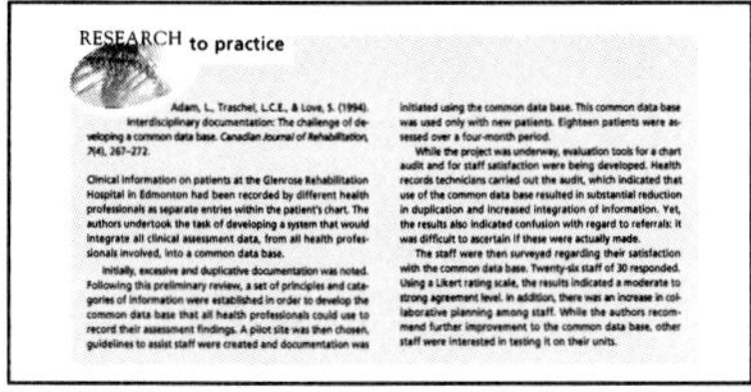

- **Research to Practice Boxes** in Units 2, 3, 4, 5, 6, and 7 illustrate how nursing research leads to improvements in clinical practice.

Tables and generic **Boxes** in every chapter provide additional details to support the discussion in the text.

Figures and **Photos** illustrate the discussions throughout the book.

An **In Review** section near the end of each chapter provides a summary in point form.

Critical Thinking Exercises near the end of each chapter provide a wide range of exercises.

Additional Readings and **References** at the end of each chapter guide users to other sources.

Supplements

The following supplements have been carefully prepared to accompany this new edition:

An **Instructor's Manual** provides a wealth of material for each chapter, including an overview, a set of central questions, ideas for classroom teaching, answers to all the critical thinking exercises in the text, ideas for clinical/laboratory experience, and list of additional resources. It also provides a set of 4 Video Cases relating to the special set of CBC videos that have been selected to accompany the book.

A set of **Transparency Masters** provides a selection of important Figures, Tables, and Boxes from the textbook for display in the classroom. These Transparency Masters are also available in a package that includes a set of blank acetates.

A **Test Item File** provides more than 2000 multiple-choice questions, organized by chapter.

Test Manager consists of a special computerized version of the *Test Item File* that enables instructors to create and distribute tests and analyze the results electronically.

CBC The **CBC/Prentice Hall Canada Video Library for Nursing** is a special compilation of 4 video segments selected from CBC broadcasts of *The Health Show*. These videos focus on some important issues of current concern, namely, Multicultural Health, Internet Medicine, Community and Health, and Informed Consent. A Video Case associated with each of these segments is provided in the *Instructor's Manual.*

Acknowledgements

We are grateful to the following instructors for providing formal reviews of parts of the manuscript for the new edition:

Cathy Colley RN, BSN, MEd
Professor
Practical Nursing Program
Conestoga College

Paula Donahoe RN, BScN, MEd
Professor
School of Applied Arts and Health Sciences
Centennial College

R. Marjorie Drury, RN, MN
Assistant Professor
Nursing Department
Trinity Western University

Penny K. Ericson, RN, MScN
Dean
Faculty of Nursing
University of New Brunswick

Janice Lander, PhD
Professor and Associate Dean Research
Faculty of Nursing
University of Alberta

Edna McKim, RN, MN
Associate Professor
School of Nursing
Memorial University of Newfoundland

Sandra Madorin, RN, BScN, MScN
Assistant Professor
School of Nursing
The University of Western Ontario

Della M. Mills, BA, RN
Professor
Health Sciences Division
Northern College of Applied Arts and Technology

Sharon Nield, RN, BN, MA
Nursing Policy Consultant
Canadian Nurses Association

Barbara L. Paterson, RN, PhD
Associate Professor
School of Nursing
The University of British Columbia

Judith Pearce, RN, BN, MSc(A), EdD
Professor
School of Nursing
Ryerson Polytechnic University

Lynnette Leeseberg Stamler, RN, PhD
Associate Professor
School of Nursing
University of Windsor

Olive Yonge, RN, PhD. CPsych
Professor
Faculty of Nursing
University of Alberta

In the preparation of the second Canadian edition of this text we have had the help of a great many nursing colleagues and other individuals whom we would like to acknowledge here. First of all, we would like to thank Emily Knor who did the preliminary work for changes incorporated into this edition. We would also like to thank all of the nursing teachers who took the time to complete our questionnaire critiquing the first edition and make suggestions for ways to make this edition better suited to student needs. Then there are the colleagues who contributed content for various chapters, and the people we consulted on specific topics, each of whom enriched the subject matter with their specialized expertise. Their names are listed on the preceding pages. We are indebted also to the many nursing teachers who reviewed various chapters and gave us helpful suggestions on content and organization. Their names are also listed.

Thanks are due also to the nurses who shared with us some of their experiences in day-to-day practice for incorporation into our Nurses at Work vignettes and to the community agencies who contributed content for our Community Practice boxes.

We are also grateful to Brenda Won for her invaluable assistance researching materials for the book and to Lisa Saul for her help with the administrative details that are part and parcel of the work of getting a textbook together. Thanks also to Morris Forchuk for his computer assistance, to Sharmila Lakhani for the case study used in the chapter on critical thinking, to Al Harvey, photographer, and to Casi McEvoy and Donna Claxton who agreed to be the models in our photo shoot.

We must also give thanks to the editors, artists and production staff of Prentice Hall Canada who provided helpful advice and supportive encouragement throughout the lengthy process of preparing this text and readying it for publication.

We owe additional thanks to Sandra Madorin of The University of Western Ontario for checking the entire edited manuscript.

In spite of great care, it is difficult to ensure that there are no errors in this text. Therefore, it would be helpful to hear from anyone who finds mistakes. And we would welcome any other comments about this new edition. Please write to us care of: Acquisitions Editor, Nursing, Prentice Hall Canada, Higher Education Division, 1870 Birchmount Road, Scarborough, Ontario M1P 2J7.

Beverly Witter Du Gas
Lynne Esson
Sharon E. Ronaldson

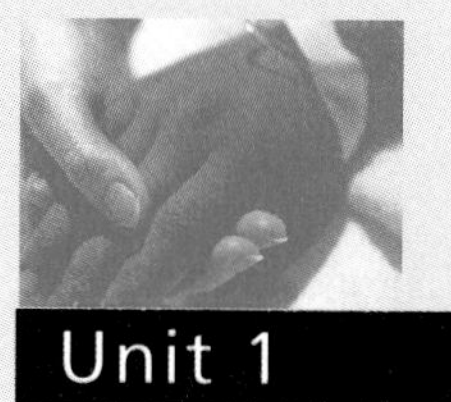

Unit 1

Health Care and the Practice of Nursing

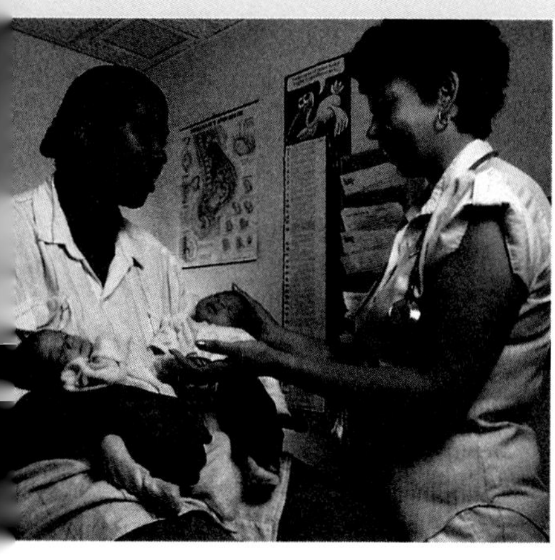

Chapter 1

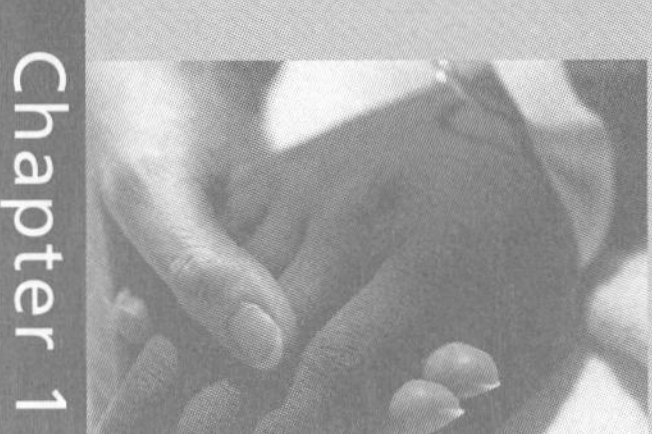

Introduction to Health Care

OUTLINE

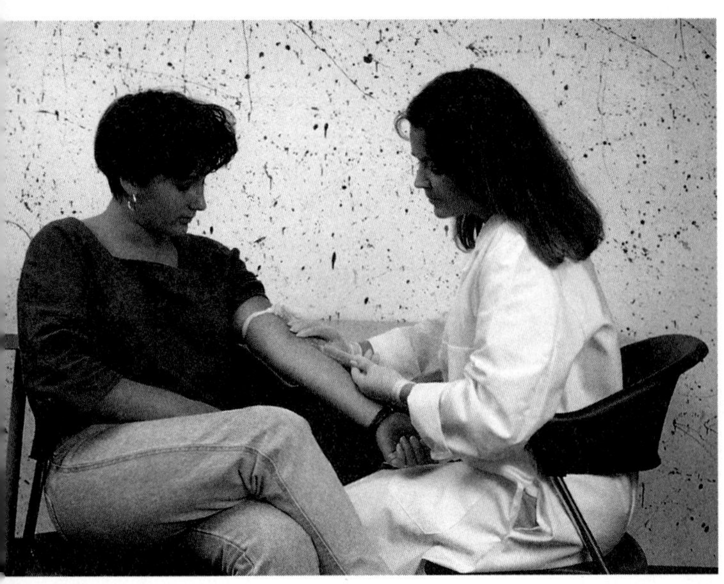

Introduction

Caring is the most common criterion of humanness . . . No discipline is seen to be so directly and intimately involved in caring needs and behaviours as nursing . . . Nursing is (in essence) the professionalization of caring.

Sister Simone Roach, 1992, p. 11

The mission of nursing is to serve humanity by assisting people in the promotion, protection and restoration of health or to comfort and support them in the event of incurable illness. In carrying out this mission, nursing responds to the needs of the people it serves, constantly modifying its practice to meet the challenges brought about by ever-changing societal forces. As beginning students in nursing, you are entering the profession at a time when nursing is taking a major role in the restructuring of health services in this country. In this chapter we will introduce some of the changes that are taking place in our society and examine the effects these changes are having on nursing.

The Changing Image of Nursing

Nursing in Canada has a long and honourable history—it has played an integral role in Canadian society from the time the first colonists arrived on the shores of New France. Long before Florence Nightingale ushered in the era of modern nursing in Britain, French nursing sisters were practising a comprehensive type of nursing care in the precarious environment of the New World.

These are exciting times for nurses—and for all who work in the health field in Canada. Major health reforms are in progress as we redefine health and reconsider what constitutes health care, how it should be managed and where and how it should be delivered. Our ponderous health care system is now shifting from one that has been disease-oriented and hospital-based to one that is focussed on health and is based in the community.

Nurses are taking a major role in the transformation of the health care system. At the time of writing, the health minister of one province is a nurse and, in increasing numbers, nurses are assuming leadership positions in health policy-making and in the planning and administration of health services at provincial, regional and community levels. In day-to-day practice, the days are long gone when the nurse was "handmaiden to the physician." Instead, we see the nurse as an equal member of the health team who shares a collegial relationship with other health professionals.

In Ontario, nurses with additional preparation are working as primary health care providers in underserviced northern and rural areas where physicians are few. They are also working in partnership with physicians in urban

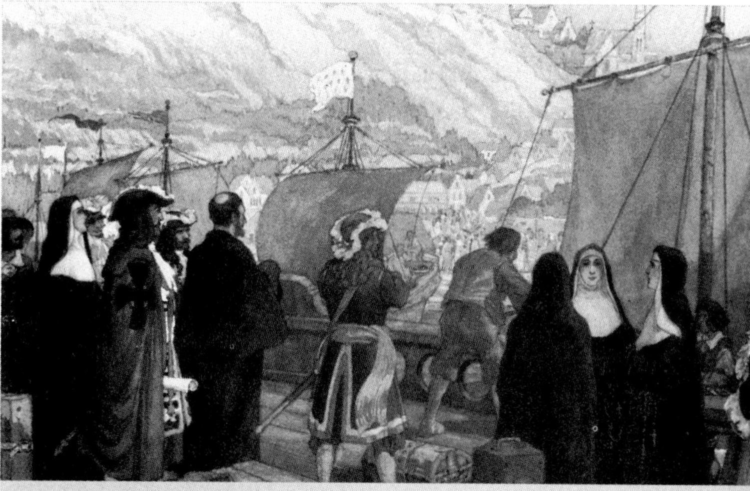

Arrival of Ursuline Nuns at Quebec, 1639.

centres. Legislation permitting them to practise in an extended role has been enacted, and preparatory courses are offered at several university schools of nursing in the province. A growing number of nurses are in independent practice in such fields as lifestyle counselling, rehabilitation, Therapeutic Touch and foot care. A number of nurses with preparation in the field are in autonomous practice as midwives.

The education of nurses is also changing and, again, the momentum has picked up in recent years. The Canadian Nurses Association in 1982 recommended the baccalaureate as the entry level requirement for professional nursing practice, and in all parts of the country this transition is now in process. In a number of provinces, colleges and universities have formed collaborative partnerships for developing and offering baccalaureate programs in nursing. Some of the programs are designed with exit points midway through the course of studies, permitting students to enter the workforce earlier, if they so wish. A common curriculum, shared by a number of institutions, facilitates re-entry into the program at a later date. The curricula for nursing education are also shifting to reflect an orientation towards health rather than illness. The baccalaureate program at the University of Prince Edward Island was the first curriculum based on principles of health promotion.

The number of graduate programs in nursing has increased at universities across Canada. Doctoral programs in nursing are offered at several Canadian universities. At the time of writing, there are doctoral programs at the Universities of Alberta, British Columbia and Toronto, and a conjoint program offered by McGill University and the University of Montreal.

The establishment of master's and doctoral level programs in nursing has spurred the development of research in the field. Nurses now sit on the esteemed Medical Research Council of Canada and, in some universities, nursing scholars are attracting more research funding than members of many other faculties. Research-based nursing practice is

LOOKING back

Jeanne Mance, 1606–1673

Jeanne Mance, nurse and extraordinary hospital administrator, was the first woman to earn an important place in the history of New France. She was founder of the Hôtel-Dieu de Ville-Marie (hospital) and is considered, along with Paul de Chomedey de Maisonneuve, cofounder of Montreal.

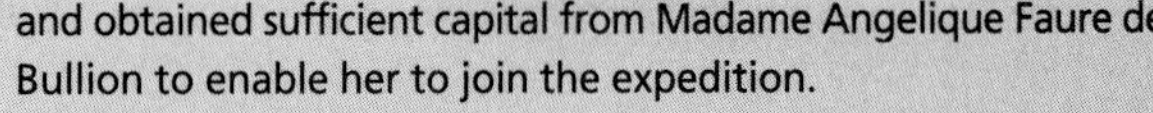

Jeanne Mance was born in 1606, the 10th child in a distinguished and well-to-do family in Langares, France. She was educated in an Ursuline convent, where she learned the basics of nursing, as befitted a woman destined to head a household, although she soon announced she would devote her life to the Church. During her young adult years, France was at war and, as her home was in a battle area, she assisted with nursing care of the sick and wounded. Then, in 1640, she heard of a proposal to found a second colony in New France, and resolved to establish a hospital there. She immediately began to raise funds for the enterprise and obtained sufficient capital from Madame Angelique Faure de Bullion to enable her to join the expedition.

After a gruelling voyage, Jeanne and the other members of the expedition were forced to remain the winter in Quebec City, where she learned more nursing skills by working with the trained Augustinian sisters who had established the first hospital in Canada. In spring 1642, the colonists journeyed on to Ville Marie, now Montreal, and Jeanne Mance built her hospital. Although the first year she did not have many patients, she soon was required to use all her nursing skills and by 1645 needed a larger building. During the next 28 years, she made three voyages to France to raise funds and to bring out trained nuns for her growing hospital. She died in 1673, in Montreal, respected and revered throughout the colony she had helped to found.

— *Glennis Zilm*

becoming a fact of life, as we will discuss more fully in Chapter 7.

Nursing still remains at the forefront of health care in Canada. Nurses constitute the largest single group of health care providers in the country. In Canada, nursing has always been held in high regard; today, nursing is a career with growing opportunities and attractive financial rewards.

From Science to Humanism and Spirituality

The latter half of this century has been characterized by a tremendous explosion of knowledge in all the sciences. The amount of knowledge in the biomedical field alone was said to have more than doubled in the 25 years between 1950 and 1975—and the field has continued to expand. During the 1950s and 1960s and well into the following decade, we were enamoured with science and all the technological wonders that were becoming part of our everyday lives. In the biomedical field, increasingly complex surgery, such as organ transplants and micro-optic and laser surgery, became possible. From the end of the 1970s, however, we have been witnessing a growing disenchantment with science. The technological age has had a tendency to depersonalize many aspects of our lives, as machines have taken over so many tasks that people used to do. Patients tell us they feel dehumanized and alienated as they are hooked up to various bottles and machines and surrounded by faceless people in masks and gowns. They long for a human touch and some recognition of their existence as people—not just appendages at the end of a machine. At the same time, nurses often feel as if they are spending their time caring for machines rather than people, and they feel frustrated that they cannot give patients the personal care they know they should give.

While science has provided answers to many questions in the health field, it has, in many cases, ignored the human component of care. This has brought about a return to *humanism*—an approach that puts the human being back at the centre of care. Along with the return to humanism has come a renewed interest in—one might almost say a revival of—spirituality. In our rapidly changing, often depersonalizing society, people are looking for something to hold onto; they are searching for meaning in their lives. In their quest, they are turning not only to the established religions but, also, to different ways in which to express their spirituality. We discuss this topic more fully in Chapter 12.

The shift towards humanism and renewed interest in spirituality has been particularly evident in health care. The traditional values on which nursing is based—those of caring and nurturing—are becoming universally recognized as essential ingredients in the process of healing. Health care providers are also increasingly aware that people's beliefs about health and illness are intimately intertwined with their spiritual beliefs, and that tending to spiritual needs is as important as looking after physical needs—and sometimes is even more important.

Our Changing Population

The face of Canada has changed dramatically during this century. We have become a nation with a rapidly growing older segment and an increasing diversity of ethnic origins among our people. Family patterns have altered. While the nuclear family, composed of a mother, a father and two or more children, is still the standard in Canadian households, the traditional situation in which the father was breadwinner and the mother was homemaker has changed. The new family structure is one in which both parents pursue careers and share equal responsibility in the home. Many other family patterns have also emerged, including single-parent, blended, cohabiting, and gay and lesbian families.

We no longer live in the small, close-knit communities that once characterized most of this country. The majority of the population now live in increasingly large cities. Our economic base has also shifted. From one that was built on logging, fishing, farming and mining, it moved first to manufacturing as we developed a strong industrial base in Central Canada, and now it is shifting again. A major restructuring of the Canadian economy is currently going on as we move from the industrial to the information age.

Aging

The aging of populations is a worldwide phenomenon. Much of it is expected to occur in the developing world over the next 20 years, as life expectancy is lengthened in many countries as a result of improvements in health. But, we are also seeing a rapid growth in the number of older persons in the population of Canada. From approximately 10 percent of the population in 1986, the number of persons over the age of 65 is expected to grow to 16 percent by the year 2016 and 23 percent by 2041, with the biggest increase coming after 2011, when members of the baby boom generation begin to reach retirement age (Chui, 1996). The increasing number of older adults is already posing a challenge to our health services. The impact will be even greater in the years to come. Particularly important in this regard is the fact that the fastest-growing segment of the older population is the group over the age of 85, whose numbers are expected to increase to 11 percent by the year 2031. This is the group who consume the most hospital days of all age groups in the country and almost all of the long-term care facilities (Beckingham, 1993).

Family Patterns

The aging of the Canadian population is occurring at a time when there has been increasing fragmentation of the family unit. Grownup children now often live thousands of kilometres away from their parents. With more women working outside the home, there is often no one at home to look after an aging mother or father. As people are living longer, many women in their middle years are being caught caring for children at home and having to look after aging parents who also need care. Alternative services have had to be developed to assist older people to remain independent as long as possible, and facilities have had to be built to care for them when they are no longer able to care for themselves.

The number of single-parent families represented 13 percent of all families in Canada in 1991 (Statistics Canada, 1996). This situation, combined with the increased numbers of women in the workforce, has meant that social institutions such as day care centres, schools, churches and community centres must provide many services that once were provided by parents in the home. The day-to-day management of many transient and chronic problems of children's illnesses may be delegated to the day care worker, the teacher or the school nurse. For example, the school nurse or the teacher may be asked to give a child medication at specified times after the acute phase of an illness is past and the parent must return to work.

Urbanization

We have also had to cope with the need for rapid expansion of health services in our cities, as new immigrants came into the country and more people migrated to urban centres in search of employment. All too often, the number of people moving into the city far outstrips the capacity of its health services. This is particularly true in inner-city neighbourhoods, where overcrowding and poverty frequently compound the situation. It is the inner-city neighbourhoods, too, that usually have the most new immigrants. This situation results in a rich cultural mix among inhabitants, but often poses problems for health workers both in terms of overcoming language barriers and in understanding different beliefs and customs about health and illness.

The trend towards increasing urbanization is beginning to change, however. As cities become more crowded, and the pace of life more hectic, many people are seeking an alternative lifestyle and are moving to the suburbs or to smaller communities. We are seeing this shift among the older population as retirement villages and other housing options for elders are developed in small communities. But, we are also seeing the trend among young people who can afford houses in small towns that they could never hope to afford in a big city.

Changes in the Economy

Although Canada's economy appears to be recovering from the restructuring necessitated by the transition to the information age and globalized trade, thousands of Canadians are still unemployed and are having to learn new skills to compete in the labour market. Poverty exists in the midst of plenty in many parts of the country. Along with poverty come its resultant social problems, not the least of which is the effect on people's health. Despite Canada's universal health care system, surveys have shown that ill health is more common among the poor, and that access to needed health services is more difficult for them. Poverty also breeds crime, and there has been a distressing increase in violent crime in Canadian cities in recent years. Our health services have had to learn to cope with gunshot wounds and stabbings in increasing numbers. There is a growing need for

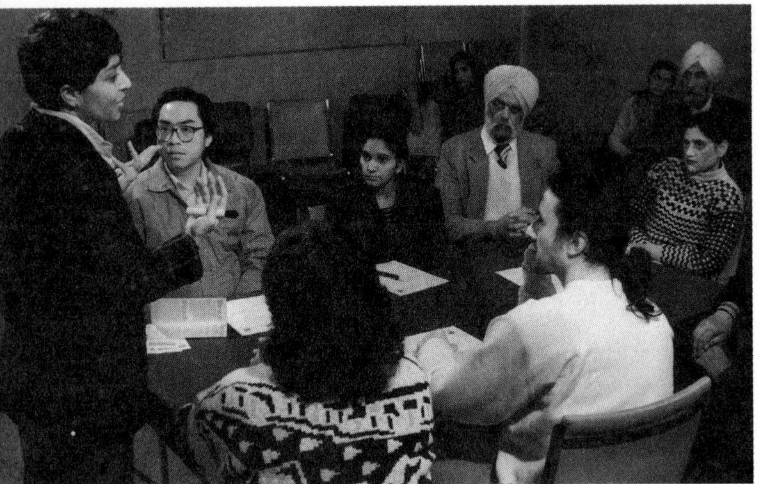

A health educator discusses health issues with community residents.

mental health and social services to help victims deal with the trauma of violent acts.

Multiculturalism

The remarkable ethnic diversity of our population is one of the most interesting challenges faced by workers in the health field as they try to tailor care to meet the needs of patients. Canada has been called a nation of immigrants. Beginning with the ancestors of our First Nations people, followed by the French and then the British, Canada has seen wave after wave of immigration, and the population has become increasingly diverse.

Today, there are more than 100 distinct ethnic groups among our population. Most Canadians (82%, according to a 1991 Angus Reid survey) live in neighbourhoods with persons of different ethnic or racial backgrounds, and nearly three-quarters of us can name people of different ethnic or cultural backgrounds among our close friends. Intermarriage between different racial and ethnic groups—once a social taboo—has become common, with 40 percent of Canadians stating that they have family members of different ethnic or racial backgrounds. (Royal Bank Reporter, 1992)

Immigration continues to swell our numbers as people from every corner of the globe come in the hope of a better life. Canada is seen as a growing nation with great economic potential, where people can be free to worship as they choose and where political diversity is tolerated. Along with Sweden, the United States and Australia, we are among the world's leaders in refugee resettlement.

Changing Patterns of Disease

The nature of the illnesses that affect us has changed dramatically over the years, and this too has had an impact on health services. The tremendous advances in medical science in the 20th century have radically altered disease patterns in Western societies and have revolutionized health care. Most of the communicable diseases that necessitated lengthy hospitalization and took such a toll on human lives at the beginning of the century, such as smallpox, diphtheria, typhoid and scarlet fever, have been virtually eliminated by improvements in public health measures coupled with the discovery and widespread use of specific immunity-producing agents. Of growing concern, however, is the resistance to antibiotics developed by a number of disease-carrying organisms. Tuberculosis, once thought to have been conquered, has resurfaced and is a major problem again in many parts of the world, particularly in crowded, poverty-ridden neighbourhoods, where it spreads rapidly through a vulnerable population. Other diseases, such as the worldwide epidemic of acquired immunodeficiency syndrome (AIDS), continue to come forward to plague us.

The massive migration of refugees, the increase in global travel, and the influx of immigrants from all over the world, have also brought different patterns of disease. Even in our northern part of the globe, we need to be aware that our patients may recently have come from a country where malaria, dengue, yellow fever and the like are common. The care of people with tropical diseases is no longer something for study only by missionaries going off to foreign lands. All Canadian health workers need to know how to identify the symptoms of these diseases and how to care for people suffering from them.

The miracle drugs of the 1940s and 1950s, the sulfonamides and the antibiotics, radically changed methods of patient care by hastening recovery and lowering fatality rates from infections. The rapid advances in surgical techniques in the latter half of the century have made procedures simpler and safer, with day surgery and home recovery possible for many operations that used to require lengthy hospital stays. The advances in medical and surgical techniques have also contributed to increasing the life span of people in our society. The longer people live, however, the more likely they are to suffer from chronic and degenerative diseases—heart conditions, cerebrovascular accidents (strokes) and cancer are among the leading causes of death in Canada today. These diseases also figure prominently on the list of chronic conditions from which people suffer.

Many of our present-day health problems are directly attributable to the way we live. Faster cars, driven at high speeds, have contributed to making the care and treatment of accident victims a major portion of the workload in hospitals. External causes of death, including accidents, violence and poisonings, are the third leading cause of death for men in Canada, and the fourth for women. Many hospitals have trauma units staffed with physicians and nurses who have taken specialist courses in the field. Rehabilitation services are needed to help restore people who have had accidents to an active, functioning role in society. The number of people permanently handicapped as a result of accidents and other acts of violence adds to the demand for long-term care services.

The heightened tempo of life in today's world has led to many stress-related health problems. There has been a marked increase in the incidence of mental illness, especially among young people, and we are also seeing much evidence of the tragic effects of alcohol and drug abuse. Suicide, homicide and other acts of violence are on the increase.

Alternative Modes of Treatment

Until fairly recently, most Canadians relied solely on Western scientific medicine to cure their ills. An increasing number of Canadians today, however, are making use of alternative or complementary therapies and practices. Acupuncture, herbal remedies, massage, therapeutic touch, hypnotherapy, aromatherapy and reflexology are among the different types of alternative medical practices that are available in most communities in Canada today.

Also new in Canada—although not in most of the rest of the world—is the recognition of midwifery as a legitimate field of practice. Legislation permitting the practice of midwifery as an autonomous health profession has been enacted in Ontario and in British Columbia, and is pending in most other provinces and the territories. Meanwhile, the only province offering preparation in midwifery is Ontario. The course provides for direct entry to the profession; that is to say, the person need not be a nurse before entering the program, although opportunity is available for registered nurses to be admitted with advanced standing to the program. Many nurses who have completed midwifery programs in other jurisdictions are practising in Ontario and British Columbia.

Changing Perspectives on Health and Health Care

Our ideas about health and the factors affecting health have undergone considerable change over the past century. We have moved from looking at health and illness from a purely biological point of view to a perspective that includes the effects of individual behaviours and, more recently, social, economic and environmental factors as major contributors to health (Health & Welfare Canada, 1987).

Today's view portrays health as a part of everyday living and as an essential dimension of the quality of life. "Quality of life" in this context implies the opportunity to make choices and to gain satisfaction from living. Health is envisaged as a resource that permits people to manage and even change their surroundings. Today's view of health recognizes freedom of choice and emphasizes the role of individuals, families, groups and communities in defining the meaning of, and in making decisions about, their health (Epp, 1986). With this view comes a change in health care from a focus on the cure of disease to an emphasis on the promotion and protection of health. "Armed with the knowledge that health goes beyond lifestyle and medical care, we can insist that policies in housing, education, justice, taxation and other areas take health into account" (Government of Ontario, 1993).

In keeping with the changing perspectives on health, there is a shift in the relationship between the nurse (and other health professionals) and the individual, family, group or community for whom health services were established. No longer is it one in which the nurse or other health professional is provider of care and the individual, family, group or community is the passive recipient. The relationship is viewed as an equal partnership—where the nurse or other health professional and the recipients collaborate to achieve the best level of health possible for them.

Typical of the health-focussed, community-based approach to health care are the "one-stop health centres" developing in various provinces under the direction of regional and community health boards. These centres offer a variety of health services under one roof, such as family doctors, nutritionists, nurses, physiotherapists, occupational therapists, dentists and social workers. The Al Ritchie Health Action Centre in Regina, Saskatchewan, provides an excellent example of the shift from a traditional service approach, with planning and direction by health professionals, to one in which community members are actively involved and pool their collective skills and expertise to address health issues. The Centre focusses on the broad determinants of health. Programs include many diverse activities, such as the development of social support networks, helping young people with résumés and job searches, sessions on education/health practices and coping skills, and access to health services (Lemon, 1998).

The shift to community-based services has resulted in the closure of hospital beds across the country. We are moving to a new type of health system in which hospital stays are shorter and reserved for the acutely ill. Many surgical procedures that used to require lengthy hospital stays are now being done on an outpatient basis. Those who are admitted to hospital are being discharged earlier for posttreatment recovery and rehabilitation, as well as chronic care in the home or in less costly inpatient facilities. These changes have led to a considerable need for the expansion of home care services, which all provinces and territories are now trying to establish.

What Does All This Mean for Nursing?

As we move from the industrial age into the information age, nurses and other health care providers are learning to use the new technologies to provide better care for their patients. Computers are used in all facets of health care, and the new field of informatics is vitally important to nurses. *Informatics* is not just about computers and the Internet, but how best to utilize these to improve patient care. In clinical practice, through informatics, nurses can gather up-to-date information on the latest research in order to make care-related decisions. They can also have access to up-to-the-minute patient data and can confer with experts worldwide. Informatics also provides nurses with the tools to document their effectiveness in providing evidence-based, cost-effective care (Sibbald, 1998).

The redefinition of health to include socioenvironmental determinants as well as biological factors and lifestyle has changed the direction of health care policy and the nature of health care services in Canada. In addition to their traditional caring functions, nurses' roles now encompass those of facilitator, advocate, community organizer, political activist and lobbyist. These roles involve collaboration with other health professionals as well as professionals from other sectors of society, such as economists, urban planners and environmentalists (RNABC, 1990). In order to undertake these new roles, nurses need highly developed skills in the caring aspects of nursing. Additionally, nurses need to be able to work with individuals and groups to enable them to determine their own needs and take control of their own health. For example, a nurse may now be asked to assist a group working to improve housing for low-income families in the community.

The realignment of our health care system, with the shift towards more ambulatory and home-care services, has increased the number of nurses working in the community. Here, nurses are playing an increasingly large role in identifying patient needs, coordinating the various services available and providing care. Community health nurses require skills in assessing the health status of individuals and families, enabling them to promote their health and to cope with the effects of illness or disability. Nurses' practice takes them into homes, schools, industry and clinics in the community.

People coming into acute care hospitals are usually very ill. Many, such as the accident victim with multiple injuries or the person who has just suffered a heart attack or a stroke, require intensive nursing care. The complexity of care and the highly sophisticated machinery used require specialized skills. Many nurses are taking advanced training to become clinical specialists in various fields.

As so many of the diseases prevalent in our society today are attributable to high-pressure urban living, it is important for nurses to have a good understanding of the nature of stress and ways of coping with it. Nurses are as vulnerable to the effects of stress as their patients are. Nurses must examine their own health practices carefully to make sure that their daily activities include sufficient rest, exercise and recreation in order to offset stress encountered in the work environment.

An increasingly large number of nurses are involved in working with older people, who now constitute such a large part of our society. Many nurses are providing health services for people in senior citizen housing units, helping them to keep well and as active and independent as possible, for as long as possible. Nurses are also the principal providers of care in nursing homes and extended-care facilities, where so many of the sick elderly are in residence.

What Does All This Mean for Nursing Students?

The only constant in the emerging world is change—and the accelerating rate of that change.

Burton, 1992, p. xv

As nursing responds to the changes occurring in society, it is important to remember that the traditional values on which nursing was founded—those of caring, nurturing, compassion and commitment—have withstood the test of time. As beginning students, you should have a sense of the rich history of nursing in this country, and in this context we introduce some of the illustrious pioneers of Canadian nursing. We start in this chapter with Jeanne Mance, who is honoured as the first nurse in Canada. You should also know something about the profession you have chosen, its mandate in society and how this mandate is carried out in practice.

The rapid and extensive changes in health care will inevitably have an impact on you, the nursing student. First, you need a good grounding in the scientific basis of nursing. The underlying foundation for nursing lies in its theoretical underpinnings—the theories that have been articulated about the phenomenon of nursing and the processes by which nursing is carried out in practice. Second, you will need a broad base of knowledge in the social sciences, as well as in the biological sciences. Third, you will have to develop critical thinking skills in problem solving, decision making and the like as part of the process of giving care. And finally, you will need to gain skills in communication, human interaction and group process. These requirements are, of course, in addition to the basic competencies that are the traditional foundation of nursing practice.

The provision of expert nursing care is a highly developed skill acquired over time with experience and continued learning. As first-year students you will develop the beginning skills necessary for nursing practice. You will learn to give care to people in their homes, in community clinics, in long-term care facilities and in acute care hospitals. The basic knowledge and skills you gain from your introductory course in nursing will provide you with a solid foundation on which to build.

But you need more than just the basic skills. You will also need an understanding of health; the factors that affect the health of individuals, families, groups and communities; and of the perceptions people have of health in general and their own health in particular. Not everyone views health in the same way. As immigrants have come to settle in Canada, they have brought customs and traditions from their native lands, and sometimes traditional practitioners of the healing arts have emigrated as well. It is often a challenge for health workers to practise culturally sensitive care and adapt interventions to meet the needs of people with backgrounds different from their own. It is helpful, then, to know something about spiritual beliefs and the health beliefs and practices of some of the major ethnic groups who have made Canada their home. A particular case in point for Canadian nurses is health care of First Nations people. This field of nursing, and particularly the challenges of nursing in Canada's North, has not only attracted Canadian nurses but has also lured nurses from around the globe.

As well as understanding health, you, as future health practitioners in Canada, need to know something about the health care system in which you will be working. We mentioned the shift to community-based care that is occurring. It makes sense, then, to learn something about the direction community-based care is taking and how nurses can work effectively with people in the community, both on an individual and a group basis. With the focus on health rather than illness, nurses need skills in health promotion and health protection—skills that depend to a large extent on communication and teaching abilities. The interpersonal skills that enable nurses to collaborate with other health professionals and with people from other sectors of the community are invaluable in making our communities healthy places in which to live.

References

BECKINGHAM, A. (1993). Aging in Canada. In A.C. Beckingham & B.W. Du Gas (Eds), *Promoting healthy aging: A nursing and community perspective*. St. Louis: Mosby.

BURTON, L.E. (Ed.). (1992). *Developing resourceful humans.* New York: Routledge.

CHUI, T. (1996, August). Canada's population: Charting into the 21st century. *Canadian Social Trends, 42,* 3–7.

EPP, J. (1986). *Achieving health for all: A framework for health promotion.* Ottawa: Ministry of Supply & Services. (Catalogue no. H39 – 102/1986E)

GOVERNMENT OF ONTARIO. (1993). *Nurturing health.* Report of the Premier's Council on Health, Well-being and Social Justice (1987–1991). Toronto: Queen's Printer. (Catalogue no. 01 – 93 – 20M)

HEALTH & WELFARE CANADA. (1987). *The active health report: A framework for health promotion.* Ottawa: Ministry of Supply & Services. (Catalogue no. H39 – 106/1987E)

LEMON, D. (1998). Personal correspondence containing excerpts from a paper prepared for presentation to the Board of the Al Ritchie Health Action Centre.

REGISTERED NURSES ASSOCIATION OF BRITISH COLUMBIA (RNABC). (1990). *Health promotion: A discussion paper.* Vancouver: Author.

ROACH, S.M. (1992). *The human act of caring: A blueprint for the health professions.* Ottawa: Canadian Hospital Association Press.

SIBBALD, B. (1998, April). Nursing informatics for beginners. *Canadian Nurse, 94*(4), 22–30.

STATISTICS CANADA. (1996, Summer). Family indicators for Canada. *Canadian Social Trends, 41,* 32–34.

A NATION WITH A DIFFERENCE. (1992). *Royal Bank Reporter,* Spring Edition.

Chapter 2

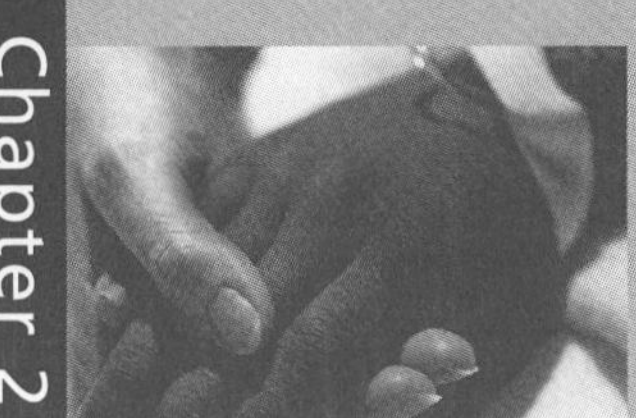

OUTLINE

Introduction

The Meanings of Health, Wellness, Illness and Disease

Chronic Illness and the Concept of Health Within Illness

Holistic Health and the Healing Process

Changing Perspectives on Health

Determinants of Health

The Health of Canadians

Health, Wellness and Healing

Central Questions

1. What are the meanings of health, well-being, wellness, illness and disease?
2. What does the concept of health within illness mean?
3. What do the terms healing and holistic health mean?
4. How have ideas of health changed over the past century?
5. How does the socioeconomic model of health differ from its predecessors—the biomedical and behavioural models?
6. What are the major factors that determine a person's health?
7. How does the World Health Organization define health?
8. What are the main indicators of health status used by most countries?
9. How does the health status of Canadians compare with that of people in other countries?
10. What are the leading causes of death in Canada?
11. What are the most common illnesses experienced by Canadians?
12. What are the most common disabilities among Canadians?
13. What are the main causes of hospitalization in Canada?
14. How do Canadians perceive their own health status?

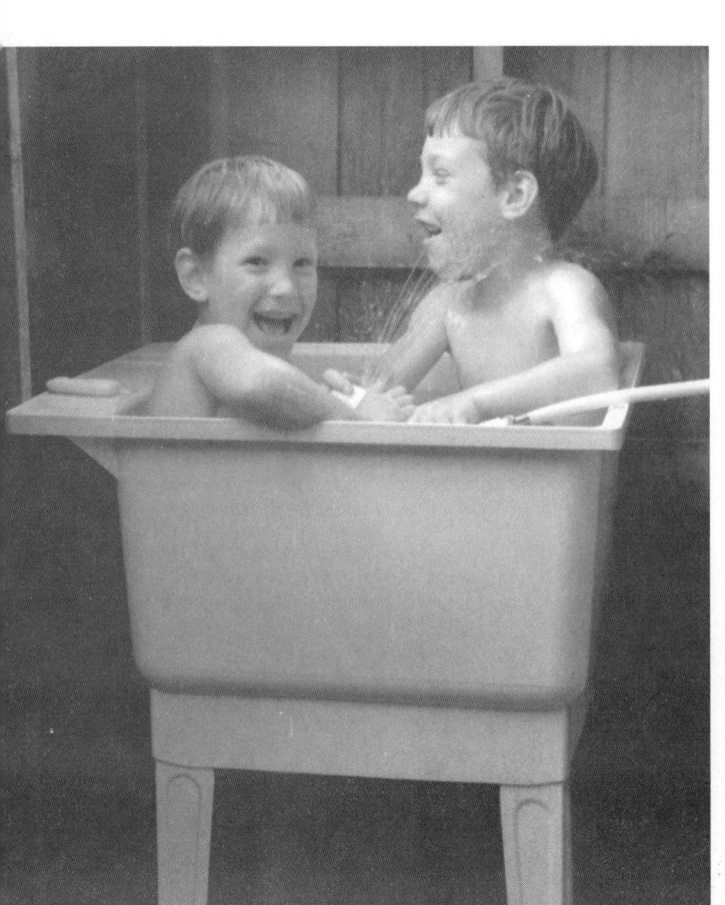

Introduction

Good health is the bedrock on which social progress is built. A nation of healthy people can do those things which make life worthwhile and, as the level of health increases, so does the potential for happiness.

Lalonde, 1974

Canadians today are a highly health-conscious people. It is health, rather than illness, that is becoming the focus of our health care system. Over the past two decades, there has been a major change, a "paradigm shift," in the philosophy of health care in Canada, in the United States and, indeed, in most countries of the world. We appear at long last to have swung towards a more positive approach. It is an approach that stresses the promotion of health and the prevention of illness as matters of primary concern, and one that focusses on restoration to optimum health (or a peaceful death), not merely on the curing of disease, as the goal of therapeutic care.

As knowledgeable professionals to whom other people turn for advice on health matters, nurses need a good understanding of what health and illness are all about. They also need to be aware of current thinking in regard to the factors that contribute to good health and those that predispose a person to illness—what are referred to in today's terminology as the determinants of health.

The Meanings of Health, Wellness, Illness and Disease

Health is a complex phenomenon which cannot be simply defined. There is a wide variation in definitions of health and in personal meanings and perceptions of health. Older people might accept a few aches and pains as a normal part of the aging process, whereas runners may feel that they are not in good health unless they can cover 25 km easily. The concept of health has been viewed from a variety of perspectives and has been interpreted in many ways. Broadly defined, **health** is a positive state of being that includes physical fitness, mental (or emotional) stability and social and spiritual ease. It is not a constant or absolute entity but rather an ever-changing and evolving state in which people actively strive to achieve the highest level of functioning that is possible for them. In order to describe the concept of health more fully, we must first define the terms *disease* and *illness*, as well as *wellness* and *well-being*.

The word *health* conveys a positive meaning, whereas *disease* and *illness* have negative connotations. We prefer to talk of a person as having a "health challenge," "health problem" or a "health deficit," rather than to say that he or she is ill. **Disease** is seen from this perspective as an interruption in the continuous process of health, manifested by abnormalities or disturbances in the structure and function of body parts, organs or systems. When these abnormalities appear clustered together, they become recognizable as the signs and symptoms of a particular disease. For example, a high temperature, cough and chest pain are commonly seen in people with pneumonia. Pneumonia is a medical label or diagnosis that the physician assigns to the complex of symptoms manifesting the disease process.

An **acute illness** is one in which the onset is rapid, the symptoms are severe and the patient usually recovers fairly quickly, for example, a bout of influenza. **Chronic illness** is the term used for illnesses of long duration. This type of illness usually progresses slowly, often with little change over long periods of time. Some examples of chronic illness include diabetes, chronic obstructive lung disorders and arthritis (Lubkin, 1998; Lindsey, 1996). **Illness** is the personal experience of feeling unhealthy.

A person may feel ill because of a disease, or may just not feel well. However, a person may also not feel ill even though disease is present. For instance, a man may have a serious illness, according to his physician, and yet feel very healthy because he is able to carry out his normal activities for daily living. On the other hand, another man may wake up in the morning with a headache and may feel so ill that he decides he is not well enough to go to work. In either case, illness involves changes in the person's state of being and in social function (Clarke, 1990). What is important in the experience is how people feel and what they do because of those feelings (Leddy & Pepper, 1993).

A term associated with disease and illness is sickness. **Sickness** is a status, defined as the social actions or roles assumed by individuals who experience illness or are diagnosed with a disease (Clarke, 1990). When a person is considered to be sick, certain behaviours are sanctioned that otherwise might not be acceptable. For instance, someone who is sick with the flu is expected to stay at home in bed. But staying at home in bed is not socially acceptable for someone who stayed out late the night before and is simply tired.

Well-being is defined as "a subjective perception of ability, harmony and vitality" (Leddy & Pepper, 1993, p. 221). Like illness, well-being is a relative, changing state experienced in the course of everyday living. When it is experienced at the lowest levels, people perceive themselves as ill, but when it is experienced at the highest levels, they feel maximum satisfaction, understanding and a sense of contribution in life (Leddy & Pepper, 1993). Often, physical symptoms of illness (headache, tiredness, etc.) may be negated—or reinforced—by environmental conditions. Well-being fluctuates towards illness or towards health depending on various factors that influence the individual at a particular time.

Well-being may be viewed on a continuum that ranges from extreme illness when death is imminent to peak or high-level wellness (Dunn, 1959a). Dunn describes a health (well-being) grid that analyses the possible interaction of environment with health and the resulting degrees of well-being and illness (see Figure 2.1). The grid consists of a health axis and an environmental axis, which intersect to make the health and wellness quadrants. The quadrants are labelled as follows: poor health in an unfavourable environment; protected poor health in a favourable environment; emergent high-level wellness in an unfavourable environment; and high-level wellness in a favourable environment. The environmental axis includes the physical and biological aspects of the environment as well as the socioeconomic conditions affecting an individual's health. The health grid ranges from death at the extreme left through serious illness, minor illness, and good health to peak wellness at the right. According to Dunn, high-level wellness can occur only in a favourable environment because people are never isolated from the effects of the world in which they live (Dunn, 1959a).

Wellness is a basic concept that underlies the framework for modern-day health care. Simply defined as a state of optimal health or optimal functioning, this concept is based on the assumption that individuals possess their own optimal level of functioning, which represents the best state of well-being that is possible for them. This definition allows for the fact that most people have some type of minor health deficit. They may have a minor physical problem, such as an allergy to certain foods, or a small speech impediment, or they may be "shy" and have a problem meeting people. Some

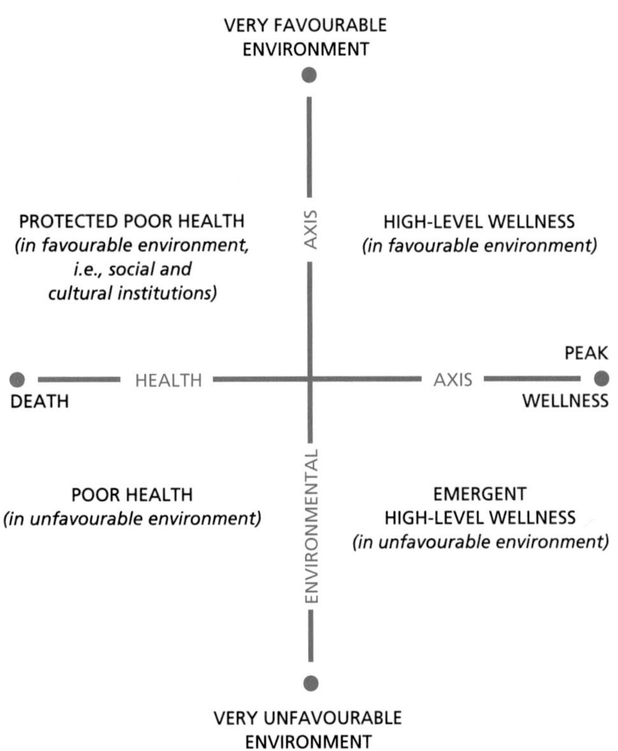

FIGURE 2.1 Dunn's health (well-being) grid, its axes and quadrants

SOURCE: Dunn, 1959a, p. 788. © APHA-American Public Health Association.

people have an unreasonable fear of heights or of cats—problems in the psychological realm of functioning. People rarely attain perfection in all aspects of their health—physical, mental, spiritual and social—and certainly do not achieve it all the time, but each individual has a unique optimal level of functioning that is attainable for him or her.

Wellness is described by Dunn as "an integrated method of functioning which is oriented toward maximizing the potential of which the individual is capable. It requires that the individual maintain a continuum of balance and purposeful direction within the environment where he [or she] is functioning" (1959b, p. 447). Dunn viewed high-level wellness not as an optimum state but rather as a progression or growth towards an ever-higher potential of functioning and an open-ended and ever-expanding challenge to live at a fuller potential. *Potential* in this sense means the best a person is capable of doing within the confines of his or her physical or mental limitations. High-level wellness involves a progressive integration (or maturation) of the whole being of the individual—one's body, mind and spirit—at increasingly higher levels throughout the life cycle. In optimum health, individuals function at a high level within a dynamic and ever-changing environment (Dunn, 1959b, 1973; Pender, 1987).

Leddy and Pepper (1993) conceptualize wellness as "an actively continuing process that involves initiative, ability to assume responsibility for health, value judgements and integration of the total person" (p. 222). While wellness is difficult to evaluate objectively, there are a number of indicators that can be used. These include:

- the capacity of people to perform to the best of their ability
- the ability to adjust and adapt to varying situations
- a reported feeling of well-being
- a feeling that "everything is together" and "harmonious."

Chronic Illness and the Concept of Health Within Illness

Sixty to 73 percent of people with a chronic illness consider their health to be good or excellent, according to a survey conducted by Health Canada in 1994–1995 (Statistics Canada, 1995). This finding necessitates a rethinking of our ideas about health and illness. Pender (1987) suggests that health is the primary life experience and that illness is superimposed upon it. Chronic illness or long-term disability, looked at in this context, then, becomes a facet of one's life rather than the dominating force in that life. This is what people with chronic health problems appear to be telling us.

The concept of **health within illness** is one that is currently receiving considerable interest from nurses and others in the health care field. In this concept, illness is regarded as "an event that can expand human potential" (Moch, 1989, p. 23). It is seen not as an enemy the patient is expected to fight against but as an opportunity for personal growth and transformation. Many people in our society have serious chronic health problems, yet they are able to live normal, healthy lives, often of a better quality than before they became ill. It is not unusual to hear people with conditions such as diabetes, for example, say that they have "never felt better" or "more alive" once their diabetic state was regulated and they have learned to live with the limitations of the disease. To use another example, a young woman afflicted with multiple sclerosis who has lost the function of one side of her body may never regain total functioning of her affected arm and leg, but may nonetheless be able to achieve independence in daily activities and maintain an active role in society. In the course of daily living, such a person would not see herself as being ill, unless she had a cold or a case of the flu. For people with a chronic illness, health means living with and mastering the disabilities imposed by the disease process, while focussing on activities that increase the quality of life and maximize the physical, mental, emotional and social potential of which they are capable.

There is an expanding body of evidence indicating that people grow and become stronger as human beings, particularly in the psychological, social and spiritual dimensions, during the experience of illness (Lindsey, 1996; Jones & Meleis, 1993; Jaffe, 1980; Siegel, 1986). They may develop a heightened sense of self and of their personal potential, feel a greater spiritual inner peace and discover new meaning and purpose in life. They may also experience changes in themselves, their personal goals, their values and their relationships with others. As well, the experience of illness may bring an increased awareness of nature and the environment in which they live. Through the experience of illness, people "may emerge healthy rather than vulnerable" (Jones & Meleis, 1993, p. 3). A wonderful example of a person who made life a healthy, positive experience in the face of terminal illness was Terry Fox, of Coquitlam, British Columbia. His 1980 "Marathon of Hope," in which he ran across Canada, despite having bone cancer, to increase awareness of cancer and raise funds for research into this life-threatening disease, has been immortalized in statues, plaques and public edifices throughout the world. More importantly, it has inspired annual fund-raising marathons around the country.

Holistic Health and the Healing Process

Holistic Health

Holistic health is an approach to wellness that recognizes the interaction between the whole person and his or her

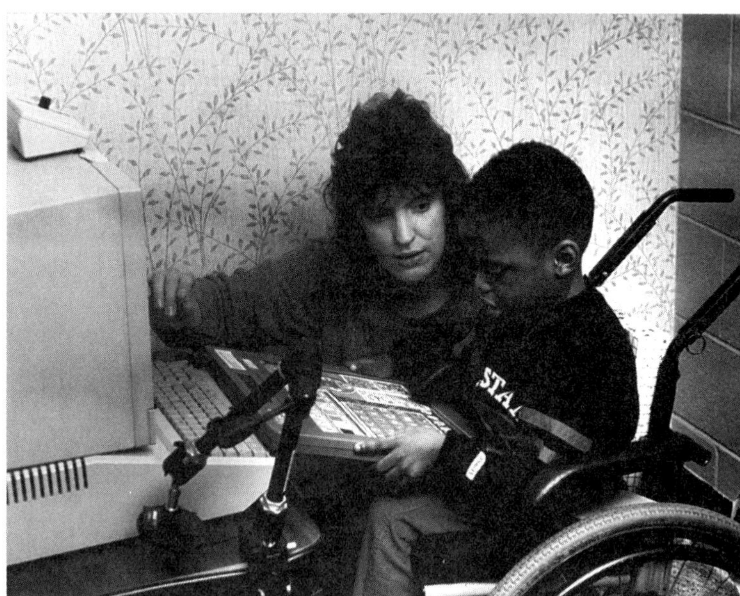

This individual is able to live a healthy life and maintain an active, fulfilling role in society.

environment, and emphasizes harmony with oneself, with nature and with the world (Flynn, 1980). This approach is based on the premise that "things and events cannot be analyzed by reducing them to component parts without destroying or distorting the integrity of the whole" (Flynn, 1980, p. 9). That is to say, an individual's health must be considered in terms of his or her total functioning. One cannot separate the physical, social, spiritual and emotional components of health; nor can one separate the whole person from his or her environment. This interaction works in both directions—an illness, even a minor one, such as influenza or a short-lived gastrointestinal upset, can affect a person's mental outlook and interactions with other people; and an emotional problem, such as anxiety over examinations or an argument with someone, can affect appetite, digestion and other aspects of physical functioning.

Flynn (1980) considers holistic health to be synonymous with Dunn's "high-level wellness" and sees wellness as "an ever-changing growth toward fulfilling an individual's potential considering individual needs, abilities and disabilities" (p.12). Holistic health care focusses on the individual rather than on the disease. Learning about the person who has the disease is considered more important than finding out about the disease itself. The ill person is viewed as having a "dynamic disturbance in the equilibrium of the body–mind–spirit environment. Health requires a harmonious integration of the body, mind, spirit and the environment, while illness indicates a degree of imbalance among them" (p.12). Illness, while often painful and frightening, is regarded as having a positive potential, providing an opportunity "to further clarify values, affirm individual priorities and direction and deepen a sense of the meaning and value of life" (p. 28).

To return to the example of the young woman with multiple sclerosis, it is easy to see that her physical disability will interfere with both her emotional and social well-being. She will undoubtedly feel grief over the loss of physical functioning. She may feel that she is no longer the person she used to be, or that she is a burden to a partner. Her illness may require lengthy hospitalization from time to time when she will be cut off from normal social activities with family and friends. Holistic care for this woman will extend beyond the therapeutic intervention needed for the physical problems caused by the disease itself. Her feelings and her relationships with her partner and others will have to be explored, and she will need help to restore harmony, balance and a sense of meaning and direction in her life.

The Process of Healing

Closely tied to the concept of holistic health is that of **healing**. The term *heal* comes from the old English word *hael*, for whole. Thus, to heal means to make whole. Just as holistic health encompasses the dimensions of body, mind and spirit, the healing of a person from illness or injury involves much more than just the physical aspects of getting better. The individual must be restored to normal, healthy functioning in all aspects of his or her being. This is a complex process that requires active participation on the patient's part, and involves a building up of new tissues, perhaps new patterns of living and sometimes a new perspective on one's philosophy of life. Take the case of an individual who has had a heart attack: not only must the damaged tissues in the heart be allowed to heal, but the person must also learn to live with a lifelong "heart condition" and will probably need to incorporate into his or her daily living pattern new dietary habits to reduce the risk of further heart attacks, an exercise regimen to strengthen heart functioning and activities to reduce stress. The person must also come to terms with the fact of mortality.

Healing takes time. Whether it be the healing of a surgical wound, recovery from a bout of influenza or a heart attack, the convalescent period is always slower than the onset of the problem. Someone who has had a surgical repair of muscles in the shoulder will probably be told that it will take at least a year to heal. There will likely be a two-week period of total immobilization of the body part, followed by several months of physiotherapy and rehabilitation exercises.

For healing to take place there are certain antecedents or prerequisites that need to be present. In the case of physical healing, such as the healing of damaged tissues in a wound, the body must have adequate energy, that is, it needs nutritional support and adequate oxygenation of the tissues. For other types of healing, it is psychic energy that is required. This energy comes from within the person. Wendler (1996) suggests it stems from one's relationships with self and others.

Certainly, there is increasing evidence that caring is an essential component of the healing process (Wendler, 1996; Cannon, 1997; Wilderquist & Davidhizer, 1994). "The purpose of human caring in the context of healing encounters is to facilitate growth in wholeness" (Cannon, 1997, p.42). Important in this process, Cannon states, in addition to competence, are good communication skills, the ability to develop good interpersonal relationships with patients, a gentle manner in carrying out the skills component of nursing, and intuition. These aspects of nursing will be discussed later in this text.

Changing Perspectives on Health

Over the years, our ideas about health and illness have changed considerably. At one time, health was defined simply as the absence of illness; people were considered healthy as long as they were not sick. Health care focussed on determining the causes of disease and on developing new and better ways to treat it. We subsequently went through a period when we put considerable emphasis on people's own behaviour—smoking, overeating, lack of exercise—as a cause of many illnesses. Health care began to focus on encouraging people to change lifestyles in order to promote their health. Today, we recognize that health is affected not only by physiological and lifestyle factors, but also by the social and economic conditions in which people live. The World Health Organization states that "health begins at home, in schools and factories. It is there where people live and work, that health is made or broken" (WHO, 1981).

In order to improve health, then, it is necessary not only to treat disease and encourage healthy habits, but also to improve living and working conditions, for as these conditions improve, so does health (Epp, 1986). In this section of the chapter, we explore the evolution of our current definition of health as exemplified in the biomedical, behavioural and socioeconomic models of health. We will discuss the models chronologically, in the order in which they have dominated the health field in Canada.

The Biomedical Model

As we noted in Chapter 1, tremendous advances have been made in the biomedical and physical sciences over the past 100 years. The application of these sciences in medicine and medical technology has dominated health care in Western cultures for the better part of this century. This purely empirical approach to health, based on scientific research and teaching, is known as the **biomedical model**. It focussed on the physiological determinants of health and disease. The body was likened to an intricate machine, with disease considered to be the result of a breakdown somewhere in the mechanism. Restoration to health required first, a diagnosis to determine the cause, and second, intervention to remedy the condition. Medications and physical or surgical measures were the common treatments. Efforts to prevent illness concentrated on measures to control or eradicate the physical causes of disease, by such means as mosquito control to prevent malaria or immunizations for communicable diseases such as typhoid, tetanus, diphtheria, smallpox and polio. Considerable progress was made in the areas of diagnosis and therapeutic treatments for disease during the time the biomedical model dominated the health field. Gradually, it was realized, however, that not all ills could be solved through the use of diagnostic and therapeutic measures alone.

The first challenge to the biomedical model came in 1948 when the World Health Organization defined health as "a state of complete physical, mental and social well-being and not merely the absence of disease or infirmity" (WHO, 1948, p. 1). This definition set the stage for a new perspective on health, which moved beyond looking only at the physiological basis of illness. As with all new ideas, the more holistic approach to health, which incorporated an individual's social and mental attributes as well as physical well-being, took time to be accepted. The WHO definition was criticized for being too vague and all-inclusive—critics claimed that it would be difficult to measure a person's health by quantitative scientific means using this definition.

The Behavioural Model

In Canada, the next major challenge to the biomedical model of health came with publication in 1974 of a working document prepared by the Research and Planning Division of the Department of Health and Welfare (Lalonde, 1974). The document was aptly entitled *A New Perspective on the Health of Canadians* (also referred to as the Lalonde Report). It suggested that health should be looked at in terms of a *health fields* approach. The basic premise of this concept was that there were four principal factors affecting both individual and group health, namely, human biology, environment, lifestyles and health care organization. Because of this emphasis, it became known as the **behavioural model**. (See Figure 2.2.)

The *New Perspective* document also suggested that the goal of health care should be to increase freedom from disability, as well as to promote a state of well-being sufficient to perform at adequate levels of physical, mental and social activity, taking age into consideration (Lalonde, 1974).

While acknowledging the contribution of medical science and technology to improvements in the health of Canadians since the turn of the century, the Lalonde Report pointed out that further improvements would come about not from further advances in medical science, but from strategies such as improving our environment, moderating self-imposed risks and adding to our knowledge of human biology. The *New Perspective* document was a landmark in Canadian health care. It not only extended the boundaries of the health field, but also suggested that the *outcomes of care* were more important than *accessibility to care*, which was seen as a variable that might or might not improve one's health (Crichton, Hsu & Tsang, 1994).

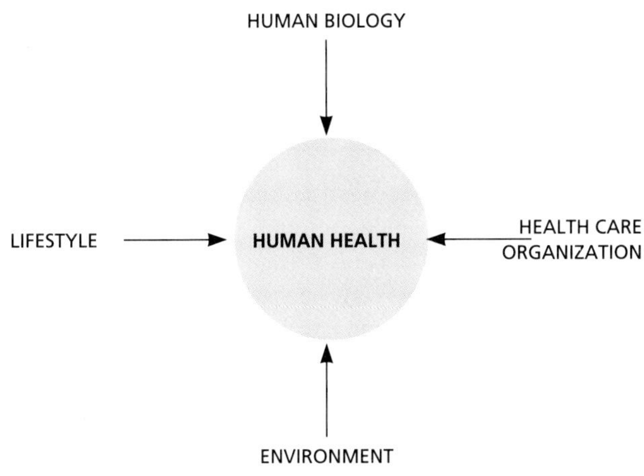

FIGURE 2.2 Behavioural model of health

SOURCE: World Health Organization, 1974, p. 8.

The *New Perspective* document put considerable emphasis on the importance of lifestyle as a contributing factor in most of the five leading causes of death in Canada—heart disease, cancer, strokes, chronic obstructive lung disease and accidents. Following this report, a Health Promotion Directorate was established in the Federal Department of Health and Welfare. Programs were subsequently initiated by federal, provincial and municipal governments and by voluntary agencies, including the Canadian Heart Association and others, to encourage us to improve our lifestyles. There is no doubt that the programs have achieved a certain amount of success. The *Active Health Report* on the findings of a 1985 study on the health and health behaviour of Canadians indicated that many of us had improved our health habits—we were exercising more, we were more conscious of the benefits of eating a healthy diet, and a great many people had stopped smoking. There has been a considerable reduction, too, in the number of accidents due to the deadly combination of drinking and driving (Health & Welfare Canada, 1987).

Although the health fields concept (behavioural model) was seen to be an improvement over the biomedical model, its usefulness was limited by the fact that it failed to take into consideration the impact of the socioeconomic environment on health.

The Socioeconomic Model

Addressing these limitations and looking back at several earlier reports on the effect of social and economic conditions on health, the World Health Organization expanded the health fields concept to include socioeconomic factors. In 1977, the Thirtieth World Health Assembly stated that "the main social target of governments and WHO in the coming decades should be the attainment by all citizens of the world by the year 2000 of a level of health that will permit them to lead a socially and economically productive life" (cited in WHO, 1985, p. 14). At the 1978 International Conference on Primary Health Care in Alma-Ata, Russia, the importance of the relationship between health and the economic and social dimensions of a community was once again emphasized. The WHO publication *Health for All by the Year 2000* (1981) outlined strategies to implement the socioeconomic, or "healthy people," vision of health espoused at the Alma-Ata conference. The deliberations of the Alma-Ata Conference also led WHO to propose the following definition of health:

> *Health is defined as the extent to which an individual or group is able, on one hand, to realize aspirations and satisfy needs; and, on the other hand, to change or cope with the environment. Health is, therefore, seen as a resource for everyday life, a dimension of our "quality of life," and not the object of living; it is a positive concept emphasizing social and personal resources, as well as physical capabilities.*
>
> (World Health Organization, 1984a)

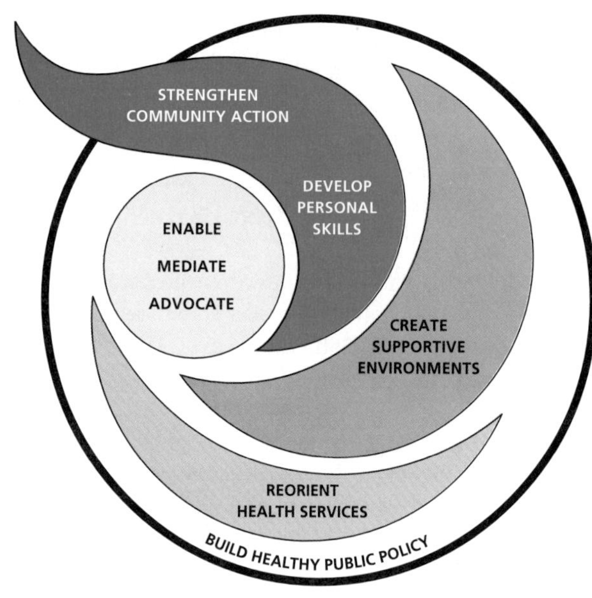

FIGURE 2.3 Ottawa Charter for Health Promotion

SOURCE: Canadian Public Health Association, 1986.

At the time of writing, the WHO is recommending that the definition of health be redefined to include two new words: dynamic and spiritual (International Nursing Review, 1998).

All countries belonging to the World Health Organization were urged to work towards the goal of "health for all by the year 2000" using ways and means best suited to their particular situation to implement the new vision of health. In Canada, the strategies to implement the new vision emerged from the findings of two studies, a *National Health Survey* which was undertaken from 1977 to 1979 and the *Health Promotion Survey* of 1985. The findings from both studies clearly showed the role of poverty, unemployment and pollution in health. These findings led to the development of Health and Welfare Canada's discussion paper entitled *Achieving Health for All: A Framework for Health Promotion* (Epp, 1986). The paper was presented at an international conference on health promotion, held in Toronto in 1986, which was sponsored jointly by the World Health Organization, Health and Welfare Canada, and the Canadian Public Health Association. From this conference came the *Ottawa Charter for Health Promotion* (see Figure 2.3).

The Epp Report and the Ottawa Charter recommended the reduction of health inequities caused by socioeconomic and environmental factors. They identified the prerequisites of health as "peace, shelter, food, income, a stable eco-system, sustainable resources, social justice and equity." These documents were another landmark in Canadian health care, signifying a major shift in thinking about both health and health care. We have moved to a **socioeconomic model** in which our ideas about health have broadened to include social and economic factors, as the list of prerequisites for health cited above indicates. The emphasis has shifted away from therapeutic care to health promotion and health protection, aimed at getting at the causes of ill health, rather than only at its cure. Actions to improve health are community based and **multisectoral**, involving collaboration between the health care sector and the business, education, justice and law enforcement sectors. The pivotal concepts in the socioeconomic model of health are **empowerment** and **community**. Use of the term "empowering" indicates a shift in the power base in public health from bureaucracies to the community (Green & Raeburn, 1988). It also implies that individuals should take an active role in making decisions as well as in creating and using resources to achieve their health potential. We will discuss these concepts further in subsequent chapters throughout the book.

The primary responsibility for administration and management of our National Health Insurance Program is vested in the provinces. Following the Epp Report, studies have been undertaken in all provinces to look at ways and means

A Vision of Health for Ontario

We see an Ontario in which people live longer in good health, and people are empowered to realize their full health potential through a safe, non-violent environment, adequate income, housing, food and education, and a valued role to play in family, work and the community.

We see people having equitable access to affordable health care regardless of geography, income, age, gender or cultural background. Finally, we see everyone working together to achieve better health for all.

SOURCE: Government of Ontario, 1993.

of implementing its recommendations and, at the time of writing, the provinces are at various stages of implementing the findings of these studies. A province-by-province comparison is made in Chapter 3.

In Ontario, the Premier's Council on Health, Well-being and Social Justice (1987–1991) published a summary of its research on the factors that determine our health. The summary was entitled *Nurturing Health* (1993), and it embodies many of the precepts of the socioeconomic model of health.

Determinants of Health

The Ontario nurturing health model (see Figure 2.4) identifies four key factors, or *determinants*, of health:

1. living and working conditions
2. social support
3. genetic makeup
4. individual behaviours.

You will notice that two of these factors—individual behaviours and genetic makeup—are essentially the same as the lifestyles and heredity factors of the behavioural model. The other two factors, which have the most influence on health, according to the Ontario report, relate to two aspects of the environment—living and working conditions, and the social support available to people. You will notice, too, that the fourth factor identified in the behavioural model—health care organization—is missing from the Ontario nurturing health model. In the approach outlined in this version of the socioeconomic model, health care is viewed as a part of both living and working conditions (community and occupational health) and as a component of social support (emergency services, and therapeutic, rehabilitative and palliative care). The integration of health care organization into living and working conditions and social support is not intended to devalue the importance of health care. Nor does it mean that there will be less need for doctors and nurses. Rather, it underscores the need for the coordination of efforts by all sectors to improve the health of people in our society. Let us take a look at each of the elements in the nurturing health model.

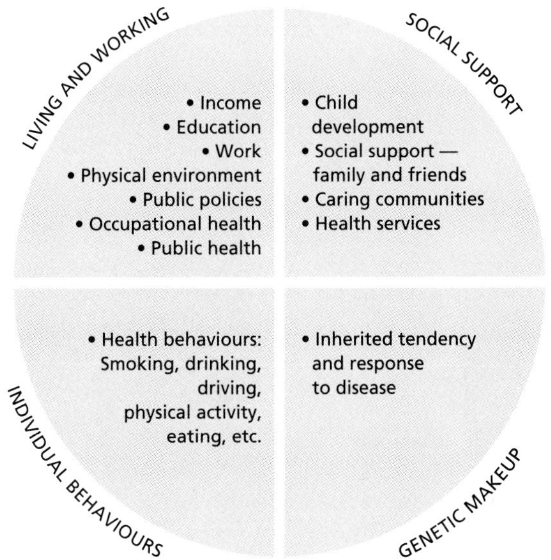

FIGURE 2.4 Beyond lifestyle: the Ontario nurturing health model

SOURCE: Government of Ontario, 1993, p. 4.

Living and Working Conditions

The *Nurturing Health* report suggests that the factors with the greatest influence on people's health are their living and working conditions and the social support available to them. Lifestyle is determined as much by circumstance as by the decisions made, consciously or unconsciously, by people about the way they choose to live. Single parents on welfare, for example, may be at a disadvantage in terms of their health if they cannot afford to join a health club or a local community centre. They also need considerable social support from family, friends, and health and social services in order to maintain their family. A good income, on the other hand, can make life more comfortable and go a long way towards enhancing one's quality of life, even for people with health problems.

In looking at living and working conditions, we will consider such elements as income, education, work (including occupational health), the physical environment (including public health) and public policies.

INCOME

Recent studies on health have shown some very interesting findings about the relationship between income and general health. The *Active Health Survey* (1987) showed that people's health is directly related to income. Men in the upper income groups can expect to live six years longer than men with lower incomes; slightly less difference (three years) was found for women. People with higher incomes can also look forward to more disability-free years—14 more for men and eight for women.

In much of the developing world, many health problems are directly attributable to a lack of the basic essentials of life (such as adequate nutrition and housing), resulting from widespread poverty among large segments of the population. In countries with a small gap between the rich and the poor, such as Japan, the Netherlands and Norway, people have a greater overall life expectancy than in countries such as the United States and France, where there is a large gap between rich and poor (Government of Ontario, 1993).

Poor people are more likely to have poor health. They have a higher incidence of mental health disorders, high blood pressure and disorders of the joints and limbs than do people with higher incomes. They are also more likely to die from accidental falls, chronic respiratory conditions, pneumonia, tuberculosis and cirrhosis of the liver. And unfortunately, Canada, despite its wealth, is not entirely exempt from the influence of poverty on the health of its people. Particularly vulnerable are certain groups within the low-income bracket, namely, older people, the unemployed, welfare recipients, single women supporting families, First Nations People and immigrants. Among the First Nations People, where the rate of poverty is more than twice the national average, the infant mortality rate is also more than double the average Canadian rate (Government of Ontario, 1993; Epp, 1986).

Although Canada is considered a rich country by international standards, it is estimated that a million Canadian children live in poverty, that is, in families with incomes below the poverty line. Given the established connection between poverty and ill health, this situation is of great significance to all health care workers.

EDUCATION

The more highly educated people are, the better equipped they are to look after their health. WHO, for example, has found that teaching mothers to read is one of the most effective ways to improve the health of families (UNICEF, 1992). In Canada, more people with post-secondary education rate their health as good or excellent (72%) than those with less than secondary education (49%).

Education contributes to good health in many ways. The *Nurturing Health* document lists the following health benefits:

- Education increases job and income security and job satisfaction
- Education equips people with the skills they need to identify and solve individual and collective problems
- Education can unlock the innate creativity in people, thereby adding to our collective ability to generate wealth
- Education improves "health literacy"—the ability to gain access to information and services that keep you and your family healthy. (Government of Ontario, 1993)

WORK

Most adults spend about one-quarter of their lives at work, so a healthy workplace is an important component of conditions for healthy living. A healthy and safe physical environment is essential and, in our country, provincial Workers' Compensation Boards are very concerned with

LOOKING back

Marguerite d'Youville, 1701–1771

Marie-Marguerite Dufrost de Lajemmerais d'Youville was the founder of the Order of the Sisters of Charity of Montreal, commonly known as the Grey Nuns. This order became one of the pioneering nursing orders, mainly involved as visiting nurses in the community; its members introduced both hospitals and district nursing throughout Canada, especially on the frontiers of the west and the north.

Marguerite de Lajemmerais was born in 1701 into one of the great and wealthy families of New France, but the death of her father when she was seven left the family financially insecure. Her marriage to François d'Youville in 1722 was not a happy one and was marked by the death, in early infancy, of four of her six children. Her husband died in 1730, leaving a debt-burdened estate. Following his death, Madame d'Youville, who had turned increasingly to her religion during the latter years of her marriage, worked actively with the established sisterhoods and soon was applying herself to service of the poor and the ill.

In 1737, with two other women, she established a lay order both to care for the sick poor and to raise money for their care, drawing on her own needlework skills as a means of raising money. The women chose a simple grey habit and, because it was not a cloistered order, did mainly visiting nursing. However, they also took into their house many abandoned children and ill elderly. Their reputation as district nurses grew rapidly. In 1747, the Governor asked Marguerite d'Youville and her Sisters of Charity to take over the running of the bankrupt and filthy general hospital of Montreal, which she soon had running smoothly and well. This became the main headquarters for their care, although the Grey Nuns continued their community nursing. The hospital was all but destroyed in a fire a few years later, but despite that and despite epidemics, war (during which they nursed both French and English soldiers), poor harvests and government interference, Madame d'Youville managed to establish a firm foundation for the growing and increasingly respected nursing sisterhood. In 1755, the Order of the Sisters of Charity was accepted as a religious order by the Roman Catholic Church.

Despite increasing ill health, Mother Marguerite d'Youville was a tireless worker and remained a remarkable administrator until her death in 1771. The Order she founded continued to grow and, in the 1800s and 1900s, established branches throughout Canada, the United States and other parts of the world. Marguerite d'Youville was personally credited with several miraculous cures, and in December 1990 she was canonized by the Roman Catholic Church. Saint Marguerite became Canada's first Canadian-born saint.

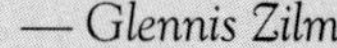

— *Glennis Zilm*

this aspect of working conditions (see Chapter 4). Also, it is increasingly being recognized that stress is one of the major contributors to decreased productivity and absenteeism. This topic is discussed further in Chapter 30, where we talk about the role of the occupational health nurse.

Employers are coming to recognize that they can positively influence the health of their employees by improving working conditions. Many are offering ongoing education and training programs, incentives for work well done, job security, employee involvement in decision making, working as a member of a team and adjustments to accommodate employees with both home and workplace responsibilities. Because many firms now offer health promotion and wellness programs in the workplace, the need for occupational health nurses can be expected to increase over the next few years.

THE PHYSICAL ENVIRONMENT

The physical environment includes both the natural and the artificial aspects of the physical world that surrounds us. Considerable research is currently being done on the effects of weather (an important part of our natural environment) on people's health. We know that many people, particularly those with rheumatism, arthritis or asthma, are sensitive to atmospheric changes. With impending changes in the weather, some individuals experience a variety of symptoms including severe pain, breathing difficulties, fatigue and depression. It has been observed that the rate of suicide is considerably greater in the northern coastal areas of British Columbia, where the rainfall is highest, than in other parts of Canada.

Many other aspects of the physical environment have been created by human beings, and are now beginning to be controlled by us as well, in order to make our surroundings more conducive to healthy living. One of the major factors in the improvement of health in the Western world during the past century and a half has been the reduction of known environmental hazards through the application of public health measures. These have included such basic measures as establishing standards for housing; provisions to ensure safe water, food and milk supplies; safety standards for places where people work; and the control of communicable disease.

Although we have greatly reduced the effect of environmental factors on health in Canada, there is still a lack of uniformity in the application of basic public health measures across the country. Housing for many people is still inadequate or even unsafe. Access to a safe water supply is not guaranteed to all. In some homes, there is still no running water or indoor plumbing. Raw sewage still pours into many of our lakes and rivers, and insects, rats and other disease-carrying pests infest many poverty-stricken neighbourhoods.

Then, too, other environmental problems have emerged in recent years, many as a result of industrialization and increasing urbanization. The contamination of our waterways by industrial pollutants is a matter of major concern. There is growing alarm about the threat to health of air pollution, particularly in large urban centres. Many cities have installed monitoring devices and have instituted controls to curb industrial activity when air pollution reaches a level considered harmful to health.

The effect of increasing urbanization on both the physical and social environment is also causing considerable concern to health professionals in the health field. In many instances, cities and new communities have grown too rapidly to cope with the housing, sewage and other basic services needed by the population. Overcrowding, lack of recreational facilities, excessive noise, violence and solitude are among the social factors resulting from urbanization that contribute to the health problems of city-dwellers.

PUBLIC POLICY

At every level of government—national, provincial and municipal—health programs are based on policies that the prevailing government either initiated or endorsed from a previous government.

"Public policy has the power to provide people with opportunities for health, as well as to deny them such opportunities. All policies, and hence all sectors, have a bearing on health" (Epp, 1986, p. 10). Many policies outside the health sector have a direct bearing on health; examples of these include regulations for safe housing, the control of agricultural pesticides, high taxation on alcohol and tobacco and regulations for a smoke-free environment. Politicians are becoming more aware and are accepting greater accountability for the effect that policies in their sectors have on health. The role of public policy on health is explored in more detail in Chapter 3.

Social Support

In looking at the determinants of health, we must remember that human beings are social animals. Their relationships with other people are very important to the satisfaction of many of their basic needs. Relationships with other people in the home, in the work or school setting and in the numerous other activities in which people engage contribute positively or negatively to their health. A number of studies have shown the influence of a supportive social environment on good health and a long life (Epp, 1986; Government of Ontario, 1993). Social support is a lifelong need. Essential to this social support is the positive interaction with others that gives a person a sense of belonging and fosters self-esteem. We will be talking about the importance to health of supportive social relationships when we discuss health and the individual, health and the family and health and the community in subsequent chapters.

Under the rubric of social support, the nurturing health model includes child development, the support given by family and friends and that provided in caring communities. In our consideration of social support, we also include the emergency, restorative and palliative care services that provide a network of health support for people in our society. These were included in the original nurturing health model.

Social support, in the form of health and social programs administered by different levels of government, also provides a buffer to help people cope with stresses faced in everyday living. Canada is called a "welfare state" because of the network of social and economic supports built into our governmental system. These include the National Health Insurance Program, Old Age Pension and other social assistance programs, Employment Insurance, Child Tax Credit, Workers' Compensation and the Canada and Quebec Pension Plans. While these resources are available to all Canadians, not everyone makes the best use of them. In fact, it is often those who are most in need of social assistance who do not use the services, either because they do not know that they are there or they do not know how to access them. Furthermore, a lack of self-esteem or low self-image all too frequently prevents people from taking the initiative to mobilize these resources for their own needs (Grant, 1988).

Genetic Makeup

Biological factors that influence human health include an individual's genetic inheritance, the processes of maturation and aging and the complex network of structures and systems that compose the human body. The role of genetics, in particular, is the subject of much recent health research.

A number of specific diseases are now known to be passed down through families. One example is Huntington's chorea, a progressive degenerative disorder of the nervous system that is transmitted through a single dominant gene and may affect both males and females in a family. Another is hemophilia, which has afflicted several generations of males in the Hapsburg family and other royal families. A more common disease, diabetes, is also believed to have an inherited component, although its exact mode of transmission is still not well understood. Down's syndrome (mongolism) is thought to be caused by a defective chromosome, which may or may not be inherited.

Although many disorders present at birth may have a genetic component, others may result from problems encountered by the unborn infant *in utero*. These are called **congenital** problems and include such things as heart malformations, cleft palate (a division in the roof of the mouth) and spina bifida (a defect in the spinal canal). Other disorders present at birth are caused by difficulties during delivery; cerebral palsy (an involuntary muscular disorder) is an example.

In many other disorders that affect human beings, the effect of genetic inheritance is suspected but the relationship has not yet been fully established. We do not know for certain at this time, for example, the extent of the role of heredity as a causative factor in heart trouble, or in hypertension, or in a number of other health problems. Nor do we yet know why some diseases seem to afflict people of one ethnic group more than another, for example, the high prevalence of diabetes among Jewish women, or of glaucoma (increased tension within the eyeball) among people in many of the West Indian ethnic groups.

Individual Behaviours

The ways of life of people in a community, and their individual lifestyles, also have a significant impact on health. Lifestyle is determined in part by circumstance and in part by the decisions made, consciously or unconsciously, by people about the way they choose to live. Lifestyle depends to a large extent on the occupations of household members, their income level, and the things that income can purchase.

In addition to circumstantial factors, the element of personal decision making that enters into an individual or family lifestyle plays an important role in determining health. One of the by-products of affluence in the developed world has been obesity, which is considered a major health problem in North American society. Although other factors contribute to obesity—many of which are not yet fully understood—individual choice of diet has a great deal to do with it. Obesity has been linked to many diseases, such as heart conditions, hypertension and diabetes. At the other end of the spectrum, malnutrition can occur even in the midst of a plentiful food supply, as indicated by the eating patterns of some adolescent females who starve themselves because they think that being thin is beautiful. Malnutrition in wealthy nations may also result from poor food choices, such as the eating of too many snack foods and sweets instead of regular, well-balanced meals.

The sedentary way of life among many people in Canada (and among people in higher socioeconomic groups in other parts of the world) must also be considered a lifestyle factor affecting health. It too is a by-product of the affluent society, in which most people rely on cars for transportation and television sets for entertainment. A lack of exercise contributes to a generally lowered state of physical fitness. When the body is deprived of physical activity, the accompanying physical decline includes decreased muscle strength, stiffened joints, increased brittleness of the bones, impaired digestion and a general decline in endurance, strength and physical skills. This "atrophy through disuse" may occur at any age. It is encouraging to see so many young—and older—people today engaging in programs of regular exercise.

Another example of individual behaviour that has an enormous impact on health is the terrible toll on human lives caused by excessive speed and careless driving on the highways. A very heavy burden is put on our health care system for the care, treatment and rehabilitation of countless victims of automobile accidents.

Numerous other major problems of increasing concern in the health field today can also be attributed to individual lifestyle factors. These include tobacco use, drug and substance abuse, sexually transmitted diseases and suicide. It is especially troubling that such problems are affecting increasing numbers of young people (see Table 2.1 for statistics on the drinking habits of Canadians).

The Health of Canadians

In this section, we are going to discuss the health of Canadians as measured by objective standards using statistical data that have been collected over the years. Then, we will look briefly at how Canadians perceive their own health, as documented in recent studies undertaken by the federal government and by the Government of Ontario. The objective standards we will examine include commonly used health status indicators; the perceptions of health status come from the findings of two surveys.

Health Status Indicators

In this chapter we have discussed comparisons between the health status of different groups of people within Canada and between that of people in different countries. We said, for example, that the poor are at a disadvantage healthwise, and that certain low-income groups are especially vulnerable to illness. We also said that the health status of people in some developed countries, for example, Japan, Norway and the Netherlands, is better than that in other countries. In Canada, Statistics Canada (an arm of the federal government) regularly undertakes surveys, collects data and compiles information about the health status of Canadians. The governments of most countries in the world routinely collect data about illness and death among the people living in their countries. The kinds of statistical information usually compiled on an annual basis by national governments include:

1. the average life span of people (*life expectancy*)
2. the number of deaths relative to the population (*mortality rates*)
3. the reasons for these deaths (*causes of death*)
4. the incidence of illness (*morbidity data*).

These statistical measures are considered four of the main health status indicators for a given population. They provide a base for identifying major health problems, that is, those problems responsible for the most deaths and those causing the greatest amount of disability to people. They also help to give some insight into the principal factors affecting the health of the population. Because virtually every country in the world collects information on these four indicators, it is possible to look at differences between countries, and where statistical information has accumulated over a number of years, to look at trends over time.

In Canada, health care for the First Nations People has been a responsibility of the federal government, which

TABLE 2.1 Drinking status, drinking level and number of heavy drinking occasions among current drinkers by gender and age

	Drinking Status			*Level and Heavy Drinking Occasions, Among Current Drinkers*			
VARIABLE	NEVER	FORMER	CURRENT DRINKERS	DRINKS/ WEEK	% ANY HEAVY OCCASIONS*	MEAN # OF HEAVY OCCASIONS†	TOTAL SAMPLE SIZE
Overall	7.7%	18.0%	74.4%	4.2	46.2%	15.7	10 385
Gender							
Male	4.8%	14.6%	80.6%	5.9	58.0	19.4	4 789
Female	10.4%	21.2%	68.4%	2.3	33.1	8.4	5 596
Age (years)							
15–17	17.8%	24.9%	57.3%	2.3	56.2	12.2	383
18–19	9.0	12.5	78.6	5.0	76.9	17.2	300
20–24	6.0	9.4	84.6	5.2	68.8	19.2	805
25–34	5.5	12.2	82.3	4.3	57.4	14.5	2 500
35–44	4.6	15.0	80.4	3.7	46.5	15.2	2 222
45–54	7.4	16.9	75.6	4.5	36.3	16.2	1 416
55–64	8.9	24.2	66.9	4.5	25.9	13.9	1 118
65–74	11.1	27.7	61.3	3.6	16.7	19.2	985
75+	14.3	42.6	43.0	3.8	9.8	4.5	656

* Percent of current drinkers reporting consumption of five or more drinks on at least one occasion in the previous year.
† Mean number of occasions in the previous year on which five or more drinks were consumed, among those reporting at least one occasion.
Data should be interpreted with caution owing to high sampling variability.

SOURCE: Statistics Canada, General Social Survey, 1993.

has kept separate statistical information on the health status of this segment of Canadian society. There are many differences in the health status of the First Nations People vis-à-vis that of other Canadians as measured by the various indicators listed above. In this chapter, we will simply note differences. In Chapter 12, we discuss some of the causes of these discrepancies and look at health services for the First Nations People.

LIFE EXPECTANCY

The average life span of people in a given country reflects, among other things, the total effect of its economic development and its health care programs. In the developed countries of the world, such as Canada, life expectancy has increased dramatically since the turn of the century—from a little under 50 years in 1900 to 78.3 years in 1995. The biggest changes in life expectancy occurred during the first half of the century, with smaller but still significant gains made since 1950 (Statistics Canada, 1996).

The remarkable extension of the life span in Canada—and in most countries of the developed world—during this century can be attributed to a constellation of factors. These include the general overall raising of standards of living, improved sanitation, the development and widespread use of immunity-producing agents to protect people from communicable disease, improvements in health care services and advances in medical science and technology. In Canada, there is an upward east-to-west gradient in life expectancy, as can be seen in Table 2.2. The difference is less pronounced than it was in earlier years—the introduction of universal health insurance is considered to be a factor in lessening the gap. It is now felt that socioeconomic characteristics of the population in each province may be the most important factor in interprovincial differences in life expectancy in the future (Nault, 1997).

TABLE 2.2 Life expectancy at birth,† by sex, Canada, provinces and territories, 1995.

	Years			
	BOTH SEXES	MALE	FEMALE	DIFFERENCE
Canada	**78.3**	**75.4**	**81.3**	**5.9**
Newfoundland	77.3	74.4	80.6	6.2
PEI	77.7	74.1	81.5	7.4
Nova Scotia	77.9	74.9	80.8	5.9
New Brunswick	77.8	74.2	81.5	7.3
Quebec	78.0	74.6	81.3	6.7
Ontario	78.5	75.8	81.2	5.4
Manitoba	77.7	74.8	80.5	5.7
Saskatchewan	78.2	74.9	81.6	6.7
Alberta	78.6	75.8	81.5	5.7
BC	79.0	76.2	81.9	5.7
Yukon	72.4	69.5	76.5	7.0
NWT	74.3	72.8	76.0	3.2

†Based on one year of mortality data.

SOURCE: Nault, 1997, p. 37.

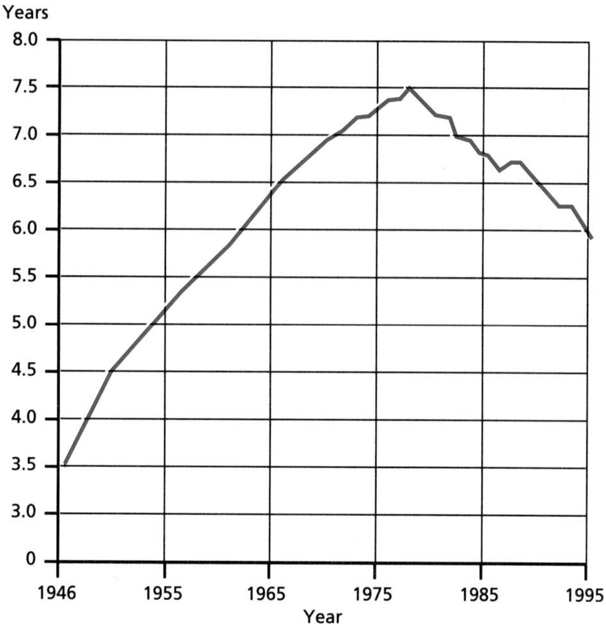

FIGURE 2.5 Gap in life expectancy at birth between males and females, Canada, 1946–1995

NOTE: Annual data from 1971 to 1995; earlier data presented at five-year intervals.

SOURCE: Canadian Vital Statistics Data Base. As cited in Nault, 1997, p. 37.

One interesting trend in the statistics on life expectancy in Canada is the widening gap between men and women (see Figure 2.5). In 1900, women outlived men by an average of approximately two years. By 1995, this figure had increased to approximately 5.9 years. The average life span for men is now 75.4 years and for women it is 81.3 years (Chui, 1996). Comparable figures from the United States are 72.3 years for men and 79.0 years for women. A major factor in the lengthening of the life span for women has been the reduction in maternal death rates.

Among the reasons women live longer than men do is the fact that they have not until fairly recently smoked as much as men have. Additionally, it is only in the past two decades that women have participated in such great numbers in the labour force, where stress is thought to contribute to ill health. The increased stress created for women by having to balance career and family demands may reduce the life expectancy gap between men and women in the future.

Although the 1995 figures appear to indicate that the gap in life expectancy between men and women is lessening, the existing imbalance between the sexes, particularly in the older age group, has brought about changes in the structure of our society. One of the unfortunate results of this trend is that widowhood and loneliness all too often contribute to the health problems of many of our senior citizens. It can be difficult to maintain a well-balanced,

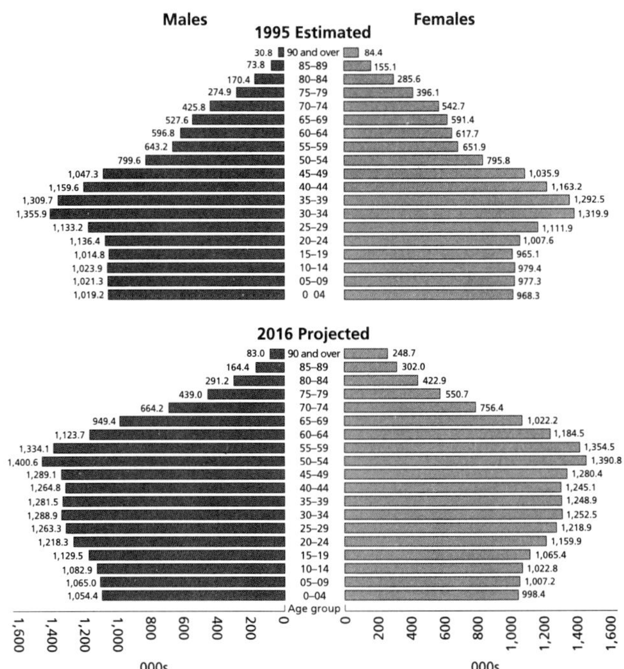

FIGURE 2.6 Canada's population, 1995 and 2016

SOURCE: Statistics Canada (1996), Catalogue nos. 91-213-XPB and 91-520-XPB.

nutritious diet when cooking for one. Many older women find it difficult to take the initiative to go out with friends. Depression is common, affecting a sizable minority of older adults (Ross & Casey, 1993; Du Gas, 1993).

There is a considerable gap between the life expectancy of people in developed countries and that of people in many developing countries. One cannot group all developing countries into the same bracket, however, as great strides have been made in improving health conditions in many countries over the past 40 years.

Equally important in both developed and developing countries is the difference that exists between various groups within the population. The figures quoted above for Canada represent average life expectancies at birth for Canadians. Through data collected by Statistics Canada, it is possible to compare differences in life expectancies for various groups within the population. The findings of such comparisons show, as was noted in the Epp Report, that there is considerable difference in life expectancy between rich and poor, and among certain groups within the low-income category. The same discrepancy holds true for people in developing countries where the rich, who enjoy a much higher standard of living, better educational opportunities and easier access to health care, are much healthier than the poor. According to Statistics Canada reports, the differences in all-cause mortality among different income groups in Canada have diminished between 1971 and 1986—perhaps as a result of the introduction of our National Health Insurance Program, which provided easier access to health care for all citizens.

MORTALITY RATES

People in Canada today have a much better chance of living to old age than did the early immigrants to this country, whose estimated life span in the 18th century was only 35 years (Charbonneau, 1970). Although life became a little less perilous during the 19th century, it was not until the 20th century that we began to see the remarkable extension in the life span that we discussed above. This increased longevity is reflected not only in the statistics on average life span, but also in the annual figures compiled on death rates in the country. The proportion of deaths to the population (**mortality rate**) is now a minimal 7.1 per 1000 population—in the United States, the figure was 8.20, and in Latin America the current level of overall mortality is equivalent to the level that existed in Canada and the United States 50 years ago (1995 figures as quoted in Statistics Canada, 1995; Pan American Health Organization, 1992; WHO, 1996).

Among Canada's First Nations, death rates have declined in recent years, falling by 21 percent between 1979 and 1993, although they still remain higher than the national level. These rates are about 1.6 times that of the general population. Young people of the First Nations, under 35 years of age, appear to be more at risk; the death rate for this group was three times that of other Canadians. In contrast, the rate for older adults, between 70 and 74 years of age, was lower than the general rate for older adults the same age in Canada (Bobet, 1989; Medical Services Branch, Health Canada, 1996).

A major factor in the lengthening of the average life span in Canada among the general population and among the people of the First Nations has been the dramatic reduction in the number of maternal and infant deaths.

Maternal Mortality

Maternal mortality has shown a remarkable decline in Canada during this century, particularly since 1921, as shown in Figure 2.7.

Not many women in Canada die as a result of childbirth these days; the maternal mortality rate was 6.3 per 10 000 live births in 1991. This is down from the 1988 figure of 7 per 10 000 in Canada, which was considerably lower than the rate of 13 per 10 000 in the United States for the same year (Statistics Canada figures as reported in Nair, Karim & Nyers, 1992; PAHO, 1992).

Maternal deaths are considered to be largely preventable. The importance of early and adequate prenatal care cannot be overstressed. The reduction in maternal death rates in Canada is attributed mainly to improved prenatal care for pregnant women and to improved care during and after delivery. Although Canada's record is very good, there are still differences in the extent of care received by women in different socioeconomic groups. Unfortunately, it is often the women at highest risk who delay prenatal care until late in pregnancy. These include First Nations women, recent immigrants, adolescents and those with low incomes.

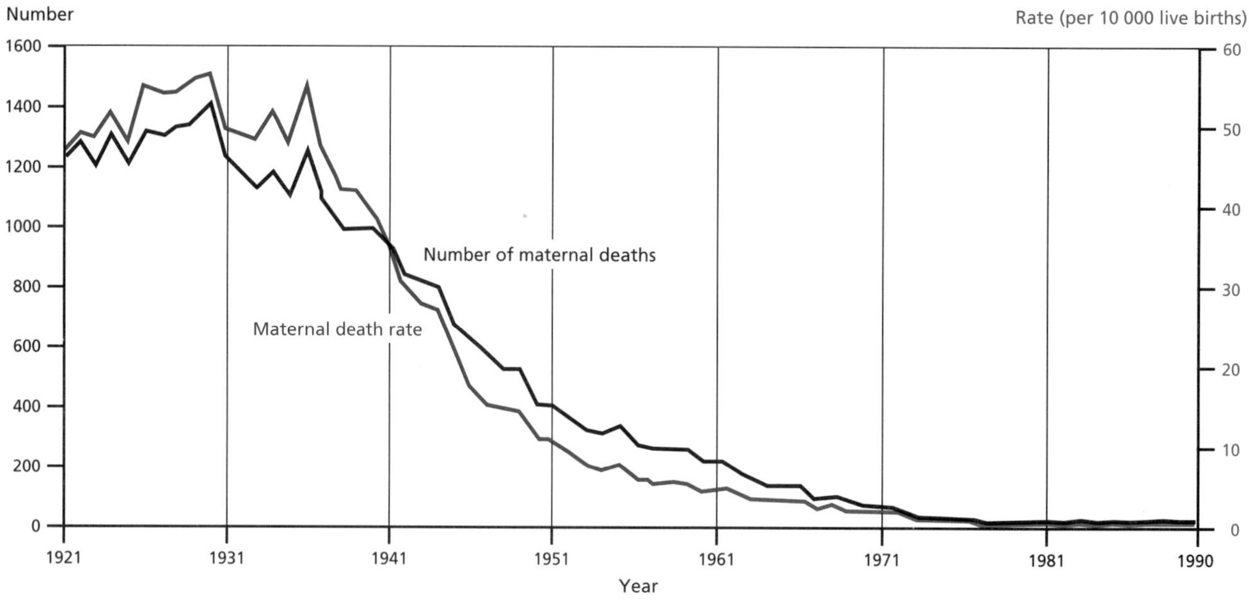

FIGURE 2.7 Number of maternal deaths and maternal death rate, Canada, 1921–1990

SOURCE: Wadhera & Strachan, 1992.

In many developing countries, maternal mortality rates are considerably higher, sometimes as much as 10 times higher than in developed countries. The high maternal mortality rates in developing countries is felt in part to be the result of discrimination against women in predominantly male-dominated societies. The International Conference on Maternity without Risk held in Nairobi, in 1987 issued a "Call for Action," stating that "high maternal death rates (particularly in developing countries) are a reflection of underlying disadvantages for and discrimination against women. This is particularly true in regard to their legal status, and their access to education, adequate nutrition, dignified employment, financial resources and satisfactory health care, including family planning services" (PAHO, 1992, pp. 121–122; WHO, 1995).

Infant Mortality

Infant mortality is considered one of the most sensitive indicators of a nation's health status. In Canada, major accomplishments in this area are reflected in the significant drop in infant mortality rates, from 102 deaths per 1000 live births reported in 1921 to 6.1 per 1000 in 1995. However, as with most of the other health status indicators we have discussed, there is much room for improvement in the differences between segments of the population divided on socioeconomic and geographic lines. Infant mortality rates are considerably higher among the lowest income groups in Canada—9.9 per 1000 live births in 1986, as compared to 6.0 per 1000 in the highest income group (King, Gartrell & Trovalto, 1991). Despite considerable improvement in the infant mortality rate among the First Nations People (see Figure 2.8), which has helped to lower the overall rate for Canada from approximately 25 per 1000 live births during the late 1950s and 1960s to 6.1 per 1000 today, the infant mortality rate for First Nations' people is still almost double the average Canadian rate (Medical Services Branch, Health Canada, 1996).

The majority of early infant deaths (neonatal) are associated with the status of the infant at birth. Later infant deaths (postnatal), with the exception of those caused by congenital anomalies, are more likely to be associated with

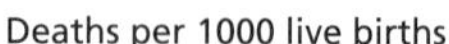

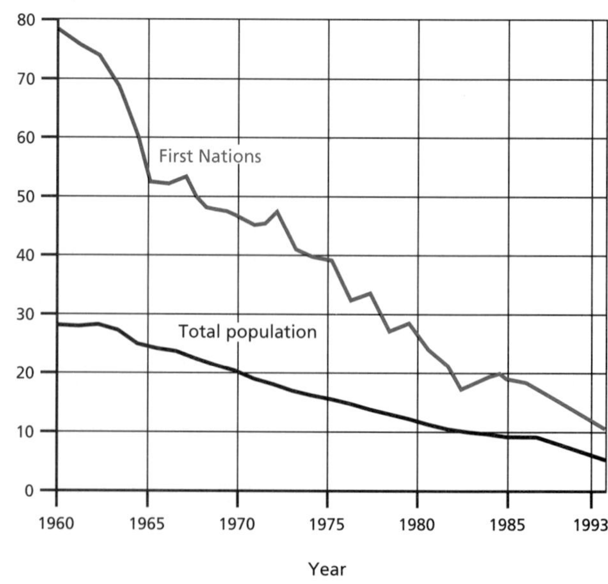

FIGURE 2.8 Infant mortality rates for First Nations people and total population (Canada), 1960–1993

SOURCES: Statistics Canada, Catalogue no. 84-206, and Medical Services Branch, Health Canada, 1996.

environmental factors. In Canada, the decrease in infant mortality has shown a continuous decline in both neonatal and postnatal deaths. In other words, babies are both getting a better start in life (an important factor here is better prenatal care for mothers) and having greater chances of survival through the first year, owing to improved environmental factors including improved nutrition and better infant health care.

In many developing countries, infant deaths remain excessively high, although considerable improvement has been made in many countries in recent years. The infant mortality rate varies from 4.8 per 1000 live births in developed countries to a high of 161 in developing countries—a 33-fold difference (UN, 1996). There is no doubt that a large number of infant deaths could be prevented by further improvements in disease prevention and environmental sanitation and by better programs of maternal–child health care.

Early Childhood Deaths

The mortality rate for children under the age of five years is another indicator that is frequently used to assess the relative health status of people in different countries. It is considered to reflect the overall socioeconomic and environmental conditions in a country. Here, again, there is a wide gap between developed and developing countries. In Canada, deaths among young children have declined dramatically since the beginning of the century, particularly for the age group one to five years. As the infectious diseases that caused so many deaths among young children in the early 1900s have been brought under control (primarily by immunization), noninfectious diseases and conditions have taken over as the leading cause of death among young children. Accidents are the most common cause of early childhood deaths in Canada today, with congenital anomalies and neoplasms next highest on the list. This is a considerable change from the 1920s, when the primary cause of early childhood death in Canada was infectious diseases.

In Canada, the United States and most other industrialized countries, early childhood death rates are now very low. Infectious diseases continue to take their toll in many developing countries, however, and the number of early childhood deaths remains high. The mortality rate for children under age five is less than 5 per 100 000 in Canada, whereas in some parts of the developing world the rate is over 200 per 1000 live births—up to 320 in one country. Most early childhood deaths in developing countries are the result of infectious diarrheal diseases, with poverty and resultant malnutrition, poor sanitation and inadequate access to health services combining to make life tenuous for small children (PAHO, 1992).

PRINCIPAL CAUSES OF DEATH

Statistical data on the leading causes of death help to identify the major health problems in a country. The pattern in leading causes of death in Canada has changed considerably since the turn of the century. In 1900, deaths from infectious diseases headed the list. These included pneumonia/influenza, tuberculosis and diarrhea/enteritis. Also on the list of major killers at that time were nephritis (for the most part, postinfectious) and diphtheria. By 1940, the noninfectious disorders of heart disease, cancer and cerebrovascular accidents had become the three leading causes of death, although tuberculosis, pneumonia and nephritis were still among the major causes. By the early 1970s, influenza/pneumonia was the only infectious disease still a major cause of death in Canada.

The leading causes of death in Canada are now circulatory disorders and cancer, which between them cause more than two-thirds of all the deaths each year. These are followed by respiratory diseases, accidents and violence; diseases of the digestive system; and endocrine, nutritional and metabolic diseases, of which diabetes mellitus is the most frequent contributor (Wilkins, 1996). Death rates for leading causes of death from 1950 to 1995 are shown in Figure 2.9; Table 2.3 shows death rates broken down by gender for 1979 and 1995.

TABLE 2.3 Deaths per 100 000 population by selected causes, Canada, 1979 and 1995

	1979			*1995*			
CAUSES	MALE	FEMALE	DIFFERENCE	MALE	FEMALE	DIFFERENCE	CHANGE IN DIFFERENCE 1979 TO 1995
Cardiovascular diseases	526.4	311.7	214.7	316.9	193.8	123.1	91.6
Diseases of the heart	394.7	212.0	182.7	238.7	134.8	103.9	78.8
Cancer	239.0	150.2	88.8	234.7	150.3	84.4	4.4
Lung cancer	71.6	16.3	55.3	72.1	31.1	41.0	14.3
Accidents and adverse effects	73.3	29.0	44.3	39.9	18.5	21.4	22.9
Motor vehicle accidents	33.8	12.7	21.1	15.5	6.7	8.8	12.3
Chronic obstructive pulmonary disease	43.1	10.4	32.7	44.7	19.3	25.4	7.3

NOTE: Age-standardized to the 1991 Canadian population.

SOURCE: Nault, 1997, p. 38.

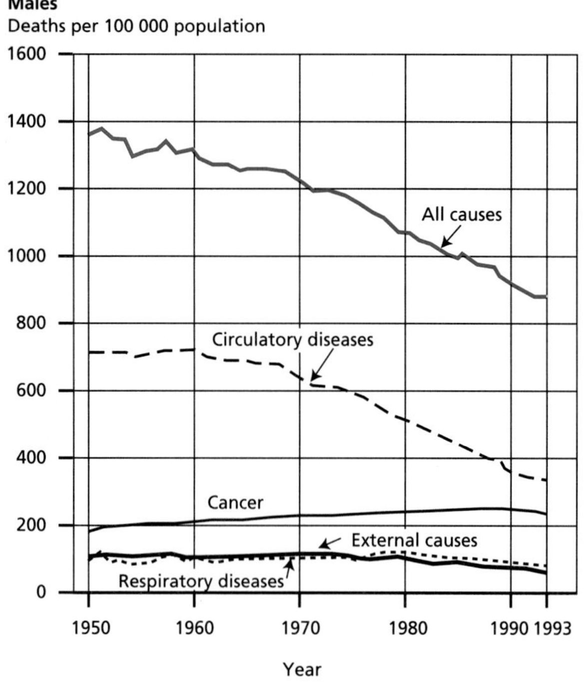

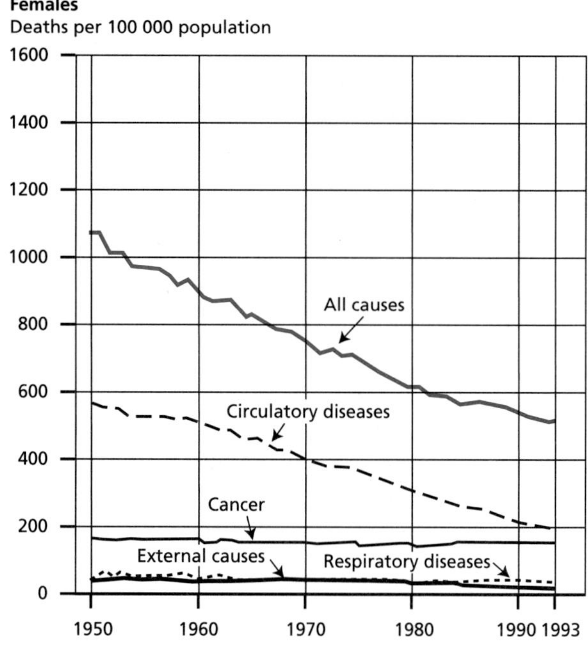

FIGURE 2.9 Age-standardized death rates* for leading causes in Canada, 1950–1993

*Age standardized to the 1991 Canadian popuation.

SOURCE: Statistics Canada, Catalogue no. 82-003-XPB, in Wilkins, 1996, p. 14.

Among our First Nations population, the major causes of death are similar to those in the overall population, but the proportion of deaths due to various causes is different. As shown in Figure 2.10, they are much more likely to die as a result of injuries than are the rest of the population. There has been a decline in recent years in the number of deaths due to accidents/violence, but it is still much higher than for the general population. Motor vehicle accidents account for almost one-third of these deaths; shootings and drownings account for another 10 percent each. Respiratory diseases also continue to be a major cause of death, particularly among First Nations infants and people over 55 years of age (Bobet, 1989; Medical Services Branch, Health Canada, 1996).

CIRCULATORY DISORDERS Cardiovascular diseases, which include both heart disease and stroke, accounted for the largest number of deaths in Canada in 1995. The number of deaths from cardiovascular disease declined considerably during the 1970s and continued to decline through the 1980s—in fact, the decline accelerated during these years. A number of factors are felt to have contributed to this. Fewer people are smoking, and our dietary habits have improved; we no longer eat as much saturated fat as we used to, and we include more fibre in our diet. More of us are exercising regularly. Emergency medical services have improved in their ability to respond quickly. There are better methods for the treatment of people with hypertension, and we have a greater number of coronary care units better equipped to handle acute cases. Still, heart disease and strokes continue to account for the greatest source of acute illness and major disability among the total population (Brancker, 1992).

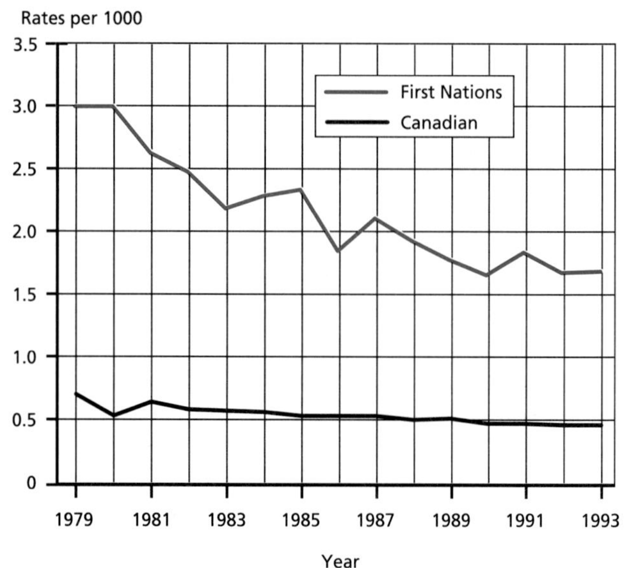

FIGURE 2.10 Age-standardized death rates from injuries, 1979–1993, First-Nations and Canadian populations

SOURCE: Medical Services Branch, Health Canada, 1996.

CANCER Cancer is the second leading cause of death in Canada. Cancer strikes people of all ages and becomes a principal cause of death and disability among people from the latter half of the young adult years onward. Lung cancer was responsible for nearly one-third of deaths in men in 1995. While the number of deaths from lung cancer has levelled off in the past few years, the number of deaths in women from lung cancer has increased (Wilkins, 1996). At the same time, there has been a decline in the number of men smoking. Among young people, aged 15–24, approximately one in five people (both genders) are smokers (Canadian Centre on Substance Abuse, 1994).

The figures for breast cancer have remained fairly constant over the past few decades. Breast cancer accounted for the largest proportion (one-fifth) of all deaths among women (Wilkins, 1996). While there is a reduced incidence of breast cancer among younger women, it is now showing up in older women much more than it did a few years ago.

There have been improvements in the methods of treating various types of cancer, such as Hodgkin's disease (a malignant disease of the lymph glands and nodes) and childhood leukemia. These advances have also helped to cut the incidence of cancer mortality among young people.

RESPIRATORY DISEASES Despite our progress in the control of infectious diseases, influenza/pneumonia continues to show up among the leading causes of death in Canada. It is a principal cause of death in infants under one year of age and remains an important cause of death and a major cause of acute illness throughout the life span. Chronic obstructive lung problems are the third leading cause of death for both men and women (Wilkins, 1996). The primary respiratory diseases are pneumonia and influenza, chronic bronchitis, emphysema and asthma and other chronic obstructions of the airway (Brancker, 1989). These diseases are also a major cause of illness throughout the life span.

ACCIDENTAL AND VIOLENT DEATHS Accidental and violent deaths are the fourth leading cause of death for men and women in Canada. Of these deaths, more than half are the result of motor vehicle accidents, while suicides make up the largest portion of remaining deaths in this category. Accidents are the leading cause of death for the male population from one to 44 years of age and for women from one to 34 years. Motor vehicle accidents and suicides are the leading causes of death in young adults from age 15 upwards (Wilkins, 1996). They are also a major cause of acute hospitalization. The residual effects of accidents in the form of long-term disability constitute a major health problem.

DISEASES OF THE DIGESTIVE SYSTEM Among the disorders included under this category are chronic liver disease and cirrhosis of the liver, noninfectious enteritis and colitis, peptic ulcer (with and without hemorrhage) and gastrointestinal hemorrhage. The proportion of deaths from digestive disorders in Canada is relatively small, although they are listed as the fifth leading cause of death and are among the 10 leading causes of acute-care hospitalization (Brancker, 1989; Statistics Canada, 1993).

ENDOCRINE, NUTRITIONAL AND METABOLIC DISEASES The largest portion of deaths in this category were caused by diabetes mellitus. The rate of deaths attributed to this cause has declined to 18.6 for males and 18.5 for females per 100 000 population in 1993 (Statistics Canada, 1995).

ALL OTHER CAUSES Among the disorders included in this category, Acquired Immune Deficiency Syndrome (AIDS) is a major cause of death among 20- to 44-year-old males in Canada. The rate was 18 per 100 000 deaths in 1993, higher than cancer for this age group but lower than the number of deaths from suicide and motor vehicle accidents (Statistics Canada, 1993).

MORBIDITY DATA

The list of leading causes of death alone does not give us a full picture of all the major health problems in Canada today. A large amount of data is collected on the prevalence of illness (**morbidity**), which helps to enlarge our perspective on the health of Canadians. Three major sources of information on morbidity are the data collected on hospitalization, on communicable diseases and on people with disabilities. Data on communicable diseases is discussed in Chapter 32.

HOSPITALIZATION We have mentioned, in the sections on mortality data and on causes of death above, some of the major causes of acute illness and hospitalization. To recapitulate, the major causes of acute-care hospitalization in Canada (as measured by total number of days spent in hospital by all persons in 1992–1993) are shown in Table 2.4.

PEOPLE WITH DISABILITIES A little over one-half of the total population reported that they had at least one chronic health problem. Among the most common chronic conditions were allergies (20%), back problems (15%), arthritis

TABLE 2.4 Causes of hospitalization in Canada, 1992–1993 (number of days)

	MALE	FEMALE
Cardiovascular diseases	3 424 090	3 886 975
Mental disorders	2 184 669	3 362 450
Respiratory disease	1 379 621	1 226 553
Neoplasms	1 558 806	1 676 907
Nervous system	1 257 012	1 707 500
Injury/poisoning	1 300 553	1 521 969
Digestive disorders	1 211 197	1 401 505
Complications of pregnancy	—	1 852 719
Musculoskeletal	659 421	1 139 591
Ill-defined	581 417	899 258

SOURCE: *Hospital Morbidity 1992–1993*. Statistics Canada, Catalogue no. 82-217.

TABLE 2.5 Population with a disability,* by nature of disability, Canada, the provinces and territories, 1991

	CDA	NFLD	PEI	NS	NB	QUE	ON	MB	SASK	AB	BC	YUKON	NWT
Any disability	17.0	10.9	19.3	23.81	19.6	13.7	17.59	19.4	20.0	18.69	18.0	12.1	14.04
Mobility	10.4	7.4	12.1	14.90	11.8	8.4	11.21	11.7	11.4	10.57	9.8	5.3	6.24
Agility	9.6	6.4	11.1	14.28	10.4	7.8	10.14	11.2	10.7	9.31	9.9	5.4	5.46
Seeing	2.7	1.9	3.0	3.18	3.2	2.4	2.85	3.5	3.6	2.58	2.5	0.9	1.60
Hearing	5.3	3.4	6.3	7.26	7.1	3.4	5.37	7.2	7.0	6.16	6.7	4.4	5.33
Speaking	1.5	1.1	1.7	1.66	2.1	1.4	1.49	1.5	1.9	1.29	1.6	0.8	0.91
Other	5.6	3.2	6.4	6.71	7.2	4.7	5.87	5.3	6.7	6.03	5.6	3.8	4.48
Unknown	1.0	0.3	0.7	1.20	0.5	0.8	1.03	0.7	1.4	1.54	1.5	1.2	0.90

*Any restriction or lack of ability to perform an activity in the manner or within the range considered normal for a human being not fully corrected by a technical aid and lasting or expected to last six months.

SOURCE: Statistics Canada (1991), Catalogue no. 82-602.

and rheumatism (13%) and high blood pressure (9%). A large number of people with chronic health problems also reported that they suffered from chronic pain. A little over one-fifth of the population over the age of 15 years reported that they had a long-term activity limitation (see Table 2.5). Among younger people, this was more likely to be due to an injury. The incidence of long-term activity limitation rose with age and, with the older group, it was more likely to be due to disease (Millar & Beaudet, 1996).

An earlier survey by Statistics Canada indicated that approximately 7.5 percent of people with disabilities resided in long-term care facilities and homes for older people. The remainder lived in households in the community. Of the disabled persons living in households, there were approximately 275 000 children under the age of 14. Among people residing in institutions, most were over 65 years of age (78.9%) and were severely disabled (72.9%). Women with disabilities were more likely to reside in an institution than men with disabilities: 9.1 percent of women with disabilities were institutionalized, whereas only 5.6 percent of men were.

The most frequently reported types of disability were agility and mobility disabilities (Table 2.5). Less common but still disabling for many people were vision, hearing and speaking problems. Other types of disabilities such as mental and emotional, psychiatric and learning disabilities were much more prevalent in people living in institutions than those living in the community.

Three out of four severely disabled adults were living in the community, where it appears clear that they receive a high degree of social support. Approximately 40 percent received help with meal preparation and with personal finances and approximately 60 percent received help with shopping and housework, as shown in Table 2.6. The availability of social support to help people with these activities is quite likely an important factor in making it possible for severely disabled adults to stay in their own homes.

Among severely disabled adults, those who were in long-term care facilities were more likely to be more severely disabled than those living at home. There is, in these cases, a resultant higher degree of dependence on others for help with personal care and with moving about within the residence (Adams, Dowler, Lafleur, Jordan-Simpson, & Wilkins, 1991).

TABLE 2.6 People with disabilities* residing in health care institutions in Canada, 1991

	PERCENTAGE
Long-term care residents (% of people with disabilities)†	7.5
Children with disabilities who live at home††	99.1
Disabled persons > 65 years old living in institutions	78.9
Persons in institutions who are severely disabled	72.9
Persons at home who are severely disabled	19.9
Disabled women who are institutionalized	9.2
Disabled men who are institutionalized	5.6
Disabled persons at home who need help with:	
Meal preparation	38.9
Personal finances	41.7
Shopping	62.5
Housework	59.0

* Total no. of Canadians with disabilities = 3 316 875
† Total number = 247 275
†† Total number = 275 050

SOURCE: Statistics Canada, 1991.

Perceived Health Status

As the data discussed throughout the chapter indicate, the health of Canadians (measured by objective standards) has improved considerably during this century. Although there are still areas for improvement, particularly with respect to certain segments of the population, Canada's record in increasing life expectancy and in reducing maternal and infant mortality and the number of deaths in early childhood is highly commendable. According to international comparisons, the health of people in this country is good.

Most studies on the health of Canadians, such as those discussed above, have focussed on illness and recognizable health problems. We have come to realize, however, that health is not merely the presence or absence of disease, but rather, "a resource for everyday living" (WHO, 1985).

As such, health is a concept that professionals have found difficult to define and to measure. In an attempt to obtain a portrait of Canadians' view of their health, the federal government undertook a Health Promotion Survey in 1985, and the Ontario Ministry of Health carried out an extensive Health Survey in 1990. The most recent study, the National Health Population Survey, is a longitudinal study initiated by Statistics Canada for Health Canada in 1994–1995. This survey was designed to measure the health of Canadians and to find out more about what makes people healthy. The survey will collect information from some 26 400 households every two years over the next 20 years. Results from the first round of interviews indicate that almost one-quarter (25%) of all adult Canadians consider their health to be excellent or very good. This is similar to the results found in earlier studies and has been unchanged since 1985 (Health Canada, 1996). (See Figure 2.11.)

People with higher incomes and people with more education rated their health higher than those with less income or education. Almost three-quarters (72%) of people with college or university education reported their health as excellent or good, compared with a little less than half (49%) of those with less than a high school diploma. Similarly, those with higher incomes reported better health, with 77 percent of men and 74 percent of women in the highest income bracket reporting excellent or very good health and 52 percent of men and 51 percent of women in the lowest income group (Statistics Canada, 1995).

According to the report of the 1990 Ontario Health Survey, numerous studies indicate that the way people assess their own health status is very similar to the physical and social well-being assessments made by objective measures. "People who rate their health as poor tend to have poor physical health and to engage in fewer health maintenance and promotion practices. They are also more likely to experience higher rates of social isolation, depression and unhappiness" (Government of Ontario, 1992, p. 9). Findings from the Ontario Survey were much like those of the National Health Promotion Study in finding that most people rate their health as good, very good or excellent.

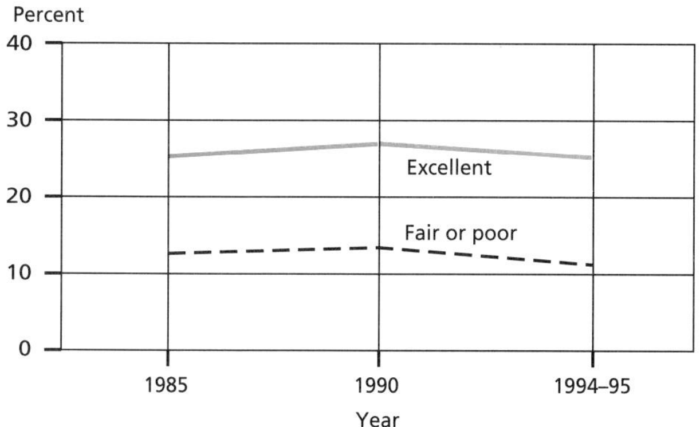

FIGURE 2.11 Self-rated health status, age 15+, Canada

SOURCE: Stephens & Fowler Graham, 1993.

The Ontario Health Survey found that, although there was not much difference in perceived health status between the genders, the ratings of this indicator did vary with age, with older people (over 65 years) reporting more frequently (almost one in four) that their health was only fair or poor and less than half reporting it as good or excellent. The number of health problems reported by respondents also increased with age. Almost three in four people over the age of 65 reported two, three or more health problems. It should be noted, however, that 13 percent of people over 65 reported that they were free of even minor health problems (Government of Ontario, 1992).

The Ontario survey also found that two out of every three people in the province had had one or more health problems in the 12 months preceding the survey. The most common problems reported were musculoskeletal (25%), respiratory (23%), injuries and poisonings (12%) and circulatory (12%) (Government of Ontario, 1992).

The Ontario Health Survey looked at health behaviours in addition to self-rated health reports, as well as several other aspects of health, including perception of pain, suffering, social support and family functioning. The findings provided valuable information about the role of social and psychological factors on health. We will discuss some of the findings of both surveys in later chapters.

IN REVIEW

- Health is an ever-changing and evolving state of being.
- Well-being is a subjective perception of ability, harmony and vitality. It exists on a continuum from extreme illness to high-level wellness.
- High-level wellness involves progressive integration (maturation) of the whole being—body, mind and spirit—throughout the life cycle.
- The concept of health within illness views illness as an opportunity for growth and transformation, particularly in the psychological, social and spiritual dimensions of being.
- Holistic health considers an individual's health in terms of his or her total functioning.
- Illness is viewed as a disturbance in the dynamic equilibrium among body, mind, spirit and environment. Care focusses on restoring harmony, balance and a sense of meaning in life.
- Healing means to make whole. It is a complex process that requires active participation on the individual's part. It takes time, requiring that the body have adequate nutritional support and oxygenation for the physical aspects and sufficient psychic energy for other types of healing.

- Our ideas about health and what promotes good health have changed over the past century. We have moved from a biomedical view of health, through one focussing on lifestyle to the present socioeconomic model.
- The major determinants of health are now considered to be:
  - living and working conditions
  - social support
  - genetic makeup
  - individual behaviours.
- The Epp Framework for Health Promotion set the stage for major health care reform in Canada based on the socioeconomic model. All provinces have subsequently embarked on new directions in health care to implement this model. The Ontario nurturing health model is one example of provincial guidelines for these new directions.
- Key points of the Ontario model include the following two points:
  - emphasis on health promotion and health protection through community and personal empowerment
  - a shift away from the disease and hospital orientation of the past.
- The health of Canadians is good according to international standards:
  - life expectancy has greatly increased in this century
  - infant, maternal and early childhood mortality rates are among the best in the world
  - most communicable diseases have been brought under control
  - new diseases such as AIDS are causing concern
  - there is still room for improvement among certain segments of the population, including the economically disadvantaged, elderly on low incomes, single mothers, immigrants and First Nations peoples.
- Leading causes of death in Canada are:
  - circulatory disorders
  - cancer
  - respiratory diseases
  - external causes (accidents and violence).
- These same conditions are also responsible for a large proportion of hospitalization, although mental illness is now the second most frequent cause.
- Most Canadians consider their health to be good, even those with a chronic health problem.
- Most people with a chronic disability live at home, requiring and receiving social support.

Critical Thinking Activities

1. Explore personal meanings of health. Ask a number of people of different ages what health means to them. How are personal meanings of health similar? How are they different? How do people's views of health change as they grow older?
2. Explore how people with a chronic health condition perceive their state of health. Talk with two or three people who have a chronic health condition (for example, arthritis, emphysema, diabetes, Parkinson's disease or hypertension). Do they consider themselves to be healthy or ill? How do they maintain their optimal level of functioning?
3. Go to the library and find out the main health status indicators in your province and community. Determine the infant and maternal mortality rates and causes of death, morbidity and disability. How do these compare with the rest of Canada?
4. From a hospital in your area, find out the major reasons for hospital admissions for infants, children, adults and older adults.
5. Talk to a community health nurse about the number of people on the nurse's case load who have chronic conditions and disabilities. What is the nature of these conditions or disabilities?

KEY TERMS

health p. 11
disease p. 11
acute illness p. 11
chronic illness p. 11
illness p. 11
sickness p. 11
well-being p. 11
wellness p. 12
health within illness p. 12
holistic health p. 13
healing p. 14
biomedical model p. 14
behavioural model p. 15
socioeconomic model p. 16
multisectoral p. 16
empowerment p. 16
congenital p. 20
mortality rate p. 23
morbidity p. 27

References

ADAMS, O., DOWLER, J., LAFLEUR, L., JORDAN-SIMPSON, D.A., & WILKINS, R. (1991). *Profile of persons with disabilities residing in health care institutions in Canada.* (Vol. 6). Prepared for Statistics Canada. Special topics from the Health and Services Canada Catalogue No. 82-615. Ottawa: Canadian Centre for Health Information.

BOBET, E. (1989). Indian mortality. *Canadian Social Trends, 15,* 11–14. (Supply & Services Canada Catalogue No. 11–008E)

BRANCKER, A. (1989). Causes of death 1987. *Health Reports, 1*(1), 97–105. (Statistics Canada Catalogue No. 82-003)

BRANCKER, A. (1992). Highlights: Causes of death 1990. *Health Reports, 4,* 185–189. (Statistics Canada Catalogue No. 82–003)

CANADIAN CENTRE ON SUBSTANCE ABUSE/ADDICTION RESEARCH FOUNDATION. (1994). *Canadian profile of alcohol, tobacco and other drugs.* Ottawa: Authors.

CANADIAN PUBLIC HEALTH ASSOCIATION. (1986). Ottawa Charter for Health Promotion. *Report of the International Conference on Health Promotion.* Ottawa: Author.

CANNON, N.J. (1997). A quest for health. In M.S. Roach, *Caring from the heart.* Mahwah, NJ: Paulist Press.

CHARBONNEAU, H. (1970). *Tourouvre-au-perche aux XVII et XVIII siècles: Etude de démographie historique.* Paris: Presses universitaires de France, 424 pages (Travaux et documents, published by l'Institut national d'études démographiques, cahier 55). As cited in Duman and Lavoie (1992), 111.

CHUI, T. (1996). Canada's population: Changing into the 21st century. *Canadian Social Trends,* 42, pp. 3–7. Statistics Canada Catalogue 11-008-XPE.

CLARKE, J.N. (1990). *Health, illness, and medicine in Canada.* Toronto: McClelland & Stewart.

CRICHTON, A., HSU, D., & TSANG, S. (1994). *Canada's health care system: Its funding and organization.* Ottawa: The Canadian Health Association.

DU GAS, B.W. (1993). Healthy lifestyles. In A. Beckingham & B.W. Du Gas (Eds.), *Promoting healthy aging* (pp. 129–160). St. Louis: Mosby.

DUNN, H.L. (1959a). High-level wellness for man and society. *American Journal of Public Health, 49*(6), 786–792.

DUNN, H.L. (1959b). What high-level wellness means. *Canadian Journal of Public Health, 50*(11), 447–457.

DUNN, H.L. (1973). *High-level wellness.* Arlington: R.W. Beatty Ltd.

EPP, J. (1986). *Achieving health for all: A framework for health promotion.* Ottawa: Minister of Supply & Services. (Catalogue No. H39–102/1986E)

FLYNN, P.A.R. (1980). *Holistic health.* Bowie, MD: Robert J. Brady.

GOVERNMENT OF ONTARIO. (1992). *Ontario health survey 1990.* Toronto: Ontario Minister of Health.

GOVERNMENT OF ONTARIO. (1993). *Nurturing health.* Report of the Premier's Council on Health, Well-being and Social Justice (1987–1991). Toronto: Queen's Printer. (Catalogue No. 01–93–20M)

GRANT, K.R. (1988). The inverse care law in Canada: Differential access under universal free health insurance. In Bolaria, B. Singh and H.D. Dickinson (1988), *Sociology of health care in Canada* (pp. 118–134). Toronto: Harcourt, Brace Jovanovich.

GREEN, L.W., & RAEBURN, J.M. (1988). Health promotion: What is it? What will it become? *Health Promotion* (Oxford), *3*(2), 151.

HEALTH CANADA. (1996). Report on the health of Canadians. [on line]. Available at http:www.hc-sc.gc.ca/hppb/nhrdp/healthofcanadians/index-e.html. (1998, Aug 10)

HEALTH & WELFARE CANADA. (1987). *The active health report: Perspectives on Canada's health promotion survey 1985.* Ottawa: Minister of Supply & Services. (Catalogue No. H39–106/1987E)

JAFFE, D.T. (1980). *Healing from within.* New York: Knopf.

JONES, P.S., & MELEIS, A.I. (1993). Health is empowerment. *Advances in Nursing Science, 15*(3), 1–14.

KING, M., GARTRELL, J., & TROVALTO, F. (1991). Early childhood mortality, 1926–1986. *Canadian Social Trends, 21*(9), 6–11. (Supply & Services Canada Catalogue No. 11–008E)

LALONDE, M. (1974) *A new perspective on the health of Canadians.* Ottawa: Information Canada.

LEDDY, S., & PEPPER, J.M. (1993). *Conceptual bases of professional nursing.* (3rd ed.) Philadelphia: Lippincott.

LINDSEY, E. (1996). Health within illness: Experiences of chronically disabled people. *Journal of Advanced Nursing, 24,* 465–472.

LUBKIN, I.M. (1998). *Chronic illness: Impact and interventions.* (4th Ed.) Boston: Jones & Bartlett.

MEDICAL SERVICES BRANCH, HEALTH CANADA. (1996). *Diagnostic on the health of First Nations and Inuit people. A draft paper.* Ottawa: Author.

MILLAR, M., & BEAUDET, M.P. (1996, Spring). Health facts. *Canadian Social Trends, 41,* 24–27. (Statistics Canada Catalogue No. 11-008-XPE)

MOCH, S.D. (1989). Health within illness: Conceptual evolution and practice possibilities. *Advances in Nursing Science, 11*(4), 23–31.

NAIR, C., KARIM, R., & NYERS, C. (1992). Health care and Health status: A Canada–United States statistical comparison. *Health Reports, 4*(2), 175–183.

NAULT, F. (1997, Summer). Narrowing mortality gaps, 1978 to 1995. *Health Reports, 3*(1), 35–41. (Statistics Canada Catalogue No. 82-003-XPB)

NO AUTHOR. (1998). International Nursing Review. Vol. 45, #2, issue 338, p. 36.

PAN-AMERICAN HEALTH ORGANIZATION (PAHO). (1992). *Health-Conditions in the Americas, 1990.* Washington, DC: Pan-American Sanitary Bureau, World Health Organization.

PENDER, N.J. (1987). *Health promotion in nursing practice.* (2nd ed.) Norwalk, CT: Appleton & Lange.

ROSS, M., & CASEY, A. (1993). Health concerns associated with aging. In A. Beckingham & B.W. Du Gas (Eds.), *Promoting healthy aging.* St. Louis: Mosby.

SIEGEL, B. (1986). *Love, medicine and miracles.* New York: Harper & Row.

STATISTICS CANADA. (1991). Catalogue No. 82-602.

STATISTICS CANADA. (1991). *Profile of persons with disabilities residing in health care institutions.* (Catalogue No. 82-615)

STATISTICS CANADA. (1993). *Hospital Morbidity, 1990–1991.* Ottawa: Minister of Science & Technology. (Catalogue No. 82–217)

STATISTICS CANADA. (1993). General Social Survey. Ottawa: Author.

STATISTICS CANADA. (1995). *National Health Population Survey. Overview, 1994–1995.* (Ministry of Industry Catalogue No. 82-567)

STATISTICS CANADA. (1996). Age-standardized mortality rates by selected causes, by sex. (Catalogue No. 82-221-XDE).

STATISTICS CANADA. (1996). Canada's population, 1995 and 2016. (Catalogue No. 91-213-XPB and 91-520-XPB).

STEPHENS, T., & FOWLER GRAHAM, E. (Eds.). (1993). *Canada's Health Promotion Survey 1990: Technical report.* Ottawa: Statistics Canada.

UNICEF. (1992). *The state of the world's children.* New York: Oxford University Press for UNICEF.

UNITED NATIONS. (1996). *Demographic Yearbook 1994.* New York: The United Nations Secretariat. Department of International, Economic, & Social Affairs, Statistics Section.

WADHERA, S., & STRACHAN, J. (1992). Selected infant mortality and related statistics, Canada, 1921–1990. *Health Reports, 4*(4), 429–433. (Statistics Canada Catalogue No. 82–003)

WENDLER, M.C. (1996). Understanding healing: A conceptual analysis. *Journal of Advanced Nursing, 24,* 838–842.

WILDERQUIST, J., & DAVIDHIZER, R. (1994). The ministry of nursing. *Journal of Advanced Nursing, 19*(4), 647–652.

WILKINS, K. (1996, Summer). Causes of death. How the sexes differ. *Canadian Social Trends, 41,* 11–18. (Statistics Canada Catalogue No. 11-008-XPE)

WORLD HEALTH ORGANIZATION. (1948). *Constitution of the World Health Organization.*

WORLD HEALTH ORGANIZATION. (1974). Community health nursing. Report of a WHO Expert Committee. Technical Report Series 558. Geneva: Author.

WORLD HEALTH ORGANIZATION. (1978). *Alma Ata 1978: Primary health care.* Geneva: Author.

WORLD HEALTH ORGANIZATION. (1981). *Global strategy for health for all for the year 2000.* (Health for All series No. 3). Geneva: Author.

WORLD HEALTH ORGANIZATION. (1984a). *Health promotion glossary.* Copenhagen: WHO Regional Office for Europe.

WORLD HEALTH ORGANIZATION. (1985). *Health manpower requirements for the achievement of health for all by the year 2000 through primary health care* (Report of a WHO Expert Committee). (Technical Report Series 717). Geneva: Author.

WORLD HEALTH ORGANIZATION. (1995). *The World Health Report. Bridging the gaps.* Report of the Director General. Geneva: Author.

WORLD HEALTH ORGANIZATION. (1996). *World health statistics annual.* Valletta, Malta: Author.

Additional Readings

DHARI, R., PATEL, I., FRYER, M., DHARI, M., BILKU, S., & BAINS, S. (1997). Creating a supportive environment for Indo-Canadian women. *Canadian Nurse, 93*(3), 27–31.

LANE, N.J. (1992). A spirituality of being: Women with disabilities. *Journal of Applied Rehabilitation Counselling, 23*(4), 53–58.

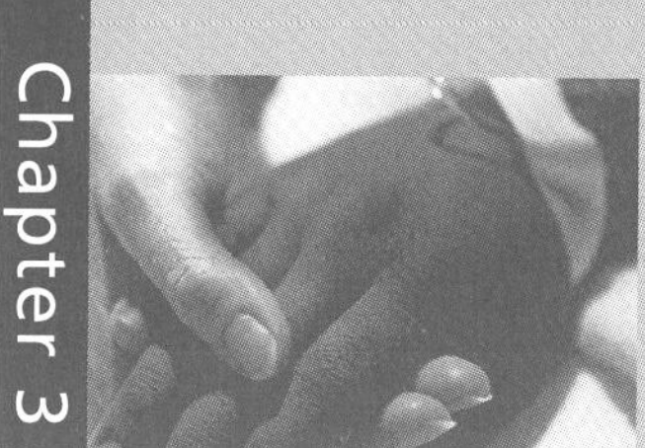

Chapter 3

Health Care in Canada

OUTLINE

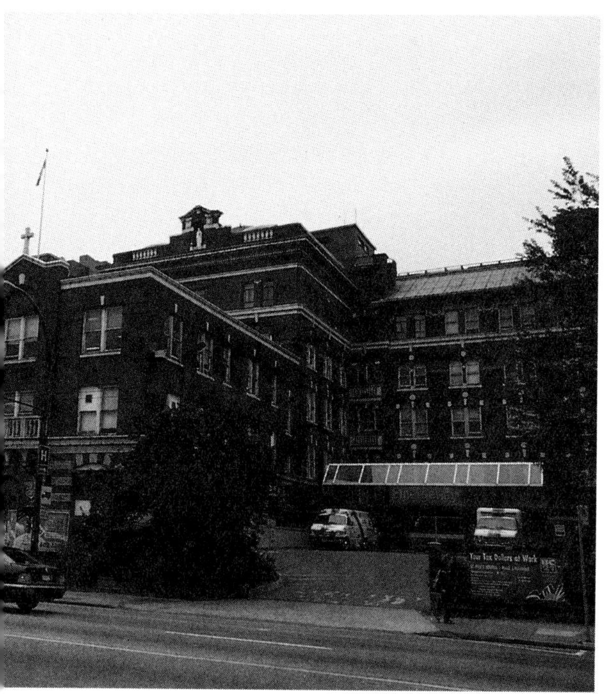

Central Questions

1. What do the terms welfare state, welfare society, healthy public policy and social safety net mean?
2. What were some of the major events leading to the National Health Insurance Program Canada has today?
3. How does Canada's national health care model differ from those of Great Britain and the United States?
4. What are the five principles on which the Canadian model was founded? How are these principles carried out in practice?
5. Why is each provincial and territorial health insurance program different from those of other provinces?
6. What specific hospital, outpatient, extended care and medical services are included in all provincial and territorial health care insurance programs?
7. What other services are included in each of the provinces and territories?
8. Why is everyone concerned about health care costs?
9. Why has every province and territory in Canada embarked on major health care reforms?
10. What are some of the commonalities of these reforms across provinces?
11. What are some of the specific changes taking place in the various provinces and the territories that are of particular interest to nurses?

Introduction

Health is said to be a human right, that is, a condition to which everyone has a just claim. The very acceptance of the notion of human right implies that society assumes a responsibility and will give high priority to carrying it out.

Lalonde, 1974

The provision of adequate health services is an essential component of a country's overall social policies. The impact of all public policies on health is powerful. The Epp Report (1986) identified healthy public policy as one of the principal strategies for reforming the health care system in Canada.

Today we view health as encompassing social, economic and environmental factors, as well as biological and lifestyle factors. This enlarged understanding of health has led us to broaden our concept of what is involved in the "right to health." The South Fraser Valley Regional Health Board (1996) provides an example of this broader view. "The vision of the South Fraser Valley Regional Board is a region of healthy individuals contributing to and arising out of healthy communities" (p. 11). To attain this vision the Board has four goals: "... healthy communities and citizens, equitable access to services (continuum of care), financial accountability (balanced budgets) and consumer and community participation" (p.13).

Canada is seen as a **welfare state** because of its **social safety net** that provides a wide range of health and social support services to its citizens. Crichton, Hsu and Tsang (1994) suggest that the welfare state is becoming a **welfare society** characterized by:

1. a multisectoral approach to promoting health
2. the participation of consumers in the formulation of health and social policies
3. partnerships between business, government, educational institutions and health agencies in research and training.

They claim that we have moved beyond the basic health policy goals of equal access to care and promotion of income security for those most in need to the recognition of the importance of human rights (or equality of condition) in health care issues (Crichton, Hsu & Tsang, 1994).

In this chapter, we will discuss the concept of *healthy public policy*, as well as the development of the Canadian social safety net that has emerged as a result of our social policies, especially the National Health Insurance Program and its administration in the different provinces and territories. Lastly, we will consider the health care reforms that are currently being initiated in every province and territory. Because of our close social and economic ties to both Great Britain and the United States, a brief comparison of their health care systems will also be included.

Policy-Making

A **policy** represents a decision or action taken in an organization. "[Policies] are not recommendation ... [but] statements of what is to be done" (Sutherland & Fulton, 1988, p.118). They provide guidelines for the actions of people within an organization. As a student, you were probably introduced to school policies in your orientation classes, for example, in regard to the dress code for class and for clinical experiences.

According to Blum (1981), **public policy** is "an established and legislatively enacted proposal by a public body duly constituted to make policy in the area of concern. It stipulates ends and it may provide resources. It may spell out specific means to reach these ends" (cited in Pederson, Edwards, Marshall, Allison & Kelner, 1989, p. 11). For example, the Royal Commission on Health Services (Government of Canada, 1964), in examining health and health services in Canada, found that there was an acute shortage of qualified health professionals across the country. Each year, increasing numbers of health professionals were immigrating to Canada to meet our needs. In response to recommendations of the Royal Commission, a policy decision was made by the prevailing government, in consultation with the provinces, to increase the Canadian supply of health professionals so that Canada would become self-sufficient in the production of qualified health professionals. To this end, the federal government passed the Health Resources Act (1966), allocating resources totalling $500 million to be expended over a 15-year period to help the provinces develop educational facilities and clinical practice areas to prepare needed health professionals. The money was to be distributed to the provinces by means of matching grants (whereby the federal government and the provincial government shared equally in the cost). A Health Manpower Directorate was established within the Department of National Health and Welfare to administer the fund. A Manpower Planning Division was incorporated to develop strategies for planning the country's future needs.

The enactment of policy decisions in legislation is a complex and lengthy process. In our democratic Canadian society, we believe that everyone should be given the opportunity to voice opinions on the issues through public forums, written briefs in reaction to "White Papers" or other means. A formal policy statement of the government's intent, for example the Nova Scotia Ministry of Health's *Health Strategy for the Nineties: Managing Better Care* (1990) or Saskatchewan's *Vision of Health* (1992), was drafted. Consensus needs to be attained through public forums or meetings with all stakeholders. With federal legislation, this may be done through federal–provincial meetings. Proposals must go through the parliamentary (or legislative) committee process. Following these steps, during which many changes may be made, proposed legislation is re-drafted and debated in Parliament or the Legislative Assembly. If proposed legislation is passed, the Senate then takes a "second look" at the bill in the case of federal legislation. This step is followed by official signing of the bill by the Governor-General, or the Lieutenant-Governor of the province, at which stage the bill becomes law.

Healthy Public Policy

A relatively new term that has come into use in recent years is **healthy public policy**. This has been defined as "policy enacted by the various levels of government that is characterized by explicit concern for health and equity, and by accountability for health impact" (Government of B.C., 1991b, p. 1). According to Pederson et al. (1989), the goal of this concept is "to suggest a new way of thinking about health and government policy that is participatory, multisectoral and ecological" (p. 5) in order to make health a higher priority on the political agenda.

An example of a healthy public policy that has been enacted at the national level of government is the Tobacco Control Act (1987), which included strengthening of the government's smoking prevention program by adding efforts to achieve cessation and a regulatory strategy (Pederson et al., 1989). The enactment of this legislation required collaboration between the Ministers of Health, Justice, Labour and the Secretary of the Treasury. An example of a provincially enacted healthy public policy is the mandatory seat belt legislation that almost all provinces have now passed (which has required the cooperation of health, justice and transport ministries). Healthy public policies can also be enacted at municipal levels. In January 1991, the Richmond (B.C.) City Council passed a by-law (subsequently approved by the Ministry of Health) requiring licensed bars and restaurants to post signs warning that drinking alcoholic beverages during pregnancy can cause birth defects (see Figure 3.1).

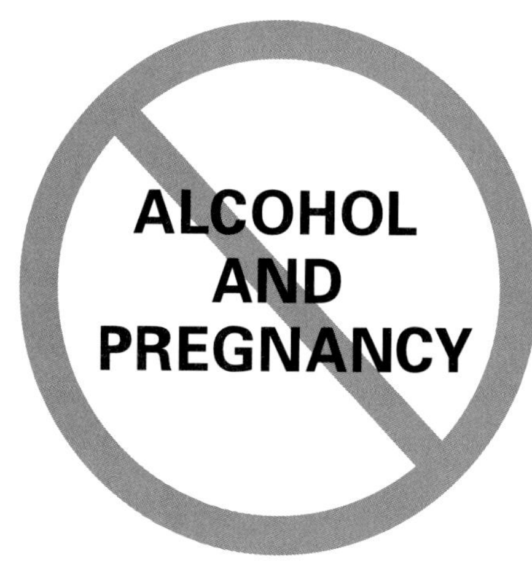

FIGURE 3.1 Fetal alcohol syndrome warning sign.

SOURCE: Government of B.C., 1991a, p. 23.

Sometimes, governments do not explicitly espouse certain policies, but may demonstrate support for them through the allocation of funds or other resources such as space. Many interested groups try to influence both policy decisions and the form and substance of proposed legislation by lobbying members of the law-making body. The use of advertisements on radio, in the newspapers and on television, or the staging of demonstrations, are means to gain public support and the attention of politicians. Nursing organizations in Canada have in recent years become aware of their influence on the political process by virtue of their numbers. We are the largest group of health workers, numbering over 264 305 at the latest count (CNA, 1996). Nursing's involvement in the political process has increased greatly in recent years (Larsen & Baumgart, 1992; Lefort, 1993). We will discuss the topic of nurses and politics further in Chapter 5. Meanwhile, it should be noted that everyone can participate in bringing about healthy policy changes. At the community and neighbourhood level, local residents can often introduce changes such as getting the city to install a traffic light at a busy intersection for public safety. Canadians can also attend public forums, and express their opinions through letters to newspaper editors, Members of the Legislative Assembly (MLAs) or Members of Parliament (MPs).

The Canadian Social Safety Net

As pointed out in the Epp Report, health cannot be separated from the social conditions in which people live (Epp, 1986). In discussing the Canadian health care system, then, we will also consider the role of Canada's social welfare programs, which ensure income security for those in need. These programs include employment insurance, old age pension, Canada and Quebec contributory pension programs for working people, and child tax benefit and social assistance programs for those in financial need. The combination of our national health plan, which includes both hospital and medical care, and our social welfare programs is frequently referred to as the Canadian social safety net. Canadians today view these social programs as a right to which all are naturally entitled, but they came about through a long, slow process of policy development, consensus building, policy finalization, endorsement by the provinces, drafting and debating of legislation and the final step of enactment into law.

Historical Perspective

Early Health Care in Canada

The early immigrants who settled in this land, although fiercely independent, accepted the reality of having to band together for mutual aid when someone was ill or in need. Until late in the 19th century, health and welfare were seen as primarily the responsibility of individuals and their families—with help from church and community in times of need. In French Canada, the tradition of church involvement in health and social welfare was established by the early settlers who sent back to France for members of the religious orders to care for the sick. In the English-speaking colonies, municipalities passed legislation similar to the English Poor Law of 1598, in which they accepted responsibility for the care of those in need.

During these early years, sisters of the Roman Catholic Church set up hospitals and provided nursing services. As the country opened up, these sisters began following the settlers westward. After the British conquest of Canada in 1767, the French nursing sisterhoods continued their work in the parishes of the Roman Catholic Church. The British set up military hospitals with male nurses. Some secular hospitals developed in the larger towns but, for the most part, these were dirty and poorly managed. In those times, it was considered part of a woman's role to look after anyone who was ill in the household, with only the homeless having to seek refuge in a hospital.

For a number of years, secular hospitals in Canada remained very primitive. The massive wave of immigrants into the country in the early 1800s brought an increased number of health problems and stimulated the development of health professionals. A number of both French- and English-speaking nursing sisterhoods were established. In addition to the Roman Catholic Church, other religious groups became involved in the provision of health services, including the Eastern Orthodox and Anglican churches as well as the Home Mission Boards of the Methodist, Presbyterian and United churches. English-speaking hospitals began to emerge, operated by these religious groups, for example, the Anglican and United Church Mission hospitals that dotted the coasts of Labrador, Newfoundland, British Columbia and the Far North (Victorian Order of Nurses, 1983).

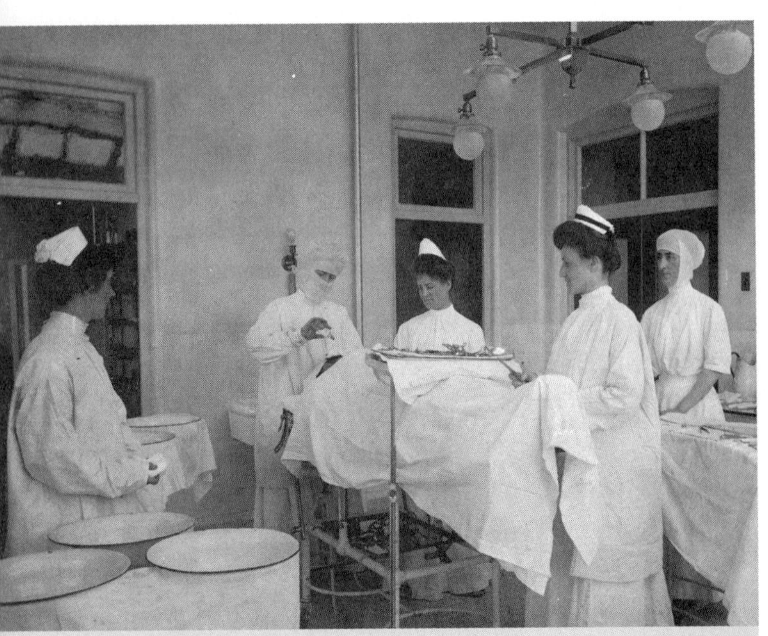

Early hospital.

"Poorhouses," which sheltered the indigent sick, the mentally ill and older people without families to care for them, were under municipal jurisdiction. Maternity care was generally undertaken by lay midwives, except in rare cases when physicians were available.

With the passage of the British North America Act in 1867, Canada became a confederation. The act carefully laid out the respective powers of the federal and provincial governments, assigning the responsibility for health and welfare matters to the provinces. Jurisdiction over the collection of the revenue necessary to pay for these services, however, was invested primarily with the federal government—a situation that has been a major source of federal–provincial conflict ever since.

Increasing urbanization and industrialization marked the post-Confederation years. Towns were often unable to cope with the floods of farm labourers seeking work in the new factories and immigrants coming from other lands to seek a better life in the "New World." Crowded conditions, poor housing, lack of health services and inadequate sewage and garbage disposal combined to make disease rampant and mortality rates high. The poor health conditions brought about the passage of a Public Health Act in each of the provinces, modelled after a British act passed in 1875. These acts established provincial and local boards of health and provided for the appointment of medical health officers and sanitary inspectors.

Hospitals and care of the needy were, however, still mainly the responsibility of the church and charitable organizations. The secular hospitals were, regrettably, "generally distinguished by a prevalence of rats, dirt, stale air and lack of order and good management" (Victorian Order of Nurses, 1983, pp. 8, 9). Nursing in the secular hospitals was carried out by poorly educated young women who were paid a miserable wage. Nursing was not something that young women from good families did.

Florence Nightingale can be given credit for changing the image of nursing. She improved hospital conditions in Great Britain, North America and throughout the western world. During the Crimean War (1850s), her work saved the lives of hundreds of British soldiers and brought her acclaim from a grateful nation. In return, the British raised funds to enable her to establish a training school for nurses (VON, 1983; Canadian Nurses Association, 1968). We will discuss the Nightingale model of nursing further in Chapter 5.

In addition to her work in hospitals, Florence Nightingale was concerned about the unsanitary conditions and ignorance of health matters of people living in the crowded slums of London and in the rural villages of England. She was emphatic that "the nurse must combat in the home, 'dirt, drink, diet, damp, draughts, drains' " (VON, 1983, p. 12). Her influence was felt in the development of the Queen's Own Visiting Nurse service in Great Britain and, subsequently, the Victorian Order of Nurses in Canada.

By the turn of the century, hospitals were beginning to flourish. People who could not afford to pay for the services of a hospital were, however, still dependent on charity. To provide an alternative to charity, fraternal societies like the Masons, the Foresters and the Knights of Columbus began to emerge. Each member contributed to a common fund which was used to help members and their families who were sick, unemployed or otherwise in need. Because government scholarships and bursaries were offered to only a select few, many students received financial assistance from one of the fraternal societies to go through normal school (teacher training), nurses' training or university.

By the end of the 19th century, medical and nursing schools were well established, standards had been raised for the qualifications of health professionals, and hospital conditions had improved considerably. Institutions were built for the mentally ill, people with tuberculosis, the blind and the deaf. In addition, a number of voluntary organizations had been established, among them the Children's Aid Societies, the Red Cross Society and the Victorian Order of Nurses (Government of Canada, 1989; VON, 1983).

Industrialization in the latter part of the 19th century also brought about the development of unions. Like the fraternal societies, they were interested in the welfare of their members. In addition to being concerned with raising living standards, they also wanted to protect workers from losing their income if they were ill, unemployed or had been injured on the job. The Ontario Workmen's Compensation Act, passed in 1914, and those subsequently passed in other provinces, were the first modern social security programs in Canada. (See Chapter 4 for a discussion of services provided by Workers' Compensation Boards.)

LOOKING back

Lady Aberdeen, 1857–1939

The founding of the Victorian Order of Nurses of Canada, like many historical firsts in nursing, was the work of a "woman of influence"—one of those women of earlier centuries who were denied access to the political and employment arenas but who applied their energies and positions to the promotion of better health care. Countess Ishbel Aberdeen was the wife of the Governor General of Canada during the years 1894 to 1898 and used her position during those years to bring into being a visiting nursing order that continues to the present day. The Victorian Order of Nurses of Canada is a voluntary charitable organization that has initiated many major advances in public health care for almost a century.

The third daughter in the wealthy Marjoribanks family, Ishbel Maria married John Gordon, seventh Earl of Aberdeen, in 1877. He was politically active, and the young couple soon had a brief viceregal appointment in Ireland. On their return to England, she began to take an active role in current events and accepted the presidency of the newly formed International Council of Women. When her husband was appointed Governor General of Canada, she immediately began to work for the Canadian National Council of Women. During a tour of Canada, members of western branches of the Council stressed the hardships of sick women and children in isolated settlements, where there was no medical assistance and no hospitals. Lady Aberdeen was familiar with the Jubilee Institute of District Nurses, formed in Britain for such work, and believed a project of home helpers would be ideal for Canada.

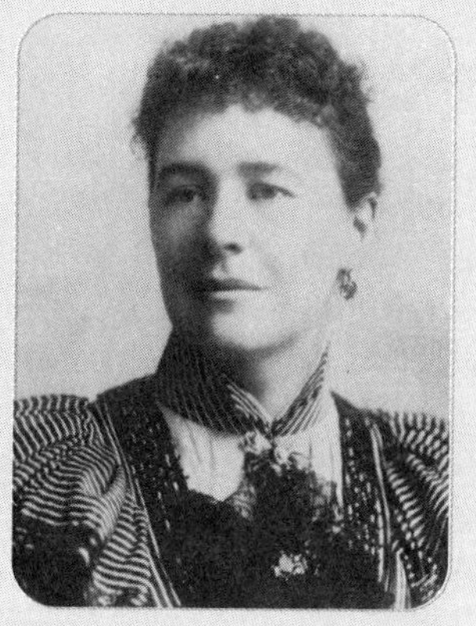

Nora E. Livingston, Lady Superintendent of the Montreal General Hospital, proposed to Lady Aberdeen that the Order should consist of qualified nurses, with extra preparation in district nursing. Once convinced, Lady Aberdeen set out to raise the funds for such an undertaking and to lay the political groundwork for it to be a success. Her proposal was at first strongly opposed by the medical profession, especially the powerful Ontario Medical Association, which was concerned that the nurses would practise midwifery and thus cut into their incomes. Through some well-placed lobbying efforts, aided by Dr. Alfred Worcester, founder of the Waltham Training School for District Nurses in the United States, she managed to gain medical endorsements and the support of the Canadian government. She also managed to convince Charlotte Macleod, a Canadian who was superintendent at Waltham, to return to Canada to become the national director. Lady Aberdeen herself became the first president of the VON Canada national board.

Four VON branches were established in 1897, in Halifax, Montreal, Ottawa and Toronto. These were, as they are now, run by local, voluntary, charitable, not-for-profit boards in each community. The boards raised money and then recruited nurses through the VON national director. Communities decided on the services to be offered, but these generally included district nursing care for those with infectious diseases, care of women and their newborns, and care for the elderly and poor who could not afford medical or hospital care. Education was a vital part of the role.

Lady Aberdeen continued her mentorship of the project, taking care that the VON received favourable publicity whenever possible. She was responsible for arranging for four VON nurses to travel to the Yukon to provide care during the Klondike Gold Rush of 1898 as one means of making the service known throughout Canada. The Victorian Order of Nurses of Canada is a tribute to her political acumen, hard work and influential support.

— *Glennis Zilm and Kirstine Griffith*

The War Years

Canada's entry into World War I, in 1914, accelerated the trend towards industrialization and urbanization. There was a demand for assistance to widows and children, as well as to older family members who had lost sons who would have supported them in their old age. Manitoba responded to this demand by passing a Mothers' Pension Act in 1916, which was followed soon after by similar legislation in other provinces. The Mothers' Pension was not available to everyone, but only to those in financial need. Receiving charity of any kind was considered a sign of personal failure. To have to admit that you were in need of assistance (whether from government, church or other charitable organization) by undergoing a means test in order to qualify for the Mothers' Pension was demeaning.

During the war years, people in rural towns and villages in Saskatchewan had a problem enticing doctors to set up practice because so many people could not pay for the doctor's services. They began to pool their resources to employ a physician for the community. Passage of the Rural Municipality Act in 1916 legitimized this practice, giving towns and villages the power to raise taxes by local levy to pay for a physician's services.

Between World War I and World War II, provincial and municipal governments began to get more involved in providing medical care for the needy and in financing hospitals for the sick. Agitation for social legislation by veterans looking for work as they returned to their homes stimulated the first policy proposals for national health insurance, unemployment insurance (now known as employment insurance) and old age pensions. These proposals were incorporated as components of the Liberal election platform in 1919—but the Liberals did not win. The federal government collaborated with the provinces in sharing half the costs for an old age pension program in 1927. The program paid 20 dollars a month, again only to those determined to be in need by a means test.

During the Depression of the 1930s, British Columbia and Alberta both made unsuccessful attempts to bring in health insurance legislation. Saskatchewan, always the pioneer, passed a Municipal Medical and Hospital Services Act in 1939, which extended the rights of municipalities to allow them to collect a levy for both hospital and physicians' services (Taylor, 1978, 1990; Guest, 1985).

In 1941, the federal government brought in an unemployment insurance program to forestall some of the social unrest anticipated when the soldiers came home. The federal government also commissioned an extensive study on the feasibility of national health insurance, but the recommendations of the Heagerty Commission were not implemented because of disputes over money during federal–provincial consultations. Parliament did, however, pass a **Family Allowance** Act in 1945, which was the first universal social program in Canada. There was no means test—every family with children received a certain allowance, according to the number of children. The National Health Grants Act, passed in 1948, helped the provinces through matching grants to improve hospitals and community health services.

The Beginnings of Medicare

Saskatchewan introduced the first province-wide universal hospital insurance in 1948, followed by British Columbia and Alberta in 1949. After several rounds of federal–provincial negotiation, Parliament finally passed a Hospital Insurance and Diagnostic Services Act in 1957, based on a 50–50 sharing of costs with provinces who met the criteria for entry into the program. All provinces had qualified and were enrolled by 1961.

During the 1950s, the federal government expanded its social service network to include cost-sharing programs with the provinces, such as universal **Old Age Security** (OAS), established in 1951, and programs for the disabled and the blind. Revisions were also made to the Unemployment Insurance Act.

The 1960s saw the birth of **Medicare** after a lengthy battle with physicians who objected to the idea of "socialized medicine" and would have preferred privately sponsored medical insurance. Saskatchewan took the lead once again, introducing a provincial Medical Care Act in 1962. A number of doctors left the province, although many returned before the year was out. Meanwhile, doctors were recruited from Great Britain during the strike, mostly coming over just for the few weeks of the strike, although some stayed on. To explore the feasibility of going ahead with plans to implement a national health program, the federal government had appointed a Royal Commission on Health Services. The Report of the Commission recommended that, although the country was short of the needed health professionals, the government should proceed with its plans (Government of Canada, 1964). To overcome the shortage of human resources in the health field, the government enacted the Health Resources Act (mentioned earlier in the chapter) in 1966. Also in 1966, Parliament passed the Medical Care Act, in which the federal government agreed to share the cost of the programs with the provinces (it was implemented in 1968). By 1972, all provinces and territories had joined Medicare.

The 1960s also saw great strides in the development of other social programs. In the Vocational Rehabilitation of Disabled Persons Act of 1961, the federal government shared with the provinces the cost of comprehensive vocational rehabilitation services for physically and mentally disabled persons. The **Canada Pension Plan** (CPP) was introduced in 1966. Contribution to this plan is compulsory for all employed persons in Canada, with the exception of Quebec, which has its own pension plan. The plan was intended to augment income in the event of retirement, disability or loss of a spouse. In 1966, Parliament passed the Canada Assistance Plan Act to provide subsidies to provinces and municipalities for social assistance and other welfare services.

Many of our older adults were in the labour force before generous retirement pension programs were made an integral component of most employee benefit packages. Those who were not able to save enough money when they were working are now having a hard time living on the government old age pension. Women who stayed at home to look after their families were in a particularly vulnerable position. Only those women who worked outside the home and who contributed could benefit from a company's pension. Additionally, a man's pension often died with him, leaving a widow in dire circumstances. Older people receiving the OAS who have a low income can apply for the Guaranteed Income Supplement introduced in 1967. In 1975, a Spouse's Allowance was added to the OAS for spouses aged 60–64 to augment the income of low-income families. By the end of the 1960s, a fairly comprehensive social safety net for Canadians was in place. All citizens had access to required medical and hospital services, regardless of their income, and a minimum income was guaranteed to those in need (Taylor, 1990; Guest, 1985).

Restructuring the Safety Net

The 1970s was a time for refining the system. The rapid rise of hospital costs prompted reconsideration of the national health program by both federal and provincial governments. It became evident that, under the National Health Grants program, too many hospitals had been built (Rachlis & Kushner, 1989; Sutherland & Fulton, 1988). By the end of the decade, it was also acknowledged that

Canada's Social Safety Net Time-Line

1867	British Parliament	British North America Act
1882	Ontario	First provincial Bureau of Health
1890s	Private sector	VON, Red Cross, Children's Aid societies established
1914	Ontario	First provincial Workmen's Compensation Act
1916	Saskatchewan	Rural Municipality Act
1916	Manitoba	Mothers' Pension Act
1927	Federal Government	Old Age Pension Act
1939	Saskatchewan	Municipal Medical and Hospital Services Act
1941	Federal Government	Unemployment Insurance Act
1945	Federal Government	Family Allowance Act
1946	Saskatchewan	Universal hospital insurance introduced
1948	Federal Government	National Health Grants
1951	Federal Government	Old Age Security Act (OAS)
		Programs for the disabled and blind
1957	Federal Government	National Hospital Insurance and Diagnostic Services Act
1961	Federal Government	National Fitness and Amateur Sport Act
1962	Saskatchewan	Medical Care Insurance Act
1962	Federal Government	National Welfare Grants
1964	Federal Government	Hall Commission Report
1966	Federal Government and Quebec	Canada/Quebec Pension Plans (CPP/QPP)
	Federal Government	Canada Assistance Plan (CAP)
	Federal Government	Health Resources Act
1966	Federal Government	Medical Care Act
1974	Federal Government	Lalonde Report
1975	Federal Government	Spouse's Allowance
		National Health Research and Development Program (NHRDP)
1977	Federal Government	Established Programs Financing Act
1980	Federal Government	Hall Commission Report on Canada's national health insurance program
1984	Federal Government	Canada Health Act

NOTE: You will sometimes find different dates for the passage of legislation in different sources. Acts of Parliament are sometimes passed in one year but not promulgated until the next. We have chosen to use the dates given in an official publication by Health and Welfare Canada (Government of Canada, 1989).

SOURCES: Du Gas & Beckingham, 1993; Government of Canada, 1989; Gibbon & Mathewson, 1947. Adapted from Canada's Social Security Network Time-Line, in Beckingham & Du Gas, 1993.

the capacity of medical schools had perhaps been increased too much and we were heading for a surplus of doctors. The Lalonde Report of 1974 set the tone for a new direction in health care in Canada. The report pointed out that further gains in the health of Canadians were not likely to come from a sickness-oriented system, but rather from measures such as improving people's lifestyles and physical environment. The provinces began to seek more control of the health care dollar, demanding relaxation of federal control over spending. This would allow them to experiment with innovative ways of delivering health care, such as community health centres, home care programs and the utilization of nurse practitioners.

Negotiations, which went on for several years, resulted in the passage of the Established Programs Financing Act in 1977. Provincial governments traded the 50–50 open-ended cost-sharing of programs with the federal government for a significant number of personal income and corporate tax benefits. The federal government's contribution was to be in the form of block grants, with an equalization formula for provinces designated as low-income provinces — all but British Columbia, Alberta and Ontario have been so designated. In 1977, the federal Extended Health Care Services program was also introduced, providing funds of 20 dollars per person so that the provinces could experiment with lower-cost alternative services, such as community health centres and home care.

By the end of the decade, health care services were taking an increasingly large share of provincial budgets. There was also concern about the erosion of the system by practices such as extra billing by doctors and a daily hospital charge. Another Royal Commission on Health Services, chaired once again by Justice Emmott Hall, was appointed to study the system. The 1980 Report pointed out that the principles (public administration, comprehensiveness, universality, portability and accessibility) on which the National Health Insurance Program had been based were indeed being eroded, and recommended a return to the original intent of the program. A new Canada Health Act was passed in 1984, which placed controls on extra billing and additional provincial levies for basic services. This act replaced the Hospital Insurance and Diagnostic Services Act of 1957 and the Medical Care Act of 1966, and remains the basis of health care in this country. As costs of maintaining the system continue to increase, many Canadians are questioning whether we can keep our national health care system intact. We will discuss this topic further in a later section of this chapter.

National Health Care

Major National Health Care Models

Sutherland and Fulton (1988) describe three basic models for the organization of health care services in a country:

1. the national health services model, in which services are provided and organized by a national government
2. the national (public) insurance model, in which the government is the insuring agency. People pay the government (or a **quasi-governmental agency***) a predictable sum, either through a premium or through taxes, to cover health care costs.
3. the entrepreneurial model, in which health services are provided by private agencies and paid for by the consumer of these services.

Canada's health care system is basically a public insurance model, although it contains elements of the other two.

The system in Great Britain is a **national health services model**, and you will often hear British people refer to it as "the NHS." In this model, health services are organized and delivered by the government, most often through a Ministry of Health. In Britain, all services are under the direct control of the national Ministry of Health; the service is therefore considered a centralized system. In some countries—Sweden and Finland are examples—the services are decentralized. Most Canadian health services are not operated by government agencies, although some are. These services in Canada include community health services, provincial hospitals, services for the mentally ill, provincial laboratory services and provincial ambulance systems. The federal government also provides direct services to certain groups within the Canadian population. We will discuss the services provided by different levels of government in Chapter 4.

In Canada, we have opted for a **national insurance model** in which the government funds most services. This model is sometimes referred to as a "one-payer system." National health insurance operates on the same principle as any other type of insurance. That is to say, people pay a predictable sum on a regular basis to cover unpredictable expenses for health care. Payments are made directly by individuals to the insuring agency, through a payroll deduction (usually on a cost-sharing basis with employers), or they may be included in the provincial tax system, where the payment is correlated with the individual's income. The insuring agency in some cases is the government. In others it is an agency closely associated with and accountable to the government, such as a Crown corporation like the Workers' Compensation Board (sometimes spoken of as quasi-governmental). In some provinces the Ministry of Health is the insuring agency; in others a Crown corporation has been established to administer the plans.

Although funded primarily by provincial governments, with contributions from the federal government, most health services in Canada are administered and delivered independently from government. For example, most hospitals

* A quasi-governmental agency is one that is closely related to government and is responsible to it, but operates autonomously. Crown corporations are quasi-governmental agencies.

are called "public general hospitals" but are run by a private "hospital society." In national health insurance systems, the government may fund, regulate and plan health services but these services may be carried out by employees of nongovernmental, non-profit agencies or by nongovernmental agencies for profit. For example, the Ontario and Nova Scotia governments contract out home nursing services to the Victorian Order of Nurses (a nonprofit voluntary agency). The B.C. Ministry of Health hires private agencies such as Comcare to provide home care services to people, in addition to those provided by employees of the Ministry's own community health agencies. The majority of the physicians in Canada are in private practice and people are free to choose their own physicians. Government is the sole payer for all insured services, including those provided by physicians. The physicians are paid for carrying out these services on a fee-for-service basis, according to a schedule for different services negotiated between the provincial medical association and the government (Sutherland & Fulton, 1988).

In the **entrepreneurial model**, services are provided by private agencies and paid for by the consumer so that market forces control the supply and demand aspects of health care. The government does not play a role in either the funding or provision of services. The health care system in the United States is closer to this model, although it has elements of each of the other two (Sutherland & Fulton, 1988). The U.S. federal government does fund services for older people through its Medicare program and services for the poor through **Medicaid**. State Departments of Health also fund and deliver some health services, for example, community health programs. Municipal governments usually plan, fund and deliver school health programs. In the United States, private health insurance is the principal method of health care financing for people under the age of 65. Much of the insurance is employer-paid as a fringe benefit of employment.

The Canadian Model

Although the federal government contributes funding, the health care system in Canada is administered by provincial and territorial governments. The National Health Insurance program was founded on the following five principles:

1. public administration
2. comprehensiveness
   a. hospital services
   b. outpatient services
   c. extended care services
   d. medical services
3. universality
4 portability
5. accessibility.

These five principles provided the basis for both the Hospital Insurance and Diagnostic Services Act of 1957 and the Medical Care Act of 1966. These principles were

Criteria Required to Obtain Federal Funding

1. **Public Administration** The plan must be administered and operated on a nonprofit basis by a public authority, responsible to the provincial government and subject to audits of its accounts and financing transactions.
2. **Comprehensiveness** The plan must insure all insured health services provided by hospitals, medical practitioners or dentists, and, where permitted, services rendered by other health care practitioners.
3. **Universality** One hundred percent of the insured persons of a province must be entitled to the insured health services provided for by the plan on uniform terms and conditions.
4. **Portability** Residents moving to another province must continue to be covered for health services by the home province during any minimum waiting period imposed by the new province of residence, not to exceed three months. For persons temporarily absent from their home provinces:
   a. Out-of-province (but within Canada) insured services are to be paid for by the home province at the rate of the host province unless other fiscal arrangements have been made between the provinces. Prior approval may be required for elective services.
   b. Out-of-country services are to be paid, as a minimum, on the basis of the amount that would have been paid by the home province for similar services rendered in-province. Prior approval may also be required for elective services.
5. **Accessibility** The health care plan of a province must provide for:
   a. insured health services on uniform terms and conditions and reasonable access by insured persons to insured health services unprecluded or unimpeded, either directly or indirectly, by charges or other means;
   b. reasonable compensation to physicians and dentists for all insured health services rendered;
   c. payments to hospitals in respect of the cost of insured health services.

SOURCE: Government of Canada, 1996.

reaffirmed in the Canada Health Act of 1984. The criteria that provincial health insurance plans must meet in order to receive full cash contributions for their plans from the federal government were derived from these principles.

Certain conditions were spelled out in the Canada Health Act which the provinces and territories must meet in order to be eligible for full cash payments for insured health services, as well as extended care services. These include keeping Health Canada informed regarding operation of the provincial and territorial plans and appropriate recognition for federal contributions. Provisions were also built into the 1984 act to ban extra billing and user charges for insured services. The federal minister of health is empowered to withhold cash payments to the provinces if the criteria and conditions are not met. Indeed, until some provinces succeeded in banning extra billing or discontinued the practice of user fees for some insured services, cash payments were withheld. At the time of writing, all provinces have complied, although from time to time, these practices tend to recur.

The insured health services covered by the Canada Health Act include all necessary hospital, physician and surgical-dental services carried out in a hospital. The act also includes provisions for extended care services. These include nursing homes, intermediate care, adult residential care, home care and ambulatory care. Within this broad framework, provincial and territorial governments are free to develop their own health care plans and, as we will discuss in the next section, each is different.

Provincial and Territorial Health Care Plans

All provinces and territories must conform to the guidelines set out in the Canada Health Act. However, the guidelines are broad and allow for considerable flexibility. The result of this flexibility is that we essentially have 10 health care plans, each one slightly different from the other. Each province or territory has the responsibility for financing its program (with contributions from the federal government). Provinces and territories can, almost as much as they wish, set their own priorities, select the policies they want to follow and plan their own health services. In looking at provincial plans, we will discuss similarities and differences under each of the principles on which the National Health Insurance Program was founded.

PUBLIC ADMINISTRATION In all provinces and territories, hospital and medical insurance are operated by the Ministry of Health and/or a public body that is responsible to it, for example a quasi-governmental insurance agency.

COMPREHENSIVENESS Bearing in mind the conditions of the Canada Health Act regarding compulsory payments for insured services, provinces are free to allocate resources, to set standards for services, to administer the services and to evaluate them. They may also deliver services. These services include physician's and dental services, ambulance services, hospital and other inpatient services such as nursing homes, as well as community health services (Sutherland & Fulton, 1988). The specific services covered by all provinces are as follows:

Hospital services

- accommodation and meals at standard ward level
- necessary nursing services, including private duty if required
- radiological and other diagnostic services (laboratory, x-ray or other)
- drugs, biologicals (medicinal compounds prepared from living organisms) and related procedures performed in hospitals
- routine surgical supplies
- use of Operating Room, Case Room and anesthetic facilities
- use of radiotherapy and physiotherapy services, where available.

Outpatient services

- laboratory, diagnostic and radiologic procedures, where available
- radiotherapy and physiotherapy
- the hospital component of other outpatient services, for example, Plaster Room and Operating Room services.

Extended care services

- nursing home intermediate care (care requiring some nursing service)—daily room service charge may be levied for this service
- assistive devices, such as wheelchairs, prostheses and hearing aids for people with disabilities or long-term incapacitating illness (in Alberta and Saskatchewan assistive devices come under a separate plan, called the Aids for Independent Living).

Medical services

- extensive scope of health and social services offered by community and institutional programs and facilities
- basic services as outlined in the Canada Health Act.

Some provinces provide payment for the services of other practitioners, such as optometrists and podiatrists or chiropodists,* either on the same basis as for physicians or with a user fee. For example, one may have to pay a ten-

* Podiatrists and chiropodists are both foot care specialists — the difference between them is that podiatry is taught in university degree programs, and chiropody in college programs.

dollar user fee per visit for physiotherapy treatment (in the physiotherapist's office), over and above the fee that the practitioner receives from the government plan for the service. The number of visits per year permitted under the plan may also be limited. Some provincial plans have a Seniors' Drug Plan under which older people do not have to pay for prescription drugs or may be charged only for the pharmacist's dispensing fee. Drug plans may be extended to other specific groups, for example, to people with diabetes. Ambulance services must be provided by all provinces. All charge a small user fee except Ontario, the Yukon and the Northwest Territories. Emergency transportation by ambulance may be exempted from the user fee. For any or all of the medical, dental and hospital services not covered by the provincial plan, insurance may be obtained from a third party. Many employee health benefit plans, for example, contain options for semi-private or private room hospital coverage, for dental plans and for other services.

UNIVERSALITY All insured persons of each province are entitled to coverage. Not eligible for coverage are people who are looked after under other health programs. For example, the federal government provides direct service for members of the armed services and members of the Royal Canadian Mounted Police, and also has special programs for First Nations Peoples and the population of prisons. Some provinces collect a premium for health insurance but, in most provinces, money comes from general tax revenues.

PORTABILITY Most provinces entitle a person to become a beneficiary on the first day of the third month following their arrival in the province. First-day (immediate) coverage is extended to certain specific groups, such as landed immigrants, in some provinces.

ACCESSIBILITY Additional charges (user fees) may be levied on services not performed in hospital, such as physiotherapy in a therapist's office, and on services provided by practitioners other than physicians or dentists — podiatrists, for example. No person is denied access to services because of inability to pay. A distinguishing number on an individual's health care identification card enables agency receptionists to identify that person as eligible for additional benefits, such as exemption from user fees for people on social welfare, low-income seniors or people with certain chronic diseases.

Table 3.1 provides a comparison of the differing aspects of the various provincial health insurance plans.

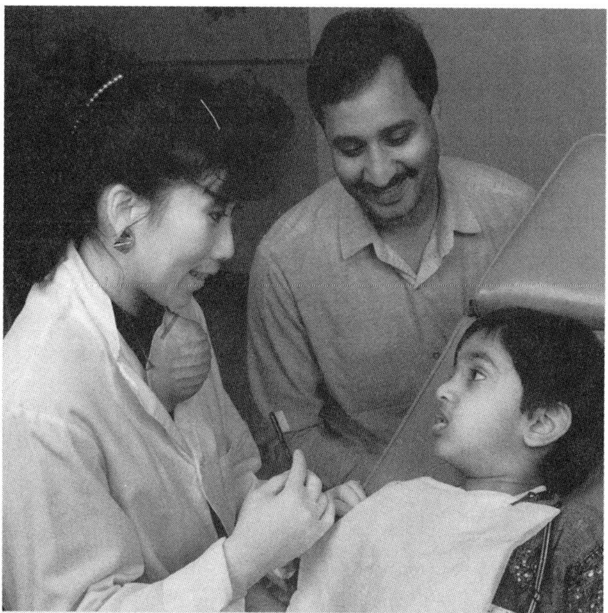

A dental hygienist teaches a boy proper use of a toothbrush.

Health Care and the Money It Costs

Canada's health care plan is basically a publicly funded health insurance program that provides remuneration for private providers (Rachlis & Kushner, 1989). When the national hospital and medical insurance programs were introduced, the federal government agreed to sharing costs with the provinces on a 50–50 "open-ended" basis. In other words, there were no limits on the amount the federal government was required to contribute. Under the Established Programs Financing Act of 1977, these arrangements were changed, as the provinces negotiated successfully for a transfer of some tax credits (that is, the right to impose certain taxes on personal and/or corporate income) together with a cash grant. This grant was to be given as a block of money for health, welfare and education services. Provinces were free to allocate these funds as they wished. Quebec opted for a larger share of tax credits and a smaller cash grant than the other provinces—a choice that later developments have shown to have been a wise one.

The Expenditures

In 1960, Canada was spending 5.5 percent of its gross domestic product (GDP) on health care. By 1991, this figure had increased to 9.9 percent of the GDP, an increase of 67 percent. Figures for the United States show that its increase in health expenditures was 135 percent from 1960 to 1996 (from 5.2 percent of GDP to 14.4 percent). In 1995, Canada consumed 9.5 percent of its GDP on health (National Forum on Health, 1997). "Canada ranks fourth among the G-7 nations for health to GDP ratios, behind the United States, Germany and France" (Canadian Institute for Health Information, 1997, p. 1). Figure 3.2 shows that the rise in Canada's spending on health as a proportion of GDP is close to the average for most of the countries in the Organization for Economic Cooperation and Development (OECD).

TABLE 3.1 A comparison of provincial and territorial health insurance plans, selected points

CRITERIA	NFL	PEI	NS	NB	PQ	ONT	MAN	SASK	ALTA	BC	YUK	NWT
Public Administration												
Hospital Plan												
MOH	✓	x	✓	✓	✓	✓	x	✓	✓	✓	x	✓
Other public body	x	✓	x	x	x	x	✓	x	x	x	✓	x
Medical Plan												
MOH	x	x	x	✓	x	✓	x	✓	✓	x	x	✓
Other public body	✓	✓	✓	x	✓	x	✓	x	x	✓	✓	x
Comprehensiveness												
Additional services:												
Children's dental plan	✓	✓	✓	x	✓	x	x	✓	x	x	x	x
Prescription drugs												
• Seniors' plan	✓	✓	✓	✓	✓	✓	✓	✓	✓	✓	✓	x
• For other groups	x	✓	✓	✓	✓	✓	✓	✓	✓	✓	✓	✓
Other practitioners												
Chiropractors	x	x	x	x	x	✓	x	✓	✓	✓	x	x
Podiatrists/chiropodists	x	x	x	x	x	✓	x	✓	✓	✓	x	x
Naturopaths	x	x	x	x	x	x	x	x	x	✓	x	x
Physiotherapists*	x	x	x	x	x	✓	x	x	✓	✓	x	x
Massage therapists	x	x	x	x	x	x	x	x	x	✓	x	x
Osteopaths	x	x	x	x	x	✓	x	x	x	x	x	x
Universality												
Premiums	x	x	x	x	x	x	x	x	✓	✓	x	x
Portability												
Day 1, third month	✓	✓	✓	✓	✓	✓	✓	✓	✓**	✓	✓**	✓**
First-day coverage for landed immigrants	✓	✓	✓	x	x	x	✓	✓	✓	x	✓	✓
Accessibility												
Reasonable access	✓	✓	✓	✓	✓	✓	✓	✓	✓	✓	✓	✓
Extended Care Services												
Home care	✓	✓	✓	✓	✓	✓	✓	✓	✓	✓	✓	✓
Extramural hospitals	x	x	x	✓	x	x	x	x	x	x	x	x

* For services performed outside of hospital or home care services.
** Not to exceed 3 months. Day not specified in report.

✓ = Yes
x = No

SOURCE: Government of Canada, 1996.

The health care systems of Canada and the United States share some similarities, although the structure of services differs to meet the respective needs of the two countries. As noted, Canada spends less per capita on health than does the United States. Canadian hospitals operate with proportionately less staff than U.S. hospitals; this helps to account for the fact that hospital expenditures are also lower in Canada, despite higher admission rates and longer average length of stay. The health status of Canadians and Americans also varies on a number of health status indicators. We noted some of these in Chapter 2; for example, life expectancy is greater in Canada and infant and maternal mortality rates are lower (Nair, Karim & Nyers, 1992).

In 1997, Canadians spent roughly $2525 per capita on health care (CIHI, 1997). Where, you may ask, does the money go? The largest share of the health care dollar goes to hospital care. In 1996, expenditures for hospitals and other institutional services took almost one-half of the total national expenditures on health care. Physician services took 14.4 percent and professional services by dentists

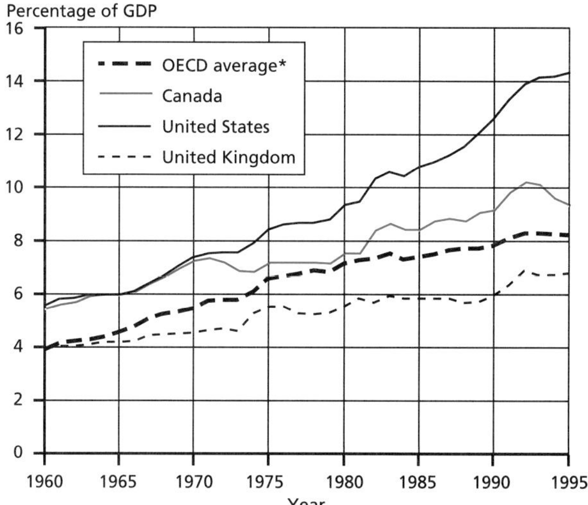

FIGURE 3.2 Health expenditures as a percentage of GDP, 1960–1995: Canada, U.S., U.K. and OECD

*OECD average does not include Luxembourg, Portugal and Turkey (incomplete data) and New Zealand, Mexico, Czech Republic, Hungary and Poland (staggered entry into OECD).

SOURCE: National Forum on Health, 1997, p. 32.

and other health professionals took 8.8 percent. Drugs, including both prescribed and nonprescribed, took almost 14.4 percent. Other health expenses, including administration, public health, capital expenses, research and miscellaneous items, accounted for the rest. See Figure 3.3.

Concerns about Health Spending

Economists tell us that our health care costs have been controlled reasonably well (Rachlis & Kushner, 1989). But this contradicts the media and general public's perception that there is a crisis in Medicare. The concern over health care costs started almost as soon as our social programs were established at the end of the 1960s. During the 1970s, the federal government began to go into deficit spending in order to finance its health programs. The Lalonde Report (1974) was developed primarily as a result of the government's desire to curb health expenditures in general, and hospital spending in particular. The report advocated less emphasis on the "sickness" side of health care and more on community health measures and public education.

As you can see from the pie chart on health care expenditures shown in Figure 3.3, community services continue to consume a very small portion of the health care dollar, being relegated to the category "other expenditures" along with other items that consume relatively small proportions of the total expenditure on health. Hospitals and physicians are still responsible for the largest part of expenditures. The national deficit continued to grow during the 1970s but it was not until the middle of the 1980s that the federal government began to take action to reduce it—in large part by cutting transfer payments to the provinces for health and welfare programs, which resulted in increased financial burdens on the provinces (Boothe & Johnston, 1993; Rachlis & Kushner, 1989; Crichton, Hsu & Tsang, 1994).

The provinces are justifiably concerned about the spiralling cost of health care. Health care reform initiatives continue to be implemented throughout the country. Recent figures indicate that during 1993–1996, hospital expenditures declined by 3.8 percent. Over the past few years, there has been an increase of 5 percent annually in private health spending while public health expenditures have remained stable (Government of Canada, 1997). The federal transfer payments remained frozen until 1996. This control of health transfer payments has required all the provinces and territories to find more innovative ways to control health care costs.

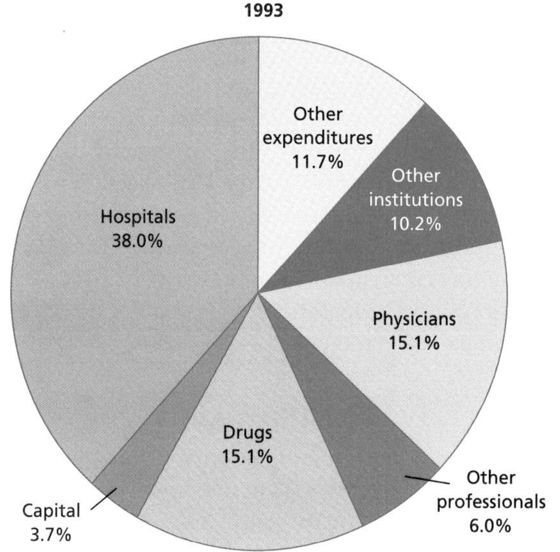

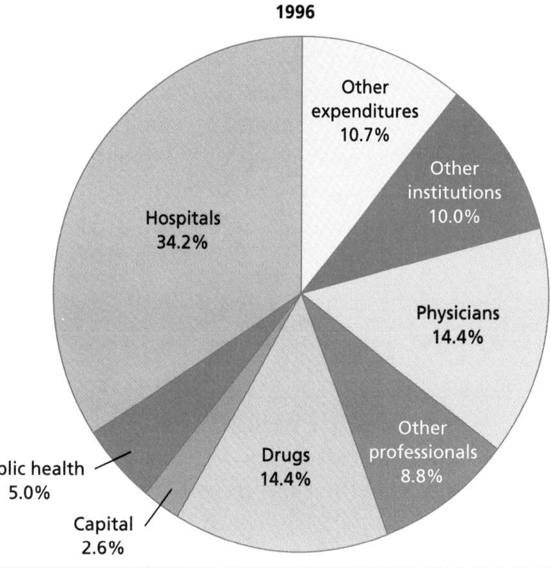

FIGURE 3.3 Percentage federal distribution of health expenditures by category

SOURCE: Government of Canada, 1994, p. 15; 1997, p. 4.

Health Care Reform Across the Country

The need for changes in the health care system in Canada was acknowledged in the early 1970s, both because the system was beginning to cost more than we could afford to pay and, as the Lalonde Report pointed out, we could not expect much more improvement in health status from pouring more money into the system. The need for trimming costs became more urgent during the 1980s, but provincial enquiries into health care reform at the time tended to focus on cost containment, rather than on severe cost cutting.

As we began to change our ideas about the determinants of health (discussed in Chapter 2), the federal government and the provinces realized that radical changes were needed in the system—simply tinkering with it to lower costs was not enough. It was realized that further improvements in the health of Canadians required "not so much ... attempts to diagnose and cure diseases and remedy disabilities as ... non-medical efforts to improve social and economic ills" (Government of Ontario, 1987a, p. 127). In other words, it was time to spend less money on the detection and treatment of disease and more on remedying some of the social and economic ills that were major contributors to health problems.

Publication of the Epp Report (1986), which outlined strategies for promoting health, set the stage for provincial enquiries into ways of reforming the system both to promote better health and, at the same time, to lower costs. The result has been an unprecedented number of reports and papers on health care reform in each province. Some provinces have moved more quickly than others and are busy implementing the changes recommended in the reports. We talked earlier in this chapter about public participation in the process of policy formulation. In all provinces, people have had the opportunity to voice their opinions. The Canadian Nurses Association and its provincial counterparts have been active in presenting briefs, speaking at public forums and developing position papers. Each province has come up with different reform packages, but the following common trends have emerged:

1. a strong movement to home- and community-based care
2. a reduction in the number of hospital beds
3. regionalization or decentralization of services
4. increasing public participation in policy-making, planning and management of care
5. increased intersectoral collaboration (that is, collaboration between health and other sectors of the community, such as business or justice)
6. attempts to reduce inequities existing between regions within a province as well as between specific groups within the population
7. more effective utilization of health personnel
8. attempts to control hospital costs
9. efforts to decrease the rapid rise in the number of physicians in the country
10. a cap on expenditures for medical care.

We will now attempt to give you a brief outline of the changes in health care reform planned or being implemented in all the provinces at the time of writing.*

Newfoundland

In attempts to improve management and to control costs, three commissions were set up:

1. the Royal Commission on Hospital and Nursing Home Costs, 1983–1984
2. an Advisory Committee on Nursing Workforce
3. the Green Paper entitled "Our Health Care System Expenditures and Funding, 1986."

In response to the reports of these commissions, the Newfoundland government initiated a plan in 1991–1992 to regionalize community health services, and had four regional boards in place by 1993. The government has also moved to decrease the number of acute care beds and to increase the number of long-term care beds. The role of small community hospitals has also been changed—they have become integrated health care centres, combining community health care services with traditional hospital services. A precedent-setting primary health care (PHC) project, planned and initiated by nurses in 1990, was the first complete nurse-run PHC pilot project in Canada and proved the cost-effectiveness and capability of nurses as primary health care providers (Hall, 1989; "Nurses prove themselves," 1994).

Currently, the Government of Newfoundland and Labrador has the lowest per capita spending on health in Canada. There are four community health boards that are responsible for five areas of health delivery—health promotion, protection, continuing care, mental health and alcohol/drug dependency. In 1995, the administration duties of home support services were transferred from the Department of Social Services to the Department of Health. In 1996, the government announced the establishment of the Newfoundland and Labrador Centre for Health Information. Its primary goal is to integrate existing health information into a comprehensive system for health and social services (Government of Nova Scotia, 1997).

Prince Edward Island

Prince Edward Island did not set up any commissions or public enquiries. The government did, however, establish a

* This summary is based on the following sources: Government of Canada, 1996; "Primary health care has arrived," 1992; "Nurses as a point of access," 1993; "Nurses prove themselves in primary health care," 1994; Crichton et al., 1994; and Government of Nova Scotia, 1997.

health care task force that reported during 1991–1992 on directions and approaches to addressing current trends and pressures in health care in the province. This document was called *Health Reform: Vision for Change*. As a result of the Health and Community Services Act, the Health and Community Services System now incorporates four areas—Department of Health and Social Services, Provincial Health Policy Council, Health and Community Services Agency (a Crown corporation governed by a provincial board) and five health regions governed by regional boards. Each of these areas has specific roles and responsibilities in the delivery of health care services in the regions (Government of Nova Scotia, 1997). A review of women's health was sponsored by consumers. A 1990 needs assessment study of people in the west central part of the island resulted in a community-initiated Farm Heart Health project. An Active Living Program is also underway to encourage healthier lifestyles. In 1995, the government developed a three-year provincial plan for ongoing health care reform initiatives. This plan focusses on community decision making, which allows community members, in collaboration with health professionals, to determine needed health services (Government of Nova Scotia, 1997).

New Brunswick

In 1988, a Commission on Selected Health Care Programs was established to review escalating health care costs, and it proposed a number of recommendations (Government of New Brunswick, 1989). The 1992 document, *An Ounce of Prevention*, was prepared, emphasizing health promotion and prevention. A number of guiding principles emerged from this report, which provided the government with a framework for health policy and an implementation plan.

The Health and Community Services Plan (1992) was designed to help with the regionalization process and to restructure the delivery of health and community services. Hospital boards soon were regionalized, and seven public health regions were created. Family and Community Social Services Regions were restructured to fit with the public health regions. Further health plans continue to be tabled in the legislature in order to evaluate the goals of the province's health care reform established in 1992 (Government of Nova Scotia, 1997).

Nova Scotia

A Royal Commission on Health Care was established in 1987 to examine the financing and delivery of health care in the province (Nova Scotia Royal Commission on Health Care, 1989). In responding to the 103 recommendations of the Commission, the Health Ministry contracted advisory services to prepare intersectoral communication and comprehensive health planning guidelines. The Nova Scotia Ministry of Health subsequently published a policy paper entitled *Health Strategy for the Nineties: Managing Better Care* (1990). Action has been taken to start the process of **regionalization**—decentralizing the health care system by giving local authorities the power to make decisions about health care (Crichton et al., 1994). During the 1991–1992 year, the Minister of Health announced a commitment to reduce the number of hospital beds to five per thousand by 1993–1994 and to control expenditures with tight budgetary restrictions. Ministerial task forces were appointed to look into physician policy development, nursing and primary health care. A community-based care pilot project was initiated in late 1992, operated out of the Sacred Heart Hospital in Cape Breton. A nurse coordinator was appointed to head the project ("Primary health care has arrived," 1992). In 1994, a working committee of the Ministry of Health released a document entitled *Nova Scotia's Blueprint for Health System Reform*. The Department of Health continues to use this document as a framework for health reform. Currently, there are four Regional Health Boards established by the Minister and 20 Community Health Boards. Evaluation of the health care restructuring system is ongoing (Government of Nova Scotia, 1997).

Quebec

The Quebec (Castonguay) model developed in the early 1970s was based on the principles of universal access, preventive medicine and community development. It set a health-outcomes model that has influenced the rest of Canada. A province-wide system of community clinics with community advisory boards was established. The CLSCs (*Centres locaux de services communautaires*), as they are known, provide health and social services and have a mandate for community development. During the 1980s the Quebec government appointed the Rochon Committee to review the progress made in implementing the Castonguay model and to assess its current appropriateness.

The Commission made a number of recommendations on better ways to promote health and prevent social and health problems. Strategies were also recommended to improve the participation of community members in care for one another and to encourage consumer involvement in policy-making and in participative management of health and social services. It also recommended that each CLSC become more streamlined to deal with the medical and social problems of their locality. Subsequent enquiries have been conducted on mental health policy (Boudreau, 1987), on the work of nurses and on the new technologies of human reproduction. Responding to the recommendations of these committees, the Ministry published a document entitled *Improving Health and Well-being in Quebec: Orientations* (1989). Another paper, published in 1990, suggested reforms for primary care services (Gouvernement du Québec, 1990). During 1992, broad public consultation was held on the major stakes involved in financing health and social services. The discussion identified objectives to be pursued and suggested ways of containing increases in health and social services expenditures. In June 1992, the Quebec Legislative Assembly passed legislation about social services and about amending previous legislation. This bill is considered a major step in the implementation of reform in the health care system in Quebec. It sets out the fundamental objectives of health and social services and the rights of users. It also outlines the services to be performed by the various providers of health and social services and redefines certain procedures regarding health personnel, health facilities and other resources. The bill also sets out new organizational structures for agency boards to facilitate mergers in order to streamline services.

In 1995, the Department of Health and Social Services asked each Regional Health Board to evaluate and reorganize the health and social services needs of their communities. As a result, action plans were developed to assess the accessibility of surgery services and institutional laboratory services. Currently, Regional Health Boards have authority to implement these action plans (Government of Nova Scotia, 1997).

Ontario

Ontario has conducted a series of studies looking into health care. Three committees were set up between 1985 and 1987:

1. to look into health promotion
2. to investigate goals
3. an overview committee to build on the other two and come out with recommendations.

The recommendations included more emphasis on health promotion and disease prevention, to be accomplished without too much remodelling of the system. A Premier's Council on Health Strategy (later changed to the Premier's Council on Health, Well-being and Social Justice when the New Democratic Party was elected to power) was established as a new mechanism for policy development. Its task was to sift data from the studies mentioned above and prepare proposals. In response to these proposals, the Ministry of Health prepared a discussion paper called *Deciding the Future of Our Health Care* (1989). The health goals subcommittee of the Premier's Council identified five goals:

1. shift emphasis to health promotion and disease prevention
2. foster strong and supportive families and communities
3. ensure a safe, high-quality physical environment
4. increase the number of years of good health by preventive measures
5. provide accessible, affordable and appropriate health services for all.

Other studies have been done on mental health, long-term care, hospital deficits and the use and provision of medical services and health promotion. The Premier's Council outlined the research done on the factors which determine our health in *Nurturing Health*, and these have been summarized in a publication by the same title (1993). Ontario is currently embarking on reforming its system to implement these goals. A major study was undertaken to assess the health behaviours and health status of people in the province (1992).

Ontario has already moved to initiate decentralization of the system, with local boards functioning with regional funding envelopes so that they control the funds for health services in their local area. Rachlis and Kushner (1989) suggest that the delegation of financial responsibility, as well as decision-making authority, to the regional boards makes local communities more accountable for the funds spent on health care. The provincial ministries of health retain overall control through the establishment of minimum standards for personnel and facilities, such as the number of acute care beds per population.

A comprehensive regional planning demonstration in the London and South West Region is in progress and a restructuring of the delivery system is taking place. Examples of the restructuring include reorganizing mental health services, initiating community clinic pilot projects, reforming long-term care organization, controlling independent health facilities, restructuring local government operations and conducting a corporate government review. The public also is involved in discussions on the health care system.

Manitoba

Manitoba set up a Health Advisory Steering Committee in 1988. Recommendations coming from the various Task Force groups of this committee were incorporated into a policy paper entitled *Quality Health Care for Manitobans: The Action Plan* (1992). The paper specified that the health services system must be directed by the health needs and active participation of Manitobans. The province is embarking on a two-year plan to shift from institutional to community-based care. It is compressing acute care drastically by cutting beds and removing services from the hospital setting and transferring resources to more appropriate prevention and home care services in the community. Of particular interest to nurses is the store-front, nurse-operated Youville Clinic, which has been highly successful in providing community health care services. A satellite outreach program was established in 1986 at the Indian/Métis Friendship Centre in downtown Winnipeg (Crichton et al., 1994; Government of Canada, 1996; "Primary health care has arrived," 1992).

In 1996, the Department of Health presented a document entitled *Next Steps: Pathways to a Healthy Manitoba.* This document outlines five pathways:

1. management and governance—system-wide structures
2. eliminating overlap and duplication—sharing support services

3. evolving roles of hospitals—a Winnipeg plan
4. community-based services—a neighbourhood focus
5. health information—a bridge to the future (Government of Nova Scotia, 1997).

Saskatchewan

Saskatchewan is busy restructuring its health services. The impetus for change came with the 1988 commission on health care, which identified major problems in Saskatchewan. A policy paper soon followed issued by the prevailing government (Government of Saskatchewan, 1990). The government was not re-elected, and *A Saskatchewan Vision of Health* (1992) was issued by the new government. This document stressed a wellness approach and suggested five strategies, which the Ministry of Health has begun to implement. A shift in emphasis was initiated, moving away from institutional care and towards a more holistic approach with the provision of a wide range of services. The community is to be the base, but the emphasis on services will be on noninstitutionalized care. Strategies to reach the wellness goal include:

1. public policies to promote good health with a provincial health council to advise on policies
2. emphasis on health promotion and disease prevention
3. the integration and coordination of services
4. the support of community-based services
5. better utilization of health services.

Already, a number of small hospitals (some with as few as nine beds) have been closed. The closures created a furore among people in the rural areas who had very strong feelings about what they saw as "*our* hospital" and a valuable asset to the community. Activities to provide more preventive care have resulted in a permanent breast cancer screening clinic, which opened in Regina in 1991, and two mobile units to service the southern and central parts of the province. Another permanent clinic was opened in Saskatoon, with a satellite clinic in North Battleford. In addition, health boards were established in the cities of Regina and Saskatoon to operate health care services. The new boards replace those of hospitals, special care and home care. A pilot project with nurses playing a central role was recommended for Eastend, a community of 600 in rural southwest Saskatchewan ("Primary health care has arrived," 1992). In 1996, a report entitled *Making Choices* revealed that the residents of Saskatchewan placed health as a priority. As a result, Saskatchewan Health has expanded community-based services and is more aware of community needs (Government of Nova Scotia, 1997).

Alberta

A broad general study of the social needs of the province was followed by the establishment in 1988 of a Royal Commission on Future Care for Albertans. Its report, entitled *Rainbow Report: Our Vision for Health* (1990), made 22 recommendations. A policy paper entitled *Partners in Health* (November 1991) suggested five initiatives to be implemented immediately:

1. a health unit/health facility partnership initiative
2. establishment of a health services innovative fund to support research and evaluation for new ways of delivering services
3. establishment of the Alberta Family Life and Substance Abuse Foundation
4. development of a collaborative process to develop health goals for Alberta
5. commencement of a major initiative in coordination.

Another policy statement, called *Future Directions for Mental Health Services in Alberta* (1992), emphasized the coordination of services across a continuum of care. Emphasis is being placed on ensuring that people requiring mental health service will have access to the most appropriate services. A series of public forums in different areas of the province was held in 1992 for the purpose of discussing the reform process and health goals. At the present time, there are 17 Regional Health Authorities responsible for the delivery of health care to Albertans (Government of Nova Scotia, 1997; Crichton et al., 1994).

British Columbia

The Report of the Royal Commission on Health Services, *Closer to Home* (1991b), was followed by a round of public consultations on its recommendations. In 1993, a policy document entitled *New Directions for a Healthy British Columbia* (1993) was published. The policy's outline was based on the principles of equity, partnership (with all participants in the health system), financial responsibility and sensitive implementation. The New Directions paper set out five goals for future health services in British Columbia:

1. better health through fostering health promotion and disease prevention by such strategies as strengthening community action, creating supportive environments, developing personal health skills and targeting screening programs for high-risk groups
2. greater public participation and responsibility at three levels: provincial, regional and community
3. bringing health closer to home through more local management of health services and the provision of more services in people's homes, local communities and regional areas
4. respecting the care provider, with paid and volunteer care providers involved in planning health services
5. effective management of the new health system, with clearly defined goals at all levels of service.

A Ministerial Advisory Committee and six working groups were established to advise on strategies for change: Better Management, Regionalization, Governance of Property and Financing, People with Special Needs, Services, and Care Delivery. Again, the stakeholders—professional organizations, administrators of service facilities and volunteer organizations — are being consulted.

In 1996, The new Minister of Health placed a temporary freeze on New Directions pending a review. The Ministry proposed several changes to regionalization:

1. the term New Directions was changed to Better Team Work, Better Care
2. the number of Regional Health Boards (RHBs), which are designated to represent urban areas, was reduced from 20 to 11
3. Community Health Councils (CHCs) representing rural areas were also reduced, from 82 to 34
4. memberships of the Boards/Councils vary, depending on the needs of the area
5. there are now two appointed voting members—one physician and one health care union representative on each RHB and CHC
6. each RHB and CHC must sign a contract with the Ministry (Stone, 1997).

The number of acute care hospital beds is being decreased and community services, particularly home care, greatly expanded.

The Yukon and Northwest Territories

Until fairly recently, health care services in the Yukon and the Northwest Territories have been handled primarily by the federal government, which provided direct care to First Nations people. We will discuss these services in Chapter 4. Meanwhile, the winds of change are also blowing in the North, as services are being taken over by territorial governments and by First Nations communities themselves.

IN REVIEW

- Canadians today consider the social safety net as a basic right. It includes:
  - a national health insurance program that covers both hospital and medical care
  - social welfare programs, which include employment insurance, old age pension, contributory pensions for working people, family allowance and social assistance.
- The British North America (BNA) Act of 1867 delegated responsibility for health and welfare matters to the provinces. At that time:
  - hospital care and care of the needy were mainly the responsibility of religious and charitable organizations
  - conditions in secular hospitals were very poor.
- By the turn of the century, medical and nursing schools were established and hospital conditions improved considerably
  - a number of voluntary organizations provided services for the sick and the poor, including the Children's Aid Societies, the Red Cross Society and the Victorian Order of Nurses.
- A hospital insurance program was started in Saskatchewan in 1948.
- Federal legislation for universal hospital insurance was enacted in 1957, with the federal and provincial governments sharing costs equally.
- Medicare started in the 1960s.
- By the end of the 1960s, the social safety net was fairly comprehensive. New programs that were initiated include:
  - Old Age Security
  - a rehabilitation program for the disabled
  - Canada Assistance Plan (which provides minimum income for those in need).
- The 1970s and 1980s saw a restructuring of the social safety net in response to concerns over the high cost of health care.
- The Canadian National Health Insurance Program was founded on five principles that were reconfirmed in the Canada Health Act of 1984. These principles are:
  - public administration
  - comprehensiveness
  - universality
  - portability
  - accessibility.
- Currently, all provinces in Canada are engaged in restructuring their health services. The direction of change is towards more community-based care.
- Key components in all provincial health care plans include:
  - regionalization
  - increased public participation in policy-making, planning and management.

Critical Thinking Activities

1. The interest of nurses in preserving the heritage of nursing has resulted in the development of both

provincial history of nursing groups and a Canadian Association for the History of Nursing (CAHN). Explore what is happening in your province. Is there a provincial history of nursing group? If so, what is the group doing to preserve the history of nursing in your province? Who were some of the early nursing leaders in your province? When were the first hospitals established? Where? By whom? Who provided the nursing care? What were the conditions like in these early hospitals? Who carried out the first community health nursing in the province? When? Where?

2. What is the amount of the current budget for health services in your province? How much of the money for health services comes from the federal government? How much from the provincial treasury? How much has the budget increased in the past ten years? What portion of the provincial budget for health goes to hospitals? other institutions? physician services? the services of other health practitioners? drugs? community health? home care? other items?
3. What health care reforms are currently taking place in your province?
   a. To what extent has there been a movement to home- and community-based care in your province? What home and community services have been developed, extended or planned? Have additional funds been allocated for expansion of home and community services?
   b. Are hospital beds being closed? hospitals? If so, where in the province? What is the community reaction to these closures?
   c. Are regional health boards being established? If so, where? How will they be formed?
   d. What is your provincial government doing to foster public participation in policy-making, planning and management of health care? Are public meetings being held? Have community health planning groups been established?
   e. Are there examples in your province of intersectoral collaboration? For example, do you have mandatory seat belt legislation? If so, what departments of government were involved in passage of the legislation? Can you think of other examples of intersectoral collaboration?
   f. What efforts are being made in your province to reduce inequities between regions within the province and between specific groups within the population? For example, increasing services to northern regions; or setting up community clinics or other services in low-income neighbourhoods?
   g. What attempts are being made to utilize health personnel more effectively? Are there pilot projects, such as primary health care projects, nurse-operated clinics or health centres, community health centres, extramural hospitals? If so, where are they? What stage are they at — planning, implementation, evaluation?
   h. What efforts are being made to control hospital costs?
   i. What is being done to decrease the rise in the number of physicians if this is a problem in your province? What is being done to cap expenditures on medical care?

KEY TERMS

welfare state p. 34
social safety net p. 34
welfare society p. 34
policy p. 34
public policy p. 34
healthy public policy p. 35
Family Allowance p. 38
Old Age Security (OAS) p. 38
Medicare p. 38
Canada Pension Plan (CPP) p. 38
quasi-governmental agency p. 40
national health services model p. 40
national insurance model p. 40
entrepreneurial model p. 41
Medicaid p. 41
regionalization p. 47

References

BECKINGHAM, A., & DU GAS, B. (1993). *Promoting healthy aging*. St. Louis: Mosby.

BOOTHE, P., & JOHNSTON, B. (1993, March). Stealing the emperor's clothes: Deficit offloading and national standards in health care. C.D. Howe Institute *Commentary, 41*.

BOUDREAU, F. (1987). The making of mental health policy: The 1980s and the challenge of sanity in Quebec and Ontario. *Canadian Journal of Mental Health, 6*(1), 24–47.

CANADIAN INSTITUTE FOR HEALTH INFORMATION (CIHI). (1997, November 12). *1997 Health expenditures highlights* (pp. 1–30). [Online.] Available at http://www.cihi.ca/facts/canhe.htm

CANADIAN NURSES ASSOCIATION. (1968). *The leaf and the lamp*. Ottawa: Author.

CANADIAN NURSES ASSOCIATION. (CNA) (1996). *Registered nurse database*. Ottawa: Author.

CRICHTON, A., HSU, D., & TSANG, S. (1994). *Canada's health care system: Its funding and organization*. Ottawa: Canadian Health Association.

DU GAS, B., & BECKINGHAM, A. (1993). The emergence of gerontological nursing. In A. Beckingham, & B. Du Gas (Eds.) *Promoting healthy aging* (pp. 70–79). St. Louis: Mosby.

EPP, J. (1986). *Achieving health for all: A framework for health promotion*. Ottawa: Ministry of Supply & Services.

GIBBON, J.M., & Mathewson, M.S. (1947). *Three centuries of Canadian nursing*. Toronto: Macmillan of Canada.

GOUVERNEMENT DU QUEBEC (Ministère de la santé et des services sociaux). (1990). *Une reforme axée sur le citoyen*. Québec: Auteur.

GOVERNMENT OF ALBERTA. (1988). *Caring and responsibility*. From the office of the Minister for Special Projects. Edmonton: Government Printer.

GOVERNMENT OF ALBERTA. (1990). *Rainbow report: Our vision for health*. Edmonton: Government Printer.

GOVERNMENT OF ALBERTA. (1991). *Partners in health*. Edmonton: Government Printer.

GOVERNMENT OF ALBERTA. (1992). *Future directions for mental health care in Alberta*. Edmonton: Government Printer.

GOVERNMENT OF BRITISH COLUMBIA. (1991a). *A guide for communities to enact health-promoting policies*. Victoria: Queen's Printer. Prepared by the B.C. Ministry of Health Office of Health Promotion in collaboration with the Social Planning and Research Council of B.C. (SPARC).

GOVERNMENT OF BRITISH COLUMBIA. (1991b). *Closer to home: Summary of the Royal Commission on Health Care and Costs*. Victoria: Crown Publishing.

GOVERNMENT OF BRITISH COLUMBIA. (1993). *New directions for a healthy British Columbia*. Victoria: Ministry of Health & Ministry Responsible for Seniors.

GOVERNMENT OF CANADA. (1964). *Royal Commission on Health Services* (E. Hall, Chairman). Ottawa: Queen's Printer.

GOVERNMENT OF CANADA. (1989). *Health and welfare in Canada*. Ottawa: Ministry of Supply & Services. (Catalogue No. H21–102/1989E)

GOVERNMENT OF CANADA. (1994). *National health expenditures in Canada, 1975–1993*. Ottawa: Health Canada, Policy & Consultation Branch. (Catalogue No. H21-99/1993)

GOVERNMENT OF CANADA. (1996). *Canada Health Act Annual Report 1995–1996*. Ottawa: Ministry of Supply & Services. (Catalogue No. H1–4/1996)

GOVERNMENT OF CANADA. (1997, November 12). *National health expenditures in Canada, 1975–1996: Fact sheets*. [Online.] Available at http://www.hc-sc.gc.ca/main/hc/web/datapcb/datahesa/hex97/ Ehex97.htm

GOVERNMENT OF MANITOBA. (1992). *Quality health care for Manitobans: The action plan*. Winnipeg: Government Printer.

GOVERNMENT OF NEW BRUNSWICK. (1989). *Report of the Commission on Selected Health Care Programs*. Fredericton: Government Printer.

GOVERNMENT OF NEW BRUNSWICK. (1992). *An ounce of prevention*. Fredericton: Government Printer.

GOVERNMENT OF NOVA SCOTIA (Ministry of Health). (1990). *Health strategy for the nineties: Managing better care*. Halifax: Government Printer.

GOVERNMENT OF NOVA SCOTIA. (1997). *Regionalization of health care systems in Canada. An overview*. Halifax: Department of Health.

GOVERNMENT OF ONTARIO. (1987a). *Health promotion matters in Ontario*. A report of the Minister's Advisory Group on Health Promotion. Toronto: Government Printer.

GOVERNMENT OF ONTARIO. (1989). *Deciding the future of our health care*. Toronto: Government Printer.

GOVERNMENT OF ONTARIO. (1992). *Ontario health survey 1990*. Toronto: Ontario Minister of Health.

GOVERNMENT OF ONTARIO. (1993). *Nurturing health*. Toronto: Government Publisher. Prepared by the Premier's Council on Health, Well-being and Social Justice. Other publications by the Premier's Council include: *A vision in health; From vision to action; Bringing health and social services together; Cooordination and integration of health policies; Community services study; Funding and incentives study.*

GOVERNMENT OF QUEBEC. (1989). *Improving health and well-being in Quebec: Orientations*. Quebec City: Author.

GOVERNMENT OF SASKATCHEWAN. (1990). *Directions in health care*. Regina: Saskatchewan Health.

GOVERNMENT OF SASKATCHEWAN. (1992). *A Saskatchewan vision of health*. Regina: Saskatchewan Health.

GOVERNMENT OF SASKATCHEWAN. (1996). *Making choices*. Regina: Saskatchewan Health.

GUEST, D. (1985). Social security. In the *Canadian encyclopaedia* (pp. 1723–1724). Edmonton: Hurtig.

HALL, D.C. (1989). *Primary health care — A nursing model*. A Danish–Newfoundland (Canada) project. St. John's, Newfoundland: Association of Registered Nurses of Newfoundland.

HALL, E.M. (1980). *Canada's national health program for the '80s*. Ottawa: Health & Welfare Canada.

LALONDE, M. (1974). *A new perspective on the health of Canadians*. Ottawa: Ministry of Supply & Services.

LARSEN, J., & BAUMGART, A. (1992). Overview: Shaping public policy. In A. Baumgart & J. Larsen (Eds.), *Canadian nursing faces the future: Development and change*. (2nd ed., pp. 469–494). Toronto: Mosby.

LEFORT, S.M. (1993). Shaping health care policy. *Canadian Nurse, 89*(3), 23–30.

NAIR, C., KARIM, R., & NYERS, C. (1992). Health care and health status. A Canada–United States statistical comparison. *Health Reports 1992, 4*(2), 175–183. (Statistics Canada No. 82–003)

NATIONAL FORUM ON HEALTH. (1997). *Canada health action: Building on the legacy*. Volume II. Ottawa: Minister of Public Works & Government Services. (Catalogue No. H21-126/5-2-1997E)

NOVA SCOTIA ROYAL COMMISSION ON HEALTH CARE. (1989). *Towards a new strategy*. Halifax: Government Printer.

NURSES AS A POINT OF ACCESS. (1993). *CNA Today, 3*(2), 1.

NURSES PROVE THEMSELVES IN PRIMARY HEALTH CARE. (1994, April). *CNA Today, 4*(2), 1.

PEDERSON, A.P., EDWARDS, R.K., MARSHALL, V.W., ALLISON, K.R., & KELNER, M. (1989). *Coordinating healthy public policy: An analytic literature review and bibliography*. Ottawa: Health & Welfare Canada. (Available from the Ministry of Supply & Services)

PRIMARY HEALTH CARE HAS ARRIVED. (1992). *CNA Today, 2*(3), 4–5.

RACHLIS, M., & KUSHNER, C. (1989). *Second opinion*. Toronto: Collins.

SOUTH FRASER VALLEY HEALTH BOARD (SFVRHR). (1996). *Health Management Plan*. Delta, BC: Author.

STONE, S. (1997). Clearing the air about health care restructuring. *Nursing BC, 29*(5), 31–32.

SUTHERLAND, R., & FULTON, J. (1988). *Health care in Canada*. Ottawa: The Health Group.

TAYLOR, M.G. (1978). *Health insurance and Canadian public policy: The seven decisions that created the Canadian health insurance system*. Montreal: McGill-Queen's University Press.

TAYLOR, M.G. (1990). *Insuring national health care*. Chapel Hill: University of North Carolina Press.

VICTORIAN ORDER OF NURSES FOR CANADA (VON). (1983). *Missioners for health*. Unpublished manuscript on the history of the VON.

Additional Readings

ARMSTRONG, H., ARMSTRONG, P., CHOINIERE, J., FELDBERG, G., & WHITE, J. (1994). *Take care: Warning signals for Canada's health system*. Toronto: Garamond Press.

BENNETT, A.I., & Adams, O. (1993). *Looking north for health: What we can learn from Canada's health care system*. San Francisco: Jossey-Bass.

McARTHUR, W., RAMSAY, C., & WALKER, M. (1996). *Healthy incentives: Canadian health reform in an international context*. Vancouver: Fraser Institute.

NATIONAL FORUM ON HEALTH. (1997). Canada health action: Building on the legacy. Volume I. Ottawa: Minister of Public Works & Government Services. (Catalogue No. H21-126/5-2-1997E)

RACHLIS, M., & KUSHNER, C. (1994). *Strong medicine: How to save Canada's health care system*. Toronto: HarperCollins.

STINGL, M., & WILSON, D. (1996). *Efficiency versus equality: Health reform in Canada*. Halifax: Fernwood.

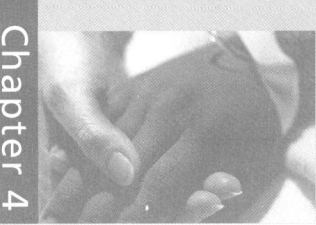

Chapter 4

Health Services: The Continuum of Care

OUTLINE

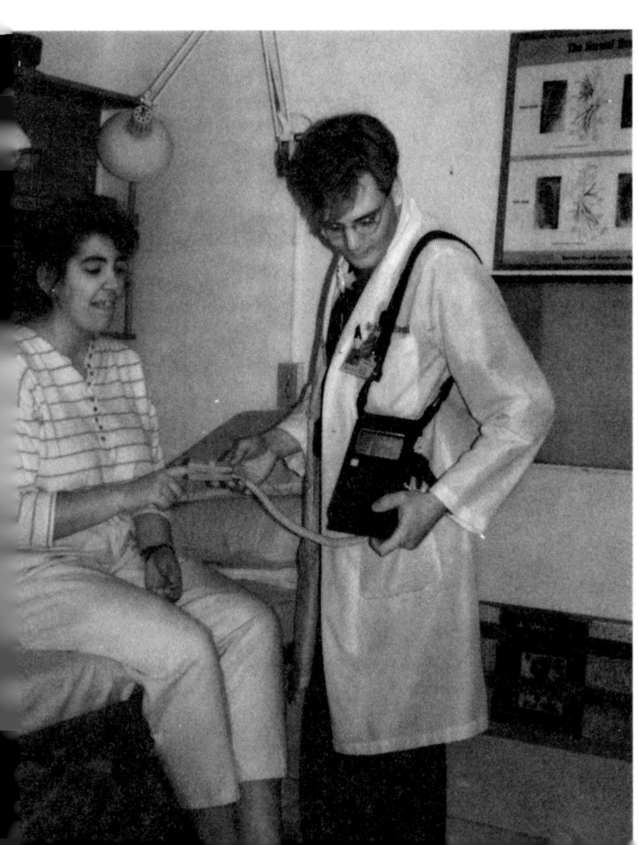

Central Questions

1. What is meant by the continuum of health care?
2. What is the philosophy underlying primary health care?
3. What strategies and mechanisms are outlined in the Epp Framework for Health Promotion?
4. What are the major responsibilities of federal, provincial and municipal governments and of the voluntary sector in health and welfare in Canada?
5. How do family and friends contribute to the health and welfare of people in our society?
6. What services are available for home care of people who are ill?
7. What is the role of voluntary and religious agencies in health and welfare?
8. What types of agencies provide health services in Canadian communities?
9. What are the differences among the following types of inpatient services:
    - acute care hospitals
    - rehabilitation agencies
    - long-term care facilities
    - personal care facilities
    - hospices/palliative care units?
10. What roles do federal and provincial governments play in health and welfare?
11. Why do we need Workers' Compensation Boards when we have national health insurance?
12. Does the private sector play a role in health and welfare in Canada?
13. What are the functions of the principal members of the health team?

Introduction

We have the foundations upon which to build. Let us continue our efforts to achieve health and improve the quality of life of the people and communities of Canada.

Epp, 1986

At the present time, health care reform is sweeping the country. In every province and territory, the structure of health services is undergoing rapid change as our health care system shifts from a disease-oriented, hospital-based system to one with a wellness orientation. The description of health services in this country used to be very straightforward—there were hospitals that cared for the sick and community health agencies that were concerned with health promotion and disease prevention. This dichotomy no longer holds true. Collaborative partnerships are being forged between community and inpatient health agencies to avoid duplication of services and to provide people with a continuum of care. This continuum includes services to promote and protect health through disease prevention and risk reduction, to restore patients' health and to provide supportive services to individuals and their families.

The **continuum of care**, you will recall, was identified in the health care reform packages put forward by all provincial and territorial governments. As the word *continuum* suggests, the range of health services can no longer be divided into neat compartments, because each phase of care merges into the others. Let's look at the example of a person who is hospitalized briefly for a cholecystectomy (removal of the gall bladder). During the period when the individual's health is being restored (convalescence), the nurse will help the patient to establish better dietary habits to promote health and to reduce the risk of further digestive problems. No doubt, the patient's family will also be encouraged to adopt healthy nutritional habits, both to help the patient and to reduce the risks for themselves of developing similar problems.

In this chapter, we begin with a discussion of the philosophy of primary health care, which is providing the foundation on which health services are being restructured. Then we will discuss the mechanisms and strategies outlined in the Epp Framework for Health Promotion (1986), which gives direction for implementing the philosophy. We will then look at the overall structure of health services in Canada—the foundation that is already in place—and go into more detail regarding the role of family and friends, the voluntary sector, the private sector and various community agencies in promoting and protecting our health. We will devote some time to a discussion of the role of hospitals and other inpatient facilities for care of the ill and will conclude with a discussion of the people who provide the services.

The Philosophy of Primary Health Care

In Canada, the term **primary health care (PHC)** was used in the *Report of the Committee on Nurse Practitioners* (the Boudreau Report, 1972) to refer to the first level of service in a comprehensive health care system. Subsequently, the meaning of the term has broadened to include an emphasis on a philosophy of care as well as on services. Primary health care was identified at an international conference sponsored by the World Health Organization in Alma-Ata in the former U.S.S.R. in 1978 as an approach to ensure delivery of essential health care to the world's population (Shestowsky, 1992).

Primary Health Care

Primary health care (PHC) is essential health care made universally accessible to individuals and families in the community by means acceptable to them, through their full participation and at a cost that the community and the country can afford.

SOURCE: World Health Organization, 1978, p. 3.

The Alma-Ata Declaration states that "primary health care is essential health care based on practical, scientifically sound and socially acceptable methods and technology made universally accessible to individuals and families in the community through their full participation and at a cost that the community and country can afford to maintain at every stage of their development" (WHO, 1978, p. 3). The Declaration goes on to say that primary health care is the initial point of contact for individuals and families with the health care system, and the first element of a continuing health process. It is seen as the central function and main focus of the health system, and an integral part of the overall social and economic development of a community (WHO, 1978). Figure 4.1 illustrates the comprehensive nature of primary health care as it is envisioned today.

Shestowsky (1992) explains the principles of primary health care as follows:

1. health services should be equally accessible to all
2. there should be maximum individual and community involvement in the planning and operation of health care services
3. the focus of care should be on prevention and promotion rather than on cure
4. appropriate technology should be used, i.e., methods, procedures, techniques and equipment should be scientifically valid, adapted to local needs and acceptable to users and to those for whom they are used
5. health care is regarded as only part of total health development; other sectors, such as education, housing and nutrition, are all essential for the achievement of well-being.

Examples of PHC Nursing Projects in Canada

- **Newfoundland.** A total of six PHC nurses meet the needs of 8800 people in 21 communities along the 240-km south coast.
- **New Brunswick.** Nursing students from the University of New Brunswick have brought a wide variety of PHC projects to communities across the province. The students assess community needs, then plan, implement and evaluate a PHC project such as a drop-in program at a shopping mall for fitness testing, blood pressure testing and health assessment.

  A clinic that opened in 1993 to serve the 2500 residents of McAdam, N.B., combines a 24-hour emergency facility with a community health clinic. Nurses are the entry point for both the emergency service and a health promotion and disease prevention public health program operated from the clinic, as well as one of five possible entry points for the shared care or community health clinic component.
- **Nova Scotia.** A PHC project with a nurse coordinator is being operated out of Sacred Heart Hospital in Cape Breton. Intended to meet the needs of residents of Cheticamp, a small, isolated Acadian community, it will be run by a community committee.
- **Prince Edward Island.** A Farm Heart Health Project has been established to meet the health needs of farming residents in the west central part of the island. As well, an Active Living Program is being adapted to meet the stated needs of farming residents.
- **Quebec.** The Local Community Services Centres (Centres locaux de services communautaires, or CLSCs) were established in the early 1970s to provide primary health care for residents of communities in the Province of Quebec. They operate with a community board of directors and provide a wide range of health and social welfare services. Nurses in the CLSCs offer walk-in clinics that serve as a point of access to the health care system.
- **Ontario.** Street clinics operate in Toronto, serving the needs of inner-city residents. One example is "Street Health," which we will describe later in this chapter. Another example of a PHC project is the Centretown Community Health Centre in Ottawa.
- **Manitoba.** The storefront, nurse-operated Youville clinic, which is located in an urban shopping mall, has successfully offered PHC services since 1984. A satellite outreach program was opened in 1986 at the Indian/Métis Friendship Centre to meet the specific needs of the aboriginal community where parenting classes, pre- and postnatal programs and individual counselling are among the services offered.
- **Saskatchewan.** An innovative pilot PHC project was announced for the rural community of Eastend in response to an assessment of the health needs of its 600 residents. The project includes a Wellness Centre in which nurses are the key people in programs promoting healthy lifestyles.
- **Alberta.** The Boyle-McCauley Health Centre is an independently operated, inner-city streetfront, walk-in clinic with a community board of directors. The total staff is 17, three of whom are nurses involved in a variety of programs, including maternal and child care, foot care, psychological assessment, alcohol recovery and nutrition.
- **British Columbia.** The nurse at a street clinic in Kamloops is involved in education, screening and some treatment for sexually transmitted diseases, HIV/AIDS, hepatitis B, tuberculosis and other health problems. She also does outreach work at the food bank and needle exchanges, first aid and referral to other services on the street. Street clinics also operate in Vancouver, with nurses in blue jeans providing health care to hard-to-reach "street people," much as the nurse in Kamloops does (Banks & Loftus, 1991).

  The Comox Valley Nursing Centre, located in a house in Courtney, B.C., opened in May 1994. This project was designed to demonstrate and evaluate the effect on the health of individuals, groups and communities when registered nurses are enabled to practise the full scope of their profession. At time of writing, funding from the B.C. Ministry of Health is ongoing. In 1995 funding was obtained as a "closer to home project" for a Substance Abuse Intervention Program (SAIP) in the Comox Valley. This program is staffed by two registered nurses who provide a seven-day-a-week mobile program that has two goals: education and clinical intervention (Andron, Greene & Ingram, 1998).
- **Northwest Territories.** Aboriginal people serve as members of regional health boards and as community health representatives (front-line workers in First Nations communities) working with nurses in community health promotion, disease prevention, community development and related activities. The 43 outpost nursing stations operate on the PHC model.
- **Yukon.** Community health nurses provide primary health care to all residents outside Whitehorse. The Kwanlin Dun First Nation in Whitehorse opened its own health clinic in 1990 using a PHC model. It employs one nurse and two First Nations community health representatives and offers various programs geared to the needs of the local community.

SOURCES: "Primary health care has arrived," 1992; St. Michael, 1993; "Nurses prove themselves," 1994; RNABC, 1994.

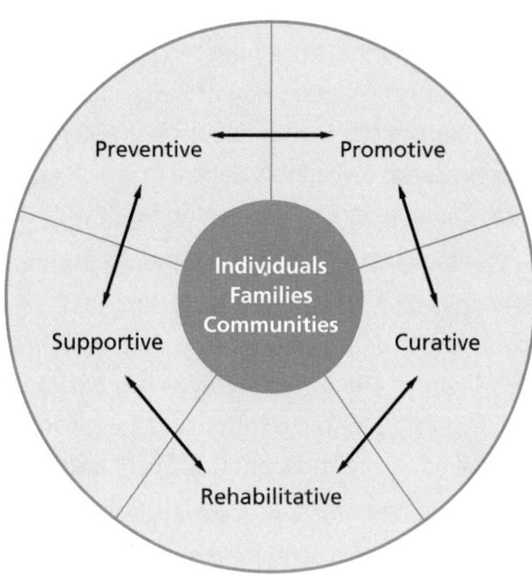

FIGURE 4.1 Primary health care: Comprehensive health services (essential health services)

SOURCE: Association of Registered Nurses of Newfoundland, 1990.

If these principles sound familiar to you, they should. They are the same basic tenets enunciated in the Epp Report (1986), in *Nurturing Health* (Government of Ontario, 1993a) and in all the health reform policy papers developed in various provinces. You will remember that WHO recommended the "healthy people" vision of the Alma-Ata Conference be implemented by all member nations. We noted, in Chapter 2, that the ways and means to do this in Canada became clear with the two reports on the health status of Canadians—The National Health Survey (1977–1979) and the Health Promotion Survey (1985). The strategies and mechanisms to implement the approach were set out in the Epp Report, *Achieving Health for All: A Framework for Health Promotion* (1986), which we will discuss further in this chapter.

Implications of Primary Health Care for Nursing

Dr. Halfdan Mahler, the Director-General of WHO at the time of the Alma-Ata Declaration, foresaw an important role for nurses in the implementation of primary health care and he challenged them to "lead the way." Because they work so closely with people, nurses, according to Mahler, are the key to acceptance and expansion of primary health care. Mahler envisioned nurses becoming resources to people rather than assistants to physicians (Mahler, 1985).

In many countries of the world, nurses are, indeed, leading the way. They are the ones out in the villages working with the people. Fiji is a country that has won awards for its PHC projects in various communities. Nurses staff the outpost nursing stations and health centres on the remote islands that make up the South Pacific country of Vanuatu (formerly the New Hebrides). Guyana had "sick nurse dispensers" (nurses with additional training in pharmacy) providing PHC services for people living in the jungles of that South American country long before the term "primary health care" was used. In Suriname, outpost nursing stations dot the hinterland. Nurses in these stations provide essential health care for the people of several villages — descendants of runaway slaves who re-established their African communities in the interior of the former Dutch colony. Case studies on the new and expanded role of nurses in the delivery of primary health care in Botswana, Colombia, Republic of Korea, Jamaica, Sudan and Thailand are documented in *Health Manpower for Primary Health Care: The Experience of the Nurse Practitioner* (Maglacas, Ulin & Sheps, 1987).

In Canada, medical services nurses in the North have been providing PHC services for First Nations people since the 1950s. Now, these services are being transferred to the communities themselves, in keeping with the philosophy of primary health care as it is being extolled today and, also, with the movement to self-government by First Nations' populations. There are numerous examples of nursing projects in primary health care across Canada. We mentioned some of these in Chapter 3, in connection with innovative health care programs in the various provinces.

The Five Basic Principles of Primary Health Care

- accessibility
- public participation
- promotion of health and prevention of illness
- intersectoral cooperation
- appropriate technologies.

SOURCE: "Making primary health care work for Canadians," 1992, p. 1.

Implementing the Philosophy: The Epp Framework for Health Promotion

In Chapter 2, we talked about the Epp Framework for Health Promotion (1986) as a landmark document signalling a major shift in our thinking about health and health care. We also said that this framework outlined the ways and means for implementing the new vision of health. We will examine the framework in more detail now because it is the basis on which health care services in Canada are being restructured. Figure 4.2 illustrates the Epp Framework for Health Promotion.

Epp saw three major health challenges facing Canadians today:

- to reduce inequities between high- and low-income groups in our society

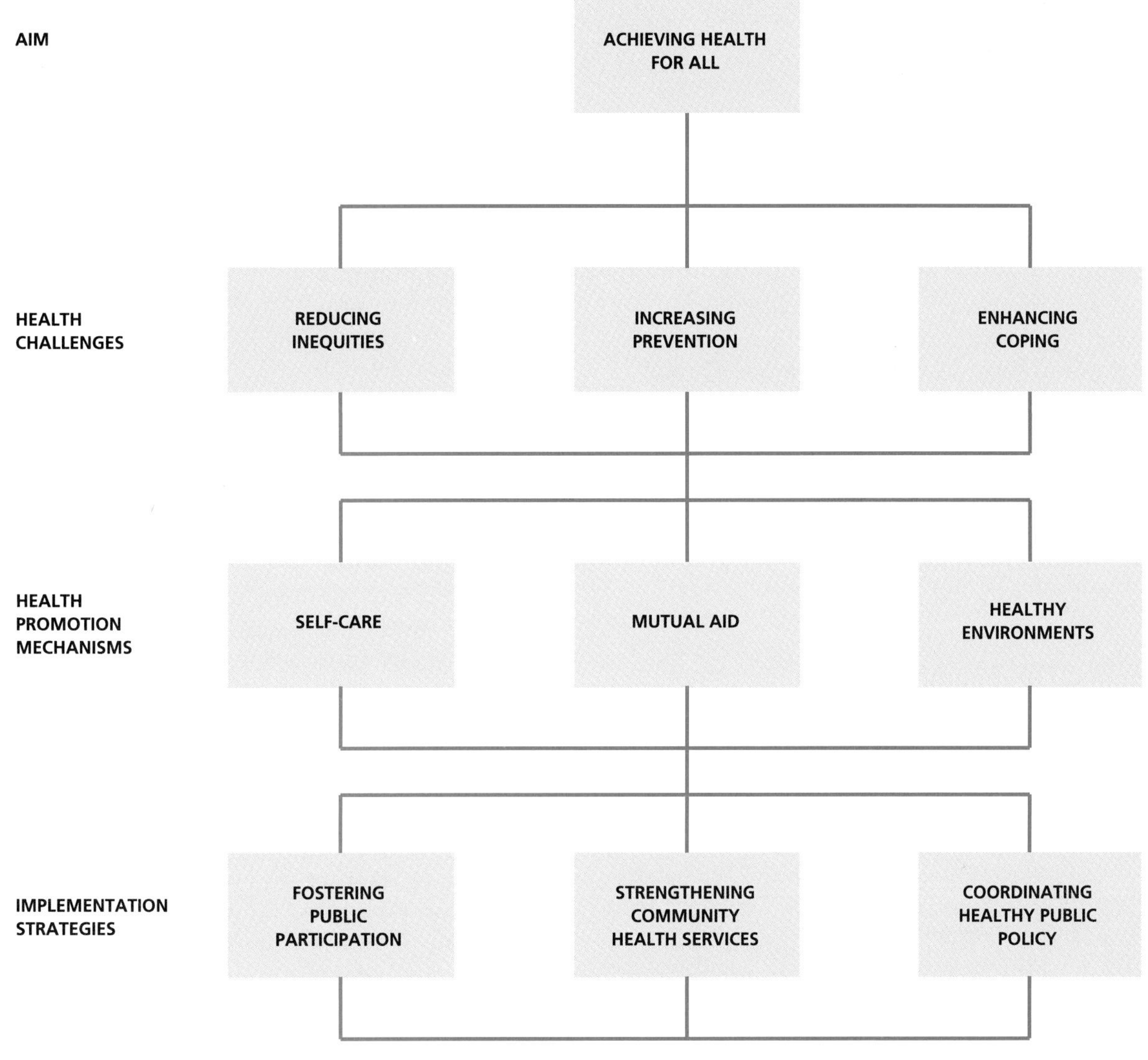

FIGURE 4.2 The Epp Framework for Health Promotion

SOURCE: Epp, 1986.

- to increase efforts towards prevention
- to enhance people's capacity to cope.

The Epp Report suggests a way of addressing these challenges through an expansion of traditional health promotion strategies and mechanisms to complement and strengthen the existing system of care. **Health promotion**, used in this context, is defined by the World Health Organization as "the process of enabling people to increase control over, and to improve, their health" (WHO, 1984). In other words, it is helping people to help themselves to gain better health—for example, helping a group of older adults to organize a tai chi program to improve their physical health, or helping a community to mobilize its resources to build and staff a centre for teenagers (Government of British Columbia, 1992).

The focus in health promotion has shifted, then, from promoting the health of the individual to helping communities to create environments to promote health (RNABC, 1990).

The Epp Report suggests three mechanisms as intrinsic to health promotion:

1. self-care—the decisions and actions taken by individuals in the interest of their own health; for example, the decision you make to join a fitness class or the choices you make in the foods you eat
2. mutual aid—the actions people take to help each other; for example, in Alberta, a group of older adults runs a program called Food for Life, designed to improve their nutritional status. The program includes Smart Shoppers' Tours to help people select the best nutritional food value for their dollar and a Nutritious

Meal Program organized by volunteers but prepared, served and hosted by a group of older adults (Du Gas & Beckingham, 1993)

3. the creation of healthy environments—communities and regions working together to create environments that are conducive to health. Activities may be as diverse as working with people in the community on a cleanup campaign to get rid of litter on the streets; ensuring that policies and practices are in place to encourage mothers of young children to participate in fitness programs, through the availability of child care, for example; or lobbying for legislation to enforce stricter standards for food handlers (Government of British Columbia, 1992).

Three strategies to provide direction for promoting the health of Canadians are suggested in the Epp Report:

- fostering public participation
- strengthening community health services
- coordinating healthy public policy.

FOSTERING PUBLIC PARTICIPATION

Helping people to take control over the factors that influence their health is an essential component of all the provincial health care reform packages discussed in Chapter 3. We mentioned there the regional and community health boards that are being established to decentralize and, hopefully, de-bureaucratize the system by putting the responsibility for and management of health services into the hands of people in the community.

The concept of empowering people to help themselves is illustrated in the description by Labonte (1987, 1989) of the experience of a group of young single mothers in a large Toronto housing project. The group decided to tackle the problem of healthful food and nutrition and determined that they had a problem getting nutritious food for their families because of a lack of control. Prices were too high in the local stores, there were no greengrocers in the neighbourhood, rents were excessive and welfare payments insufficient to cover rent and nutritious food. The group developed its own objectives, which included a community garden, community dinners, pick-your-own farm trips and a food co-op feasibility study. The project was so successful that it was expanded to other housing projects. One goal of the expanded project is to increase the political strength of low-income groups so that they can lobby for policies to reduce hunger and end their dependence on foodbanks.

In Chapter 11, we will look at the "Healthy Communities" concept and some of the projects that have been going on across the country in the past few years. These projects provide excellent examples of public participation in health care. One example is the case of Granisle, British Columbia. The community was coping with the threat of closure of the mine that provided its economic base, and was concerned about the effect of these tensions on their young people. The community worked to establish the Granisle Youth Centre so that they could have a place to call their own (Government of British Columbia, 1992). During the 1980s, the VON initiated a number of community development projects in Ontario to promote elders' participation in determining their own needs and developing programs to meet these needs. The project, given the acronym PEP

Principles of Health Promotion

1. Health promotion involves the population as a whole in the context of everyday life rather than focussing on people at risk for specific diseases. This principle is the foundation of many public health programs, such as maternal and child health programs.
2. Health promotion is directed at the determinants of health, such as poverty and environment.
3. Health promotion combines diverse but complementary approaches including communication, education, legislation, fiscal measures, organizational change, community development and spontaneous local activities against health hazards.
4. Health promotion aims particularly at effective public participation with a view to having individuals take greater responsibility for their health and to empowering communities to take greater responsibility for and control over those things that affect health.
5. Health professionals have an important role in nurturing and enabling health promotion. This means that health professionals will work beyond the normal patient–provider relationship and participate in a more diverse range of activities.

SOURCE: WHO, cited in RNABC, 1990, p. 3.

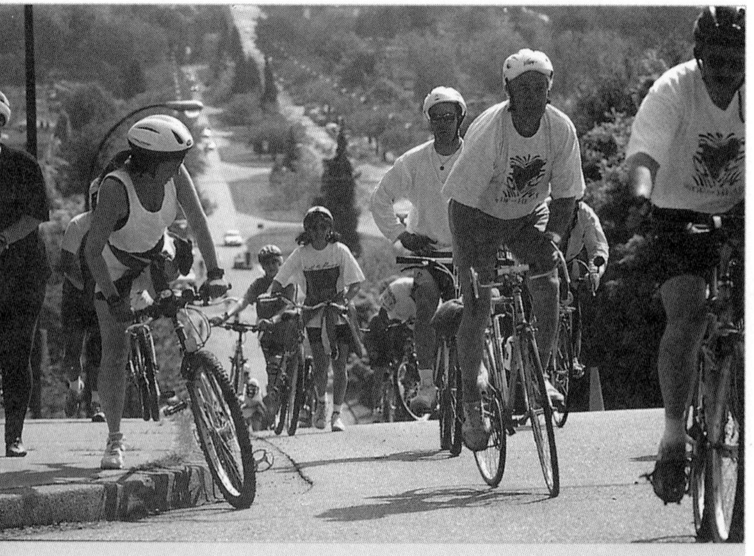

Individuals participating in an organized bike-a-thon.

(Promoting Elders' Participation), was targeted particularly at rural and underserviced areas. Programs developed included a drop-in centre for seniors, Meals-on-Wheels, a grief reaction support group, Friendly Visitors, Handy Helpers, sitters for family relief, evening entertainment, volunteers for the rest home and a transportation network (VON, 1988).

STRENGTHENING COMMUNITY HEALTH SERVICES

The major shift in health care towards a health promotion and health protection orientation requires that more resources—funds and people—are allocated to community health services. For example, a four-million-dollar initiative was launched in Victoria, British Columbia, to improve the health of residents, particularly the elderly, living in the Capital Regional District. Programs that have ensued include a series of seniors' wellness centres, an expanded Quick Response Team to prevent hospitalization of the elderly and programs to support family caregivers (RNABC, 1990).

The strengthening of community services means providing more services for disadvantaged groups and taking more responsibility for planning and directing the community's own health care. It also implies greater intersectoral cooperation as communities work on fostering self-care, mutual aid and the creation of healthy environments. Such cooperation may include health and social services personnel working together with the business sector and with the police, fire and other departments in community projects (for example, neighbourhood police stations) to promote health and protect people (Epp, 1986; Government of British Columbia, 1991; Government of Ontario, 1993a).

COORDINATING HEALTHY PUBLIC POLICY

As we discussed in Chapter 3, Canadians have become aware of the need for assessing the health impact of policy decisions made in all sectors of the economy. Epp suggests that "all policies—and hence all sectors—have a bearing on health" (1986, p. 10) and he further states that all policies that bear directly on health should be coordinated. This includes a long list of policies in different sectors of our society, such as income security, employment, education, housing, business, agriculture, transportation, justice and technology. Policies in the agriculture sector—for example, on pesticides—have a direct bearing on the health not only of agriculture workers who apply the pesticides but also of people who eat the sprayed fruit and vegetables.

The Overall Structure of Health Services

In Canada, as in all democratic societies, individuals are considered to be responsible for their own health and welfare. Primary support for both health and welfare comes from family and friends, who care for and support you when you are ill. Backup is provided by religious and voluntary organizations and by municipalities through their community services. Over and above these layers protecting our health and welfare, we have the provincial and federal governments. The provincial governments have primary responsibility for providing health and welfare services. However, the federal government has considerable influence through legislation and its sharing of the costs of health care services (Health & Welfare Canada, 1989). Figure 4.3 outlines the major responsibilities of the federal, provincial and municipal layers of government and of the voluntary sector in health and welfare in Canada.

Health and Welfare in the Home

Role of Family and Friends

We cannot overemphasize the role of family and friends in helping one another to promote and maintain health and to care for those who are ill. *Nurturing Health*, the summary report of the Premier's Council on Health, Well-being and Social Justice in Ontario, suggests the following ways families and friends influence health:

- provide the basic prerequisites of health (housing, food, etc.)
- look after family members who are ill (90% of informal health care is provided in the home)
- provide mental, physical and emotional support in times of distress
- protect other family members (for example, buckle up a child's seat belt)
- provide love and respect
- support individual members in lifestyle changes (Government of Ontario, 1993a).

Home Care Services

Anderson (1990) states that the current emphasis on home care and self-care is consistent with the ideology in Western culture that people should be self-reliant and productive members of society. Indeed, the care of people at home when they were ill was the usual method of care and the principal area of practice for graduate nurses in Canada until the Depression years of the 1930s, when people could not afford the services of nurses at home and went to hospitals for care (CNA, 1968).

During World War II, graduate nurses left the hospitals to join the armed services, and hospitals were staffed mainly with student nurses. After the war, when hospitals again had a full complement of graduate nurses and rapid advances were being made in medical and surgical treatment, the

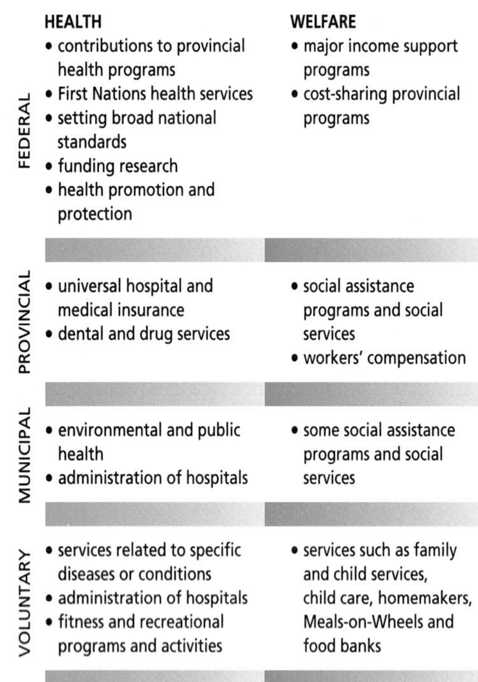

HEALTH
WELFARE
FEDERAL
• contributions to provincial health programs
• First Nations health services
• setting broad national standards
• funding research
• health promotion and protection
• major income support programs
• cost-sharing provincial programs
PROVINCIAL
• universal hospital and medical insurance
• dental and drug services
• social assistance programs and social services
• workers' compensation
MUNICIPAL
• environmental and public health
• administration of hospitals
• some social assistance programs and social services
VOLUNTARY
• services related to specific diseases or conditions
• administration of hospitals
• fitness and recreational programs and activities
• services such as family and child services, child care, homemakers, Meals-on-Wheels and food banks

FIGURE 4.3 Distribution of major responsibilities for health and welfare

SOURCE: Health & Welfare Canada, 1989. p. 11.

hospital was seen as the best place for care. The introduction of health insurance supported this view. Provincial insurance plans covered the costs of hospital care and care in physicians' offices, but not home care.

The present return to home care is due to a number of factors. First, there is a trend towards making care less impersonal and more humanistic—patients have more control at home over the care they receive and they are able to enjoy a better quality of life with family and friends. Second, the cost of hospital care has escalated rapidly over the years, and it is now considered less expensive to look after people at home. Finally, home care is becoming a part of essential health services covered by health insurance programs in most provinces and territories (Sutherland & Fulton, 1988).

Home care services usually include nursing, personal care and homemaker services, respite care and family relief.

NURSING SERVICES Services may be provided by a registered nurse (RN), or a licensed practical nurse (LPN) (Registered Practical Nurse in Ontario), depending on the level of service required. Virtually the whole range of nursing services can be provided in the home except those requiring equipment or services available only in a hospital. Thus, home nursing care may include health promotion as well as such diverse nursing interventions as intravenous therapy, dressings, catheterization, enemas, administration (and control) of medications, nursing care for mothers and infants, postoperative care for early discharge patients or palliative care for the terminally ill.

PERSONAL CARE AND HOMEMAKER SERVICES A wide range of care assistance is available, ranging from light housekeeping and meal preparation to personal care. Personal care includes assistance with bathing, grooming, dressing, walking, eating, oral medications, maintenance of dentures and glasses, and care of feet and nails. Depending on the level required, a homemaker, nurse's aide or health care aide may perform these services.

RESPITE CARE AND FAMILY RELIEF Staff will come into the home to provide care and give relief to family caregivers. Some hospitals and other agencies provide adult day care, and some agencies provide inpatient respite beds.

Home care services may also include one or more of the services listed below.

1. household maintenance services, such as meal delivery, shopping, snow shovelling and heating (furnace) maintenance
2. health maintenance services, such as nutrition counselling, physiotherapy, occupational therapy, podiatry (care of the feet), health teaching and speech therapy
3. health support services, including diagnostic services, transportation services, home equipment services, wheelchair and prosthetic appliance services
4. individual and family social services, such as the provision of information about services and benefits available, counselling and referral as well as financial, employment and volunteer opportunity services
5. community liaison services, such as educational services for school-age children, library services, visiting services, telephone assurance and telecheck services, child care, programs in seniors' centres and recreational activities (Sutherland & Fulton, 1988).

SOURCES OF CARE IN THE HOME

In Canada, home care programs are major providers of care. A number of agencies and services may provide these programs:

1. provincial, metropolitan and regional community (public) health agencies. Manitoba, for example, has a province-wide home care program operated by the provincial government; so does British Columbia, except for the metropolitan areas of Vancouver and Victoria, where home care services are provided by Regional Health Boards. In Ottawa, home care services are provided through the Ottawa– Carleton Regional Health Department
2. voluntary agencies such as the Victorian Order of Nurses, the Arthritis Society, the Canadian Red Cross Society, the Greater Vancouver Mental Health Service
3. private agencies such as ComCare, Paramed and others. Often, the services of private agencies like ComCare are contracted by government agencies to provide services

4. Community Health Centres. In the Province of Quebec, home care is carried out by staff of the CLSCs. However, in some communities it has become a separate program
5. extramural hospitals. In New Brunswick, under the Extramural Hospital Program, home care services are provided by hospital personnel (Sutherland & Fulton, 1988).

ISSUES IN HOME CARE

A wide range of services are available to assist with the care of people at home, yet there are differences in the utilization of these services by different groups in our society. Studies conducted in Great Britain showed that inequalities in health continued to exist, even after 15 years of the National Health Service. It was clear that people in higher-income groups knew how to access the system better and made better use of it than people in lower-income groups (Grant, 1988). Both the Epp Report (1986) and the Ontario document, *Nurturing Health* (1993a), point out the need to redress similar health inequities that exist in Canadian society.

Anderson (1990), reporting on research studies conducted to address policy issues in home care management and self-care, states that, despite the services available, the burden of care—that is, the ongoing monitoring and management of illness—still rests with families. She notes that new Canadians often find caring for ill family members particularly difficult for several reasons. For example, there is a dearth of services to help families who do not speak English. Often, they are not aware of the services that are available. Many newcomers struggle to survive in their new environment. This often requires that both parents in a family work, leaving no one at home to care for an ill child or an aged parent.

Roberts (1988), in reviewing the literature on social supports/networks and help-seeking, suggests that the social network (of family, friends and trusted others) is an important influence on the process of seeking help for health-related problems. She further states that nurses in their day-to-day practice can and do provide the support needed to encourage people to utilize available services.

Role of Voluntary and Religious Agencies

Voluntary agencies are established by the people in a community in response to a particular need. They are usually supported by donations, and the services they provide supplement or augment the functions performed by official agencies. In many instances, new services are pioneered by voluntary agencies and later taken over by government agencies. For example, the Victorian Order of Nurses, a voluntary agency established in 1898 to provide home nursing services in Canada, pioneered a number of home care programs that have subsequently been taken over by provincial and/or municipal government services (Du Gas & Beckingham, 1993).

Voluntary agencies usually provide services of a specific nature. They may be concerned with the preventive, curative and rehabilitative aspects of one disease, for example, provincial Heart and Stroke Foundations, the Canadian Liver Foundation and the Greater Vancouver Mental Health Service. Some voluntary agencies confine their attention to a particular segment of the population, such as the Volunteers for Seniors in Continuing Care, or the Shriners, who operate hospitals for children. Dedicated volunteers have set up shelters for battered women in numerous communities. Volunteers also provide food, shelter and clothing in times of crisis for families in need—not only to battered women but, also, to the old and the young who are homeless.

Voluntary agencies also play a large role in the support of fitness and recreation programs. Many agencies today are concerned about environmental health hazards, spearheading movements to reduce pollution, to protect our waterways and to preserve our wildlife habitats. Voluntary agencies may develop at the local, provincial or national level. In Canada the major visiting nurse service has until recently been the Victorian Order of Nurses, a national voluntary agency. These services have been taken over in some provinces by government agencies, and the VON has moved on to develop other innovative programs, such as foot care clinics and day care centres for the **frail elderly** (people who require nursing care or supervision). The role played by volunteers and by voluntary agencies in health and welfare in Canada is a very large one, and we will be discussing it further later in this chapter.

Religious organizations have played a large role in the development of health and welfare services in Canada from the time of the early French settlers. They continue to play a very large role, for example, in the Grace Hospitals run by the Salvation Army in most large cities in Canada, and the hospitals run by orders of the Roman Catholic Church and other denominations. A large number of the hospitals formerly operated by religious groups are now under secular management. Most religious denominations, however, support and many operate, a variety of services in their communities. The basements of many churches are used for daycare centres for pre-schoolers and after-school care for older children. In inner-city neighbourhoods, religious organizations often provide shelter for the homeless at night. Religious groups work with alcoholics and provide meals for the hungry. In Vancouver, the Anglican Church helped to get a rehabilitation program started for "street kids," training and giving them practical experience in staffing and managing a restaurant that is open to the public five days a week.

Community Health Services

Community health services are much more difficult to fit into neat categories than are hospital and other inpatient services. They are delivered in "homes, offices, clinics, the street, shopping centres, schools, workplaces, jails and recreation sites" (Sutherland & Fulton, 1988, p. 219). Community health services need to work closely with other social networks in the community. These other social networks may include those involved with housing, urban planning, recreation, protective services and education.

Official Community Health Agencies

The local governmental agency responsible for community health services is usually a municipal or regional health board. Outside large cities, the local governmental agency may be operated directly by a unit of the provincial health ministry. Other branches of a local government (for example, a school board) may also provide health services. Some municipalities and provincial governments also administer social assistance programs and provide social services. The health board of a municipality or a region usually develops its own health program, based on the needs of the people in the community and the resources available to meet those needs. The general community program usually includes the control of communicable diseases, a number of environmentally related health protection measures and a health promotion program. Many communities also provide other services.

Local governmental community health agencies also put great emphasis on health promotion. Traditionally, this has involved health education and such services as prenatal, postnatal and well-baby clinics for mothers and infants, school health programs, and wellness centres for older adults. The health promotion role now encompasses community development and empowering people to assume more control over their own health services. We will discuss this concept in more detail in Chapter 11.

Environmentally Related Health Protection Measures Carried Out by Local Official Community Health Agencies

- examination of selected aspects of air and water quality
- testing of rural water and sewage systems
- food testing
- inspection of restaurants and other eating places and food premises
- control of insects and animals
- maintenance of cleanliness of public beaches and swimming pools
- inspection of public and residential buildings and spaces.

SOURCE: Sutherland & Fulton, 1988.

LOOKING back — Georgina Fane Pope, 1862–1938

Georgina Fane Pope, first matron of the Canadian Army Medical Corps, was also Canada's first recipient of the Royal Red Cross. The award, for conspicuous service in the field, was awarded in 1903 by the British Government for her outstanding work as a nursing sister in South Africa during the Boer War.

Cicely Jane Georgina Fane Pope was born in Charlottetown in 1862 to one of Prince Edward Island's most prominent families. Her father, W.H. Pope, was Colonial Secretary and became a Father of Confederation when Canada was formed in 1867. Georgina Pope trained as a nurse at Bellevue Hospital in New York, graduated in 1886, and worked in the United States for several years. During the Boer War, she was one of four nursing sisters who accompanied the first Canadian volunteer force to South Africa in 1899. The Canadian nurses served with great distinction in several locations at or near the front lines. In December 1900, after more than a year in South Africa, Sister Pope nursed the wounded on a troop ship returning to Canada. When fighting resumed in 1902, she returned once more with another band of nursing sisters and another contingent of troops.

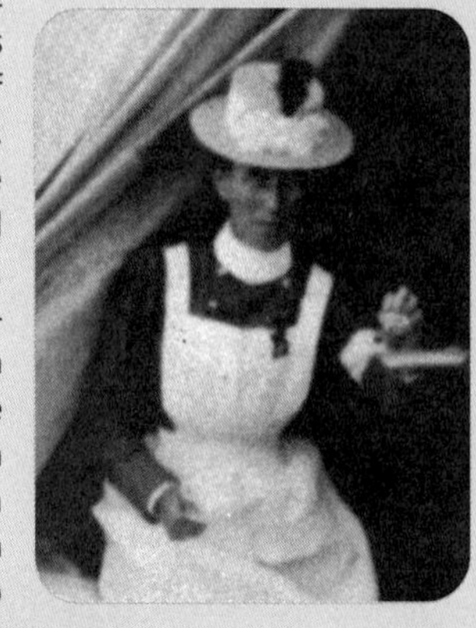

Following the war, reorganization of the Canadian services was announced, first with a reserve unit of 25 nursing sisters, and then in 1906 with a permanent military nursing service. Nursing Sister Pope was selected from the reserves for this permanent group and in 1908 was named the first matron of the Canadian Army Medical Corps. In World War I, Matron Pope (age 52) went overseas with the first group of nurses and served in Canadian army hospitals in the United Kingdom. In December 1917 she went with the No. 8 Canadian Hospital to France, where she fell ill and had to be invalided home. Despite a pensionable disability, Georgina Pope lived to age 76, died in her beloved PEI and was buried with full military honours.

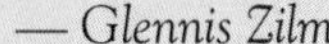

Many official agencies at the local level also provide a number of specialized health services in addition to the general community programs. These services frequently include maternal and child care services, immunization clinics and, often, diagnostic, treatment and rehabilitative services for people on low incomes. Some municipalities also operate hospitals and other inpatient services for people who are ill or who need long-term care.

Community Health Centres

Community health centres (CHCs) provide primary health care services in an ambulatory setting. The common features of CHCs are shown in the box below.

Common Features of Community Health Centres

- emphasize health promotion
- are community oriented
- offer a broad range of services
- are multidisciplinary
- do not rely on fee-for-service payments as primary source of income.

A number of different models have developed in Canada over the past 30 years. These include those designated as CHCs: health services organizations (HSOs) and comprehensive health organizations (CHOs), Health and Human Resources Centres (in British Columbia), Local Community Services Centres (CLSCs—in Quebec), multiservice centres, hospital-affiliated centres and physician-based centres. Most are funded by provincial governments and operate on a global budget—one that includes all services and salaries. Exceptions are the physician-based clinics you might find in local neighbourhoods (sometimes in shopping malls) that offer walk-in and after-hours services.

Because most CHCs do not depend on fee-for-service as the major source of income, they can utilize the talents of nurses, social workers and whomever is best suited to do the work to achieve an integrated approach to assessment, care planning and service delivery. Most centres have a fairly extensive health team comprising registered nurses, community health nurses, nurse practitioners and social workers as well as physicians. The larger centres may have nutritionists, physiotherapists and occupational therapists, psychologists, mental health therapists and counsellors, pharmacists, health educators, optometrists, podiatrists or chiropodists, community developers, health records analysts and chiropractors (Sutherland & Fulton, 1988).

MULTISERVICE AGENCIES

As provincial governments begin restructuring their health services, CHCs are being considered as a viable option for providing care that is convenient and comprehensive, and allows greater consumer participation and control of services. In Ontario, intersectoral cooperation between the Ministry of Health, the Ministry of Community and Social Services and the Ministry of Citizenship has resulted in the development of **multiservice agencies (MSAs)** to provide coordinated services for the following three groups:

1. adults with physical disabilities
2. elderly persons who need long-term care and support services
3. people of any age who require health services at home or at school, for example, people who need care at home after being hospitalized, those needing longer-term personal care at home and children who need professional health services to go to school.

The MSAs will serve as the single entry point (point at which an individual enters the health care system) for people needing long-term care services at home or in the community. The range of services to be delivered by MSAs includes visiting nurses, supportive housing, homemaking, friendly visiting, security programs, physiotherapy, nutrition counselling, meal programs and transportation as well as palliative care either at home or in the community. Care will be coordinated with other services such as hospitals (Government of Ontario, 1993b).

HEALTH MAINTENANCE ORGANIZATIONS (U.S.)

The **health maintenance organizations (HMOs)** in the United States are essentially a form of prepaid group practice. They provide a comprehensive range of services on a fixed contract basis, which is paid for in advance by people enrolling in the organization. The emphasis in the HMOs, as in the Canadian CHCs, is on health promotion and protection. The range of services provided by HMOs covers both preventive and curative care and includes physician services, health counselling, inpatient and outpatient hospital services, and diagnostic and therapeutic services, including home care. Many nurses are employed in HMOs, including nurse practitioners in various fields, including midwifery (Frankel, Speechley & Wade, 1996).

STREET CLINICS

Street clinics, known also as "storefront" or "free" clinics, developed in the 1960s and 1970s in both Canada and the United States. Set up in poor or ghetto neighbourhoods, they provide services for the homeless, "street kids," alcoholics, prostitutes and drug addicts who are reluctant to use traditional agencies. The clinics offer readily accessible care, usually on a 24-hour free basis in a setting that is as devoid of "red tape" as possible. In the beginning, the clinics were staffed mainly by volunteers, but many of these clinics are now operated by official or other types of community health agencies. An example is Street Health, a community-based nursing organization in Toronto, currently operating four nursing stations in various drop-in centres and shelters for women and men who are homeless or underhoused. In order to document both the health problems and the barriers to services encountered by their patients in traditional health agencies, a comprehensive, rigorously executed research study was undertaken by Street Health. Findings of the study point to inadequacies in both the health and social services systems, providing the nurses with hard, reliable data that can be used to lobby for policy changes to improve the situation for the people they serve (Crowe & Hardill, 1993).

In Vancouver, an alternative approach to primary health services is offered at the Portland Hotel, which is home to many of the residents of the downtown east side. These residents experience such health problems as substance, physical and psychological abuse; poverty; mental health concerns; hepatitis; tuberculosis; and HIV and AIDS. Two home care nurses and one physician make twice-weekly visits to the hotel to provide primary care. The success of this approach has seen improved outcomes with wound healing, along with reduced emergency admissions. Because of the positive response, other services have been considered, such as primary health services to street-involved women (Griffiths, 1996).

MENTAL HEALTH CENTRES AND OTHER COMMUNITY MENTAL HEALTH SERVICES

Mental health services have undergone tremendous change since World War II in Canada and elsewhere in the Western world. Most of the large asylums have been closed, the patients discharged and the care of people with mental illness transferred to the community. There has been a large and rapid increase in the number of psychiatric units within general hospitals, and a network of community-based services, such as mental health clinics, has developed. The hospital-based services provide treatment for the acutely ill under the care of psychiatrists. Community-based services are dominated by non-physician health professionals, such as psychologists, social workers and nurses (Dickinson & André, 1988). The types of services offered include the following treatments and supports:

- screening and referral
- assessment, diagnosis and treatment
- medication
- individual, couple, group and family therapy
- coordination of services
- rehabilitation services in self-care, leisure and work-related areas
- emergency services
- residential care.

Concerns have been expressed in Ontario, British Columbia and other provinces that there are many gaps in the services provided for the mentally ill. Wickens (1998) states that, often, individuals with a mental illness are discharged from the hospital prematurely. As a result, these individuals receive little or no follow-up health care. Some individuals, who become unstable, commit crimes and end up within the criminal justice system rather than receiving appropriate treatment. Most provinces are currently looking into this issue, with a view to providing individuals with more mental health care support in the community.

PHYSICIANS' OFFICES

A great deal of ambulatory care is provided in physicians' offices. The majority of physicians in Canada are in private practice. They are reimbursed for their services on a fee-for-service basis by provincial or territorial government medical insurance programs. Physicians may work in either solo or group practice; the latter is becoming more common. In group practice, several physicians work together to provide more comprehensive care for individuals and families. For example, there may be one or two family practitioners in the group, an obstetrician, a pediatrician and a surgeon. Frequently, there is also a psychiatrist, and there may be other specialists as well. A large number of nurses are employed in physicians' offices.

HOSPITAL AMBULATORY SERVICES/ OUTPATIENT DEPARTMENTS

Five to 10 percent of ambulatory health care is provided by hospitals (Sutherland & Fulton, 1988). The many services performed in emergency departments and outpatient departments have led to the latter being renamed "ambulatory care departments" in many institutions. These departments provide diagnostic, screening and treatment services, and often rehabilitative services. Many hospitals offer day programs for specific groups, such as those for seniors who are being cared for at home when caregivers need to work or have other commitments. They are also providing such services as one-day surgery and pre-admission clinics so that patients do not have to be admitted one or two days before surgery but can be admitted on the day of their surgery (LeNoble, 1993).

EMERGENCY SERVICES

We have become increasingly conscious in the past few years of the need for highly skilled personnel to deal with medical emergency situations in the community. Most large hospitals, and many small community hospitals, have well-staffed, well-equipped emergency rooms that are open 24 hours a day. Accidents and sudden attacks of illness may occur at any time and in any place. The first few minutes of care that individuals receive are often crucial to their survival and subsequent recovery.

All provinces must provide ambulance services under their health insurance programs. In most provinces, the services are subsidized, so people pay only a small fee; in some, there is no charge. Ambulance drivers are being trained in emergency measures to provide initial treatment and in life support measures for people who have suffered an acute attack until they can be treated in an acute care agency. Regrettably, not all ambulance drivers are fully trained as yet, particularly in rural areas.

Inpatient Services

Hospitals, which began to flourish in the latter part of the last century, continue to dominate the health care scene. Despite the rapid de-institutionalization of services currently in progress, it is likely that there will always be people who are best cared for in a hospital or other inpatient facility. Those who require major surgery and those who need intensive care or recovery-room services, for example, need to be in a facility that has high-technology equipment and teams of specialized personnel to provide skilled care. People whose aggressive behaviour threatens their own or others' safety also need the supervision available in an inpatient facility. The list of those who cannot be cared for in the community grows shorter, however, as alternative treatment delivery modes replace the dependence on hospital care for many people with health problems (Sutherland & Fulton, 1988).

Historically, older adults have utilized most hospital services and, as this segment of the population increases, it can be argued that the demand for hospital services will also increase. In 1984, 51 percent of all hospital bed-days in this country were used by the elderly. Projections based on an extrapolation of current trends anticipate that it will be 74 percent by 2036, with a corresponding demand for more hospital beds (Hamilton & Trepanier, 1989). There are some indications, however, that the anticipated future demand for hospital beds may be offset by improvements in the health of people, particularly older adults, and by a reallocation of resources, including both money and people, to community-based services (Trepanna, 1990).

At the present time, in Canada, there are a number of different levels of inpatient services, including community, regional and teaching hospitals, rehabilitation centres, extended- or long-term care facilities and supervised residences. Nurses are the largest component of professional staff in all inpatient services, with the exception of supervised residences, which may have predominantly lay staff, with nursing services provided on a reduced basis. The need for skilled nursing care is often the major reason for admitting an individual to an inpatient facility.

Hospitals

The basic purpose of hospitals is the care of ill and injured people. Hospitals have traditionally performed curative, rehabilitative, preventive and restorative functions, and are also involved in two additional areas of commitment: research and education. Hospitals provide a clinical environment for students in the health disciplines. The hospital's role in research has expanded in recent years, from providing a field of study for health scientists to collaborating with universities and government research teams. Most large hospitals now have a head of nursing research on staff.

Hospitals vary considerably in size. In Canada we have had general hospitals of up to 1600 beds and psychiatric hospitals that housed 4000 or more people. Today, most hospitals are closing beds. Many small communities have had a hospital with 10 to 20 beds, but there is a trend towards making these small hospitals into multiservice community health centres. When affiliated with a medical school, a hospital is designated as a teaching hospital. Examples of teaching hospitals include the Ottawa General Hospital, the Ottawa Civic Hospital and the Children's Hospital of Eastern Ontario, all of which are part of the University of Ottawa Faculty of Health Sciences.

CONTROL AND FINANCING OF HOSPITALS

Every province has a Public Hospitals Act and most also have a Private Hospitals Act. In Canada, most hospitals are nonprofit (public) general hospitals. The few private, for-profit or **proprietary hospitals** are usually small and provide specialized mental health or addiction-related services. In 1991, 57 private, for-profit hospitals were in operation (Tholl, 1994). The Canada Health Act specifies the services that hospitals must provide, although they may offer additional services. The **public general hospitals** vary in their ownership; they may be owned by religious groups, by municipalities, by a provincial government (for example, some hospitals in New Brunswick) or by the federal government (Tholl, 1994).

Provincial and territorial governments have both legal and financial control over public hospitals. The provincial statutes regulate the conduct of hospitals, and provincial hospital insurance provides the funding, usually through a global budget. The government also sets standards for all inpatient facilities, including those that are privately run. However, with the movement towards regionalization of health services, the control and operation of hospitals is being delegated in many instances to Regional Health Boards (Stone, 1997).

Rehabilitation Centres

Rehabilitation is the restoration of an individual who has been ill, from any cause, to the most complete level of social, physical and mental functioning that is possible for him or her. Rehabilitation should not begin when the patient has recovered from the acute phase of illness, nor should it be the responsibility of specialized agencies only. It should begin with the patient's admission to an agency for the care and treatment of an illness. The restoration of the individual to an active, functioning role in society, insofar as this is possible, should be the aim of all who care for that person.

Today, with the increasing prevalence of chronic and degenerative diseases and the vast numbers of people suffering injuries as a result of accidents, there is a growing need for long-term restorative services. For many people injured in accidents or disabled with degenerative disorders, restoration to their optimal level of functioning is a lengthy process that may take years of specialized care. Frequently these people need the help of members of a variety of health disciplines—physicians, nurses, occupational and physiotherapists, clergy, social workers and others—to assist in their rehabilitation. Often, they require facilities such as gymnasiums, swimming pools and outdoor recreation areas, as well as nursing units specially adapted to facilitate increasing independence in the activities of daily living.

In response to the growing need for these types of services, specialized agencies have developed whose primary purpose is rehabilitation, for example, the Rehabilitation Centre that forms part of the Health Sciences Complex in Ottawa and the B.C. Rehabilitation–G.F. Strong Centre in Vancouver.

A rehabilitation centre coordinates the efforts of many disciplines in order to plan an approach designed to meet individual needs. The rehabilitation team meets regularly to discuss the patient's progress and revise the plan to the individual's changing needs. Family and patients may participate in team meetings.

Nurses play a key role in rehabilitation both while the patient is in an acute facility and afterwards, in a rehabilitation unit. When people are acutely ill, good nursing care supports their own resources in all areas of functioning and helps prevent the development of complications that can delay or prevent full recovery. For example, a person with a spinal injury who is paralyzed from the waist down can develop foot drop if adequate preventive measures are not taken during the acute stage of illness. In both the acute care setting and in specialized rehabilitation units, nursing is the one constant in a variety of services needed to restore the individual to an optimal level of health. Nursing is there on a round-the-clock basis, whereas other health professionals come and go, spending varying amounts of time with the patient. It is frequently up to the nurse to ensure that all aspects of the rehabilitation plan for the individual are carried through, and that there is continuity and consistency in the approaches used by all members of staff.

Extended/Long-Term Care Facilities

People with chronic or degenerative diseases and conditions need care over an extended period of time, and therefore need more long-term services. However, most older adults are functioning fully in the community—fewer than eight percent are in residential facilities. Older adults are in good health mentally, physically and socially, according to recent national and provincial health surveys, and are taking better care of themselves than are younger Canadians (Statistics Canada, 1997). The findings of Canada's Health Promotion Study (1985) suggest that "to an even greater extent than among younger Canadians, positive preventive health measures are the norm among the older population" (Health & Welfare Canada, 1987, p. 4).

Most older people consider themselves well even if they have a chronic disease such as arthritis. Such individuals need monitoring to make sure that their arthritis is not interfering with their activities of daily living. There are other groups in the population who also need long-term care, such as children and adults with disabilities and people with long-term mental health problems. All need a continuum of care. An increasing number of services in the community provide skills to allow patients to live outside an institution. At the time of writing, a review of institutional and community mental health services is underway.

The philosophy of residential long-term care has also changed. The "warehousing" of older people in nursing homes and hospitals, where physical needs were looked after but psychosocial needs were neglected, is disappearing. Experts on aging contend that we still have a long way to go to accommodate the needs of today's older population who are "healthier, better educated, more knowledgeable and therefore can be expected both to know their rights and to make them known to the service system" (Seymour, 1991, p. 27).

A philosophy of restorative care for older adults was pioneered by Vera McIver at four extended care hospitals operating in Victoria in the mid-1970s. She introduced a method of care based on the belief that the older adult is still a unique individual, working towards growth and self-fulfillment, and that a therapeutic and restorative environment can be achieved if this attitude is kept in mind (McIver, 1978). The **priory model**, as it has come to be called, has won international acclaim and has formed the philosophic background for gerontological nursing as it has developed in Canada (Mantle, 1992).

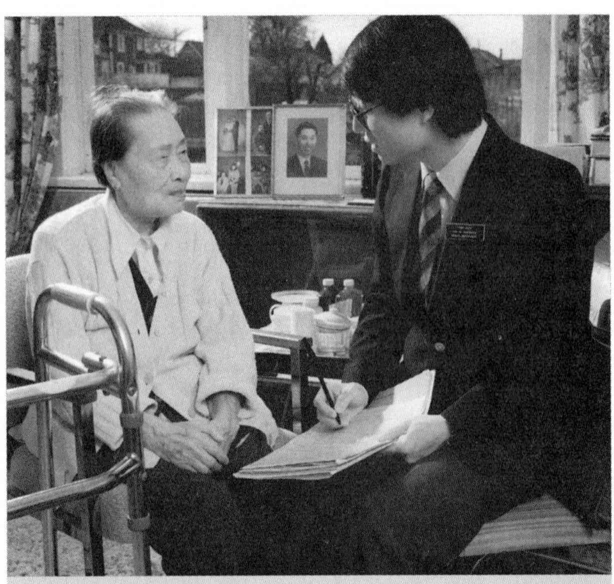

A case manager assessing the long-term care needs of an older patient.

Implementation of the concept of restorative care is not equal across the country, but changes in our thinking about health and health care, as well as an increase in the number of nurses and other health professionals with additional preparation in gerontological nursing, is a positive step forward. The experience of the Queensway–Carleton Hospital in Nepean, Ontario, provides an example of how the concept of restorative care can be put into practice on an extended care unit within an acute care hospital. An interdisciplinary psychosocial approach was used to care for elderly on the unit, which made the resident "the centre of a caring community that fosters individual rights, respect and self-determination" (Carson & Ross, 1993, p. 35).

A variety of new types of residential facilities are developing to meet the progressive needs of people for long-term care. The range of facilities includes:

- communal residences, such as the Abbeyfield residences for small groups of nine to 10 older adults who can look after themselves, but who need the companionship and security of living in a residence
- group homes for the mentally challenged and for disabled adults and children
- senior citizen apartment complexes designed to provide the safety and security measures needed by older people, such as grab bars in the bathroom and emergency call bells
- personal care homes for people who need help with dressing, grooming and other activities of daily living
- nursing homes and extended care units for people who need skilled nursing care
- multilevel facilities such as the Unitarian House (Centre) in Ottawa, which combines single-room and small apartment accommodation for people who are independent and a nursing unit for those needing skilled care, dining room service for those who want it, and kitchen facilities for people who wish to prepare meals or snacks for themselves.

Hospices/Palliative Care

The purpose of both **hospices** and **palliative care units** (the terms are nearly interchangeable) is to care for people who are dying, while enabling them to live as normally and with as much freedom from pain as possible. The terms *palliative care* and *hospice* are used to express both a philosophy of care and an agency for inpatient and home care services. Care is provided so that the dying person can be maintained at home as long as feasible, with nurses, physicians, clergy and social workers on the palliative care team providing the assistance and support required by patients and their families. When it is no longer feasible to maintain dying patients at home, they are transferred to an inpatient facility, where they may move in and out as their condition warrants. (See Chapter 37 for further discussion.)

The Role of Provincial and Territorial Governments

The primary responsibility for administering the National Health Insurance Program in Canada is vested in the provinces. They are the insuring agencies, and they are responsible for all aspects of the delivery of care. This includes setting standards for hospitals and long-term care agencies, negotiating fees and salaries for health professionals and determining the financial resources for hospitals and all other service agencies. Many provinces also have dental plans and programs that eliminate or defray the cost of prescription drugs for senior citizens.

Provincial governments assume a leadership and advisory role for health boards who, for the most part, operate the services. The provincial governments provide many direct services such as the operation of laboratories, the licensure of individuals and agencies, the dissemination of information and the provision of financial assistance. Outside large metropolitan areas, community health services have traditionally been organized and operated by provincial governments in Canada. As we noted in the previous chapter many provinces are in the process of decentralizing. Regional Health Boards and Community Health Councils are assuming increasing responsibility for the management and control of local health services. Provincial governments still operate some hospitals, such as psychiatric facilities (Frankel, et al., 1996).

Workers' Compensation Boards

Each province and territory has its own Workers' Compensation Act, but all are based on the same model. The Canadian model was derived from the German Accident Insurance Act, passed in 1884, which historians tell us was developed by Chancellor Bismarck as a political ploy to keep followers of Karl Marx from being elected to the German parliament. Be that as it may, the results have benefited workers in many countries. Considered the first legislation in social welfare, Workers' Compensation laws are based on the principle that production costs should include the cost of any injuries sustained by workers in the making of a product. These costs should then be incorporated into the selling price—in this way, the consumer bears the cost burden (Eades, 1965).

Although earlier versions were passed in British Columbia (1902), Alberta (1908) and Quebec (1909), it was the Workers' Compensation Act of 1914 in Ontario that provided the present basis for Canadian legislation (Eades, 1965). The legislation was, in effect, a compromise between labour and management, with labour giving up the right to sue an employer for negligence (the right of individuals under common law) in return for receiving benefits regardless of who was at fault. An exception is made where the injury was caused by serious and willful misconduct on the part of the worker, unless the individual is permanently or seriously disabled.

Workers' Compensation Boards (WCBs) in Canada operate under provincial statute, as quasi-governmental agencies. The Boards both collect and dispense funds. Money is collected from employers through an assessment designed to cover the costs involved in a particular industry. The rate of assessment for employers is determined by the Board. Under the scheme, industries are divided into rate groups reflecting industry and/or cost similarities. For example, logging has a higher cost history than does retail sales. Therefore, companies in the lumber industry would be assessed at a higher rate than department stores. The assessment levied on employers in each rate group is intended to cover the cost of health care, income replacement and survivor benefits for workers, including administrative costs and costs for accident prevention* and the rehabilitation of workers.

Most workers in Canada, except the self-employed, are covered by workers' compensation, although agricultural workers are not yet covered in all provinces. Workers' benefits include medical coverage, rehabilitation and income continuity for personal injury, disease or death arising out of and in the course of employment.

In the United States, as in Canada in the provinces, each state has its own Workers' Compensation legislation. The model that developed in the U.S., however, requires employers to be individually liable for providing coverage, as opposed to the Canadian system of collective liability. In some states, this is done through private insuring agencies; in others, the state is the insuring agency; and still others have both private insurance carriers and a State Board (Workers' Compensation Board of British Columbia, 1997).

The Federal Government's Role

The federal government exerts considerable influence over both health and welfare services in Canada through national legislation and through its financial contribution to the programs operated by the provinces. The federal government both funds and operates the national security program, which includes Old Age Pensions, the Canada Pension Plan, the Child Tax Credit and Employment Insurance. It also funds and operates health protection programs.

Through its numerous agencies, the federal government provides advisory and consultative services to provincial health ministries. Another federal responsibility is the maintenance of a national information service about health and social welfare matters. Statistics Canada is the agency with primary responsibility for collecting and disseminating information on a wide variety of topics. The individual ministries also collect and share information with their provincial counterparts across the country—through federal–provincial meetings of Health Ministers and meetings of government nursing consultants; through the publication of papers on different topics; and through news bulletins and journals such as *Canadian Social Trends*.

The federal government's role in research in all aspects of health and social welfare is also significant. The Extramural Research Programs Directorate is responsible for management of the National Health Research and Development Program (NHRDP). This program is the principal source of support for scientific research on national health issues. It also provides support for the development of research protocols and for the training and career development of health researchers. Some of your professors may be career scientists or career scholars whose positions are funded by the NHRDP.

At the direct services level, the federal government is concerned with interprovincial hazards such as pollution, with the control of communicable diseases and with the setting of standards for drug control. The federal government is also directly responsible for the provision of health care services to certain segments of the population such as armed services personnel and their families, war veterans and the members of First Nations populations. Health Canada, through its Medical Services Branch, is currently in the process of transferring the provision of health care services to First Nations people (Health & Welfare Canada, 1989). We will be discussing this move in Chapter 12.

The Private Sector's Role

Although we tend to think of our health care system as being run by the government, the private sector is very much involved in the provision of health and welfare services in Canada. Many of these services, such as homemaker and home nursing services, as well as long-term care, are purchased by governments from private companies. Among the services provided by private companies are pharmaceuticals, home care, homes for the elderly, residential services for the disabled and day care services. The services of many health professionals (such as physicians), also in private practice, are purchased by governments on a fee-for-service basis (Health & Welfare Canada, 1989). A number of hospitals have nonprofit foundations that raise funds for the hospital. This appears to be a growing trend in an effort to increase noncapital funds.

* In some provinces, the Board funds accident prevention directly; in other provinces, it provides the funds to another agency for this purpose.

Providing Services to Multicultural Communities

Families of different ethnic origins are often perceived by service providers as being difficult to reach. They do not respond to traditional services that are in place for most English-speaking communities. For example, health nurses working in the Sunset neighbourhood of Vancouver, B.C., noticed a considerable decline in attendance at their local drop-in program for parents and infants. This group of health professionals recognized that their service needed to be more ethnically relevant for the population they wished to serve. Therefore, they collaborated with other community agencies in an effort to create a program for Punjabi- and Hindi-speaking families.

This new program appears to be extremely successful, and is in the process of formal evaluation. In the meantime, preliminary evaluation has suggested that a successful program must involve multi-agency partnerships and be culturally sensitive to the defined community.

SOURCE: Bhagat, Biring, Pander, Quong & Triolet, 1997.

The People Who Provide the Services

The provision of health care in Canada is estimated to employ between seven and eight percent of the labour force. In many communities, the health care sector is one of the largest employers (Trepanna, 1990). Thirty-one occupational groups of health professionals are listed by Health and Welfare Canada. In 1992, 234 128 were employed as RNs, 83 749 as LPNs/RNAs. If you add nursing orderlies (47 763) to this group, nursing personnel account for the majority of health personnel. The next largest group of health professionals is physicians, whose numbers total 61 649, followed by laboratory technologists (19 367) and pharmacists (18 969). Approximately 27 517 people practise in the dental field, including 14 897 dentists, 10 529 dental hygienists and 2091 dental assistants (Statistics Canada, 1992).

Collaboration—An Essential Component of Nursing Practice

Regardless of where nurses practise, even if they are engaged in independent practice, they work in collaboration with other members of the health team. The health team of today is composed of a variety of personnel representing professional disciplines concerned with the health and welfare of people.

In addition to the traditional health professions of medicine, nursing, dentistry and pharmacy, a number of other, highly specialized positions in health care have developed. Many of the people in these specialties, such as physical and occupational therapists, provide direct care services to patients that are complementary to medical and nursing care. Some are technologists, such as respiratory technologists and renal dialysis (artificial kidney) technicians, whose occupations have evolved because of the need for people with specific skills in handling the complex machinery used in the care of patients. Several of the newer groups have emerged as a result of the delegation of certain functions by the major professionals. These include licensed practical nurses, RNAs (registered nursing assistants), dental hygienists, dental nurses, dental assistants and pharmacy assistants.

The provision of health care today requires a multidisciplinary team approach. In some instances, the team may consist of only three members—the physician, the nurse and the patient; in others, there may be a dozen or more health professionals involved in the care of one individual, a family or a community. All members of the team possess knowledge and skills unique to their discipline, and all contribute their special expertise to the care of the patient. There are also many areas of shared knowledge and skills. Students who have all or part of their educational program in the health sciences division of a community college, or in a university health sciences centre, may find themselves sharing common core courses with students in several other health disciplines. Most of the health professions require that their practitioners have a good foundation in the biophysical and social sciences; frequently, students from several health sciences programs take classes together in such subjects as anatomy, physiology, microbiology, psychology and sociology.

The essence of the collaborative team concept is that all members work cooperatively with the patient—whether an individual, a family or a community. Together, they are able to make a concerted effort towards their common goal of attaining the highest level of health possible for that patient. The nursing team is an integral part of the overall health team; we will discuss the various members of the nursing team in Chapter 5. In the following pages, we will look at other members of the health team with whom the nurse collaborates in community-based and in institution-based health services. We will also discuss the role of volunteers as part of a large and growing group of people working in the health field.

MEMBERS OF THE MEDICAL TEAM

Patients are admitted to a hospital in most instances under the care of their own private physician or a physician on the staff of the agency to which they have been admitted. The physician is usually responsible for directing the diagnostic and therapeutic plan of care for the patient. Most teaching hospitals and their related community agencies also have interns and resident physicians. Interns are recent graduates of medical school who have a planned program of clinical experience in the various services of these agencies in order to complete requirements for licensure as practising physicians. Residents are qualified medical practitioners who are preparing for practice in a medical specialty. If an agency is affiliated with a medical school, there will also be medical students receiving clinical instruction and experience in the various units of the agency. In Canada the numbers of specialist and family practice physicians are almost equal, with the balance slightly in favour of those in family practice.

In the United States (and in some other countries) a **physician's assistant** category of worker has developed. Designated by various titles, such as medex, primex or simply physician's assistant, he or she is usually employed by a physician and performs traditional medical tasks under the supervision of the physician. These may include taking the medical history and undertaking the initial physical examination of a patient, assisting in primary care and monitoring the progress of patients. Many physicians' assistants work in rural areas (where there is a scarcity of doctors) with physicians in solo practice, where they help to extend the range of medical coverage. Many are former military corpsmen; some are nurses; others enter the educational programs for preparation as physicians' assistants without previous experience in the health field. The course of studies, which is usually offered in a university setting in conjunction with a medical school, ranges from one to five years, depending on the individual's previous training and experience in the health field. The physician's assistant category did not develop in Canada.

MEMBERS OF THE HEALTH TEAM INVOLVED PRIMARILY WITH HEALTH PROMOTION

Health educators are responsible for the development of health education programs in the community. A large part of their work is in community development, working with people to identify community health needs and to take action to improve health conditions. The nurse and the health educator collaborate on many health promotion programs. The health educator usually has a baccalaureate or higher degree.

Recreation specialists are also members of the health team concerned with promoting health and physical fitness. Their responsibilities include the development of recreation, sports and physical fitness programs in the community. The recreation specialist is usually a graduate of a baccalaureate program in human kinetics (or recreation).

Nutritionists are on the staff of many community health agencies. They advise people about good dietary habits, counsel them about their nutritional problems and undertake nutrition education programs in the community. The nutritionist has usually had a four- to five-year program of studies at university, followed by a year of internship in various health agencies. The nutritionist who works in a hospital or other institutional setting is called a **dietitian**. The dietitian is usually responsible for planning meal service for patients and staff, supervising other workers in the preparation of food and counselling patients about their nutritional problems.

ENVIRONMENTAL HEALTH WORKERS

Environmental health workers have as their primary concern the improvement, control and management of our environment. **Public health inspectors** are the traditional workers in this field (called **sanitarians** in the United States). The responsibilities of these workers are principally the elimination or control of **nuisances** — factors in the environment that may endanger health, such as excessive noise or offensive odours; ensuring the safety of water, milk and food supplies; ensuring that garbage and sewage disposal is properly carried out; enforcing public health laws with regard to sanitation; and assisting in the control of communicable diseases. In Canada, programs for public health inspectors are usually offered in institutes of technology or in community colleges. The sanitarian in the United States usually has a baccalaureate degree in the biological, physical or sanitary sciences.

A large number of new workers have emerged in the field of environmental health. There is, for example, the **industrial hygienist**, whose main concern is the detection and control of hazards in the work environment. There are also technologists specializing in water, in pollution and in other facets of environmental health.

OTHER HEALTH SERVICE PROVIDERS

Some of the other health professionals with whom the nurse will collaborate are the social worker, pharmacist, physiotherapist, occupational therapist, respiratory technologist, medical laboratory technologist and radiology technologist.

Social workers assist in evaluating the psychosocial situation of the patient and help people with their social problems. They usually have extensive knowledge of community agencies and frequently make arrangements for the patient to be cared for by the appropriate agency. The majority of social workers hold a bachelor's or master's degree in social work; many community colleges are now offering courses for assistant social workers.

The **pharmacist** is an individual whose primary area of responsibility is the preparation and dispensing of drugs and other chemical substances used in the detection, prevention and treatment of illness. Because drug therapy is an important part of the treatment of many illnesses, most hospitals and other health agencies in the community usually employ a staff of pharmacists. The pharmacist is an excellent source of information for nurses on the nature of medications—their composition, mode of action, method of administration, dosage and possible side effects. Most pharmacists in North America complete a four-year course of studies at a university. A number of community colleges are developing courses for pharmacy assistants. In many

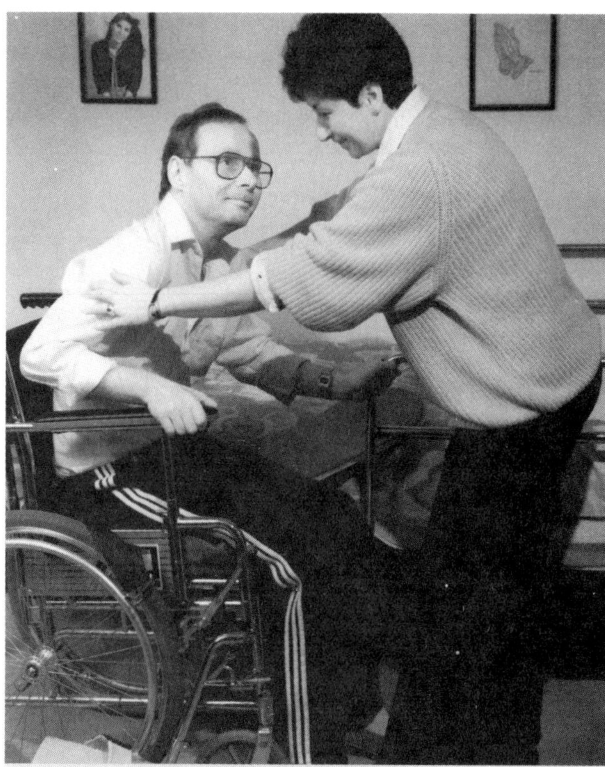

Physiotherapist teaching a patient how to transfer from bed to chair.

countries of the world, new programs to prepare pharmacists (to replace the old apprenticeship type of training) are being located in community colleges and technological institutes as well as in universities.

Physiotherapists have specialized preparation in physical therapy in a three- to four-year program of studies, usually in a university. They assist in assessing the patient's functional ability, strength and mobility; carry out therapeutic treatments, particularly those dealing with the musculoskeletal system; and teach families and individuals exercises and other measures that can contribute to the patient's recovery and rehabilitation.

Closely allied to the physiotherapist are two other occupational groups, the **remedial gymnast**, whose specialty is rehabilitation through exercise, and the **kinesiologist**, who is a specialist in human movement and human performance. Kinesiology is offered in baccalaureate programs, usually of four years' duration, in a university setting. Remedial gymnasts are often trained by kinesiologists in a certificate or diploma program at the community college or technological institute level.

Occupational therapists have a background similar to the physiotherapist's. Many individuals, in fact, hold a combined degree (or certificate) in physical and occupational therapy. The occupational therapist, however, is primarily concerned with the restoration of bodily functions through specific tasks or skills, rather than exercises and treatments. Occupational therapists frequently play a large role in rehabilitation by helping people to develop new skills or to relearn skills lessened or lost through illness.

Respiratory technologists (therapists) are experts in diagnostic procedures and therapeutic measures used in the care of patients with respiratory problems. They are skilled in handling oxygen therapy equipment. Programs in respiratory technology are usually two to three years long and are offered in community colleges or other postsecondary educational institutions.

Many **clinical laboratory technologists** (also called *medical technologists*) assist in patient care in both the institutional and the ambulatory care settings. The medical technologist is responsible for collecting many of the specimens needed for laboratory tests; he or she treats and analyses these specimens and advises physicians and nurses on the results of these tests. The technologist is also helpful in advising nurses on the nature of tests and the specific procedure for carrying out tasks. In Canada, courses in medical laboratory technology are offered in community colleges and technological institutes, and generally last two to three years. In the United States, clinical laboratory technologists are usually required to have a baccalaureate degree in medical technology, chemistry or a biological science.

Radiology technologists carry out diagnostic and therapeutic measures involving the use of radiant energy. The radiology technologist's preparation is usually a two- to three-year program of combined academic work and clinical experience. The programs are usually conducted by postsecondary educational institutions, such as a community college or technological institute, with hospital affiliation.

Speech-language pathologists carry out diagnostic and therapeutic measures with individuals who have language and speech difficulties. The programs are conducted by postsecondary educational institutions such as universities. Most programs are four to five years in length.

Pastoral care is a ministry of compassionate individuals who offer emotional and spiritual support to patients, family and staff. Some services include prayer, rituals, morgue viewing, and grief or loss counselling. Most hospitals provide an in-house training called clinical pastoral education. The course consists of approximately 400 hours of clinical experience and classroom instruction (Mauley, 1998).

MEMBERS OF THE HEALTH TEAM PRIMARILY CONCERNED WITH EMERGENCY SERVICES

Personnel in agencies providing emergency medical services require training that ranges from basic first aid to professional-level training in emergency care. In Canada, the St. John's Ambulance Society offers a 16-hour basic first aid course, which is often a pre-entrance requirement for nursing students. An advanced-level course is also offered in some provinces. Virtually all health professionals and others working in the clinical field today are required to become certified in cardiopulmonary resuscitation (CPR). As student nurses, you will probably take the six-hour CPR training followed by a 3-hour recertification every year, as part of your introductory nursing course, unless this was a pre-entrance requirement. The CPR course is often taught by local branches of St. John's Ambulance, the Canadian Heart Association and the Canadian Red Cross, and is also a regular offering of in-service educational programs in most health agencies today.

In Canada, people working as first aid personnel in industry (e.g., in industrial plants, canneries, logging or mining operations) are usually required to have an Industrial First Aid Certificate. The program leading to this certificate consists of a 50-hour course which may be given in a concentrated two-week period, or extended over a period of several weeks. A "survival first aid" course of eight hours may be given to first aid attendants in work settings where the services of an industrial first aid attendant are not warranted (for example, when there are a small number of employees or when the probability of accidents requiring additional skills is minimal).

An advanced first aid course that includes CPR training is frequently incorporated into the basic training programs for police officers and fire fighters who, by the nature of their work, are often first on the scene in an emergency. This training is also often required for civil defence workers, who volunteer to assist in case of emergencies or civil disaster in their community.

Ambulance drivers and attendants in Canada are increasingly being trained as **emergency medical technicians (EMTs)**. Programs leading to a certificate as an EMT are offered in many community colleges in Canada. They provide training in advanced life support skills so that the EMT can do CPR and basic and advanced first aid, and can start intravenous infusions.

Nurses and physicians working in emergency services also need to have specialized training to be able to react quickly and without hesitation to carry out competently the care that is required. Emergency or trauma medicine has become a recognized specialty in the medical field. For nurses, a variety of continuing education courses are now being offered to assist those working in emergency units. The courses may be given on an in-service basis in a health agency, or offered as part of a continuing education program for nurses by an educational institution or other agency.

All emergency health professionals need to have their skills updated regularly. Most agencies granting certificates require that individuals be recertified annually.

PRACTITIONERS OF COMPLEMENTARY/ALTERNATIVE MEDICINE

Today we are seeing a blending of Western and traditional medicine. A number of practitioners of alternative medicine are being recognized by the mainstream medical community as legitimate healers. For example, the services of **naturopaths** (practitioners of natural medicine) are covered under provincial health insurance in at least one province (British Columbia). We will discuss the topic of traditional—also called *alternative* or *complementary*—medicine more fully in Chapter 12. Massage, music, art and pet therapy are other complementary health promotion treatments.

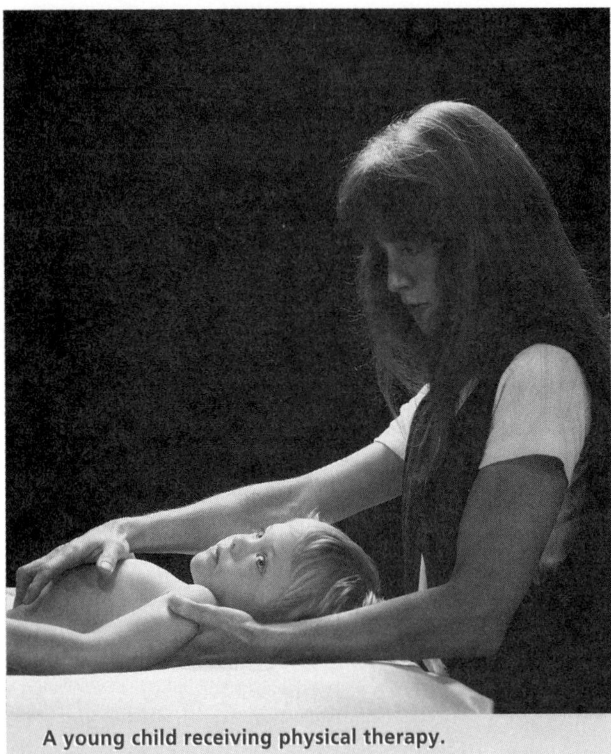

A young child receiving physical therapy.

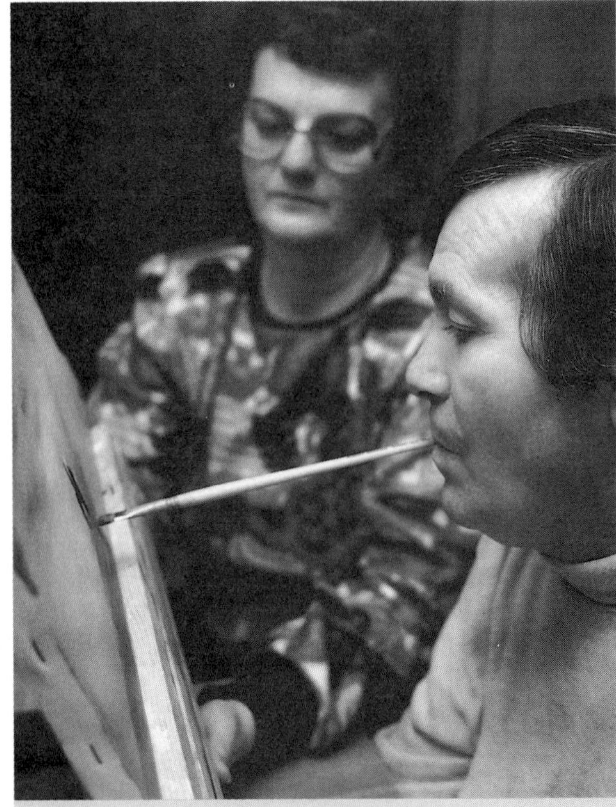

A nurse exploring the use of therapy with a patient.

Homeopathy is a holistic system of therapeutics in that it takes a broad view of illness and how individuals express illness. Practitioners prescribe minute quantities of natural substances that, in strong doses, would produce in healthy persons symptoms like those of the disease to be treated. Homeopaths are registered, and their services are not covered under provincial health insurance.

VOLUNTEERS IN HEALTH CARE

Each year, volunteers contribute thousands of hours in unpaid services in the health field. According to a study undertaken by Statistics Canada, the factors motivating people to volunteer their services include: a desire to help others; working for a cause they believe in; doing something they like to do; and feeling that they have accomplished something (Duchesne, 1989). At the time of writing, major restructuring of the health care system is taking place, and this may affect the roles and responsibilities of volunteers.

Hospitals have traditionally looked to hospital auxiliary groups to furnish the funds for extra equipment. Volunteers provide enormous amounts of time and money to hospitals and, indeed, to all types of health agencies. The services they provide for patients are invaluable.

Services Provided by Volunteers on Palliative Care Units

- support to patients and families
- night sitters — sitting with patients during the night so patient is not alone if there is no family, or to provide respite to family
- marking of special events, such as birthdays, anniversaries
- outings, such as drives, visits to home or other special events.

Services Provided by Volunteers in Acute Care Hospitals

- pre-admitting escort service
- admitting/discharge escort service
- flower delivery
- book/library service
- shopping carts
- craft carts
- activity assistants, especially with geriatric care, in occupational therapy
- one-to-one visiting
- emergency and outpatient departments—escort services and tea and coffee for patients and those waiting with them
- gift shops
- support aide services in surgical day care and cardiac units
- baby photos in maternity units
- recreational assistance in rehabilitation hospitals and children's hospitals, such as swim and exercise programs, arts and crafts, entertainment, meetings.

Services Provided by Volunteers in a Community Agency

- visit isolated seniors
- provide transportation and assistance to appointments
- assist at agency clinics
- provide labour support to pregnant teens
- organize shopping programs
- give public presentations
- participate in community organizations such as stroke clubs, adult day cares, neighbourhood houses, community centres and early childhood centres
- participate in planning new programs and facilitate community action and health promotion programs.

Services Provided by Volunteers in Long-Term Care Agencies

- program assistant—may help with crafts, general activities (e.g., bingo, checkers, bowling), outings (group and one-to-one), gardening, special events such as parties, lunches, teas, swim programs, exercise programs
- one-to-one visiting
- mealtime helper
- hair care, manicure and pedicure
- entertainment—music, singalong programs
- music therapy
- pet therapy
- church services
- shopping service
- driving van or bus
- cooking programs with residents.

SOURCE: Boggan, 1998.

IN REVIEW

- The Epp Report (1986) outlined strategies and mechanisms for implementing the concept of primary health care (PHC). The mechanisms identified included:
  - self-care
  - mutual aid
  - creation of healthy environments.
- The strategies involved:
  - fostering public participation
  - strengthening community health services
  - coordinating healthy public policy.
- As health care reform sweeps the country, health services are being restructured to provide a continuum of care that includes:
  - health promotion programs
  - health protection programs
  - health restorative services
  - supportive care.
- Primary health care, the foundation for this restructuring, encompasses both a philosophy of care and the services provided at the first level of the continuum. The basic principles of primary health care are:
  - accessibility
  - public participation
  - health promotion and prevention of illness
  - intersectoral cooperation
  - usage of appropriate technologies.
- Primary health care includes:
  - preventive and health maintenance
  - diagnostics, therapeutic and rehabilitative services.
- These services are provided:
  - in patients' homes
  - in ambulatory departments
  - in the community.
- In Canada, most health care and support for individuals is provided in the home by family and friends. Numerous services are available through governmental and nongovernmental agencies and organizations. These include:
  - nursing care
  - personal and homemaker services
  - respite care and family relief.
- Voluntary agencies provide services that are supplemental to those provided by government.
- Health services in the community develop to meet the specific needs of individuals in a geographic area. They include services provided by:
  - governmental agencies
  - community health centres
  - street clinics
  - mental health centres
  - physicians' offices and clinics
  - hospital ambulatory and emergency services.
- Agencies providing inpatient services are regulated and funded, for the most part, by the government. They include:
  - hospitals that provide acute care services
  - rehabilitative centres
  - long-term care facilities
  - hospices and palliative care units.
- A variety of independent-living residences have also developed to meet the individual needs of people who do not wish, or are unable, to maintain their own homes.
- The federal government plays a major role in health and welfare in Canada, both through national legislation and through its financial contribution to programs. It also provides:
  - advisory and consultative services
  - a national health information service
  - research and educational funds
  - standards for drug control
  - standards for the control of communicable diseases and other hazards.
- The federal government also provides direct health services to certain segments of the population.
- The administration of health care and social assistance programs is vested in provincial and territorial governments. These governments are responsible for:
  - allocating funds
  - setting standards of care
  - regulating facilities
  - negotiating salaries of health professionals.
- Workers' Compensation Boards (WCBs) operate under provincial or territorial statute as quasi-governmental agencies. Under legislation, most workers except for the self-employed are covered by WCBs.
- WCBs are financed through levies on employers provide the following to workers:
  - health care
  - rehabilitation services
  - income replacement
  - survivor benefits.
- WCBs also participate in injury prevention programs.
- The private sector provides many services in the health and welfare area. Some are purchased by government; others are paid for on a fee-for-service basis.

- Health professionals make up approximately eight percent of the total Canadian labour force. Over one-half of these are nurses, with physicians as the next largest group. Volunteers also make a major contribution to health care.
- In health care today, a multidisciplinary team approach is essential. Each member can contribute his or her unique knowledge, experience and skill to achieve the common goal of promoting the highest level of health possible for each individual.

Critical Thinking Activities

Nettie McLeod and her sister, Jean, live together in a small house in one of the suburbs of a large Canadian city. Nettie, who is 84, is a retired teacher. Jean (81 years old) was an accountant in a small business. Since her retirement, Nettie has devoted herself to looking after her sister, who has had a series of health problems and has become a semi-invalid. Nettie herself had surgery for removal of a cancerous growth five years ago. She requires monitoring as well as occasional chemotherapy, which necessitates an overnight stay at the cancer clinic in the city. Nettie does the shopping and manages most of the housework, including meal preparation for herself and her sister. She still drives the car, but only around the small community where they live. The two women do not have any family living in the province, although they have a wide circle of friends—mostly older women like themselves, or older couples whom they have known for a long time.

From time to time, one or the other of the sisters falls ill. Jean was hospitalized recently for removal of a kidney stone, but has recovered quite well from that episode.

1. If Nettie and Jean lived in your community, what services would be available to help them to maintain their health and to stay in their own home as long as possible?
2. If Nettie or Jean developed a minor illness, sufficient to incapacitate but not to require hospitalization, how would they obtain care to help them in the home? What services might this include? Would they have to pay for these services? If so, what is the cost?
3. Once, Jean, who had a bout of diarrhea for several days and was not eating her meals, collapsed on her way to the bathroom in the middle of the night. What services could Nettie call on to get help? Where are the nearest emergency services in your area? How large is the nearest hospital? What services does the hospital provide?
4. Jean spent a week in hospital. What types of health workers would have been involved in her care? in the emergency department? when she was on the nursing unit? If she needed home care after her discharge, who would arrange for the services?
5. When Nettie feels she can no longer cope with the house and the meal preparation, the two sisters will have to consider alternative living arrangements. What is available in your community that might suit them? What would it cost these women per month? If the cost is more than they can afford, what other options are available for them?

KEY TERMS

continuum of care p. 54
primary health care (PHC) p. 54
health promotion p. 57
frail elderly p. 61
community health centre (CHC) p. 63
multiservice agency p. 63
health maintenance organization (HMO) p. 63
street clinic p. 63
proprietary hospital p. 65
public general hospital p. 65
rehabilitation p. 65
priory model p. 66
hospice p. 67
palliative care unit p. 67
physician's assistant p. 70
health educator p. 70
recreation specialist p. 70
nutritionist p. 70
dietitian p. 70
public health inspector p. 70
sanitarian p. 70
nuisance p. 70
industrial hygienist p. 70
social worker p. 70
pharmacist p. 70
physiotherapist p. 71
remedial gymnast p. 71
kinesiologist p. 71
occupational therapist p. 71
respiratory technologist p. 71
clinical laboratory technologist p. 71
radiology technologist p. 71
speech-language pathologist p. 71
pastoral care p. 71
emergency medical technician (EMT) p. 71
naturopath p. 72
homeopathy p. 73

References

ANDERSON, J.M. (1990). Home care management in chronic illness and the self-care movement: An analysis of ideologies and economic processes influencing policy decisions. *Advances in Nursing Science, 12*(2), 71–83.

ANDRON V., GREENE, A., & INGRAM, D. (1998). Comox's little program that could. *Nursing BC, 10*(1), 6–8.

ASSOCIATION OF REGISTERED NURSES OF NEWFOUNDLAND. (1990). *Primary health care: A nursing model.* St. John's, Newfoundland: Author.

BANKS, J.W., & LOFTUS, P. (1991). Street smarts. *Canadian Nurse, 87*(7), 25–27.

BHAGAT, R., BIRING, D., PANDHER, P., QUONG, E., & TRIOLET, K. (1997). Partners in health. *Nursing BC, 29*(4), 16–19.

BOGGAN, S. (1998, March 9). Personal communication with Director of Agency Services, Volunteer Vancouver, B.C.

BOUDREAU, T. (1972). *Report of the committee on nurse practitioners*. Ottawa: Health & Welfare Canada.

CANADIAN NURSES ASSOCIATION (CNA). (1968). *The leaf and the lamp*. Ottawa: Author.

CARSON, M.M. and ROSS, M.M. (1993) Changing the model of practice: Geriatric extended care in an acute care hospital. *Canadian Nurse, 89*(2), 35–38.

CROWE, C., & HARDILL, K. (1993). Nursing research and political change: The street health report. *Canadian Nurse, 89*(1), 21–24.

DICKINSON, H.D., & ANDRE, G. (1988). Community psychiatry: The institutional transformation of psychiatric practice. In B.S. Bolaria & H.D. Dickinson (Eds.), *Sociology of health care in Canada*. Toronto: Harcourt Brace Jovanovich.

DUCHESNE, D. (1989). *Giving freely: Volunteers in Canada*. Labour Analytic Report No. 4. Ottawa: Minister of Supply & Services. (Catalogue No. 71–535)

DU GAS, B.W., & BECKINGHAM, A.C. (1993). The emergence of gerontological nursing. In A.C. Beckingham and B.W. Du Gas (Eds.), *Promoting healthy aging: A nursing and community perspective*. St. Louis: Mosby.

EADES, J.E. (1965). *Workmen's compensation in Canada and the United States*. Vancouver: Workers' Compensation Board of British Columbia.

EPP, J. (1986). *Achieving health for all: A framework for health promotion*. Ottawa: Minister of Supply & Services. (Catalogue No. 39–102/1986E)

FRANKEL, B.G., SPEECHLEY, M., & WADE, T.J. (1996). *The sociology of health and health care: A Canadian perspective*. Toronto: Copp Clark.

GOVERNMENT OF BRITISH COLUMBIA. (1991). *Closer to home: Summary of the royal commission on health care and costs*. Victoria: Crown Publishing.

GOVERNMENT OF BRITISH COLUMBIA. (1992). *Healthy communities 1991 yearbook*. Victoria: Office of Health Promotion, British Columbia Ministry of Health and Ministry Responsible for Seniors. (Catalogue No. QP 92835 03/92)

GOVERNMENT OF ONTARIO. (1993a). *Nurturing health: Report of the Premier's council on health, well-being, and social justice (1987–1991)*. Toronto: Queen's Printer. (Catalogue No. 01–93–20M)

GOVERNMENT OF ONTARIO. (1993b). *Highlights: Partnerships in long-term care*. Toronto: Ontario Ministries of Health, Community and Social Services and Citizenship.

GRANT, K.R. (1988). The inverse care law in Canada: Differential access under universal free health insurance. In B.S. Bolaria and H.D. Dickinson (Eds.), *Sociology of health care in Canada* (pp. 118–134). Toronto: Harcourt Brace Jovanovich.

GRIFFITHS, H. (1996). Nursing in the urban core. *Nursing BC, 28*(5), 14–16.

HAMILTON, K., & TREPANIER, H. (1989, Winter). Hospital care in the 21st century. *Canadian Social Trends*, 31–34.

HEALTH & WELFARE CANADA. (1987). *The active health report: Perspectives on Canada's health promotion survey*. Ottawa: Minister of Supply & Services. (Catalogue No. H39–106/1987E)

HEALTH & WELFARE CANADA. (1989). *Health and welfare in Canada*. Ottawa: Minister of Supply & Services. (Catalogue No. H21–102/1989E)

LABONTE, R. (1987, Summer). Community health promotion studies. *Health Promotion*, 5–10; 32.

LABONTE, R. (1989). Community and professional empowerment. *Canadian Nurse, 85*(3), 23–26; 28.

LENOBLE, E. (1993). Preadmission clinics gaining ground. *Nursing BC, 25*(4), 20–24.

MAGLACAS, A.M., ULIN, P.R., & SHEPS, C.G. (1987). *Health manpower for primary health care: The experience of the nurse practitioner*. Chapel Hill, NC: World Health Organization / University of North Carolina.

MAHLER, H. (1985, June). Nurses lead the way. *WHO Features, 97*.

MAKING PRIMARY HEALTH CARE WORK FOR CANADIANS: A CNA PRIORITY. (1992). *CNA Today, 2*(3), 1.

MANTLE, J. (1992). Nursing practice in long-term care agencies. In A. Baumgart & J. Larsen (Eds.), *Canadian nursing faces the future* (pp. 135–151). St. Louis: Mosby.

MAULEY, C. (1998, March 10). Personal communication with Director of Pastoral Care, St. Paul's Hospital, Vancouver, B.C.

McIVOR, V. (1978). Freedom to be, Part two: The priory method. *Canadian Nurse*, 74(3), 23–26.

NURSES PROVE THEMSELVES IN PRIMARY HEALTH CARE. (1994). *CNA Today, 4*(2), 1–2.

PRIMARY HEALTH CARE HAS ARRIVED. (1992). *CNA Today, 2*(3), 4–5.

REGISTERED NURSES ASSOCIATION OF BRITISH COLUMBIA (RNABC). (1990). *Health promotion: A discussion paper*. Vancouver: Author.

REGISTERED NURSES ASSOCIATION OF BRITISH COLUMBIA (RNABC). (1994). *Creating the new health care: A new nursing perspective*. Vancouver: Author.

ROBERTS, S.J. (1988). Social support and help seeking: Review of the literature. *Advances in Nursing Science, 10*(2), 1–11.

SEYMOUR, M.D. (1991). Too old to care. *Canadian Nurse, 87*(11), 26–27.

SHESTOWSKY, B. (1992). Primary health care: Still relevant after 14 years. *CNA Today, 2*(3), 3.

ST. MICHAEL, M. (1993, September). Letter to the editor. *Nursing BC*.

STATISTICS CANADA. (1992). *Health professionals and population per professional*. Table 32.1. Ottawa: Author.

STATISTICS CANADA. (1997, August 8). *A portrait of seniors*. [Online.] Available at: http://www.statcan.ca/english/seniors/link.htm

STONE, S. (1997). Clearing the air about health care restructuring. *Nursing BC, 29*(5), 31–32.

SUTHERLAND, R., & FULTON, J. (1988). *Health care in Canada*. Ottawa: The Health Group.

THOLL, W.G. (1994). Health care spending in Canada: Skating faster on thinner ice. In A. Blomqvist & D. Brown (Eds.), *Limits to care: Reforming Canada's health care system in an age of restraint* (pp. 53–90). Toronto: C.D. Howe Institute.

TREPANNA, K. (1990). *A view of the horizon: Regional trends*. Ottawa: Institute for Health Care Facilities of the Future.

VICTORIAN ORDER OF NURSES. (1988, March). *VON Health promotion project for seniors*. Final Report. Ottawa: Author.

WICKENS, B. (1998). Unwell and untreated. *Maclean's Canadian Weekly Newsmagazine. 11*(32), 44–45.

WORKERS' COMPENSATION BOARD OF BRITISH COLUMBIA. (1997). Discussion with senior officials of WCB in Richmond, B.C.

WORLD HEALTH ORGANIZATION. (1978). *Alma-Ata 1978: Primary health care*. Geneva: Author.

WORLD HEALTH ORGANIZATION. (1984). A discussion document on the concept and principles of health promotion. Geneva: Author.

Additional Readings

ARNOLD, J. (1996). Rethinking grief: Nursing implications for health promotion. *Home Healthcare Nurse, 14*(10), 777–785.

BERLAND, A., WHYTE, N.B., & MAXWELL, L. (1995). Hospital nurses and health promotion. *Canadian Journal of Nursing Research, 27*(4), 13–31.

CAMILETTI, Y.A., & MARCHUK, B. (1998). How men learn about health. *Canadian Nurse, 94*(1), 29–31.

DORLAND, J.H., & DAVIS, M.S. (1995). *How many roads...? Regionalization and decentralization in health care*. Ottawa: Renouf.

JONES, F., & GREEN, M. (1996). The B.C. baby-friendly initiative. *Nursing BC, 28*(5), 7–8.

MASS, H., & WHYTE, N. (1997). Primary health care in action. *Nursing BC, 29*(2), 13–16.

MCARTHUR, W., RAMSAY, C., & WALER, M. (1996). *Healthy incentives: Canadian health reform in an international context*. Vancouver: Fraser Institute.

SULLIVAN, J., & VAIL, S. (1997). Issues and trends: It's a small world. *Canadian Nurse, 93*(5), 59–60.

SUTHERLAND, R.W. (1996). *Will nurses call the shots? A look at the delivery of health care twenty years from now*. Plevna, ON: Author.

SUTHERLAND, R.W., & FULTON, M.J. (1994). *Spending smarter and spending less: Policies and partnerships for health care in Canada*. Ottawa: The Health Group.

TENN, L. (1995). Primary health care nursing education in Canadian university schools of nursing. *Journal of Nursing Education, 34*(8), 350–358.

Chapter 5

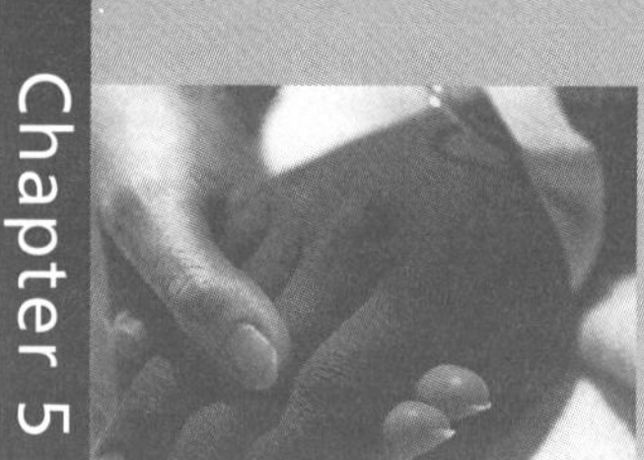

OUTLINE

Introduction

Nursing Resources in Canada

Registered Nursing Education in Canada

Nursing's Role in Health Care

Career Choices for Nurses

Modes of Practice

Nurses and the Political Process

Nursing in Canada

Central Questions

1. What categories of nursing personnel are there in Canada?
2. How are nurses currently prepared?
3. What is meant by scope of practice?
4. How has registered nursing education developed in Canada?
5. Why has the baccalaureate been recommended as entry level for professional nursing practice?
6. What continuing education opportunities are available for nurses in Canada?
7. How does Benner's "domains of practice" explain the nurse's role?
8. What are some of the career options nurses have?
9. Where are some of the various places nurses work?
10. What is primary nursing?
11. What are some of the new models for practice and structures for delivery of care?
12. How are nurses involved in the political process?

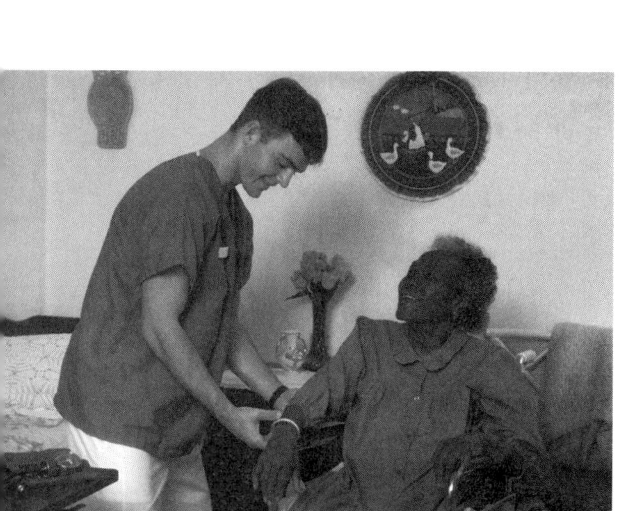

Introduction

Changes in all phases of life, including health care, are inevitable. Beneficent changes in the field of health care will be those reflecting the knowledge and experience injected through the political action of nurses.

Mussallem, 1977

Nursing is a dynamic profession, and its practice is constantly changing. Throughout their relatively short history in North America, nurses have played an important role in providing needed health services for people, a role that has been continuously reshaped by the changing needs of society. In the preceding few chapters, we have discussed some of the changes that are affecting the current practice of nursing. Among these are:

1. population changes that include more older adults as well as a more ethnically diverse society
2. a revision of our thinking about health and illness
3. recognition of the need to empower people so that they can participate in planning, managing and evaluating their own health care
4. a change of focus that is shifting health care from an illness orientation to one stressing health promotion and the prevention of illness
5. a trend away from institutionalized and towards community-based services
6. the integration of services to provide a continuum of care
7. a more collaborative and multidisciplinary approach
8. a shift to patient-centred care driven by patient need rather than by supply and availability of providers.

These changes are having a profound effect on the practice of nursing. Nurses are being challenged to assume new roles, to work in new and different health care settings and to accept increasing responsibility in the provision of comprehensive health care.

In this chapter, we will discuss nursing resources in Canada. We will start with a look at the structure of the nursing workforce, and at the various categories of nursing personnel and their relative numbers and educational level. We will touch upon the scope of practice for nurses. A discussion of the development of registered nursing education in Canada from Confederation to the present will follow. Next, we will describe briefly the educational programs currently preparing nurses for practice, highlighting opportunities for continuing education, as well as a variety of career options. Then we will explore the domains of practice and several modes of practice, and will also look at nursing's changing role in the current country-wide health care restructuring. Finally, we will discuss the relationship between nurses and the political process.

Nursing Resources in Canada

Nurses constitute the largest single group of health professionals in the health field in Canada. Of the approximately three-quarters of a million people employed in health occupations, over 60 percent are in nursing (Statistics Canada, 1993).

Nursing personnel include registered nurses (RNs), registered psychiatric nurses (RPNs), in Ontario, registered practical nurses (RPN), licensed practical nurses (LPNs), and nursing aides, orderlies and other attendants. Registered nurses alone constitute almost one-third the total number of persons employed in health care. The largest component of nursing personnel is made up of RNs (see Figure 5.1). There were an estimated 264 305 RNs in Canada in 1996, of whom 227 830 were employed in nursing. In most countries, nursing is still predominantly a female profession. Although the number of male RNs has increased in Canada in recent years, men still account for only four percent of the total number of RNs in the country, up from one percent in 1966 (CNA, 1996).

In Canada, there has been some movement towards the integrated development of health human resources (Integrated Health Human Resources Development Project, 1995). This approach requires planning across disciplines and sectors, so that the right person is in the right place doing the right thing at the right time for the right person. The appropriate **skill mix** on a health care team is one example of planning to meet the needs of the community that the team intends to serve: each team member's knowledge, skills and judgement are maximized, duplication of effort is reduced and quality of care is enhanced.

Among the types of workers who represent nursing resources, some are regulated (RNs, RPNs and LPNs) and

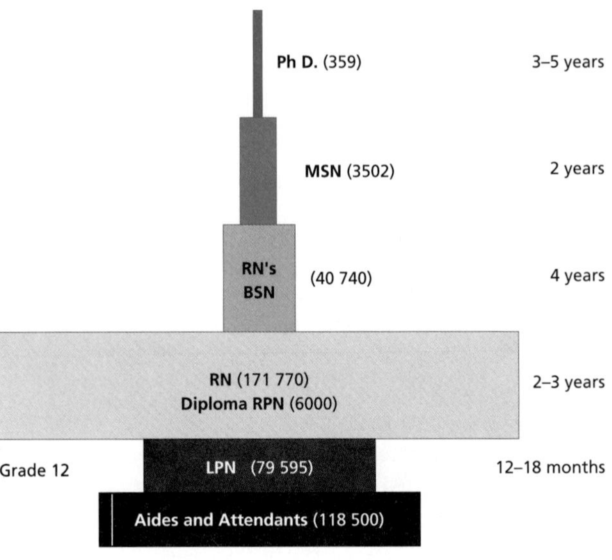

FIGURE 5.1 Nursing resources in Canada, 1996

SOURCES: Statistics Canada, 1996; CAPNNA, 1996; PNAC, 1996; CNA, 1996; Human Resources Development Canada, 1996.

others are unregulated (aides and attendants). The major goal of regulation is to protect the public from the risk associated with unqualified practitioners. Unregulated health workers may support the provision of care by performing some of the tasks associated with nursing practice, provided that certain conditions (e.g., training, supervision, safety) are met (CNA, March 1995). There will be more discussion on the topic of regulation later in this chapter (see Scope of Practice) and also in Chapter 6.

Registered Nurses

In 1964, the Royal Commission on Health Services reported that there was a severe shortage of skilled health personnel needed to implement the proposed national health care plan (Mussallem, 1965). Subsequently, educational programs for health professionals were expanded with the assistance of federal grants from the Health Resources Fund. Since then, the number of registered nurses in Canada has risen sharply, from 115 000 in 1966 to more than double that figure in 1996. To date, the rate of growth of the nursing profession has been faster than the rate of growth of the population, so that the proportion of nurses to population has increased. In 1996, Canada was in a very favourable position with regard to nursing resources vis-à-vis most other countries in the world. Our ratio of nursing personnel to population gave us one registered nurse for approximately 127 people (Statistics Canada, 1996; CNA, 1996). However, a future nursing shortage is predicted unless we begin to recruit and retain RNs (CNA, 1997b). Given that the most common age for an RN in 1996 was around 44 years, the majority of nurses will retire over the next 15 to 20 years. In addition, the current intake into professional nursing is not enough to replace those nurses who will leave the profession because of age. The baby boomer cohort that is now moving through the system will not only ensure a large elderly population by the year 2011, but will also mean that a large number of experienced practitioners will be leaving the workforce just when they will be most needed.

The proportion of nurses holding baccalaureate or higher university degrees in nursing has also increased steadily, from only 5.0 percent in 1966 to 10.1 percent in 1981, with a more rapid gain during the 1980s to 17.7 percent in 1996 (see Figure 5.1).

The number of nurses with master's level preparation is still relatively small, at a little over one percent of the total RN population. The numbers have, however, shown a steady increase in the past decade, growing from 1960 in 1987 to 3980 in 1996, of whom 3502 were employed in nursing.

The first Canadian nurse to earn a doctoral degree was Sister Denise Lefebvre, who received a Docteur de Pédagogie from the Université de Montréal in 1955. Since then, the number of nurses in Canada holding earned doctoral degrees has grown, albeit slowly. In 1989, there were 257 nurses with doctoral degrees in Canada (Stinson, MacPhail & Larsen, 1992). By 1995, the number had grown to at least 359, with about 100 more enrolled in doctoral programs (CNA, 1996).

REGISTERED PSYCHIATRIC NURSES

Registered psychiatric nurses (RPNs) are recognized in the four western provinces (British Columbia, Alberta, Saskatchewan and Manitoba). In 1997, there were just over 6000 RPNs in Canada (Psychiatric Nurses Association of Canada, 1997). The primary role of the RPN is to provide psychiatric nursing care for individuals, families and groups at all stages of life in a variety of institutional and community settings. The RPN may enter practice after qualifying for licensure. Qualifications include completion of an approved diploma or university program (two to four years) and success in a written examination.

At Douglas College in British Columbia, graduates of the two-year RPN program also have the option of taking a third year of studies that leads to an Advanced Diploma in Psychiatric Nursing. They are then eligible to complete requirements for a Bachelor of Health Sciences degree (in psychiatric nursing) from the Open Learning Agency of British Columbia. A Bachelor of Science Mental Health Program is also available for graduates of RPN programs at Brandon University in Manitoba. As of 1997, Brandon also offers a generic baccalaureate program for entry to practise as an RPN.

LICENSED PRACTICAL NURSES

The total number of licensed practical nurses (LPNs) employed in Canada in 1996 was 79 595 (Canadian Association of Practical Nurses and Nursing Assistants, 1996). LPNs are called registered practical nurses (RPN) in Ontario and certified nursing assistants (CNA) in Alberta. LPNs are prepared, for the most part, in one-year educational programs in a community college or in a vocational school. Many nursing schools provide access for graduates of these programs to enter registered nursing programs without loss of credit. LPNs perform standardized nursing procedures and treatments, most frequently working under the direction of a registered nurse or physician in hospitals as well as other health care settings. They also provide nursing care in patients' homes, with RNs giving direction and assuming responsibility for the care they give. The specific roles and procedures that LPNs perform are detailed in provincial standards of practice established by their provincial nursing associations. LPNs are licensed by their provincial licensing body after completing an approved educational program and passing a licensure examination.

Nurse's Aides and Attendants

The number of other nursing attendants has increased considerably in the past five years—from 77 000 in 1985 to more than 118 500 in 1996 (Statistics Canada, 1996). One reason for the rapid increase has been the expansion of home care as an insured service in various provinces (see Chapters 3 and 4). Designated by a variety of names, such as **nurse's aide**, *nursing orderly*, *nursing attendant*, *personal* *care attendant* or *health care aide*, workers in this category are frequently trained on the job or in a formal course of a few weeks' duration. The nature of the tasks assigned to the nurse's aide varies considerably from one agency to another. In some agencies, nurse's aides perform tasks that are essentially housekeeping in nature, while in others they assist with the care of patients.

Scope of Practice

The regulation of professionals can be done via a defined **scope of practice**, title protection, or both. For example, in every province the title of the person working in a registered nurse's role is protected by law, and the names of qualified practitioners are registered annually. However, the scope of nursing practice for which an individual is licensed is not uniformly legislated across the nation. In some jurisdictions, the scope of practice is defined and exclusive. In others, the definition of practice is general in nature, but specific activities (i.e., those considered potentially harmful to the public if performed by unqualified persons) are restricted to certain professionals. If an act is not restricted, it can be performed by anyone, whether that person is a health professional or not.

Legislation that facilitates overlapping scopes of practice increases the opportunity for patient choice and the appropriate utilization of professional skills. With flexible scopes of practice, the evolution of professional groups is promoted and the cost of service delivery is decreased. Further, employer assignment of practitioners is more flexible. However, the potential exists for the proliferation of unlicensed workers, and for underprepared workers to be assigned, and to assume, inappropriate responsibility — with resulting risk to the client, the worker and the employer (Cutshall, 1994; Sibbald, 1997a; CNA, 1993c, March 1995, August 1996).

MULTISKILLING

Multiskilling (also known as *multitasking*) is the consolidation of responsibilities for diverse work assignments within a single job description (Pischke-Winn, 1995). Personnel are retrained and redeployed to assist with patient care. In most instances, multiskilling has focussed on workers who handle non-nursing duties. For example, housekeeping duties could be combined with food services and central supply activities to produce a worker who could assist the nurse by keeping the patient's environment clean, helping with meal delivery and feeding, and restocking necessary supplies.

Registered Nursing Education in Canada

In Canada today, the education of the registered nurse for entry to practice takes place in two different types of educational program: (a) in two- to three-year diploma programs in a community college or technological institute and (b) in four-year baccalaureate programs in colleges and universities that grant a baccalaureate degree in nursing. In 1996 there were a total of 94 diploma programs and 29 generic baccalaureate programs in universities in Canada. There was also one generic master's program, at McGill University, for people holding a baccalaureate degree in another field (CNA, 1996).

Rapid change is occurring not only in health care in Canada today, but also in the education of nurses. Individuals familiar with the process of change maintain that it takes almost a full century to bring about a major revision in an educational system, and they cite as an example the incorporation of kindergarten into the public school system—which is still not an accomplished fact in all provinces (Du Gas, 1991). In nursing education, the change from hospital-based, service-oriented schools to programs integrated into the general educational system of the country has also taken 100 years—from the first insights into the need for change to the ultimate full-scale adoption of the change.

Historical Perspective

THE HOSPITAL SCHOOLS

At the time of Confederation (1867) in Canada, care of the ill was carried out mainly in the home as the responsibility of the women in the family. Hospitals were basically charitable institutions operated by religious groups or other organizations for care of the poor, the homeless or those who, for one reason or another, could not be looked after at home. With the exception of the religious orders, nursing in Canada, as in other parts of the world at the time, did not attract a very high calibre of candidate. Most of the nurses in secular hospitals were poorly educated country girls who, in many instances, had never seen a hospital before. It was said of their situation that "the pay was a mere pittance, the work so repulsive and hopeless that there was little to attract a different class" (VON, 1983, p. 9).

The nursing sisterhoods of the Roman Catholic and other churches had an apprenticeship system for training new recruits, but it is Florence Nightingale who must receive credit for ushering in a training system that permitted the eventual development of professional nursing education (CNA, 1968). She raised the standards for women entering nursing and insisted on satisfactory evidence of good moral character. The elements of a basic educational program were prerequisites for admission to the Nightingale School of Nursing at St. Thomas's Hospital in London, England.

The first school of nursing in Canada based on the Nightingale model was the Mack Training School at the General and Marine Hospital in St. Catharines, Ontario, in 1874. Schools of nursing followed in other cities across the country in rapid succession (Gibbon & Mathewson, 1947; CNA, 1968). There was no lack of candidates for the schools. Young women from good families considered it a

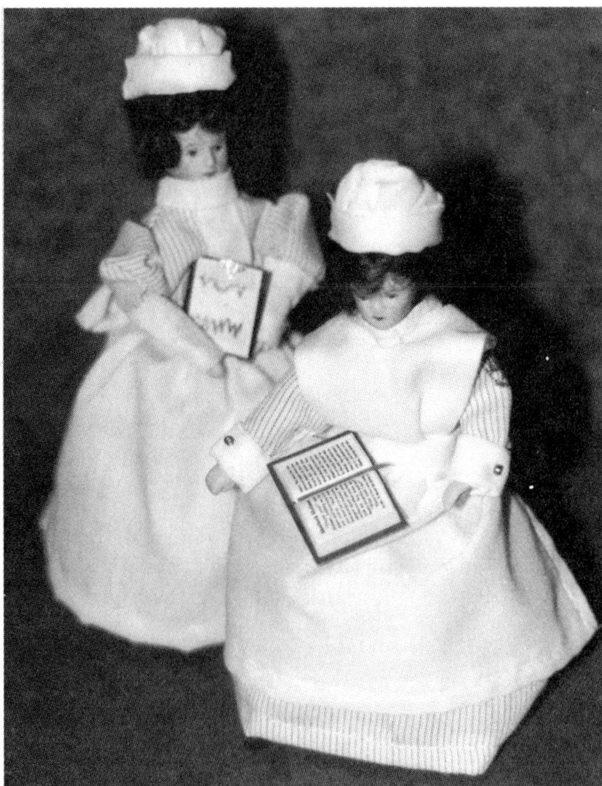

The student nurses' uniforms of the Winnipeg General Hospital, 1895 and 1897, as would have been worn by Ethel Johns.

privilege to be selected for the opportunity to enter their chosen vocation and cheerfully endured the rigorous, militaristic training imposed by their teachers. The students were well groomed, neatly uniformed, trained to be obedient and were well supervised. Nursing service was considerably improved by their presence. The graduates were proud of their "trained" status and, in the 1890s and early 1900s, the matter of professionalism was a serious issue concerning nurses. With the advent of the training schools, nursing entered a new phase as graduate nurses became part of the medical missionary movement, taking their skills to the still sparsely populated settled areas of the country. In one highly publicized endeavour, four VON nurses travelled to the Klondike in 1898 to provide health services for the people flocking there for the Gold Rush (VON, 1947). By the turn of the century, the nurse had an established role in Canadian society as an essential person in the care of the sick in hospitals and at home (VON, 1983).

DISSATISFACTION WITH THE SYSTEM

Regrettably, the Nightingale model for a school of nursing did not survive its cross-Atlantic voyage intact. Administrators of the rapidly proliferating hospitals in North America were quick to see the financial advantages of having a ready source of cheap labour in the nursing students. The schools, instead of being autonomous, as the Nightingale School had been, became an integral part of the hospital establishment (Mussallem, 1960). Dissatisfaction with the improperly imported system of nursing training started early. It was first vocalized in 1893, when nursing leaders in Canada and the United States came together in a historic meeting in Chicago to share their concerns. The result of this meeting was the formation of the American Society of Lady Superintendents of Training Schools. Its purpose was to promote the exchange of ideas and the establishment of high educational standards. Its main undertaking was to work for higher standards of nurse preparation. The Society later divided to become, in Canada, the Canadian Society of Superintendents of Training Schools for Nurses. In 1908, this became the Provisional Society of the Canadian Association of Trained Nurses — the forerunner of the Canadian Nurses Association. The first president of the Society, Mary Agnes Snively, took the Association into the International Council of Nurses in 1909 (CNA, 1968).

The desire to differentiate between trained and untrained nurses led to the development of provincial nursing acts regulating the preparation for and practice of nursing. Voluntary registration began in 1910 in Nova Scotia, followed by other provinces within the next few years (Gibbon & Mathewson, 1947). Detailed standard curricula for schools of nursing were established in different provinces, and committees were set up by graduate nurses' associations (forerunners of present-day provincial registered nurses' associations) in attempts to improve training programs for nurses. Prominent nurses spoke out against the exploitation of nursing students. Ethel Johns, for example, when reporting on the findings of a Committee on Standardization of Training Schools at a national meeting in 1917, stated, "Anyone may start [a training school]. All that is necessary is to gather some sick people under a roof and call it a hospital. . . . There are no standards at all. . . . You just start a training school, and providence and the patients do the rest" (Johns; cited in Street, 1973, p. 90). Many of the small schools that had proliferated during and after World War I were closed during the 1920s and 1930s in response to the lobbying efforts of the nurses.

THE WEIR REPORT

The problem of nursing education was of concern to nurses all across Canada. In 1927, the CNA struck a joint committee with the Canadian Medical Association to look into the problem of "the nurse in her relationship to the hospital, the medical profession and the public at large" (Cameron; cited in Weir, 1932, p. 5). This committee appointed Dr. George Weir, head of the Department of Education at the University of British Columbia, to conduct a survey of nursing education in Canada. In his report, published in 1932, Dr. Weir recommended that nursing education be integrated into the general education system.

LOOKING back

Mary Agnes Snively, 1847–1933

Mary Agnes Snively was responsible for organizing nurses in Canada and making them a part of the international body of nurses. A teacher before she entered nursing, the Ontario-born woman graduated from New York's Bellevue Hospital School of Nursing in 1884 at age 37. She then accepted the position of Lady Superintendent of the Toronto General Hospital, where she remained until her retirement at age 63. One of her first priorities as superintendent was to improve the three-year-old nurses' training program; within 10 years the Toronto School's reputation was so high that there were 600 applicants for the 22 places in the program. To respond to the demand, the hospital became the largest in Canada and maintained a remarkable reputation for quality nursing care.

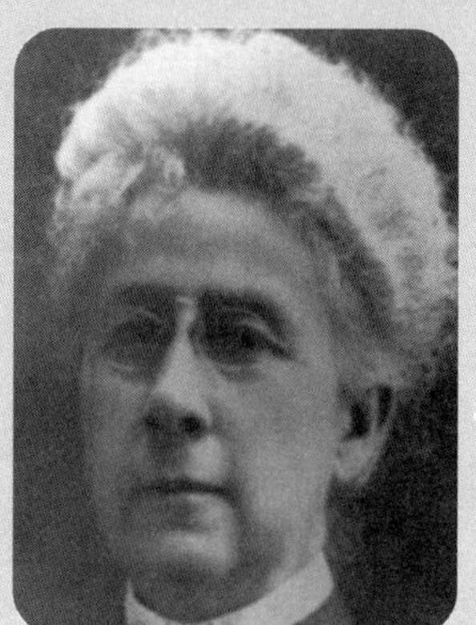

Through her friendships and professional networks with nurses in the United States, Mary Agnes Snively was a founding member of the American Society of Superintendents of Training Schools for Nurses (a joint Canadian–American group) and was a member of its first Board. She also was interested in a British proposal for an international organization. In 1899, she represented Canada as one of the leaders from countries still without national associations at the founding meeting of the International Council of Nurses (ICN) and was named its first honorary treasurer. After five years in that position, she became the Council's vice-president.

At home in Toronto, she had already formed an alumnae association and worked to form a Graduate Nurses' Association of Ontario from the various alumnae groups in the province. Through this organization, Mary Agnes Snively and others persuaded the provincial government to secure registration for nurses. She forged ahead with the idea of a national organization and, in 1908, was instrumental in bringing together representatives from 16 alumnae associations from all parts of Canada to form the Canadian National Association of Trained Nurses (CNATN), which later changed its name to the Canadian Nurses Association (CNA). Mary Agnes Snively was elected its first president, from 1908 to 1912, shepherded it into full membership in the ICN and established a sound professional infrastructure for Canadian nursing.

—*Glennis Zilm*

Thus, some 40 years after the need for change in the education of nurses was voiced in Chicago, the direction of the needed change was determined (Weir, 1932). Sixteen years were to pass before an acceptable way was found to implement the recommendations of the Weir Report. Again, the Canadian Nurses Association took the lead and, with financing from the Red Cross, established a demonstration school of nursing in Windsor, Ontario. The Metropolitan School of Nursing (1948–1952), as it was called, pioneered the independent school of nursing in Canada. The school was separated financially and physically from the hospital, and the clinical practice of the students in hospitals and other institutions was under the direction of school authorities (CNA, 1968).

In the United States, a different solution was tried as Mildred Montag, in 1952, launched a two-year junior college program on an experimental basis (Donahue, 1996). This program set the pattern that came to be adopted throughout North America. Nursing education had finally found a niche in the educational system. The development of community colleges and the subsequent incorporation of nursing education into them took place a little later in Canada. Meanwhile, Dr. Helen Mussallem (1965) was asked to undertake a study of nursing education for the Royal Commission on Health Services. The Report of the Commission reinforced Weir's recommendation to transfer nursing education to postsecondary institutions (Hall, 1964). The first nursing education program in a postsecondary institution in Canada was established at the Ryerson Institute of Technology in 1963, but widespread acceptance of the idea had to wait for the development of the community college system in various provinces. Saskatchewan, in 1967, was the first province to transfer authority for schools of nursing from hospitals to the Department of Education (CNA, 1968). Quebec began the process in 1967, and by 1972, all hospital schools were closed and nursing education programs were offered in the community colleges (CEGEPs). Ontario transferred all diploma nursing education programs to the Colleges of Applied Arts and Technology in 1973. Community college programs developed rapidly in most other provinces during the 1970s and 1980s. By 1996 there were only nine hospital diploma programs; by 1997, there were none (CNA, 1997b).

DEVELOPMENT OF UNIVERSITY PROGRAMS FOR REGISTERED NURSES

Nursing education . . . cannot remain permanently apart from the stream of invigorating life and inspiration which the university can best supply. Sooner or later, the university, in affiliation with the well-equipped hospital, must face the problem of educating the nurse. Evolutionary trends all point in this direction.

Weir, 1932

When the Victorian Order of Nurses was founded in 1897, it was recognized that the nurses would need additional preparation to work effectively in the community. There were no programs providing this education in Canada at the time, so the VON set up its own programs in various cities across the country (VON, 1983).

Subsequently, the vision of a broader role for nurses, not only doing home nursing but also carrying out health promotion and disease prevention in the community, led to the establishment of a program for the preparation of public health nurses at the University of British Columbia. By 1919, the Department of Nursing and Public Health was established at UBC, with Ethel Johns holding dual responsibilities as the head of the program and Lady Superintendent of the Vancouver General Hospital. The first class graduated from this program in 1920. The Bachelor of Applied Science in Nursing program was added as demand grew. The first three nurses graduated from this program in 1923 (Green, 1984). The program included two years on campus in university studies, followed by 24 (later 28, then 32) months at the Vancouver General Hospital. The final year of the six-year program was spent on campus, where the students had the option of taking either public health nursing, or teaching and supervision. Graduates of diploma schools of nursing could also enroll in the public health nursing or teaching and supervision courses, where they received a diploma in their respective field on successful completion of the one-year program. Similar "sandwich" type programs developed in other universities across the country (Gibbon & Mathewson, 1947).

Gradually, however, the university schools of nursing began to want more control over their students, instead of handing them over to the hospital for the entire clinical portion of the program. The Integrated Basic Degree Program was pioneered by E. Kathleen Russell in 1942 at the University of Toronto. This program gave students a broad foundation in the humanities and sciences as well as in nursing (Bajnok, 1992). During the 1950s and 1960s, other universities began to follow suit. The Report of the Royal Commission on Health Services (1964), reflecting findings from the studies of nursing education by both Mussallem (1960; 1965) and Weir (1932), accelerated the movement by recommending expansion of university programs and criticized the "sandwich" program of studies. The integrated five-year (later reduced to four years) basic baccalaureate programs came to be the norm. In addition to generic baccalaureate programs, post-basic baccalaureate programs have also developed. These programs leading to a degree are for registered nurses who have already received their basic nursing diploma through a hospital or community college. Graduate education in nursing is also available at both the master's and doctoral levels. In 1993, there were 29 basic degree, 32 post-basic baccalaureate, 19 master's and eight doctoral degree programs in Canadian universities (CNA, 1996).

THE BACCALAUREATE AS ENTRY TO PRACTICE

Concerned about the increasing responsibilities that RNs were expected to assume in response to the changing demands of health care, the Canadian Nurses Association in 1982 recommended the baccalaureate as entry level for professional practice. Since then there has been a tremendous amount of activity in all provinces as nurses at all levels debated the issue and explored ways and means of accomplishing the target date of 2000 advocated by the CNA.

The result has been a rapid increase in the number of baccalaureate programs in Canada. Some are new programs at universities, but many are collaborative programs that combine diploma and baccalaureate programs. Some of the collaborative programs provide the option of diploma-level exit; some do not. Students exiting at the diploma level may write the examination for registration as a nurse and enter the workforce at that point, with the option to complete their baccalaureate studies at a later date. The goal of the baccalaureate as entry level for professional nursing practice is at varying stages of realization across the country. Five provinces have government support for degree as entry (Manitoba and the four Atlantic Provinces) (CNA, 1993a).

Prince Edward Island has the distinction of having been the first province to move to baccalaureate preparation for all new graduates with the opening of a four-year baccalaureate program at the University of Prince Edward Island in 1992. The first collaborative program in Canada was established by the University of British Columbia and the Vancouver General Hospital Schools of Nursing in 1989. Now, all diploma nursing programs in British Columbia are involved in collaborative programs with a university. The majority of programs will offer both a diploma and a baccalaureate degree. The one exception in British Columbia is the program at Trinity Western University, which initiated a four-year baccalaureate program in nursing in September 1993. The RNABC has issued a policy statement to the effect that the diploma exit is to be phased out as soon as possible (RNABC, 1994).

The University of Alberta has collaborative programs with five diploma programs, and the University of Calgary has collaborative programs with one. The collaborative programs in Alberta provide diploma level exit at the end of two years at the University of Alberta and at the end of three at the University of Calgary.

In Saskatchewan, a collaborative model has been developed for a four-year baccalaureate program that provides for a diploma exit after three years of study. It is offered collaboratively by the University of Saskatchewan and the two nursing programs at the Saskatchewan Institute of Applied Sciences and Technology.

In Manitoba, with government support, the Health Sciences Centre and St. Boniface Hospital have entered into collaborative arrangements with the University of Manitoba School of Nursing so that all students will graduate with a baccalaureate in nursing from the university. The University of Manitoba also offers a Northern Bachelor of Nursing Program in The Pas at Keewatin College. The remainder of Manitoba's diploma nursing programs are being phased out.

In Ontario, both university and community colleges offer programs in nursing education. Discussions have taken place on a province-wide approach to the restructuring of nursing education programs. However, to date, only isolated activities have been undertaken, such as the collaboration of some community colleges with nearby universities.

In Quebec, during the Quiet Revolution of the 1960s and 1970s, colleges and universities were restructured to form an educational continuum, with university programs building on those of the colleges. Students graduating from CEGEP diploma programs in nursing have access to degree programs at the Universities of McGill, Montreal, Sherbrooke, Laval and five campuses of the Université de Québec. The Order of Nurses of Quebec (the professional voice and regulating authority for registered nurses) recognizes the need for baccalaureate preparation for RNs in order to meet evolving health needs, and is supporting the development of basic nursing programs at universities that do not already have one. The University of Quebec at Hull opened a basic program in 1994; one at the University of Quebec at Trois-Rivières admitted its first class in the fall of 1995. Sherbrooke, Rimouski, Chicoutimi and Abitibi-Temiscamingue are also sites for basic programs.

In New Brunswick, the government has given support to baccalaureate education for nurses. Seven schools worked together to develop a curriculum. There is an English multisite program by the University of New Brunswick and a French multisite program by L'Université de Moncton.

In Nova Scotia, a university degree is the only entry to practice. A collaborative baccalaureate program is in effect among Dalhousie University, Queen Elizabeth II Health Science Centre, IWK Health Centre–Grace, the Reproductive Care program of Nova Scotia, and the Western Regional Health Centre (Yarmouth).

In Newfoundland, with government support, a single, province-wide nursing program that all schools deliver has been developed. Under this program, students are able to take courses at one of three sites and graduate with a baccalaureate degree in nursing from Memorial University. The last diploma students graduated in 1998.

Nursing Programs for the First Nations People

There are approximately 263 000 registered nurses in Canada, but only about 400 are of aboriginal ancestry (CNA, April 1995). During the past decade, a number of programs have developed to help the First Nations People to access nursing education. A diploma program opened in September 1994 at Arctic College in the Northwest Territories to bring the programs closer to home for people of the Territories. Upgrading courses to prepare students for the first year of the course were started in September 1993. The program lasts two years, followed by a one-semester practicum. Students who wish to take further studies may do so at one of the southern universities. The University of Manitoba established a Northern Bachelor of Nursing Program for registered nurses at Keewatin College in 1990 and a generic baccalaureate program at Norway House in 1996. The Keewatin program's goal is to provide aboriginal and northern nurses with the opportunity to gain advanced clinical and communication skills in order to meet the health care needs of isolated communities. In order to get more First Nations People involved in the health field, a National Nurses Access program was also developed. This program lasts nine weeks and is intended to orient First Nations students to nursing and to the intensity of a university progam. On successful completion of the program, access to a diploma or degree program of the student's choice is negotiated. Access programs are offered at the University of Saskatchewan and at Lakehead University in Northern Ontario. Other programs that provide special support for First Nations students include John Abbott College in St. Anne-de-Bellevue, Quebec, and the Indian Diploma Nursing Progam at the Saskatchewan Institute of Technology in North Battleford (CNA, 1993b; April 1995).

Continuing Education

"The Canadian Nurses Association considers continuing nursing education as vital to nurses in the maintenance of professional competence throughout their careers" (CNA, 1992, p. 1). Continuing education includes self-study—the professional reading of journals, new texts and other literature and the gaining of new and varied clinical experiences—as well as the in-service educational programs run by agencies for their staff; short continuing education programs sponsored by various agencies, professional associations and educational institutions; and formal educational programs offered by educational institutions. These formal programs are often referred to as **post-basic education**, particularly when they lead to a certificate, diploma or degree.

Early in the development of nursing education in Canada, nurses recognized that post-basic education was necessary to practise in specialized fields. The earliest post-basic programs that developed were in community health nursing and in teaching and administration. Hospitals also felt the need for nurses to have additional knowledge and skills in areas such as obstetric and neurosurgical nursing and the operating room. Most of the larger hospitals across the country developed post-basic courses in clinical nursing specialties. Graduates of the programs received a certificate attesting to their competence in a particular field. These hospital postgraduate courses unfortunately had the same flaw as the early hospital diploma programs and were accused of exploiting students. Although there were some very good programs, in many of them the postgraduate students were used simply as extra staff and given little in the way of education. When the diploma nursing programs moved into community colleges and other postsecondary educational institutions, the postgraduate programs were also transferred there, a move that has provided them with a more sound educational base.

A relatively recent movement has seen the predominantly college-based programs being accorded university transfer credit, and, in some instances—as at the University of Ottawa—incorporated into basic and post-basic baccalaureate programs (Du Gas & Casey, 1989). Another interesting program is a collaborative one between the B.C. Institute of Technology and the Open Learning Agency of British Columbia, which permits nurses holding advanced diplomas in various clinical specialties to complete requirements for a baccalaureate degree in health sciences, with full transfer of credits (the equivalent of one year) for the post-basic program. Another development was the transfer of the Introduction to Nursing Management Distance Education Program, jointly operated by the CNA and the Canadian Hospital Association, to McMaster University in the fall of 1993 ("Collaborative project in Nova Scotia," 1993).

CNA CERTIFICATION PROGRAM

The many changes in nursing and in health care in Canada have made it very difficult for nurses to acquire all the knowledge required to practise in all settings. Because of this, nursing practice is becoming increasingly specialized. There has been a lack of agreement and some confusion, however, over just what is a specialty, what the requirements to practise in the specialty should be and how continued competence in the specialty can be assessed and assured. In order to address some of these issues, the CNA (1982) developed a policy statement on specialization and certification. In its statement, a **specialty** is defined as "a specifically defined area of clinical and functional nursing with a narrowed, in-depth focus, necessary for the safe delivery of the full range of services required in that area of nursing" (CNA, 1982, p. 1). Since 1991, when only 47 nurses were certified in one specialty (neuroscience), the CNA's certification program has grown rapidly. As of 1997, over 5500 registered nurses hold certification in one of eight specialties: critical care, emergency, nephrology, neuroscience, occupational health, oncology, perioperative and psychiatric mental health. In addition, work is underway on a gerontology examination, which will be offered for the first time in Spring 1999.

The CNA's **certification** process includes the designation of a specialty, the development of an examination by Assessment Strategies Incorporated and the certification of individuals. Candidates must meet the eligibility requirements established for that specialty. On passing the examination in their selected specialty through the CNA certification program, an individual is certified for a period of five years. Recertification normally requires a specified minimum amount of time in practice, a certain number of continuing education hours and a satisfactory performance appraisal. The CNA distinguishes the nurse who acquires certification through this process from the clinical nurse specialist, who is a registered nurse with advanced preparation in a clinical area at the master's or doctoral level (CNA, 1993d).

POST-RN BACCALAUREATE

An increased demand by registered nurses across the country for access to post-basic baccalaureate programs has led to the expansion of these programs by university nursing schools and to new and innovative ways of delivering courses. Currently, post-basic baccalaureate programs are offered at 32 universities, and many offer courses by distance education (CNA, 1996). Information is available from provincial nursing associations. The Registered Nurses Association of Ontario produces an annual publication listing offerings by various schools, the association and other agencies in the province.

GRADUATE EDUCATION FOR NURSES IN CANADA

Master's-Level Programs

In 1996, programs leading to a master's degree in nursing, or in nursing science, were offered at 19 universities in Canada. The programs are two years in length if taken on a full-time basis; provision is also made for those who wish to study on a part-time basis. Prior to 1965, the emphasis in master's-level nursing programs in Canada was on teaching and administration—mainly in the hospital field. Since the early 1970s, the focus has changed to include the opportunity to gain increased knowledge and skills in clinical specialties.

The number of applicants for master's-level programs far exceeds the number of places available, with the result that many nurses pursue graduate studies in other disciplines. In 1996, of the 8463 master's-prepared nurses in Canada, approximately one-half held master's degrees in disciplines other than nursing, such as in education and social sciences (CNA, 1996).

Doctoral Programs in Nursing

Doctoral programs in nursing were slow to develop in Canada. Nurses wishing to pursue studies at the doctoral level have until recently enrolled either in doctoral programs outside Canada, or in doctoral programs in other disciplines, such as education, the social sciences and epidemiology. The first person to complete requirements for a PhD in nursing at a Canadian university graduated from a conjoint program offered by McGill University and the Université de Montréal in 1990 (Field, Stinson & Thibaudeau, 1992). By 1996, there were eight programs offering a research degree with a focus on nursing at the doctoral level—Université de Montréal with McGill University; University of Alberta; University of British Columbia; University of Toronto; McMaster University; University of Calgary; University of Victoria; and University of Sherbrooke. The program of studies, which includes formal course work and a major research study, usually requires three to five years for completion (CNA, 1996).

Nursing's Role in Health Care

The International Council of Nurses has stated that "the fundamental responsibility of the nurse is fourfold: to promote health, to prevent illness, to restore health, and to alleviate suffering" (ICN, 1975).

In carrying out their responsibilities, nurses assist individuals, families and communities in the promotion of health and the prevention of illness; they minister to the needs of the sick, helping them to the fullest restoration of health compatible with their illness, or providing comfort and support in the event of incurable disease. In so doing, nurses work in close collaboration with patients and their families, with the members of other health disciplines and, increasingly, with people in sectors of the community other than health.

Domains of Nursing Practice

Dr. Patricia Benner identifies seven aspects of the nurse's role, which she calls "domains of nursing practice":

- the helping role
- the teaching–coaching function
- the diagnostic and patient monitoring function
- the effective management of rapidly changing situations
- the administering and monitoring of therapeutic interventions and regimes
- the monitoring and ensuring of the quality of health care practices
- the organizational and work-role competencies (Benner, 1984, p. 46).

To this list of nursing practice domains, we would add an eighth, relating to the nurse's role in primary health care: community development.

HELPING

From its inception, nursing's nurturing quality has been best evidenced in the helping aspects of the nurse's role. In the home and in the community, the nurse is a resource for patient and family, providing information about health matters and helping people to cope with developmental and emotional changes in their lives as well as the changes that illness brings. In caring for people who are ill, in the home or in an inpatient facility, the nurse assists patients to carry out those activities that they would do for themselves if they were capable. Much of nursing action is thus concerned with the daily living of patients, helping them to meet their basic needs for water, food, rest and sleep and to maintain normal body functioning. A large part of the helping function is the provision of comfort and support for patients and their families.

Comfort and support may be offered through touch. Sometimes, it is just a matter of taking the other person's hand or helping him or her to walk down the hall. The gentle art of listening is also part of the provision of comfort and support. Just being with patients is enough to convey that you are there to help—for example, when they have to undergo a painful procedure.

A large part of the nurse's helping role is concerned with assisting the person and the family to cope with illness and the stress and anxiety that accompany even the slightest deviations from health. In all these activities the nurse works with the patients, helping them to regain their independence as rapidly as possible and to take control of their own health. Carrying out nursing activities with compassion, with empathetic understanding and with respect for the patient as an individual of worth and dignity is essential in the helping role of the nurse.

TEACHING–COACHING

Teaching is a very important part of nursing care. It may involve such diverse activities as advising new mothers how to breastfeed their babies, teaching hygiene and nutrition to school children, helping people with diabetes to plan a diet compatible with their health problem, teaching deep-breathing exercises to a patient before surgery to prevent postoperative complications or helping a person to cope with the activities of daily living after he or she has been handicapped by illness. The nurse also teaches the patient and family members to carry out care at home.

DIAGNOSTICS AND PATIENT MONITORING

Many of the nurse's activities are concerned with the detection and treatment of illness. In the initial examination of an individual, the nurse assesses the patient's potential for wellness. Nurses prepare patients for diagnostic tests, many of them involving complex procedures. They must be able to explain the nature and purpose of the tests to the patient. Because nurses understand the particular demands and usual experiences of various illnesses, they are able to anticipate the patient's needs. They become very skilled at detecting significant changes in a patient's condition and taking appropriate action, either by intervening themselves or by alerting those who need to be made aware of the changes. The nurse's careful documentation of observations is invaluable for the continuity of care for the patient, as well as providing a legal record.

EFFECTIVE MANAGEMENT OF RAPIDLY CHANGING SITUATIONS

Nurses often find themselves in life-threatening emergencies that require a rapid grasp of the situation and an ability to carry out emergency measures with skill and competence. Identifying and managing a patient crisis until physician assistance is available is something you will learn to do and will become comfortable in doing as you gain knowledge, skills and experience.

ADMINISTERING AND MONITORING THERAPEUTIC INTERVENTIONS AND REGIMENS

Nurses carry out a number of therapeutic measures that are part of the plan of care for each patient. The administration of medications and the carrying out of treatments are therapeutic measures typically undertaken by nurses. Nurses also monitor the effects of therapeutic measures and must be alert to untoward reactions that the patient may have to drugs or treatments. Today, the nurse is responsible for carrying out and monitoring increasingly complex therapeutic regimens. Nurses are expected to start and maintain intravenous therapy with minimal risks to the patient, to administer total parenteral nutrition and to interpret the readings from cardiac monitors. They must also be skilled in the care of wounds and in combatting the hazards of immobility (all these techniques are detailed in later chapters of this text).

MONITORING AND ENSURING THE QUALITY OF HEALTH CARE PRACTICES

In this domain of practice, the nurse acts as the patient's advocate. As the health care system has become more complex with a multitude of different agencies and an increasing variety of workers concerned with different aspects of health care, patients need someone who can help them speak for themselves. Sometimes nurses intercede on their patients' behalf. This advocacy is an important role in nursing care.

In the community people often do not know about (or if they do know, they have difficulty accessing) the services that are available to help them with their problems. This is particularly true of people in low-income groups and new immigrants. The nurse, with knowledge of the services offered by government and various community agencies, can facilitate access to appropriate resources.

In an inpatient facility, the multitude of health professionals who do things for and to a patient seems never-ending. Some patients have reported as many as 50 employees who were in and out of their hospital room during one day. The patient needs one person to whom he or she can relate in a meaningful way and who can act as the patient's spokesperson with other members of the health team.

ORGANIZATIONAL AND WORK-ROLE COMPETENCIES

The coordinating aspects of the nurse's role have become increasingly important as health agencies have become decentralized. As a result, more responsibility and authority have been given to the individual nurse. It is the nurse who establishes a plan of care for the patient and serves as coordinator for all activities. In this, the nurse works in close collaboration with the patient, his or her family, the patient's physician and all other members of the health team. The nurse plans and supervises the care given by auxiliary nursing personnel, such as the LPN, the nurse's aide, and the various people who help with the provision of home care services. In addition, the nurse consults with other health professionals regarding the delivery of care.

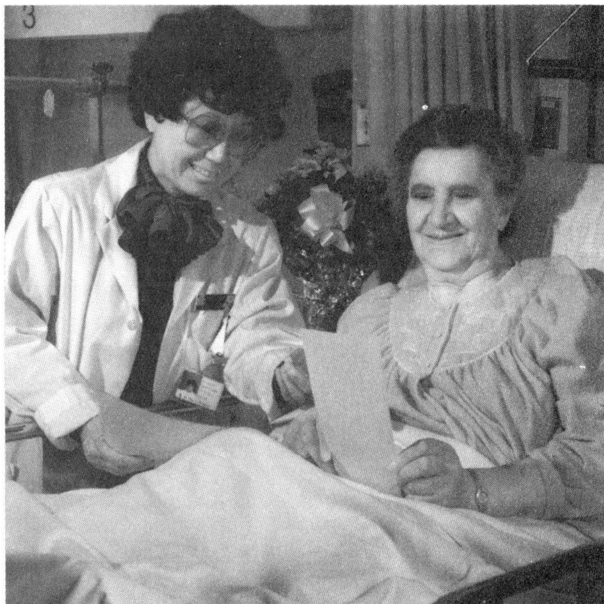

Community health nurse discussing home care services with a patient who is about to be discharged.

COMMUNITY DEVELOPMENT

Many nurses are now functioning in a community development role, helping people to identify their health concerns and to plan and organize actions relating to their concerns. In this role, the nurse works as a partner with community groups, rather than as a "doer-provider" of services, facilitating the process of identification of health needs and serving as a resource for information about programs and services to help communities meet their health needs. In order to carry out this role, nurses identify and work with social networks in the community and with lay support groups (e.g., the Multiple Sclerosis Society) and other volunteer organizations and agencies in the community.

Career Choices for Nurses

At the present time, the majority (61.3%) of professional nurses in Canada are employed in general and psychiatric hospitals. Another large number (11.5%) are employed in nursing homes and in rehabilitation centres that provide residential care. Approximately 10.3% work in nursing stations, in home care or in community health agencies. The expansion of community health services in every province has meant that more nurses are working outside of hospitals (see Figure 5.2 and Table 5.1)—in home care, in community health centres and clinics, and in other types

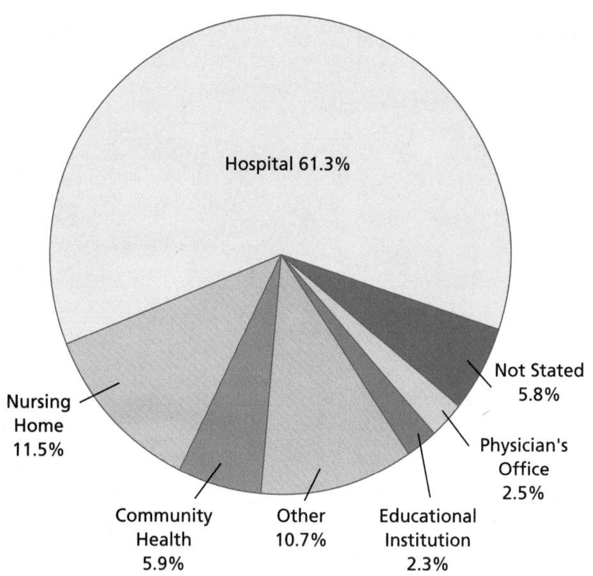

FIGURE 5.2 Settings for practice: Registered nurses in Canada, 1996

SOURCE: Statistics Canada, 1996. Prepared by: Policy, Regulation and Research Division, CNA, 1997b.

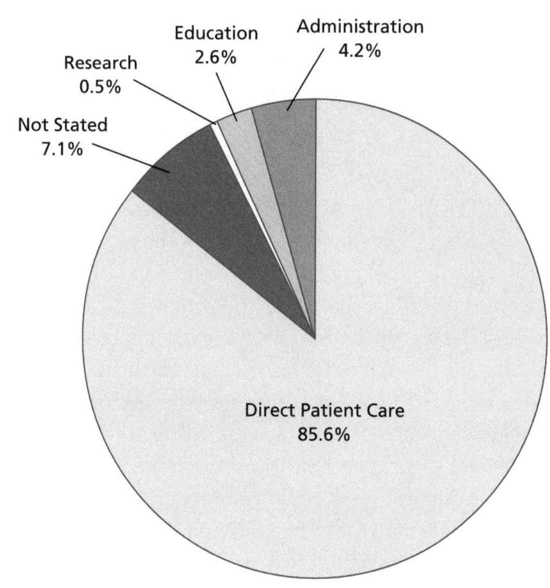

FIGURE 5.3 Registered nurses employed in nursing in Canada by primary area of responsibility, 1996

SOURCE: Statistics Canada, 1996. Prepared by: Policy, Regulation and Research Division, CNA, 1997b.

TABLE 5.1 Registered nurses employed in nursing in Canada by place of employment and education, 1996

Place of Employment	*Education*					
	TOTAL	RN DIPLOMA	BACCALAUREATE	MASTER'S	DOCTORATE	NOT STATED
Total	227 830	171 770	40 740	3 502	164	11 654
Hospital	139 680	116 665	21 298	1 685	32	0
Nursing Home	26 254	22 965	3 053	228	8	0
Community Health	13 379	6 238	6 852	286	3	0
Physician's Office	5 615	5 014	579	21	1	0
Educational Institution	5 265	1 748	2 642	776	99	0
Other	24 357	17 835	6 033	471	18	0
Not Stated	13 280	1 305	283	35	3	11 654

SOURCE: Statistics Canada, 1996. Prepared by: Policy, Regulation and Research Division, CNA,1997b.

TABLE 5.2 Registered nurses employed in nursing in Canada by type of employment and education, 1996

Position	*Education*					
	TOTAL	RN DIPLOMA	BACCALAUREATE	MASTER'S	DOCTORATE	NOT STATED
Total	100.0%	100.0%	100.0%	100.0%	100.0%	100.0%
Director	1.8	1.4	3.5	10.6	7.9	0.0
Supervisor	3.8	3.4	6.1	6.6	0.6	0.0
Clinical Specialist	0.8	0.6	1.1	11.7	1.8	0.0
Head Nurse	3.6	3.4	5.5	5.9	3.7	0.0
Staff Nurse	69.8	77.9	59.5	22.8	13.4	0.0
Instructor	2.2	0.8	6.8	20.5	52.4	0.0
Other	7.7	6.9	12.2	15.6	15.9	0.0
Not Stated	10.4	5.6	5.3	6.3	4.3	100.0

SOURCE: Statistics Canada, 1996. Prepared by: Policy, Regulation and Research Division, CNA, 1997b.

of health services. Many nurses (approximately 1% of the total of employed nurses in the country) work in business and industry. Around five thousand nurses (2.3% of employed RNs) work in educational institutions, and an almost equal number in physicians' offices. A growing number of nurses are employed by private, for-profit and nonprofit entrepreneurial agencies that furnish home care and hospital replacement services, and still others are self-employed (Statistics Canada, 1996).

Most of the nurses with baccalaureate or higher degrees work in hospitals, but many are employed in community health. The majority are involved in direct patient care, either as general duty or staff nurses, or as clinical specialists. Many are employed in administrative positions such as directors, nurse managers, supervisors or coordinators, or assistants (see Figure 5.3 and Table 5.2).

Nurses graduating from educational programs in Canada today have a promising future. According to Employment and Immigration Canada projections, the demand for nurses, which has been growing steadily over the past 30 years, will continue to surpass employment opportunities for people in most other fields.

The continually increasing demand for registered nurses is the result of a number of factors. There has been an increase in all-RN staffing in hospitals. The role of RNs in health care delivery is expanding, and the increasing technical complexities of patient care require the services of a growing number of highly skilled nurses. Although the current downsizing of hospitals, combined with the effects of a nation-wide recession, has caused some concern over job opportunities for nurses, projections anticipate a marked increase in the number of nursing positions becoming available over the next few years. Nurses holding university degrees and those with specialty training, such as intensive care, gerontological nursing and surgical nursing, will be in great demand (CNA, 1997b).

Nurses today have the opportunity to choose from a wide range of career options. We have selected a few to discuss here. These include hospital nursing, clinical nursing, administration, education, research, long-term care, community health nursing, outpost nursing, office nursing, occupational health nursing, military nursing, midwifery, independent practice, consultancy in international development, and provision of expanded health services.

Hospital Nursing

Almost two-thirds of all employed nurses in Canada work in general or psychiatric hospitals, most as general staff nurses (Statistics Canada, 1996). The duties and responsibilities of staff nurses vary, depending on the agency in which they are employed, although all are guided by the standards of practice established by regulating authorities. In hospitals, nurses may work in any one of a number of areas, such as medical-surgical nursing, maternal-newborn, critical care or extended (long-term) care nursing, pediatric nursing, psychiatric nursing or in specialized units such as emergency, the operating room or intensive care.

Clinical Nursing

Many nurses who want to have a career in clinical nursing are choosing to increase their knowledge and skills in a particular field through further education. Numerous courses are available in fields such as gerontology (care of the older adult), psychiatric/mental health nursing, critical care nursing, advanced obstetric nursing, nursing of the high-risk newborn and palliative care nursing (care of people with terminal illness). Increasingly, these courses are carrying university credits for transfer towards a degree in nursing. Nurses who wish to advance further in their chosen field through the clinical ladder may opt to become clinical specialists. In 1996, there were a total of 400 clinical nurse specialists holding a master's or doctoral degree employed in Canadian health services (Statistics Canada, 1996).

> "The **clinical nurse specialist (CNS)** is a registered nurse who holds a master's or doctoral degree in nursing with expertise in a clinical nursing specialty. An expert practitioner, the CNS provides direct care, education and consultation to clients, as well as education and consultation to the health care team."
>
> **SOURCE:** CNA, 1993d, p.1.

Administration

Some nurses opt to advance in nursing through the administrative ladder. More than 10 percent of employed nurses are in management or administrative positions as managers, supervisors or coordinators. They usually start as **nurse manager**, or charge nurse of a nursing unit. If they wish to advance further in administration, as a director/assistant director of nursing, a vice-president, or chief executive officer of nursing, a baccalaureate or higher degree in nursing (or in administration of health services) is becoming the expected qualification, although at the present time about one-half (44%) of the nurses in CEO/director positions hold an academic degree (Statistics Canada, 1996).

Education

Just over 5000 nurses, roughly 2.3 percent of the number of employed nurses in Canada, are engaged in education (Statistics Canada, 1996). The field of education has three distinct sub-fields — all involve teaching, but to different groups of people:

1. patient education
2. in-service education for employees of health agencies
3. nursing education (i.e., teaching students).

All three areas are growing. The emphasis on health promotion today, as well as on teaching people to protect their health and to cope with the complex therapies used when they are ill, has made patient education one of the most important aspects of care for people. In-service education in a health agency involves a wide range of activities, including hosting orientation programs for new employees, teaching new knowledge and skills to keep nurses and other health workers up-to-date with advances in their field, and holding conferences, teaching programs and other short, continuing education programs for people working in the agency and, often, in other agencies as well. For example, a regional hospital, such as the Prince George Regional Hospital in central British Columbia, will often have in-service education programs for their nurses, which they will share with nurses from smaller hospitals in the region. The majority of nurses engaged in teaching are, however, in schools of nursing. As the preparation of nurses has moved into colleges and universities, the academic credentials of nursing teachers have needed to meet the standard set for teaching faculty in other disciplines. This standard is usually a minimum of a baccalaureate degree, preferably a master's degree in colleges and, increasingly, doctoral preparation in university programs.

Research

Although research is a part of every RN's practice, a steadily increasing number have dedicated their career to nursing research. While nurse researchers are still few in number in Canada, it is becoming evident that research is no longer the domain of academics only. Nurses in service agencies are questioning traditional nursing practices and are seeking to validate their actions through research (Brown, 1993). The benefits of research are also being recognized by hospitals and other health agencies. Administrators are encouraging nurses to use research as a method of developing more efficient and more effective nursing interventions. Of the 1006 nurses who consider themselves researchers, fewer than one-half (47.3%) were employed in general and psychiatric hospitals (Statistics Canada, 1996). These figures are slightly misleading, however, because research is also an essential component of the role of nurses on university faculty who consider themselves primarily to be teachers. At the present time, there are still few nurses qualified at the master's or doctoral level in Canada—the usual educational requirement considered necessary for research—but many hospitals and other agencies are making use of the few who have had preparation in research by having them act as research facilitators to enable staff nurses to conduct studies. The role of research in nursing practice is discussed further in Chapter 7.

Long-Term Care

The field of long-term care is an expanding one, first, because of the increased number of older persons in our society and second, because of the devastating number of people injured in motor vehicle and other accidents who require long-term care and rehabilitation. Long-term care includes both inpatient nursing services in nursing homes and rehabilitation centres and the provision of nursing services in the community to those who require direct care or monitoring over an extended period of time. The nurse's role in long-term care has many facets. In both community and inpatient facilities, it is usually registered nurses who undertake the initial assessment of the health care needs of individuals (and of family members); and it is the RNs who develop the plans of care, in conjunction with the members of other health disciplines, such as physicians, physiotherapists and social workers. Registered nurses provide high-level technical and complex care for those who need it, as well as palliative and bereavement care for individuals with terminal illnesses and their families. They also often have to sort out and manage the multiple medications taken by people in long-term care. They have a major teaching role with both the individual's family and with other care workers, teaching them to carry out a plan of care and to monitor procedures such as intravenous therapy. Another important function of nurses in long-term care is that of patient advocate (Blunt, 1992).

Community Health Nursing

The community health field is also one that is growing rapidly. At the present time, approximately 13 379 nurses are employed in community health agencies, and another 9064 in home care (Statistics Canada, 1996). These numbers are expected to increase considerably in the next few years. As hospitals are downsized and community services expanded, provincial governments are encouraging nursing schools to offer specific courses to enable hospital nurses to make the transfer to community services. They are also encouraging nurses to enrol in post-basic courses. The role of the nurse in the community is discussed further in Chapter 11. This is an exciting field in which nurses have an opportunity to be involved in a much broader role in the implementing of primary health care.

In recent years, nurse-managed health clinics have been established in urban centres in a number of provinces (Attridge et al., 1997). Initiated as pilot projects, these clinics allow RNs to be the access point to the health care system. Assessment, treatment or referral, follow-up, illness prevention and health promotion are the major areas of emphasis for these nurses.

Public health nurses (PHNs) play a major role in our society in health promotion and illness prevention throughout the life span. These nurses work in homes, schools and communities, assisting parents with newborns, immunizing and screening school children, dealing with infection control, and participating in other activities such as supporting independence in the elderly.

Although relatively new in Canada, *parish nursing* is felt to be an effective component of community health care. A parish nurse is a registered nurse who delivers primary health care in congregations and is on the ministerial team. The nurse focusses on the physical, mental and spiritual wellness of the individual or family.

Outpost Nursing

Working in Canada's North and other isolated areas has always had a special attraction for Canadian nurses—and for nurses from many other countries. On outposts in the North and elsewhere, community health nurses are employed in nursing stations and in health centres with and without treatment facilities. These nurses have a much broader scope of practice than in communities in southern Canada. In nursing stations and in health centres that provide treatment services, community health nurses are required to be knowledgeable and skillful in recognizing and managing common medical disorders and pediatric problems, as well as common obstetric conditions throughout the maternity cycle for low-risk obstetric patients. They are also responsible for acute emergency care and initial management of problems requiring medical and surgical intervention, for the temporary management of people with psychiatric problems, and for temporary management of patients with more serious medical, pediatric or obstetric problems. They also prepare patients for and manage them during emergency evacuations, when a medical or nursing escort is required. Further discussion of RNs' provision of expanded health services appears at the end of this section.

All community health nurses in nursing stations or health centres are expected to be able to provide the appropriate care, including referral, for an extensive list of community health program areas. Responsibilities include health education, promotion and prevention services in communicable disease control, maternal/child health, preschool health, school health and adult health, plus such areas as family violence, substance abuse, dental health and environmental health. Proficiency is also required in nutrition, physical fitness, injury prevention, occupational health, disaster management and home nursing care.

Preparatory programs to enable nurses to practice in the expanded role required by isolated health services are available through Lakehead University in Ontario and at the University of Manitoba. For nurses in Quebec who are hired by the province or by First Nations Councils, the University of Quebec at Trois-Rivières offers a program (Cruikshank, 1997).

Office Nursing

A few more nurses (5615) work in physicians' offices than in teaching (Statistics Canada, 1996). The usual pattern is for the nurse to work in collaboration with one physician in solo practice or with two or more physicians in a group practice in the community. At the present time, most nurses play a traditional role, assisting the physician in his or her practice. We can anticipate, however, that an increasing number of nurses will become employed in collaborative practice (rather than purely as assistants) with physicians in the community, in doctors' offices, community health centres and health service organizations as these develop.

Two factors facilitate an expanded role for nurses in collaborative roles with physicians and in independent practice: first, the changes occurring in Health Practice Acts in various provinces that legitimize an expanded scope of practice for nurses; and second, a clause in the Canada Health Act (1984) permitting "qualified health practitioners other than physicians and dentists" (Adaskin, 1988, p. 475) to be reimbursed for their services, providing this does not conflict with provincial legislation. This clause makes it possible for services provided by nurses to be insurable.

Occupational Health Nursing

Approximately 2400 nurses are employed in business or industry in Canada. Traditionally, the role of the **occupational health nurse (OHN)** has included rendering emergency care to people who are injured or become ill at work, as well as providing health counselling, health promotion and health protection services for employees. An important aspect of these nurses' work has always been participating in safety programs in the working environment. Although accident prevention, health protection and emergency care are still regarded as important, increasing attention is being paid to stress—both home- and work-related—as a major factor in employee productivity and absenteeism. This recognition of the role of stress, along with today's emphasis on health promotion, has shifted the emphasis in occupational health to wellness programs. Many corporations are hiring "wellness coordinators," whose role is to design and implement health promotion programs for employees. Professionals from other disciplines, such as teachers, social workers and fitness experts, are vying for these positions too. Nurses, particularly community health and occupational health nurses, are in a good position vis-à-vis candidates from other disciplines, because of their preparation in health promotion and their broad background in health matters. Courses in occupational health nursing are offered at various schools across the country—at the University of Ottawa as a concentration in Community Health/Occupational Health Nursing at the baccalaureate level, and as a post-basic diploma or certificate program at some other schools. A 16-week post-diploma certificate program in Wellness and Lifestyle is offered at Centennial College in Toronto (Farr, 1990; Thomas, 1993).

Military Nursing

A total of 246 registered nurses and 58 nurses' aides are currently serving with the Canadian armed services (Gagné, 1998). They work in Department of National Defence hospitals and in field units in Canada and abroad. Canada has the distinction of being the first country to confer officer status on nurses serving with the armed forces. A Canadian nursing service became an integral part of the Army Medical Corps in 1901, and nursing sisters were accorded the rank, status and pay of lieutenant (Nicholson, 1975).

The distinguished history of Canadian nurses in the Riel Rebellion, the Boer War, World Wars I and II and the Korean War makes for fascinating reading (Feasby, 1946; Gibbon & Mathewson, 1947; McPhail, 1925; Nicholson, 1975; Wilson-Simmie, 1981). Nurses also served with Canadian forces in the Gulf War.

Midwifery

Midwifery is the care of women and their families throughout the maternity cycle, which begins before pregnancy and ends approximately six weeks after birth. Its mandate is to provide care for normal, rather than high-risk pregnancies. Midwives refer high-risk women to family practice physicians or obstetricians for care. Until recently, Canada was one of the few countries in the world where midwifery was not a legal practice. Up to now, educational programs in midwifery have focussed mainly on preparing nurses to work in the missionary field abroad, in outpost nursing stations in the Canadian North or in other isolated parts of the country. At the present time, two university schools of nursing offer midwifery courses for registered nurses. At the University of Alberta, a Midwifery Certificate is offered in conjunction with the master's degree in nursing. At Dalhousie University in Halifax, a 15-month Outpost Nursing Program includes midwifery preparation, with emphasis on comprehensive care throughout the maternity cycle.

The practice of midwifery has now been legalized as an autonomous discipline in the provinces of Manitoba, Ontario, Alberta and British Columbia. There is no doubt that other provinces will follow suit. The Midwifery Act in Ontario permits the practice of midwifery by direct-entry practitioners as well as by RN-midwives. The term "single-trained midwife" is also sometimes used instead of "direct-entry practitioner" to refer to an individual who has entered a midwifery program without having first qualified as a nurse. In some countries, midwives must be qualified nurses before they can enter a midwifery program; in other countries, there may be both direct-entry practitioners of midwifery and nurse-midwives. McMaster University's Faculty of Health Sciences, Laurentian University in Sudbury and Ryerson Polytechnic University in Toronto have collaborated on a program that will lead to a Bachelor of Health Sciences in midwifery. The first students were enrolled in the program in September, 1993.

Independent Practice

"A job is not only about money. A job is also about satisfaction and what you can do with your knowledge" (Mongeon-Meredith; cited in Brown, 1993, p. 15). Entrepreneurship is attracting a growing number of nurses in Canada. There were an estimated 1533 self-employed registered nurses in Canada in 1996. These nurses offer counselling, educational and administrative services on a consulting basis, as well as providing direct nursing care to the public on a fee-for-service basis. They offer a wide range of services, such as midwifery, mental health counselling, family counselling, sexual counselling, holistic nursing care and wellness education. They also offer consultant services in education (as curriculum development consultants, for example), in nursing administration and in research. Many Canadian nurses have served, and continue to serve, as consultants in various fields in international nursing with agencies such as the World Health Organization and the Canadian International Development Association.

International Development

The most familiar form of nursing work related to international development is assignments to developing countries. Such postings through agencies like the Red Cross and Canadian International Development Agency (CIDA) usually attract nurses for the adventure and because of a concern for humanity. Assignments can be for emergency relief to a war zone or natural disaster area, or to implement public health and primary health care initiatives such as immunization, maternal/child care and development of community health workers.

Another area for international involvement is liaison between countries that are at a similar stage of development and economy. Practice issues are compared and projects established to examine and improve nursing care in all partner nations. A third focus for international work is supporting the development of the nursing profession. Typically, many countries participate in any one nation's project, with nurse consultants offering expertise in a variety of areas such as education, development of an association, political action, legislation and regulation. Most overseas positions require education at the university level (Sibbald, 1997b).

Provision of Expanded Nursing Services

Over the past few decades, expanded practice roles have evolved for registered nurses. Familiar examples of such roles are clinical nurse specialist and nurse practitioner. A variety of other titles and roles have also been developed in response to local needs (e.g., expanded role nurse, case manager, physician's assistant, clinician nurse). Whatever the title, the role usually involves an increased emphasis on health assessment, health promotion and illness prevention, for which the knowledge and skills are obtained through additional educational preparation.

A recent ruling by the B.C. Ministry of Health, which does not contravene the Hospital Act, allows nurses who take first call to admit and discharge patients with minor health problems from the emergency department at Ashcroft District General Hospital (Griffiths, 1997).

Nurse Practitioners

The development of the position of **nurse practitioner** that took place in the United States in the 1970s was not paralleled in Canada. The Report of the Committee on Nurse Practitioners (Boudreau, 1972) viewed the Nurse Practitioner's role as "an extension of the present nursing role with [the nurse's] unique skills in the care of the patient being developed and utilized more effectively" and as "complementary to that of the physician and other members of the health team" (p. 5). Although a number of nurse practitioner programs were established in Canada in the early 1970s, these programs were viewed as temporary measures until such time as preparation for an expanded role could be incorporated into basic educational programs.

There are, however, a number of graduates of nurse practitioner programs who have continued to practice and have formed an association. The Nurse Practitioner Association of Ontario defines the nurse practitioner as:

> *. . . a nurse specializing in primary health care, with advanced knowledge and decision-making skills, built on basic nursing education preparation, and emphasizing health promotion and disease prevention.*

In the same document, primary health care was defined as:

> *. . .[the patient's] first contact with the health care system and offers comprehensive and continuous care. Comprehensive primary health care may require collaboration with and referrals to other health professionals and health resources.* (Standards of Practice for Nurse Practitioners, March 1993. Cited in Marchand & Goodine, 1993, p. 10.)

There has recently been interest by provincial governments in the re-establishment of nurse practitioner programs. The Ontario Government has worked with universities to implement programs to prepare registered nurses for this role. In June 1997, the Expanded Nursing Services for Patients Act was passed, allowing a greater scope of practice for these nurses. It is expected that the nurse practitioners will usually be the first point of contact for people with the health care system and may work independently or as part of a health team (Haines, 1993b).

Modes of Practice

The vast majority of nurses in Canada still work in hospitals—and it is on the hospital wards that you will have much of your clinical practice as students. It is helpful, then, to understand how nurses function in hospitals. The most common mode of practice for nurses in hospitals today is primary nursing, although other patterns are developing for the organization of nursing services.

Primary Nursing

Primary nursing is "a system of delivering nursing services where the nurse is responsible for planning complete 24-hour care for each patient" ("What's the difference?" 1992, p. 2). It has become a fairly standard mode of practice in hospitals in this country in the last decade. In this type of nursing, each patient is assigned, on admission, to a specific (primary) nurse. Originally, this nurse was responsible for the patient's care throughout the hospital stay; in practical terms, however, the nurse cares for this patient throughout a tour of shifts, which may be three, four or five days depending on rotation patterns. The primary nurse plans for the patient's needs over the 24-hour period and gives direct care when on duty. Through the use of nursing care plans, conferences, referrals and collaboration with other nurses, the primary nurse guides and supervises the patient's care when not on duty. The primary nurse sees the patient with the physician when he or she is making rounds, confers with the physician about the patient's care and confers with other health team members, such as the physical therapist, who may be involved in the patient's care. The usual caseload varies depending on the area and the complexity of patient care.

Modular Nursing

In **modular nursing**, the nurse is assigned a group of patients, usually eight to 12 (in acute care settings), whose beds or rooms are close together in the nursing unit. The nurse may have the same group of patients over a period of time. Often other personnel, such as a licensed practical nurse or registered/certified nursing assistant, are also assigned to the module so that it becomes, in essence, a small team. This method may be used in long-term care settings.

Shared Governance

Shared governance is a term used for the organization of hospital patient services in which staff nurses have more autonomy and decision-making authority than in the traditional structure. Sometimes called *participatory management*, shared governance involves general staff nurses in making management decisions. The McKellar General Hospital in Thunder Bay provides one example of a hospital that has successfully implemented shared governance. Its process of change involved staff nurses from the outset, with staff and managers identifying together the changes they wanted made and then creating the desired structure. In the process, they learned to appreciate the special knowledge and skills each brings to patient care. The manager's role has shifted from one of controlling, planning and directing to one of coaching and facilitating. Staff nurses have gained skills in speaking up and expressing their opinions and have learned to take an active role in making management decisions.

Patient-Centred Care

Another new mode is evolving at Sunnybrook Hospital in Toronto. The reorganization of patient services at this hospital was the first of its kind in Canada. It involves three components: decentralization of authority, the establishment of patient service units and the development of multiskilled employees. To reflect the philosophy of **patient-centred care**, decision making is being decentralized and put into the hands of those closest to the patient. There are no middle management (supervisory) positions. The hospital is organized around the patient, rather than around departments, with a small number of clinical units, basically encompassing medicine, surgery, long-term care and psychiatry. Each clinical unit is composed of four or five patient service units. The patient service units are made up of like groups of patients, such as patients undergoing circulatory surgery. Each patient service unit becomes, in effect, a mini-hospital, with its own laboratory and basic x-ray equipment, where this is economically feasible, and its own budget. It is felt that nurses can coordinate their work better and get more satisfaction from their work in smaller care teams that focus on patients with similar health problems. The plan includes a system whereby a nurse and a multipurpose worker are assigned to care for a group of patients. The multipurpose worker sees to all the non-nursing, non-professional activities that were carried out by a number of different workers, such as delivering meal trays to the patients, washing the floors and collecting the garbage. There would also be multiskilled administrative personnel and clinical staff who can assist the nurse by doing tasks such as helping patients to ambulate ("Hospitals in transition," 1993).

Program management is a relatively new approach to organizing the delivery of clinical services to specific patient groups in the hospital or the community. Each program or product line (e.g., pediatrics, renal, mental health) has its own budget so that costs can be tracked. The goal is more effective and efficient health care (Haines, 1993a). The program management team is usually composed of a physician, a nursing director and an administrator. The chair of the team usually reports to the chief executive officer or a vice-president. With program management, the traditional line authority and discipline-specific infrastructure often disappear and practitioners are absorbed into the larger structure of the program.

Another approach to organizing the delivery of care is **case management**. Each patient is assigned a case manager who is responsible for coordinating multidisciplinary services to assist the patient to achieve standardized expectations (Lynn & Kelley, 1997). Care maps or pathways guide the service delivery and the appropriate utilization of resources. A care map is a framework that outlines the expected outcomes patient behaviours) at specific times for a particular type of case (e.g., newly diagnosed diabetic). Once a care pathway is in place, the case manager receives reports on any variance and takes action to correct the problem(s). Indicators for the next level of care (e.g., discharge to home or admission to hospital) are preset and clearly outlined.

Nurses and the Political Process

Larsen and Baumgart (1992) likened the nursing profession to a sleeping giant in Canadian public life. The fact that nursing is "the largest nationally organized group in Canadian society made up predominantly of women" (p. 469) provides it with the potential to wield a considerable amount of power. Nurses have traditionally been uncomfortable with power; it is only recently that they have begun to appreciate the importance of taking an active part in the political process to influence public policy.

Dr. Helen Glass (1985) suggested three approaches whereby nursing can influence public policy in the health field. The first is increased public representation by nurses, that is to say, getting nurses elected or appointed to positions on local, provincial and national committees and boards, and electing nurses to city councils, provincial legislatures and Parliament. The second is the integration of nurses into high-level government positions, for example, as Chief Nursing Officer in Ministries of Health. There are also nursing consultants in various branches of Health Canada who wield considerable influence in their areas of expertise, for example, in the development of national guidelines for infection control in hospitals. The third approach suggested by Glass was the use of professional power strategies to influence government decision making. The Canadian Nurses Association and the various provincial associations are becoming much more skilled in using professional power strategies and in encouraging local groups and individual nurses to get involved in the political process.

Canadian nursing's political "coming of age" occurred in 1984 when the Canadian Nurses Association, in collaboration with the provincial nursing associations, succeeded in obtaining passage of a clause amending the Canada Health Act to permit nurses to have a broader role in primary health care (Adaskin, 1988). Since then, the CNA has joined with six other national organizations to form a Health Action Lobby (HEAL) to preserve and protect the principles of the Canadian health care system. The other members of the alliance are the Canadian Hospital Association, the Canadian Medical Association, the Canadian Long-Term Care Association, the Canadian Public Health Association, the Canadian Psychological Association and the Consumers Association. Members of the seven national HEAL organizations discuss issues that affect health care with consumers, politicians and government officials. They were involved, for example, during the 1993 election campaign when it appeared that some parties would institute user fees for Medicare if elected. The Canadian

Nurses Association also published an election handbook entitled *Nurses Know Nurses Can*, which outlined why nurses should be involved in the political process and how they can get involved; gave some facts about nursing that could be helpful in presenting opinions to candidates; and suggested questions to ask of candidates (CNA, 1993b). The CNA has also published a new self-help document, *Getting Started: A Political Action for Registered Nurses* (CNA, 1997a). As nursing at the national level continues to press for health care reform, provincial nursing associations are making their voices heard and their influence felt in the restructuring of health services in their jurisdictions.

IN REVIEW

- Nursing is a dynamic profession whose practice is constantly evolving in response to societal needs. The rapid change in today's health care system requires a change in the nurse's educational preparation and role.
- In Canada, nurses are the largest group of health professionals. Nursing personnel include:
  - registered nurses
  - psychiatric nurses
  - licensed practical nurses
  - nurse's aides
- Practice settings include:
  - hospitals (acute/psychiatric)
  - extended care homes
  - rehabilitation centres
  - communities (home care/prevention)
  - physicians' offices
  - private industry.
- From apprenticeship-like training to baccalaureate preparation in colleges and universities, continuing education is vital for the maintenance of professional competence.
- Benner (1984) identifies seven domains of nursing practice:
  - helping
  - teaching-coaching
  - diagnostics and patient monitoring
  - management of changing situations
  - administration and monitoring of therapeutic interventions and regimes
  - monitoring and ensuring quality of health care and practices
  - organizational and work-role competencies.
- An eighth domain includes community development.
- Career choices for nurses include:
  - hospital nursing
  - clinical nursing
  - administration
  - education
  - research
  - long-term care
  - community health nursing
  - outpost nursing
  - office nursing
  - occupational health nursing
  - military nursing
  - midwifery
  - independent practice
  - international development
  - expanded nursing services (nurse practitioners).
- Modes of nursing practice include:
  - primary nursing
  - modular nursing
  - shared governance
  - patient-centred care
  - program management
  - case management.
- Today the Canadian Nurses Association, provincial nursing associations and nurses at the local level are becoming involved in the political process in order to press for health care reform.

Critical Thinking Activities

1. Explore the history of nursing education in your province:
   a. When were the first hospital schools of nursing started?
   b. Where were they located?
   c. What was the educational program like?
   d. Who were the most notable early nurse educators in the province?
   e. When did the educational preparation of nurses move from hospital schools and where did they move to?
   f. What changes are currently taking place in nursing education in your province?

2. You have been asked to talk at a career day for high school students in your community on basic education for nursing, specialty preparation and career options for nurses. You will be allowed 30 minutes. Outline your presentation.
3. Talk with two nurses—an older retired nurse and one who is in active practice in your community. Explore with each their education for practice and the nature of their practice in terms of the eight domains of practice discussed in the chapter.
4. What role is your provincial nursing association taking with regard to the restructuring of health care in the province? Are there particular issues affecting nursing?

KEY TERMS

skill mix p. 78
nurse's aide p. 79
scope of practice p. 80
multiskilling p. 80
post-basic education p. 84
specialty p. 85
certification p. 85
clinical nurse specialist (CNS) p. 89
nurse manager p. 89
public health nurse (PHN) p. 90
occupational health nurse (OHN) p. 91
midwifery p. 92
nurse practitioner p. 93
primary nursing p. 93
modular nursing p. 93
shared governance p. 93
patient-centred care p. 94
program management p. 94
case management p. 94

References

ADASKIN, E.J. (1988). Organized political action: Lobbying by nurses' actions. In A.J. Baumgart & J. Larsen, *Canadian nursing faces the future* (pp. 474–487). Toronto: Mosby.

ATTRIDGE, C., BUDGEN, C., HILTON, A., MCDAVID, J., MOLZAHN, A., & PURKIS, M. (1997). The Comox Valley Nursing Centre. *The Canadian Nurse, 93*(2), 34–38.

BAJNOK, I. (1992). Entry-level educational preparation for nursing. In A.J. Baumgart & J. Larsen (1992), *Canadian nursing faces the future*, 2nd ed., (pp. 383–420). Toronto: Mosby.

BENNER, P. (1984). *From novice to expert.* Menlo Park, CA: Addison-Wesley.

BLUNT, A. (1992). The registered nurse in long-term care. *Registered Nurse, 4*(3), 7.

BOUDREAU, T.J. (1972). *Report of the committee on nurse practitioners.* Ottawa: Health & Welfare Canada.

BROWN, L. (1993). Making it on her own. *Nursing BC, 25*(1), 15.

CANADIAN ASSOCIATION OF PRACTICAL NURSES AND NURSING ASSISTANTS (CAPNNA). (1997, July). Written communication with Canadian Nurses Association.

CANADIAN NURSES ASSOCIATION. (1968). *The leaf and the lamp.* Ottawa: Author.

CANADIAN NURSES ASSOCIATION. (1982). *Credentialling in nursing: Policy statement and background paper.* Ottawa: Author.

CANADIAN NURSES ASSOCIATION. (1992). *Continuing nursing education position statement.* Ottawa: Author.

CANADIAN NURSES ASSOCIATION. (1993a). *Entrance requirements for nursing education programs in Canada 1993.* Ottawa: Author.

CANADIAN NURSES ASSOCIATION. (1993b). *Nurses know nurses can: An election handbook.* Ottawa: Author.

CANADIAN NURSES ASSOCIATION. (1993c). *The scope of nursing practice: A review of issues and trends.* Ottawa: Author.

CANADIAN NURSES ASSOCIATION (1993d). *Policy statement: Clinical nurse specialist.* Ottawa: Author.

CANADIAN NURSES ASSOCIATION. (1995, March). *Policy statement: Unregulated health care workers supporting nursing care delivery.* Ottawa: Author.

CANADIAN NURSES ASSOCIATION (1995, April). *Health in Canada: Perspectives of urban aboriginal people.* Ottawa: Author.

CANADIAN NURSES ASSOCIATION. (1996). *Registered nurse database.* Ottawa: Author.

CANADIAN NURSES ASSOCIATION. (1996, August). *Policy statement: Necessary support for safe nursing care.* Ottawa: Author.

CANADIAN NURSES ASSOCIATION. CNA (1997a). *Getting Started: A political action for registered nurses.* Ottawa: Author.

CANADIAN NURSES ASSOCIATION (1997b). *The future supply of registered nurses: A discussion paper.* Ottawa: Author.

COLLABORATIVE PROJECT IN NOVA SCOTIA. (1993). *Edufacts: The News in Nursing Education, 3*(3), 3.

CRUIKSHANK, P. (Nursing policy consultant, Medical Services Branch). (1997). Personal communication.

CUTSHALL, P. (1994). Megatrends in professional regulation: Toward the year 2000. *Nursing BC, 26,* 16.

DONAHUE, M.P. (1996). *Nursing the finest art: An illustrated history.* (2nd ed.). St. Louis: Mosby.

DU GAS, B.W. (1991). *The development of nursing education in BC.* Paper presented at the First Annual General Meeting of the History of Nursing Professional Practice Group of the RNABC.

DU GAS, B.W., & CASEY, A. (1989). Baccalaureates for RNs. *Canadian Nurse, 85*(2), 31–33.

FARR, M. (1990). Wellness at work. *Registered Nurse, 2*(4), 13–17.

FEASBY, W.R. (1946). *Official history of the Canadian medical services 1939–1945. Volume 1: Organization and campaigns.* Ottawa: MDN.

FIELD, P.A., STINSON, S.M., & THIBAUDEAU, M.F. (1992). Graduate education in nursing in Canada. In A.J. Baumgart & J. Larsen (1992), *Canadian nursing faces the future,* 2nd ed., (pp. 421–445). Toronto: Mosby.

GAGNÉ, (1998). *Personal Communication.* Department of National Defense.

GIBBON, J.M., & MATHEWSON, M.H. (1947). *Three centuries of Canadian nursing.* Toronto: Macmillan.

GLASS, H. (1985). *The future of health care in Canada and nursing's role within it.* Ottawa. (Available from the Canadian Nurses Association)

GREEN, M.M. (1984). *Through the years with public health nursing.* Ottawa: The Canadian Public Health Association.

GRIFFITHS, H. (1997). First call. *Nursing BC, 29*(5), 16–18.

HAINES, J. (1993a). *Leading in a time of change: The challenge for the nursing profession—A discussion paper.* Ottawa: Canadian Nurses Association.

HAINES, J. (1993b). *The nurse practitioner: A discussion paper.* Ottawa: Canadian Nurses Association.

HALL, E.M. (1964). *Report of the Royal Commission on Health Services.* Ottawa: Queen's Printer.

HOSPITALS IN TRANSITION, (1993) *CNA Today, 3*(1), 1–2.

HUMAN RESOURCES DEVELOPMENT CANADA (HRDC). (1996). *National occupation classification data.* Ottawa: Author.

INTEGRATED HEALTH HUMAN RESOURCES PROJECT. (1995). *National framework.* Ottawa: Canadian Nurses Association.

INTERNATIONAL COUNCIL OF NURSES (ICN). (1975). *Ethical concepts applied to nursing 1973.* ICN News Release No. 6.

LARSEN, J., & BAUMGART, A.J. (1992). Overview: Shaping public policy. In A.J. Baumgart & J. Larsen (Eds.) *Canadian nursing faces the future,* 2nd ed., (pp. 469–492). Toronto: Mosby.

LYNN, M., & KELLEY, B. (1997). Effects of case management on the nursing context: Perceived quality of care, work satisfaction, and control over practice. *Image: Journal of Nursing Scholarship, 29*(3), 237–241.

MacPHAIL, SIR ANDREW. (1925). *History of the Canadian forces medical services 1914–1919*. Ottawa: MDN.

MARCHAND, J., & GOODINE, W. (1993). Non-traditional roles for nurses. *Registered Nurse, 5*(5), 10–12.

MUSSALLEM, H.K. (1960). *Spotlight on nursing education: The report of the pilot project for the evaluation of schools of nursing in Canada*. Ottawa: Canadian Nurses Association.

MUSSALLEM, H.K. (1965). *Royal Commission on Health Services: Nursing education in Canada*. Ottawa: Queen's Printer.

MUSSALLEM, H.K. (1977). Nurses and Political Action. In B. Le Sor and M.R. Elliott (1977), *Issues in Canadian nursing*. Scarborough: Prentice Hall Canada, 154–181.

NICHOLSON, G.W.L. (1975). *Canada's nursing sisters*. Toronto: Samuel Stevens Hakkert. Historical publication 13. Canadian War Museum, National Museum of Man, National Museums of Canada.

PISCHKE-WINN, K., CATRAMBONE, C., & MINNICK, A. (1995). Regulatory requirements and the multitask worker. *Nursing Management, 26*(12), 39–41.

REGISTERED NURSES ASSOCIATION OF BRITISH COLUMBIA. (1994). *Position statement: Education requirements for future nurses*. Vancouver: Author.

PSYCHIATRIC NURSES ASSOCIATION OF CANADA (PNAC). (1997). Written communication with Canadian Nurses Association.

SIBBALD, B. (1997a). Delegating away patient safety. *Canadian Nurse, 93*(2), 22–26.

SIBBALD, B. (1997b). Beyond our borders: How to get involved in international development. *Canadian Nurse, 93*(5), 24–30.

STATISTICS CANADA. (1993). Population 15 years and over with employment income by sex, work activity and detailed occupation (selected tables). *The Nation*. Ottawa: Author. Catalogue no. 93–332.

STATISTICS CANADA. (1993, November). Health personnel in Canada. *Registered nurses*. 1992. Ottawa: Author. Catalogue no. 83–243.

STATISTICS CANADA. (1996). *Registered nurses management data*. Ottawa: Author.

STINSON, S.M., MacPHAIL, J., & LARSEN, J. (1992). *The Canadian nursing doctoral statistics: 1989 update*. Ottawa: Canadian Nurses Association.

STREET, M.M. (1973). *Watch-fires on the mountains: The life and writings of Ethel Johns*. Toronto: University of Toronto Press.

THOMAS, G. (1993, June). Working can be harmful to your health. *Canadian Nurse, 89*(6), 33–38.

VICTORIAN ORDER OF NURSES FOR CANADA. (1947). *The Victorian Order of Nurses for Canada 50th anniversary 1897–1947*. Montreal: Southam Press.

VICTORIAN ORDER OF NURSES FOR CANADA. (1983). *Proud achievement: A history of the Victorian Order of Nurses*. (Unpublished).

WEIR, G.M. (1932). *Survey of nursing education in Canada*. Toronto: University of Toronto Press.

WHAT'S THE DIFFERENCE? PRIMARY NURSING, PRIMARY HEALTH CARE, PRIMARY CARE. (1992) *CNA Today, 2*(3), 2.

WILSON-SIMMIE, K.M. (1981). *Lights out! A Canadian nursing sister's tale*. Belleville, ON: Mika.

Additional Readings

CANADIAN NURSES ASSOCIATION. (1993, March). *Policy statement: Future educational requirements*. Ottawa: Author.

GRAKIST, D. (1997, May–June). The changing face of public health nursing. *Registered Nurse Journal*, 13–14.

LANDSMAN, A. (1996). Restructuring hospitals, restructuring nursing. *Canadian Nurse, 92*(2), 27–30.

MARTIN, L.B. (1996). Parish nursing: Keeping body and soul together. *Canadian Nurse, 92*(1), 25–28.

McNEIL, J., & AFFARA, F. (1996a). *The value of nursing in a changing world*. Geneva: International Council of Nurses.

McNEIL, J., & AFFARA, F. (1996b). *Professional and socio-economic welfare responsibilities within NNAs*. Geneva: International Council of Nurses.

MOREWOOD-NORTHROP, M. (1994). Nursing in the Northwest Territories. *Canadian Nurse, 90*(3), 26–31.

PYKE, J. (1996). Case management and mental health services. *Canadian Nurse, 92*(7), 31–35.

RAIWET, C., HALLIWELL, G., ANDRUSKI, L., & WILSON, D. (1997). Care maps across the continuum. *Canadian Nurse, 93*(1), 26–30.

ROATH, T. (1997). Parish nursing: A spiritual path to healing. *Nurscene, 22*(2), 8–9.

SIMMINGTON, J., OLSON, J., & DOUGLAS, L. (1996). Promoting well-being within a parish. *Canadian Nurse, 92*(1), 20–24.

STEADY PROGRESS TOWARD BACCALAUREATE PREPARATION (1996). *Edufacts: CNA Today—The National News in Nursing, 6*(1), 4.

Wearing, J. (1994). The new emphasis of home care. *Canadian Nurse, 90*(2), 22–26.

Chapter 6

The Legal and Ethical Foundations of Nursing Practice

OUTLINE

Introduction

Professional Nursing Associations

Nursing Unions

Regulating Authorities

Nursing Practice Acts

The Legal Status of the Nurse

Accountability, Safety to Practise and Quality Assurance

Consumers' Rights in the Health Care System

Legal Issues of Interest to the Nurse

Ethics in Nursing Practice

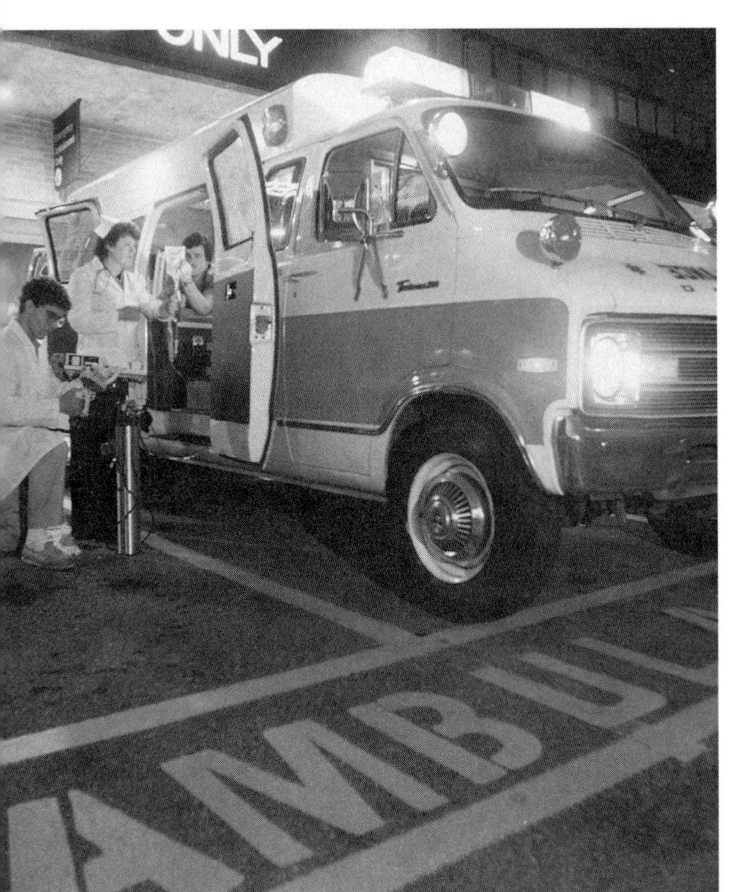

Central Questions

1. What are the objectives of professional nursing associations at the provincial, territorial, national and international levels? Of nursing unions? Of Regulating Authorities?
2. What is the difference between licensure and registration?
3. How are decisions made regarding the functions nurses are legally permitted to carry out?
4. What is the legal status of nurses?
5. What mechanisms are in place to ensure that the quality of nursing care is maintained at a high standard?
6. What rights do Canadians have with regard to health care?
7. What are the most common acts of negligence committed by nurses, and how can they be prevented?
8. What is a Good Samaritan law?
9. What is meant by informed consent?
10. What responsibilities do nurses have when dealing with confidential information? With wills?
11. What is the nurse's role regarding narcotic drugs and other controlled substances?
12. What does ethics have to do with nursing practice?
13. What are nurses' ethical responsibilities?
14. Why do we have codes of nursing ethics?
15. What kind of ethical problems do nurses face in practice?
16. How can nurses deal with ethical problems?
17. What are fundamental concepts of ethical theory?
18. How can nurses clarify their own values?

Introduction

The Code of Ethics for Registered Nurses gives guidance for decision-making concerning ethical matters, serves as a means for self-evaluation and reflection regarding ethical nursing practice, and provides a basis for peer review initiatives. The code not only educates [registered] nurses about their ethical responsibilities, but also informs other health care professionals and members of the public about the moral commitments expected of nurses.

Canadian Nurses Association, 1997
Part of the Preamble to the Code of Ethics for Registered Nurses

We all place a great deal of trust in health professionals. We expect them to be qualified to practise their profession, and to provide safe and competent care while respecting our basic rights as human beings. Although nurses are not responsible for all aspects of health care, they have a responsibility to ensure that, insofar as the nursing component is concerned, patients are assured of safe and competent care and that their fundamental rights, such as the right to courtesy, to privacy and to information, will be safeguarded during the process of care.

Most of the developed countries of the world have laws that regulate the practice of health professionals; these laws are intended to protect the public from unqualified practitioners. In some cases, the laws also define the scope of professional practice—that is, they specify the functions that the qualified practitioner may undertake. In many instances, the law has been vague and therefore more flexible in this respect, particularly in regard to the practice of nursing and medicine. Often it has been the professional associations that have undertaken to define the role and functions of the practitioner, based on currently accepted standards of practice.

In most democratic countries, an individual's basic human rights are protected, either in the constitution of the country or in its legally enacted laws. **Consumers' bills of rights** developed both in Canada and in the United States have sought to clarify an individual's basic rights as these are applicable to health care. Safeguarding the patient's rights is also an important aspect of the ethical codes adopted by each of the major health professions. These codes extend beyond the legal basis for practice and into the realm of social values to which members of the particular profession are committed. The professional associations have also become increasingly concerned with the need to develop standards to ensure that patients will receive safe and competent care. Both the Canadian Nurses Association and the provincial nursing associations, for example, have developed statements regarding standards that must be maintained in various fields of nursing practice in order to assure the consumer of quality nursing care.

Nurses should be familiar with the Canadian Nurses Association **Code of Ethics for Registered Nurses** (1997), which describes values and obligations considered important in nursing practice. (The complete text is given in Appendix A.) They should also be familiar with the laws in their province concerning the provision of health care to the public, and particularly with the acts that control the practice of nursing. Nurses should be aware of their functions and responsibilities, both as defined by law and as delineated by their professional nursing associations. It is also important for nurses to be familiar with the various charters that outline consumers' rights in the health care system, and they should be aware of how the law protects the patient in this regard. Nurses should also be cognizant of their own legal status, both as students and as graduate nurses.

All professions must organize themselves to achieve three primary functions: to protect the public, to promote the profession and to advance the socioeconomic welfare of the professional. While these functions may overlap, in most professions unions have as their major mandate the socioeconomic welfare of their members, while the public interest is the main focus of regulating authorities. Promotion of the profession is primarily done by professional associations, which set policy, lobby governments and move the profession forward.

Professional Nursing Associations

Professional nursing associations in Canada and other countries, as well as the International Council of Nurses, have been instrumental in developing and promoting a sound legal and ethical basis for nursing practice. We will be referring throughout this chapter to statements made by the professional associations. It would seem important, then, for the beginning student of nursing to know a little about these organizations.

International

INTERNATIONAL COUNCIL OF NURSES

The International Council of Nurses (ICN) is a nonpolitical, self-governing organization, with headquarters in Geneva, Switzerland. It was founded in 1899 as a federation of national nurses' associations and has two primary objectives: (a) to develop and enhance the national nursing organizations and (b) to promote favourable working and other conditions for nurses. The ICN holds an international congress once every four years that provides an opportunity for nurses from all member associations, now including about 100 countries, to meet to share common interests and discuss common problems. The 1997 Congress was held in Vancouver, British Columbia. In 2001, Denmark will be the host.

Each member association has one representative (usually its current president) on the Council of National Representatives, which is the policy-setting body of the ICN. The Council meets every two years. Its president, three vice-presidents and board of directors are elected at the previous ICN Congress (Splane & Splane, 1991).

National

CANADIAN NURSES ASSOCIATION

The Canadian Nurses Association (CNA) is the member association for Canada at ICN. The CNA had its origins in a joint American–Canadian association called the American Society of Superintendents of Training Schools, which was concerned with the need to improve educational programs for student nurses. This group was established in 1894 and worked closely together for a number of years until 1908, when it divided to form the Provisional Society of the Canadian National Association of Trained Nurses (CNATN)—forerunner of the Canadian Nurses Association—and the National League for Nursing Education (in the United States).

The Canadian association was established at first to represent Canada at the International Congress of Nurses. It became a truly national organization only when the subsequently developed provincial associations joined. These provincial associations originally came into being in response to the need to differentiate between trained and untrained nurses. By 1922, all provinces had some form of Registration Act that set out educational requirements for admission to schools of nursing and delegated responsibility for maintaining the standards of practice in the province to the provincial nursing associations. By 1924, each province had a nurses' organization with membership in the CNATN, which in that year changed its name to the Canadian Nurses Association (CNA, 1968).

The CNA has retained its interest in the improvement of nursing education but has broadened its scope, as befitted a national nursing association. The CNA is a professional nursing association that is a federated model of 11 provincial and territorial professional nursing associations representing over 260 000 registered nurses in Canada. The province that is not represented is Quebec. All 11 jurisdictional members strive to advance the profession of registered nursing. Ten of the jurisdictional members are also the regulating authority for registered nurses in their province or territory. The exception is Ontario, where the professional association and the regulating authority are separate. Membership in the professional association is voluntary in Ontario.

The CNA's mission is to advance the quality of nursing in the interests of the public. The CNA values:

- health for all as a primary and fundamental goal
- excellence in nursing practice, health care delivery and association services
- inclusiveness through partnership, collaboration and respect for diversity.

These values are enacted through advocacy, representation and leadership.

The CNA's stated objectives are:

- to promote high standards of nursing practice, education, research and administration in order to achieve quality nursing care in the public interest
- to promote uniform and high-quality regulatory practices in the public interest and in collaboration with nursing regulatory bodies
- to act in the public interest for Canadian nursing and nurses, providing national and international leadership in nursing and health issues (CNA, 1993).

The Canadian Nurses Association is a trilevel organization, that is, it has national, provincial and regional levels. The provincial associations are subdivided into district chapters, which provide all members with the opportunity to participate in the affairs of their professional association. An interesting trend is the increasing need for nurses in specialized areas of practice to keep up to date with the latest developments in their area by exchanging views with other nurses in the same field. This trend has resulted in the proliferation of interest groups within the provincial associations. These groups consist of nurses engaged in a specific area of practice, such as neurological nursing, critical care nursing and other specialized areas. In British Columbia, the interest groups have become Professional Practice Groups within the RNABC and, as of September 1994, had an elected representative on the board of directors of the association.

In many instances, specialty practice interest groups at the provincial level have joined to form national interest groups. The purpose for amalgamation is usually based on sharing of information related to the area of practice (e.g., conferences, journals, research, education). At the national level, many have become associate or affiliate members of the CNA. To date the CNA has 29 such members. These national groups select a representative to the CNA's board of directors.

The Canadian Nurses Association represents registered nurses and serves as the official voice of nursing in relations with allied national and international organizations, governmental bodies and the public. The provincial associations function similarly within their jurisdictions. The CNA publishes a monthly professional journal, *The Canadian Nurse/L'Infirmière Canadienne*. This journal serves as the principal resource for Canadian registered nurses in regard to national and international affairs affecting nursing. It also helps to keep nurses up to date with new developments in nursing through articles reporting on the latest in nursing research and clinical practice. The provincial nursing associations also publish monthly or bimonthly journals. Many of the provincial association journals started out as newsletters but they are rapidly becoming polished journals, along the lines of *The Canadian Nurse*.

CANADIAN NURSING STUDENT'S ASSOCIATION

Canada also has a student organization, the Canadian Nursing Student's Association/L'Association des étudiant(e)s infirmiers et infirmières du Canada (CNSA/AEIC). This association, to which students in all diploma and baccalaureate nursing programs may belong, is concerned with fostering high standards of nursing education to promote the highest quality nursing care. CNSA is an Affiliate Member of the CNA.

CNSA/AEIC holds an annual national conference at which the association's business is accomplished and speakers on various topics are heard. Topics addressed have included women in health care, empowerment and assertiveness. At least two provincial nursing associations, the Registered Nurses Association of British Columbia and the Registered Nurses Association of Ontario (RNAO), permit undergraduates enrolled in RN programs to hold student membership in the Association for a nominal fee. Student members elect a student to sit on the board of directors and may participate in chapter and provincial activities, serve on committees and represent chapters as voting delegates to annual and special meetings.

CANADIAN REGISTERED PSYCHIATRIC NURSES ASSOCIATION

The Canadian Registered Psychiatric Nurses Association (CRPNA) is composed of only four provincial associations, because there are preparatory programs for RPNs only in British Columbia, Alberta, Saskatchewan and Manitoba. These four provinces are also the only ones that recognize RPNs. The objectives of the CRPNA, however, are similar to those of the CNA—the promotion of high standards of psychiatric nursing care and the welfare of psychiatric nurses are its main purposes.

CANADIAN ASSOCIATION OF PRACTICAL NURSES AND NURSING ASSISTANTS

The Canadian Association of Practical Nurses and Nursing Assistants (CAPNNA) is a national organization composed of provincial associations to promote practical nursing in Canada. As such, it is analogous to the CNA and CRPNA. Its purposes include promotion of the welfare of the licensed practical nurse and the nursing assistant as well as promotion of the highest standards of health care. Membership is made up of all nurses who belong to their provincial association of practical nurses.

Nursing Unions

In 1973, the Supreme Court of Canada ruled that the professional association could not act as the bargaining agent for salaried nurses because the professional association was "management dominated." This meant that unions must become separate from associations. At present, there are provincial nursing unions and a union for nurses employed by the federal government, whose primary objective is to advance the social, academic and general welfare of the nurse (Jensen, 1992).

Regulating Authorities

The protection of the public from risk or harm is the primary purpose of any **regulating authority** (or licensing authority). The authority to self-regulate a profession is delegated to specific professional organizations by each provincial or territorial government. In Canada, each jurisdiction has a regulating authority for registered nurses and licensed practical nurses. Registered psychiatric nurses are recognized and regulated in the four western provinces. Each regulating body has the authority to:

- issue a licence and/or maintain a register of qualified practitioners
- set standards of practice
- discipline its members.

In other words, regulating authorities promote good practice, prevent undesirable practice, protect the public and intervene when practice is below standard.

Government legislation—such as the Nurses (Registered) Act in British Columbia and the Nursing Profession Act in Alberta—is the framework for the activities of a regulating authority. Self-regulation is a privilege; it means that the government believes the profession is best suited to set standards of practice and ensure that practitioners comply with those standards. In the public interest, only qualified and competent individuals who meet the standards of professional conduct and competence are permitted to practise. If the licensing organization is seen as self-serving, public trust is eroded and self-regulation in the public interest is questioned. Legislation in most provinces stipulates the inclusion of public representatives on the governance board or working committees of the regulating body and/or on advisory councils to government.

Nursing Practice Acts

The laws in Canada derive from two main sources: the statutes passed by law-making bodies, such as Parliament, and the decisions of the courts. The latter are collectively known as common law. The law is a reflection of public opinion and of civic and social movements within a community. The law therefore is not static—it is constantly changing. Changes in the statutes and the decisions of the courts in cases involving nursing reflect changes in public thinking about nursing. In recent years, there has been an increasing awareness by nurses and by the public of the need to standardize the laws concerning the practice of both the RN and the LPN. The authority to control nursing, together with various other professions and occupations concerned with health and welfare, has been vested in the provinces. Thus, each province has enacted its own laws to control the practice of nursing. These laws are generally termed **nursing practice acts**, although the exact title of the statute varies in the different jurisdictions. Because each province has set up its own law, it is understandable that the statutes vary somewhat. Nevertheless, the purpose of these laws is the same—that is, to protect the health and safety of the public through the establishment of minimum standards that a qualified health professional must meet in order to practise as a nurse.

Nursing practice, as we have already noted, is constantly changing in response to societal needs. Guidance on what constitutes nursing practice has come principally from two sources, the nursing practice acts and the statements of the professional nursing associations. Because of the interdependence of nursing and other health care professions, these professions frequently consult one another and often make joint statements on functions nurses may undertake. The opinions of provincial attorneys generally provide some additional assistance from the legal point of view, although these opinions usually pertain to specific situations (Philpott, 1985).

In the past few years, there have been an unprecedented number of changes in nursing practice acts in Canada, as nurses have felt the need to have embedded in the law a more precise definition of nursing practice and a clearer description of their role and functions than previous statutes contained. Most nursing (and medical) practice acts in the past were written in broad, general terms. The general nature of the wording permitted both disciplines to enlarge the scope of their practice without the need for changes in the law each time and, also, made possible the orderly transfer of many procedural functions from medicine to nursing without recourse to the law. Not too many years ago, for example, only physicians were permitted to start intravenous infusions, yet today this is an accepted nursing procedure. One of the principal reasons for the need for a more precise definition of nursing practice has been the development and rapid proliferation of expanded roles for nurses. In some aspects of expanded role practice, for example, when a nurse practitioner initiates treatment on his or her own, the question of the legality of these actions has arisen. Another reason for precise definition has been the increasing concern by governments for legislation pertaining to all health personnel and government suggestions

LOOKING back

Eunice Henrietta Dyke, 1883–1969

Toronto's first "tuberculosis nurse" and first director of the Division of Public Health Nursing for the Toronto Department of Public Health was Eunice Henrietta Dyke. When she took on this challenge in May 1911 at age 28, she was committed to bringing under control the dreaded "white plague" — tuberculosis. Her first major duties were to "register" the cases of TB which, for the first time in Toronto, was made a "notifiable disease." Under her capable administration, she identified some 800 cases in the first year alone and soon had arranged for herself or another nurse to visit all positive and suspected cases.

Soon a small team of nurses was working under her direction, not only to carry out care in the home but also to educate the family and neighbours to prevent the spread of this highly contagious disease. Her public health nurses also visited schools and began to attack the serious problems of high infant mortality and morbidity. She introduced district offices both to cut down on transportation costs and to increase the presence of the health professionals in the neighbourhood. Under her capable and frequently outspoken direction, the city's public health service grew rapidly, soon becoming a model for other cities in North America.

Born in Toronto, Eunice Dyke graduated in 1909 from Baltimore's highly respected Johns Hopkins Hospital School of Nursing, which had an excellent reputation for preparing nurses to carry out public health nursing duties. Her nursing education was interrupted by a bout with tuberculosis, and she spent a year as a patient in the Muskoka Sanatorium. Following graduation, she worked as a private nurse in Baltimore, then returned home to Toronto to care for an aunt who was dying of cancer.

Eunice Dyke's innovations as head of the nursing division led the League of Red Cross Societies in Geneva to second her for a four-month consultancy on public health nursing services in 1923. She then returned to Toronto's Department of Public Health until 1933, when she was forced to resign by the newly appointed medical director, with whom she had a serious dispute over the assignment of nurses. The local Council of Women appealed her dismissal to City Hall. Despite strong public support and a close vote in Council, she was not reinstated. However, the immediate offer of a Rockefeller Scholarship indicated the high regard in which she was held by the nursing and health communities nationally and internationally. Following her Rockefeller year and a cross-Canada tour to study public health nursing, she was appointed for a brief period to the Canadian Council of Child and Family Welfare in Ottawa as secretary of the maternal and child division.

After her retirement, she turned her attention to the needs for social and recreational services for the elderly. In 1946, she was instrumental in organizing the "Second Mile Club," where Toronto seniors were offered organized activities and a place to socialize and contribute to the community. Such a service marked her awareness of social needs and was considerably ahead of its time. In 1960, the Canadian Public Health Association made her an honorary life member. After several years of ill health and recurring episodes of cancer, Eunice Henrietta Dyke died in 1969.

—*Glennis Zilm*

for changes in existing statutes. Following are some examples of some definitions of nursing practice found in provincial nursing practice acts:

Quebec: "Every act the object of which is to identify the health needs of persons, contribute to methods of diagnosis, provide and control the nursing care required for the promotion of health, prevention of illness, treatment and rehabilitation, and to provide care according to a medical prescription constitutes the profession of nursing."

Nurses Act RSQ, Chapter 1–8
Quebec, 1994

British Columbia: "The 'practice of nursing' means the performance for others of health care services that require the application of professional nursing knowledge and skills and includes (a) promoting, maintaining or restoring the health of the general public, (b) teaching nursing theory or practice, (c) counselling persons in respect of health care, (d)coordinating health care services, and (e) engaging in administration, supervision, education, consultation, teaching or research for any of the foregoing."

Nurses (Registered) Act, Rules Part 2,
British Columbia, 1988

In addition to the definitions of nursing practice in provincial laws, the provincial nursing associations have issued guidelines from time to time regarding the additional functions that may be performed by nurses when these are delegated by a physician. Although statements made by professional associations lack the authority of legally enacted statutes, they are generally persuasive in that they reflect common practice (Philpott, 1985).

Licensure and Registration

In Canada, with the exception of Ontario, provincial governments have delegated administration of the nursing acts to the provincial professional nursing associations. In Ontario the responsibility rests with a College of Nurses, which is separate from the professional nursing association. In Canada, nurses are not licensed; they are, rather, registered by their provincial nursing association and in Ontario by the College of Nurses of Ontario. A **licence** is a permit granted by a government agency to an individual to engage in the practice of a profession and to use a particular title. The term **registration** means the listing of an individual's name on the official roster. Nurses who are registered are permitted to use the title "registered nurse"; nurses who have failed to register are not permitted to do so. In order to be registered, the nurse must have completed a basic course of nursing studies in a program approved by the registering body, and have passed the national qualifying examinations with an acceptable grade (see Appendix B for CNA Registration/Licensure Examinations). Nurses from other provinces in Canada may be granted registration by endorsement, as may nurses from other countries, providing their qualifications meet the criteria established by the provincial registering body. Nurses wishing to return to practice after an absence from the professional workforce may have their registration reinstated. Provincial agencies are beginning to demand that nurses take refresher courses to update their knowledge and skills if too many years have elapsed since they were last in active practice. Registration must be renewed on an annual basis in order to be valid.

In the past few years, there have been a number of changes in registration regulations in Canada. Most of the provincial registered nursing acts now require that the nurse be registered with the provincial association/College of Nurses in order to use the term "registered nurse" or the initials "RN." In addition to the laws controlling registered nurses, all provinces have other nursing laws. Licensed practical nurses (LPN), called Registered Practical Nurses (Ontario) or Certified Nursing Assistants (CNA) are in some jurisdictions granted licensure by provincial licensing bodies that administer the provisions of the act regulating practical nursing in that province. LPNs are licensed by their provincial licensing body after completing an approved educational program and passing a licensure examination. Psychiatric nursing is regulated under separate provincial legislation, and registration is mandatory for psychiatric nurses in the four provinces that recognize it as a separate branch of nursing. The regulatory body for psychiatric nursing is the provincial professional association. Graduates of RPN programs write the registration examinations for psychiatric nurses set by the provincial associations.

Professional Conduct Review

As previously suggested, the protection of the public from risk or harm is the primary purpose of any regulating or licensing authority. **Professional conduct review (PCR)** is the process (or processes) used by a regulating authority to respond to a complaint about a registrant or licensee. Nursing practice acts usually outline the scope of practice, the concepts of professional misconduct (i.e., unethical behaviour), incompetence (i.e., lack of knowledge, skills and/or judgement) and incapacity (i.e., inability to perform well owing to health reasons), as well as the structure to be used to manage a complaint. The regulating authority establishes committees (of members and the public) to deal with the various stages of PCR (intake of complaint, investigation and, if necessary, hearing and appeal), and strives to ensure that principles of administrative fairness are applied to all parties at every stage.

If, upon investigation, a disciplinary hearing is warranted, both the registrant and the regulating authority have the opportunity to present evidence. If the registrant is found to be in error, various sanctions can be imposed by the discipline committee. These range in severity and may involve an oral reprimand, remedial education, suspension for a specific period, or even revocation of a licence. A nurse's registration is usually revoked if, in the opinion of the discipline committee, it is not safe to permit him or her to practise nursing.

In certain cases, such as complaints of incapacity, an alternative (and perhaps more appropriate) mechanism may be used to resolve complaints within the process of professional conduct review. A mediated or negotiated agreement is an alternative to a formal investigation and enquiry. The regulator acts as a facilitator and ensures that the outcomes and resolutions are consistent with the public interest. This approach often allows the practitioner the opportunity to regain his or her health and continue to be a productive worker. It is less adversarial and more likely to resolve the problem.

Continuing Education Requirements

The speed with which new knowledge and technology are becoming available in nursing has created problems in keeping the health professional up to date with the latest developments in the field. In Canada, although there has been considerable discussion about mandatory continuing education as a requirement for continued practice, no province to date has incorporated this requirement into its registration renewal process. However, many jurisdictions are beginning to address the issue of competence assurance. This means that the regulating authorities, in the public interest, are examining various mechanisms through which a registered nurse can demonstrate that he or she has the professional competence to qualify for (annual) renewal of registration. The College of Nurses of Ontario has implemented a quality assurance program in which RNs will be randomly selected to provide evidence of continuing competence. For example, the RN may submit a self-assessment or a professional portfolio that would outline, among other items, continuing education activities. In B.C., the Registered Nurses Association of British Columbia (RNABC) has implemented a similar continuing competence program. Most regulating authorities require nurses to have practised a minimum number of hours in the preceding year as one of the criteria in order to renew their registration. Ultimately, it is up to the individual nurse to maintain an up-to-date level of knowledge and skill.

The Legal Status of the Nurse

The nurse in his or her practice can be classed as either an independent contractor or an employee. Private duty nurses, that is, nurses who are engaged by the patient to perform nursing service, come under the category of independent contractors. Nurses who are working in independent practice in the community (not in the employ of a community agency) would also be considered independent contractors. Nurses who work in hospitals or clinics, in public health agencies, in industry or for private physicians are considered employees. The distinction is a matter of authority. While all nurses are responsible to society, their professional association and their patients, independent contractors develop and are responsible for following their own policies and procedures. Employees, however, are also responsible to the employing institution and must follow the institution's policies. Nursing students, when assigned for clinical experience to a hospital or other health agency, are usually considered employees, since they are subject to the authority of nurse managers, clinical instructors and staff nurses and physicians (Philpott, 1985). Students in college or university schools of nursing may, however, be entirely under the supervision of the faculty of their school while in the practice area.

It is helpful for students to remember that even though they may be responsible to others, they are still responsible for their own actions. Anyone who gives nursing care, whether student or graduate, assumes certain duties, and it is expected that these will be carried out with **reasonable prudence** under the circumstances. Reasonable prudence is taken to mean that the individual acts with the care that any reasonable person with his or her knowledge, education and experience would take. It is important to determine the status of the nurse because, under the law, not only are individuals liable for their own actions but their employers are also liable under the rule of *respondeat superior* (let the master answer). Thus, if a nurse is negligent and a patient is harmed, both the nurse and the employer can be sued. Nurses are not absolved of responsibility for their actions simply because they may be carrying out the orders of a physician. The law states that the nurse must understand the cause and effect of the treatment that is undertaken. If nurses carry out orders that they know are wrong, they are guilty of negligence. At all times the patient's safety must be paramount. If nurses undertake work that they know is beyond the scope of their education or experience—for example, performing an action or treatment that is defined as being within the province of medical practice—they may again be considered negligent or guilty of malpractice (Philpott, 1985).

Accountability, Safety to Practise and Quality Assurance

One of the most pressing concerns of individual nurses and of professional nursing associations at present is to ensure that patients receive safe and competent nursing care regardless of the setting or the circumstances under which that care is given. Health professionals have long been concerned about the need to maintain high standards of practice. However, the growing rise of consumerism in the health field and the generally increased sophistication of the public in relation to health care matters have put additional emphasis on the accountability of health professionals to the public they serve. Also, elected representatives in government are becoming increasingly concerned about the quality of health care, since health care is taking more and more of provincial budgets. They, too, are demanding that the work of health professionals be monitored to ensure that high-quality standards are maintained. We are hearing a lot these days about accountability, about safety to practise and about quality assurance. As beginning students, you are probably wondering what these terms mean, and how they affect you.

Accountability means that a person is answerable (or accepts responsibility) for his or her own actions. Health professionals must be able to account for the care they give, that is, to tell precisely what they did and why they did it. The term was initially used in the business world, but has now taken on a much broader meaning. Individual practitioners and health care institutions are being held accountable for both what they do and what they have said they will do, as well as for the process by which it is done (Quinn & Smith, 1987).

Safety to practise means simply what it says — the nursing profession, along with other health professions, makes sure that beginning health professionals have the knowledge and skills necessary to practise their profession competently and without harming the people to whom they render care. Ensuring that the health professional remains safe to practise has become of increasing concern to the health professions. It used to be that once nurses, physicians or dentists had completed a basic educational program and passed qualifying examinations, their names would be inscribed on a permanent roster and they could practise throughout their lifetime—providing, of course, that they did not commit some flagrant offence that caused them to have their licence or registration revoked. The rapidity with which health care is changing, however, and the increasing emphasis on accountability have made it imperative that the professions develop mechanisms to ensure that practitioners remain competent and safe to practise throughout their professional careers. The issue of competence assurance has already begun to be addressed by the regulating authorities for registered nurses.

Quality assurance, another term borrowed from the business world, refers to a program designed to ensure that health care provided to patients is consistently of good quality. In any situation in which health professionals are providing services for the public, the quality of care the patient receives depends on at least the following four variables:

1. the providers of the care—the nurses, physicians and all others who contribute to patient care
2. the standards that are maintained in the agency providing care
3. the environment, or setting, in which the care is given
4. the recipient of care—the patients themselves.

In attempting to ensure that patients receive good nursing care at all times, the nursing profession has given a great deal of consideration to each of these four variables and has developed a number of mechanisms to try to ensure that the practice of nursing is consistently safe and of good quality.

The Providers of Nursing Care

We have already mentioned several ways in which the registered nursing profession tries to ensure that its health professionals are competent and safe to practise. Perhaps it is time, however, to pull all these together with some others that we have not discussed so far. The quality of the providers of care (the nurses themselves) is assured by the following controls:

1. **Accreditation/Approval of Basic Nursing Education Programs.** Minimum standards for basic nursing education programs have been established in each province in Canada. All programs preparing candidates for registration are carefully monitored by the provincial regulating authority. Provincial approval is granted to schools of nursing meeting the minimum criteria.
2. **Accreditation of schools of nursing.** The Canadian Association of University Schools of Nursing (CAUSN) is concerned with optimum, rather than minimum, standards. In other words, voluntary accreditation by CAUSN certifies that an educational program has not only met minimum standards, but is considered "good" by national standards. It indicates a level of excellence.
3. **National qualifying examinations.** The Canadian Nurses Association provides national testing services, which are used by provincial registering bodies for the examination of candidates for the registered nursing profession and the practical nursing profession. These examinations are available in both French and English. Appendix B contains further information on the CNA Nurse Registration/Licensure Examinations.
4. **Licensing/registration.** The licensing/registration mechanism is the basic safeguard protecting the public from unsafe practitioners and assuring employers that the individual has met certain standards established by the licensing or registering body as minimum requirements for entry to practise or renewal of registration.
5. **Code of ethics.** *The Code of Ethics for Registered Nurses* (CNA, 1997) provides guidance for decision making on ethical issues, allows for self-reflection about practice, and is used as a basis for professional conduct review initiatives. The Code informs nurses, other health care providers and the public about the expected ethical behaviour of a registered nurse.

6. **Standards of practice.** In assessing the quality of care provided by individual health professionals, it is essential to have objective criteria by which to judge whether the care given is good, adequate or unsafe. Such objective criteria both protect the public and regulate the practice of nurses. The CNA and provincial regulating authorities have developed standards for nursing practice. An example of such standards are those from the Registered Nurses Association of British Columbia, which are classified according to the characteristics of a profession (see box).

The Standards statements are broad in nature, capturing the varied practice settings and roles in which nurses practice. They are:

- **Responsibility and Accountability:** Maintains standards of nursing practice and professional behaviour determined by RNABC and the practice setting.
- **Specialized Body of Knowledge:** Bases practice on nursing sciences and humanities.
- **Competent Application of Knowledge:** Determines client status and responses to actual or potential health problems, plans interventions, performs planned interventions and evaluates client outcomes.
- **Code of Ethics:** Adheres to the ethical standards of the nursing profession.
- **Provision of Service to the Public:** Provides nursing services and collaborates with other members of the health care team in providing health care services.
- **Self-Regulation:** Assumes primary responsibility for maintaining competence, fitness to practice and acquiring evidence-based knowledge and skills for professional nursing practice.

SOURCE: RNABC, 1998, pp. 5, 6.

Many of the specialty practice groups have developed standards of practice as part of the process of being designated a specialty for the purpose of certification. These focussed standards guide the practice of nurses working in that specific area. Since certification is a voluntary process, the nurse voluntarily assumes the specialty standards to guide his or her practice.

7. **Professional conduct review.** In the public interest, the professional conduct review is used by a regulating authority to respond to a complaint about a practitioner. Committees (composed of members and the public) deal with the complaint, the investigation and, if necessary, a hearing and appeal. If the registrant is found guilty, various sanctions can be applied, depending on the severity of the infraction.
8. **Continuing education.** The rapid expansion of knowledge in the health field means that all practitioners need to update their knowledge and skills on a continuing basis throughout their professional careers.
9. **Certification.** Certification provides yet another mechanism for ensuring the competence of practitioners — at a level higher than licensure. The Canadian Nurses Association has established a certification program for nurses who have achieved expertise in practice in specialized fields of nursing.
10. **Assessment of clinical competence.** A number of mechanisms have been developed that attempt to judge a nurse's competence in clinical practice:
    a) *employer performance appraisal* is a method of rating the nurse's performance in the work setting. Although numerous performance-rating scales have been tried to make the ratings as objective as possible, it is difficult to eliminate the subjective bias from an assessment of one person's work by another.
    b) *peer review* is a method of assessing the quality of care provided by a practitioner through a review of his or her work by a group of peers. Methods used in this review may include looking at care plans or patient records written by the nurse, gathering evaluations from patients cared for by the nurse and from professional co-workers, and reviewing evidence of attendance at continuing education programs.
    c) *nursing audit* is a method of evaluating nursing care through a review of patient records that document the care given. It may be used for evaluating a single nurse's clinical performance, or for assessing the quality of care on a given nursing unit or in an agency.
11. **Competence assurance.** Regulating authorities are examining ways by which an RN can demonstrate professional competence in order to qualify for renewed registration (e.g., submitting a portfolio listing continuing education courses and other professional activities).

Agency Standards of Care

Individual health agencies have been attempting to determine standards that nurses in their agency consider important in the care of patients. This work has resulted in the development of standard nursing care plans for the care of patients with particular health problems, for example, patients who have had a cerebrovascular accident (stroke), who are unconscious, or who are undergoing different types of surgery. We will be discussing this topic at greater length in connection with the nursing process in Chapter 14. There may always be additional nursing care required because of individual needs of a patient. The important point here is that these standard plans provide guidelines for nurses to assess, through reviewing documented records of patient care, whether everything that should have been done routinely in the way of nursing care for a patient with a particular health problem was indeed done.

The Practice Setting

In order for nurses to give good care to patients, the environment in which they work must permit and encourage good nursing care. In reviewing the physical and social environments as determinants of health (in Chapter 3), we discussed some of their effects on individual and group health. Similarly, in considering the environment in which nursing is practised, one must take into account both the material things necessary to provide care and the social environment of the agency that encourages or discourages the maintenance of high standards of nursing care. Individual nurses and their professional nursing organizations have become increasingly concerned about such matters as ensuring that nurses have a safe environment in which to practise, that they have sufficient equipment in good working order to work with, that nursing units and community health units are adequately staffed with competent personnel and that nurses are not required to work in areas for which they are not prepared, or in situations that conflict with their values.

In some jurisdictions, practice setting requirements have been identified and employers have volunteered to be evaluated against those standards. The practice setting review is done at the corporate and not individual level, and all feedback is confidential. The review provides the employer with the opportunity to improve the professional practice environment and enhance the ability of the practitioners to meet their standards of practice.

In many legislated practice acts for health professionals, the employer has a legal obligation to report, to the appropriate regulating authority, the termination of an employee for reasons related to unprofessional conduct, incompetence or incapacity. This gives the professional's regulating body, in the interest of the public, the opportunity to investigate and, if necessary, assist or sanction the member. Without the employer's cooperation, the problem will not be addressed, and the public may be placed at risk—when the employee finds another place of employment.

The Patient

The fourth variable in any health care situation is the patient. Because patients are human beings, in all their infinite variety, this is probably the least predictable element in the situation—and the most difficult to provide with adequate safeguards. The best prepared practitioner working in an agency with the highest standards and under the best possible conditions of work can still not guarantee the patient's response to care. The elderly woman whose mouth needs attention may spit out the mouthwash that the nurse has given her. A "helpful" patient may lend his salt shaker to a neighbour who is on a salt-free diet. The emergency patient "high" on drugs or alcohol may lash out at anyone who comes near, foiling the attempts of health professionals to provide the needed care.

Consumers' Rights in the Health Care System

The art of healing has, from ancient times, been imbued with an aura of mystery, and magical powers have been attributed to those who practise the healing arts. Even modern practitioners of "scientific Western medicine"—nurses, physicians and other health professionals—have,

Consumer Rights in Health Care

1. Right to be informed
   - about preventive health care, including education on nutrition, birth control, drug use, appropriate exercise
   - about the health care system, including the extent of government coverage for services, supplementary insurance plans and the referral system to auxiliary health and social facilities and services in the community
   - about the individual's own diagnosis and specific treatment program, including prescribed surgery and medication, options, effects and side effects
   - about the specific costs of procedures, services and professional fees undertaken on behalf of the individual consumer
   - about the policies and procedures of the health care facility or program
2. Right to be respected as the individual with the major responsibility for his or her own health care
   - right that confidentiality of his or her health records be maintained
   - right to refuse experimentation, undue painful prolongation of his or her life or participation in teaching programs
   - right of adult to refuse treatment; right to die with dignity
   - right to considerate and respectful care
3. Right to participate in decision making affecting his or her health
   - through consumer representation at each level of government in planning and evaluating the system of health services, the types and qualities of service and the conditions under which health services are delivered
   - with the health professionals and personnel involved in his or her direct health care
4. Right of equal access to health care regardless of the individual's economic status, gender, age, creed, ethnic origin and location
   - right of access to adequately qualified health personnel
   - right to a second medical opinion
   - right to prompt response in emergencies
   - right to expect continuity of care.

SOURCE: Consumers' Association of Canada, 1989 (under review).

until fairly recently, tended to perpetuate the belief that the average layperson could not possibly understand the complex workings of the human body or have the knowledge and experience to choose the best treatment. Through the use of technical jargon that is incomprehensible to anyone outside the health field, and in many other subtle (and some not-so-subtle) ways, health professionals usually managed to convey to patients that they should not question what was being done for them but simply trust in the experts to cure them of their ills. There is no doubt that trust is still an important ingredient in the relationship between health professional and health consumer, but today's patient is viewed as an active member of the health team rather than a passive recipient of care. People today are often well informed, thanks to the popular media (including the Internet), about the latest advances in surgery and medicine. They are also conscious of their right to question the treatment they receive, to have a say in that treatment and to be kept informed of their progress.

There has been an active and growing consumer movement in the health field in recent years. Increasing public awareness of health issues, increased knowledge about health and illness, and the rising costs to the consumer of health services are three major factors that have contributed to this movement. Further, the fact that people have become more conscious of their rights generally—particularly women, First Nations people and members of minority ethnic groups—have had repercussions in the health field. Consumer Bills of Rights have been developed and widely publicized, in Canada by the Consumers' Association of Canada and, in the United States, by the American Hospital Association.

Charters on the rights of members of special groups have also been developed and made public. For example, declarations on the rights of the mentally and physically challenged were adopted by the General Assembly of the United Nations in 1971 and 1975, respectively; the Dying Person's Bill of Rights was developed in 1975 at a workshop in Lansing, Michigan, on care of the terminally ill; and the Pregnant Patient's Bill of Rights was published by the International Childbirth Education Association in 1975. While these charters do not have the force of legally enacted statutes, they have been influential in raising the consciousness of consumers of health services so that they feel freer to express their dissatisfactions with the health care system and are less reluctant to demand their rights. The charters have also increased the awareness of health care workers of the fundamental rights of patients as human beings and as citizens.

Legal Issues of Interest to the Nurse

Torts and Crimes

In addition to understanding their ethical responsibilities as health professionals, nurses should be aware of their legal responsibilities as well. Nurses often become witnesses or defendants in various types of legal proceedings. Generally speaking, there are two types of court actions in which nurses may be involved. The first is called a tort. A **tort** is a legal wrong committed by one person against the person or property of another. The injured party may sue for damages and, if the suit is successful, is usually awarded money to be paid by the other party. Sometimes this is spoken of as a civil suit, as opposed to a criminal action.

A **crime** is also a legal wrong but, in general, it refers to a wrong committed against the public and is punishable by the Crown. The punishment for a crime is either a fine or imprisonment. In a criminal action, the case is designated in the form *Regina versus Mary Jones*; in a tort, the form used is *John Doe versus James Jones*, or *Mary Doe versus the Blank Hospital*. Acts such as murder, manslaughter and robbery are considered crimes, whereas negligence and malpractice are usually torts. The case against Susan Nelles is an example of a criminal action. Nelles was a nurse at the Hospital for Sick Children in Toronto and was wrongfully accused of a number of infant deaths on one of the wards at the hospital. After a lengthy investigation, she was cleared of all wrong-doing (Charbonneau, 1985; Grange, 1984; Dubin, Gilchrist, McDonald & Nadler, 1983; RNAO, undated; Hamilton, 1993).

Negligence and Malpractice

It has already been noted that each individual is responsible for his or her own actions and that nurses can be held liable for their own negligent actions. **Negligence** is legally defined as the omission to do something that a reasonable person, guided upon those considerations that ordinarily regulate the conduct of human affairs, would do, or doing something that a prudent and reasonable person would not do. The standards of care that a reasonable and prudent nurse would use in a particular situation are established by the courts through the review of nursing texts, nursing curricula, nursing standards and the testimony of expert witnesses.

The term **malpractice** is virtually synonymous with professional negligence. As a general rule, nursing negligence usually means failure by the nurse to take the appropriate action to protect the patient from harm. Negligence may involve either doing something that ought not to be done or failing to do something that ought to be done. If the nurse does not assess a patient's heart rate prior to giving digoxin, for example, and the patient dies, the nurse may be considered negligent. Similarly, failure to put up side rails on the bed of a confused patient could also be considered negligence on the nurse's part. Any individual, professional or nonprofessional, may be sued for negligence; when the negligence is on the part of a professional person, it is deemed malpractice. It should be noted that, although the term is most frequently used in connection with cases involving negligence, malpractice may include other claims against a professional person (for example, breach of contract).

Because of the increase in the number of malpractice suits in general, and against nurses in particular, many authorities now recommend that each nurse carry malpractice insurance to cover the cost of lawyers' fees and possible damages. Several of the provincial nursing associations in Canada have made malpractice insurance available to their members at a reasonable cost or as one of the benefits of membership. Many nurses have the mistaken belief that, because they are employees, their employer will carry the burden of responsibility for their negligent actions. This is not so; the nurse can be sued as an individual as well.

COMMON ACTS OF NEGLIGENCE

Professional nurses may be called upon to testify in a legal proceeding in regard to some matter pertaining to their work. The most common incidents leading to legal proceedings involving a patient and a nurse are those in which negligence is a factor. The most common of such acts of negligence that have resulted in suits for damages involve burns, falls, medication, malfunctioning apparatus and abandonment. We shall look at each of these in turn.

BURNS Hot water bottles, heating pads, inhalators, steam radiators, enemas, douches and sitz baths can all cause a patient to be burned. Nurses may be held responsible if they have neglected to take the usual safety precautions, such as taking the temperature of the water used in a solution administered to a patient or keeping articles that might burn the patient out of reach.

FALLS Another common type of accident that may result in injury to the patient and subsequently a suit for damages is falling from bed. The usual safety precautions against falls include the use of side rails. Most health agencies have rules regarding the use of side rails for patients at risk of falling, for example, those who are recovering from anesthesia and those under sedation. The nurse should remember, though, that the competent, alert patient has the right to refuse side rails as long as he or she has been informed about and understands the risks involved. The risk of falling must be balanced against the risk to the patient's dignity.

WRONG MEDICINE, WRONG DOSAGE, WRONG PATIENT, WRONG CONCENTRATION, WRONG TIME Another common area in which negligence occurs is in giving medications. Labels can be misread or may not be read at all. The nurse may fail to identify the patient correctly and consequently give a medication to the wrong person. Numerous errors are made in giving medications. With the tremendous increase in the number of medications taken by patients and the numerous commercial names commonly used for the various drugs, safety precautions assume greater importance in ensuring that the right patient gets the right drug in the proper concentration at the right time and in the proper manner.

DEFECTS IN APPARATUS OR SUPPLIES Patients can be injured by the use of defective equipment. Nurses are not held responsible if patients are injured as a result of hidden defects, but if equipment or supplies are known to be faulty, nurses may be held liable. The use of unsterile gauze for a surgical dressing might be an example of negligence relating to defective supplies.

ABANDONMENT Instances in which patients have been left unattended and have injured themselves as a result have led to suits for negligence. If a nurse left a baby on a table and the baby fell in the nurse's absence, this might result in a negligence suit.

The above are by no means all the acts of negligence that have resulted in suits for damages. To guard against negligence, nurses should always use knowledge and judgement in providing care and follow established professional and agency guidelines and policies.

INCIDENT REPORTS

The nurse has an ethical and a legal responsibility to report to the health agency any accidents, losses or unusual incidents. Most health agencies have special forms for this purpose. The primary purpose of reporting these incidents is to protect the patient and the nurse by ensuring that there is a record of the details of the incident and the subsequent action taken, in the event that legal proceedings are instituted. Incident reports are also useful as a source of information in research to improve the quality of care and the effectiveness of policies.

GOOD SAMARITAN LAWS

Some provinces have enacted legislation designed to protect the health professional from all practice suits arising from care given to the injured at the scene of an accident or other emergency. Some of these statutes cover physicians only; others cover all health professionals. In some instances, the law covers any individual who renders first aid at the scene of an accident, with the exception of persons who receive compensation for such acts, for example, ambulance workers or other emergency personnel. The laws are provincial rather than national; therefore, they tend to vary from one jurisdiction to another. These laws are usually referred to as **Good Samaritan laws** and are intended to encourage qualified people to give aid in an emergency. In general, these laws protect the individual who renders emergency care from civil liability for this care, unless he or she is guilty of gross negligence or extreme malpractice in giving the care.

In some provinces, there is specific legislation stipulating that no one may leave the scene of an automobile accident without first giving aid to those injured in the accident. The Ontario Highway Traffic Act also places an obligation on people directly or indirectly involved in an accident to render assistance to those who have been injured. In the absence of such a law, there is no legal compulsion for the nurse, or anyone else for that matter, to give assistance in an emergency. If aid is given voluntarily, the person giving the aid is under an obligation to give the best care possible under the circumstances, commensurate with his or her knowledge, training and experience. Thus, if a nurse stops at the scene of an accident and gives emergency care as she or he has been taught (for example, applying pressure to stop bleeding), the nurse would be acting within accepted standards (Philpott, 1985).

Assault and Battery

In some instances, nurses have been involved in legal proceedings as a result of a charge of assault and battery by a patient. **Assault** refers to a threat to do physical harm to another, together with an apparent ability to carry out that threat. **Battery** is the actual touching of another person without consent. Assault and battery are considered criminal offences as well as torts. At all times, undue force is to be avoided in caring for patients. The law protects every individual against bodily harm by another person and also against any form of assault due to interference with his or her person. Therefore, a nurse cannot take a blood sample from a patient without consent. Nor may a person be operated on for any condition unless consent for the procedure has been obtained and the patient understands the significance of the procedure. Force-feeding a patient who refuses to eat may also be considered an assault.

The nurse may be the victim of assault by a violent patient. If the assault results in injury, the nurse has a legal right, just as any other person, to sue the person who committed the assault. Although the problem of nurses (and other staff) being assaulted by patients is by no means new, it is receiving increased attention as health agencies become more concerned about safety in the workplace. Support services are being developed to assist staff who have been assaulted by patients.

Recognizing that an unsafe environment undermines the quality of care, many health care agencies have developed written policies, offered educational programs and implemented documentation systems, all focussed on the prevention and management of aggression in the workplace. These employers also ensure that a variety of medical, psychological and legal supports and services are available to nurses and other staff who have been assaulted. Nova Scotia offers one excellent example of how a government agency, nursing and other partners have come together "to develop programs and materials that support individual health care organizations in addressing aggression in their workplace" (Whitehorn & Nowlan, 1997, p. 24).

Informed Consent

One of the most fundamental rights of patients is the right to consent to treatment. It is a well-established principle of law and ethics that competent individuals have the right to make their own decisions—including decisions about whether or not to have even life-saving treatment. Respect for this principle has led to the legal doctrine of informed consent. Informed consent is based on the ethical principle of autonomy.

Health professionals' belief that certain treatment is desirable for a person does not give them the right to go ahead with that treatment without the consent of the patient, except in an emergency. In an emergency, when treatment is a matter of life and death *and* the patient is unable to give permission, consent may be implied. In the past few years a number of lawsuits have centred on the issue of a patient's lack of consent to treatment. Although suits of this nature usually involve physicians or health agencies, the nurse may be called upon as a witness, for example, to attest to the patient's mental condition at the time consent was given to treatment. The nurse is also frequently asked to obtain the patient's signature on a consent form. She or he should be aware of the implications of these actions from a legal and ethical point of view.

Legally, **informed consent** means that the consent must be freely given, informed and specific to both the treatment and the caregiver (Philpott, 1985). In order for a consent to be valid, the patient must be of such mental capacity that he or she is capable of deciding whether or not to have the proposed treatment. In order to make that decision, the patient must be given sufficient information (in a language the patient understands) to give an informed consent. It is the physician's direct responsibility to inform patients about medical or surgical treatment—this is not a responsibility that can be delegated. The nurse may, however, present the form granting permission for medical or surgical treatment to the patient for a signature. In doing so, the nurse is simply verifying the identity of the patient—his or her signature does not require the nurse to determine whether the patient has had sufficient information to make a rational decision.

All health professionals should know, however, that the mere existence of a signed consent form does not by itself constitute a legal informed consent. Legally, there must be evidence that the patient is, indeed, informed. The ethical implications of witnessing a patient's signature on a consent form are different from the legal implications. As a patient advocate, the nurse should ensure that the patient understands what is being consented to. This does not mean that the nurse must supply the information—unless it is within the scope of nursing knowledge—but the nurse has an ethical obligation to make sure the patient gets the necessary information from the appropriate professional.

Professional nursing associations are concerned about the nurse's ethical responsibilities with respect to informed consent, and some have issued guidelines for nursing action in the form of policy statements. In their position statement on informed consent, the Registered Nurses Association of British Columbia (1994) states:

While registered nurses are responsible for explaining to the patient the care and treatment they give, physicians are legally responsible for informing patients of impending medical or surgical treatment. If a nurse should witness a consent form, this does not constitute obtaining the patient's consent. Nevertheless, nurses are ethically obliged to assess the patient's understanding of the proposed treatment and to inform the physician and/or the appropriate agency representative if there is reason to believe the patient has any misunderstanding regarding the nature, purpose, inherent risks or alternatives of his or her treatment.

RNABC, 1994

In the case of children, either parent may give permission for treatments and operative procedures. The age when individuals are no longer considered minors and can give their own consent to medical treatment varies in different jurisdictions, from 14 years of age (in the province of Quebec) to 21 years. Canadian law is increasingly recognizing that age by itself does not signify competence; rather, it is an individual's ability to understand the information and weigh the alternatives that matters. While it is unlikely that someone under the age of 13 would be able to demonstrate this, an older teenager may be able to do so. A teenager who no longer lives at home and is self-supporting may be legally deemed an **emancipated minor** and, as such, is considered an adult for the purpose of giving consent for medical treatment (Sneiderman, Irvine & Osborne, 1995). A **mature minor** is one who has demonstrated that he or she has the intelligence, understanding and independence to make decisions in regard to the acceptance or rejection of medical treatment.

Many hospitals are in the process of revising both their procedures for obtaining consent from patients and the forms that are used. Nurses should familiarize themselves with those that are being used in their agencies. A consent form used for specific operations or other special procedures is shown in Figure 6.1.

False Imprisonment

Individuals who are unjustifiably detained, or confined against their will and without a legal warrant for detention, may bring charges of **false imprisonment** against the individual or the agency that detained them. Most instances in which nurses have been involved in court proceedings on charges of false imprisonment have been in relation to patients with mental health problems. Canadian law provides for the detention without a warrant of persons who are mentally ill and who may hurt themselves or others. In addition, the law allows for the confinement of persons with selected communicable diseases that present a danger to society, for example, a person with tuberculosis in the highly contagious stage.

People cannot be prevented from leaving health agencies if they are of sound mind, even if health professionals feel that leaving would be inadvisable. If the patient insists on leaving, most agencies require that the patient sign a release stating that the agency will not be held responsible for any resulting harm. As with all patient decisions, the nurse and other health professionals should try to inform the patient in this situation of the risks and alternative courses of action. The use of force to hold someone against his or her will, or even the threat of forcible restraint made in order to detain a person, is considered assault. The nurse must therefore exercise caution in the use of restraints (see Chapter 30).

Invasion of Privacy

Under Canadian law, every individual has the right to withhold both self and property from public scrutiny. The right does not hold, however, if the individual has given consent for exposure; nor is there a tort when the person is a public figure or one who does acts of public interest (Philpott, 1985). A common instance in which the nurse must guard against invasion of a person's right to privacy is in the taking and use of photographs of patients. Consent must be obtained if these are to be used in any way not connected with the patient's treatment. Care must be taken by nurses also to avoid the exposure of a patient to roommates, visitors or others during the process of nursing care or when the patient is being transported from one area to another in the health agency.

Technology makes it more important than ever to take precautions to safeguard privacy. The use of tape recorders, videotapes and two-way mirrors without the patient's knowledge and consent could be taken as invasion of privacy.

Defamation of Character

Another area of the law the nurse should be aware of is that of suits arising from defamation of character. **Defamation of character** occurs when a person's reputation is damaged by written or spoken words that tend to lower his or her esteem in the eyes of other people. If the defamation is in a published article or a letter to a third party, or is depicted in a cartoon that causes the person to be the subject of ridicule or contempt, the term **libel** is used (Picard, 1978). **Slander** refers to defamation of character through spoken words. The nurse should always be careful not to discuss patients except with others who are involved with their care. Not every negative mention of a patient is slander or libel, of course; these terms are used only when there is a threat to the individual's reputation. To state that a patient had a broken leg would not be defamatory. If, however, one added that the broken leg was the result of a fall down the stairs because the patient was intoxicated, this might be considered defamation of character.

The Nurse and Confidential Information

The right to privacy extends also to information about the patient. The patient's record contains confidential information; it should not be left where it might be read by unauthorized persons. In using information from patients' records (or any

St. Paul's Hospital

1081 Burrard Street
Vancouver, B.C. V6Z 1Y6
(604) 682-2344

CONSENT FOR OPERATION/PROCEDURES

I, ____

(name of patient or person legally authorized to give consent)

do hereby authorize ____

(name of attending physician(s))

and the staff of St. Paul's Hospital to perform

____

(name of operation / procedure to be performed)

on ____

(name of patient)

the nature of which as been explained to me by Dr. ______________________

I further authorize the attending physician(s) and the staff of St. Paul's Hospital to perform such additional operations and/or surgical procedures as required or deemed advisable to safeguard life or health during surgery. In addition, I am aware that St. Paul's Hospital is a research and teaching hospital and give my consent that tissue removed for treatment and/or diagnostic evaluation may be used for research and educational purposes, with the understanding that all information concerning these tissues will be treated confidentially.

I further consent to the administration of a general or other anaesthetic for the purpose of this operation.

______________________ ______________________

(signature of patient) (signature of attending physician or delegate)

OR

______________________ ______________________

(signature of person legally qualified to give consent) (relationship to patient)

DATE ______________________

FORM NO. NF081 (Rev 8/96)

FIGURE 6.1 Consent for operation/procedures

SOURCE: St. Paul's Hospital, Vancouver, B.C.

information obtained from the patient) for case studies or other types of classroom work, the student nurse should be careful not to reveal the patient's identity; nor should information about a patient be discussed carelessly with people who are not entitled to that information. The nurse should always be discreet in giving out information about patients. Care should also be taken to limit access to computerized information about patients.

The CNA *Code of Ethics for Registered Nurses* (1997) specifically states that "nurses safeguard the trust of clients that information learned in the context of a professional relationship is shared outside the health care team only with the client's permission or as legally required" (p. 15). Legally, the betrayal of a patient's confidence is covered under the area of professional misconduct and may result in discipline by the professional organization. Whether confidential information entrusted to the nurse by the patient is considered to be a privileged communication and therefore inadmissible as evidence in court proceedings has not been definitely settled. In Canada, the rule of privilege for confidential information is not absolute. Although the nurse and the physician should not disclose confidential information entrusted to them, they may be directed to do so if this is justified by public policy or if the law requires reporting of the matter, or if the individual consents. The law requires that a witness in a court proceeding answer all questions that are relevant, whether or not the answer is incriminating. In certain cases, the witness can invoke the protection of the Canada Evidence Act. Mark Siegler, an ethicist, reminds us that it is the small indiscretions that the principle of confidentiality arose to prevent (Siegler, 1982). For example, the nurse should take care not to discuss patients in elevators, in the cafeteria, at home and so forth.

Wills

Nurses are often asked to witness a will for a patient. A **will** is a declaration of an individual's wishes regarding what is to be done with his or her property after death. The individual making the will is called the **testator**. A will must ordinarily be in writing and must be signed by the testator. The law usually requires the signature of two or three competent witnesses. Because an individual who may expect to benefit from a will should not act as a witness to its signing, the family and close friends of a patient are naturally reluctant to be witnesses. The nurse is therefore frequently called upon to act in this capacity, as the nurse is not an interested party. The nurse who is a minor should not agree to act as a witness, however. Minors—persons under the legal age as defined by the law of the particular province—are not usually acceptable as witnesses.

In most jurisdictions, all witnesses are required to be present at the same time and to sign the will in the presence of the person making it. Prior to signing the will, the witness should see the testator sign the will. If, however, the will has already been signed, the witness should either ask the testator to sign again or to declare that this is his or her will and signature and that the testator was competent to sign. It is not necessary for the witness to know the contents of the will, nor in most jurisdictions is it necessary for the witness to be told that the document is a will.

For a will to be valid, the person making it must be capable of understanding what he or she is doing. If the patient dies and the validity of the will is questioned, a nurse may be called upon to testify in court concerning the mental capacity of the individual at the time the will was made, even if the nurse was not a witness to the will. If the nurse is aware that a patient has made a will while in the hospital, it is a good practice to note on the patient's record the fact that a will was made, the date and time that it was signed, and the nurse's observations regarding the mental state of the patient at the time the will was made.

A **living will** is a form of what is called an *advance directive* in which an individual writes down preferences for treatment in the event that he or she cannot decide for him- or herself. Advance directives are increasingly common because people are afraid of what might happen if they become unable to make decisions for themselves. They often fear that they will be "hooked up to machines" when they would prefer to be allowed to die. At present, living wills have no legal authority in Canada, although there is considerable effort on the part of consumer groups to enact living will legislation. Nonetheless, a living will is often considered to be some evidence of a person's wishes. Patients should be counselled to discuss with their family members and physicians their preferences for treatment. Some agencies have policies about including a patient's living will in the patient's record.

Controlled Substances Legislation

Another area of the law in which the nurse is involved is in the control and administration of narcotics and other potentially harmful drugs. In Canada, the control of narcotic drugs is under federal jurisdiction as set out in the Controlled Drugs and Substances Act and Regulations (1997). This legislation controls the use of a number of drugs classified as **narcotics** (substances that induce drowsiness, sleep, stupor or insensibility). Certain other drugs, for example, barbiturates, have also been designated **controlled drugs**—those drugs which, under Canadian law, only certain persons are authorized to prescribe and dispense. These persons include physicians, dentists and veterinarians, but not nurses. Agencies develop policies based on these laws that nurses and other health professionals are responsible for upholding. Nurses are considered to be acting as agents of the physician when they administer controlled drugs. Nurses functioning as nurse practitioners in areas with few doctors usually prescribe and dispense medications (including controlled drugs) under *standing orders* from the physician, who is providing medical supervision, albeit on a remote basis. With changes in legislation to permit nurses to provide expanded health services, it is likely that the authority to prescribe certain narcotics and controlled drugs will be given to specific nurses in the near future.

It is unlawful for nurses to have narcotic drugs in their possession. The attempt to obtain narcotic drugs by fraud or deceit is a violation of the law. Penalties for violation include fine or imprisonment, or both. The nurse must be careful when handling narcotics to see that they have been ordered in writing by a duly licensed physician and that careful records are kept of their use.

Ethics in Nursing Practice

What Do Ethics Have to Do with Nursing Practice?

The law helps us to understand our rights, duties and obligations as nurses (Keatings & Smith, 1995). While legal judgements may appeal to ethical principles, and while the law may evolve towards higher ethical standards, the law is different from ethics (Storch, 1982). The law gives us the bottom lines for our practice, while ethics give us the horizons. Having explored the legal foundations of nursing practice, we now turn to its ethical foundations.

Ethics is a branch of philosophy that focusses critical reflection upon "actions and events from the standpoint of right and wrong, good and evil, moral value and moral disvalue, and ... the resolution to seek the truly valuable in life" (Kelly, 1980, p.13). Ethics give us horizons because it help us to know what is right, good and/or valuable. In other words, ethics give our practice a sense of direction. Since the 1960s, a great deal of attention has been paid to ethics in questions of health and health care. The specialized field known as *health care ethics* (or bioethics or biomedical ethics) is continuing to evolve, and has a strong multidisciplinary focus (Roy, Williams, & Dickens, 1994).

Within nursing, we have come to understand ethics in terms of good practice—practice that comes from good character and good action (Aristotle, ca. 320 BCE; cited in Benner, Tanner & Chesla, 1996). Thus, ethics is part of our daily work as nurses, not just the kind of life-and-death situations we read about in newspapers. As Benner and her colleagues state:

> *... even in clinical situations, where the ends are not in question, there is an underlying moral dimension: the fundamental disposition of the nurse toward what is good and right and action toward what the nurse recognizes or believes to be the best good in a particular situation.*
>
> Benner, Tanner & Chesla, p. 6

In the illustrations given in the box at the right, Tim Wong's concerns about an inadequate discharge plan for Sarah James and her family and Mary Danieli's desire to maintain trust with the Dickson family are significant ethical—not just clinical—concerns. Tim and Mary are trying to find the best good in the particular (and complex) situations in which they find themselves.

Nurses' Ethical Responsibilities

Central to our identity as nurses is the notion of ourselves as advocates for patients and families (Storch, 1992). Being an **advocate** means "to see that the patient's rights and interests are protected in health settings" (Davis, Aroskar, Liaschenko & Drought, 1997, p. 76). Over the years there have been different formulations of what advocacy in nursing

Illustrations: Ethics in Nursing Practice

Sarah James

Sarah James is a 79-year-old woman with severe arthritis. Over the past 10 days, she has been hospitalized in an acute medical unit for pneumonia and a urinary tract infection. She is due to be discharged home tomorrow, but she is still unable to walk or care for herself without extensive assistance. She is to be discharged home to the care of her son-in-law, who is also looking after his 58-year-old wife (Sarah's daughter). Sarah's daughter is seriously ill with cancer.

Tim Wong is the nurse assigned to care for Sarah. He is concerned that there is no adequate discharge plan for Sarah and her family. His workload on the ward is such that he has had almost no opportunity to meet with the physician or social worker to discuss his concerns.

SOURCE: Adapted with permission from Rodney, 1997.

The Dickson Family

Mary Danieli is a public health nurse. Her caseload includes the members of the Dickson family, who are being seen because two of the three children have significant health problems. The family includes a baby with cerebral palsy and a school-age girl with a genetic condition necessitating psychiatric care. Other family problems include drug and alcohol abuse, poor parenting skills and marital conflict. The family's experience with health care providers in the past has not been good, and they were initially guarded in their interactions with Mary. For example, they let Mary into their home only because she specializes in the care of children with disabilities. Over several months, Mary has worked hard at developing a good rapport with the family, and is beginning to see positive results from her efforts. However, a home support aide working with the baby noticed some problems which the aide interprets as neglect, and which she believes need to be reported to the Children's Aid Society. Mary is concerned about reporting the family because she knows that such an action will destroy the trust she has built with the family, and would make it difficult for any health care providers to enter the home in future.

SOURCE: Adapted with permission from MacPhail, 1996.

practice is, and although there is not theoretical consensus about the notion, it remains central to our identity. In the illustrations given above, for example, Tim Wong and Mary Danieli are acting as advocates by trying to protect the rights and interests of their patients and the patients' families. In the case of Sarah James, this means trying to ensure a proper plan for her and her family upon discharge; for the Dickson family, this means trying to protect the children's welfare while continuing to develop the parents' coping skills.

It should be noted that nurses are not the only possible advocates. Physicians, social workers, pastoral care workers, physiotherapists and others also believe in protecting the rights and interests of their patients and the patients' families. For example, the physician, social worker and physiotherapist caring for Sarah James are also concerned about her welfare. The problem is that they are not always available, and Tim has little time to consult them. The home support aide working with the Dicksons' baby is certainly trying to protect the children of the family. The problem is that calling in outside help from social services may worsen their long-term welfare.

Codes of Nursing Ethics

Nurses' ethical responsibilities, including the central notion of patient/family advocacy, are delineated in professional **codes of ethics**. "As creeds, codes of nursing ethics provide a valuable reminder of the special responsibilities incumbent upon those who tend the sick. Nurses often deal with people who, because of their illness or injury, are especially vulnerable and must depend upon the professional's special knowledge and skills. Hence, it is important that the nursing profession formulate and adhere to high ideals of conduct in order to assure the public that individual nurses will not exploit their advantaged position" (Benjamin & Curtis, 1992, p. 6).

Codes of ethics set the standards for moral decency by which the profession and the public can evaluate (and potentially discipline) individual members. Further, codes provide guidance for individual members about their own conduct (Benjamin & Curtis, 1992). Codes also "inform the public about what they can expect from professional practitioners" (Yeo, 1996, p. 3). Each profession has its own code, and individual countries usually have their own form of each professional code. Within the nursing profession, the International Council of Nursing also has a code of ethics to address nursing across countries.

Codes of ethics are not static documents, and must be reviewed at regular intervals. The Canadian Nurses Association *Code of Ethics for Registered Nurses* (reprinted in Appendix A) has been newly revised on the basis of "the consequences of economic constraints; increasing use of technology in health care; and, changing ways of delivering nursing services, such as the move to care outside of the institutional setting" (CNA, 1997, p. 1). While codes of ethics cannot be used to solve the particulars of complex situations, they can provide significant direction, particularly if they are kept current (Storch, 1992; Yeo, 1996). To illustrate, in the new CNA Code (1997), under the value of "health and well-being," Tim Wong would find the statement: "Nurses support and advocate a full continuum of health services ..." (p. 8). This delineation of responsibility would validate his desire to facilitate a proper discharge plan for Sarah James. Under the value of "choice," Mary Danieli would find the words: "Nurses seek to involve clients in health planning and health care decision-making." This statement of responsibility would support her wish to work with the Dickson family's strengths (p. 10). However, under the same value, Danieli would also find the statement: "Nurses respect the informed decisions of competent persons to refuse treatment and to choose to live at risk.... [N]urses are not obliged to comply with clients' wishes when doing so would require action contrary to the law" (p. 11). If the Dickson children are, in fact, suffering from neglect, Mary would be obligated to report the family to social services.

Mary's situation demonstrates the complexity and ambiguity of many ethical problems. While the Code would be a good starting place for her, she would also need a number of other ethics resources. Some possible resources will be explored later in this chapter.

Ethical Problems Faced by Nurses in Practice

Ethical problems* are issues that:

- cannot be resolved solely through an appeal to empirical data
- involve conflicts of values and uncertainty about the amount or type of information needed to make decisions
- have profound relevance for several areas of human concern (Curtin, 1982a, pp. 38–39).

The past three decades have seen much research on the types of ethical problems that nurses face in their daily practice. These problems include prolongation of life, lack of informed consent, violations of confidentiality, questionable practices of professionals within and outside the field of nursing, team conflict, allocation of scarce resources and inadequate nursing staffing (Rodney & Starzomski, 1993). Recently, research has increasingly emphasized problems of resources and staffing (Rodney, 1997; Sibbald, 1997).

Nursing is not the only profession concerned with ethics. Physicians, social workers, and professionals in

* The term *ethical dilemma* is often used in place of "ethical problem." Technically, a dilemma is a choice between two mutually exclusive alternatives. In nursing, the realities of practice are such that we often face more than two mutually exclusive alternatives. "Ethical problem" will therefore be the preferred term in this chapter.

other disciplines share similar problems. However, what seems to be unique to nursing is the morally "in between" position that we occupy (Bishop & Scudder, 1990). Nurses are often caught between their obligations to patients and families, our employing institutions, and physicians and other health professionals (Davis, et al., 1997; Storch, 1992). These multiple obligations can conflict, and may leave us in situations where we cannot implement the moral choices that we wish to make (Liaschenko, 1993; Yeo & Ford, 1996).

For example, in the illustration given above, Tim Wong has a moral obligation to Sarah James and her family to facilitate a safe and well-planned discharge, but he also has an obligation to the hospital to care for a number of other ill patients. These conflicting obligations are going to make it difficult for Tim to initiate the multidisciplinary team meeting that is required to help Sarah and her family. Indeed, the heavy workload that Tim is carrying and the inaccessibility of the physician and social worker are significant situational constraints. **Situational constraints** are "aspects of our structural and interpersonal work environments that impede our implementation of the standards of our practice and thus jeopardize the quality of patient and family care" (Rodney & Starzomski, 1993, p. 24).

Furthermore, when we are unable to implement our moral choices because of our morally in-between position and situational constraints, we often suffer moral distress. **Moral distress** leaves us with feelings of guilt, anger, frustration and powerlessness (Wilkinson, 1987/1988). For example, during the research interviews that led to their stories being used as illustrations for this chapter, Tim Wong expressed anger and frustration about his difficulty in initiating a team meeting for Sarah James and her family. Mary Danieli expressed guilt and powerlessness when the home support aide wanted to call social services about the Dickson family. Mary's moral distress was all the more acute because the consequences of her moral choices were unclear. The Dickson family might have continued to improve in their parenting with her interventions, but it was unclear what immediate risk the children were at. Nor was it clear what would happen if social services were brought in. The past experiences of Mary and other public health nurses indicated that social services intervention, if not well coordinated, could worsen family conflict and leave the nurse unable to continue in a therapeutic relationship with family members (MacPhail, 1996).

Dealing with Ethical Problems

MAKING GOOD DECISIONS

Mary Danieli's concerns about the Dickson family indicate that she needs a process by which to sort out the relevant facts, examine possible courses of action, and generate ethically sound solutions. She will not be able to do this alone, no matter how expert she is, and she will need time and strong communication skills to involve the family and other health care team members. What she needs is an ethical decision process.

There are several models of ethical decision making, and most of the models follow a process of rational deliberation not unlike the nursing process. For an ethical decision-making model to be effective, it must be used in a team* context, and it must include a sociocultural assessment of the patient and family. Furthermore, ethical decisions cannot be made in a one-shot, linear process. They require time, and decisions should be subject to revision as the facts of a particular situation are further discovered or as they change. The guiding light for any model is the best interests of the patient (as closely as can be determined).

Curtin's model (1982b) incorporates the major elements of the various decision-making models, and is expressed succinctly:

- Background information or data base. Relevant information should be gathered, organized, and sorted.
- Identification of ethical components. The information should be analysed to determine the nature of the ethical problem(s).
- Individuals involved in decision making. All persons affected by the decision should be identified and involved.
- Options or possible courses of action. A range of options, and their projected consequences, should be identified.
- Reconciling facts and principles. The options should be examined in light of relevant ethical theory in order to come up with a rational and defensible solution.
- Resolution. A decision should be generated that all members of the team have been party to and can understand even if they do not all agree with it (pp. 60–63).

In the resolution phase, solutions may be generated that are time-limited and thus scheduled for re-evaluation. For example, with the Dickson family the team might agree to a month's period of more intense intervention by Mary and the social workers, followed by a re-evaluation of the children's well-being at a designated point. The collection of facts must be continuous, because the facts will matter a great deal for each phase of the process. Discovering that the Dickson children have poor hygiene, for example, would be quite different from discovering that they are being physically abused.

INDIVIDUAL ETHICAL RESOURCES

One of the most important ethical resources for individuals is the clinical expertise of the various team members. For

* The team includes the patient (or the patient's designated spokesperson, if the patient is no longer competent), family members (those individuals identified as family by the patient, which may or may not include next of kin), and health professionals/providers involved in the care of the patient.

example, Tim Wong's expertise in nursing the elderly will help him to understand, and explain to others, what kind of care Sarah James will require when she returns home. The physician will need to be able to project how Sarah's lungs and kidneys will function; the social worker will need to know the scope of community resources available for the James family; and the physiotherapist will need to devise a progressive mobilization regime for Sarah.

Secondly, the personal values and sensitivities of the individual team members are an essential resource. Ethical problems can be addressed only if they are noticed. As Canadian philosopher Michael Yeo (1996) explains:

> *The Socratic injunction "know thyself" names the task at the entrance to the moral life. Through our upbringing and acculturation—the influence of family, peers, and so on—we acquire numerous beliefs about right and wrong and good and bad. Beliefs thus acquired are deeply constitutive of who we are as adults, and may manifest themselves in our actions without our ever having reflected upon them. We may not realize how these beliefs express themselves in our lives until challenged by others. The choice of the ethical life as expressed in the injunction "know thyself" commits one to bringing such unreflected beliefs to light and, having clarified them, to explicitly and responsibly embrace, reject, or modify them.* (p. 11)

Being able to notice, and subsequently respond to, ethical problems thus necessitates an ongoing commitment to critical self-reflection. Health professionals need to understand their own values so that they do not inadvertently use them to arrive at decisions that ought to serve the best interests of the patient. Critical self-reflection means understanding the differences between the values held by the self, the values held by others and professional values.

Indeed, Tim Wong's values pertaining to the elderly mean that he is sensitive to the need to come up with a plan that maximizes Sarah James's independence. Mary Danieli's values about equity mean that she will try to make economic and personal resources available to the Dickson family. The values that Tim and Mary hold come from their family backgrounds, their peers and past experiences, and have been thoughtfully refined over time. While reflecting on their own values, they have tried to make them congruent with their professional values, which are articulated in the CNA *Code of Ethics for Registered Nurses*.

For example, if Mary previously held the belief that individuals who use drugs and alcohol are less worthy than those who do not, she will have refined this belief over time. Knowledge about the traumas that lead to problems with substance use will have helped her to modify this belief. Mary will also have realized that this personal belief is incongruent with the value of "fairness" defined in her nursing code, which tells her that "nurses provide care in response to need regardless of such factors as race, ethnicity, culture, spiritual beliefs, social or marital status, gender, sexual orientation, age, health status, lifestyle or the physical attributes of the client" (CNA, 1997, p. 17).

Thirdly, in order to deal with ethical problems in their practice, nurses (and other members of the health care team) require a knowledge base in ethical theory. That is, they need a "philosophical understanding of the fundamental concepts used in moral analysis and the tensions between them" so that they may "sort out confusions, clarify disagreements, and promote creative problem-solving" (Yeo, 1996, pp. 15–16).

The reader is directed to the references listed in the back of this chapter for sources on ethical theory. However, five fundamental concepts will be identified here. These concepts provide important direction in the fifth phase of Curtin's (1982b) model ("reconciling facts and principles"). They are *autonomy*, *beneficence/nonmaleficence*, *justice*, *fidelity* and *care*. The first three concepts are well-established principles that have become a foundation for health care ethics. Ethical theory has evolved to address the context in which health care is delivered, including the nature of health care team relationships (Winkler, 1993; Wolf, 1994). Fidelity and care are two important contextual/relational concepts.

Fundamental Concepts of Ethical Theory

- **Autonomy** can be defined as self-governance by the individual, or "personal rule of the self while remaining free from both controlling interferences by others and personal limitations ... that prevent meaningful choice" (Beauchamp & Childress, 1989, p. 68).
- **Beneficience/nonmaleficence** directs us to prevent or remove evil or harm, do or promote good, and not inflict evil or harm (Beauchamp & Childress, 1989, pp. 122–123).
- **Justice** is defined as fairness— giving persons what they are entitled to or can legitimately claim. Distributive justice refers to the just distribution of goods and services in society. This distribution is structured by various moral, legal and cultural rules and principles that form the terms of cooperation for society (Beauchamp & Childress, 1989, pp. 257–258).
- **Fidelity** is based on trust, and generates rules for promise-keeping based on respect for autonomy (Beauchamp & Childress, 1989, pp. 341–342). Given the trust that patients and family members must put in professionals, fidelity is an important feature in relationships between health care providers and their clients (Cooper, 1988; Sokolowski, 1991).
- **Care** is the basis for ethical decision making in health care. That is, health professionals should strive to do good in the context of relationships between themselves and patients and their family members (Fry, 1991).

Knowledge Needed for Ethical Problems

- KNOWLEDGE OF THE SITUATION: A case history and knowledge of the roles and opinions of major participants help to clarify the facts and the nature of the problem.
- KNOWLEDGE OF ONESELF AND ONE'S VALUES: An understanding of one's own philosophy of nursing helps to clarify one's options and sometimes the nature of the problem.
- KNOWLEDGE OF THE PROFESSION'S VALUES: In Canada, the CNA *Code of Ethics for Registered Nurses* defines the profession's expectations.
- KNOWLEDGE OF THE LAW: While ethical behaviour is not always consistent with legal behaviour, knowledge of the laws impinging on the problem aids in identifying consequences of alternative actions.
- KNOWLEDGE OF PHILOSOPHY: Application of ethical principles as well as ethical theories provides a broader philosophical perspective to the problem at hand.

SOURCE: Perry & Ericksen, 1993, p. 367.

Together, these five concepts can provide comprehensive direction for ethical decision making. To return to Sarah James's situation:

- Autonomy would remind team members to respect Sarah's choices about her independence.
- Beneficence/nonmaleficence would remind them to prevent injury to Sarah.
- Justice would remind them to come up with a solution for Sarah that they would be happy with if Sarah were the mother of any of the team members.
- Fidelity would remind them to treat Sarah on the basis of her best interests and not on the basis of the hospital's need for her bed.
- Caring would remind them to ensure that Sarah's daughter and son-in-law were considered.

In conclusion, it can be seen that the individual resources needed to make good decisions are substantial (see Knowledge Needed for Ethical Problems, above).

Other individual resources include knowledge of the law, and knowledge of relevant professional and institutional policies and procedures. However, ethical problems take place in complex health care contexts. Institutional resources are also required.

INSTITUTIONAL ETHICAL RESOURCES

Since the late 1970s, institutional ethics committees have become a feature in many hospitals, and are beginning to appear in long-term care and community settings. Institutional ethics committees are multidisciplinary in their function and assist health professionals with education, policy development and/or case consultation. It is generally acknowledged that ethics committees take time to become functional in an institution. Unfortunately, not all health professionals know about their institutional ethics committee or are comfortable accessing it, and this is particularly true for nurses (Storch, 1994). Nevertheless, institutional ethics committees are an important resource, and usually have an open-door policy for staff as well as patients and families. They serve in an advisory capacity and can help staff with difficult deliberations such as those faced by Tim Wong and Mary Danieli.

Members of an ethics committee could, for example, attend a team meeting with Mary Danieli, the home support aide, the social workers, psychiatrist and other professionals/providers involved with the Dickson family to help initiate an ethical decision process. Sometimes the ethics committee will have available a health care ethics consultant, who is a professional philosopher well versed in ethical theory, clinical practice and group process (Baylis, 1994).

Nurse managers also have responsibilities for ethics at the institutional level. They need to work to set up a positive moral climate for practice (Storch, 1994). Clearly, this is a task that requires the support of their staff, their institutional administration and their professional association. For example, a nurse manager who listened to Tim Wong's concerns about inadequate staffing and poor discharge planning could collect supportive data from other staff, set up interdisciplinary meetings to look for solutions and approach hospital administration and/or the ethics committee about the seriousness of the problems. At a broader level, the nurse manager could also speak to the provincial nurses' association to address societal issues about health care resource allocation.

Values Clarification

A principal foundation of professional behaviour is understanding why we do what we do—that is, making conscious rational decisions. Our values are one factor that shape our behaviour. "A value is an affective disposition towards a person, object, or idea" (Steele & Harmon, 1983, p. 1).

You have probably acquired your values from many sources—family, friends, society. As well, your values may change over time in response to your life experience. Stopping to clarify your values facilitates critical reflection, ethical decision making and moral development—and thus your growth as a health professional and as a person.

Values clarification is a process of choosing, prizing, and affirming. The process uses strategies and exercises to engage you in:

- becoming aware of your own set of values
- choosing among alternative values
- matching your stated values with actions.

SOURCE: Steele & Harmon, 1983.

Looking to the Future

Ethics establishes horizons for our practice. Every nurse needs to enact ethics as part of nursing practice, and groups of nurses and nursing associations need to make ethical practice possible. This has implications for nursing education and research. Education in ethics is an ongoing venture, partly because ethical theory itself continues to evolve. Ethics education must include a focus on multidisciplinary collaboration. As was clear with Sarah James and the Dickson family, the solutions to ethical problems cannot be achieved by any one profession alone.

Study guides called *Everyday Ethics: Putting the Code into Practice* (1998) and *Ethics in Practice* (1998) are currently being produced by the Canadian Nurses Association to assist nurses to use the Code within their practice.

Ethics and Nursing Research

Research about ethics in nursing practice is just beginning to flourish. While we need to attend to ethics in the way we conduct any research, we also need to devise ways to make our ethical horizons in practice achievable.

One area of practice that has been of considerable concern to nurses from an ethical point of view is research that involves human beings as subjects. The Canadian Nurses Association (1994) has developed a position paper, *Ethical Guidelines for Nursing Research*, addressing this issue. The relationship of trust between patient and nurse has always been an essential element of the professional code of ethics. In research, the relationship of trust between subject and investigator requires that the investigator assume special obligations to safeguard the subject in several ways. Subjects in a research study must consent voluntarily to participate. Before obtaining this consent, the researcher must make sure that the subject understands the nature and purpose of the study and is fully aware of his or her role in it. The subject needs to know the risks involved and any potential physical or psychological discomfort that may ensue from participating. For example, in a study to examine the grieving process, asking the participant to discuss his or her reactions to the death of a loved one may bring back painful memories. Subjects also need to be made aware of the extent of any anticipated invasion of privacy. For example, when the study involves asking personal questions, the individual should know the areas to be covered by the questions and the amount of detail required in the answers. Additionally, the investigator must guarantee that no risk, discomfort, invasion of privacy or threat to personal dignity beyond that initially stated in describing subjects' roles in the study will be imposed without further permission being obtained. Finally, subjects must be assured that if they do not wish to participate in the study, neither will they be subjected to harassment nor will the quality of their care be influenced by this decision.

To close with the words of a philosopher who has written extensively about ethics in nursing practice, "we want, as participants in institutional culture, to be able to notice our moral problems and to cope with them with sensitivity and integrity and to keep our health care institutions responsive to their moral goals" (Jameton, 1990, p. 450).

IN REVIEW

- Nurses have a responsibility to provide safe and competent care to their patients and to respect their patients' fundamental rights while doing so.
- Professional nursing associations represent nursing and serve as the official voice for the profession. These associations include:
  - International Council of Nurses (ICN)
  - Canadian Nurses Association (CNA)
  - Canadian Nursing Students Association (CNSA)
  - Canadian Association of Practical Nurses and Nursing Assistants (CAPNNA)
  - Canadian Registered Psychiatric Nurses Association (CRPNA).

  At all levels, these associations are concerned with promoting the profession and advocating high standards of nursing care in the interest of the public.
- Nursing unions serve as the bargaining agents for salaried nurses. These organizations are concerned with the social and financial welfare of their members.
- Nursing is regulated by provincial and territorial nursing practice acts. These acts protect the health and safety of the public by:
  - registering nurses to practise
  - setting standards for practice
  - intervening when practice falls below standard (i.e., determing competency to practise).
- Nurses are legally responsible to:
  - society
  - their professional association
  - their patients.
- Reasonable prudence is expected of all nurses, and each nurse is accountable for his or her own actions.
- The Canadian document, *Consumer Rights in Health Care* (1989), states that consumers have the right to:
  - be informed
  - be respected as the persons having the major responsibility for their own health decisions
  - participate in decision making that affects their health
  - have equal access to health care.

- Legal matters relevant to nursing include:
  - torts
  - crimes
  - negligence
  - malpractice
  - assault
  - battery
  - invasion of privacy
  - false imprisonment
  - defamation of character.
- Informed consent is the fundamental right of the patient, and the nurse has the ethical responsibility to ensure that the patient is informed before the consent form is signed. To be legally valid, consent must be:
  - informed
  - consensual
  - freely given
  - specific to both the treatment and the caregiver.

  Further, the patient must be mentally competent to comprehend the information and make decisions based on it.
- A will is a declaration of an individual's wishes regarding the disposition of property after death.
- Although not a legal document in Canada, a living will is an advance directive regarding treatment when a patient is unable to make decisions for himself or herself.
- Narcotics and certain other substances are controlled under the federal Controlled Drugs and Substances Act and its regulations. Under this Act, nurses must:
  - not prescribe or dispense narcotics or controlled drugs
  - keep careful records on the administration of these substances.
- Ethics focusses on critical reflection on what is right, good and valuable. Ethics gives health professionals a direction in which to move their practice.
- The CNA *Code of Ethics for Registered Nurses* commits its members to certain ethical values. Ethical principles of particular concern to nurses are:
  - autonomy
  - beneficence/nonmaleficence
  - justice
  - fidelity
  - care.

  When faced with an ethical problem, nurses have a responsibility to use sound reasoning based on the CNA *Code of Ethics*.
- Values clarification is a three-step process that allows an individual to identify personal values. These steps are:
  - choosing
  - prizing
  - acting.

Critical Thinking Activities

1. What issues are currently of concern to the ICN, the CNA, your provincial professional association, regulating authority, your district chapter and the nursing union in your province?
2. Do you have a student association at your nursing school? Is it affiliated with the provincial/territorial nursing association? Does your class have a representative on it? What issues are of current concern to the student association?
3. What are the titles of the provincial statute(s) regulating nurses in your province? When was it (were they) passed? How does it (do they) define the functions of nurses? Does your professional association have guidelines delineating nurses' functions? Compare the scope of practice of registered nurses, registered psychiatric nurses (if applicable in your province) and licensed practical nurses as these are specified in nursing acts and in professional association guidelines in your province/territory. Check out the Web site of your provincial association.
4. Discuss the two major regulating processes (i.e., registration and professional conduct review) of your province/territory as they relate to the public interest.
5. Discuss with your classmates the Susan Nelles case, using the following questions as a basis for your discussions:
   a) Why was Susan Nelles charged with the murder of infants at the Hospital for Sick Children in Toronto?
   b) What evidence led to her arrest?
   c) What were the findings of the Grange Inquiry?
   d) What were the recommendations of the Dubin Commission?
   e) How did the professional nursing association respond?
   f) What new evidence/theories have been put forth to explain the deaths of the infants?

KEY TERMS

consumers' bill of rights p. 99
Code of Ethics for Registered Nurses p. 99
regulating authority p. 101
nursing practice act p. 101
licence p. 103
registration p. 103
professional conduct review (PCR) p. 103
reasonable prudence p. 104
accountability p. 105
safety to practise p. 105
quality assurance p. 105
tort p. 108

KEY TERMS

crime p. 108
negligence p. 108
malpractice p. 108
Good Samaritan laws p. 109
assault p. 110
battery p. 110
informed consent p. 110
emancipated minor p. 111
mature minor p. 111
false imprisonment p. 111
defamation of character p. 111
libel p. 111
slander p. 111
will p. 113
testator p. 113
living wil p. 113
narcotics p. 113
controlled drugs p. 113
ethics p. 114
advocate p. 114
code of ethics p. 115
situational constraints p. 116
moral distress p. 116
autonomy p. 117
beneficence/ nonmaleficence p. 117
justice p. 117
fidelity p. 117
care p. 117

References

BAYLIS, F.E. (1994). A profile of the health care ethics consultant. In F.E. Baylis (Ed.), *The health care ethics consultant* (pp. 25–44). Totowa, NJ: Humana Press.

BEAUCHAMP, T.L., & CHILDRESS, J.F. (1989). *Principles of biomedical ethics.* (3rd ed.). New York: Oxford University Press.

BENJAMIN, M., & CURTIS, J. (1992). *Ethics in nursing.* (3rd ed.). New York: Oxford University Press.

BENNER, P.A., TANNER, C.A., & CHESLA, C.A. (1996). *Expertise in nursing practice: Caring, clinical judgment, and ethics.* New York: Springer.

BISHOP, A.H., & SCUDDER, J.R. (1990). *The practical, moral, and personal sense of nursing: A phenomenological philosophy of practice.* New York: State University of New York Press.

CANADIAN NURSES ASSOCIATION. (1968). *The leaf and the lamp.* Ottawa: Author.

CANADIAN NURSES ASSOCIATION. (1993). *The scope of nursing practice: A review of issues and trends.* Ottawa: Author.

CANADIAN NURSES ASSOCIATION.(1994). *Ethical guidelines for nurses in research involving human participants.* Ottawa: Author.

CANADIAN NURSES ASSOCIATION. (1997). *Code of ethics for registered nurses.* Ottawa: Author.

CANADIAN NURSES ASSOCIATION. (CNA) (1998a). *Everyday ethics: Putting the code into practice.* Ottawa: Author.

CANADIAN NURSES ASSOCIATION. (CNA) (1998). *Ethics in practice.* Ottawa: Author.

CHARBONNEAU, L. (1985). The Grange Report: Nurses criticize commission's report for lack of answers. *Canadian Nurse, 81*(3), 14–18.

CONSUMERS ASSOCIATION OF CANADA. (1989). *Consumer rights in health care.* Toronto: Author. (Under review)

COOPER, M.C. (1988). Covenental relationships: Grounding for the nursing ethic. *Advances in Nursing Science, 10*(4), 48–59.

CURTIN, L. (1982a). Human problems: Human beings. In L. Curtin & M.J. Flaherty (Eds.), *Nursing ethics: Theories and pragmatics* (pp. 37–42). Bowie, MD: Prentice Hall.

CURTIN, L. (1982b). No rush to judgement. In L. Curtin & M.J. Flaherty (Eds.), *Nursing ethics: Theories and pragmatics* (pp. 57–63).Bowie, MD: Prentice Hall.

DAVIS, A.J., AROSKAR, M.A., LIASCHENKO, J., & DROUGHT, T.S. (1997). *Ethical dilemmas and nursing practice.* (4th ed.). Stamford, CT: Appleton & Lange.

DUBIN, C.L., GILCHRIST, J.M., McDONALD, H.D., & NADLER, H.L. (1983). *Report of the Hospital for Sick Children Review Committee.* Toronto: Alan Gordon, Queen's Printer of Ontario.

FRY, S.T. (1991). A theory of caring: Pitfalls and promises. In D.A. Gaut & M.M. Leininger (Eds.), *Caring: The compassionate healer* (pp. 161–172). New York: National League for Nursing.

GRANGE, S.G.M. (1984). *Report of the Royal Commission of Inquiry into certain deaths at the Hospital for Sick Children and related matters.* Toronto: Ontario Ministry of the Attorney General. (Available by mail through Publications Services, 5th Floor, 880 Bay Street, Toronto, Ontario)

HAMILTON, G. (1993). The nurses are innocent. *Canadian Nurse, 89*(11), 27–32.

JAMETON, A. (1990). Culture, morality, and ethics: Twirling the spindle. *Critical Care Nursing Clinics of North America, 2*(3), 443–451.

JENSEN, P.M. (1992). The changing role of nurses' unions. In A.J. Baumgart & J. Larsen (1992). *Canadian nursing faces the future.* (2nd ed., pp. 557–573). Toronto: Mosby.

KEATINGS, M., & SMITH, O.B. (1995). *Ethical and legal issues in Canadian nursing.* Toronto: W.B. Saunders.

KELLY, E. (1980). The search for values. In L.E. Navia & E. Kelly (Eds.), *Ethics and the search for values* (pp. 3–22). New York: Prometheus Books.

LIASCHENKO, J. (1993). Feminist ethics and cultural ethos: Revisiting a nursing debate. *Advances in Nursing Science, 15*(4), 71–81.

MacPHAIL, S.A. (1996). *Ethical issues in community nursing.* Unpublished master's thesis, University of Alberta, Edmonton, Alberta.

Nurses (Registered) Act Rules, Part 2. (British Columbia,1988).

Nurses Act RSQ, Chapter 1–8. (Quebec, 1994).

PERRY, J., & ERICKSEN, J. (1993). Legal and ethical issues. In A. Beckingham & B.W. Du Gas (Eds.), *Promoting healthy aging* (pp. 353–369). St. Louis: Mosby.

PHILPOTT, M. (1985). *Legal liability and the nursing process.* Toronto: W.B. Saunders.

PICARD, E. (1978). *Legal liability of doctors and hospitals in Canada.* Toronto: Carswell.

QUINN, C.A., & SMITH, M.D. (1987). *The professional commitment: Issues and ethics in nursing.* Toronto: W.B. Saunders.

REGISTERED NURSES ASSOCIATION OF BRITISH COLUMBIA. (1994). *Position statement: Informed comment.* Vancouver: Author.

REGISTERED NURSES ASSOCIATION OF BRITISH COLUMBIA (RNABC). (1998). *Standards for nursing practice in British Columbia.* Vancouver: Author.

REGISTERED NURSES ASSOCIATION OF ONTARIO (RNAO). (undated). *RNAO responds. A nursing perspective on events at the Hospital for Sick Children and the Grange Inquiry.* Toronto: Author.

RODNEY, P.A. (1997). *Towards connectedness and trust: Nurses' enactment of their moral agency within an organizational context.* Unpublished doctoral dissertation, University of British Columbia, Vancouver, British Columbia.

RODNEY, P., & STARZOMSKI, R. (1993). Constraints on the moral agency of nurses. *Canadian Nurse, 89*(9), 23–26.

ROY, D.J., WILLIAMS, J.R., & DICKENS, B.M. (1994). *Bioethics in Canada.* Toronto: Prentice Hall.

SIBBALD, B. (1997). Delegating away patient safety. *Canadian Nurse, 93*(2), 22–26.

SIEGLER, M. (1982). Confidentiality in medicine: A decrepit concept? *New England Journal of Medicine, 301*, 1518–1521.

SNEIDERMAN, B., IRVINE, J.C., & OSBORNE, P.H. (1995). *Canadian medical law: An introduction for physicians, nurses and other health care professionals.* (2nd ed.). Toronto: Carswell.

SOKOLOWSKI, R. (1991). The fiduciary relationship and the nature of professions. In E.D. Pellegrino, R.M. Veatch & J.P. Langan (Eds.), *Ethics, trust, and the professions: Philosophical and cultural aspects* (pp. 23–43). Washington, DC: Georgetown University Press.

SPLANE, R., & SPLANE, V.H. (1991). International nursing: Looking beyond our borders. In J. Kerr & J. MacPhail (Eds.), *Canadian nursing: Issues and perspectives.* (2nd ed., pp. 353–365). Toronto: Mosby.

STEELE, S., & HARMON, V. (1983). *Values clarification in nursing.* New York: Appleton-Century-Crofts.

STORCH, J. (1982). Patients' rights: *Ethical and legal issues in health care and nursing.* Toronto: McGraw-Hill Ryerson.

STORCH, J.L. (1992). Ethical issues. In A.J. Baumgart & J. Larsen (Eds.), *Canadian nursing faces the future.* (2nd ed., pp. 259–270). Toronto: Mosby.

STORCH, J.L. (1994). Ethical dimensions of nursing management. In J.M. Hibberd & M.E. Kyle (Eds.), *Nursing management in Canada* (pp. 142–158). Toronto: W.B. Saunders.

WHITEHORN, D., & NOWLAN, M. (1997). Towards an aggression-free health care environment. *Canadian Nurse, 93*(3), 24–26.

WILKINSON, J.M. (1987/88). Moral distress in nursing practice: Experience and effect. *Nursing Forum, 23*, 16–28.

WINKLER, E.R. (1993). From Kantianism to contextualism: The rise and fall of the paradigm theory in bioethics. In E.R. Winkler & J.R. Coombs (Eds.), *Applied ethics: A reader* (pp. 343–365). Oxford, U.K.: Blackwell.

WOLF, S.M. (1994). Shifting paradigms in bioethics and health law: The rise of a new pragmatism. *American Journal of Law & Medicine, 20*(4), 395–415.

YEO, M. (1996). Introduction. In M. Yeo & A. Moorhouse (Eds.), *Concepts and cases in nursing ethics.* (2nd ed., pp. 1–26). Peterborough, ON: Broadview Press.

YEO, M., & FORD, A. (1996). Integrity. In M. Yeo & A. Moorhouse (Eds.), *Concepts and cases in nursing ethics.* (2nd ed., pp. 267–306). Peterborough, ON: Broadview Press.

Additional Readings

AFFARA, F., & STYLES, M. (1993). *Nursing regulation guidebook: From principle to power.* Geneva: International Council of Nurses.

CANADIAN NURSES PROTECTIVE SOCIETY. (1993). Confidentiality of health information: Your client's right. *InfoLaw: A Legal Information Sheet for Nurses, 1*(2). Ottawa: Author.

CANADIAN NURSES PROTECTIVE SOCIETY. (1994a). Negligence. *InfoLaw: A Legal Information Sheet for Nurses, 3*(1). Ottawa: Author.

CANADIAN NURSES PROTECTIVE SOCIETY. (1994b). Consent to treatment: The role of the nurse. *InfoLaw: A Legal Information Sheet for Nurses, 3*(2). Ottawa: Author.

CANADIAN NURSES PROTECTIVE SOCIETY. (1996). Medication errors. *InfoLaw: A Legal Information Sheet for Nurses, 5*(2). Ottawa: Author.

MASS, H. (1998). Telephone advice. *Nursing BC, 30*(1), 31–32.

McNEIL, J., & AFFARA, F. (1996). *The value of nursing in a changing world.* Geneva: International Council of Nurses.

OTT, B.R., & HARDI, T.L. (1997). Readability of advance directive documents. *Image, 29*(1), 53–57.

REGISTERED NURSES ASSOCIATION OF BRITISH COLUMBIA (RNABC). (1995). *Nursing self-regulation.* Vancouver: Author.

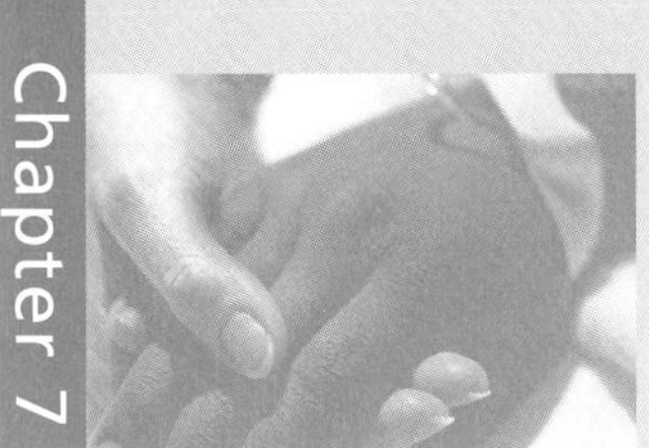

Chapter 7

Research and Nursing Practice

OUTLINE

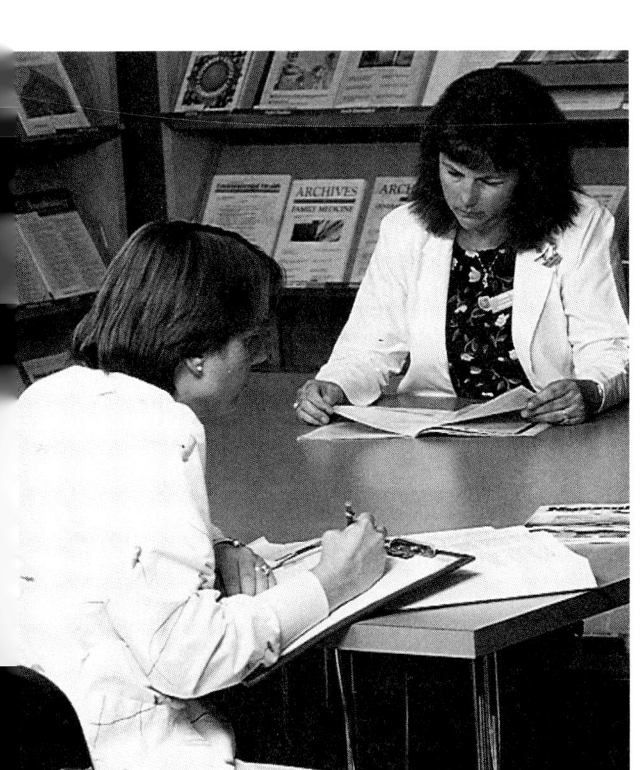

Central Questions

1. What is meant by research-based practice?
2. What is my role as a student in research-based practice?
3. How do we know things?
4. Why do nurses do research?
5. What kinds of research are Canadian nurses doing?
6. What is involved in critiquing a research report?
7. How can I understand research reports?
8. What is the purpose of the abstract?
9. What is a problem statement? Hypothesis? Assumption?
10. What kind of research designs are there?
11. What do the terms "sample," "population," "independent variable" and "dependent variable" mean?
12. How do I interpret the results of research findings?
13. What is the purpose of a statistical analysis of data?
14. How can I tell from the analysis whether the findings of the study are valid?
15. What can I learn from the discussion section of a report?
16. What does "clinical significance" mean?
17. What does the term "scientific merit" mean?

Introduction

Research is central to the development of theories for nursing practice. It stimulates growth of the body of knowledge upon which the practice of nursing is built.

Canadian Nurses Association, 1990

We said at the beginning of this text that research-based practice is an imperative for all who practise nursing in Canada today. You will, no doubt, have one or more courses on research methodology and on statistics at a more senior level in your program. In this chapter, we are concerned with helping you to gain an appreciation of the role of research in nursing practice, so that you can base practice on a solid research foundation from the first clinical assignment. In order to do this, it is essential to have some understanding of the research process and of the kinds of research that nurses in Canada and in other parts of the world are doing. You must also develop beginning skills in reading research reports, interpreting the findings and assessing the usefulness of these for your practice.

In this chapter, we will talk first about the meaning of the term **research-based practice**, and your role as students in regard to its various components. We will then discuss some basic concepts, such as ways of knowing, the goals of research and the kinds of research nurses are doing in Canada. The major portion of this chapter will be devoted to learning to read and understand research reports. As you gain skill in reading reports, you will also gain some understanding of the process a researcher follows in conducting a study.

Components of Research-Based Practice

"Research-based practice" includes three components:

1. the conduct of studies
2. the dissemination of research findings
3. the utilization of research in practice.

Research-Based Practice

Historical Perspective

The idea of basing one's clinical practice on nursing research has begun to take on increasing importance as research focussing on nursing practice grows and expands. Nursing researchers have not always focussed on nursing practice. The development of nursing research in Canada, like that in the United States and the United Kingdom, followed the evolution of nursing education in universities. Nursing programs initially focussed on preparing nurse educators and administrators, and researchers followed this lead by directing their attention to conducting investigations that would strengthen nursing education programs and help solve the problems that nurse administrators faced. It was not until the mid-1970s that a shift to research that was focussed on clinical nursing practice was observed in Canada (Stinson, 1986). There were several developments that precipitated this shift. One key development was the initiation of a series of national nursing research conferences. The first, cohosted by the University of British Columbia School of Nursing and National Health and Welfare, was held in Ottawa in 1971. These meetings provided an important stimulus for research designed to improve practice. By 1975 the national nursing research conference included five studies focusing on nursing practice in the program and by 1985 this increased to 39 studies (MacPhail, 1988). This trend has continued and augmented as nurses have begun to appreciate the importance of knowledge gained from research to improving nursing care.

The introduction of research courses in nursing undergraduate programs and the expansion of graduate programs in nursing have also facilitated the development of nursing research. The first master's-level program in nursing at a Canadian university was established at the University of Western Ontario in 1959. Nurses wishing to undertake graduate studies prior to that time entered programs in other disciplines such as education or public health, or they went to American schools of nursing (Field, Stinson & Thibaudeau, 1992). Now we have 19 master's-level programs in nursing in Canada. And with recent developments we have six Canadian universities with formal doctoral programs in nursing (Wood, 1997).

Now more than ever before, there is an increasing focus on nursing research as a strategy for enhancing nursing practice. There are many nurses in both hospital and community agencies who have varying levels of preparation in research. Baccalaureate graduates understand the research process and how to read and use research to guide their practice. Master's-prepared nurses are skilled in conducting systematic reviews of the research literature to determine the most up-to-date scientific information that should be used to guide patient care. Large hospitals and community health agencies often have doctorally prepared nurse researchers on staff to carry out studies, and to help other nursing staff review nursing research reports to identify the "best practice" to address clinical problems; to formulate research questions; and to undertake studies relevant to their practice concerns. The link between nursing research and practice has also been strengthened in health care organizations through the formation of nursing research committees, educational sessions for staff nurses, strategic plans for nursing research, and programs that encourage research-based decisions by staff nurses (Davis & Simms, 1992; Olson, 1992, 1993; Simpson, 1997). The development of closer links between researchers and practising nurses has acted as an important stimulus for nursing research. When faculty researchers are cross-appointed to clinical or community agencies, they collaborate with practising nurses to design and conduct research projects that address clinical problems.

LOOKING back Dr. Shirley M. Stinson, b. 1929

Shirley Stinson, one of Canada's most distinguished nurses, has a number of "firsts" among her many contributions to health care generally and to nursing and nursing research in particular. In 1972, she was the first nurse (and the first woman) to receive a Senior National Health Scientist Award (National Health Research and Development Program [NHRDP]). She completed only one year of the term of the award as she took a position as Acting Director of the University of Alberta's nursing program. However, she was then selected to serve on several NHRDP Review Committees that helped select those to receive the Senior National Health Scientist Award.

Dr. Stinson also was the founding chair of the first nursing research foundation in Canada to be funded by provincial or federal monies, the Alberta Foundation for Nursing Research, which was established in 1982. This foundation was the culmination of her efforts between 1972 and 1982 to achieve such status for nursing.

Born in Arlee, Saskatchewan, Shirley Stinson was raised in Alberta and received a bachelor of science in nursing from the University of Alberta in 1953. She took a master's degree in nursing service administration from the University of Minnesota in 1958 and a doctorate in higher education in nursing from Columbia University, New York, in 1969. Except for a four-year stint as Associate Director of Nursing Services with the Hospital for Sick Children in Toronto, she was associated for most of her career with the University of Alberta. In 1969, she was the first nurse in Canada to be given a joint appointment to teach in both the Nursing and the Health Sciences Administration departments. During her appointment with the Faculty of Nursing at the University of Alberta, she served for various terms as Acting Director and Associate Dean for Graduate Education. She was the principal developer of Canada's first doctoral nursing (PhD Nursing) program in 1991, and in 1988, she started working with three "special case" nursing students who were working towards this doctoral degree.

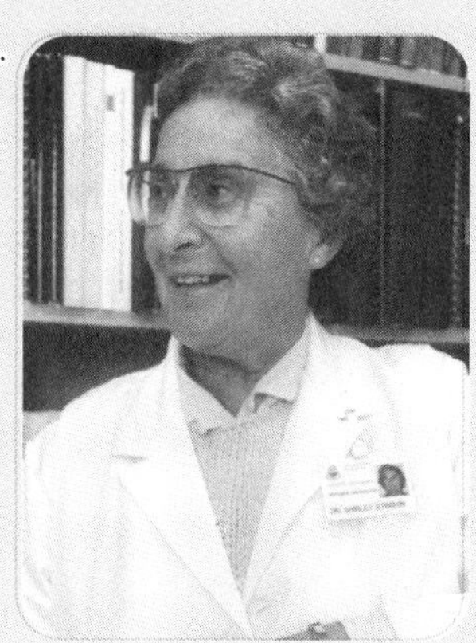

While teaching at the University of Alberta, she also held several other joint teaching appointments, with the Faculty of Medicine at the University of Alberta and with the Faculty of Nursing at the University of Calgary. She also carried out much nursing research of her own, including major studies on nursing education needs in Canada and investigations into doctoral preparation for nursing, including several national studies on doctoral preparation for nurses. During this time, she also served as an officer with nursing associations provincially, nationally and internationally, including a term as president of the Canadian Nurses Association from 1980 to 1982.

Upon her retirement from the University of Alberta at the end of 1993, she was described as "Alberta's most distinguished nurse." Her honours and awards are many, including the Jeanne Mance Award from the Canadian Nurses Association, the Ross Award for Leadership from the Canadian Nurses Foundation, and the Alberta Achievement Award for Excellence from the Government of Alberta. She holds honorary doctorates from the University of Calgary and Memorial University. Following her retirement, she had plans to serve as visiting professor at various universities, including at least one appointment in Australia.

— *Glennis Zilm*

The importance of nursing research has also been bolstered by national and provincial nursing organizations. For example, these organizations have explicated nurses' roles related to research and undertaken a variety of strategies to support the use and conduct of nursing research through the development of educational materials and sponsorship of nursing research workshops and conferences (Clarke, 1995, 1997; CNA, 1993; RNABC, 1990, 1997, 1998; CNO, 1996). Nursing leaders have also worked to strengthen nursing research by arguing for stronger links between research and practice (Thurston, 1995; Wuest, 1995).

Finally, coordinated efforts to systematically review research evidence and disseminate the findings are underway worldwide. For example, the Cochrane Collaboration is an international initiative created to facilitate the review, maintenance and dissemination of systematic overviews of the effects of health care. Access to information on its activities can be obtained through its home page (http://hiru.mcmaster.ca/COCHRANE/DEFAULT.HTML). Nurses at McMaster University, as part of the Cochrane Collaboration, have completed several systematic overviews of relevant research to determine the effectiveness of public health nursing interventions such as home visiting (e.g., Ciliska et al., 1994), adolescent suicide prevention programs (Ploeg et al., 1995) and parent-child health promotion activities (Hayward et al., 1996). Others at the University of Alberta have systematically reviewed the research literature to determine the most effective strategies for managing the symptoms of Alzheimer's Disease (Forbes & Strang, 1997). The dissemination of these reviews as full reports or as articles in nursing journals provides the opportunity for all nurses to learn about the findings of these reviews and move towards evidenced-based decision making in nursing.

Conducting Nursing Research

One of the questions frequently asked by students is, "Are all nurses expected to do research these days?" The answer is that not all nurses design and conduct research studies, but all nurses are expected to be aware of research being done in their area, to be able to read and interpret research findings and to use relevant findings in their practice. Because one of the basic societal functions of a university is to push back the boundaries of knowledge, it is understandable that a considerable amount of research in nursing is being conducted by people in university schools of nursing—master's- and doctoral-level students and faculty. Completion of an original research project (either as a thesis or as a smaller study) is often one of the requisites for a master's degree in nursing, as it is in most other disciplines. The doctorate (in any field) is considered a research degree; completion of a dissertation (the report of a major research study) is always a requirement and the major focus of doctoral studies. Except in a few instances, all university faculty members are required to undertake research in their field as an ongoing part of their workload. In addition, there are the research scholars and fellows who have received funding to enable them to devote themselves full-time or part-time to conducting studies.

As we mentioned in our discussions on the role of government in Chapter 4, one source of funding for nurses is Health Canada's National Health Research and Development Program. Other major sources include the Canadian Nurses Foundation, provincial governments and provincial nursing association foundations as well as private organizations. The Medical Research Council and the Social Sciences and Humanities Research Council of Canada (SSHRC) are also potential sources of funds for nursing research. There is considerable competition, however, and nurses must compete with scientists from other fields. The increasing number of nursing research fellows and scholars attests to the quality of studies being undertaken by nurses.

In addition to nursing studies conducted in universities, a considerable amount of research is taking place in clinical agencies and by staff nurses with the help of agency staff who are skilled in research methodology, or with the help of faculty members from a university school of nursing.

SOLO AND COLLABORATIVE RESEARCH

Doctoral students and many master's students are required to undertake **solo research**—research that is done independently by one person. Other nurses may conduct their own studies as independent researchers or they may do **collaborative research**—research done in teams with colleagues, people in other agencies, people in other provinces or countries or with members of other disciplines. Research teams are becoming common in nursing, as in many other disciplines, with the faculty and associated clinical staff of one agency collaborating on one particular area of enquiry and several people undertaking studies on various aspects of it. For example, at the University of Ottawa School of Nursing several colleagues have been involved in research in patient decision making, exploring beliefs, values and social influences on decisions to quit smoking or decisions concerning suicide, toxic cancer treatments, immunization for hepatitis B and influenza and the duration of breast feeding (CNA, 1991).

A large amount of interagency research is also being done; collaboration between university faculty and staff of an affiliated hospital is very common, as are university and community agency research teams. Collaboration between hospitals is also occurring more and more, as in the case of the Calgary District Hospital Group, which has completed several studies on different aspects of caring for the elderly. We are also seeing interprovincial collaboration on research projects, as for example, the Western Consortium of Cancer Nurses, which has carried out a project on the prevention and treatment of chemotherapy-induced mouth sores with researchers from all four western provinces examining various aspects of the problem (CNA, 1991, 1992; Church, Thurston, Tenove & Weisgerber, 1991).

INTERNATIONAL COLLABORATION

Many Canadian University and Collegiate Schools of Nursing are engaged in international projects to help with the development of nursing education in Third World countries. For example, the University of Ottawa School of Nursing has had a project with the Tienjin Medical College School of Nursing in China for several years to help faculty with their baccalaureate program. The School of Nursing at Dalhousie University has had a project with a school in Tanzania, and the University of Manitoba School of Nursing has had one in Chengdu, China—and there are many more. Many faculty from Canadian universities are collaborating on research with their colleagues in these countries.

Some collaborative international research is done by students meeting requirements for a master's or doctoral degree. A student from China studying at the University of Manitoba may wish to do research for a master's degree on a nursing problem in China or, as travelling fellowships for nurses become more common, Canadian nursing students may undertake to collect data for their study in another country. There may also be collaboration between experienced researchers in different countries as in, for example, the Denmark–Newfoundland project on primary health care (Hall, 1989). Participating in this project were the Nurses Association of Denmark and the Association of Registered Nurses of Newfoundland (CNA, 1991, 1992; Church et al., 1991).

Many Canadian nurses are also seconded by international agencies to undertake studies in other countries, in collaboration with nurses in that country. To cite one example, Dr. Linda Ogilvie (1993) of the University of Alberta undertook a study for the World Health Organization to examine forces shaping nursing contributions to primary health care in Nepal.

MULTIDISCIPLINARY COLLABORATION

Also becoming more common is multidisciplinary research. One example of a multidisciplinary research project is a study directed towards reducing the pain and distress experienced by children undergoing venipuncture for blood collection or intravenous (IV) cannulation. This study involved nurse researchers and pharmacists in evaluating the effectiveness of using a topical anesthetic prior to these procedures (Lander et al., 1996). Another example of a multidisciplinary research project is a study directed towards the prevention of pre-term births, which looked at the health promotion practices of health professionals in eastern Ontario. This study involved nurse researchers, a public health physician and a statistician (Davies et al., 1993).

THE STUDENT'S ROLE IN CONDUCTING RESEARCH

As beginning students, you are able to examine the practice of nursing uninfluenced by the dogmas and rituals of the past. From your first clinical experience, you should begin to think of ways of improving nursing practice and articulate your ideas. The ideas may seem unconventional at first but often can be developed into original ideas for research.

In some senior courses, you may be expected to undertake a small study; probably it will be a small group project. As beginning students, you are not likely to be asked to do research. You should, however, be aware of and begin to develop an appreciation for the research that has been done in the area of practice in which you are having clinical experience. You should also be aware of completed research that has contributed to the knowledge you are gaining from other courses you are taking. In this, you will be guided by reading lists for each course, but you will also want to explore other avenues. You will find research articles in all refereed and many other professional journals. **Refereed journals** contain articles that have been reviewed, assessed for accuracy, scholarliness and scientific merit and accepted for publication by an editorial board of nursing experts (RNABC, 1990). The two major Canadian refereed journals that publish nursing research reports are *Canadian Journal of Nursing Research (Nursing Papers)* and *Canadian Journal of Public Health.* You will also find articles reporting on nursing research in *The Canadian Nurse* and in many of the provincial nursing journals and the journals of interest groups, such as the *Canadian Journal of Nursing Administration*. You may also look at the American, British and Australian journals you will find on your reading lists.

Some students, especially those who are interested in going on to complete graduate degrees, seek experiences as research assistants during the summer vacation period or as part-time assistants during the term. This type of work experience is not only interesting, it also provides valuable insight into the actual process of research, strengthens students' applications to graduate school and increases their competitiveness for graduate scholarships. Working under the supervision of experienced researchers, students gain important skills and make important contributions to the research programs they are involved with. For example, two nursing students working with Dr. Janice Lander at the University of Alberta completed preliminary work to establish research techniques that would be used in an investigation on reducing the pain associated with injections and then later participated as research assistants in that study. They published their preliminary work (Givens, Oberle & Lander, 1993) and the study they assisted with was also subsequently published (Lander et al., 1996).

As students at any level, you may be asked to participate in research being conducted by others. Your participation may take the form of being a **subject**, that is, a member of a given population under study, or you may be asked to assist in collecting data. Most of you will have considerable clinical practice in teaching hospitals and community agencies affiliated with a university Health Sciences Centre. There may, therefore, be numerous research projects involving your patients. You can use this situation as an additional learning experience by finding out the nature of the research being undertaken and the methodology being used. Researchers and their assistants are usually very willing to share what they are doing with an interested student.

The ethical guidelines developed by the Canadian Nurses Association (1994) stress that the relationship between subject and researcher is the most important component in the ethical dimension of the study. The relationship must be one of mutual trust in which the subject is aware of and satisfied with his or her involvement and protection during the course of the study.

The guidelines point out that, although researchers have the primary responsibility to build a trusting relationship with subjects in their study, it is every nurse's responsibility to collaborate in fostering relationships that will facilitate the ethical conduct of research.

If you are involved in a particular study, as a data collector or as a subject's caregiver, you should be aware that the investigator is obligated to provide you with information that clarifies the roles of everyone involved, that is, the researcher, the research subject, the data gatherer and the caregiver. You will also want information about the purpose of the study.

It is the responsibility of all nurses to ensure that the health and the rights of the patient who is a subject in a research study are safeguarded. All universities and most hospitals and other health agencies now have an ethics committee that reviews all research proposals to ensure that patient rights are not jeopardized by the conduct of a study.

Dissemination and Use of Research Findings

The process of disseminating, and subsequently using, research findings in practice has been studied in many fields including education, anthropology and rural sociology. Two of the most eminent researchers in the diffusion and adoption of innovations, as this branch of research has been called, are E.M. Rogers and R.G. Havelock. Rogers maintains that people in any social system go through a similar process from first awareness of a new idea or practice, through seeking information about it, to making a decision to adopt it in practice. Both Rogers and Havelock have used the concept of **change agents** in their theories. These are outside consultants who are called in to assist with the dissemination of information about new ideas and/or practices in an organization (or in a social system) and with their adoption in practice (Burns & Grove, 1993).

A classic Canadian nursing study showed that nurses in a given community did, indeed, follow a definable pattern similar to that found in other groups as they sought information about new ideas and practices and made decisions to adopt or not adopt the innovation. The channels of communication used by nurses to find out about new ideas and practices may be expected to vary somewhat from one jurisdiction to another. In this study, the channels used included the nursing journals, continuing education courses (conferences, seminars or formal courses), and nursing consultants from government and from the professional nursing association, as well as nursing faculty from schools of nursing and other colleagues. One of the most important findings in this study, and in diffusion and adoption studies in all disciplines, is the importance of personal communication — nurses talking to other nurses about their work (Du Gas, 1969).

The RNABC has developed a *Workbook on Nursing Research* (1990) which lists various ways to interest nurses in research. These ways include a good sampling of "channels of communication" that may be used by nurses to disseminate information about nursing research activity, as well as ways to encourage the conduct of research in agencies and the utilization of research findings.

Examples of Ways to Motivate Nursing Research Activity

1. Nursing research committees in health care agencies
2. Research interest groups
   - agency-based, interagency–based
   - nursing and interdisciplinary
   - brown bag discussions on research topics
3. Journal clubs
4. Research awareness days in agencies
   - nursing units can submit problems and questions that might be studied
   - competitions between nursing units for examples of how research was used to solve a problem
5. Professional association annual research days
   - paper and poster presentations
   - colloquia or workshops on research and practice
6. Professional practice group activities
   - newsletters
   - meetings
   - networking

Source: RNABC, 1990, p. 2.

THE STUDENT'S ROLE IN THE DISSEMINATION OF RESEARCH FINDINGS

As students, you have a wonderful opportunity to learn about the latest findings of nursing research. You can attend the research seminars, "brown bag" lunch discussions of research and many other continuing education programs that are held regularly by different departments in health sciences centres including university facilities or schools and teaching hospitals. You can also attend nursing conferences where research reports are given — registration for students is usually at a much reduced rate from that charged other registrants. The annual meetings of provincial nursing associations and the Canadian Nurses Association are also good places to find out about new ideas and practices, to exchange information with students from other schools and to talk with experienced nurses about their views on some of the new ideas.

The most reliable way of disseminating new knowledge and practices in nursing, as in any other field, is through the education process. Many heads of nursing departments in clinical agencies will tell you that they always question new graduates, particularly those coming from other parts of the province and other provinces or countries, on new practices they have been taught in their basic nursing programs. As students you and your faculty guides are sources of new knowledge for staff of the agency in which you are gaining experience.

USING RESEARCH FINDINGS

Much of nursing research focusses on resolving problems nurses have encountered in practice or on ways to improve practice. For example, a major concern of nurses caring for people in an inpatient facility is the problem of patients falling out of bed, or falling while walking on legs made unsteady by age, illness or infirmity. Dr. Janice Morse and her colleagues in Alberta set out to identify the risk factors associated with patients' falls in acute and long-term care (Morse, Prowse, Morrow & Federspeil, 1985; Morse, Tylko & Dixon, 1985; Morse, Black, Oberle & Donahue, 1989). A six-item scale that can be used by nurses to identify individuals at risk for anticipated physiological falls (falls that occur primarily in confused patients with mobility problems) was developed out of this work (Morse, 1997). In another study, researchers in British Columbia were concerned about the high rate of smoking relapse among mothers who had quit smoking during their pregnancies. They designed and evaluated an intervention provided by nurses to help new mothers remain nonsmokers after their babies were born (Johnson, Ratner, Bottorff, Hall & Dahinten, 1997). The smoking relapse prevention intervention, consisting of a short in-hospital counselling session and follow-up telephone support, was found to be effective in reducing smoking relapse during the first six months postpartum.

The findings of all of these studies can be used by nurses in numerous health agencies. If nurses can identify the risk factors associated with patients' falls, for example, they can take preventive measures to eliminate (or minimize) the factors wherever possible (Morse, 1997). Similarly, the findings of the study on preventing smoking relapse during the postpartum period could be useful to nurses on maternity units in hospitals and in community health settings all across the country, where nurses are in contact with new mothers.

Unfortunately, the adoption of new ideas and practices is a lengthy process that usually takes a number of years. In seeking to help nurses to use research findings in their practice, Grinspun, MacMillan, Nichol and Shields (1993) at Mount Sinai Hospital in Toronto found that several barriers to the use of research in clinical practice have been identified. These include: "(1) limited access to research findings, (2) difficulty interpreting published research reports, and (3) attitudes" (p. 46). Believing that organizational support and a knowledgeable staff are necessary to promote the utilization of nursing research, the nursing research committee at Mount Sinai made the use of research their priority, rather than the conduct of research itself.

A very effective tool for finding out about current research is the Internet. Many research journals are now on line (e.g., the *American Journal of Preventive Medicine* can be found at the following Internet address: http://www-east.elsevier.com/ajpm/). University departments (e.g., Schools of Nursing) and research centres have home pages where you can read about research that is completed or underway. For example, research being conducted through the Health Canada funded Centres of Excellence on Women's Health can be found on the Internet at (http://www.hc-sc.gc.ca/datapcb/datawhb/cewheng.htm).

THE STUDENT'S ROLE IN THE UTILIZATION OF RESEARCH FINDINGS

In an educational program, you reap the benefits of others' research in learning up-to-date nursing interventions which, increasingly, are being based on research findings. It is important to know which of the nursing interventions you are learning are based on sound research, which are **empirically** (experience) based and which are unsubstantiated.

You can also offer a fresh outlook on the way things are done and can question your professors on the rationale behind various nursing interventions and routines. Don't hesitate to ask your professors, "Why do they do it this way?" Usually, there is a valid reason. If not, you may have a potential researchable question. During your clinical experience in various agencies, you will want to look for possible researchable questions that you may be able to develop into a study later in your program.

Basic Concepts

Ways of Knowing

Nursing research is the scientific investigation of nursing practice problems to generate new knowledge that is essential to the quality of nursing care (CNA, undated). The knowledge generated by research is important, but Benner points out that "mere techniques and scientific knowledge are not enough" in nursing (Benner, 1984, p. 4). She suggests that *caring* is what makes the nurse take note of those interventions that help the patients and guide their future actions. Nor has all of the body of knowledge that nursing encompasses been derived from research. Henderson suggests that clinical nurses develop knowledge through the practice of nursing (Henderson, cited in Benner & Wrubel, 1980).

Much of our knowledge has come from the experience of nurses who have gone before us, some of it from common sense, some learned by trial and error in the process of giving care, some passed on by tradition and some from scientific enquiry. As the number of clinical nursing studies has expanded, many traditional nursing techniques have been questioned—often resulting in the discovery that there is, indeed, a scientific basis for traditional nursing interventions. For example, the evening back rub has been used in hospitals by many generations of nurses who found that it helped patients to relax in preparation for sleep. Nowadays, we are aware that there is a scientific reason for the back rub; the slow, gentle massage has the effect of stimulating the thick nerve fibres in the spinal cord that help to mitigate pain. In other cases, research has led to new knowledge and to new nursing interventions. Dr. Dolores Krieger's research on faith healing, for example, led to the development of therapeutic touch techniques, which are being used by many nurses today.

Feldman and Millor (1994) suggest that the numerous ways of gaining knowledge can be classified into two broad categories: structured and unstructured. Unstructured ways of gaining knowledge include empathy, intuition, trial-and-error experience, tradition and authority and meditation. Structured ways include scientific enquiry, critical thinking and logical reasoning.

The scientific enquiry or research approach is not unlike the nursing process (see Table 7.1). Both are used to solve problems using a systematic approach. The information derived from the research process adds to the discipline's knowledge base. The nursing process serves to advance nursing practice in specific contexts or situations (Feldman & Millor, 1994). The research process and the nursing process both involve observation and recording of empirical information, analysis and classification of that information (data), and conclusions that are derived from the data.

Like the nursing process, scientific enquiry or research is a complex process that involves a series of tasks. These tasks, however, are often not completed as discrete sequential

TABLE 7.1 Comparison of the scientific enquiry/research process and the nursing process

The Scientific Enquiry/Research Process	*The Nursing Process*
1. statement of problem	assumption that patient needs nursing assistance
2. review of the literature to determine what is already known and what gaps exist	widely known scientific information and past experience guide data collection to identify specific patient problems (stated as a nursing diagnosis)
3. identification of a theoretical framework or perspective, statement of the hypothesis or research question, and the selection of a research design (blueprint for conducting a study)	development of a plan of care (using up-to-date, scientifically sound information to guide selection of the "best" patient care interventions)
4. implementation of the research plan (data collection and analysis)	implementation of plan
5. intepretation of the results of the study	evaluation of patient outcomes
6. conclusions about the problem or phenomenon under study	conclusions
7. wide communication of findings	communication to other member of health team

SOURCE: Feldman, 1990, p. 29.

steps. Researchers may work simultaneously at several tasks and, especially during the early stages, may revisit some tasks to make changes based on new insights or developments.

Goals of Generating Research-Based Knowledge

In conducting research, nurses use their curiosity, imagination and reasoning to adapt the methodology of scientific enquiry to gain fresh knowledge and to find solutions to practical problems.

Some authors make a distinction between *nursing research* and *research in nursing* (Gortner, 1975). Nursing research, these authors feel, is a systematic, logical enquiry into the processes of health care, and the clinical problems and issues encountered in the practice of nursing. It is a process by which the knowledge base for nursing practice grows. Research in nursing, on the other hand, they feel, is the broader study of people and the nursing profession, including historical, policy and ethical studies. Others feel that dividing the research that is being done in the nursing field into two categories is an arbitrary distinction; in the final analysis, research into all aspects of nursing will strengthen nursing practice.

The position of the Canadian Nurses Association (CNA, 1985) is that the results of research provide guidance to nurses in all practice areas and indicate what nurses

The Goals of Nursing Research

1. **Building the Knowledge Base**
   Nursing must build its own knowledge base, rather than falling back on tried and true practices. The search for new knowledge is part of nursing's commitment to high-quality care. What is learned through nursing research can be used to:
   - help people and their families develop constructive lifestyles
   - promote the maintenance and restoration of health
   - care for individuals and families through periods of health crisis
   - improve the quality of community health care delivery.
2. **Prediction and Control**
   Along with other scientific disciplines, nursing research aims to *describe* and *explain* phenomena, *predict* the results of interventions and *control* undesirable outcomes.
3. **Accountability**
   Nurses who base their clinical decisions on scientifically documented evidence are nurses who are being accountable to the patients they serve.
4. **Quality of Life**
   The ultimate goal of nursing research is to improve the quality of human life by helping people to learn healthier lifestyles, restore their health or deal positively with terminal illness.

SOURCE: CNA, n.d.

should do, what they could try and what they should question and research.

The four principal goals of nursing research, as set forth by the Canadian Nurses Association, are:

1. building the knowledge base of nursing
2. describing and explaining phenomena, predicting the results of interventions and controlling undesirable outcomes
3. strengthening accountability in patient care
4. ultimately improving the quality of human life.

Research Being Done by Canadian Nurses

Nursing is a dynamic profession and its knowledge base is constantly changing as new information is discovered. The motivation for this search for new information comes from recognition of the gaps that exist in current knowledge. Research plays a critical role in enlarging the scientific foundations of nursing knowledge. Much of the early research in nursing in Canada was on nursing education. As graduate programs began to develop in nursing administration, nursing education and community health in Canadian universities, these areas became the main foci for research by nurses. From the early 1970s, however, the principal focus has been on issues related to nursing practice (Ritchie, 1992). In looking at current trends in Canadian nursing research, the CNA (1991) identified that a considerable amount of research is currently being carried out in the following areas:

1. women's health
2. HIV infections
3. nurses' roles in the health of Canadians
4. care of families with chronically ill children
5. promoting and maintaining health in the elderly
6. systems to deliver health care
7. the development of nursing.

Learning to Read and Interpret Research Reports

As beginning students, your primary role in nursing research is that of research consumer. As a research consumer you will want to read research reports so that you have up-to-date scientific information you can use to provide the "best" patient care. For example, if you are caring for a child who is experiencing pain, you will want to read research reports that provide information on the usefulness of pain assessment tools and on children's pain management.

In order to become an intelligent consumer of research literature and, ultimately, to be able to use research findings in your clinical practice, you need to develop skills in reading research reports and in assessing research for scientific merit and clinical applicability. These skills require learning to critique research reports—an activity you will be given plenty of practice in during your nursing courses. The following section is an introduction to critiquing research reports.

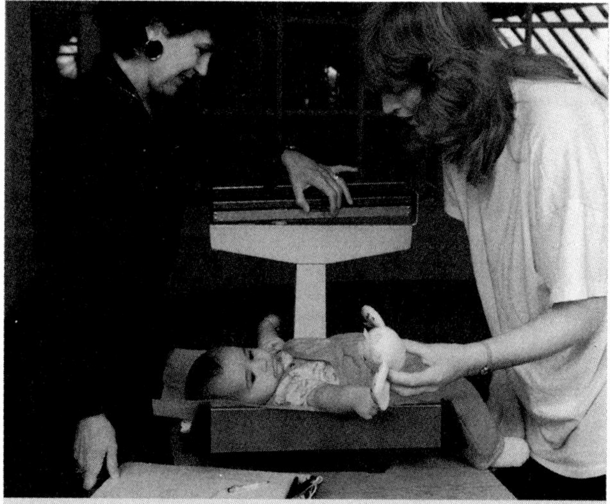

A considerable amount of research is being done in maternal and child health.

What Is a Critique?

A **critique** is a critical assessment of a piece of research involving a systematic appraisal according to specified criteria (Woods & Catanzaro, 1988). Conducting a good critique of a research study, proposal or report of findings requires not just a list of pertinent questions to ask, but criteria or standards against which to evaluate answers to the questions and comprehension of the rationale for asking them in the first place (Ryan-Wegner, 1992; Downs, 1984; Burns & Grove, 1993). In order to critique a research study, you will need to engage in three activities:

1. analysis of the study to identify the component parts and the procedures used by the researcher, as well as to understand the reasons given for their use
2. evaluation of the study by appraising the strengths and weaknesses of those areas identified in the analysis
3. expression of your judgement about the merit or worth of the study. This assessment should be based on the analysis and evaluation. Remember, a critique identifies both strengths and weaknesses.

As you can see, a critique is not a summary of the study, although the opening sentence or paragraph of a critique should briefly summarize the whole article and emphasize a major strength. Nor is a critique a checklist identifying whether an element of a study is present or absent. While these two aspects are part of a critique, the main focus should be on providing evidence to support your evaluation and on determining whether the findings are ready for use in practice. Critiquing research reports is an important activity for nursing students because it helps increase your understanding of the research process and ensures that you are learning the most up-to-date information in nursing in order to provide the "best" nursing care. Nurses also need to be involved in this activity because, like all professionals, they need to update their knowledge and repertoire of interventions constantly in response to new research evidence.

A critique is an objective evaluation of the quality of the written report or article, the strength of the research design and the adequacy of the author's interpretation of the findings.

Typical Headings in a Research Report

1. Title
2. Abstract
3. Introduction
4. Review of the literature and theoretical framework
5. Hypotheses, assumptions and objectives
6. Research methods, design and procedures
   - sample
   - data collection
7. Data analysis and results
8. Discussion.

Guidelines for Writing a Critique

Although the terms *critique* and *evaluation* are frequently perceived as having negative connotations, when used to describe research procedures, they imply only an objective assessment. The tone of a critique can convey either a negative or a positive view. The term **evaluation** implies a comparison against accepted standards that apply to all types of research. Objectivity is important in a critique. Always keep in mind that you are making evaluative comments about the study and not about the researchers.

In a critique you should strive to be readable, concise, rational, accurate, sensitive and impartial; explanations for the judgements that you make must always be given. You should convey respect for the investigator's activities; it is often easier to critique than to create. To soften the tone of your delivery, use conditionals such as *could, would, should, might*.

To start the process of critiquing a research report or research article, it is helpful to read the entire report through once, quickly and objectively, to gain a perspective of what was done, why and how it was done, and the results of the study. Following this first assessment, a more in-depth evaluation of each section of the research report can then be accomplished.

Elements of a Research Report

The headings commonly used to divide a research report can be useful in organizing a critique of a research study or report of findings. These usually follow the steps the researcher followed in conducting the study. Understanding the logic behind the organization of the report, whether you are merely critiquing the research or contemplating its use in practice, is important. As a reader, you must raise critical questions and find satisfactory answers from the information communicated in the report.

At the end of each section below describing the content of elements in a research report, we have suggested some basic questions that should be asked about each particular element and could be used as a guide for critiquing that section of the report. A summary of these questions is included at the end of the chapter. In addition to the questions, Table 7.2 provides an excellent framework prepared by Clarke (1995) to assist nurses (and others) in using research in their clinical practice.

There are two main types of research designs or overall plans for organizing a study: quantitative and qualitative. **Quantitative designs** involve the analysis of numbers to answer research questions. These studies are based on the tenets of the scientific method, measurement theory, statistical principles and ethical standards. Quantitative designs include a variety of experimental and nonexperimental designs (Brink & Wood, 1998). **Qualitative designs** involve the analysis of words instead of numbers for their meanings to answer the research questions. Ethical standards still apply, but in this case there is no statistical analysis of data. Qualitative studies are often undertaken when little is known about the topic under study and relevant theory does not exist. For example, qualitative designs have been used to learn more about patient comfort (Morse, Bottorff & Hutchinson, 1994) and nurses' use of touch (Estabrooks, 1989). Qualitative studies may also follow quantitative studies to examine or extend the quantitative findings. There are important differences between these two designs that are reflected in research reports. Since these differences should be taken into consideration when you read and critique a research report, we will draw your attention to them in the sections that follow on each component of the research report.

Let us examine each of the components of a research report more closely.

Title and Abstract

Typically, a research article begins with a title to introduce the major topic or area of study. Following the title is an

abstract, which is intended to give the reader a brief summary of the entire study. An abstract usually provides the following information about the study: its purpose, objectives or hypotheses; a description of the subjects or sample members; a brief explanation of the data collection methods and analysis procedures; and a summary of important findings.

Questions to Ask About the Title and Abstract

1. Does the title of the research accurately reflect the problem under study?
2. Does the abstract present a succinct overview of the study?

Introduction

The introduction provides a brief overview of the research topic. It is a summary statement of what the research is about, why it was done and how it is important to nursing. The introduction describes the nature of the research and should briefly explain why the study was undertaken. It also usually includes a short rationale for addressing the topic, which should let the reader know whether the research is relevant to his or her area of practice.

In the introductory section, the investigator also describes the preliminary research steps that specify the general focus of the study, presents background information and the need for the study, and then states the purpose of this particular investigation. Consider, as an example, a large hospital that is planning to introduce primary nursing, which, it is hoped, will help nurses in their clinical practice. Some nurses like the idea; others have expressed doubts about it. In order to develop a relevant teaching program for the nurses, the nursing education unit of the hospital would like to investigate why some nurses like and some do not like the idea of primary nursing. They hope to use their findings to plan a program to overcome negative attitudes and foster interest and enthusiasm among all the nurses for primary nursing. The purpose of the research would be to examine (investigate) the reasons for nurses' anxiety towards primary nursing in order to design a program to help them to feel comfortable in learning how to implement it. From the stated purpose (also called a **problem statement** or **research question**), the reader should be able to identify clearly the general problem under study.

Questions to Ask About the Introduction

1. Do you have a clear idea of what the research is all about?
2. Do you understand why the research is being done?
3. Is the significance of the problem discussed and the research justified?
4. Is the problem substantiated with adequate background information?
5. Is the problem statement clear? Concise?

Review of the Literature and Theoretical Framework

A literature review is the next section of a research report (and next step in the research process). It is a discussion of previous relevant studies that the investigator or others have conducted, as well as a review of the current knowledge about the concepts under study. The literature review serves multiple purposes and provides essential information for many of the other components of the research process. In general, there are three purposes of the literature review:

1. to validate knowledge
2. to avoid unintended duplication
3. to review methods used in previous research.

The first purpose of a literature review is to allow the researcher to **validate the knowledge base** (assess the extent of current knowledge about the subject). The literature

Questions to Ask About the Literature Review

1. Does the literature review support the significance of the selected problem?
2. Is the relationship of the problem to previous research clear?
3. What is the theoretical base for this study? What are the major concepts used? For example, change theory, diffusion/adoption theory and theories on attitudinal change are all possibilities to use as a foundation for the study on nurses' anxieties and attitudes about the introduction of primary nursing.
4. Does the researcher indicate how previous knowledge has been used in developing this study?
5. Is the literature review well organized? What topics are addressed?
6. Is there a sufficient review of the literature so that the reader can be assured that the investigator has considered a broad spectrum of possibilities for investigating the problem?
7. Are the references up to date, that is, are most of them less than 10 years old?
8. Has reference also been made to classic studies (early studies in an area of research), to original and up-to-date work by experts in the field, as, for example, Leininger's work over the years in studies involving cross-cultural nursing?

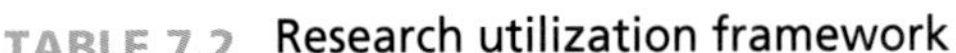

TABLE 7.2 Research utilization framework

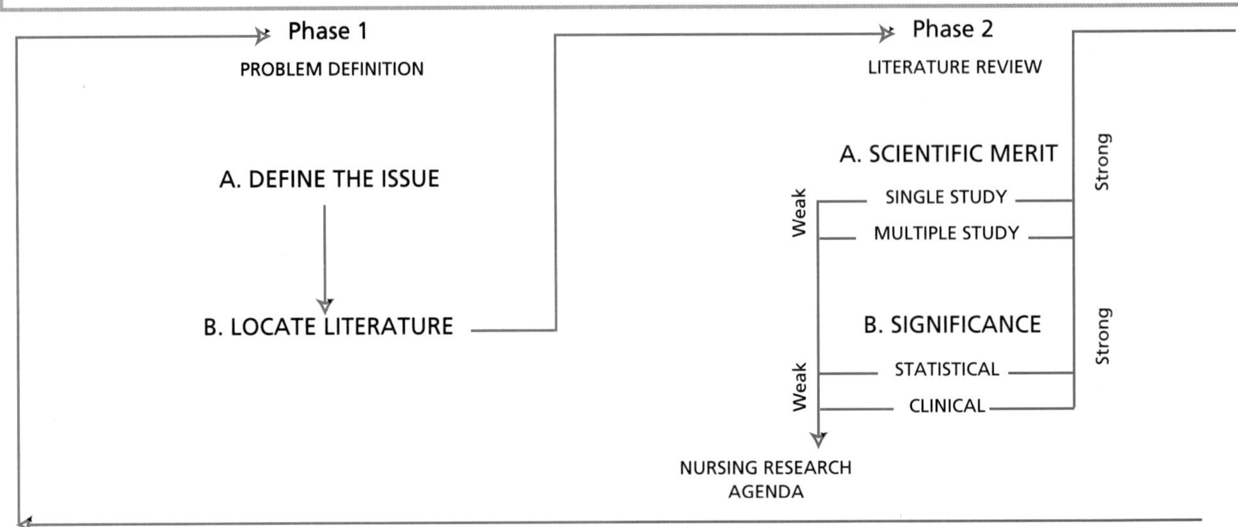

Phase 1

PROBLEM DEFINITION

A. DEFINE THE ISSUE

State your issue or problem as questions. This helps to define the problem clearly and identify important gaps in your knowledge. Consult with others who are closest to the problem and most affected by it.

B. LOCATE LITERATURE

Find literature related to your problem. Reviewing this literature helps to identify various factors associated with the issue. Then you can be more precise about your questions. Although anecdotal, theoretical or opinion articles may be useful, it is important to focus your search on research articles. RNABC's Helen Randal Library is a good place to start your search. Use the *Cumulative Index of Nursing and Allied Health Literature* (CINAHL), or the computerized data base in the library's book and file holdings, or (for a fee) have a librarian do a broader search. Other resources include university, college and public libraries, the Ministry of Health library in Victoria, and perhaps your agency library.

Phase 2

LITERATURE REVIEW

A. REVIEW FOR SCIENTIFIC MERIT

- Analyse the study to identify and understand component parts and procedures used by the researcher.
- Appraise the strengths and weaknesses of those areas identified in the analysis.
- Judge the merit or worth of the study. (Davies & Logan, 1997.)

Once you have completed these activities for one study, you will need to do the same with the other studies and compare results. Similar results lend strength to the findings. On the other hand, conflicting results may be difficult to interpret and not be ready to use in practice. To evaluate the overall impact of findings from multiple studies about a single issue, meta-analysis can be used to integrate the findings. An experienced nurse researcher or statistician can help with this.

B. REVIEW FOR SIGNIFICANCE

- Statistical significance refers to whether the result(s) could have just happened by chance, or were due to the study.
- Clinical significance relates to the importance or potential importance of a finding when the "whole picture" is taken into account. It may be clinically important that an intervention caused some change towards normal, even though the small change was not statistically significant.

(Continued)

SOURCE: Clarke, 1995, pp. 20–21.

forms the background and framework for the study. This background information helps the reader to understand how the study relates to and builds on previous research and theory in the field. Gaps in existing knowledge should become apparent as you read the literature review.

The second purpose of a literature review is to determine if the proposed study has already been done. Prior to conducting the study, the researcher needs to identify how different or similar other studies are to the proposed study, and determine whether replication with a different sample and in a different setting is needed. Replication is the repetition of a study in different settings with different samples taken from the same or different populations (Burns & Grove, 1995). If the researcher finds that the proposed study differs significantly enough from previous studies to warrant pursuing the project, the researcher may use the previous studies to build the framework for the proposed study. If, to return to our example, it had been established in a previous study that a large number of nurses employed in the hospital were worried about the introduction of primary nursing, the proposed study to identify reasons for anxieties could build on the framework of the previous study.

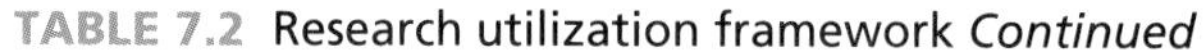

TABLE 7.2 Research utilization framework *Continued*

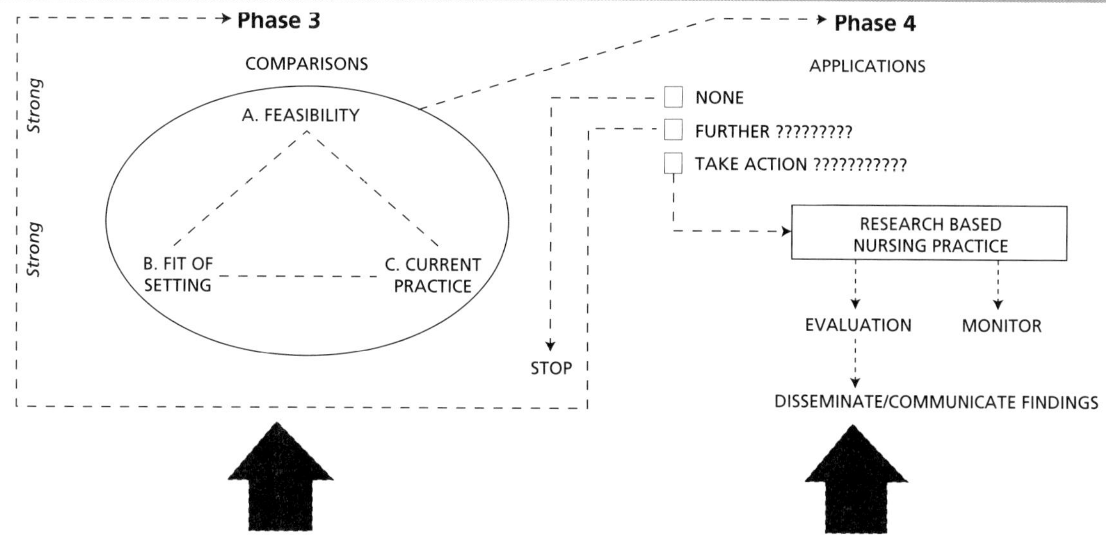

Phase 3

COMPARISONS

Compare studies to your specific setting and nursing problem.

A. FEASIBILITY

- What are the risks of changing or not changing from current practice?
- What are the costs and benefits of change?

B. FIT OF SETTING

- How similar are characteristics of those studied to those of your setting?
- What are the differences or similarities of the research to your setting?
- Are the resources (human and material) you'll use similar to those of the research?

C. CURRENT PRACTICE

- How effective is your current practice?
- Is your nursing practice based on a nursing model or philosophy similar to that of the research, if there was one? How will this affect using the findings in your setting?
- How will differences affect application of findings?
- Is the type of organization or management of nursing practice critical to the implementation of the findings?

Phase 4

APPLICATION

A. DETERMINE THE CONTRIBUTIONS OF THE RESEARCH FINDINGS TO THE NURSING PRACTICE PROBLEM IDENTIFIED IN PHASE 1.

The decision about using the research findings may be to:

- Not use because of risks or costs involved or lack of consistent, strong findings.
- Consider for future use, but not now, because research findings and/or comparisons are tentative only.
- Use to inform colleagues that current practice is evidence-based.
- Use to plan for change or to provide new options in practice.

B. IF THE PRACTICE IS TO BE CHANGED, YOU MAY NOW HAVE TO INVOLVE OTHERS IN THE PROCESS SUCH AS SENIOR MANAGEMENT, A QUALITY IMPROVEMENT PROGRAM, AND/OR A RESEARCH COMMITTEE. YOU MAY WISH TO CONDUCT A PILOT PROJECT BEFORE BRINGING ABOUT AN AGENCY-WIDE CHANGE.

C. APPLYING RESEARCH FINDINGS REQUIRES ATTENTION TO THREE KEY PROCESSES:

- change and adopting innovations
- evaluation
- dissemination

Finally, the third purpose for performing a literature review is to identify methods other researchers have used in their investigations on the topic of interest. The researcher may uncover new research tools or measures that can be used for data gathering in the proposed study, variables he or she had not considered or unanticipated problems in data collection or analysis. A careful look at these aspects of previous work can help the researcher to avoid problems others have had, thus strengthening his or her own research.

The literature review also helps the reader to determine how the study being reported relates to current theoretical knowledge on the topic. Knowledge of the literature available on a subject allows subsequent placement of the problem in a theoretical context—an important step in the eventual integration of findings.

In reports of qualitative studies, there may not be an extensive data base for literature review. Because there is little or no theoretical foundation on which to build, qualitative studies are exploratory and are completed for the purpose of in-depth description or generation of theory. Thus, a theoretical framework is not included in the research report. However, researchers usually identify a broad perspective or philosophical position from which they are addressing the research question. For example, in a qualitative study, a cultural perspective may be used to explore and describe the beliefs of South Asian women related to breast health practices.

Hypotheses, Assumptions and Objectives

From the review of the literature, the researcher narrows down the field of enquiry and refines the problem statement into one or more research questions. In qualitative studies, the research questions are often broad questions about human experiences and realities that are studied through contact with people in their natural environments.

In quantitative research studies, the research problem is expressed in a clear, specific statement or research question that expresses a relationship between two or more variables (concepts) of interest. When concepts are operationally defined, they are called variables. An **operational definition** specifies all the relevant aspects of the concept to be measured. It defines a concept so that later researchers will be able to measure the same thing in the same way. Thus, the concept of "stress" might be operationally defined as self-ratings of current and usual levels of anxiety as measured by The State-Trait Anxiety Inventory (Spielberger, Gorsuch, & Lushene, 1970), which consists of two separate 20-item scales for measuring state (current) and trait (usual) anxiety. Stress arousal could also be operationally defined by using physiological measures such as blood pressure, heart rate or urinary measures of cortisol and catecholamines.

As the word suggests, a **variable** is something that changes. In quantitative research the term is used to designate a quality, characteristic or property of an object, a person or a situation that can and does change in different circumstances (Burns & Grove, 1993). The fact that it changes implies that it can be measured. A variable may be concrete and directly measurable—for example, height, weight or pulse rate—or it may be abstract and only indirectly observable—for example, anxiety, pain or grief.

Research often attempts to determine the relationship between variables, that is, whether differences in one variable are related to differences in another (for instance, whether a person's age is related to the number of close friends he or she has). Relationships between variables do not necessarily imply **causality**, that is, that one variable is the cause of the other. However, if there is no relationship between the variables (if a study showed that there was no difference in the number of close friends older and younger people had), the researcher can rule out the possibility of a causal relationship. Conversely, the possibility of a causal relationship increases as the relationship strengthens, although it should be noted that two variables can be closely related without one being the cause of another (Burns & Grove, 1993).

Variables are categorized as *dependent*, *independent* or *intervening*. The **dependent variables** are also sometimes called the *outcome* variables. It is the characteristic that the study or experiment intended to measure. In the case of the nurses' anxiety about the introduction of primary nursing, the dependent variable is their level of anxiety. The dependent variable is related to (depends on) the independent variable.

The **independent variables** are also sometimes called *experimental* variables or *intervention* variables. These are the characteristics that may be changed (manipulated) by the investigator. Many drug experiments involve giving different groups of subjects varying amounts of a medication. In this case the amount of medication would be the independent variable. Independent variables can also refer to things that the experimenter cannot change, but which nonetheless differ—the subjects may themselves vary in certain characteristics. Age and gender are two important (demographic) independent variables that play a role in many studies. The values of independent variables are established by the researcher ahead of time. They constitute the input of an experiment and precede the measurement of the dependent variable. It is possible to have both more than one dependent variable and more than one independent variable, but all must be operationally defined. The variables (including the population under study) to be examined, and others that may affect the study, should be introduced in the hypothesis section of the report.

Extraneous variables are factors that might influence the measurement of study variables and the relationships between them (e.g., age, gender, amount spouse smokes, number of days post-op). These are characteristics that are not under study but might influence the results of the study. The researcher tries to think of all the variables that might possibly have an influence and tries to negate their effect through the design of the research or through statistical techniques (Davies & Logan, 1997). The extraneous variables that are not recognized until the study is in progress or that cannot be controlled are referred to as **confounding variables**.

In the case of the nurses' anxieties about the introduction of primary nursing, a nurse's employment status (permanent or casual) and/or personal problems that are causing anxiety might be extraneous variables that could affect the results of the study. The former could be controlled by having only permanent staff members participate in the study, but it would be difficult to control for personal circumstances that could be influencing a nurse's attitude to something new in the work situation.

Once the variables have been identified, the researcher normally formulates a hypothesis (or hypotheses), develops objectives or assumptions, or states the research questions in more precise detail than the general statement made in the introductory section of the report. Researchers formulate two types of hypotheses: scientific hypotheses and null hypotheses. The scientific or research **hypothesis** indicates what the researcher expects will be the outcome of the study

Questions to Ask About Hypotheses, Assumptions, Objectives and Research Questions

Quantitative Studies

1. Are the research objectives, questions or hypotheses expressed clearly?
2. Are the research objectives, questions or hypotheses logically linked to the research purpose?
3. Are the research objectives, questions or hypotheses derived from the theoretical framework?
4. What are the independent and dependent variables specified in each of the research objectives, questions or hypotheses?
5. What possible extraneous variables has the researcher considered? Can you think of others?

Qualitative Studies

1. Is the phenomenon of interest clearly identified?
2. Are the research questions logically linked to the research purpose?

(e.g., "If nurses receive inservice training they will have less anxiety about the introduction of primary nursing than will those who do not receive inservice training"). The **null hypothesis** is the hypothesis that is tested by statistical methods and is stated to suggest that there is *no* difference between groups (e.g., "There will be no significant difference in anxiety between those groups who received extra instruction and those who did not").

Assumptions, objectives and research questions are used in more descriptive studies where precise prediction of results is not the ultimate goal. **Assumptions** are provisional suppositions; the researcher might assume, for example, that there is a relationship between age and response to medication.

When the primary purpose of the research is to gather new knowledge about a phenomenon, objectives may be developed to provide guidance for the study, or the original research question (problem statement) may be refined into more precise questions. For example, is age related to response to medication? Is gender related to it? Are expectations about results a factor? By developing hypotheses, assumptions, objectives or specific questions prior to the conduct of a study, the researcher provides specific direction for subsequent aspects of design, as well as data collection and analysis.

Methodology (Design or Procedures)

In the section of a research article entitled *Methodology* (or *Design* or *Procedures*), the investigator explains, in detail, exactly how the study was conducted. The investigator should provide an explanation of the type of research design used in conducting the study, who participated in the study, what tools or instruments were used to collect data, what data were collected, what procedures the participants were required to do, and the methods used for data analysis.

THE RESEARCH DESIGN

The **research design**, as described earlier in this chapter, refers to the overall structure of an investigation. The design, in conjunction with the methods and procedures, provides the mechanisms for answering research questions. Within the two broad types of research designs, qualitative and quantitative, there are numerous types. While none is perfect (Davies & Logan, 1997), all have been useful in addressing research questions of interest to nurses. As you read a research report you will need to evaluate whether the results of the study are valid or credible. If we are to use the results of a study to guide practice decisions or as a basis for further research, then the results must be believable and dependable (LoBiondo-Wood, 1994). The issue of design bias is important in both qualitative and quantitative studies. When there is evidence of substantial bias, caution will need to be taken in interpreting and using the results of the study (Davies & Logan, 1997).

When using a quantitative design, the researcher attempts to maintain control over all variables. However, the amount of control that a researcher has over variables varies with the different types of quantitative designs and, in turn, this influences the credibility and dependability of the study findings. Two criteria are used to evaluate quantitative designs: internal validity and external validity.

Internal validity refers to factors (extraneous variables) within a particular study design that may have influenced the findings apart from the independent variable (or intervention variable). Problems with internal validity are related directly to issues of control. For example, scores on a post-test may be higher simply because of experience gained through taking the pretest. When a comparison group is used, it is possible to separate the effect of taking the pretest from the effect of the independent variable or treatment in post-test measures. The use of a comparison group (or groups), random assignment of subjects to groups, and consistent data collection procedures are examples of measures that researchers use to control factors (extraneous variables) and enhance the internal validity of their studies. To assess internal validity, one should ask if the researcher has introduced sufficient controls to minimize threats to it.

External validity relates to things that happen in a study that make it difficult to apply the findings to other samples or other settings (often referred to as the problem of generalizability). For example, the way that subjects are selected for a study and their characteristics affect the extent to which one can generalize study findings to other groups. The artificiality imposed by some study procedures may also pose a threat to the generalizability of findings to individuals in more natural settings. In assessing the external validity of a study, it is important to determine under what circumstances and with what types of subjects the same results can be expected to occur (LoBiondo-Wood, 1994).

Studies that make use of qualitative designs also need to be evaluated for credibility or trustworthiness. To enhance trustworthiness, qualitative researchers use a variety of strategies, including prolonged contact or observation with informants and attempts to identify their own biases through such devices as memo writing. Although it is difficult to arrive at one set of criteria for evaluating the whole range of qualitative designs, four general criteria have been proposed that can be used to judge qualitative research studies: *credibility*, *audibility*, *fittingness* and *confirmability* (Sandelowski, 1986).

Credibility or truth value refers to the degree to which the researcher has captured, accurately interpreted and faithfully described human experiences. When informants recognize the description as representing their experiences, a study is credible. Credibility is also achieved when other researchers or readers recognize the experience on the basis of what they have read about it.

The criterion of **audibility** refers to the adequacy of information about the researcher's decisions, choices and insights that directed each step of the research. On the basis of this information, a reader should be able to follow the researcher's thinking during the entire research process.

Fittingness is the criterion against which the applicability of qualitative findings be evaluated. It refers to whether the results provide a meaningful picture of the phenomenon under study (e.g., "Are relationships among the concepts clearly expressed? Are the findings well-grounded in the life experiences under study? Is the resulting theory trivial, or are new insights revealed?"). If the results are clearly presented, others are able to determine if they are applicable to their own experiences. Rather than relying on objectivity, a qualitative researcher looks to **confirmability** in establishing the value of the data. Here neutrality refers to the findings themselves, and not to the objective stance of the researcher. Confirmability is achieved when the other criteria have been met.

Morse and Field (1995) state that although the purpose of both quantitative and qualitative research is to generate nursing knowledge, there is a basic difference in the approach of the two methodologies. In quantitative research, knowledge is derived **deductively**, that is to say, the investigator works from existing theory and hypothesizes relationships that are then tested by experimental or nonexperimental means. An example of an experimental study is one that was done by a multidisciplinary team at the University of Ottawa. The research team evaluated the effectiveness of a diabetic education program for nurses to assist patient self-care in the community. Two randomly selected teams of nurses were used, with one group receiving a one-hour briefing and the other a two-day workshop with additional case management assignments. Both groups had access to the same resources in the agency (Davies, et al., 1993). The numerous health surveys undertaken by Statistics Canada are examples of quantitative studies done on a nonexperimental basis. We have referred to a number of these in earlier chapters. Another example, on a smaller scale, was a study by nurses in Fort McMurray and district in northern Alberta who used a survey to collect data on the health behaviours of pregnant women (Ali, Dow-Clarke & MacCalder, 1993).

In qualitative research, on the other hand, knowledge is developed **inductively** from the data. The studies are usually descriptive and are used when not much is known about a topic. In the course of the study, phenomena and concepts are identified and possible relationships are suggested. In other words, qualitative research identifies variables in order to generate a theory, which may subsequently be tested in further quantitative studies. There are three major types of quantitative studies: experimental (randomized controlled trial), quasi-experimental (pretest/post-test control group, no randomization) and non-experimental designs (survey and correlational studies).

EXPERIMENTAL STUDIES Experimental studies are usually used to determine cause-and-effect relationships between variables (i.e., when X occurs, is it likely Y will result?). There are three criteria for experimental designs. First, the researcher must manipulate the independent variable (e.g., an intervention). This means that the researcher has control of who administers the intervention, how it is administered, and who will receive it. Secondly, the study must include at least one experimental and one control or comparison group. Finally, random assignment must be used to allocate subjects to the experimental and control groups. The randomized controlled trial is a commonly used experimental design and includes randomized clinical trials, a term used to describe the same research design when it is used for evaluating the effectiveness of medical, pharmaceutical or nursing interventions. Johnson, Ratner, Bottorff, Hall and Dahinten (1997) wanted to see if nurses could reduce the high rate of postpartum smoking relapse among women who had quit smoking during pregnancy. They designed a randomized clinical trial to evaluate the effectiveness of a nurse-delivered smoking relapse prevention intervention specifically targeted towards postpartum women. Women who met the eligibility criteria for the study were randomly assigned to either an experimental or a control group. All women in the experimental group received the same smoking relapse prevention intervention, consisting of an in-hospital counselling session, printed materials and telephone support following discharge. Women in the control group received usual hospital care. At six months postpartum the resumption of daily smoking was lower in the experimental group than the control group.

Quantitative Design

Experimental and Nonexperimental

Experimental designs have three essential characteristics:

- randomization (random assignment of participants to groups)
- a control group for comparison with the experimental group
- manipulation of a special treatment (e.g., early discharge, teaching program).

Nonexperimental designs lack one or more of the above three characteristics.

Common Quantitative Designs

Experimental

- randomized controlled trial
- clinical trial
- quasi-experimental pretest–post-test control group (no randomization)

Nonexperimental

- survey
- correlation

Qualitative Design

There are some important differences between qualitative and quantitative design. The standards for choosing a sample, sample size and data analysis methods are not the same.

The sample is selected by different means to get the best possible information. For example, purposive (not random) or nominated (named by knowledgeable others) samples are used. The sample in a qualitative study will be much smaller, about 12 to 20 participants (usually not called subjects). Since there is no statistical analysis of numbers to be done, large samples are not required. A case study design may use only one participant or single organization. The procedures to ensure reliability and validity should be described, but the terms used may be different (e.g., credibility, audibility, fittingness and confirmability).

Analysis of qualitative data involves coding and categorizing to form themes and generate theoretical concepts. The categories must be defined. Quotes or examples from the data would be provided to support the investigator's interpretation.

Common Qualitative Designs

- grounded theory—to develop theory
- phenomenology—to describe experience
- ethnomethodology—to examine cultures

SOURCE: Davies & Logan, 1997, p. 8.

Questions to Ask About the Study Design

1. What research design was used in this study? Quantitative: experimental? or nonexperimental? Or qualitative: grounded theory? phenomenological? or ethnomethodological?
2. Is the method appropriate for studying the problem? Does it follow clearly from the problem statement and research questions?
3. Quantitative studies: Are important extraneous variables adequately controlled (internal validity)? What are the limitations to generalizing the results of this study (external validity)?
4. Qualitative studies: Is there sufficient demonstration of the researcher's concern for the credibility, audibility and fittingness of the study findings?

QUASI-EXPERIMENTAL STUDIES When researchers are unable to randomly assign subjects to study groups or a comparison group is not available for some reason a quasi-experimental design is used. There are several different designs that fit into the category of quasi-experimental design. One common quasi-experimental design, the pretest post-test nonequivalent group design, involves an experimental intervention (independent variable) and two or more groups of subjects (nonrandomly assigned). Studies using this design often take place in natural settings, where it is difficult or impractical to deliver an experimental intervention to individuals who have been assigned to the experimental group on a random basis. For example, Dr. Joy Johnson and her colleagues at St. Paul's Hospital evaluated a nurse-administered smoking cessation intervention for cardiac patients (Johnson, Budz, Mackay & Miller, in press). At the time of the study patients who met the eligibility criteria were recruited for the study from two cardiac units in the hospital. Rather than using subjects randomly assigned to the experimental and control groups, the researchers worked with intact groups. Patients on unit #1 received the smoking cessation intervention (experimental group), while patients on unit #2 received usual care (comparison group). Administering the smoking cessation intervention to patients who were on one unit helped to ensure that patients who were in the control group were not exposed to the smoking cessation materials or provided with additional encouragement to stop smoking beyond that normally provided by nursing staff. The two groups were compared six months following the intervention to determine smoking rates. The strength of this design depends on whether a strong case can be made for the similarity of the study groups before the experimental intervention is given.

NONEXPERIMENTAL STUDIES Many problems and questions of interest to nursing researchers do not lend themselves to experimental or quasi-experimental designs. Two main types of nonexperimental studies are surveys (sometimes referred to as descriptive research) and correlational research. The main purpose of survey research is to describe aspects of a situation. There are a variety of survey designs. Key elements of these designs are the procedures used to select subjects and the sample size. When small convenience samples are used, the results of the study may apply only to the individuals in the sample. The researcher's confidence in generalizing the findings beyond the study sample can, therefore, vary considerably depending on the sampling procedures used. A good example of survey research involves a telephone survey of 406 randomly selected married (including common law) women in Edmonton, Alberta (Ratner, 1993). The survey was conducted, in part, to determine the incidence and type of wife abuse. In this study 10.6 percent of the sample reported physical abuse and 13.1 percent reported being psychologically abused. Nearly all of the respondents who reported being physically abused were also psychologically abused.

Correlational designs are used to determine the relationship between two or more variables. The extent to which one variable (X) is related to another variable (Y) is referred to as a correlation. In a simple correlational study, one group of subjects is measured onthe variables of interest (X and Y) to describe the relationships between these variables. This design was used to describe the relationship between symptom distress at the time of diagnosis (X) and survival five years later (Y) among a consecutively selected sample of 82 newly diagnosed patients with lung cancer (Degner & Sloan, 1995). The correlation between symptom distress and the length of time of survival was –.49, a negative relationship indicating that as symptom distress scores increase survival time decreases. In other words, patients with high symptom distress had short survival times. Based on the results of this study, it appears a simple measure of symptom distress could be useful in identifying those patients with high distress who may be at risk for shortened survival times irrespective of medical treatment.

There are three major types of qualitative studies: *grounded theory* (used to develop theories), *phenomenology* (used to describe experience) and *ethnomethodology* (used to examine cultures).

GROUNDED THEORY STUDIES The term **grounded theory** refers to theory that has been grounded in reality. The theory is derived from data systematically obtained from social research and must provide an explanation of events as they occur (Morse & Field, 1995).

An example of a study using grounded theory methods is one undertaken by Wilson and Morse (1991). Concerned about the negative impact that diagnosis and treatment of cancer may have for spouses, they wanted to understand a husband's experience of living with a wife undergoing chemotherapy for cancer. Analysis of in-depth interviews revealed that the main way husbands coped with their wives' reactions to chemotherapy was by "buffering." By using a variety of buffering strategies, husbands were able to continually filter and reduce the stresses of day-to-day living to protect their wives. For example, the husbands designed buffering strategies to "resist disruption" to the household. These strategies included disguising their feelings, avoiding discussions about their distress at their wives' appearance and maintaining self-control (e.g., by hiding their sadness and fear). A three-stage model describing the process of buffering was developed to depict the way husbands reacted to their wives' response to chemotherapy.

PHENOMENOLOGICAL STUDIES The purpose of **phenomenological** studies is "to describe experience as it is lived" (Munhall & Oiler, 1986, p. 70). They are not done for the purpose of generating theory or developing general observations. The researcher, rather, is concerned with how people perceive experiences such as being in pain, recovering from an illness or giving birth (Morse & Field, 1995).

The phenomenological investigator starts with no preconceived notions, attempting only to describe accurately the phenomenon being studied. It has been suggested that empathy could be studied by phenomenological methods because it is so little understood and yet is considered a very important trait for nurses to have (Morse & Field, 1995).

Phenomenological methods have been used to study the meaning of pain during labour (Kelpin, 1992), the meaning of surgery for a small child (Smith, 1992) and the meaning of patient comfort (Bottorff, 1991; Morse, Bottorff & Hutchinson, 1994). These studies and others using phenomenological methods provide important insights for the reader. For example, Kelpin's (1992) study helps us understand that the pain of labour is not experienced from a state of passive suffering, but rather demands the kind of endurance that reveals previously unrecognized stamina and strength. The offer of analgesics for pain during labour, therefore, needs to be made in ways that do not undermine a woman's confidence that she will be able to "stand" the pain.

ETHNOMETHODOLOGICAL STUDIES **Ethnography** is the scientific description of cultural groups. The research methodology developed by anthropologists to generate cultural theory through the examining of different cultures has begun to be used in nursing as transcultural nursing has come into prominence. The purpose of **ethnomethodological** (ethnographic) studies is to undertake a descriptive analysis of a culture or subculture that can be used as a basis to develop theories about that culture. For example, Dr. Madeleine Leininger, who is recognized as the founder of transcultural nursing, has studied human care phenomena in 54 cultures (Cohen, 1992). From these studies she developed her theories of the diversity and universality of cultural care, which we will discuss further in Chapter 12.

In nursing, the ethnomethodological approach is also used to look at questions such as "What does it mean to be a member of a mixed-ethnic family?" "What are the rules for appropriate behaviour among teenage girls in Indo-Canadian society?" and other questions that are relevant to holistic nursing. In ethnomethodological studies, the researcher has to become to a certain extent a part of the community under study for a while in order to gather the data and gain insight into the behaviours of people in the group. Methods used to gather data include interviewing people in the community who are knowledgeable about the culture and willing to talk with the researcher, and **participant observation**, in which the researcher takes part in the activities of the group. The participation may range from full involvement to pure observation (Liehr & Marcus, 1994; Morse & Field, 1995; Munhall & Oiler, 1986).

THE POPULATION UNDER STUDY

The term **population** refers to a well-defined group of people who have certain characteristics in common; they may be nurses who work in the Intensive Care Unit of a hospital, for example, or people with a specific disease. In some studies, a *total population* may be used, for example, all the senior nurse administrators in public general hospitals in a province. Most times, however, it is not feasible to survey a total population and it is necessary to use a **sample** of the total. The way the sample is selected is a critical aspect in determining the extent to which the findings from a study sample may be generalized to the larger population. The procedures for selecting the sample of study subjects should be carefully described by the investigator, as should the size and the characteristics of the sample. Failure to report sampling procedures greatly weakens any research report.

There are several appropriate and legitimate ways in which samples can be selected from a population. The population that is a feasible source of sample members is termed the **accessible population**. In most types of quantitative studies, the investigator wants to ensure that each element in the accessible population has an equal and independent chance of being selected. In order to ensure this, **probability sampling**, in which participants are selected randomly from within the accessible sample, is used. Probability sampling is also called **random sampling**. **Simple random sampling**, using a table of random numbers, is the most widely used and acceptable method of obtaining a random sample for quantitative studies. However, there are many variations that may be used.

Stratified sampling involves making a random selection from each of different subgroups within the population (for example, diploma RNs, baccalaureate graduates and nurses with master's and higher degrees among a population of nurses). **Cluster sampling** involves taking progressively larger random samples from different units within a population. **Systematic sampling** is done by taking every *n*th member of the population (for example, every 10th name on the list of RNs in the various counties of eastern Ontario). In experimental research, the investigator selects a **control** group that can be compared with the experimental group; the characteristics of the control group should be similar to those of the experimental group. The control group is not part of the experimental manipulation; it is used only as a basis for comparison, to ensure that the effects of the research variables are genuine. For example, if recovery rates for a control group were just as high as for a group that received increased medication, it would be clear that it wasn't the medication that was improving recovery, but some other factor altogether.

In qualitative research, it is important to ensure that participants are knowledgeable about the information the investigator wants to collect, so nonprobability (nonrandom) methods of sampling the population are used. Convenience, quota and purposive sampling are three types of nonprobability sampling.

Convenience sampling (or **accidental sampling**) allows the entry of any available (convenient) subjects into the study until the desired sample size is reached. A study of health perceptions of homeless people (McCormack & Gooding, 1993) used a convenience sample of 29 individuals from among the homeless who made use of shelters and hostels.

Quota sampling is done by selecting participants by proportional representation of different groups or strata within the total population. For example, in a hypothetical study of the adjustment to school of new-Canadian children in Toronto, one might want to use quota sampling to be sure to include in the sample children of different ethnic groups, with the sample size for each group proportionate to their numbers in the total population of newcomers to the school system. That is to say, if 100 children from different ethnic groups entered the Toronto public school system in a given year and 30 came from China, 25 from Korea, 20

Questions to Ask About the Population Under Study

1. What are the common characteristics of the population under study?
2. How was the study sample selected—were sampling techniques employed?
3. If sampling was used, what method was used for obtaining the sample? Is it appropriate for the type of study that was done?
4. Is the number in the sample sufficient? How does the researcher justify the sample size? The selection process?
5. Quantitative studies: In your opinion, is the sample representative of the defined population?
6. Qualitative studies: Are the participants appropriate to inform the research?

from the Philippines, 15 from Peru and 10 from Scotland, the quota sample of the population would be proportionate, with 30 percent Chinese children, etc.

In **purposive sampling** investigators use their knowledge of the population and its elements to select subjects to be included in the study. This type of sampling differs from convenience sampling, in that convenience sampling is not purposeful or strategic. A purposive sampling approach is often used in qualitative studies to include individuals who have had the particular life experience that is under study. For example, a purposive sample of family members who are caring for an elderly relative would be used in a qualitative study of the experiences of family caregivers because they have important first-hand experiences that are relevant to the study. Purposive sampling may also be used in some quantitative studies. For example, if a researcher was investigating the relationship between older adults' cognitive functioning and health status, past education could be regarded as an important factor. Since a proportionately small number of seniors have a university education, a convenience sample or random sample may not provide the researcher with a sufficient number of seniors with university education. Purposive sampling would allow the researcher to select enough highly educated seniors to ensure that they were adequately represented in the study sample.

Finally, **theoretical sampling** is used in grounded theory studies as a process for generating theory (Morse & Field, 1995). In this approach, the collection and analysis of data are closely linked. As initial data are collected and analysed, questions and tentative hypotheses that are linked to the emerging theory are used to decide what data need to be collected next. The criteria for selection of individuals to participate in the study, therefore, change as the study progresses, according to what has been learned from previous sources. As such, researchers using theoretical sampling methods do not select their participants before the study begins.

Safeguarding the Rights of the Population Under Study

Ethical issues require careful attention when research of any type is conducted. These issues relate to the rights of research subjects, the recruiting of subjects, the confidentiality of responses and the disclosing of the actual purpose of the research to the respondents. Today, research proposals are under close scrutiny by human-subject review committees in most hospitals, other health agencies and universities. Such committees are made up of groups of representatives of various departments or disciplines with the purpose of reviewing ethical concerns about research proposals. The major concern is the protection of the rights of the participants in the research study. The role of the researcher is to communicate clearly in writing to the review committee how subjects will be used in the research and whether subjects are at any risk as a result of participating in the research. The researcher is responsible for carrying out these plans as directed or approved by the committee. The Research Committee of the Canadian Nurses Association has developed *Ethical Guidelines for Nursing Research Involving Human Subjects* (1994), which all introductory nursing students would do well to read.

In addition, the Tri-Council Policy Statement on Ethical Conduct for Research Involving Human Subjects descrbes the common policies of three major Canadian research councils and is available on the Internet (http://ncehr.medical.org/English/mstr_frm.html).

Questions to Ask About Measures to Safeguard the Rights of Subjects in the Study

1. What measures were taken to ensure that the rights of subjects were protected (e.g., informed consent, protection of confidentiality)?
2. Does the researcher make available to the reader the information given to subjects about the research?
3. Does the researcher discuss possible benefits of the research for the subjects in the study?

DATA COLLECTION

The term **data** is used to describe the information the researcher (also called the *investigator*) collects from subjects or participants in the research study, or about objects in a nonhuman study (note that *data* is a plural noun). To collect data for quantitative studies where one wants to obtain numerical values, the investigator will use some sort of **instrument**. This might be a questionnaire, a structured interview (in which all participants are asked the same questions) or an instrument such as a sphygmomanometer (to measure blood pressure).

In qualitative research, both interview and observation methods are used. In an interview, the researcher gathers information from the research subject by means of verbal communication. The interview may be unstructured, or "open-ended," or it may be guided by the interviewer. The interview may or may not be recorded on audio- or videotape. Short-answer questionnaires are used in some studies. A variety of observational strategies may also be used.

Measurement by observation tends to be more subjective than measurement by other means (using a sphygmomanometer, for example). Hence, the researcher needs to include safeguards to ensure consistency. As with interviews, observations may range from totally unstructured, with the researcher simply observing the subjects' behaviour in their natural setting, to structured. Structured observation techniques include the use of tools such as categories, checklists and rating scales. In using categories, observed behaviours are recorded in previously defined categories of activity. With checklists, the observer indicates simply whether listed

Questions to Ask About Data Collection Methods Used in the Study

1. What data were collected?
2. Were the right data collected to answer the research question?
3. How were the data collected?
4. Were the measures used to collect data appropriate for the study?
5. Did the researcher use a standard protocol for gathering data during the research?
6. If others besides the principal investigator collected data (e.g., interviewed subjects or informants, administered questionnaires or other instrument), how were they trained?
7. Quantitative studies: Does the researcher show evidence of having established the reliability and validity of the procedures used for data gathering?
8. Qualitative studies: Is saturation of the data described?

behaviours occurred or did not occur. With rating scales, the observer judges the behaviour observed on a predetermined scale (Burns & Grove, 1993). In studying other cultures, participant observation is commonly used.

Videotapes may also be systematically reviewed to study different behaviours—for example, the pain responses of postoperative neonates (Côté, Morse & James, 1991), nurses' use of touch (Bottorff, 1993) or the response of cognitively impaired elderly to restraints (Morse & McHutchion, 1991). Other methods of gathering data for qualitative studies include studying life histories. In historical research on nursing, there is usually considerable perusal of old records, as well as interviews with people who were practising in the early years of the century and/or with their daughters, sons or grandchildren. Letters are also a rich source for historical research. For example, in one aspect of an International Council of Nurses Centennial Project (the ICN will be 100 years old in 1999), Barbara L. Brush of the University of Pennsylvania and Dr. Meryn Stuart of the University of Ottawa School of Nursing examined international women's history theory and the concepts of "difference" and "unity." Focussing on the ICN's longevity and power and reviewing its purpose, the study used ICN Board minutes, financial records, Congress notes and personal correspondence, as well as numerous secondary source materials (Brush & Stuart, 1992).

In quantitative research studies, whatever instrument or procedures are used to collect the data, the researcher should describe exactly how the measurements were done and report on the validity and reliability of the procedures (see page 147). If modifications to an instrument are made for the purpose of the study, the researcher should explain how the original instrument was modified.

In qualitative studies, it is also important for the researcher to provide a clear description of the data collection strategies that were used. Qualitative researchers are interested in individuals' reports or perceptions of situations or events. Although individuals may report different versions of the same event, for a qualitative researcher this is part of the problem to be studied. Morse and Field (1995) explain: "A patient's perspective on and report of a visit to the doctor may be quite different from the doctor's account of the visit, and both of these reports may differ from an objective observer's report. However, the purpose of qualitative research is not to determine objectively what actually happened (as in a court of law) but rather to objectively report the perceptions of each participant in the setting" (p. 142). Data collection in qualitative studies should continue until the categories being used for analysis are saturated (i.e., there are no "thin" areas about which little is known and they "make sense"), the relationships between the categories are clear and no new information is being revealed during interviews.

Data Analysis and Results

The data analysis section of a research report explains how the data that were collected were processed and interpreted. In qualitative studies, the process of data analysis occurs as data are collected. There are few or no numbers to be analysed or reported. Instead, analysis is focussed on categories or themes and may suggest possible causal relationships that can be tested in further studies. A number of computer programs have been developed to assist people with qualitative analysis. These programs help the investigator to process, store, retrieve, catalogue and sort data that have been collected. The researcher does the actual analysis. You may note in the data analysis section of a qualitative study, for example, that the investigator has used CATS (Computer Assisted Topical Sorting) or another program to assist with one of the tasks mentioned above (Davies & Logan, 1997; Burns & Grove, 1993).

In quantitative studies, data are collected and then subjected to analysis. The data collected are numerical and, therefore, lend themselves to statistical analysis. The term **statistics** refers to the "systematic collection, organization, analysis and interpretation of numerical data" (*Taber's Cyclopedic Medical Dictionary* [16th ed.], 1989, p. 1744). Most basic nursing education programs today include a course in statistics as well as courses in research methodology. We will not, therefore, go into a detailed description of statistical techniques in this chapter. Instead, we will talk about the purpose and methods of using statistics to assist in data analysis. We have also provided, at the end of the chapter, an explanation of some of the more common statistical terms you may find in reports. A knowledge of these terms is basic to understanding how data were handled in many research studies and in other professional reports.

In quantitative research studies, statistics are used to find those numbers that most accurately communicate the nature of attitudes, processes, events and achievements that need to be described; using statistics makes numbers more manageable and casts light on data. Statistical methods assist researchers in describing data, in drawing inferences to larger bodies of data and in studying causal relationships. There are two types of statistical analysis that are done on numerical data. The first type is **exploratory** or **descriptive data analysis**. This type of analysis is usually performed first, to get an overall impression of the data. The second type is called **confirmatory data analysis.** At this stage, inferential statistics are used. Researchers make an inference (generalization) about a population or a process based on data collected during the study.

Exploratory or **descriptive statistics** represent the end result of the tabulating, depicting and describing of collections of data. The data might include measures of blood pressure, anxiety, weight, medical diagnosis, gender or nationality or any other type of data that have been systematically collected and can be represented numerically. Generally speaking, large masses of data must undergo a process of summarization or reduction in order to make them more comprehensible. For example, the large masses of data collected by Statistics Canada about university students in the country are much easier to understand when they are put into tables, graphs or histograms (as exemplified in Figure 7.1) than in the original *raw data* form, which is also available from Statistics Canada. Descriptive techniques serve as tools to describe, summarize or reduce to a manageable form the properties of an otherwise unwieldy accumulation of data. In some studies, descriptive analysis is all that is done.

Confirmatory statistical treatment of data (using inferential statistics) involves the use of various techniques in order to:

- test proposed relationships between variables
- ascertain (infer) that the findings from a sample are representative of the total population
- examine causality (that a specific change in *a* caused reaction *b*)
- predict (that under similar circumstances, *a* will probably cause *b* again)
- infer from the sample to a theoretical model. (Burns & Grove, 1993)

The results of a study are translated and interpreted, a process that yields the study *findings*—in statistical form (Burns & Grove, 1993). These may be reported in the text, summarized in tables or presented visually in figures or graphs.

In quantitative studies of a nonexperimental nature, the findings of the study are often shown in tables, graphs or histograms. Because it is difficult to interpret the findings from inferential statistical techniques without a course on statistics, we will not go into great detail here. However, at the very least, you will need to be able to understand from reading research reports whether the findings show that there is a significant relationship between the variables. Davies and Logan (1997) suggest that, for consumers of research, the key point to look for in the report is the p (for probability) value of statistical significance of the results. These are stated in terms of p, which indicates the probability of the results being *not true*. If p is less than 0.05 (or less

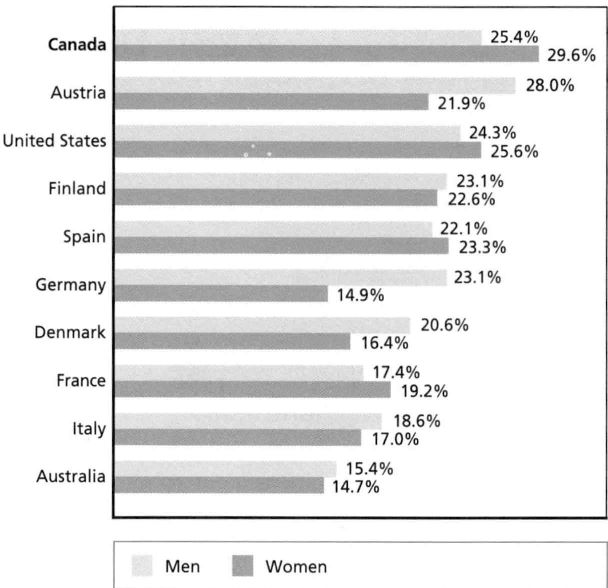

FIGURE 7.1 A Histogram: Ten OECD (Organization for Economic Cooperation and Development) countries with the highest percentage of young adults enrolled* in university, 1988

* Full-time and part-time enrolment converted to full-time equivalents. Population is those of theoretical university enrolment age (18–25 in Canada).

SOURCE: OECD, 1992. As cited in Oderkirk, 1993 p. 9.

Questions to Ask About Data Analysis and Results

1. Does the researcher inform you of the steps taken to process and interpret the data?
2. Do the methods selected to analyse the data seem appropriate?
3. Are reasons given for decisions to analyse the data in the manner in which they were analysed?
4. Are the primary findings of the study clearly presented?
5. Are the results clear?
6. Are conclusions logical?
7. Did the researcher identify methodological problems?

than 0.01), it means that the probability of the results being *not true* is less than five percent (or one percent). To put that statement in the positive, a low *p* value indicates more likelihood that the findings from the study were due to the experimental manipulation of the variable by the researcher—that is, that the experimental manipulation did have an effect.

In experimental studies, the investigator should report on whether or not the hypothesis was supported. When support for the hypothesis is obtained, the researcher must be cautious in generalizing the results. Factors related to validity, methodological problems and limitations of the research design must be taken into account when generalizing study results. Often, however, hypotheses are not supported, or findings are contradictory to those of similar studies. In such cases, the researcher should attempt to identify probable reasons for the findings.

Contradictory findings may be the result of lack of precision or methodological problems. A common problem is the imprecise definition of variables. If this is the case, it may well be that the method of measuring variables has affected the results. Finally, there may be nothing wrong with the study, but contradictory findings may have identified an intriguing aspect of ambiguity that opens a whole new field of investigation. The important point to remember is that, while it may be difficult to identify the actual basis for the unusual findings because of lack of information, the investigator should always discuss them.

In qualitative research, the researcher analyses textual narrative (e.g., transcribed interviews), written field notes of observations, and reflections or ideas recorded in a researcher's diary. Although the procedures for data analysis vary depending on the qualitative research method being used, there are some common processes. Qualitative data analysis requires that the researcher be very familiar with—often—hundreds of pages of data. Thus, the process of data analysis can be lengthy and require continual review and questioning of data collected.

The researcher begins by having all interviews transcribed verbatim and checks these for accuracy. Persistent words, phrases or themes in the data are then identified and sorted into categories or groups. In this way, categories are derived directly from the data. Usually, researchers begin with a few categories. As more data accumulate, categories may be divided into subcategories (Morse & Field, 1995).

Computer programs specifically designed for qualitative data analysis are now used by many researchers to facilitate the coding, sorting and analysis of large amounts of data. As the data analysis proceeds, the researcher begins to make sense of the data and to learn what is going on. At this point, the researcher is able to identify what stories are part of the topic under study as well as some of the patterns in this experience. However, further analysis of commonalties and differences among participants or events helps the researcher begin to see links and relationships in the data and between the data and emerging concepts. Sometimes matrices, taxonomies or diagrams are used to help order the data and to depict relationships. Sometimes a theory or model is developed that provides the best explanation of the experience or event under study. The results of a qualitative data analysis are often verified with study participants (or sometimes other people). If the analysis accurately reflects the participants' experience, they should be able to recognize it as their own.

Qualitative researchers may present their findings in several ways. Usually it is in the form of a narrative report that includes excerpts from the data (e.g., quotations) to support conclusions about the nature of the human experience under study. The general goal is to provide a vivid description so that the reader shares the participants' experiences (Morse & Field, 1995). Sometimes, the new findings are discussed in relation to the work of other researchers or established theories when results are presented. If this is done well, it will be clear how the results of the study are supported by the literature and where they make a new contribution.

Discussion

Whereas the section on results presents a report of how the statistical analysis turned out, the discussion section explains what the results mean with regard to the purposes of the study and relates them to a theoretical context. Sometimes the discussion section is called *Conclusions*.

In reading a research report, you must decide whether the discussion and conclusions articulated represent a logical outcome of the procedures, methods, design and analysis of data; they should also be consistent with the focus of the problem and variables under study. In the discussion section, the researcher points out what the results mean in terms of the problem being studied and identifies the extent to which additional knowledge about the purpose of

Questions to Ask About the Discussion

1. Is the discussion clearly presented?
2. Is it reported logically? Is it well organized?
3. Are conclusions drawn from the data rather than the speculation of the researcher?
4. Are omissions and limitations of the study noted by the researcher?
5. Are the implications of the study clearly stated?
6. Do they seem plausible to you?
7. Is it clear how the study will extend previous findings?
8. Does the author give a concise, inclusive summary?

The Scientific Merit of a Study

Funding agencies who allocate monies for proposed research projects use *scientific merit* as one criterion in their evaluation of the worth of a project. Experts at the RNABC have identified the following as the basic elements for judging the scientific merit of a research project:

- the proposal must be grounded in previous knowledge and relevant literature
- the hypothesis and/or research question must be relevant, clear and crisp
- the research design must be elegant—complete yet direct and simple
- the methods proposed to test the hypothesis or answer the questions must be clearly described and appropriate
- the study must be scientifically valid
- the study must generate knowledge not yet articulated, or corroborate previous findings that need further study.

SOURCE: RNABC, 1990.

the study has been gained. Thus, the investigator relates the findings to the theoretical position in the study. At this time, findings should be discussed in light of results from related research. One must keep the research problem in mind when writing the discussion section in order to ensure that no subtle reinterpretation of the problem has taken place. As readers of research reports, you should be aware of these considerations as well.

In addition to the statistical significance of the findings of a study, you will want to consider their **clinical significance**—whether the study is going to be useful in clinical practice. Looking at a specific example, Rosenbaum's 1991 study on *Widowhood Grief* among older Greek-Canadian women should enable community health nurses to provide more culturally sensitive care to older women members of the Greek-Canadian community in Canada.

Sometimes, the clinical significance is reported in a separate section entitled *Implications*, in which the investigator explains in more specific terms how the findings can be implemented. Clinicians would want to know the area of practice where the findings could be used, for instance, in the assessment of patients, in the improvement of nursing interventions or interpersonal relationships, or in the modification of factors in the environment or in the work life of nurses. For example, the research may have involved the trial of a new procedure for skin care. The researcher would indicate the specific situations in which this procedure might be used, such as the protection of skin around a wound, the prevention of decubitus ulcers (bedsores) and other situations where there is a risk of skin breakdown.

In the section discussing clinical significance, the researcher should also indicate the ease with which the findings can be implemented. Does the implementation involve changes in routines or in record forms, for example, or will it involve an extensive educational program—for example, teaching all staff a new procedure. The clinician will be concerned also with whether the findings are compatible with the agency's present policies, procedures and standards—or do they require major changes in these areas? Above all, clinicians will want to know about safety. Can the findings be implemented without jeopardizing the safety of patients, staff or visitors? Do they provide more safeguards than present procedures?

The resources required to implement the change(s) suggested in the findings of the study are also of concern. Would the implementation require the purchase of new equipment, more staff or a major investment of time or money (Davies & Logan, 1997)?

It is also important to consider whether or not the study contributes to the general body of nursing knowledge. Some studies in nursing—historical studies, for example—may not be directly applicable in clinical practice but they contribute to our base of nursing knowledge. In the discussion section of the report, the investigator should show how the findings of the study contribute to the field (Burns & Grove, 1993).

Most investigators identify areas where knowledge is inadequate and further research is required. These recommendations for further research should arise directly from the problem and findings. Such recommendations either are included in the discussion section of the article, or these may appear in a separate section.

It is a convention in research to present a general summary of the study at the end of the article or report. It may be labelled *Summary*, or it may be included in a section entitled *Conclusions*. This section is very similar to the abstract found at the beginning of the study, although the summary frequently emphasizes the findings more than the methodology. It is important to ensure that the summary is consistent with the focus of the study and that no deviations from the original purpose have taken place.

Selected Research Terminology

HYPOTHESIS A hypothesis is the statement of relationships the researcher expects to find between independent and dependent variables in a study. The hypothesis is usually a declarative statement and may be designated by the symbol H. If the researcher is going to test the reverse of his or her hypothesis, H_0 represents the null hypothesis, which is a statement that no relationship other than chance exists between or among a study's concepts or variables.

INSTRUMENTS Instruments are the devices used to record the data obtained from subjects. Two important qualities of research instruments used to measure variables in a research study are their reliability and validity. **Reliability** means that the instrument will produce consistent results, or data, on repeated use. For instance, if temperature is measured several times under unchanged conditions and the same readings are obtained, the measure is said to be reliable. **Validity** refers to the property or characteristic of a psychosocial instrument that means the instrument measures what it purports to measure.

FREQUENCY DISTRIBUTIONS A **frequency distribution** is an analysis method that involves determining how often scores or values appear in a data set. This procedure produces a **graph** showing how many times each score has occurred, that is, displaying the frequency of each score. The graph illustrates what is called the distribution of scores. An example of a frequency distribution is a **histogram**, which is a graphic display of a frequency table using rectangular bars with heights equal to the frequency in a particular class. Figure 7.2 shows a histogram and a polygon. The range is the simplest measure of dispersion. It represents the difference between the smallest and largest numbers in a distribution.

MEASURES OF CENTRAL TENDENCY A **measure of central tendency** is a statistic that summarizes the data into one representative value. There are three measures of central tendency: the mean, median and mode.

- **Mean** (also called the average) is the measure of central tendency derived by dividing the sum of the values in a data set by the total number of values, scores or subjects in it. It is represented by the symbol *x*, read as *x bar*. The mean score is a balance point. If the scores were weights on a scale, the mean would be the spot at which the scale would balance.
- **Median** is the measure of central tendency that corresponds to the middle score. The median is obtained by rank ordering the scores. If there exists an uneven number of scores, exactly 50 percent of the scores are above the median, and 50 percent are below the median. If there is an even number of scores, the median is the average of the two middle scores. Thus, the median may not be an actual score in the data set.

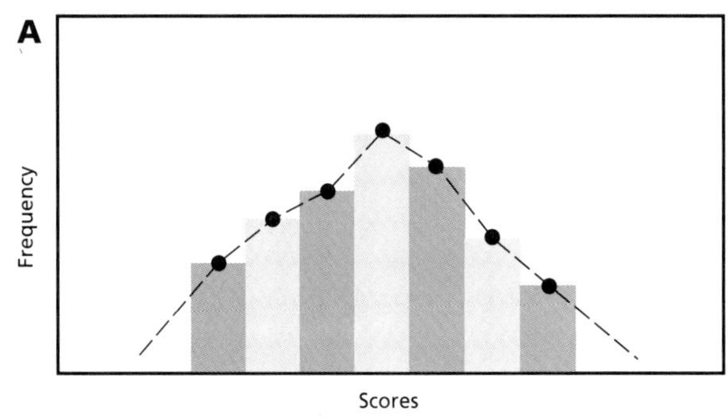

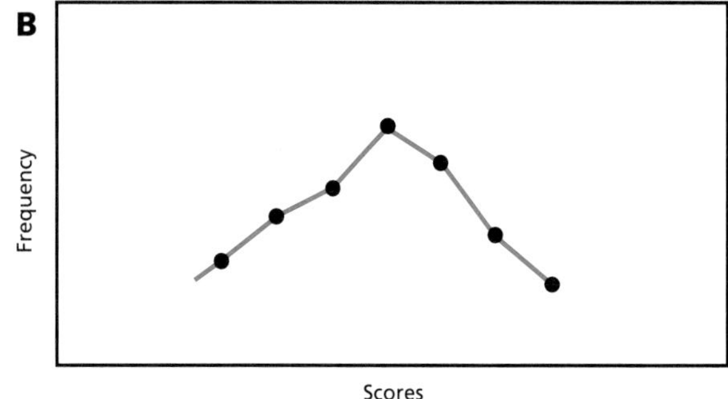

FIGURE 7.2 A. A histogram B. A frequency polygon

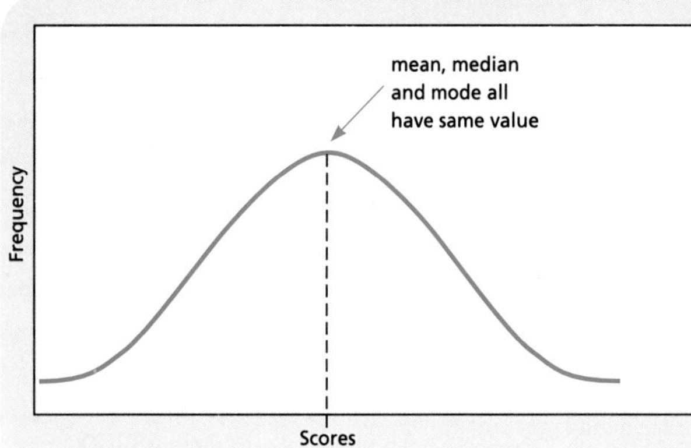

FIGURE 7.3 Measures of central tendency in a normal distribution

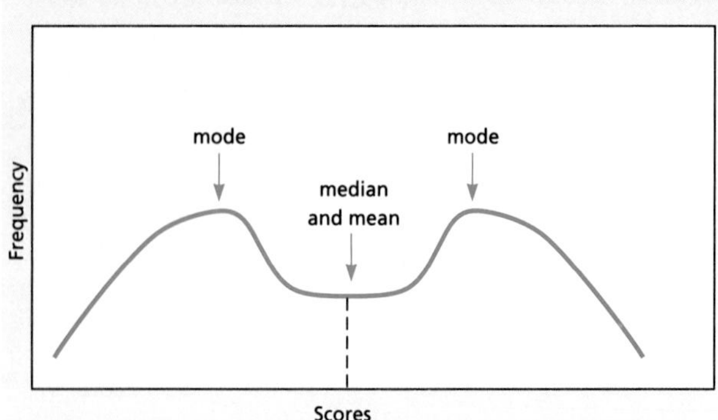

FIGURE 7.4 Bimodal frequency distribution

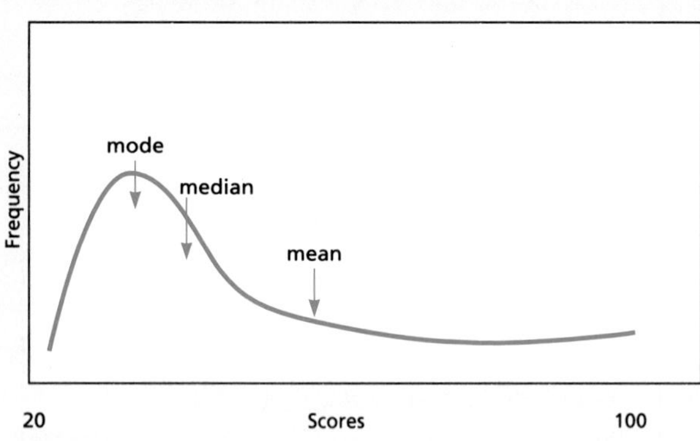

FIGURE 7.5 Skewed frequency distribution of scores*

* In this situation, a very few students received extremely high scores, whereas the majority received very low scores. This means that the mean tends to give too high a picture of the typical score, and the mode gives a marked underestimate of the typical score. The median is the best indication of the typical score.

- **Mode** is the category or class that has the highest frequency. It is the simplest measure of central tendency. The mode is the score or numerical value that occurs with the greatest frequency. A data set can have more than one mode. If two modes exist, the data set is referred to as bimodal. Thus, the mode does not necessarily indicate the centre of the data set. Figure 7.3 shows the mean, median and mode all having the same value in a normal distribution. Figure 7.4 shows a bimodal frequency distribution where there are two large clusters of scores, one at the upper end of the curve, the other at the lower end. Figure 7.5 shows a skewed curve, where a few high scores distort the value of the mean.

STANDARD DEVIATION The **standard deviation** is the most widely used measure of variability when a frequency distribution approximates a normal curve. It is the average of the deviations from the mean. The standard deviation of a group of scores is a number indicating whether most of those scores cluster closely around their mean or are spread out along the scale.

CORRELATION The Pearson moment correlation (*r*) is a statistic that shows the extent to which values of one variable are related to values of another variable. A **correlation** can be described in terms of the direction of the relationship. For example, a direct relationship is a positive correlation between two variables. On the other hand, an indirect relationship (inverse relationship) is a negative correlation between two variables.

Guidelines for a Research Critique

Title and Abstract

1. Does the title of the research accurately reflect the problem under study?
2. Does the abstract provide a succinct overview of the study?

Introduction

1. Do you have a clear idea of what the research is all about?
2. Do you understand why the research is being done?
3. Is the significance of the problem discussed and the research justified?
4. Is the problem substantiated with adequate background information?
5. Is the problem statement clear? Concise?

Review of the Literature and Theoretical Framework

1. Does the literature review support the significance of the problem?
2. Is the relationship of the problem to previous research clear?
3. What is the theoretical base for this study? What are the major concepts used?
4. Does the researcher indicate how he or she has used previous knowledge in developing this study?
5. Is the literature review well organized? What topics are addressed?
6. Is there a sufficient review of the literature to assure the reader that the researcher has considered a broad spectrum of possibilities for investigating the problem?
7. Are the references up to date, that is, are most of them less than 10 years old?
8. Has reference been made to classic studies in the area being investigated?

Hypotheses, Assumptions and Objectives

Quantitative Studies

1. Are the research objectives, questions or hypotheses expressed clearly?
2. Are the research objectives, questions or hypotheses logically linked to the research purpose?
3. Are the research objectives, questions or hypotheses derived from the theoretical framework?
4. What are the independent and dependent variables specified in each of the research objectives, questions, or hypotheses?
5. What possible extraneous variables has the researcher considered? Can you think of others?

Qualitative Studies

1. Is the phenomenon of interest clearly identified?
2. Are the research questions logically linked to the research purpose?

The Research Design

1. What research design was used in this study? Quantitative: experimental? or nonexperimental? Or Qualitative: grounded theory? phenomenological? or ethnomethodological?
2. Is the method appropriate for studying the problem? Does it follow clearly from the problem statement and research questions?
3. Quantitative studies: Are important extraneous variables adequately controlled (internal validity)? What are the limitations to generalizing the results of this study (external validity)?
4. Qualitative studies: Is there sufficient demonstration of the researcher's concern for the credibility, auditability, and fittingness of the study findings?

The Population Under Study

1. What are the common characteristics of the population under study?
2. How was the study sample selected—were sampling techniques employed?
3. If sampling was used, what method was used for obtaining the sample? Is it appropriate for the type of study that was done?
4. Is the number in the sample sufficient? How does the researcher justify the sample size? Selection process?
5. Quantitative studies: In your opinion, is the sample representative of the defined population?
6. Qualitative studies: Are the participants appropriate to inform the research?

Safeguarding the Rights of Subjects in the Study

1. What measures were taken to ensure that the rights of subjects were protected in this study?
2. Does the researcher make available to the reader the information given to subjects about the research?
3. Does the researcher discuss possible benefits/risks of the research for the subjects in the study?

Data Collection

1. What data were collected?
2. Were the data collected the right data to answer the research question?
3. How were the data collected?
4. Were the measures used to collect data appropriate for the study?
5. Did the researcher use a standard protocol for gathering data during the research?
6. If others besides the principal investigator collected data, how were they trained?
7. Quantitative studies: Does the researcher show evidence of having established the reliability and validity of the procedures used for data gathering?
8. Qualitative studies: Is saturation of the data described?

Data Analysis and Results

1. Does the researcher inform you of the steps taken to process and interpret the data?
2. Do the methods selected to analyse the data seem appropriate?
3. Are reasons given for the methods used to analyse the data?
4. Are the primary findings of the study clearly presented?
5. Are the results clear?
6. Are conclusions logical?
7. Did the investigator identify methodological problems?

Discussion

1. Is the discussion clearly presented?
2. Is it reported logically? Is it well organized?
3. Are conclusions drawn from the data rather than the speculation of the researcher?
4. Are omissions and limitations of the study noted by the researcher?
5. Are the implications of the study clearly stated?
6. Do they seem plausible to you?
7. Is it clear how the study will extend previous findings?
8. Does the researcher give a concise, inclusive summary?
9. What recommendations would you make to the author to improve this research? Note: These recommendations should follow logically and clearly from your assessment of the study.
10. How can you utilize this research in your studies or in your clinical practice?

IN REVIEW

- Canadian nursing research was slow to develop for several reasons:
  - scarcity of qualified nurse researchers
  - paucity of graduate programs offering methodology courses
  - lack of incentive for practising nurses to do research.
- Until recently, most research was limited to the academic environment. Today, a large number of research studies are ongoing, in a variety of health care settings.
- The goals of nursing research are to:
  - increase the knowledge base of nursing
  - describe and explain phenomena
  - strengthen accountability in patient care
  - improve the quality of human life.
- Over the past decade, research-based practice has become an essential aspect of nursing. The components of this practice include:
  - conduct of studies (solo, international, multidisciplinary)
  - dissemination of findings
  - utilization of research in clinical practice.
- Nursing knowledge is gained through unstructured means such as:
  - empathy
  - trial and error
  - intuition
  - tradition

  and through structured research using:
  - scientific enquiry
  - critical thinking
  - logical reasoning.
- The scientific enquiry/research process adheres to the following sequence:
  - develop a statement of the problem
  - review the literature
  - identify a theoretical framework
  - select a research design
  - implement the research plan
  - interpret the results of the study
  - draw conclusions
  - disseminate research findings.
- As students, you can begin to identify researchable nursing problems early in your program. Areas in which you may be involved include:
  - gathering data for studies
  - evaluating research reports
  - using findings of studies in your practice
  - sharing the findings of research with colleagues
  - protecting the rights of patients who are part of a research study.
- As a beginning student your primary role is that of research consumer. This role includes learning to read and interpret research reports using the critiquing approach.
- A critique is a critical assessment of a piece of research involving a systematic appraisal according to specific guidelines. In order to critique a research study you need to engage in three activities:
  - analysis of the study to identify component parts and procedures used
  - evaluation of the study by appraising its strengths and weaknesses
  - expression of your judgement about the merit or worth of the study.

Critical Thinking Activities

1. Explore the research being done in your school and in the clinical agencies affiliated with your school of nursing.
   a) What research projects are currently being carried out by school faculty? By graduate students? By nursing staff in the clinical agency (agencies)?
   b) Do the projects involve solo, collaborative or multidisciplinary research? International collaboration?
2. Compare the ethical guidelines suggested by the Canadian Nurses Association with those established by the research committee of your school/university or of a clinical agency with which the school is affiliated.
3. What sources are available to you for information on recent nursing research findings? What research journals are available in the library? Are there research seminars or conferences to which you can go? Is there a research interest group in the school or health agency? What other sources are available on the Internet?
4. Select a research article on a topic of interest to you from one of the nursing research journals in the library. Do a critique of the article, using the guidelines at the end of the chapter.

KEY TERMS

research-based practice p. 124
solo research p. 126
collaborative research p. 126
refereed journal p. 127
subject p. 127
change agent p. 128
empirical p. 129
critique p. 131
evaluation p. 132
quantitative design p. 132
qualitative design p. 132
abstract p. 133
problem statement p. 133
research question p. 133
validate the knowledge base p. 133
operational definition p. 136
variable p. 136
causality p. 136
dependent variables p. 136
independent variables p. 136
extraneous variables p. 136
confounding variables p. 136
hypothesis p. 136
null hypothesis p. 137
assumptions p. 137
research design p. 137
internal validity p. 137
external validity p. 137
credibility p. 138
audibility p. 138
fittingness p. 138
confirmability p. 138
deductive p. 138
inductive p. 138
grounded theory p. 140
phenomenological p. 140
ethnography p. 140
ethnomethodological p. 140
participant observation p. 141
population p. 141
sample p. 141
accessible population p. 141
probability sampling p. 141
random sampling p. 141
simple random sampling p. 141
stratified sampling p. 141
cluster sampling p. 141
systematic sampling p. 141
control p. 141
convenience sampling (accidental sampling) p. 141
quota sampling p. 141
purposive sampling p. 142
theoretical sampling p. 142
data p. 142
instrument p. 142
statistics p. 143
exploratory (descriptive) data analysis p. 144
confirmatory data analysis p. 144
exploratory (descriptive) statistics p. 144
confirmatory statistical treatment of data p. 144
clinical significance p. 146
reliability p. 147
validity p. 147
frequency distribution p. 147
graph p. 147
histogram p. 147
measures of central tendency p. 147
mean p. 147
median p. 147
mode p. 147
standard deviation p. 148
correlation p. 148

References

ALI, D., DOW-CLARKE, A., & MacCALDER, L. (1993). Health behaviours of pregnant women. In M. King, S.M. Stinson & K. Mills (Eds.), *Proceedings of the First International Conference on Community Health Nursing Research. Edmonton, AB, Canada, September 26–29.* Edmonton: Edmonton Board of Health.

BENNER, P. (1984). *From novice to expert.* Menlo Park, CA: Addison-Wesley.

BENNER, P., & WRUBEL, J. (1980). *The primacy of caring.* Menlo Park, CA: Addison-Wesley.

BOTTORFF, J.L. (1991). The lived experience of being comforted by a nurse. *Phenomenology and Pedagogy, 9,* 237–252.

BOTTORFF, J.L. (1993). The use and meaning of touch in caring for patients with cancer. *Oncology Nursing Forum, 20,* 1531–1538.

BRINK, P.J., & WOOD, M.J. (1998). *Advance design in nursing research.* (2nd ed.). Newbury Park, CA: Sage.

BRUSH, B.L., & STUART, M. (1992). Unity amidst difference? The ICN project and writing international women's history. In *Visionaries: Proceedings of the First International Nursing History Conference, June 17–20, Saint John, NB, Canada.* The Canadian Association for the History of Nursing and the American Association for the History of Nursing.

BURNS, N., & GROVE, S.K. (1993). *The practice of nursing research. Conduct, critique and utilization.* (2nd ed.). Philadelphia: Saunders.

BURNS, N., & GROVE, S.K. (1995). *Understanding nursing research.* Philadelphia: Saunders.

CANADIAN NURSES ASSOCIATION. (Undated). *Nursing research: A solid foundation for nursing practice.* Ottawa: Author.

CANADIAN NURSES ASSOCIATION. (1985). *Statement on research in nursing.* Ottawa: Author.

CANADIAN NURSES ASSOCIATION. (1990). *Submission to the Royal Society of Canada University Research Committee.* Ottawa: Author.

CANADIAN NURSES ASSOCIATION. (1991). *Current trends in Canadian nursing research.* Ottawa: Author.

CANADIAN NURSES ASSOCIATION. (1992). *Index of Canadian nursing research. Including 1992 supplemental data.* Ottawa: Author.

CANADIAN NURSES ASSOCIATION (CNA). (1993). *The role of nurses in research: A policy statement.* Ottawa: Author.

CANADIAN NURSES ASSOCIATION. (1994). *Ethical guidelines for nursing research involving human subjects.* Ottawa: Author.

CHURCH, J., THURSTON, N., TENOVE, S., & WEISGERBER, R. (1991). *Nursing research in Canadian teaching hospitals.* Calgary: Foothills General Hospital Department of Nursing and Faculty of Nursing, University of Calgary.

CILISKA, D., HAYWARD, S., THOMAS, H., MITCHELL, A., DOBBINS, M., UNDERWOOD, J., RAFAEL, A., & MARTIN, E. (1994). *The effectiveness of home visiting as a delivery strategy for public health nursing interventions: A systematic overview.* Hamilton, ON: McMaster University Nursing Effectiveness Utilization and Outcomes Research Unit.

CLARKE, H.F. (1995). Using research to improve the quality of nursing care. *Nursing BC, 27*(5), 19–22.

CLARKE, H.F. (1997). Nursing and research: Getting the most out of RNABC's position statement. *Nursing BC, 29*(5), 21–22.

COHEN, J.A. (1992). Janforum: Leininger's culture care theory of nursing. *Journal of Advanced Nursing, 17.* 1149.

COLLEGE OF NURSES OF ONTARIO (CNO). (1996). *Standards for nursing practice.* Toronto: Author.

CÔTÉ, J.J., MORSE, J.M., & JAMES, S.G. (1991). The pain response of the postoperative newborn. *Journal of Advanced Nursing, 16,* 378–387.

DAVIES, B., & LOGAN, J. (1997). *Reading research. A user-friendly guide for nurses and other health professionals.* (2nd ed.) Ottawa: Canadian Nurses Association.

DAVIES, B., LEITERMAN, J., DULBERG, C., DONBROOK, C., CLOSS, C., & McDONALD, B. (1993). In M. King, S.M. Stinson & K. Mills (Eds.), *Proceedings of the First International Conference on Community Health Nursing Research. Edmonton, AB, Canada, September 26–29.* Edmonton: Edmonton Board of Health.

DAVIES, B., NIDAY, P., NIMROD, D., STEWART, P., SPRAGUE, A. & DULBERG, C. (1993). Prevention of preterm birth: A population survey of health professionals. In M. King, S.M. Stinson and K. Mills (Eds.), *Proceedings of the First International Conference on Community Health Nursing Research. Edmonton, AB, Canada. September 26–29.* Edmonton: Edmonton Board of Health.

DAVIS, B., & SIMMS, L.C. (1992). Are we providing safe care? *Canadian Nurse, 88*(1), 45–47.

DEGNER, L.F., & SLOAN, J.A. (1995) Symptom distress in newly diagnosed ambulatory cancer patients and as a predictor of survival in lung cancer. *Journal of Pain & Symptom Management, 10,* 423–431.

DOWNS, F.S. (1984). *A source book of nursing research.* (3rd ed.). Philadelphia: F.A. Davis.

DU GAS, B.W. (1969). *An analysis of certain factors in the diffusion of innovations in nursing practice in the public general hospitals of the province of British Columbia.* Unpublished doctoral dissertation, the University of British Columbia, Vancouver.

ESTABROOKS, C.A. (1989). Touch: A nursing strategy in the intensive care unit. *Heart & Lung, 18,* 392–401.

FELDMAN, H.R., & MILLOR, G.K. (1994). The scientific approach to the research process. In G. LoBiondo & J. Haber (Eds.), *Nursing research: Methods, critical appraisal, and utilization.* (3rd ed., pp. 33–54). St. Louis: Mosby.

FELDMAN, J.R. (1990). The scientific approach to the research process. In G. LoBiondo & J. Haber (Eds.), *Nursing research: Methods, critical appraisal, and utilization* (2nd ed., pp. 21–36). St. Louis: Mosby.

FIELD, P.A., STINSON, S.M., & THIBEAUDEAU, J. (1992). Graduate education in nursing in Canada. In A.J. Baumgart & J. Larsen (Eds.), *Canadian nursing faces the future* (pp. 421–445). Toronto: Mosby.

FORBES, D., & STRANG, V. (1997). Managing the symptoms of individuals with Alzheimer's disease: A systematic overview. Abstract. *AARN Newsletter, 53*(10), 7–8.

GIVENS, B., OBERLE, S., & LANDER, J. (1993). Taking the jab out of needles. *Canadian Nurse, 10,* 37–40.

GORTNER, S.R. (1975). Research for a practice profession. *Nursing Research, 24*(3), 193–197.

GRINSPUN, D., MacMILLAN, K., NICHOL, H., & SHIELDS, D.(1993). Using research findings in the hospital. *Canadian Nurse, 89*(1), 46–48.

HALL, D.C. (1989). *Primary health care—A nursing model.* A Denmark–Newfoundland (Canada) project. Report available from Registered Nurses Association of Newfoundland, St. John's, NF.

HAYWARD, S., CILISKA, D., DOBBINS, M., THOMAS, H., & UNDERWOOD, J. (1996). *The effectiveness of public heath nursing in parent-child health: A systematic overview of review articles.* Hamilton, ON: McMaster University Nursing Effectiveness Utilization and Outcomes Research Unit.

JOHNSON, J.L., BUDZ, B., MACKAY, H., & MILLER C. (in press). Evaluation of a nurse delivered smoking cessation intervention for hospitalized cardiac patients. *Heart & Lung.*

JOHNSON, J.L., RATNER, P.A., BOTTORFF, J.L., HALL, W., & DAHINTEN, S. (1997). *Evaluation of a smoking relapse prevention intervention for postpartum women.* Report submitted to Health Canada's National Health Research and Development Program, Ottawa, Canada.

KELPIN, V. (1992). Birthing pain. In J.M. Morse (Ed.), *Qualitative health research* (pp. 93–103). Newbury Park, CA: Sage.

LANDER, J., HODGINS, M., NAZARALI, S., McTAVISH, J., OUELLETTE, J., & FRIESEN, E. (1996). Determinants of success and failure of EMLA. *Pain, 64*(1), 89-97.

LIEHR, P.R., & MARCUS, M.T. (1994). Qualitative approaches to research. In G. LoBiondo-Wood & J. Harber (Eds.), *Nursing research: Methods, critical appraisal, and utilization* (3rd ed., pp. 253–285). St. Louis: Mosby.

LOBIONDO-WOOD, G. (1994). Introduction to design. In G. LoBiondo-Wood & J. Harber (Eds.), *Nursing research: Methods, critical appraisal, and utilization* (3rd ed., pp. 192–230). St. Louis: Mosby.

MacPHAIL, J. (1988). Scope of nursing research. In J. Kerr & J. MacPhail (Eds.), *Canadian nusing: Issues and perspectives* (pp. 123–133). Toronto: McGraw-Hill Ryerson Limited.

McCORMACK, D., & GOODING, B.A. (1993). Homeless persons communicate their meaning of health. *Canadian Journal of Nursing Research, 25*(1), 33–50.

MORSE, J.M. (1997). *Preventing patient falls.* Thousand Oaks, CA: Sage.

MORSE, J.M., BLACK, C., OBERLE, K., & DONAHUE, P. (1989). A prospective study to identify the fall-prone patient. *Social Science & Medicine, 28,* 81–86.

MORSE, J.M., BOTTORFF, J.L., & HUTCHINSON, S. (1994) The phenomenology of comfort. *Journal of Advanced Nursing, 20,* 189–195.

MORSE, J.M., & FIELD, P.A. (1995). *Qualitative research methods for health professionals.* (2nd ed.). Thousand Oaks, CA: Sage.

MORSE, J.M., & McHUTCHION, E. (1991). The behavioral effects of releasing restraints. *Research in Nursing and Health, 14,* 187–196.

MORSE, J.M., PROWSE, M.D., MORROW, N., & FEDERSPEIL, G. (1985). A retrospective analysis of patient falls. *Canadian Journal of Public Health, 76,* 116–118.

MORSE, J.M., TYLKO, S.J., & DIXON, H.A. (1985). The patient who falls ... and falls again: Defining the aged at risk. *Journal of Gerontological Nursing, 11*(11), 15–18.

MUNHALL, P.L., & OILER, C.J. (1986). Nursing research. A qualitative perspective. Norwalk, CT: Appleton-Century-Crofts.

OGILVIE, L. D. (1993). Nurses and primary health care in Nepal. In M. King, S.M. Stinson & K. Mills (Eds.), *Proceedings of the First International Conference on Community Health Nursing Research. Edmonton, AB, Canada, September 26–29.* Edmonton: Edmonton Board of Health.

OLSON, K. (1992). Strengthening the link between research and practice. *Canadian Nurse, 88*(1), 42–47.

OLSON, K. (1993). Creating the impetus for research-based practice. *Canadian Nurse, 89*(1), 36–39.

PLOEG J., CILISKA, D., DOBBINS, M., HAYWARD, S., THOMAS, H., & UNDERWOOD, J. (1995). *A systematic overview of the effectiveness of public health nursing interventions: An overview of adolescent suicide prevention programs*. Hamilton, ON: McMaster University Nursing Effectiveness Utilization and Outcomes Research Unit.

RATNER, P.A. (1993). The incidence of wife abuse and mental health status in abused wives in Edmonton, Alberta. *Canadian Journal of Public Health, 84,* 246–149.

REGISTERED NURSES ASSOCIATION OF BRITISH COLUMBIA (RNABC). (1997, Nov./Dec.). Position statement. Nursing and research. *Nursing BC, 28,* 19–20.

REGISTERED NURSES ASSOCIATION OF BRITISH COLUMBIA (RNABC). (1990). *Nursing research: From question to funding. A workbook.* Vancouver: Author.

REGISTERED NURSES ASSOCIATION OF BRITISH COLUMBIA (RNABC). (1998). *Standards for nursing practice in British Columbia.* Vancouver: Author.

RITCHIE, J.A. (1992). Research issues. In A.J. Baumgart & J. Larsen (Eds.). *Canadian nursing faces the future.* (2nd ed., pp. 307–324). Toronto: Mosby.

ROSENBAUM, J.N. (1991). Widowhood grief: A cultural perspective. *Canadian Journal of Nursing Research, 23*(2), 61–76.

RYAN-WENGER, N.M. (1992).Guidelines for critique of a research report. *Heart and Lung, 21*(4), 394–401.

SANDELOWSKI, M. (1986). The problem of rigor in qualitative research. *Advances in Nursing Science, 8*, 17–37.

SIMPSON, B. (1997). Evidence-based nursing practice: The state of the art. *Canadian Nurse, 92*(10), 22–25.

SMITH, S.J. (1992). Operating on a child's heart: A pedagogical view of hospitalization. In J.M. Morse (Ed.), *Qualitative health research* (pp. 93–103). Newbury Park, CA: Sage.

SPIELBERGER, C.D., GORSUCH, R.L., & LUSHENE, R.E. (1970). *The State-Trait Anxiety Inventory (STAI).* Palto Alto, CA: Consulting Psychologists Press.

STINSON, S.M. (1986). Nursing research in Canada. In S.M. Stinson & J.C. Kerr (Eds.), *International issues in nursing research* (pp. 236–258). London: Croom Helm.

TABER'S CYCLOPEDIC MEDICAL DICTIONARY. (16th ed.). (1989). Philadelphia: F.A. Davis.

THURSTON, N. (1995). Hospital research comes of age. *Canadian Nurse, 91*(4), 34–38.

WILSON, S., & MORSE, J.M. (1991). Living with a wife undergoing chemotherapy. *Image: Journal of Nursing Scholarship, 23*, 78–84.

WOOD, M.J. (1997). Canadian Ph.D. in nursing programs. *Clinical Nursing Research, 6*, 307–309.

WOODS, N.F., & CATANZARO, M. (1988). *Nursing research.* St. Louis: Mosby.

WUEST, J. (1995). Breaking the barriers to nursing research. *Canadian Nurse, 91*(4), 29–33.

Additional Readings

CLARKE, H. (1996). Integrating evidence-based clinical tools with practice. *Nursing BC, 28*(5): 19–22.

HILL, M.N., BONE, L.R., & BUTZ, A.M. (1996). Enhancing the role of community health workers in research. *Image, 28*(3), 221–226.

JOHNSON, J.L., RATNER, P.R., BOTTORFF, J.L., HALL, W., & DAHINTEN, S. (in press). Preventing Smoking Relapse in Postpartum Women. *Nursing Research*

LINCOLN, Y.S., & GUBA, E. (1995). *Naturalistic enquiry*. Newbury Park, CA: Sage.

MOCH, S.D., ROBIE, D.E., BAUER, K.C., PEDERSON, A., BOWE, S., & SHADICK, K. (1997). Linking research and practice through discussion. *Image, 29*(2), 189–191.

MORSE, W., OLESON, M., DUFFY, L., PATEK, A., & SOHR, G. (1996). Connecting the research and nursing processes: Making a difference in baccalaureate students' attitudes and abilities. *Journal of Nursing Education, 35*(4), 148–151.

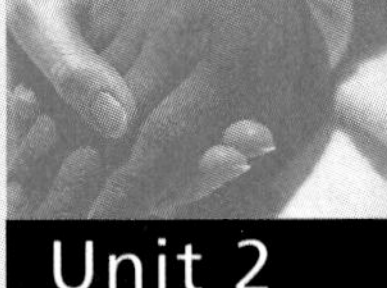

Dimensions of Health

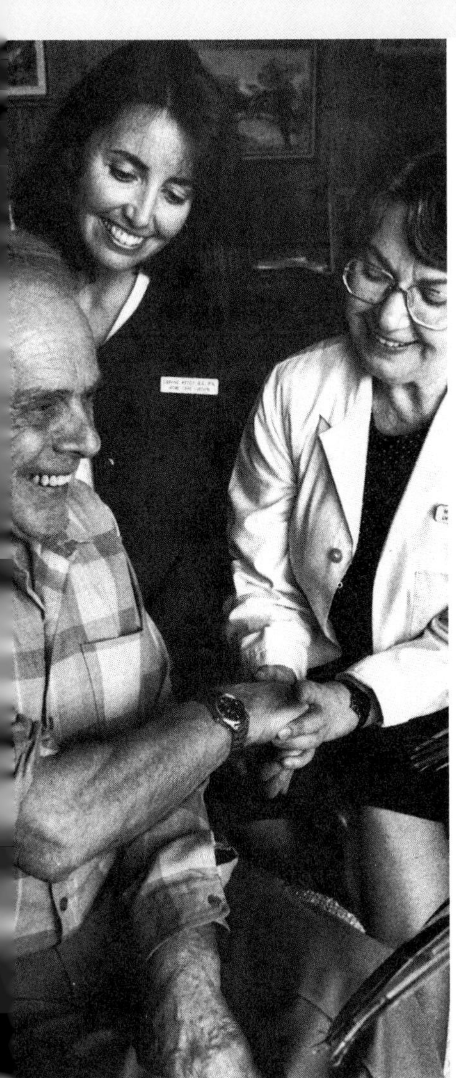

Chapter 8

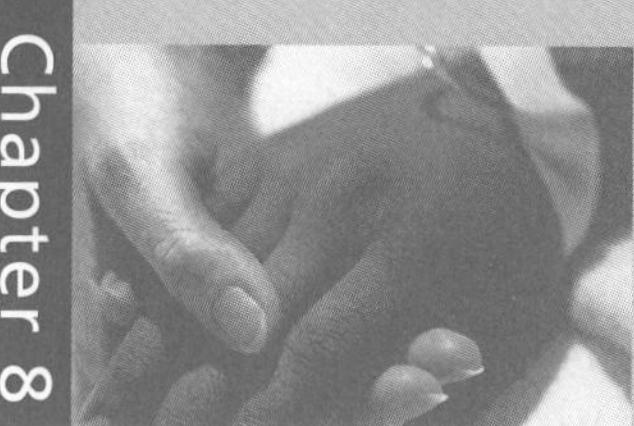

Health and Human Development

OUTLINE

Central Questions

1. What is the nature of Maslow's hierarchy of needs?
2. What five basic needs did Maslow postulate?
3. Describe briefly Freud's theory of psychosexual development.
4. What are the four stages of Piaget's theory of cognitive development?
5. Describe briefly Kohlberg's theory of moral development.
6. Describe briefly Gilligan's theory of moral development.
7. What are the stages and conflicts in each stage of Erikson's theory of psychosocial development?
8. What are the different passages of adulthood described by Sheehy?
9. What are Peck's developmental tasks of middle-aged and older adults?
10. How do cultural values and beliefs influence social and psychological growth and development?
11. What are the stages of fetal growth and development?
12. What needs require special attention during pregnancy, and what factors affect these needs?
13. Outline the development of an individual through the various stages of the life cycle, from birth to old age.
14. What factors affect basic needs during each stage of the life cycle?

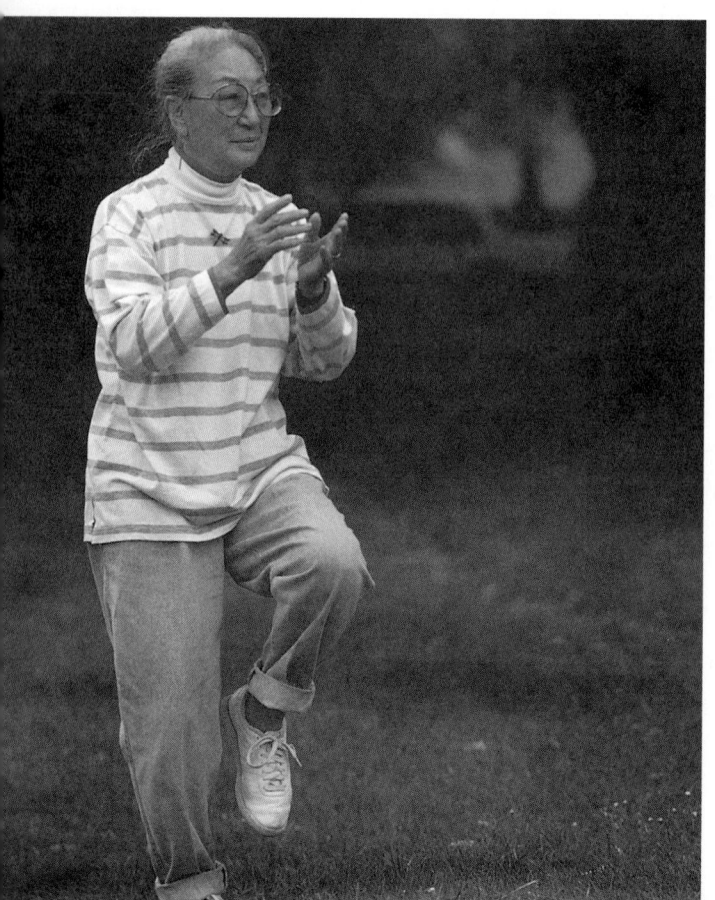

Introduction

In Unit 1, we discussed some of the basic concepts that underlie our current beliefs about health and illness. If we accept the premise that optimal health, or wellness, is the ability to function at one's highest level physically, mentally, spiritually and socially, it seems appropriate to look at the conditions that foster optimum functioning. What is needed for individuals to attain their optimal level of well-being? This leads us to a consideration of basic human needs.

There are certain basic needs common to all human beings which must be fulfilled if individuals are to attain their optimal level of well-being. The subject of basic needs has been studied in depth by social scientists looking for the motivating forces underlying human behaviour, and by people in the health field seeking to identify factors causing health problems. Early theorists felt that all human needs could be categorized under two headings: physiological and psychological. Another group of theorists classified needs on the basis of whether their origin was internal or external. Still others felt that basic human needs could not be categorized, and simply identified long lists of them.

Much of nursing is concerned with helping people to meet their basic needs and to achieve optimal health or wellness. This part of nursing is embodied in the caring aspects of the nursing role and includes basic nursing measures that are applicable in the care of individuals of all ages.

It is generally agreed that people have the same basic needs throughout the life span. However, the expression of these needs and their relative importance to an individual's well-being vary with a person's age and stage of physical and psychosocial development. A growing child's nutritional needs are different from those of a middle-aged adult; the child needs more protein, for instance, to build bones and muscle tissue.

Both the very young and the very old have increased safety needs. The very young have not yet learned to be aware of danger, and so need the help of others to protect them from harm. The elderly have bones that are more fragile and break more easily than those of younger people. Their sensory faculties may deteriorate, especially in the presence of a health problem such as Alzheimer's disease.

In this chapter, we will explore the nature of human development, beginning with the basic needs. We will also look at some of the theories of growth and development that contribute to our understanding of differences in basic needs at various stages in the life cycle. Finally, we will discuss changes that occur as individuals grow and develop throughout life.

The Nature of Basic Needs

Maslow's Hierarchy of Needs

Abraham Maslow's (1970) theory of a hierarchy of needs is used in many nursing schools as a conceptual framework for the consideration of human needs. Not everyone agrees with all aspects of his theory, and some have suggested modifications to his hierarchy, but the basic principles outlined in the theory are fairly well accepted.

Maslow suggested that there are five basic categories of human needs and that these may be arranged in order of priority for satisfaction. The types of needs identified by Maslow, in order of priority, are:

1. physiological
2. safety and security
3. love and belonging
4. self-esteem
5. self-actualization.

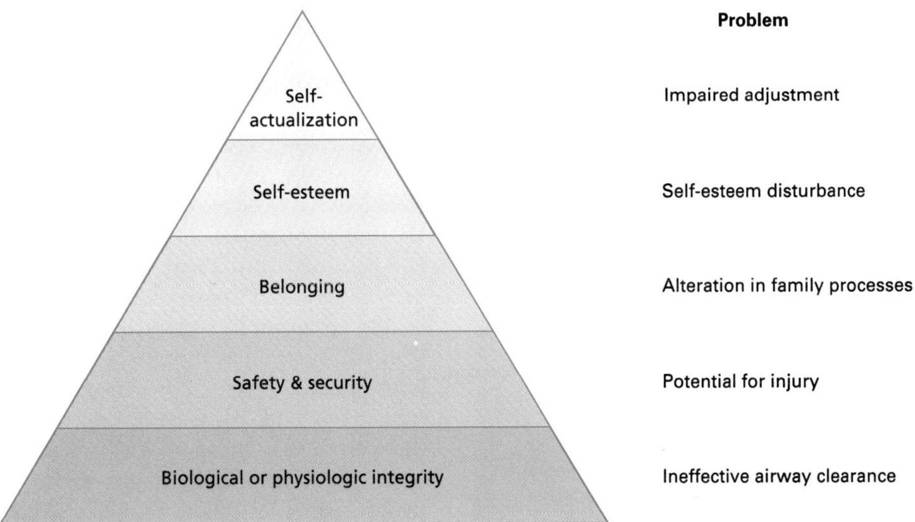

FIGURE 8.1 Correlation between Maslow's hierarchy and Gordon's functional pattern of nursing diagnosis

SOURCE: Ebersole & Hess, 1998, p. 108.

Maslow believed that there is a hierarchy of needs according to priority, in the form of a pyramid (Figure 8.1). According to Maslow, the more fundamental needs must be satisfied before a person can proceed to seek satisfaction for needs of a higher order (Murray & Zentner, 1997).

Physiological needs take precedence over all others because they are essential for survival. These include the need for water, food, air, elimination, rest and sleep, temperature maintenance and the avoidance of pain. When a person is starving, life revolves around the need to obtain food. Similarly, a person deprived of water for a long period of time is concerned above all else with relieving his or her thirst. The fulfillment of certain physiological needs is so essential that if there is interference with the attainment of them, life itself is threatened. If there is interference with breathing, for example, prompt measures must be initiated to restore adequate respiration or the person will die. The relief of pain is also a primary physiological need. If pain is severe, the sufferer cannot rest, sleep or think of anything else until the pain is relieved.

Next in order of priority are the **safety and security** needs. These include adequate shelter from the elements and protection from harmful factors in the environment. But people must also *feel* that they are secure and protected from both real and imagined dangers. People usually feel more secure when they are in familiar surroundings, with accustomed routines and with those they can trust. Conversely, they feel threatened when they are in strange places or when their usual pattern of living is disturbed. Often, inanimate objects assume a symbolism that represents safety and security for an individual. Linus's blanket (in Charles Schulz's cartoon "Peanuts"), which he carries everywhere with him, has become a symbol of security that is recognized by most North Americans. Many children have a toy or other object that gives them a sense of security. They often like to take their favourite toy or object with them wherever they go. Many adults have lucky charms, talismans or other objects that they feel give them special protection against harm. Maslow has suggested that many of our religious rituals, superstitions and traditions have their origins in this basic need for safety and security.

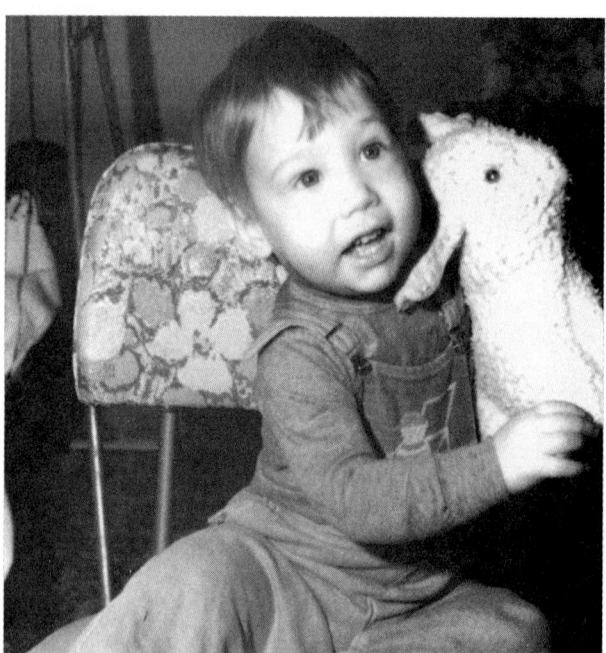

Most children have a favourite toy that gives them a sense of security. This little boy takes "Bubby," his favourite lamb, wherever he goes.

The need for **love and belonging** are placed next on the hierarchy. "From infancy, every human being has a need for love and caring" (Rambo, 1984, p. 8). Infants deprived of love and affection do not thrive, even if all their physiological and safety needs are met.

Higher on the pyramid is the need for **self-esteem**. Individuals seek to be valued and respected by others. Maslow has suggested that many of the problems in our depersonalized society, particularly in big cities, are due to failure to satisfy the needs of love and belonging and of self-esteem. If these needs are not satisfied, people may experience feelings of inadequacy, frustration, alienation and hopelessness (Rambo, 1984; Murray & Zentner, 1997).

At the peak of the pyramid is the need for **self-actualization**—attaining one's full potential. This includes the need to seek knowledge, to appreciate harmony and beauty and to explore one's spiritual and emotional being (Murray & Zentner, 1997).

Growth and Development

Theories About Growth and Development

In Maslow's hierarchy, individuals are seen as constantly striving to fulfill their basic needs. As one set of needs is gratified, others of a higher order emerge and become more powerful. People who have fulfilled the first four levels of needs may spend their lives developing their need for self-actualization.

The concept that is presented in Maslow's theory, then, is not of human beings as static entities, trying simply to maintain their equilibrium in a changing world, but of individuals as developing beings, constantly reaching for things beyond their immediate grasp. This concept embodies the idea of continuous growth and development of the human organism, which begins at the moment of birth and continues until death.

The study of human development has received a great deal of attention in recent years from educators and social scientists, as well as from people in the health field. Our knowledge of physical growth and development has increased tremendously with advances in scientific technology that permit us to measure, with great accuracy, the changes occurring in most body tissues and processes throughout the life span. Our understanding of social and psychological development, however, has to be derived from studies of observable behaviour. A wide variety of theories exist to account for our social and psychological development.

FREUD AND PSYCHOSEXUAL DEVELOPMENT

One of the pioneers in the field of personality development was Sigmund Freud. His theory of psychosexual development shocked the scientific and lay community of the early 1900s and still evokes controversy today. According to Freud, individuals progress through five stages of development from infancy through puberty, and it is the quality of their experiences in each stage that determines their adult personality. Deprivation, or overindulgence, of the individual's needs in any one of the stages may cause him or her to become "fixated" at that stage. The five stages identified by Freud were:

- **Oral stage** (birth to 1 year). Freud believed that during this stage infants derive their greatest sensual satisfaction through their mouths. Behavioural traits that may develop as a result of too little or too much oral satisfaction in infancy, he felt, included aggression, a preoccupation with food or drink, cigarette smoking and nail biting.
- **Anal stage** (1 year to 3 years). Freud felt that toddlers' greatest pleasures come from moving their bowels. The management of toilet training during this stage is therefore crucial to one's development. If this training is not handled correctly, the individual may show behavioural characteristics as an adult that include hoarding, an obsession with cleanliness, or conversely, a tendency towards slothfulness. If training is too rigid, Freud felt, the parent might stifle the child's creativity.
- **Oedipal stage** (3 to 6 years). During this stage, according to Freud, the child identifies with and derives sensual satisfaction from the parent of the opposite sex, and views the parent of the same sex as a rival. Behavioural traits that Freud felt may develop from overindulgence or deprivation at this stage include competitiveness, seductiveness and a preoccupation with older partners.
- **Latent stage** (6 to 12 years). The child at this stage identifies with the parent of the same sex, and learns to assume his or her appropriate social role. Behavioural characteristics that Freud believed were formed at this stage include the development of a conscience as well as the seeds for later rebellion if this stage is not handled properly by parents.
- **Genital stage** (12 to 19 years). Freud believed that adolescents derive their most pleasurable experiences through their genital organs. Personality traits felt to result from mishandling of this stage include a tendency to rationalization and a preoccupation with sex.

The terms coined by Freud are still widely used, although most people feel that his theory of psychosexual development is too restrictive, focussing as it does on only one aspect (sexual) of growth and development (Freud, 1972).

PIAGET AND COGNITIVE DEVELOPMENT

Looking at growth and development from a different perspective, Jean Piaget formulated a theory of cognitive, or intellectual, development based on four sequential stages. Subsequent studies have confirmed that although the rate of development may vary, children do indeed seem to progress through the stages of intellectual development in a sequence similar to the one Piaget outlined. These stages are briefly described as follows:

- **Sensorimotor stage** (birth to 2 years). During this stage children are concerned mainly with actions and sensations that affect them directly. They begin to relate to outside events, at first tentatively, then actively experiment with their environment. They develop *object permanence* (knowledge that an object exists even when it is not visible to them). At birth, the infant's response range is basically limited to reflex actions. By the age of two he or she is capable of thinking through a problem before taking action.
- **Preoperational stage** (2 to 7 years). At this stage a child's thinking is still *egocentric*. That is, children are concerned mainly with themselves. They believe that everyone sees the world as they do. Language becomes an important vehicle of communication. Piaget has divided this stage into two distinct periods:
  - **Preconceptual period** (2 to 4 years). Children at this point are not yet capable of reason, although they are able to form general concepts. They may call all soft, stuffed toys "bear," for example, or they may use a face cloth (with which they have just wiped their face) to polish the furniture.
  - **Perceptual (intuitive) period** (4 to 7 years). Children at this stage are capable of reason, yet it is not a logical, adult form of thinking. They can concentrate on only one aspect of an object or idea at a time. For example, if a child at this stage put an equal number of candies in two jars, one tall and narrow, the other short and stout, he or she would think there were more candies in the tall narrow jar because the level of candies would be higher.
- **Concrete operational stage** (7 to 11 years). During this stage, children's reasoning becomes logical but is limited to their own experiences. They are now able to understand concepts and to concentrate on more than one aspect of an object or idea. For example, if you asked a seven-year-old boy to describe a coin, he could probably tell you that it is round, that it is shiny and that it is a form of money. At this point children acquire the ability to reverse their thinking, learning the relationship of cause and effect.
- **Formal operational stage** (11 to 16 years). During this stage individuals acquire the ability to develop abstract concepts for themselves. Their thinking is oriented

towards problem-solving and transcends concrete experience. They no longer have to experience things before they can understand them. Science fiction has a great appeal for people at this stage (Piaget, 1963, 1969).

Piaget's theory of cognitive development is currently well accepted, although some feel that it is incomplete because Piaget believed that the highest level of cognitive development is reached by the end of adolescence. Subsequent studies indicate that individuals do not reach their full mental capacity until about age 25, and that they continue to learn throughout their life span. Another criticism of Piaget's theory is that he does not give enough consideration to the effects of environmental factors on intellectual development. Piaget's theory also ignores the impact of motivation on behaviours (Wong, 1995).

KOHLBERG AND MORAL DEVELOPMENT

Looking at a different aspect of psychological development, Lawrence Kohlberg presented a theory of *moral* development, defining three levels that, like Piaget's, are inflexibly sequential, but are attained at varying rates. According to Kohlberg, the individual's progression through these levels occurs as conflict is encountered, often through interaction with a person at a higher level. Progression through these levels of moral development is not necessarily age-related. Kohlberg's levels are as follows:

- **Preconventional.** At this level, individuals are primarily concerned with themselves (egocentric focus). They are occupied only with satisfying their own needs, without regard to others. An individual at this level will obey an authority figure, although only to avoid punishment.
- **Conventional.** At this level, individuals are concerned mainly with pleasing others and maintaining order (societal focus). They show great respect for rules and socially accepted authority figures, such as police officers.
- **Postconventional.** At this level, an individual's morality is based on personal conscience, dictated by the desire to avoid self-condemnation. The individual shows a profound respect for human dignity and life (universal focus). He or she is able to think abstractly and to take another's point of view (Kohlberg, 1984).

GILLIGAN AND MORAL DEVELOPMENT

Carole Gilligan's research on the theory of moral development has focussed on women, in comparison with Kohlberg's focus on men. Gilligan identified that moral development proceeds through three levels and two transitions. Each level represents a more elaborate awareness of the association between oneself and others, and each transition allows for a review of the conflict between egocentrism and duty. In her studies Gilligan identified that women define a moral problem in terms of human relationships. Their moral judgement proceeds from "initial concern with survival, to a focus on goodness, to a principled understanding of others' need for care" (Murray & Zentner, 1997, p.231). Further research done by Friedman et al. (1987) does not support Gilligan's claim that men and women differ in moral judgements. Gilligan theorizes that the roots of moral behaviour—kindness and fairness—begin in childhood (Gilligan, 1982). Table 8.1 outlines Gilligan's theory of moral development.

TABLE 8.1 Gilligan's Theory of Moral Development

Level	*Characteristics*
1. Orientation of Individual Survival	*Concentrates on what is practical and best for self;* selfish; dependent on others.
Transition 1: From Selfishness to Responsibility	Realizes connection to others; thinks of responsible choice in terms of another as well as self.
2. Goodness as Self-Sacrifice	*Sacrifices personal wishes and needs to fulfill others' wants* and to have others think well of her; feels responsible for others' actions; holds others responsible for her choices; dependent position; indirect efforts to control others often turn into manipulation through use of guilt; aware of connectedness with others.
Transition 2: From Goodness to Truth	*Makes decisions on personal intentions and consequences of actions rather than how she thinks others will react;* takes into account needs of self and others; wants to be good to others but also honest by being responsible to self; increased social participation; assumes more responsibilities.
3. Morality of Nonviolence	*Establishes moral equality between self and others; assumes responsibility for choice in moral dilemmas;* follows injunction to hurt no one, including self, in all situations; conflict between selfishness and selflessness; judgement based on view of consequences and intentions instead of appearance in the eyes of others.

SOURCE: Murray & Zentner, 1997, p. 233.

ERIKSON AND PSYCHOSOCIAL DEVELOPMENT

Erik Erikson formulated a theory of psychosocial development that, like Kohlberg's theory of moral development, is based on conflicts. According to Erikson's theory, people encounter the conflicts within themselves. Although, ideally, individuals resolve each conflict as it is encountered, failure to do so does not mean that they will be forever burdened with it. It is possible to resolve the conflict at a later stage. According to Erikson, there are a number of developmental tasks related to the principal conflicts that an individual must complete at each stage.

Resolution of the conflicts during the stages of infancy through the preschool years is largely dependent on one's parents. During middle childhood and the adolescent years this responsibility is shared with the child's teachers. Beginning in adolescence and continuing through the adult years, individuals assume responsibility for their own development. A brief outline of Erikson's stages of development, including the principal conflict and some related developmental tasks, is given below.

- **Infancy** (birth to 1 year)

  Principal conflict: Trust vs. mistrust. During this stage infants develop either a basic trust or mistrust of others, depending on the relationship they develop with their mothers (or other principal caregivers) and the quality of care they receive.

  Tasks: Primary caregiver and infant adjust to each other. Infant learns to take solid foods, to walk and to talk.

- **Toddlerhood** (1 year to 3 years)

  Principal conflict: Autonomy vs. shame. During this stage children either develop a sense of pride in their independence and new accomplishments or they develop feelings of shame and doubt concerning their abilities to deal with other people and the world.

  Tasks: The child seeks independence in his or her actions, learns to control elimination, learns to communicate through language and learns to differentiate between right and wrong.

- **Early childhood** (3 to 6 years)

  Principal conflict: Initiative vs. guilt. In this stage children learn to initiate activities, and it is the response they receive to these activities that determines whether their sense of initiative will remain intact or whether they will feel a sense of guilt for their actions.

  Tasks: The child establishes relationships with his or her peers, begins to form concepts based on reality, refines his or her motor control and learns a social role based on gender identification.

- **Middle childhood** (6 to 12 years)

  Principal conflict: Industry vs. inferiority. During this stage children divide their time between home and school. A negative response received at home to their new sense of industry can be neutralized by a positive response at school, or vice versa. If children encounter consistent failure or discouragement, they will experience feelings of inferiority.

  Tasks: The child learns autonomy, refines his or her coordination, learns cooperation and self-control, develops social skills, learns to view the world objectively and forms values.

- **Adolescence** (12 to 19 years)

  Principal conflict: Identity vs. role confusion. During this stage adolescents ideally develop a positive and stable sense of identity, or self-image, in relation to their past and future. Lacking this, they will experience a sense of confusion with regard to their social role.

  Tasks: The adolescent accepts his or her changed physique, seeks and achieves independence from adults, forms close peer relationships, defines his or her social role and reasons logically.

- **Early adulthood** (19 to 35 years)

  Principal conflict: Intimacy vs. isolation. During this stage individuals establish close relationships with others of the same and opposite gender. If individuals develop no close emotional ties they will experience feelings of isolation.

  Tasks: The individual decides on a career path, chooses a marriage partner, raises children and assumes social responsibilities.

- **The middle years** (35 to 65 years)

  Principal conflict: Generativity vs. self-absorption. Generativity means being concerned with the future of society and the world in general. Persons lacking in this quality are overly concerned with themselves.

  Tasks: Individuals adjust to physical and physiological changes, accept the needs of their children and of their aging parents and attain their career and social goals.

- **The later years** (over 65 years)

  Principal conflict: Integrity vs. despair. During this stage most adults take stock of their lives and their accomplishments. If they are content with what they have done, they experience what is called "integrity," or a sense of "wholeness." People who are dissatisfied with life, who wish they could do it over again, yet know that it is impossible, succumb to despair.

  Tasks: The individual accepts the aging process, adjusts to retirement and adjusts to the death of his or her spouse and friends (Erikson, 1963).

  Table 8.2 summarizes the major themes described above.

SHEEHY AND THE PASSAGES OF ADULTHOOD

Erikson was one of the earliest of the developmentalists to go beyond the realms of childhood to incorporate changes

TABLE 8.2 Summary of personality, cognitive, and moral development theories

STAGE/AGE	PSYCHOSEXUAL STAGES (FREUD)	COGNITIVE STAGES (PIAGET)	MORAL JUDGEMENT STAGES (KOHLBERG)	PSYCHOSOCIAL STAGES (ERIKSON)
1. Infancy Birth to 1 year	Oral sensory	Sensorimotor (birth to 2 years)		Trust vs. mistrust
2. Toddlerhood 1–3 years	Anal–urethral	Preoperational thought, preconceptual phase (transductive reasoning, e.g., specific to specific) (2–4 years)	Preconventional (premoral) level Punishment and obedience orientation	Autonomy vs. shame and doubt
3. Early childhood 3–6 years	Phallic–locomotion	Preoperational thought, intuitive phase (transductive reasoning) (4–7 years)	Preconventional (premoral) level Naive instrumental orientation	Intiative vs. guilt
4. Middle childhood 6–12 years	Latency	Concrete operations (inductive reasoning and beginning logic) (7–11 years)	Conventional level Good-boy, nice-girl orientation Law-and-order orientation	Industry vs. inferiority
5. Adolescence 12–19 years	Genitality	Formal operations (deductive and abstract reasoning) (11–16 years)	Postconventional or principled level Social-contract orientation Universal ethical principle orientation (no longer included in revised theory)	Identity and repudiation vs. identity confusion
6. Early adulthood				Intimacy and solidarity vs. isolation
7. Young and middle adulthood				Generativity vs. self-absorption
8. Later adulthood				Ego integrity vs. despair

SOURCE: Wong, 1995, p. 119.

occurring during adulthood into his life cycles theory of growth and development. His work has subsequently been extended by others in the field. Notable among those who followed Erikson is Gail Sheehy (1976), who has contributed much to our understanding of the nature of the inner changes taking place as a person passes through the various turning points of adulthood. Sheehy preferred to call these turning points **passages**, rather than crises, because *crisis* has negative connotations. The passages, Sheehy felt, are very normal and highly predictable. Although individuals experience a period of instability as they pass each turning point, it is not necessarily a "bad" experience. Rather, each passage represents an essential factor in their growth and development.

Early Adulthood

In her research, Sheehy found that, although men and women both reported going through the same passages in adult life, they did not necessarily do so at the same ages or in the same sequences. A woman who has spent her young adult years at home raising a family, for example, may be just entering the labour force at the age of 40. On the other hand, a man who has been the bread-winner of the family since his early 20s may feel that he has reached just about the peak of his career at age 40 and will be looking for something else to round out and enrich his life. Sheehy divides the early adult period (from 18 to 35 years) into four stages or passages:

1. **Pulling up roots** (after age 18). Moving away from the family and family home for higher education or career and beginning independence
2. **The trying 20s**. A time of goal achieving, career, relationships, child bearing and rearing
3. **Catch 30** (approaching age 30). The need to reassess and change the direction of one's life—a marriage or divorce, a child where there was a decision to be childless, a promotion or a new career
4. **Rooting and extending** (to age 35). Stabilizing and putting out roots. Community involvement and family promotion, plus all-out career efforts.

Later Adulthood

Erikson grouped together the years from age 35 to 65, calling them the "middle years." Sheehy, however, divides these years into two distinct "passages." The period from age 35 to 45 she calls the "deadline decade." It is a crossroads, a time when individuals must come to terms with themselves and set a life course before time runs out. Levinson (1978) has coined the term "BOOM" (becoming one's own man) to describe this maturational crisis stage. According to Sheehy, women often feel this push around age 35, and men feel it around age 40.

"Renewal or resignation" is the term Sheehy uses to describe life after age 45. If individuals have felt and responded to the urge to reorganize life during the preceding decade, they will experience a feeling of happiness or renewal during the remainder of adult life. If they have simply continued on in an unsatisfactory course set earlier, they may experience a feeling of stagnation, becoming resigned to the idea that now it is too late to change.

PECK'S DEVELOPMENTAL TASKS OF MIDDLE AGE AND OLDER

Robert Peck's (1960) research shows that the middle-aged are more concerned with a reassessment of self than with Erikson's concepts of intimacy and generativity. To Peck, middle-aged and older individuals are faced with four additional developmental tasks:

1. **Valuing wisdom vs. valuing physical power**. Finding identity from values and judgements based on wisdom from life experiences as one's physical strength declines
2. **Socializing vs. sexualizing**. Redefining the male–female relationship away from sexual objectives
3. **Cathectic or emotional flexibility vs. cathectic impoverishment**. Adjusting to the losses of middle and older age and investing in new interpersonal adventures
4. **Mental flexibility vs. mental rigidity**. Problem-solving and finding new solutions to old problems; option-hunting versus doing things from habit.

OTHER THEORISTS

Neugarten (1968), Gould (1975), Berger (1993) and Schuster & Ashburn (1992) all offer other theories about the developmental stages of the middle-aged and older person. Healthy development through involvement in continuing education, extending family pursuits, second careers and changing lifestyle patterns are discussed. Retirement planning in early adulthood is proving to be another key to healthy, happy and active aging.

Cultural Influences on Growth and Development

It is essential to consider cultural differences as they relate to health behaviours and thus to the growth and developmental patterns of individuals. Each culture has different emphases on family, child-rearing practices, nutrition, health care and education.

There may be health-related differences among races of people. For example, people of Asian descent may have a predisposition to adult lactose intolerance, whereas sickle cell anemia is most common among people of African heritage (Eschelman, 1996).

It is part of the nurse's assessment to determine the impact of cultural values and beliefs on a person's health practices. The nurse must never make assumptions about a person's culture.

In the young, growth and development tests commonly used must be applied only when culturally specific. Although some would dispute the possibility of developing tests that are entirely "culture-free," it is possible to use tests that are not culturally biased. In a verbal test, for example, a picture-matching technique may be used when the child's first language is not English. At the other end of the age spectrum, the elderly tend to depend on and get comfort from their traditions and practices. No matter what the age, in times of stress, illness, loss and separation, it is not unusual for people to call on all their cultural values and beliefs to sustain them.

Prenatal Growth and Development

There is a great deal of controversy about the point in human development at which a fetus becomes a human being. Regardless of one's views on this matter, **gestation**—the term used to describe the development of new life that takes place in the womb between conception and birth—begins at conception when the male sperm unites with the female ovum (or ova) during its journey down the fallopian tube. This development normally takes 40 weeks and is divided into three trimesters.

Zygote Stage (Fertilization to 2 Weeks)

During this stage, the cells of the fertilized ovum, now called a **zygote**, multiply rapidly and the new cell mass moves down the fallopian tube and into the uterus. Approximately two weeks after fertilization the zygote attaches itself to the uterine wall (Pillitteri, 1995; Reeder, Martin & Koniak-Griffin, 1997).

Embryonic Stage (2 to 8 Weeks)

After the zygote has attached itself to the uterine wall, the cells continue to multiply, forming three distinct layers. The **ectoderm**, or outer layer, will later form the nervous system and sense organs; the **mesoderm**, or middle layer, becomes the skeletal, muscular and circulatory systems; the **endoderm**, or inner layer, becomes the digestive system.

It is during the embryonic stage that the amniotic sac and the placenta are formed. The **amniotic sac** is a protective membrane filled with fluid that surrounds the developing embryo, providing warmth, moisture and relative freedom of movement. The **placenta** is an organ that attaches to the uterine wall and to the fetus by means of the **umbilical cord**. Through the umbilical cord, the unborn child receives nourishment and oxygenated blood, and disposes of wastes. The placenta serves as a barrier, protecting the developing child from potentially harmful agents.

By eight weeks, the embryo is recognizably human, with distinct arms, legs, fingers and toes, although the head comprises about half its length. It is only about two and a half centimetres long, but already its systems are beginning to function (Pillitteri, 1995; Reeder et al., 1997).

Fetal Stage (8 Weeks to Birth)

The most striking change that occurs during the fetal stage is the dramatic increase in size from approximately two and a half centimetres to an average length of 45 to 50 cm at birth. The systems that began to form in the embryonic stage increase in complexity and maturity. The fetus begins to move by the 12th week, although this is not usually felt by the mother until the 16th to 20th week, when its actions become more vigorous. By the 24th week, the eyelids open and the fetus begins to take amniotic fluid into its lungs as a rudimentary form of breathing.

A fetus is capable of surviving outside the uterus (Pillitteri, 1995). The 28-week fetus is neurologically mature enough to survive in the extrauterine world in a controlled environment such as an incubator. It can breathe, although the lungs are not fully developed until approximately 36 weeks. The fetus at 28 weeks has not accumulated the layers of fat so noticeable in a full-term baby. These layers protect the fetus from temperature changes and enable him or her to go without nourishment for the first day or two after birth (Pillitteri, 1995; Reeder et al., 1997).

The 36th to 40th weeks of fetal development are devoted primarily to maturation of the lungs and nervous system and to the accumulation of fat. Towards the end of the 40th week, activity often diminishes as the fetus becomes cramped for space. Shortly before the onset of labour the fetus becomes "engaged" in the pelvic cavity, normally with its head down, in preparation for birth (Pillitteri, 1995).

During its period of development inside the womb the fetus is totally dependent on the mother to satisfy its basic needs. She provides nutrients, oxygen, warmth and protection and disposes of fetal wastes. Although the placenta provides some protection from harmful agents, many others pass through the placental barrier to the fetus. As the fetus is very vulnerable to infection and the effects of noxious stimuli, particularly in its early developmental stages, the mother must take care to protect her unborn child from such dangers. Studies have suggested that maternal emotions might affect the developing fetus too and can have long-range effects on personality. To date, the results of such studies have been inconclusive, largely owing to the difficulty of collecting data over a period of several years, and of separating out other influences that may affect a person's psychological make-up (Reeder et al., 1997).

Pregnancy

Pregnancy can occur any time in a woman's childbearing years, usually from the age of 13 to the late 40s. Just as there are three stages of growth and development of the fetus, there are three stages of pregnancy for the mother-to-be. While the unborn child grows and develops inside the womb, many other changes are occurring that affect the pregnant woman herself. The duration of an average pregnancy is 38 weeks from conception (or 40 weeks from the last menstrual cycle), divided into trimesters.

First Trimester (Last Menstrual Cycle to 13 Weeks)

The newly pregnant woman usually (but not always) misses a menstrual period. She may feel tired and her breasts may swell, tingle and feel tender as the milk glands prepare to produce milk. She may experience nausea and vomiting, especially upon arising in the morning (usually called *morning sickness*). During the first trimester of pregnancy there is a marked increase in the production of hormones, particularly estrogen and progesterone. These hormonal changes account for many of the early signs of pregnancy.

At this stage, the pelvic structure begins to widen to accommodate the growing uterus. During pregnancy, the uterus will increase in weight from approximately 60 g (pre-pregnant weight) to approximately 1100 g at full term. Many women feel the need to urinate more frequently, owing to pressure of the uterus on the bladder as well as to hormonal changes. The increase in progesterone has a

Pregnancy

Needs Requiring Particular Attention	Factors Related to These Needs
Nutrition	Growth of new tissue, requiring additional nourishment Fetal nutritional needs are met through proper maternal intake
Elimination	Hormonal changes affecting kidney, bowel function and digestion Expansion of uterus into abdominal cavity
Circulation	Increase in total fluid volume Increased body mass
Comfort, rest and sleep	Weight gain, increasing body bulk making some resting positions difficult
Pain management	Medications may cross placenta and have harmful effects on the fetus
Movement and exercise	Awkwardness due to weight gain; increase in fluid volume; shift in centre of gravity, affecting balance; relaxing of ligaments Slowing down of body processes
Safety	Fetal well-being dependent on mother Shift in centre of gravity, affecting balance
Hygiene	Hormonal changes affecting skin texture and secretions
Infection control	Placenta only a partial barrier to harmful agents
Love, security and self-esteem	Possibility that strong emotions may affect the fetus
Sexuality	Hormonal and psychological changes as well as altered body proportions, affecting sexual expression New motherhood role requires psychosocial adaptation

relaxing effect on smooth muscle, which causes bowel irregularity and, in many cases, constipation (Pillitteri, 1995).

The degree to which these changes are felt depends on the individual—on her physiological make-up and on her emotional response to her pregnancy. While one woman may experience nausea every day for the first trimester, another may simply feel tired, while yet another may feel no change at all. No two pregnancies are exactly alike.

Second Trimester (14th Week to 27th Week)

During the 14th to the 27th week of pregnancy, the future mother usually experiences a feeling of overall well-being. Her body has adjusted to the hormonal changes and she has more energy. She can now feel the baby move, which usually has a positive effect.

By the 14th week, weight gain is usually evident. There is a thickening of the waist as the uterus expands and rises out of the pelvis. Blood volume increases up to 50 percent during pregnancy. The cervix softens and is closed by a mucous plug. The breasts, including the nipples, enlarge and may begin to produce **colostrum** (a thin, yellowish substance rich in maternal antibodies). The nipples may become darker, and a vertical line of dark pigment, called the **linea nigra**, appears between the pubic area and the navel. Some women develop **stretch marks** (reddish streaks) on their breasts and abdomen (Pillitteri, 1995; Reeder et al., 1997).

Third Trimester (28th Week to 40th Week)

During the third trimester, the future mother again often experiences fatigue and a new feeling of heaviness. A general relaxation of all body ligaments occurs in late pregnancy, and the continually enlarging uterus pushes the woman's centre of gravity backward. The enlarged uterus is responsible for much of the discomfort a woman feels at this time. It may press on the lungs or diaphragm, causing shortness of breath; on the bladder, causing urinary frequency; or on the stomach, causing indigestion.

Approximately two weeks before birth the baby "drops" as its head settles into the pelvic cavity. This makes the mother generally more comfortable, although the uterus may now be pressing on the bowel, causing constipation. During this stage **Braxton-Hicks contractions**, that is, tightening of the uterine muscles in preparation for labour, often occur.

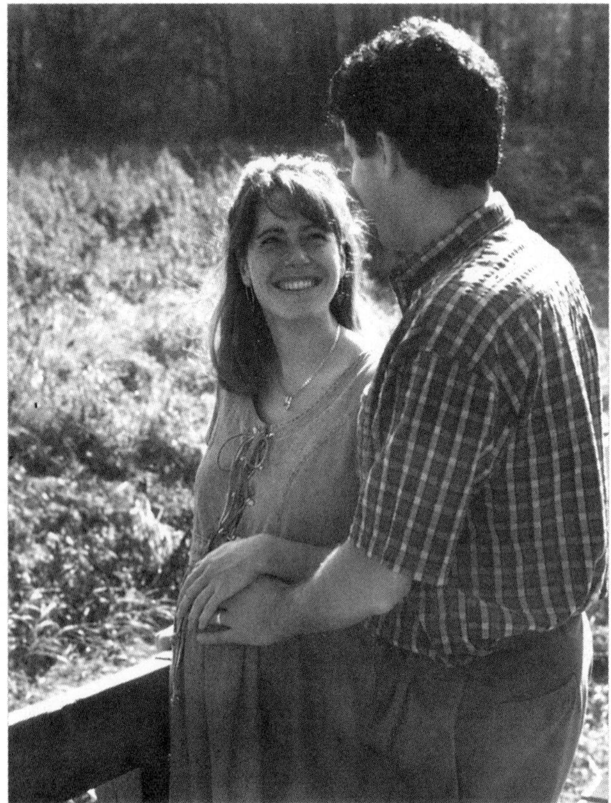

The expectant couple share the joy of pregnancy as they anticipate the birth of their baby.

The loss of the mucous plug (often called a "show") and the appearance of amniotic fluid are generally good indications that labour is imminent. Labour may start with the rupture of the membranes, which can be a gush or a slow flow of clear fluid from the vagina. **Labour** is the process by which the baby is expelled from the uterus. It consists of a series of strong contractions, and can be divided into four stages (Reeder et al., 1997).

During *first-stage of labour* the cervix shortens and becomes thinner **(effacement)** and opens **(dilation)** to allow the baby to pass through. *Second-stage of labour*, also known as the "pushing stage," begins from full dilatation of the cervix (10 cm)—when the head becomes visible ("**crowning**")—to the birth of the baby. During *third-stage of labour* the placenta is expelled. The *fourth stage of labour* is a time of critical adaptation and bonding of the mother and father and newborn. Physiological stability is restored during the first four hours postpartum (Reeder et al., 1997).

During pregnancy and labour many women sense a diminution of their self-image, a loss of respect from others for their needs and wishes. All too often, especially during labour, the pregnant woman's wishes have been overruled or ignored in favour of the convenience of hospital personnel. It should be remembered that while the health and safe delivery of the infant are important, so are the needs and wishes of the parents. For these reasons, many couples are seeking alternative birthing arrangements, either in the hospital setting or at home. The recent regulation of midwifery care in Ontario and British Columbia has increased the options for birth support for low-risk women. The provision of midwifery services has decreased intervention rates and increased couples' satisfaction with their birth experiences.

Infancy (Birth to 12 Months)

The first sight of a newborn baby comes as a shock to most of us. Expecting to see a plump, rosy-cheeked, bright-eyed infant (as often depicted on television), we are instead presented with a squalling bundle with reddish or blue-tinged wrinkled skin, a puffy face, a flat nose and, often, a misshapen head. Newly born infants are covered with a creamy white substance called *vernix,* which protected their skin in the womb and eased their passage through the birth canal. They may also be covered with **lanugo**, thick downy hair, and they may be slightly bloody from their passage through the birth canal. Upon closer inspection you may notice that their skin is peeling in some places, or they may be bruised from a forceps delivery. In addition, their legs may be bowed and their toes bent in odd ways from their cramped position in the womb.

At birth, newborns must make immediate adjustments in order to survive. Accustomed to having their needs met automatically in the womb, they are now forced to rely on

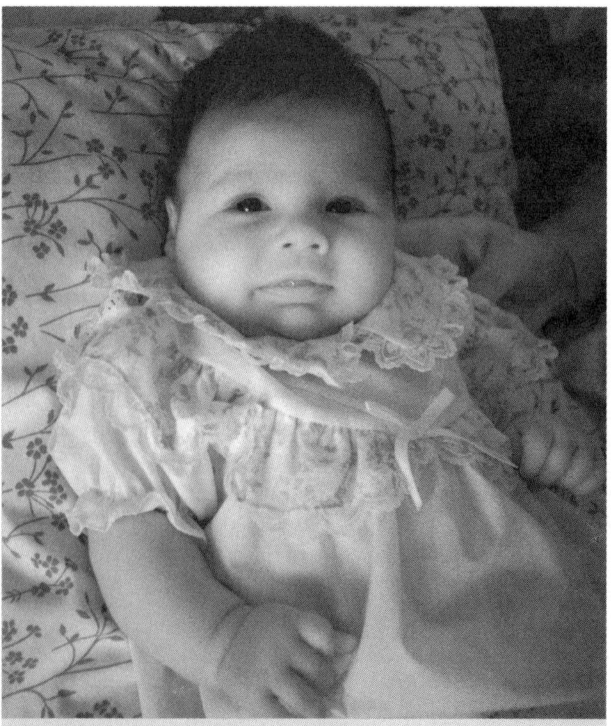

Emily relates to the world primarily through the use of her senses.

Infancy

Needs Requiring Particular Attention	Factors Related to These Needs
Nutrition	Immaturity of gastrointestinal system Rapid growth of all body tissues, requiring increased nutrition Appearance of teeth, requiring dental hygiene
Elimination	Immaturity of gastrointestinal system Immaturity of neuromuscular structures necessary for control
Temperature regulation	Immaturity of temperature regulation system
Comfort, rest and sleep	Rapid growth, requiring increased rest and sleep
Sensory stimulation	Quality of environment Mobility status
Movement and exercise	Neuromuscular development Opportunity for exploration of environment
Protection and safety	Lack of experience to perceive danger Inability to protect self
Hygiene	Vulnerability to infection Sensitivity of skin
Infection control	Maternal antibodies in young infants—prolonged by breastfeeding Immunization schedule
Security and self-esteem	Mother (caregiver)–infant adjustment of primary importance
Love and belonging	Mother (caregiver)–infant "bonding" important Quality of care, extent of cuddling, affection important

their own systems to satisfy many of their basic needs, such as nutrition, elimination, oxygen and circulation. Newborns typically fall into a deep sleep shortly after birth, and this sleep can last up to 12 hours. During the first few months of life, many babies spend most of their time sleeping and feeding.

The first 12 months of life are a period of rapid growth. By the end of their first year, most infants have tripled their birth weight and increased their length again by half. Normally born without teeth, they begin teething at around five or six months. Most infants have six to eight teeth by one year. Babies have a relatively immature gastrointestinal system at birth. For the first few months they can handle only breast milk or formula; anything else passes through them without being absorbed.

Newborns and young infants generally have very sensitive skin. It breaks down easily, providing an ideal site for bacteria and other organisms to grow. Skin rashes on the face and especially in the diaper area are common. Young babies are also very sensitive to even mild fluctuations in temperature, as their temperature-regulating system is immature and does not adapt quickly. They do not shiver; instead, they produce heat when they are cold by increasing their metabolic rate and burning calories.

Infants receive some protection from disease during their first two to three months through the mother's antibodies that remain in their system. It is also possible to confer some passive immunity through breastfeeding, as some maternal antibodies are present in breast milk.

In Canada, the recommended immunizations are usually begun at two months of age for diphtheria, pertussis, tetanus, inactivated poliomyelitis and *Haemophilus influenzae* type B (HIB) vaccine. The first injection of hepatitis B vaccine (HBIG) is given as soon after birth as possible, with the second at one month and the third at six months of age. The follow-up schedules vary from province to province, but boosters of these vaccines continue throughout infancy and childhood. The measles-mumps-rubella (MMR) vaccine is given at 12 months of age. Children are also given regular boosters of this vaccine throughout the preschool and school years.

Newborn babies have very little motor control; most of their movements are **reflexes**, that is, automatic responses to stimuli. They will withdraw from a pinprick, turn towards a sound, grasp your fingers or startle at a loud noise. When their cheeks are stroked babies will turn their heads in the direction the stroking is coming from and begin

Age and Motor Skill

Birth (full term)
- sucks, breathes and swallows in a coordinated fashion

Three months
- absence of grasp reflex
- hands often open, able to pull at blankets and clothes
- directs vision, "reaching" for objects with eyes

Six months
- holds bottle
- grasps feet and pulls up to mouth
- can localize sounds
- rolls from back to abdomen
- able to lift head

Nine months
- crawls on hands and knees
- pulls self to standing position with help from furniture
- dominant hand preference evident
- sits unaided indefinitely
- grasps, using opposition of thumb and fingers (pincer grasp)

Twelve months
- walks with one hand held
- can turn pages in a book
- can sit unaided from standing position

SOURCE: Wong, 1995; Pillitteri, 1995.

sucking movements. This reflex is called **rooting**, and allows babies to begin sucking when they come in contact with the breast. Many of the reflexes present at birth disappear as the infants achieve control over their actions. They progress from simple movements, such as watching their mother move around a room, to complex skills within a relatively short time. Development of motor skills appears to progress in a head-to-foot, central- to-peripheral direction. By 12 months most infants have learned to walk.

In the area of communication, infants progress from crying to smiling in a few short weeks. Soon they begin to vocalize. By one year, most infants have two or three words with many meanings. Infants can understand their own name by about eight months, and by one year they know and can say the names of those close to them. They are capable of understanding more than they can say and enjoy being read to, although their attention span is very short (Wong, 1995).

Erikson identified the principal conflict of this stage as *trust vs. mistrust*. Perhaps the most important task during infancy is the adjustment that mother (and father) and child must make to each other. The **bonding**, or attachment, that occurs between parent and newborn is important in creating a sense of security in the infant. When the parents care for their infant in a loving and consistent manner, meeting his or her needs as they arise, the infant develops a sense of trust in others (Murray & Zentner, 1997).

Toddlerhood (12 Months to 3 Years)

During the toddler stage, children continue to grow, although not quite so rapidly as during infancy. The proportions of their body begin to change—the head does not appear quite so large, and the limbs begin to lengthen in relation to the trunk. The body systems continue to mature, and mental functions increase in complexity.

By the beginning of toddlerhood the digestive process is complete; toddlers can handle most adult foods and can follow the usual schedule of three meals a day. By three years, dentition is complete (20 teeth) and oral hygiene is essential.

Between 18 and 24 months, most children have the neuromuscular capacity for sphincter control; that is, they are capable of controlling elimination. This is the time when most parents initiate toilet training (Wong, 1995).

Language plays an important role for children at this stage. They are learning to make their wants and needs understood by others. At 18 months they may have an "understandable" vocabulary of about a dozen words. By two years of age, children have a vocabulary of approximately 300 words; by the age of three they are capable of forming complex sentences to express their ideas (Wong, 1995).

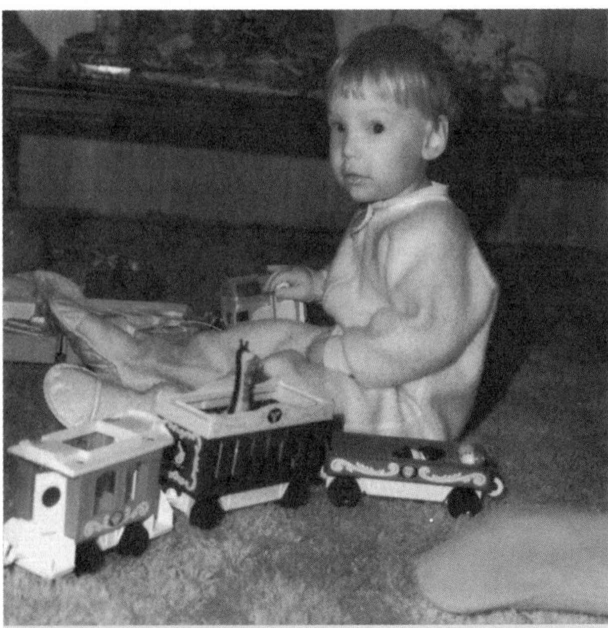

Toddlers enjoy toys that are active and that they can play with independently.

Toddlerhood

Needs Requiring Particular Attention	Factors Related to These Needs
Nutrition	Continued growth and maturation of systems Abandonment of bottle and/or pacifier (usually)
Elimination	Proportional fluid constituency of body is great compared with that in adults Achievement of control of elimination
Sensory stimulation	Increased mobility and improved motor control, making exploration further afield possible Developing sense of autonomy Independence of movement
Movement and exercise	Increasing neuromuscular maturation Improved motor control Development of motor skills
Protection and safety	Developing independence Insatiable curiosity Improved motor control Inability to understand danger
Hygiene	Parental teaching Toilet training Oral/dental hygiene
Infection control	Increased contact with other children Immunization schedules
Security and self-esteem	Developing sense of autonomy Home atmosphere
Love and belonging	Quality of parent–child interactions Stability of relationships with parents and siblings Development of trust
Sexuality	Gender identification

Motor coordination improves greatly during this stage. By 18 months, infants are capable of negotiating stairs, for example, or turning the pages in a favourite book. Children can hold a crayon to draw, and they can manipulate buttons to put on and take off their clothes. There is a new sense of mobility as they learn to run and climb, ride a tricycle or push themselves on the swings.

Small wonder, then, with all their new abilities, that children seek to employ them. This stage is often referred to as the "terrible twos" as the charming and compliant one-year-old child is transformed into a veritable monster. At this stage children seem to have limitless energy. Their new abilities, combined with an insatiable curiosity about their world, turn them into little dynamos, busily exploring everything within their reach. They want to do things themselves, without another's help, and they can be very vocal when expressing their disapproval of interference. Unfortunately, children of this age have little concept of danger, and even less understanding of cause and effect. It is often necessary to curtail their activities for their own protection.

Erikson identified the principal conflict of this stage as *autonomy vs. shame*. Children are actively seeking independence, yet they also need approval for their actions. It is important, then, in setting limits, to help children to understand the distinction between right and wrong, without discouraging them in their activities.

Before age three, children take little notice of one another. They will play side by side (*parallel play*), but there is little interaction. Around age three, however, children begin to have more contact with others their age, and they learn to play together as a sense of cooperation emerges. The primary influence on children of this stage, however, is still the immediate family. They learn mainly through observation and imitation of their parents and siblings. The home atmosphere has a profound effect on a child's image of him- or herself (Wong, 1995; Murray & Zentner, 1997).

Early Childhood (3 to 6 Years)

During the early childhood (preschool) years, the rate of growth begins to slow down, although children will continue to gain two to three inches a year until they reach puberty. In appearance, their proportions resemble more closely those of an adult. Their bones become harder and their muscle control and coordination improve noticeably. By age four a child is able to climb stairs without holding onto railings, can climb and jump without difficulty and is able to dress him- or herself in simple clothing.

Most children have all their primary teeth by the age of three. Their body systems have reached functional maturity. For example, they can handle adult foods, and they are capable of controlling their elimination and taking care of their various toilet needs. Although infants are capable of seeing at birth, full visual maturity does not occur until about age five.

At this stage, children begin to develop active immunity through exposure to disease. From the time they start playing with other children on a regular basis, at preschool or kindergarten, for example, they seem to catch whatever is going around, be it a cold, flu or childhood diseases such as chicken pox. As stated earlier, immunization programs, usually begun in infancy, continue throughout the childhood years. Although inoculations do not guarantee that a child will not succumb to a particular disease, they usually mean a less severe attack and a quicker recovery.

The preschool stage is a time when children begin to socialize actively with one another. Many children attend day care, preschool or nursery school at age three or four, and almost all school systems now incorporate a kindergarten class for five-year-olds. The child's world expands beyond the home and family, although the family is still a major influence on his or her development. During this stage, children begin to identify with the parent of the same gender, learning a social role based largely on imitation of this parent. They practise these new-found social skills during play with their peers; the physical differences between the genders become apparent.

The Childhood Years

Needs Requiring Particular Attention	Factors Related to These Needs
Nutrition	Continued growth and maturation of systems
Elimination	Functional maturity of systems
Sensory stimulation	Maturation of vision Improved muscle control, making exploration easier
Movement and exercise	Improved neuromuscular control Developing motor skills
Protection and safety	Lack of awareness of danger Expanding horizons
Infection control	Increasing contact with others Development of active immunity to infection Immunization schedule for communicable diseases Nutritional status affects vulnerability to infection
Sexuality	Gender identity with parent of same gender
Love and belonging	Home environment Development of initiative Parents' and siblings' attitudes towards child
Security	Development of initiative Support and guidance from parents Stability of home Accustomed routines
Self-esteem	Interaction with peers Family atmosphere Relationships with parents and siblings important

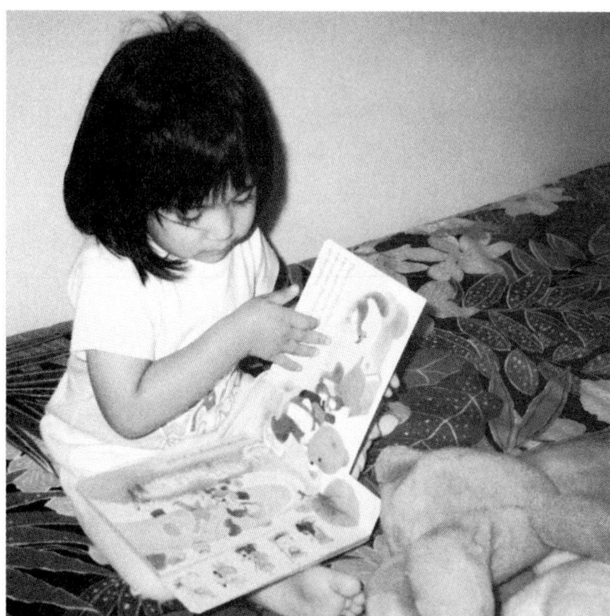

Preschoolers enjoy experiences in which they can use their active imaginations.

Language development continues to play a major role throughout this stage. It is a means by which children can capture the attention of others and assert themselves. As their horizons broaden and they are capable of doing more and more for themselves every day, children want to tell people about it. Sometimes children of three and four cannot seem to stop talking. They have fertile imaginations and often get reality and fantasy mixed up. Children at this stage are highly impressionable; that is, they will take to heart what others, particularly adults, tell them. It is important to recognize, in talking with young children, that they are not always capable of detecting sarcasm.

According to Erikson, the principal conflict of this stage is *initiative vs. guilt*. The delight of children as they explore the world and discover their own emerging capabilities is truly wonderful to see. They are so proud of their accomplishments. However, not all their endeavours may fall into the category of acceptable behaviour, and often it may be necessary to redirect their energies. Children of this age are mainly motivated by a sense of discovery, and it is important to discourage unacceptable behaviour without discouraging initiative or making the child feel guilty (Wong, 1995; Murray & Zentner, 1997).

Middle Childhood (6 to 12 Years)

During middle childhood (school age), the child's growth continues at a slow and steady rate. Boys are generally heavier and taller than girls of the same age. The child's body is now in proportion to that of an adult. There is further maturation of the body's systems, and brain development is virtually complete by puberty. Neuromuscular coordination is further refined, and team sports become a major activity for children of this age. As they continue to develop their active immunity, school-age children are prone to various childhood diseases. Immunization schedules generally continue throughout this stage (Wong, 1995).

In the schoolroom and through participation in team activities, children develop an attitude of cooperation and self-control. Their thinking and actions are no longer so completely self-centred as they learn that not everyone shares their viewpoint. They begin to think about things that do not necessarily affect them directly and to express their thoughts and feelings about themselves and others. They learn that there is a relationship between cause and effect.

The period of middle childhood is a critical one in terms of psychosocial development. During this time children firmly establish their sense of independence and define their social role. According to Erikson, the principal conflict of middle childhood is *industry vs. inferiority*. Children are on a quest of discovery throughout both their inner and outer selves. They ask many questions, seeking to understand every aspect of the world. They may want to know where they came from, for example, or who made the world. They might enjoy taking things apart to see what makes them work. (They may not be so successful in putting things back together again, though.)

If children are encouraged to try new things and taught to learn from their mistakes, they will develop a positive image of themselves and their capabilities. If, on the other hand, they are continually discouraged in their endeavours through failure or negative comments from others, they will

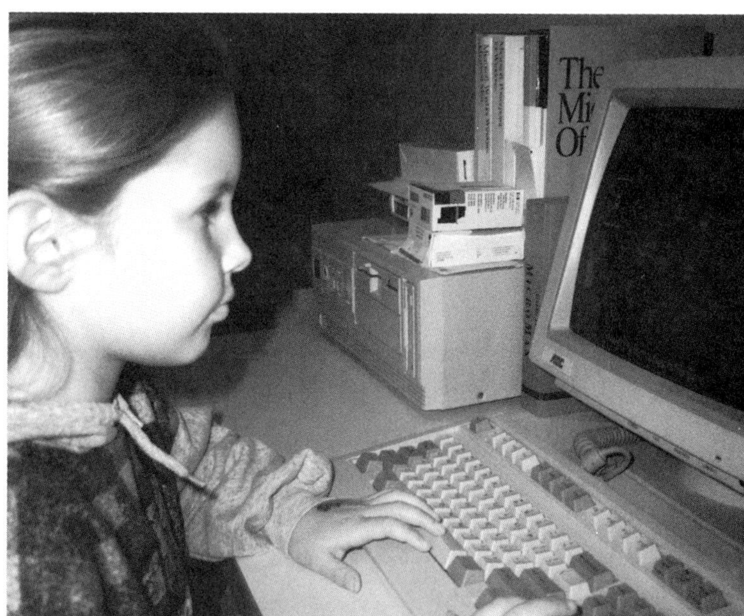

Today's school-age children enjoy high-tech games.

Middle Childhood

Needs Requiring Particular Attention	Factors Related to These Needs
Nutrition	Continued growth and maturation of systems
Movement and exercise	Further refinement of neuromuscular control
Protection and safety	Understanding of relationship of cause and effect
Infection control	Increased contact with others (school and extracurricular) Development of active immunity Immunization schedule Nutritional status
Sexuality	Adoption of social role based on gender Development of social role based on gender Role model (parent or parent-substitute of same gender)
Self-esteem	Establishment of independence Home atmosphere and school atmosphere Relations with peers, adults outside home Success in endeavours
Security	Parental support Teachers' support
Love and belonging	Stability of home environment Continuity of school environment Routines and schedules

soon feel incapable of anything worthwhile, assuming what is commonly called an "inferiority complex." Success in any endeavour, no matter how small, is necessary for individuals to feel good about themselves.

As mentioned above, children during this stage establish their independence from their family. They spend a large part of their day now away from home. As well as attending school, they may also participate in community activities or team sports. Although the home and family remain a primary factor in their development, other adults and their peers are beginning to play an important role in their life, too (Wong, 1995; Murray & Zentner, 1997).

Adolescence (12 to 19 Years)

Much has been written about the turbulent adolescent years. The notion that adolescence is an unsettling (or unsettled) period in one's life, however, seems to be peculiar to the modern Western world. In many other parts of the world, for example, Samoa, where adult roles are clearly defined, the transition from childhood to adulthood is gradual and serene (Papalia & Olds, 1986). Even in our own society less than a century ago, children gradually assumed adult responsibilities at home and then apprenticed at an early age in a vocation that was chosen for them. Perhaps it is the number of options available to adolescents today that can be unsettling.

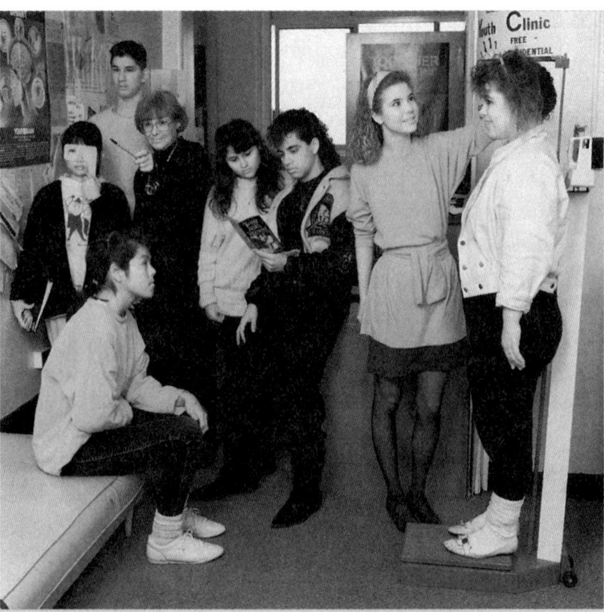

These students appear to be enjoying their visit to the school health room.

Adolescence is a maturational time during which individuals become capable of reproduction. Owing to a secondary physical growth spurt, there are height and weight changes, as well as the appearance of secondary sexual characteristics (Olds, London & Ladewig, 1996). Girls usually attain their maximum height earlier, but boys are generally taller. There is also a rapid increase in the vital capacity of the lungs during adolescence, greater in boys than in girls (Murray & Zentner, 1997).

During adolescence, body proportions change—girls develop breasts and hips, and boys' shoulders become broader. Other physical changes are apparent as the reproductive system matures. There is an increased production of the hormones testosterone in males and estrogen in females, which are primarily responsible for the appearance of the secondary sex characteristics. **Puberty** is marked by **menarche** (the onset of the menstrual cycle) in girls, and by the production of sperm in boys. The increased production of hormones also results in the secretion of excess amounts of *sebum*, a thick, oily substance that can plug the hair follicles, often resulting in skin eruptions called *acne*.

Most adolescents enjoy general good health, having already established immunity to most contagious diseases. The principal infections suffered by adolescents these days are sexually transmitted. Chlamydia is the most frequently reported sexually transmitted disease. In Canada the reported rate was 123 per 100 000 in 1995. The population that reported the highest incidence was young women under the age of 25. Despite the reported decrease in cases of gonorrhea since 1980, the rate among 15- to 24-year-olds is still two to four times higher than the overall average. The decline of syphilis in Canada is equal to that of gonorrhea. Both chlamydia and gonorrhea cause long-term health problems, such as pelvic inflammatory disease and its complications (Patrick, 1997).

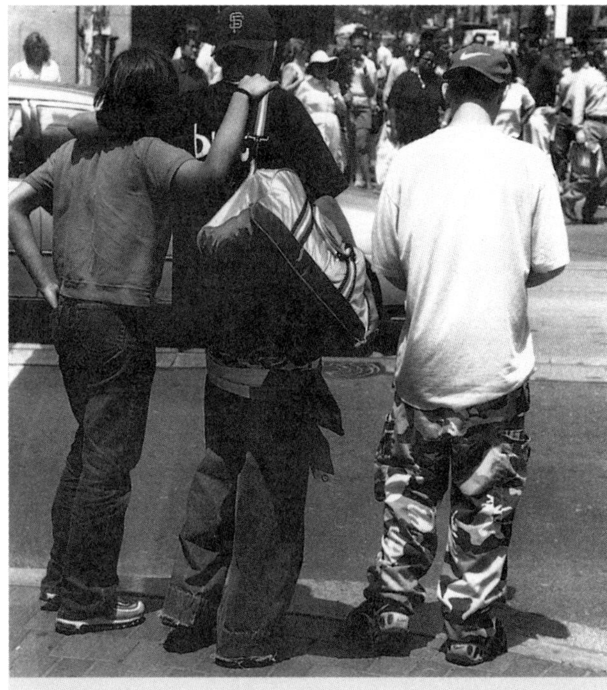

Adolescents' appearance and the clothes they wear are important in establishing their sense of identity.

As adolescents take on the appearance of adults they want to be treated as adults. They can be very critical of

Adolescence

Needs Requiring Particular Attention	Factors Related to These Needs
Nutrition	Growth spurt Maturation of systems
Oxygen	Rapid increase in vital capacity of lungs
Movement and exercise	Change in body proportions
Safety	Risk-taking behaviour
Hygiene	Excessive sebum production Attainment of puberty
Infection control	Sexual experimentation
Sexuality	Maturation of reproductive system Establishment of social role
Self-esteem	Physical appearance Peer relations Attainment of independence Establishment of identity

TABLE 8.3 Growth and development during adolescence

EARLY ADOLESCENCE (11–14 YEARS)	MIDDLE ADOLESCENCE (14–17 YEARS)	LATE ADOLESCENCE (17–20 YEARS)
Growth		
Rapidly accelerating growth Reaches peak velocity Secondary sex characteristics appear	Growth decelerating in girls Stature reaches 95% of adult height Secondary sex characteristics well advanced	Physically mature Structure and reproductive growth almost complete
Cognition		
Explores newfound ability for limited abstract thought Clumsy groping for new values and energies Comparison of "normality" with peers of same gender	Developing capacity for abstract thinking Enjoys intellectual powers, often in idealistic terms Concern with philosophic, political, and social problems	Established abstract thought Can perceive and act on long-range operations Able to view problems comprehensively Intellectual and functional identity established
Identity		
Preoccupied with rapid body changes Trying out various roles Measurement of attractiveness by acceptance or rejection of peers Conformity to group norms	Modifies body image Very self-centred; increased narcissism Tendency towards inner experience and self-discovery Has a rich fantasy life Idealistic Able to perceive future implications of current behaviour and decisions; variable application	Body image and gender role definition nearly secured Mature sexual identity Phase of consolidation of identity Stability of self-esteem Comfortable with physical growth Social roles defined and articulated
Relationships with Parents		
Defining independence-dependence boundaries Strong desire to remain dependent on parents while trying to detach No major conflicts over parental control	Major conflicts over independence and control Low point in parent–child relationship Greatest push for emancipation; disengagement Final and irreversible emotional detachment from parents; mourning	Emotional and physical separation from parents completed Independence from family with less conflict Emancipation nearly secured
Relationships with Peers		
Seeks peer affiliations to counter instability generated by rapid change Upsurge of close idealized friendships with members of the same gender Struggle for mastery takes place within peer group	Strong need for identity to affirm self-image Behavioural standards set by peer group Acceptance by peers extremely important—fear of rejection Exploration of ability to attract the opposite gender	Peer group recedes in importance in favour of individual friendship Testing of male–female relationships against possibility of permanent alliance Relationships characterized by giving and sharing
Sexuality		
Self-exploration and evaluation Limited dating, usually group Limited intimacy	Multiple plural relationships Decisive turn towards heterosexuality (if homosexual, knows by this time) Exploration of "self-appeal" Feeling of "being in love" Tentative establishing of relationships	Forms stable relationships and attachment to another Growing capacity for mutuality and reciprocity Dating as a male–female pair Intimacy involves commitment rather than exploration and romanticism
Psychologic Health		
Wide mood swings Intense daydreaming Anger outwardly expressed with moodiness, temper outbursts, and verbal insults and name-calling	Tendency towards inner experiences; more introspective Tendency to withdraw when upset or feelings are hurt Vascillation of emotions in time and range Feelings of inadequacy common; difficulty in asking for help	More constancy of emotion Anger more apt to be concealed

SOURCE: Wong, 1995, p. 843.

their parents, partly because they are frustrated at still being dependent on them, partly because they feel parents do not understand them. This is a common complaint of adolescents. And yet, as they seek independence, they also desire parental guidance and approval.

Communication with parents is often difficult at this stage, and adolescents tend to turn to their peers. The importance of peer relations during adolescence cannot be overemphasized. The peer group provides the individual with a sense of belonging. Conformity is the order of the day, as no one wants to be "different." Peer pressure is an important influence on an adolescent, affecting many aspects of his or her life. For example, the attitude of the group usually decides the degree to which individuals will engage in sexual experimentation, the leisure activities in which they will participate, how long, or short, they will wear their hair and what style of clothes they will buy. Adolescents are particularly concerned with their physical appearance, often spending hours in front of a mirror. Problems with body image may have a negative impact on adolescents, and many struggle with eating disorders such as anorexia and bulimia, which can have serious health consequences.

Adolescence is characterized by experimentation as individuals seek to gain knowledge about themselves and about the world around them. During this stage, many adolescents engage in risk-taking behaviour, often pushing themselves and others to test their limits. For example, they may drive at high speeds, experiment with drugs or alcohol or engage in sex without taking precautions against pregnancy or disease. Experimentation with their new-found sexuality is a major concern of most adolescents, both boys and girls, although boys have the stronger sex drive at this stage of development.

Adolescents also experiment with their self-image, trying on various roles in an effort to establish a true sense of self. For example, parents may watch their teenage son drive off with his friends in a great roar on his motorcycle one moment, and find this same son strumming his guitar and singing quiet folk songs the next. Erikson has defined the principal conflict of this stage as *identity vs. role confusion.* The individual who does not have the opportunity to try on different roles may ultimately be unable to settle on one identity. This leads to role confusion and can disrupt one's relationships with others.

In the area of intellectual development, adolescents differ from younger children in their ability to think and reason in a logical manner. Also, they are capable of understanding and forming abstract thoughts. Values acquired in childhood are questioned and new ones are formed. Adolescents are often critical of the state of the world in general, and actively seek to change it (Wong, 1995; Murray & Zentner, 1997).

Table 8.3 summarizes growth and development during adolescence.

Early Adulthood (19 to 35 Years)

As they enter adulthood, most people have reached their physical maturity and their body systems are functioning at their optimum level. Sensory and intellectual perception and muscular strength are at their peak.

Young adults comprise the healthiest segment of our population. They rarely succumb to contagious diseases, and when they do, their illness is generally brief and without complications. As with adolescents, however, the major causes of infection are sexually transmitted diseases. A major concern for young adults is acquired immune deficiency syndrome (AIDS). In Canada, the total number of AIDS cases reported for 1997 was 15 101. The number of men diagnosed was 13 962; the number of women, 980. Canada appears to have an increasing number of human immunodeficiency virus (HIV) transmissions among injection drug users and young gay men. However, available data also suggest increasing rates of HIV infection among heterosexuals (especially women) and First Nations people (Health Canada, 1997). Data from HIV testing programs in British Columbia from January to September 1997 indicate that 83 women tested positive for HIV; 23 of these women reported heterosexual contact as their only risk (B.C. Centre for Disease Control, 1997).

Young adults have a tendency to view themselves as indestructible and as having limitless physical capabilities. The feeling that "it won't happen to me" is very prevalent among this age group. Consequently, as with adolescents, there is much risk-taking. High-risk activities may also provide a release for individuals from the many stresses they encounter at this stage of their life.

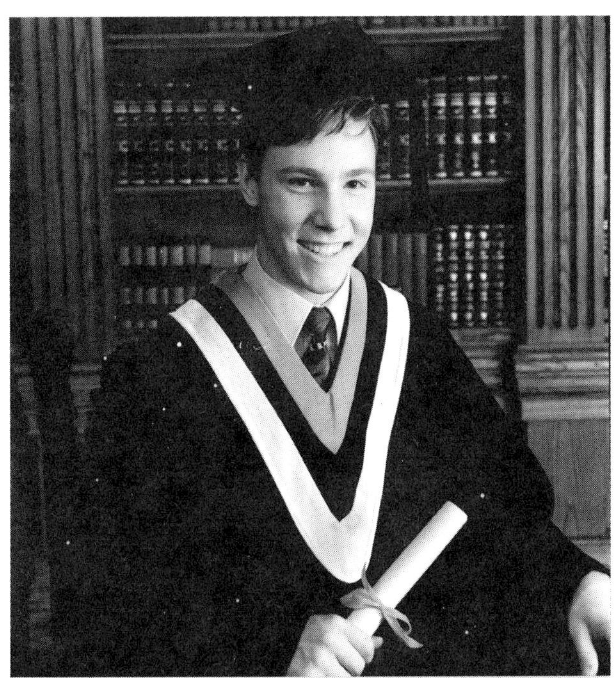

Young adult poised to begin his career.

Early Adulthood

Needs Requiring Particular Attention	Factors Related to These Needs
Nutrition	Continued growth and development in early adult years Establishment of own dietary habits (early training and habits formed in childhood important here) Time and work pressures
Movement and exercise	More sedentary lifestyle Development of own lifestyle Gradual decline in physical performance from peak fitness
Safety	Feelings of indestructibility Risk-taking behaviour common
Infection control	Strength of sexual drive Choice of sexual partners
Sexuality	Self-image Ability to establish close relationships Choice of marriage partner
Security and self-esteem	Decline in physical performance Relationships with others Ability to make major decisions
Love and belonging	Ability to form close ties with others

Initiation into adulthood involves many major decisions. Young adults, often for the first time, set goals for the future. Whether to continue one's education, to find a job immediately after high school, to remain at home or move out are but a few of the decisions facing young adults. They are also faced with the questions of whether to settle down, choose a marriage partner and have children.

The numerous major decisions young adults must face can make this stage of life an extremely stressful one. Often young people have to leave their home, family and friends as they move to a different city to pursue their education or a career goal. Others may be unable to make a definitive career choice. They may want to travel, yet feel pressured by their family and friends to settle down and get married. A major factor contributing to the stress individuals experience at this stage is their own conviction that the decisions they make at this time, once made, are irrevocable. They want to be sure to make the right decision now.

Another cause of stress for individuals in the later years of this stage may be the realization that their physical performance is diminishing. They can no longer match the strength and endurance of which they were capable just a year or two ago. If they are unwilling to accept these new physical limitations in their activities, they may push themselves too far, causing more harm than good in many cases. Acceptance of such limitations may make people feel that they have compromised their self-image.

According to Erikson, the principal conflict of this stage is *intimacy vs. isolation*. Individuals need to establish a close relationship with one or more persons with whom they can share their innermost thoughts and feelings, and who will accept them as they are. Many individuals achieve such closeness only with their marriage partner. Others may have several good friends on whom they can rely for emotional support. A person who has no one with whom to share his or her intimate thoughts may experience a feeling of profound loneliness or isolation. He or she may feel worthless and lacking in positive qualities. Individuals' relationships with others, that is, family and especially friends, during this stage are important in the development of their self-esteem. They look to others for advice and support as they seek to establish their own personal lifestyle (Murray & Zentner, 1997).

The Middle Years (35 to 65 Years)

During the first decade of this period (Sheehy's "deadline decade"), the physical changes accompanying the aging process may be almost imperceptible. Individuals who have participated in a regular exercise program, maintained good nutritional habits and had a generally healthy lifestyle throughout their young adult years often look, feel and are remarkably fit in their late 30s and early 40s. Many young adults, however, are too busy—climbing the corporate ladder, raising children or just earning a living—to look after their health. They are often suddenly brought up short by the realization that the waistline has thickened or that wrinkles have suddenly appeared around the eyes or mouth. People may also notice a decrease in the perception of taste and smell, or find that they need to wear glasses for the first time in their life. Sometimes, the change in health status is more serious. For example, there has been an alarming incidence of heart attacks among men around the age of 40. As part of the general reassessment of one's lifestyle that is often faced some time between the ages of 35 and 45 years, health is usually an important consideration. An increasing number of people in this age group are joining fitness programs as they begin to realize that their health is not indestructible and that it is time to take action to safeguard it.

The physical changes of the aging process inevitably catch up with people in the late middle years. The "change of life" may occur as early as the mid-40s in some women and as late as the mid-50s in others. Generally, this means **menopause** or end of the childbearing years for women. The onset and duration of menopause varies with each individual. It may start and end abruptly, or it may be a gradual process. There is a decrease in the production of estrogen, causing the ovaries to cease releasing ova. Other changes directly related to decreased estrogen production are "hot flashes," a thinning of the vaginal lining and urinary dysfunction (Pilletteri, 1995).

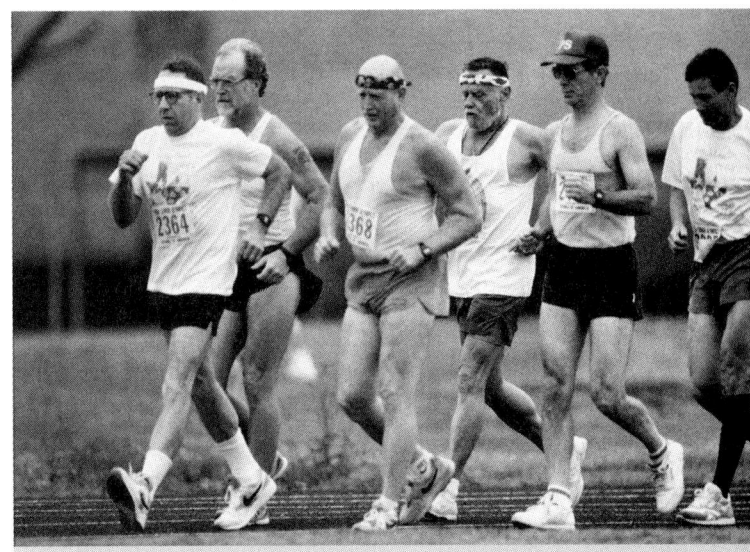

Employees enjoy a noontime power walk competition.

Some women experience other symptoms such as fatigue, dizziness or nervousness which—although not directly attributable to estrogen reduction—may result from a combination of factors at this stage in a woman's life. Many women, indeed, look forward to the cessation of menstruation.

The phenomenon of "male menopause" occurs when men experience a decrease in the production of testosterone,

The Middle Years

Needs Requiring Particular Attention	Factors Related to These Needs
Nutrition	More sedentary lifestyle
Sensory	Greater intensity of stimulation required
Movement and exercise	Decline in physical performance Awareness of preventive value of regular exercise program Availability of programs
Hygiene	Decrease in skin integrity
Sexuality	Elimination of fear of pregnancy for women Decrease in fertility Self-image
Self-esteem	Attainment of career and social goals Decline in fertility and sexual function
Security	Visual signs of aging process Mid-life transition
Love and belonging	Decline in sexual function Adolescent children Aging parents

decreased fertility and ability to achieve orgasm. Impotence can also be a problem. In our youth-oriented North American society, many men seem to have difficulty accepting the "change of life" process. They may feel the need to compensate by driving flashy sports cars and seeking involvement with younger people—particularly of the opposite gender. It is not unheard of for a man in this age group to abandon his wife of many years and all he has worked hard to achieve for a new life with a younger woman (Murray & Zentner, 1997; Bomar, 1996).

There are other adjustments associated with the middle years. Often, individuals at this stage are caught in the middle of three generations. While coping with the problems of teenaged children and adjusting to their eventual independence, the middle-aged individual is often faced with the realization that his or her own parents are aging. They may now need help and support with their physical, emotional or financial problems.

In spite of the many changes and adjustments one experiences, the late middle years are often referred to as the "prime of life." It can be a time of general good health and relative stability, when individuals attain the goals they have set for themselves. This is often the most productive period in a person's life. Through their various life experiences, individuals have achieved a measure of self-assurance and will feel satisfied as they reach the peak of their career and earning power and attain their most influential role in society. As the children grow up and leave home, many married couples find that they have more time to devote to leisure activities and more time for each other. Many women report having a renewed interest in and considerably more enjoyment from sex at this time of their lives than at any other (Bomar, 1996).

The Later Years (Over 65 Years)

The final stage in an individual's development has been called the "golden age." It is a time when individuals no longer have to strive to achieve, when they can relax and enjoy the fruits of their labour. In Canada, we believe that the state has a responsibility to care for its older adults, who have already made their contribution to society. Through our social security program, older people are assured an income at least minimally sufficient to meet their basic needs.

Social security may be at risk as the large cohort of baby boomers reach retirement. Registered retirement savings plans and other means of planning for one's retirement are an important issue for this generation of seniors.

Senior citizens in Canada are also provided with health care, largely at government expense. This is particularly important because our health typically diminishes as we get older. This is characterized by a general decline in the functioning of all body systems. The body, in this respect, is

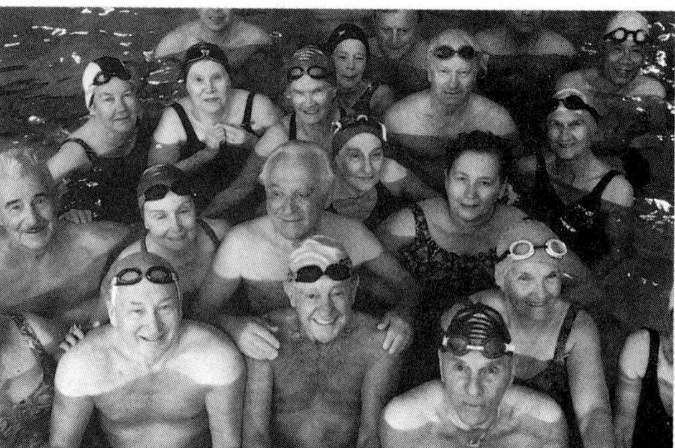

Older adults having a group photo taken after a Masters competition.

rather like a motor that begins to show the effects of long usage. Body parts start to wear out (luckily, an increasing number of them can be replaced these days) and our internal systems become unable to tolerate the wear and tear they once did. Individuals may have to be more selective in the foods they eat, or pay the penalty of indigestion. Like a vintage model car, the older person's body needs gentle handling and preventive maintenance to ensure that all systems are kept functioning as well as possible, for as long as possible. Physiological needs, then, assume a great deal of importance for people in their later years. Figure 8.2 illustrates the hierarchy of needs and tasks for older adults.

Protection and safety needs are also increased during the later years. Sensory perceptions and reflexes diminish with aging. The elderly react more slowly to dangerous situations, and have less ability to cope with them. Combined with these changes is an increased fragility of the bones. This is due to a loss of cartilage (which in many parts of the body provides a cushion to protect bony structures) and a loss of calcium from the bones. The elderly are more likely to suffer fractures when they fall than younger people are. Healing is also slower, largely because circulation is less efficient, and the elderly do not recover from illness as rapidly as younger adults do (Ebersole & Hess, 1998).

In the psychosocial realm, the later years are marked by many lifestyle changes. "Retirement has become the major normative event of the second half of life" (Ekerdt, Vinick & Bosse, 1989, p. 5). Retirement no longer lasts just a few years, but is a developmental stage that may encompass up to 20 years of one's life, perhaps into early retirement (Ebersole & Hess, 1998). Retirement involves a major adjustment. Most companies in Canada require that their employees retire by age 65. Even though it is expected, many people find retirement a traumatic experience. Often, it means reduced income, loss of self-esteem (as one no longer feels useful) and diminished social status—ours is, unfortunately, not a culture in which the elderly are revered for their wisdom. It may also mean dependence on one's family or on the state for financial, physical or emotional assistance.

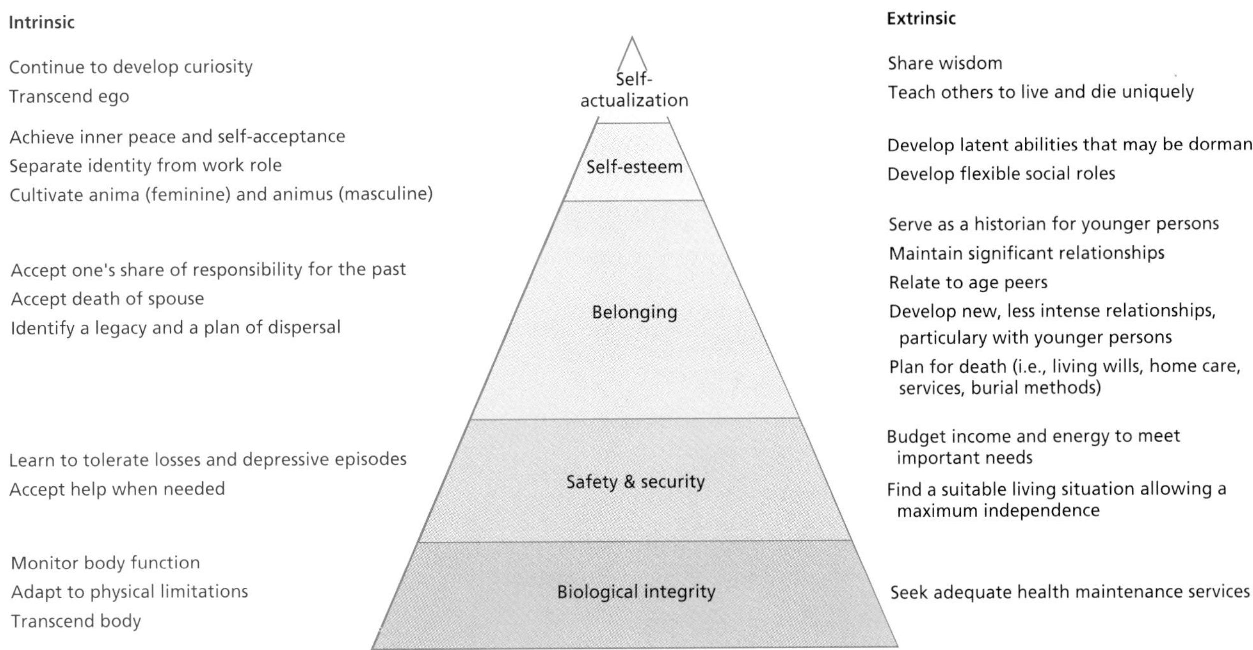

FIGURE 8.2 Developmental tasks of late life in hierarchic order

SOURCES: Peck, 1968; Havighurst, 1972; Ebersole, Butter & Lewis, 1977, in Ebersole & Hess, 1998, p. 641.

Increasingly, however, companies are helping their employees to prepare for retirement. Those who have prepared for their withdrawal from the work force can find it a very rewarding period. Topics for retirement education include the following:

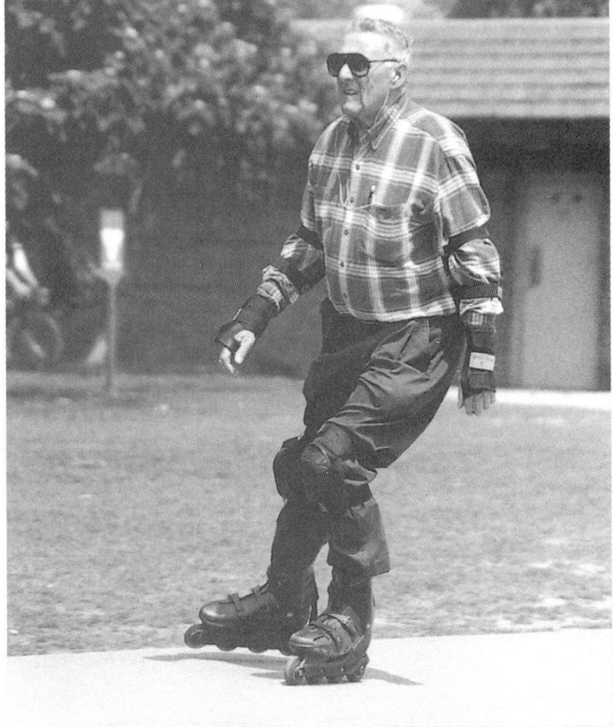
This gentleman remains active by in-line skating.

- financial planning (budgeting)
- health care services
- legal and estate planning
- living arrangements
- leisure and recreational activities
- role transitions.

Income affects many aspects of a person's life—the food one eats, the activities in which one participates and one's self-esteem, to name a few. Most people contribute to pension or retirement plans during their working years in order to supplement the state-provided pension. In most communities in Canada, senior citizens also benefit from a number of financial concessions, such as reduced fares for transportation; special rates for admission to movies, concerts, sports events and other entertainment; and reduced (or waived) tuition fees at colleges and universities. Financial considerations such as these help people to stretch a fixed income and also enable them to participate in a great many activities they would otherwise not be able to afford. The secret of a happy retirement, according to many, is to keep active and involved.

Living arrangements are also an important consideration for older adults. It is important for them to retain their independence as long as they are physically capable of doing so. An increasing number of services are helping people to remain in their own homes, such as Meals-on-Wheels, homemaker services, and "good neighbour" programs. Inevitably,

The Later Years

Needs Requiring Particular Attention	Factors Related to These Needs
Nutrition	Fixed or diminished income Reduced caloric intake Oral problems Loneliness, depression
Elimination	More sedentary lifestyle Loss of muscle tone Poor eating habits
Circulation	Slowed heart rate Fatty deposits around heart Chronic conditions
Oxygen	Decrease in vital capacity of lungs Chronic conditions
Temperature regulation	Diminished adaptation to extremes of heat and cold
Comfort, rest and sleep	Alteration of sleep patterns
Pain management	Reduced sensitivity to pain
Sensory	Diminished perception in all areas
Movement and exercise	Loss of muscle tone, mass Loss of cartilage Limited range of motion Slower coordination
Safety	Loss of cartilage Bones more fragile Presence of osteoporosis Slower reflexes Diminished sensory perception
Hygiene	Loss of skin integrity Loss of teeth Dentures, gum disease
Infection control	Loss of skin integrity Decreased immunity Immunosuppressive drugs Chronic conditions
Sexuality	Privacy Past sexual patterns
Self-esteem	Financial status Leisure, social activities Dependency status Attitudes of family, others
Security	Financial, social status Dependency status Death of spouse, friends Attitudes of family, others
Death, loss and grieving	Death of spouse, friends Inevitability of own death

LOOKING back

Dorothy Percy, 1901–1992

Dorothy Percy was the first nurse to be hired in Canada's fledgling Department of National Health and Welfare when it was set up in 1947, and the first to become Canada's chief nursing consultant in 1954. This chief nursing officer (CNO) position represented the increasing importance of nursing in the government bureaucracy. The position was created partly as a response to lobbying efforts by the Canadian Nurses Association and partly in response to the increasing importance of the nursing role in provincial health care systems. Until Dorothy Percy's appointment, advisory roles to government on health care had been filled mainly by physicians. Her sound knowledge, frankness, clarity of thought and diplomacy made her a key contributor in the development of Canada's social service programs, including the implementation of nation-wide hospital insurance and later, medical care insurance. Her role went largely unrecognized because she believed wholeheartedly that public service employees should remain in the background.

After undergraduate study at Queen's and Carleton universities, she graduated in nursing from Toronto General Hospital in 1924 and obtained a diploma in public health nursing from the University of Toronto. She then returned to her home town of Ottawa to be a nurse at the Ottawa Civic Hospital and with the Victorian Order of Nurses, moving quietly up the administrative ladders. In 1934, she was appointed lecturer at the University of Toronto School of Nursing.

She volunteered for duty as a nursing sister during World War II, serving overseas in Britain, and was discharged in 1945 with the rank of captain. Among her awards for duty overseas are the Red Cross Medal of Honour, the Defence of Britain Medal, and the Jubilee and Coronation medals. Following the war, she took the position of executive secretary for the Welfare Council of Toronto before joining government service.

In 1953, she received a one-year fellowship from the World Health Organization and took a leave of absence to observe and study nursing throughout the world. During her years as chief nursing consultant, she acted as a liaison between the national and provincial nursing organizations in Canada. She also established strong international ties with her counterparts in other nations, as well as with the World Health Organization and the International Council of Nurses. Upon her retirement, the position of chief nursing consultant was discontinued, but reinstated as a Principal Nursing Officer position under the Deputy Minister of Health.

Dorothy Percy's 43 years of service to nursing were acknowledged in 1967 when she was the first recipient of an honorary Doctorate of Nursing awarded by the University of Ottawa. That same year, the University of Toronto established a scholarship in her name. In 1977, Governor General Jules Léger presented her with the Florence Nightingale Medal, given by the International Committee of the Red Cross—one of the highest international awards in nursing. She was the 13th Canadian to be so honoured. She died peacefully in Ottawa in 1992.

— *Glennis Zilm*

the older adult is no longer able to manage alone. Many people, at this stage, decide to move into a smaller house or an apartment, or they may move in with relatives. A wide variety of alternative housing arrangements for senior citizens have developed in recent years, including expensive, privately developed "retirement communities" complete with golf course, swimming pool and other amenities. In addition, there are publicly financed low-rent apartment complexes; housing projects sponsored by church groups and service clubs; and personal care homes, both private and public, available to seniors. Regardless of the type of accommodation, the move is always a difficult one for the elderly. It is less painful if the individual can retain an essence of privacy and if steps are taken to ensure that he or she is always treated with dignity and respect (Ebersole & Hess, 1998).

One of the major adjustments for the older adult is the reversal of roles that takes place with one's children, as the older individual becomes more dependent on them. Another role change that many elderly must face is that of being widowed. The sense of loss experienced by the elderly at the death of a spouse is often overwhelming. Although the support of family and friends can be a great comfort, the surviving spouse may never recover from his or her despair. Many who have become widowed do, however, recover and remarry, and indeed weddings in senior citizen communities are becoming quite common.

As people age, they must accept not only the death of those close to them, but the inevitability of their own death. In preparation for this eventuality, many individuals make out a will. Often, older adults are able to discuss the disposal of their worldly assets with relative equanimity, but their family may become upset at the thought of the parent's death. Many older individuals like to have a "squaring up" of their accounts, to get all their affairs in order (Ebersole & Hess, 1998).

Often, too, there is a renewed interest in religion as one gets older and faces the prospect of death. The individual's spiritual counsellor can usually provide much solace and support. Counselling in matters related to death and dying has been developed in recent years largely as a result of work done by Elisabeth Kübler-Ross. This matter will be further discussed in Chapter 37. As science continues to extend the time we mortals spend on this earth, we are becoming wiser about how to enrich the later years.

In your clinical experiences on the medical-surgical wards of acute care hospitals, in nursing homes and extended care units and in your work in community agencies, you will undoubtedly meet many 90-year-olds and even 100-year-olds. If you take the time to talk with some of your older patients, you will find that a rapidly growing number of people continue to lead full, active and interesting lives long after the traditional retirement age of 65 years.

IN REVIEW

- There are certain basic needs common to all human beings that must be fulfilled if individuals are to attain health or wellness. Nursing is concerned with helping people to meet their basic needs and to achieve their full potential.
- Maslow's theory of a hierarchy of needs states that fundamental needs take priority and must be met before a person can proceed to higher needs.
- Maslow's hierarchy of needs takes the form of a pyramid:
  - physiological (base)
  - safety and security
  - love and belonging
  - self-esteem
  - self-actualization (top).
- Growth and development in the physiological sphere is well understood. However, various theories have been put forward to explain the spheres of personality, psychosocial, cognitive and moral development.
  - Freud identified stages of psychosocial development
  - Piaget formulated a theory on cognitive development
  - Kohlberg developed a theory of moral development
  - Gilligan developed a theory of moral development
  - Erikson formulated a psychosocial theory that embodies a person's whole life
  - Sheehy described "passages" through which each adult passes during early and middle adult years
  - Peck refined Sheehy's theory for middle age and later years by adding new developmental tasks.

Critical Thinking Activities

1. Reflect on the basic needs of a patient you recently cared for in clinical practice. How did the person's illness alter his or her basic needs? How did these compare with Maslow's priority of needs? How did the patient's illness and/or the constraints of the hospital environment affect the patient's fulfillment of their psychosocial needs?
2. Think about your own growth and development through the years. What were some of the major influences on your social, psychological, moral and spiritual development? In what ways did your family's cultural values and beliefs influence your growth and development?
3. From your own family or the family of friends or neighbours, select an individual from each of the different age groups and observe his or her physical, psychosocial, psychosexual, cognitive, moral and spiritual development. Compare your observations with the theories discussed in this book.
4. Visit a preschool or playground in your neighbourhood. Observe the social interactions of the children. Describe behaviours that characterize the emotional and social development of preschool children. What is the importance of social interactions in the preschool child's psychosocial development?
5. Talk to a school nurse about working with school-age and adolescent children. What are the common health problems of school-age children and adolescents? Ask the nurse to share strategies he or she finds effective in working with children in these age groups.
6. Talk with young or middle-aged adults and ask them to share some of their current problems and concerns. As a young or middle-aged adult, what are your concerns? How would illness or injury disrupt the psychosocial development of young and middle-aged adults?
7. Visit a community centre in your neighbourhood. What programs and activities are offered to promote healthy living for older adults?

KEY TERMS

physiological p. 158
safety and security p. 158
love and belonging p. 158
self-esteem p. 158
self-actualization p. 158
passages p. 162
gestation p. 163
zygote p. 164
ectoderm p. 164
mesoderm p. 164
endoderm p. 164
amniotic sac p. 164
placenta p. 164
umbilical cord p. 164
colostrum p. 165
linea nigra p. 165
stretch marks p. 165
Braxton-Hicks contractions p. 165
labour p. 166
effacement p. 166
dilation p. 166
crowning p. 166
lanugo p. 166
reflexes p. 167
rooting p. 168
bonding p. 168
puberty p. 173
menarche p. 173
menopause p. 177

References

BERGER, K.S. (1993). *The developing person through the life-span.* (3rd ed.). New York: Worth Publishers.

BOMAR, P. (Ed). (1996). *Nurses and family health promotion.* (2nd ed.). Baltimore: Williams & Wilkins.

BRITISH COLUMBIA CENTRE FOR DISEASE CONTROL. (1997, third quarter). *AIDS update: Quarterly report.* Victoria: Author.

EBERSOLE, P., & HESS, P. (1998). *Toward healthy aging: Human needs and nursing response.* (5th ed.). St. Louis: Mosby.

EKERDT, D.J., VINICK, B.H., & BOSSE, R. (1989). Orderly endings: Do men know when they will retire? *Journal of Gerontology, 44*(1), 5–8.

ERIKSON, E.H. (1963). *Childhood and society.* (2nd ed.). New York: Norton.

ESCHELMAN, M.M. (1996). *Introductory nutrition and nutrition therapy.* (3rd ed.). Philadelphia: Lippincott.

FRIEDMAN, W., ET AL. (1987). Sex differences in moral judgement: A test of Gilligan's theory. *Psychology of Women Quarterly. 7*(1) p. 87.

FREUD, S. (1972). *A general introduction to psychoanalysis.* New York: Pocket Books.

GILLIGAN, C. (1982). *Mapping the moral domain.* Cambridge, MA: Harvard University Press.

GOULD, R. (1975). Adult life stages: Growth towards self tolerance. *Psychology Today, 8*(9), 74–78.

HEALTH CANADA. (1997, August). *AIDS in Canada: Quarterly surveillance update.* Ottawa: Author.

KOHLBERG, L. (1984). *The psychology of moral development.* New York: Harper & Row.

LEVINSON, D.J. (1978). *Seasons of a man's life.* New York: Ballantine Books.

MASLOW, A.H. (1970). *Motivation and personality.* (2nd ed.). New York: Harper & Row.

MURRAY, R.B., & ZENTNER, J.P. (1997). *Health assessment and promotion strategies through the life span.* Norwalk, CT: Appleton & Lange.

NEUGARTEN, B.L. (1968). *Middle age and aging.* Chicago: University of Chicago Press.

OLDS, S., LONDON, M., & LADEWIG, P. (1996). *Maternal–newborn nursing: A family-centered approach.* (5th ed.). Menlo Park, CA: Addison-Wesley.

PAPALIA, D.E., & OLDS, S.W. (1986). *Human development.* (3rd ed.). New York: McGraw-Hill.

PATRICK, D.M. (1997). The control of sexually transmitted diseases in Canada: A cautiously optimistic overview. *Canadian Journal of Human Sexuality, 6*(2), 79–87.

PECK, P.F. (1960). *The psychology of character development.* New York: Wiley.

PIAGET, J. (1963). *The origin of intelligence in children.* New York: Norton.

PIAGET, J. (1969). *The theory of stages in cognitive development.* New York: McGraw-Hill.

PILLITTERI, A. (1995). *Maternal and child health: Nursing care of the childbearing and childrearing family.* (2nd ed.). Philadelphia: Lippincott.

RAMBO, B.J. (1984). *Adaptation nursing: Assessment and intervention.* Philadelphia: W.B. Saunders.

REEDER, S.J., MARTIN L.L., & KONIAK-GRIFFIN, D. (1997). *Maternity nursing, family newborn and women's health care.* (18th ed.). Philadelphia: Lippincott.

SCHUSTER, C.S., & ASHBURN, S.S. (1992). *The process of human development: A holistic life-span approach.* (3rd ed.). Philadelphia: Lippincott.

SHEEHY, G. (1976). *Passages: Predictable crises of adult life.* New York: Bantam Books.

WONG, D.L. (1995). *Whaley & Wong's nursing care of infants and children.* (5th ed.). St. Louis: Mosby.

Additional Readings

ALLEN, K.M., & PHILLIPS, J.M. (1996). *Women's health across the lifespan: A comprehensive perspective.* Philadelphia: Lippincott.

BARROW, G.M. (1996). *Aging, the individual and society.* (6th ed.). New York: West Publishing.

BECKINGHAM, A.C., & DU GAS, B.W. (1993). *Promoting healthy aging: A nursing and community perspective.* St. Louis: Mosby.

BERGER, K.S. (1991). *The developing person through childhood and adolescence.* (3rd ed.). New York: Worth Publishers.

BOYD, M.A., & NIHART, M.A. (1998). *Psychiatric nursing: Contemporary practice.* Philadelphia: Lippincott.

DROEGEMULLER, H.A., MISHELL, D., & STENCHEVER, M. (1997). *Comprehensive gynecology.* (3rd ed.). St. Louis: Mosby.

ELIOPOULOS, C. (1997). *Gerontological nursing.* (4th ed.). Philadelphia: Lippincott.

KAPLAN, P.S. (1993). *A child's odyssey, child and adolescent development.* (3rd ed.). New York: West.

KELLER, M.L., DUERST, B.L., & DUERST, J. (1996). Adolescents' view of sexual decision-making. *Image, 28*(2), 125–130.

MATTESON, M.A., McCONNELL, E.S. & LINTON, A.D. (1997). *Gerontological nursing: Concepts and practice.* (2nd ed.). Philadelphia: W.B. Saunders.

McLAREN, P., MALLESON, R., & KLEIN, M. (1998). Teenage pregnancy and adolescent sexuality: Present status, practice issues, effective strategies. *BC Medical Journal, 40*(2), 64–67.

McPHERSON, B.D. (1998). *Aging as a social process.* (3rd ed.). Toronto: Harcourt Brace.

MURPHY, A., & TONKIN, R.S. (1998). Health status and concerns of adolescents in British Columbia. *BC Medical Journal, 40*(2), 61–63.

NOVAK, M. (1997). *Aging and society: A Canadian perspective.* (3rd ed.). Toronto: ITP Nelson.

RICE, P.F. (1992). *Human development: A life-span approach.* Toronto: Maxwell Macmillan Canada.

SCHROEDER, B.A. (1992). *Human growth and development.* New York: West Publishing.

SCHUSTER, C.S., & ASHBURN, S.S. (1992). *The process of human development: A holistic life-span approach.* (3rd ed.). Philadelphia: Lippincott.

SHEEHY, G. (1995). *New passages: Mapping your life across time.* New York: Random House.

Chapter 9

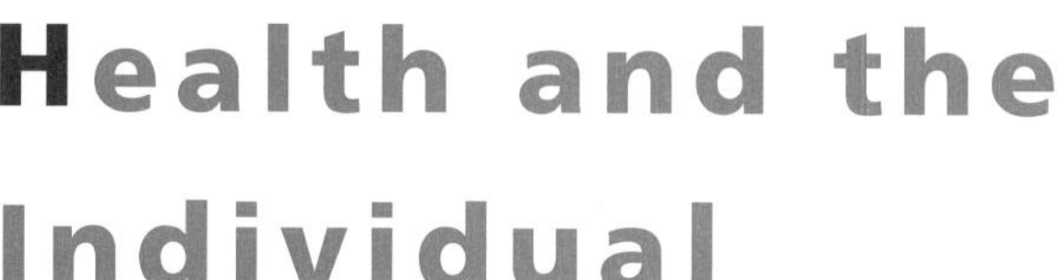

Health and the Individual

OUTLINE

Central Questions

1. Why is a person's health viewed as a spiral?
2. How is systems theory used to explain the structure and functioning of the human body?
3. What do the terms "equilibrium" and "homeostasis" mean?
4. What is involved in physiological homeostasis? Psychosocial equilibrium? Environmental equilibrium? How do they interact on an individual's health?
5. What is stress? Is all stress harmful?
6. What are the common stressors affecting an individual's health?
7. How do people react to stress?
8. How can a person minimize the emotional and physiological effects of stress?
9. What is "learned resourcefulness"?
10. What personality characteristics differentiate stress-resistant people from others?
11. How do people determine their health status?
12. What is the nurse's role in the admission of an individual to a health agency? In the discharge of an individual?
13. What is the nurse's role in the care of the individual in health promotion? In health protection? In health restoration and supportive care?

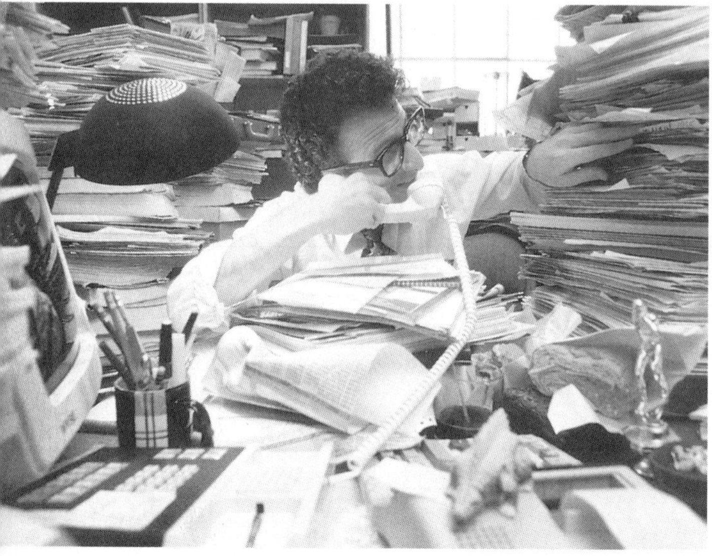

Introduction

An individual's health is more than a personal phenomenon. As we discussed in Chapter 2, health is affected by many interrelated aspects of our lives, including living and working conditions, social support networks, genetic endowment and individual behaviours.

Health can be depicted in terms of a spiral. In this analogy, human beings are seen as a system composed of numerous subsystems that interact internally. The system is also constantly interacting with external forces in the surrounding environment, in a series of ever-widening circles that include an individual's family, school, workplace, community and country.

In order to understand the health of the individual, then, it is essential to have some knowledge of systems theory. We will, therefore, deal with this concept at the beginning of the chapter. Then we will look at some of the other basic concepts that are important to an understanding of health. These include the concepts of equilibrium and homeostasis, stress and stressors and an individual's coping capabilities. In connection with coping we will explore hardiness, which is considered an important factor in rendering some people more resistant to stress than others.

The next section of the chapter deals with the personal experience of health and illness as it affects the individual. In connection with the experience of illness, we will also discuss admission to and discharge from an inpatient health care facility. In the last section of this chapter we will discuss the role of the nurse in health care.

General Systems Theory

In recent years there has been a renewed interest in systems theory as a theoretical basis for examining the phenomenon of the individual as a human system interacting with other systems in the environment. Systems theory has been particularly useful in our understanding of the individual as a member of a family and of the community.

General systems theory provides a way of examining knowledge pertaining to the world or to certain phenomena of interest. A **system** consists of two or more connected elements or parts that mutually interact to form an organized whole. Each part has a function, and the system as a whole has a function. The focus in systems theory is on the interaction among the various parts rather than on describing the functions of the parts themselves (Auger, 1976; von Bertalanffy, 1968). The human individual can be viewed as a system whose parts interact as a unified whole, which in turn interacts with the environment. A change in one part of the individual will create a change in the whole individual. For example, if a person undertakes a weight reduction program, the resulting loss of weight will affect physical appearance. This, in turn, may enhance the individual's self-esteem, which may increase confidence in social interactions with others. This view of the whole person interacting with the environment forms the basis of holistic health care.

General systems theory was introduced by Ludwig von Bertalanffy in the 1960s as a universal theory that could be used in many fields of study. Indeed, general systems theory provides the framework for understanding a large number of physical as well as social and psychological phenomena. Principles of systems analysis are being used in the behavioural, social and physical sciences, and have been applied to educational systems, cybernetics (the science of systems of control), information theory and computer sciences.

In nursing, systems theory provides an approach to understanding the multitude of elements that make up the individual human system—the biological and physiological functions, as well as the interaction of the psychological, cognitive, social and spiritual dimensions that constitute a unified whole. It also allows an examination of the individual interacting as part of a larger system, namely the family, the community and society. This aspect will be dealt with further in Chapter 10.

In systems theory, the human system is seen as comprising parts with specific structure and function. **Structure** refers to the arrangement of the specific parts of the system (what it is). For example, the body is made up of cells, organs and organ systems. **Function** is the dynamic interaction among these component parts (what it does). In a smoothly functioning system, all the body systems (for example, the respiratory, cardiovascular and nervous systems) interrelate and affect one another, such that we are not consciously able to distinguish the function of one part from that of another (Auger, 1976).

The parts of living systems exist in a hierarchy of order. At each level, a part may be examined as a separate system having a specific function with regard to the whole, or as a

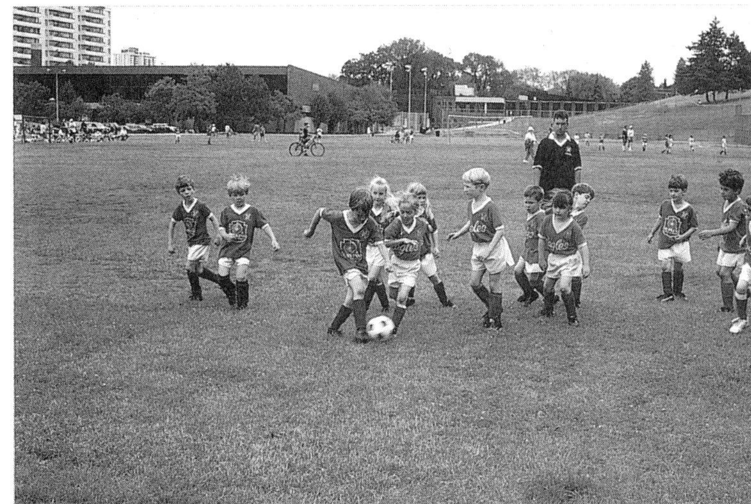

As these children compete in a soccer match, changes occur constantly as their bodies adjust to the demands of running interspersed with waiting.

component of another system at the same level of functioning, called a **subsystem**. In human beings, for example, the respiratory system may be examined as a separate system made up of cells, tissues and organ structures all interrelating for the effective exchange of oxygen and carbon dioxide. The respiratory system, in turn, may be examined along with the circulatory system, endocrine system, nervous system and others as subsystems of the larger physiological system. Each of these subsystems, then, may be scrutinized as whole entities with interrelated parts that have functions specific to the subsystem, functions specific to the other subsystems and functions that relate to the physiological system as a whole (Auger, 1976). At a higher level, the whole individual is viewed as a part of larger systems, such as the family or the community. These are called **macrosystems**. Figure 9.1 depicts the hierarchical nature of living systems.

The parts of a system are surrounded by imaginary or actual lines, called **boundaries,** that separate the system from its environment. A boundary may be a cell membrane that separates structures within the body, the skin that physically separates the body from the external environment or abstractions like attitudes, values and beliefs that regulate human interaction with other systems in the environment. Boundaries regulate the exchange of information, energy and matter between the individual and the environment. A boundary might be envisioned as a filter that permits varying degrees of exchange between the system and the environment (Auger, 1976; Loomis, 1960). Systems that freely exchange energy, matter and information are termed **open systems**. All living systems are open systems because their survival depends on a continuous exchange of energy, matter and information with the environment. The more porous the boundary, the greater the degree of interaction between the system and its environment. Conversely, systems that limit interaction with their environment are **closed systems**. A family that isolates itself from the community in which it lives by building a fence around its property and by avoiding social contacts is an example of a closed system (von Bertalanffy, 1968).

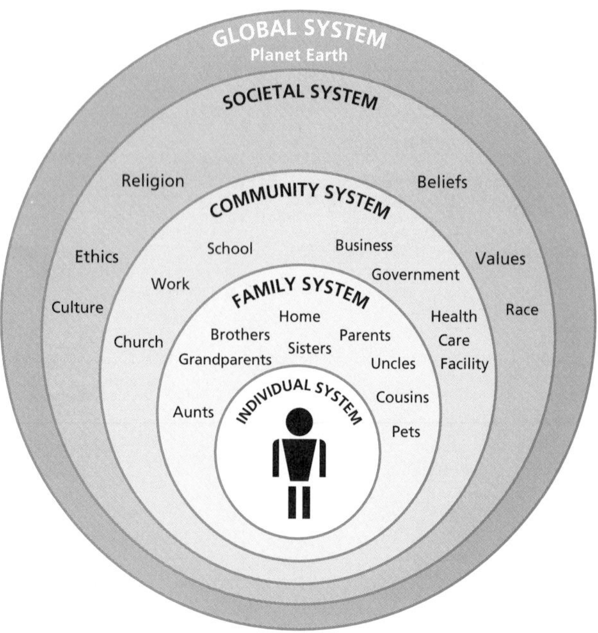

FIGURE 9.1 The hierarchy of living systems

SOURCE: Berger & Williams, 1992, p. 144.

In order to function effectively, open systems receive energy, matter and information from the environment, known as **input**. The system must then transform the input into meaningful forms that it can use for its survival. This process is termed **transformation**. For instance, food taken into the body must first be transformed, through the process of digestion, into carbohydrates, proteins and fats that the body can use. The system not only takes input from the environment; it gives similar forms of energy, matter and information back to the environment. This is called **output**. For example, energy and intestinal wastes are the output from the intake and digestion of food. Figure 9.2 illustrates three separate views of systems—a basic systems model, the patient as input and staff as input to the system model.

The output of a system creates a process of **feedback**, which permits the system to maintain stability of its internal function (shown in Figure 9.3). In the body, the constant interplay between the sympathetic and parasympathetic nervous systems in regulating heart rate is but one example of the use of feedback.

Open systems function to maintain a constant state of equilibrium or balance between the system and its surroundings. Disruption in the stability of the system results in tension or stress, which triggers an adjustment in function and energy distribution. For example, when body temperature rises above normal for any reason, the thermoregulatory mechanisms are mobilized to bring the temperature back to its normal limits (Watzlawick, Beavin & Jackson, 1967).

Equilibrium and Homeostasis

Throughout life, individuals must continuously adjust to changes both within themselves and in their relationships with the world around them. Their basic needs must be met, and at the same time they must maintain equilibrium in a constantly changing world.

Physiological Homeostasis

The 19th century French biologist Claude Bernard is credited with being the first to understand the body's need to maintain a certain consistency in its internal environment. He described the process of physiological homeostasis, although he himself did not use the term. It was Walter Cannon, an American physiologist of the 20th century,

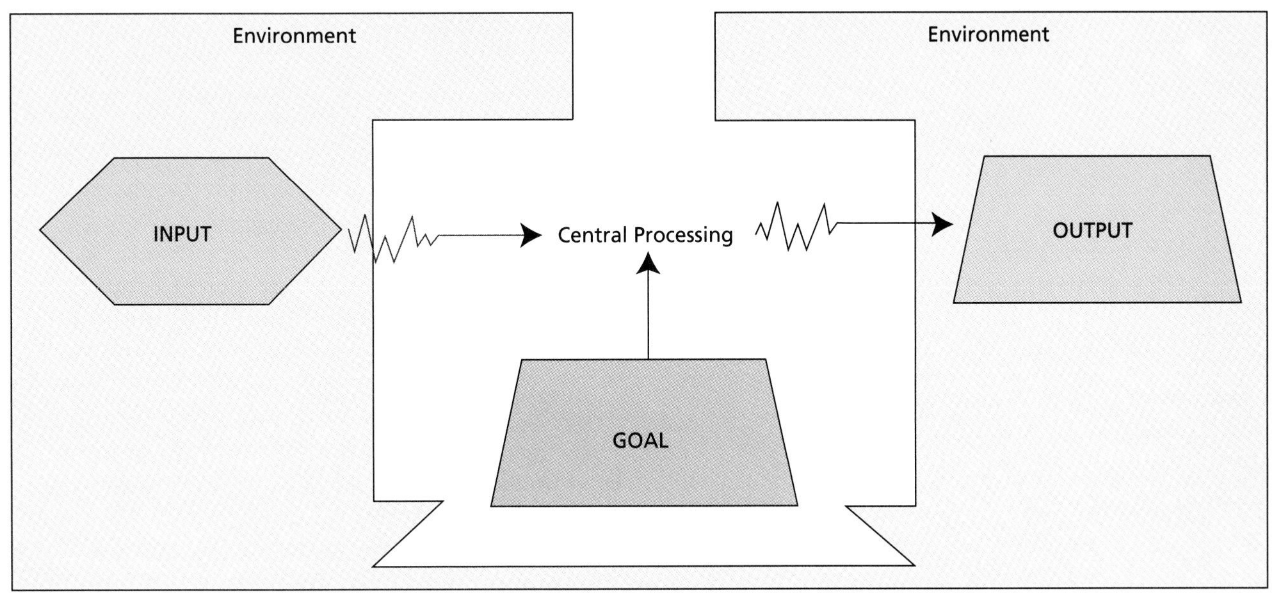

A. Basic systems model

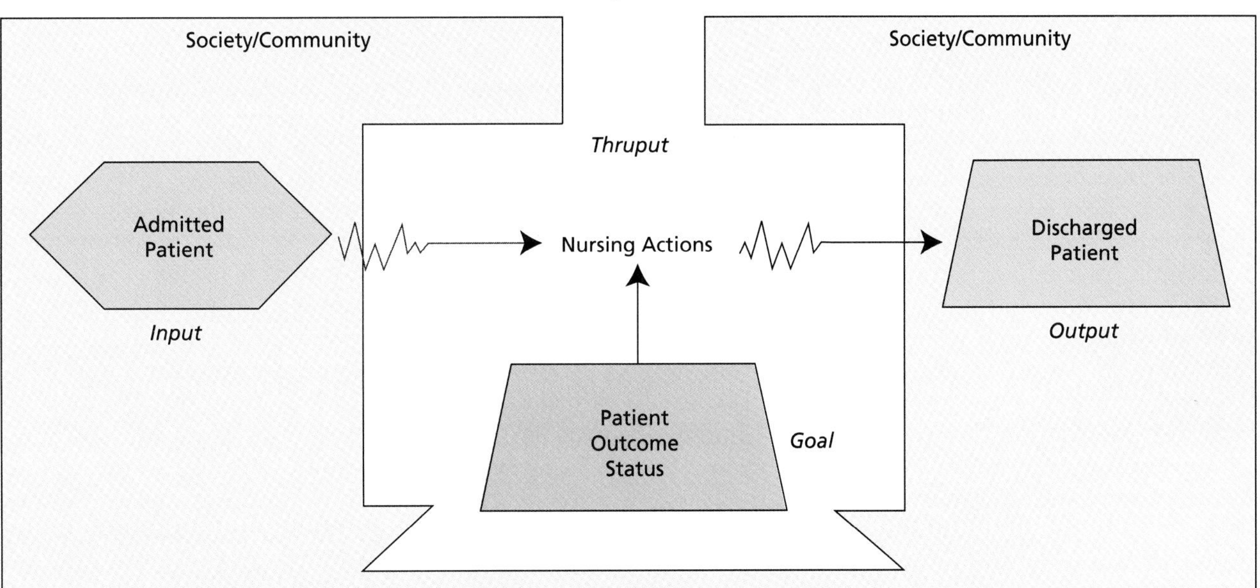

B. Patient as input to the nursing system

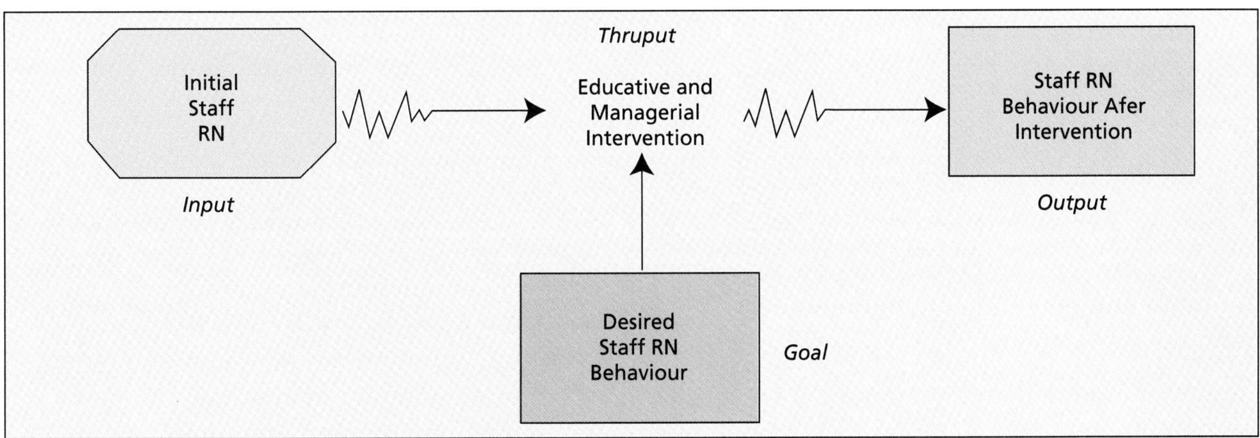

C. Staff as input to the systems model

FIGURE 9.2 A. Basic systems model; B. Patient as input to the nursing system; C. Staff as input to the systems model

SOURCE: Barnum & Kerfoot, 1995, pp. 222 & 223.

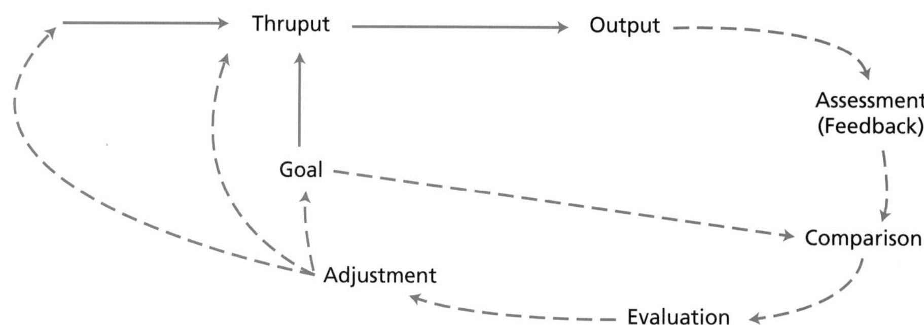

FIGURE 9.3 Systems model with a cybernetic loop

SOURCE: Barnum & Kerfoot, 1995, p. 223.

who coined the word *homeostasis*. Cannon (1932) wrote of the "wisdom of the body" in bringing into play certain mechanisms if changes in its internal environment threaten to go beyond safe limits. These are frequently referred to as "adaptation mechanisms"; they are the body's counterbalances.

As people carry out the functions of daily living, changes are constantly occurring within the body as it adjusts to demands made upon it. One's temperature, for example, rises during waking hours and falls again during sleep. The heart beats faster when a person exercises, and returns to a lower rate when at rest. Muscles alternately tense and relax as individuals engage in various activities. In fact, an infinite number of minor adjustments are continuously being made in the body during the normal process of living. However, these adjustments must be kept within certain limits if the individual is to survive. The process whereby the body maintains a state of relative balance of the internal environment is called **homeostasis.** Homeostasis is an automatic, self-regulating process that occurs within the cells, organs and organ systems of the body. Its purpose is to maintain the internal environment (McCance & Shelby, 1996).

If body temperature threatens to go too high, the individual usually becomes very flushed and diaphoretic. Both these reactions are attempts on the body's part to lower its internal temperature. Increased circulation to the tissues underlying the skin (which causes the appearance of flushing) helps to expose more blood to the cooling effects of the surrounding atmosphere. The perspiration from the profuse sweating evaporates on the surface of the skin and, in the process, also helps to carry heat away from the body. The body has a number of adaptation mechanisms, and we will be discussing many of these in later chapters of this text in conjunction with specific body processes.

Psychosocial Equilibrium

Contact with other human beings is essential to our well-being. We are constantly interacting with family, friends and neighbours—all the people who inhabit our social world. Most of us have learned to achieve a balance in our relationships with other people, so that our **psychosocial equilibrium** remains intact. We have learned to use emotional outlets when stress becomes too great. We may use physical exercise, yoga or meditation, for example, to get rid of tension caused by an unpleasant day with people at work or at school. We may go to a movie to forget temporarily our troubles with the family.

Environmental Equilibrium

Just as the body must maintain a relatively constant internal environment and the individual must maintain equilibrium in the psychosocial sphere, the human organism must also achieve a balance in its interactions with the physical environment. The physical environment consists of natural elements, such as the land we inhabit, as well as the structures that we have built upon the earth.

We have learned both to adapt to the physical environment and to change the environment to suit human needs. In a cold climate, for example, the human basal metabolic rate increases in order to maintain body temperature at a constant level. People living in such climates must eat more energy-giving foods and wear warm clothing to protect themselves from the cold. We have also modified the environment to meet our needs by building well-insulated and heated houses for cold climates and well-ventilated houses for hot climates.

There are many aspects of our interaction with the physical environment that are currently giving cause for concern. **Ecology**, the study of organisms and how they relate to their environment, is a major area of study in universities across the country. Many people fear that the delicate balance between human beings and nature is being disturbed. Assessing the ecological implications of large projects such as the building of hydroelectric dams is now a mandatory requirement prior to approval of these projects. We will discuss the environment in more detail in Chapter 11.

THE INTERPLAY OF FACTORS

In discussing health and the individual, it is impossible to separate physiological homeostasis from psychosocial

LOOKING back Alice Girard, 1907–1998

The first Canadian to become president of the International Council of Nurses (ICN) was Alice M. Girard, taking office at the meeting in Frankfurt, Germany, in 1965 and serving until 1969. As Canada's representative to this prestigious post, she was a dynamic leader. But this was just one of a number of "firsts" for this diplomatic, yet outspoken nursing leader. She was the first woman to be appointed a dean at the University of Montreal, when she became "doyenne fondatrice" (founding dean) of the Faculty of Nursing Education (1963–1972). She was also the first bilingual president of the Canadian Nurses Association (1958–1960) and she was the only woman named to the seven-member 1961 Royal Commission on Health Services.

Born in Waterbury, Connecticut, she received most of her education in Canada and graduated in nursing from the St. Vincent de Paul Hospital in Sherbrooke, Quebec. After several years as a staff nurse with the Metropolitan Life Insurance Company and then as a nurse assistant to a physician, she took a public health nursing certificate at the University of Toronto in 1939, a baccalaureate in nursing science from the Catholic University of America in Washington, D.C., and a master's degree in nursing education from Columbia University in New York. She returned to Metropolitan Life as the national director of nursing service. During her travels across Canada, she encouraged the development of municipal and provincial public health services, effectively putting herself out of a job as the company gradually decreased the nursing services it had offered for more than 40 years.

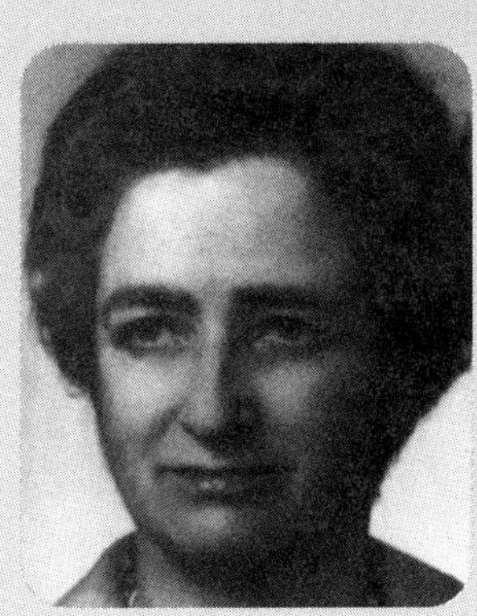

Alice Girard was then approached to help set up a university hospital at the French-language Université de Montréal. When political pressures delayed this project, she took further courses in hospital administration at Johns Hopkins University in Baltimore, then became Director of Nursing and, later, Assistant Administrator at St. Luke's Hospital in Montreal. In 1962, the Université de Montréal once again called upon her to establish the nursing program. She proceeded to establish not only a basic program but, in 1965, the world's first master's-level nursing program in the French language. She retired in 1973.

Always active in provincial and national nursing organizations, Alice Girard was named an honorary member of both the Ontario and Saskatchewan registered nurses associations and, in 1974, was honoured by the Canadian Nurses Association for her long and outstanding career in nursing. She received the Florence Nightingale Medal from the International Red Cross and is a Commander of the Order of St. John and Dame Commander of the Order of St. Lazarus. She has received two honorary doctorates from the universities of Toronto and Montreal. She is an honorary citizen of the City of Montreal and has been a member of the Order of Canada since 1968.

— *Glennis Zilm & Kirstine Griffith*

equilibrium and **environmental equilibrium**. Each affects the others. A computer programmer, for example, may be under considerable pressure at work. His or her psychosocial equilibrium may be disturbed by constant pressure at the office—but the hypertension that the programmer develops indicates a resultant disturbance in physiological equilibrium. On the other hand, when a person is physically ill, relationships with other people undergo a change. A person who is ill is less inclined to interact socially with others. The physical environment also affects physiological equilibrium and psychosocial equilibrium. A lack of adequate housing, for example, can be a major contributing factor in both physical and mental illness (Ambrosio, 1991).

Stress and Stressors

The late Hans Selye, a professor of endocrinology at the University of Montreal, is internationally renowned for his work on stress. He used the term **stress** to refer to the response to any demand, physical or mental, made upon the body (Selye, 1976). Demands of any kind upset the delicate balance of the human organism, which reacts by altering certain structures, processes or behaviours to restore equilibrium. A person may restore physical equilibrium, for example, by increasing fluid intake after perspiring profusely on a very warm day.

The term **stressor** is used to designate any factor that disturbs equilibrium. There are a number of ways of categorizing stressors. We have opted to classify them as physiological, psychological, sociocultural and environmental. Common stressors in each category are shown in the box on the following page (Selye, 1976).

Major Life Events and Life's Daily Hassles

The various types of stressors and the physiological and psychosocial responses to them have been investigated by many medical scientists and social psychologists over the years. A number of lists of stressful major life changes and the irritating, distressing and frustrating demands of everyday life (daily hassles) have been developed, along with rating scales to assess stress load.

The popular Social Readjustment Rating Scale on the following page, developed by Holmes and Rahe, ranks major life events on a scale from 0 to 100. The death of a spouse is considered to be the change causing the greatest disturbance in a person's life. Other stressful events include losing one's job, changing jobs, moving from one part of the country to

Potential Physiological, Psychological, Sociocultural and Environmental Stressors

Physiological

- drugs, poisons, alcohol
- heat, cold, radiation, electric shock, trauma
- bacteria, viruses, fungi
- poor nutrition, hunger
- pain, discomfort
- sleep disturbances

Psychological

- interpretation of events, perceptions, thoughts
- personal significance of events
- worry
- fear
- anger
- happiness

Sociocultural

- job loss or promotion
- conflict at work or at home
- loss of spouse
- interpersonal conflict

Environmental

- pollution (air/noise)
- earthquake, flood, other natural disasters
- inadequate housing
- crowding
- time pressures

SOURCES: Brunner & Suddarth, 1996; DeLaune & Ladner, 1998; Government of British Columbia, 1992.

another, or even from one neighbourhood to another, and changes in lifestyle. Happy events, such as marriages, getting a promotion, taking a vacation and even Christmas, also bring their stresses. If people have too many changes in their lives in too short a period of time, they may become candidates for major illness (Holmes & Rahe, 1967). Although the scale has been found not to correlate as significantly as originally thought to illness (Kobasa, 1979), it can be used to get an indication of the amount of stress a person has experienced.

Lazarus (1981), a social psychologist, was particularly interested in the effects of **daily hassles** on a person's health. He postulated that these daily stressors are more likely to cause illness than are major life events, possibly because the minor frustrations and irritations tend to accumulate to create a chronic state of stress. Lazarus felt that there are things in a person's daily life that help to balance these stressors, circumstances such as relating well to one's spouse or lover, relating well to friends, completing a task or feeling healthy. He called these buffers **daily uplifts** (Monat & Lazarus, 1991).

Social Readjustment Rating Scale

Rank	Life Event	Mean Value
1	Death of spouse	100
2	Divorce	73
3	Marital separation	65
4	Jail term	63
5	Death of close family member	63
6	Personal injury or illness	53
7	Marriage	50
8	Fired at work	47
9	Marital reconciliation	45
10	Retirement	45
11	Change in health of family member	44
12	Pregnancy	40
13	Sex difficulties	39
14	Gain of new family member	39
15	Business readjustment	39
16	Change in financial state	38
17	Death of close friend	37
18	Change to different line of work	36
19	Change in number of arguments with spouse	35
20	Mortgage over $10 000	31
21	Foreclosure on mortgage or loan	30
22	Change in responsibilities at work	29
23	Son or daughter leaving home	29
24	Trouble with in-laws	29
25	Outstanding personal achievement	28
26	Wife begins or stops work	26
27	Begin or end school	26
28	Change in living conditions	25
29	Change in personal habits	24
30	Trouble with boss	23
31	Change in work hours or conditions	20
32	Change in residence	20
33	Change in schools	20
34	Change in recreation	19
35	Change in church activities	19
36	Change in social activities	18
37	Mortgage or loan less than $10 000	17
38	Change in sleeping habits	16
39	Change in number of family get-togethers	15
40	Change in eating habits	15
41	Vacation	13
42	Christmas	12
43	Minor violations of the law	11

Life Crisis Categories and LCU Scores*

Category	Score
No life crisis	0–149
Mild life crisis	150–199
Moderate life crisis	200–299
Major life crisis	300 or more

*The LCU score includes those life event items experienced during a 1-year period.

SOURCE: Holmes & Rahe, 1967.

Ten Most Frequent Hassles and Uplifts*

Hassles

1. Concerns about weight
2. Health of a family member
3. Rising prices of common goods
4. Home maintenance
5. Too many things to do
6. Misplacing or losing things
7. Yard work or outside home maintenance
8. Property, investment or taxes
9. Crime
10. Physical appearance

Uplifts

1. Relating well to spouse or lover
2. Relating well to friends
3. Completing a task
4. Feeling healthy
5. Getting enough sleep
6. Eating out
7. Meeting your responsibilities
8. Visiting, phoning or writing someone
9. Spending time with family
10. Home (inside) pleasing to you

* N=100; items listed by frequency

SOURCE: Black & Matassarin-Jacobs, 1997, p. 24.

Stress, Distress and Eustress

Not all stress is unhealthy. Selye (1974) coined the term **eustress** to refer to "good" stress and used **distress** to refer to harmful stress. Other writers differentiate between necessary or appropriate stress (for example, the kind that makes one study for an exam) and unwanted, undesirable or excess stress. Existential philosophy suggests that, because life is constantly changing, stress is an integral part of life and, further, that "persons can rise to the challenges of their environment and turn stressful life events into opportunities for growth and benefit" (Kobasa, 1982, p. 6).

Life would indeed be very dull if we did not have some challenges. Boredom has, in fact, been called the worst enemy of wellness (Martin, 1993). Most of us like some excitement in our lives. Some people seem to enjoy a high level of stress and deliberately seek it out. Often they have high achievement needs and set themselves increasingly difficult goals. Sometimes referred to as **type A personalities** or "workaholics," these people often drive themselves to the brink of exhaustion by ignoring the need for rest and relaxation. Individuals who suffer from chronic episodes of stress are at risk of becoming ill. Selye (1976) refers to chronic stress as "dis-ease," which happens in the exhaustion stage of the general adaptation syndrome (see Figure 9.4).

The Individual's Response to Stressors

Each individual responds differently to stressors. Physiological responses to stress are modulated by the emotions attached to the stressor. This individual reaction is called the **stress response.** The physiological aspects of the stress response were first studied by Hans Selye who, in his early work, was looking only at the body's reaction to physiological stressors. He postulated first the *general adaptation syndrome* to account for the generalized reaction of the body, then the *local adaptation syndrome* to explain the localized reaction when a specific area of the body is affected. Although Selye's early work focussed only on the body's general response to physiological stressors, subsequent studies have indicated that the stress response is evoked by psychological and social factors as well as physical ones. More recent research has explored the specific physiological changes that occur in the body and the mind–body interaction that modulates the individual's responses to stress.

THE GENERAL ADAPTATION SYNDROME

In his research on stress, Selye found that there is a general response that occurs when the body's equilibrium is disturbed. He described this originally as the phenomenon of "just being sick" and later elaborated on it in his theory of the **general adaptation syndrome** (GAS). This syndrome, he believed, is the response of the body to any agent that causes physiological stress. The response may be divided into three stages: the **alarm reaction**, in which the body's defence mechanisms are mobilized; the **stage of resistance,** when the battle for equilibrium is most active; and the **stage of exhaustion,** which occurs if the stressor is severe enough, or is present over a period of time long enough to deplete the body's resources for adaptation (Selye, 1972).

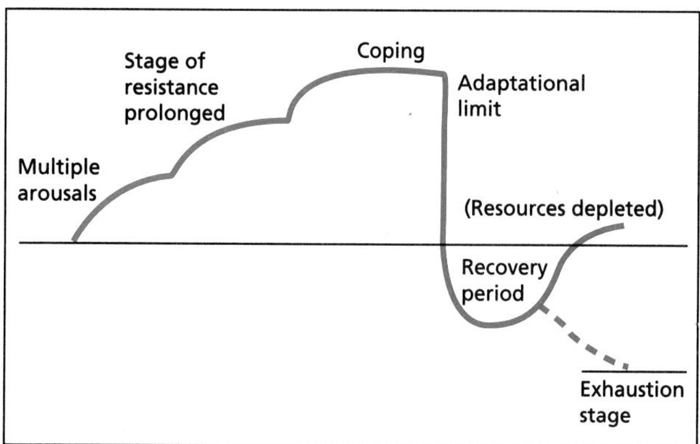

FIGURE 9.4 Reaction pattern in chronic stress

SOURCE: Murray & Huelskoetter, 1991.

Stage of Alarm Reaction

- initial reaction to a stressor when the central nervous system is aroused
- body's defence mechanisms are mobilized
- body activates physiological responses that prepare it for fight or flight.

Stage of Resistance

- body reacts and makes an effort to return to a homeostatic state
- if stressor is removed, body should return to homeostatic balance.

Stage of Exhaustion

- stressor continues and body is no longer able to adapt
- often caused by prolonged exposure to a stressor.

The Physiological Response to Stress

Stressor

↓

Stimulates the Hypothalamus

Sympathetic Response

- ↑ blood pressure
- ↑ heart rate
- ↓ gastric secretion
- ↑ pupil dilation
- ↑ sweat production
- ↑ rate of breathing
- ↑ production of blood glucose
- ↓ digestive activity
- ↑ catabolism for energy production
- shutdown of nonessential body mechanisms

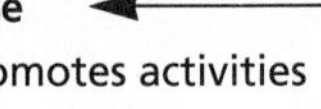

Parasympathetic Response

- rest response system promotes activities to restore and conserve energy
- provides opposite response to sympathetic system
- maintains smooth muscle control

The early signs and symptoms of disease are remarkably similar for many illnesses; this fact may account for Selye's original "just being sick" phenomenon. These symptoms usually include a slight rise in temperature, a loss of energy, a lack of interest in food and a general feeling of malaise. It is in the second stage of this syndrome, the "stage of resistance," that the signs and symptoms of the body's reaction to specific disorders are seen: a rash may erupt on the skin of the child with measles, or localized pain in the chest and difficulty in breathing may occur in pneumonia. If the stress is not relieved, or if it is of sufficient intensity to cause extensive damage to tissues, the body's adaptive mechanisms may not be able to restore equilibrium, and exhaustion will set in.

THE LOCAL ADAPTATION SYNDROME

In addition to the generalized reaction that occurs in the body as a result of stress, localized reactions occur when a specific part or organ is affected. Probably the most common example of a localized reaction is inflammation, which represents an attempt on the part of the body to barricade or "wall off" the area that has been damaged to prevent the spread of a harm-producing agent to other healthy sections of the body. Thus, if you prick your finger with a contaminated needle, you will probably soon have a swollen, painful finger. The finger may be very uncomfortable, but the localization of the inflammation will help to prevent the infection from entering the blood stream and travelling to other parts of the body (Selye, 1972).

Selye called this local reaction the **local adaptation syndrome** (LAS). It follows the same three-stage pattern as the GAS. First, there is a generalized reaction—in the case of a swollen finger, the whole hand becomes slightly reddened and a little swollen. This is followed by a more localized reaction in the specific finger, which becomes very painful, reddened and swollen. The inflammation will gradually subside unless the infection is sufficiently potent to overcome the defences marshalled to stop it. In the latter case, it will overcome the "barricade" and travel up the arm, spreading to other parts of the body.

COGNITIVE APPRAISAL

Evidence suggests that we become ill not so much from the presence of the stressor itself but, rather, from the way we react to it. As Selye himself put it, "it is not so much what happens to you but the way you take it" that is important in producing stress (1977, p. 35). Lazarus and Folkmann (1984) coined the term **cognitive appraisal** to describe this phenomenon. They suggested that the individual's perception of a situation as harmful or potentially harmful is the stimulus that triggers the chemical changes that occur in the brain and the body. "The brain appears to be the mediating physical structure between the body and the mind" (Black & Matassarin-Jacobs, 1997, p. 74). The cognitive appraisal of a situation involves both an interpretation of a situation as threatening or nonthreatening and the assessment of an individual's capacity to deal with it. Lazarus and Folkmann (1984) saw this process essentially as a transaction between the person and the environment. The process is as follows:

- Let us suppose that you are hiking up Mount Seymour and you see a brown bear on the trail farther up the mountain.

- The stimulus (visual image of a brown bear) is received in the cortex, the centre of logical thinking in the brain that interprets it as a potentially harmful stimulus.
- A message is sent to the limbic system, which adds an emotional tone (fear). The limbic system is a series of brain structures that influence both the endocrine system and the autonomic nervous system.
- A message is sent by the limbic system to the hypothalamus, which regulates the autonomic nervous system and sets into motion a chain of reactions to prepare the body to respond to the threat. Messages are sent:
  - to the pituitary gland that regulates hormones
  - to the medulla of the adrenal glands to release adrenaline and noradrenaline, which contribute to increased heart rate, elevated blood pressure, dilated pupils, palpitations and pain and tightness in the chest
  - to the pons in the lower brain, which regulates heart beat, respiration and other basic body functions.
- The hypothalamus also stores neuropeptides, the special proteins in the brain that turn physiological responses on or off in response to a stimulus and the emotion it provokes.
- The anterior lobe of the pituitary gland secretes ACTH, which travels to the outer cortex of the adrenal glands.
- The posterior lobe of the pituitary gland releases ADH, the antidiuretic hormone that causes the retention of water in the kidneys, thereby raising blood volume and blood pressure.
- The adrenal cortex releases corticosteroids into the circulation, including the mineralocorticoids, of which aldosterone is the principal one, and the glucocorticoids, mainly cortisol. Together, these have the effect of decreasing urinary output, increasing blood pressure and increasing the amount of sucrose in blood serum. In addition to raising blood sugar levels, the glucocorticoids increase fat in the blood, increase protein metabolism, reduce inflammation and reduce the responsivity of the immune system (Green & Shellenberger, 1991; Lazarus, 1991).

This is a rather simplified version of the stress response, dealing with the short-term effects of stress, which are instantaneous and extensive. There is a mobilization of the body's physiological defence mechanisms as the body prepares for instant action, either **fight or flight**. The heart beats more forcefully and faster, breathing is increased in rate and depth, blood is withdrawn from surface vessels and the viscera and is shunted into the muscles, the unneeded gastrointestinal tract goes into a temporary slowdown, blood pressure increases and the muscles become tense in preparation for action. This is the body's emergency mechanism, designed to protect the individual from real or imagined danger.

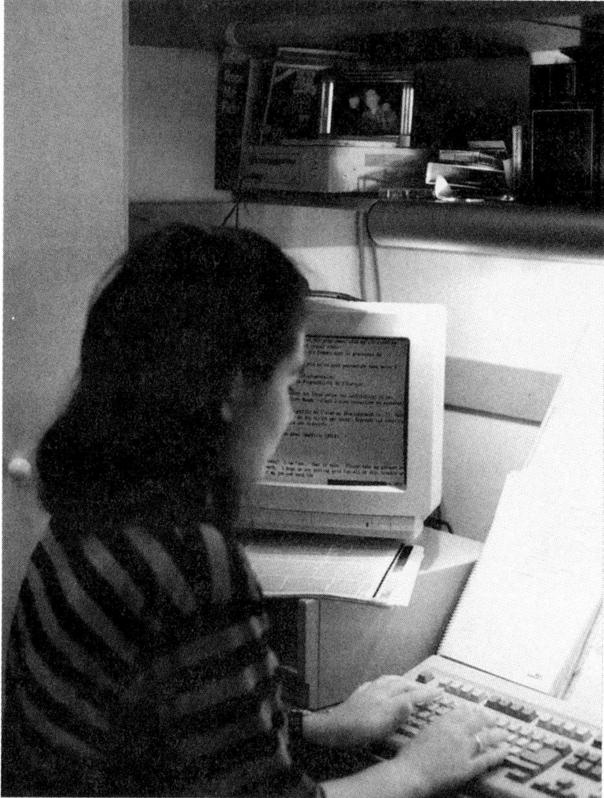

The pressure of writing term papers is a major source of stress for many students.

Manifestations of Stress

People react to stress in different ways. If you are having lunch in the cafeteria, for example, and one of your classmates comes along and says, "The mid-term exam results are posted," you may suddenly find that your appetite is gone. You leave your lunch until after you have seen the grade you received—and, if the grade is not up to your expectations, you may find that you still have no interest in eating. On the other hand, most of us know of people who eat to relieve tension. We also know people who chatter incessantly when they are tense. They feel they just have to talk to someone immediately about the grade they received. Other people just want to withdraw and be alone.

Reactions to stress are highly individualized. They include physical, emotional, spiritual, mental and interpersonal relationship symptoms. Everyone, of course, does not exhibit all of these symptoms. A person's reaction depends on his or her cognitive appraisal of the situation, on basic personality characteristics and on past experience in coping with stressful situations (Stuart & Laraia, 1998).

The physical manifestations may be readily apparent, for example, drumming the fingers on the table or foot-tapping, or they may be internal responses such as digestive upsets, headaches and fatigue. Emotional reactions to stress may vary from mild anxiety and irritability to profound depression. In the spiritual realm, people under stress often say that they are discouraged, or they may show lack of direction and express self-doubt.

Although mild stress may increase alertness, prolonged stress may dull the mental processes and the sufferer may complain of lethargy, of boredom or of feeling "spaced out." Some patients say their mind is "going in a dozen different directions" and they have trouble concentrating. Often people who are under a great deal of stress want to isolate themselves to work out their problems and they may be intolerant of others (Martin, 1993).

Coping Strategies

Lazarus and Folkmann (1989) define coping as "constantly changing cognitive efforts to manage external and/or internal demands that are appraised as taxing or exceeding the resources of the person" (p.179). The stress management process is two-pronged: first, to minimize, avoid, tolerate or accept the situation and second, to achieve control over the situation. The first is a problem-oriented approach to resolve the situation by doing something about it. The second approach suggests an emotion-focussed mode of attacking the problem, by relieving it of its harmful meaning and minimizing its impact on the body. For example, if you are worried about a mid-term examination coming up, you want to modify your anxiety (the emotional reaction) so that it does not overwhelm you. You will want to take some action to resolve the problem by taking control of the situation, for example, by setting up a study schedule.

The Emotional Buffers

All people develop individual coping strategies that work for them. Some of the strategies that people commonly use in their day-to-day lives to buffer the emotional impact of a stressful situation are well known to psychologists as **defence mechanisms**. These are often referred to as "mental mechanisms" because they represent intellectual processes, or changes in thought behaviour; we use them to protect ourselves from stressors that threaten our self-esteem. If people are frustrated in attempts to fulfill their basic needs, they usually become angry and may retaliate with aggression towards the person or object that is thwarting their goal-attainment. Open aggression is not generally acceptable in our society, and by the time we have reached adulthood, we have usually learned to control hostility. Adults seldom attack people in a physical sense, as children often do, but they resort to more subtle forms of aggression, such as verbal attacks, against the person or group of persons blocking them from attaining their goals (Stuart & Laraia, 1998; Boyd & Nihart, 1998).

If a person fails to gain an objective on the first attempt, he or she may try again, fighting a little harder this time or seeking alternative means to achieve the same goal. A person who wants to be promoted, for example, may not get the coveted position on first application. This person may then decide to upgrade his or her qualifications and enrol in an evening course to improve chances for the next opening. Such a person may decide to use every means available, fair or unfair, to get the next promotion. Alternatively, of course, he or she may decide to stop trying and move to a different company, or to settle for a less prestigious position in the same company.

If people have used socially unacceptable means to achieve their goals—for example, the executive who has ridden roughshod over others to reach the top—or if they have failed to achieve their goals either by withdrawing from the field completely or by accepting a lesser, more achievable goal, they must somehow find a way to protect their self-esteem. In order to make their behaviour acceptable to themselves and to others, they frequently make use of defence mechanisms.

RATIONALIZATION One of the most commonly used defence mechanisms is **rationalization**, in which a person gives socially acceptable reasons for a particular behaviour. A student who goes to a movie, for example, instead of staying in to study for exams, may rationalize the behaviour by saying that, after all, everyone needs a little relaxation.

DISPLACEMENT OF AFFECT If the individual later gets angry at the teacher for not assigning a high enough grade, the student may not be able to express hostility directly at the teacher. Instead, he or she may become annoyed with a best friend, or go home and take the anger out on parents or siblings. This is a form of **displacement of affect**, in which emotional reactions associated with experiences (affect) are not directed at the offending person (or object), but are shifted to a substitute. If the hostility is frequently directed at one particular person or group of people, it is called **scapegoating**. In a family situation, there is often one member, child or adult, who seems to bear the brunt of the other members' anger. He or she is the family scapegoat.

PROJECTION Oftentimes, we ascribe our own unacceptable feelings or attitudes to other people. We may say, for example, that somebody else doesn't want a group home for people with mental health problems in the neighbourhood when, in actual fact, these are our own feelings that we dare not admit to ourselves. This is called **projection** and is another form of defence mechanism by which we protect our feelings of self-worth.

IDENTIFICATION When people have not achieved their own goals, they may tend to identify themselves with someone who has. They may adopt this person's form of dress or mannerisms and suffer acute distress when their idol is attacked. Children, of course, identify with parents of the same gender as themselves, and this is a necessary part of their development. Students, too, will frequently select one particular teacher as an example of the person they want to become when they graduate, and then try to model themselves upon the image they have of this person. **Identification**, like the other defence mechanisms we use, is often very helpful in goal achievement (Stuart & Laraia, 1998).

COMPENSATION **Compensation** can also be a constructive defence mechanism. With compensation we attempt to make up for real or imagined inferiorities by becoming highly competent in a sphere of endeavour different from the one in which we feel we are not competent. The child who has poor motor coordination and does badly at sports in the early school years, perhaps because of growth patterns, may compensate by achieving success in the academic field.

Sometimes, compensation takes place in the same sphere as the inferiority. This same child may feel that he or she has to make good at sports whatever the cost in time and energy, and will practise night and day to overcome physical problems and become skilled at some form of sports. Such a child may choose a highly individualized sport where skills can be developed at his or her own rate, and become an expert tennis player, a ping-pong champion or a long-distance runner. This person may become a physical education teacher with an unconscious (or expressed) desire to help children with problems similar to the ones he or she had (Stuart & Laraia, 1998).

DENIAL When we have feelings or desires that we cannot accept consciously, or when we encounter problems that we do not feel capable of resolving, there are a number of defence mechanisms we use to deal with the situation. We may deny that we have the forbidden motive or problem and unconsciously refuse to acknowledge that it is there, in which case we are using **denial**. We may state, for example, "I would never do that sort of thing," when we may subconsciously be tempted to do just that. A person's first reaction on learning of a serious health problem may be to deny that the words they are hearing are true. Sometimes the denial persists for a long time, and the person has to work through the acceptance of the diagnosis before undergoing treatment. Denial is the simplest and most primitive of all defence mechanisms (Stuart & Laraia, 1998).

REACTION FORMATION At times, a person may attempt to remove a subconscious, and forbidden, motive or desire by vigorously attacking it. Witness the ex-smoker who denounces the evils of smoking to those who are still smoking. The person who jokes about unacceptable feelings—for example, fear—thereby gives the impression that only the weak are afraid, and that he or she certainly is not. Such behaviours as proclaiming too loudly against other people's sins and temptations and joking about unacceptable feelings or actions are termed **reaction formation** (Boyd & Nihart, 1998).

SUBLIMATION Socially unacceptable motives are, however, often channelled into acceptable forms of behaviour. This is called **sublimation**. A person may sublimate strong aggressive feelings by participating in sports where these feelings are acceptable, for example, football, where kicking the ball and attacking opponents physically are within the rules of the game (Boyd & Nihart, 1998).

REPRESSION When we have problems that we cannot resolve or experiences we would prefer to forget, we may unconsciously put them out of our minds; this is called **repression**. Without knowing we are doing so, we forget all about the appointment we do not want to keep, or completely eliminate from our minds all memory of unpleasant events. This has sometimes been called the "old oaken bucket" phenomenon, from the song in which fond memories of the songwriter's childhood are recalled. Unpleasant memories, for most of us, are often removed from memory by the subconscious mechanism of repression, the primary ego defence mechanism (Stuart & Laraia, 1998).

SUPPRESSION If, however, we consciously decide to forget about something, the behaviour is called **suppression**. An example of suppression is Scarlett O'Hara in *Gone With the Wind*, saying "Tomorrow is another day," clearly putting off focussing on her present problems (Stuart & Laraia, 1998).

FANTASY Most of us use **fantasy** in the form of daydreaming to escape temporarily from the realities of our everyday problems. In fantasy we can indulge our secret desires, achieve our goals and forget our troubles. Daydreaming can, of course, be very productive. When lost in reverie, we may work out the solution to an apparently impossible problem or develop long-range plans to achieve our goals; sometimes it is very difficult to separate thoughtful reverie from unproductive daydreaming (Boyd & Nihart, 1998).

REGRESSION On occasion, in attempting to reach our goals, we may revert to a form of behaviour that was acceptable at one stage of our development but is no longer considered appropriate. The expression "you are acting like a child" succinctly describes this type of mental mechanism, which is called **regression**. People, when they are ill, are often forced to sacrifice their independence in regard to caring for themselves. Having someone else do for them the things they are accustomed to doing, such as feeding or bathing, is often seen as a form of regression to an earlier dependent stage of development (Stuart & Laraia, 1998).

SOMATIZATION Emotional discomfort or psychosocial stress, rather than being expressed openly, is often channelled into bodily symptoms or physical language. This behaviour is called **somatization.** The child who does not want to go to school because some bigger children are bullying him or her on the schoolground may develop a stomachache, which offers a legitimate excuse for not going to school. The stomachache is real; the child may vomit and have diarrhea, but its cause is emotional. Sometimes, somatization involves both vocal expression of emotion and body language, as when you hold your nose and turn away from a disgusting sight (Boyd & Nihart, 1998).

THE USEFULNESS OF DEFENCE MECHANISMS

Psychological defence mechanisms serve a useful purpose. They help to reduce the anxieties caused by conflicts or frustration in our attempts to fulfill basic needs; they help us to maintain our equilibrium. If, however, defence mechanisms are overused, or used inappropriately, illness may ensue. As with disturbances of physiological functioning, abnormalities in the use of defence mechanisms may be viewed as quantitative changes that blend imperceptibly into one another and into the normal.

Measures to Minimize the Stress Response

As we noted in talking about the cognitive appraisal of stress, a number of physiological reactions are triggered in the stress response, including elevated blood pressure, increased heart rate and other manifestations to prepare the body for emergency action. If the stress is prolonged, these manifestations become destructive and render the person vulnerable to serious illness, such as a stroke (cerebrovascular accident) or a heart attack (myocardial infarction), to name just two of the many stress-related illnesses. Activities that are particularly useful in helping to minimize the harmful effects of stress are physical activities and exercise. Exercise can release much of the muscle tension and generalized physical readiness to "fight or flight" that accumulates when the stress response is prolonged (Charlesworth & Nathan, 1984). Often a brisk walk is enough to lower stress level after a difficult day. Many people find physical fitness activities helpful, for example, a workout at the gym. Other activities many people enjoy are swimming, cycling, dancing, gardening and games such as tennis, volleyball and basketball, all of which are good tension-reducers. As students, you will want to ensure that you take time to engage in a regular program of physical activity to relieve the stresses of studying (Boyd & Nihart, 1998).

There are also specific *relaxation techniques*, such as meditation, deep breathing, progressive relaxation, massage and biofeedback training, which are all widely used today to combat stress. Some relaxation techniques, such as deep breathing and progressive relaxation, are incorporated into physical fitness programs for people of all ages. Stress has been called the disease of the 90s, and we are all beginning to appreciate the importance of learning to relax to preserve well-being (Martin, 1993; Green & Shellenberger, 1991; Boyd & Nihart, 1998).

Emotional Buffers—Psychological Defence Mechanisms

- Rationalization: giving socially acceptable reasons to defend one's actions
- Displacement: the type of behaviour in which one transfers anger at one person to another person or object
- Projection: ascribing one's own unacceptable feelings to others
- Identification: modelling oneself on a successful person
- Compensation: overachieving in the same sphere or one different from that in which we feel inferior
- Denial: refusal to acknowledge a threat
- Reaction formation: protesting too much against something for which one secretly yearns
- Sublimation: channelling socially unacceptable motives into acceptable forms of behaviour
- Repression: unconsciously forgetting that which we do not want to remember
- Suppression: deliberately putting something unpleasant out of one's mind
- Fantasy: daydreaming
- Somatization: expression of emotional and psychosocial discomfort through physical symptoms or body language

NEGATIVE COPERS

Some people choose ineffective coping strategies, which have been called **negative copers**. Some of these are listed here:

- Physical: smoking tobacco, using drugs (caffeine, alcohol, tranquillizers, sedatives, etc.), overeating (fats, sugars, etc.), overspending, becoming physically ill
- Mental: blaming, criticizing (self or others), punishing
- Emotional: throwing a tantrum, taking revenge, worrying, becoming stubborn, sulking, pouting, becoming depressed
- Social: fighting, abusing, withdrawing, being passive
- Spiritual: blaming God, withdrawing (Tubesing, 1983).

HEALTHY COPING STRATEGIES

Rosenbaum (1983) has suggested that there is a learned repertoire of skills that people use to regulate their lives and overcome the stresses of life. He coined the term **learned resourcefulness** to cover this repertoire of skills, which he felt was a major factor in health and wellness. They include (1) cognitive coping skills, (2) problem-solving skills, (3) delayed gratification and (4) self-efficacy.

COGNITIVE COPING SKILLS These skills are the mental processes used to regulate the emotional and physiological responses to stress by attempting to see at least some part of a stressful situation in a positive way (Martin, 1993). They include using positive imagery and positive thoughts, setting positive expectations for oneself and engaging in positive

LOOKING back

Lyle Morrison Creelman, b. 1908

Canada's first nurse to serve with the World Health Organization (WHO) was Lyle Morrison Creelman, whose dedication to health for all at the international level remains an inspiration to Canadian nurses two generations later. In 1950, she was invited to become a nursing consultant in maternal and child health in WHO's newly formed Nursing Unit and, in 1954, she became WHO's second Chief Nursing Officer, a position she held until her retirement in 1968.

Her international role began at the end of World War II, when she was invited by the United Nations Relief and Rehabilitation Administration (UNRRA) to be chief nurse in the British Zone of occupied Germany. Her job was to organize nursing services to help care for millions of people of many nationalities who had been displaced during the war. After an intense two-year period in this work, she returned to working with public health services in British Columbia.

Born in Nova Scotia, she moved with her family to British Columbia as a child. Her first brief career was as a teacher, but when she graduated from the nursing program at the University of British Columbia in 1936, she immediately entered the pubic health sector. A Rockefeller scholarship in 1938 took her to Teachers College at Columbia University in New York for a master's degree. During the early 1940s, she worked with Metropolitan Health in Vancouver, first as a supervisor then as director, and served on the board of directors and as President of the Registered Nurses Association of British Columbia. Following her work with UNRRA, she was the field director for an extensive study of public health services in Canada conducted by the Canadian Public Health Association and was co-author, with Dr. J.H. Baillie, of a highly acclaimed report used for many years as a reference for public health professionals in Canada.

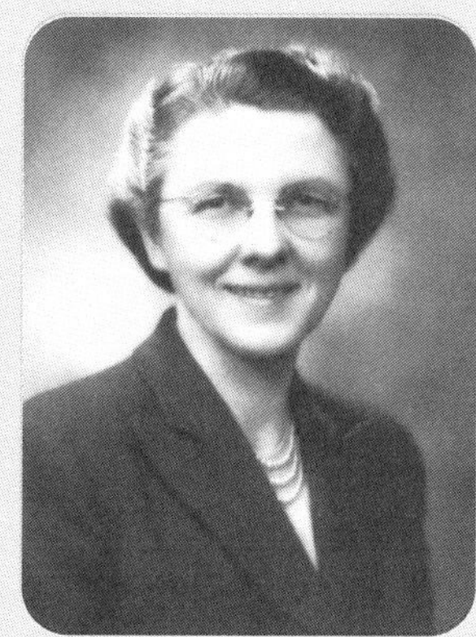

During her work with WHO, she visited many countries and collaborated with nurses from many nations. She also recruited many well-prepared nurses to initiate international projects that could later be carried on independently by the host country. She recognized the importance of national self-sufficiency in health care and used her superb administrative abilities to put this philosophy into practice. She was a frequent advisor to the International Council of Nurses and on her retirement from WHO, an editorial in *ICN Calling* recognized her many contributions, stating: "In these fourteen years, she has probably achieved more for nursing throughout the world than any other nurse of her time."

Following her retirement, she was commissioned by WHO to help study maternal and child health services in South-East Asia. Although she now lives quietly, she continues to be consulted by visitors from other countries. She has received many tributes, including recognition from nurses associations at provincial, national and international levels and honorary doctorates from the universities of British Columbia and New Brunswick. The Government of Canada awarded her the Canada Centennial Medal and the Medal of Service – Canada, and she is a member of the Order of Canada.

— *Glennis Zilm*

self-talk. For example, regarding the mid-term exam you are worried about, you might say to yourself, "I am going to get an 'A'" or "I can do it if I try"—expressions that include both a positive expectation and some positive thinking. Your chances of being successful in achieving the grade you desire will be much better than if you had started with the negative "That teacher never gives me better than a 'C+' anyway, so why should I bother trying?" Indeed, negative thinking hinders achievement (Green & Shellenberger, 1991; Martin, 1993).

PROBLEM-SOLVING SKILLS Problem-solving skills include being able to:

1. acknowledge that a problem exists and assess its dimensions
2. plan a course of action
   a) identify possible alternative courses to resolve the problem
   b) anticipate the possible consequences of carrying out each of these alternative courses of action
   c) select one course of action that would best resolve the problem with the most beneficial and least harmful consequences
3. implement the plan
4. evaluate the results of your action
5. if necessary, revise the plan and try again (Green & Shellenberger, 1991; Martin, 1993).

DELAYED GRATIFICATION **Delayed gratification** is the ability to put off immediate rewards in order to achieve long-term goals. You have probably all learned to do this in order to enter the school of nursing. For example, you probably denied yourself the pleasures of spending all the money you made in your job in order to save enough for your expenses at college or university. You probably stayed in many nights to study in order to get good grades to meet the school's admission criteria when your friends were out socializing. The ability to delay gratification is essential if you are to achieve long-term goals; it is also important in health and wellness. For example, if you want to achieve physical fitness, you usually have to suffer a few minor muscular aches and pains when you start an exercise program.

SELF-EFFICACY "**Self-efficacy** is a belief in personal responsibility for one's own behaviour and in one's ability

Healthy Coping Skills

Healthy people use a repertoire of skills to regulate their lives successfully and to cope with the stresses of everyday life. Termed *learned resourcefulness*, these skills include:

- **cognitive skills—using positive thinking**
- **problem-solving**
- **delayed gratification**
- **self-efficacy.**

to influence events" (Martin, 1993, p. 324). One of the leading researchers in the field of self-efficacy is Albert Bandura, a psychologist at Stanford University in California (1977; 1986). He maintains that when people feel that they have some control over a situation, their efforts are much more likely to be successful. They will work longer and harder to get something done and they can successfully overcome their fears. The feeling of self-efficacy enables us to have confidence that we can accomplish what we set out to do (Green & Shellenberger, 1991; Martin, 1993; Boyd & Nihart, 1998).

Physical Health and Stress Resistance

People who are physically healthy are better able to resist stress than those who are not. In our discussions of stress and ways of coping with stress, then, we should not overlook the importance of physical fitness. To maintain good physical fitness requires good nutrition, a regular program of exercise, adequate amounts of rest and relaxation and the avoidance of known health risks. In this connection, our own personal behaviours and health practices are important. These behaviours include the choices we make in the food we eat, the amount of exercise we do, the amount of rest we get and the health risks we take or avoid such as smoking, the excessive use of drugs or alcohol, driving recklessly or taking unnecessary risks in sports.

Social Support and Coping

The Premier's Council on Health, Well-being and Social Justice in Ontario has said, "The support we get from family and friends from birth throughout life is an important determinant of a healthy long life" (1993, p. 18). Many studies in recent years have demonstrated the positive relationship between social support and good health. Social support has many dimensions, as we noted in Chapter 2. It includes our social networks—our family and friends, the people we work with and go to school with and a supportive community. Social support can also buffer some of the economic stresses and strains of everyday life, through such systems as national health insurance, Employment Insurance, Workers' Compensation and the Canada and Quebec Pension Plans.

Of all the components of social support, the one that has been found to have the highest correlation with health and longevity is the number of social ties that a person has (Green & Shellenberger, 1991). In Chapter 4, we discussed the role of families and friends in exerting a positive influence on health. Of particular importance in our discussion of stress and coping strategies is the role of family and friends in providing mental, physical and emotional support in times of distress. When something does not go well, it is to family and friends that we look for support. They can often help to relieve the stressor of its emotional force so that we are able to look at it from a different perspective. Frequently, it helps just to talk things through with a family member or a close friend. As you talk about the stressful situation, you very often work through the problem-solving process to find your own solution to a dilemma, or to allay your fears (see Chapter 17).

Much of the research on social support has focussed on the role of social support in directly protecting a person, and in serving as a buffer from the effects of life's stressors.

The Concept of Hardiness

Some people seem to be able to resist stress much better than others. They never become ill or collapse when faced with life's challenges; instead, they seem to grow stronger. The question of why some people are more stress-resistant than others has intrigued social psychologists and people involved in stress research in the health field for many years. Much of the work on stress has shown that there is a definite link between stress and illness. Studies by psychologist Suzanne Kobasa (in 1979, 1982, 1983 [Pucetti] & 1991), and by others, found low correlations between scores (Pucetti) on one of the popular social readjustment rating scales and illness. Indeed, some people had high scores and yet few illnesses (Kobasa, 1979; Neugebauer, cited in Green & Shellenberger, 1991).

In the course of subsequent studies, Kobasa identified a particular constellation of personality characteristics that helps people to stay healthy despite facing stressful life events

Promoting Stress Resistance

1. **Eat a well-balanced diet**
2. **Engage in a regular exercise program**
3. **Develop a regular pattern of daily activities for:**
    - **eating**
    - **sleeping**
    - **activity and rest**
    - **recreation**
4. **Avoid known health risks, such as smoking, excess consumption of caffeine or alcohol or the use of drugs**
5. **Develop a positive outlook on life**
6. **Practise stress management skills**
7. **Maintain your social contacts with friends and family**
8. **Maintain spiritual/religious connections such as:**
    - **prayer**
    - **meditation**
    - **forgiveness of self and others.**

Personality Characteristics Associated with Hardiness

- commitment: a belief in the rightness and importance of one's actions
- the ability to view change as a challenge
- a sense of personal control over one's life.

(Tartasky, 1993). She coined the term **hardiness** to describe these characteristics. Hardiness includes:

1. **Commitment.** This is a belief in the rightness and importance of what one is doing that gives a person a sense of purpose in life. People who feel they have a purpose in life are better able to make decisions than those who do not. The commitment may be to work, family, friends, religion, a political party, an altruistic endeavour or other major interest.
2. **The ability to view change as a challenge.** People who are hardy can turn change into a challenge. When faced with stressful life changes, they feel confident rather than helpless that they can handle situations.
3. **A sense of personal control over their lives.** This is essentially the same as Bandura's concept of self-efficacy. People who have a sense of having some control over events feel they can make their own decisions; they are not passive recipients of whatever life deals out. These people can incorporate stressful life events into their ongoing life plans. For example, a pregnant student in a master's program in nursing decided in consultation with her faculty adviser that, rather than drop out of the program completely, she would forgo summer school and also stay at home with her new baby (expected in September) during the fall term. She would then return to school in the winter term to complete her course work and her master's thesis. She graduated that summer—a little later than originally planned but with all course work and thesis completed.

If nurses have a better understanding of the concept of hardiness, then patients with hardy or less hardy personalities could be differentially diagnosed. As well, nursing interventions could then be initiated and tested to ascertain whether strategies to promote hardiness would contribute to the reduction of illness from stressful life events (Lindsey & Hill 1992).

The Personal Experience of Health

We all interpret our own health status according to a particular perspective. The way we view our health status tends to vary with a number of factors. These include cultural background, religion, socioeconomic status, educational level, experience, gender, role and situational factors.

CULTURAL BACKGROUND Personal perspectives on health are considerably influenced by social and cultural factors. In assessing a person's health, it is important to understand the social context in which he or she lives. All societies, as well as subgroups within these societies, have certain norms, or standards, with regard to health and illness. In some cultures, for example, obesity is considered a healthy and desirable state, whereas in others it is regarded as unhealthy.

The customs, traditions and mores of a society also dictate acceptable behaviours in regard to health. Individuals are expected to take all measures necessary, as approved by that society, to promote and protect their health. The beliefs about health and about ways of preventing and treating illness in other cultures do not always coincide with those of Western medicine. In the culture of First Nations people, for example, a healthy individual is seen as one who is in harmony, or balance, with the universe. The traditional Oriental medicine belief in the principles of Yin and Yang is also based on a theory of balance. Differing health beliefs and practices are discussed in Chapter 12.

RELIGION In many cultures, health behaviours are closely intertwined with religious beliefs and practices. Many religious groups hold strong beliefs about a number of things that affect a person's health. Some have strict dietary rules, for example, that forbid the use of tea, coffee or other beverages containing caffeine. Many prohibit the eating of pork. In some religions, the giving or receiving of organ transplants is not permitted. Some religions, for example, the Roman Catholic Church, prohibit abortion and permit only natural contraceptive methods. A belief about the cause of illness common to many religions is that the afflicted individual is being punished for his or her sins. This belief will, of course, affect a person's reaction to illness. Such people may feel guilty about being sick, or feel that they have to atone for their sins through suffering. They sometimes may feel that they do not deserve to get better. Some religious sects believe in the total efficacy of prayer to help the individual either overcome or accept illness, and do not believe in intervention by physicians or other health practitioners. We will discuss the intertwining of religious and health beliefs in more detail in Chapter 12.

SOCIOECONOMIC STATUS AND LEVEL OF EDUCATION Socioeconomic status (SES) influences the way people perceive their health, as does their level of educational attainment. People in higher socioeconomic brackets are usually much more knowledgeable about the signs and symptoms of illness than are people in lower socioeconomic brackets. They are also much more inclined to seek the help of a health professional on the basis of symptoms. People in lower socioeconomic groups are just as concerned about health as those in higher socioeconomic groups, but often they lack knowledge about health and about the services available. Often, they do not trust the prevailing health care system.

Sociologists point out that there is a wide social gap between physicians, who are at the top of the socioeconomic scale, and most of their patients. This social disparity makes it difficult to achieve the "partner" relationship that is being advocated today (Grant, 1988; Epp, 1986).

AGE Age has a great deal to do with how we view our health. Healthy young people tend to take good health for granted and often take more risks than older people do. Older people usually value health as one of the most important assets in life, but they do not expect to enjoy the same level of health as they did when they were younger. The findings of Canada's Health Promotion Survey indicated that older people are much more likely to engage in positive health promotion practices than are younger people. Older people are more likely to eat breakfast regularly, less likely to smoke or drink excessively, less likely to drink and drive and more likely to use seat belts (Government of Canada, 1989).

GENDER In most cultures, men are not encouraged to express pain as much as women are permitted to; hence, they may tend to ignore the early signs and symptoms of illness. Women may have more access to health-related information as they are often the ones who attend well-baby clinics and other health sessions. It is usually the mother in the family who sets the tone for health care, and her attitudes and practices greatly influence those of her children.

SITUATIONAL FACTORS Situational factors also play a role in the perception of health. The mother in a family, for example, frequently does not become ill, even when one after another of the children, and the father, take to their beds with a cold or the flu; she is literally too busy looking after everyone else to become ill. Often, it is after a crisis is past that a person succumbs to illness, when the stresses and strains that have forced the body to maintain its healthy status have subsided and the individual has time to rest.

CRITERIA FOR JUDGING HEALTH

We all have our own standards for assessing the state of our health. The World Health Organization defines health as a dimension of our "quality of life"—a resource for everyday living that enables people to satisfy their needs, achieve their aspirations and cope with the environment (1984). Indeed, people tend to view their health mainly in terms of the way they feel and their ability to carry out their daily activities. In Canada's Health Promotion Survey of noninstitutionalized adults over the age of 15 years (1985), respondents were asked to rate their health on four measures: (1) their perceptions of their health status vis-à-vis that of others of their age, (2) their health-related activity limitations, (3) their assessment of the level of stress in their lives and (4) their assessment of their happiness. The survey indicated that most Canadians, including most older adults, perceived themselves as healthy, despite reported problems that limited their activity. Adults over the age of 55 tended to report lower stress levels than did younger adults. They were also less likely to say they were very happy and a little more likely to say they were not happy than younger adults (Government of Canada, 1989).

The Personal Experience of Illness

The Sick Role

Numerous studies have been undertaken by sociologists and social psychologists about the health and illness behaviours of people. There appears to be general agreement that health and illness behaviours are socially learned responses. Society has established acceptable and unacceptable behaviours for sick people. In most societies, the sick person is not expected to carry out usual responsibilities; for example, he or she can be excused from work or school. Usually, sick people are not considered responsible for their illnesses, although we are learning more and more about the role we can play in protecting our health. People who are ill are expected to take "appropriate" action to restore themselves to a healthy state; they are expected to want to get well. If they solicit help from a health professional, they are also expected to cooperate with the treatment suggested (Parsons, 1979; Bolaria, 1988).

Many of the studies on health and illness behaviours have focussed on the stages of illness. Some researchers divide illness into three stages, some into five. For ease of discussion, we have opted to use a three-stage approach, which includes: (1) the experience of symptoms, (2) the dependent role and (3) recovery and rehabilitation.

STAGE 1: THE EXPERIENCE OF SYMPTOMS

During the initial stages of an illness, sufferers may experience many of the discomforts that Selye described as "just being sick." They usually do not feel well, they may have distressing symptoms and they often find that they cannot keep up with their normal workload without tiring or, perhaps, cannot enjoy their usual leisure-time activities. People are usually irritable when they do not feel well. This irritability may show itself in tears that come at the slightest provocation or in anger.

People react to the early signs of illness in a variety of ways. Some attempt to deny that they are ill and "keep

Characteristics of the Sick Role

- exempted from usual responsibilities
- not considered responsible for the illness
- expected to want to get better
- expected to take appropriate action to get better
- expected to cooperate with treatment.

going" despite their fatigue, or may even try to do more than usual to prove to themselves that they are not really sick. Some people respond to the threat of illness with anger; others become very quiet and withdrawn. A few seem to enjoy their symptoms and the attention they receive from other people. The individual's reaction depends to a large extent on the way the person perceives the situation and the social ramifications that go with it (Bolaria, 1988).

STAGE 2: THE ACUTE PHASE OF ILLNESS

The acutely ill have disturbances in all areas of functioning. If the problem is a physical one, not only are they physiologically in a state of disequilibrium; their emotional balance is also threatened, and their relationships with other people are upset. Physically, they are often weakened by the illness and simply do not have the strength to cope with the daily activities of living, let alone withstand additional stress. Individuals are particularly vulnerable, then, to assault by such stressors as shock, fluid and electrolyte imbalance, or infection. Particular care must be taken to protect the patient from further harm. Extra precautions must be taken against infection, and the patient's physiological responses must be carefully monitored to assess progress of the disease and the effects of therapy.

Mentally, the patient's energies are focussed on the illness. He or she will likely be much more concerned with bodily processes and will anxiously await the outcome of tests and examinations. The interests of the acutely ill are narrowed; the patient is much more concerned with the immediate environment than with anything that goes on outside that environment. Frequently, defence mechanisms the individual has found useful in coping with the initial stages of illness, such as denial, rationalization and repression, continue to be used. It is important that the nurse respect these behaviours and not challenge them. It is essential that the patient maintain integrity and a feeling of having some control over the situation. The nurse, the patient and the patient's family work together as partners to enable the patient to get better.

In the social realm, there are certain expectations that go along with being ill. For example, people are expected to stay at home and to cooperate with those who are helping them get better. They are also expected to assume increasing responsibility for their own care.

Acutely ill patients often find themselves highly dependent on others for things they used to do on their own. They may need help to bathe, to change position in bed or to have a dressing reinforced. They may even need help in maintaining such a vital body function as breathing. People who have been independent all their lives may find it difficult to accept this help, and the nurse will need to be very careful to ensure that the person is able to maintain self-respect and dignity. It is very important that the individual be allowed to retain a sense of control over the situation. Often, the patient's family can be very helpful during the acute stage in helping the sick person, and the nurse should support them in their efforts.

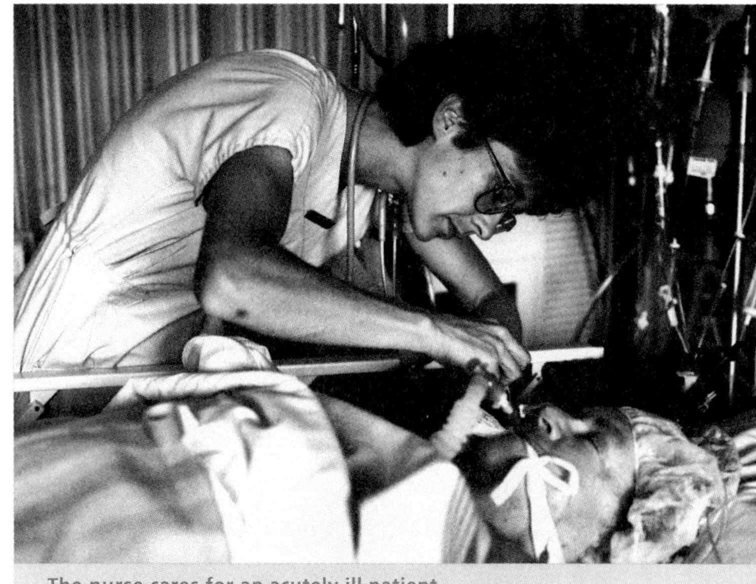
The nurse cares for an acutely ill patient.

STAGE 3: RECOVERY AND REHABILITATION

The Convalescent Stage

During the convalescent stage of an acute illness, the patient is recovering physical and psychosocial balance. Soon, he or she will leave the hospital and move back into the everyday world. This is a transition period and, for many patients, a difficult time. Most people recovering from an acute illness are irritable. Their strength has not fully returned, yet often new demands are being put upon them. Patients recovering from hospitalizations for such conditions as diabetes will probably have to adjust to many lifestyle changes. They may have to learn to give themselves insulin injections, to do various tests to estimate their insulin needs and to modify their eating habits to keep the diabetes under control. Often, people worry about their ability to learn everything they need to know to look after themselves. They may be fearful about resuming their normal activities.

The primary focus of nursing during the convalescent stage is to enhance the patients' ability to care for themselves. The nurse's teaching role is important at this stage. Not only must the nurse help the patient to gain new knowledge and skills; he or she must also provide the support and encouragement needed to foster a good learning environment. The patient's family or significant others are resources that should be tapped for assistance during the convalescent stage. This effort involves the nurse in working with the family, as well as the patient, and supporting them in their efforts to help. Many people require a lengthy rehabilitation program to restore their health to an optimal level. As we mentioned in Chapter 4, much rehabilitation takes place in the community with the patient at home, but there are

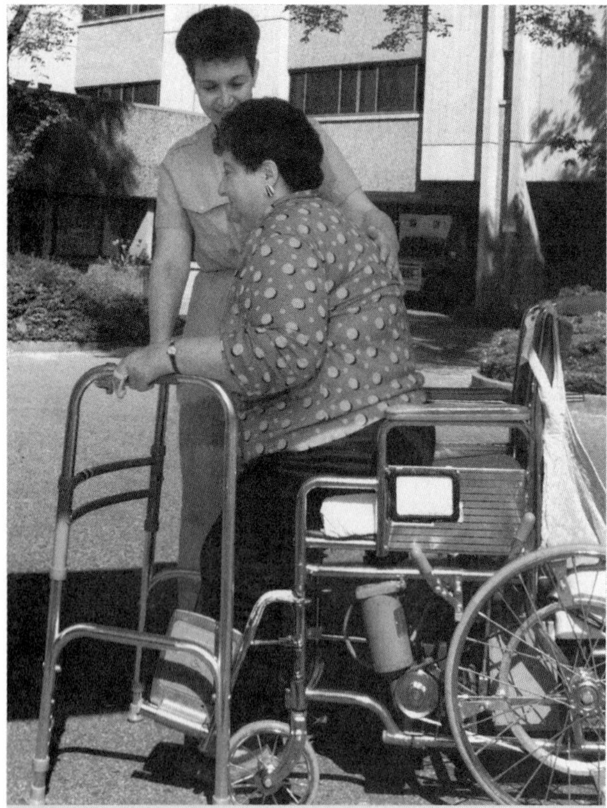
A convalescent patient learns to use a walker.

also specialized rehabilitation units—sometimes a unit within a general hospital and sometimes a separate facility—where programs are tailored to each individual's needs for physical and social rehabilitation.

The Stage of Restored Health

After the convalescent stage is over and the recovered patient returns to normal activities, he or she enters a stage of restored health. For people who have had a self-limiting illness, such as a bout of pneumonia or surgery to remove a diseased gallbladder, restoration to health ideally means a return to a state of balance in all areas of functioning. For those who have a chronic health problem, such as newly diagnosed diabetes, and those with a terminal illness such as leukemia (often called cancer of the blood), it means restoration to a state of optimal functioning for that individual.

All will, however, require continued supervision by health professionals to make sure that health, once restored, is maintained. The person who has had an episode of acute illness, with no residual problems, will probably need a check-up in a few weeks and then, perhaps, another in a few months to make sure that all is going well with the healing process. After that, he or she can usually return to a regular health maintenance program. A person with a long-term health problem will require supportive health care throughout the remainder of his or her lifetime—to assess responses to therapeutic regimens, to help institute changes as needed and to detect the early signs of any developing imbalance before it reaches critical proportions. The person with a terminal illness requires supportive care to help maintain an optimal level of functioning for as long as possible and to provide comfort and support for the individual (and family) as health deteriorates.

In the stage of restored health, the nurse's focus is again primarily on enhancing the patient's self-care abilities. Once the patient is discharged from a health agency and begins to resume normal daily activities, doubts and fears may arise. The person with diabetes, who was doing well with injections under the nurse's supervision, may lose self-confidence when he or she is at home, and require reinforcement of those skills learned while the patient was an inpatient. Convalescing patients may also need help in fitting an exercise schedule into their daily routine, or assistance in utilizing health information services in the community. For example, many communities have "Dial-a-Dietitian" services to help with any uncertainties about diet. The nurse should alert patients to the services available.

Today, many services in the community can help people with long-term health problems and those who have been discharged from the hospital—some still in the acute stage. We discussed a number of these when we reviewed the structure of health services in Chapter 4.

Sectors of Health Care

Helman (1994) describes three sectors of health care that are used by people in any society when they feel ill: (1) the popular sector, (2) the folk sector and (3) the professional sector.

THE POPULAR SECTOR

The majority of minor illnesses are diagnosed and treated in the home, which Helman states is where primary health care is provided (1994). Most people who think they are coming down with an illness follow similar patterns. They first try to treat themselves. People can buy a wide variety of medicines in drugstores to treat themselves. They may take extra vitamin C and drink more fluids. There are numerous folk remedies that are tried before further help is sought, for example, eating a clove of garlic to cure a cold, wearing a copper bracelet to ward off arthritis or taking echinacea to ward off the flu. The treatments people use vary considerably, depending on their beliefs about the structure and functioning of the body and the causes of health and illness.

If the self-treatment is not effective, certain family members or friends may be consulted who, primarily because of their experience, are considered good resources. Among them are nurses and pharmacists who are family members or friends, as well as people with relevant experience, such as a mother who has had several children. If the ill person has a long-term condition, such as diabetes or arthritis, he or she may consult with someone else who has the same health problem. Self-help groups such as the

RESEARCH to practice

Martinson, I.M., Liu-Chiang, C., & Yi-Hua, L. (1997). Distress symptoms and support systems of Chinese parents of children with cancer. *Cancer Nursing, 20*(2), 94–99.

The purpose of this study was to determine the physiopsychological reactions to the stress of Chinese parents whose children were diagnosed with cancer in China. The sample consisted of 89 families who had a child with cancer. These 89 families were then divided into four groups: group A consisted of children who were newly diagnosed with cancer, group B included children who were under treatment for cancer, group C consisted of children who had relapsed and were not expected to live and group D were children with cancer who had already died.

The parents were interviewed using a semistructured format. Interviews were conducted in Cantonese, either in the hospital or at home. The focus of the interview questions was the extent of reported colds, headaches, dizziness, loss of appetite and weight loss by the parents. The Parent Stress Rating Scale (PSRS) and the Parent's Support Scale (PSS) were administered to all parents.

The findings of this study revealed that parents most often reported symptoms of loss of appetite, weight loss and sleeping difficulty, followed by headache and dizziness. Colds were the symptom least reported by parents. Mothers experienced more symptoms than fathers. Fathers reported having more colds than mothers in the newly diagnosed group.

Parents rated the child's death as having caused the highest stress. Spouses received the highest rating for being supportive, across all groups.

This research identified a lack of support within the health care system in China. Previous studies identified that, within the Chinese population, emotions are suppressed by social conditioning. This observation gives rise to the following practice implications:

- development of childhood cancer foundation to provide support to parents
- development of educational materials
- development of parent support groups.

diabetes and arthritis societies are good resources. The leaders of such groups are usually very knowledgeable and a good source of information. In some religious sects and churches, people share experiences about their illnesses, as in some Pentecostal religions and spiritualist churches where there is a belief in "occult" or "divine" healing (Helman, 1994).

If self-treatment and remedies suggested by friends fail to cure, an ill person will usually seek the advice of healers from the folk or professional sector. Some of the specific situations that encourage a person to seek a higher level of health advice include:

1. other people calling attention to symptoms (e.g., remarking about a rash, a raspy cough or a limp)
2. the symptoms interfering with social activity
3. other people sanctioning the person's need to consult someone
4. the person perceiving the symptoms as threatening
5. comparing the nature and quality of present symptoms with those experienced previously or with those of other people indicating the need for further advice (Zola, cited in Bolaria, 1988, p. 7).

THE FOLK SECTOR (ALTERNATIVE/COMPLEMENTARY)

After the popular sector, people turn to the folk sector. This sector includes practitioners who deal with the spiritual world and those who heal by secular means. The first group includes the shaman (medicine man/woman or "witch doctor") and the "divine healers" of some religious groups, such as the healers of the Christian Science Church. The secular practitioners include herbalists; people who practise acupuncture, acupressure and other forms of Eastern medicine; lay midwives and others whom we discuss in Chapter 12. Practitioners in the folk sector have had special training in their fields or are believed to have been appointed by divine authority.

Although practitioners in the folk sector have been widely consulted in many countries for thousands of years, Western medicine has until recently been highly skeptical of these healers. For many people growing up in rural parts of developing countries where Western medicine is not widely available, folk medicine is often the only type of medical care they have known. Many recent immigrants to Canada from developing countries in Asia, Africa and Central America have brought with them traditional health practices and practitioners to whom they turn when they are ill. An increasing number of nonimmigrant Canadians are also turning to practitioners such as herbalists, naturopaths and homeopaths.

In addition to treating people with noninvasive techniques, practitioners in the folk sector provide other advantages. They usually use a more holistic approach than many traditional physicians do. That is to say, they tend to look at the whole person, rather than only at the problem. They look at social environment and interpersonal relationships; they involve the whole family in diagnosis and treatment. Usually, the practitioner in the folk sector is from the same culture as the patient and has the same social background, which can make patient–practitioner relationships more satisfactory (Helman, 1994).

NURSES at work

Case Manager, Continuing Care

Our aging population and philosophy of deinstitutionalization are changing the face of our communities and, as a result, the roles of community nurses. As a case manager (community nurse assessor) in the Continuing Care Division of the Ministry of Health, I help patients with chronic health problems to remain independent as long as it is possible for them to do so. Working with patients, I assess needs and plan how and what resources families and communities can provide. I use the services of health care providers such as home nursing care, rehabilitation services, home support, adult day care, respite or mental health services. I use these services in conjunction with community organizations such as Meals-on-Wheels, Handidart (which is a subsidized bus service for those who cannot easily use regular public transportation), community volunteer organizations and seniors' centres. I frequently link patients to the services of specific groups such as the Multiple Sclerosis Society and social, recreational and cultural resources. I also help patients access information about other provincial and federal government services that are available to help with their financial, housing or legal needs.

When patients and their families feel they can no longer cope, or when available home resources cannot meet their needs, I help them work through the difficult process of having to place a family member in a care facility. I provide information and counsel them about what care facilities might best meet the patient's needs. After the patient and family have viewed and selected a future home, I place the patient's name on the waiting list of the chosen care facility.

My patients range from 19 to 96 years of age. The greatest percentage of them are elderly women over the age of 80, who have minimal resources and supports. I help them learn to cope with physical disabilities, memory loss and social isolation. I have developed expertise in helping patients cope with chronic illness or disabilities such as strokes, Parkinson's disease, Alzheimer's and osteoporosis. I help patients to realize their strengths and personal coping styles or strategies. I also help them to use these skills to meet the challenges they face as they try to remain independent and live with dignity.

My role involves educating patients about their disease process, counselling them about lifestyle changes they might need to make. I help them access the services that can best assist them to cope and be independent. I am ever mindful of the potential for patient abuse and neglect. My practice is greatly influenced by family dynamics and societal expectations about women's roles as caregivers. I find that wives and daughters carry the largest burden for providing support and, thus, need to be proactive about their right to receive help to prevent burnout.

I frequently have to educate family members and other health professionals about patients' rights to self-determination and the right to choose how and where they want to live. I strive always to respect the reality of what the patient is experiencing and to see the person rather than the disease or the disability. I respect and support the choices that patients make. I have patients who have experienced ageist, sexist and racist barriers in their efforts to access services and health care. I am a strong advocate of my patients' rights to receive appropriate assessment, treatment and services.

— *Cherry Nettleton, RN, BScN*

THE PROFESSIONAL SECTOR

The professional sector is made up of the organized health care system. It includes physicians, dentists, nurses, physiotherapists and other health professionals.

Although some people use the folk sector to meet most of their health needs, not everyone does. The majority of people in Canada still turn to the professional sector when self-treatment and home remedies fail to effect a cure. Often, both the folk and the professional sectors are used; a person may take vitamins recommended by a naturopath and go to a physician for major health problems.

Admission of an Individual to a Health Agency

The changes taking place rapidly in the health care system across the country are having an impact on all aspects of care. The admission of patients to a health agency and their discharge from an agency is no exception.

ADMISSION TO A COMMUNITY AGENCY

In the community, people may or may not take advantage of health promotion services that are available. Expectant parents may register for prenatal classes being given by the community health nurse, but they do not have to do so; the choice is theirs. Similarly, with health restoration and supportive services, the individual has the right to decide whether or not to take advantage of them. Referrals for home care of an individual may come from any one of a number of sources: the physician, the community liaison nurse in a hospital or the patient's family, friends or concerned neighbours. Patients may also make the initial contacts themselves (Government of Ontario, 1993). Whatever the source of the original contact, it is important to remember that the patient has the right to self-determination. Unless the patient has been declared incompetent, he or she must make the decision to receive care.

Once this decision has been made, a case manager usually goes into the home to undertake an initial assessment. The case manager is most often a nurse but, in some situations, may be someone from another discipline such as a social worker. The case manager assesses the patient and the home situation, decides on the type and amount of care needed and makes arrangements for the various services. These include nursing, physiotherapy, homemaker services and other types of services, as described in Chapter 4. In

Services Commonly Provided in Preadmission Clinics

- clerk interviews for patient demographics
- nursing interviews/preoperative assessments
- diagnostic preoperative testing—blood tests, electrocardiograms, x-rays, respiratory tests, etc.
- screening of test results for early detection and treatment of abnormalities
- discharge planning
- patient teaching and support
- anesthetic consultations and medical examinations.

the case of nursing services, the case manager specifies the level of care required. For example, the situation may require a registered nurse to do dressings, injections or other interventions or, on the other hand, may involve only bathing and other activities of daily living, which could be done by a home support worker. Waring (1994) points out that "the responsibility for admission, discharge and the amount and kind of care [an individual receives] is held by the primary Home Care nursing and rehabilitation staff" (p. 24).

ADMISSION TO AN ACUTE CARE HOSPITAL

Patients are usually admitted to acute care hospitals through either the admitting or emergency departments. In the case of elective surgery, however, an increasing number of hospitals have preadmission clinics for people who are slated for day care, short-stay or inpatient services. The clinics serve as surgical outpatient units. People report to the clinic seven to 14 days before surgery for various administrative procedures, laboratory tests and preadmission assessment and counselling. Some of the services that may be included are shown in the box above.

Some preadmission clinics also admit patients on the day of surgery and prepare them for the operating room. They are transferred postoperatively to another surgical unit. The preadmission clinics have many advantages. Family members are welcomed. Patients and families become familiar with the hospital surroundings, routines and procedures, which helps to reduce stress and anxiety. Teaching sessions are a major focus in most preadmission clinics, and these also help to relieve anxiety. Patients are taught postoperative exercises and have a chance to practise them. Some units have generalized teaching sessions for all patients, followed by specialized sessions for specific types of surgery (LeNoble, 1993).

For people entering hospital through the usual routes, that is, through the admitting or emergency departments, there are also certain admitting formalities. Although each agency has its own admission procedure, there are some commonalities that the nurse will find in all agencies. The patient's first impression of a hospital is often formed in the admitting department. It is essential that nurses and other admitting staff treat patients as people of worth and dignity and do what they can to make them feel welcome. Hospitals are busy places and personnel are often rushed, but it does not take extra time to be kind or to convey welcome.

Staff in the admitting department usually explain hospital policy to the patient and/or family regarding personal effects and advise that clothing and valuables be sent home whenever possible. Specific information is gathered from the patient (or from the person accompanying, if the patient is unable to communicate). The information usually requested includes: medical insurance number and additional coverage; demographic data, such as full name and address, date of birth, next of kin, religion and usual employment; as well as physician's name and the reason for admission. Most hospitals have an admission form that becomes part of the patient's record. Most require patients to sign a consent form during the admitting procedure. This form usually gives the hospital staff permission to perform any diagnostic and treatment procedures considered necessary during the patient's stay.

After the admission formalities are completed, the patient is taken to a nursing unit. The reception provided by the staff here is, again, of the utmost importance. A sincere welcome helps to ease adjustment to the new environment. The new patient should be greeted by name and asked how he or she would like to be addressed. Nurses should also introduce themselves. Any family or friends who have accompanied the patient to the hospital should also be made welcome.

The patient's room or bed unit should be ready, so that he or she feels expected. The nurse admitting the patient to the unit should explain the use of equipment such as the call system, the bed controls and over-bed table, and, if the patient is to be up and walking around, show them the location of bathrooms and showers, as well as other facilities,

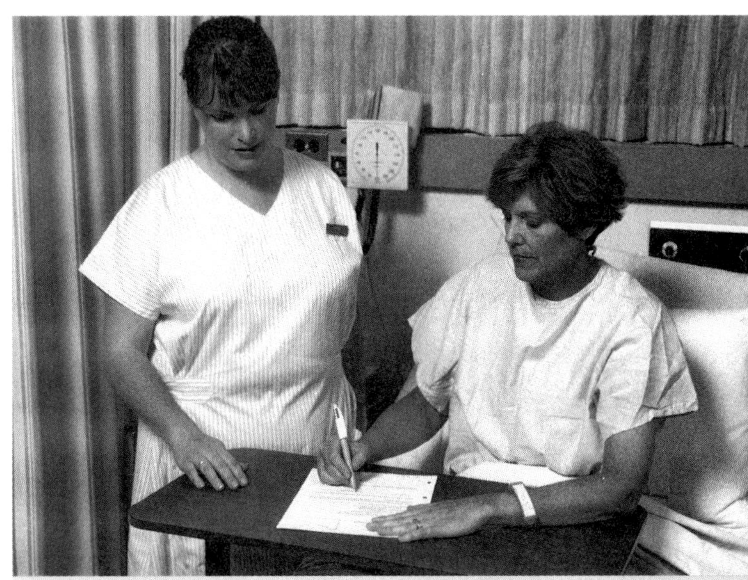
An individual signing a consent form on admission.

such as telephones and the patients' lounge. It is also helpful to give directions to the cafeteria or coffee shop, and to describe other services for patients and visitors. The nurse should also explain hospital routines such as meal times, visiting hours and restrictions on smoking. Many hospitals have patient information pamphlets.

Introductions to staff are important. All nurses who enter the patient's room should introduce themselves, and it is also helpful if the admitting nurse tells the patient who will be looking after him or her. If the patient is in a room with other people, introductions are in order.

The nurse should also find out if the patient has any particular needs or wishes that would make the stay in hospital more comfortable. A detailed nursing history will be taken later, but it is useful to know right away whether the patient has any specific dietary requests so that the dietitian can be alerted. If applicable, an allergy alert should be posted on the patient's record and entered into the computer file (if the agency has a computer-based information management system).

Once the initial orientation to the hospital has been completed, the patient is usually examined by the hospital physician. This examination includes a medical history, a physical examination and routine screening tests. In many hospitals, these tests include a urinalysis and routine blood work. The nurse should explain to the patient what to expect and who will be coming in to do the various tests.

Discharge from a Health Agency

Preparation for discharge begins with the patient's admission to an agency. Whether the individual is being cared for in a home situation or an inpatient facility, the goal of care is to enable the patient to take control of his or her own health. This does not negate the provision of supportive care as required; it does, however, mean helping patients to gain the knowledge and skills needed to provide this self-care insofar as this is possible to develop confidence in their ability to do so.

Hospitals provide a protective environment for patients, and many are genuinely concerned about their discharge. They wonder how they will manage at home. They worry about being a burden to their families and about their ability to contribute as a functioning member of the family and the community. Patients are usually discharged from the hospital when they no longer need the services it offers. If they need the services of another agency, such as a rehabilitation unit, a long-term care agency or home care, arrangements are made prior to discharge. Most hospitals have a nurse or other staff member who is responsible for making arrangements and coordinating the services needed by patients upon discharge. The social worker may also see the individual if there is a need for financial assistance or for homemaker service. Discharge planning rounds are held weekly by the multidisciplinary team. This ensures that all services are in place prior to discharge.

The Nurse's Role in the Care of Individuals

The nurse works in all phases of the health care continuum—helping people to promote health, to protect themselves from illness and disease and, if need be, to restore health in the case of an acute episode of illness or to provide supportive care in the case of long-term or terminal illness.

Nursing and Health Promotion

In keeping with the World Health Organization's definition of health promotion as "the process of enabling people to increase control over, and to improve their health" (WHO, 1984), the nurse's role in health promotion for the individual is one of helping people to help themselves to attain their optimal state of health and wellness. In health promotion, the nurse, individual and family work as partners, with the process based on the specific needs of the individual as they are perceived. Health promotion, then, is patient-driven, rather than controlled by the nurse. In health promotion, the nurse is a resource for the patient. In this capacity, the nurse may:

1. assist in procuring information. For example, in one hospital, computer programs are available for patient (and family) use in the hospital library so that patients can learn about their condition. This may include learning about the disease process, its possible causes, recommended treatment and home care. Nurses direct patients and/or families to the library to study these.
2. encourage patients to explore health habits and practices and to look at possible alternatives to maximize patients' potential for wellness
3. assist in making healthy choices from the alternatives available
4. assist in planning a course of action to implement patients' choices, if requested to do so by the patient.

Nursing and Health Protection

Health protection has always been a core component of the work of community health nurses, but it is an equally important part of the nurse's role in caring for people in inpatient facilities. The traditional role of the nurse in health protection in the community is to help healthy people to prevent illness through such measures as:

- the control of communicable diseases, for example, immunization programs for protection against those diseases for which there are known vaccines or other immunity-producing agents

- screening programs to detect illness in its early stage
- environmental safety programs.

The nurse is responsible for helping patients (both at home and in inpatient facilities) to protect their health by:

- maintaining their regular patterns of functioning. This includes a nutritious diet, good hygiene practices, normal patterns of elimination and sufficient rest and sleep to increase stress resistance. In so doing, the nurse helps patients to maintain normal activities of daily living insofar as this is possible within the limitations of their illness
- implementing measures to prevent complications such as infection, constipation and the loss of muscle tone due to bed rest.

Many nursing interventions for people who are ill are basically health protection measures—to ensure that general health does not deteriorate during the course of treatment for an illness. For example, someone who has had a fall that necessitates hospitalization with surgery to correct a fracture in one wrist may have difficulty using the other hand as well because of painful bruises and swelling. This patient will need help with meals to prevent development of a nutritional deficit. The hazards of bed rest are discussed in Chapter 29, as are measures the nurse can take to prevent these. Interventions to protect the health of the individual are included in the chapters dealing with basic needs (Chapters 20 to 37).

Nursing and Health Restoration

The nurse's role in health restoration includes not only helping a patient to recover from episodic illness but, also, providing supportive care for those with long-term or terminal illnesses. As we discussed in Chapter 4, health restoration services in the community blend imperceptibly with those for health support. To try to separate them would seem to be an exercise in semantics, rather than being helpful in the provision of nursing care. We have therefore not attempted in this text to separate nursing measures for health restoration from those for supportive health care.

What is more important is the reorientation of nursing care to a health promotion model that permeates all aspects of nursing care from health promotion and health protection through health restoration and supportive care. This implies that the nurse and the individual work together in a collaborative (rather than provider/recipient) relationship.

HOME CARE

The focus in home care is on helping patients and their families to learn to manage the acute, chronic, rehabilitative and palliative care needs of the individual. The case manager in the initial home visit and, subsequently, the nurses and other health professionals involved in care of an individual assess the capacity of the patient (or the family) to manage his or her own care or to learn to manage it. The nurses and other clinicians in home care work in a collaborative role with patients and their families, serving as consultants on health matters, rather than as "doer–providers" of care. They share their knowledge with patients and explain their professional perspective, encouraging patients to share with them their own view of their health and their health goals (Waring, 1994; Government of Ontario, 1993).

Waring (1994) describes the changing role of the nurse in home care with the Vancouver Health Department. In this home care program nurses act as case managers and are the "gatekeepers" to services. They are responsible for admission and decisions as well as the amount and kind of care the patient receives. The care focusses on health and health promotion. It is provided within a family–community context in which the nurse is "ally and consultant" to the patient, and the patient's family members provide much of the "hands-on" care. The nurses foster a climate in which the patient's ability to take control of health-related decisions is nurtured. To undertake their role as independent practitioners, Waring feels that nurses need a strong generalist clinical background and that they must be sensitive to cultural issues. At the time of writing, home care departments in British Columbia are undergoing major restructuring. This restructuring includes changes to jurisdictional boundaries, job descriptions and titles.

ACUTE CARE

In Chapter 5, we discussed the various aspects of the nurse's role, using Benner's "domains of nursing practice" as a framework (1984). These domains can be used to explain the nurse's role in health restoration and supportive care for people in an acute care facility. However, these roles are not limited to acute care.

THE HELPING ROLE The helping role involves helping people who are ill to carry out those activities that they would do for themselves if they were capable, such as feeding and bathing. It also means letting people make as many decisions and retain as much independence as possible. It involves helping patient and family to come to terms with illness and helping the patient to regain as much independence as possible and to take control of his or her own health.

THE TEACHING–COACHING FUNCTION People who are ill have many learning needs, and patient teaching is one of the nurse's major functions in acute care. We mentioned earlier the teaching sessions that are part of the preadmission clinics for surgical patients. Nurses on the nursing unit follow up on these, and incorporate other teaching as needed, as does the nurse who goes into the home on follow-up visits. People with medical conditions such as heart disease must learn to cope with their illness which, in many cases, means

COMMUNITY health practice

Using Humour to Decrease Stress in Home Care

Humour may be used by home care nurses as an intervention to relieve individual and family stress. Humour can help create supportive relationships and establish trust. The opportunity to share laughter with another can be an uplifting experience. Laughter can decrease stress, and has a measured physiological and psychological response—for example, increasing blood pressure, pulse and respiration. Humour and laughter can also be used as tools to increase communication. A sense of humour can assist the individual and family to cope with the changes that accompany an acute or chronic illness.

The use of humour, however, may not be appropriate for all situations; therefore, wise selection and use are imperative. The nurse must also be sensitive to language and cultural barriers that may cause clients to misunderstand an attempt at humour.

The therapeutic use of humour is not limited to the home care setting, and can be used by all health professionals in a variety of settings (Davidhizar & Shearer, 1996).

restructuring their lives. Far too often in the past, patient teaching was based on the nurse's perceptions of what the patient needed to know. The emphasis has changed to focus on the patient's perceptions, which are often quite different from those of the nurse and other health professionals. We discuss this aspect of the nurse's role further in Chapter 18.

THE DIAGNOSTIC AND MONITORING FUNCTION Nurses today are responsible for carrying out many complex diagnostic procedures. They also monitor the condition of patients in situations where highly technical equipment is being used, for example, in the intensive care unit. In order to carry out these tasks, the nurse needs considerable skill in manipulating equipment and in interpreting the readings on various machines (such as cardiac monitors), as well as the knowledge base required to take appropriate action when necessary. It is important to note, however, that, in the midst of all the machines and highly specialized equipment, it is the nurse who provides the human link for patients and their families, always remembering that the patient is a person, not an inanimate object in a bed. The nurse is alert to the feelings of the patient and family and sensitive to their reactions to all that is going on.

EFFECTIVE MANAGEMENT OF RAPIDLY CHANGING SITUATIONS People are unpredictable and, as you go about your daily work on clinical assignments, you will find you have to adjust your plans innumerable times in many situations. As you become more experienced you will learn to handle the unexpected with calm assurance and to take charge in emergency situations with skill and competence.

ADMINISTERING AND MONITORING THERAPEUTIC INTERVENTIONS AND REGIMENS People tend to think of the nurse as the person who gives medications and injections and, indeed, this is an important aspect of nursing care. Equally important, however, is monitoring the reactions of people to medications and treatments. Another aspect of this part of the nurse's role—which is receiving increasing attention—is teaching people (patients and families) to administer their own medications and treatments at home.

MONITORING AND ENSURING THE QUALITY OF HEALTH CARE PRACTICES In home care, the case manager coordinates all aspects of the individual's care. This concept is also being tried in the acute care hospital. The case manager is in an ideal position to monitor the care the patient receives from all health professionals. Every nurse, however, has a responsibility to the patient to see that they receive the best care possible. In doing so, the nurse frequently acts as the patient's advocate, speaking for the patient or interceding with others on his or her behalf.

ORGANIZATIONAL AND WORK-ROLE COMPETENCIES In the busy acute care hospital, the nurse needs good organizational skills. Often responsible for the care of several patients, the nurse must juggle several roles: seeing to patients' personal care needs, administering medications and treatments, monitoring the work of other staff and responding to unexpected interruptions and special requests from patients or families.

LONG-TERM CARE

Many people do not need the services of an acute care hospital but, because of physical or mental frailty or disability, are unable to function in the community. These individuals require long-term care. The majority of these people are older adults, most of whom require care for months or years until they die (Mantle, 1992).

Nursing in long-term care agencies has changed dramatically in recent years. Formerly patterned on the acute care hospital model, the focus was on physical care of the patients. Nursing homes and other long-term care agencies were essentially custodial institutions. Today, these agencies are considered communal residences that take the place of the individual's own home when he or she can no longer maintain independent living. A major player in bringing about change in the long-term institutional care field was Vera McIvor, who introduced the Priory Model in four extended care hospitals operated by the Juan de Fuca Hospital Society in Victoria (Du Gas & Beckingham, 1993). The Priory Model is based on the belief that the older person is still a unique individual, working towards growth and self-fulfillment, and that a therapeutic and restorative environment can be achieved if this attitude is kept in mind (McIvor, 1978). The Priory Model has become a standard for care of the elderly across the country.

In long-term care agencies today, people are called *residents*, rather than *patients*. As Mantle aptly describes it: "A primary goal of long-term caregivers is to create environments that facilitate healthy living and dying even though the residents are experiencing varying degrees of illness" (1992, p. 142).

PALLIATIVE CARE

Another term for **palliative care** is *hospice care*, a term derived from the original model at St. Christopher's Hospice in London, England. Both terms refer to the provision of humane, compassionate care of the dying. "It is the link between the needs of the terminally ill and their families and a staff that employs the medieval concept of hospitality in which a community assists the traveller at dangerous points along his journey" (Ebersole & Hess, 1998, p. 962). In this analogy, the dying are the travellers at a point in their journey along the continuum of life when they need the comfort and support of their community of family and friends, and the specially trained palliative care team. These teams may be community- or institution-based, with the individual often moving from one to the other as needed. The role of nurses in palliative care is discussed in Chapter 37.

IN REVIEW

- Systems theory provides a theoretical basis for examining the phenomenon of the individual as a human system interacting with other systems in the surrounding environment.
  - physiological homeostasis and psychosocial and environmental equilibrium play a role in maintaining an individual's balance
  - alterations in any one of these areas affect the individual's interaction with others
  - physiological, psychosocial and environmental stressors upset the delicate balance that is maintained in the human system.
- Stressors can be positive or negative and vary from minor to major in their effect on the human system:
  - a person who experiences many life changes in a short period of time or an individual with constant "daily hassles" may become a candidate for major illness
  - these stressors need to be balanced by interspersed uplifts
  - stressors in themselves do not cause illness; an individual's reactions to them can.
- Cognitive appraisal is an individual's perception of a situation as harmful and his or her assessment of how to cope with the particular situation.
- When danger threatens, a number of physiological changes occur as the body prepares for fight or flight.
- Stress reactions are individualized and depend on:
  - an individual's cognitive appraisal of the situation
  - basic personality characteristics
  - past experiences
  - previous coping strategies.
- The response of the body to physiological stress was described by Hans Selye. He referred to this response as the general adaptation syndrome (GAS). GAS consists of three stages:
  - alarm reaction stage
  - stage of resistance
  - stage of exhaustion (when the body has depleted its ability to adapt and can no longer restore its equilibrium).
- A local reaction to stress was described by Selye as local adaptation syndrome (LAS).
- Individuals use a variety of coping strategies to protect themselves from the emotional impact of stress.
- Some individuals are better able to cope with stress than others. Characteristics associated with a hardy (stress-resistant) personality include:
  - sense of commitment
  - ability to view change as a challenge
  - sense of personal control over one's life.
- Effective stress coping strategies (learned resourcefulness) include:
  - physical activity
  - relaxation
  - cognitive coping, problem-solving
  - support from family, friends.
- Ineffective coping strategies include:
  - use of tobacco and alcohol
  - withdrawal
  - worrying.
- Defence mechanisms are used constantly to protect an individual's self-esteem. They help to reduce anxiety and maintain equilibrium; however, overuse may lead to illness.
- Perceptions of health are influenced by:
  - cultural background
  - religion
  - socioeconomic status (SES)
  - education
  - age
  - gender
  - situational factors.

- Illness behaviour is socially based. Learned behaviours guide individuals through the stages of:
  - symptoms awareness
  - acute illness
  - recovery
  - rehabilitation.
- Individuals often engage in self-treatment when they begin to feel ill. If self-treatment is ineffective, individuals may seek other resources from:
  - the popular sector: friends, family, neighbours
  - the folk sector: spiritual and traditional healers
  - the professional sector: health professionals.
- Individuals may be admitted to a community health or acute care agency. Discharge teaching and planning begins during the admission phase and continues throughout the stay, with follow-up in the community.
- The nurse's role in the health of the individual includes:
  - health promotion
  - health protection
  - restorative and supportive care.
- In the health promotion domain, nurses work in partnership with individuals by helping them attain optimal health.
- In the health protection domain, nurses are involved in:
  - control of communicable diseases
  - screening programs
  - environmental safety.

  Nurses also help individuals maintain normal body functioning and prevent complications when they are ill.
- In the restorative and supportive domain, nurses:
  - carry out interventions to help individuals recover from illness
  - provide support to family when illness becomes chronic or terminal.

Critical Thinking Activities

1. Think of one of the most stressful events in your life.
   a) What physical signs and symptoms do you remember having?
   b) What emotional response did you have?
   c) What action did you take?
   d) Do you think you coped well?
2. What defence mechanisms are you aware of having used? What ones have you seen friends, family members or other people using?
3. Think of two people among your friends or acquaintances who have undergone a considerable amount of stress in the past few years, one who has coped well and one who has coped not so well. Compare the characteristics of the two individuals, using as a basis for comparison Kobasa's characteristics of a "hardy" personality.
4. Talk with someone who has had an illness requiring medical care in the past few weeks or has recently undergone surgery. Ask about their experience of illness.
   a) What made them think that they were ill?
   b) What self-treatment did they try?
   c) Whom did they consult in the early stages of their illness?
   d) What made them seek further consultation?
   e) Did they consult anyone in the folk sector? If so, whom did they consult? Did they try herbs or other remedies or treatments?
   f) What made them seek professional help?
   g) What professional help did they choose?
5. Discuss with a patient in hospital his or her thoughts and feelings about the admission procedure in the admitting or emergency department or in the preadmission clinic and about his or her preparation for discharge.
6. Talk with a community health nurse and with a hospital nurse. What do these nurses see as their roles in health promotion? Health protection? Health restoration and/or health support?

KEY TERMS

system p. 185
structure p. 185
function p. 185
subsystem p. 186
macrosystems p. 186
boundaries p. 186
open systems p. 186
closed systems p. 186
input p. 186
transformation p. 186
output p. 186
feedback p. 186
homeostasis p. 188
psychosocial equilibrium p. 186
ecology p. 188
environmental equilibrium p. 189
stress p. 189
stressor p. 189
daily hassles p. 190
daily uplifts p. 190
eustress p. 191
distress p. 191
type A personalities p. 191
stress response p. 191
general adaptation syndrome (GAS) p. 191
alarm reaction p. 191
stage of resistance p. 191
stage of exhaustion p. 191
local adaptation syndrome (LAS) p. 192
cognitive appraisal p. 192
fight or flight p. 193
defence mechanisms p. 194
rationalization p. 194

KEY TERMS

displacement of affect p. 194
scapegoating p. 194
projection p. 194
identification p. 195
compensation p. 195
denial p. 195
reaction formation p. 195
sublimation p. 195
repression p. 195
suppression p. 195
fantasy p. 195
regression p. 195
somatization p. 195
negative copers p. 196
learned resourcefulness p. 196
delayed gratification p. 197
self-efficacy p. 197
hardiness p. 199
palliative care p. 209

References

AMBROSIO, E. (1991). Poor housing, poor health. *Canadian Nurse, 87*(5), 22–24.

AUGER, J.R. (1976). *Behavioural systems and nursing*. Englewood Cliffs, NJ: Prentice Hall.

BANDURA, A. (1977). Self-efficacy: Towards a unifying theory of behavioral change. *Psychological Review, 84*, 191–215.

BANDURA, A. (1986). *The social foundations of thought and action*. Englewood Cliffs, NJ: Prentice Hall.

BARNUM, B.S., & KERFOOT, K.M. (1995). *The nurse as executive*. (4th ed.). Gaithersburg, MD: Aspen.

BENNER, P. (1984). *From novice to expert*. Menlo Park, CA: Addison-Wesley.

BERGER, K.J., & WILLIAMS, M.B. (1992). *Fundamentals of nursing: Collaborating for optimal health*. Norwalk, CT: Appleton & Lange.

BLACK, J.M., & MATASSARIN-JACOBS, E. (1997). *Medical–surgical nursing: Clinical management for continuity of care*. (5th ed.). Philadelphia: W.B. Saunders.

BOLARIA, B.S. (1988). Sociology, medicine, health and illness. In B.S. Bolaria & H.D. Dickinson (Eds.), *Sociology of health care in Canada* (pp. 1–14). Toronto: Harcourt Brace Jovanovich.

BOYD, M.A., & NIHART, M.A. (1998). *Psychiatric nursing: Contemporary practice*. Philadelphia: Lippincott.

BRUNNER, L.S., & SUDDARTH, D.S. (1996). *Textbook of medical–surgical nursing*. (8th ed.). Philadelphia: Lippincott.

CANNON, W.B. (1932). *The wisdom of the body*. New York: Norton.

CHARLESWORTH, E.A., & NATHAN, R.G. (1984). *Stress management: A comprehensive guide to wellness*. New York: Atheneum.

DAVIDHIZAR, R., & SHEARER, R. (1996). Using humour to cope with stress in home care. *Home HealthCare Nurse, 14*(10), 825–830.

DELAUNE, S.C., & LADNER, P.K. (1998). *Fundamentals of nursing: Standards and practice*. Boston: Delmar Publications.

DU GAS, B.W., & BECKINGHAM, A. (1993). The emergence of gerontological nursing. In A. Beckingham & B. Du Gas (Eds.), *Promoting healthy aging*. St. Louis: Mosby.

EBERSOLE, P., & HESS, P. (1998). *Toward healthy aging: Human needs and nursing response*. (5th ed.). St. Louis: Mosby.

EPP, J. (1986). *Achieving health for all: A framework for health promotion*. Ottawa: Health & Welfare Canada.

GOVERNMENT OF BRITISH COLUMBIA. (1992). *Health indicator workbook*. (1st ed.). Victoria: Office of Health Promotion, B.C. Ministry of Health and Ministry Responsible for Seniors. (Catalogue no. QP 91029)

GOVERNMENT OF CANADA. (1989). *The active health report on seniors*. Ottawa: Health & Welfare Canada.

GOVERNMENT OF ONTARIO. (1993). *Nurturing health*. Premier's Council on Health, Well-being and Social Justice, 1987–1991. Toronto: Queen's Printer. (Catalogue no. 01.93.20M)

GRANT, K.R. (1988). The inverse care law in Canada: Differential access under universal free health insurance. In B.S. Bolaria & H.D. Dickinson (Eds.). *Sociology of health care in Canada* (pp. 118–134). Toronto: Harcourt Brace Jovanovich.

GREEN, J., & SHELLENGBERGER, R. (1991). *The dynamics of health and wellness: A biopsychosocial approach*. Philadelphia: Harcourt Brace.

HELMAN, C.G. (1994). *Culture, health and illness*. (3rd ed.). London: Guildford–Butterworth–Heinemann.

HOLMES, T.H., & RAHE, R.H. (1967). The social readjustment rating scale. *Journal of Psychosomatic Research, 11*,(8) 213–218.

KOBASA, S.C. (1979). Stressful life events, personality and health: An enquiry into hardiness. *Journal of Personality & Social Psychology, 37*, 1–11.

KOBASA, S.C. (1982). The hardy personality: Toward a social psychology of stress and health. In G.S. Sanders & J. Suls (Eds.), *Social psychology of health and illness* (pp. 3–32). Hillsdale, NJ: Erlbaum.

KOBASA, S.C. (1991). Stressful life events, personality and health: An inquiry into hardiness. In A. Monat & R. Lazarus (Eds.), *Stress and coping: An anthology*. (3rd ed.). New York: Columbia University Press.

KOBASA, S.C., & PUCETTI, M.C. (1983). Personality and social resources in stress resistance. *Journal of Personality & Social Psychology, 45*, 839–850.

LAZARUS, R.S. (1981, July). Little hassles can be hazardous to health. *Psychology Today*, 58–62.

LAZARUS, R.S. (1991). *Emotion and adaptation*. New York: Oxford University Press.

LAZARUS, R.S., & FOLKMANN, S. (1984). *Stress, appraisal and coping*. New York: Springer.

LAZARUS, R.S., & FOLKMANN, S. (1989). *Stress appraisal and coping*. New York: Springer.

LENOBLE, E. (1993). Preadmission clinics gaining ground. *Nursing BC, 25*(4), 20–24.

LINDSEY, E., & HILLS, M. (1992). An analysis of the concept of hardiness. *Canadian Journal of Nursing Research, 24*(1), 39–50.

LOOMIS, C.P. (1960). *Social systems*. New York: Van Nostrand.

MANTLE, J. (1992). Nursing practice in long-term care agencies. In A.J. Baumgart & J. Larsen (Eds.). *Canadian nursing faces the future* (2nd ed., pp. 134–151). Toronto: Mosby.

MARTIN, L. (1993). Stress, distress and eustress. In A.C. Beckingham & B.W. Du Gas (Eds.), *Promoting healthy aging* (pp. 303–331). St.Louis: Mosby.

MARTINSON, I.M., LIU-CHIANG, C., & YI-HUA, L. (1997). Distress symptoms and support systems of Chinese parents of children with cancer. *Cancer Nursing, 20*(2), 94–99.

McCANCE, K.L., & SHELBY, J. (1996). Understanding pathophysiology. In S.E. Huether & K.L. McCance (Eds.), *Stress and disease* (chap 8). St. Louis: Mosby.

McIVER, V. (1978). Freedom to be (Part 2): The priory method. *Canadian Nurse, 74*(3), 23–26.

MONAT, A., & LAZARUS, R.(1991). *Stress and coping*. New York: Columbia University Press.

MURRAY, R.B., & HEULSKOETTER, M. (1991). *Psychiatric/mental health nursing: Giving emotional care*. (3rd ed.). Norwalk, CT: Appleton & Lange.

PARSONS, T. (1979). Definitions of health and illness in the light of the American values and social structure. In E.G. Jaco (Ed.), *Patients, physicians and illness* (3rd ed., pp. 107–127). New York: Free Press.

ROSENBAUM, M. (1983). Learned resourcefulness as a behavioral repertoire for the self-regulation of internal events: Issues and speculations. In M. Rosenbaum, C.M. Franks, & Y. Jaffe (Eds.), *Perspectives on behavior therapy in the eighties*. New York: Springer.

SELYE, H. (1972). Stress and the nation's health. In *Proceedings of the National Conference on Fitness and Health, Ottawa, December 4–6, 1972*. Ottawa: Health & Welfare Canada.

SELYE, H. (1974). *Stress without distress*. New York: New American Library.

SELYE, H. (1976). *The stress of life*. (Rev ed.). New York: McGraw-Hill.

SELYE, H. (1977). A code for coping with stress. *AORN Journal, 25* (1), 35–42.

STUART, G.W. & LARAIA, M.T. (1998). *Stuart and Sundeen's Principles and Practice of Psychiatric Nursing*, (6th ed.). St. Louis: Mosby.

TARTASKY, D.S. (1993, Fall). Hardiness: Conceptual and methodological issues. *Image, 23*(3), 225–229.

TUBESING, D. (1983). *Stress talk worksheet*. Duluth, MN: Aid Association for Lutherans.

VON BERTALANFFY, L. (1968). *General systems theory: Foundations, development, applications*. New York: Braziller.

WARING, J. (1994). The new emphasis of home care. *Canadian Nurse, 90*(2), 22–26.

WATZLAWICK, P., BEAVIN, J., & JACKSON, D. (1967). *Pragmatics of human communication*. New York: W.W. Norton.

WORLD HEALTH ORGANIZATION (WHO). (1984). *Health promotion glossary*. Copenhagen: WHO Regional Office for Europe.

Additional Readings

BOLARIA, B.S., & DICKINSON, H.D. (1994). *Health, illness and health care in Canada*. Toronto: Harcourt Brace.

GERDNER, L.A., HALL, G.R., & BUCKWALTER, K.C. (1996). Caregiver training for people with Alzheimer's: Based on a stress threshold model. *Image, 28*(3), 241–245.

GOTTLIEB, B.H., KELLOWAY, E.K., & MARTIN-MATTHEWS, A. (1996). Predictors of work–family conflict, stress and job satisfaction among nurses. *Canadian Journal of Nursing Research, 28*(2), 99–117.

HAMBLY, K., & MUIR, J.A. (1997). *Stress management in primary care*. Oxford/Boston: Butterworth–Heinemann.

HOLLISTER, R. (1996) Critical incident stress debriefing and the community health nurse. *Journal of Community Health Nursing, 13*(1), 43–49.

HUANG, C. (1995) Hardiness and stress: A critical review. *Journal of Maternal–Child Nursing, 23*(3), 82–89.

MOORE, S., & KATZ, B. (1996). Home health nurses: Stress, self-esteem, social intimacy, and job satisfaction. *Home Healthcare Nurse, 14*(12), 963–969.

PAPPAS, S.H. (1995). Creating an environment to support hardiness and quality patient care. *Seminars for Nurse Managers, 3*(3), 115–118.

STETSON, B. (1997). Holistic health stress management program: Nursing student and client health outcomes. *Journal of Holistic Nursing, 15*(2), 143–157.

Chapter 10

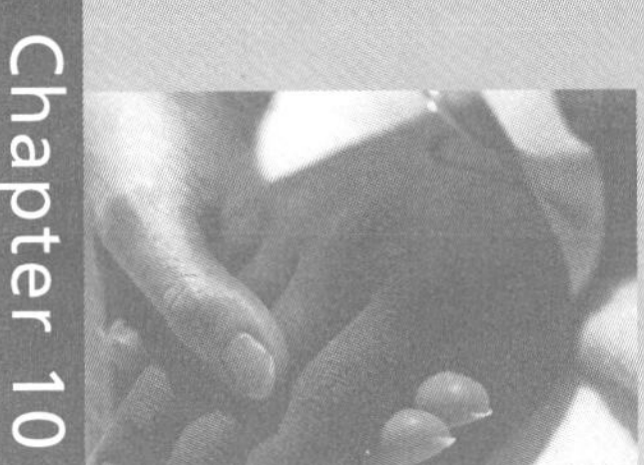

Health and the Family

OUTLINE

Central Questions

1. What is the meaning of family?
2. What is the relationship between health of the individual and health of the family?
3. What are the different types of family forms in Canada?
4. What are the theoretical perspectives of the family systems framework, the structural-functional framework and the family developmental framework?
5. How can nurses use concepts from the selected frameworks when working with families?
6. How does the meaning of family health differ from the meaning of health?
7. What are the main determinants of family health?
8. What are the criteria for judging family health?
9. What is family stress and crisis?
10. What impact does illness in a family member have on family functioning?
11. How is the family conceptualized in the three types of nursing practice with families?
12. What are the categories of the Calgary Family Assessment Model, and how is it used in family assessment?
13. What intervention strategies can nurses use in assisting families to promote and protect family health?
14. What intervention strategies can nurses use in helping families to cope with family stress and crisis?

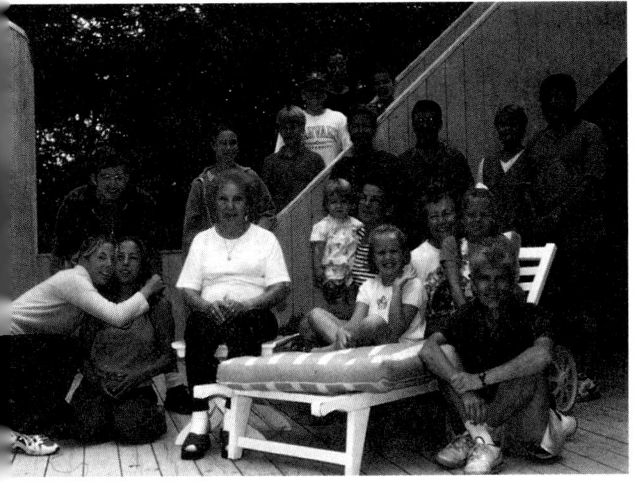

Introduction

Behavioural scientists tell us that few people can live in isolation. By interacting and associating with other human beings, we develop our personality and our humanness. Our initial interactions with others most often occur within the family. How we lead our lives, and give meaning to all that happens to us, is usually rooted in experiences we have had with our families. When we are in need of human support and affection, it is often our families that we turn to because we know that they will give us unconditional love and accept us for who we are.

In many parts of the world, the family is recognized as society's most basic institution. Consisting of individuals bound together by emotional ties and a sense of belonging, the family persists as the major unit for reproduction, socialization and the perpetuation of sociocultural traditions. As a social unit, the family is believed to exert the greatest influence on the growth and development of its members, namely its children. It is through the family that children first learn about the social world into which they are born, and it is with the family's continuous nurturing and support that they grow up to be productive and self-sustaining members of society. Children develop their sense of identity and self-worth, and learn rules of conduct, values and adult social roles, largely through the family. How we behave socially, our sense of self and our career choices are the result of family influences.

The family is viewed by some as a mediating agent or a "buffer" between society and the individual. It transmits and modifies social values, goals and expectations, and at the same time fosters the growth of individuals so that they will become capable members of society. Other groups, such as school, church or youth clubs, may also have a mediating function. But it is the family that provides transportation, lunches, proper clothing and footwear to ensure the child's physical well-being. In addition, the family fosters attitudes and values that ensure positive, productive learning behaviours (Friedman, 1998).

The family plays a vital role in the health of its members. Some health professionals believe that the family is "probably the most significant factor in the state of health and well-being of individuals" (Ramshorn, 1978, p. 248) and "constitutes perhaps the most important social context within which illness occurs and is resolved" (Litman, 1974, p. 495). The family is a significant factor in the health of individuals because it provides the physical and social environment in which health and illness occur.

A family's health beliefs, practices and socioeconomic capabilities influence the lifestyle and living conditions for individual members. It is difficult to maintain a healthy lifestyle if one does not have enough money to afford good housing and nutritious food. Individuals whose families live in poverty often lead unhealthy lifestyles, lack adequate social support and generally experience more illness than do those individuals who come from a family of higher socioeconomic status (SES). Poverty is a significant threat to health because it limits options available to the family for creating living conditions that promote health and prevent illness (Roberge, Berthelot & Wolfson, 1995).

The family is also a primary resource for its members in its ability to provide support and care. Family members care for one another. Parents care for their children, spouses care for each other, and adult children become caregivers for their aging parents. The support and care that a family gives to an ill member can be powerful factors in that person's ability to cope with illness and to recover. For example, educating a diabetic patient about diet would not achieve a successful outcome unless his or her spouse was committed to choosing and preparing foods that are low in sugar content. Individuals have shown that they respond to treatment and heal more effectively when they have the support of a caring family.

There is a reciprocal relationship between the health and well-being of the family and its members. The health or illness status of one family member affects all other family members, which in turn affects the health and well-being of the family as a whole.

Sometimes the family itself is at the root of problems for the individual. For instance, poor family communication and interaction may lead an adolescent to adopt unhealthy behaviours. In this case, care for the individual would involve an assessment of family dynamics and intervention for the whole family. Because of this interrelationship between family health and the health of family members, nurses often care for families as well as individuals. In this chapter we will outline the nature of Canadian families and discuss concepts of family life as a foundation for nursing care. Family health will be defined and described, along with family stress and the impact of illness on the family. We will present a model for family assessment, as well as nursing interventions for helping families promote family health and cope with family stress and illness.

The Canadian Family

There was a time in Canada when the word *family* was synonumous with an immediate household comprising a married man and woman living with their children or other kinfolk related by blood, marriage or adoption. This no longer is the case. Even though the family is the fundamental social unit of society, its form and character vary greatly throughout the world. Because Canadian families are made up of Canadian-born descendants of immigrants, recent migrants and First Nations people, family structure is diverse. In addition, a number of changes have taken place—and are still taking place—in Canadian society that are influencing family form. For instance, the women's movement, high cost of living, rising divorce rates, increased

LOOKING back

Sister Denise Lefèbvre, 1907–1993

The first Canadian nurse to obtain a doctoral degree was Sister Denise Lefèbvre, who received a Docteur de Pédagogie from the Université de Montréal in 1955. Although nursing education had moved into universities in Canada in 1919, a lack of advanced academic qualifications for nurses had plagued the profession. Without doctorally prepared academics, nursing could not achieve status within universities; and without status in the campus communities, the discipline could not introduce programs to enable nurses to achieve academic qualifications. Sister Lefèbvre was the first to break this cycle and pioneer the movement to doctoral preparation for Canadian nurses.

The first doctoral nursing program (PhD Nursing) did not open in Canada until the University of Alberta began enrolling students in January 1991. At that time, three "special case" students (Joan Bottorff, Joy Johnson and Paulette Paul) and one direct admission student (Ginette Rodger) were admitted to the Alberta program. The "special case" programs—with three students at McGill University and three at the University of Alberta—started in 1988. These programs were a direct result of strong lobbying by the nursing profession to ensure that doctoral education in nursing was finally available in Canada.

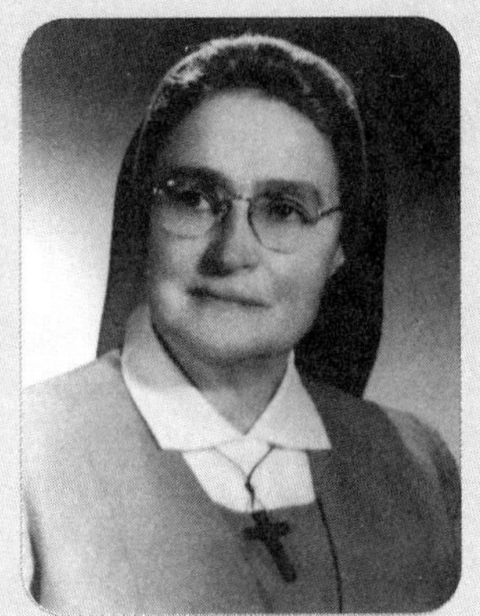

Marie-Denise Lefèbvre was born in Saint-Benoît, Quebec, into a staunch Catholic family that already had several members in the Grey Nuns Community. She was admitted to the novitiate at the Mother House of the Grey Nuns of Montreal in 1926. During the latter part of her career, from 1973 to 1981, she was Superior General of the Order. Beginning in 1981, she was assigned to preparing the case of Marguerite d'Youville, the founder of the Order, for canonization, which was realized in 1991. Sister Lefèbvre graduated as a nurse from St. Boniface (Manitoba) Hospital School, then attended the University of Saint Louis, Missouri, for a bachelor of science in nursing. She also held a baccalaureate degree in nursing education from St. Louis University in Missouri and a master of science in nursing education from the Catholic University of America in Washington, D.C.

For 20 years, she was director of the Institut Marguerite d'Youville, a French-language nursing school, which soon developed a baccalaureate program in conjunction with the Université de Montréal. In 1967, this program was integrated with the newly created Faculty of Nursing Science at the University of Montreal. Following this integration, the Institut Marguerite d'Youville closed after 33 years, although Sister Lefèbvre remained on faculty at the university. Sister Lefèbvre also worked with the World Health Organization as a member of several of its committees, including one on nursing specialists. She wrote numerous articles, especially in the areas of advancement of nursing science and improvement of teaching methods in nursing.

Among the many awards for her contributions to the education of nurses and to the improvement of care for the ill was a Centennial Medal of Confederation in 1967 from the Government of Canada. In 1984 the government also awarded Sister Lefèbvre the Thérèse Casgrain prize and appointed her to the Order of Canada. Also in 1984, the Canadian Nurses Association presented her with the Jeanne Mance Award, its highest honour. She also holds an honorary doctorate from the University of Moncton and has been recognized by the nursing departments at Université de Montréal and McGill University for her services to nursing.

— *Glennis Zilm*

personal freedom, growing acceptance of out-of-wedlock births, and increased disclosure of sexual preference are contributing to the evolution of family structure and the resulting diversity in form.

Because of this diversity, a definition of family must encompass a broad meaning. Therefore, **family** is defined as two or more people, who may or may not be related by blood, marriage or adoption, bound by strong emotional ties, a sense of belonging and a commitment to live with and care for one another over time (Friedman, 1998; Bomar, 1996; Clemen-Stone, McGuire & Eigsti, 1998). This broad definition covers the wide range of forms the family can take. It includes, for example, a family comprising an unmarried mother and her offspring, a married but childless couple or two gay males and their adopted child. Each family form has its own set of distinctive characteristics that may help or hinder family life. Nurses must have an awareness and an understanding of the characteristics of the various family forms so that we can assess, plan and implement care to meet their unique needs. The family forms that are common in Canada today are outlined in the following pages and summarized in Table 10.1.

Typical Family Forms

NUCLEAR FAMILY

The **nuclear family** consists of a husband and wife with their own or adopted children, who share a residence, divide their labour and cooperate economically (Baker, 1990). This form had traditionally been accepted as the "ideal" family, in which the father was the sole provider and the mother was the full-time homemaker. The mother was primarily devoted to supporting her husband in his career and bringing up the children. However, owing to increased costs of food, shelter and education, and increased choice for women to pursue their own careers, many married women have made the transition to working outside the home.

In 1991, 68 percent of mothers with children at home were in the labour force, up from 52 percent in 1981 (Logan & Belliveau, 1995). The largest increases in participation

TABLE 10.1 Types of families and their defining features

Family Type	*Defining Features*
Nuclear	Husband and wife who are married with biological or adopted children
Dual-career	Nuclear family in which husband and wife pursue active careers, in a relationship of equal power and decision making, and shared economic and domestic responsibility
Nuclear-dyad	A married couple who are childless because of choice or infertility, or because their children have left home
Extended	Network of relatives of the nuclear family such as grandparents, aunts, uncles, cousins
Single-parent	A mother or father living alone with biological or adopted children
Blended	Husband and wife, one or both of whom were previously married, living with children from previous marriages and/or children from the new union
Cohabiting	Unmarried heterosexual couple living together, with or without children
Gay or lesbian	A cohabiting couple of the same sex living together, with or without children
Communal	An intimate network of unrelated adults and their children who make a commitment to live together as one large family

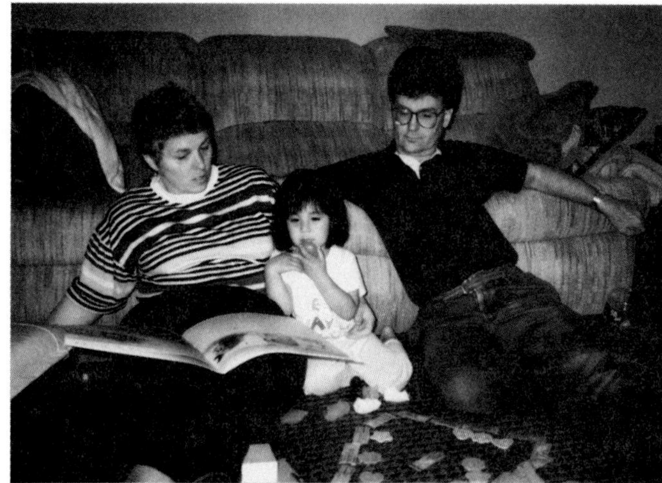

The nuclear family remains the predominant family form in Canada.

rates occurred among women aged 35 to 44 and those aged 45 to 54 with preschool-age children. This movement created a new family structure called the dual-career family. Rapaport and Rapaport (1971) define the **dual-career family** as "the type of family in which both heads of the household pursue careers and at the same time maintain a family life together" (p. 18). In this new family structure the traditional husband–wife roles of provider and homemaker give way to a contemporary relationship of equal power and decision-making along with shared economic and domestic responsibility. The careers of husband and wife are viewed as equally important. Similarly, housekeeping duties and childrearing are equally divided. While dual-career families enjoy the economic advantages of two incomes, they also face a number of difficulties. For example, there might be competition in relation to career importance, as well as conflict and strain in assuming family versus career roles. Women, in particular, sometimes find that it is not easy trying to be a wife, a mother and a worker, along with maintaining a household. When a child is ill, for example, it is often the mother who must take time off work to provide necessary care. While she fulfills her role as mother, she feels guilty because her work-related tasks are put on hold. Dual-career couples may need support and assistance in establishing a balance in their pursuit of a satisfying family life and fulfilling careers. One form of dual career family is called the **commuter family**, in which spouses live in separate cities or countries on a voluntary basis (Friedman, 1998).

Not all nuclear couples have children. Known as the **nuclear-dyad**, this type of family comprises a couple without children. Some married couples choose not to have children; others are childless because of infertility or because their children have grown up and left home. While the nuclear-dyad does not fit the definition of nuclear family because of the absence of children, these couples are recognized as families.

The nuclear family still predominates as the most common family form in Canada. However, fewer Canadians are living in nuclear families today than were 30 years ago. At the same time, those living in single-parent families, blended families and cohabiting (common-law) families are gradually increasing.

EXTENDED FAMILY

The **extended family** is a wider network of two or more related nuclear families, known in everyday language as *relatives* or *kinfolk*. This family unit consists of grandparents, aunts, uncles and cousins, who may live near or far away. Regardless of proximity, it is a network of relatives who visit or correspond regularly, and who, in good times or bad, give social, emotional, physical and economic support to one another. In some cultures, extended families live together in a single household. In South Asia, for example,

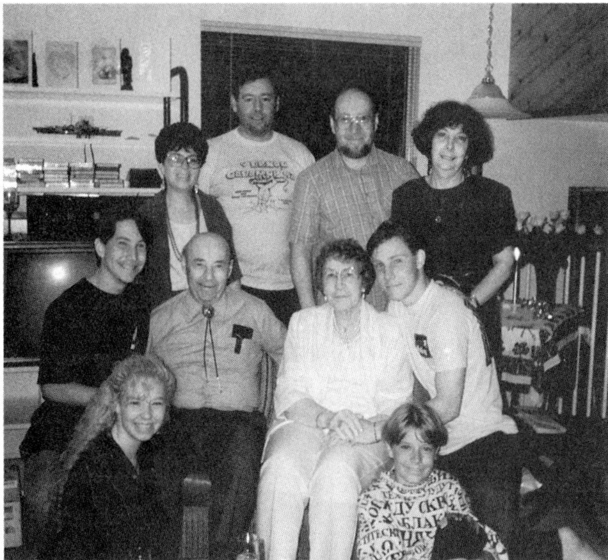

Relatives get together for special occasions such as this 50th wedding anniversary party.

often brothers and their nuclear families live with their parents, sharing economic resources and living a collective lifestyle (Assanand, Dias, Richardson & Waxler-Morrison, 1990). Extended family units, with three or more generations living together, also predominate in certain Canadian communities such as the Inuit, Cree, Hutterites and Amish (Ramu, 1993).

SINGLE-PARENT FAMILY

A **single-parent family** refers to a mother or a father living with one or more dependent children. According to Statistics Canada, lone-parent families account for a growing proportion of families in Canada, and the overwhelming majority of them are headed by lone mothers. In 1994, one in six children under the age of 12 (15%) lived in lone-mother families, created primarily as a result of marital separation or divorce. Widowed and never-married mothers make up the balance of female-headed single-parent families (Statistics Canada, 1997a).

Having to assume responsibility as both provider and homemaker, single mothers, in particular, often encounter financial burdens and other difficulties in providing adequate food, housing and child care. Because of their dual role, single parents spend less time with their children than do married parents. They may also feel stress, weakened self-esteem and loneliness in a couples-oriented society. All of these conditions can combine to create a negative influence on the health and well-being of the family as a whole. Single parents often need help and support from their extended families (particularly their parents) and from the communities in which they live in order to succeed as parents and achieve satisfaction in other facets of their lives.

BLENDED FAMILY

The **blended** or **reconstituted family**, also known as the *step-family*, consists of a husband and wife, at least one of whom has been married before. Owing to the increasing divorce rates in Canada, blended families are becoming more common (Boyd & Norris, 1995). The blended family can include one or more children from a former marriage as well as offspring from the new union, creating a constellation of step-children, step-parents and step-siblings. Also associated with the blended unit is the **binuclear family**, in which children are members of two family households as a result of joint-custody arrangements by their parents following divorce (Bohannan, 1985). Blended families may experience the same kinds of problems faced by nuclear families, particularly if both adults work. In addition, blended families encounter the challenges of integrating family members and establishing satisfying relationships. For example, children do not always accept their step-parents right away. They need time to adjust to new patterns of interaction and authority, which can create stress and disharmony in the family unit.

COHABITING FAMILY

The **cohabiting family** consists of a man and a woman living together without being legally married. Also known as *common-law* relationships, these unions are common among young adults as a prelude or "trial run" to marriage. Cohabiting unions can provide the social, emotional and economic support provided by legal marriages but without the binding commitment of marriage. There is also testimony suggesting that common-law unions are a growing alternative to marriage and remarriage following divorce or death of a spouse. For some Canadians, particularly those who have gone through the emotional trauma and financial burden of divorce, a common-law union may be more desirable than a legal marriage. Overall, cohabitation rates doubled in Canada between 1981 and 1995. By 1995, approximately 12 percent of all couples in Canada were in common-law relationships. Much of the increase in common-law living was accounted for by increases in Quebec, where the rate is 21 percent (Statistics Canada, 1995).

GAY OR LESBIAN FAMILY

The **gay** or **lesbian family** is a form of cohabitation in which individuals of the same sex live together, with or without children, and share a sexual relationship (Caudle & Grover, 1992). While the nature of homosexuality is becoming more clearly understood and social acceptance of homosexual coupling is increasing, gay and lesbian families still encounter a number of problems. The first is stigmatization. Because of continued homophobia (the strong, irrational fear of homosexuals), lesbian women and gay men may be the subjects of jokes, disparaging remarks and verbal and even physical abuse. Gay men and lesbians may face isolation and lack of support from their families of origin (their parents and siblings), who, for personal, cultural or religious reasons, do not regard homosexuality as an acceptable lifestyle.

A second problem that gay and lesbian couples may experience relates to the law. Although this area is in a state of flux, these couples may have difficulty obtaining benefits for each other because the Canadian legal system still does not recognize gay and lesbian unions. Moreover, gay or lesbian couples cannot legally marry.

However, significant changes are underway, because sexual orientation is increasingly being recognized as grounds for legal protection under the Canadian Charter of Rights and Freedoms and various federal and provincial laws. Many employers throughout Canada now grant health benefits to same-gender partners if the couples have been living together for two years. In addition, at the time of writing, several court challenges are underway in relation to the inclusion of same-gender couples in family law and pension plans (Yogis, Duplak & Trainor, 1996).

The law also discriminates against lesbians and gay men in cases of child custody and adoption. Courts make decisions about where children will go with "the best interests of the child" in mind. The courts tend to find that it is in the "best interests" of the child not to be placed with a gay or lesbian applicant for custody. Most Canadian provinces do not allow same-gender couples to adopt as couples, but only as individuals (Yogis, Duplak & Trainor, 1996).

Concerns about custody often revolve around unfounded fears that children of gay or lesbian parents will become homosexuals and around the worry that the children will be harassed by their peers (Baker, 1990). Evidence reveals, however, that this is not the case. Parental homosexuality has been shown to have no effect on the sexual identity of children. Children of homosexual parents develop their sexual identities and orientations in the same manner that all children do (Williamson, 1986). Furthermore, Harry (1983) found that, while the lives of gay and lesbian parents and their children are not without problems, harassment of the family is uncommon, and is manageable when it does occur. It is important for nurses working with gay and lesbian families to realize that sexual orientation is only one aspect of these individuals' lives, and that they have the same physical and emotional needs as do all human beings.

COMMUNAL FAMILY

The **communal family** is an intimate network of unrelated adults and their children who make a commitment to live together as one large family unit. Communal families are like extended family systems in that they fulfill similar functions of affection, interdependence, and social, physical and economic support (Scanzoni, 1976). "People choose to belong to communes because of some common attraction, which may vary from a desired geographic location to a strong commitment to a particular ideology or religious doctrine" (Logan & Dawkins, 1986, p. 421). Control over communal members can be so strong that friendships and relationships outside the group may be difficult or even impossible. Communal families can vary in structure and function. For example, in some communes married couples may retain their nuclear structure, sharing separate dwellings and economic independence, whereas in others, all adults are considered to be married to one another. The children belong to the whole group. Personal possessions are relinquished and economic resources are pooled for use by all.

Although communal living may be seen as a reasonable alternative to the traditional nuclear family, such forms may have negative consequences for their members. For example, decision making can be very complicated, leading to resistance, rivalries and conflicts of interest. Multiple caretaking and sharing of tasks may need continual negotiation and clarification of roles. Children, although they may benefit from having various teachers and socializing agents, may suffer from the lack of someone special to care for them, to stand up for them or simply to be there when they are in need. Communal family members may also experience lack of privacy and feel they are constantly under scrutiny, making it hard to resolve problems (Logan & Dawkins, 1986).

Culture and the Family

The family has been called society's transmitter of cultural practices and traditions. Traditions, attitudes, values and beliefs are passed down from one generation to the next. Family structure, communication patterns, coping strategies, lifestyles, dietary habits, health practices and religious beliefs are reflected in one's cultural and ethnic background. Nurses must be sensitive to the influence of cultural values and beliefs on the family's personal views of health and family functioning. A nurse's culturally based health beliefs and values can help or hinder his or her work with families. Nurses must be culturally aware of their own health beliefs and values and avoid imposing these on the patient and family. The influences of culture and ethnicity on health, and the implications for nursing care, are examined in Chapter 12.

Conceptual Frameworks of the Family

Conceptual frameworks are used to guide nursing practice. In family nursing, conceptual frameworks give us a perspective on family life. They also provide a basis for assessing families, interpreting their needs and planning their care. The conceptual frameworks of family that we use in nursing practice come from a variety of disciplines, such as sociology, anthropology, public health and family therapy. Each framework provides a distinct perspective on family life. For instance, the structural-functional framework looks at how family members are arranged and at the relationships among them, whereas the developmental framework looks at the life cycle of the family and the changes that occur as members grow and mature. As much as the frameworks focus on different aspects of family, they also overlap in some of their concepts. For example, concepts such as communication patterns and interaction among members run through all the frameworks.

Depending on their focus of practice, nurses working with families may select a single framework, or they may use a combination of concepts from several frameworks to guide their care. Some nurses prefer a pluralistic approach, in which they use selected concepts from a number of frameworks. This is because they often find that not all aspects of a particular framework explain the relevant phenomena of the families they work with. Three frameworks that are commonly used in family nursing will be described. These are the *systems*, *structural-functional* and *developmental* frameworks.

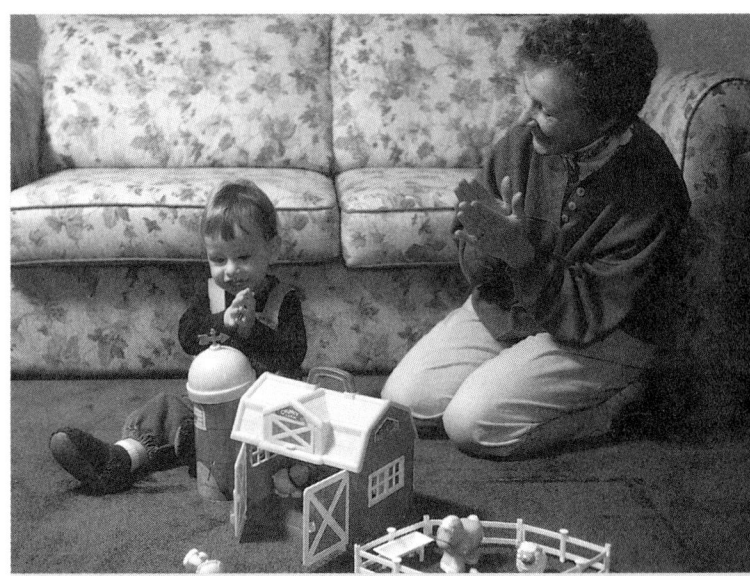

A grandmother looks forward to a visit with her grandchild.

Family Systems Framework

The family systems framework was derived from the general systems theory introduced by von Bertalanffy (1968). He defined a system as "a complex of elements in interaction" (p. 83). While various authors have altered this definition somewhat, it is generally agreed that "a system consists of two or more connected components or subsystems which form an organized whole and that interact with each other to achieve desired goals" (Clemen-Stone et al., 1998, p. 166). Further, the actions of a system are goal-directed. In order to achieve its goals, the system functions in a dynamic state of adaptive interaction with its environment. In Chapter 13 we note that a number of general conceptual models of nursing are based on systems theory, for example, the Roy and Neuman models. In this section we will discuss the basic concepts of general systems theory as they apply to family.

The family systems framework characterizes the family unit as it relates and interacts with itself and with other units in a larger society. In the systems framework, the family is viewed as a social system comprising a small group of people who share common goals and functions, and who interact with one another and their environment as a whole.

The interrelationships among family members are characterized by mutual dependence. Children are dependent on their parents for food, shelter, affection and education. At the same time, parents may be dependent on their children for personal gratification or the satisfaction gained from watching their sons' and daughters' achievements as they grow and develop. Elderly parents may rely on their adult children for physical and emotional support. The relationships among family members are intertwined in such a way that whatever happens to one member will invariably affect the entire family. For example, when a mother is hospitalized, her husband may have to take time off work to care for their preschool son, placing the family under financial stress.

According to family systems theory, a family is made up of members who interrelate as subsystems or hierarchies. Two or more interrelating family members can form **subsystems**, such as the spousal subsystem, the parent–child subsystem or the sibling subsystem. "Any one family member is a part of several subsystems in which the members have different functions and levels of power and influence" (Janosik & Miller, 1979, p. 7). For example, parents usually hold the power in the family and have substantial influence over their children. The subsystems keep the family organized and provide the capacity to carry out its functions. The family system, in turn, is part of a wider social system that includes, for example, school, church and community, all of which make up the suprasystem. The **suprasystem** comprises the physical, social and cultural environment with which the family interacts in order to sustain its life, continuity and growth (Friedman, 1998).

Boundaries encompass the family, individual family members and the subsystems within it. **Boundaries** are physical demarcations such as the family's property line or a member's bedroom. They can also be abstract entities, such as rules, norms, attitudes and values, that separate families and subsystems from their environment. These boundaries regulate human interaction inside and outside the family. Boundaries filter the flow of inputs from the environment and output to it. **Input** refers to the energy, information and resources that the system receives and then processes in order to achieve its goals. **Output** refers to the energy, information and resources that are released back into the environment. For example, Mary Martin is a community health nurse in Halifax who wants to return to work but who is having difficulty finding after-school child care. She brings her concern to the school's Parents' Association, where it is discovered that there are a number of families who would support an after-school care program. For Mary, the *input* was the knowledge of inadequate child care facilities in her community. Her decision to approach the Parents' Association in support of her family's need constituted the *process*. The *output* was the establishment of an after-school care program that met not only the Martins' needs but also the needs of other families in the community. This exchange of energy is crucial to the survival of the system. Boundaries promote equilibrium in the system and allow the exchange of energy with the environment.

Systems are typified by the degree of interaction with their surrounding environment. The family is viewed as an **open system**, because it exchanges energy, resources and information with its environment. As an open system, the family takes in what is needed from the environment for its own survival and growth and, in turn, gives back energy, information and materials to support the environment's more global needs.

An important element in the functioning of family systems is **feedback**. Janosik and Green (1992) describe feedback as "a continuous process of input and output exchanges between families and the community that surrounds them" (p. 14). An example of feedback might be neighbours reacting negatively to heavy-metal band practices next door. Feedback fosters family functioning and stability by alerting the family to behaviours that comply with or deviate from community norms. It is an important process that helps a family identify its strengths and evaluate how well it is achieving its goals. Feedback may be informal, such as a neighbour's reaction to loud music, or it may be formal, such as a phone call to the police. These are examples of negative feedback, but feedback can be positive as well. Positive feedback tells the family to carry on with its existing standards and patterns of behaviour. Negative feedback indicates to the family that it needs to modify its current behaviours. The family can adapt by accepting or rejecting the incoming feedback, or by modifying it to suit its particular needs.

While the family is an open system, the degree of openness varies according to the nature of its boundaries. Open families, for example, invite people into their home, encourage their children to bring friends in and interact freely with neighbours. These families welcome change as a normal process in life, and reach out to the larger community for support in solving their problems and maintaining their well-being. Closed families, on the other hand, resist change. They believe that people are not trustworthy and that interactions and relationships must be kept under strict control. Closed families avoid discussing matters with people outside their immediate family. Families who keep highly rigid boundaries are often isolated and deprived of necessary information and resources required for optimal growth and well-being (Friedman, 1998).

Nurses can use concepts from the family systems framework to assess family functioning and determine family needs. Because the systems framework considers the family as a whole, it provides the basis for a holistic approach to nursing practice. Functional and dysfunctional patterns of behaviour are regarded as the result of systems functioning as opposed to individual members' functioning. Family structure, functions and processes are examined for adaptive or maladaptive behaviours within families. Blame is shifted away from individual members, while attention is centred on the family system and how it must change in order to function successfully.

Structural-Functional Framework

The structural-functional framework was developed by anthropologists and sociologists, who viewed the family as a social system interacting with other social systems such as the school or the health care system (Duvall, 1977). The essence of this framework is family structure and function.

Family structure refers to the way a family is organized. It identifies how family members are arranged and how they relate to one another as a unit.

Friedman (1998) identifies four basic components of family structure:

1. role structure
2. value systems
3. communication processs
4. power structure.

The first component, family **role structure**, defines the behaviours expected of members in designated positions. For example, the oldest child in the family has expectations placed upon him or her, by virtue of being the first born. The oldest child might be the one who carries the money, buys the tickets and treats, and looks out for the younger siblings when they all go to a Sunday afternoon movie. Roles are important in family functioning because it is through the execution of family roles that family functions are fulfilled.

The second component of family structure is the value system. Every family creates its own system of values, primarily from its culture and secondarily from the society in which it lives. **Values** are the ideas, attitudes and beliefs about the worth of an entity or concept that consciously or unconsciously bind together the members of a family in a common culture (Parad & Caplan; cited in Friedman, 1998, p. 328). Family values serve as guides to judge behaviour and develop norms and rules for conduct. For example, families who believe in self-responsibility for problem solving actively seek out information and necessary resources to deal with their problems. On the other hand, families who believe in fate might accept and cope with problems as "God's will." Family values are affected by such variables as religion, spiritual beliefs, social class, age and developmental stages of family members. A family's value system is not static. Rather, it is a dynamic system that evolves over time as the family and its members interact with different subcultures, adjust to changes in society or respond to particular needs in their lives. For example, a family belonging to the Jehovah's Witnesses faith, which prohibits blood transfusions, might grant permission for a life-saving blood transfusion if their child sustained a near-fatal injury in an accident.

Values are important in the context of family structure because a family's attitudes and beliefs affect the behaviour of family members. Thus, it is important for nurses to identify a family's value system in order to understand the behaviours of family members. As nurses, we must also be aware of our own value system. Differences in values between the nurse and the family can interfere with the nurse–family relationship and will ultimately affect the care a family receives (Friedman, 1998; Ross & Cobb, 1990).

Communication patterns and processes are key components in family structure. **Communication** is the process by which individuals transmit information to one another through verbal and nonverbal messages or cues. The meaning of these messages is influenced by the roles and value systems of the members. Communication patterns directly influence family interactions and family functioning. When messages among members are clearly conveyed and understood, the family communication patterns are considered to be functional. Conversely, communication patterns are dysfunctional when messages are ambiguous or blocked, or when there is no communication among family members at all.

Power structure, the fourth component of family structure, is defined as the actual or potential ability of individual members to control, influence or change the behaviour of other family members (Friedman, 1998). The power structure of a family determines who makes the decisions and who has the most influence in the family. In other words, it defines the authority figure and the "pecking order" of family members. **Authority** is the status attributed to individuals or groups, giving them the power and right to command and be obeyed. In the family, authority is often vested in a particular member on the basis of family and cultural values and social factors. For example, in traditional mid-European and Asian families, the father is usually the authority figure who makes decisions unilaterally and holds firm control over family behaviour. This highly patriarchal family structure is becoming less common in Canada, but in many nuclear families it is still the husband or male partner who, as head of the family, holds the major decision-making power.

However, with changing social influences, a more egalitarian distribution of power in Canadian families is becoming common. Power and decision making are often shared jointly by parents, with the participation of family members. The power structure is important for family functioning because it affects communication patterns and interactions inside as well as outside the family unit. That is to say, families who interact openly and freely among themselves are more apt to interact in the same manner with other social institutions or groups.

Family functions are those activities a family performs in order to meet the needs of both individual family members and society as a whole. Friedman (1998) has identified five basic family functions:

1. affective function: for meeting the psychological needs of family members for affection and understanding
2. socializing and social placement function: primarily for teaching children how to function, making them productive members of society; and conferring status on family members, that is, passing on values, traditions and social class privileges
3. reproduction function: for ensuring family continuity over the generations and producing new members for society
4. economic function: for providing sufficient economic resources and allocating them effectively
5. health care function: for providing physical necessities, such as food, clothing, shelter and health care.

The structural-functional framework provides a valuable guide for assessing families because it analyses the internal and external forces that influence individual members as well as the family as a whole. The nurse in a medical setting, for instance, can use the structural-functional approach to assess the impact of illness on family functioning. She or he could evaluate how illness of the husband/father, which required a lengthy hospital stay, would affect the family's economic resources and the role of the wife/mother. Would she have to obtain employment outside the home to maintain the family financially and, if so, what assistance would she need for child care? How is the family adjusting to the father's illness? Does it continue to function effectively, or is it experiencing stress? Answers to questions such as these would determine the nursing interventions, for example, support and mobilization of resources, that this family may require to meet its needs.

Family Developmental Framework

The developmental framework examines the family as it continues over time, following the chronological and sequential changes in growth and development throughout the entire life cycle of the family (Duvall, 1977). This framework describes the changes that occur in family roles and relationships as individual members grow and mature, moving from one life stage to the next. Duvall developed an eight-stage model of the family life cycle, each stage of which has a set of distinctive developmental tasks.

The family developmental tasks refer to the growth responsibilities that must be accomplished by a family during each stage of its development in order to fulfill its biologic function, its cultural obligations and its own aspirations and values (Duvall, 1977). Family developmental tasks parallel individual developmental tasks, such as Erikson's stages of emotional development (Erikson, 1963). Like individual developmental tasks, family developmental tasks must be successfully achieved in each stage before proceeding to the next. Further, family members must achieve both individual and family developmental tasks in order to function effectively as a family unit. Failure to achieve a developmental task leads to unhappiness in the family, social disapproval and difficulty accomplishing later developmental tasks (Duvall, 1977). Duvall's family life cycle and developmental tasks are outlined in Table 10.2. In this model, Duvall uses the age and school placement of the oldest child to define life-cycle stages.

The developmental framework is a very useful guide for assessing families and determining their health needs. The common, general features of family life for the different stages of the life cycle provide a basis for knowing what to expect. These common features, however, are based on the premise of the nuclear childbearing family. As we discussed earlier, not all families fit into these typical family life-cycle stages (Friedman, 1998). For example, the never-married single-parent family begins with Stage 2, the early childbearing stage. Parental adaptation includes the performance

TABLE 10.2 Family life cycle and developmental tasks

Family Stage	*Time Period*	*Developmental Tasks*
1. Married couple	Marriage to birth of first child	Establishing a mutually satisfying marriage Adjusting to the kin network Family planning
2. Childbearing	Birth of oldest child to 30 months of age	Adjusting to parenthood Maintaining a satisfying home Facilitating infant's developmental tasks
3. Preschool-age	Oldest child is 2 to 5 years of age	Promoting growth and nurturing children Integrating new children Learning to separate from children Coping with energy depletion and lack of privacy as parents
4. School-age	Oldest child is 6 to 13 years of age	Socializing children and promoting educational achievement Fitting into the community of school-age families Maintaining a satisfying marriage
5. Teenage	Oldest child is 13 to 20 years of age	Balancing teenage freedom with responsibility Establishing postparental interests
6. Launching	From time first child leaves home to time last child leaves home	Releasing children as young adults Extending the family upon marriage of children Developing postparental interests Assisting aging and ill parents
7. Middle-age	From time last child leaves home to retirement	Rebuilding marital relationship Enhancing leisure activities Maintaining a healthy environment Maintaining family ties with older and younger generations
8. Aging	Retirement to death	Maintaining satisfying housing Adjusting to retirement, reduced income, aging, loneliness, death

SOURCES: Duvall, 1977; Janosik & Green, 1992; Spradley & Allender, 1996.

of both maternal and paternal roles, while providing a healthy environment for family growth and development. Family life-cycle patterns are altered for childless couples, single-parent families and reconstituted families. Nurses working with these families need to be aware of the modifications in the respective family life cycles in order to make accurate assessments of their health needs.

Family Health

What Is Family Health?

Family health can be defined from the perspective of a number of theories and frameworks dealing with the family. For example, if we were to use the developmental framework as a perspective, which identifies family developmental tasks that must be accomplished according to the family life cycle, family health would be defined as the ability of family members and the family as a whole to achieve stage-specific developmental tasks. Or, if we subscribed to Roy's (1984) nursing model, family health would be viewed as a state and a process of being or becoming an integrated and whole family system.

In this book, our perspective on family health is reflected in the World Health Organization's (1984) definition of health. Health is defined as the extent to which an individual or group is able to realize aspirations, to satisfy needs and to change or cope with the environment (WHO, 1984). The family, as society's most basic unit, provides the physical, cultural, spiritual, psychological and social foundation for the health and well-being of individual members. Since health and illness behaviours are primarily learned and, for the most part, performed within the family, the family is both a resource and an environment for the health and well-being of individual members.

Family health, like health in general, is not static in nature. It is a dynamic process in which family members create adaptive patterns of interaction with one another and with an ever-changing physical and social environment. This is done in order to manage stress, survive crisis, handle conflict and organize individuals so as to satisfy their needs and achieve their goals. Family health is an enabling process with a focus on the quality of life. For example, a family who has effectively adapted its lifestyle around nurturing a child with diabetes may not see itself as having a health problem—even though others might view it that way because of the child's disease.

Determinants of Family Health

Wellness and illness do not happen on their own. An individual's health is influenced by sociological and environmental factors, as well as health-promoting and health-protecting beliefs and practices of his or her family. Social and environmental factors are instrumental in family health because they affect the family's economic resources and housing and its family dynamics. **Family dynamics** are the interrelationships among members, namely their roles, relationships and communication patterns.

Social factors play a large role in family health. Families in which parents are well educated and have ample financial resources to afford adequate housing, transportation and good nutrition tend to practise healthier lifestyles. These families are often located towards the wellness end of the wellness–illness continuum. On the other hand, families who live in poverty because of unemployment or low-paying jobs often lack the resources for adequate housing, nutrition and family care. They are therefore at risk for location at the illness end of the continuum (RNABC, 1992).

The family environment influences the health of family members. Danielson, Hamel-Bissell and Winstead-Fry (1993) reviewed a number of studies dealing with family influences on individual health and illness behaviours. They found that a family's ethnic background, social class and satisfaction with life influenced nutritional status and health-promoting practices. Obesity in children was attributed to family nutrition and eating patterns. Another study showed that children as young as four years of age understood health behaviours and practised them. Furthermore, parents who, as children, were taught and encouraged to engage in self-care practices were especially effective in bringing up children who actively promoted their own health. The families' ability to solve problems was an indicator as to whether adolescents engaged in negative behaviours. Research indicated that "excessive demands within the family may have caused stress for the adolescent and could be ameliorated if the adolescent and family could communicate and resolve conflicts and differences" (Danielson et al., 1993, p. 12). It is interesting to note that adolescent peer support did not prevent negative behaviours, nor did complaining about family members to others. The important factor was the ability of the adolescent and his or her family to communicate and resolve differences in a satisfying manner (Danielson et al., 1993).

Family values also influence health-protecting practices and use of health care services. For example, whether an infant is immunized or taken to the community health clinic for health assessments depends on the parent's beliefs and attitudes regarding use of health care services.

The health status of family members and the family mutually influence each other. Illness of one member affects the whole family and its interactions, while the family in turn affects the health status and course of illness of its members (Friedman, 1998). The following case depicts this relationship.

> *Irfan Virani is a 28-year-old self-employed truck driver who sustains traumatic injury, including loss of a leg in an accident. Irfan's family will play a large part in his healing and return to health; in turn, his recovery will influence the health of the whole family. The family can help Irfan directly by*

giving care and providing support, or indirectly by participating with health professionals in decisions regarding treatment and care. For example, Irfan's healing process requires prolonged convalescence. In collaboration with the health care team, Irfan and his wife, Mina, decide that he will convalesce at home. Mina will be taught necessary physical care and, in addition, will drive Irfan for daily physiotherapy. Clearly, this father's injury has affected the whole family. In order to care for Irfan, Mina has to make adjustments in family schedules and routines. The children's swimming lessons are put on hold, and alternative transportation is arranged to get the children to and from their weekly religion classes. The family is now without a regular income because Irfan was the sole wage earner. Mina finds little time to spend with her children and even less time for herself. This, combined with the financial burden of lost income, leaves her feeling tired and depressed.

How well this family can support Irfan's recovery and at the same time facilitate the growth and well-being of its members will depend on its coping strategies and its strengths and capabilities as a unit. We will follow Irfan and Mina in the next section to see how they mobilize their strengths to cope with this health challenge.

Criteria for Judging Family Health

Research on families and family behaviour points to a number of similarities in how healthy families maintain their health and cope with life's problems. Spradley & Allender (1996) outline six important characteristics exhibited by healthy families:

1. there is a facilitative process of interaction among family members
2. they enhance individual member development
3. their role relationships are structured effectively
4. they actively attempt to cope with problems
5. they have a healthy home environment and lifestyle
6. they establish regular links with the broader community.

These characteristics of healthy families will be described more fully.

FACILITATIVE PROCESS OF INTERACTION In healthy families, communication is open and supportive. Ideas, feelings and concerns are shared with one another on a regular basis, through a variety of forms. Verbal communication is often used—healthy families telephone or write to one another when they are separated. These families also use nonverbal means to transmit feelings, thoughts, love and affection or show consideration for one another. For example, a mother smiles warmly and gives her son a hug when he achieves an A in mathematics. On the other hand, she frowns in disapproval when he asks to play out on the street. Spradley & Allender (1996) maintain that in healthy families, members are sensitive to one another. They watch for cues and confirm messages so as to ensure understanding. These families also recognize and resolve conflicts and problems as they arise. Members learn to share and to work cooperatively in order to meet individual and family needs.

Open and facilitative patterns of interaction enable families to meet their needs and achieve their goals. Families must communicate in order to show affection and acceptance, to promote identity and affiliation and to guide behaviour through socialization and social controls. Families who communicate openly and effectively with one another will also be better prepared to communicate with other families and groups, or with society as a whole (Spradley & Allender, 1996).

ENHANCEMENT OF INDIVIDUAL DEVELOPMENT Healthy families are responsive to the needs of individual members and provide the freedom and support that is necessary to foster the growth of each member. In the case of Irfan Virani, the truck driver who lost his leg in an accident, family responsiveness and support would be shown through efforts to aid his emotional and physical adjustments and by encouraging him to move forward with a new career opportunity.

The healthy family understands and promotes the growth and developmental needs of children. This kind of family provides opportunities for increasing freedom and autonomy and permits differences in opinions and lifestyles. It shows unconditional love, affection and approval, as well as respect for the unique rights of each member. Families vary in how they promote the development of individual members, depending on their cultural orientation. For example, the Virani family, being Indo-Canadian, may express autonomy differently than an Italian-Canadian family would. Nonetheless, each family facilitates freedom and autonomy of its members in some way (Spradley & Allender, 1996).

EFFECTIVE STRUCTURING OF ROLE RELATIONSHIPS Healthy families are adaptive and flexible. That is, they can alter their roles and tasks to meet changing needs over time. The needs of families change according to their life-cycle stages or because of forces such as loss of a job, illness or sudden death of a member. Healthy families are able to adapt their roles and tasks in response to forces beyond their control. The Virani family, for example, are adjusting to the effects of Irfan's accident by changing their roles and tasks. Mina obtained a job outside the home, while Irfan took on more of the household and child care duties. This family shows flexibility and the ability to restructure its roles and relationships in order to meet the demands of its situation.

In healthy families, roles and tasks are also altered to fit the developmental needs of members. For example, children are given increasing responsibility and assigned more complex household tasks as they become more mature.

Parents may adapt the rules of conduct, giving children more freedom as they learn to manage their own behaviour in a positive, constructive manner.

EFFECTIVE COPING WITH PROBLEMS Families who try to solve their problems in an effective, creative manner are considered to be healthy. Not only do these families take responsibility for problem solving, but also they ensure mutual involvement of family members in identifying problems and making decisions (deChesnay, 1986). Healthy families try to find solutions and overcome their problems by themselves; however, they may seek outside help if necessary. Using the Virani family as an example once again, Irfan and Mina dealt with their financial difficulty by deciding that Mina would get a job until Irfan was established in a new occupation. Irfan enrolled in evening courses at the community college so that he was free to care for the children after school. Because money was still a problem, they decided to move into a suite in Irfan's parent's home, while renting out their own house in order to keep up mortgage payments.

HEALTHY HOME ENVIRONMENT AND LIFESTYLE Healthy families maintain a safe, healthy home environment and lifestyle. For example, a young childbearing family removes potential hazards such as sharp objects or toxic solutions from the reach of infants and toddlers. These families also ensure good hygiene and cleanliness in order to reduce infection and the spread of disease. Healthy families foster a healthy family lifestyle. They advocate a nutritious diet along with adequate rest, exercise and relaxation. The emotional environment of a healthy family is positive and supportive, and one in which members feel welcome and accepted. Members share a strong sense of values, which may or may not be coupled with a religious orientation (Spradley & Allender, 1996). The home environment provides a strong influence on health practices and lifestyles of individuals. It is not unusual for young adults to continue eating nutritiously and living healthy lifestyles after they leave home.

MAINTAIN LINKS WITH THE BROADER COMMUNITY Families do not live in isolation but are members of a suprasystem—the neighbourhood in which they live, the school their children attend, the church they choose for religious affiliation and the larger community from which they derive services. Healthy families maintain regular, open ties with the broader community. They are active participants in community groups, such as the school's parents' association, the church choir or the local Boy Scouts group. They select external resources most suited to the family's needs. For example, a family that recognizes its daughter's talent in playing the saxophone might join the local youth band, in which one of the parents might serve as secretary-treasurer.

It is not unusual for healthy families to assume leadership positions in the community groups they join. Healthy families keep themselves informed of events in the world around them. They attempt to know and understand current social, economic and political issues that affect their lives. As a result, healthy families possess a wide range of options and a variety of resources that are available to them for meeting their needs (Spradley & Allender, 1996).

Family Stress and Illness

All families face a certain degree of stress as they strive to meet their needs for everyday living and cope with changes in their physical and social environments. Some stress-producing events, such as loud music or traffic noise, may be mild and even go unnoticed, whereas illness in the family, divorce or death of a family member may be devastating. The family's perception of the stressful event, the availability of resources and its coping abilities determine the degree of stress a family actually experiences. When families cannot resolve stressful events because of inadequate coping abilities or lack of appropriate resources, they experience crisis.

Family Stress and Crisis

Family stress is defined as a state of imbalance in the family, or as Boss (1987) identifies, "an upset in the steady state of the family . . . anything that . . . causes uneasiness or pressure on the family system" (p. 695). Life events or demands that affect the family and disturb its equilibrium are called **family stressors**. Family stressors may emerge from within the family system itself or from external sources.

Internal family stressors originate from individual members or from relationships between and among family members. The developmental transition of children from school age to adolescence is an example of an internal stressor. This transition imposes a change on all other family members, particularly the parents who must now adjust their control over the adolescent as they allow increasing freedom and responsibility so as to foster individual growth and development. Other examples of internal stressors include financial pressures when a parent becomes unemployed, birth of a baby with a congenital defect, children leaving home, family adjustments in newly blended families, arguments between family members or illness of a family member.

External family stressors originate outside the family. They involve situations such as conflicts at work, disagreements with neighbours or friends and social stressors such as racism or prejudice.

A stressor produces tension—a response in the family that signals the need for change. "Stress emerges when this tension is not reduced or brought within manageable limits" (Danielson et al., 1993, p. 30). The amount of stress varies, depending on the family's perception of the stressor, the resources and capabilities of the family to handle stress, and the physical and psychological well-being of individual members at the onset of the stress-producing event. Families respond to stress in the same way that individuals do. That is, when the stressor is perceived as an unpleasant or hazardous event that creates hardships, the family experiences **distress**. An example of distress might be the changes required in family functioning when the mother is absent from the home for a few days because of travel responsibilities associated with her work. Events that are perceived as pleasant bring **eustress**, or good stress, to the family. For example, even though the birth of a baby is a joyous occasion for most families, there is a certain amount of stress brought about by the challenges of integrating this new person into the family unit.

The family's ability to resolve stress depends on its strengths or resources for managing a stressor. Crucial resources include economic stability, family cohesiveness, flexibility, hardiness, shared spiritual beliefs, open communication, traditions, family routines, patterns of problem solving and coping strategies. Family problem solving refers to the process of organizing a stressor into manageable parts, identifying alternative courses of action and initiating steps to resolve the issues. Family coping refers to the strategies and behaviours designed to maintain or strengthen the family as a whole, to maintain emotional stability and well-being of members, to use family and community resources and to resolve the hardships created by the stressor. The goal of family adaptation to stress is to manage the stressor without creating major or lasting changes in the family's established patterns of functioning (Danielson et al., 1993).

Effective family adaptation to a stressor is exemplified by the case of Sara, a single parent who has lost her evening babysitter. This is particularly problematic because Sara, who is a waitress, works morning and evening shifts. She deals with this situation by inviting a cousin, who is a college student, to live with her in exchange for evening babysitting. This arrangement proves effective because it causes minimal disruption to the family's usual routines.

In many situations, families are able to respond to stressors with minimal adjustments in the family unit. Some stressors, however, such as loss of family home and belongings by fire, create numerous problems that demand significant change. Families in these situations often face difficulty resolving the stressor. Stress that is unresolved progresses to crisis. **Family crisis** is defined as a state of disorganization in the family unit (Danielson et al., 1993).

Stressors such as loss of a family home or sudden death of a family member move quickly into crisis because families do not have enough time to mobilize their adaptive resources. Emotional turmoil and disorganization quickly follow and, as a result, the family's usual approaches to problem solving and decision making may not be effective. Boss (1987) states that when families can no longer cope, they exhibit the following characteristics:

- they cannot perform their customary roles
- they are unable to maintain their structural boundaries
- they become immobilized as a system.

Danielson et al. (1993) state that crisis signals family disorganization and a demand for changes in patterns of family functioning in order to restore stability, order and a sense of coherence and well-being. The family's move to begin changes in its patterns of functioning indicates the start of family adaptation to the crisis. When the crisis is resolved, families may not necessarily return to their pre-crisis level of functioning. Some, having been weakened from the experience, will function below their pre-crisis state, whereas others, having developed strengths because of it, will function at a higher level (Boss, 1987).

Impact of Illness on the Family

Illness in the family is a stressful event that may lead to crisis if the family is not able to adjust its coping strategies. When a family member is ill, the total family unit is affected.

If the ill person is the breadwinner, there is a natural concern about the loss of ability to maintain financial responsibility for the family. Both patient and family may worry about how long the patient will be unable to work and the using up of sick leave from the place of employment. There may be additional concern over the costs of illness, such as medications, equipment, medical supplies and surcharges for diagnostic and medical services. The head of the household may not be in a position to make decisions about family matters while ill. Someone else may have to take over the responsibility for this.

When the single mother is sick, not only does the family encounter financial worry, but household routines and child care are also disrupted. Other family members must take over the shopping, the planning and cooking of meals, the washing and the ironing in addition to looking after the children. Relatives are often many miles away, and the family may have to rely on friends or homemaker services for help.

There is also much concern when an older member of the family is ill. It may be the first member of the household to be seriously ill, and the family is reminded of the fragility of human life. There may be additional worries over who will care for the patient, and again the costs, particularly of prolonged illness, may be a matter of concern.

When one of the children is sick, parents are usually very anxious. They may feel guilty of being in some way responsible for the child's illness. Often they feel helpless, and their anxiety and feelings of helplessness may be expressed in hostility and criticism directed towards those who are caring for the child. Hospitals today permit open visiting on children's wards and encourage parents to share in the care of their children. If nurses understand some of the reasons behind the parents' behaviour and that of family members, and also realize that their own feelings about this behaviour are normal, they are better able to accept hostility and criticism without showing anger and hostility in return.

Admission to hospital has many implications for patients and their families. While they were at home, responsibility for their care probably fell to other family members. After they enter a hospital, the responsibility for care is transferred from the family to health professionals. This transfer of responsibility often produces emotions of mixed relief and guilt on the part of the family. They feel relief because trained people will now provide professional care, and perhaps guilt because they think that the patient would be happier at home or that they have passed on responsibilities that they should accept as a family. These feelings are sometimes expressed verbally to health professionals, or they may be expressed in activities such as bringing food to the patient or by criticizing the personnel and the institution. If the nurse recognizes the needs of family members and solicits their help in appropriate areas of patient care, such as assisting the patient to eat, the family will feel more comfortable and will be better able to assist in the patient's healing.

Nursing Care of the Family

Nurses care for families in almost every area of nursing practice. This may be in hospitals, extended care agencies, old age homes, hospices, clinics and doctor's offices, and in the workplace, the home and the community. Regardless of where it is practised, nursing of families focusses on involving families in health care and on helping families to promote, protect or restore their family health. Various terms are used to describe nursing care of the family. Some of these are *family-centred nursing* (Wright & Leahey, 1994), *family-focussed nursing* (Janosik & Miller, 1980), *family interviewing* (Wright & Leahey, 1994), *family nursing* (Wright & Leahey, 1990; Gilliss, 1991; Friedman, 1998), *family systems nursing* (Wright & Leahey, 1990) and *nursing of families* (Feetham, Meister, Bell & Gilliss, 1993; Wright & Leahey, 1994).

Types of Nursing Practice with Families

According to Friedman (1998), there are four types of family nursing practice. These are conceptualized as *family as context*, *family as sum of its members*, *family subsystem as patient*, and *family as patient* (see Figure 10.1).

FAMILY AS CONTEXT

In the first type of nursing practice with families, the family is conceptualized as the social environment or context for the individual. The nurse is concerned primarily with the needs of the individual family member. The family, as the patient's primary social group, can act as either a stressor or a resource to the patient. For example, in one family, parents taught their adolescent son the dangers of using drugs and alcohol and discouraged him from using these substances. Yet, they openly related stories of their own social use of marijuana. When the son was discovered to be using marijuana, he argued that this was acceptable because his parents used the substance, too. In this case, the family, specifically the behaviour of the parents, is initially the stressor. But, the family can then become a resource, a source of support, if the parents participate in a drug rehabilitation program with their son. Many nursing theories and most of the nursing specialties view the family as a crucial social environment and a primary resource for the patient (Friedman, 1998). Pediatric nursing is one specialty that ". . . considers and treats the child in the context of the family and recognizes the family as the primary and continuing provider of care for the child" (Friedman, 1998, p. 32).

FAMILY AS SUM OF ITS MEMBERS

In the second type of nursing practice with families, the family is viewed as the sum of the individual family members. Thus, "care is made available to or provided for all of the family members" (Friedman, 1998, p. 33). This type of nursing might be carried out in an intensive care unit where

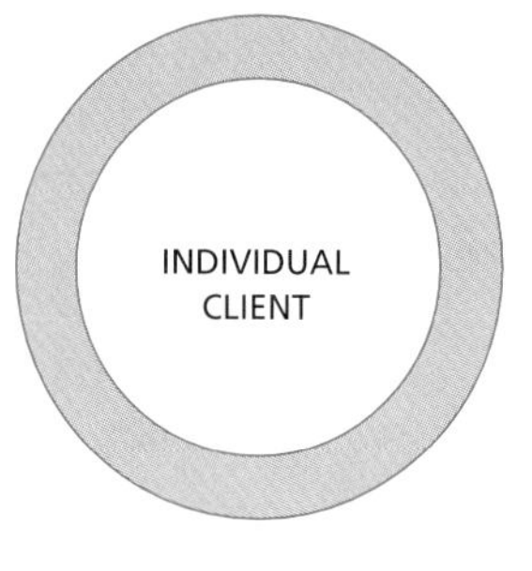

Level I
Family as Context

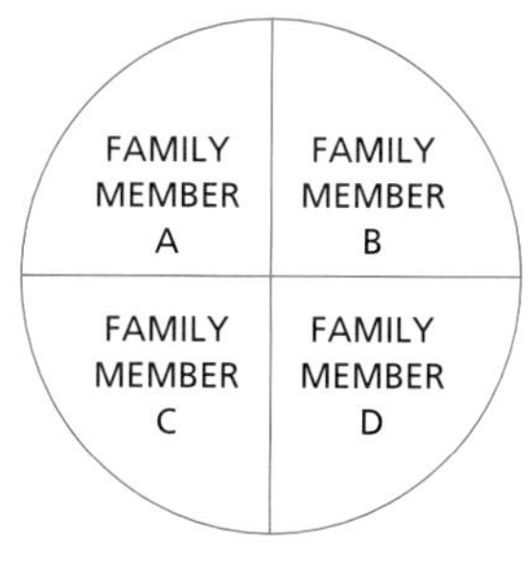

Level II
Family as Sum of Its Parts

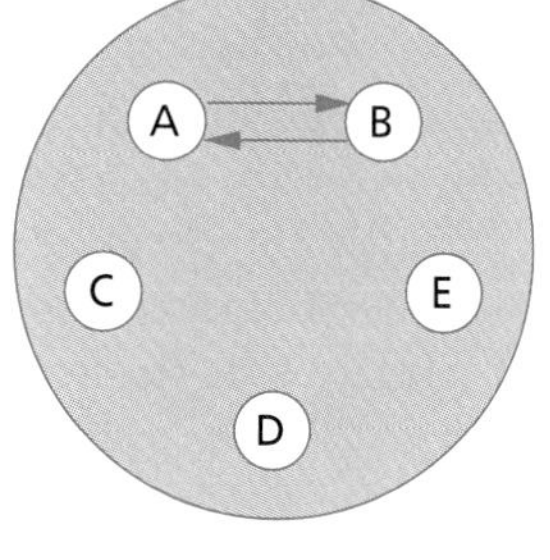

Level III
Family Subsystem as Client

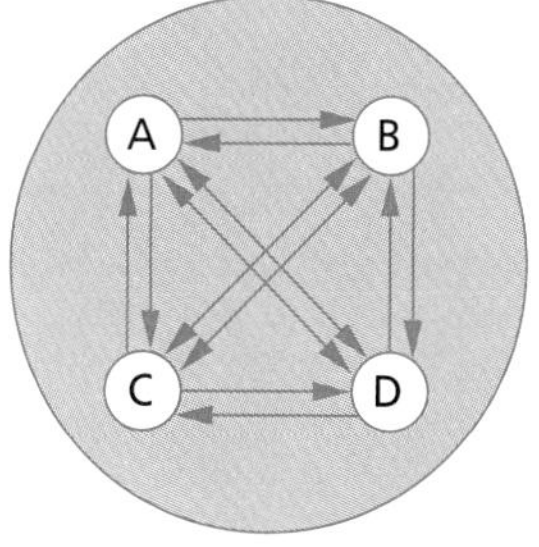

Level IV
Family as Client

FIGURE 10.1 Levels of family nursing practice

SOURCES: Adapted from Friedman, 1998; Wright & Leahey, 1994.

NURSES at work — Staff Nurse, Pediatric Hospital

I'm a staff nurse at the British Columbia Children's Hospital. During the course of a day at my job, I interact with many different people, employ a wide range of nursing skills and enjoy the rewards of "hands-on" care. In this tertiary care hospital, children come to our neurosurgical unit from all over the province, with a wide variety of diagnoses such as head injury, seizure disorders, non-accidental trauma, spina bifida (a tumour caused by a defect in the walls of the spinal canal, resulting in a protrusion of the membranes of the spinal cord) and brain tumours. Frequently, they have already been seen or treated in a community hospital and come to Children's Hospital for more specialized care.

A typical shift on our unit begins at 07:00 or 19:00 hours and lasts 12 hours. Each nurse is assigned three to five patients, depending on the complexity of each child's care. After studying my assignment for the shift and participating in a detailed nursing report, I spend about 15 minutes assessing each patient's condition briefly while taking vital signs. Pouring and administering medications is followed by breakfast and morning care. Our patients range in age from birth to 17 years and within this span, development varies from severely delayed to normal. The task of feeding four infants at once can be overwhelming! On the other hand, it is much easier to bathe an infant than to convince a toddler that she needs a bath, or to manoeuvre a comatose teenager into a Century tub.

It is a particular challenge to meet children's nutritional needs. Hospital food may be unfamiliar or unappealing to them. We keep a large stock of popsicles, ice cream, yogurt, pudding and juice, and we also encourage parents to bring favourite treats from home. During the day, I do ongoing assessment of nutritional and fluid intake, seizure activity, intravenous sites and rates, dressings, level of consciousness, as well as arranging school and playtimes. Probably the hospitalized child's greatest need is for love and security. To this end, the hospital actively promotes family-centred care. Parents and siblings are a constant presence on the ward. Because of this, I do a lot of teaching and a lot of listening.

This large teaching hospital attracts specialists and students from around the world. As a staff nurse, it is my job to facilitate their work while acting as an advocate for the client and family. I make decisions about when to contact the physician about the client's condition and which physician to contact. I ensure that orders are carried out safely and on time. I intervene when the family is overstressed from too many visitors or is attempting to cope with a catastrophic diagnosis. As the family nurse, I also coordinate the activities of physiotherapists, the Child Life Department, social services and pastoral care.

I see many sick children during a day. The rewarding part of my job is watching so many of them heal so quickly. Most children don't lie in bed for long. They are in a hurry to get out of bed and get on with the business of growing.

— *Anne Gasson, BA, RN,*
Staff Nurse, B.C. Children's Hospital

the nurse is concerned about the response of family members to their father's heart attack. The family's coping strategies and care-giving abilities, in addition to the father's needs, become the focus of assessment and planning for optimal care of the father once he goes home.

Community health nurses also practise this second type of family nursing, but a distinction has to be made in their target of practice. In community health nursing, the target of practice is the health of a community. Community health nurses attempt to enhance and maintain the health of the community by providing care to families. In the community health setting, the nurse would still be attentive to the health needs of the family, but the focus would be on common community problems that are relevant to the particular family. For example, in caring for a young childbearing family, the community health nurse would be concerned with such aspects as immunizations and family planning, along with the unique health needs of the family (Friedman, 1998).

FAMILY SUBSYSTEM AS PATIENT

The third type of nursing practice with families, looks at family subsystems as the focus of assessment and care. This model is the basis of interpersonal family nursing. (Friedemann 1993; Robinson 1995). The unit of analysis and care may be parent-child relationships, marital connection and care-giving issues.

FAMILY AS PATIENT

The fourth type of nursing practice with families is called *family systems nursing*. Family systems nursing views the whole family as a unit of care, such that the family *is* the patient. "Family systems nursing is the integration of nursing, systems, cybernetic and family therapy theories" (Wright & Leahey, 1990, p. 149). The focus of assessment and care is on family interactions and relationships, and on the reciprocity between family functioning and health and illness. The impact of illness on the family and the influence of family interaction on health, illness and healing are primary factors considered in plans for care. In family systems nursing, the nurse concentrates on the family system and individual systems simultaneously, and may also include the interaction of the community and society. Wright and Leahey offer a clear example of the nurse's involvement at all systems levels. They state:

> *... if the presenting problem is electrolyte imbalance, then the primary unit of treatment would be the individual patient with attention to the cellular level. If the presenting concern is a husband's understanding of the diabetic regimen, then the primary unit of treatment would be the family for health*

teaching about diet, exercise and insulin. If the patient is a school-age child, then the primary unit of treatment might also include, in addition to the family, the community (i.e., school) because this is where the child spends a large majority of time (1990, p. 150).

The type of family care the nurse chooses to practise depends largely on the clinical setting, the context of the health challenge and his or her expertise as a practitioner. For instance, when the primary focus of care is the illness or health challenge of a family member, as may occur in emergency rooms, intensive care units or medical-surgical areas, the conceptualization of family as context would be the appropriate choice for practice. This type of nursing with families is typically used by nurse generalists at the baccalaureate level. Wright and Leahey prefer the term *nursing of families* to describe this level of practice (1994). On the other hand, when the focus of care is the interaction and reciprocity of family members, family systems nursing would be more suitable. For example, family systems nursing might be used in helping a family resolve problems created by the pregnancy of an unwed adolescent daughter. According to Wright and Leahey (1994), family systems nursing requires specialization at the graduate (master's or doctoral) level.

As a beginning graduate, you will need interviewing theory and skills in order to work with families. The communication skills and interviewing techniques that you will need for family interviewing are outlined in Chapter 17. Here, we will outline a family assessment model and discuss nursing interventions for enabling families to promote their health and cope with stress and crisis in their lives.

Family Assessment

There are several assessment frameworks that can be used for assessing family health and well-being. Many combine family theory and nursing conceptual frameworks in order to identify the unique focus of family health in relation to nursing practice. Here we will present one such framework—The Calgary Family Assessment Model (CFAM).

THE CALGARY FAMILY ASSESSMENT MODEL

The Calgary Family Assessment Model, developed by Lorraine Wright and Maureen Leahey, is an integrated conceptual framework that combines concepts from nursing and family therapy to provide a clear, systematic model for assessment. The model, which was originally adapted from the assessment model produced at the Family Therapy Program, University of Calgary, places emphasis on a method of continuous family assessment rather than on family diagnosis. Thus, it focusses on the use of an open-ended and changing problem list rather than a finite schema of family classification (Tomm & Sanders, 1983).

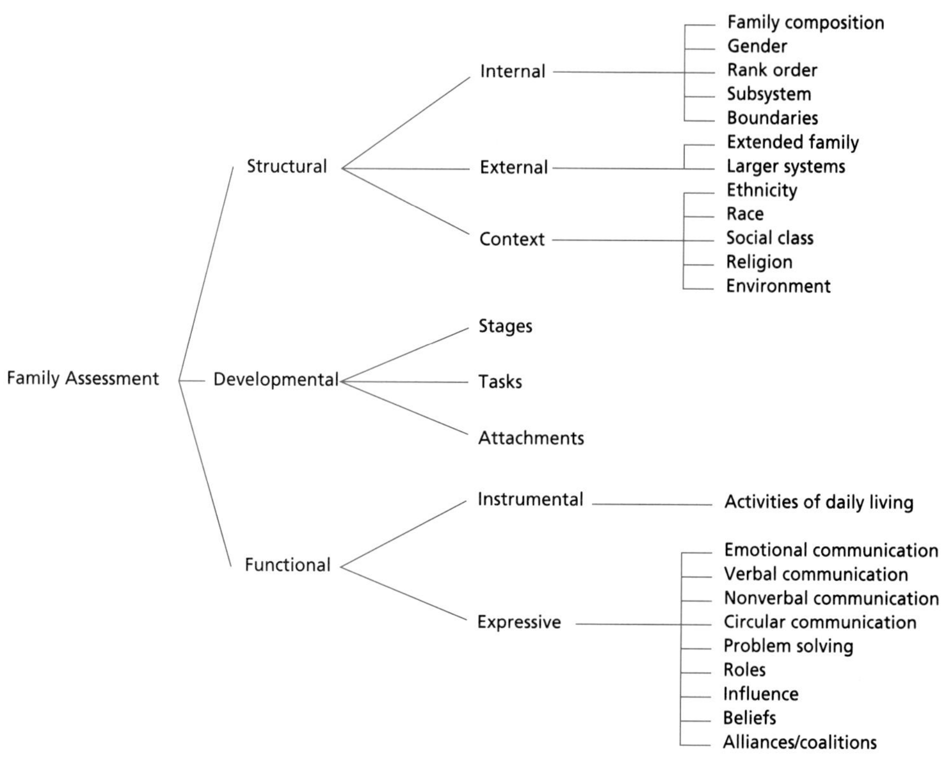

FIGURE 10.2 Branching diagram of CFAM

SOURCE: Wright & Leahey, 1994, p. 38.

The CFAM is a multidimensional model that incorporates structural, functional and developmental theory and is based on a systems–cybernetics–communication–change theory foundation. Individuals are viewed as bio–psycho–social–spiritual beings, and the person as a whole is seen to be greater than, and different from, the sum of his or her parts.

Five predominant systems concepts are used in the CFAM:

- a family system is part of a larger subsystem and is also composed of many subsystems
- the family as a whole is greater than the sum of its parts
- a change in one family member affects all family members
- the family is able to create a balance between change and stability
- family members' behaviours are best understood from a view of circular rather than linear causality.

There are two primary cybernetics concepts in the CFAM:

- families possess self-regulating ability through the process of feedback
- in families, feedback processes can occur simultaneously at several different systems levels.

At this point, it is necessary to differentiate cybernetics from systems theory. Conceived by mathematician Norbert Weiner, the term **cybernetics** refers to the science of communication and control theory. In cybernetics, both

The Calgary Family Assessment Model

Structural Assessment

Internal Structure

This includes the notions of family composition, rank order, subsystems and boundaries.

- *Family composition* refers to all members living in the home. This definition includes nuclear families, single-parent families, homosexual couples, boarders, grandparents, step-parents and children. A family is a small social system made up of individuals related to one another by reason of strong reciprocal affections and loyalties and comprising a permanent household that persists over years.
- *Gender* refers to the set of beliefs about or expectations of male and female behaviour and experiences that have developed by cultural, religious and family influences. Gender is an important consideration, because differences in how males and females experience the world is at the heart of therapeutic conversation.
- *Rank order* refers to the position of the children in the family with respect to age and gender. It is believed that sibling position influences personality and levels of motivation and achievement as well as vocational choices.
- *Subsystems* in a family are delineated by generation, sex, interests and function, according to Minuchin (1974). Each family member belongs to several subsystems that differentiate the level of power and skills. Examples of nontypical subsystems include a step-parent who lacks power over the children, or a child who has power over the parent.
- *Boundaries* refer to the rules defining which family members participate in functions and how. Boundaries protect family members by obtaining, containing, retaining and disposing of information, products or people. For example, a family may prevent members from bringing in drugs or using vulgar language, or it may prevent members from divulging family information to outsiders. Boundaries can be diffuse or rigid, and the degree of permeability may change over time.

External Structure

This includes two subcategories: extended family and larger systems.

- The *extended family* includes grandparents, aunts, uncles and cousins who may live near or far away.
- The subcategory of *larger systems* refers to social agencies and personnel with whom the family has meaningful contact. Such systems generally include work systems. For some families they may include welfare, child care, foster care, courts and ambulatory clinics. They may also include services for special populations such as people with mental or physical disabilities or frail older adults.

Context

This term describes the whole situation or background relevant to the family. Each family system is part of broader systems such as neighbourhood, social class, religion, community and country.

- *Ethnicity* refers to the concept of a family's "peoplehood," which is derived from a blend of cultural heritage, race and religion. It pertains to the ancestral roots or origins of a population and depicts a commonality of conscious and unconscious processes that are transmitted by the family over generations. Ethnicity is an important factor influencing family life as well as family health beliefs and practices.
- *Race* refers to a distinct group of people who share certain physical characteristics such as skin colour or body frame that are transmitted genetically. Its influence on family life is mediated by variables such as social class, religion and ethnicity. Racial attitudes, stereotyping and

discrimination are powerful influences on family interaction, and if they are not addressed, they can have negative effects on nurse–family relationships.

- *Social class* status and mobility strongly influence the family value system. The adults' educational attainment, income and occupation usually determine values that influence the family's lifestyle and behavioural patterns.
- *Religion* refers to the family values, size, health care practices and socialization practices. It includes level of community involvement and maintaining of certain traditions, both religious and hygienic.
- *Environment* refers to both the general neighbourhood and the home. The type of neighbourhood, proximity of stores, transportation, recreation and health facilities are considered. In the home, the amount of space and privacy, along with access, safety and security, are important.

Developmental Assessment

The family development level is based on the family developmental framework, outlined earlier in this chapter, and on Falicov's definition of family development. According to Falicov, "... family development is an over-arching concept, referring to all transactional evolutionary processes connected with the growth of the family ..." (cited in Wright & Leahey, 1994, p. 57). In addition, she states:

> Although there is a regularity and internal logic to many of the processes subsumed under family development ... each family is different precisely because each can be said to have its own developmental path, which evolves from all the different settings in which development takes place, including each family's construction of its past and present (cited in Wright & Leahey, 1994, p. 58).

Stages

There are eight stages to the family development assessment. The term *stages* refers to the identifiable periods that occur during the length of marriage and are noted by the age of the eldest child. The cycles are repeated as later children reach the identified stages. Family theorists stress that families do not move smoothly or automatically through one stage to another and that there are stressful transition points along the way.

Tasks

Tasks include general maintenance responsibilities such as employment, spending, education and socialization, which are necessary to achieve a satisfactory resolution of the stages. The tasks are outlined for each of the stages.

Attachments

Attachments are the unique and relatively enduring emotional ties between two family members. They are looked at from an adaptive and maladaptive perspective at each of the eight stages.

Functional Assessment

Family functions include the actual behaviours of family members in relation to daily activities and their emotional interactions. There is an instrumental function and an expressive function.

Instrumental Functioning

Instrumental functioning includes activities of daily living in a family.

Activities of daily living are the patterns of functioning such as working, eating, sleeping and cooking meals. These are what the family members do together and what they do alone, and they constitute the more frequent everyday activities. The instrumental function may include the tasks involved in caring for an ill or elderly family member.

Expressive Functioning

Expressive functioning involves emotional communication, verbal communication, nonverbal communication, circular communication, problem solving, roles, influence, beliefs and alliances/coalitions.

Communication between family members includes verbal and nonverbal exchanges, as well as the range and types of emotions and feelings expressed in interaction. Circular communication refers to the reciprocal communication between members or the patterns they establish in the relationship that are adaptive or problematic.

Problem solving refers to the family's method of identifying and solving problems, that is, how decisions are made and who is called upon to make them.

Roles of family members are their established patterns of behaviour as they interact with one another. Each member can have overlapping roles. These roles may be assumed or assigned, formal or informal. What function have these roles in family interaction?

Influence refers to the methods that family members use to affect one another's behaviour. Instrumental influence refers to the use of objects or privileges (for example, the use of money, watching television or going to a movie) as reinforcers. Psychological influence refers to communication and feelings (for instance, words, affection or the withholding of these) to control members.

The term *beliefs* refers to the expectations, attitudes, values and priorities that the family holds. Are different views tolerated by other family members? What are the family myths?

The term *alliances/coalitions* refers to the direction, balance and intensity of relationships among family members.

SOURCE: Wright & Leahey, 1994.

parts and wholes are looked at in terms of their patterns of organization (Keeney, 1982). **Systems theory**, you will recall, is a science of wholeness. As such, it examines the interconnections of two or more parts that form an organized whole and that interact with each other. The whole is greater than the sum of its parts.

Even though systems theory speaks of feedback from a similar perspective, cybernetics distinguishes feedback as positive or negative. Positive or negative feedback occurs in a family system as information about the output. With positive feedback, information serves to increase the output, whereas with negative feedback, the same information serves to decrease the output. For example, if nagging a withdrawing husband increases his withdrawal behaviour, then positive feedback has occurred. On the other hand, if nagging causes the husband to withdraw less, then negative feedback has occurred (Wright & Leahey, 1994). With cybernetics, feedback may occur at several levels simultaneously. Therefore, the communication pattern between a nagging wife and withdrawing husband, for example, would be examined in greater scope and involve the couple's relationship to their families of origin.

The four communication concepts used in the CFAM are:

- all verbal communication is meaningful
- all communication has two major channels for transmission: digital and analogic. **Digital** refers to verbal communication and **analogic** refers to usual nonverbal communication such as body posture, facial expression and tone, as well as creative expression such as music, poetry and painting. If there are discrepancies between the digital and analogic channels, then the analogic is seen as more valid and reliable
- a dyadic relationship has varying degrees of symmetry and complementarity. A relationship is symmetrical when the two people behave as if they have equal status, for instance, a preadolescent peer relationship. In a complementary relationship, the two people are of unequal status, where one appears to initiate action and the other follows. A basic example of a complementary relationship is a mother and an infant
- all communication consists of two levels: content and relationships. Content refers to what is being said. Relationship defines the nature of the connection between those interacting, for example, whether it is loving or conflictual.

The CFAM uses seven change concepts. These are:

- change is dependent on the perception of the problem
- change is dependent on context
- change is dependent on coevolving goals for treatment. Goals are set collaboratively between the nurse and the family once the family has gained a different view of its problem and the changes it desires
- understanding alone does not lead to change
- change does not necessarily occur equally in all family members
- facilitating change is the nurse's responsibility
- change can be due to a myriad of causes.

In the CFAM, families are seen to be a group of individuals who are bound by attributes of affection, strong emotional ties and a sense of belonging. A family evolves an ecology of beliefs that helps each individual to define thoughts (cognitions), behaviours and emotions. Individuals and families are seen to be unique and autonomous, possessing the strengths and abilities necessary to solve their own problems. The focus is on "family" even when only one person is involved in treatment, because individuals are best understood within the context of their families.

Health is viewed through relationships and communication with other human beings. Distinctions such as "health" and "illness" are believed to be subjective judgements made by observers about adaptation. When individuals or families are seen with problems that have been identified, this model seeks to invite new ways to view the situation (in order to broaden the choices for solution) without making judgements about the problem or solution.

We mentioned earlier in this section that the CFAM incorporates structural, functional and developmental theory. CFAM considers each of these approaches separately, and consists of the following three major categories:

1. structural
2. developmental
3. functional.

Each assessment category contains several subcategories. It is important for the nurse to decide which subcategories are relevant and appropriate for families at particular times. That is, not all subcategories need to be assessed at the first meeting and some may never have to be used. Wright and Leahey (1994) conceptualize the three assessment categories and the many subcategories as a branching diagram adapted from the work of Tomm and Sanders (1993, see Figure 10.2 on page 229). Although the family may be examined by looking at specific parts, each part interacts with others and changes the whole family configuration.

The CFAM is very useful during assessment because it can be applied to various types of families such as single-parent, blended and communal families. It also includes extended-family members. Another advantage of this model is that it integrates sociocultural, ethnic and community data. The nurse poses questions to the family to assess each of the categories.

The Genogram and the Ecomap

The genogram and the ecomap are two tools commonly used in working with families. They are particularly helpful to the nurse in outlining the family's internal and external structures.

RESEARCH to practice

Grandine, J (1995). Embracing the family. *The Canadian Nurse. 91*(9) pp. 31–35

Family nursing has been a component of nursing but until recently family care has received little attention in publications and academic and clinical practice settings. Nurses are in an ideal situation to assist families experiencing health problems. This task is difficult to accomplish due to the changing health care system and the skill level of nurses working with families. At Peel Memorial Hospital in Brampton Ontario. A course called Family Systems Nursing was developed to increase the nurses theoretical and practical knowledge of family nursing. The course included an overview of the theoretical foundations of family nursing, the Calgary Family Assessment Model(C-FAM), interviewing skills and family intervention strategies. Initial outcomes identify that nurses had increased job satisfaction, gained confidence when working with a model, that enhances partnerships. In assessing the effectiveness of the course, from the families perspective, they revealed that they communicated more effectively, increased their understanding of ways to cope and improve their family situation and had an overall sense of well being.

IMPLICATIONS FOR PRACTICE

As a result of this established program there has been:

- increased collaboration with other health professionals
- established scheduled family interviews
- ongoing seminars
- annual workshops with updated content
- increased sense of self worth
- a shift to a more holistic nursing perspective
- a reduction of family complaints
- an increase in family/nursing collaboration

The **genogram** is a diagram of the family constellation that shows the structure of the intergenerational relationships of a family. The **ecomap**, on the other hand, is a diagram of the family's contact with others outside the immediate family. It pictures the important connections between the family and the world. Both the genogram and the ecomap are simple to use and require only paper and pencil.

GENOGRAM

The skeleton of the genogram tends to follow conventional genealogical charts. It is useful to include at least three generations. Family members are placed on horizontal rows that signify generational lines. For example, a marriage or common-law relationship is denoted by a horizontal line. Children are denoted by vertical lines that are rank-ordered from left to right beginning with the eldest child. Each individual is represented. Ages are noted, as are illnesses and deaths. A blank genogram is shown in Figure 10.3.

Authors differ slightly in the symbols that they use for details of the genogram. The symbols depicted in Figure 10.4 are generally agreed upon by the majority of family therapists (Wright & Leahey, 1994). The person's name and age should be noted *inside* the square or circle. Significant data, such as "depressed" or "overinvolved at work," should be noted *outside* the symbol.

The genogram is an important tool that can be used when conducting a family interview. At the beginning of the

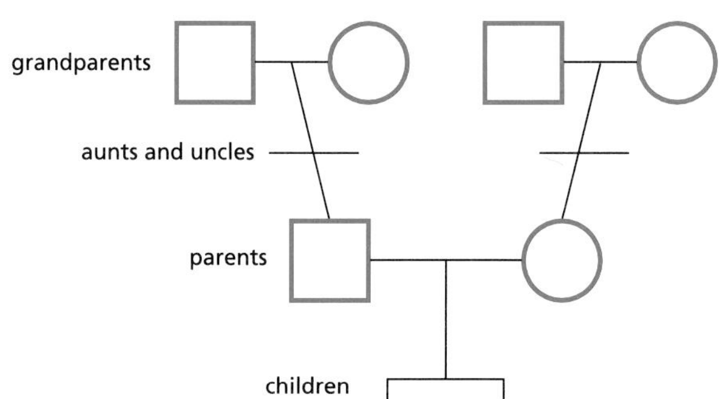

FIGURE 10.3 Sample of a blank genogram

SOURCE: Wright & Leahey, 1994, p. 50.

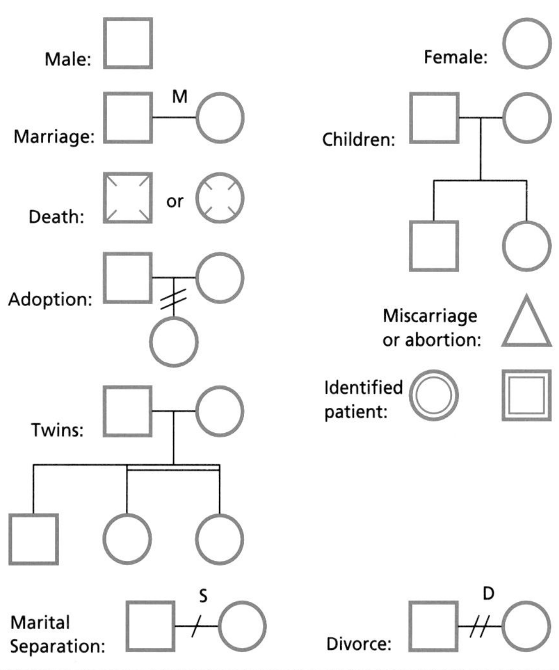

FIGURE 10.4 Symbols used in genograms

SOURCE: Wright & Leahey, 1994, p. 51.

interview, the nurse can tell the family that they will be asked a few background questions that will help to gain an overview of their situation. The nurse uses the structure of the genogram to spell out the family's composition and boundaries. The interviewer starts with a blank sheet of paper and draws a square or circle for the first person with whom he or she is talking. After enquiring about the immediate family, the nurse continues to ask about the extended family. It is important to gain an overview of the family structure without getting sidetracked and inundated by a volume of information. Most families are extremely cooperative and interested in completing the genogram.

ECOMAP

As with the genogram, the primary value of the ecomap is in its visual impact. The purpose of the ecomap is to depict family members' contact with their outside world. It demonstrates the flow of resources or the lack of deprivations. The mapping procedure highlights the points of conflict to be mediated, bridges to be built and resources to be sought and mobilized. As with the genogram, family members can actively participate in working on the ecomap during the assessment. An ecomap is depicted in Figure 10.5.

The family genogram is placed in the centre of the ecomap (see the circle in the centre of Figure 10.5). The outer circles represent significant people, agencies or institutions within this family's context. Lines are drawn between the family members and the outer circles to show the nature of the connections. Straight lines depict strong connections, dotted lines depict tenuous connections and slashed lines depict stressful relationships. Arrows can be drawn beside the lines to indicate the flow of energy and resources.

Family Intervention

FAMILY HEALTH PROMOTION AND PROTECTION

In keeping with the Ottawa Charter for Health Promotion (WHO, 1986), family health promotion is defined as the process of enabling families to increase control over and improve the quality of life and well-being. Families promote health by creating living conditions in which family members' experiences of health and well-being are increased. They do this by teaching and fostering good health practices, such as washing hands before handling food or eating, and

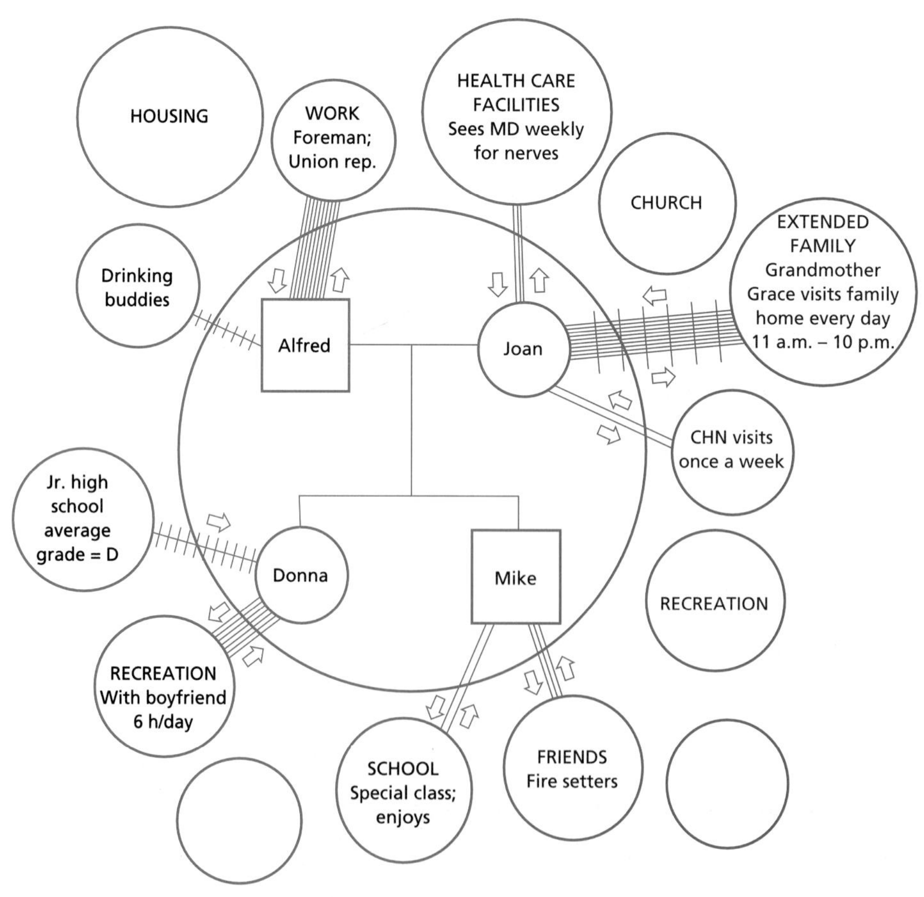

FIGURE 10.5 Ecomap

SOURCE: Wright & Leahey, 1994, p. 57.

by managing health resources, such as providing a safe, clean dwelling. Families also protect their health by promoting activities that prevent or decrease the risk of disease, for example, avoidance of smoking, alcohol or drugs. Nursing interventions for family health promotion and health protection are based on the assumptions that families are the best judges of their health needs and that they are capable of assuming responsibility for health and those things that affect their health. Thus, families are seen as collaborative partners with health professionals in promoting health and wellness of members. Collaboration implies the sharing of information and equal participation in decision making and assumption of responsibilities (Lancaster, McCance & Vanderschmidt, 1986). Families are asked what their health care needs are as opposed to being told. In addition, their opinions regarding health care are considered along with those of the health professional.

The nurse's role in family health promotion is to help in enhancing family resources (that is, their strengths and capabilities) so that members can increase control over and improve their health. Nurses do this by identifying families' personal meanings of health, determining their strengths and capabilities and educating them about health and healthy living. Nurses also promote family health by facilitating use of health resources and fostering active family involvement in health-promoting programs and policies in the community.

IDENTIFYING FAMILY MEANINGS OF HEALTH In order for nurses to intervene effectively in family health promotion, they must understand a family's personal definition of *health*. Health means different things to different families. For a retired couple, health might mean having the finances and the physical capabilities to live in their own home, drive their automobile, get out and visit with friends and relatives and continue with leisure activities such as walking, swimming or golfing. A young childbearing family, on the other hand, might define its health as the ability of all members to eat nutritiously, to express themselves freely, to be actively involved in school activities and sports and to participate together in leisure activities. These examples point to the fact that a family's view of health changes as it progresses through the family life cycle. A family's personal meaning of health is also influenced by its health beliefs, its past experiences with health and its cultural and ethnic background.

Some families have a clear idea of what health means to them; others do not. It is not unusual to find people who say that they do not really think about their health beliefs or practices. They simply behave according to past traditions and norms without too much thought about the effects these might have. It is not until they have reflected upon and considered their personal beliefs and practices that they might see a need for improvement or change. Therefore, an appraisal of the family's personal definition of health assists both nurse and family. This appraisal helps the family become aware of its own health beliefs and practices, and at

Social Trends of Canadian Families

Children

- 1 in 4 children under 12 lived in low-income families (1994)
- 32% of children aged 0–11 were in child care (1994)
- 2% of children under age 15 lived with relatives (1991)
- 53% of females and 31% of males had been victims of unwanted sexual acts. Most of these acts occurred when they were children or adolescents.

Seniors

- most seniors lived at home
- 28% of seniors over the age of 65 lived alone; 8% lived with extended family
- 38% of senior women lived alone.

First Nations Peoples

- birth and fertility rates were twice the Canadian average (1993)
- 33.4% of First Nations Canadians were unemployed, compared with 10% of the Canadian population
- 23% of all First Nations families were headed by a single parent, compared with 13% of the Canadian population
- 62% reported alcohol abuse; 49% reported drug abuse
- 22% of youth reported chronic solvent abuse
- suicide rates were 3 times higher than in the general population
- 39% believed family violence was a concern
- 4% of children were in the care of child and family services (1993–94)
- 5% of children lived with relatives.

Canadians

- marriage occurred later in life (in 1992, average ages for women and men were 27 and 29, respectively)
- one-half of women over the age of 16 reported violence by an intimate partner
- women were 4 times more likely to be injured by a male partner than by a motor vehicle accident
- stalking and harassment of women by spouses were common after separation
- 43% of injuries inflicted by spouses required medical intervention (1993)
- 27% of births occurred outside marriage (1991)
- two-thirds of men and women aged 20–24 lived with a parent
- 67% of young adults lived with their mother (1990).

SOURCES: Statistics Canada, 1996, 1997a, 1997b; National Forum on Health, 1997; Health Canada, 1996; Oderkirk, 1994; Zukewich Galam, 1996; Boyd & Norris, 1995.

the same time helps the nurse gain knowledge of the family's views and perceptions. The nurse can view the family through their own eyes, so to speak.

Communication and interviewing techniques such as discussion, exploration, values clarification and critical reflection are tools that the nurse uses in helping families define health. These are discussed in Chapter 17.

DETERMINING FAMILY STRENGTHS AND CAPABILITIES

Family strengths and capabilities are central to interventions that enable families to take responsibility for and control over the health of their members. Duffy (1988) states that "health promotion in the family is the result of an interaction between the internal environment of the family and the external environment which impinges upon it" (p. 112). The internal environment mainly refers to structure and function. Family structure includes composition, subsystems, boundaries, social class, roles, power, occupation and income of adult members. Family function refers to things like activities of daily living, allocation of tasks, communication, problem solving and decision making.

The external environment involves a wide range of influences outside the family, for example, the kinship network, religious affiliations, type of neighbourhood and community resources, including health promotion facilities. A study done by Blaxter and Patterson (1983) found that an environment of poverty, rather than the health attitudes and behaviours of mothers, contributed to accidents in families. Poverty is said to be "the greatest threat to health promotion since it decreases the family's options, thus contributing to many of the health problems faced by the poor" (Duffy, 1988, p. 112).

An analysis of family structure and function will determine a family's strengths and capabilities for healthy living as well as its weaknesses. Once these are established, the nurse and the family can work together to plan activities that support existing strengths. In addition, resources can be appropriated to fulfill health needs within the economic constraints of the family.

EDUCATING FAMILIES ABOUT HEALTH AND HEALTHY LIVING

In order for people to analyse their health behaviours and determine their health needs, they must have knowledge about health and healthy living conditions. For instance, many people considered eggs to be an excellent dietary source of protein until researchers learned of their high fat and cholesterol content. Similarly, a pregnant woman may think an occasional social drink is acceptable until she learns of the potential harmful effects of alcohol on her growing fetus.

Dunn (1980) identified education of individuals and families about health and healthy living as an important approach for promoting high-level wellness. Through education, families are provided with information that assists them to cope more effectively with life, life changes and stresses of daily living. Having useful information helps families feel a sense of control and enables them to explore options and solve their own problems (Watson, 1985). Because nurses interact directly with families in hospitals, in community clinics and at home, they play a large role in educating families about health and self-care. Using the principles of teaching and learning outlined in Chapter 18, nurses educate families in a number of ways. They can give information through verbal interaction, handouts or pamphlets. They may suggest books or videos that the family can obtain from the library. Nurses also teach caregiving skills through role modelling or demonstration, for example, instructing a new childbearing family in bathing techniques and infant care.

FACILITATING FAMILY USE OF HEALTH RESOURCES "Many families are in need of supportive services at various points of their lives; at other times a supportive environment is all that is necessary to enable a family to function effectively" (Lundy, 1992, p. 4). Many healthy families actively seek out health resources in their community, with little need for assistance from health professionals. There are others, however, who are not able to do this for themselves. These people either lack knowledge of available resources or perceive themselves as being unable to pursue assistance. They also may not know how to go about obtaining needed resources.

Nurses provide support to these families by helping them find and then access the resources they require to meet their needs. Because these people often feel helpless, it is important for the nurse to bolster their sense of self-esteem and self-confidence so that they feel empowered to take action for themselves. To illustrate, one nurse helped an elderly family find respite care to ease the burden of the spouse in caring for his wife.

> *Cora, who has been living with diabetes and Parkinson's disease for the past 20 years, is no longer able to look after herself. Her spouse, Elmer, takes care of her and maintains the household. He doesn't go out very often because he can't leave Cora alone. When Cora is in hospital, Elmer confides to the nurse that he is finding it more and more difficult to care for Cora. In further discussion with Elmer, the nurse finds out that he is not aware of services in the community that may be able to provide assistance, such as adult day care or respite programs. When the nurse suggests some options to Elmer, he is reluctant to pursue them because he does not know how to go about doing such things. With Elmer's consent, the nurse places a phone call that starts the process of arranging respite care.*

In this case, all that was needed was a community support worker who would come into the home and spend time with Cora so that Elmer could get out for some exercise, do the shopping or spend time with friends at the recreation centre.

There is a wide range of resources in the community that offer education and support to families in meeting their health needs. Local, regional or provincial social services and human resources agencies provide financial assistance, housing and child care. In addition, health services, such as adult day care for seniors or homemaker services for families in need, are often available.

Community organizations offer educational programs dealing with family life, such as marriage counselling and positive parenting. There are supportive networks for new parents, adolescent parents and gays and lesbians. Community health agencies also provide well-baby clinics, which offer programs for screening infant growth and development, immunization and teaching of infant needs and care. There are also a host of educational programs such as "quit smoking" or "eating for heart health" directed towards preventive health.

Many communities provide drop-in centres for all age groups—seniors, women, teens and families. Transition houses for battered and abused women and children are available in urban centres in Canada. In large cities where language and cultural beliefs of different ethnic groups may pose problems to families, interpreters and other resource persons for new immigrants are available through neighbourhood and community centres, local drop-in centres or churches. Communities often modify programs and facilities to meet the ever-changing health needs of individuals and families. Therefore, it is important for nurses to keep up to date with the various health resources in their communities.

FOSTERING ACTIVE INVOLVEMENT OF FAMILIES IN HEALTHY COMMUNITIES Canadian families have the opportunity to participate in decision making and public policy regarding health promotion issues in their communities. Through what is known as the Healthy Communities initiative, municipal governments and residents can work together to resolve their health issues and create supportive environments for health (B.C. Ministry of Health, 1992). Providing safe streets and roads, adequate and affordable housing, recreational activities for teens and clean and smoke-free environments are but a few examples of health issues for which communities created solutions and set policies that would promote healthy living for their residents.

The Healthy Communities concept arose from the World Health Organization's emerging definition of health and health promotion (WHO, 1986), which recognized the importance of public policy, particularly at the municipal level, in creating a physical and social environment that promotes health for the community as a whole (B.C. Ministry of Health, 1992). Families may become directly involved in the health of their communities by identifying issues and by participating in the development of programs and public policies. Nursing's participation in health promotion at the community level will be discussed in Chapter 11.

In family nursing, the nurse's role is to give information, and to nurture and empower families to take action on health issues in their communities. Information and guidelines on the process of establishing health-promoting policies in communities may be obtained from the Office of Health Promotion, Ministry of Health, in each province.

CRISIS INTERVENTION WITH FAMILIES

The family has a very distinct position in our society. It is the most common source of support and understanding when we are in trouble, yet it can also be the domain in which we encounter our most intense distress. All families have problems at one time or another, and all families deal with problems in their own ways. Some are more successful than others in solving their problems. Much of their success depends on the resources available to them and their usual strategies for coping (Hoff, 1995). Nursing intervention for families experiencing stress and crisis in their lives focusses on helping them to identify their strengths and resources and mobilize their coping strategies. This involves establishing communication and rapport, determining the family's understanding of the stressors, facilitating use of social supports and resources and supporting family coping strategies. **Empowerment**—that is, enabling families to assume control over their stressor, meet their needs and re-establish their health and harmony—is central to crisis intervention with families.

ESTABLISHING COMMUNICATION AND RAPPORT Interventions for family stress and crisis depend upon the establishment of rapport and effective communication. Hoff argues that crisis interventions are not likely to work unless nurses can establish rapport and communicate effectively with families. She maintains that communication is the medium through which:

- we struggle to survive (for example, by giving away prized possessions or saying "I don't care anymore" as a cry for help after a serious loss)
- we develop meaningful human communication and maintain it (such as giving and receiving support during stress and crisis)
- we bring stability and organization into our lives (such as by sorting out the chaotic elements of a traumatic event with a caring person)
- we negotiate social and political struggles at the national and international level (Hoff, 1995, p. 106).

Hoff also maintains that when communication fails, people may feel alone, abandoned, worthless and unloved, or in conflict. "The most tragic result of failed communication is violence toward self and others; at the societal level it translates into war. Such destructive outcomes of failed communication are more probable in acute crisis situations" (Hoff, 1995, p. 106). Nurses need good communication skills in order to work with families in stress and crisis.

Nurses must also establish a relationship in which the family will accept their help. The quality of the relationship, in particular the empathy, caring and sincerity displayed by the nurse, has been shown to affect the outcome of work with people in crisis (Hoff, 1995). Hoff says that in trying to establish rapport with people in crisis we should strive for two objectives:

1. we should make the distressed person feel understood. We can convey understanding by using reflective statements such as, "You seem to be very hurt and upset by what has happened" and "Sounds like you're very angry." If our perception of what the person is feeling is incorrect, the words "seem to be" and "sounds like" provide an opening for the person to explain his or her perception of the traumatic event. The expression "I understand" should generally be avoided, as it may be perceived as presumptuous; there is always the possibility that we do not truly understand. Parents who suffer the loss of a child say that no one but a similarly grieving parent can truly understand
2. if we are unclear about the nature or extent of what the person feels or is troubled by, we should convey our wish to understand by asking, for example, "Could you tell me more about that?" or "How do you feel about what has happened?" or "I'm not sure I understand—could you tell me what you mean by that?" (Hoff, 1995, p. 110).

DETERMINING FAMILY UNDERSTANDING OF THE STRESSOR

A family's ability to cope with a stressful event is influenced by its perception of the problem. Even though family responses to stressful events vary, there is evidence to support the theory that distress increases:

- when people encounter a number of stressors all at once
- when they experience the stressor for a prolonged period of time
- when they are exposed to a stressor with little time to anticipate problem solving.

Distress also increases when people encounter events that are highly ambiguous, or when they present hardships or serious consequences, such as death. As stress increases, people develop a distorted view of the stressor. They often experience such feelings as helplessness, hopelessness, anxiety, fatigue and depression (Clemen-Stone et al., 1998).

In order for a stressor to become problematic, "it must be perceived as a threat or loss to needs satisfaction or as a challenge" (Caplan, 1964, pp. 42–43). Caplan believes that there are two major variables that affect how people perceive life events. These are personality and sociocultural factors. "These variables determine the type of life experiences one has, prescribe the limits of acceptable behaviour when dealing with stress, and influence how one feels about one's abilities to handle changes in life" (cited in Clemen-Stone et al., 1998, p. 208). By way of example, let's consider two childrearing families, both of whom lost the father, about six months ago. Both fathers were the families' sole providers.

> *In the first family, the Whites, the mother is distraught. She can barely look after her two school-aged children. Her home is untidy, she cries all the time and cannot see how she will cope with the future. Her husband made all decisions for the family. Mrs. White is concerned because her husband's insurance is not adequate for the family's needs. She married at a young age and has never worked because it was the family belief that women should stay at home and care for the family. She is afraid to consider work outside the home because she thinks she is not capable of doing anything besides cleaning the house, cooking meals and raising a family.*
>
> *In the second family, we see a different picture. Five months after her husband's death, Mrs. Storly perceives that while she is still grieving, she is managing well. She arranged day care for her preschool daughter and obtained a job at a local A&W restaurant, where she had worked as a teenager. She is planning to enroll in nursing at a community college. Money will be a problem; however, she will seek financial assistance from her municipal social services. In addition, Mrs. Storly's parents have offered to help pay for her education.*

Both these families have experienced similar stressor events in that both lost a significant other who was the sole family provider. In the White family, the mother was immobilized by sociocultural beliefs regarding her role and a lack of confidence in her abilities to work outside the home. Mrs. Storly, on the other hand, took control of her situation and became actively involved in assuming her provider role.

COMMUNITY health practice: Street Youth and Gangs

A report written for the Ministry of the Solicitor General of Canada (1993) revealed that youth got involved in gangs because of perceived need for personal safety, escape from an abusive home environment, peer pressure, and social or financial need. A predominant theme that emerged while interviewing these street-involved youth was that they perceived themselves to be members of a family. Moreover, they describe this family form as dysfunctional and, at times, more dangerous to be part of than their biological family.

McCarthy (1996) prepared a report about youth who live on the streets of Vancouver. In his study, street youth reported physical and sexual abuse in their home environment as reasons for leaving home. Much of their time was spent unsuccessfully searching for food, shelter and employment. As a result, these youth often turned to crime to obtain the basic necessities of life.

SOURCES: McCarthy, 1996; Mathews, 1993.

Having worked as a teenager, she was more confident in her abilities. The life experiences of both women provided them with differing perceptions of their roles, which influenced their sense of control over the stressor events.

FACILITATING USE OF FAMILY SOCIAL SUPPORT AND RESOURCES "Whether or not stressful events lead to crisis depends on a family's resources for handling such events" (Hoff, 1995, p. 138). In times of difficulty, many people turn to someone with whom they have a meaningful relationship for strength and support. The network of social relationships through which resources may be derived is known as *social support* (Kane, 1988). A family's social support network may include relatives, friends, neighbours, colleagues, health professionals, social workers, employers, teachers, school counsellors, clergy and lawyers.

Kane maintains that "family social support is a pattern of social interaction characterized by interdependence in social relationships" (1988, p. 20). For example, when Janice's husband suffered a near fatal heart attack at the age of 44, she sought help from her younger sister, Julie, someone with whom she shares a special relationship. Both sisters have always "been there" for one another in times of need. For families, social support comes from long-term relationships and the things they have in common (Kane, 1988). Social supports provide a *buffer* against stressor events and have a *mediating effect*, which fosters effective coping strategies (Clemen-Stone et al., 1998).

Nurses can assist families by helping them to identify and obtain social supports. When first confronted with a situational crisis—for example, when a family member is admitted to the emergency or critical care unit—families often experience a period of distress and disorganization. During this time, a calm, sensitive manner, reassurance and an atmosphere that enables expression of feelings will help reduce tension and foster a sense of control. The nurse might also help the family contact their support people by providing access to a telephone or making the call for them.

SUPPORTING FAMILY COPING STRATEGIES During times of disequilibrium, people need supportive relationships that enable them to verbalize feelings, sort out the realities of their situation and begin to solve their problems (Clemen-Stone et al., 1998). When first confronted with a crisis, people often have a distorted view of the situation and want to place blame on someone else. Furthermore, initial shock and anxiety can cause difficulty in understanding and storing information accurately. Clear, simple explanations, focussing only on aspects that will relieve immediate concerns, are necessary at this point. The nurse should give family members time to ventilate feelings and help them place their circumstances into perspective. Reassure families that their reactions are common and predictable. Figley (1989) maintains that "normalizing" a family's situation is an effective supportive technique. Avoid and discourage blaming behaviours, as these only inhibit family growth and successful problem solving.

Effective support for family coping strategies is based on the assumption that families possess a "natural resourcefulness" for solving their own problems. All families have strengths and resources to help them deal with stressful events. Nurses can support families in crisis by empowering them to identify their strengths and coping strategies. We can explore coping mechanisms that the family has found effective in the past. If these are not adequate for the current situation, then we can assist further by exploring new coping mechanisms. Help might also be needed in mobilizing community resources such as financial assistance or home care services. Figley explains the benefit of empowerment in crisis intervention:

> *I try to empower the family by creating the kind of intervention context that results in the resolution of the traumatizing experience but, just as importantly, that results in the family's giving themselves most of the credit for the accomplishment. Moreover, this approach makes the family feel more confident to face any future traumatic experience equipped with the necessary information, skills, and problem-solving methods. (1989, p. 42).*

IN REVIEW

- In most societies, the family is the basic unit for reproduction, socialization and perpetuation of sociocultural traditions. Factors that influence a family's health include:
  - family role
  - health beliefs and practices
  - culture and ethnicity
  - socioeconomic conditions
  - environment (internal/external)
  - communication and coping skills
  - links with the community.
- The family is considered a primary resource for its members in times of trouble or illness. Research has demonstrated that family support and involvement are crucial to healing.
- Family stress, or a state of imbalance in the family, signals a need for change. Continuing unresolved stress can lead to:
  - health problems
  - crisis, disorganization of the family unit
  - a state of immobilization.
- There are many types of families, including:
  - nuclear
  - extended
  - single-parent
  - blended

- cohabiting
- gay or lesbian
- communal.

- Conceptual frameworks of the family give a perspective on family life and provide a basis for:
  - assessing families
  - interpreting their needs
  - planning interventions.
- Three frameworks commonly used in family nursing include:
  - the family systems framework
  - the structural-functional framework
  - the family developmental framework.
- In working with families, nurses must:
  - be aware of the characteristics of the various family forms
  - identify strengths and resources of the family
  - promote family health through education
  - empower the family to create living conditions conducive to a good quality of life
  - facilitate family support and use of community resources
  - assist families to function effectively.

Critical Thinking Activities

1. When working with families, the nurse brings along a unique set of beliefs about family based on personal life experiences. It is important for the nurse to be aware of his or her values and attitudes about family and effective family functioning and to ensure that these are not unconsciously imposed on the patient. Clarify your beliefs and values of family through reflection, talking with classmates and reading professional literature on the subject. Find a values clarification tool in the literature (Pender, 1987, pp. 162–181 gives one) and, by yourself or in a group, complete a values clarification exercise.
2. Explore the concept of family health. How does the meaning of family health differ from the meaning of health? In what ways do families promote and protect the health of family members? What health practices did you learn from your family? What programs are available in your community aimed at family health promotion (for instance, positive parenting classes at the neighbourhood community centre)?
3. Complete an assessment of a family using the CFAM. You might consider doing this over three visits and explore one major category per visit. Then draw the information together into an integrated data base of the family. What family strengths and problems are evident in the data?
4. Using sources in the reference list (Wright & Leahey, 1994; Danielson, Hamel-Bissell & Winstead-Fry, 1993; Friedman, 1998), explain and illustrate with examples the difference between nursing intervention with families and family therapy.

KEY TERMS

family p. 215
nuclear family p. 215
dual-career family p. 216
commuter family p. 216
nuclear-dyad p. 216
extended family p. 216
single-parent family p. 217
blended or reconstituted family p. 217
binuclear family p. 217
cohabiting family p. 217
gay or lesbian family p. 217
communal family p. 218
subsystems p. 219
suprasystem p. 219
boundaries p. 219
input p. 219
output p. 219
open system p. 220
feedback p. 220
family structure p. 220
role structure p. 220
values p. 220
communication p. 221
power structure p. 221
authority p. 221
family functions p. 221
family health p. 223
family dynamics p. 223
family stress p. 225
family stressors p. 225
distress p. 226
eustress p. 226
family crisis p. 226
cybernetics p. 230
systems theory p. 232
digital p. 232
analogic p. 232
genogram p. 233
ecomap p. 233
empowerment p. 237

References

ASSANAND, S., DIAS, M., RICHARDSON, E., & WAXLER-MORRISON, N. (1990). The South Asians. In N. Waxler-Morrison, J. Anderson & E. Richardson (Eds.), *Cross-cultural caring* (pp. 150–152). Vancouver: University of British Columbia Press.

BAKER, M. (1990). *Families: Changing trends in Canada.* (2nd ed.). Toronto: McGraw-Hill Ryerson.

B.C. MINISTRY OF HEALTH (Office of Health Promotion). (1992). *Healthy Communities 1991 Yearbook*. Victoria: British Columbia Ministry of Health and Ministry Responsible for Seniors. (Catalogue no. Q 92835)

BLAXTER, M., & PATTERSON, E. (1983). The health behaviours of mothers and daughters. In N. Madge (Ed.), *Families at risk* (pp. 174–196). London: Heinemann.

BOHANNAN, P. (1985). *All the happy families: Exploring the variety of family life*. New York: McGraw-Hill.

BOMAR, P.J. (1996). *Nurses and family health promotion: Concepts, assessment and interventions.* (2nd ed.). Toronto: W.B. Saunders.

BOSS, P.G. (1987). Family stress. In M. Sussman & S. Steinmetz (Eds.), *Handbook on marriage and the family* (pp. 695–723). New York: Plenum.

BOYD, M., & NORRIS, D. (1995). Leaving the nest? The impact of family structure. *Canadian Social Trends.* Ottawa: Minister of Supply & Services. (Catalogue no. 11-008E)

CAPLAN, G. (1964). Principles of preventive psychiatry. New York: Basic Books.

CAUDLE, P., & GROVER, S. (1992). Care of the family patient. In Clark, M.J. (Ed.). *Nursing in the community* (pp. 396–417). Norwalk, CT: Appleton & Lange.

CLEMEN-STONE, S., McGUIRE, S.L. & EIGSTI, D.G. (1998). *Comprehensive family and community health nursing.* (5th ed.). St. Louis: Mosby.

DANIELSON, C.B., HAMEL-BISSELL, B., & WINSTEAD-FRY, P. (1993). *Families, health and illness.* St. Louis: Mosby.

DeCHESNAY, M. (1986). Promoting healthy family functioning in acute care units. *Journal of Pediatric Nursing, 1*(2), 96–101.

DUFFY, M.E. (1988). Health promotion in the family: Current findings and directives for nursing research. *Journal of Advanced Nursing, 13,* 109–117.

DUNN, H.L. (1980). *High level wellness.* Thorofare, NJ: Charles B. Slack.

DUVALL, E.M. (1977). *Marriage and family development.* (5th ed.). Philadelphia: Lippincott.

ERIKSON, E.H. (1963). Childhood and Society. New York: Norton.

FEETHAM, S.L., MEISTER, S.B., BELL, J.M., & GILLISS, C.L. (1993). *The nursing of families: Theory, research, education and practice.* Newbury Park, CA: Sage.

FIGLEY, C.R. (1989). *Helping traumatized families.* San Francisco: Jossey-Bass.

FRIEDEMANN, M.L. (1993). Closing the gap between ground theory and mental health practice with families. In G. Wegner & R. Alexander (Eds.), Reading in family nursing. Philadelphia: Lippincott, pp. 41–56.

FRIEDEMANN, M.M. (1998). *Family nursing: Theory and practice.* (4th ed.). Norwalk, CT: Appleton & Lange.

GILLISS, C.L. (1991). Family nursing research, theory and practice. *Image: Journal of Nursing Scholarship, 23*(1), 19–22.

GRANDINE, J. (1995). Embracing the family. *Canadian Nurse, 91*(9), 31–36.

HARRY, J. (1983). Gay male and lesbian relationships. In E. Macklin and R. Rubin (Eds.), *Contemporary families and alternative life-styles.* Beverly Hills, CA: Sage.

HEALTH CANADA, MEDICAL SERVICES BRANCH. (1996). *Diagnostic on the health of First Nations and Inuit people.* Draft for discussion. Ottawa: Author.

HOFF, L.A. (1995). *People in crisis.* Understanding and helping. San Francisco: Jossey-Bass.

JANOSIK, E.H., & GREEN, E. (1992). *Family life: Process and practice.* Boston: Jones & Bartlet.

JANOSIK, E.H., & MILLER, J.R. (1979). Theories of family development. In D.P. Hymovich and M.U. Barnard (Eds.), *Family health care: Volume I* (2nd ed.), pp. 3–15. New York: McGraw-Hill.

JANOSIK, E.H., & MILLER, J.R. (1980). *Family-focused care.* New York: McGraw-Hill.

KANE, C.F. (1988). Family social support: Toward a conceptual model. *Advances in Nursing Science, 10*(2), 18–25.

KEENEY, B. (1982). What is an epistemology of family therapy? *Family Process, 21,* 153–168.

LANCASTER, J., McCANCE, K., & VANDERSCHMIDT, H. (1986). A curriculum project for clinical prevention: The role of the nurse. *Family, Community and Health, 8*(4), 48–53.

LITMAN, T.J. (1974). The family as a basic unit in health and medical care: A social-behavioral overview. *Soc Sci Med, 8,* 495. In S. Clemen-Stone, D.G. Eigsti, & S.L. McGuire (Eds.), *Comprehensive family and community health nursing.* (3rd ed.). St. Louis: Mosby.

LOGAN, B.B., & DAWKINS, C.E. (1986). *Family-centered nursing in the community.* Menlo Park, CA: Addison-Wesley.

LOGAN, R., & BELLIVEAU, J. (1995, Spring). Working mothers. *Canadian Social Trends* (pp. 24–28). Ottawa: Minister of Supply & Services.

LUNDY, T. (1992). *Healthy families in healthy communities: Tools for action.* Vancouver: British Columbia Council for the Family.

MATHEWS, F. (1993). *Youth gangs on youth gangs: User report.* Ottawa: Ministry of Supply & Services. (Catalogue nos. JS4/1-1993-24E & JS4/1-1993-24-1)

McCARTHY, B. (1996). *On the streets: Youth in Vancouver.* Victoria: B.C. Minister of Social Services; Research, Evaluation and Statistics Branch.

MINUCHIN, S. (1974). *Families and family therapy.* Cambridge, MA: Harvard University Press.

NATIONAL FORUM ON HEALTH. (1997). *Canada health action: Building on the legacy.* Synthesis reports and issues papers. Final report (vol. II). Ottawa: Author.

ODERKIRK, J. (1994, Summer). Marriage in Canada: Changing beliefs and behaviours, 1600-1990 (pp. 2–7). *Canadian Social Trends* (#33). Ottawa: Minister of Supply & Services. (Catalogue no. 11-008- XPE)

PENDER, N.J. (1987). Health promotion in nursing practice (2nd ed.). Norwalk CT: Appleton & Lange.

RAMSHORN, M.T. (1978). The individual in the family system. In L.A. Hall & D. Collins (Eds.). *Psychiatric nursing: Theory and application.* New York: McGraw-Hill.

RAMU, G.N. (1993). *Marriage and the family in Canada today.* Toronto: Prentice Hall Canada.

RAPAPORT, R., & RAPAPORT, R.N. (1971). *Dual-career families.* Harmondsworth, U.K.: Penguin Books.

REGISTERED NURSES ASSOCIATION OF BRITISH COLUMBIA (RNABC). (1992). *Determinants of health: Empowering strategies for nursing practice.* (RNABC Publication no. 24). Vancouver: Author.

ROBERGE, R., BERTHELOT, J.M., & WOLFSON, M. (1995). Health and socioeconomic inequalities (pp. 14–17). *Canadian Social Trends.*(#38). Ottawa: Minister of Supply & Services. (Catalogue no. 11-008E)

ROBINSON, C.A. (1995). Unifying distinction for nursing research with persons and *Journal of Family Nursing, 1*(1), 8–29.

ROSS, B., & COBB, K.L. (1990). *Family nursing.* Redwood City, CA: Addison-Wesley.

ROY, S.C. (1984). *Introduction to nursing: An adaptation model.* (2nd ed.). Englewood Cliffs, NJ: Prentice Hall.

SCANZONI, L. (1976). *Men, women and change: A sociology of marriage and family.* New York: McGraw-Hill.

SPRADELY, B.W., & ALLENDER, J.A. (1996). *Community health nursing: Concepts and practice.* (4th ed.). Philadelphia: Lippincott.

STATISTICS CANADA. (1995). *General social survey.* Ottawa: Author.

STATISTICS CANADA. (1996, Summer). Family indicators (pp. 32–33). *Canadian Social Trends* (#41). Ottawa: Minister of Supply & Services. (Catalogue no. 11-008-XPE)

STATISTICS CANADA. (1997a). Canadian children in the 1990s: Selected findings of the national longitudinal survey of children and youth. *Canadian Social Trends* (#44). Ottawa: Minister of Supply & Services. (Catalogue no. 11-008-XPE)

STATISTICS CANADA. (1997b, August 8). A portrait of seniors. [Online]. Available at http://www.statcan.ca/english/seniors/link.htm

TOMM, K., & SANDERS, G. (1983). Family assessment in a problem oriented record. In J.C. Hansen & Keeney (Eds.), *Diagnosis and assessment in family therapy* (pp. 101–122). London: Aspen Systems Corporation.

VON BERTALANFFY, L. (1968). *General system theory: Foundations, development, applications.* New York: Brazillier.

WATSON, J. (1985). *Nursing: The philosophy and science of caring.* Denver, CO: Colorado Associated University Press.

WILLIAMSON, M. (1986). Lesbianism. In J. Griffith-Kenney (Ed.), *Contemporary women's health.* Menlo Park, CA: Addison-Wesley.

WORLD HEALTH ORGANIZATION. (1984). *Health promotion glossary.* Copenhagen: WHO Regional Office for Europe.

WORLD HEALTH ORGANIZATION. (1986). *Ottawa Charter for Health Promotion.* Geneva: Author.

WRIGHT, L.M., & LEAHEY, M. (1990). Trends in nursing of families. *Journal of Advanced Nursing, 15*, 148–154.

WRIGHT, L.M., & LEAHEY, M. (1994). *Nurses and families: A guide to family assessment and intervention.* Philadelphia: F.A. Davis.

YOGIS, J.A., DUPLAK, R.R., & TRAINOR, J.R. (1996). *Sexual orientation and Canadian law: An assessment of the law affecting lesbian and gay persons.* Toronto: Emond Montgomery.

ZUKEWICH GALAM, N. (1996, Autumn). Living with relatives (pp. 20–24). *Canadian Social Trends* (#42). Ottawa: Minister of Supply & Services. (Catalogue no. 11-008- XPE)

Additional Readings

BAKER, M. (1996). *Families: Changing trends in Canada.* (3rd ed.). Toronto: McGraw-Hill Ryerson.

BRADLEY, P.J., & ALPERS, R. (1996). Home healthcare nurses should regain their family focus. *Home Healthcare Nurse, 14*(4), 281–288.

CLARK, M.J. (1996). *Nursing in the community.* (2nd ed.). Norwalk CT: Appleton & Lange.

COORDINATED LAW ENFORCEMENT UNIT. (1993). *Lower mainland gangs: Review of criminal history and country of origin.* Victoria: B.C. Ministry of the Attorney-General.

DAVIES, B. (1995). Windows on the family. *Canadian Nurse, 11*, 37–41.

FINK, S.V. (1995). The influence of family resources and family demands on the strains and well-being of caregiving families. *Nursing Research, 44*(3), 139–146.

FORCHUK, C., & DORSAY, J.P. (1995). Hidegard Peplau meets family system nursing: Innovation in theory-based practice. *Journal of Advanced Nursing, 21*, 110–115.

FRIEDEMANN, M.L. (1995). *The framework of systemic organization: A conceptual approach to families and nursing.* London: Sage.

GRACE, J.J. (1995). Families and nurses: Building partnerships for growth and health. *Journal of Obstetric, Gynecologic & Neonatal Nursing, 24*(4), 298–300.

HANSON, S., & BOYD, S. (Eds.). (1996). *Family health care nursing: Theory, practice, and research.* Philadelphia: F.A. Davis.

HARTRICK, G. (1995). Transforming family nursing theory from a mechanism to contextualism. *Journal of Family Nursing, 1*(2), 134–147.

HARTRICK, G., LINDSEY, A.E., & HILLS, M. (1994). Family nursing assessment: Meeting the challenge of health promotion. *Journal of Advanced Nursing, 20*, 85–91.

LARSON, L.E., GOLTZ, J.W., & HOBART, C.W. (1994). *Families in Canada: Social context, continuities and change.* Toronto: Prentice Hall Canada.

LEE, H.J. (1993). Health perceptions of middle, "new middle," and older rural adults. *Family Community Health, 16*, 19–27.

LIMANDRI, B.J., & TILDEN, V.P. (1996). Nurses' reasoning in the assessment of family violence. *Image, 28*(3), 247–252.

NETT, E.M. (1993). *Canadian families: Past and present.* Toronto: Butterworths.

RICHARD, B.S. (1996). Gerontological family nursing. In S. Hanson & S. Boyd (Eds.), *Family health care nursing: Theory, practice, and research.* Philadelphia: F.A. Davis.

ROBINSON, C.A. (1995). Beyond dichotomies in the nursing of persons and families. *Image, 27*(2), 116–120.

ROBINSON, C.A. (1996). "Health care relationships revisited." *Journal of Family Nursing. 2*(2), pp. 152–173.

ROBINSON, C.A. & WRIGHT, L.M. (1995). Family nursing interventions: What families say makes a difference. *Journal of Family Nursing. 1*(3), 327–345.

SPENCER, M. (1996). *Foundations of modern sociology.* (7th ed.). Toronto: Prentice Hall Canada.

VOSBURG, D., & SIMPSON, P. (1993). Linking family theory and practice: A family nursing program. *Image, 25*(3), 229–233.

WARD, M. (1994). *The family dynamic: A Canadian perspective.* Toronto: Nelson Canada.

Chapter 11

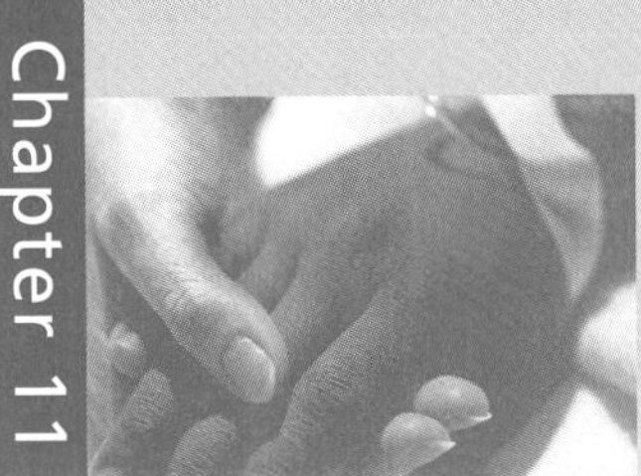

Health and the Community

OUTLINE

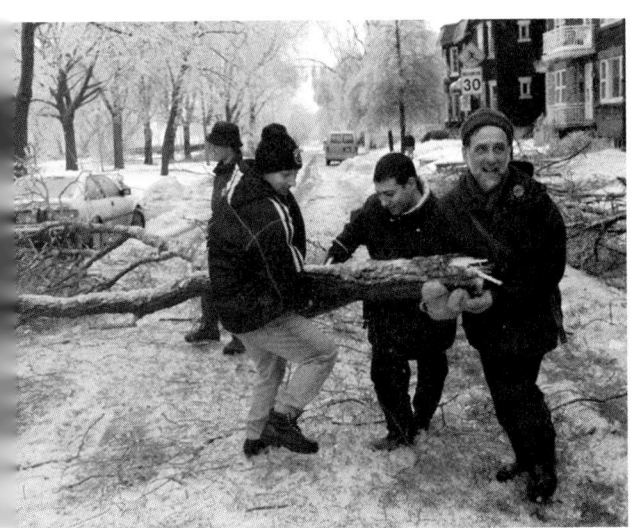

Central Questions

1. How has the concept of community developed in Canadian society?
2. How is the science of epidemiology used to assess the health of a community?
3. What is the Healthy Communities concept, and how does it differ from the epidemiological approach in looking at the health of a community?
4. Why do people live in communities?
5. What factors affect the healthy functioning of a community?
6. What are the major stressors affecting the health of communities?
7. What community ills can result from these stressors?
8. What is the nurse's role in community health?

Introduction

One of the major factors in the improvement of health in Canada and, indeed, in all of the developed world in the past century and a half has been the reduction of environmental hazards brought about by the application of known public health measures. These measures have traditionally been instituted at the local level in organized communities by municipal or city councils. They include provisions to ensure safe water, food and milk supplies, sewage treatment, standards for housing and the control of communicable diseases. All too often, a lack of safe drinking water, inadequate sewage disposal and improper handling of food and milk supplies are major contributors to high infant and early childhood mortality rates as well as the spread of communicable diseases—problems that still plague many developing countries.

In Canada today, the emphasis in health care is once again on the community. As our health care system struggles to shift from a disease orientation to a focus on health and its socioeconomic determinants, the base for services is shifting from hospitals to the community. Nurses at all levels are expected to be able to function in community settings as well as in hospitals. It is important for you as students to develop an understanding of how communities function and of the factors that affect the health of the people in communities, as well as the various facets of the nurse's role in community health.

In this chapter, we will examine the concept of community and the reasons for its prominence in the restructuring of health services in the provinces and territories. We will look at methods for assessing the health of communities, at the various functions of a community and at the factors affecting these functions. We will also discuss the stressors that can disrupt the healthy functioning of a community and the ills that can result. Finally, we will explore the nurse's role in community health as it is being practised in Canada today.

Historical Perspective

Human beings are social creatures. We know from written and archeological evidence that humans have always lived in family-like units and in larger organized groups for mutual protection, social support and the sharing of resources and skills. In Canada, we developed a strong sense of community as an integral part of our social structure. Ours is a vast country with grand expanses of land and a relatively small number of inhabitants. Until well into the middle of this century, most Canadians lived in small, rural communities in which they were often cut off from their neighbours during the severe winters. The people in these small communities were dependent on one another for food, protection from the elements, social interaction and health care. Neighbour had to help neighbour in order to survive. As a result, a strong sense of community developed and, along with it, an assumption that matters such as health and social welfare were the collective responsibility of community members. On the other hand, in some urban areas, some Canadians currently feel a "lack of community" in spite of the fact that they are surrounded by people. The reasons for this are numerous, including the fast pace of life and, perhaps, increased diversity in languages and cultures (Du Gas & Beckingham, 1993).

The assumption of collective responsibility for the common good is evident in many aspects of Canadian life. For example, it is evident in the cooperatives that developed in fishing communities in the Maritime Provinces, in the farming cooperatives of the Prairies and, today, in credit unions that provide an alternative to the chartered banks for financial services. In the health field, the principle of collective action for the common good is illustrated in the passage in Saskatchewan of a Rural Municipality Act in 1916, which enabled communities to raise funds by local levy to pay for the services of a physician for people of the community. This legislation, a forerunner of our National Health Insurance Program, was pioneered by the same province that has initiated many of our health care reforms.

In Canada, the community is now being viewed as the basic unit for health care. *Closer to Home* is the title of a Royal Commission report on health services in the province of British Columbia (1991), which strongly recommended shifting health care from an institutional to a community base. In Ontario, the report of the Premier's Council on Health, Well-being and Social Justice, entitled *Nurturing Health: A Framework of the Determinants of Health*, states that "Health is created in our homes, schools, workplaces and communities" (1993, p. 20).

The potential of communities for dealing with health matters in a democratic way is being explored in all provinces. Community members participate in the planning and management of their health care, rather than merely accepting the provision of community health services guided and directed exclusively by bureaucratic departments of health. We will explore the concept of participation in more detail when we discuss the Healthy Communities approach to community health. First, however, we will talk about types of communities and then discuss two conceptual frameworks for looking at health in the community—the epidemiological model and the Healthy Communities model. We will also look at the stressors and subsequent illnesses that afflict communities, the role of the nurse in community health care and measures to promote, protect or restore the community to a healthy state.

Types of Communities

We often think of community as a group of people living in one locality, but there are other types of communities. The term **community** is broadly used in the English language to refer to any group of people with a common bond, who interact with one another and share collective responsibility for common concerns. The communities most familiar to us are those with defined geographical and jurisdictional boundaries, that is, villages, towns and cities. The term *community* can, however, also be used to refer to smaller, local areas such as neighbourhoods, which may or may not be defined in municipal by-laws. If you live in a large city or town, your community may be a specific neighbourhood. Conversley, if you practise in a rural area, you may have many kilometres to cover to service your community in your daily rounds.

A community can also be made up of people who may not necessarily live in the same area but who share a common interest. A university, for example, is often referred to as a "community of scholars." Or, you might use the term "nursing community" to refer to all the nurses who practise in Canada. A large hospital often is like a community, almost like a small town, with a wide diversity of workers and patients sharing common goals, as well as all the services and amenities needed to meet their needs.

In our discussions of health and the community we will be using *community* in its most familiar sense, as a group of people living in a given geographical area (which may not necessarily be defined by legislation) who interact with one another and ideally work collectively on matters of common concern.

Conceptual Frameworks for Looking at Community Health

The two conceptual frameworks we will discuss for looking at community health are the *epidemiological model* and the *Healthy Communities model.* The Healthy Communities model is being widely used across the country as nursing moves beyond the Lalonde "health fields concept" (introduced in Chapter 2) to a broader approach to community health.

The Epidemiological Approach

The traditional way of looking at the health of a community has been through an epidemiological approach. **Epidemiology** is "the study of the distribution and determinants of various health-related states or events in specified populations and the application of this study in the control of health problems" (Last, 1988, p. 42). Historically, epidemiology has been concerned primarily with the study of disease. In the 19th century, it was the communicable diseases such as cholera, typhoid, plague, smallpox, and yellow and typhus fevers that posed the most serious threats to human life. As the incidence of communicable diseases decreased, more attention was focussed on the frequency and determinants of noninfectious chronic diseases and other health problems. Examples of prevalent noninfectious chronic diseases are heart conditions, diabetes, cancer, respiratory diseases and arthritis. Accidents and suicides are examples of major causes of morbidity and mortality that would be classified as other health problems.

The field of epidemiology has now been expanded to include the study of the health status of people and the factors that determine health. The federal government's *Active Health Report* (1987) presented the results of the first national survey on how Canadians felt about their own health. Whereas previous surveys had studied the nature and causes of health problems, this report provided a comprehensive picture of the health knowledge, attitudes, behaviours and intentions of Canadians (Health & Welfare Canada, 1987).

The use of an **epidemiological model** in community health has served us well in the past and continues to do so. The basic components of an epidemiological model are the systematic collection of health data through surveys and the search for causes of various states of health. The methodology used includes descriptive, analytical and experimental studies.

Descriptive studies measure the amount and distribution of a health concern within a given population by looking at the number of persons affected, where the cases are located and when they occur (that is, they look at person, place and time). For example, 40 percent of the elementary school children were absent with the flu during the week of January 18–25 in Weyburn, Saskatchewan, and no cases were reported during the week of May 3–7. From these observations, one would gather that there was a flu epidemic in January.

Surveys in which people gather data about various characteristics of the population are the most common type of descriptive study done in epidemiology. Health departments routinely gather information on illnesses occurring among the school-age population and the incidence of communicable diseases in that community. Statistics Canada regularly collects a large amount of information about the health of Canadians, such as births, deaths and the occurrence of illness in the population, as we discussed in Chapter 2. It also undertakes special surveys at the request of Health Canada on particular aspects of health such as, for example, the data reported in the *Active Health Report.* A second type of epidemiologic approach is the **analytic study.** This approach investigates data obtained from descriptive studies and attempts to identify relationships with other factors. In other words, the characteristics, exposures or behaviours that might account for the differences in the observed patterns of the health problem are researched. For example, investigating the number of automobile accidents in relation to increasing speed or use of alcohol is a type of analytic study.

In **experimental studies**, the researcher intervenes and changes one variable, then observes what happens. For example, in order to find out if flu shots are effective, a possible study might involve giving one group of older people in a community flu shots at the beginning of winter. The question under study would be, "Do people who had the flu shots report fewer cases of flu than a comparable group of older people who did not have the preventive inoculations?" The investigators would, of course, have to take into consideration the ethical dimension of giving some people and not others the opportunity to protect themselves from the flu. Given the ethical concerns regarding witholding the flu shot, the research team may instead choose to collect observational data on the number of cases of flu among those who voluntarily chose to have or not to have the flu shots.

Another common type of experimental study in epidemiology is a **demonstration project** that involves studying a new method of delivering health care in the community. For example, the Ministry of Health in British Columbia funded a two-year demonstration project of a nursing centre to serve as a point of entry for the public into the health care system. The centre, located in the Comox Valley on Vancouver Island, opened in 1994. Using a primary health care approach, the centre provides an alternative method for delivering health care in line with the New Directions for Health Care program in the province (Mass & Whyte, 1997). Other examples of demonstration projects involving nurses in key roles in the delivery of health services include the McGill Workshops, which were based on the Allen family-oriented nursing model, and the Denmark–Newfoundland project, "Primary Health Care—A Nursing Model" (Hall, 1989).

At some point in your career you are likely to participate in epidemiological studies, either as part of a population under study and/or as a member of an investigative team. You will also want to be able to interpret data stemming from these studies. Therefore, you need to understand the meaning of the key terms used. We discussed some of the common terms, such as mortality and morbidity rates, causes of death and number of potential years of life lost, in Chapter 2. A few more are listed in the box on p. 247.

EPIDEMIOLOGY AND ITS USES

The systematic collection of health data and the search for causation of health and illness have been of inestimable value in helping us to tackle health issues for a number of reasons.

DEVELOPMENT OF A HEALTH PROFILE The systematic collection of health data enables us to develop profiles of the health status of people living in various community groups. With this information, we can compare, for example, the health of communities in different geographical areas, or of differing socioeconomic groups within the same community. In Chapter 2 we discussed some comparisons between countries on a few of the common health status indicators such as life span, causes of death, and infant and maternal mortality rates. We also looked at trends over time, such as, for example, the lengthening of the life span in Canada. Canada's 1985 Health Promotion Survey provided data for comparisons between different socioeconomic groups in the country. The *Active Health Report* on the findings of this survey showed clearly that "not all Canadians have equal likelihood of being healthy or have equivalent access to the resources required for health" (Health & Welfare Canada, 1987, p. 7). In particular, the socially disadvantaged are "less happy, more anxious and depressed, suffer more disease, live shorter lives and experience more physical disability" (RNABC, 1996, p. 13).

IDENTIFICATION OF HEALTH PROBLEMS Epidemiology also enables us to identify health problems. This knowledge helps in the determination of priorities for the allocation of resources, including the need for continuous monitoring as well as the need for specific programs. For example, data collected on the incidence of communicable diseases have alerted health authorities to the alarming increase in the number of cases of hepatitis B in Canada over the past 10 years. This has led to widespread immunization programs for people who are most at risk, namely, children and health workers. Most nursing schools now require students to be immunized against hepatitis B before beginning clinical practice.

CONTROL OF EPIDEMICS The continuous monitoring of communicable diseases enables health authorities to take quick action to avoid epidemics. An outbreak of measles at Simon Fraser University in 1996 alerted the Health Department to inform the residents of Vancouver, since the students lived throughout the lower mainland. One of the outcomes was the reimmunization for measles of all students in the province. The systematic collection of data about health-related problems in a population also provides scientists with a more complete picture of the manifestations of disease. Further, it enables them to differentiate among variations of a disease, for example, the identification of the different types of hepatitis—A, B, C, D and E (Tyler & Last, 1992).

IDENTIFICATION OF RISK FACTORS Epidemiology enables us to identify the risk factors associated with specific health problems and to take appropriate action. For example, the high incidence of low birth weight infants among women who smoke during pregnancy and the incidence of fetal alcohol syndrome in infants of mothers who consume excessive alcohol have stimulated the development of programs advocating the avoidance of smoking and consuming alcohol during pregnancy.

EVALUATION OF HEALTH SERVICES Direct cause-and-effect relationships (causalities) are difficult, some say impossible, to establish when dealing with the multiplicity of variables involved in a person's health. Still, it is possible, by means of epidemiological surveys, to assess the impact

Epidemiological Research Terminology

Causality—the "relating of causes to the effects they produce" (Last, 1988, p. 21). The establishment of a link between specific factors (such as smoking or eating a high-fat diet) and the development of health problems might be an example of causality.

Through the ages, disease has been attributed to many causes including divine intervention, malevolent mists or other harmful substances in the environment and, more recently, to single, specific agents such as bacteria or foods (Clark, 1996). We now believe that disease is caused by a multiplicity of factors. Many people in a room may be exposed to tuberculosis germs, for example, but only one, or perhaps none at all, will develop the disease, depending on a number of factors including each individual's resistance and state of health at the time of exposure. The recent resurfacing of TB as a major health problem is felt to be due to many factors, including poverty, overcrowding and poor nutrition, as well as inadequate immunization and control measures (Friedman, 1994). Causality is therefore often hard to determine, and is rarely, in the case of disease, attributable to a single source.

Risk—"the probability that an event will occur, for example, that an individual will become ill or die within a stated period of time, or [at a specific] age" (Last, 1988, p. 115).

Although a variety of factors is involved, as we noted above, if there is diabetes in your family, you are more at risk for developing the disease than others without such a family history. Fatigue and stress render you more vulnerable to, or at risk for developing, a cold or the flu than when you are in good physical and emotional condition.

Populations at risk—groups of people who, because of certain risk factors, are more likely to develop a disease or condition.

Nurses and other health workers are more at risk for developing tuberculosis than people in the general population because of their close contact with patients and the potential exposure to the disease from undiagnosed cases. They are also at risk for such diseases as hepatitis B and AIDS (acquired immunodeficiency syndrome) that can be transmitted through body fluids and may enter the bloodstream through a puncture of the skin with an infected needle.

Incidence—"the number of instances of illness commencing, or of people falling ill, during a given period in a specific population" (Last, 1988, p. 63). For example, the first case of AIDS was diagnosed in Canada in 1979. Since then, the annual incidence, or number of new cases, has risen rapidly.

Prevalence—"the number of instances of a given disease or other condition in a given population at a designated time" (Last, 1988, p. 103). In other words, prevalence tells us the total number of people in a specific group who are affected at any given time. Malaria, for example, is still prevalent in many provinces in China (and in many other parts of the world), and travellers are advised to take precautionary measures when going into these areas.

of health programs on overall health, some more definitively than others. For example, widespread immunization programs for children have dramatically reduced the incidence and number of deaths from communicable diseases in most countries. Although heart disease is still the leading cause of death in Canada, mortality from both heart disease and stroke was reduced by half over a period of 20 years (1971–1991), as found by Statistics Canada (see Chapter 2). The reduction may be largely due to people changing their lifestyles in response to health promotion programs.

Although a number of factors must be taken into consideration in the reduction of infant mortality rates in any country, including improvements in the overall socioeconomic well-being of people, there is no doubt that community health nursing services play a large role. Primary health care provided by nurses in the rural villages and on the outer islands of Fiji, for example, includes prenatal monitoring, midwifery services and well-baby clinics. These services have been a significant factor in cutting the infant mortality rate in half in less than 20 years (Government of Fiji, 1986).

In Canada, First Nations infant mortality rates have declined from 28 percent per 1000 live births in 1979 to 11 percent per 1000 live births in 1993 (Health Canada, 1996). The expansion of the Northern nursing program that was started in the 1950s and continued during the 1960s and 1970s by the Medical Services Branch of Health and Welfare Canada is credited with being a significant factor in lowering the infant mortality rates in the North. As recommended by the Royal Commission on Health Services (the Hall Report) of 1964, each community of 150 persons or more was allocated a nursing station, with at least one registered nurse assigned to carry out primary health care (Health Canada, 1993).

PUBLIC POLICY DEVELOPMENT "Epidemiology is essential to the development of scientifically responsible public health policy" (Tyler & Last, 1992, p. 37). Surveillance of the health status of a community and investigation into specific problems provide the baseline data needed for decisions by policy makers. For example, differences in health indicators such as higher-than-average infant mortality rates and a shorter life span in rural and remote areas of British Columbia have led to policies designed to provide better health service to these parts of the province (Government of British Columbia, 1993).

The search for the causes of disease and other health states has enabled us to take action to eliminate many causes of poor health and to reinforce those factors that contribute to good health. For many years, the search for causality focussed on disease entities, and the resulting research has been of inestimable value in helping to reduce many health problems. The majority of communicable diseases have been brought under control in large part because epidemiologists have traced the **etiology** (science of the causes of disease) of the different diseases. For example, knowledge of the etiology of cholera, which caused thousands of deaths in Canada in the early 20th century, stimulated changes in environmental policy to assist in drastically reducing the incidence of the disease. These policies involved strict guidelines for the maintenance of a safe water supply.

The *New Perspective on the Health of Canadians* (Lalonde, 1974) was based on findings from epidemiological studies. Now, studies such as those discussed in the *Active Health Report* are showing that "...health is affected by social and environmental concerns as well as lifestyle and medical factors. Health is inextricably linked to the living and working conditions Canadians enjoy" (Health & Welfare Canada, 1987, p. 3). Our attention is turning to ways and means of improving the living and working conditions of the socially disadvantaged as a health priority.

The Healthy Communities Concept

The *Active Health Report* emphasized that health is affected by social and environmental concerns as well as lifestyle and medical factors. As we discussed in Chapter 2, we tend today to look at health as a much broader concept than we did 20 years ago. Health is now viewed more as a social issue than as a biological phenomenon. An individual's health is determined not only by biological inheritance and health services but also by the circumstances of our daily lives, our culture and beliefs and by social, economic and physical aspects of our environment. The WHO definition states that health is "the extent to which an individual or group is able, on one hand, to realize aspirations and satisfy needs; and, on the other hand, to change or cope with the environment. Health is, therefore, seen as a resource for everyday life, a dimension of our 'quality of life,' and not the object of living; it is a positive concept emphasizing social and personal resources as well as physical capabilities" (WHO, 1984).

Recognizing the importance of public policy, particularly at the municipal level, in creating a physical and social environment that promotes health for the community as a whole, the World Health Organization in 1985 launched a five-year Healthy Cities project in Europe as a vehicle for achieving its health promotion goal of "Health for All by the Year 2000" (Boothroyd & Eberle, 1990). In 1988, a similar project was initiated in Canada, entitled the Canadian Healthy Communities Project. The project was funded for a three-year period by Health and Welfare Canada. Some Canadian cities, such as Toronto, have kept the WHO terminology of Healthy Cities for their project. However, the Healthy Communities framework is common to all.

The philosophy behind the Healthy Communities concept is that communities have the ability to identify their own health needs and to plan and manage their own health care—and to do so in a democratic way that involves the whole community. In British Columbia, the management of health services has been delegated to "Community Health Councils" and "Regional Health Boards." At the present time, all provinces and territories are involved in major reforms to shift health care to the community. (See Chapter 3.)

THE HEALTHY COMMUNITIES PROCESS

In many neighbourhoods, towns and cities across the country, people are using the Healthy Communities process to identify and resolve local health issues. In this context, the community is seen not as the focus of action for health providers but as the *agent* of action. The emphasis is on the democratic process so that people, health professionals and community organizations can work together to bring about change. Collaboration between different departments of government, voluntary and official health agencies, professional associations and citizen groups is crucial to the successful implementation of change.

The key to the Healthy Communities process is that the nurse is present not as the service provider, or the one who holds the power, but rather as a resource and a partner in an egalitarian process.

The **Healthy Communities process** is illustrated in Figure 11.1. In the *entry phase*, attention is focussed on

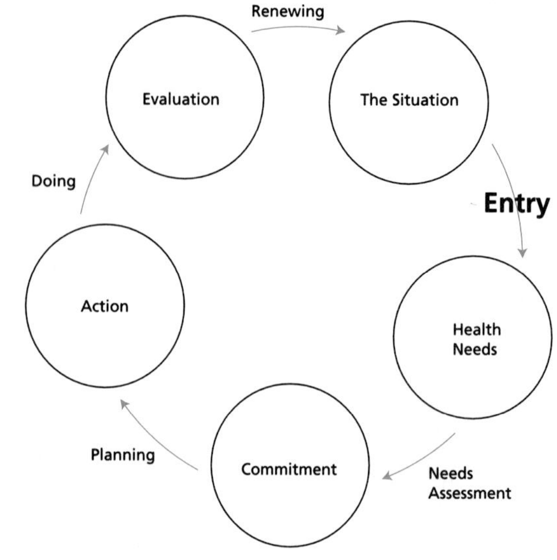

FIGURE 11.1 The Healthy Communities process

SOURCE: Government of British Columbia, 1992a.

LOOKING back

Helen Kathleen Mussallem, b. 1915

One of the most dominant, distinguished, and influential of Canada's nurses in the latter half of the 20th century was Helen K. Mussallem of Ottawa. Born in Prince Rupert, B.C., she graduated from the Vancouver General Hospital School of Nursing, then earned a diploma in teaching, supervision and administration from the University of Washington in Seattle. She served overseas during World War II with the Royal Canadian Army Military Corps (RCAMC) from 1943 to 1946, mainly as operating room supervisor, often under threat of air and missile raids. Following the war, she earned a baccalaureate in nursing from McGill University, then attended Teachers College, Columbia University in New York for master's and doctoral work.

After work in both administration and teaching at the Vancouver General Hospital, she was chosen to head a Canadian Nurses Association (CNA) pilot project for Evaluation of Schools of Nursing in Canada from 1957 to 1960. Her research report on the project, *Spotlight on Nursing Education*, became a landmark in nursing education, identifying serious deficiencies in standards that led to closure of several hospital schools. She was then hired as director of special studies for the CNA, during which time she was seconded to the federal government's Royal Commission on Health Services as part of that Commission's investigation into nursing education.

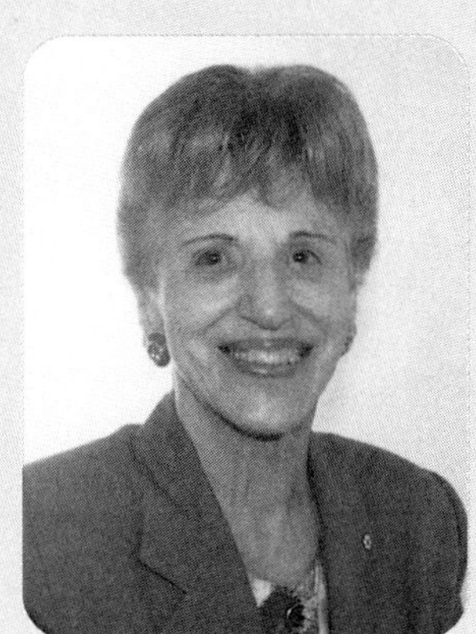

In 1963, she became the CNA's Executive Director, a position she held for 18 years. During this time, she was instrumental in establishing the Canadian Nurses Foundation and served as its secretary-treasurer from 1966 to 1981. She also established a national library for nursing at the CNA, which was named in her honour on her retirement in 1981. She then was elected and served as a member of the International Council of Nurses Board of Directors from 1981 to 1985.

Her educational credentials, outgoing personality and diplomatic skills made her an influential leader throughout her career, recognized by government ministries and by senior professional organizations. For example, she was the first nurse to be named to the prestigious Economic Council of Canada (1971–1980) and was instrumental in affecting policy decisions related to health care for all Canadians. She was frequently sought as a consultant and adviser by international health organizations such as the World Health Organization, Pan-American Health Organization and Commonwealth Foundation, and she carried out assignments in more than 40 countries.

Following retirement, Mussallem was president of the Victorian Order of Nurses for Canada, and served on several national non-nursing boards, such as those of the St. John Ambulance Association of Canada and the Human Rights Institute of Canada. She holds many honours, including honorary doctorates from five Canadian universities (New Brunswick, Memorial, Queen's, McMaster and British Columbia) and the Medal of Distinguished Service from Columbia University. She has the Florence Nightingale Medal from the International Red Cross, and the Queen's Silver Jubilee Medal. She was named an officer of the Order of Canada in 1969 and was promoted to Companion of the Order in 1992, Canada's highest award to its citizens.

— *Glennis Zilm*

identifying the current situation of the community. The nurse introduces him- or herself and then learns about the community. The health needs are identified in the *needs assessment phase*. Members of the community are asked their opinions, and current research is utilized, in this part of the process. Once the needs are identified, then public acceptance is sought. It is crucial that commitment from community members is attained at this point. The third phase—*planning*—is undertaken, and methods of responding to health needs are identified. The necessary resources must also be acquired or activated during this phase. The *doing phase* follows, in which the plans are implemented. Finally, the *renewal phase* focusses on evaluation and rejuvenation. The task force must examine what did or did not work, and what was learned. Also, a sense of self-renewal of involved individuals is fostered. The process is circular; thus, the entry phase resumes when the existing situation is re-examined.

The Healthy Communities process includes conducting surveys, neighbourhood discussions, public forums and interviews with key leaders to gather information on health needs and to monitor progress towards the goal of a healthier community (Government of British Columbia, 1992b, 1992c).

Between June 1989 and June 1990, the town of Princeton, B.C. experienced an unusual increase in suicide. In response, the town mounted a crisis line staffed by volunteers. The committed response from volunteers is what has made the crisis line work. Unemployment rates in Princeton are high. Making the crisis line work is one way that the residents of the town have banded together to support one another. The challenge now is to build partnerships with other sectors in the community to develop a comprehensive approach to suicide prevention. This has started with discussions between crisis line workers and the hospital health committee.

Determinants of Community Health

A healthy community is "one in which all organizations—from informal groups to governments—are working effectively together to improve the quality of all people's lives" (Boothroyd & Eberle, 1990, p. 7). This definition of the healthy community was formulated in line with the WHO (1984) definition of health as "the ability to realize aspirations and satisfy needs and, on the other hand, to change or cope with the environment."

In order to look at the determinants of health in a community we need to examine first the functions of a community. We need to ask ourselves such questions as: Why is it that most people prefer to live in communities rather than in isolation? What is the purpose of a community? Why does it exist? When we understand the functions, then we can look at the factors that affect the health of a community by supporting or hindering its ability to perform its various functions. The following sections of this chapter—on functions of a community (and factors affecting these functions) and on community stressors—were developed from material contained in the *Health Indicator Workbook: A Tool for Healthy Communities*, published by the Office of Health Promotion of the B.C. Ministry of Health and Ministry Responsible for Seniors (Government of British Columbia 1992c).

Functions of a Community and the Factors Affecting These Functions

The Healthy Communities projects in British Columbia have identified the following six functions of a community: (1) production, (2) consumption, (3) maintenance of the physical environment, (4) management, (5) growth and development and (6) social support (Government of British Columbia, 1992c).

PRODUCTION

Communities produce the goods and services needed to promote good health. A healthy community supports people in their ability to obtain the necessities of life and provides opportunity for them to gain the knowledge and skills needed to cope with and/or change the environment. A thriving business sector and the availability of goods and services contribute to the health of a community by providing employment opportunities and a sound economic base for community development.

A community's production capacity is enhanced by the presence of schools, colleges, universities and libraries and by the availability of other educational programs. We live in a knowledge-based society, so it is increasingly apparent that education is one of the most powerful tools at our disposal in developing and maintaining a healthy economy in our communities. A well-educated workforce is essential in the competitive environment of the global economy. It is education that provides us with the skills to manage our environment—for example, developing better ways of controlling and reusing our human and industrial waste to enhance rather than pollute our environment.

Factors Affecting the Production Function of Communities

- the soundness and extent of a community's economic base
- the availability of a wide range of educational services.

Further, an individual's level of education improves his or her overall health status. A 1990 Canada Health Promotion Survey (Government of Canada, 1994) noted that as the level of education increases, self-rated health status improves and activity limits decrease. In addition, people with higher levels of education have fewer sick days per year: university-educated persons averaged fewer than four sick days, while those with an elementary education averaged seven.

CONSUMPTION

A community not only produces goods and services; it also uses them. Our physical and social abilities are strongly influenced by the availability and affordability of goods and services. Adequate food, housing and energy to heat our homes in winter are essential for good health. There are, however, items that community members purchase which are detrimental to health. Cigarettes, alcohol, foods with a high fat content and illegal drugs are but a few examples. In looking at the factors affecting health in a community, then, one must consider both aspects of consumption, that is to say, things we consume that promote health and those that are detrimental to health.

Factors Affecting Consumption in a Community

- the availability and affordability of goods and services that contribute to good health, for example, nutritious food and adequate housing
- the availability of goods and services that are detrimental to health, for example, alcohol, drugs and high-fat foods.

MAINTENANCE OF THE PHYSICAL ENVIRONMENT

As we mentioned in Chapter 2, our physical environment affects our health in many ways, both directly and indirectly. We are directly affected by our community's quality of air, water, food supply and waste disposal. Nurses must be vigilant about assisting efforts to decrease air, water and soil pollution. The soil, where much of our food supply originates, must be monitored for radioactive material or animal excreta.

Appropriate maintenance of the physical environment goes far beyond simple adequate disposal of waste products. We must consciously work to incorporate the principles of recycling into a community.

Other factors, which at first may appear to have less direct effect, must be considered in the physical environment. Noise, psychological stressors, the general state of the physical environment, availability of recreational sites and the diversity of wildlife also affect the overall health and integrity of the community.

Factors Affecting Maintenance of the Physical Environment

- the quality of the air we breathe
- the safety of food and water supplies
- the safe disposal of waste
- the availability of recreational sites
- wildlife preservation
- noise control
- recycling.

MANAGEMENT

Good management is essential for the smooth, efficient functioning of all aspects of community health. A well-managed community identifies its priorities, adapts services to the needs of changing situations and makes the most of resources. In a democratic society, it is essential that members take an active part in local government to ensure that wise and effective decisions are made to meet their needs and to promote a healthy community. We cannot all be city councillors or other elected officials, but we can all vote in elections and on referendums. We can express our opinions at town meetings and through participation in local action groups, on local planning committees and on community boards.

It is easy to express our views on what is wrong, but much more difficult to promote positive change. In order to tackle health problems in the community, priorities must be established and a plan of action developed if goals are to be accomplished. For example, long-range planning in a community is important in order to protect green space, for example, or to ensure the maintenance of water and sewage systems. A community also has to make plans to cope if disaster strikes. Planning is also needed to ensure safe, affordable housing for people, and to see that health and education services are maintained at a high level. The list of planning needs is long; communities have to set priorities for action based on what is possible within a given time frame, and with the resources of the community.

Factors Affecting the Management of Communities

- citizen participation in governance
- short- and long-range planning.

GROWTH AND DEVELOPMENT

A very important function of any community is the promotion of the growth and development of those who live there. Most communities include a diversity of age groups. Healthy, well-nourished children who are growing and developing normally are essential for the continued renewal of a community.

Equally important is a healthy economy that attracts new business into the community. Nor should we forget the importance of the cultural sector in contributing to the intellectual and spiritual growth and development of a community. Early immigrants to Canada knew the importance of cultural stimulation when they established the Chatauqua program that took eminent speakers, well-known musicians and theatrical offerings to rural communities and frontier towns in the late 1890s and early 1900s as part of a continuing education program for people living in rural areas.

Factors Affecting the Promotion of Growth and Development of Communities

- the availability and accessibility of health promotion and health protection services for people of all ages
- a business climate conducive to attracting new businesses
- an active cultural sector.

SOCIAL SUPPORT

As pointed out in the Epp Report (1986) and in the *Nurturing Health* document (1993), health is considerably affected by social relationships. After family and friends, it is the community in which we live that provides us with the most important source of social contacts. A supportive, nurturing community also provides people with opportunities for social interaction through recreation programs, clubs, churches, libraries and schools. In healthy communities, there is generally no problem recruiting volunteers for community projects. You will probably also find numerous community associations and projects such as Neighbourhood Watch and Block Parents advertised in the windows of various houses in residential areas.

Community support is also evident in the accessibility of adequate health services—emergency, restorative and palliative—and in the range of social services that are

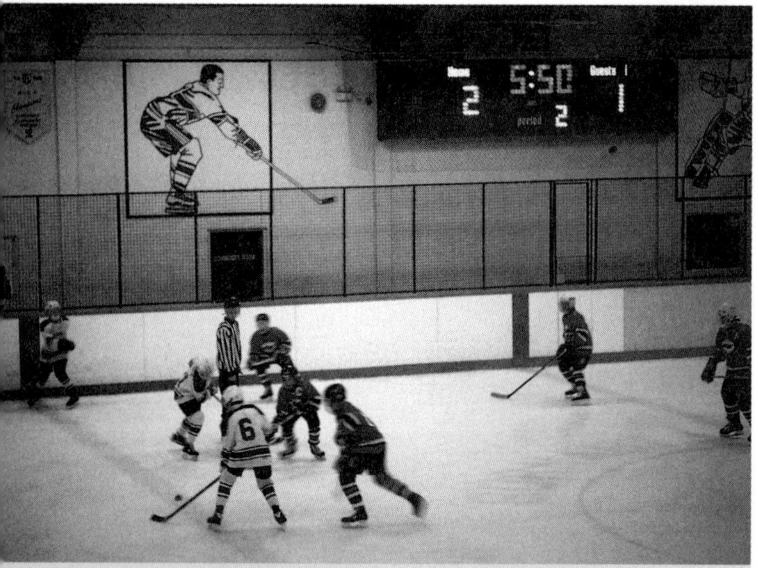

Communities need adequate recreation facilities.

available and accessible to all citizens. A supportive community protects its citizens from violence and other criminal activities. In addition, the healthy population movement has a mandate to strengthen social supports by including initiatives to maintain strong families, decrease discrimination and promote social tolerance (Government of Canada, 1994).

Factors Affecting the Support Function of Communities

- the availability of affordable and accessible recreation facilities
- opportunities for social interaction (clubs, churches and adult education programs)
- adequate and accessible emergency, restorative, rehabilitative and palliative health services
- an effective social services network
- effective law enforcement.

Community Stressors

We all know communities that are healthy, thriving places where people like to live and bring up their children. Most of us have also seen communities that people are anxious to move away from as soon as they can. What makes the difference? Why do some communities seem to grow and develop at a rapid rate while the streets of others are lined with empty houses, closed stores and playgrounds where there are no children playing?

There are many stressors that can affect communities and many ways to categorize these stressors. We have opted to discuss the following stressors that can have a negative impact on communities: (1) economic stressors, (2) population pressures, (3) excessive consumption of harmful substances, (4) physical and chemical stressors and (5) biological stressors.

Economic Stressors

Tough economic times can have a devastating effect on every one of the six major functions of a community. The Great Depression of the 1930s virtually crippled North America. The recession that Canadians experienced in the early 1990s also had a major impact on the functioning of communities. When markets slump, the production of goods and services declines. Factories and stores close and people lose employment. They cannot afford to buy the things they need to maintain their health—let alone luxuries—and the consumption of goods and services is decreased. This causes more stores and manufacturing plants to close, creating a further downward spiral of the economy.

When the economy is poor and people are out of work, a strain is put on the support services in a community. Governments have to make more funds available for employment insurance and for social assistance. Money left over for environmental services is decreased and the renewal of highways, the development and maintenance of the water supply system, and even the building of needed sewage disposal plants may be postponed. When budgets are tight, all departments, including the health department of a community, must share in cost-cutting. The growth and development function of a community may be jeopardized by the cutting of health promotion and protection services. Schools and cultural sectors are often very hard hit during times of economic strife. For example, "nonessential" staff may be laid off, buildings may not be upgraded or maintained, and portable classrooms may be used more extensively. Cultural sectors suffer at several levels: basic support services, such as translation services, may become unavailable; the development of cultural facilities and "green space" may be postponed; and people's ability to enjoy leisure activities may be curtailed. Such cutbacks in funding can add to health problems within the community.

Unemployment is a detriment to a person's health (Government of Canada, 1994). Health suffers, not only because of lessened income, but also because of the loss of self-esteem. Unemployment affects not only the worker but also the family. Children are likely to worry about who will pay the bills, and whether they will lose their home. Even the insecurity caused by the threat of unemployment can be enough to cause ill health (Government of Ontario, 1993). As we noted in Chapter 2, poor people have more health problems than people with an adequate income. There are also more mental health problems among the children of the poor (Sutherland & Fulton, 1988). Some people turn to alcohol or drugs to provide temporary solace from their problems. In addition, crime often increases as people become desperate for money.

Potential Community Problems Resulting from Economic Stressors

- poverty
- crime and violence
- mental and physical illness
- decaying community infrastructure (highways, water supply systems, etc.)
- less development of green space
- fewer resources invested in arts.

Potential Community Problems Resulting from Population Increases

- lack of affordable housing
- crowded schools
- insufficient postsecondary educational facilities
- racial tensions and conflicting values
- mental health problems
- insufficient services, for example, water and sewage lines, telephone and hydroelectric services, transportation services.

Population Pressures

POPULATION INCREASES

In Canada we have seen rapid increases in population in many of our cities and towns in the past few years. Two factors have contributed to this growth. One is the trend towards urbanization, which we mentioned in Chapter 1. The other is immigration. The growth of a community has both positive and negative effects. Urbanization and immigration have put tremendous pressure on all community services from the sheer increase in number and diversity of people to be served. Population growth benefits the economy by contributing to the number of new houses and to the establishment of more shops and factories that cater to the needs of the increased population. Thus, there is a positive effect on both the production and consumption capacities of communities. Also, many newcomers bring with them specialized skills and knowledge that contribute to the economy.

On the other hand urbanization and immigration have strained our health, education, social and protection services, to name a few. There is a great need for more inpatient and community health services, as well as a need to offer these services in different languages, to people coming from a variety of cultures (see Chapter 12). Schools are pressured to keep up with the demand for classrooms and for qualified teachers. One of the greatest needs is for courses in English as a second language (ESL). There is currently also a great need in most parts of the country to expand postsecondary educational facilities to prepare the skilled workforce needed for today's economy. Immigrants often need help to adjust to their new environment; thus the demand for social services grows. With the influx of immigrants into communities of long-time residents, there arises a mutual need for adjustment to living together. Ideally, each group should develop tolerance and respect for other people's customs and beliefs. However, prejudices often develop. Nurses can assist communities to achieve a state of tolerance, understanding and strength.

POPULATION DECREASES

As some communities grow, others get smaller. One of the major reasons for the exodus of people from a community is loss of its economic base. In many parts of Canada, the economy is still largely resource-based. When the mines run out, when crops are poor several years in a row, or there are no more fish on the cod banks, people must leave their home community to seek work elsewhere. You have probably all visited a "ghost town" that was once a thriving community. When the economic base of a community is lost and people have to move elsewhere, it is the younger people who go first, the older ones being more reluctant to give up their homes. The result is a smaller community with an older population. This puts great pressure on those who stay to maintain all community functions. The tax base created by businesses and working people for the funding of services is decreased, and the human resources to staff services are no longer there.

Potential Community Problems Resulting from Population Decreases

- decreased production capacity
- decreased consumption of goods and services
- decaying infrastructure due to loss of tax base.

Excessive Consumption of Harmful Substances

Cigarettes, alcohol, drugs and high-fat foods are all detrimental to health. The dangers of smoking have been well documented in a multitude of studies. Although there has been a tremendous reduction in the number of smokers in Canada, the number of teenagers, particularly girls, who smoke is a concern. Still, many people continue to smoke, and our health care system is burdened with individuals whose health has been damaged by smoking.

Damage resulting from the excessive consumption of alcohol affects not only the individual but also the family and the wider community in which they live. Previously, we discussed the effect of alcohol-related accidents and the increase in morbidity and mortality rates. Alcohol abuse also increases hospital admissions and rehabilitation needs, and contributes to family violence, loss of self-esteem and loss of trust within families. Ultimately, these effects may permeate an entire community. The abuse of illegal drugs not only undermines the individual user's health, but is also devastating to families and is a major factor in promoting crime.

With regard to the overconsumption of harmful foods, many people have changed their eating habits in recent years and are consciously purchasing foods that are lower in fat and cholesterol content and higher in fibre (Health & Welfare Canada, 1987; Government of Ontario, 1993). Still, French fries and gravy are a common lunch, as you can observe in many hospital and school cafeterias. However, these "comfort foods" offer only momentary palliation from the stresses of daily life. As we have pointed out in earlier chapters, poor dietary habits are an important factor in a number of health problems, such as diabetes, heart disease and other circulatory problems that put a strain on health services.

When we talk about the problems resulting from the excessive consumption of harmful substances, however, we must be careful not to fall into the trap of "blaming the victim." The underlying causes are complex. People who drink too much alcohol, continue to smoke, are dependent on drugs or overeat all need support from the community, not condemnation. We need to ask why people make these choices and what can we do to help them make healthier choices. As pointed out in the Epp Report (1986), lifestyles cannot be changed in isolation without considering the social, economic and environmental context in which people live.

Potential Community Problems Resulting from Excessive Consumption of Harmful Substances

- crime and violence
- excessive mortality and hospitalization rates
- family disintegration
- excessive number of health problems, such as heart conditions, stroke, lung cancer and chronic lung disorders, obesity, diabetes.

Physical and Chemical Stressors

Among the physical stressors affecting communities are factors such as pollution, radiation, noise, workplace hazards, severe weather conditions and the forces of nature.

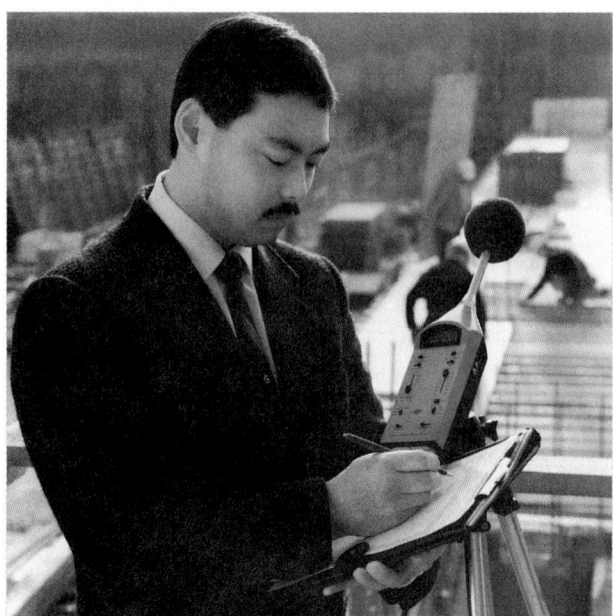

A public health inspector monitoring noise levels at a construction site.

Most of us are aware of the dangers of environmental degradation. Indeed, it is frequently a leading topic in newspapers, on television and on radio. Both indoor and outdoor atmospheric pollution are problems in many communities. Heavy traffic on the highways, and smoke from mills, manufacturing plants and incinerators combine to create the smog that hangs over many cities. This smog can become so bad that people with asthma or other respiratory problems may experience difficulty in breathing. Our water, food and milk supplies can also become polluted. On the West Coast, it is not unusual for a warning to be issued, advising people not to eat the shellfish harvested from specific areas because of contamination. The emptying of waste products from lumber mills into the ocean near fishing grounds has been blamed in some instances for contamination of fish. All levels of government have a responsibility to control pollution in areas under their jurisdiction. The federal government, for example, sets standards in regard to such matters as the content of water supplies, foods and drugs. Provincial governments are taking steps to restrict the amount of chlorine and other noxious substances in the effluent of mills and manufacturing plants. There is a need for the establishment and constant monitoring of regulations regarding the safe disposal of noxious products to ensure that manufacturing plants, mills and other industries adhere to regulations. Many municipalities have established safety levels for air pollution and building standards for allowable smokestacks and other possible sources of air pollutants. The enforcement of these standards, though, is often difficult. Large companies may choose to pay fines rather than change their practices.

People are concerned about the depletion of the ozone layer, a phenomenon that results in increased levels of harmful ultraviolet (UV) rays. Overexposure to UV rays is linked to skin cancer. As a result, many weather-monitoring stations now report the UV index (a measure of the strength of UV rays) on a daily basis during the summer and advise people on the length of time they can stay in the sun before skin starts to burn.

Radiation is an increasing problem in our technological age. The use of atomic fuel as a source of energy is a controversial issue. It is a clean and efficient fuel source, but there are worries about its manufacture and use. Although we have been assured that the production process in atomic energy plants in Canada is safe, there is concern that a disaster like the one at Chernobyl in the Ukraine or at Three Mile Island in the United States may occur here as well. There is also concern about the health risks involved in the disposal of nuclear wastes.

At this time, the effects of computers, microwaves, cellular telephones and other common factors in our daily lives are unknown. Too much radiation can cause genetic defects. People who work with radioactive materials must constantly be monitored to ensure that they do not receive too much radiation. Nurses and other health workers also need to take special precautions when caring for patients who are receiving treatments involving radiation, or the use of radioactive substances. The hydroelectric lines running over residential communities are also a concern to many because of the unknown long-term effects of electromagnetic fields. In newer communities, these are now installed underground.

Noise, which is a common characteristic of many workplaces and city streets, is another pollutant that must be controlled. The hustle and bustle of city streets and the noise of traffic on the highways are things we have learned to live with. However, excessive noise can be harmful in that it destroys some of the 15 000–20 000 sensitive hair cells lining the cochlea. Repeated noise will destroy the nerve fibres leading to these cells, causing deafness. One should be aware, then, of the dangers of turning the volume too high on radios and CD players.

There are also hazardous chemical products that we encounter in everyday living—in the home and in the workplace. There are numerous other workplace hazards besides noise, radiation and air pollution that are of concern to workers, unions, employers and health authorities. The Workers' Compensation Boards, or in some provinces, the Department of Labour, have developed safety standards for most industries, and these are enforceable by law.

Lastly, we must not forget about the effects of severe weather conditions and natural phenomena such as earthquakes, hurricanes (typhoons) and floods that can cause enormous stress on communities. In Canada we have learned to dress appropriately to withstand the bitter cold of our northern winters and to build houses that will keep us warm in the winter and cool in the summer. Still, a prolonged "cold snap," a heavy snowfall, torrential rains or a prolonged hot spell can cause havoc in a community. Severe weather can cause floods, violent windstorms and the like.

Currently, there is concern about the effects of the weather on people's health. Infants, the elderly, people with cardiovascular disease and the chronically ill are particularly at risk when environmental temperatures are extremely high or low. The problem is more acute when there is a prolonged period of heat combined with high humidity. Many people find that moods are affected by the weather; most of us feel more cheerful on a sunny day than on one that is dull and grey. **Seasonal affective disorder (SAD)** is the term given to a depression induced by insufficient exposure to sunlight.

Potential Community Problems Resulting from Physical and Chemical Stressors

- atmospheric pollution
- pollution of water, food and/or milk supplies
- health problems—respiratory, gastrointestinal, genetic and other problems
- civic disaster.

Biological Stressors

Biological stressors are those caused by living organisms. Included in this category are plants, insects and animals, and the infectious agents that cause disease.

Plants are an essential element in renewal of oxygen in the atmosphere and, thus, the promotion of a healthy environment. Many plants are used in the preparation of medicines, prescription and over-the-counter drugs as well as herbal remedies. However, some plants are poisonous. Poison ivy and poison oak, for example, can cause severe skin reactions. Other plants are poisonous when eaten, such as some varieties of mushrooms, holly, honeysuckle and the spider plant (Clark, 1996).

Insects and animals frequently serve as both reservoirs and carriers of disease-causing agents. Flies, fleas, cockroaches, mosquitoes and animals such as rats, cats and dogs often bring disease into a community. The malaria that caused so many deaths among soldiers building the Rideau Canal from Ottawa to Kingston in the early 1800s was carried by the swarms of malaria-carrying mosquitoes that infested the marshy lands through which the canal was built. Rats were the principal carriers of the plague that devastated Europe in the Middle Ages.

The draining of swampy marshes and other measures used to eradicate mosquitoes have rid Canada of malaria, but the disease is still a problem in many parts of the world. Rats and other rodents still infest some communities in Canada, particularly the seaports. We should not forget that dogs, cats and other household pets can also be **vectors** (carriers) of disease. Not only are there insects that can bring disease, but some, such as grasshoppers and locusts, can destroy crops, which can destroy the economic base of a farming community. Destruction of crops can devastate both the production and consumption functions of a community as well as the physical environment.

Other biological factors are the infectious agents that cause disease. They may be transmitted by air currents, by person-to-person contact, by animals and insects (as noted above) or by other vectors. It is estimated that, world-wide, 80 percent of all communicable diseases are transmitted by infectious agents in water (Page, 1987).

Potential Community Problems Resulting from Biological Stressors

- pestilence
- disease
- epidemics
- economic distress.

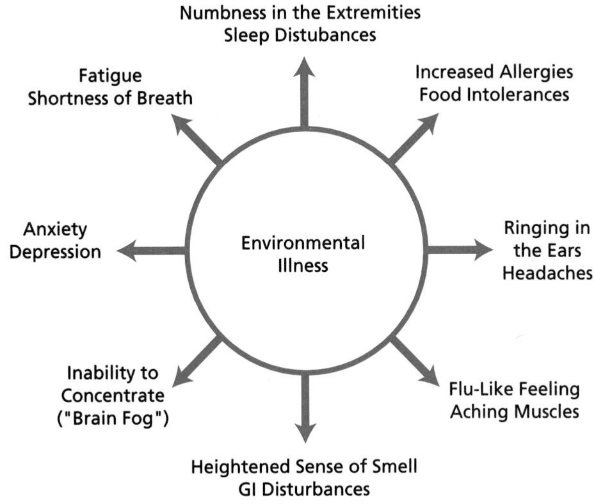

FIGURE 11.2 Symptoms of environmental illness

SOURCE: Millar & Millar, 1998.

Environmental Illness

Today, the environment has become an important influence in the practice of nursing. Recent developments have demonstrated the significant role it plays in the illness–health equation. Many patients now manifest illnesses that are a direct result of hypersensitivity to our changing environment. To keep pace with evolution of these illnesses, the nursing profession must incorporate the assessment and treatment of environmentally related illnesses into daily practice. The link between the environment and the health of the Canadian population will be a major factor in the transition of nursing into the 21st century.

Environmental illness is one manifestation of hypersensitivity to the environment. Twentieth-century environmental practices have led to a growing incidence of this condition. Nurses will observe more of this illness in the future and thus need to be familiar with its clinical manifestations and the factors that contribute to precipitating this hypersensitivity. As shown in Figure 11.2, environmental illness affects multiple body systems, causing the patient to become sensitive to the environment and unable to tolerate "normal" levels of everyday chemicals that pose no problems to the general population. Because these chemicals are present everywhere, it is difficult to escape them. Common sensitivities include reactions to such substances such as perfume, paper, ink, vehicle exhaust, tobacco smoke, paint, new carpeting, pesticides, cosmetics or foods and food additives (Rea, 1992).

Both outdoor and indoor pollution have contributed to the escalating number of patients suffering from environmental illness. Outdoor pollution has affected the health of Canadians over a long period of time, from the earliest days of heavy industry. However, the sheer increase in the number of industries that produce toxic waste has had serious health ramifications. Indoor pollution is a much more recent problem that has evolved over the last 20 years. Although outdoor pollution cannot be ignored, indoor pollution is also having a detrimental effect on the health of Canadians.

INDOOR POLLUTION

In examining the effects of indoor pollution, the nurse's assessment seeks to determine whether a particular location or facility is toxic, and also explores the lifestyle of the individual.

There are four factors that are associated with environmentally related health conditions:

1. increase in the manufacture and use of synthetic chemicals
2. decrease in nutritional status of the population
3. effects of endocrine-disrupting chemicals
4. creation of energy-efficient buildings and use of synthetic building materials (Meggs, 1992; Amdur, Doull & Klaassen 1991; Shils & Young, 1988; Rea, 1994; Colborn, Vomsaal & Soto, 1993; Stancel et al., 1995; Soto et al., 1995; Teeuw, Vandenbroucke-Grauls & Verhoef, 1994).

In our quest to reduce cost and to design efficient, contemporary surroundings, two harmful variables have been factored into the environmental equation: energy-efficient buildings and synthetic construction materials. These factors are important because the populations of the industrialized countries spend more than 90 percent of the time indoors (Hope, 1993). One-third of newly constructed or remodelled buildings are estimated to have the potential to induce illness in the occupants, thus creating a new diagnostic label: sick building syndrome (SBS) (Teeuw et al., 1994).

Sick building syndrome is defined by the World Health Organization (cited in Tamblyn et al., 1994) as "an increase in the frequency of building occupant reported complaints associated with acute, non-specific symptoms in non-industrial environments that improve while away from the building" (p. 603). Modern technology has fostered the use of large amounts of synthetics in the manufacture of fabrics, building materials, clothing, cleaning products, fragrances and pesticides. Thus, a wide range of chemicals enter our homes, schools, offices and industrial settings, where they emit toxic vapours that contribute to SBS. These substances also affect air quality in hospitals, airlines, automobiles and shopping centres (Sherin, 1993; Mikatavage et al., 1995).

The design and construction of energy-efficient building features—such as sealed windows and doors, insulated walls and roofs, and specialized ventilation systems—dramatically reduce the exchange and flow of outside air (Sherin, 1993). As well, construction materials have changed dramatically over the past decade. Wood, metal and glass have been replaced with synthetic substitutes that often emit chemicals not found in natural building products (Ruhl, Chang, Halpern & Gershwin, 1993). In addition, other factors in the building can precipitate SBS: exceeding the occupancy limit, using industrial cleaners, and applying pesticides and carpet cleaners (Sherin, 1993). The creation of this serious health problem is the consequence of saving energy, utilization of synthetic building materials and certain unhealthy events within the building.

OUTDOOR POLLUTION

Although the effects of pollution on the outdoor environment are well known, Canadians have not adequately addressed the growing degradation of air quality caused by vehicle exhaust and industrial effluents and emissions. Further, we are exporting harmful environmental practices to developing nations where few regulations are enforced. Studies have shown that harmful environmental practices are not locally contained; rather, they create a global environmental emergency, as shown by the worldwide mutation and extinction of plant and wildlife species.

Canadians are thus an integral part of an ecosystem that is deteriorating. Along with the rest of the world, we must concern ourselves with the effects of current practices and policies on the health of present and future generations.

The challenge for the nurse is to become knowledgeable about the relationship between environmental practices in a region and the possible health consequences to its residents. An environmental assessment, in addition to the standard community assessment, can enable the nurse to demonstrate a relationship between the specific health problems of residents and local environmental practices. Examples of community health consequences related to environmental practices are:

1. pollution of air and water
2. pollution of the food chain
3. long-term health effects on children of exposure to chemicals
4. increased use of farm chemicals to combat resistant weeds and insects
5. segmentation of community over environmental degradation (Donald & Syrgiannis, 1995; Rea, 1994; Birnbaum, 1995; Labonte, 1989).

THE ROLE OF THE NURSE

The nurse can contribute to the new field of environmental medicine by becoming knowledgeable about environmental illness and its implications for the nursing process. Comprehensive nursing skills must include:

- self-education about environmental illness and its complexities
- recognition of the clinical manifestations of environmental illness
- inclusion of environmental history as part of a community assessment
- identification of precipitating events and exposures that place patients and communities at risk
- development of counselling skills specific to environmental illness
- design of care plans tailored to community needs.

Environmental factors are precipitating changes in the illnesses that the nurse will encounter, and these changes are dictating the addition of new principles to the practice of nursing. Adopting new concepts in the nursing care plan is the foundation of progressive nursing care.

Health Care in the Community

The following was written by a nurse currently practising in the field of community health in Vancouver, British Columbia:

The role of the nurse in community settings requires continual consideration of the overall health of the community, and the strengths and capabilities of those within it.

Health is now understood to be a resource for everyday living, and health promotion as "a process which enables people to increase control over, and improve their health" (Canadian Public Health Association, 1986). Community health nurses who understand their primary role to be one of promoting health have good success when they build on the capacity of the local community to support an acceptable quality of life for individuals, families and neighbourhoods. The nurse must consider the ability of the community to support healthful living. The most effective strategies for health promotion in the community focus on forming partnerships. Collaboration with citizens, professionals, associations, agencies, and other individuals and groups help to identify and resolve health issues. The process increases opportunities for people to have control over their health.

Nurses work in a variety of community settings such as homes, workplaces, community health centres, public health units, clinics and schools. Nursing interaction in each of these settings includes working with individuals, families, groups and the community as a whole. A nurse's role in promoting health varies with the setting, the health issues identified, the level of interaction (individual or group) and the strengths and abilities of those involved. Despite these variables, however, the common role is that of the skilled facilitator who may, for example, be working in partnership with a person who is managing a chronic disease, or a group of citizens who are concerned about the safety of the streets in a neighbourhood. Utilizing additional health promotion strategies in community settings further builds on the strengths of those involved, and in turn, increases resources for everyday living.

P. Lynn Buhler, RN, BSN, MSc
Manager
Health Promotion and Prevention Programs
Vancouver Health Department
West Main Health Unit
October 1993

Assessment of the Health of a Community

In your nursing program you will have courses on community health nursing. This chapter is intended as merely an introduction to the field of community health nursing. We will not, therefore, describe a detailed assessment tool but will, instead, suggest ways in which you, as a student, can look at the health of a community. The basic methods you can use include gathering information by (a) reviewing statistical data and literature related to the community, (b) direct observation and (c) talking with people who live and/or work in that community. Other methods that are used in the Healthy Communities process to gather information on a community's health needs and to monitor its progress towards a healthier state include surveys, neighbourhood discussions, public forums and interviews with community leaders.

When gathering information about a community, it is also useful to focus on how well it is carrying out its major functions of production, consumption, maintenance of the physical environment, management, growth and development and social support.

GATHERING BASELINE DATA ABOUT A COMMUNITY

The data collected, compiled and analysed by Statistics Canada and by the Vital Statistics Departments of provincial ministries of health can provide a lot of valuable information about a community. Census data, for example, give basic information about a given population, such as total number of people, age and gender distribution, ethnic origin of inhabitants, population density (number of people per square kilometre) and birth rates. These statistics are summarized in community profiles that provide an abundance of specific information in defined geographical areas. Government health departments—federal, provincial and municipal—usually collect and publish basic health statistics, such as life expectancy rates; maternal, infant and child mortality rates; leading causes of death and major illnesses. These statistics are often broken down to the county or municipal level, or in sections of a city. A useful source of information on specific topics such as the health of people who live in the North or trends in child mortality is the Statistics Canada quarterly *Canadian Social Trends*.

COLLECTING INFORMATION BY DIRECT OBSERVATION

You can also learn a lot about a community by walking about the streets. If you keep in mind the community functions we talked about and look for evidence of the factors affecting these functions discussed above, you will easily develop a focus for your observations.

The factors affecting the *production function* of a community are the soundness and extent of the community's economic base and the availability of a wide range of educational services. Businesses, manufacturing plants, shops, offices, banks and other places of employment are all relevant. Large city cores are often dominated by financial exchanges, whereas tourist areas have many restaurants and retail outlets. A drive or walk through the area will provide the nurse with an abundance of information. Important, too, are the number and types of schools and colleges in the area. Regarding the *consumption function*, the price of groceries, for example, and whether there is a good supply of fresh foods and vegetables can be very revealing. The type of housing in the area—single-family homes, apartments, high-rises, etc.—their state of repair and the number of "for rent" and "for sale" signs can also be important indicators of the consumption function within a community. The state of the physical environment of the community can also be assessed on a preliminary basis by walking around. How clean are the streets? Are there trees in residential areas, parks and other recreational sites? Are these clean or littered with empty bottles, beverage cans, paper and the like? A public health inspector would be able to provide specific information about the safety of food and water supplies. You can assess, on your own, the cleanliness in stores, restaurants and fast-food outlets in the neighbourhood—and you can note garbage on the streets or in the alleyways. Indications of a healthy physical environment can also be observed from the parks and other recreation sites in the community, as well as the wildlife living in them.

LOOKING back

Evaline Mary Pemberton, circa 1875–1949

Canada's first registered nurse was Evaline Mary Pemberton of Halifax; hers was the initial signature on the official Register when Nova Scotia enacted the first nursing legislation in Canada in April 1910. As president of the Graduate Nurses Association of Nova Scotia, she had been one of the growing number of nurses in Canada who, in the early 1900s, lobbied their provincial governments for protection of the public through registration. Before that time, no legislation in Canada had recognized the need for standards for nursing practice.

Although nursing education had shown great strides in the preceding 35 years, legislation to register nurses and have nurses set standards for practice was something entirely new in Canada. The Graduate Nurses Association of Nova Scotia was not the first provincial organization of nurses; the Graduate Nurses Association of Ontario had been formed from hospital nurses' alumnae groups in 1904, and by 1910 several provinces had associations. However, the small group of Nova Scotia nurses organized in 1909 under president Evaline Pemberton was determined to achieve official status for properly educated "graduate" nurses who would be certified as safe practitioners. They were the first to get a provincial body to act.

Little is documented about Evaline (also spelled Eveline) Pemberton's personal life. She graduated in 1894 in the sixth class of the School of Nursing of Western Hospital of Montreal (later part of Montreal General) and was immediately placed in charge of the Women's Hospital in Montreal. Her records show that she also at some time received a certificate in Home Economics from Battle Creek (Michigan) Sanatorium and took a course at New York's Bellevue Hospital. She then moved to England, where she attended Queen Victoria's Jubilee Institute for Nurses and was appointed a Queen's Nurse in 1897. She stayed at least eight years in England, finally working as nurse-in-charge of the Victoria Nursing Station in Grantham, Lincolnshire. When she returned to Canada, she became matron of the Edgehill Church School for Girls in Windsor, Nova Scotia, at which time she became active in forming the Graduate Nurses Association of Nova Scotia. She remained active in the Association for many years. In 1922, when the Act of 1910 was amended, the Association issued official Certificates of Registration and awarded Certificate Number One to Evaline Pemberton as first president and charter member, thus making her Canada's first RN.

— *Glennis Zilm*

How well the *management function* of a community is operating can be difficult to assess just by walking around a community. However, attending, as an observer, a meeting of the community/town council or other elected body can provide some information.

Although more precise data from other sources should be gathered, one can also observe in "walkabouts" the *growth and development function* of the community. Are there many mothers with small children in the grocery stores, strolling the streets or playing in the parks? Are there a lot of older people in the neighbourhood? Do you see notices regarding health promotional activities such as the services of a health unit, well-baby clinics or "wellness centres" for older people? Many large grocery stores now have "smart shopper" or similar programs with a nutritionist helping people select the most nutritious foods from the choices available. In the context of cultural growth and development, is there evidence of cultural activities in the community—art galleries, theatres, playhouses? Is there advertising for concerts or plays by a local theatrical group in neighbourhood stores or on bulletin boards in the grocery store? Does the community look prosperous enough to support cultural activities?

With regard to the *support function*, is there a community centre? If so, what sorts of programs do they have for different age groups in the community? Is the community centre busy with groups of people doing different things, such as a group of older adults playing cards, a preschool group colouring, older children playing basketball in the gym or swimming in the pool? Are there many churches or synagogues in the neighbourhood? Do you see "Neighbourhood Watch" or "Block Parent" signs in the windows of many houses?

The location of health services in the community is also an important indicator of a community's overall functioning. Are there other health agencies in the community—physicians' offices and those of other health practitioners such as physiotherapists, massage therapists, naturopaths? Do you see any local social service agencies? Are there many police officers on the streets and/or patrolling the neighbourhood in cars or on bicycles? In Canada, there are three levels of police: municipal, provincial (in some provinces) and the Royal Canadian Mounted Police (RCMP), who serve communities and rural areas that do not have a provincial or municipal constabulary. At all levels, police officers work in partnership with community groups. For example, they may visit schools to talk to students about street and road safety.

GATHERING INFORMATION BY TALKING WITH PEOPLE

A good way to learn how people perceive the community's ability to carry out its major functions is to meet and talk with them informally—in the community centre, in the grocery store, in the coffee shop. As you gain skills in interpersonal relationships and in communication, you will find it much easier to elicit information from people about business and educational facilities in the community. You will want to find out about the availability of affordable housing, for example, and the cost of living in that community. You will want to find out where people go when they are sick. How do they feel about the health services that are available? Once you have gained their trust, people will usually talk about their concerns.

Many of these will probably not be "traditional" health concerns. In 1993, the South Fraser Valley Health Council (an interim committee formed prior to regionalization) conducted a health needs survey in four communities. The survey found that the issues varied in the different communities. The major concerns were similar; the issue of affordable and accessible health care was the most important concern (see Figure 11.3). You will note, however, in Figure 11. 4, that some issues were of more concern than others in each of the four communities (SFVHC, 1993). It should be noted that this survey was not an official research project, but provides an example of what a community group can do to get the "feel" of its community regarding health issues.

INTERPRETING THE RESULTS

Once you have collected the data, you will want to try to identify challenges and problems in the community. If you are acting as a resource person for people in a community in a Healthy Communities or similar project, analysis of the data might be accomplished by the group. Statistical data for individual communities can be compared with national and provincial data and with that of other communities in the province. For example, you will probably find a difference in infant mortality rates in regions across a province, and different rates of crime and violence in specific communities. Average income of families in the community will certainly vary, as will the number of people with high school completion or postsecondary education. You can compare your community with that of other communities in the city (if you live in a major urban centre), in the province and also with the national average.

You can also collate the impressions you have gained by walking around the neighbourhood or community and the data you have picked up from talking with people. These can be grouped under the six major functions of the community to create a community profile.

For those working in Healthy Communities projects wishing to do a more specific analysis, the Office of Health Promotion of the B.C. Ministry of Health and Ministry Responsible for Seniors has developed a *Health Indicator Workbook* (1992c) as a tool to assist communities to gather information about their health needs and to monitor the community's progress towards a healthier community; it is available to other provinces as well. They point out that there are numerous criteria that could be developed. The ones shown in the workbook are examples of criteria that have been found useful in Healthy Communities projects. Another community assessment tool, using Gordons Functional Health Patterns is shown on the following page.

Nursing Interventions in the Community

The distinction is rapidly blurring between institutional and community health care. Many hospitals are becoming "hospitals without walls," as nurses and other health professionals take services to people in their homes. For example, an enterostomy service that has been strictly hospital-based may be extended to have the nurses doing preoperative counselling and follow-up visits to teach people to care for their "ostomies" at home. Another example is the Early Postpartum Discharge program at the Lions Gate Hospital in North Vancouver, British Columbia. Patients who meet specific criteria are discharged home within 24 hours of giving birth. Nurses employed at Lions Gate Hospital make home visits on postpartum days 2 and 3.

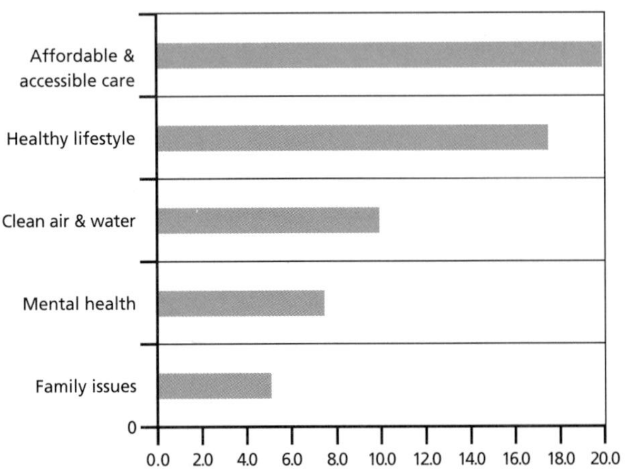

FIGURE 11.3 Most important health issues

SOURCE: SFVHC, p. 12.

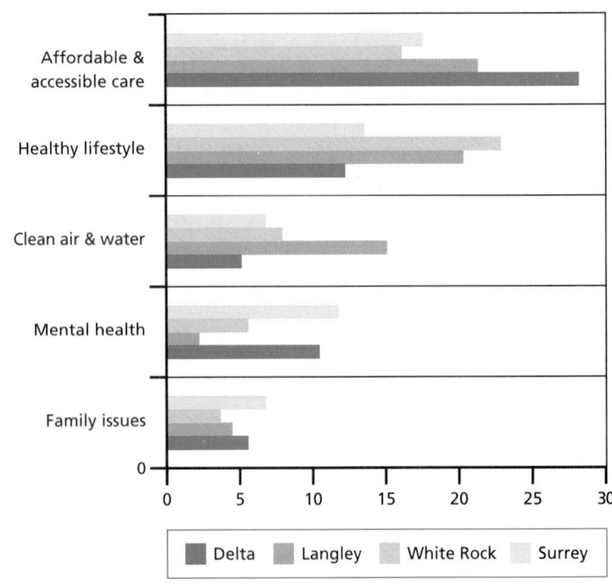

FIGURE 11.4 Most important health issues, by community

SOURCE: SFVHC, p. 12.

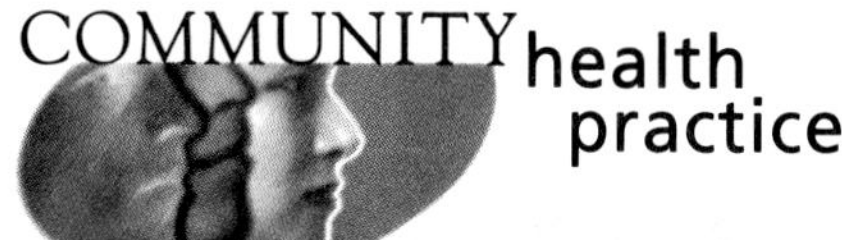

Community Assessment Using Functional Health Patterns

Health Perception–Health Management Pattern

- health facilities
- availability of health professionals (traditional/complementary)
- promotion and prevention programs
- usage rates
- perceived level of wellness/health problems

Nutrition–Metabolic Pattern

- food supplement programs (food banks, Meals-on-Wheels)
- availability of natural resources
- number of grocery stores/markets
- water supply and quality of water
- water restrictions
- climate

Elimination Pattern

- types of wastes, sewage systems
- waste/recycling programs
- pest control
- perception of problems

Activity–Exercise Pattern

- employment opportunities
- transportation
- shopping malls
- community centres, athletic/social clubs, organizations
- communication system
- hiking/walking trails, golf courses, playgrounds

Sleep–Rest Pattern

- usual business hours
- activity levels
- noise levels (busy/quiet areas)

Cognitive–Perceptual Pattern

- opportunities for education
- language
- effects of outside system on community

Self-Perception–Self-Concept Pattern

- community history (published descriptions)
- local newspapers
- ethnic/cultural composition
- visibility/acceptability of marginalized populations
- pride indicators
- museums/zoos, educational and cultural/arts facilities

Role–Relationship Pattern

- fire/safety programs (Neighbourhood Watch, lighting)
- police/community relationships, patrol system
- traffic/highways/public works programs
- inspection programs
- budgets
- perception of roles/responsibilities and problem-solving ability
- relationship with other communities

Value–Belief Pattern

- the priority of health issues, community-identified health problems
- religious denominations; number of churches, synagogues, mosques
- limits of acceptable behaviour
- housing/zoning laws
- political, social issues
- ethnic groups

Sexuality–Reproductive Pattern

- male/female ratio
- population changes/growth patterns (family size/form)
- changes in fertility rates (maternal age)
- teenage pregnancies
- prevalence of pornography, abortion, prostitution

Coping–Stress-Tolerance Pattern

- delinquency
- drug/alcohol abuse
- child/spouse/elder abuse
- unemployment rate
- immigration rate
- community occupational stress
- crime
- socioeconomic levels
- number of parks and recreational facilities
- divorce
- suicide rates/patterns
- incidence of mental health problems
- presence of telephone help lines/support groups

SOURCE: Gikow & Kucharski, 1987.

During their visits, they assess the health status of both mother and baby, provide education on aspects of self and infant care, and provide emotional support and counselling to the new parents as they cope with integrating a new baby into the family. This usually involves a reintegration of the family, a redefinition of the roles of members, and changes in their relationships as they return to family lifestyles and the activities of daily living.

Community agencies and hospitals are also getting together in partnerships to offer people more continuity of care. We have come a long way since 1955, when the VON assigned the first "liaison nurse" to the Montreal General Hospital to discuss discharge plans with patients and coordinate the services needed (VON, 1983).

In the community, nurses work in all phases of the health care continuum. They carry out health promotion and health protection activities, provide restorative services in the home, and may also extend home support to people with chronic and terminal illnesses.

HEALTH PROMOTION ACTIVITIES

A major portion of the community health nurse's work has always been in health promotion activities—helping people learn how to live a healthier life. Traditionally, this has involved such activities as prenatal classes for pregnant women (fathers are now included), visits to new mothers, well-baby clinics, and school and employee health programs. Since the Lalonde Report in 1974 pointed out the link between lifestyle and the major causes of death (heart disease, strokes and accidents), health promotion has become a large part of the work of national, provincial and municipal health agencies. A Health Promotion Directorate at Health Canada and similar units in provincial ministries of health and municipal departments have been established.

As we mentioned in Chapter 3, our ideas about health promotion have broadened considerably over the years since the Lalonde Report (1974). By the mid-1970s, health promotional activities had expanded from teaching people to adopt a healthy lifestyle to include education, training and research, legislation, policy coordination and community development. The Ottawa Charter defined health promotion as "the process of enabling people to increase control over, and to improve, their health" (Canadian Public Health Association, 1986, p. 426). A key word here is *enablement*: the health professional's task is to help people to take control of their own health. It is essential that people take an active role in developing programs that suit individual and community needs. It is also important for people to be able to make choices regarding the programs they want to participate in to improve their health (Epp, 1986, p. 3). The Epp Report suggests three mechanisms for promoting health:

1. self-care, the decisions and actions individuals take in the interest of their own health
2. mutual aid, the actions people take to help one another

NURSES at work — Community Health Nurse

I am a Community Health Nurse (CHN) with the City of Vancouver Health Department. Three years ago, the West Main Health Unit in Vancouver made a decision to assign a Community Health Nurse to work with residents in the Little Mountain neighbourhood. This is a middle-class neighbourhood in which many recent immigrants have settled over the past few years. The role of this CHN was to work with local residents to address issues affecting the livability of Little Mountain. I volunteered to undertake the project.

In the first few months, I identified key informants who could provide me with some background information about the area and activities that were taking place. The steering committee for a Community Awareness Survey invited me to become a member. This survey was a tool to collect demographic data and to identify interested residents who would like to participate in organized actions aimed at strengthening community networks.

After completion of the survey, I helped to establish the Little Mountain Healthy Communities Initiative and to secure funding from the Ministry of Health. Residents decided to use the funds to hire a community development worker. I then worked closely with the residents and the community development worker to set up community meetings. At these meetings, the residents debated issues that were important and formulated action plans to address some of these concerns. Examples of these included:

1. traffic
2. the need to increase community cohesiveness
3. a business sector that was not reflecting the needs of the residents
4. petty crime.

The residents set up small committees to examine some of these issues more closely. Many of these neighbourhood concerns have been solved through cooperation among residents, social agencies and civic government.

In this project, I maintained the role of a facilitator at community meetings and a resource person to liaise with the different levels of government. The community identified the issues and decided on the approach to address them. This approach differs from the traditional medical model that employs a top-down approach to problem-solving. In the Healthy Communities framework, the role of health professionals changes depending on the needs of the community in question. This bottom-up approach allows residents to become experts in their particular communities and permits me to maintain a supportive role.

— *Vanessa Lam, BScN, RN*

3. healthy environments, the creation of conditions and surroundings conducive to health.

The implementation of these three mechanisms involves nurses in many nontraditional activities to promote the health of people in the community. The Victorian Order of Nurses has been instrumental in pioneering many programs for various groups in the community. One example is the foot care clinics that have enabled many older adults with painful feet to participate in walking and other exercise programs. Another program initiated by the VON, but taken over in many communities now by official or other voluntary agencies, is Meals-on-Wheels, which ensures the recipient of at least one good, hot meal a day. In line with the newer definition of health promotion to enable people to take control of their health, the VON initiated community development programs to encourage older adults to participate in developing their own programs. This program was titled Promoting Elders' Participation (PEP) and was targeted primarily for rural and underserviced areas. The VON provided a coordinator to establish the group. The PEP undertakes needs assessments and explores ways and means of supplying the needed services (Du Gas & Beckingham, 1993; VON, 1988, 1991).

HEALTH PROTECTION ACTIVITIES

Among the activities of nurses in the health protection segment of the health care spectrum are those involving the control of communicable disease, screening programs to detect the early development of health problems in at-risk populations for specific disorders and environmental safety programs.

Control of Communicable Diseases

Nurses are very involved both in preventing the spread of infection of communicable disease and in carrying out immunization programs to increase the resistance of people to these diseases. The nurse is very often the person who identifies the disease, for example, when examining school children. The nurse is often responsible for identifying people who have been exposed to a disease, informing them that they have been exposed and referring them to the appropriate agency for testing and treatment (Clark, 1996). Nursing interventions in the prevention of communicable disease include teaching people precautions that should be taken to prevent other members of a family and other people from developing the disease. As we mentioned in Chapter 2, most of the infectious diseases that were the leading causes of death at the beginning of this century have been virtually eliminated. One of the main reasons has been the development and widespread use of vaccines and other immune-producing agents. Today, immunization is available for many communicable diseases including the childhood diseases of measles, mumps, rubella, diphtheria, pertussis and polio. Immunization is also available for hepatitis B and for diseases caused by the *Hemophilus influenzae* type B bacteria (Clark, 1996). Nurses carry out the majority of immunization programs in most communities.

Screening Programs

Screening is done to detect disease in its early stages. It is a "preliminary examination or testing of a person to determine whether or not he or she might have a particular condition and whether further diagnostic testing is indicated" (Clark, 1996, p. 405). A woman with a family history of cancer of the breast may be advised to have a mammogram (an x-ray of the breast) on a yearly basis as a screening procedure whereas other women without family histories of the disease would not have this diagnostic procedure done as often. The screening, which includes a thorough physical examination of the breast, is often carried out by nurses. For many years, a routine chest x-ray was included in the admission procedure to hospitals to screen for tuberculosis (the procedure is no longer part of the admissions routine). Screening may also be carried out for sexually transmitted diseases, for example, in people who have been exposed to chlamydia, gonorrhea or HIV, the human immunodeficiency virus that causes AIDS (Clark, 1996).

Eye examinations and hearing tests carried out on children starting school in the public school system are other examples of screening programs.

Environmental Safety Activities

The nurse collaborates with a number of other health workers and with workers from other sectors in carrying out environmental safety activities in the community. Among the others concerned with environmental safety are public health inspectors, whose main focus is environmental safety; the medical officers of health, whose mandate concerns all possible sources of ill health in the community; social workers concerned with the living conditions of people (among other things); and the fire department, which carries out fire prevention programs in the community. In the workplace, the nurse (OHN) and the occupational safety officer work in collaboration. During home visits, nurses have a good opportunity to observe conditions in the household and to advise on measures to make the house a safer place. In families with young children, for example, parents may want some help in "child-proofing" their house. A great many devices are available to make home environments safer for older people and those with disabilities. These include grab-bars for bathtubs, handrails for walls and numerous other adaptations to normal household equipment.

NURSING INTERVENTIONS IN RESTORATIVE AND SUPPORTIVE CARE

The interventions nurses carry out in the community to help people to restore their health or to cope with long-term or terminal illness include direct care, monitoring the health of people with various illnesses, counselling and providing emotional support for patients with long-term and terminal illness and their families, coordinating care given by others and teaching and supervising other caregivers (Bullough & Bullough, 1990).

Direct Care

Home nursing has been part of community nursing in Canada from the early 1700s, when the Grey Nuns began visiting the sick in their homes in Montreal. However, it did not become an integral part of secular nursing until the establishment of the VON in the latter part of the19th century. Today, with early hospital discharge, the tremendous increase in "day surgery," and the increased provision of services in the home, there has been considerable expansion of the need for highly skilled nurses in the community (Bullough & Bullough, 1990).

Direct nursing care is also needed by many people with long-term illnesses and by people who are terminally ill. In providing direct care in the home, nurses may assist patients with hygiene measures; they may carry out treatments, such as dressings or injections; and they may administer medications. Many patients have intravenous and other types of therapy that the nurse administers, or teaches patients or family members to administer (Bullough & Bullough, 1990).

Monitoring Health Status

Many people with acute or long-term illness need a nurse to check on their progress at regular and frequent intervals. A postoperative patient's incision needs to be assessed for wound healing, and a new mother and infant need to be monitored. The nurse can use the visit to answer questions, perhaps incorporate some new health teaching and follow up on the teaching begun in the hospital. People with chronic illnesses, such as hypertension, diabetes and arthritis, need occasional home visits. In the case of the hypertensive patient, the nurse would visit to check the blood pressure; with the diabetic patient, to monitor blood glucose results; and with the arthritic patient, to assess pain, coping and ability to carry out activities of daily living. Once the nurse has the data, he or she can then take appropriate action to have the problem taken care of before expensive hospitalization is needed.

Counselling and Emotional Support

Part of the goal in nursing is to assist patients and their families to live as fully as possible with long-term or terminal illness—if possible, in their home environment. When illness is prolonged, patients and families will experience varying levels of stress, frustration and emotional trauma.

Nurses are in a key position to provide the emotional support and counselling that are necessary with long-term or terminal illness. The nurse can assist patients and families with coping strategies to deal with the peaks and valleys of long-term and terminal illness. In addition, the nurse can refer family members to appropriate community groups that may also offer support.

People with long-term or terminal illness and their families need help in coping with the illness. In addition to the physical problems associated with both long-term and terminal illness, the mental anguish that accompanies them needs to be addressed. There is a need for people to come to terms with illness—to adjust to decreasing physical, and sometimes mental, ability. If patients have to depend on others to do things for them, they undoubtedly feel the loss of the independence they have cherished. People need to be able to talk through their feelings. Often, they do not want to distress family members by discussing these feelings with them and feel more comfortable talking with a nurse. We will be returning to this topic in Chapter 17 and also in Chapter 37. Many nurses work on palliative care teams, providing comfort and support to people who are terminally ill and to their families.

Coordinating Home Care Services

Many nurses serve as coordinators, or case managers, for people needing care in the home. In this capacity, they undertake the initial assessment of the patient's needs and develop a plan of care. They also make arrangements for the services of nursing, physiotherapy, occupational therapy, homemaking or other areas as needed. They monitor the care given and intervene if problems occur. Here, it is the nurse, rather than the physician, who acts as a "gatekeeper" for health care services (Bullough & Bullough, 1990; Clark, 1996).

Teaching and Supervising Other Caregivers

Paid caregivers in the home include a variety of workers: registered nurses, licensed practical nurses (called Registered Practical Nurses [RPNs] in Ontario), long-term care aides, attendants and sitters/companions. In addition, a family member or a friend may be the principal caregiver for a person needing nursing care, personal care or supervision in the home. The registered nurse is often responsible for teaching basic nursing techniques to paid caregivers who have not had formal preparation, such as attendants and sitters/companions, before they are assigned to cases. The nurse is also available to teach the family member or friend who is a principal caregiver. Family members providing care in the home are not infrequently on 24-hour duty, seven days a week, as in the case of someone caring for a spouse who has Alzheimer's disease (a chronic organic mental disorder). It is important to remember that volunteer caregivers need relief or they too will become ill. A variety of caregiver relief services are available, including day care centres and day programs for the elderly and the handicapped. We discussed a number of these programs in Chapters 3 and 4. The nurse who is going into the home is well suited to assess the caregiver's needs, suggest ways and means for respite and, if needed, make the necessary referrals.

IN REVIEW

- A major factor in the improvement of health in the Western world over the past 150 years has been the reduction of environmental hazards through the institution of public health policy measures by local governments.
- Until recently, concerns over environmental factors that adversely affect health have focussed mainly on outdoor pollution. However, indoor pollution also has a major effect on the health of the population (e.g., sick building syndrome).
- Community is viewed as the basic unit in health care. It is important for nurses to understand:
  - community function
  - determinants of health
  - nursing's role in community health.
- The science of epidemiology has been used extensively to assess the health of communities. The methodology of epidemiology includes:
  - systematic assessment of data (descriptive, analytic, experimental)
  - determination of the causes of health and illness
  - manifestations of specific diseases
  - identification of risk factors
  - establishment of a community health profile
  - control of epidemics
  - determination of the impact of health programs
  - assistance in formulating public health policy.
- The Healthy Communities approach looks at the health of a community by assessing its ability to carry out its various functions. Functions include:
  - production
  - consumption
  - maintenance of the physical environment
  - management
  - growth and development
  - social support.

  Healthy communities are those in which all functions are carried out well.
- The nurse's role in community health includes:
  - health promotion (e.g., encouragement towards self-care, mutual aid and community development)
  - health protection (e.g., control of communicable diseases, establishment of screening programs and environmental safety programs)
  - provision of restorative and supportive care (e.g., direct care, monitoring of acute and long-term illness, counselling of individuals and families, coordination of home care services, teaching and supervision of other caregivers in the home)
  - promoting responsibility for one's own health (e.g., with individuals, families and communities)
  - collaboration (e.g., with individuals, professional agencies and governments).

Critical Thinking Activities

Select a city neighbourhood or a small rural community to which you have access and see what you can find out about the health of that community from a literature search, from direct observation and from talking with people in the community. Some questions are suggested to help you to organize your plan for gathering information (you may want to add more).

1. Review statistical data and literature in the area.
   a) How many people live in the community?
   b) What is the approximate age distribution of the population?
   c) What is the population density?
   d) What are the predominant ethnic groups?
   e) What statistical data have been collected on the health status of people in this community?
   f) Are there brochures or pamphlets about the community in the library or a community centre?
2. Walk around the streets and look around. Look for evidence of community functioning in regard to:
   a) *Production*
      - What businesses, manufacturing plants, shops and offices do you see?
      - Do these look prosperous or shabby?
      - What types of schools and colleges are there? What other educational programs exist there?
      - Is there a public library? If so, is it busy?

   b) *Consumption*
      - Is there a good supply of fresh fruits and vegetables in the local shops?
      - Is the price of groceries high, average or low in the shops?
      - What type of housing is there in the area: single family dwellings, apartment blocks, townhouse complexes?
      - What is the state of repair of the residences?
      - How many "for rent" and "for sale" signs do you see?

   c) *Maintenance of the Physical Environment*
      - How clean are the streets?
      - Are there trees in the residential areas? Are there parks or green spaces or other recreational sites?
      - How clean are the shops, restaurants and fast-food outlets? The parks and recreational areas?

d) *Management*

If possible, attend a meeting of the community council.

- Is there a good representation of both men and women, people of different age groups, various ethnic groups and people representing different interests?
- What issues are of concern?

e) *Growth and Development*

- Are there many parents with small children in the grocery stores, in the parks or strolling on the streets?
- Are there notices regarding health promotional activities?
- Does the community have an art gallery, a theatre or any other evidence of cultural activity?

f) *Social Support*

- Is there a community centre? If so, what types of programs does it offer?
- Is there a seniors centre?
- Are there many places of worship in the area?
- Do you see many "Neighbourhood Watch" or "Block Parent" signs in the windows of residences?
- Are there police officers on the streets?
- What health services are available in the community?

3. Talk with some residents of the community informally to supplement the information you have obtained from your literature search and your observations. Some of the questions you might ask are:
   - Do you think this is a good neighbourhood to live in?
   - What are your reasons for saying yes (or no)?
   - What are business opportunities like here?
   - Are there good educational facilities?
   - What are real estate prices like?
   - Where do you go when you are ill?
   - How do you feel about the health services and the recreational facilities in the community?
   - Is there much crime in the community?
   - Do you think this is a healthy community? Why or why not?
   - Do you think the community is well run?
   - What are your major concerns about this community?
4. Summarize your impressions of the health of the community. Compare your findings with those on other communities done by your classmates.

KEY TERMS

community p. 245
epidemiology p. 245
epidemiological model p. 245
descriptive study p. 245
analytic study p. 245
experimental studies p. 245
demonstration project p. 246
causality p. 247
risk p. 247
populations at risk p. 247
incidence p. 247
prevalence p. 247
etiology p. 248
Healthy Communities Process p. 248
seasonal affective disorder (SAD) p. 255
vector p. 255
Environmental illness p. 256
sick building syndrome p. 257
screening p. 263

References

AMDUR, M., DOULL, J., & KLAASSEN, C. (1991). *Casarett and Doull's toxicology: The basic science of poisons.* New York: McGraw-Hill.

BIRNBAUM, L. (1995). Developmental effects of dioxins. *Environmental Health Perspectives, 103*(7), 89–94.

BOOTHROYD, P., & EBERLE, M. (1990, August). Healthy communities: What they are, how they're made. *CHS Research Bulletin.* British Columbia: UBC Centre for Human Settlements.

BRITISH COLUMBIA ROYAL COMMISSION ON HEALTH CARE AND COSTS. (1991). *Closer to home.* (Vols. 1–3). Victoria: Crown Publications.

BULLOUGH, B, & BULLOUGH, V. (1990). *Nursing in the community.* St. Louis: Mosby.

CANADIAN PUBLIC HEALTH ASSOCIATION (1986) Ottawa charter for health promotion. *Report of the International Conference on Health Promotion.* Ottawa: Author.

CLARK, M.J. (1996). *Nursing in the community.* (2nd ed.). Stanford, CT: Appleton & Lange.

COLBORN, T., VOM SAAL, F., & SOTO, A. (1993). Developmental effects of endocrine-disrupting chemicals in wildlife and humans. *Environmental Health Perspectives, 101*(10), 378–384.

DONALD, D., & SYRGIANNIS, J. (1995). Occurrence of pesticides in prairie lakes in Saskatchewan in relation to drought and salinity. *Journal of Environmental Quality, 24*(2), 266–270.

DUGAS, B.W., & BECKINGHAM, A. (1993). The Emergence of Gerontological Nursing. In A. Beckingham & B. Dugas *Promoting healthy aging.* St. Louis: Mosby.

EPP, J. (1986). *Achieving health for all: A framework for health promotion.* Ottawa: Minister of Supply & Services.

FRIEDMAN, G.D. (1994). *Primer of epidemiology.* (4th ed.). New York: McGraw-Hill.

GIKOW, F.F., & KUCHARSKI, P.M. (1987). A new look at the community: Functional health pattern assessment. *Community Health Nurse, 1*(4), 21–27.

GOVERNMENT OF BRITISH COLUMBIA. (1992a). *Healthy communities: The process.* Victoria: Office of Health Promotion, B.C. Ministry of Health & Ministry Responsible for Seniors. (Catalogue no. QP 82437)

GOVERNMENT OF BRITISH COLUMBIA. (1992b). *Healthy Communities Yearbook 1991.* Victoria: Office of Health Promotion, B.C. Ministry of Health and Ministry Responsible for Seniors. (Catalogue no. QP 92835 03/92)

GOVERNMENT OF BRITISH COLUMBIA. (1992c). *Health indicator workbook.* (1st ed.). Victoria: Office of Health Promotion, B.C. Ministry of Health and Ministry Responsible for Seniors. (Catalogue no. QP 91029 01/92)

GOVERNMENT OF BRITISH COLUMBIA. (1993). *New directions for a healthy British Columbia*. Victoria: Ministry of Health & Ministry Responsible for Seniors.

GOVERNMENT OF CANADA. (1994). *Strategies for population health: Investing in the health of all Canadians.* Ottawa: Minister of Supply & Services. (Catalogue no. H39-316/1994E)

GOVERNMENT OF FIJI. (1986). *Ministry of Health annual report for the years 1985–86.* Suva: Ministry of Health.

GOVERNMENT OF ONTARIO. (1993). *Nurturing health. Report of the Premier's Council on Health, Well-being and Social Justice.* Toronto: Queen's Printer. (Catalogue no. 01–93–20M)

HALL, D. (1989). *Primary health care—a nursing model: A Denmark–Newfoundland (Canada) Project.* (Report available from the Registered Nurses Association of Newfoundland.)

HEALTH CANADA. (1993). Telephone conversation with Ann Wiehler, Acting Regional Nursing Advisor, October 3, 1993.

HEALTH CANADA MEDICAL SERVICES BRANCH. (1996). *Diagnostic on the health of First Nations and Inuit people.* Draft for discussion. Ottawa: Author.

HEALTH & WELFARE CANADA. (1964). *Report of the Royal Commission on Health Services. (Hall Report).* Ottawa: Author.

HEALTH & WELFARE CANADA. (1987). *Active health report—Perspectives on Canada's health promotion survey 1985.* Ottawa: Minister of Supply & Services. (Catalogue no. H39–106/1987E)

HOPE, P.R. (1993). Indoor climate. *Experientia, 49*(9), 775–779.

LABONTE, R. (1989). Pesticides and healthy public policy. *Canadian Journal of Public Health, 80*(4), 238–242.

LALONDE, M. (1974). *A new perspective on the health of Canadians.* Ottawa: Information Canada.

LAST, J.M. (1988). *A dictionary of epidemiology.* (2nd ed.). Toronto: Oxford University Press.

MASS, H., & WHYTE, N. (1997). Primary health care in action. *Nursing BC, 29*(2), 13–16.

MEGGS, W. (1992). Health effects of indoor air pollution. *North Carolina Medical Journal, 53*(7), 354–358.

MIKATAVAGE, M., ROSE, V., FUNKHOUSER, E., OESTENSTAD, R., DILLON, K., & REYNOLD, K. (1995). Beyond air quality—Factors that affect prevalence estimates of sick building syndrome. *American Industrial Hygiene Association Journal, 56*(11), 1141–1146.

MILLAR, H., & MILLAR, M. (1998). *Environmental health nursing: Planning patient care for environmental illness and multiple chemical sensitivity.* Vancouver: NICO Environmental Health Strategies.

PAGE, G.W. III. (1987). Water and health. In M.R. Greenberg (Ed.), *Public health and the environment.* New York: Guilford Press. As cited in M.J. Clark (1992), *Nursing in the community.* Norwalk, CT: Appleton & Lange, p. 348.

REA, W. (1992). *Chemical sensitivity.* (Vol. 1). Boca Raton, FL: Lewis Publishers.

REA, W. (1994). *Chemical sensitivity: Total body load.* (Vol. 2). Boca Raton, FL: Lewis Publishers.

REGISTERED NURSES ASSOCIATION OF BRITISH COLUMBIA (RNABC). (1996). *Creating the new health care: A nursing perspective.* Vancouver: Author.

RUHL, R., CHANG, C., HALPERN, G., & GERSHWIN, M. (1993). The sick building syndrome. II. Assessment and regulation of indoor air quality. *Journal of Asthma, 30*(4), 297–308.

SHERIN, K. (1993). Building-related illness and sick building syndrome. *Journal of the Florida Medical Association, 80*(7), 472–474.

SHILS, M., & YOUNG, V. (1988). *Modern nutrition in health and disease.* Philadelphia: Lea & Fegriger.

SOTO, A., SONNENSCHEIN, C., CHUNG, K., FERNANDEZ, M., OLEA, N., & SERRANO, F. (1995). The E-screen assay as a tool to identify estrogens: An update on estrogenic environmental pollutants. *Environmental Health Perspectives, 103*(10), 113–122.

SOUTH FRASER VALLEY HEALTH COUNCIL. (1993). *Regional and community health profile: An initial perspective July 1993.* White Rock, B.C.: Author.

STANCEL, G., BOETTGER-TONG, H., CHIAPPETTA, C., HYDER, S., KIRKLAND, J., MURTHY, L., & LOOSE-MITCHELL, D. (1995). Toxicity of endogenous and environmental estrogens: What is the role of elemental interaction? *Environmental Health Perspectives, 103*(10), 29–33.

SUTHERLAND, R., & FULTON, J. (1988). *Health care in Canada.* Ottawa: M.O.M. Printing. (Distributed by the Canadian Public Health Association, Ottawa.)

TAMBLYN, R.M., MENZIES, R., TAMBLYN, R.T., FARANT, J., & HANLEY, J. (1992). The feasibility of using a double-blind experimental cross-over design to study interventions for sick building syndrome. *Journal of Clinical Epidemiology. 45*(6), 603–612.

TEEUW, K.B., VANDENBROUCKE-GRAULS, C., & VERHOEF, J. (1994). Airborne gram-negative bacteria and endotoxin in sick building syndrome. *Archives of Internal Medicine, 154*(10), 2339–2345.

TYLER, C.W., & LAST, J.M. (1992). Epidemiology. In Maxcy, Rosenau, & Last, *Public health and preventive medicine.* (13th ed.). Norwalk, CT: Appleton & Lange.

VICTORIAN ORDER OF NURSES FOR CANADA. (1983). *Missioners for health.* Unpublished manuscript.

VICTORIAN ORDER OF NURSES FOR CANADA. (1988, March). *VON health promotion project for seniors: Final report.* Ottawa: Author.

VICTORIAN ORDER OF NURSES FOR CANADA. (1991, May). The VON Footcare Project: Keeping Canadians on their feet: Final report. Ottawa: Author.

WORLD HEALTH ORGANIZATION (WHO). (1984). *Health promotion glossary.* Copenhagen: WHO Regional Office for Europe.

Additional Readings

CLEMEN-STONE, S., McGUIRE, S.L. & EIGSTI, D.G. (1998). Comprehensive Community Health Nursing. (5th ed.). St. Louis: Mosby.

LABONTE, R. (1987, Summer). Community health promotion strategies. *Health Promotion, 26*(1), 5–10.

REGISTERED NURSES ASSOCIATION OF BRITISH COLUMBIA (RNABC). (1993, April). Government backs plan for new nursing centre. *RNABC Newsline.*

Chapter 12

Ethnicity, Spirituality and Health

OUTLINE

Central Questions

1. How is the ethnic composition of the Canadian population relevant to health care?
2. What do the terms culture, ethnicity, socialization and acculturation mean?
3. What is the difference between the integration of immigrants in the United States and those in Canada?
4. Why is spirituality important?
5. What are some of the beliefs about health, illness and death held by major religious groups?
6. What are the basic tenets of some of the more commonly used types of alternative medicine?
7. What are some of the barriers to health care for nonimmigrant and new Canadians?
8. How can these barriers be crossed?
9. What are some of the health care concerns for people of the First Nations?
10. What is the role of nurses in health services in Canada's North?

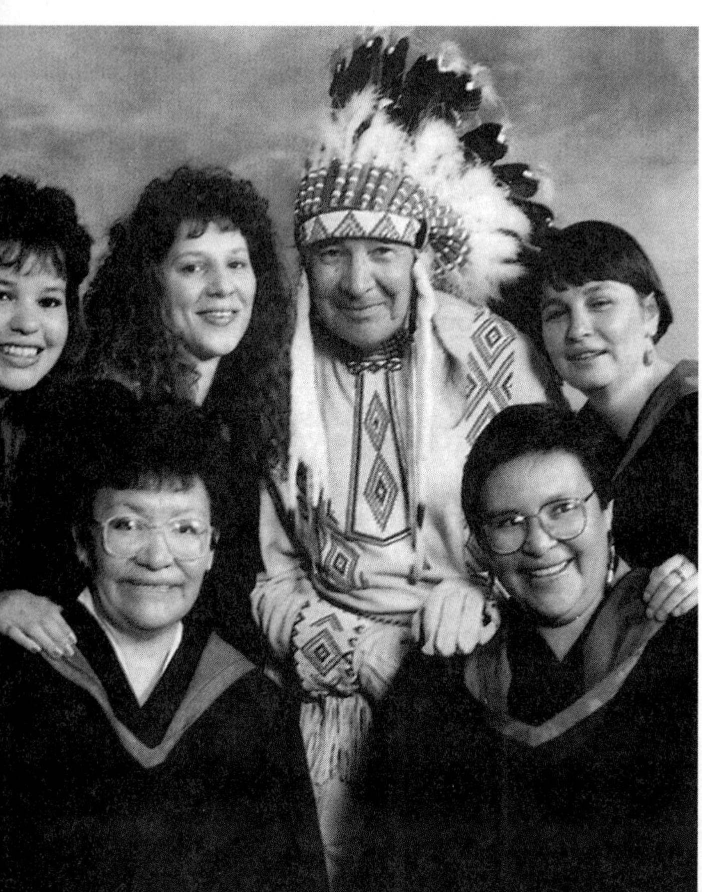

Introduction

Confederation was built on the concept of cultural plurality, and from the outset diversity was acknowledged to be integral to its continuation.

Masi, 1993, p.11

Diversity has characterized the Canadian people ever since the first French and, later, British settlers joined the country's long-established aboriginals—the North American Indians and the Inuit—to form the fledgling nation that would become Canada. As wave after wave of immigration populated its shores, Canada's ethnic diversity became more pronounced. Today, there are over 100 distinct ethnic groups among the Canadian population (Badets, 1993).

As people have come, they have brought customs and traditions from their native lands. Healers and traditional practitioners of the healing arts have come as well. It has been the policy of the Canadian government to help people retain and take pride in their heritage, and Canadian culture has been enriched by the contributions of people from many different lands.

The latest wave of immigration poses many challenges for nurses as they try to practise culturally sensitive care and adapt interventions to meet the needs of people of various ethnic backgrounds. Particularly important is a knowledge of patients' spiritual beliefs and religious customs, and of the types of medical treatment in which they have faith. Many religious customs have a direct bearing on health care, as for example, the dietary restrictions followed by Muslims and many other religious groups. It is also helpful to know if patients come from communities where non-Western medicine is the common mode of practice, and to know about treatments they have received.

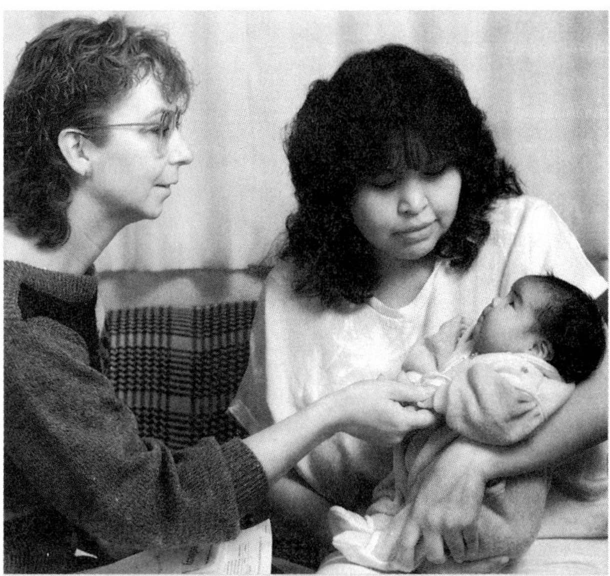

Learning to practise culturally sensitive care can be very rewarding.

Of particular interest to Canadian nurses is health care for First Nations peoples. This field of practice has always attracted Canadian nurses, and the adventure of nursing in the North has lured nurses from around the globe. In line with the movement towards self-government for First Nations peoples, the federal government is rapidly transferring control of health care to the people—a process that will permit the incorporation of traditional customs and healing practices into their health programs.

In this chapter, we will first define the basic concepts of culture and ethnicity. Then we will look at the ethnic composition of the Canadian population. We will then turn our attention to some of the spiritual beliefs held by people of different cultures and to the religious customs they follow, particularly as these pertain to their beliefs about health and illness. We will also look at some of the forms of alternative or complementary medicine that are used by increasing numbers of Canadians. Then, we will discuss some of the barriers to health care both for segments of the general population and for new Canadians, and we will look at ways to overcome these barriers. Finally, we will discuss health care for First Nations peoples.

Basic Concepts

Ethnicity

Statistics Canada defines **ethnicity** as "the ethnic or cultural group(s) to which an individual's ancestors belonged; it pertains to the ancestral roots or origins of the population and not to place of birth, citizenship, nationality or language" (Renaud & Badets, 1993, p. 280).

Culture

The word culture has many different meanings in the English language. We are using **culture** in our discussions as it is used in sociology and anthropology, to refer to the basic beliefs, values and lifeways of groups of people. These are the characteristics that differentiate one group from another (Leininger, 1978). Cultural characteristics are transmitted from generation to generation through the process of learning. Change occurs constantly through cultural diffusion, for example, through immigration, widely accepted innovations and changing family patterns. Trying to interact with others of a different culture can be disorienting, as familiar patterns are not present. This experience is common among immigrants and also, to a lesser degree, when a person starts a new occupation (Ferrar, 1995).

We have mentioned in earlier chapters some of the beliefs and values shared by people in our country that distinguish us as Canadians. We believe that everyone has the right to adequate health services regardless of race, colour, creed or ability to pay and we value the health care system that provides universal access to health services. As

Canadians, we also believe in free speech and the democratic process, and value the political system that enables everyone to voice opinions.

These are just a few of the many characteristics Canadians have in common. Within the overall common culture that identifies us as Canadians, however, there are numerous subcultures in which people have differing ideas on nutrition, hygiene, child-rearing, and other health-related issues. As people have come from other lands, it has been the policy of the Canadian government to help them to retain their cultural identity within the overall Canadian whole. Often, we tend to view people from unfamiliar ethnic groups or cultures from our own cultural perspective. This tendency is called **ethnocentricity,** and it can be a major obstacle to understanding another's point of view and culture. Nurses should strive to see the individual within the context of his or her own culture, which is neither superior nor inferior to their own—just different. This perspective is called **cultural relativism** (Ferrar, 1995).

Socialization

The process by which people learn the beliefs, values and lifeways of a culture is called **socialization**. The process starts in the home as children are socialized into behavioural patterns that are acceptable in the family. It continues through school, work and social settings as people move into different environments and learn the customs and conventions (the social mores) characteristic of the new community. As a person becomes socialized into each new environment encountered, personal behaviour is modified so that relationships with others can be established and maintained. This is a two-way process; the outcome depends on the willingness of all those involved to adapt.

Acculturation

Acculturation refers to the process whereby individuals learn the beliefs, values and lifeways of a culture other than the one into which they were born, and accept these as their own. As newcomers settle into Canada, they learn one or both of the two official languages, and they gradually adopt behavioural patterns similar to those of other people in the community. Children adapt very quickly; older people sometimes find it more difficult to become accustomed to Canadian ways. Particularly troublesome are situations where there is a conflict of cultural values. For example, in families coming from a culture where young women are not allowed to mix with members of the opposite gender except in closely chaperoned situations, the free and easy comradeship of adolescent boys and girls in this country is often a cause of dissension in the family.

Assimilation and Integration

The United States has been called a **melting pot**, and Canada a **cultural mosaic**, or an *ethnically plural* society, because of the different ways the two countries have absorbed immigrants. The United States has encouraged the blending of the various nationalities into a homogeneous American identity. Canada, on the other hand, has opted to assist people to retain a more distinct sense of their own cultural identity. This policy was formalized and incorporated into legislation in the Canadian Multiculturalism Act (1988), which states:

> *The Government of Canada recognizes the diversity of Canadians...as a fundamental characteristic of Canadian society and is committed to a policy of multiculturalism designed to preserve and enhance the multicultural heritage of Canadians while working to achieve the equality of all Canadians in the economic, cultural and political life of Canada.*
>
> Multiculturalism & Citizenship Canada, 1990

Porter (1979) suggests that neither *melting pot* nor *cultural mosaic* is entirely appropriate for these two countries. In the United States, many immigrant groups are beginning to assert their cultural heritage. In Canada, intermarriage between racial groups is becoming more common, so that a blending of cultures would appear to be inevitable (Porter, 1979).

It is useful to reflect that the process of assimilation also occurs when a person moves to a different job, city or lifestyle—for example, from secondary school to college or university, or from a rural area to city life.

The Composition of the Canadian Population

The composition of the Canadian population can be looked at from a number of different perspectives. In discussing the multicultural nature of our society, we are concerned particularly with the following aspects: (a) the immigration patterns that have shaped the present composition of our population, (b) the ethnic origins of people in our society, (c) their languages and (d) their religions.

Immigration Patterns

The first immigrants to this country were the ancestors of First Nations peoples who, it is believed, migrated to North America from Asia. Anthropologists believe that various waves of migration occurred over the centuries. In a well-researched and carefully documented text on the Dene and the Na-Dene, Stewart (1991) presents an interpretation of the history of the Athapaskan or Dene people whom early European explorers found living from Alaska to New Mexico, and the Na-Dene people living on the coastal islands of British Columbia. The ancestors of these linguistically related people originated from a region in northwest

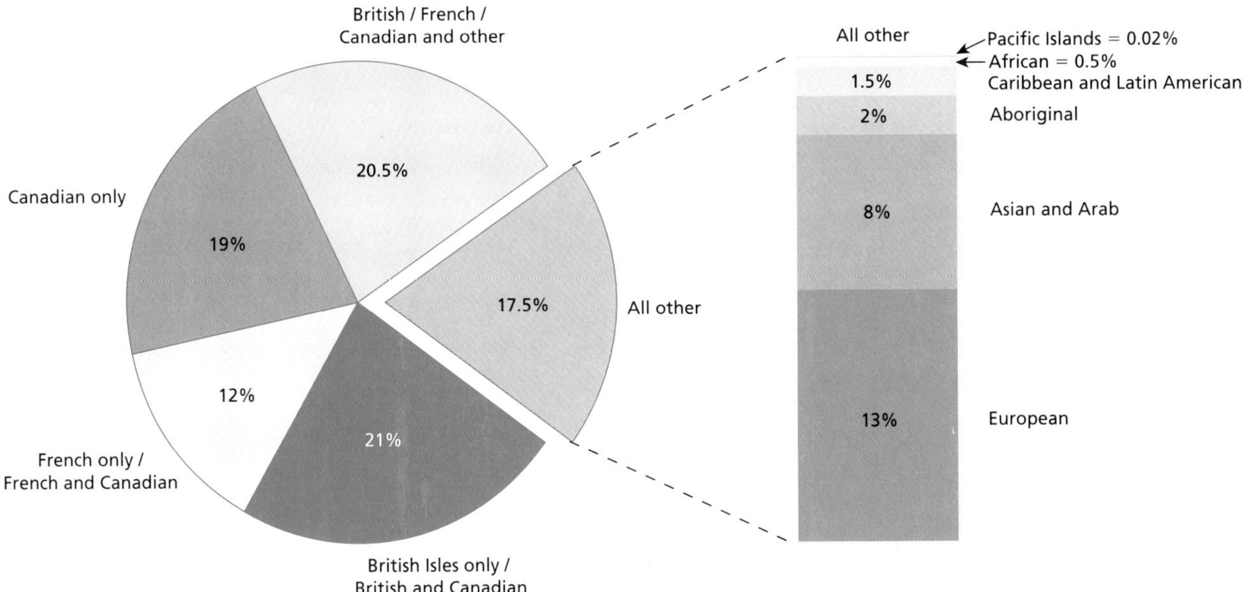

FIGURE 12.1 Ethnic composition of Canada's population, 1996

Note: A considerable increase in the reporting of "Canadian" ethnic origins on the 1996 Census (based on 20% sample data) appears to have affected the reporting of many ethnic origin groups, particularly the British and French.

SOURCE: Adapted from Renaud & Badets, 1993, with data from Statistics Canada, 1996–1997.

China, near the border of present-day Kazakhstan. They reportedly followed early routes of the fur hunters from northeast Asia along the Aleutian Island chain as they fled from the Mongol armies of Genghis Khan in the 13th century. Many were from royal descent or the ruling classes, or were military leaders or caravan traders. These disparate groups joined together for the expedition to the Great Land. Coming from multiethnic groups and from a highly developed region, they had to learn to become hunters and gatherers in the new undeveloped area where they settled. As their numbers grew, they dispersed southward and eastward in search of grazing lands (Stewart, 1991).

The next group of settlers to come to Canada were the French. Although they settled mainly in Quebec, New Brunswick and Nova Scotia, they also moved westward, establishing settlements in various parts of Ontario, the Prairie provinces and British Columbia. The defeat of Montcalm on the Plains of Abraham above Quebec City in 1769 put Canada under British rule and stimulated a wave of settlement by people from England, Ireland, Scotland and Wales. During the 19th century, immigrants came mainly from Britain and other parts of Western and Eastern Europe to help open up the land.

During the 20th century, there have been three major waves of immigration, which have helped to shape the present composition of the population. The first occurred in the early years of the century, between 1901 and 1912, when almost three million people arrived, mainly from the British Isles, and other countries in Europe. The second wave came after World War II, when hundreds of thousands of people were displaced from their homeland or were refugees. Canada accepted a total of 1 222 000 immigrants between 1946 and 1955, with most of them coming from the British Isles and other European countries.

The third wave started in 1977 and continues today. Between 1991 and 1996, more than one million immigrants were accepted into Canada. The largest group have come from Asia, with smaller numbers from Poland, the United States, the United Kingdom and other countries. This latest wave of immigration is rapidly changing the demographics of Canada, as shown in Figures 12.1 and 12.2 (Renaud & Badets, 1993; Badets, 1993; Statistics Canada, 1996–97).

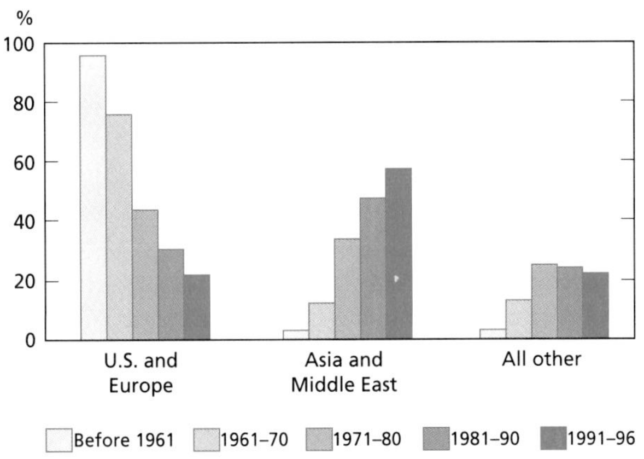

FIGURE 12.2 Place of birth of immigrants by period of immigration, 1996

SOURCE: Statistics Canada, 1997, p. 4.

TABLE 12.1 Top 10 countries of birth for immigrants before 1961, recent immigrants and all immigrants

	IMMIGRATED BEFORE 1961		RECENT IMMIGRANTS*		ALL IMMIGRANTS	
	No.	%	No.	%	No.	%
Total	**1 054 930**	**100.0**	**1 038 995**	**100.0**	**4 971 070**	**100.0**
United Kingdom	265 575	25.2	25 425	2.4	655 540	13.2
Italy	161 730	15.3			332 110	6.7
Germany	107 270	10.2			181 650	3.7
Netherlands	88 810	8.4				
Poland	57 820	5.5	36 965	3.6	193 375	3.9
United States	45 050	4.3	29 020	2.8	244 695	4.9
Hungary	33 215	3.1				
Ukraine	27 640	2.6				
Greece	21 555	2.0				
People's Rep. China	17 545	1.7	87 875	8.5	231 055	4.6
Hong Kong			108 915	10.5	241 095	4.8
India			71 335	6.9	235 930	4.7
Philippines			71 325	6.9	184 550	3.7
Sri Lanka			44 235	4.3		
Taiwan			32 140	3.1		
Viet Nam			32 060	3.1		
Portugal					158 820	3.2

*Recent immigrants are those who immigrated between 1991 and the first four months of 1996.

SOURCE: Statistics Canada, 1997, p. 4.

REFUGEES

Since the end of World War II, a considerable proportion of immigrants—more than half a million in total—have been refugees from various troubled countries. They came from Hungary in 1956, Czechoslovakia in 1968, and, more recently, from Southeast Asia, the Middle East, South and Central America and from Africa; from countries such as Vietnam, Lebanon, Poland, Iran, Chile, El Salvador, Sri Lanka, Guatemala, and more recently from Bosnia and Somalia. Table 12.1 shows the 10 leading countries of birth for immigrants before 1961, for recent immigrants and for all immigrants.

PROVINCIAL DISTRIBUTION OF IMMIGRANTS

In 1996, the immigrant population of Canada, that is, those who were not born here, accounted for 17.4 percent of the population, the largest share in more than 50 years. The provinces of Ontario, British Columbia and Quebec continue to attract the largest number of immigrants. More than 90 percent of all immigrants, according to 1991 census figures, live in these three provinces. With regard to the ethnic composition of the population of specific provinces, the Atlantic Provinces are the only ones where people of British origin are now the majority ethnic group, while Quebec retains French as the dominant ethnic origin of the majority of its population. Figure 12.3 shows the provincial distribution of immigrants to Canada in 1996.

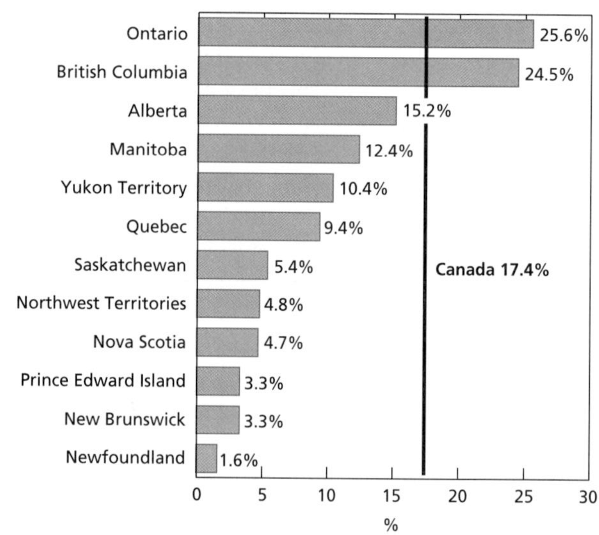

FIGURE 12.3 Immigrants as a percentage of census population of provinces and territories, 1996

SOURCE: Statistics Canada, 1997, p. 3.

Most immigrants live in urban, rather than rural parts of Canada, with more than one-half in the three largest metropolitan areas of Canada—Toronto, Montreal and Vancouver. Toronto is the most multicultural, with 41.9 percent of its population (1.5 million) composed of immigrants, although Vancouver runs a close second (Statistics Canada, 1997). Figure 12.4 shows the percentage of immigrants in the census population of metropolitan areas.

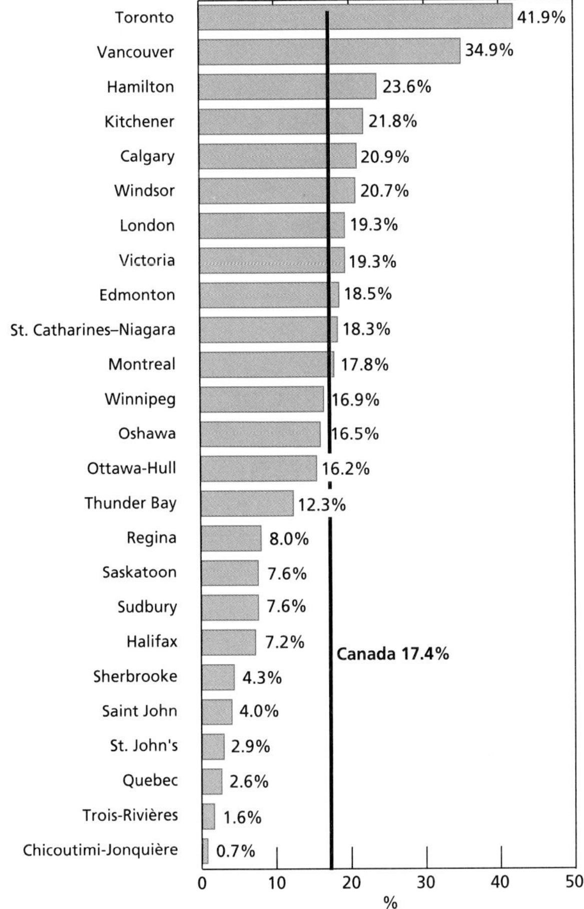

FIGURE 12.4 Immigrants as a percentage of census metropolitan areas, 1996

SOURCE: Statistics Canada, 1997, p. 3.

Ethnic Origins

PEOPLE OF THE FIRST NATIONS

The small bands who originally found their way across the Bering Sea flourished in the new land, growing to an estimated 200 000 in Canada by the time the first French settlers arrived. Although Canada did not have the Indian wars that decimated the aboriginal people in the United States, the numbers of First Nations people dwindled considerably during the 18th and 19th centuries due, in large part, to the new diseases the Europeans brought with them. During the past half century, the aboriginal population has begun to grow again as infant and child mortality rates have declined. At present, the growth rate of First Nations peoples is greater than the overall Canadian rate (Bobet, 1989).

In the 1996 census, approximately one million people reported that they were North American Indians, Métis or Inuit (Statistics Canada, 1998). The aboriginal population cannot be looked upon as a single, homogeneous group. According to a 1991 Aboriginal Peoples Survey, there are over 15 languages spoken among First Nations people. The **First Nations** population includes approximately 41 000 Inuit, who live mainly in the Arctic, a little more than half a million North American Indians (status or single origin) and more than 200 000 Métis (of mixed ethnic origin). There are also those who name another ethnic group as their primary origin but claim some First Nations people among their ancestors (Statistics Canada, 1998). The North American Indian group includes some 600 tribes. The **Inuit** occupy small communities north of the treeline in Canada, stretching from the Mackenzie River Delta, through the Arctic Islands and Baffin Island, along the coast of Hudson Bay and Ungava Bay in Quebec, to the east coast of Labrador (Siggner, 1989).

THE FRENCH

The first French colonists arrived on Canadian shores in the early 1600s and established settlements in the areas we know as Quebec, Nova Scotia and New Brunswick. The large families that were common in Quebec up until the Quiet Revolution of the 1960s helped to ensure perpetuation of the French language and culture in Canada. The current low birth rate in Quebec is, however, causing concern as it is now below replacement level. In 1991, the population reporting ethnic origin as French was an estimated 17 percent of the total population, down from 24 percent in 1986. Because of changes in the collection of census data, it is impossible to compare figures for ethnic origin from year to year. The greatest number of people claiming French as their ethnic origin or as one of their ethnic origins are concentrated in Quebec; the next largest group is in New Brunswick, although communities of ethnic French people are found in almost all provinces (Statistics Canada, 1997).

THE BRITISH

The British conquest of Canada in 1769 marked the beginning of wide-scale settlement by people from England, Ireland, Scotland and Wales. A century later, at the time of Confederation, 61.5 percent of the estimated 5.7 million people in Canada were of British origin. Today, the percentage of people of British origin, including both single and multiple origin, has dwindled to 21 percent reporting British only or British and Canadian.

VISIBLE MINORITIES

The 1996 census collected information on people who are members of a visible minority in Canada, defined by the Employment Equity Act as "persons, other than Aboriginal peoples who are non-Caucasian in race, or non-white in colour" (Statistics Canada, 1997). In 1996, 3.2 million persons identified themselves as visible minorities, a figure that represents 11.2 percent of the population of Canada. Ontario and British Columbia together accounted for almost three-fourths of the visible minority population.

The largest visible minority population were Chinese (3% of Canada's total population). The next largest groups were South Asians (2.4%) and Blacks (2%). The remainder

TABLE 12.2 Visible minority population, 1996

	TOTAL POPULATION	TOTAL VISIBLE MINORITY POPULATION	VISIBLE MINORITIES AS % OF TOTAL POPULATION	GEOGRAPHIC DISTRIBUTION OF VISIBLE MINORITIES
			%	%
Canada	**28 528 125**	**3 197 480**	**11.2**	**100.0**
Newfoundland	547 155	3 815	0.7	0.1
Prince Edward Island	132 855	1 520	1.1	0.0
Nova Scotia	899 970	31 320	3.5	1.0
New Brunswick	729 625	7 995	1.1	0.3
Quebec	7 045 085	433 985	6.2	13.6
Ontario	10 642 790	1 682 045	15.8	52.6
Manitoba	1 100 295	77 355	7.0	2.4
Saskatchewan	976 615	26 945	2.8	0.8
Alberta	2 669 195	269 280	10.1	8.4
British Columbia	3 689 760	660 545	17.9	20.7
Yukon Territory	30 650	1 000	3.3	0.0
Northwest Territories	64 125	1 670	2.6	0.1

SOURCE: Statistics Canada, 1998, pp. 5–6.

included Filipinos, Southeast Asians, Latin Americans, Japanese, Koreans, Arabs and West Asians. Almost all visible minority persons lived in urban areas, mostly in the large metropolitan areas, with Toronto and Vancouver having the largest numbers, followed by Calgary. The distribution of visible minorities by province is shown in Table 12.2 and as a percentage of census metropolitan areas in Figure 12.5.

LANGUAGE

During the 1991 and the 1996 censuses, all Canadians were asked to identify their mother tongue, defined as "the first language that a person learned at home in childhood and still understands" (Statistics Canada, 1997). A total of 126 languages were reported, including 23 aboriginal languages. English was the most common language, with nearly 60 percent of the population reporting it as either their first language (mother tongue) or one of their mother tongues. Second most common was French, which approximately 24 percent of the population reported. A single mother tongue other than English or French was reported by 16 percent of the population. Almost one in every 10 people in Canada was an **allophone** (i.e., spoke a language other than English or French most of the time). Chinese was the most common, followed by Italian and Punjabi (Statistics Canada, 1996–97). Table 12.3 shows the most common primary languages in Canada and the approximate number of people in the country speaking them. Table 12.4 shows the 10 most frequently used home languages other than English or French and all aboriginal languages in Canada.

According to the 1996 census, almost half a million people (a little more than one percent of the total population)

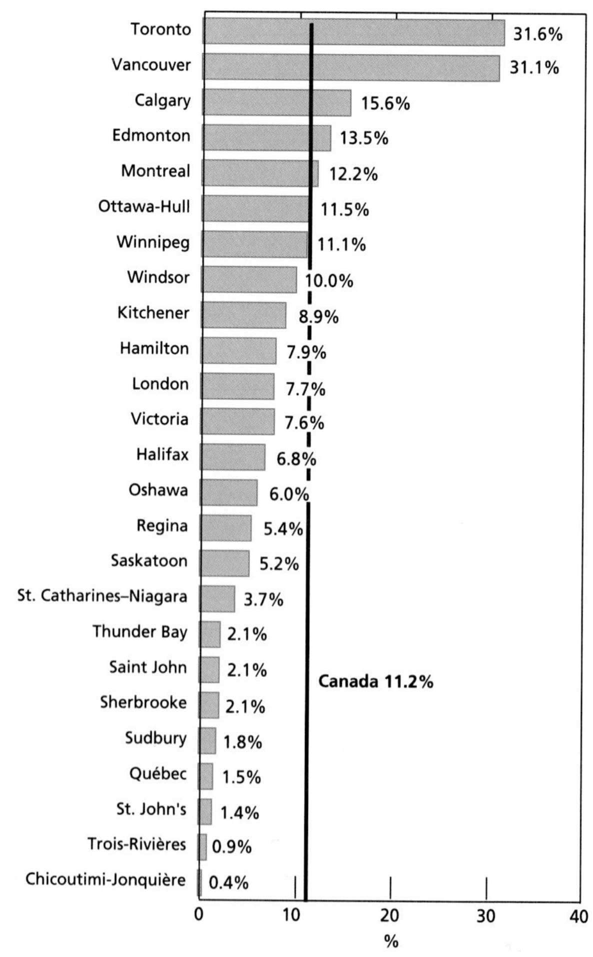

FIGURE 12.5 Visible minority population as a percentage of census metropolitan areas, 1996

SOURCE: Statistics Canada, 1998.

TABLE 12.3 Most common primary languages of Canadians

Canada	Population 28 528 125
Single language —	
English	16 890 615
French	6 636 660
Non-official	4 598 285
Multiple language —	
French and English	107 940
English and other	249 545
French and other	35 840
English, French and other	9 225

SOURCE: Statistics Canada 1996–1997.

TABLE 12.4 The 10 most frequently used home languages other than English or French and all aboriginal languages

Home Language	Number	%
Chinese	630 520	2.2
Italian	258 050	0.9
Punjabi	182 895	0.6
Spanish	173 040	0.6
Portuguese	142 975	0.5
Polish	137 330	0.5
German	134 615	0.5
Arabic	118 605	0.4
Tagalog (Filipino)	111 865	0.4
Vietnamese	102 905	0.4
Aboriginal languages	146 120	0.5

SOURCE: Statistics Canada, 1997, p. 7.

over the age of five were unable to speak either one of the two official languages (Statistics Canada, 1997). This is a larger number than at any other time in the century, a situation that puts a strain on services, such as English/French language training and translation services, and can cause problems in the delivery of health care. Most people who cannot speak either one of the two official languages live in large households in urban areas where there is a sizeable ethnic community. Many have been in the country for over 10 years. They are mainly women who, because of domestic responsibilities and limited labour force participation, have not had many opportunities to meet with other people outside their own ethnic community or to have access to language training programs.

Religion

More than 100 denominations were named by Canadians as religious affiliation on the 1991 census. Historically, the major religions in this country have been Christian, either Catholic or Protestant. A 1990 General Survey undertaken by Statistics Canada indicated that a larger proportion of Canadians (46.5% of the population) were Roman Catholic than Protestant (30%). The most common other religions reported were: Judaism (1%), Islam, Hinduism, Sikhism and Buddhism. The last four named constitute the majority of the three percent reporting other than Christianity or Judaism. Approximately 12 percent of the people in Canada reported that they had no religious affiliation (Colombo, 1992; *Canada's Family Tree: Celebrating our Diversity*, 1992; Griffith, 1996).

Ethnicity, Culture and Health

As health professionals in a country with such a diverse population as Canada, nurses must consider both ethnicity and culture to be important variables in the provision of health care. However, ethnicity is not the same as culture: just because people belong to the same ethnic group, it may not be assumed that they all share the same cultural characteristics.

Ethnicity refers to a person's ancestral roots or racial origin; *culture* refers to the beliefs, values and lifeways of groups of people. Any given ethnic population may contain numerous subcultures, each with its own beliefs, values and lifeways.

People at the same socioeconomic level in different ethnic groups may have more in common than they share with people from a different socioeconomic level in their own ethnic group (Masi, 1993). Besides socioeconomic status, other variables might include the length of time people have been in Canada, and their educational level, age, gender and country or place of origin. For example, a Canadian of Chinese ancestry could be: (a) a fifth- or sixth-generation Canadian who cannot speak a word of either Cantonese or Mandarin, (b) a recently arrived entrepreneur from Hong Kong, (c) an ethnic-Chinese refugee from a village in the Meikong Delta in Vietnam, or (d) an eminent heart surgeon from Mauritius. Thus, people who belong to the same ethnic group may have little in common in their lifestyles, beliefs and values.

This example illustrates the importance of not stereotyping people on the basis of their ethnic origin. However, there are genetically acquired biological traits that may have a bearing on a person's health. There are differences in skin pigmentation, body build and facial structure, as well as differences in metabolism. For example, black people, with their dark skin pigmentation, are more sensitive to cold and, hence, more vulnerable to hypothermia than people with fair complexions. A large percentage of the Southeast

Asian population (80%) are lactose intolerant, an important factor to consider when caring for such patients (Masi, 1993).

Further, people of some ethnic groups are more at risk for certain genetically transmitted disorders. For example, sickle cell anemia is more common among blacks, and there is a high incidence of cervical cancer among aboriginal women (Freeman, cited in Masi, 1993, p. 15).

Spiritual Beliefs and Health

Health professionals in a multicultural society such as Canada must also take into account the beliefs, values and traditional lifeways of people. There is often a close relationship between people's spiritual beliefs, their beliefs about health and their health practices.

Spirituality

The word **spirit** comes from the Latin word for *breath* (Davidson, 1986, p. 41). Newborns come to life when they take their first breath. When someone ceases to breathe, it is said that the spirit has left the body—the person is no longer alive. The *Concise Oxford Dictionary* (1995) defines "spirit" as "the vital animating essence of a person or animal ... the intelligent non-physical part of a person; the soul" (p. 1341). Other terms used for the spirit in different healing and medical traditions include *prana, chi, Holy Spirit* or *life force* (Chow, 1997).

In ancient times, the spirit or soul was believed to be located in the heart. For Christians and Muslims, the heart is still considered the location of a person's spiritual force. In other traditions, the soul may be located elsewhere. Traditional Vietnamese believe that it is located in the mind; people in Melanesian cultures of the South Pacific Islands believe the spirit is encompassed in the total human body (Leininger, 1995).

The term **spirituality** has been defined in many different ways. Philosophers tell us that spirituality is "our capacity for self-transcendence, a capacity demonstrated in our ability to know the truth, to relate to others lovingly, and to commit ourselves freely to persons and ideals" (Conn, 1986, p. 3). Psychologists see spirituality as that part of ourselves that gives us power, energy and motivating force. Theologians consider spirituality as the "actualization of human transcendence by whatever is acknowledged as the ultimate or holy" (Conn, 1986, p. 3)—the ultimate or holy being specific for each religion. McCulloch (1997) sees spirituality as having a number of other dimensions, such as "love, faith, hope, trust, generativity, inner meaning, mystical experience, and religious behaviours" (p. 139).

The term **transcendence** should also be explained here. It refers to an experience that is outside normal sensory phenomena. Often used to describe a classical mystic experience of God, transcendence is not reserved for religious experience alone; it may also be applied to an aesthetic response to art or music, or to an overwhelming feeling of wonder and awe at the majesty of creation. Maslow (1970) called these "peak experiences." People in all societies and cultures have reported such experiences, which usually have a profound effect, often causing them to alter their lives (Johnstone, 1990).

Variations in the meaning, form, expression and interpretations of spirituality can be found in almost all cultures (Leininger, 1997). Roach suggests that "for all people of whatever faith or persuasion, spirituality is an integral, holistic, dynamic force in human life, for the individual and for the community" (Roach, 1997, p. 11). It has become a universal expression of the search for meaning in a largely materialistic society. We know there is something beyond our biophysical experience, and we keep searching for it. We are continually searching for the meaning not only of our individual identity but, also, "for the meaning of our personhood, our interconnectedness with others" (Roach, 1997 p. 12).

Common Themes of Spirituality

- It is an attribute of the human person.
- It involves a search for the meaning and purpose of life.
- It relates to the inner core of a person's being.
- It includes acceptance of oneself, and feeling at ease with others, with the world around us and with an Ultimate Other.
- It is the integrating force of the human person.

SOURCES: Nagai-Jacobson & Burkhart, 1989; Balzer-Riley, 1996; Roach, 1997; Conn, 1986.

Spirituality and Religion

Spirituality must be differentiated from religion. According to Hall (1997), **religion** implies adherence to a belief system (or doctrine), whereas spirituality is a quality of human life. Hall states that all persons are spiritual beings—one does not need to adhere to a specific religious doctrine in order to have a spiritual component to one's being. She suggests that the link between religion and spirituality lies in the search for meaning in our lives. People look for an understanding of themselves, of other people and their connectedness to them, and of God. Davidson (1986), an Anglican priest, believes that the task of the church is "to help people who are trying to make sense of apparently senseless lives to rediscover their own dignity and worth and place in the scheme of things" (p. 87). Religious rituals are one way of expressing spirituality; thus, it is important that religious patients have the opportunity to practise their rituals.

Recent years have seen a resurgence of interest in spirituality, and there are probably many reasons for this. The accelerated pace of change in the past few decades has left many people feeling confused and frightened. Changes in family structure and a loss of traditional family values have shaken the foundations of society. Stress and burnout are among the most common disorders of the workplace. The depersonalization accompanying the increased use of technology in our daily lives—for example, the recorded menu of directions we encounter when we telephone a company or agency—makes us long for a human connection. Many people have become disillusioned with science, realizing that it does not have all the answers. People are looking for something to believe in—to provide a sense of structure to the universe, and to give meaning to life.

THE ROLE OF SPIRITUALITY IN HEALTH

The ancient Greeks believed that human beings were composed of three parts: the physical body (**soma**), the mind (**mensa**) and the spirit (**pneuma**). Hippocrates, the father of medicine, emphasized in his teachings the wholeness of the human person, and stated that all three components must be in harmony for good health. He also believed that the human being is capable of generating powerful responses to combat disease. In other words, the body is not just the passive recipient of medical treatment, but a powerful force in its own healing (Cousins, 1994).

The Code of Ethics for Registered Nurses (CNA, 1997; reprinted as Appendix A of this text) states that "nurses value and advocate the dignity and self-respect of human beings." In implementing this value statement, "nursing care is designed to accommodate the biological, psychological, cultural and spiritual needs of clients" (p. 13).

For a time Western medicine lost sight of the spiritual aspects of health, relying instead on science and technology to cure physical ills. But many other traditions emphasize the need for attention to the spiritual aspects of health. For example, the traditional health practices of First Nations peoples were holistic in that they formed "part of an integrated belief system in which the individual ... was in harmony with [the] community and with nature" (Shah & Dubeski, 1993, p. 74). They believed that health depends not only on physical characteristics, but also on the social, psychological and spiritual aspects.

The concept of body, mind and spirit as aspects of an indivisible whole is the essence of the philosophy behind holistic nursing theory (Chow, 1997). It is a concept that has gained rapid acceptance among nurses. The medical community also appears to be returning to the teachings of Hippocrates, recognizing that the body's healing system is closely tied to a person's belief system (Cousins, 1994).

THE ROLE OF SPIRITUALITY IN ILLNESS

Who am I? Why am I here? What kind of a world is this? Many people who never asked these questions when they were healthy have found that they suddenly become urgent at times of serious illness. Some ill people are led to question their entire system of values. A man who is recovering from a heart attack may ask, "What is the purpose of working so hard to accumulate money when I could be spending more time with my family? Where are my priorities?" It is also not unusual for people to seek reasons for their illness. A woman with a diagnosis of breast cancer may ask, "Why me? What have I done to deserve this?"

The paradoxical bond that seems to exist between suffering and its meaning—between **pathos** and **machos**—has long concerned care providers, philosophers and theologians. Spiritual beliefs, whether they stem from religious doctrine or a person's secular values, can help patients to maintain a realistic perspective of themselves and their relationship to the world around them. Religious rituals and philosophical and theological discussions often help them to work through the meaning of suffering (Johnstone, 1990).

THE ROLE OF SPIRITUALITY IN OLDER ADULTS

Although physiological needs assume an increasingly important role as people grow older, it has been said that the spiritual aspects are even more important (Bianchi, cited in McCulloch, 1997). As the years begin to take their toll, people must contend with more illness and disability. Many live with chronic diseases such as arthritis, hypertension or cardiovascular disease. Older adults also fear the loss of their independence—for example, that they will be unable to care for themselves and will become a burden on their children.

Growing old threatens the personhood of an individual. As we mentioned in Chapter 8, the older adult often has reduced income, loss of self-esteem and diminished social status after retirement from the workforce. Older people look for meaning in their lives as their functional abilities decline and their dependence on others increases (McCulloch, 1997).

The belief and value systems that people have built up through the years can help to sustain them through the trials and tribulations of old age. Many older people find they have a renewed interest in religion. Spirituality, whether religious or secular, takes on new dimensions for older adults and for the terminally ill, helping them to cope with their daily lives and providing a source for forgiveness and hope (McCulloch, 1997).

Helping People to Meet Their Spiritual Needs

Caring of the whole human being presupposes that we understand and accept the patient's spiritual experiences irrespective of his way of expressing them. A professional nurse should be able to recognize and, to a certain extent, meet the patient's spiritual needs and demands irrespective of her own personal attitude to spirituality and religion.

Eriksson, 1997, pp. 78–79

What, then, are the spiritual needs of people? Based on common themes that run through the literature, we can identify some of these as follows.

Spiritual Needs

Common spiritual needs include:

- acceptance of oneself without criticism or self-reproach
- a sense of meaning and purpose to one's life
- harmonious relationships with others
- feeling comfortable in the world around us; being at ease in our place within the scheme of things
- trust in God or an Ultimate Other.

How can the nurse help people to meet their spiritual needs?

Spiritual needs are personal to each individual. Most people go through a period of self-reflection as they struggle to come to terms with their illness, disability, approaching death or other crisis in their lives. The role of the caregiver, and that of the pastoral counsellor, is to provide support for the person during this period of self-reflection (Johnstone, 1990).

To provide care that is sensitive to the patient's spiritual needs, Griffith (1996) suggests that one must be aware of "one's own religious identity and [acknowledge] the integrity and value of other people's religions" (p. 10). Further, theories and abstract frameworks of spirituality can be a hindrance rather than a help, because they tend to block intuition and lead us to routinize care for the person who needs our help and support. That is, we tend to view the person within the theoretical framework of spirituality, rather than through the person's own framework of values (Hall, 1997). Individuals have unique life experiences that have contributed to the development of their own system of values, spiritual beliefs and religious rituals. Before we can help a person, we need to know what these are. We can learn that only from the individual, and only when that individual has sufficient trust in us to talk freely, knowing that we will treat the discussion seriously and with respect for his or her beliefs and values (Johnstone, 1990).

Assessment of Spiritual Needs

Stoll (1979) suggests four areas for assessment of a person's spiritual needs:

1. the person's concept of God or deity, elicited by asking simply, "Is religion or God significant to you? If so, can you give me a simple description of [your God or deity]?"
2. the sources of hope and strength for the individual. For example, "To whom do you turn when you need help?"
3. religious practices, particularly as these affect care. For example, "Do you have any special dietary rules, or customs of prayer or devotion that you follow?"
4. the person's conception of the relationship between spiritual beliefs and health. For example, "What do you think is the cause of your illness? What will help you to get better?"

SOURCE: Stoll, 1979; Johnstone, 1990.

Eliciting information about a person's spiritual needs is a delicate matter, highly personal and usually charged with emotion. The nurse must tread gently in this area. A set of guidelines drawn up by Ruth Stoll (1979) emphasizes the need to recognize patients' right to their own beliefs and, also, their right to remain silent about them if they choose to do so.

Differing Beliefs and Health Care Practices of Major Religions

The nurse should support and assist [the patient] in maintaining traditional religious practices important to that person.

Griffith, 1996, p. 11

People acquire beliefs about health and health practices for the most part in the home as part of their cultural heritage. Although these beliefs and practices may be modified by education and by exposure to other beliefs and practices in later life, there is a tendency when one is ill to revert to the beliefs and practices that were learned first. As the influence of thoughts and beliefs on healing is increasingly recognized, it is essential that nurses and other health workers are aware of the health beliefs and practices of people coming to them for care. Since a person will heal more quickly when he or she believes in the effectiveness of the remedy, regardless of what that remedy is, rituals play a large part in the psychological aspects of cure (Frideres, 1988).

Health beliefs and practices are more closely tied to religion and to medical philosophy than to country of origin or ethnicity. But, in caring for people of different cultures, it is important to remember that no matter the country of origin or the religious beliefs, the patient must be assessed and treated as an individual; the diversity between people of similar backgrounds is likely to be greater than the similarities (Wexler-Morrison, Anderson & Richardson, 1990).

Religious beliefs tend to reflect the different wants and needs of different people. Based on faith and, perhaps, extended study, these beliefs are not always well understood by nonbelievers. Among the major world religions, there are many minor divisions with great differences in belief and practice. Many of these beliefs and practices have implications for health care. As a nurse, for example, you will want to know if the religion your patient subscribes to has any particular beliefs or practices regarding such matters as hygiene, modesty, diet, burial and faith healing, as well as any taboos that might interfere with the acceptance of treatment.

The religions of the world can be divided basically into two major groups—Western and Eastern. The birthplace of the Western group of religions was the Near East; in Palestine, the Arabian Peninsula and Iran. The Western religions include Christianity, Judaism, Islam, Baha'i and Zoroastrianism. People adhering to these religions believe that each person has an individual relationship with God, and they believe in a life after death. The major Eastern religions in Canada are Hinduism, Sikhism and Buddhism. Common beliefs of people adhering to these religions include a belief in reincarnation and in nonviolence (Bentley, 1986).

Western Religions

Although different in many respects, the Western religions all share some common themes or beliefs, such as the following:

- God is the creator of the world
- God is the final judge of the world's people
- God forbids the worship of false gods
- human beings were created by God and have a duty to obey God
- humans have only one life to live in this world
- prophets reveal God's will
- the Holy Books or Scriptures contain revealed truth
- a moral code, or code of conduct (for example, the Ten Commandments), must be adhered to (Bentley, 1986).

We will look at the Western religions in the order in which they developed historically.

ZOROASTRIANISM

This religion is not among those with a large number of members in Canada. It is, however, the oldest monotheistic religion practised today. It originated in Persia (now Iran), predating both Christianity and Islam, and has many followers in India and Iran. **Zoroastrianism** provides an interesting bridge between the religions of the West and the East. It has a highly moral belief system where salvation is the reward for those who follow "good thoughts, good words and good deeds." There is one god, Ahura Mazda. Immortality in heaven is believed to be attained by striving for spiritual and physical perfection through expanding one's knowledge and understanding. The spiritual leaders are ordained priests whose titles are inherited. They worship in the Fire Temple. Their Holy Scriptures are the Gathas Khirdeh and Avesta. After initiation into the religion, followers wear a **sudreh** (a white muslin vest), which symbolizes purity and humility, and a **kusti** (a woven cord around the waist), which symbolizes good thoughts, good words and good deeds. These are worn at all times and should be removed only with the consent of the individual.

Although no special diet is prescribed, many Zoroastrians abstain from eating meat or poultry. Followers pray five times a day with the head covered. Their holy days commemorate each stage of creation, New Year's Day and the birthday and death date of the prophet Zoroaster. After death the body is given a ritual bath, and the sudreh and kusti remain with the body before either burial or cremation. (Griffith, 1996).

JUDAISM

Judaism is the mother religion of both Christianity and Islam. It began before written history in the Eastern Mediterranean. There are over 15 million Jews in the world. There are three main branches of Judaism: Orthodox, whose adherents maintain traditional ways of worship and rituals, including dietary laws; Reform, whose members are not as strict and may not adhere to dietary and other rules; and Conservative, which falls between the Orthodox and the Reform.

The Jewish place of worship is the **synagogue**; the spiritual leader (a teacher, not a priest) is called a **rabbi**. Jewish people set aside Saturday as their holy day (from sunset Friday to sunset Saturday). Festivals include: Rosh Hashanah (New Year's Day), Yom Kippur (Day of Atonement—considered the most holy day), Hanukkah (Festival of Lights) and Passover (Festival of Freedom). Their Holy Scriptures are: the Tanach (the Old Testament of the Bible), the Torah (teachings of Moses) and the Talmud (oral law). During prayers, Jewish men may wear a prayer shawl and a **yarmulke** (skull cap). The Jewish holy days follow the Jewish calendar, which predates the Gregorian calendar used in Canada.

Sacraments include: (a) prayers, which precede meals, and grace, which follows; (b) a glass of wine is taken with the main meal on holy days (a religious act); (c) Bar Mitzvah (for boys at age 13) and Bat Mitzvah (for girls at age 12 or 13).

Beliefs and practices affecting health care include:

1. **Food**: for Orthodox and others who maintain dietary laws, food must be specially prepared in a kosher kitchen, according to ritual:
    - meat must come only from animals with a split hoof who chew cud (no pork); only certain cuts are kosher; only fish with fins are eaten (no shellfish); no predatory birds are eaten
    - animals must be killed in a kosher manner by a specially trained person and prepared by ritual
    - dairy products and meat cannot be served at the same meal
    - two sets of dishes are used for preparing and serving food—one for meat, one for dairy dishes

- it should be noted that kosher-style meat has a high sodium content. In hospital, many Jewish people prefer a vegetarian diet if kosher food is not available. They may also prefer disposable dishes and cutlery to avoid mixing dairy foods and meat.

2. **Contraception** is limited to females and allowed only for medical reasons
3. **Circumcision**: all male infants are circumcised on the eighth day of life
4. **Burial**: the right to die is not recognized. The body is buried intact within 24 hours of death; neither autopsy nor cremation is permitted. Transplants and the donation of body organs or parts are also prohibited. After death, a special group prepares the body ritually for burial (Bentley, 1986)
5. **Procedures/treatments:** consultation between rabbinical authorities and medical practitioners may be necessary for certain medical procedures or for scheduling treatments (Griffith, 1996).

CHRISTIANITY

Christianity has more followers than any other religion of the world, with an estimated one billion adherents. Christians believe that Jesus is the Messiah and the son of God. He is called the prophet of the Christian religion, who proclaimed a New Covenant between God and all humankind. There are over a thousand different denominations within the Christian Church, with Roman Catholicism the largest, claiming over 600 million members.

Christians share many beliefs, including the belief in Jesus as the son of God. Their Holy Scriptures are the Bible, both Old and New Testament. God is perceived to be a God of mercy and grace, which are mediated through the church. The sacraments are signs and seals of God's expressions to His people, and through them a believer attains forgiveness of sins or salvation through God's grace. In response to God's forgiveness, Christians are meant to forgive those who sin against them.

All Christians celebrate Christmas as the birthday of Christ and Easter as the day of His resurrection. There are many variations in the sacraments performed in the different denominations of the Christian Church. The two principal sacraments, shared by Roman Catholics and by most Protestants, are baptism and communion. **Baptism** is considered by most to be essential for salvation, although the age for baptism varies. In this ritual, the individual is immersed in or sprinkled with water as a sign of purification and of admission to the Church; it is usually accompanied by the giving of a name. **Communion**, or Eucharist, is a ritual in which believers partake of bread and wine or grape juice. The bread represents the body of Christ; the wine or grape juice His blood. Some consider this rite to be a cleansing of sin from the soul. The sacraments vary in the different denominations, as do many of the beliefs and practices pertaining to health (Bentley, 1986; Griffith, 1996).

The Roman Catholic Faith

The Roman Catholic faith originated in the first century and has evolved into the largest of the Christian denominations in the world. Roman Catholics celebrate Sunday as the holy day of the week. A number of other days are celebrated as well. Fasting and penitence are practised during Lent in commemoration of Christ's fasting in the wilderness. Lent lasts for 40 days, from Ash Wednesday until Easter Eve. The rosary is an important religious symbol to all Catholics and is used for saying prayers. Some Roman Catholics wear a religious medal, which may be a cross or a medal of one of the saints.

There are seven sacraments in the Roman Catholic Church: baptism, communion, confession, confirmation, anointing (or unction) of the sick, matrimony and holy orders. Those of most concern to nurses are baptism, communion and the anointing of the sick.

Baptism is the first of the sacraments to be administered; it is usually performed when an infant is one to several months of age. As Roman Catholic doctrine states that an infant has a soul from the moment of conception, a fetus at any stage of development must be baptized in order to receive salvation. In an emergency, a nurse can perform a baptism by pouring water on the head of the fetus or child and saying, "I baptize thee in the name of the Father, and of the Son and of the Holy Spirit." Most hospitals have forms to record baptism.

Holy communion is often requested by people who are ill or dying. When it is requested, a priest from the church the patient attends should be notified or, if the patient is in an inpatient facility, the sacrament can be performed by the Roman Catholic chaplain of the agency. A clean white cloth, such as a towel, is used as a cover for the bedside table on which the nurse places a glass of water and a spoon. Because people may wish to confess their sins at this time, it is important to ensure that the patient and the priest have privacy for the sacrament. Dietary rules regarding fasting before communion are not as strict as they once were; it is sufficient for the patient to abstain from food and alcohol for 15 minutes prior to receiving communion.

The **anointing of the sick** is a sacrament many people request when they are ill. Formerly known as extreme unction, or last rites, it used to be given only to the person who was dying. Now, however, it is interpreted as an aid to healing and a source of strength. It may therefore be received by a patient one or more times during an illness. Prayers, the anointing with oil and faith are believed by Catholics to restore health, but these do not rule out medical treatment. It is felt that the sacrament of anointing the body should be administered when the patient is conscious, although it can be administered to an unconscious person. It can be performed any time of the day or night. In this sacrament, the priest anoints the eyes, ears, nostrils, lips, hands and feet with oil, for which cotton balls have been provided. Even if a patient of the Roman Catholic faith dies without receiving the anointing of the sick, a priest should be called. He can administer the sacrament immediately following death. Nothing should be done to the body until all sacraments have been completed. The body is treated with respect and honour. All body parts must be left intact for burial or cremation.

The Roman Catholic Church does not permit abortion, nor does it allow artificial contraception (Griffith, 1996).

The Protestant Denominations

The sacrament of baptism is practised in most Protestant denominations. In some, baptism is performed in infancy; others baptize at the age of understanding, often when a child is 12 years old; some baptize adults. For a few Protestant denominations, baptism is a necessity before death. Some Protestant denominations hold communion. A few also practise the ritual of anointing. Some groups have dietary customs. Some forbid the eating of certain meats or espouse vegetarianism, and some prohibit the drinking of tea and coffee. Others have religious doctrines that prohibit tobacco products and the consumption of alcoholic beverages. During Lent, some Protestants practise a variety of dietary restrictions. Generally, however, most Protestants' eating habits are not restricted by religious doctrine. Particular denominations whose beliefs and practices affect health care are noted below.

CHURCH OF CHRIST THE SCIENTIST Christian Science was founded in 1879 by Mary Baker Eddy because of a personal healing experience. A fundamental belief of this religion is that healing occurs through divine power. There is no need, therefore, for medical intervention except in the case of births or fractures, for which conventional medical care is sought. Members decide individually what care they will accept if they should find themselves in a health care facility. They prefer to be free from the use of drugs, medicines and surgical interventions. The church has its own health practitioners who devote themselves full-time to healing. Members do not believe in physical examination or immunization, although they will comply with the law in this regard (Bentley, 1986; Griffith, 1996).

THE BAPTIST CHURCH The Baptist Church was one of the earliest Protestant denominations. It was founded in 1525, shortly after the beginning of Protestantism. It is the largest Protestant group in the United States, where many Baptists fled in the early 1600s to avoid religious persecution in Europe. Although the beliefs and practices of most Baptists do not affect health care, it is helpful to know that many Baptists like some quiet time to read the Bible. Many Baptists believe in healing by the laying on of hands. The artificial prolongation of life is discouraged (Zumbro Valley Medical Society, 1975).

JEHOVAH'S WITNESSES This religion was founded in 1884 by Charles Taze Russell and has over two million followers throughout the world. Jehovah's Witnesses withdraw from society to a certain extent, refusing to salute the flag or participate in worldly politics. There are no holy days, no sacraments and no belief in faith healing. Because the Bible says that people should not "eat blood," Jehovah's Witnesses refuse blood transfusions and will not eat foods with blood added or the meat of animals from which the blood has not been properly drained. They do, however, accept albumin, clotting factors and immune globulins. Provided it is not stored, blood by autotransfusion is acceptable. Medications and therapy are acceptable when necessary. Abortion and artificial insemination are both prohibited. Autopsy is permitted only if legally necessary. Euthanasia and the receiving or giving of organ transplants are not permitted (Bentley, 1986; Griffith, 1996).

MORMON CHURCH (CHURCH OF THE LATTER-DAY SAINTS)
The Mormon Church was founded in the United States by Brigham Young in 1830. It is estimated that there are over five million followers. Laws in this religion are very strictly adhered to. The Mormon diet consists mostly of fruits, vegetables and grains, with few animal products. The use of alcohol, tobacco products and other addictive substances, including tea, coffee and cola drinks, is prohibited. Some members wear short-sleeved, knee-length undergarments for God's protection. Mormons believe in baptism by immersion and in the laying on of hands to heal the sick by those who have the authority to act in Jesus Christ's name. They also believe that spiritual growth continues after death. They do not permit euthanasia or birth control. The Mormons have extensive libraries for genealogical research so that ancestors can be recorded and brought into the faith. These libraries are open to the public (Bentley, 1986; Zumbro Valley Medical Society, 1975; Griffith, 1996).

ISLAM

Islam means "peaceful submission to the will of God" (Bentley, 1986). A **Muslim** is one who practises Islam. Muslims believe that life is but a stay on earth during which people are tested, purified and developed. This religion began in Arabia over 1400 years ago and it has spread throughout the world. It teaches the equality of all humans in the eyes of God. The Muslim name for God is **Allah**, and Mohammed was His prophet.

The Holy Scriptures of the Islamic religion are the **Koran**, containing the revelations of God, and the Hadith, which is an interpretation of the Koran by the Prophet Mohammed, containing his wisdom and explorations. There are two major sects in the Islamic religion—the Sunni and the Shiites. There are no priests and no baptism in this religion. The **mosque** is the house of worship; when **muezzins** issue the call to prayer five times a day, the faithful must kneel, if possible, facing Mecca. The sabbath day is Friday. Muslims celebrate Eid El Fita, which is the first day of Ramadan (the ninth month of the Islamic year) and Eid El Adha, the Feast of Sacrifice, for the pilgrimage to Mecca, which all Muslims are required to make at least once in a lifetime.

Islamic dietary laws prohibit the eating of pork, pork products and any seafood without fins and scales. The **halal** (lawful), or ritually slaughtered, meat of the Muslims has a high sodium content. Intoxicants and tobacco products are prohibited. Muslims usually use the right hand for eating and rinse the mouth with water after eating. During the month of Ramadan, Muslims fast from dawn to sunset. The local imam (spiritual leader) may be helpful with dietary or fasting practices that interfere with a patient's medical regime.

Modesty is very important to Muslims. If at all possible, their health care should be given by people of the same gender. Orthodox Muslim women must always be covered from neck to ankles and men from waist to knees. The typical hospital gown is therefore considered indecent. During medical examinations, only a small portion of the body should be uncovered at one time. Most Muslim women cover their hair and many wear a veil; in some countries, women do not go outside the home. They need the consent of the family leader (a man) for treatment, medications and the like.

Muslims always wash, preferably with running water, in preparation for prayers and after going to the bathroom. The importance of cleanliness requires that Muslims have a full shower after seminal discharge or menstruation.

Muslims are fatalistic, accepting what happens (for example, the birth of a crippled child) as the will of God. Circumcision is performed on all male Muslim children. Muslims believe in life after death and in burial, rather than cremation. After death, the body should be handled only by Muslims; it is usually looked after by family members. If it is necessary for a non-Muslim to handle the body, gloves must be worn. The body is not washed and hair and nails are not cut. Burial should take place within 24 hours after death. Faith healing may be used to supplement a physician's efforts. The "right to die" is not accepted, nor is autopsy, unless required by law (Bentley, 1986; Zumbro Valley Medical Society, 1975; Griffith, 1996).

BAHA'I

Baha'i is a relatively new religion, founded in 1844 in Persia (Iran) by Baha'u'llah, whom Baha'is believe is the latest of God's prophets. The fundamental belief of the Baha'i is that everyone is a part of one human race; they teach the unity of all religions and the unity of all human beings. The world centre for this religion is Mount Carmel in Haifa, Israel. The sacred Baha'i literature was written by the founder in the mid-1800s. There are no clergy or other spiritual leaders. Rather, there is a spiritual assembly, democratically elected by the congregation. They read the scriptures of all religions and pray daily.

Baha'is have a special meeting on the first day of each month. They follow a calendar of 19 months, each of 19 days, with the New Year starting with the spring solstice. There are no dietary requirements, although they fast from sunrise to sunset during the last month of the year.

The use of alcohol and narcotics is prohibited. Canadian Baha'is have been active in international affairs to promote world unity. At the local level, they are active in community development projects (Bentley, 1986; Martin, 1985; Griffith, 1996).

Eastern Religions

The three most common Eastern religions in Canada are Hinduism, Sikhism and Buddhism.

HINDUISM

Hinduism is more than a religion to 80 percent of India's population; it is a social system and a way of life. There are many Hindu gods and goddesses; the main ones are Vishnu, Shiva and Brahma. A number of holy days are observed. The most important festival is **Dewali** (Festival of the Lights). There are holy writings—the four oldest being the Vedas, which were written in Sanskrit and are believed to be more than 4000 years old. There are no major prophets and many ways to follow one's religion. However, the following beliefs are common to all Hindus:

- there is one Supreme Spirit
- there is an immortal soul in all living beings
- people are reincarnated after death
- **karma** (the law of cause-and-effect) is the reward or punishment for one's acts and thoughts
- there is a clear code of dutiful and righteous behaviour
- violence is unacceptable
- the supreme duty is to seek truth.

The Hindu family is often an extended one, with several generations living together. The obligation for all family members to care for those who are ill or elderly is very strong. It is usually the eldest granddaughter who looks after the grandmother when she is ill or incapacitated. The father is traditionally the breadwinner and the mother custodian of family beliefs, values and religious teaching.

Many Hindu practices and beliefs are relevant for health care. Hindus are modest about their bodies. Women keep their upper arms, legs and breasts covered in the traditional **sari** and blouse or long tunic and loose trouser (**salwar kameze**). A long scarf is usually worn as well, which can be used as a head covering. Hospital gowns are embarrassing for devout Hindus, who should be provided with a long gown, or gown and pyjama bottoms. A man's body must be covered from waist to knees. For examinations, only one part of the body should be exposed at a time. It is considered improper to touch the body of a member of the opposite gender, except one's spouse.

Washing is done before prayers and after using the toilet. Food is eaten with the fingers, and Hindus wash their hands both before and after meals. Running water is necessary to purify the body; still water is believed to be unclean.

Many Hindus are vegetarian. The cow is considered sacred; therefore, beef is not usually eaten and milk and milk products are also not consumed. A devout Hindu may refuse food if he or she does not know what the ingredients are. Fasting is common, and may be done several times a week.

Most Hindus require privacy twice daily for their prayers. They may use prayer beads. Many men wear a thread over the right shoulder and around the waist, and women may wear a thread around the neck and a red mark on the forehead. Family members often wish to stay with someone who is ill regardless of visiting hours.

Death at home is preferred, if at all possible. After death, relatives wash and prepare the body. Non-Hindus should not touch the dead body of a Hindu person unless necessary, and then only using disposable gloves. The body is not washed and is covered with a plain sheet. The dead are cremated rather than buried. Cremation occurs as soon after death as possible in a special ceremony. In India, the ashes of the dead are often scattered on the holy Ganges River (Henley, 1983a; Griffith, 1996).

SIKHISM

Sikhism is an offshoot of Hinduism that originated in the 16th century. There are now 10 to 12 million Sikhs in the world, most of whom are from Punjab State in northern India. Sikhs believe in one God and in reincarnation. Their New Year is April 13 (Baisakh), celebrated with special sweets prepared in the temple. There are no ordained priests; any initiated Sikh can lead prayers and readings, as all Sikhs are equal. Prayers are usually recited morning and evening. The Holy Scriptures are those of the Guru Granth Sahib, the founder of Sikhism. A code of conduct is contained in the Rahab Maryada.

Family ties are strong—extended families often live together, and duty to all family members is emphasized. Sikh men wear a turban to cover their long hair, which the faith requires not be cut.

In addition to the turban worn by men, there are five signs of Sikhism worn by all Sikhs, both men and women:

- ***kosh***—uncut hair. Hair must be kept clean and neat. If shaving is necessary, the patient should be consulted; a depilatory cream may be preferred
- ***kanga***—a comb worn in the hair
- ***kara***—a steel bangle, worn on the right wrist, that should never be removed (in hospital it should be taped, if possible)
- ***kirpan***—a symbolic dagger, worn under the clothes, as a symbol of readiness to fight
- ***kaccha***—special undershorts. These are worn day and night by members of both genders. They are a reminder of modesty and sexual morality. During childbirth and surgery, women often prefer to keep kaccha on one leg or one ankle.

Modesty is very important to Sikhs. Upper arms, legs and breasts are covered by a sari and blouse or salwar kameze. A long scarf is usually worn by Sikh women. Washing is done before prayers, after lavatory and before and after eating.

The Sikh diet is often vegetarian. Pork is not eaten as the pig is considered a scavenger, and beef is seldom eaten. Fasting is not usual. Tobacco products and alcohol are prohibited.

Death is considered a part of life. Hymns and prayers are said for the dying person. After death, family members wash and prepare the body. Cremation is done as soon as possible (Henley, 1983b; Griffith, 1996).

BUDDHISM

Buddhism is a worldwide religion that was founded by Siddhartha Gautama (Buddha) in the fifth century BC in the area now known as Nepal. It has spread throughout Asia to the rest of the world. Buddhism is nontheistic and has no sacraments; however, men and women may take either monastic or lay ordination. In Canada, Sunday is usually observed as the sabbath. There are several holy days, depending on the sect, but most denominations celebrate Vesak (the full-moon day in May), which commemorates the birth, enlightenment and death of the Buddha.

Buddhists follow the Eightfold Path, which sets down guidelines for moral behaviour. Their sacred writings are the Tripitaka. Prayers are usually said five times a day, and prayer beads may be used. A quiet place is preferred for meditation. Most Buddhists adhere to a vegan or semivegetarian diet and do not use alcohol or tobacco products.

A central belief common to all branches is that the ultimate state is one of self-enlightenment. Buddhists are agreeable to all pursuits that enhance one's ability to attain enlightenment. They believe in faith healing, and feel that the spiritual peace and liberation from anxiety that comes from awakening to Buddha's wisdom will hasten healing and recovery, but most will take medications and treatment as needed. Buddhists are fatalistic, accepting life's events with imperturbable calm. Death is likewise accepted. Since the body is considered only a shell after death, most denominations have no restrictions on handling it; however, Tibetan Buddhists believe that the body should remain untouched (or touched as little as possible) for three days after death, during which an unenlightened person may still attain enlightenment. Burial may be by cremation or internment (Zumbro Valley Medical Society, 1975).

Alternative Medicine

In caring for people from different ethnic groups, it is helpful for nurses to know if a patient adheres to a particular religion. While this is a useful frame of reference for establishing a plan of care, it is not predictive from individual to individual. Thus, the nurse must also determine the patient's health beliefs, including the therapies he or she uses, before a treatment regime can be established. Frequently, the patient and the health professional will need to compromise to determine the best course of treatment acceptable to both (O'Connor, 1995).

People have very different ideas about health, illness and treatment for a variety of reasons, including their cultural heritage, religious beliefs (e.g., regarding fasting), philosophy of life (e.g., deciding to become a vegetarian), desire for treatment options for specific illnesses (e.g., cancer) and dissatisfaction with conventional medical treatments (O'Connor, 1995).

Millions of people throughout the world rely on traditional healers when they are ill or injured. Although many people who immigrate to Canada are city dwellers who have been exposed to Western medicine, many others have never known anything but the folk medicine used in their villages. Many of these folk medicines, remedies and traditions have survived because they work.

In North America and Europe, an increasing number of people are using alternative medical therapies and practices. **Alternative medicine** can be described as any approach to solving a health problem that is different from that used by conventional Western practitioners. The term **complementary** is applied when alternative medicine is used in conjunction with, or to supplement, Western medicine.

Alternative medicine attempts to promote the self-healing capacities of the body, amplify natural recuperative processes and augment the energy upon which the patient's health depends. The many practices of alternative medicine share commonalties that differentiate them from Western medicine (see box).

Watson (1996) postulates that nursing may form the bridge between conventional Western medical practice and the nonconventional practices that are converging in present-day health care. She has stated that nursing practice has a "long history of noninvasive, naturalistic care modalities and nursing therapeutics which encompass comfort measures, pain control, symptom management and healing arts which seek to promote well-being and potentiate wholeness and healing" (Watson, 1996, p. 1). Many of the practices now termed "alternative medicine" have been central to quality nursing for many years.

Commonalties of Alternative/ Complementary Therapies

Practices focus on:

- self-responsibility
- nutrition
- balanced lifestyle
- detoxification of the body
- treatment of the whole person, rather than treatment of symptoms or disease.

SOURCE: Adapted from Burton-Goldberg Group, 1995, p.14.

Types of Alternative Medicine

There are many practices and therapies available outside conventional Western medicine. Some have a better basis of scientific research than others. The Office of Alternative Medicine in the U.S. National Institutes of Health classifies alternative/complementary medical practices into the following categories:

1. alternative systems of medical practice
2. diet, nutrition and lifestyles changes
3. manual healing
4. pharmacological and biological treatments
5. bioelectromagnetic applications
6. herbal medicine
7. mind/body control.

The section that follows describes some of the better-known of these.

ALTERNATIVE SYSTEMS OF MEDICAL PRACTICE

ACUPUNCTURE Originating in China, **acupuncture** is now practised extensively in Canada. It is based on **chi,** which is the finite amount of energy with which we are endowed at birth. Chi flows throughout the body from one **meridian** (channel) to another and is determined by heredity and lifestyle. Many factors can slow or block its flow, thus creating an energy imbalance. To correct the imbalance, the acupuncturist inserts fine needles on the meridians and stimulates (rotates) the needles. This is done by hand in China, while many Western practices use electrical charges to pulse the needles (electroacupuncture) (Olson, 1990; Grossman, 1985). One safety factor, which needs careful scrutiny, is the sterility of the needles because of the danger of infection. Acupuncture is used extensively to relieve pain. It has some merit in combating substance abuse (e.g., tobacco) and is often helpful in cases of nausea from seasickness, pregnancy and chemotherapy.

AYURVEDIC MEDICINE This the oldest form of health care that considers natural phenomena—rather than spirits—to be the cause of illness. Records go back 2500 years in India, where **Ayurvedic medicine** is believed to have originated. Treatment is based on a belief in the body's innate ability to heal itself. Illness is felt to result from internal disharmony resulting from improper diet, activities inappropriate for the season (such as swimming in the midst of winter), or other lifestyle indiscretions. There is a dual emphasis in Ayurvedic medicine on treatment and prevention.

Treatment is carried out by trained physicians and can involve a wide range of therapies, including herbal remedies and **pancha karma**, which includes many means to cleanse the body of wastes. Prevention is initiated on noting a disturbance in functioning, and can involve altered diet or exercise routines, or initiating changes in thought and emotional patterns to restore balance in the body. Many people of East Indian descent in Canada make use of both Ayurvedic and Western medicine (Guinness & Rutherford, 1993).

NATUROPATHY OR NATURAL MEDICINE The practice of **naturopathy** includes discovering and eliminating the cause of disease; using the most natural, nontoxic and least invasive therapy available when treatment is necessary; treating the whole person; teaching the person to develop a healthy diet and lifestyle; and trusting in the healing power of Nature (Olson, 1990; Murray & Pizzoromo, 1991). At the time of writing, British Columbia is the only province in Canada to license naturopaths.

SHAMANISM The **shaman** uses traditional rituals to exorcise spirits, which are considered to be the cause of health problems. Shamans have great stature within their societies because they act as intermediaries with the spirit world (Frideres, 1988). Shamanism is found in many areas worldwide. Medical practices of First Nations people who use shamans are discussed later in this chapter.

TRADITIONAL CHINESE MEDICINE A preventive rather than curative approach, **traditional Chinese medicine** revolves around theories of energy flow and elements. Treatments include acupuncture, herbal medicine, acupressure and qui gong, as well as exercise, of which the most common in Canada is t'ai chi. **Qui gong** is based on the principle of energy flow and uses visualization, movement and breathing exercises to unblock the channels and enhance the flow of vital energy in the body (Olson, 1990; Shaw, 1986). This increases both circulation and immune functioning. A practitioner moves from simple relaxation to very deep relaxation through practice (Burton-Goldberg Group, 1995). At the time of writing, British Columbia had established the Tzu Chi Institute for Complementary and Alternative Medicine, which is housed on the grounds of Vancouver Hospital and Health Sciences Centre.

DIET, NUTRITION AND LIFESTYLE CHANGES

DIET The importance of nutrition is emphasized by both conventional and nonconventional practitioners. There is concern that many Canadians today eat too much fast food and snacks that have high fat content, meet too few of the body's nutritional needs and contain too little fibre. Proper nutrition can help one to live longer and, even more important, to stay healthy. Chapter 20 of this text discusses *Canada's Food Guide for Healthy Eating.*

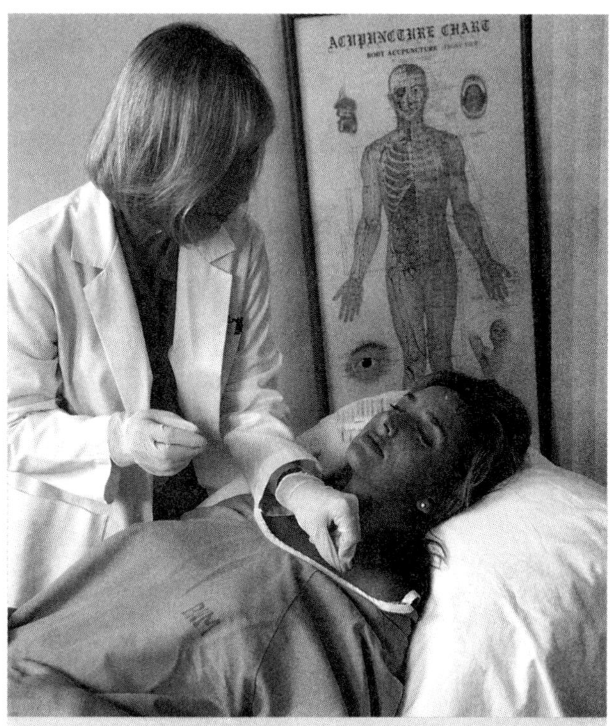

Acupuncture physician applying alcohol rub.

LIFESTYLE CHANGES The most common lifestyle change is an increase in exercise. Many Canadians live rather sedentary lives, and this is often reflected in their health. Exercise can decrease the risk of developing coronary heart disease, protect against strokes, decrease the risk of adult-onset diabetes, lower the risk of cancer and prevent and treat anxiety and depression (Fugh-Berman, 1996). Exercise is something everyone can afford to do. Walking is one of the best exercises and costs the least. There are many different types of exercise programs, varying from sports for youngsters to adults, fitness clubs, and special exercise groups for pregnant women, adults, seniors and for those with specific health problems, such as heart conditions, arthritis and urinary incontinence.

YOGA **Yoga** originated in conjunction with Ayurvedic medicine and is considered important in preventive medicine. It uses *asanas* (postures), breathing and visualization exercises to improve mobility, circulation, digestion and energy level.

TAI CHI Many people, especially the Chinese, practise **tai chi** as a form of meditation in motion. Regular practice loosens the joints and spine and relaxes tension points. Because it does not involve jarring movements, t'ai chi can be practised by people of any age and with varying degrees of disability (Olson, 1990; Shaw, 1986).

MANUAL HEALING

ACUPRESSURE Employing the same channels and points as acupuncture, **acupressure** uses massage (light to moderate manual pressure) to stimulate energy flow through the body. **Shiatzu** is a Japanese form of acupressure that combines the use of touch with a traditional form of Oriental massage. Both are helpful for muscle tension and relaxation. A seaband—an elasticized band applied to a specific point above the wrist—uses the principles of acupressure to help prevent nausea in chemotherapy patients and others.

AROMATHERAPY This approach uses aromatic oils or essences extracted from plants for therapies similar to those used in herbal medicine (see below). **Aromatherapy** oils are administered by massage, through baths or by inhalation and produce a wide range of therapeutic responses, including relaxation and decreased anxiety. Some studies claim a reduction in pain (Olson, 1990).

CHIROPRACTIC MEDICINE The third largest primary health care specialization in the Western world (after medicine and dentistry), this approach originated in the United States. **Chiropractic medicine** is primarily concerned with the examination and manipulation of the spinal column "to rehabilitate normal nervous system functioning" (Olson, 1990, p. 119). Some practitioners confine their practice to manual manipulation and others use a wide range of therapies (excluding surgery). Chiropractic medicine is especially helpful for people with acute lower-back pain (Fugh-Berman, 1996). (Note that there is an important distinction between chiropractic medicine and osteopathy. Osteopaths are medical doctors with additional preparation in disorders of the musculoskeletal system and the structural elements of the body.)

MASSAGE THERAPY There are many varieties of massage, some of which originated in ancient times. **Massage therapy** involves the systematic use of friction, stroking and kneading to improve circulation and mobility, drain lymph, and release tension. It has also been found to facilitate the growth and development of premature babies and to help reduce some types of pain (Fugh-Berman, 1996).

THERAPEUTIC TOUCH Developed by Dolores Krieger after observing the effects of faith healing (discussed below), Therapeutic Touch has become a popular nursing tool in conjunction with other therapies (Krieger, 1975, 1979; Guinness & Rutherford, 1993). In experimental studies, Krieger found that the laying on of hands increased relaxation and reduced anxiety. Further, there was a significant rise in hemoglobin levels. **Therapeutic Touch** practitioners hold their hands lightly on the skin or a short distance away from the patient to sense and smooth out the patient's energy field (Fugh-Berman, 1996). The healing process is potentiated by the transfer of energy from practitioner to patient. Because it is noninvasive, Therapeutic touch can be helpful to patients who cannot tolerate massage therapy.

PHARMACOLOGICAL AND BIOLOGICAL TREATMENTS

CHELATION THERAPY **Chelation therapy** treats poisoning from toxic metals by removing these from the body with a chemical agent. The technique has been used experimentally to remove plaque from blood vessels (Burton-Goldberg Group, 1995).

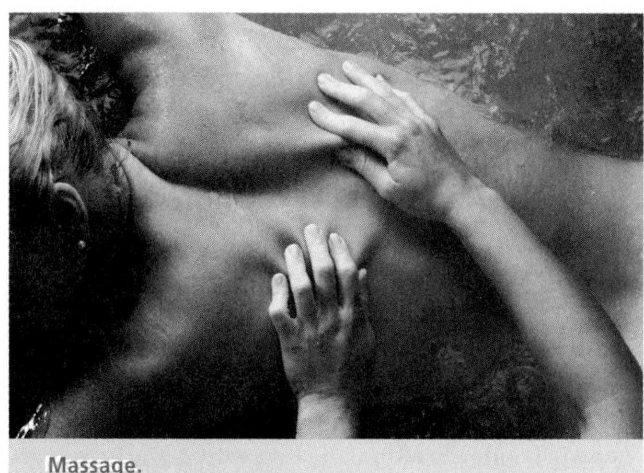
Massage.

BIOELECTROMAGNETIC APPLICATIONS

ELECTROACUPUNCTURE Producing the same results as acupuncture, **electroacupuncture** uses electrical charges to pulse the needles rather than manual rotation (Burton-Goldberg Group, 1995).

STIMULATION DEVICES A variety of instruments are used to relieve pain or promote wound healing. A common method is **TENS** (transcutaneous electrical nerve stimulation), which uses a small machine that can be operated by the patient at home (Fugh-Berman, 1996).

HERBAL MEDICINE

Herbs are plants or parts of plants that may be used for their medicinal effects as well as for food or flavouring. The effects of **herbal medicine** vary according to the age, weight, genetics, gender and biochemistry of each individual. Herbs can interact with drugs and should be used only under the supervision of a knowledgeable health practitioner.

There is considerable controversy over the effects of many herbs. Some may be effective in only one form; the active ingredient may be destroyed by commercial processes; or the herb may be ineffective for the use promoted by folklore or propaganda. The lack of standardization of herbal preparations, with respect to both the contents of the mixture and the dosage, makes it essential that only reputable brand names are used. (Information about herbal medicine may be found in Tyler, 1993; Fugh-Berman, 1996; and Burton-Goldberg Group, 1995.)

The World Health Organization notes that of 119 plant-derived pharmaceutical medicines, about 74 percent are used in modern medicine in ways that correlate directly with their traditional uses as plant medicines by native cultures (Farnsworth et al., 1985).

Some of the more common herbs used in Canada are:

ALOE VERA A gel made from this plant is used widely in cosmetics and in skin lotions for its softening effect. The fresh gel of a broken leaf is an effective home remedy for minor burns, abrasions and skin irritations. Aloe vera latex is used in laxatives.

BRAN The outer husk or hull of the wheat grain provides an excellent dietary source of fibre. Adequate dietary fibre reduces colonic diseases and ischemic heart disease.

CRANBERRY The juice from this berry may help to reduce bladder infections through its antiadhesive properties, which reduce the ability of bacteria to adhere to the bladder wall.

ECHINACEA This herb boosts the immune system and is also used as an anti-inflammatory agent and for wound healing. It is often taken for the common cold and for influenza.

GARLIC Well known for its antibiotic, antifungal and antiviral activity, garlic is used in the prevention and treatment of the common cold and influenza as well as their complications. It has an antioxidant effect that helps to protect arteries, lower cholesterol and thin blood. It is also used to prevent and treat intestinal worms.

GINGER Used to reduce or alleviate nausea and vomiting, especially in motion sickness, ginger also aids digestion and has cardiotonic properties.

GINKO This herb helps increase peripheral blood flow without changing the blood pressure. It is often used to treat intermittent pain in the legs from walking (claudication). It may also relieve memory problems and confusion resulting from cerebral insufficiency. It tends to reduce anxiety, dizziness and asthma.

GINSENG Widely used in Asia as a tonic, ginseng is called an adaptogen as it helps the body to resist and endure stress.

MIND/BODY CONTROL

FAITH HEALING Used from time immemorial, **faith healing** is based on a belief in the healing power of an individual, object or place. Examples of faith healing include the New Testament stories of Jesus healing the sick, the shaman's healing power, the Roman Catholic sacrament of anointing the sick, healing by practitioners of the Christian Science Church, and the miraculous cures at the Roman Catholic shrine at Lourdes (Frank, cited in Kennison, 1987). Touch is often used in conjunction with faith healing. The term **laying on of hands** is sometimes used to refer to both faith healing and therapeutic touch.

SUPPORT GROUPS **Support groups** exist in many communities, often linked throughout the world, to assist people with a variety of specific problems and illnesses. They reassure people that they are not alone and offer contact with others who have similar problems. Also called **mutual aid groups,** they serve a wide range of needs, such as those of new parents or of caregivers to the disabled or the chronically ill. Two of the best known support groups include Alcoholic Anonymous (AA) for alcoholics and Al-Anon for relatives of alcoholics. Support groups are usually formed in communities as a need becomes known. They serve their memberships through meetings, telephone calls and newsletters.

BIOFEEDBACK A relatively new technique in which a person learns to control body systems by self-monitoring, **biofeedback** is particularly helpful for chronic muscle tension in the neck and lower back, headaches, urinary and fecal incontinence, stroke rehabilitation and improving circulation (e.g., in diabetics). It does not work in all cases, but can be beneficial in many (Fugh-Berman, 1996).

MUSIC THERAPY It is well known that listening to music lowers blood pressure and stress levels. **Music therapy** is often used to reduce anxiety and increase relaxation.

MEDITATION A safe and simple way to balance a person's physical, emotional and mental states, **meditation** is used to treat stress and manage pain, and in the overall plan of care for hypertension and cardiac disease.

HYPNOSIS Used in both physical and psychological disorders, **hypnosis** employs an artificially induced state characterized by greater receptivity to suggestion. Its aim is to quiet the patient's conscious mind and make the unconscious mind more accessible. Hypnosis can create shifts in behaviour and enhance well-being. It can reduce stress and pain and has been used instead of anesthesia for surgery in a few cases (Guinness & Rutherford, 1993).

Barriers to Accessing Care

The Epp Report (1986) documented the poor health status of certain segments of the Canadian population. Particularly at risk are people in low socioeconomic groups, new immigrants and other minority groups, including the people of the First Nations. One major cause is poverty and the inability to purchase the things needed for good health, such as nutritious food or good housing. We have discussed this aspect in previous chapters. Other factors contributing to the poor health of various groups are the barriers they meet when they seek health care. In Canada, although we have universal health care, for various reasons, many people find it difficult to access this care.

Attitudes of Health Professionals

A major barrier to accessing health care for some people is the attitude of health professionals. Even though an increasing number of health professionals in this country are second-, third- and fourth-generation Canadians of both European and non-European descent, their backgrounds are considerably different from those of new immigrants.

Most health professionals have gone through the Canadian educational system and are well socialized into Canadian ways. Many have lost their heritage language; it may not have even been spoken in the home in which they were raised.

Although many physicians came from other countries to Canada in the middle years of the century, when we were short of Canadian-trained physicians, few are admitted now that we have a more than adequate supply. Those who are admitted have difficulty obtaining licensure to practise in Canada because of qualifying examinations, language proficiency and a shortage of internship placements for foreign-trained doctors. Nurses coming from other countries are often required to take additional clinical courses and sit qualifying examinations. Another problem in nursing is the difficulty in recruiting students into nursing schools whose families have come from countries where nursing has a low status. Brisson and Deslauriers (1992), in a study on the proportion of immigrants in nursing in Canada, found that the proportion had dropped from 7.7 percent to 0.4 percent between 1967 and 1977. This trend appears to be changing since this research was done.

Physicians, nurses and other health professionals in this country have all been educated in the Western medical model, with its emphasis on the biophysical causes of disease and the scientific treatment of it. It is only in very recent years that alternative forms of medicine have been accepted in Canada as having some validity—even so, they are greeted with much scepticism by many. The biomedical model assumes certain attitudes towards health care and those who come for care. These attitudes are deep-rooted; their foundations are in cultural values and beliefs that have been acquired in the home and moulded by education, religion and personal experience. We are often not aware of our own values and beliefs because they are obtained subconsciously. They determine, however, the way in which we view the world and the way we relate to other people (Grypma, 1993).

SPECIAL PROBLEMS FOR THE GENERAL POPULATION

UNEQUAL DISTRIBUTION OF RESOURCES Some problems people have in accessing health care are due to disparities in the health care system itself. Tertiary care hospitals and most of the highly qualified health professionals, such as specialist physicians and nurses with advanced preparation, are located in major urban centres in the southern parts of Canada. People living in northern and rural areas have long been underserved. Provincial governments, in planning health care reforms, are aware of the problem, and in several provinces, steps are already underway to address the disparities.

OTHER REASONS The poor, the homeless, people with mental health problems and those who are mentally challenged, alcoholics and drug addicts frequently experience difficulties accessing care regardless of whether they live in urban Toronto or in Inuvik. The barriers to care for these groups come in part from the attitude of health professionals towards them and the low self-esteem they often have. All barriers to health care are compounded by a lack of information about available health care resources and a lack of information about accessing these. People need to learn how to use the information that is available about health matters. Many things can interfere with a person's ability to understand health information, including language difficulties, fear of authority, distaste for charity, lack of ability to follow through and cultural conflict. Some very promising results have occurred as a result of teaching mothers in infant care groups with a leader who understands the culture of origin of the mothers and speaks their language.

SPECIAL PROBLEMS FOR IMMIGRANTS AND REFUGEES

HEALTH INSURANCE REGULATIONS People coming into the country in most provinces are not eligible for health insurance until they have completed three months' residency. Meanwhile, their immigration sponsors are responsible for their welfare, so they need to take out private insurance. In the case of refugees, financial help is available from Citizenship and Immigration Canada in the event of a critical situation.

LANGUAGE In many cases, there is a language barrier to overcome when immigrants seek the help of health professionals. As we noted above, a large number of immigrants can speak neither English nor French, which are often the only languages the health care workers do speak (Non parlo ne inglese ne francese, 1993).

LOW SELF-ESTEEM Many immigrants, even people who have been professionals in their home country, often have to take low-paying, low-status jobs in Canada. Many of the people who have come from Central or South America, Somalia or Bosnia, for example, are refugees who were victims of torture for their political or religious beliefs, or for their ethnic identity. Both situations can contribute to feelings of low self-esteem. Any lack of sensitivity on the part of health professionals can cause further insecurity in people whose self-esteem is already low.

LACK OF CULTURALLY RELEVANT TREATMENT In our Western medicine-oriented health agencies, people from different cultures may experience conflict with their religious beliefs or cultural values. One example is a Chinese man who was admitted to the emergency department of a large hospital. The patient did not speak English and became very agitated when the nurse tried to take a sample of blood that had been ordered. The patient eventually had to be restrained and was put in isolation. When an interpreter arrived on the scene, it was learned that the patient was objecting to the invasion of his body and he was not going to submit to it. When the procedure and the reasons for it were explained, he relaxed and allowed the nurse to take the blood sample.

Culturally sensitive care is particularly important for people with mental health problems. Often hidden because of the stigma attached to them, mental health problems are common among immigrants for many reasons. One is the instability caused by moving to another part of the world and getting settled in a new community. Another is the stress of the immigration process itself. The problems are more pronounced in refugees who often suffer from depression and anxiety, constantly wondering if they are ever going to be safe.

CULTURAL DIFFERENCES IN ATTITUDE TOWARDS TREATMENT
In some cases, services such as social assistance are considered unacceptable because any form of charity is a disgrace. Community health services may also be looked upon as charity because in the person's home country, one has to pay for health care. Wife-beating is considered a family matter in some cultures and not a matter for health authorities or the police. In most Eastern cultures, it is the duty of the family to care for aging parents, aunts and uncles. Having to put them in an extended care facility—because there is no one at home to care for them, or for any other reason—causes the family a tremendous burden of guilt.

INCONVENIENT HOURS FOR SERVICES The nine-to-five office hours of physicians and clinics are often a deterrent for people who work long hours and are unable to take time off because they are paid on an hourly basis. Not infrequently, both husband and wife work to make enough money for the family to survive. In these situations, it is difficult for parents to take a child to the clinic for immunization or to make time to go to the physician themselves.

RACIAL TENSIONS Sometimes, racial conflict can create a barrier to health care. A patient may not want to be cared for by a physician or nurse of a certain race or colour. Or, a visiting health professional may be reluctant to go to the home of a person of a different race (Hong Fook Mental Health Association, 1986).

Crossing the Barriers

Dr. Madeline Leininger, the acknowledged founder of transcultural nursing, believes that nursing is basically a transcultural care profession. Its primary focus is the provision of "human care to people in a way that is meaningful, congruent and respectful of cultural values and lifestyles" (Luna & Cameron, 1989, p. 228). The transcultural nursing concepts and cultural care theory developed by Leininger over the past three decades have given nurses a new insight into better ways to understand individuals, families and cultures (Leininger, 1978).

Numerous researchers have subsequently extended Leininger's work through comparative studies of cultural care patterns, values and practices of people of different cultures to add to our nursing knowledge and thereby improve nursing practice. The terms **cultural sensitivity**, *cross-cultural competence*, *intercultural effectiveness* and *ethnic competence* have all been used to describe the ability to work effectively with people of different cultures in a way that people of these cultures find acceptable.

Lynch and Hanson (1992), in their book *Developing Cross-Cultural Competence*, have suggested that this competence includes five elements: awareness of one's own cultural limitations; openness, appreciation and respect for cultural differences; a view of intercultural interactions as learning opportunities; ability to use cultural resources in interventions; and acknowledgement of the integrity and value of all cultures. We will look at each of these in turn.

Cultural Sensitivity

"Cultural sensitivity, cultural competence, intercultural effectiveness and ethnic competence . . . all refer to ways of thinking and behaving that enable the members of one cultural, ethnic or linguistic group to work effectively with members of another. . . . it does not mean knowing everything there is to know about another culture. It is, instead, respect for the difference, eagerness to learn and a willingness to accept that there are many ways of viewing the world."

SOURCE: Lynch & Hanson, 1992, p. 357.

AWARENESS OF ONE'S OWN CULTURAL LIMITATIONS The first step in overcoming the barriers in caring for people of other cultures is to become aware of our own beliefs and values. Most of these we have acquired subconsciously and they may therefore be difficult to identify. What, for example, are your beliefs about abortion? Breastfeeding? The right to die? How do these influence your reaction to a patient who has just had an abortion, refuses to breastfeed her infant or has requested "do not resuscitate" orders?

OPENNESS, APPRECIATION AND RESPECT FOR CULTURAL DIFFERENCES Cultural values, customs and beliefs are an integral part of an individual. If each patient is to receive "humane, personalized culturally sensitive care with due regard for spiritual, physical and emotional needs in addition to the full spectrum of patients' rights," as suggested by Berube (1990, p. 1), we must first establish the role of the patient's ethnicity in their beliefs about health and illness. Does the patient belong to a group that follows strict rules in regard to diet, bathing, clothing, prayers and the like?

There is a tremendous diversity of beliefs and practices within each major religious/cultural group. It is necessary, then, to ask the patient about individual preferences in order to determine whether there are any differences in views about health and illness and, if so, what these are. Some religions have strong views on medical-surgical procedures such as blood transfusions, abortion, transplants and the prolongation of life; some have none. Holy days have varying meanings for each individual and their significance should be ascertained. Respect for the patient's beliefs is essential and, insofar as possible, the patient should be assisted to maintain traditional rituals of prayer, washing and diet. Religious objects, such as scriptures and prayer beads, should be handled with respect.

A VIEW OF INTERCULTURAL INTERACTIONS AS LEARNING OPPORTUNITIES There is a wealth of knowledge about different cultures among patients in all health care agencies in Canada today. In the process of caring for your patients, you have a wonderful opportunity to expand your knowledge about the world.

ABILITY TO USE CULTURAL RESOURCES IN INTERVENTIONS Both in Vancouver and in Toronto, health departments have established a separate division to assist in providing culturally sensitive health care to people of different ethnic groups. A number of cultural resources have been developed in different centres across the country. These include health promotion material, such as pamphlets and videotapes, in a number of languages, and the use of cultural media for health education programs. Additionally, there is the important task of training interpreters for hospitals and other health care needs.

Continuing education sessions are being held to sensitize health care professionals to the needs of people of different cultures. Health education can be incorporated into English as a second language (ESL) classes with the cooperation of the teacher. Ethnic community organizations can be approached for people to help, for example, with interpretation. Volunteers can also be useful in helping with the organization of clinics for pregnant women and new mothers or for seniors and the establishing of health education programs. With some ethnic groups there are now third and fourth generations in Canada who are also usually willing to assist newcomers, although many may have lost their mother tongue and cannot be called upon as interpreters.

ACKNOWLEDGMENT OF THE INTEGRITY AND VALUE OF ALL CULTURES As you learn more about the beliefs, values and customs of others, you will gain a greater appreciation of the heritage of people coming from different lands. Koreans will proudly tell you that their ancestry goes back four thousand years as a race separate from the Chinese and the Japanese. Our Canadian heritage is a brash newcomer, compared to the cultures of people from the Middle East, Asia and Europe (Lynch & Hanson, 1992; Berube, 1990; Wexler-Morrison, Anderson & Richardson, 1990; Vancouver Health Department, 1993).

LOOKING back

Alice Katherine Smith, 1910–1998

Alice Katherine Smith, the first Chief Nursing Consultant with Indian Health Services (later renamed Indian and Northern Affairs and, still later, the Medical Services Branch of Health and Welfare Canada), was a major contributor to the development and success of the health care programs for Canada's remote areas from 1950 to 1975 and a major force behind the development of Canada's northern health services.

Alice Katherine Smith was born in Cartwright, Manitoba, in 1910, the eldest daughter in a family that lost the father during World War I. She received her nursing diploma from the Winnipeg General Hospital in 1933 and took a certificate in public health nursing at the University of Toronto in 1938. She then joined the Manitoba Department of Health as a staff nurse in rural areas, eventually becoming the nursing consultant responsible for rural cancer education programs from 1942 to 1948. As a young public health nurse in rural and northern areas, she recognized the importance of primary nursing services in the many areas of Canada where doctors are not available.

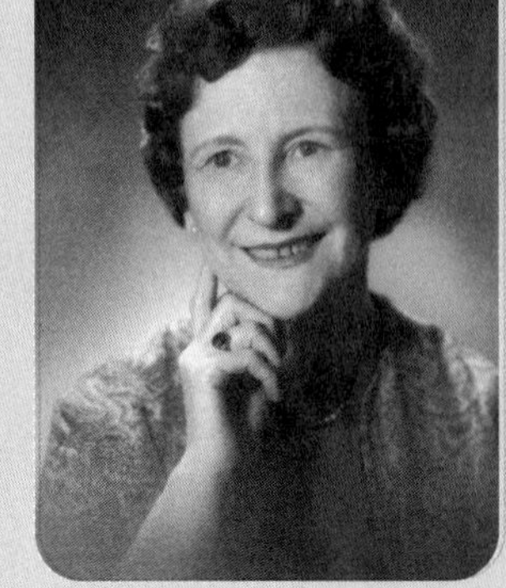

In 1948, she was asked by the Canadian Nurses Association to go to Great Britain to study the effects on nursing of the new national health insurance plan that had been launched in that country. She received her baccalaureate degree in nursing education from Teachers College, Columbia University, in 1950. She then joined the newly reorganized Indian Health Services, part of the Department of National Health and Welfare, in Winnipeg. She took her master's degree in public health at Yale University in 1957.

In her 25 years with the federal government, during which she achieved increasing influence as a Chief Nursing Consultant, she initiated continual refinements in the medical services under her supervision. She saw drastic improvements in health care for the Inuit and the North American Indian peoples, especially the dramatic decreases in maternal and infant mortality rates and the reductions in incidence of tuberculosis. She found many practical ways for northern nurses to upgrade their credentials and improve practice in their remote health facilities. As well, she provided opportunities for universities to work with remote nursing stations to increase their field experience and understanding of primary nursing needs. Her efforts helped establish ever-better guidelines for health care delivery in Canada's remote areas.

— *Glennis Zilm*

Health Care for People of the First Nations

Historical Perspective

The traditional health care system of First Nations peoples was rooted in their religious beliefs. It was felt that people brought illness upon themselves by actions such as breaking a taboo, thus allowing an evil spirit to enter the body. There were basically three types of illness:

1. those that were visible, such as a fracture or a bleeding leg resulting from physical injuries
2. those caused by an invisible external agent such as infectious agents including smallpox, pneumonia and measles
3. a group of residual diseases that did not fit into either of the other two categories, for example, mental illness (Frideres, 1988).

First Nations peoples had a wide variety of medicines, including many herbal remedies, that were developed to treat different diseases. Acting on the belief that most illnesses had a biological basis, the medicines were administered at the onset of an illness. If the ill person did not respond to the medications, it was assumed that the disorder in question was rooted in spiritual, rather than biological causes. Shamanistic methods might then be tried. The task of the shaman or medicine man (or woman) was to drive out the foreign object or evil spirit that had invaded the ill person's body. These methods might involve such practices as incantations and/or prayers to the spirits, as well as purification by sweetgrass ceremonies or by having the ill person spend time in a sweat lodge (Frideres, 1988; Jilek, 1982; Tucker, 1965).

Regrettably, the traditional health care system of the First Nations peoples disintegrated as colonization by the Europeans proceeded. The new settlers brought not only Western-style medicine but also a new way of life and new diseases. First Nations peoples were decimated by epidemics of smallpox, diphtheria, measles and influenza, along with the ever-present tuberculosis. In addition, high rates of mental illness and alcoholism resulted from attempts to cope with the rapid changes that were taking place in their society (Frideres, 1988).

In 1945, the Department of Health and Welfare assumed responsibility for the provision of direct health care services to all First Nations peoples. At first, this was in a separate unit called "Indian Health." In 1962, this unit was merged with other federal health programs to form the Medical Services Branch of the Department. During the 1960s and 1970s, a network of hospitals, nursing stations and community health centres were developed by Medical Services to provide health care to First Nations peoples, including those living on reserves within provincial boundaries and those

NURSES at work: Nursing in Canada's North

It's a crispy, cool Saturday afternoon in Arctic Red, one of the satellite towns our nursing station is responsible for. It's October, and I've been here now for almost two weeks. Arctic Red will be completely cut off from civilization for the seven or eight weeks when the road is closed. The road depends on ferry crossings in the summer and ice roads in the winter. During the between-times, there is no way into Arctic Red except by Ski-doo or helicopter.

It finally happened yesterday. I went to work as usual and watched the first ferry crossing while I ate my breakfast at the health centre. It seemed to be having a bit of trouble dodging the big pieces of ice that floated down the river. Some of these "floaters" are nearly half a kilometre long with jammed-together pieces of ice. Anyway, the ferry got hit broadside by a "floater," which apparently did some damage, and for about an hour, I watched a most interesting drama of "rescue the ferry." By afternoon, it was running normally again. According to the ferry patrol, today is the last day it is in the water. Tonight they will be down there winching the ferry up onto the shore. I guess that should be worthy of a few pictures. Right now, I can see the ferry has a "cat-digger" on board and he's hanging over the edge, breaking up the ice for the ferry as it goes along.

My nursing duties are mainly preventive in nature—that is, until a medical emergency occurs that I must deal with. This week, I was invited to the school feeding program. They had a Thanksgiving dinner with all the trimmings for the kids and all the town. There must have been 100 people there.

The next day I was invited to the adult education pot-luck lunch that they do every Wednesday. I had no warning, so I had no one to take but my dog, Misha. The kids had a splendid time with her.

I also went to the school this week to do the physicals and the eye and hearing checks. My problem is that the kids all seem to have several names. At the school, they are registered under one name, and in the health care system, they are under their birth-registered name, so it gets pretty confusing sometimes.

The coldest we have had here in Arctic Red so far is –28° C. People here don't seem very conscious of the temperatures, but one old-timer told me you can tell how cold it is by watching the birds. He went into an amazing spiel about how they fly differently in different temperatures, how they huddle, how they eat. I found it amazing when all we do is look at a thermometer. He did say that beyond –45°C it was hard to know 'cause the birds don't move at all.

— *Caroline Wiebe**

* This excerpt was taken from a letter contributed to an ongoing research project into Northern nursing experiences. Research and analysis of descriptions of experiences in the many letters collected by this project will be used to document and validate the role of nurses in Canada's North.

living in the northern territories. The structure is still in place, with services provided by physicians, nurses, health educators, dental therapists and community health representatives.

The Current Situation

Nurses have played the greatest role in the delivery of these health services—first with the missionary services provided by church groups and later by the federal government (Keith, 1971). The network of services consists of base hospitals from which satellite nursing stations and community health centres (also staffed by nurses) fan out, supported by community health workers at the local level. The standard nursing station has two or more nurses, and may have a few inpatient beds, cribs and bassinets.

The nurses are responsible for providing primary health care for a community of 200 to 800 people and possibly the people in one or two surrounding smaller communities. The nurses provide treatment services for those who are ill and promotive and preventive services for people in the community, including school health services, pre and postnatal clinics and home visits. The nurses diagnose and treat common illnesses and follow certain standard protocols. They also have access to medical support at the hospital through telephone and can evacuate patients if necessary to the base hospital or to other centres for treatment. Physicians make regular visits to all the nursing stations to see people who require additional care.

By 1988, Medical Services Branch staff had peaked at more than 200 doctors (11 of them First Nations people), over 1000 nurses (150 of whom were First Nations) and over 500 community health workers (Frideres, 1988). In addition to the nursing and medical services described above, the Indian and Northern Health Services provide noninsured health benefits to Inuit and registered Indians. These services include drugs, medical supplies, medical equipment, vision care, dental care, medical transportation, health insurance premiums and co-insurance fees.

The governments of the Northwest Territories and the Yukon have taken over administration and delivery of services and health benefits for Inuit and registered Indians in the territories under agreements with the federal government. Other programs include a National Native Alcohol and Drug Abuse Program which was established to provide culturally relevant, community-based preventive and treatment services, as well as a program directed at minimizing family violence. Medical Services also has a Native Career Development Program to prepare First Nations peoples for careers in the health field.

The aboriginal population is growing more rapidly than the general population in Canada. It is also an average of 10 years younger than the general Canadian population. Figure 12.6 shows the age distribution of the First Nations population. Life expectancy has increased considerably over the past two decades but is still less than that for the rest of the

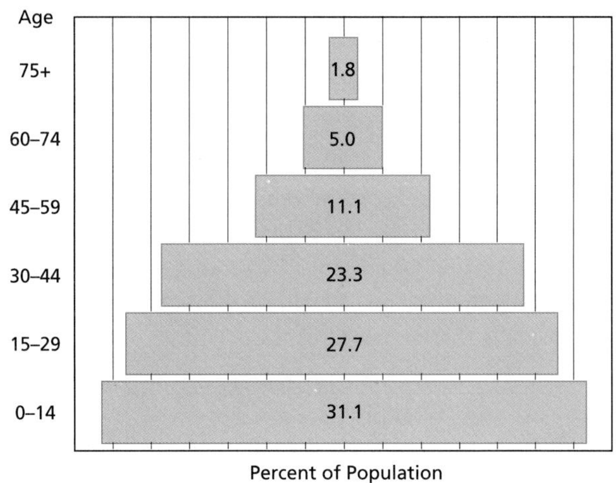

FIGURE 12.6 First Nations population by age

SOURCE: Medical Services Branch, Health Canada, 1996.

Canadian population (see Figure 12.7). There is no doubt that the health care provided by Medical Services did a great deal to improve the health status of First Nations peoples—one has only to look at the considerable decline in infant and child mortality from the 1950s to the 1980s to appreciate this fact. However, the rate is still more than double that of the rest of Canada, and other health statistics strikingly attest to the need for improved health and living conditions.

Keeping in mind the *Active Health Report* (1987), which documented the poor state of health of people in low-income brackets, it is important to note that First Nations peoples as a group occupy the lower-status positions in Canadian society. In 1991, only 37percent of people living on reserves had completed high school, compared with 62 percent in the general Canadian population. Only 3 percent had university education vis-à-vis 13 percent of the general population (Health Canada, 1996).

The unemployment rate among First Nations peoples has been excessively high (around 60 percent, ranging to 90 percent in some parts of the country). Income is corres-

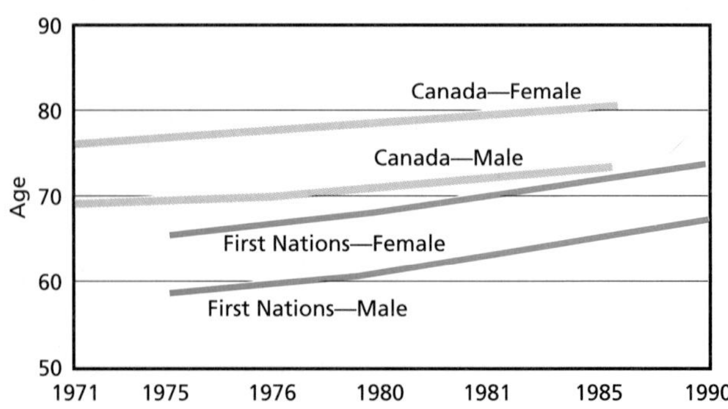

FIGURE 12.7 Life expectancy at birth—First Nations and total Canadian population

SOURCE: Medical Services Branch, Health Canada, 1994.

LOOKING back

In memory of Jean Goodwill 1928–1997

Jean Goodwill, founder of what is now known as the Aboriginal Nurses Association of Canada, recipient of the Order of Canada and long-time advocate for health, passed-away in Regina, Saskatchewan on August 25. She was 69.

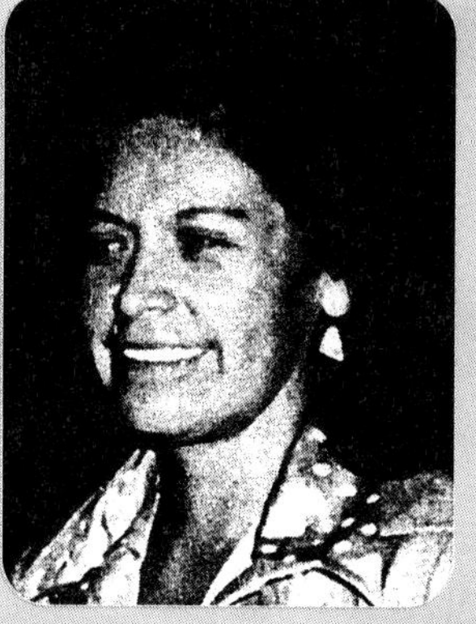

Jean Ida Goodwill Wapasini Apewis devoted her life to advancing the role of Aboriginal nurses in Canada and improving health care services for Aboriginal people. She entered the health field in 1955 as a general duty nurse at the Indian Hospital in Fort Qu'Appelle, Saskatchewan and went on to become a Northern nurse, then Executive Director of the Winnipeg Indian and Métis Friendship Centre. In 1966 she moved to Ottawa, where she started out as co-editor of *Indian News* for the Department of Indian and Northern Affairs, and ended up as special advisor on Indian health to then federal Minister of Health, Monique Bégin in 1980. During her 20 years as a civil servant, Goodwill helped push through programs for Aboriginal people that promoted careers in health, and prevented alcohol and drug abuse. One of her main goals was to convince Ottawa that it should provide financial support to allow Aboriginals greater control of health care in their own communities.

The author of four books, Goodwill was a founding member of both the Native Women's Association of Canada and the National Organization for Indian and Inuit Nurses, which became the Aboriginal Nurses Association of Canada (ANAC). She was the association's president from 1983 to 1990, and was one of the first recipients of the National Aboriginal Achievement Award.

In the mid-1980s, Goodwill retired to the Dakota (Sioux) Standing Buffalo Reserve in Qu'Appelle Valley. She is survived by her husband, Ken.

SOURCE: Canadian Nurses Association 1998

pondingly low, with most of those who work occupying low-status jobs. More than one-half of those living on a reserve, off a reserve and the Inuit population had incomes in the lowest bracket in 1995 (see Figure 12.8). Much of the income comes from government transfer payments, although the income figures do not include income-in-kind from hunting, fishing and similar activities. Housing, which is looked upon as one of the main determinants of the level of welfare of a population, is well below that of the average non-First Nations Canadian (Frideres, 1998; Health Canada, 1996).

The Transfer of Services

The transfer of health services to First Nations peoples can be viewed as part of a devolutionary process that has been going on for the past 25 years. This process started in the 1970s when the federal government turned educational control over to local First Nations authorities. It continued through the 1980s and into the 1990s with the transfer of child and family services and with the development of economic institutions for people of the First Nations that have continued to progress (Gibbons & Associates, 1992).

The push for a transfer of health services was accelerated by passage of the Constitution Act of 1982 and the subsequent movement towards self-government. Between 1983 and 1986, Medical Services funded community health demonstration projects in 31 communities as an experiment with the administrative transfer of health services. The Health Transfer Initiative was announced by Health Minister Jake Epp in 1986. Following a period of consultation with all North American Indian bands in the country, the Treasury

Health Care Transfer

Health transfer enables First Nations to:

- design and manage health programs according to specific community priorities
- mobilize community participation, leading to improved health status
- become recognized as equal participating health care providers within the Canadian health care system
- be autonomous and accountable to their memberships
- enhance self-government.

SOURCE: Health & Welfare Canada, 1992.

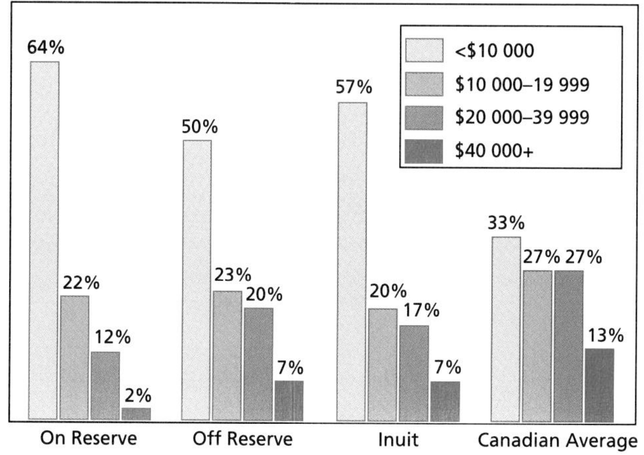

FIGURE 12.8 Income status

SOURCE: Medical Services Branch, Health Canada, 1996

Board of Canada in June 1989 approved authorities and resources for the transfer of Indian health services from the federal government to First Nations wishing to assume responsibility. The long-term goal of the transfer, as stated in a discussion paper that was sent to all Indian chiefs in Canada, is "a more integrated, culturally relevant community health program and improved health conditions for Indian people" (Health & Welfare Canada, 1986; Gibbons & Associates, 1992).

The transfer process was designed to have three phases:

1. research into the health needs of the community and the resources available to meet these needs, with subsequent development of a community health plan
2. negotiation between the First Nations community and government. During this phase, any outstanding issues are resolved and a transfer agreement is signed
3. the actual transfer implementation. As part of the agreement, the community must prepare an annual report for community members and an evaluation of the program to be used for future planning. (Health & Welfare Canada, 1992)

The whole process takes approximately one to two years, or more, in some cases. The health transfer process is going on at the same time as many Indian bands are becoming self-governing. The health transfers appear to be most successful in communities where the two processes are taking place together or where self-government is already in effect. First Nations peoples may also take control of their health services through other funding arrangements with the Medical Services Branch of Health Canada. Contribution agreements, stacked agreements and integrated agreements allow First Nations communities to take increasing control over their own health service delivery. All these agreements can lead to self-government or transfer arrangements.

Early reports indicate that most communities feel they have benefited from the transfer process. At the local level, there has been a development of new skills in planning and management and few negative consequences. First Nations people are involved in the health care of their own communities as members of community and regional health councils and they are involved as front-line workers, as community health representatives and, increasingly, as professional health workers in these communities.

IN REVIEW

- Canada is a multicultural society whose people have come from many different countries in successive waves of immigration:
  - the earliest settlers were the First Nations people (the North American Indian and the Inuit)
  - from the 17th century onward, settlers arrived from France, then Britain, then other European countries
  - from the 1970s, most immigrants have come from Asian countries.
- Canadians speak a total of 126 mother tongues. Of these:
  - 60% speak English
  - 23% speak French
  - 16% speak other languages.
- Canadian policy on multiculturalism:
  - encourages immigrants to retain their own culture
  - creates the need for culturally sensitive nursing care.
- Beliefs about health and health care are closely tied to personal, family and cultural beliefs, including spiritual values and traditional health practices.
- Spirituality has different meanings for different people. In its broadest sense, it denotes the search for meaning in our lives.
  - spirituality is different from religion, which implies adherence to a particular belief system or doctrine
  - spirituality is important for all people but becomes increasing so for the ill and for older persons
  - nurses should be able to assess and, to a certain extent, meet patients' spiritual needs
  - nurses should support and assist patients to maintain their traditional religious practices.
- In Canada, the most common of these are:
  - Western religions—Catholic (46.5%); Protestant (30%); Judaism (1%)
  - Eastern religions—Hinduism; Sikhism; Buddhism (combined, total 3% of population).
- Religious groups differ on such matters as:
  - holy days
  - scriptures
  - permissible foods
  - clothing
  - cleanliness
  - sacraments and rituals
  - transplantation of body parts
  - abortion
  - autopsy
  - care of the dead.

  Nurses must familiarize themselves with the customs and taboos of their patients in order to provide culturally sensitive, comprehensive care.
- Many Canadians today use alternative or complementary medicine and therapies in addition to, or instead of, traditional Western medicine. Types used include:
  - alternative systems of medical practice (e.g., acupuncture, Ayurvedic medicine, naturopathy, shamanism, traditional Chinese medicine)
  - nutrition and lifestyle changes
  - manual healing (e.g., acupressure/shiatzu, aromatherapy, chiropractic medicine, massage therapy, Therapeutic Touch)

- pharmacological and biological treatments (e.g., chelation therapy)
- bioelectrical applications (e.g., electroacupuncture, TENS)
- herbal medicine (e.g., aloe vera, bran, cranberry juice, echinacea, garlic, ginger, gingko, ginseng)
- mind/body control (e.g., faith healing, support groups, biofeedback, music therapy, meditation, hypnotherapy).

- Problems in accessing health care differ for different groups of people.
  - for people in the general population: unequal distribution of health resources geographically; negative attitudes of some health professionals towards the poor, the homeless, substance abusers, people from other cultures or those having other healing traditions
  - for immigrants and refugees: problems with health insurance regulations; lack of common language; low self-esteem or insecurity; conflict with traditional beliefs and practices; cultural prejudices; inconvenient hours for health services; racial tensions with health providers.
- Crossing the barriers to effective health care involves:
  - awareness of one's own cultural limitations
  - openness
  - appreciation and respect for other points of view
  - viewing intercultural interactions as learning experiences
  - using cultural resources as interventions
  - acknowledging the integrity and value of all cultures.
- Health care issues regarding the First Nations people include the facts that:
  - traditional health practices used shamanism and herbal medicine
  - the population was decimated by diseases brought by European colonization
  - traditional health practices were gradually discontinued
  - responsibility for health care was gradually assumed by the federal government
  - a network of hospitals, nursing stations and community health centres has been established across the North
  - there has been considerable improvement in health, but more needs to be done
  - the current transfer of services to First Nations people is intended to provide more culturally relevant services to meet community needs.

Critical Thinking Activities

1. Who were the first members of your family to settle in Canada? What country did they come from? When did they arrive in Canada, and where did they settle first?
2. Examine your own health beliefs and practices.
   - What do you think causes illness?
   - What health practices (preventive and curative) are traditionally used in your family?
   - Are there religious traditions or taboos that might influence a hospital stay by someone in your family?
   - What influence has your background (ethnicity, religion and education) had on your health beliefs and practices?
   - Do your beliefs and practices concur or conflict with concepts being taught in your nursing program?
3. In discussion with classmates, compare backgrounds of ethnic origin, religion, health beliefs and practices and modifications with those that have occurred or are occurring.
4. If possible, talk with someone among your friends or acquaintances who comes from a different ethnic background than your own. Explore with this individual:
   a. what it was like growing up, either in his or her homeland or in Canada, as a member of an ethnic group different from your own.
   b. what experiences family members have had with the Canadian health care system:
   - How did the individual enter the health care system? Through a family physician? The emergency department? A clinic or hospital visit? A community health nurse?
   - How did the person and the family feel about the experience?
   - What comparisons did they make to the care they were used to receiving in their country of origin?
     - Did they encounter any difficulty getting care? If so, what were the problems? How were these problems resolved?
5. Talk with a nurse who has worked or is working in the North about his or her experiences there. If this is not possible, read the articles in the March 1994 issue of *The Canadian Nurse* on nursing in the North (Bates; Brumwell & Janes; Edgecombe; Graham; and Morewood). Write a short report outlining the benefits and drawbacks of working in a nursing station, community health centre or hospital in the North.

KEY TERMS

ethnicity p. 269
culture p. 269
ethnocentricity p. 270
cultural relativism p. 270
socialization p. 270
acculturation p. 270
melting pot p. 270
cultural mosaic p. 270
First Nations p. 273
Inuit p. 273
allophone p. 274
spirit p. 276
spirituality p. 276
transcendence p. 276
religion p. 276
soma p. 277
mensa p. 277
pneuma p. 277
pathos p. 277
machos p.277
Zoroastrianism p. 279
sudreh p. 279
kusti p. 279
Judaism p. 279
synagogue p. 279
rabbi p. 279
yarmulke p. 279
Christianity p. 280
baptism p. 280
communion p. 280
anointing of the sick p. 280
Islam p. 281
Muslim p. 281
Allah p. 281
Koran p. 281
mosque p. 281
muezzins p. 281
halal p. 282
Baha'i p. 282
Hinduism p. 282
Dewali p. 282
Karma p. 282
sari p. 282
salwar kameze p. 282
Sikhism p. 283
kosh p. 283
kanga p. 283
kara p.283
kirpan p. 283
kaccha p. 283
Buddhism p. 283
alternative medicine p. 284
complementary p. 284
acupuncture p. 284
chi p. 284
meridian p. 284
Ayurvedic medicine p. 284
pancha karma p. 285
naturopathy p. 285
shaman p. 285
traditional Chinese medicine p. 285
qui gong p. 285
yoga p. 285
tai chi p. 285
acupressure p. 285
shiatzu p. 286
aromatherapy p. 286
chiropractic medicine p. 286
massage therapy p. 286
therapeutic touch p. 286
Chelation therapy p. 286
electroacupuncture p. 286
TENS p. 286
herbal medicine p. 286
faith healing p. 287
laying on of hands p. 287
support/mutual aid groups p. 287
biofeedback p. 287
music therapy p. 287
meditation p. 287
hypnosis p. 287
cultural sensitivity p. 289

References

BADETS, J. (1993, Summer). Canada's immigrants: Recent trends. *Canadian Social Trends, 29*, 8–11.

BALZER-RILEY, J.W. (1996). *Communications in nursing: Communicating assertively and responsibly in nursing—A guide book.* (3rd ed.). St. Louis: Mosby.

BATES, V. (1994). What is a northern nurse? *The Canadian Nurse. 90*(3), 26–31.

BENTLEY, S. (1986). *Religions of our neighbours.* (Vols. 1–8). Coquitlam, B.C.: Bentley West.

BERUBE, J. (1990). *Delivering culturally sensitive care.* Vancouver: B.C. Health Association.

BOBET, E. (1989, Winter). Indian mortality. *Canadian Social Trends, 15*, 11–14.

BRISSON, D.P., & DESLAURIERS, C.L. (1992). Les groupes minoritaires visibles. *Canadian Nurse, 88*(3), 33–35.

BRUMWELL, A. & JANES, C. (1994). Primary healthcare in Rac-Edzo. *The Canadian Nurse. 90*(3), 37–38.

BURTON-GOLDBERG GROUP. (1995). *Alternative medicine: The definitive guide.* Fife, WA: Future Medicine Publishing.

CANADA'S FAMILY TREE: CELEBRATING OUR DIVERSITY. (1992, Spring). *Royal Bank Reporter.*

CANADIAN NURSES ASSOCIATION. (1997). *Code of ethics for registered nurses.* Ottawa: Author.

CHOW, J.A.D. (1997). *Nursing beyond duality: The integrated practice of wholeheartedness.* Unpublished major paper submitted in partial fulfilment of the requirements for the degree of Master of Science in Nursing. Vancouver: University of British Columbia.

COLOMBO, J.R. (Ed.). (1992). *1993 Canadian global almanac.* Toronto: Macmillan.

CONN, J.W. (Ed.). (1986). Women's spirituality: Resources for Christian development. Mahwah, NJ: Paulist Press.

COUSINS, N. (1994). *Healer within: The Parabola book of healing* [an expanded edition of the "Healing" issue of *Parabola* magazine (Spring, 1993), pp. 125–127].

DAVIDSON, P. (1986). *A faith of our own: Living and believing in an age of change.* Toronto: Anglican Book Centre.

EDGECOMBE, N. (1994). Northern nurses' petition. *The Canadian Nurse. 90*(3), 39.

EPP, J. (1986). *Achieving health for all: A framework for health promotion.* Ottawa: Minister of Supply & Services.

ERIKSSON, K. (1997). Caring, spirituality and suffering. In M.S. Roach (Ed.), *Caring from the heart: The convergence of caring and spirituality* (pp. 68–84). Mahwah, NJ: Paulist Press.

FARNSWORTH, N.R., et al. (1985). Medical plants in therapy. *Bulletin of the World Health Organization, 63*(6), 965–981. Reprinted in Classical Botanical Reprint No. 212. Austin, TX: American Botanical Council.

FERRAR, G. (1995). *Cultural anthropology: An applied perspective.* New York: West.

FRIDERES, J.S. (1988). Racism and health: The case of the native people. In B.S. Bolaria & H.D.Dickinson (Eds.), *Sociology of health care in Canada*, (pp. 135–147). Toronto: Harcourt Brace Jovanovich.

FUGH-BERMAN, A. (1996). *Alternative medicine: What works.* Tucson, AZ: Odonian Press.

GIBBONS, A. & ASSOCIATES. (1992). *Short-term evaluation of Indian health transfer.* Victoria, BC: Author.

GRAHAM, K. (1994). Inservice education for northern nurses. *The Canadian Nurse. 90*(3), 33–36.

GRIFFITH, K. (1996). *Religious aspects of nursing care.* Vancouver: Author (Box 172072, Vancouver, BC V6R 4P2).

GROSSMAN, R. (1985). *The other medicines.* Garden City, NY: Doubleday.

GRYPMA, S. (1993). Culture shock. *Canadian Nurse, 89*(8), 33–36.

GUINNESS, A.E., & RUTHERFORD, A.P. (1993). *Family guide to natural medicine.* Montreal: Reader's Digest Association (Canada).

HALL, B.A. (1997, March). Spirituality in terminal illness: An alternative view of theory. *Journal of Holistic Nursing, 15*(1), 82–96.

HEALTH & WELFARE CANADA. (1986). *A discussion paper on the transfer of Indian health programs for consultation with the Indian people.* Ottawa: Author.

HEALTH & WELFARE CANADA. (1987). The Active Health Report: Perspective on Canada's Health Promotion Survey, 1985. Ottawa: Ministry of Supply & Services. (Catalogue no. H39-106/1987E)

HEALTH & WELFARE CANADA. (1992). *Health transfer. Year-end report, 1991–1992.* Ottawa: Medical Services Branch, Health & Welfare Canada.

HEALTH CANADA. (1994). Life expectancy at birth. First Nations and total Canadian population. Ottawa: Medical Services Branch.

HEALTH CANADA. (1996). Diagnostic on the Health of First Nations and Inuit People (draft document). Ottawa: Medical Services Branch.

HENLEY, A. (1983a). *Asians in Britain: Caring for Hindus and their families—Religious aspects of care.* Cambridge, UK: National Extension College.

HENLEY, A. (1983b). *Caring for Sikhs and their families: Religious aspects of care.* Cambridge, UK: National Extension College.

HONG FOOK MENTAL HEALTH ASSOCIATION. (1986). *Assessment and treatment of Chinese patients: A holistic model.* Toronto: Author.

JILEK, W.G. (1982). *Indian healing.* Surrey, BC: Hancock House.

JOHNSTONE, C.B. (1990). *Spiritual aspects of palliative cancer care.* Working paper prepared for the Expert Committee on Cancer Pain Relief of the World Health Organization. Vancouver: B.C. Cancer Agency.

KEITH, C.W. (1971). Leadership in nursing north of sixty. *Nursing Clinics of North America, 6*(3), 479–488.

KENNISON, M.M. (1987). Faith: An untapped health resource. *Journal of Psychosocial Nursing, 25*(10), 28–30.

KRIEGER, D. (1975). Therapeutic touch: The imprimateur of nursing. *American Journal of Nursing,* 784–787.

KRIEGER, D. (1979). *Therapeutic touch: How to use your hands to heal.* Englewood Cliffs, NJ: Prentice Hall.

LEININGER, M. (1978). *Transcultural nursing: Concepts, theories and practices.* New York: Wiley.

LEININGER, M. (1995). *Transcultural nursing: Concepts, theories, research and practices.* (2nd ed.). New York: McGraw-Hill.

LEININGER, M. (1997). Transcultural spirituality: A comparative care and health focus. In M.S. Roach (Ed.), *Caring from the heart: The convergence of caring and spirituality* (pp. 99–118). Mahwah, NJ: Paulist Press.

LUNA, L., & CAMERON, C. (1988) Leininger's transcultural nursing. In J.J. Fitzpatrick & A.L. Whall, *Conceptual models of nursing.* Norwalk, CT: Appleton & Lange, 227–240.

LYNCH, E.W., & HANSON, M.J. (1992). *Developing crosscultural competence.* Baltimore: Paul H. Brooks.

MARTIN, J.D. (1985). Baha'i faith. *The Canadian Encyclopaedia.* Edmonton: Hurtig.

MASI, R. (1993). Multicultural health: Principles and Policies. In R. Masi, L. Mensah, & K.A. McLeod (Eds.), *Health and cultures: Policies, professional practice and education.* (Vol. 1, pp. 11–31). Oakville, ON: Mosaic Press.

MASLOW, A.H. (1970). *Motivation and personality.* (2nd ed.). New York: Harper & Row.

McCULLOCH, C.H. (1997). The care of older persons. In M.S. Roach (Ed.), *Caring from the heart: The convergence of caring and spirituality* (pp. 135–148). Mahwah, NJ: Paulist Press.

MOREWOOD, N. (1994). Nursing in Northwest Territories. *The Canadian Nurse. 90*(3), 26–31.

MULTICULTURALISM & CITIZENSHIP CANADA. (1990). *The Canadian Multiculturalism Act—A guide for Canadians.* Ottawa: Author.

MURRAY, M., & PIZZOMO, J. (1991). What is natural medicine? *Encyclopedia of Natural Medicine.* Rockland, CA: Prima.

NAGAI-JACOBSON, M.G., & BURKHARDT, M.A. (1989). Spirituality: Cornerstone of holistic nursing practice. *Holistic Nursing Practice, 3*(3), 18–26.

NON PARLO NE' INGLESE NE' FRANCESE. (1993, Winter) *Canadian Social Trends, 31,* 26–28.

O'CONNOR, B.B. (1995). *Healing traditions: Alternative medicine and the health professions.* Philadelphia: University of Pennsylvania Press.

OLSON, K.G. (1990). *The encyclopedia of alternative health care.* New York: Simon & Shuster.

PORTER, J. (1979). *The measure of Canadian society: Education, equality and opportunity.* Toronto: Gage.

RENAUD, V., & BADETS, J. (1993, Fall). Ethnic diversity in the 1990s. *Canadian Social Trends, 30,* 17–22.

ROACH, M.S. (Ed.). (1997). *Caring from the heart: The convergence of caring and spirituality.* Mahwah, NJ: Paulist Press.

SHAH, C.P., & DUBESKI, G. (1993). First Nations peoples in urban settings: Health issues. In R. Masi, L. Mensah, & K.A. McLeod (Eds.), *Health and cultures. Policies, professional practice and education.* (Vol. 1, pp. 71–93). Oakville, ON: Mosaic Press.

SHAW, E. (1986). *60 second Shiatzu.* New York: Mills & Sanderson.

SIGGNER, A.J. (1989, Winter). The Inuit. *Canadian Social Trends, 15,* 8–10.

STATISTICS CANADA. (1996–1997). Ethic composition of Canada's population, 1996. (Catalogue no. 93F0026XDB96002 in the Nation Series; available at http://www.statcan.ca/english/census96/Feb17/e02can.htm)

STATISTICS CANADA. (1997). *The daily 1996 census: Immigration and citizenship.* Ottawa: Author. (Catalogue no. 11-001E)

STATISTICS CANADA. (1998). *The daily 1996 census: Ethnic origin, visible minorities.* Ottawa: Author. (Catalogue no. 11-001E)

STEWART, E. (1991). *The Dene and Na-dene Indian migration, 1233 AD: Escape from Ghenghis Khan to America.* Columbus, GA: Institute for the Study of American Cultures.

STOLL, R. (1979, September). Guidelines for spiritual assessment. *American Journal of Nursing,* 1574–1577.

THE CONCISE OXFORD DICTIONARY (1995). Oxford: Oxford University Press.

TUCKER, P. (1965). *Cultures of the North Pacific Coast.* San Francisco: Chandler.

TYLER, V.E. (1993). *The honest herbal: A sensible guide to the use of herbs and related remedies.* (3rd ed.). New York: Pharmaceutical Products Press.

VANCOUVER HEALTH DEPARTMENT. (1993). Discussions with G.C. Mumick, Multicultural Health Education Consultant, Vancouver, B.C.

WATSON, J. (1996). Nursing perspectives on alternative medicine. Lecture presented at the Harvard Medical School, Department of Continuing Medicine.

WEXLER-MORRISON, N., ANDERSON, J. & RICHARDSON, E. (1990). *Cross-cultural caring.* Vancouver: University of British Columbia Press.

ZUMBRO VALLEY MEDICAL SOCIETY. (1975). *Religious aspects of medical care.* Rochester, MN: The Catholic Hospital Association.

Additional Readings

ANDREWS, M., & BOYLE, J. (1996). *Transcultural concepts in nursing care.* Glenview, Il: Scott Foresman.

BHIMANI, R. & ACORN S. (1998). Managing Within a Culturally diverse environment. *Canadian Nurse. 94*(8), 32–36.

BRONSTEIN, J.G., CHESNEY, A.P. & SALCIDO, R. (1995). Health and Organizational issues in managing a multicultural work force. *Family & Community Health, 18* (2), 1–8.

BRUHN, M. (1996). Healing hands. *Canadian Nurse, 92*(1), 32–34.

BRYANT, J. (1996). Therapeutic touch in home healthcare: One nurse's experience. *Home Healthcare Nurse,* 14(8), 580–586.

CAMPINHA-BACOTE, J. (1995). The quest for cultural competence in nursing care. *Nursing Forum, 30*(4), 19–24.

CLARKE, H.E. (1997). Research in nursing and cultural diversity: Working with First Nations peoples. *Canadian Journal of Nursing Research, 29*(2), 11–25.

DOWD, S.B., GIGER, J.N., & DAVIDHIZAR R. (1998). Transcultural assessment model by health professions. *International Nursing Review, 45*(4), 119–122.

FEHRING, R.J., MILLER, J.F., & SHAW, C. (1997). Spiritual well-being, religiosity, hope, depression and other mood states in elderly people coping with cancer. *Oncology Nursing Forum, 24*(4), 663–671.

GIGER, J.N., & DAVIDHIZAR, R.E. (1995). *Transcultural nursing assessment and intervention.* (2nd ed.). St. Louis: Mosby.

GIGER, J.N. & DAVIDHIZAR R.E. (1998). *Canadian transcultural nursing: Assessment & intervention.* St Louis: Mosby Yearbook.

GURUGE, S., & DONNER, G. (1996). Transcultural nursing in Canada. *Canadian Nurse, 92*(8), 36–40.

KAYE, J., & ROBINSON, K.M. (1994). Spirituality among caregivers. *Image, 26*(3), 218–221.

LANE, N.J. (1992). A spirituality of being: Women with disabilities. *Journal of Applied Rehabilitation Counselling, 22*(4), 53–58.

NARAYAN, M.C. (1997). Cultural assessment in home healthcare. *Home Healthcare Nurse, 15*(10), 663–670.

NARAYAN, M.C., & REA, H. (1997). The South Asian client. *Home Healthcare Nurse, 15*(7), 461–469.

PETERSON, B. (1996). The mind–body connection. *Canadian Nurse, 92*(1), 29–31.

POLASCHEK, N.R. (1998). Cultural safety: A new concept in nursing people of different ethnicities. *Journal of Advanced Nursing, 27*(3), 452–457.

REIMER, S. (1995). Nurses' descriptions of caring for culturally diverse clients. Unpublished masters thesis, Vancouver: University of British Columbia.

SHESTOSKY, B. (1995). Health-related concerns of Canadian aboriginal people residing in urban areas. *International Nursing Review, 42*(1), 23–26.

SHULMAN, B. (1997). The connection between culture and family medicine. *B.C. Medical Journal, 39*(7), 418.

SPECTOR, R. (1996). *Cultural diversity in health and illness.* (4th ed.). Norwalk, CT; Appleton & Lange.

SPRUHAN, J.B. (1996). Beyond traditional nursing care: Cultural awareness and successful home health care nursing. *Home Healthcare Nurse, 14*(6), 444–449.

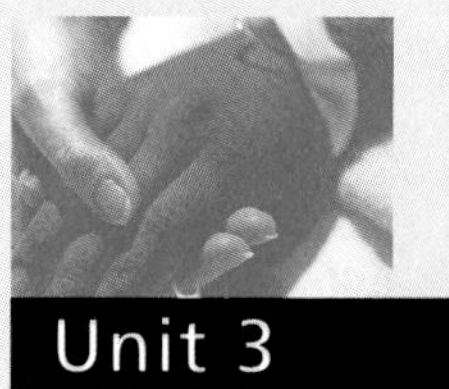

Unit 3

Skills Basic to Nursing Practice

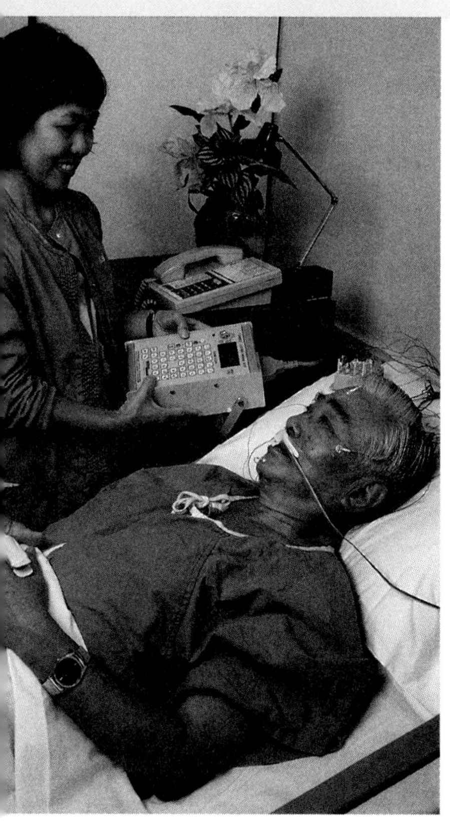

Chapter 13

Theories and Conceptual Frameworks for Nursing Practice

OUTLINE

Central Questions

1. What do the terms theory, model, conceptual model, conceptual framework, grand theory, mega-theory and metaparadigm mean?
2. What is the difference between a concrete and an abstract concept?
3. What concepts are considered central to nursing?
4. What are the three levels of nursing theory?
5. How have developments in the humanities and in the biological and physical sciences influenced the development of nursing theory?
6. What differentiates one conceptual model of nursing from another?
7. What is the value of nursing theories for nursing practice, education and research?
8. How do you use a nursing model in clinical practice?

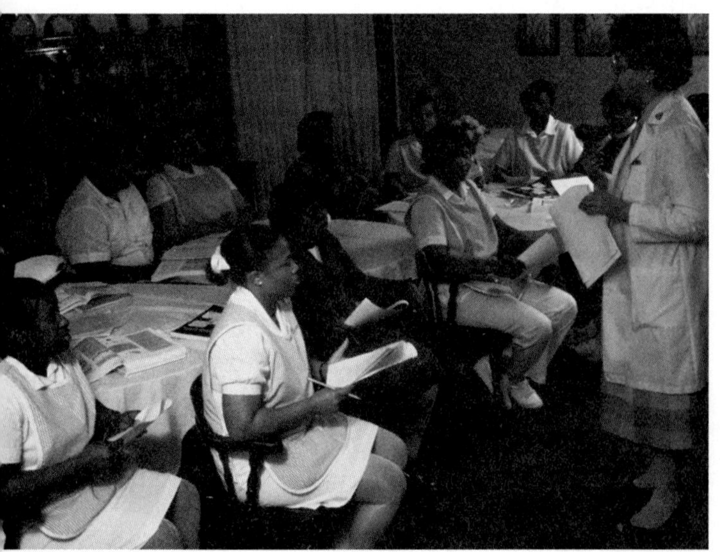

Introduction

Theory is the process by which nursing becomes a science and a special way of human caring.

Roach, 1992

The caring professions are as old as humankind. There have always been healers, wise men and wise women who assisted in the birth of infants, cared for the sick and gathered medicinal herbs from which they concocted medicines to heal ailments. In some societies, the healer and the caregiver were one and the same. In others, the healers became a specialized group known variously as *wizards*, *witches*, *shamans*, and later, *doctors* or *physicians*. Those who nurtured the sick—the caregivers—became another specialized group: the *nurses*, from the Greek word for *nurture*.

Behavioural psychologists tell us that the knowledge and skills of both groups were probably learned initially through a process of trial and error, with medicines and techniques found to be effective passed down from one generation to the next. There are others who believe that there is a collective consciousness, or "collective knowing," that is imprinted in the subconscious memory of the human race and that provides us with an intuitive understanding of what needs to be done for the survival of the species. Those who subscribe to the latter theory believe that we can tap into this archetypal knowledge if we open ourselves up to it (Agan, 1987).

Whichever theory you subscribe to, there is evidence to support the view that, as the knowledge and skills of healing and of caring for the sick became more clearly defined, an apprenticeship form of training evolved. Self-selected, chosen by the master or, sometimes, by the community, apprentices learned by observing, by listening and, then, by carrying out procedures and preparing medications themselves under the watchful eye of their role model. Both nursing and medicine went through the same process.

In nursing, apprenticeship as preparation for practice lasted well into the second half of the 19th century, when Florence Nightingale opened the first truly educational program for nurses at St. Thomas' Hospital in London, England, in 1860. For the better part of a century, most nurses were prepared in hospital schools modelled on the Nightingale school. There are many who say that nursing did not progress from the apprenticeship method of training until the middle of the 20th century. Hospital schools that followed in the wake of the Nightingale school gave higher priority to service by students than to the educational component of the programs.

Nursing managed finally to move from the apprenticeship mode and into the realm of professional education based on an emerging nursing science. As with the evolution of knowledge in other fields, the development of nursing science is a history of shifting ideas. Many traditional nursing procedures have been discarded, others have been modified and the value of some reaffirmed in studies undertaken by nurse researchers.

An example of a modified traditional procedure is the back rub—a nursing intervention used over the years by thousands of students and practitioners. Nurses used to rub the patient's back with alcohol after a bed bath and also as part of the "evening care" routine in most hospitals. There was probably good reason to use rubbing alcohol in the days when infections were rampant and there was a need to cool the skin of feverish patients. This practice has long since been replaced by back rubs for bedridden patients using emollient creams or lotions that do not have such a drying effect on the skin. Practitioners no longer do things simply because it is the traditional way of doing them but, rather, with an understanding of the rationale behind their actions. Students learn not only to carry out nursing interventions with skill and dexterity; they also learn why these interventions are implemented, through a process of logical reasoning.

The importance of certain traditional practices has been reaffirmed in the current emphasis on the caring aspect of the nurse's role. We now realize that the human aspect of caring is just as important as developing knowledge and skills. This caring aspect, historically passed from expert to novice in apprenticeship programs, was almost overshadowed by the emphasis placed on the science of nursing.

Leininger (1988) says that human caring is a universal phenomenon which, she feels, is the "central, dominant and unifying feature" for the body of nursing knowledge (p. 152). The focus of nursing is on people and on how people cope with their state of health, while the focus of medicine has historically been on people's illnesses. Nursing theory is what differentiates the focus of nursing from that of medicine and other disciplines. It also facilitates the identification of health problems and provides nurses with a rational basis for their actions. Nursing theory guides the nurse in making clinical decisions. Increasingly, nurses in clinical practice are using theoretical models not only to provide direction for their practice, but also to develop standards for evaluating the quality of care (Campbell, 1987; Casey, 1989).

Credit for the tremendous advances in nursing, over the past few decades, belongs to the nurse researchers who have pushed back the boundaries of knowledge in the field, to the nurse clinicians whose expertise provides us with clues about the nature of nursing practice and to the nurse theorists who have contributed the framework on which to base further nursing knowledge. In this chapter, we explore the nature of nursing knowledge, the evolution of nursing theories and the value of theories for education, research and practice.

The Nature of Nursing Knowledge

In your readings, you will come across a number of different terms used in discussing nursing theories. *Theory*, *model*, *conceptual model*, *conceptual framework*, *grand theory*, *mega-theory* and *metaparadigm* are all terms that are used to describe theoretical frameworks. Different theorists ascribe different meanings to some of these terms. We will discuss the terms and provide you with workable definitions.

Theories and Conceptual Models

The terms *theory* and *conceptual model* are used interchangeably in much of the nursing literature; however, they are not the same. According to Watson (1988), "A theory is an imaginative grouping of knowledge, ideas and experience that are represented symbolically and seek to illuminate a given phenomenon" (p. 1). In other words, a **theory** is a supposition, or system of ideas that has been proposed to explain a given happening in the world. For example, Newton proposed the theory of gravity concerning the gravitational pull of the earth's centre to account for the apple's always falling from tree to ground rather than the other way around.

A **conceptual model** is the diagrammatic representation of a theory. You have probably seen a number of conceptual models, particularly in courses such as chemistry and physics, where models have been used for many years to describe various theories. Most nurse theorists develop diagrams of their theories, and the term *conceptual model*, or simply, *model*, refers to both the diagram and the theory. The models are also referred to as **conceptual frameworks**.

Sometimes you will see conceptual models in nursing referred to as *grand theories* or *mega-theories*. Some theorists, for example, Fawcett (1989), use the term *metaparadigm* to refer to the grand theories (conceptual models), reserving the term *theory* for smaller, testable suppositions. We prefer to use the generic term *theory* as defined above. The term *metaparadigm* comes from two Greek words, *meta* meaning *with* and *paradigm* meaning *pattern*. Thus, **metaparadigm**, **grand theory** and **mega-theory** are terms used to describe the essential pattern of a discipline. Basically, they imply a global statement that identifies phenomena (concepts or ideas) that are of interest to the discipline.

Theories and conceptual models are found in all disciplines. They can be classified into three levels:

1. **descriptive**—these theories classify or describe phenomena of concern to a discipline, for example, the descriptions of person, health, environment and nursing stated explicitly or implicitly inferred in all conceptual nursing models. They are needed when there is nothing or not much known about the phenomenon
2. **explanatory**—these specify relationships among phenomena. Orem (1995), for example, identifies linkages between person, environment and nursing when she talks about the role of the nurse in helping the person to cope with developmental changes
3. **predictive**—these move beyond explaining relationships to predicting precise relationships among certain characteristics of a phenomenon or specific differences among groups. Predictive theories deal with the principle of cause and effect. This type of theory may be used to suggest interventions. Nursing does not as yet have very many prescriptive theories that tell us what interventions are best in which situation because much basic descriptive research on phenomena and their relationships still needs to be done (Fawcett, 1989; Fawcett & Downs, 1986).

The concepts that are considered central to nursing—the ones discussed in all nursing theories (although not always explicitly defined)—are:

1. **person**—the individual, family, group or community that is the recipient of nursing care
2. **environment**—includes both the social and the physical environments
3. **health**—the patient's state of wellness/illness
4. **nursing**—the actions taken by the nurse on behalf of, or in conjunction with, the patient (Fawcett, 1989, p. 21).

Concepts

In discussing theories and conceptual models, it is important to have a clear understanding of the term *concept*. A **concept** is a complex mental formulation of an object, a property (characteristic) or an event that is derived from an individual's perceptual experience. Some concepts, such as *chair*, *apple* and *book*, are concrete. They can be observed, touched or seen, and there is a high level of agreement on their meaning. For example, a chair is a chair to most people, whether it is a rocking chair, a folding chair or an office chair. **Empirical** concepts "are ... precise and include measurable concepts, such as hours of sleep and body temperature" (McKenna, 1997, p. 57).

Other concepts are **abstract**; their meaning is inferred from direct or indirect evidence in the real world. Abstract concepts are more general in nature and are related to an event or to a property of something. Examples of abstract concepts include the emotions—*love*, *hatred*, *prejudice*; events—*Christmas*, *Passover*, *Ramadan*; and properties—*normalcy*, *abnormality*. Some abstract concepts can be observed directly and some are more intangible. *Pain* is an example of an abstract concept that can be observable—from the patient's facial expression, or attempts to protect an injured part of the body. As we discussed in Chapter 2, health is an intangible concept that each individual views according to his or her own perspective.

There is usually less agreement about the meaning of abstract concepts than there is about concrete concepts. There is a need to confirm, or validate, with people exactly what they mean when they use an abstract term. The concepts central to nursing—person, environment, health and nursing—are abstract concepts. Like other abstract concepts, the terms have different meanings for different people. Later in the chapter, we will take a look at the different meanings ascribed to the basic concepts of person, environment, health and nursing by some theorists.

The Evolution of Nursing Theories

Numerous authors have traced the development of nursing theory, and it is not the purpose of this text to duplicate their work. Nor do we believe that, as beginning students, you need exposure to all the nursing theories that have been articulated over the past few decades. We will, therefore, limit our discussion to major trends in the development of nursing theory, illustrating these with conceptual frameworks that have been adopted in Canadian nursing schools and health agencies.

Florence Nightingale is often spoken of as the first modern nurse theorist. Long before the nurses of this century began questioning what nursing is and is not, Nightingale had articulated her views on the subject. These views are recorded in her well-known *Notes on Nursing*, first published in 1859 following her experience in the Crimean War. In these *Notes*, Nightingale (1859) proposed a philosophy for nursing that outlined the basic premise on which nursing should be practised and the functions nurses should undertake. Nightingale felt that nursing was quite distinct from medicine, the focus of nursing being to put "the patient in the best condition for nature to act upon him" (Nightingale; cited in George, 1990, p. 36).

The nurse's responsibility was to provide a clean, safe, quiet, pleasant environment and to provide an adequate diet to promote the patient's recuperative powers. Nightingale's emphasis on a clean, sweet-smelling environment is understandable when one considers that sanitary conditions in most towns and cities of the late 19th century were deplorable. Secular hospitals were with few exceptions dirty, foul-smelling places, staffed by slovenly workers who no doubt lived in deplorable conditions themselves. The first Public Health Law in England was enacted in 1875. This law established standards for sanitation, quarantine regulations for communicable diseases, and measures to ensure safe water and food supplies. Most Canadian provinces subsequently passed laws modelled after the English version during the latter years of the 19th century.

Using today's terminology, we might say that Nightingale focussed on the interaction between the recipient of nursing care (the patient) and the environment, with nursing interventions directed at manipulating the environment in order to promote the person's return to health.

Early 20th-Century Nursing Theory

The period following Florence Nightingale's era—the first half of the 20th century—was not always viewed as positive for nursing. It saw the hospitals become the primary focus for health care and physicians the dominant force in the provision of health services. Nursing schools, which Nightingale had envisioned as separate educational institutions, became instead part of the nursing service of hospitals. Students were looked upon as a source of cheap labour in most hospital "training schools." Most courses were taught by physicians, and most hospitals were administered by physicians—nursing was viewed simply as an extension of (and subordinate to) medicine. Nursing was considered a vocation for women, whereas the medical profession was for men, with very few exceptions. Indeed, nurses were considered to be "handmaidens to the physician."

It was not until the 1950s and early 1960s that nurses began to assert their independence. A number of factors were involved in this movement—feminism, the increasing number of nurses prepared in university schools and the emergence of graduate programs in nursing. Struggling to find their own identity separate from medicine, nurses kept asking, "What is nursing?" Eventually, some nurses began to articulate their views. Gradually, the four basic concepts emerged as common themes in the descriptions of nursing theory by the early theorists. In developing their views on nursing, these theorists also began to explore the relationships between the four concepts—for example, how the environment affected the person and his or her health, and what actions nurses could take to help bring about changes in the health status of the person they were caring for (Chinn & Kramer, 1991; Whall, 1989).

THE INFLUENCE OF THE HUMANISTS

Many of the early nurse theorists were influenced by developments taking place in the behavioural sciences of psychology, sociology and education. These disciplines provided a humanistic perspective from which to explore ideas central to nursing. Three of the humanists whose work was particularly influential in the development of nursing theory were Carl Rogers, Edward Thorndike and Abraham Maslow.

During the 1940s and 1950s, Rogers's nondirective approach to counselling had revolutionized the field of psychology. This approach was based on the premise that all people have the capacity to solve their own problems, given the opportunity to work them through with an empathetic counsellor who permits the patient to direct the therapeutic process (Rogers, 1961).

Thorndike was the author of *Human Nature and the Social Order* (1940) and is well known for his work in the field of education. He postulated a set of "laws of learning," which has been widely used in courses on the nature of learning.

Abraham Maslow's (1970) primary contribution to nursing theory is found in his hierarchy of human needs, which we discussed in Chapter 8. His prioritization of needs is directly relevant to nurses, who are responsible for attending to a patient's many, and often conflicting, needs.

Two of the most influential of the early nursing theorists of the 20th century were Hildegarde Peplau and Virginia Henderson. Peplau's work shows the influence of the humanists, in particular, that of Rogers. Her work embraces his emphasis on patient-directed therapy. Peplau (1952) saw nursing as a "significant, therapeutic, interpersonal process" and coined the term "therapeutic use of self," which has subsequently been incorporated into our nursing language. She viewed the nurse's role in the therapeutic process as assisting the individual in solving problems through increasing interpersonal and problem-solving competencies (Forchuk, 1990).

Virginia Henderson has had considerable influence on nursing in North America and around the world. She is well known for her *Textbook on the Principles and Practice of Nursing* (1955; co-authored with Canadian Bertha Harmer), subsequent texts on the nature of nursing (1966) and numerous scholarly papers. She defined nursing as assisting "... the individual, sick or well, in performance of those activities ... that he or she would perform unaided if he or she had the strength, will or knowledge, ... to gain independence as rapidly as possible" (Harmer & Henderson, 1955, p. 4).

Henderson's work reflects the influence of Thorndike and Maslow, both of whom saw the person as an integrated whole. Henderson believed in the uniqueness of the individual and in the inseparability of mind and body. Henderson's well-known definition of nursing and list of fundamental needs extended Thorndike's research in the field of psychology to apply to the person in hospital (Fitzpatrick & Whall, 1996).

Henderson identified 14 fundamental needs. These are the need to:

1. breathe normally
2. eat or drink adequately
3. eliminate body wastes
4. move and maintain desirable postures
5. sleep and rest
6. select suitable clothes—dress and undress
7. maintain body temperature within normal range by adjusting clothing and modifying the environment
8. keep the body clean and well groomed and protect the integument
9. avoid dangers in the environment and avoid injuring others
10. communicate with others in expressing emotions, needs, fears or opinions
11. worship according to one's faith
12. work in such a way that there is a sense of accomplishment
13. play or participate in various forms of recreation
14. learn, discover or satisfy the curiosity that leads to normal development and health and use the available health facilities (Adam, 1991, pp. 14–15).

The nurse's actions should be directed to promoting an individual's optimum independence in meeting these needs (Henderson, 1966). We are indebted to Evelyn Adam, a Canadian nurse theorist, for presenting Henderson's philosophy of nursing in the structure of a conceptual model (Chong Choi, 1989; Adam, 1991).

One can see in Henderson's work the foundational ideas that Dorothea E. Orem used in her self-care conceptual framework, which is also based on a needs approach. Orem is another early American nurse theorist whose work has continued to evolve over the past two decades. The major theme of Orem's conceptual theory is that human beings have self-care needs. These needs may be universal; they may be developmental, changing as the individual passes from one stage of life to the next; or they may be related to the individual's health status.

Orem saw nursing as a helping service and the nurse's role as helping individuals to achieve the maximum independence of which they are capable. She identified the following five methods nurses use for helping people:

1. acting for or doing for another
2. guiding and directing
3. providing physical or psychological support
4. providing and maintaining an environment that supports personal development
5. teaching (Orem, 1995, p. 15).

The Scientific Era

In Chapter 1, we talked about the explosion of knowledge that has characterized the biomedical sciences in the latter half of this century. We are living in a technological age, and nurses have to become skilled in many highly technical diagnostic and therapeutic procedures in the course of their work. Nursing theory has not been immune to the prevailing emphasis on science. A number of nursing theories put forth in the 1960s and 1970s were based on advances in the biomedical sciences. Nursing theories that developed in this era were also influenced by Selye's (1976) work on stress and by Dunn's (1973) ideas of "optimal wellness."

Faye Abdellah is credited with ushering in the "scientific" era in nursing theory. We are indebted to her for changing our way of thinking about nursing. She has moved nursing from the medical model's focus on the signs and symptoms of disease to a separate model with a singular focus—the patient—and a unique body of knowledge generated from nursing phenomena. The approach of Abdellah et al. to nursing, as outlined in the text *Patient-Centered Approaches to Nursing* (1960), revolutionized nursing curricula, changing the emphasis of nursing courses from a disease and body systems orientation to one focussed on patient needs. This was the beginning of patient-centred nursing practice as we know it (Fitzpatrick & Whall, 1996).

Like Henderson and Orem, Abdellah used a needs approach as her conceptual framework. She classified the problems that could be helped by nursing action into 21 categories, which she called **nursing problems**. Abdellah felt that it was the nurse's responsibility to help patients (individuals and/or families) to meet their needs using a problem-solving approach. This approach included an assessment of individual patients receiving nursing care, a determination of the nature and extent of their problems (this step is now referred to as *diagnostic reasoning*) and actions taken within the province of nursing to help to resolve these problems. The problem-solving approach is now called the *nursing process* and the steps are labelled slightly differently but, basically, it is the same process that Abdellah introduced to our thinking nearly 40 years ago (Abdellah & Levine, 1986).

Although in this book we have divided the evolution of nursing theory into separate periods to illustrate changes in ideas about nursing over the years, the divisions are not clear cut. Nurse theorists have continued to develop their original ideas, incorporating newer ways of thinking as they went along. Orem, for example, has used the more recent concept of nursing process in elaborating her conceptual model (see Figure 13.1).

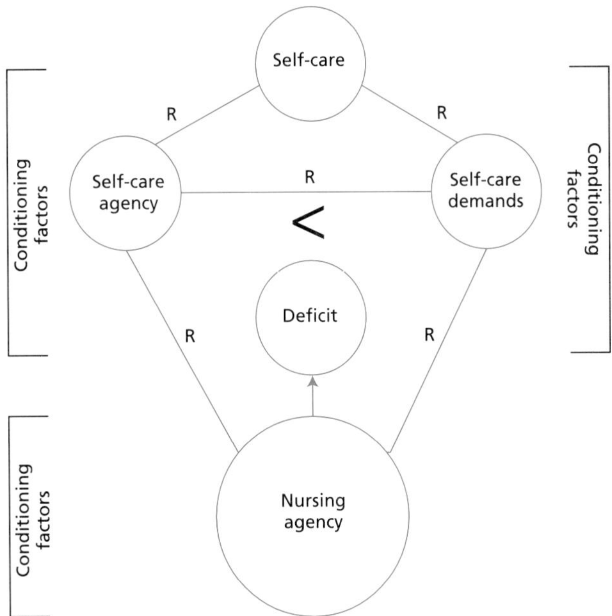

FIGURE 13.1 A conceptual framework for nursing

SOURCE: Orem, 1995, p. 435.

SYSTEMS THEORY

Among the many theorists who were influenced by the biomedical and psychosocial sciences were those who based their conceptual frameworks on general systems theory (see Chapter 9).

The University of British Columbia (UBC) model for nursing, developed in the 1970s by Dr. Margaret Campbell for the UBC School of Nursing, reflects both the humanist approach of earlier theorists and the scientific approach ushered in by Abdellah. According to this model, the patient is an individual who has the following nine basic needs:

1. mastery
2. love, belongingness and dependence
3. respect of self by self and others
4. collection and removal of accumulated wastes
5. intake of food and fluid, nourishment
6. safety and security
7. balance between production and utilization of energy
8. intake of oxygen
9. stimulation of the senses (Campbell, 1987, p. 7).

The individual can be viewed as a behavioural system with nine subsystems, each consisting of one of the basic needs and the ability to meet that need (inner personal region) and the psychological environment (need-related goals and the forces influencing their attainment).

In this model, the nurse's role is seen as nurturing "individuals experiencing critical periods so that they may develop and use a range of coping behaviours that will permit them to satisfy their basic human needs, to achieve stability, and to reach optimal health" (Campbell, 1987, p. 10). The critical period may be either maturational events, such as puberty, or unpredictable events, such as the death of a loved one. Optimal health is the highest level of behavioural system stability achieved by the individual at any given time. Figure 13.2A illustrates the interrelatedness of the various subsystems that make up the behavioural system of the individual. Figure 13.2B shows the structure of a subsystem and the interrelationship of its parts.

Betty Neuman and Sister Calista Roy are two other nurse theorists who based their models on systems theory, viewing the human being and the environment as interacting systems.

Neuman's conceptual model is often referred to as a **holistic** model, focussing as it does on the total person, the person's reaction to stress and on factors influencing the person's ability to cope with stress and restore equilibrium. Neuman uses the term **client system** to refer to either an individual or a group. Neuman (1995) sees her model as "a comprehensive, systems-based conceptual framework for nursing ... [that] illustrates the composite of five interacting variables—physiological, psychological, sociocultural,

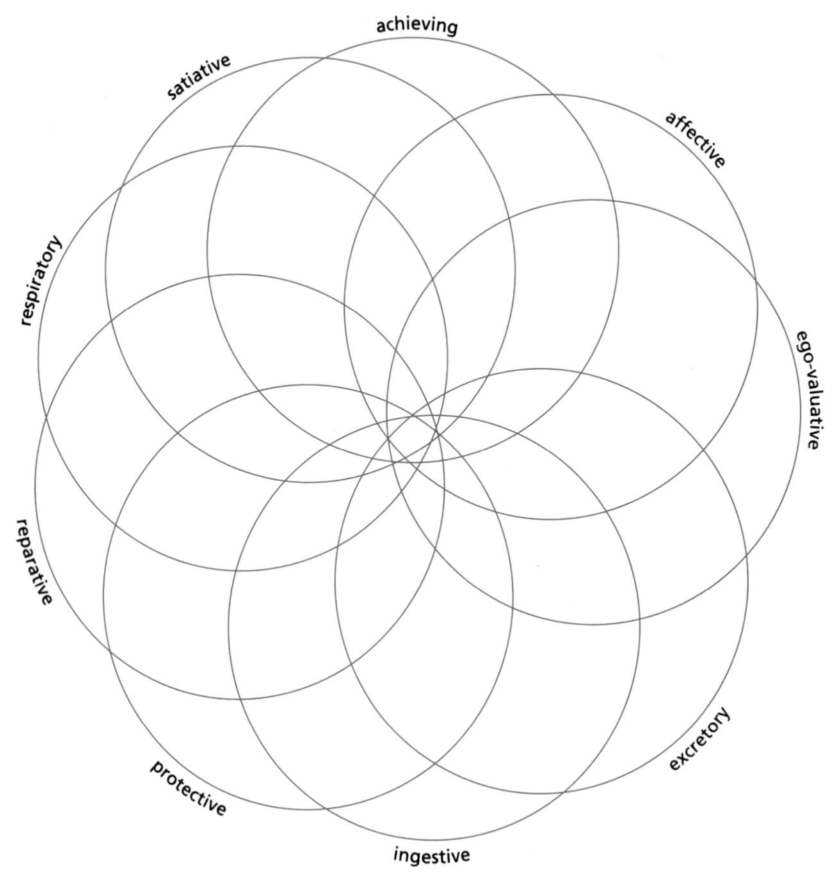

FIGURE 13.2A UBC model: The individual as behavioural system

SOURCE: Campbell, 1987, p. 32.

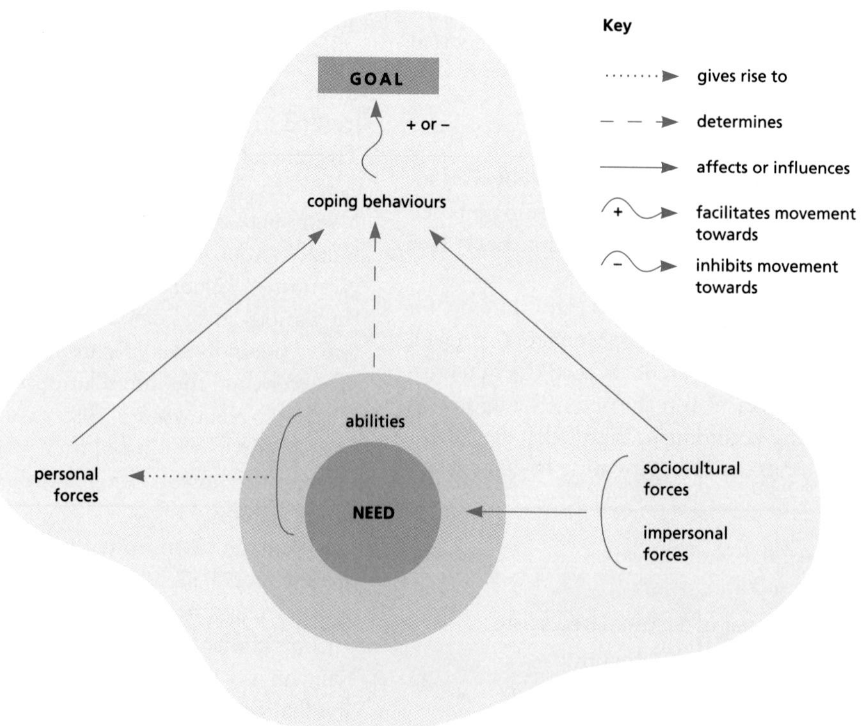

FIGURE 13.2B Structure of a subsystem: Interrelationship of the parts

SOURCE: Campbell, 1987, p. 32.

developmental and spiritual—ideally functioning harmoniously or stable in relation to internal and external environmental stressor influences upon the client, as a system, at a given point in time" (p. 24). Neuman considers nursing to be primarily concerned with appropriate nursing action to facilitate optimal client stability. Neuman's model is shown in Figure 13.3.

In her conceptual model, Roy makes use of general systems theory and of Selye's work on stress. The major theme of Roy's theory is adaptation with a holistic focus on the person in an adaptive system. According to Roy, *person* may refer to either an individual, a family or group, a community or a society. The person is also viewed as an adaptive system interacting with the external system of the environment. The person as an adaptive system is comprised of two coping mechanisms—the regulator and cognator, whose responses to stressors or stimuli are manifested in the four adaptive modes (physiological, self-concept, role function and interdependence (Andrews & Roy, 1991). Roy views nursing's role as promoting adaptation in the patient (individual or group) to promote wellness. Her model is illustrated in the Research to Practice feature at the end of this chapter, describing how the nursing staff at one hospital used a conceptual model to move into theory-based practice in their agency (Roy, 1984; Roy & Andrews, 1998). Figure 13.4 shows Roy's adaptation model.

ENERGY FIELDS

Martha Rogers and, more recently, Rosemary Parse, used developments in modern physics to take nursing theory beyond the concepts of equilibrium used in earlier systems models (Chinn & Kramer, 1991). Rogers (1970) portrays humankind as a unified whole whose fundamental unit is the human energy field. The human energy field is an open system constantly exchanging energy with the environment (Quillin & Runk, 1989). Rogers says that nursing is unique among the sciences because it is the only one that deals with the person as a whole. She sees the goal of nursing as promoting harmonious interaction between the person and the environment (Barrett, 1990).

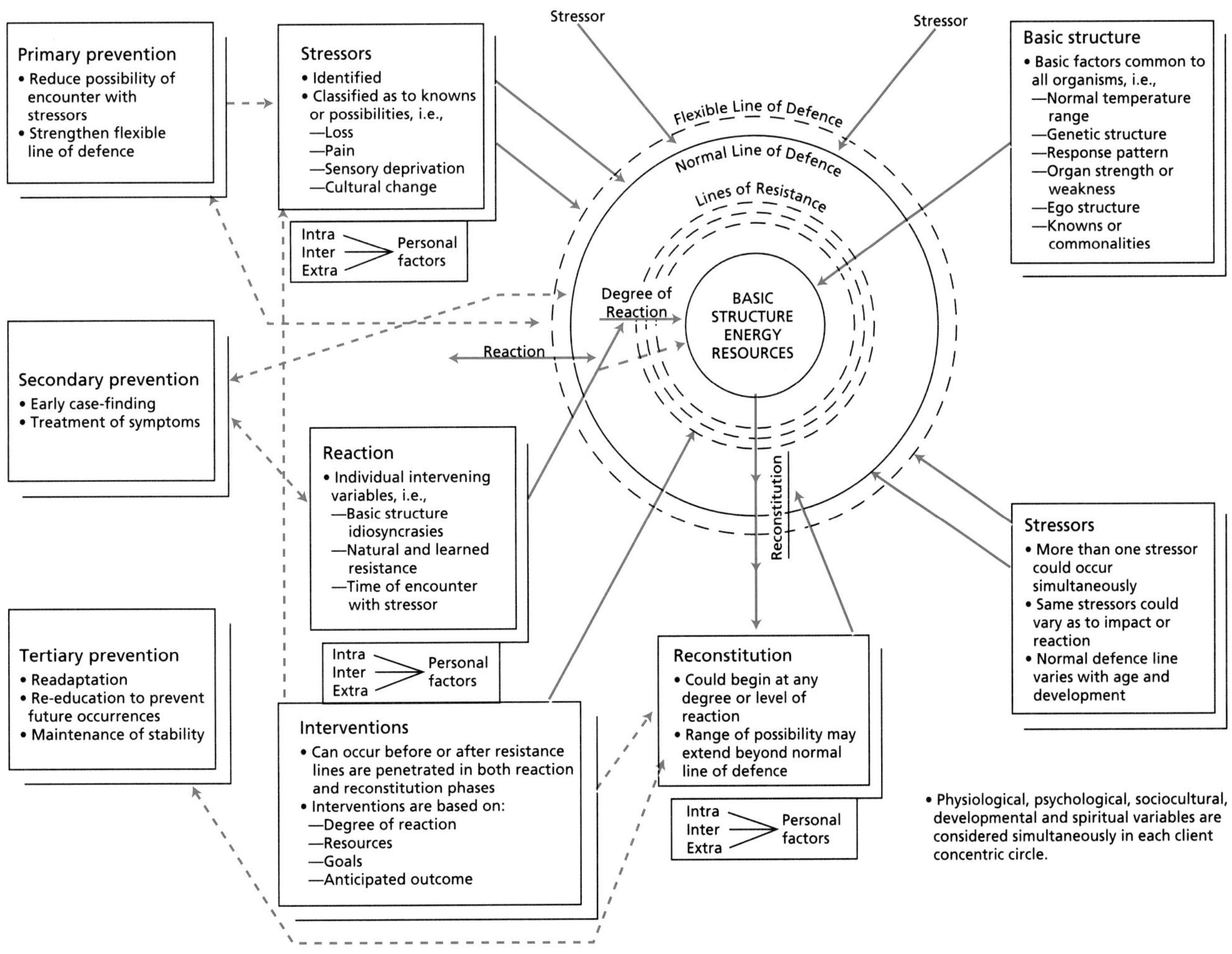

FIGURE 13.3 The Neuman systems model

SOURCE: Neuman, 1995.

Parse, in explaining her man–living–health model (1981, 1987), expresses the view that nursing is both an art and a science. She sees the individual as a unitary, indivisible human being existing together with the universe and free to make independent decisions. She sees the role of nursing as that of assisting the patient to participate in making decisions in situations involving the person's health.

Return of the Humanist Influence

By the late 1970s, nurses, and many people in other fields, were beginning to question the widespread reliance on empirical science as the sole basis for knowledge. The 1980s saw a shift towards a broader view that encompassed personal knowledge, as well as ethics and aesthetics, as a basis for nursing knowledge. From its earliest beginnings, nursing has had a nurturing quality, and it is this quality that dominates nursing literature at the present time. The caring, promotion of growth and provision of support implied by *nurturing* are referred to in the profession as the *caring paradigm*. This paradigm has been explored by numerous nurse theorists in the past decade. Theories that have emerged from these explorations include:

1. Dr. Madeline Leininger's culture care theory of nursing
2. Dr. Jean Watson's theory of human care
3. Sister (Dr.) M. Simone Roach's theoretical philosophy on the nature of human caring.

Dr. Madeline Leininger was the first of the human care theorists in nursing. In studying different cultures, Dr. Leininger found that caring is a universal phenomenon, although the nurturant activities of people in different cultures vary considerably. Leininger feels that caring is the essence of nursing and defines **care** as "action towards assisting, supporting or enabling another individual (or group) with evident or anticipated needs to ameliorate or improve a human condition or lifeway" (Leininger, 1988, p. 156). Leininger sees the person as a cultural being. She feels that human beings have survived because of their ability to care for infants, younger and older adults, and their ability to adapt to different environments and different ways. She sees the environment as a broad concept encompassing the total context in which a person lives, including the physical, social, ecological and global setting. Leininger concluded from her studies that caring is a universal trait that is essential to human survival. The focus of her research has been to discover the care phenomena (practices) of different cultures in order to provide people with culturally congruent care (Cohen, 1992; Leininger, 1995, 1991, 1977). Figure 13.5 shows Leininger's sunrise model.

Dr. Jean Watson calls her theory "human science and human care." She believes that the nurse's role is based on human caring for one who is ill and that nursing is "an art and a science directed toward the protection, enhancement and preservation of human dignity" (Watson, 1988, p. 35). To Watson, the relationship between patient and nurse is the key to helping the individual to gain more self-knowledge,

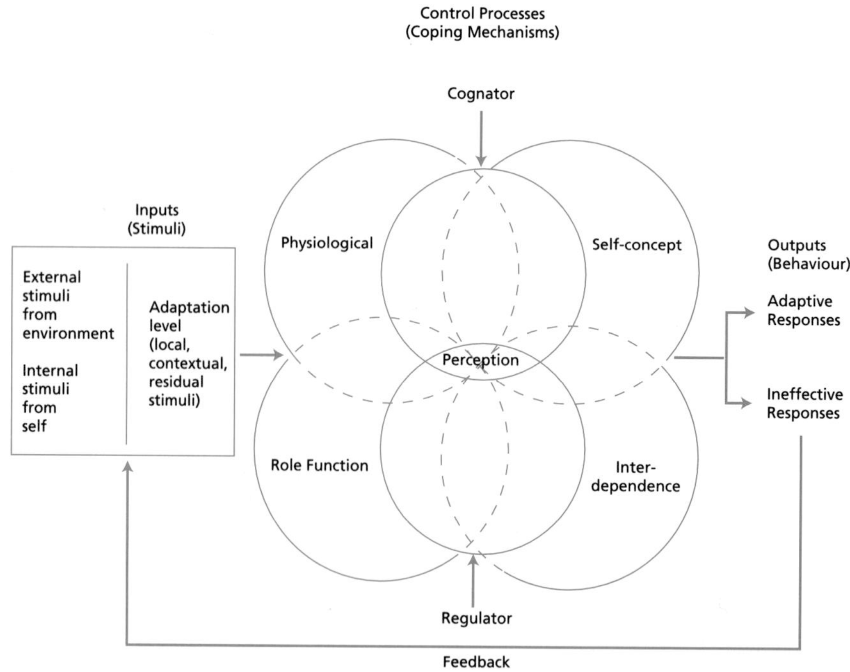

FIGURE 13.4 The Roy model: The person as adaptive system

SOURCE: Fitzpatrick & Whall, 1996.

self-control and readiness for self-healing, regardless of the person's health condition. In her work, Watson emphasizes the psychological and emotional, as well as the spiritual, dimensions of nursing care. She states that "the interventions related to the human care process require an intention, a will, a relationship, and actions. The process entails a commitment to caring as a moral ideal directed toward the preservation of humanity" (Watson, 1988, p. 75).

Dr. Simone Roach, in her 1992 philosophical treatise, *The Human Act of Caring*, states that "... the desire to care is human, it manifests itself in the human mode of being" (p. 48). Like Leininger, she sees caring as "an essential ingredient in human development and survival" (p. 2) and, like Leininger and Watson, as the essence and core of nursing (p. 11). She views nursing as the professionalization of human caring and states, as we did in Chapter 1, that most

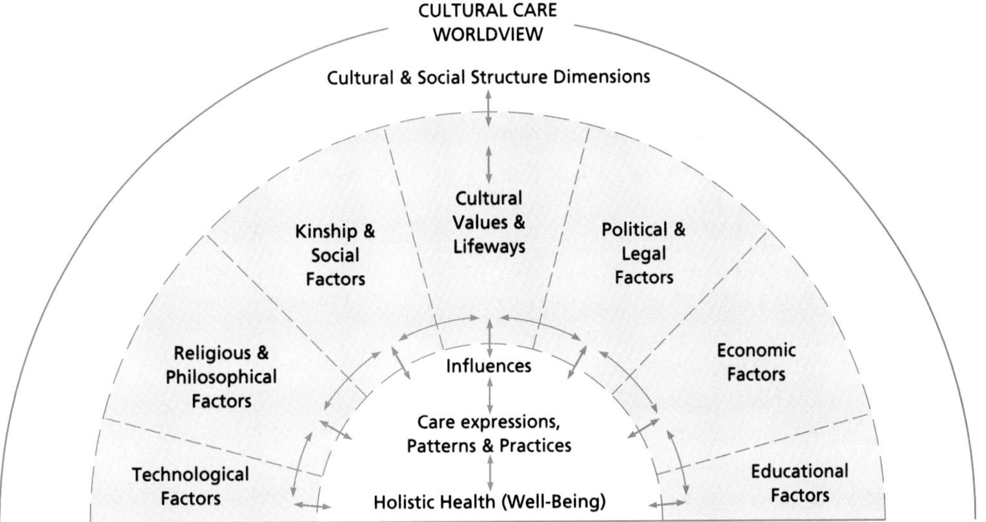

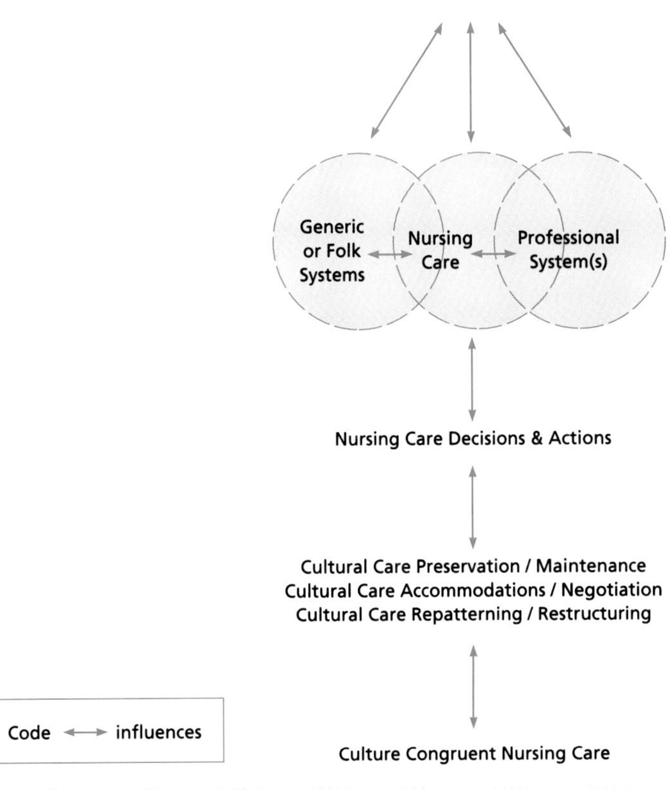

FIGURE 13.5 Leininger's sunrise model

SOURCE: Leininger, 1991, p. 43.

beginning students of nursing enter their professional schools with a sincere desire to help people. The knowledge, skills and attitudes they gain during their educational program enable them to provide the professional help people need to promote and protect their health, or to cope with health problems.

In answer to the question "What is a nurse doing when she or he is caring?" Dr. Roach suggests that in caring, nurses use the "Five Cs" of professional caring: compassion, competence, confidence, conscience and commitment.

Dr. Roach has suggested that other "C"s might be added to this list. One of these is **comportment**, used here to mean bearing, demeanour, dress and language—all of which she feels are important in conveying an attitude of caring. A neat, well-groomed appearance conveys to the patient that you regard him or her as a person worthy of respect; it also means that you respect yourself. Although the starched white uniforms and crisp nurses' caps are no longer seen in most hospitals in Canada, studies have found that the traditional uniform conveyed an image of professional competence that is lacking in the informal dress code of today (Magnum, Garrison, Lind, Thackeray & Wyatt, 1991; Joseph, 1986). Campbell-Heider and Hart (1993) go so far as to say that the informality of dress and speech by nurses in today's health care agencies reinforces negative stereotypes of nurses and diminishes the image of professional competence they wish to convey. In regard to language, the authors contend that social status is conveyed in the forms of address we use. Many people, particularly older people, do not like to be called by their first names—to them, it suggests a lack of respect and makes them feel robbed of their social status. Patients are also often confused by the implied social intimacy which they are not prepared for in a therapeutic relationship. If patients prefer to be called by "Mr.," "Mrs.," "Miss" or "Ms," nurses should respect their wishes. By encouraging patients and co-workers to call them by their first names, nurses may perpetuate a second-class role for themselves, in which they are seen as subservient to physicians who are, except in rare circumstances, always addressed by their professional title (see Figure 13.6).

In more recent times, the concept of caring has been expanded to include a critical and feminist perspective. From these perspectives, caring compels nurses to become moral, ethical and just agents in promoting effective nurse/patient relationships, and to improve health care. The assumptions underlying critical and feminist perspectives are that social and gender dominance have oppressed many patients and nurses. Critically questioning this assumed domination, and uncovering experiences of oppression, social isolation, economic, political, gender and health care inequities, will lead to a raising of consciousness. Bevis and Watson (1989) urge nurses to engage in this critical consciousness-raising; to uncover inequities and power imbalances; and to seek to act in ways that foster choice, emancipation and freedom. From this perspective, caring is defined as the moral imperative to act ethically and justly, and is the motivating power underlying all nursing realities and possibilities (Hills, et al., 1994). It should be noted that this expanded view of caring in no way negates the value of caring as nurturance, self-care and the artistic nature of enhancing human dignity. In this sense, caring is at the heart of nursing, and this broadened definition described here provides an expanded view of the very essence of nursing.

Attributes of Professional Caring—The Five Cs

- **compassion**—a sensitivity to the pain and brokenness of the other; a quality of presence that allows one to share with and make room for the other
- **competence**—having the knowledge, judgement, skills, energy, experience and motivation required to respond adequately to the demands of one's professional responsibilities
- **confidence**—the quality that fosters trusting relationships
- **conscience**—a state of moral awareness that grows with experience
- **commitment**—a complex, affective response characterized by convergence between one's desires and one's obligations and by a deliberate choice to act in accordance with them

SOURCE: Roach, 1992.

Towards a Health Orientation

Many of the nurse theorists whom we have discussed have continued to develop their conceptual models. Many of the earlier models viewed patients as being somewhat incapacitated and needing the nurse's help to regain health and independence. Now, as our health care system shifts towards a health- rather than an illness-oriented model, we see in the work of nurse theorists increasing emphasis on health promotion and health protection (rather than illness prevention—a subtle distinction, but one that underscores the changes taking place) and on the concepts of self-knowledge and self-healing. Watson's and Leininger's work both show evidence of this trend.

One Canadian theorist whose work reflects this reorientation to health is Moyra Allen. The McGill model, which has been evolving over a period of some 20 years, was designed to serve as a means for generating a knowledge base about nursing through accumulating knowledge about the nature of healthy living. Much of the data was gathered through a series of health workshops funded by Health and Welfare Canada.

Allen (1986) suggests that the search for healthy living is a natural quest of human beings, and she sees nursing as a professional response to this search. Health is viewed as a

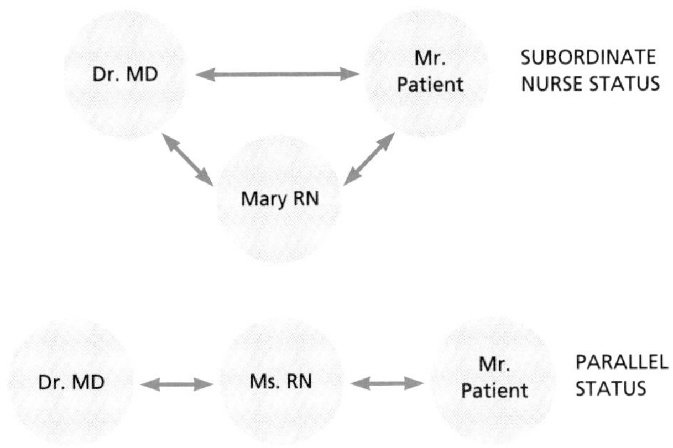

FIGURE 13.6 Communicating social status

SOURCE: Campbell-Heider & Hart, 1993, p. 135.

way of living, rather than as a state of being. It is something that is learned over time. The basic unit in Allen's model is the family or other social group in which learning about health and healthy behaviours takes place. The nurse and the patient (patient–family) are viewed as equal partners in the search for healthy living. The nurse's role is to assist families to enhance their problem-solving skills and to use their own (individual, family and community) potential to make the best decisions possible about the various options open to them. The process involves learning how to select from among available resources, when to ask for help and where and how to get it (Kravitz & Frey, 1989).

Nursing theory continues to evolve. The questioning and testing of existing knowledge by nurses, clinicians, researchers and theorists stimulate the development of new ideas. As new ideas emerge, they are used to build on previous thinking. Thus, there is a synthesis of knowledge that adds to, refines and changes the existing body of knowledge (Casey, 1989).

As we look at the evolution of nursing theory, it is easy to see the emergence of different schools of thought. The differences in conceptual frameworks that have emerged reflect the theorists' interpretations of the major concepts considered central to nursing and the linkages between them. Table 13.1 provides a comparison of how some of the different theorists view *person*, *environment*, *health* and *nursing*.

The Value of Theories and Conceptual Models for Nursing Education, Research and Practice

In any given discipline you will usually find more than one conceptual model on which people base their practice. The theories underlying an individual's pattern of practice depend on the theories espoused by teachers and practitioners, and on the situations encountered in practice.

The Canadian Nurses Association's *Standards for Nursing Practice* (1987) states that "... nursing practice requires that a conceptual model(s) for nursing be the basis for that practice" (p. 3). Most Canadian schools of nursing and many health agencies have now adopted specific nursing models or have developed their own. The acceptance of theory-based practice by both academics and clinicians has been slow and fraught with resistance. The early theories provided rather general descriptions of nursing and were criticized for presenting an overly idealistic view that did not reflect real life. They were also often couched in esoteric language that nurses found difficult to understand. Nurse educators were the first to make use of conceptual models as a framework for curriculum. As the theories have been expanded and explained by the original author or by others, they have become more widely accepted. Today, the health agency that does not base practice on a conceptual framework is the exception, rather than the rule.

The value of the models commonly used in schools and agencies across the country is first and foremost in providing nursing with its perspective. All members of the health team are concerned with the patient, but all view the patient from a different perspective. The physician, for example, sees the patient as someone with a health problem, which it is their responsibility to diagnose and treat. The nutritionist is concerned with the patient's diet and nutritional status; the physiotherapist focusses on the patient's musculoskeletal system and mobility.

The conceptual frameworks in nursing help practitioners to look at the patient as a whole person, not just as a health problem, a nutritional problem or a mobility problem. Orem views the person as an integrated whole, unity functioning biologically, symbolically and socially (Fitzpatrick & Whall, 1996); Neuman talks of five interacting variables (physiological, psychological, sociocultural, developmental and spiritual) impinging on a person's health. These are just two examples. You will find that all nursing models treat the person as a multifaceted being and acknowledge that all these facets must be taken into account in caring for that person.

In addition to providing us with a distinctive nursing perspective and helping us to look at the whole person, the assessment tools that have developed from the models provide a framework for the organization of nursing care. They offer guidance for the collection of data and the identification of health problems. The models also give us a common language that can be used to describe the patient's health status and to communicate nursing's concerns. For example, if an agency has adopted Orem's conceptual model as the basis for practice, the nurses will talk in terms of the patient's "self-care deficits." These will be identified and described in the nurse's assessment of the patient and nursing interventions planned to overcome the deficits. For ex-

TABLE 13.1 The Basic Elements of Selected Conceptual Models

	FLORENCE NIGHTINGALE	*HILDEGARDE PEPLAU*	*VIRGINIA HENDERSON*	*DOROTHY OREM*	*FAYE ABDELLAH*	*SISTER CALISTA ROY*
Major Theme	Unique Role of the Nurse	Interpersonal Process within the Nurse–Patient Relationship	Basic Needs	Self-care Requisites	Patient's/Nursing Problems	Adaptation
Person	An individual who has the recuperative powers within self to restore own health	An individual with the capacity for growth through increasing interpersonal and problem-solving competencies	A unique individual in whom mind and body are inseparable who has 14 fundamental needs	A unity functioning biologically, symbolically and socially, who has three categories of self-care requisites: 1. universal 2. developmental 3. health deviation	Patient or the patient's family with an overt or covert problem which the nurse can assist in solving through the performance of professional functions	A holistic adaptive system in constant interaction with the environment who has four modes of adaptation: 1. physiological function • five needs: oxygenation, nutrition, elimination, activity and rest, protection • four processes: senses, fluids and electrolytes, neurological function endocrine function 2. self-concept 3. role function 4. interdependence
Environment	Involves those external conditions that affect life and the development of the individual, with a focus on ventilation, warmth, odours, light and diet	Significant others with whom the person interacts	Not defined specifically	Environmental elements are seen as external to the person and composed of both physical and psychosocial components	Societal and environmental needs are contributing factors to actual and/or anticipated problems. These include not only need-satisfaction problems the patient has in hospital but also at home in the community	All conditions, circumstances and influences surrounding and affecting the development and behaviour of persons or groups, having both internal and external components and constantly changing
Health	Absence of disease and the ability to use one's own abilities to the highest potential, with emphasis on the reparative process of getting well	Health is represented by forward growth of personality	Optimum health is achievement of the desired measure of independence in carrying out activities of daily living	A state of being sound and whole	An optimum state of need satisfaction, including the ability to satisfy one's own needs	"A state and a process of being and becoming an integrated, whole person." (Andrews & Roy 1991, p. 69)

BETTY NEUMAN	*MARTHA ROGERS*	*ROSEMARY PARSE*	*MADELEINE LEININGER*	*JEAN WATSON*	*MOYRA ALLEN*	*MARGARET CAMPBELL (UBC MODEL OF NURSING)*
Systems	Interaction Between Person and Environment	Man-Living-Health	Transcultural Care Diversity and Universality	Human-to-Human Process of Caring	Nature of Healthy Living	The person as a behavioural system with interacting and interdependent subsystems, each representing a basic human need
An interacting open system that is dynamic and composed of five interacting variables — physiological, psychological, sociocultural, developmental and spiritual	A four-dimensional energy field characterized by organization and pattern that functions as a unified whole within an open system, exchanging energy with the environment	May be an individual or family. The person as a unitary, indivisible human being in constant interchange with the environment, who is free to make decisions and choices about health behaviours based on past or present experience	Human beings (individuals, families and cultural groups) who have survived because of their ability to care for infants, young and older adults in a variety of ways and places	A living, constantly growing totality comprising mind, body, emotion and soul	The family or other social group in which learning is initiated, nurtured and directed	An individual with nine basic human needs, constantly striving to satisfy these needs by using a range of coping behaviours, both innate and acquired
Has both external and internal components: the external environment consists of forces external to the client system, e.g., inter-/extra-personal stressors; the internal environment consists of forces found within the client's own boundaries and that correlate with interpersonal stressors	Also a four-dimensional energy field, with organization and pattern, that is specific for each individual and includes all that is outside the person's own energy field	A constantly changing energy field that surrounds the person and is an integral part of the state of being	The total context within which the individual, family or cultural group live including the physical, ecological, social and world-view aspects	The external reality of the person	The social context in which learning takes place. This may be at home, the workplace, community group, a hospital or a clinic	That which lies outside the boundary of the system
Health or wellness is equated with optimal client system stability	Health and illness are seen as cultural values denoting behaviours of high and low value as defined by individuals and cultures	A continuously changing state of being, or "becoming," as experienced by the person	Culturally determined beliefs, values and patterns of action used to preserve and maintain the well-being of persons	Unity and harmony within mind, body and soul of the person	A social process, a way of living rather than a state of being. Similar in meaning to health behaviour, it is something that can be measured and can be modified	Optimal health is the highest level of behavioural system stability perceived by an individual as achievable at any given time

TABLE 13.1 The Basic Elements of Selected Conceptual Models *(continued)*

	FLORENCE NIGHTINGALE	*HILDEGARDE PEPLAU*	*VIRGINIA HENDERSON*	*DOROTHY OREM*	*FAYE ABDELLAH*	*SISTER CALISTA ROY*
Definition of Nursing	A profession for women, separate and distinct from medicine, using nature's laws of health in the service of humanity	An interpersonal process between nurse and patient that is goal-oriented	An independent, unique health profession carrying out activities with or on behalf of the patient that contribute to health or recovery (or to a peaceful death) that the patient would perform unaided given the necessary strength, will or knowledge	A human service helping people to overcome self-care deficits related to health	An art and a science that focusses on helping people to solve their health problems	The science and practice of promoting adaptation in individuals or groups in order to help them achieve health
Goal of Nursing	To place the patient in the best condition for nature to act by providing an environment conducive to healthy living and a nourishing diet	To assist the patient to solve problems through new learning and positive change	To assist humankind to regain optimal health or, in the event of incurable illness, to achieve peaceful death	To assist the individual in achieving the maximum independence of which he or she is capable, in caring for own health and that of dependent others	Satisfaction of patient health needs is the objective of nursing function and nursing activity	The promotion of adaptation in each of the four modes, thereby contributing to the person's health, quality of life and dignified death

ample, a nurse assesses Mrs. Singh and notes a weakness of the left arm. As a result, she has difficulty dressing and feeding herself. The care plan for Mrs. Singh would describe a self-care deficit in regard to certain activities of daily living. This would direct other nurses that Mrs. Singh needs help with dressing and with cutting her food.

Using Theories and Conceptual Models in Education

As we mentioned earlier, it was nurse educators who initially adopted the theories (conceptual models), using them originally as a framework for curriculum, and later to provide structure for individual nursing courses. The use of nursing models provides a distinctive approach that serves to differentiate nursing education from medicine.

Nursing education programs up to, and including, the early 1950s had a heavy emphasis on the basic sciences and little on the social sciences. Clinical courses were taught predominantly by physicians, with follow-up lectures on nursing care of patients, with various diseases given by the nurse educator responsible for the course. The use of specific nursing models as the structure for clinical nursing courses has enabled nurse educators to change the focus of their teaching to matters that are important to nursing. The caring curriculum of the Collaborative Nursing Program (CNP) in British Columbia was developed by nurse educators from five nursing education institutions throughout the province. At the time of writing, 10 schools of nursing are part of the CNP. The concept of caring has been a guiding principle and a philosophical foundation of the program. Nursing theories of caring guided the development of each nursing course, and different dimensions of caring are articulated and actualized throughout the baccalaureate curriculum. Students are educated from a caring paradigm (Bevis & Watson, 1989) that facilitates the opportunity for nurses to "be" caring practitioners as well as to "act" in ways that promote just and ethical nursing practice. To that end, the

BETTY NEUMAN	*MARTHA ROGERS*	*ROSEMARY PARSE*	*MADELEINE LEININGER*	*JEAN WATSON*	*MOYRA ALLEN*	*MARGARET CAMPBELL (UBC MODEL OF NURSING)*
A unique profession focussing on the total person (patient system) and his or her, or group, reactions to stress and on factors influencing reconstitution	A profession with a focus on compassionate concern for the maintenance, promotion, protection and restoration of health in people	An art and a science focussing on the living unity that characterizes all people	A learned humanistic art and science concerned with personalized care behaviours, functions and processes	A human art and science directed towards the protection, enhancement and preservation of human dignity	A professional response to the person's natural search for healthy living	The nurturing of individuals experiencing critical periods in the life cycle, so that they may develop and use a range of coping behaviours that permit them to satisfy their basic human needs, to achieve stability and to reach optimal health
To promote optimal client system stability	To promote harmonious interaction between the patient and the environment	To facilitate optimal wellness in the patient by assisting him or her in achieving system stability	To assist, support or enable another person (individual or group) with existing or potential needs to ameliorate their health through preservation, accommodation or repatterning of culturally determined beliefs, values and patterns	To help people gain more self-knowledge, self-control and readiness for self-healing, regardless of the external health condition	To assist people in enhancing their problem-solving skills in dealing with health matters	To nurture the behavioural system that is the person

concept of caring is influenced by four different theoretical perspectives: phenomenology, critical social theory, feminism and humanism.

The central tenet of phenomenology is the understanding of human experience as it is lived. The aim is to gain a greater understanding of the meaning of experience. This quest for meaning requires a phenomenological attitude that compels people to raise questions about the nature of human experiences in an effort to uncover the deeper meaning structures embedded within. As Ray (1990) suggests, phenomenology offers a means by which human phenomena or the lived experiences of nurses and the people with whom they interact can be understood. This phenomenological attitude is actualized through nurses' caring relationships.

Critical social theory (CST) refers to both a school of thought and to a process of critique (Giroux, 1983). One of the central values of critical theorists is a commitment to penetrate the world of objective appearances in order to expose the underlying social relationships that are often concealed.

The concept of caring, from a socially critical perspective, directs nurses to analyse the dominant social conditions that often constrain people and their health and healing practices. This critical examination of the dominant social structures includes a critique of the health care system, the methods of health care delivery, the philosophy of equal access to health care, and issues of power and control. As nurses begin to examine and critique these dominant social structures, they become aware of social and economic inequities and power imbalances, and seek to act in ways that foster choice, emancipation and freedom.

Another theory, feminism, has historically focussed on valuing women and confronting systemic injustices based on gender. Categories of feminism identified by Sherwin (1992) include liberal, socialist, cultural and postmodernist.

Within the B.C. Collaborative Curriculum, a feminist philosophy attends to the reality of women's oppression.

Traditionally, women have been oppressed, and nursing as a predominantly female profession has been particularly affected by the oppression of women. From a feminist perspective, caring compels nurses to engage in feminist critique, and to act as change agents to enhance gender equality and the promotion of equal rights.

Humanism is a philosophical perspective based on the assumption that people have a tendency to develop all their capacities that serve to maintain or enhance them. Underlying a humanist perspective is the belief that if certain definable conditions are present in human relationships, people will gradually allow their self-actualizing capacity to overcome restrictions that they have internalized through life experiences. These relational conditions include: (a) genuineness or congruence, (b) empathic understanding and (c) unconditional positive regard (Rogers, 1961).

Caring, from a humanistic perspective, involves engaging in relationships that enhance genuineness, empathic understanding and unconditional positive regard. These qualities promote the movement towards self-actualization. As Bevis and Watson (1989) explain, caring is not a "soft" and sympathetic notion; rather, it is the driving force behind all nursing actions. As such, the attitude and action of caring provides a moral, ethical and just foundation upon which to base all forms of nursing practice and is a guiding principle upon which the profession of nursing is both recognized and actualized.

Using Theories and Conceptual Models in Research

Nursing theories have provided opportunities for nurse scholars to expand their knowledge on the original concepts. Nurse scholars have described other phenomena that are part of nursing. For example, Benner (1984) has explored the nature of caring in studies focussing on the daily practice of expert nurses.

Further research has led to the development of midrange theories that can be used more directly to guide nursing care than can the grand theories (conceptual models). Orem's model, for example, has given rise to a theory of self-care which states that the care of oneself and the care of dependent family members (or significant others) are behaviours that human beings learn in order to regulate their structural identity, functioning and development (Orem, 1995). New mothers, for example, need to learn how best to care for their babies, and a teaching program, based on this midrange theory, can be developed to help them.

There is a definite reciprocal relationship between theory and research. Nurses' practice has also generated new theories, as noted in the example cited above of Benner's work. Many other concepts with which nursing is concerned are also being explored as focusses for theory development—for example, the nature of social support, prenatal maternal attachment, pain control and coping mechanisms for stress (Chinn & Kramer, 1991).

RESEARCH to practice

Nursing Theories in Practice at Mount Sinai Hospital

Nursing care based on knowledge drawn from a nursing perspective is an essential contribution of our discipline to the health care system and to those in need of nursing services. Provision of quality care, based on a sound body of nursing knowledge, enables us to meet our social mandate and empowers us to influence health care policy. It is in this context that theory-based practice has become a popular theme in nursing practice settings throughout North America (Mayberry, 1991; Sorrentino, 1991) and elsewhere (Perry, 1985).

The use of nursing theories in the practice setting was encouraged in Ontario by the College of Nurses which, in 1984, stated that nursing practice should be guided by a conceptual framework. Several hospitals have since adopted nursing theories as guiding frameworks for their practice. In Toronto alone, the models of King, Orem, Watson, Peplau, Parse and Roy have been incorporated into different practice settings.

Nursing is a discipline that provides holistic care. Theory-based practice supports and fosters holistic care. Theory-based practice also encourages nurses to a higher level of conceptual thinking, assisting us in broadening and deepening the mental image that we have of "what nursing is" and providing some specific characteristics and direction to our nursing practice. Theories also assist us in articulating the meaning of nursing for ourselves and for others.

The process of implementing a conceptual framework at Mount Sinai Hospital began in fall 1984. A nursing theories committee explored 20 conceptual frameworks during a period of 10 months. Following this extensive review, four conceptual frameworks were chosen as possible options. These were again reviewed in five half-day workshops, with participation of outside speakers who had worked with these models. The decision to choose the Roy adaptation model was based on the belief that this conceptual framework offered the best fit with the values held by the department of nursing. In winter 1987, we began piloting the model in four units. It was only in 1994 that hospital-wide implementation was completed.

The Roy adaptation model is a highly developed and widely used conceptual description of nursing. As in all other models, the major concepts of the Roy adaptation model are *person, environment, nursing* and *health* (Roy, 1984). According to Roy, the recipient of nursing care can be an individual, a family, a group, a community or society as a whole. Roy considers nursing first in terms of its goal to promote adaptation.

Adaptation, a key concept in the model, is "a process involving holistic functioning to affect health positively" (Roy, 1984, p. 36). Adaptation is the process of promoting health. Roy defines health as a state and a process of being and becoming an integrated and whole person. Thus, Roy believes that health is a dynamic process of evolution and growth.

The following is a description of how the Roy adaptation model could contribute to the plan of care of a person who has suffered a cerebrovascular accident (CVA):

Focal stimuli for the patient who has suffered a CVA will be the impact and implications of the CVA physiologically (physiological mode), in the way this patient feels about him- or herself (self-concept mode), the patient's relationships with others (interdependence mode) and his or her ability to function effectively as a parent or in other important roles (role function mode). As the nurse, during the initial assessment phase, identifies areas of ineffective responses (for example, a poor relationship between the patient and spouse), the nurse will conduct a more in-depth, second-level assessment.

During the second-level assessment, the nurse will explore with the patient the impact of the focal stimuli (what is immediately confronting the patient), the contextual stimuli (what else is occurring in the patient's life that affects the way he or she responds) and the residual stimuli. Residual stimuli include general stimuli that have a lifelong and permeating effect on behaviours. These include culture, socioeconomic status, religion, ethnic group, education level, family structure and stage of growth and development of the patient. Some of these stimuli may contribute to promote adaptation while others may hinder it. For example, a well-constituted family structure might contribute to the patient's adaptation process. A history of addiction to drugs may hinder adaptive responses. One of the purposes of nursing assessment will be to determine which stimuli are predominant in each case. Effective adaptation will contribute to the patient's long-term quality of life, which should be the goal of nursing intervention. In order to tailor nursing intervention to promote adaptation, one must identify factors that assist in or detract from promoting adaptation in all four modes.

As we can learn from this example, nurses practising from a Roy perspective aim at assisting people to respond in a positive way to stimuli and to move to a state of health (being and becoming an integrated and whole human being). These can be done by changing the stimuli and/or by enhancing the coping mechanisms.

Our experience of practising nursing based on a conceptual framework at Mount Sinai Hospital has been a positive one. Its impact has been significant for patients and their loved ones, as well as for nurses. Formal and informal evaluations attest to a genuine change towards holistic nursing care. We have integrated theoretical thinking and the Roy adaptation model in all aspects of our practice—the nursing process documentation, unit-based primary nursing rounds (held every two weeks) and hospital-wide primary nursing rounds (held every two months). It is important to note that our focus at Mount Sinai Hospital has been on "thinking nursing," "practising nursing" and "documenting nursing." We very strongly believe that the model has contributed positively to our nursing practice and to the quality patient care we so proudly provide.

— *Doris Grinspun, RN, MSN, CRRN,*
Program Director, Nursing

IN REVIEW

- Until the middle of the 19th century, nursing knowledge was traditionally passed down from one generation to the next. Apprenticeship training was the most prevalent means of disseminating knowledge.
- Florence Nightingale was the first nursing leader to record and articulate her views of nursing and to differentiate nursing's roles and functions from those of other health professionals.
- The development of conceptual models by other nurse theorists was influenced by events in other fields.
- There are many different conceptual models, each with unique definitions of the major concepts central to nursing:
  - person
  - environment
  - health
  - nursing.
- The Canadian Nurses Association's *Standards for Nursing Practice* requires that conceptual model(s) for nursing be the basis for nursing practice.
- The value of the models for nursing education, practice and research is multifaceted. The models provide nurses with a distinctive nursing perspective:
  - some health agencies have adopted several conceptual models to direct practice
  - nursing models have been used as frameworks for curriculum and course development
  - nursing theories continue to be tested and new ones emerge from research studies.
- The concept of caring is the driving force behind all nursing actions. Caring is informed and influenced by four different theoretical perspectives:
  - phenomenology
  - critical social theory
  - feminism
  - humanism.
- Research helps guide and strengthen nursing knowledge.

Critical Thinking Activities

1. What conceptual models are used in your school of nursing as a framework for the curriculum and/or nursing courses?
2. What conceptual models are used in the clinical agencies that are affiliated with your school?
   a. in community agencies?
   b. in inpatient facilities (hospitals, rehabilitation centres or other specialized units, or long-term care facilities)?
3. Explain how the use of conceptual models in practice discussed on p. 316 are illustrated in Grinspun's description of the use of the Roy adaptation model at Mount Sinai Hospital in Toronto.

KEY TERMS

theory p. 302
conceptual model p. 302
conceptual framework p. 302
metaparadigm p. 302
grand theory p. 302
mega-theory p. 302
descriptive theory p. 302
explanatory theory p. 302
predictive theory p. 302
person p. 302
environment p. 302
health p. 302
nursing p. 302
concept p. 302
empirical p. 302
abstract p. 302
nursing problems p. 305
holistic p. 305
client system p. 305
care p. 308
commitment p. 310
compassion p. 310
competence p. 310
comportment p. 310
confidence p. 310
conscience p. 310

References

ABDELLAH, F.G., BELAND, I.L., MARTIN, A., et al. (1960). *Patient-centered approaches to nursing.* New York: Macmillan.

ABDELLAH, F.G., & LEVINE, E. (1986). *Better nursing care through nursing research.* (3rd ed.). New York: Macmillan.

ADAM, E. (1991). *To be a nurse.* (2nd ed.). Toronto: Saunders.

AGAN, R.D. (1987). Intuitive knowing as a dimension of nursing. *Advances in Nursing Science, 10*(1), 63–70.

ALLEN, M. (1986). A developmental health model: Nursing as continuous inquiry (audio cassette). In series *Theory congress—Theoretical pluralism: Directions for a practice discipline.* Markham, ON: Audio Archives of Canada.

ANDREWS, H.A., & ROY, S.C. (1991). Essentials of the Roy adaptation model. In S.C. Roy & H.A. Andrews (Eds.), *The Roy adaptation model: The definitive statement* (pp. 2–25). Norwalk, CT: Appleton & Lange.

BARRETT, E.A.M. (Ed.). (1990). *Visions of Rogers science-based nursing.* New York: National League for Nursing.

BENNER, P. (1984). *From novice to expert.* Menlo Park, CA: Addison-Wesley.

BEVIS, E.O., & WATSON, J. (1989). *Toward a caring curriculum: A new pedagogy for nursing.* New York: National League for Nursing.

CAMPBELL, M.A. (1987) *The U.B.C. Model for Nursing: Directions for practice.* Vancouver: University of British Columbia School of Nursing.

CAMPBELL-HEIDER, N., & HART, C.A. (1993, Summer). Updating the nurse's bedside manner. *Images, 25*(2), 133–139.

CANADIAN NURSES ASSOCIATION. (1987). *A definition of nursing practice: Standards for nursing practice.* Ottawa: Author.

CASEY, A. (1989). *An introduction to conceptual frameworks: Unit objectives and course notes.* Ottawa: University of Ottawa School of Nursing.

CHINN, P., & KRAMER, M.K. (1991). *Theory and nursing (a systematic approach).* (3rd ed.). St. Louis: Mosby.

CHONG CHOI, E. (1989). Evolution of nursing theory development. In Marriner-Tomey, *Nursing theorists and their work.* St. Louis: Mosby.

COHEN, J.A. (1992). Janforum: Leininger's culture care theory of nursing. *Journal of Advanced Nursing, 17,* 1149.

DUNN, H.L. (1973). *High-level wellness.* Arlington, VA: R.W. Beatty.

FAWCETT, J. (1989). Nursing knowledge and nursing practice: Essential tension. *Proceedings of the National Conference on Putting It All Together: Nursing theory, nursing diagnosis and nursing interventions.* Ottawa: University of Ottawa Service for Continuing Education, 20–29.

FAWCETT, J., & DOWNS, F.S. (1986). *The relationship of theory and research.* Norwalk, CT: Appleton-Century-Crofts.

FITZPATRICK, J.J., & WHALL, A.L. (1996). *Conceptual models for nursing: Analysis and application.* (3rd ed.). Stamford, CT: Appleton & Lange.

FORCHUK, C. (1990). Peplau's interpersonal theory. In A. Bauman, A.N. Johnston & D. Antai-Otong, *Decision-making in psychiatric and psychosocial nursing.* Hamilton, ON: B.C. Decker.

GEORGE, J.B., (Ed.). (1990). *Nursing Theories: The base of professional nursing practice.* (3rd ed.). Norwalk CT: Appleton & Lange.

GIROUX, H. (1983). Theory and resistance in education: A pedagogy for the opposition. London: Heinemann.

HARMER, B., & HENDERSON, V. (1955). *Textbook of the principles and practice of nursing.* (5th ed.). New York: Macmillan.

HENDERSON, V. (1966). *The nature of nursing: A definition and its implications for practice.* New York: Macmillan.

HILLS, M., LINDSEY, E., CHISAMORE, M., BASSETT-SMITH, J., ABBOTT, K., & FOURNIER-CHALMERS, J. (1994). University–college collaboration: Rethinking curriculum development in nursing education. *Journal of Nursing Education, 33,* 220–225.

JOSEPH, N. (1986). *Uniforms and non-uniforms: Communication through clothing.* New York: Greenwood Press.

KRAVITZ, M., & FREY, M.A. (1989). The Allen nursing model. In J.J. Fitzpatrick & A.L. Whall (Eds.). *Conceptual models for nursing.* (2nd ed., pp. 313–330). Norwalk, CT: Appleton & Lange.

LEININGER, M.M. (1977). *Caring: The essence and central focus of nursing.* New York: American Nurses Foundation.

LEININGER, M.M. (1995). *Transcultural nursing: Concepts, theories and practices.* New York: Wiley.

LEININGER, M.M. (Ed.). (1988) Leininger's theory of nursing: Cultural care diversity and universality. *Nursing Science Quarterly, 1,* 152–160.

LEININGER, M.M. (1991). *Culture care diversity and universality.* New York: National League for Nursing.

MAGNUM, S., GARRISON, C., LIND, C., THACKERAY, R., & WYATT, M. (1991). Perceptions of nurses' uniforms. *Image, 23,* 127–130.

MASLOW, A.H. (1970). *Motivation and personality.* (2nd ed.). New York: Harper & Row.

MAYBERRY, A. (1991). Merging nursing theories, models, and nursing practice: More than an administrative challenge. *Nursing Administration Quarterly, 15*(3), 44–53.

McKENNA, H. (1997). *Nursing theories and models.* New York: Routledge.

NEUMAN, B. (1995). *The Neuman systems model.* (3rd ed.). Norwalk, CT: Appleton & Lange.

NIGHTINGALE, F. (1859). *Notes on nursing: What it is and what it is not.* (Commemorative edition, 1992). D.P. Carroll (Ed.). Philadelphia: Lippincott.

OREM, D.E. (1995). *Nursing: Concepts of practice.* (5th ed.). St. Louis: Mosby.

PARSE, R.R. (1981). *Man-living-health: A theory of nursing.* New York: Wiley.

PARSE, R.R. (1987). Parse's man-living-health theory of nursing. In R.R. Parse (Ed.), *Nursing science: Major paradigms, theories and critiques* (pp. 181–204). Philadelphia: Saunders.

PEPLAU, H.E. (1952). *Interpersonal relations in nursing.* New York: Putnam.

PERRY, J. (1985). Has the discipline of nursing developed to the stage where nurses do "think nursing"? *Journal of Advanced Nursing, 10,* 31–37.

QUILLIN, S.I.M., & RUNK, J.A. (1989). Martha Rogers' unitary person model. In J.J. Fitzpatrick & A.L. Whall (Eds.), *Conceptual models for nursing.* (2nd ed.). Norwalk, CT: Appleton & Lange.

RAY, M. (1990). Phenomenological method for nursing research. In N.L. Chaska (Ed.), *The nursing profession: Turning points* (pp. 173–179). St. Louis: Mosby.

ROACH, M.S. (1992). *The human act of caring: A blueprint for the health professions.* (Revised ed.). Ottawa: Canadian Hospital Association Press.

ROGERS, C.R. (1961). *On becoming a person.* Boston: Houghton Mifflin.

ROGERS, M.E. (1970). *An introduction to the theoretical basis of nursing.* Philadelphia: F.A. Davis.

ROY, S.C. (1984). *Introduction to nursing: An adaptation model.* (2nd ed.). Englewood Cliffs, NJ: Prentice-Hall.

ROY, S.C., & ANDREWS, H.A. (1998). *The Roy adaptation model.* (2nd ed.). Norwalk, CT: Appleton & Lange.

SELYE, H. (1976). *The stress of life.* (2nd. ed.). New York: McGraw-Hill.

SHERWIN, S. (1992). *No longer patient: Feminist ethics and health care.* Philadelphia: Temple University Press.

SORRENTINO, E. (1991). Making theories work for you. *Nursing Administration Quarterly, 15*(3), 54–59.

THORNDIKE, E. (1940). *Human nature and the social order.* New York: Macmillan.

WATSON, J. (1988). *Nursing: Human science and human care.* New York: National League for Nursing.

WHALL, A.L. (1989). Nursing science: The process and the products. In A.L. Whall & J.J. Fitzpatrick (Eds.), *Conceptual models for nursing.* (2nd ed. pp. 1–14). Norwalk, CT: Appleton & Lange.

Additional Readings

ALLEN, M. (1974). Query and theory. *Nursing Papers, 6*(1), 43–44.

ALLEN, M. (1982). A model of nursing: A plan for research and development. In M. Allen, *Research: A base for the future. Proceedings of the International Conference on Nursing Research.* Edinburgh: University of Edinburgh.

ALLIGOOD, M.R., & MARRINER-TOMEY, A. (1997). *Nursing theory: Utilization and application.* St. Louis: Mosby.

BARNAM-STEVENS, B.J. (1998). *Nursing theory: Analysis, application, evaluation.* (5th ed.). Philadelphia: Lippincott.

BENNER, P., & WRUBEL, J. (1989). *The primacy of caring: Stress and coping in health and illness.* Menlo Park, CA: Addison-Wesley.

CHINN, P.L. (1995). *Theory and nursing: A systematic approach.* St. Louis: Mosby.

DALEY, B.J. (1996). Concept maps: Linking nursing theory to clinical nursing practice. *Journal of Continuing Education in Nursing, 27*(1), 17–27.

EVANS, C.A., & CUNNINGHAM, B.A. (1996). Caring for the ethnic elder. *Geriatric Nursing, 17*(3), 105–110.

FAWCETT, J.L. (1995). *Analysis and evaluation of conceptual models for nursing.* (3rd ed.). Philadelphia: F.A. Davis.

GADOW, S. (1990). The advocacy covenant: Care as clinical subjectivity. In J.S. Stevenson & T. Tripp-Reimer (Eds.), *Knowledge about care and caring* (pp. 33–40). Kansas City, MO: American Academy of Nursing.

GEORGE, J.B. (Ed.). (1995). *Nursing theories: The base for professional nursing practice.* (4th ed.). Norwalk, CT: Appleton & Lange.

HAMNER, J.B. (1996). Preliminary testing of a proposition from the Roy adaptation model. *Image, 28*(3), 215–220.

MELEIS, A.B. (1996). *Theoretical nursing: Development and progress.* (3rd ed.). Philadelphia: Lippincott.

MORSE, J.M., SOLBERG, S.M., NEANDER, W.L., BOTTORFF, J.L. & JOHNSON, J.L. (1990). Concepts of caring and caring as a concept. *Advances in Nursing Science, 13*(1), 1–14.

OERMANN, M. (1997). *Professional nursing practice.* Norwalk, CT: Appleton & Lange.

PINCH, W J. (1996). Is caring a moral trap? *Nursing Outlook, 44*(2), 84–88.

ROGERS, M.E. (1980). A science of unitary man. In J.P. Riehl & C. Roy (Eds.), *Conceptual models for nursing practice.* (2nd ed.). New York: Appleton-Century-Crofts.

ROGERS, M.E. (1986). Science of unitary human beings. In V.M. Kalinski (Ed.), *Explorations on Martha Rogers' science of unitary beings.* Norwalk, CT: Appleton-Century-Crofts.

ROLFE, G. (1996). *Closing the theory–practice gap: A new paradigm for nursing.* Boston: Butterworth-Heineman.

STRICKLAND, D. (1996). Applying Watson's theory for caring among elders. *Journal of Gerontological Nursing, 22*(7), 6–11.

ULRICH, Y.C. (1996). The relational self: Views from feminism on development and caring. *Issues in Mental Health Nursing, 17*(4), 369–380.

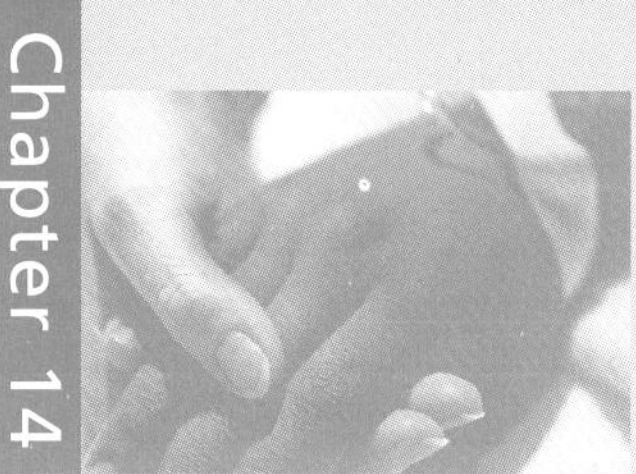

Chapter 14

Nursing Process

OUTLINE

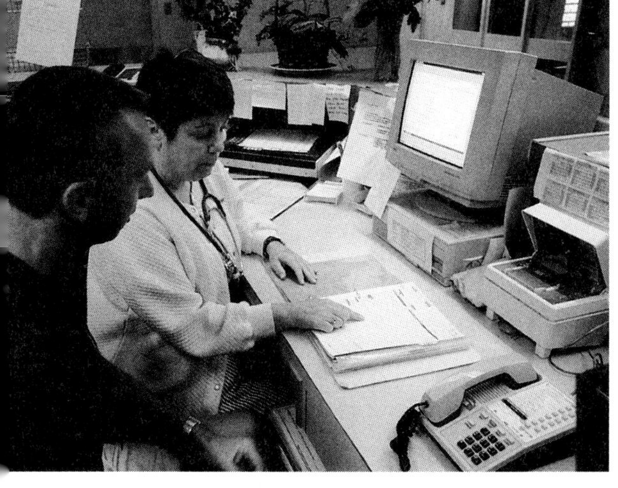

Central Questions

1. What is the nursing process, and why is it used?
2. What are the steps in the nursing process, and how do they relate to one another?
3. What are the purposes of data collection, and what information does the nurse collect during assessment?
4. What sources are used for data collection?
5. What is diagnostic reasoning, and how is it used in the assessment phase of the nursing process?
6. What is the difference between subjective and objective data?
7. What are some frameworks the nurse can use for organizing assessment data?
8. How does the nurse document and communicate the information collected?
9. How does the nurse use the diagnostic process to identify client problems and strengths?
10. How do nursing diagnoses differ from collaborative problems?
11. What are the parts of the diagnostic statement, and how would the nurse write diagnostic statements for actual, potential and possible nursing diagnoses and for collaborative problems?
12. How does the nurse determine priorities among the identified problems?
13. How are goals and expected outcomes developed?
14. What types of interventions does the nurse carry out in giving care?
15. How does the nurse determine nursing interventions?
16. What is a nursing care plan, and how does the nurse develop one?
17. What knowledge and skills does the nurse need to implement a plan of care?
18. What methods does the nurse use in evaluating the effectiveness of care?

Introduction

Nursing care may range from the simple act of cleansing and bandaging a child's cut finger to the highly complex measures involved in caring for a patient in the intensive care unit of a hospital, or in helping a family with multiple problems to meet their health needs in a community setting. The process of nursing is the same, however, whether the nursing care given is a basic first aid measure or a sequence of complicated nursing activities.

The term **nursing process** designates a systematic and organized approach to nursing practice that embodies a series of interrelated steps the nurse takes in identifying and making decisions about nursing care. Based on the problem-solving, or scientific, method, the nursing process provides a consistent framework that all nurses can use in planning and giving care. Moreover, the terminology that has evolved can be readily understood by all nurses, as well as by other members of the health team.

Nursing process is:

- planned
- patient-centred
- problem-oriented
- goal directed.

The essential elements of the nursing process are that it is planned, it is patient-centred, it is problem-oriented and it is goal-directed. The term **patient** is used here to denote the recipient of care and can mean an individual, a family or a community. Five basic steps are involved in the process:

1. assessment—gathering and organizing information
2. diagnosis—analysing and synthesizing the information to identify strengths and actual or potential problems
3. planning—establishing goals and developing a plan of action
4. implementation—carrying out the plan of action
5. evaluation—determining if the goals have been achieved.

The steps in the process follow logically one after the other. As a basis for making decisions about nursing actions, the nurse must first assess the need for action. During assessment the nurse gathers all pertinent information (commonly referred to as data) about the patient and then groups the information into meaningful categories or clusters. This prepares the information for the next step, diagnosis.

In diagnosis, the data are analysed and a judgement is made about the patient's health status. This may include a patient's strengths, level of wellness and actual or potential health problems that are amenable to independent nursing intervention or those that require referral to other health professionals. In order to diagnose accurately, the nurse must have a thorough understanding of the nature of health and illness; of the physiology, pathophysiology and signs and symptoms (clinical manifestations) of illness; and of human behaviour. Nursing diagnoses provide a focus and give direction in planning goal-directed care.

In planning, the nurse and the patient together set patient-centred goals (also referred to as *expected outcomes*) and develop a plan of action (called the *nursing care plan*) to help patients promote and protect their health or resolve problems. The next step is implementation, in which the specified measures (nursing interventions) outlined in the plan of action are carried out.

The final step is evaluation. This is when the results of the action(s) taken are reviewed to determine if the expected outcomes have been attained. The last step may result in new information that leads to modification in the nursing diagnoses, changes in the plan of action or a restatement of patient goals.

Although the nursing process is viewed as a series of deliberate steps that are separated and studied individually, it must be pointed out that, in practice, the steps are continuously interacting and overlapping with one another in such a way that one step may contain elements of the next. Or, in some situations, especially emergencies (as when a patient stops breathing), all steps may occur simultaneously. Figure 14.1 depicts the nursing process.

Assessment and diagnosis overlap significantly, as illustrated by the following example: During a physical examination, the nurse finds that the patient feels warm, looks flushed and has a rapid pulse. The patient also reports anorexia and nausea. From knowledge of pathophysiology, the nurse assumes that the patient has a fever and focusses the data-gathering activity on validating this assumption. In this example we see that, as the data were being collected, the nurse grouped the information and began to make an assumption about the meaning of this information. In other words, hypotheses or nursing diagnoses were being generated even before data gathering was complete. An assumption is "an idea or concept that you take for granted (e.g., people used to assume the world was flat). Assumptions can be true or false" (Wilkinson, 1996, p. 36). This overlap in the thinking process between assessment and diagnosis describes what a number of authors refer to as "diagnostic reasoning" (Carnevali, Mitchell, Woods & Tanner, 1984; Kelly, 1985; Gordon, 1987; Carnevali & Thomas, 1993).

Diagnostic reasoning is the process of critical thinking in which the nurse uses clinical knowledge and experience to collect information, interpret the information collected and make a judgement about the patient's health status. This judgement is the nursing diagnosis. The reasoning process will be discussed in more detail later in the chapter.

Some authors do not see assessment and diagnosis as two distinct steps of the nursing process. Rather, they view

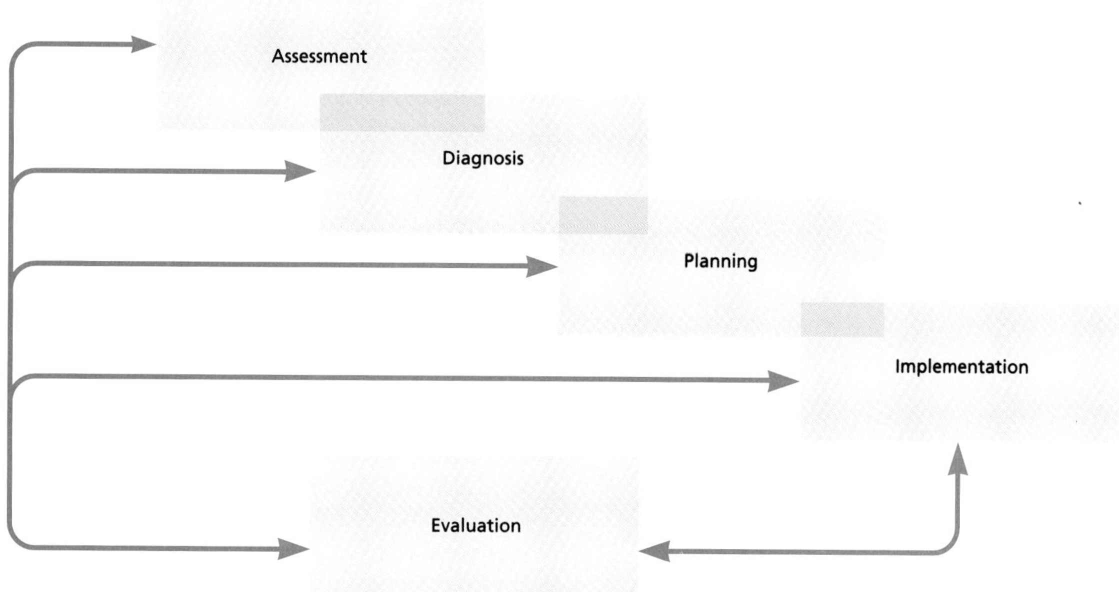

FIGURE 14.1 Relationships among the steps of the nursing process*

* Each step of the nursing process is dependent on the accuracy of the preceding step. The steps are also overlapping because you may have to move more quickly for some problems than for others. Evaluation involves examining all the previous steps, but focusses upon outcome achievement. The arrows between assessment and evaluation, and between evaluation and implementation, go in both directions because assessment and evaluation are ongoing processes as well as separate phases.

SOURCE: Alfaro-Lefevre, 1998, p. 10.

diagnosis as an integral part of assessment and advocate a four-step model in which diagnosis is seen as the conclusion of the assessment phase (Yura & Walsh, 1988). Furthermore, diagnostic reasoning is carried out with little conscious awareness of the mental activities involved, particularly as nurses become more advanced in their abilities. Students, however, with beginning levels of the knowledge and skills needed for data collection and limited experience in diagnostic reasoning, may find it easier to learn the processes involved by carrying out these steps as separate operations (Carnevali & Thomas, 1993).

Diagnosis and planning may also overlap. In the situation described above, for example, if the patient's temperature were found to be 40°C and the patient expressed severe headache, the nurse would first take action to deal with the fever and pain, and then continue with analysis and synthesis of all of the assessment data. Similarly, planning and implementation overlap because there are times when nursing interventions have to be implemented before the entire plan for care is developed. Thus, the nursing process is a dynamic series of steps that provides a framework for giving quality care, yet is open and adaptable to the unique and changing needs of the patient.

Assessment

As the first step in the nursing process, **assessment** refers to the collection and interpretation of clinical information (Gordon, 1994). The systematic collection of information for a specific purpose is called "data gathering." The information collected is used to develop a *data base*, which can be analysed in a number of different ways, depending on the purpose for which the information was collected in the

The Logical Flow in the Steps of the Nursing Process

Steps	Process	Action
Assessment	gather all pertinent data	cluster data in preparation for next step
Diagnosis	analyse data	make a judgement about the patient's health
Planning	set patient-centred goals	develop a nursing care plan
Implementation	carry out the planned nursing interventions	begin evaluation of effectiveness of interventions
Evaluation	determine if desired outcomes have been achieved (have patient-centred goals been met?)	continue with implementation of nursing care plan or reassess and begin process again

first place. Analysis is a process of studying or examining the nature of something, or of determining essential features and relationships within the data collected.

Analysis is the ability to:

- break down and classify data
- explore relationships and interactions
- distinguish fact from hypothesis
- distinguish relevant data from those that are extraneous or irrelevant
- determine what assumptions, if any, have been made
- recognize overall relationships and categories (pattern/themes).

As a nursing function, assessment focusses on the patient's health status and responses to illness—as opposed to medical assessment, which focusses on the pathology underlying illness and is the responsibility of a doctor. The information collected during assessment forms the basis on which nursing diagnoses and nursing care decisions are made. Therefore, it is essential that the information is complete and relevant to the patient's situation and that it is sorted and organized into a format that can be analysed. In addition, the information has to be recorded and communicated to other health professionals. Assessment involves three components:

1. collecting information—gathering data about the patient's health status and responses to illness
2. organizing the information—grouping or clustering the data into meaningful patterns
3. documenting the information—recording the relevant data.

These three components are described more fully in the following sections.

Collecting Information

In order to develop a solid base for identifying health problems and planning nursing care, the nurse needs to know the following five steps:

1. the purpose for which the information is being collected
2. what information is needed
3. what sources can be used to obtain data
4. how these sources can be tapped
5. how to interpret and use the information collected.

PURPOSE OF DATA COLLECTION

The nurse's objective in collecting information about a patient is to identify areas in which nursing intervention is required. There are two types of data collection for this purpose: data base assessment and focus assessment (Alfaro-Lefevre, 1998). The ***data base assessment*** (baseline assessment) is conducted on admission to a health care agency or upon initial contact with the patient. It includes the nursing history and physical assessment, the physician's report on the patient's history and physical examination, the results of diagnostic and laboratory tests, and reports from other health professionals. The information gathered in the data base assessment gives a comprehensive picture of the patient's health status and enables the nurse to begin a plan of care for the patient. Information collected by the nurse may also identify problems that require intervention by other members of the health team, such as the physician, the social worker or the physical therapist.

In addition to the data base assessment, information is collected on an ongoing basis to determine changes in the patient's health status and the consequent need for change in the plan of action. This is called a **focus assessment**. As the name suggests, data collection is directed to specific problems or needs. For example, the nurse who periodically examines the colour and respiratory pattern of a newborn baby or observes the wound drainage of a postoperative patient is conducting a focus assessment.

INFORMATION NEEDED BY THE NURSE

Virginia Henderson, in her well-known and often-quoted definition of nursing, has stated, "The unique function of the nurse is to assist the individual, sick or well, in the performance of those activities contributing to health or its recovery (or to peaceful death) that he [she] would perform unaided if he [she] had the necessary strength, will or knowledge" (Henderson, 1966, p. 15).

We might rephrase this to say that nursing care of individuals, families and groups is primarily concerned with assisting them in managing their activities of daily living in such a way as to promote their optimal functioning or, in the case of incurable disease, to cope with terminal illness. In order to identify areas in which individuals (or families or groups) require such nursing assistance, the nurse needs to know:

1. basic data about the individual as a person
2. his or her usual abilities (or lack of abilities) in managing activities of daily living (health patterns)
3. the nature of any health problems that are interfering with the ability to cope (illness patterns)
4. current status in regard to these abilities
5. health-promoting and health-protecting practices
6. potential risk factors
7. the physician's plan of care for the individual.

SOURCES OF DATA COLLECTION

The **primary source** of information is always the patient. Other sources, termed **secondary sources**, include other people such as family members or "significant others" with whom the individual has had a close relationship. In the case of a child or an unconscious or irrational patient, much of the information the nurse needs must be obtained from someone other than the patient.

The patient's chart (health record) is also a valuable source of data for the nurse, and today an increasing number of health professionals contribute to it. If a chart has already been started, or if old charts are on file, the nurse reviews these, if possible, before the first encounter with the patient. This review helps to avoid duplication in information gathering, which may unnecessarily tire or annoy the patient, and gives the nurse the benefit of data gathered by others. The physician, for example, is usually responsible for taking the patient's medical history, for identifying medical problems and for developing medical diagnostic and treatment regimes for the individual, if such are warranted. The results of the physician's findings and the medical plan of care are incorporated into the patient's chart. In addition, the nurse will find other sources, such as reports on radiography and ultrasonography, as well as laboratory and other diagnostic tests on the patient's chart. This information is necessary for developing a nursing plan of care.

Other members of the health team also contribute to the nurse's understanding of the patient's health status. Observations and interpretations may be communicated by the social worker, the nutritionist (dietitian) or the physical therapist, to name only a few, through written notes on the patient's chart, in consultations with the nurse or in conferences and other meetings of various health professionals.

If the individual has a known medical problem, the nurse may want to increase his or her knowledge of it by reading available literature in the library. Students might review notes they have taken in class or through independent study that will contribute to their understanding of the particular problem.

HOW TO COLLECT INFORMATION

Whether conducting a data base assessment or a focus assessment, the nurse uses the same methods of gathering data about a patient. These are the interview (talking to the patient, family or significant other), the physical assessment (observation and examination), consultation (with other members of the health care team) and the chart (and other written material).

Interview

The nurse conducts an interview to obtain information from patients or from their family or significant other. Interviewing goes on during every phase of the nursing process and is a component of both data base and focus assessments. An interview must be conducted in a deliberate, systematic manner to ensure that all necessary information is obtained. In order to carry out an effective interview, nurses need to have knowledge and skill in communication, such as listening, questioning and observing,

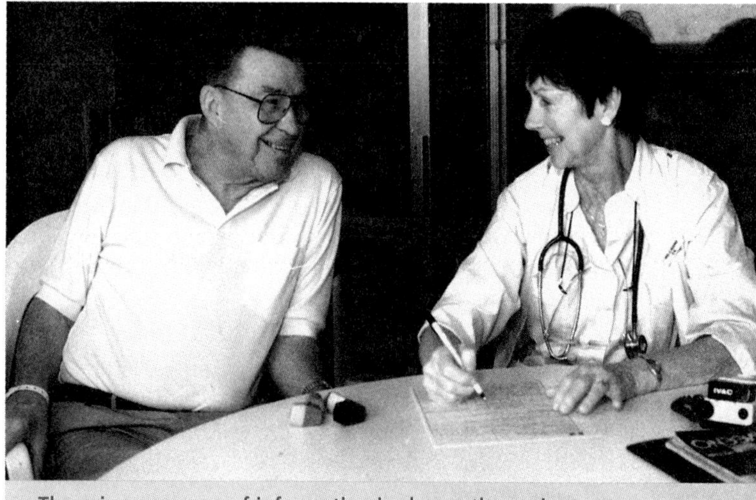

The primary source of information is always the patient.

and in basic interviewing techniques. These skills are discussed in Chapter 17.

Nursing Health History

A primary tool for collecting baseline data that relies on skillful interviewing techniques is the health history. The **health history** provides a guide for systematically obtaining information that can help the nurse to plan and modify care to suit the individual patient's preferences and usual living patterns, as well as to establish a baseline from which to evaluate the results of nursing action.

The history is taken as soon after the patient's admission to the agency as is possible, preferably by the nurse who has primary responsibility for planning the patient's care. The technique for obtaining the history is a **structured interview**, that is, one in which the nurse controls and directs the interview for the purpose of gathering specific information. Information commonly gathered in a nursing history includes:

1. events leading up to admission to the agency
2. the reasons for admission
3. basic social data about the patient
4. usual patterns of daily living—habits in regard to eating, eliminating, rest and sleep and hygiene practices
5. health and illness patterns—perception of usual patterns of physiologic, psychosocial and spiritual functioning and an exploration of changes in these patterns
6. health promotion and protection patterns—what he or she does or does not do to remain healthy
7. environmental factors that may affect health—the patient's family, where the patient lives and works
8. concerns and expectations of care—things the patient is worried about, what he or she expects to happen and the care anticipated from health care personnel.

Many agencies use a specific form commonly called a *health history*, a *nursing history*, a *patient profile* or a *nursing admission assessment* to assist nurses in gathering data and to provide a written record of the information obtained. Today, most agencies have patterned their health history form on a nursing model (see Chapter 13) to ensure that the central concepts of nursing are integrated into the data collection. The views of the nurse and the agency about the patient, the patient's environment, health and the purpose of nursing govern how the nurse will carry out the nursing process. Establishing a data base on those views sets the foundation for optimal care. Figure 14.2 gives an example of a nursing history form based on Gordon's functional health patterns.

Physical Assessment

The physical assessment is conducted by using observation and examination techniques. **Observation** refers to the collection of information through the use of the physical senses (sight, sound, touch, smell and taste). For instance, upon approaching the bedside of a postoperative patient, the nurse will look at the patient's posture and facial expression and listen to the sound of the patient's voice in order to detect signs of emotional distress or physical discomfort. The nurse might also touch the patient's skin to feel moisture and temperature. Then, the nurse will inspect the equipment (such as an intravenous line or drainage tubing) for proper functioning and visually scan the surrounding area for potential hazards to patient safety.

Skillful observation is vital in data collection. Observation provides information about patients' physical, emotional, developmental and social behaviour, as well as their physical and social environment. It is a process that occurs in every nurse–patient encounter, be it during an interview or physical examination, or when giving and evaluating care. These basic skills are discussed further in Chapter 16.

Examination is an objective, systematic assessment of the patient's physical status, performed in conjunction with, or after, the nursing interview. It involves the use of four sensory techniques: *inspection*, through critical visual observation; *palpation*, by touching and feeling with the fingers; *percussion*, by tapping with the fingers, and listening for sounds; and *auscultation*, by listening for sounds directly or with a stethoscope. These techniques are outlined in Chapter 16.

The physical examination is carried out in a systematic manner. There are a number of ways of conducting a physical examination. The nurse can use a head-to-toe format, a systems approach or a needs approach. In the head-to-toe method, the nurse begins by assessing the head and neck, and then continues down the body to the chest and thorax, the abdomen, the perineum and then the arms, legs and feet. In the systems approach, each of the body systems is examined separately. The nurse first assesses the respiratory system (nose, mouth, throat and lungs), and then continues methodically with the cardiac and circulatory system, neurological system, gastrointestinal system, genitourinary system, musculosketetal system, integumentary system and so on.

The patient-needs approach uses a biopsychosocial format that includes an analysis of biological, psychological, developmental, social, cultural, religious and spiritual factors, organized around needs such as oxygen, nutrition, self-esteem or safety. A physical examination can also be organized around a nursing model. For example, when using Orem's model the patient would be examined for self-care capabilities and deficits. Use of a nursing model is beneficial because it directs the examination towards a particular nursing perspective and clearly points out the nurse's role in patient care. The approach that a nurse uses in conducting a physical examination depends on personal preference and agency requirements.

Use of a nursing model is beneficial to guide physical assessment because it:

- organizes the data collection and the data collected
- directs the examination towards a particular nursing perspective
- clearly points out the nurse's role in patient care.

Review of Resources

Resources are reviewed to ensure that information about a particular patient is complete. The nurse should check the patient's chart, scan the baseline or focus data, review laboratory and diagnostic test results, talk to family members or significant others if appropriate or consult with other health team members for any additional information that may be required for making nursing diagnoses and planning care.

HOW TO INTERPRET AND USE INFORMATION COLLECTED (DIAGNOSTIC REASONING)

The information collected during assessment is of no value unless it means something within the context of the patient's situation. During and after data collection, the nurse assigns meaning to data and makes judgements about the patient's health status and abilities to function in daily living. Diagnostic reasoning is a basis for establishing nursing diagnoses and making decisions for care.

Diagnostic reasoning is a complex mental process that combines data collection with the deliberate use of knowledge, experience and logic to identify and classify the findings related to a patient's situation and then form a conclusion about the patient's state of health. In many cases, this process goes on without the nurse's conscious

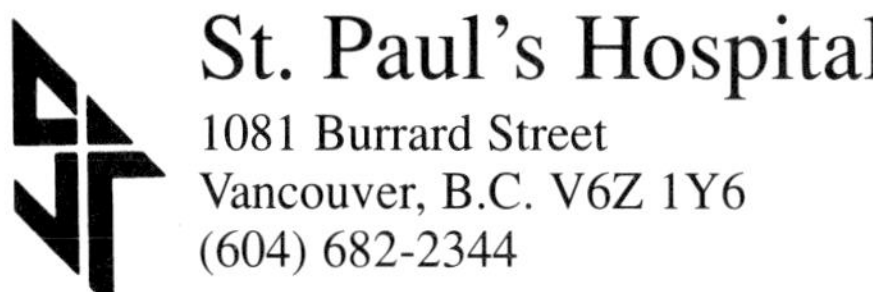
St. Paul's Hospital
1081 Burrard Street
Vancouver, B.C. V6Z 1Y6
(604) 682-2344

Department of Nursing Admission Assessment

Date: ____________ Informant: ( ) Patient ( ) Other ____________

Significant Findings

HEALTH PERCEPTION/HEALTH MANAGEMENT PATTERN

Reason for this admission and history of presenting problem (as stated by patient) ____________

Expected length of hospitalization: (as stated by patient) ____________

RELEVANT Health History: ____________

Are there any current appointments/services that need to be cancelled while you are in hospital? Describe:

ALLERGIES: Describe any adverse reactions to Food, Drugs, Tape, Other:

Describe your medication schedule: (put additional medications on separate page)

MEDICATIONS: Drug/Dose/Frequency	MEDICATIONS: Drug/Dose/Frequency

Can you tell me the purpose of your medications? ❑ Yes ❑ No

Do you have any difficulty taking medications? (Describe)

Any medications brought into hospital? ❑ Yes ❑ No ❑ Sent Home ❑ To Pharmacy ❑ Unit Lockup

COGNITIVE/PERCEPTUAL PATTERN

MENTAL STATUS: ❑ **No Problems** ❑ Alert ❑ Drowsy ❑ Confused
Oriented to: ❑ Person ❑ Place ❑ Time

EYES: ❑ **No Problems** ❑ Draining ❑ Reddened ❑ Other ____________
Pupils: ❑ Equal ❑ Unequal

VISION: **No Problems** Acuity: Can see 2 fingers at 2 feet: ❑ Yes ❑ No
❑ Glasses ❑ With Patient ❑ Contacts ❑ With Patient
Blind: ❑ L ❑ R Implants/Glass Eye: ❑ L ❑ R

HEARING: ❑ **No Problems** Impaired: ❑ L ❑ R Hearing Aid: ❑ L ❑ R

SENSATION: ❑ **No Problems** ❑ Decreased ❑ Numbness ❑ Tingling

COMMUNICATION: ❑ **No Problems** ❑ Slurred ❑ Garbled
❑ Aphasia: Expressive/Receptive (circle)
First language ____________ Speaks English ❑ Yes ❑ No
Understands English ❑ Yes ❑ No

FIGURE 14.2 Nursing health history form based on Gordon's functional health patterns

SOURCE: Nursing Department, St. Paul's Hospital, Vancouver, British Columbia.

COGNITIVE/PERCEPTUAL PATTERN (CONT'D)

Significant Findings

PAIN EXPERIENCE: ❑ **No Problems** Current Pain ❑ Yes ❑ No

If YES: ❑ Sharp ❑ Stabbing ❑ Burning ❑ Dull Aching

❑ Other:

LOCATION/PAIN SCALE RATING (0 = no pain, 10 = worst pain imaginable) RELIEF MEASURES

1. ______
2. ______
3. ______
4. ______

Other: ______

NUTRITION/METABOLIC PATTERN

DIET: ❑ **No Problems** Special diet/Supplements: ______

APPETITE: ❑ **No Problems** ❑ Increased ❑ Decreased ❑ Nausea ❑ Vomiting ❑ Mouth ulcers ❑ Distention ❑ Decreased taste

SWALLOWING: ❑ **No Problemss** ❑ Solids ❑ Liquids

DENTURES: ❑ None ❑ Upper (partial/full) ❑ With patient

❑ Lower (partial/full) ❑ With patient

WEIGHT: ❑ **No Problems**

❑ Loss ❑ Gain ______ kg/lb Since:______/______(mm/yy)

SKIN: ❑ **No Problems** ❑ Itching ❑ Rash ❑ Lesions ❑ Bruises ❑ Jaundice ❑ Edema

Describe: ______

❑ Incisions: Location ______ ❑ Skin Breakdown: ______

ACTIVITY/EXERCISE PATTERN

SELF-CARE ABILITY:

1 = dependent
2 = maximal assist.
3 = moderate assist.
4 = minimal assist.
5 = setup, supervision, cues
6 = independent with equipment
7 = independent

	CURRENT	USUAL		CURRENT	USUAL
Eating/Drinking			Bed Mobility		
Bathing			Transferring		
Dressing/Grooming			Ambulating		
Toiletting			Other		

GAIT/BALANCE: ❑ **No Problems** ❑ Unsteady ❑ Crutches ❑ Walker

❑ Cane ❑ Splint/Brace ❑ Wheelchair

❑ Other ______

RESPIRATIONS: ❑ **No Problems** ❑ Shallow ❑ Rapid ❑ Labored

Describe: ______

Any concerns about your breathing? ______

Cough: ❑ Yes ❑ No ❑ Home Oxygen

FIGURE 14.2 Continued

ELIMINATION PATTERN

BLADDER:
❑ **No Problems** ❑ Discomfort Voiding
❑ Difficulty starting stream ❑ Frequency
❑ Nocturia
❑ Incontinence (Describe) ______________
❑ Self-care ❑ Needs assistance
❑ Other (e.g., catheter, Ileal conduit) ______________

BOWELS:
❑ **No Problems** Usual Pattern: Frequency ________ Description ________
Last BM ______—______ ❑ Incontinent ❑ Ileostomy ❑ Colostomy
Aids: ❑ Laxative ❑ Enema ❑ Suppository ❑ Other
❑ Self-care ❑ Needs assistance

Significant Findings

SLEEP/REST PATTERN

❑ **No Problems** Sleep schedule: Hours/night: ______ From: ______ To: ______
Naps: ❑ Yes ❑ No
Uncommon sleep patterns/difficulty sleeping? (Describe problems/solution) ______________

SEXUALITY/REPRODUCTIVE PATTERN

REPRODUCTION: ❑ **No Problems** LMP ________ Could you be pregnant? ❑ Yes ❑ No
Using any form of contraception? ❑ Yes ❑ No Menstrual concerns? ______

SEXUALITY: Describe any concerns: ♀/♂ e.g., discharge, bleeding, sores, itching

COPING/STRESS TOLERANCE/PATTERN (SUGGESTED LEAD-IN STATEMENTS)

"What are the problems or concerns you anticipate due to your hospitalization or illness?" ______________

"How do you usually deal with stressful situations?" ______________

"Have you experienced any losses/changes/traumatic events that are still affecting you?" ______________

Tobacco use: ______ pk/day X ______ yrs ❑ Non-smoker

ALCOHOL USE: CAGE QUESTIONNAIRE:
Tell me about your use of alcohol ______________
If patient used alcohol:
Have you ever felt the need to cut down on drinking? ❑ Yes ❑ No
Have you ever felt annoyed by criticism of your drinking? ❑ Yes ❑ No
Have you ever felt guilty about your drinking? ❑ Yes ❑ No
Have you ever had a drink first thing in the morning to steady your nerves or get rid of a hangover? ❑ Yes ❑ No
When did you have your last drink? Date: ______________
Tell me about your use of street drugs? ______________

FIGURE 14.2 Continued

Significant Findings

SELF-PERCEPTION/SELF-CONCEPT PATTERN

Has this illness changed the way you feel about yourself? ❑ Yes ❑ No

If YES, How? ______

VALUES/BELIEFS PATTERN

Any religious/cultural/spiritual practices that should be considered during your hospitalization? ______

Would you like to have clergy/support person visit during your stay? Yes No ______

______

ROLE/RELATIONSHIP PATTERN

Significant other: ______

Next of kin / Emergency contact: ______

Housing arrangements (Stairs/multilevel): ______

What kind of assistance is available for you at home? ______

______

Destination upon discharge? ______

Anticipated changes because of this illness (job/family/housing?) ______

______

Previous Utilization of Community Resources: ❑ Home Care ❑ Hospice ❑ Adult day care ❑ Church Group ❑ Meals-on-Wheels ❑ Homemaker/Home Health Aide ❑ Community Support Group ❑ Mental Health ❑ Other

Discharge Transportation: ❑ Car ❑ Airline ❑ Bus/Taxi ❑ Do not know at this time

Anticipated need for financial assistance ❑ Yes ❑ No

Anticipated need for help with self-care postdischarge ❑ Yes ❑ No

What additional information (activities, routines, habits, concerns) would help us give you better care?

______

______

ADMISSION CHECKLIST

Oriented to: ❑ Room ❑ Unit

Valuables: ❑ Cashiers ❑ Security ❑ Unit Lockup ❑ Sent Home ❑ Patient assumes responsibility

Problem List (Analyse significant findings and identify nursing diagnoses/patient problems)

1. ______
2. ______
3. ______
4. ______
5. ______
6. ______
7. ______
8. ______
9. ______
10. ______

Signature/Status: Date: Time:

Signature/Status: Date: Time:

Signature/Status: Date: Time:

FIGURE 14.2 Concluded

awareness of the mental operations involved. An experienced nurse, for example, can make an observation, form a conclusion and take immediate action for the problem without thinking about the underlying reasoning process.

Diagnostic reasoning, however, is a learned skill. As in learning all skills, the beginning practitioner has first to learn the elements of diagnostic reasoning and carry out the mental operations in their logical order. To understand diagnostic reasoning, one should know something about the nature of information and how meaning is derived from this information. We will begin by looking at the types of information collected, and then move on to an examination of specific pieces of information (cues), how inferences are made and how meaning is attached to both cues and inferences.

Subjective and Objective Data

There are two types of information that the nurse gathers through assessment. **Subjective data** refers to information reported primarily by the patient, but it can also come from the patient's family or significant other. It includes feelings and perceptions about one's state of health and abilities to cope with activities of daily life. "I feel short of breath," "I feel hopeless," "I have a stomachache" are examples of subjective information expressed by the patient. Subjective data obtained from a family member, for example, may include a mother's perception of her child's stomachache and how she herself is feeling about her child being sick. Subjective data, also called *symptoms* or *covert* data, cannot be observed directly but are obtained by asking questions.

Objective data refers to information about a person that can be observed, perceived or measured by another through the use of sense organs or instruments. The colour of skin, vital signs, changes in behaviour and laboratory tests are examples of objective data—also called *signs* or *overt* data.

Recognizing Cues and Making Inferences

Interpreting information is knowing the meaning of what is being perceived from the environment. In order to do this, one has to notice a piece of information, put a name to it and attach meaning to it. The pieces of information that one perceives from the environment are called **cues**. Subjective and objective data are cues. The nurse's interpretation of these cues is called an **inference**. For instance, the nurse notices a grimace on a patient's face (a cue) and infers that the patient is anxious or in pain (the inference). Or, a patient who looks flushed and reports feeling chilled (cues) leads the nurse to infer that the patient has a fever. Inferences are subjective interpretations of cues and, therefore, are influenced by the nurse's level of knowledge and experience, as well as by personal attitudes and values. It is important to validate cues and inferences with the patient to avoid making the wrong interpretation.

Interpreting data involves two cognitive skills: recognizing the cue or inference as significant and assigning meaning to the significance (Carpenito, 1997). The nurse recognizes the significance of cues or groups of cues on the basis of his or her knowledge of patterns or characteristics of phenomena. Meaning is assigned to cues by comparing them to patterns or features of normal, healthy or abnormal, unhealthy states retrieved from memory or obtained from reference materials. The inference mentioned above about a patient's rising temperature was made by associating the cues (flushed skin and feeling chilled) to knowledge of the signs and symptoms and pathophysiology of infection.

Knowledge and experience enhance the nurse's ability to make accurate inferences about patient states. Inferences that nurses make are aided by their:

- knowledge of normal functioning, derived from courses in basic biophysical and social sciences
- understanding of normal and abnormal factors that may affect functioning in a particular area
- awareness of common problems and the signs and symptoms that accompany various health problems.

As a beginning student in nursing, you will not have an extensive knowledge base from which to draw. You will, however, be able to identify many deviations from normal and relate these to the knowledge you do have. As your knowledge increases and your clinical experience grows, you will be able to determine the significance of your

Interpreting data involves:

Subjective data / Objective data → recognizing a cue → making an inference → assigning meaning

Example of Interpreting Data

Cue	Inference	Meaning
Objective data: flushed skin Subjective data: "I feel hot and cold"	patient has a fever	patient is having an inflammatory response

findings more readily and with greater depth of understanding. At all times, however, it is important that you communicate your findings and interpret them honestly at your level of understanding.

An important feature about information cues is that they are variable and uncertain. That is to say, cues can mean different things in different situations. A single cue can have one meaning when seen by itself, and a different meaning when seen in combination with other cues. For example, a young woman who gave birth to a baby two days ago is found crying. This cue, that she is crying, could mean a number of things. Perhaps she is crying because she is overjoyed with the birth. On the other hand she may be feeling disappointment over the gender of the baby. She may be experiencing postpartum depression, a common response caused by hormonal readjustment after childbirth. Or she may be crying because she is in pain or because she just received some sad news from home. Obviously, more information is needed to make an inference about the cause of this woman's crying.

Cues can also mean different things when combined with other cues. Take, for example, the cue of hot and flushed skin. When combined with signs of infection, this cue is a fairly strong indicator of fever; whereas in a diabetic person, hot and flushed skin combined with signs of high blood sugar indicate an altered nutritional state. Thus, cues vary in relation to the patient's circumstances.

Some cues give irrefutable grounds for making inferences; for example, if a patient's temperature is 39°C, one can infer absolutely that the patient has a fever. Gordon calls this type of cue a **diagnostic cue** (Gordon, 1994). When a diagnostic cue is present in the assessment findings, the nurse can be quite sure of the condition it represents. Other cues are not so clear. The hot and flushed skin in the example above may not stand alone as a diagnostic cue, but is valuable in assuring certainty of the patient's state when combined with other cues. These variable indicators are called **supporting cues** (Gordon, 1994).

Validating Inferences

Because inferences are often based on cues that are variable and uncertain, there is a risk of error in the conclusions reached. Nurses can decrease the chance of error by validating the inferences and the information they collect. One way of doing this is by comparing objective and subjective data. For example, if a patient states, "I feel very warm" and the nurse observes a temperature of 39°C, the nurse's observation validates the inference of fever made on the basis of what the patient is experiencing. If there is a discrepancy between the nurse's observations (objective data) and what the patient states (subjective data), however, data collection must continue until a valid inference is established. Inferences may also be validated by reexamining data or reassessing the patient, by consulting other health professionals or by referring to a textbook.

Organizing the Information

In order to examine data critically in the diagnosis step of the nursing process, the nurse will find it helpful to group the information by categories, commonly referred to as **clusters**. Putting information into a logical and systematic order makes the mass of data more meaningful and manageable. It brings together related information that helps the nurse see patterns and identify problems and strengths.

There are a variety of frameworks that the nurse can use for clustering the assessment data. A nursing model provides designated categories for data that give meaning to the information from a nursing perspective. Frequently, the model used for the nursing history of a data base assessment can also serve as an organizing framework for data clustering. Frameworks based on human needs also help keep a nursing focus and, in addition, lead logically to nursing diagnoses. A body systems approach is useful because it helps the nurse identify problems that should be referred to the physician (Alfaro-Lefevre, 1998). Table 14.1 illustrates three frameworks for organizing assessment data: Gordon's model, body systems and human needs. The needs framework reflects the needs approach we have taken in this book.

Documenting the Information

The last phase of assessment is communicating and documenting the data that have been collected. Any findings that point to problems requiring immediate attention (for example, abnormal vital signs, breathing problems, severe pain) that the nurse is not qualified to deal with independently must be reported to an appropriate health team member (head nurse, physician or supervisor) before documentation occurs. As a nursing student you will want to report to your primary nurse or your teacher. In this way, significant problems can be examined by appropriately qualified health team members and treatment measures can be instituted without delay.

Documentation procedure for the patient's baseline data varies. Many agencies now use admission forms or patient profiles for recording the nursing history, as well as pertinent observations and examinations. Focussed assessments are entered onto the patient's record according to charting procedure. General guidelines for charting are presented in Chapter 19.

Diagnosis

As the second step in the nursing process, **diagnosis** is defined as a deliberate, systematic process of data analysis and synthesis that ends with a clinical judgement. During assessment, the nurse gathers and organizes data into clusters depicting patterns of health and illness. In diagnosis, these patterns are intellectually examined (analysed) and pulled

TABLE 14.1 Frameworks for organizing (clustering) data

FUNCTIONAL HEALTH PATTERNS (Gordon, 1994)	BODY SYSTEMS (Alfaro, 1990)	HUMAN NEEDS (McCain, 1965)
health perception/health management	integument	physiological needs
nutrition/metabolism	head & neck	oxygen
elimination	special senses	nutrition
activity/exercise	thorax & lungs	urinary elimination
sleep/rest	heart & blood vessels	bowel elimination
cognition/perception	breast	fluid, electrolyte & acid-base balance
self-perception/self-concept	abdomen	temperature regulation
role/relationship	extremities	comfort, rest & sleep
sexuality/reproduction	(musculoskeletal)	pain management
coping/stress tolerance	extremities	activity needs
value/belief	(neurological)	sensory
	genitourinary	movement & exercise
		protection & safety needs
		hygiene
		safety
		control of infection
		psychosocial needs
		sexuality
		security & self-esteem
		death, loss & grieving

together (synthesized) to identify patient problems and strengths. The problems form the basis of the plan of action (nursing care plan), and the strengths are used in developing the most effective plan for the patient. There are three components involved in diagnosis:

1. identifying patient problems and strengths
2. formulating the diagnosis
3. writing the diagnostic statement.

A patient problem is often identified as a health problem that has a number of defining characteristics.

Characteristics of a Health Problem

A health problem:

- is a human response to a life process, event or stressor
- is a health-related condition that both the client and the nurse wish to change
- requires intervention in order to prevent or resolve illness, or to facilitate coping
- results in ineffective coping/adaptation of daily living that is unsatisfying to the client
- is an undesirable state.

SOURCE: Wilkinson, 1996.

Identifying Patient Problems and Strengths

In diagnosis, the nurse examines the data clusters identified during assessment to determine what they mean in the context of the information available. In identifying problems and strengths, the nurse goes "beyond the information contained in the inferences, cues or cue clusters to generate a set of possible diagnostic meanings" (Gordon, 1987, p. 220). The nurse formulates hypotheses of probable nursing diagnoses by comparing observed patterns of functioning in the data clusters to knowledge of significant deviations from normal. What is unusual in the findings about this patient? In what way does the status of the patient's functional abilities compare with known health problems? How important are the deviations from normal?

Problems are identified by comparing the clusters of data to knowledge of lists or categories of signs and symptoms, (i.e., objective and subjective data) or risk factors that depict the hypothesized problems. These lists or categories are called **defining characteristics** (Carpenito, 1997). If, for example, a nurse hypothesizes that a patient's problem is dehydration, he or she will look for defining characteristics of dehydration. If the data in the cluster are similar to the defining characteristics for dehydration, the nurse will conclude that the patient has an **actual problem** of dehydration or fluid volume deficit. If the data in the cluster are not similar to the defining characteristics, the problem is rejected and alternative explanations are considered.

The presence of risk factors in a data base without the accompanying defining characteristics of a hypothesized problem indicate a **potential problem**. For instance, the patient who experiences fever, vomiting and diarrhea faces the potential problem of developing fluid volume deficit because fluid loss would likely be greater than intake. A potential problem may become an actual problem if the nurse or patient does not take action. Problems may also be defined in the absence of adequate defining characteristics. In this case, there are some data to support a diagnosis but they are insufficient to say the patient has an actual problem. For example, a nurse might consider the possibility that ineffective breastfeeding in a young mother might occur because she has not taken prenatal classes. This problem is called a **possible problem**. It indicates that more information is needed to validate that a problem actually exists.

Once a problem has been identified, the nurse's next task is to determine the causative etiology or the contributing factors of the problem (Carpenito, 1997). For example, in an identified problem of patient anxiety, the contributing factor might be "insufficient knowledge of diagnostic test procedure." It is important to determine the cause of the problem because knowing the cause helps to select appropriate nursing interventions. For example, the problem statement "anxiety" gives no indication of actions needed. But, "anxiety related to insufficient knowledge of diagnostic test procedure," on the other hand, tells the nurse what actions will be necessary to treat the problem.

Alfaro-Lefevre (1998, p. 94) offers the following questions that the nurse can ask to help identify the factors causing or contributing to a problem:

- What factors does the person (or significant others) identify as causing or contributing to the problem?
- Are there factors related to developmental age, disease or changes in lifestyle that may be contributing to the problem?
- Are there cultural, socioeconomic, ethical or religious factors that may be contributing to the problem?
- Do your other resources for data collection (e.g., medical records, other health care professionals, literature review) identify factors that might be causing or contributing to the problem?

In addition to identifying health problems, the nurse also has to determine patient strengths. **Strengths** refer to the physical and psychosocial capabilities, the cultural and religious values and beliefs and the spiritual dimensions of persons or families that enable them to cope with the challenges of daily living. Strengths can help patients and families adjust to their health problems and assume responsibility for their own care. Knowledge of patients' strengths helps the nurse determine the amount of assistance they will require in meeting their needs.

Physical strengths include good physical health, regular exercise, a nutritionally well-balanced diet, appropriate weight for body size, and strong muscles and endurance. Psychosocial strengths include effective coping abilities, strong motivation to live optimally with a chronic condition, relatives who are supportive and available to help with home care, ability to use resources in the community, or a positive health attitude (belief in eating well, balancing rest and exercise, avoiding alcohol or nicotine). Together with the patient and/or family, the nurse makes a list of strengths that will help in planning care for the identified health problems. A benefit of this process is that it may also indicate opportunities in which the nurse can assist patients and families in achieving higher levels of wellness.

Example of Problem Identification

DATA CLUSTER	DEFINING CHARACTERISTICS
Temperature 38.4° C Nausea and vomiting Not drinking or eating Diarrhea Dry skin, decreased turgor Concentrated urine	Insufficient fluid intake Less intake than output Dry skin, mucous membranes Decreased, concentrated urine

Interpretation: Data cluster similar to defining characteristics

Actual problem: Fluid volume deficit

Formulating the Diagnosis

NURSING DIAGNOSIS AND COLLABORATIVE PROBLEMS

A **nursing diagnosis** is a clinical judgement about individual, family or community responses to actual or potential health problems or life processes that provides the basis for selecting interventions to achieve desired outcomes (NANDA; cited in Carpenito, 1997). The nursing diagnosis describes a health problem that nurses are responsible for identifying and treating by nurse-prescribed interventions. In contrast, a **collaborative problem** describes "certain physiological complications that nurses manage using both nurse and physician-prescribed interventions" (Carpenito, 1997, p. 2). Nursing is the only discipline that can treat nursing diagnoses and also manage collaborative problems. As an example, if a patient were at risk for fluid volume deficit following surgery because of the possibility of bleeding, the collaborative problem would be described as *Potential Complication: Bleeding*. Table 14.2 provides a comparison of nursing diagnoses with collaborative problems and medical diagnoses.

Alfaro (1990) outlines a number of guidelines the student may use in identifying collaborative problems:

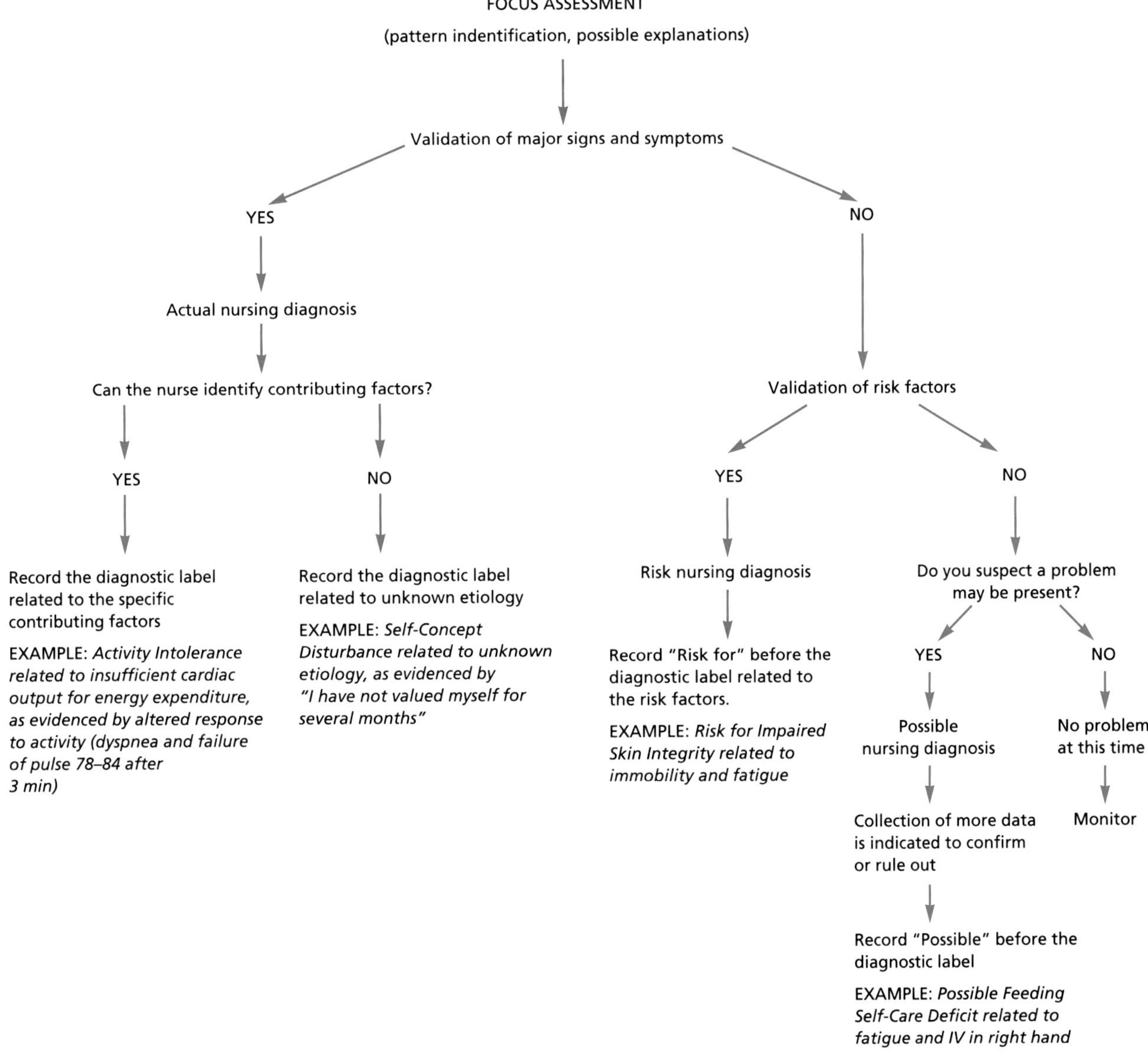

FIGURE 14.3 Decision tree differentiating among actual, risk and possible nursing diagnoses

SOURCE: Carpenito, 1997, p. 7.

- Fluid Volume Deficit related to decreased oral intake, manifested by dry skin and mucous membranes
- Fluid Volume Deficit related to decreased oral intake secondary to difficulty in swallowing, manifested by dry skin and mucous membranes; takes only sips of juice, states "it hurts to swallow."

The first statement describes the problem but tells nothing about why the nurse chose that particular diagnosis, nor does it give any direction to intervention choices. The second statement, on the other hand, describes why the patient has the particular problem and indicates what the nurse should do to treat the problem.

STATING AN ACTUAL NURSING DIAGNOSIS

An actual nursing diagnostic statement consists of three parts: the *problem*, the cause or *etiology*, and the *manifesting signs and symptoms* (defining characteristics). These three parts are linked in the written statement as:

> *Problem* RELATED TO *etiology* MANIFESTED BY *defining characteristics*.
>
> *Example: Impaired Physical Mobility* RELATED TO *pain from surgical incision* MANIFESTED BY *reluctance to move in bed, moaning and stating "it hurts."*

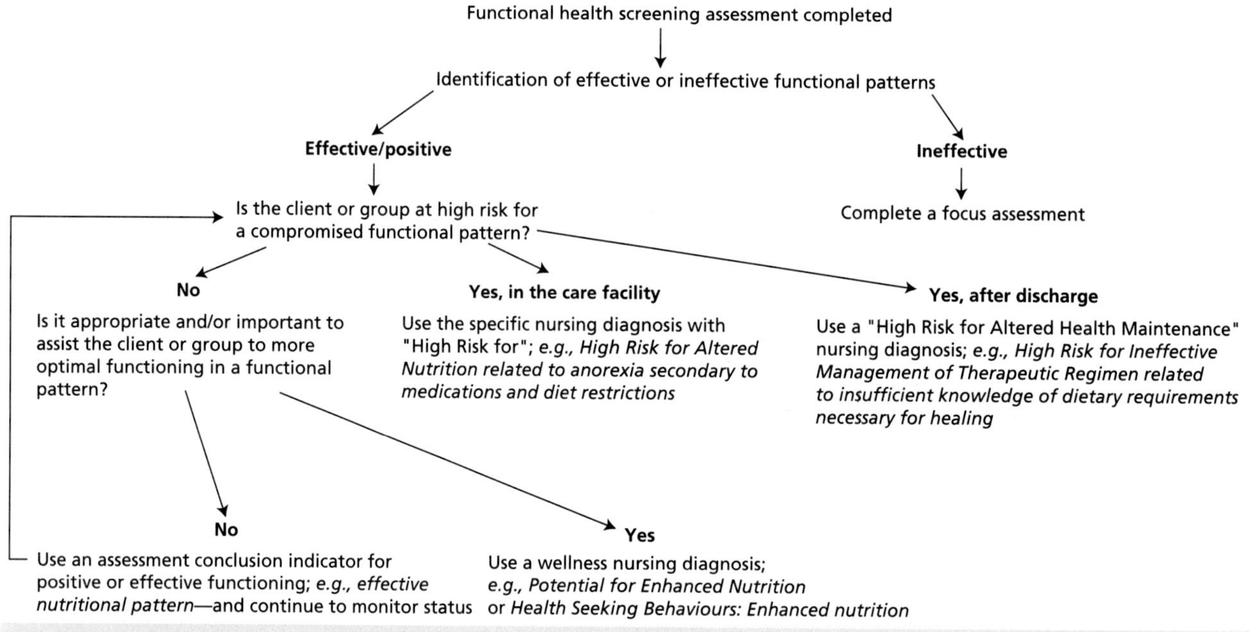

FIGURE 14.4 Decision tree for differentiating among positive/effective functioning and actual, risk and wellness nursing diagnoses

SOURCE: Carpenito, 1997, p. 20.

The **problem** should describe the state that exists as specifically as possible. For example, the diagnosis *Knowledge Deficit* does not specify in what area the patient has a learning need. However, *Knowledge Deficit in diet for diabetes* indicates exactly what it is the patient has to learn.

The **etiology** should specify one or more causes of (or contributors to) the health problem. To be useful it should not only tell why the problem is occurring but give direction in determining nursing interventions. For instance, the problem *Ineffective Family Coping* may be related to conflict between husband and wife, to lack of mutual decision making or to economic difficulties. Nursing interventions would vary considerably for these etiologies. Etiologies may include physiological, psychological, sociological, environmental and spiritual factors believed to cause or contribute to the problem.

Sometimes the cause of a problem may occur at two levels. For example, *Fluid Volume Deficit* related to decreased oral intake may be due to two (or more) factors. In this case, the etiology is stated in two parts, such that the second part explains the first. Notice how the diagnosis *Fluid Volume Deficit related to decreased oral intake* SECONDARY TO *difficulty swallowing* clearly indicates the nature of the patient's decreased intake.

The defining characteristics are the signs and symptoms of the problem that, in the diagnostic statement, serve to validate the nursing diagnosis. They should include the clinical cues, that is, the subjective and objective data that confirm the health problem exists. NANDA's defining characteristics are separated into major and minor categories. "Major defining characteristics are defined as critical indicators present 80%–100% of the time; minor defining characteristics, or supporting indicators, occur 50%–79% of the time" (Carpenito, 1997, p. 13).

STATING A POTENTIAL OR POSSIBLE DIAGNOSIS

Potential and possible diagnoses may often have no defining characteristics. Potential diagnoses are made because of factors in patient situations that may leave them vulnerable to specific problems. For example, a smoker who undergoes major thoracic surgery is at a higher risk for *Ineffective Airway Clearance*. Possible diagnoses may be made to identify suspected problems that require more investigation. Potential and possible diagnoses direct the nurse to continue assessing and monitoring the patient. These diagnoses are written in two-part statements that outline the problem and possible etiology.

> *Examples: Potential Ineffective Airway Clearance related to smoking; possible disturbance in self-concept related to chronic illness.*

STATING THE COLLABORATIVE PROBLEM

The nurse uses the collaborative problem statement to describe a potential complication that may result because of the disease process, trauma or diagnostic tests and treatment. This type of problem identification helps the nurse focus on nursing assessments and the need for referral to the physician. A collaborative problem is written as a potential complication, abbreviated as "PC," linked to its cause.

Example: PC: pulmonary edema secondary to congestive heart failure.

Planning

In the planning step of the nursing process, the nurse prepares for intervention. Goals are set and strategies are selected to achieve the goals. A care plan is written to outline the individualized care needed to promote, protect or restore the patient's health. It is based on the nursing diagnoses and collaborative problems identified in assessment and diagnosis. During planning, the nurse sets priorities, develops goals, selects strategies, collaborates with the patient and family or other health professionals and writes the plan of action. Because patients and families are now assuming greater responsibility for decisions regarding their care, their active involvement in every phase of planning is essential.

Setting Priorities

Once nursing diagnoses and collaborative problems are identified, they are prioritized. It is not possible to attend to all the patient's problems at the same time. Therefore, it is necessary to determine those problems that require treatment immediately and those that can be attended to later.

A helpful guide in priority setting is Maslow's (1970) hierarchy of needs, which was introduced in Chapter 8. Basic physiological needs are given the highest priority, followed by safety, and then love, esteem and self-actualization needs. When physiological needs are life-threatening, priority is given to them. However, in most patient situations—where physiological and safety needs are not life-threatening—equal attention is given to the physiological and psychosocial (cultural, developmental, emotional and spiritual) needs.

However, physiological and safety needs are often the most urgent. Patients may have multiple physiological and safety needs that must be prioritized. In this case, "priorities for treatment depend on 1) the urgency of the problem, 2) the nature of the treatment indicated, and 3) the interactions among diagnoses" (Gordon, 1987, p. 315). Actual or potential problems that are life-threatening are given highest priority. Examples are ineffective breathing patterns or violence directed at self or others. Similarly, when patients are physiologically unstable, intervention for physiological needs may take precedence over attending to knowledge or emotional needs. For example, the nursing diagnosis of *Knowledge Deficit of diet and drug therapy for hypertension* would not be given priority until the patient's physiological state (in this case, high blood pressure) had been stabilized.

Finally, the interaction of diagnoses also influences priority setting. For a woman who had just given birth and was diagnosed with situational low self-esteem and knowledge deficit of infant care, teaching her about infant care could help re-establish her self-esteem. Therefore, improving her knowledge and skill in caring for the baby would be a priority.

Priorities should also be set according to the patient's or family's perception of what is important. When physiological or safety problems take precedence, however, the nurse should clearly explain the rationale for these priorities. The nurse should also remain aware of the psychological and emotional needs of the patient.

Developing Goals and Expected Outcomes

Goals are the statements of expected outcomes of nursing intervention. Intervention is planned to assist or enable the patient to achieve these outcomes. The **expected outcomes** describe the behaviour the patient is expected to achieve. For example, "Mr. M. will dress himself without help every morning" might be one goal for a partially paralyzed patient. Expected outcomes provide the criteria for evaluating the effectiveness of care. Therefore, they must be observable, measurable and understandable.

GOALS FOR NURSING DIAGNOSES

A goal statement usually includes:

1. the healthy response, or desired patient behaviour (for example, "dresses himself")
2. the conditions, if any, under which it is to occur (for example, "without help")
3. a criterion of performance, or standard for judging the performance (for example, each morning).

Some agencies ask that a target date be included (for example, "by April 10, the patient will dress himself without help every morning"). By following a number of guidelines, the nurse can correctly develop a goal and its outcome criteria. These are outlined in Table 14.4 along with examples of correct and incorrect goal statements.

Goals originate from the nursing diagnoses and should reflect improvement in the identified problems. The easiest way to derive a goal is to convert the problem component

TABLE 14.4 Guidelines for writing goals and outcome criteria

Guideline	*Example*
1. Focus the goal statement on expected patient behaviours and responses	**Correct:** The patient will walk... **Incorrect:** The nurse will help the patient walk...
2. Base the goal statement on the nursing diagnosis	Nursing diagnosis: Ineffective Airway Clearance related to incisional pain **Correct:** The patient will keep his airway clear... **Incorrect:** The patient will support his incision when coughing...
3. Use observable verbs to state the outcome criteria. These must describe an expected action or response that can be seen or heard by the nurse	Goal: The patient will keep her airway clear as evidenced by: **Correct:** 1. deep breathing and coughing... 2. changing positions... **Incorrect:** 1. knowing how to cough and turn... 2. relief of incisional pain...
4. State outcome criteria in measurable terms, such that they give a standard against which the patient's activity or response can be compared. Use modifiers to describe what, when, where and how the activity or response will take place	Goal: The patient will keep his airway clear as evidenced by: **Correct:** 1. deep breathing and coughing 5 times qh without incisional pain... **Incorrect:** 1. deep breathing and coughing frequently...
5. Specify a time frame for goal achievement. This helps to keep patient priorities in perspective. Terms like "by discharge" or "continued" are acceptable	**Correct:** 1. The patient will walk down the hall t.i.d. with the aid of a walker by Friday 2. The patient will show continued intact skin

of the nursing diagnosis into a description of the state of health that would exist if the problem were absent. For example, if the nursing diagnosis is *Activity Intolerance related to dypsnea and fatigue*, then the goal should be stated as: "The patient will demonstrate progressive activity tolerance." The outcome criteria are then listed in the goal statement using the phrase "as evidenced by." Thus, a goal statement for the nursing diagnosis above might be, "The patient will demonstrate progressive activity tolerance as evidenced by sitting in the chair for 15 min t.i.d. without dypsnea by Monday."

Outcome criteria can also be derived from the etiological component of the diagnosis, because the best way to treat the problem is to reduce or eliminate the etiology or contributing factors. For example, if the patient's problem is stated as "Altered Nutrition: More Than Body Requirements related to poor eating habits and lack of physical activity," the outcome criteria would focus on the patient's learning proper nutrition and exercising.

Goals should be realistic and attainable both in terms of the patient's potential and of the ability of nurses to help. For example, to set as a goal that Mr. T. will regain complete motor functioning may not be realistic for a patient partially paralyzed by a stroke. But Mr. T. may be able to achieve independence in feeding and dressing himself, and these are goals the nurse can help him achieve. Whenever possible, goals should be set mutually with the patient and family and other members of the health team. This will ensure that the goals are compatible not only with the patient's (and family's) expectations for care but also with other treatment measures, such as physiotherapy, occupational therapy or diagnostic testing.

There are short-term and long-term goals. When expected outcomes can be met in a relatively short period of time—a week or less—they are called **short-term goals** (STGs). Those that will be achieved over a long period of time, sometimes weeks or months, are called **long-term goals** (LTGs). Long-term goals are used in discharge planning from an acute care agency and are very useful in ensuring the continuity of care when patients are discharged to home care or to community settings such as long-term care and ambulatory services. They are also used for patients receiving mental health services both in institutions and in community settings.

Because long-term goals may span weeks or months and patient progress may be slow, short-term goals are often used as stepping stones to reaching long-term goals. By breaking down the long-term goals, the nurse is better able to assess the patient's progress in achieving the final desired outcomes. Both short- and long-term goals are written in the same format as described in Table 14.4.

GOALS FOR COLLABORATIVE PROBLEMS

Goals for collaborative problems are different from goals for nursing diagnoses. Because the nurse is not responsible for diagnosing and prescribing interventions for collaborative problems, setting patient-centred goals for collaborative problems is not appropriate. Rather, collaborative problems involve nursing goals, which reflect nursing accountability in situations requiring physician-prescribed and nurse-prescribed interventions. This accountability includes:

- monitoring for physiologic instability
- consulting standing orders and protocols or a physician to obtain orders for appropriate interventions
- performing specific actions to manage and reduce the severity of an event or situation
- evaluating patient responses (Carpenito, 1997, p. 66).

Nursing goals for collaborative problems can be written to indicate that the nurse will minimize or manage the problem (Carpenito, 1997). For example, if the patient's collaborative problem is PC: *Pulmonary edema secondary to congestive heart failure*, the nursing goal would be, "The nurse will keep the head of the bed at 45° and give diuretic as ordered by physician."

Selecting Nursing Strategies

Nursing strategies are the specific actions or interventions the nurse performs to achieve patient outcomes. These include activities to assist and enable individuals to promote, protect and restore their health or to experience a peaceful death. Nursing interventions are based on the nursing diagnosis and take into account the patient's strengths, preferences and level of ability as well as the physician's orders for care.

TYPES OF INTERVENTION

Nursing interventions are any direct care measures that nurses perform on behalf of patients. These interventions include nurse-initiated measures that result from nursing diagnoses, physician-initiated treatments that result from the medical diagnosis and performance of essential daily functions for patients who are unable to do these (Bulechek & McCloskey, 1989). Bulechek and McCloskey identified six types of nursing activities the nurse carries out in the course of giving care. These are:

1. assessment activities to make a nursing diagnosis
2. assessment activities to gather information for a physician to make a medical diagnosis
3. nurse-initiated treatments in response to nursing diagnoses
4. physician-initiated treatments in response to medical diagnoses
5. daily essential function activities (for example, bed-making, help with meal trays) that may not relate either to medical or to nursing diagnoses but are done by the nurse for the patient who cannot do these things. These do not include deficits in performing the activities of daily living (ADL), such as bathing or combing the hair. When patients cannot perform these activities by themselves they would be diagnosed as having a self-care deficit and care would be done as nursing treatments in (3) above
6. assessment activities to evaluate the effects of nursing and medical treatments (p. 24).

DETERMINING NURSING INTERVENTIONS

In determining interventions for nursing diagnoses, the nurse selects activities to reduce or eliminate the cause or contributing factors; for collaborative problems the activities focus on managing or minimizing the problem. Alfaro (1990) maintains that to determine nursing interventions for actual and potential nursing diagnoses, the nurse has to identify the etiology and decide what needs to be done to eliminate or reduce it. Thus, for a diagnosis of *Fluid Volume*

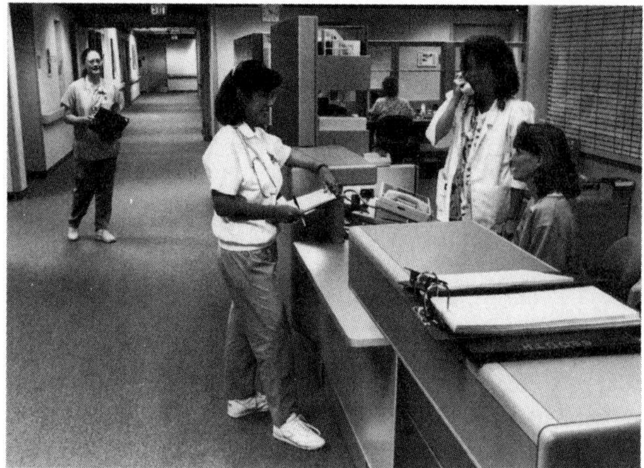

Nurses discussing plan of care for their patients.

Deficit related to decreased oral intake secondary to difficulty swallowing, the nurse would select activities to reduce or eliminate the problem with swallowing.

The selection of interventions involves critical thinking as well as collaboration with the patient and other health professionals. "*Thinking* should be the nurse's first action when planning care" (Hickey, 1990, p. 111). Critical thinking, problem solving and decision making are terms associated with the concept of thinking. These terms will be discussed in Chapter 15.

Using reflection and remembering, devising and brainstorming, the nurse generates possible ways to achieve the expected outcome. Standardized care plans and professional reference books and journals can be consulted for general solutions to the problem. The nurse must examine the general solutions in light of the patient's needs, level of ability, strengths and preferences to determine the interventions most suited to the patient. After formulating a list of possible interventions, the nurse collaborates with the patient and other health team members. Knowledgeable members of the health team—those who have cared for the patient or who have expertise in the problem area—will provide valuable information and advice on the planned interventions. The final information on the interventions most suitable for them based on their values, beliefs and preferences comes from patients and families. Involving patients and their families in selecting interventions for care will gain their commitment, promote patient and family well-being and make implementation easier for the nurse.

Nursing orders/actions are:

- detailed
- specific
- time-bound.

WRITING THE NURSING CARE PLAN

To facilitate the implementation of nursing action, many agencies have developed a system of nursing care plans. The nursing care plan is a written guideline for nursing care. It includes the nursing diagnoses, the goals and outcome criteria and the specific strategies for care. The care plan is formulated as soon after the patient's admission as sufficient data are available on which to base a plan. It is developed by the nurse who has the primary responsibility for the patient's care; or, in some agencies, it is developed jointly by the nursing team responsible for caring for the patient.

Because patients' problems may change from day to day when they are acutely ill, the nursing care plans for sick people are constantly subject to revision. Care plans for patients in ambulatory settings and for those in long-term facilities also need frequent revision but usually not as often as for patients in acute care settings.

In some agencies, the nursing strategies are written in terms of nursing orders, which are prescribed and followed through in the same way as doctor's orders. In other agencies, the terms "nursing approach," "nursing actions" or "nursing directions" may be used to identify the specific strategies prescribed for care of the patient. Nursing orders must be sufficiently detailed and specific to enable all personnel to carry them out in the same manner at the designated times.

The nursing care plan is a means of communicating in writing, to other nursing personnel and to other members of the health team, the nursing diagnoses, the expected outcomes of care and the specific actions to be taken in the care of the patient. In many agencies, the care plans are incorporated into the patient's record; in some, they form part of the Kardex report. Sometimes, a separate notebook is kept for nursing care plans. An example of a nursing care plan is presented in Figure 14.5.

STANDARD CARE PLANS

Because nurses have found that patients with similar conditions have many problems in common, a number of agencies have developed standard care plans for use with patients who have a particular condition. There might be a standard care plan for all medical patients, for example, supplemented by a plan for all patients who have suffered a stroke. There might be another standard care plan for all surgical patients, supplemented by one for patients who are having one particular type of surgical intervention.

Space is usually left on these standard plans for unusual problems—those that are not anticipated and are unique to the patient.

Over the past few years **critical** (clinical) **pathways** have emerged as a means of standardizing "daily care priorities, timely achievement of outcomes and the length of hospital stays" (Alfaro-Lefevre, 1998, p. 115). Wilkinson (1996) describes pathways as a combination of nursing, medicine and other health professions with an imposed time-line on the combined plan. See Figures 14.6 A and B for an example of a clinical pathway for the care of patients after a cerebrovascular accident (CVA).

Implementing

Once nursing care plans have been developed, the next step is to put them into action. **Implemention** is the step of the nursing process in which nurses use their knowledge and skills to carry out the planned interventions. The nurse may give direct care to patients or engage in indirect activities that contribute to their care. This may include giving patients a bath, administering their medications or supervising others in these activities. Nursing care encompasses a variety of interventions. As students progress through their educational program, they will learn many types of interventions; and they will continue to do so throughout their career.

The knowledge and skills needed for implementing a plan of care focus on:

- performing ongoing assessments to determine the status of existing nursing diagnoses and to identify new ones
- setting daily priorities to facilitate optimum treatment of a number of different problems during the course of the day
- directly performing activities for patients
- assisting patients or families in performing activities for themselves
- teaching patients and families about their health care and management of a disorder
- counselling patients and families in making decisions about their own health care and using health resources
- monitoring patients for potential complications or problems
- charting or documenting according to the legal specifications of the agency (Alfaro, 1990).

Documenting Care

Agencies vary in their requirements for documentation. In some, the nursing care plan is supplemented by a record that lists the nursing orders (taken from the care plan) and provides space for the nurse to tick off as each intervention is carried out. This type of record acts as a checklist that the nurse responsible for the patient's care on each shift can review to see what was done and what was omitted.

Another type of form, similar in purpose to the checklist described above, is the flowsheet. When a specific intervention or a group of related interventions are to be done on a regular basis, it is helpful to have a special form that details the intervention specifically and documents the results of that intervention. See Chapter 19 for more details about documentation.

Evaluating

Evaluation is "planned, ongoing, deliberate activity in which the nurse, client, significant others and other health professionals determine the extent of client outcome achievement and the effectiveness of the nursing care plan" (Wilkinson, 1996, p. 272). Implicit in this assessment is the need for constant revision of nursing care plans as new problems emerge, others are resolved and some change. Priorities may need to be reordered, goals modified and new goals established. In addition, new decisions may have to be made in light of new information, changes that have occurred in the patient's condition and success or failure of the interventions that have been tried.

Evaluation is the process of determining the extent to which the expected outcomes have been attained. It implies measurement against predetermined standards. If the outcome criteria have been carefully thought out and stated as observable and measurable standards, the nurse has a standard for comparing the patient's achievements. For example, an outcome criterion for a problem of impaired physical mobility might be stated as "Will maintain prescribed position at all times, except when necessary to turn on side for care." In evaluating the patient's achievement of the outcome criterion, the nurse checks through the points enumerated regarding the position. Is the patient (Ms. J.) flat in bed? Is she on her back? Does she have two pillows under her head? Is one supporting her shoulders? Does she have a pillow under her knees? Is she maintaining this position at all times, except when it is necessary to turn on her side for a back wash or a linen change?

In evaluating the patient's goal achievement, the nurse compares the patient's activities and responses to the

Assessment Data	Nursing Diagnosis/ Collaborative Problem	Outcome
10/20	10/20	
Health management/Health perception: Nonsmoker. Goes to aerobic 3 × wk when well. States being ill and dependent on others is very difficult on her.	1. Fluid Volume Deficit R/T Fever, diarrhea, and loss of appetite as manifested by dark concentrated urine.	Will maintain hydration by drinking at least 2000 mL per day every day.
Nutrition/metabolic pattern: 20 lb overweight. Has had no appetite since illness started 10 days ago. Has had fever of 37.5° much of the time. Skin intact—no rashes.		
Elimination pattern: BM q other day usually. Now has diarrhea 10–15 × /day. Has external hemorrhoids. Urine dark and concentrated.	2. Diarrhea R/T unknown etiology.	Will develop normal bowel movements by controlling diarrhea through medication and diet by 10/22.
Activity/exercise pattern: Has not been out of house for past 10 days. Feels she is too weak to go out.		
Cognitive perception pattern: College graduate. Alert and appropriate in communication		
10/20	10/20	
Sleep/rest pattern: Sleeps much of the time, but disturbed by having to get up to BR for diarrhea	3. Possible Altered Family Process R/T illness of mother	She and her husband will discuss how family will cope with illness by 10/22.
Self-perception/self-concept pattern: States she's an independent individual.	4. Potential Impaired Skin Integrity (rectal area) R/T diarrhea & hemorrhoids.	
Role/relationship pattern: Married. Has one child. Worried because she says husband is "not good" with daughter.		Rectal area will remain clean and without signs of irritation.
Sexual/reproductive pattern: Married. Other data collection deferred.		
Coping/stress pattern: States she's a "doer"—likes to be active doing things when she is depressed.		
Value/belief pattern: Catholic. Attends Mass most Sundays.		

FIGURE 14.5 Example of a nursing care plan using Gordon's model

SOURCE: Alfaro, R., 1990, pp. 128, 129.

Nursing Orders	Evaluation
10/20 1. Keep ginger ale with juice at bedside. 2. Force fluids (clear liq) to: 1000 mL (7–3) 750 mL (3–11) 250 mL (7–11) 3. Assess fluid intake every 2 h while awake. 4. Both nurse & pt should keep a record of I/O. 5. Monitor electrolyte studies. J. Martin RN	10/22 Fluid intake only 1500 mL last 2 days. Discussed her need to push more. JM Electrolytes WNL JM Urine output 700 mL and concentrated. JM Keeping own I/O record. JM
10/20 1. Maintain clear liquid diet. 2. Assess BMs q 3° while awake and give Lomotil prn. J. Martin RN	10/22 Diarrhea ↓ to 4 x day. Clear liquids maintained. Taking Lomotil q.i.d. JM
10/20 Spend time discussing with husband and wife together and separately to determine how the family is adapting to illness and to identify potential problems. J. Martin RN	10/22 Husband has not been to visit for longer than 10 min. and I have missed him both times. Told her to ask him to call me when he can. JM
Encourage warm sitz baths q.i.d. especially $\bar{p}$ BMs J. Martin RN	10/22 Taking sitz bath. Rectal area clean—not red. JM

FIGURE 14.5 Example of a nursing care plan using Gordon's model

SOURCE: Alfaro, R. (1990) 128, 129.

FASTRACK STREAM
CVA Clinical Pathway (Hemorrhagic & Nonhemorrhagic)
ST.PAUL'S HOSPITAL

Patient Name: ____________________

Date:				
	Day 1 Emergency	**Day 1 Admission**	**Day 2**	**Day 3**
DIAGNOSTIC	As per Emerg Lab Order Protocol: CBC & Diff, CK, Pt/INR, PTT, gluc, Na^+, K^+ Cl^+, HCO_3, BUN, CR, U/A	ECG, CXR ± ☐ CT Head ± ☐ Cardiac Echo	± ☐ Urine C&S (persistent incontinence) ± ☐ Hotler monitor ± ☐ Carotid duplex U/S ± ☐ Cerebral angiograms	
CONSULTS	• Emerg UC to notify disciplines as per the pathway distribution list. Disciplines include OT, PT, SW, Pharmacy, Dietitian. CNS, Speech. ☐ If TPA candidate, consult neurologist	• UC on ward to notify ☐ GP • Initial assessment done within 24–48 h and intervention initiated by PT, OT & SW ± ☐ Rehab Medicine referral	Consult MD to MD: ± ☐ Neurology (consider on all patients) ± ☐ Geriatrics (consider if pt ≥ 75 yrs)	☐ Pharmacist Assess medication knowledge and ability to self-medicate
ASSESSMENT/ TREATMENTS/ INTERVENTIONS	• If CVA presents within 3 h, consider TPA protocol • Nursing history • Neuro VS q1–2h • Cardiac monitoring • Foley catheter per order	• Admission history • Nursing assessment q shift (resp, skin, safety precautions, communication deficits, pain) • VS & neuro VS q4h x 24 h • IV • Monitor I/O q shift • ± ☐ Post-void residual for incontinence or when patient has not voided Where PVR ≥ 150 mL perform In/Out PVR q6–8h until res. vol. < 150 mL on two consecutive occasions (Avoid routine Foley, except if patient comatose) • Initiate bowel protocol (MAR)	→ • VS & neuro VS (NVS) q shift, if stable • D/C IV if drinking well → • If Foley in, remove if patient able to sit →	→ • VS & NVS q shift • MD reassess need for NVS → →
ACTIVITY/ MOBILIZATION	• Bedrest • Head of bed elevated 30° • Position changes q2h, as needed	• Bedrest • Head of bed elevated 30° • If unable to move, turn q2h • Assist with ADLs • Full bath	• Activity order reviewed by attending MD ± Dangle up in chair, or walking c assist (RN/PT) • If unable to mobilize, passive ROM exercises initiated • Assist ADL • Full bath	Nsq, OT, PT collaborate: • Walking with assist if able • Up in chair for meals • ADL assessment (OT) • Encourage independence with ADLs as appropriate • Exercise with PT → →
MEDICATIONS	• Per MD orders ☐ TPA ☐ Other	• As per MD orders for: ☐ Nonhemorrhagic CVA ☐ Embolic CVA • Personal meds	→ →	→ →
DIET	• NPO, unless otherwise ordered • Check cough reflex • Check gag reflex • Check ability to swallow • Diet per order	• Nsg swallowing assessment • If unable to tolerate, make NPO & initiate OT swallowing assessment • If no problem → DAT	recommendation: • OT swallowing assessment ☐ Modified diet ☐ Tube feeds • Monitor food/fluid intake ± ☐ Calorie count prn (if < 50% meal intake)	• Ongoing swallowing assessment/intervention • Patient self-feeding ± adaptations → →
DISCHARGE PLANNING/ TEACHING	• Orient patient/family to unit. Admitting MD: • Ascertain Degree of Intervention/CODE Status and document on MD orders	RN: • CP handout & stroke package given to pt/family, as appropriate, with explanation/outcomes • Orient patient/family to ward Speech: Dysarthria or aphasic pamphlet given to patient/family SW: • Discharge pamphlet given to patient/family • Family spokesperson identified	RN: CP handout information & stroke package discussed MD: • Reassess Degree of Intervention/CODE Status and document on MD orders • Ongoing education by team	• Guidelines for determining pt stream completed by team • Patient stream identified: ☐ Fastrack ☐ Regular Housestaff documents: ➢ expected day of discharge on Discharge Form & informs patient/family • Family to bring in clothes (suitable to facilitate ADLs) →

FIGURE 14.6A CVA clinical pathway form

SOURCE: Nursing Department, St. Paul's Hospital, Vancouver, British Columbia.

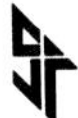

CVA Clinical Pathway (Hemorrhagic & Nonhemorrhagic)

Patient Name: ______________________

Date:				
	Day 4	Day 5	Day 6	Day 7 Discharge
DIAGNOSTIC				
CONSULTS		± ☐ Home Care	• Rehab assessment completed • Notification of consultants & GP of discharge date	
TREATMENTS/ INTERVENTIONS	• Nursing assessment q shift • VS q shift • ± NVS q shift • Invasive PVR completed • Continue bladder program • Continue bowel protocol (MAR)	• Nursing assessment q shift • VS q shift • ± NVS q shift ➜ ➜	• Nursing assessment q shift • VS q shift ➜ ➜	• Nursing assessment q shift • VS q shift ➜ ➜
ACTIVITY/ MOBILIZATION	• Continue progressive mobilization • Up in chair for meals • Ongoing ADL assessment/intervention ☐ Mat Program (PT) ☐ Functional re-education (OT) • Patient wears own clothes	➜ ➜ ➜ ➜ • Stair training if required for home (PT)	➜ ➜ ➜ ➜	➜ ➜ ➜ ➜
MEDICATIONS	• As per MD orders for: ☐ Nonhemorrhagic CVA ☐ Embolic CVA • Personal meds	➜ ➜	➜ ➜	➜ ➜
DIET	• Regular diet ± ☐ Calorie count prn	➜ ➜	➜ • D/C calorie count if adequate nutrition	➜
DISCHARGE PLANNING/ TEACHING	• Ongoing education by team • Home environment needs assessment discussed with pt/family by OT • Discharge support & education for patient/family by multidisciplinary team • Progress of medication teaching documented by pharmacist Documentation on Discharge Form • Determine need for Outpatient Services and referrals initiated: ☐ Home Care ☐ Nursing ☐ OT ☐ PT ☐ SLP ☐ Continuing Care (refer to *Criteria for Early Discharge*, Frail Elderly Program, VHB)	➜ RN: • Follow-up teaching re: ☐ risk factors ☐ preventive measures • Caregiver training ➜ Documentation on Discharge Form • Determine: ☐ Transportation ☐ Confirm discharge date	➜ • Discharge pamphlet completed with instructions for patients & reviewed by SW (including referral to Stroke Club) → • Pt has final med profile • Outpatient services arranged Discharge Form finalized: ☐ Equipment for home in place (OT/PT) ☐ Transportation home ☐ D/C order written ☐ Prescriptions written & on chart	➢ Discharge home prior to 11:00

FIGURE 14.6B Fast-track CVA clinical pathway form

SOURCE: Nursing Department, St. Paul's Hospital, Vancouver, British Columbia.

standards set out in the outcome criteria of the goal statement. Progress can be noted and, if a particular nursing strategy does not appear to be effective, an alternative course of action can be recommended. The attainment of certain short-term goals may mean that the patient is ready for more far-reaching ones. The patient who has learned to dress without assistance, for example, may be ready to learn another activity of daily living.

Stating outcome criteria in question form helps the nurse to be objective and look for specific indications that expected outcomes have been met. Questions are not always written, but beginning nurses may find that, by writing them down, it is easier to develop the habit of asking themselves the questions implicit in the outcome criteria for the patient.

Nurses evaluate the effectiveness of care through observations of the patient. Is the paralyzed arm in good anatomical position, or is the hand in a dependent position? It is also necessary to ask patients if nursing actions have been effective. Is the patient more comfortable or free from pain?

As we stated in the beginning of the chapter, the nursing process is a circular one. Evaluation means reassessment and a gathering of additional information. On the basis of reassessment, the nurse may identify new problems, modify the care plan or decide to try alternative interventions for the goals that were unsuccessful.

Revising the Plan of Care

- Does the nursing care plan contain enough information for effective nursing diagnosis and care planning?
- Were all relevant factors taken into consideration in making the nursing diagnoses?
- Were nursing diagnoses omitted for which care would have helped the patient?
- Was the plan a logical outgrowth of the nursing diagnoses?
- Were the established priorities correct?
- Were unique factors in regard to the patient taken into consideration?
- Was the plan consistent with the physician's plan of therapy?
- Were expected outcomes logical, realistic and attainable?
- Were the nursing orders clearly stated?
- Was the plan successful? If so, what factors contributed to its success? Were there factors that interfered with success?
- Is the plan current and up to date? Have some problems resolved, or new ones emerged?

IN REVIEW

- Nursing process is a problem-solving approach to practice that:
  - is used to identify, prevent and treat health problems and promote wellness
  - provides a structural framework that has several interrelated steps.
- Assessment is the collection and interpretation of clinical information using a variety of sources that enable the nurse to develop a beginning nursing care plan. Sources include:
  - interviews with patients and/or families
  - observations
  - physical examination
  - consultation with other health professionals
  - review of health records (including chart).
- A data base (baseline) assessment is performed on admission, and focus assessments are conducted on an ongoing basis. These two types of assessments provide a comprehensive picture of a patient's health status.
- Diagnostic reasoning is used to interpret data collected and to make judgements about a patient's health status:
  - subjective data include any information reported by the patient
  - objective data are observable, measurable or perceptible by another person.
- All data must be validated to decrease the chance of error. A framework based on a nursing model can be used to organize data.
- Diagnosis is a deliberative process that involves the analysis and synthesis of data to identify patient problems and strengths. A nursing diagnosis identifies a health problem, of which there are four types:
  - actual
  - potential
  - possible
  - collaborative.
- Planning involves setting priorities, establishing goals, selecting interventions and writing the nursing care plan:
  - goals are statements of expected outcomes (short- or long-term) derived from the nursing diagnosis
  - goals should be attainable, measurable, understandable and agreed upon by patient and family
  - nursing interventions include any direct care measures the nurse performs to achieve expected outcomes

- the nursing care plan is developed and updated in accordance with any changes in the patient's health status
- the nursing care plan functions as a means of communication among health professionals.

■ Implementation is the step during which planned nursing interventions are carried out. This includes:

- direct care
- ongoing assessments and monitoring
- supervision of care
- teaching and counselling
- documentation.

■ Evaluation is a planned, ongoing, deliberate activity to determine outcome achievement and effectiveness of the nursing care plan. Evaluation involves nurse, patient, family and other health professionals.

Critical Thinking Activities

In consultation with your teacher, select a patient who has recently been admitted to the agency in which you are doing your clinical practice.

1. Review the patient's record to identify how and where the steps of the nursing process are documented.
2. Examine the patient's baseline data. Identify the information that would be helpful in planning nursing care.
3. Determine how focus assessment data are recorded. How does information gathered by focus assessment differ from baseline data? What factors might determine what information is gathered in the focus assessment?
4. State the nursing diagnoses you can identify from the data in the patient's record.
5. Arrange these problems in a list according to priorities as you see them.
6. Develop expected outcomes for each of the diagnoses.
7. Compare your diagnoses and expected outcomes with those on the nursing care plan prepared by experienced nurses. Did you identify the same problems? Did you miss any? Did you identify ones not listed? Did you use similar wording in the diagnostic statements? Did you rank priorities in the same order? If not, why do you think the order was different? Were your goal statements similar?
8. Review the nursing interventions prescribed in the nursing care plan and flowsheets or other forms used to facilitate care. Relate these interventions to the nursing diagnoses and to principles underlying care.
9. Describe how you would evaluate the effectiveness of the nursing care plan.

KEY TERMS

nursing process p. 322
patient p. 322
diagnostic reasoning p. 322
assessment p. 323
data base assessment p. 324
focus assessment p. 324
primary source p. 324
secondary sources p. 324
health history p. 325
structured interview p. 325
observation p. 326
examination p. 326
subjective data p. 331
objective data p. 331
cue p. 331
inference p. 331
diagnostic cue p. 332
supporting cue p. 332
cluster p. 332
diagnosis p. 332
defining characteristic p. 333
actual problem p. 333
potential problem p. 334
possible problem p. 334
strengths p. 334
nursing diagnosis p. 334
collaborative problem p. 334
actual diagnosis p. 335
risk diagnosis p. 335
wellness diagnosis p. 335
syndrome diagnosis p. 335
problem p. 338
etiology p. 338
expected outcome p. 339
short-term goal p. 341
long-term goal p. 341
critical pathways p. 343
implementation p. 343
evaluation p. 343

References

ALFARO, R. (1990). *Applying nursing diagnosis and nursing process.* (2nd ed.). Philadelphia: Lippincott.

ALFARO-LEFEVRE, R. (1998). *Applying nursing process: A step-by-step guide.* (4th ed.). Philadelphia: Lippincott.

BULECHEK, G., & McCLOSKEY, J. (1989). Nursing interventions: Treatments for potential nursing diagnoses. In M. Carroll-Johnson (Ed.), *Classification of nursing diagnosis: Proceedings of the eighth national conference.* Philadelphia: Lippincott.

CARNEVALI, D., MITCHELL, P.H., WOODS, N.F., & TANNER, C.A. (1984). *Diagnostic reasoning in nursing.* Philadelphia: Lippincott.

CARNEVALI, D.L., & THOMAS, M.D. (1993). *Diagnostic reasoning and treatment decision making in nursing.* Philadelphia: Lippincott.

CARPENITO, L.J. (1997). *Nursing diagnosis: Application to clinical practice.* (7th ed.). Philadelphia: Lippincott.

GORDON, M. (1987). *Nursing diagnosis: Process and application.* (2nd ed.). New York: McGraw-Hill.

GORDON, M. (1994). *Nursing diagnosis: Process and application.* (3rd ed.). St. Louis: Mosby.

HENDERSON, V. (1966). *The nature of nursing: A definition and its implications for practice, research and education.* New York: Macmillan.

HICKEY, P.W. (1990). *Nursing process handbook.* St. Louis: Mosby.

KELLY, M.A. (1985). *Nursing diagnosis source book: Guidelines for clinical application.* Norwalk, CT: Appleton-Century-Crofts.

MASLOW, A.H. (1970). *Motivation and personality.* (2nd ed.). New York: Harper & Row.

McCAIN, R.F. (1965, April). Nursing by assessment—Not intuition. *AJN*, 82–84.

NORTH AMERICAN NURSING DIAGNOSIS ASSOCIATION. (1994). *NANDA nursing diagnoses: Definitions and classification 1995–1996.* Philadelphia: Author.

WILKINSON, J.M. (1996). *Nursing process: A critical thinking approach.* (2nd ed.). Menlo Park, CA: Addison-Wesley.

YURA, H., & WALSH M. B. (1988). *The nursing process.* Norwalk, CT: Appleton & Lange.

Additional Readings

CALLADINE, M.L. (1996). Nursing process for health promotion: Using King's theory. *Journal of Community Health Nursing, 13*(1), 51–57.

CARPENITO, L.J. (1995). *Nursing care plans and documentation.* (2nd ed.). Philadelphia: Lippincott.

CHRISTENSEN, P., & KENNEY, J. (1994). *Nursing process: Application of conceptual models.* (4th ed.). St. Louis: Mosby.

CONGER, M., & MEZZA, I. (1996). Fostering critical thinking in nursing students in the clinical setting. *Nurse Educator, 21*(3), 11–15.

DALY, B. (1996). Concept maps: Linking nursing theory to clinical nursing practice. *Journal of Continuing Education in Nursing, 27*(1), 17–27.

GEORGE, J.B. (1995). *Nursing theories: The base for professional nursing practice.* (4th ed.). Norwalk, CT: Appleton & Lange.

IYER, P.W., TAPTICH, B.J., & BERNOCCHI-LOSEY, B. (1986). *Nursing process and nursing diagnosis.* Philadelphia: Saunders.

LA MONICA, E.L. (1985). *The humanistic nursing process.* Monterey, CA: Wadsworth.

LEDDY, S., & PEPPER, J.M. (1993) *Conceptual bases of professional nursing.* Philadelphia: Lippincott.

LUTZEN, K., & TISHELMAN, C. (1996). Nursing diagnosis: A critical analysis of underlying assumptions. *International Journal of Nursing Studies, 33*(2), 190–200.

MILLER, E. (1989). *How to make a nursing diagnosis work.* Norwalk, CT: Appleton & Lange.

MORITZ, D.A. (1982). Nursing diagnosis in relation to the nursing process. In M.J. Kim & D.A. Moritz (Eds.), *Classification of nursing diagnoses: Proceedings of the third and fourth national conferences* (pp. 53–57). New York: McGraw-Hill.

ROY, C. (1984). *Introduction to nursing: An adaptation model.* (2nd ed.). Englewood Cliffs, NJ: Prentice Hall.

SHOEMAKER, J. (1984). Essential features of a nursing diagnosis. In M.J. Kim, G.K. McFarland, & A.M. McLane (Eds.), *Classification of nursing diagnoses: Proceedings of the fifth national conference* (p. 109). St. Louis: Mosby.

SNYDER, M., EGAN., E.C., & NOJIMA, Y. (1996). Defining nursing interventions. *Image, 28*(2), 137–141.

STOLTE, K.M. (1996a). *Nursing diagnosis for health promotion.* Philadelphia: Lippincott.

STOLTE, K.M. (1996b). *Wellness: Nursing diagnosis for health promotion.* Philadelphia: Lippincott.

Chapter 15

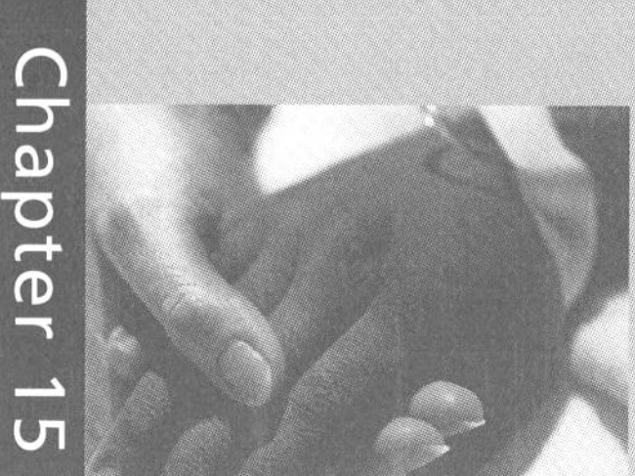

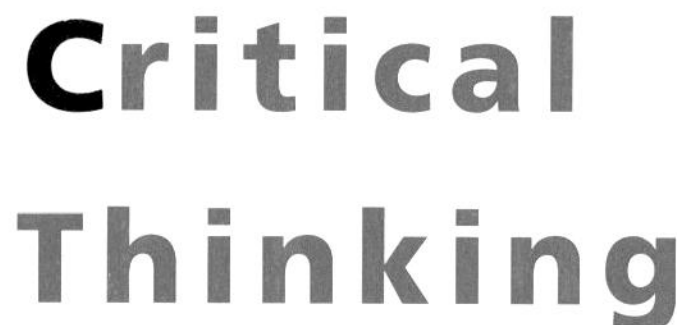

Critical Thinking

OUTLINE

Central Questions

1. What is critical thinking?
2. Why do nurses need to be able to think critically?
3. What is intuition?
4. What are the components of critical thinking?
5. What must the nurse know in order to be able to think critically?
6. What cognitive skills does the nurse need? What attitudes are important?
7. How do nurses use critical thinking in carrying out each step of the nursing process?

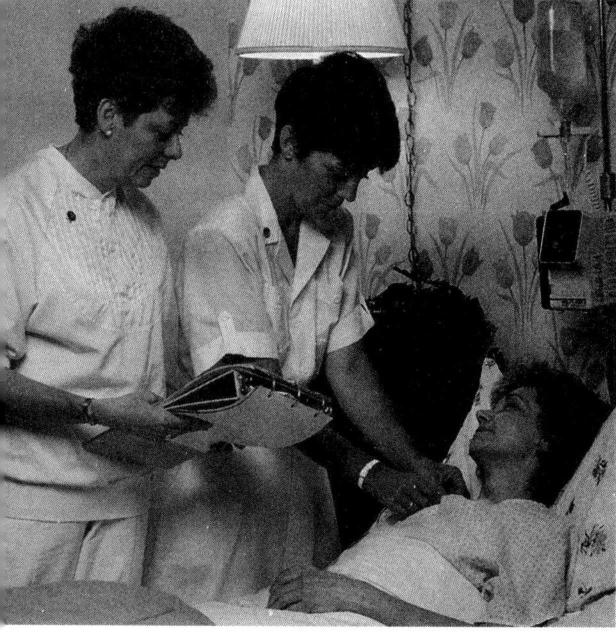

"Why" is the crucial question in the development of critical thinking skills. One must take abstract theoretical concepts and turn them into questions. This provides a framework to put things together. "How" is the beginning of a critical thinking skill question: knowing how to apply, how to put things together, how to take the material and actually start to manipulate it—in other words, to get in there and wrestle with the material. Critical skills that are absolutely necessary [to the nurse] include how to read critically, how to write critically, how to think critically.

J. Rehner, personal communication, 1997

Introduction

At the beginning of the last chapter we said that the process of nursing is the same, whether the act involved is a simple first aid measure or a sequence of complicated activities. Carrying out the nursing process in day-to-day practice requires the ability to assess a situation, to see relationships and to predict outcomes. In order to do this, the nurse must be able to engage in purposeful mental activity—to generate and evaluate new ideas, to use information in making judgements and decisions, and to solve problems (Wilkinson, 1996). In addition, the nurse must be able to apply nursing knowledge in a variety of practice settings. This requires critical thinking skills, as does almost everything a nurse does on a daily basis.

Critical thinking has been defined in many different ways. Some definitions emphasize the goals of critical thinking; others emphasize its process, its methodology or its scope. In this text we have chosen to use Miller and Babcock's (1996) definition of **critical thinking** as "purposeful thinking that takes into consideration focus, language, frame of reference, attitudes, assumptions, evidence, reasoning, conclusions, implications, and context when they matter in deciding what to believe or do" (Miller & Babcock, 1996, p. 8).

Critical thinking is the kind of thinking in which nurses are aware of the implications of the ideas they hold and the decisions they make. Many situations faced by nurses in their day-to-day practice do not require a decision about what is truth or fact, or what is the right or wrong response, but rather require a clinical judgement that takes into consideration the many options available and the ultimate effects of any one of them. For example, if a patient asks what kind of medication she is taking and what the side effects are, the nurse has the option of answering the question at length or of filtering out some of the information for fear of overwhelming the patient with too much detail. In this situation, critical thinking may, first of all, cause the nurse to wonder why the patient asked the question and, secondly, to consider the potential benefits and harms that might arise from the response.

Critical thinking means exploring a situation, phenomenon, question or problem with an open mind. It means considering all available information before arriving at a tentative conclusion, and being able to support the decision with sound facts (Brigham, 1993). Critical thinking is not a linear process, but rather a multidimensional process that includes imaginative speculation, reflective thinking, questioning of assumptions, and intuition (Brigham, 1993). Critical thinking helps the nurse move beyond objective, rational, linear thinking to a more expansive, imaginative and creative way of thinking. Overall, critical thinking helps to focus and sharpen the nurse's awareness.

Critical thinking challenges nurses to examine and clarify assumptions—our own as well as those of others. It helps us to question "the way things are" by challenging inferences and existing principles, arguments and conclusions. It suggests that even at the action or implementation stage, the nurse continues with an inquiring attitude so that if more information becomes available, thought processes or actions can change as a result. Critical thinking suggests that the nurse differentiates between good and bad arguments and seeks to confirm those facts and values from which reliable and sincere judgements and actions flow (Bandman & Bandman, 1995).

In this chapter we are going to discuss why the nurse needs to be able to think critically. Then we will talk about the components of critical thinking: the knowledge base that is needed, the cognitive skills to be acquired and the attitudes to be developed. We will then look at critical thinking as nurses apply it in their day-to-day practice. We are going to use a case study to illustrate some of the critical thinking the nurse does as he or she proceeds through the steps of the nursing process.

Mrs. Narindar Sandhu is a 60-year-old East Indian woman who was admitted to the emergency department at Adanac Hospital with a diagnosis of hyperglycemia (high blood sugar) at about 19:00 h. She was brought in by ambulance in a comatose state. Her husband and daughter accompanied her to the hospital. The physician on duty examined Mrs. Sandhu and initiated treatment. As soon as her blood sugar was normal and her condition was stable, she was transferred from emergency to a semiprivate room on the medical floor of the hospital. An intravenous infusion was begun and blood glucose monitoring was ordered four times a day. The admission information lists Mrs. Sandhu's religion as Hindu.

The Need for Critical Thinking in Nursing

One of the most important reasons for nurses to develop critical thinking skills is that many practical problems cannot be resolved by a standard set of interventions. Health care workplaces, as with many other workplaces today, require open-minded, creative, flexible individuals who have the ability to make effective, reflective, knowledge-based decisions for which they are prepared to be accountable.

Critical thinking is invaluable to nurses in developing the skills and knowledge needed to use technology in ways that are ethical and appropriate to the needs of the patient, whether that patient is an individual, a family or a community. For example, the nurse caring for Mrs. Sandhu needs a good knowledge of anatomy and physiology as well as knowledge about diabetes and about family-centred care in order to help the family. In addition, he or she needs to be able to identify deviations from the normal in laboratory test results in order to explain, to the patient and family, the purpose and results of laboratory tests and to assist the patient in learning to manage her diabetes at home.

As we saw in Chapter 12, increased immigration—as well as increased mobility of the general population—has made many areas of Canada more racially and ethnically diverse. This diversity encompasses culture, economic conditions, education, income and employment; it affects rural, urban and suburban communities. Gender, age and sexual orientation are further areas of diversity. In order to be sensitive to other cultures, the nurse must move beyond ethnocentrism—the deep-seated belief that one's own culture is superior to all others (Miller & Babcock, 1996; see Chapter 12). Recognizing our own tendency towards ethnocentrism and giving sincere thought to the beliefs of cultures other than our own require critical thinking.

Our perceptions are "shaped by our culture, our past experiences, our psychological makeup, our spiritual beliefs, as well as how we are feeling at the time" (Miller & Babcock, 1996, p. 3). In nursing, it is important to be aware of the attitudes, values and beliefs we hold, where they came from and how they influence our perceptions and behaviours, whether in personal or in professional situations. Nurses accomplish this self-awareness through critical thinking skills—that is, questioning and challenging themselves, both professionally and personally.

In hospital, Mrs. Sandhu has many concerns regarding attire, privacy and food. At home, she always wears a sari or salwar kameze (traditional dress over trousers), but was put into a hospital gown in emergency. She insists on having only female nurses. She is independent in her activities of daily living. The patient had two Hindu relics (religious objects) with her at the time of admission.

Mrs. Sandhu insists on wearing her salwar kameze during the day while in hospital. You think she should wear a hospital gown, as other patients do. You probably think this way because your previous experience created this expectation, or *mindset.* How can you get beyond this point of view? The answer is by using critical thinking—by questioning yourself, your beliefs and your assumptions. Following are some questions you might ask yourself in order to think more critically:

- Is there any specific reason why Mrs. Sandhu needs to wear a hospital gown? For example, is she having treatments or procedures—such as radiology—that require her to be in a gown?
- Why does the patient want to wear the salwar kameze? For cultural reasons? For modesty? For religious reasons?
- Would she feel more comfortable wearing her traditional dress?

Critical thinking is consistent with nursing because it implies a sense of responsibility. The outcomes of clinical reasoning can make a real difference in people's lives. In Mrs. Sandhu's case, it is important that the nurse be able to help her learn how to maintain her blood sugar at a stable level when she goes home, in order to prevent further complications. Because nurses accept this responsibility, they understand that excellent nursing will never be a matter of simply following prescribed routines, or responding the way they feel at a particular moment.

The ability to think deeply, effectively and critically promotes lifelong learning, assists the nurse to make more astute life choices, builds self-confidence, and fosters self-actualization, both professionally and personally (Miller & Babcock, 1996). Effective thinking is essential in a world where knowledge is generated exponentially on a daily basis.

Critical Thinking and Intuition

An experienced nurse might walk into Mrs. Sandhu's hospital room and immediately note several problems: her intravenous infusion has run dry, her position needs changing, and she looks both uncomfortable and apprehensive. Similarly, an experienced community nurse visiting Mrs. Sandhu after she has been discharged from the hospital will be able to assess the home situation and identify a number of problems. For example, the lunch that Mrs. Sandhu is eating does not conform to her diet instructions; she looks as if she is in dire need of rest, and the children in the household all have bad colds.

The experienced nurse's ability to assess a situation quickly, make decisions and act is often called **intuition.** We used to believe that intuition was a "sixth sense" that one acquired through years of practice, rather than a process that was rational, systematic or data-based. Largely through the work of Benner and her colleagues (1984, 1987, 1989), it is now understood that intuitive decision making is an essential and legitimate aspect of expert clinical judgement that is based on knowledge and experience gained through extensive clinical practice and the opportunity to compare and contrast symptoms and outcomes in many similar and dissimilar situations (Benner & Tanner, 1987).

Intuition is "not a mystical or accidental human capacity, but a judgement or decision that distinguishes expert human judgement from the decisions or computations that might be made by a beginner or by a machine" (Benner & Tanner, 1987, p. 23).

We might, then, view intuitive reasoning as the goal of every clinician. But how does one get there? Clinical practice is, of course, a large part of the answer, but crucial to the honing of clinical nursing expertise is the development of critical thinking skills.

Components of Critical Thinking

The ability to think critically in nursing practice requires:
- **a sound knowledge base**
- **critical thinking skills**
- **attitudes that facilitate the use of these skills.**

Knowledge Base

A basic core of nursing knowledge is necessary in order to provide quality care. In Chapter 7 we identified various sources of nursing knowledge, including research, clinical experience, common sense, trial and error and tradition. Critical thinking skills are used to apply this knowledge in each patient situation. If the knowledge base is inadequate, the nurse's ability to use cognitive, interpersonal or technical skills effectively will be adversely affected. Two "ways of knowing"—structured and unstructured—were also identified in Chapter 7. Structured ways of knowing include scientific inquiry, critical thinking and logical reasoning. Unstructured ways of knowing include empathy, intuition, trial and error, tradition and authority, and meditation or reflection. Carper's (1978) "patterns of knowing" address similar sources of knowledge.

According to Carper (1978), the basic core of nursing knowledge comprises four patterns of knowing: nursing science, nursing art, nursing ethics and personal knowledge. The *scientific pattern of knowing* is similar to that described earlier in this text as the structured way of knowing. Such knowledge is gained from research findings and from the conceptual models of nursing, as described in Chapter 13. Theoretical explanations and research findings from other disciplines, such as social work, psychology and mathematics, also form part of the scientific knowledge base for nursing. Nurses use this knowledge on a daily basis and in all aspects of patient care.

In addition, the scientific pattern of knowing includes understanding the theoretical basis of communication and of therapeutic relationships (see Chapter 17). Nurses use this knowledge to interact with patients and families and to communicate caring and support, for instance during painful technical procedures and in times of grief. Other illustrations of scientific knowledge include an understanding of the effects of sociocultural and developmental factors on patient behaviour, such as how a patient's religious or cultural beliefs may influence her willingness to engage in treatment plans. For example, Mrs. Sandhu tells you that she does not want to be disturbed for treatments during her twice-daily prayers and meditation. The nurse respects her wishes by scheduling treatments and other activities around these times. Knowledge of the principles on which skills are based, and knowledge of the use of appropriate technology, constitute additional aspects of the scientific pattern of knowing.

The way a nurse expresses his or her knowledge is called the "art of nursing," or the *aesthetic pattern of knowing*. The art of nursing involves all those things that nurses do that defy description. As Carper (1978, p. 16) puts it, "the art of nursing is expressive rather than merely formal or descriptive." Caring, sensitivity and empathy are expressed through the art of nursing. These qualities enable the nurse to be aware of cues indicating the patient's psychological state and to be sensitive to the patient's perceptions. A nurse who is able to empathize with patients has a wider range of interventions available for providing effective, supportive and satisfying nursing care (Carper, 1978).

Knowledge of ethical theory and principles, and of professional guidelines and standards of conduct (see Chapter 7), make up the *ethical pattern of knowing*. Ethical theory describes relationships among phenomena and, hence, does not determine what a nurse "should" do in a particular situation. Rather, it provides insight into what the problems and possible decisions or actions might be. The ethical pattern of knowing involves implicit knowledge about what is right or wrong and what should be done, as well as knowledge of the formal ethical principles and theories in nursing (Chinn & Kramer, 1991).

The aspect of knowledge called *personal knowledge* or *personal knowing* refers to becoming self-aware. It involves knowing the self in order to know another human being as a person (Chinn & Kramer, 1991). This ability allows nurses to establish therapeutic relationships and to interact with patients as people rather than as objects, to relate to them on a person-to-person basis rather than on a "role-to-role" basis (Wilkinson, 1996, p. 25). The more self-aware nurses are, the better their self-concept will be, together with their ability to discern patients' needs and to make responsible, unbiased decisions (Carper, 1978; Wilkinson, 1996).

You note that Mrs. Sandhu has two unusual-looking objects on her bedside table. You want to use the table to put down your blood pressure cuff, stethoscope and other items, so you put the objects away in the drawer. The patient becomes quite upset, and her daughter tells you that these objects are very important to Mrs. Sandhu—they are relics (statues or other objects of religious significance). You apologize and put the objects back on the table. You are concerned, however, because you found it distasteful to touch the objects after you discovered what they were. You hope your feelings were not obvious to the patient or her daughter. Reflecting on why you felt this way, you realize that you were brought up in a very strict Christian sect that denounced idols and virtually all religious symbols except the cross. You begin to understand your reaction to the relics, and are now in a better position to overcome your bias. As a first step, you might attempt to by learn more about Mrs. Sandhu's religion, which is Hinduism (see Chapter 12).

Critical Thinking Skills

What are the critical thinking skills that nurses need in order to make judgements in daily practice? Some of these will be familiar, such as the general skills of the scientific method, problem solving and decision making by assessment and choice of options. We introduced some of the more specific nursing skills in Chapter 14 on the nursing process. These include diagnostic reasoning, clinical inferencing, clinical decision making and, of course, skill in applying the nursing process. A list of critical thinking skills and attitudes applied in nursing is shown in Table 15.1. You will note on this list that critical thinking involves both cognition (thinking) and attitudes (feelings). In this section, we are going to explore some of the cognitive skills that we have not discussed in detail before.

REASONING SKILLS

"Reasoning is the processing and organizing of ideas in order to solve problems" (Polit & Hungler, 1997, p. 10). Logical argument, in which each point is built on the one before in order to reach a logical conclusion, is an example of reasoning. Two such processes will be discussed here: inductive and deductive reasoning.

We used the terms inductive and deductive in Chapter 7 to refer to types of research methodology. The processes are the same, whether used in research or in a clinical situation. Nurses use both inductive and deductive reasoning when looking for patterns and relationships among various pieces of data. **Inductive reasoning** begins with specific details and facts and uses them to arrive at conclusions and generalizations. The nurse who reasons inductively forms concepts by generalizing from specific experiences, impressions and knowledge. With this type of reasoning, there is an assumption that particular instances, if observed consistently, can be generalized to a larger whole or a general statement. In other words, if something is true in a sufficient number of individual cases, it can be assumed to be true of all cases having the particular attributes noted. For example,

TABLE 15.1 Critical thinking skills and attitudes applied to nursing

Focus:
- distinguish between the central issue or problem and the peripheral issues or problems
- clarify the central issue or problem
- state the central issue or problem.

Language:
- assess clarity and precision
- define key words
- identify emotive words
- assess context
- detect and explore labels.

Assumptions:
- assess patient, family, institutional and societal contexts
- analyse value, descriptive, definitional and contextual assumptions
- assess frame of reference, attitudes and assumptions
- recognize one's own frame of reference, attitudes and assumptions.

Evidence:
- create criteria for evaluating
- evaluate evidence derived from qualitative and quantitative research
- evaluate evidence derived from the assessment of patients
- make appropriate inferences based on evidence derived from research and patients
- assess research for its relevance to clinical practice
- participate in systematic and accurate data collection
- distinguish among facts, opinions and inferences.

Reasoning:
- evaluate deductive and inductive arguments
- differentiate between warranted and unwarranted inferences
- distinguish among issues, reasons, conclusions (assumptions and alleged facts)
- evaluate pertinence of the reasons
- assess for errors in reasoning
- think independently.

Conclusions:
- generate alternatives
- support conclusions and beliefs with relevant reasons
- evaluate deductive and inductive arguments
- evaluate the strength of the evidence, supporting conclusions and beliefs.

Implications:
- identify implications of conclusions and beliefs
- evaluate desirability of the implications
- anticipate consequences.

Attitudes:
- questioning approach
- independence and creativity
- reflection
- confidence in multiple ways of knowing
- intellectual honesty
- openness to other points of view
- willingness to take a position and defend it
- willingness to change one's own opinion based on evidence.

SOURCES: Miller & Babcock, 1996, p. 24, as adapted by faculty of the University of Prince Edward Island School of Nursing for use in its school curriculum planning sessions (Spring, 1996).

when you document an elevated temperature, you might assume the patient has a fever.

Deductive reasoning involves the development of specific predictions, or the generation of certain details from a major theory, generalization, fact or assumption. In deductive reasoning, one moves from the universal to the particular (Polit & Hungler, 1997; Wilkinson, 1996). For example, if we know that anger frequently accompanies grief, then we can assume that the anger expressed towards staff by a woman whose husband died recently and unexpectedly in hospital might be related to the grief she is feeling about the sudden loss of her husband, rather than to any complaint about the care he received prior to his death.

Both methods of reasoning are useful when attempting to understand phenomena. However, it is important to remember that any reasoning process is only as good as the information or premises with which one starts.

REFLECTIVE THINKING

"Critical thinking requires reasonable, reflective thinking ..." (Alfaro-Lefevre, 1995, p. 1). **Reflection** is a mental exercise used to review and reconsider ideas and situations, and is very important to the development and use of critical thinking skills. "Reflection allows one the opportunity to think carefully about an event and to discover the purpose and meaning of that event" (Miller & Babcock, 1996, p. 95). It occurs best in an unhurried atmosphere and/or during rhythmic activity such as walking, housework activities such as vacuuming or ironing, or while driving long distances. Reflection allows one the opportunity to question the assumptions that structure the way we interpret our experiences; it allows the individual to question long-held beliefs and values. Reflection sidetracks habitual thinking and consequently contributes to the autonomous, independent thinking that is so much a part of critical thinking (Mezirow, 1990). According to Mezirow, in order to have the awareness and independence associated with critical thinking, the nurse needs to be reflective.

Reflection is a process of pondering feelings and emotions. The individual looks back on an experience to determine how he or she feels about it, and may make changes in future behaviour based on that reflection. During a discussion about reflection on Nursenet (an electronic listserver), one nurse said: "I look for patterns or errors in reasoning, things that might have worked better" (Duchscher, 1997, p. 2). Gaining perspective is an important outcome of reflection.

INTERPERSONAL SKILLS

The ability to use effective interpersonal processes for problem solving and managing conflict is also characteristic of critical thinkers. In a conflict, critical thinkers examine their own experience, discuss it with colleagues, look at the professional literature and then make a decision. This process of examining evidence and critiquing courses of action contributes to "win–win" approaches (solutions in which each party gains) in resolving conflict.

ABILITY TO EMPATHIZE

The critical thinker is both a reflective and a creative thinker—able to establish relationships among thoughts and concepts that may result in the creation and evaluation of original ideas, or to imagine existing concepts in new and unusual settings or uses (Wilkinson, 1996). The critical thinker may use the creative activity of **brainstorming**—the spontaneous consideration of ideas or solutions—as one aspect of the critical thinking process.

Reflection helps one learn from experience, to look back and determine how things went and to consider whether anything could be done differently or better. The critical thinker who engages in reflection does not make hurried decisions, but takes time to think things through in a disciplined manner (Wilkinson, 1996). Learning to think deeply, creatively and reflectively helps the nurse to provide better care for patients.

Finally, nurses with critical thinking abilities have a highly developed ability to empathize. **Empathy** is that all-important ability to understand what another person is going through, and to comprehend another's behaviours and beliefs even though one has never experienced that particular situation.

Attitudes

Several attitudes are characteristic of the nurse who is a critical thinker. As you read through this section, you will notice that the concept of self-awareness appears again and again as the basis for many of the attitudes characteristic of critical thinkers.

An **assumption** is an idea or concept that we take for granted. Assumptions can be true or false. Nurses who are critical thinkers do not make assumptions. In fact, making an assumption is the antithesis of critical thinking. Once an assumption is made, the chance of error is increased because the nurse may then fail to consider all possible descriptions of a situation. The nurse examines his or her own assumptions and perspectives by first exploring thoughts and feelings. Critical thinkers examine beliefs and values acquired in childhood, questioning their validity; they keep those that they determine to be useful and discard those that are not. Because assumptions, beliefs, values and perspectives are well entrenched in experience, examining them—or becoming self-aware—is one of the greatest challenges of critical thinking.

The nurse who is a critical thinker:

- suspends judgement
- avoids oversimplification
- examines evidence and alleged facts, while recognizing the role of her or his own perspective.

Nurses who are critical thinkers look for input from other people and disciplines; they share and critique with others in order to expand their own perspective. They remain open-minded and flexible, able to explore and imagine alternatives and to change approaches and priorities as needed. They have the courage and willingness to listen to ideas that may feel foreign, and they are able to **reframe** (redefine) a situation in order to consider it from many perspectives.

Reframing a Situation

Example: Patient who frequently has his call light on

Frame #1: This is a demanding patient who is trying to control the nurses.

Frame #2: This is a very ill person who is frightened.

The perspective or frame used can positively or negatively affect the actions of the nurse. In the first instance, the nurse would possibly ignore the call light. In the second instance, she or he would answer the light, stay with the patient and provide comfort and support while talking with him about his fears.

Autonomous thinking—thinking for oneself—is another characteristic of critical thinking. Although they obtain input from others, critical thinkers do not passively or blindly accept their own beliefs or the opinions and beliefs of others; instead, they question these at every opportunity. A critical thinker examines existing claims and statements to determine their truth and validity. This does not mean rejecting ideas and opinions outright, but rather maintaining an attitude of inquiry. Critical thinkers are skeptical, but constructively so. They ask *why* and *how* questions (Wilkinson, 1996).

For the nurse who is a critical thinker, questions enter into every situation: Is this assumption or fact? What evidence supports this inference? How can I check out the validity of this conclusion? The critical thinker will compare and contrast one situation with another, looking for similarities and differences. The nurse with the ability to question deeply will question nursing activities and rituals that appear to have no scientific or rational basis. She or he will question tradition, doctor's orders and the actions of fellow health professionals when necessary.

Critical thinkers also practise **fair-mindedness,** that is, the ability to recognize bias and narrow thinking in themselves and in others. This involves examining the reasons for choices and decisions. It also requires awareness of one's own values and beliefs, as well as feelings. "The fairminded thinker consistently seeks truth and objectivity" (Miller & Babcock, 1996, p. 56).

Another important attitude of critical thinking is **intellectual integrity.** This attitude requires nurses, as critical thinkers, to be consistent in the standards they apply—that is, to apply the same rigorous standards of proof to their own evidence as they apply to the evidence of others.

Critical thinkers also have **intellectual humility.** They know they don't know everything. Further, they know that not everything is known. Most knowledge in the health care field has a very short life; what seems true this year may be disproved next year.

Critical Thinking and the Nursing Process

The ability to think critically supports and enhances the nurse's success in applying the nursing process. There are three levels of critical thinking in the nursing process as described by Alfaro-Lefevre (1995). At the first ("basic") level, the critical thinker assumes that authorities have the right answers for every problem. Answers are seen as right or wrong, black or white, and the belief is held that there is usually one right answer for each complex problem. In order to move to a higher level of thinking, the nurse must have a strong knowledge base, practical experience and efficiency in skills, along with a positive attitude and familiarity with professional standards.

The second level of critical thinking is described as "complex." At this level, the nurse begins to realize that "alternative, perhaps even conflicting solutions exist, each with benefits and costs" (Alfaro-Lefevre, 1995, p. 173). The nurse recognizes that the unique aspects of the patient and the situation (context) are important in determining the best possible approach(es).

At the third level, "commitment," the nurse chooses an action or a belief based on the alternative identified in the previous level. "If the chosen action is unsuccessful, alternative solutions are considered and used" (Alfaro-Lefevre, 1995, p. 173). After a decision is made and an intervention has been selected and initiated, the nurse nevertheless remains open to alternative solutions if the one chosen is not successful.

Table 15.2 lists critical thinking skills used at each step of the nursing process and suggests questions to check the nurse's thinking. We will use these questions to check your reasoning with respect to the case study of Mrs. Sandhu.

Assessment

The assessment phase of the nursing process includes data collection and analysis. During the first step (collection), critical thinking will help the nurse to ask appropriate questions related to the patient's perceived needs, health problems, goals, values and lifestyle. The ability to narrow the field of data collection requires the ability to think critically (Bandman & Bandman, 1995). The second step (analysis) involves giving the data some meaning, or making sense of the information gained. Here, the nurse must make reliable observations and distinguish relevant from irrelevant data. Data analysis involves the critical thinking skills of seeing relationships among pieces of data and drawing hypotheses or conclusions (Rubenfield & Scheffer, 1995). The nurse must recognize that data collection and analysis will be affected by preconceived ideas, both implicit and explicit; again, self-awareness is relevant. At this point, the nurse remains skeptical and maintains an attitude of inquiry. Both attitudes are forms of critical thinking that allow the nurse to see the blind spots

TABLE 15.2 Critical thinking and the nursing process

Step	*Critical Thinking Skill*	*Questions to Check Your Thinking*
Assessment	Making reliable observations Distinguishing relevant from irrelevant data Distinguishing important from unimportant data Validating data Categorizing data according to a framework Recognizing assumptions	• What assumptions am I making about the patient? • Are my data correct and accurate? • How reliable are my sources? • What data are important? Relevant? • What biases do I have that might cause me to miss important information? • Am I listening carefully to get the patient's/family's perspective? • Do I have all the facts? What other data might I need?
Diagnosis	Finding patterns and relationships among cues Identifying gaps in the data Suspending judgement when lacking data Stating the problem Making interdisciplinary connections Comparing patterns with norms Identifying contributing factors	• Do I know what is within normal limits for these data? • Do I have enough data to make a valid inference? • What biases might I have that could affect how I see the patient's problems? • Do I have enough data to make a nursing diagnosis, or should I make a "possible" diagnosis? • What other problems might these data suggest?
Planning	Forming valid generalizations Transferring knowledge from other situations Developing evaluative criteria Hypothesizing Making interdisciplinary connections Prioritizing patient problems Generalizing principles from other situations	• Do I need help to plan interventions? • Did I give priority to the problems the patient/family identified as important? • What are the most important problems? • What interventions worked in similar situations? • Is this situation similar enough to merit using them now? • Are there other plans that might be more agreeable to the patient and thus more likely to work? • Why do I expect these interventions to be effective? Based on what knowledge?
Implementation	Applying knowledge to formulate interventions Using interventions to test hypotheses	• Has the patient's condition changed since the plan was made? • Have I overlooked any new developments? • What is the patient's initial response to the intervention? • Are there any safety issues I have overlooked?
Evaluation	Deciding whether hypotheses are correct Making criterion-based evaluations	• What are the patient's responses after the interventions? • Have I overlooked anything? • Do the data indicate that goals were met? Does the patient feel the goals were met? • Does the patient trust me enough to give honest answers? • Am I sure the problem is really resolved? • What might the team have done that would have been more effective? • What nursing care, if any, is still needed?

SOURCE: Wilkinson, 1996, pp. 37–39.

in the team's approach to data collection (Bandman & Bandman, 1995).

The following data about Mrs. Sandhu were gathered in the nurse's initial interview, during which Mrs. Sandhu's daughter assisted.

Mrs. Sandhu immigrated to Canada from India about five years ago with her husband in order to be close to her son and daughter, who have lived in Canada for over 10 years. She was diagnosed with type II diabetes about one year ago. Since her diagnosis, she has attended the diabetic clinic with her husband several times for education sessions regarding the management of her diabetes. Mr. and Mrs. Sandhu live with their children and grandchildren in an extended family setting. Mr. Sandhu retired nearly a year and a half ago from his job as a security guard. Mrs. Sandhu is a housewife. She prepares most of the family meals and takes care of her three grandchildren, ages two, three and four years, while her daughter and daughter-in-law work in the produce store their husbands own jointly. Mrs. Sandhu's first language is Hindi, and she has limited knowledge of English. When asked what she thought the reason was for her hospital admission, she said, "I have sugar disease and they told me my sugar went out of balance."

At home Mrs. Sandhu administers Novolin 30/70 insulin, once a day before breakfast. She also does her blood sugar testing daily. The daughter says her mother understands why she has to do the testing and give herself insulin and is quite good with the techniques of administering the insulin. She also knows that she should eat all her meals.

When you arrive for your shift, you notice that Mrs. Sandhu ate only half the food on her breakfast tray. She says she wasn't hungry. Use the questions shown in Table 15.2 to check your thinking.

ARE YOU MAKING ANY ASSUMPTIONS ABOUT THIS PATIENT? The patient has attended education sessions at the diabetic clinic. Are you assuming that she therefore has a good knowledge about her medical condition? Is this a valid assumption?

ARE YOUR DATA CORRECT AND ACCURATE? You have no reason to believe that the data are not correct.

HOW RELIABLE ARE YOUR SOURCES? Your sources of data include the patient and her daughter, the brief notes written by the physician, the admitting nurse in emergency, the results of laboratory tests, as well as your own observations. You think they are reliable.

WHAT DATA ARE IMPORTANT? RELEVANT? Mrs. Sandhu was admitted because her blood sugar was too high. Information about the patient's ability to carry out the activities of daily living and her preferences in this regard are important in providing care for her in hospital. Of higher priority, however, and more relevant to the reason for her hospital admission, is information about Mrs. Sandhu's eating habits, her treatment regimen and how she carries these out at home. At present, you do not have a great deal of information about this.

WHAT BIASES DO YOU HAVE THAT MIGHT CAUSE YOU TO MISS IMPORTANT INFORMATION? You don't think you have any biases—but then, you found you did not like touching the religious objects Mrs. Sandhu brought with her. You have not had much contact with people of East Indian origin before. Perhaps you have more biases than you thought you had.

ARE YOU LISTENING CAREFULLY TO GET THE PATIENT'S AND FAMILY'S PERSPECTIVE? Communication with Mrs. Sandhu is difficult because of her limited English. It is good that her daughter is with Mrs. Sandhu when you are interviewing her, because the daughter can translate your questions and her mother's answers.

DO YOU HAVE ALL THE FACTS? WHAT OTHER DATA MIGHT YOU NEED? You would like to have more information on what Mrs. Sandhu eats on a regular basis at home and, also, how much she understands about the importance of controlling her diet and the composition of various foods.

Diagnosis

The diagnostic phase of the nursing process involves the interpretation (clustering) of the data collected during assessment. In the case of Mrs. Sandhu, the nurse clustered the data she has about the reason for the patient's admission, about her diet and her treatment regimen and makes a tentative diagnosis of *Ineffective Management of Therapeutic Regime*. Let us look at the questions suggested for critical thinking in the diagnostic phase of the nursing process.

DO YOU KNOW WHAT IS WITHIN NORMAL LIMITS FOR THESE DATA? In order to interpret the laboratory results on Mrs. Sandhu, you would have to know the normal levels for blood glucose readings.

DO YOU HAVE ENOUGH DATA TO MAKE A VALID INFERENCE? You would like to have more data on Mrs. Sandhu's eating habits at home and on the amount of exercise she gets on a daily basis. The daughter says Mrs. Sandhu knows how to give her insulin injections and understands why she has to have them, but you would like to have more information on the patient's understanding of the relationship between food intake and her diabetic condition.

WHAT BIASES DO YOU HAVE THAT COULD AFFECT HOW YOU SEE THE PATIENT'S PROBLEMS? You tried East Indian food once and the hot, spicy curry made your eyes water and burned your tongue. You didn't like it, and you don't see how anyone can eat this food every day. Will that opinion affect your judgement?

DO YOU HAVE ENOUGH DATA TO MAKE A NURSING DIAGNOSIS, OR SHOULD YOU MAKE A "POSSIBLE" DIAGNOSIS? You think you should ask the dietitian to talk to Mrs. Sandhu, preferably when her daughter is present, to find out more about the patient's eating habits at home.

On day 1 after Mrs. Sandhu's admission, the dietitian is consulted to help the patient to manage her diet and to understand the importance of this. Mrs. Sandhu's daughter is present; she tells the dietitian that her mother is not accustomed to Western food and that her diet consists of East Indian food only. Although Mrs. Sandhu was given a diet of East Indian foods in the diabetic clinic, the daughter admits that her mother does not follow it. The patient also admits to eating foods that are high in calories as well as in sugar. The patient eats rice for one meal at least once daily, and also eats roti (flatbread), samosas (small, deep-fried pastries containing vegetables and/or meat), curries and other ethnic foods. In between meals the patient snacks on fresh fruit.

The dietitian's report confirms your tentative diagnosis that Mrs. Sandhu's problem is one of ineffective management of therapeutic diet regimen. The patient's diet is the key to management of her diabetes, and it appears that she is not adhering to the diet recommended for her at the diabetic clinic.

WHAT OTHER PROBLEMS MIGHT THESE DATA SUGGEST? You note that Mrs. Sandhu is responsible for preparing the family's meals, and wonder if this is contributing to her problem. You wonder also if the dietitian has guidelines for a diabetic diet that uses East Indian foods.

Another problem may be Mrs. Sandhu's accuracy in administering her insulin. Is she consistent with her administration? Does she do the testing and administer her insulin at a regular time every day?

Also, if Mrs. Sandhu is looking after three small children, getting the family's meals and helping with the housework, you wonder if she is getting enough rest. Does she have time to exercise? (Her daughter says Mrs. Sandhu takes the children for a walk when the weather is good, but that is all the exercise she gets.)

Planning

Once a cluster is named, and you have a diagnosis, it gives direction to the next step—planning. In our case study, the diagnosis is *Ineffective Management of Therapeutic Diet Regime*. When planning action, the nurse must always ask why this action would be helpful, and how it would be implemented. Asking why and how, and providing sound rationale, demonstrates the use of critical thinking skills in this step of the nursing process (Rubenfeld & Scheffer, 1995). The goals or outcomes are then developed in collaboration with the patient, and are used as criteria for evaluating the patient's progress and the success of the nursing interventions.

When planning care with patients, nurses use knowledge and reasoning skills to develop evaluative criteria. Nurses use the skill of forming valid generalizations, explanations and predictions to develop the goals and to choose nursing interventions. The nurse uses critical thinking skills in deciding which other health professionals to involve. Nurses use a broad base of knowledge in their critical thinking to choose appropriate nursing interventions to relieve the patient's symptoms or to help the patient to achieve health goals (Wilkinson, 1996.)

Questions suggested to check your thinking in the planning stage of the nursing process include:

DO YOU NEED HELP TO PLAN INTERVENTIONS? In the case of Mrs. Sandhu, you will need the dietitian's help in planning a diet for the patient to follow when she goes home. You will also need the cooperation of the daughter and Mrs. Sandhu's husband, as well as all members of the patient's family, if she is to maintain her therapeutic regimen. Exercise is also important in the diabetic regimen. You may wish to have the physiotherapist discuss with the patient and her family the importance of exercise and the type of exercise most suitable for Mrs. Sandhu.

DID YOU GIVE PRIORITY TO THE PROBLEMS THE PATIENT AND FAMILY IDENTIFIED AS IMPORTANT? The patient and the patient's daughter say their most important concern is to get Mrs. Sandhu's blood sugar balanced. You have given this problem top priority. However, Mrs. Sandhu is also concerned about privacy, modesty and hospital attire. The charge nurse has scheduled only female nurses to look after Mrs. Sandhu. As far as wearing her salwar kameze, the charge nurse said this is fine; she understands that East Indian women find the hospital gown indecent. You have noted that Mrs. Sandhu wants privacy for her twice-daily prayers, and you respect her designated times.

WHAT ARE THE MOST IMPORTANT PROBLEMS YOU NEED TO SOLVE? The patient's diet appears to be the greatest concern at this point because she does not seem to understand the importance of diet control and the high sugar content of certain foods.

WHAT INTERVENTIONS WORKED IN SIMILAR SITUATIONS? IS THIS SITUATION SIMILAR ENOUGH TO MERIT USING THEM WITH THIS PATIENT? The dietitian tells you that there is a good diabetic diet using East Indian foods. It has worked well with other patients, and should work with Mrs. Sandhu.

ARE THERE OTHER PLANS THAT MIGHT BE MORE AGREEABLE TO THE PATIENT, AND THEREFORE MORE LIKELY TO WORK? As long as Mrs. Sandhu's family are supportive and willing to make dietary changes, the above plan would appear to be the best solution. In view of the limited English of both Mr. and Mrs. Sandhu, it would be reasonable to suggest that Mrs. Sandhu's daughter attend the diabetic clinic with her mother on a weekly basis.

WHY DO I EXPECT THE INTERVENTIONS TO BE EFFECTIVE? BASED ON WHAT KNOWLEDGE? Mrs. Sandhu's daughter is well educated and says she is willing to go to the diabetic clinic with her mother.

Implementation

Once outcomes are determined, the nursing interventions must be put into motion. This is the implementation phase. Implementation normally follows the planning phase and consists of developing a comprehensive, scientifically based patient care plan.

In this phase of the nursing process, nurses "apply the knowledge gained from nursing and other related courses to each individual patient care situation" (Wilkinson, 1996, p. 37). Implementing the care plan requires the use of critical thinking skills, such as choosing and applying relevant knowledge from all that is known, acting on a plan and keeping an open mind to alternative care measures if the plan chosen is not successful (Wilkinson, 1996).

HAS THE PATIENT'S CONDITION CHANGED SINCE THE PLAN WAS MADE? Mrs. Sandhu's condition has stabilized and her blood sugar is within normal limits.

HAVE YOU OVERLOOKED ANY NEW DEVELOPMENTS? Mrs. Sandhu's family have brought in food that is not on her diabetic diet. You explain to them that this meal is not on her diet and provide them with a copy of the diet that the dietitian has given Mrs. Sandhu.

WHAT IS THE PATIENT'S INITIAL RESPONSE TO THE INTERVENTION? Mrs. Sandhu says the Western food that was served to her at breakfast was not to her liking. She hopes that she will get some rice for lunch. She is worried about being able to adjust to her diet when she goes home, because she has to cook for the whole family. They may not like the food that she is required to eat.

ARE THERE ANY SAFETY ISSUES YOU HAVE OVERLOOKED? Friends coming to visit Mrs. Sandhu may bring in sweets. You are also concerned that Mrs. Sandhu's technique for giving her insulin may be incorrect. You plan to observe Mrs. Sandhu administering her insulin tomorrow morning.

Evaluation

The last phase of the nursing process is evaluation, which is concerned with the efficacy of the initial assessment, diagnosis, planning and implementation. Critical thinking also plays an important role in the evaluative process. Here, the nurse assesses the effectiveness of the interventions against objective measures or accepted criteria, and decides whether the outcome goals have been successfully met or whether a reassessment must be performed and different interventions implemented. Use of criterion-based measures is a critical thinking skill. During the evaluation phase, critical thinking is used when the nurse questions what he or she sees, or questions the outcomes (Wilkinson, 1996).

WHAT ARE THE PATIENT'S RESPONSES AFTER THE INTERVENTION? Mrs. Sandhu is pleased that her daughter will be going to the diabetic clinic with her. She says she is grateful to the nurse for monitoring her insulin administration. She is never sure if she is doing it correctly.

HAVE YOU OVERLOOKED ANYTHING? Have you contacted the liaison nurse from the community regarding follow-up home monitoring of insulin administration and adherence to diet, as well as more regular blood glucose testing?

Also, the physiotherapist recommended that Mrs. Sandhu have regular exercise, preferably with a member of the family. You note that the Sandhu family live close to a golf course that has a 3 km jogging path around it. You suggest that Mrs. Sandhu and a family member walk this route at least three times a week.

DO THE DATA INDICATE THAT GOALS WERE MET? DOES THE PATIENT FEEL THE GOALS WERE MET? The goals were met during Mrs. Sandhu's hospital stay. The home care nurse will need to continue with the plan in the home environment to evaluate the short-term goals for Mrs. Sandhu.

Mrs. Sandhu says that she feels more comfortable about taking her insulin and understands the need to avoid foods high in sugar content.

DOES THE PATIENT TRUST YOU ENOUGH TO GIVE HONEST ANSWERS? You think you have established a good rapport with Mrs. Sandhu and her family. You know she appreciated having privacy for her prayers. She and other family members have sought you out to ask questions about her care. You think they trust you.

ARE YOU SURE THE PROBLEM IS REALLY RESOLVED? You are satisfied that Mrs. Sandhu knows how to administer her insulin correctly and you think she understands the need to modify her diet. However, you are aware that these modifications are difficult and that she will need follow-up in the community.

WHAT MIGHT YOU HAVE DONE THAT WOULD HAVE BEEN MORE EFFECTIVE? A more comprehensive treatment plan could have been carried out if Mrs. Sandhu had been kept in hospital. The early-discharge policy of the hospital, however, allowed you to supervise Mrs. Sandhu in administering her insulin on only two occasions.

WHAT NURSING CARE IS STILL NEEDED, IF ANY? The liaison nurse from the community has put in a referral for Mrs. Sandhu to be followed by a community health nurse in her district in order to monitor her adherence to her diabetic diet, her attendance at the diabetic clinic and her exercise program. Also, further dietary teaching could be done.

In summary, nurses use critical thinking in applying the nursing process and in "achieving the purpose of nursing" (Wilkinson, 1996, p. 39). The initial steps towards critical thinking involve a belief in the importance of understanding rather than memorizing. Further steps along the path are taken when nurses begin to trust their own ability to make sense of evidence and principles. Critical thinking is involved in the ability to understand and apply the principles of nursing in a variety of settings and to use knowledge from all areas within nursing, and relevant related areas, towards positive outcomes for patients. As critical thinking abilities grow, the nurse is no longer limited by the influences of unexamined beliefs and values.

IN REVIEW

- Critical thinking is "purposeful thinking that takes into consideration focus, language, frame of reference, attitudes, assumptions, evidence, reasoning, conclusions, implications and context when they matter in deciding what to believe or do" (Miller & Babcock, 1996, p. 8).
- Nurses need to use critical thinking because:
  - many problems cannot be resolved with standard interventions
  - technology must be used in ways that are ethically sound and appropriate for each individual
  - nurses must question and challenge their own attitudes, beliefs and values if they are to give culturally sensitive care to patients
  - critical thinking implies a sense of responsibility for one's decisions.
- The ability to reason intuitively is based on knowledge and experience. It is gained by extensive clinical practice and the honing of critical thinking skills.
- The components of critical thinking include:
  - a sound knowledge base composed of the four patterns of knowing (scientific, aesthetic, ethical and personal)
  - cognitive skills, such as problem solving, decision making, reasoning, reflective thinking
  - skills specific to nursing, such as diagnostic reasoning, clinical inferences, clinical decision making and the nursing process
  - skills in the effective use of interpersonal processes
  - skills in thinking creatively and reflectively
  - skills in being empathetic
  - attitudes that facilitate critical thinking, such as suspending judgement; being open-minded and flexible; thinking autonomously; maintaining an attitude of inquiry; questioning deeply; being fair-minded, having intellectual integrity and humility.
- Three levels of critical thinking in applying the nursing process include:
  - the "basic" level, in which the nurse uses standard interventions advocated by authorities
  - the "complex" level, in which the nurse realizes that problems can have more than one solution and that care must be based on the unique aspects of each patient with respect to situation and context
  - the level of "commitment," when the nurse makes a decision, selects an intervention and initiates it, based on alternatives identified at the previous levels.
- During the assessment phase, the nurse needs to narrow the field in collecting data appropriately and make sense of the information collected. This involves distinguishing between important and irrelevant data. An attitude of skepticism and inquiry are needed.
- During the diagnostic phase, the nurse must be able to interpret the data, identify patterns and relationships and make inferences. Careful to suspend judgement if there is not enough data, the nurse must also examine assumptions about the situation and about the meaning of the data collected.
- During the planning phase, the nurse must always question why an intervention would be helpful and how it is to be implemented. The skills of collaboration and discussion with others are useful at this stage. Knowledge and reasoning skills are used to develop evaluative criteria.
- During the implementation phase, the nurse uses critical thinking skills such as choosing and applying relevant knowledge, acting on a plan and keeping an open mind to alternative measures.
- During the evaluation phase, the nurse uses the skill of measuring outcomes against established criteria. Useful attributes include an attitude of inquiry, open-mindedness and flexibility.

Critical Thinking Activities

Mr. Abdurrahman Hassan is a 50-year-old Caucasian male who came to Canada 20 years ago as a refugee from Afghanistan with his wife and two small children. He was sponsored by the Muslim community of Toronto, which helped him to settle into his new home. He enrolled in George Brown College, where he took a course in small-appliance maintenance and repair. He is presently working for a small-appliance company in the repair department. His wife works part-time in the local grocery store to supplement the family income. One daughter has just graduated from York University with a degree in business administration. The second daughter is in her third year of biochemistry studies at the University of Ottawa.

Mr. Hassan was at work when he felt unwell. His employer drove him to the hospital, where he was admitted. He complained of chest pain that radiated down his left arm. He was perspiring profusely and was short of breath. The physician in the emergency department ordered an electrocardiogram, oxygen, blood work and morphine. The physician stated that Mr. Hassan was having a heart attack. The emergency department nurse called Mrs. Hassan to let her know that her husband was in the hospital. Mrs. Hassan came from work as quickly as she could.

Based on your understanding of the cardiovascular system, reflect on the following questions:

1. What information would you give to Mrs. Hassan?

2. How would you reassure Mr. Hassan and his wife?
3. Mrs. Hassan wants to stay at her husband's bedside. Would you allow this?
4. Mrs. Hassan has been at the hospital all day and appears anxious and distressed. She has been unable to contact her daughters. How might you help her?
5. On the fourth day, Mr. Hassan is transferred to the medical unit. Both he and his wife have many questions regarding needed lifestyle changes. Mr. Hassan tells you that the doctor has said he will need to change his diet and lose 20 pounds. The doctor also told him to reduce some of the stress in his life. Mr. Hassan asks the nurse, "How am I going to do all this?" How would you respond?
6. Did you take into consideration Mr. Hassan's cultural and religious beliefs?
7. The doctor has indicated that this heart attack was a warning. Mr. Hassan is discharged home. He seems to be motivated to make the necessary changes that the doctor has recommended. Mrs. Hassan expresses concern about their financial situation, especially if her husband needs to reduce his work hours. What community resources are available to help Mr. Hassan adjust to life after a heart attack? What financial help can be provided to assist the Hassan family?
8. What other health professionals may be involved?

KEY TERMS

critical thinking p. 352
intuition p. 353
inductive reasoning p. 355
deductive reasoning p. 356
reflection p. 356
empathy p. 356
brainstorming p. 356
assumption p. 356
reframe p. 357
autonomous thinking p. 357
fair-mindedness p. 357
intellectual integrity p. 357
intellectual humility p. 357

References

ALFARO-LEFEVRE, R. (1995). *Critical thinking in nursing: A practical approach.* Philadelphia: Saunders.

BANDMAN, E.L., & BANDMAN, B. (1995). *Critical thinking in nursing.* (2nd ed.). Norwalk, CT: Appleton & Lange.

BENNER, P. (1984). *From novice to expert: Excellence and power in clinical nursing practice.* Menlo Park, CA: Addison-Wesley.

BENNER, P., & TANNER, C. (1987). Clinical judgement: How expert nurses use intuition. *American Journal of Nursing, 87*(1), 23–31.

BENNER, P., & WRUBEL, J. (1989). *The primacy of caring: Stress and coping in health and illness.* Menlo Park, CA: Addison-Wesley.

BRIGHAM, C. (1993). Nursing education and critical thinking: Interplay of content and thinking. *Holistic Nurse Practitioner, 7*(3), 48–54.

CARPER, B.A. (1978). Fundamental patterns of knowing in nursing. *Advances in Nursing Science, 1*(1), 13–23.

CHINN, P.L., & KRAMER, M.K. (1991). *Theory and nursing: A systematic approach.* (3rd ed.). St. Louis: Mosby Year Book.

DUCHSCHER, J.D. (1997). Reflection review by Internet [on-line]. Available at duchscher@sk.sympatico.ca.

MEZIROW, J. (1990) *Fostering reflection in adulthood: A guide to transformative and emancipatory learning.* San Francisco: Jossey-Bass.

MILLER, M.A., & BABCOCK, D.E. (1996). *Critical thinking applied to nursing.* St. Louis: Mosby.

POLIT, D.F., & HUNGLER, B.P. (1997). *Essentials of nursing research: Methods, appraisals, and utilization.* (4th ed.). Philadelphia: Lippincott.

REHNER, J. (1997). Personal communication.

RUBENFELD, M.G., & SCHEFFER, B.K. (1995). *Critical thinking in nursing: An interactive approach.* Philadelphia: Lippincott.

WILKINSON, J.M. (1996). *Nursing process: A critical thinking approach.* (2nd ed.). Reading, MA: Addison-Wesley.

Additional Readings

BOUD, D., KEOUGH, R., & WALKER, D. (Eds.). (1985). *Reflection: Turning experience into learning.* London: Routledge & Kegan Paul.

CASE, B. (1994). Walking around the elephant: A critical thinking strategy for decision-making. *Journal of Continuing Education in Nursing, 25*(3), 101–109.

DALY, W.M. (1998). Critical thinking as an outcome of nursing education. What is it? Why is it important to nursing practice? *Journal of Advanced Nursing, 28*(2), 323–331.

DELA CRUZ, F.A. (1994). Clinical decision-making styles of home health-care nurses. *Image, 26*(3), 222–226.

DURGAHEE, T. (1996). Reflective practice: Linking theory and practice in palliative care nursing. *International Journal of Palliative Nursing, 2*(1), 22–25.

FACIONE, N.C., & FACIONE, P.A. (1996). Externalizing the critical thinking in knowledge development and clinical judgement. *Nursing Outlook, 44*(3), 129–136.

FOWLER, L.P. (1998). Improving critical thinking in nursing practice. *Journal for Nurses in Staff Development. 14*(4), 183–187.

KOCH, F.T., & SPEARS, A.T. (1997). It is time to move from the nursing process to critical thinking. *AORN Journal, 66*(2), 318–320.

PARSE, R.R. (1996). Critical thinking: What is it? *Nursing Science Quarterly, 9*(4), 139.

PAUL, R. (1992). Why critical thinking? Why now? *Critical Thinking, 1*(1), 3.

RANE-SZOSTAK, D., & ROBERTSON, J.F. (1996). Issues in measuring critical thinking: Meeting the challenge. *Journal of Nursing Education, 35*(1), 5–11.

STARK, J. (1996). Critical thinking for outcomes-based practice. *Seminars for Nurse Managers, 4*(3), 168–171.

TANNER, C.A. (1996). Critical thinking revisited: Paradoxes and emerging perspectives. *Journal of Nursing Education, 35*(1), 3–4.

Chapter 16

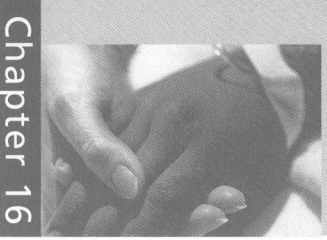

Health Assessment

OUTLINE

Central Questions

1. What are the components of a health history?
2. What are the four basic techniques used during physical examination, and how does the nurse perform these techniques?
3. What sequence might a nurse use for a head-to-toe examination?
4. What are some common positions patients are asked to assume for examination or treatment?
5. What is included in a beginning assessment of basic needs or functional abilities?
6. How does the nurse measure temperature, pulse, respirations and blood pressure?
7. What are the nurse's responsibilities when assisting with a physical examination?
8. What are the responsibilities of the nurse when assisting with diagnostic tests and examinations?

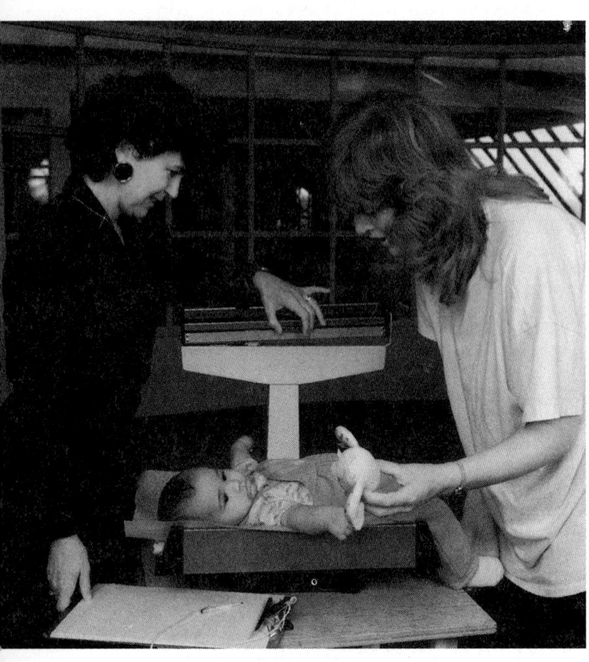

Introduction

The assessment phase of the nursing process begins with interviewing the patient and gathering information for the health history. The quality of this initial contact with the health professional forms the basis for a therapeutic relationship and partnership.

The nursing health history provides subjective data for a patient's record. It is the first component of the data base and is considered the single most important element in making an accurate assessment. Much of the data on which nursing diagnoses are made, and on which care is planned, are obtained in the health history. In addition, information about the patient's symptoms and perceptions of health problems helps to determine the focus of physical examination and the choice of assessment techniques.

Objective data are gathered through observation and physical examination. Data from the history and physical examination are combined with laboratory and diagnostic studies to form the patient's data base.

Nurses need skills in interviewing to collect a health history, and skills in observation, examination and measurement techniques to perform a physical examination. The development of these assessment skills begins early in a nurse's education program and continues to expand during the course of studies and throughout his or her professional career. The key to these skills is the ability to make intelligent observations based on the nurse's knowledge of the biomedical, physical and social sciences.

A knowledge base provides the substructure of the examination and directs the nurse to look for particular findings, rather than simply to look at body parts. Jarvis (1996) quotes the 18th century poet Goethe: "We see only what we know" (p. 162). To recognize a significant finding, the examiner needs to know what to look for (Jarvis, 1996). Moreover, assessment data are of no value unless they mean something within the context of the patient's experience. Critical thinking skills (see Chapter 15) enable the nurse to assign meaning to the significance of the data. Meaning is assigned to findings by comparing them to knowledge of patterns or features of normal/healthy or abnormal/unhealthy states and by understanding normal and abnormal factors that may affect functioning in a particular body system.

Basic interviewing skills are outlined in Chapter 17. The health history, the use of the four classical examination techniques (inspection, palpation, percussion and auscultation) and the measurement of vital signs (temperature, pulse, respirations and blood pressure) are the focus of this chapter. The assessment of specific basic needs and functional abilities are introduced here and enlarged upon in each of the basic needs chapters. For example, assessing an individual's nutritional status will be described in the chapter on nutritional needs, and similarly, assessing respiratory status in the chapter on oxygen needs. In this chapter, assessment of the adult patient is the primary focus, with age-related variations briefly discussed.

It must be noted at this point that the assessments described in this book are at an introductory level. These assessments include basic skills such as taking vital signs, observing colour or listening to bowel sounds. They depend on the student's knowledge of the structure and functioning of the body and the ability to detect readily observable deviations. More advanced skills, such as listening to extra heart sounds or conducting an internal pelvic exam, are not addressed in this text. We recommend that students purchase a book specifically on physical examination and health assessment, which they can use as a reference throughout their program.

In addition to taking health histories and conducting physical examinations, the nurse often assists other health professionals in carrying out diagnostic procedures that are part of the medical assessment of a patient's health status. It is the nurse's responsibility to prepare patients physically and mentally for the various diagnostic tests and procedures. Collection of specimens for laboratory tests may be necessary. Nurses perform many of the tests and procedures as collaborative functions on orders from the physician or as independent functions based on their own judgements. Information of a general nature about common diagnostic procedures used in the detection of illness has been included in this chapter. More detailed information about specific diagnostic tests and examinations used in assessing various body systems is included in the chapters on specific needs.

Nursing Health History

The Interview

The interview has been called a "talk with a purpose." In health assessment it is a talk between the nurse and the patient to obtain a health history and to explore the patient's symptoms and perceptions of health status. During a successful interview the nurse gathers a complete and accurate data base about a person's health and, at the same time, establishes rapport and the basis for a trusting nurse–patient relationship.

The interview is the first and most important part of data collection because it gives patients the opportunity to tell their story—their symptoms, feelings and perceptions, including their expectations regarding care and outcome. If patients are unable to speak for themselves, the interview is conducted, whenever possible, with family members or significant others. This might occur, for example, in the case of a very young child, or when a patient is critically ill, debilitated or confused.

In order to conduct a successful interview, the nurse must first establish rapport and a climate of trust with the patient. In most cases, the history-taking interview begins as an encounter between two strangers. People are not apt to share personal information or raise questions about their health with a stranger unless they feel they can trust that person. The nurse's initial encounter with the patient sets the stage for a trusting nurse–patient relationship. This begins with a warm greeting and an approach that conveys respect and genuine concern, in an environment that ensures comfort, privacy, confidentiality and mutual participation. Then, by the nurse's efforts to guide the interview, to listen and to show empathy (the capacity to understand another's feelings) and acceptance (the capacity to remain neutral and nonjudgemental), a climate of trust is created in which the patient feels at ease sharing information and asking health-related questions.

Through the interview—by the questions they ask and the answers they receive—patients develop an understanding of their health situation that better enables them to identify their health needs. They also learn that control in the relationship is shared with the nurse, and that they are equal partners with the nurse in making decisions regarding their care. The following guidelines should assist the nurse in conducting a successful interview.

HISTORY Review data from the patient's previous medical and nursing records/charts, if available. In addition, you might want to consult texts, journals or other resources for information concerning the patient's past health problems, if you have had little experience in these areas.

TIMING Select a time for the interview. In primary health care—for example, a physician's office or health clinic—a time that suits both the patient and the nurse is usually set by appointment. In the hospital setting, however, selecting a time for the interview requires a nursing judgement based on the patient and his or her health status. If the patient is well and experiencing no discomfort, schedule a time when a complete history can be obtained in one encounter. However, if the patient is seriously ill, and is having numerous tests, examinations and therapeutic interventions, it may be best to complete the health history in segments over several encounters. When a patient is in pain, very tired or emotionally upset, the health history interview should be delayed until pain relief measures have been instituted or the patient has had rest or is feeling emotionally stable.

SETTING Conduct the interview in a quiet area that is free from distractions (noise, odours, interruptions) and ensure privacy. If you are in a private room, close the door; if in a public room, draw the curtains. If family and friends (who need not speak for the patient) are present, ask them to wait outside unless the patient requests their presence.

Arrange equal-status seating. Both you and the patient should be comfortably seated so that you can make level eye contact, with a distance of approximately 1.5 m between you. This provides normal social distance, yet is close enough for eye contact and easy communication. Sitting at 90° from each another is good because this arrangement allows the patient either to look at you or to look straight ahead from time to time. It also allows you to observe the patient fully. Avoid sitting behind a desk or bedside table, because this creates the feeling of a barrier. Avoid standing, because this communicates haste and superiority.

GREETING Greet the patient warmly with a smile or a handshake. Call him or her by name. Offer a seat (in a primary care setting) or ask permission to sit down and talk (in an inpatient facility). Introduce yourself and state your role in the agency. These courtesies convey respect for the person being interviewed and help him or her feel at ease with you.

State the purpose of the interview and the length of time it will take, for example, "Ms. Gray, the purpose of this interview is to learn something about you so that we can plan care to suit your needs and preferences." Describe what will happen during the interview and discuss any concerns that the patient may have about impending procedures. Knowing what to expect will make the patient feel more comfortable. Also, at this time, assure the patient that all information will be kept confidential and will be used only by health professionals participating in that patient's care.

FORMAT Conduct the interview in a systematic manner, using the agency health history form as a guide. Use open-ended questions to introduce a general topic and to obtain a narrative account of the patient's feelings, concerns and perceptions of his or her health and problem—for example, "Tell me what brings you to the hospital today" or, "What can you tell me about the symptoms you are having?" Use closed-ended questions to obtain specific, nonexplanatory information. Such questions are meant to elicit brief responses—for example, "Where do you feel the pain?" or, "How long have you had this cold?"

Use reflection, repetition and clarification to validate information and to verify perceptions. Avoid giving opinion, unwanted advice or false reassurance. Speak clearly and distinctly. Use language that the patient can understand.

LISTENING Listen carefully to what the patient says, and pay attention to nonverbal behaviour. Observe body posturing, facial expressions, gestures and tone of voice. Often, it is not only what is said but also how it is said that provides relevant information.

Maintain cultural sensitivity to the patient's customs, beliefs and values. (See Giger and Davidhizar's Transcultural Assessment Model on the following pages.)

DOCUMENTING Record the data on the nursing history form during the interview. Validate information with the patient so that you are sure the data are accurate.

CONCLUDING When data collection is complete, summarize your mutual understanding of the information, provide opportunity for further questions and answers and then inform the patient of the events likely to occur next. End the interview using common courtesies, such as "Thank you." Tell the patient when you will see him or her again.

Giger and Davidhizar's Transcultural Assessment Model

Culturally Unique Individual

1. Place of birth
2. Cultural definition (What is ...)
3. Race (What is ...)
4. Length of time in country (if appropriate)

Communication

1. Voice quality
   A. Strong, resonant
   B. Soft
   C. Average
   D. Shrill
2. Pronunciation and enunciation
   A. Clear
   B. Slurred
   C. Dialect (geographical)
3. Use of silence
   A. Infrequent
   B. Often
   C. Length
      (1) Brief
      (2) Moderate
      (3) Long
      (4) Not observed
4. Use of nonverbal communication
   A. Hand movement
   B. Eye movement
   C. Entire body movement
   D. Kinesics (gestures, expressions or stances)
5. Touch
   A. Startles or withdraws when touched
   B. Accepts touch without difficulty
   C. Touches others without difficulty
6. Ask these and similar questions:
   A. How do you get your point across to others?
   B. Do you like communicating with friends, family and acquaintances?
   C. When asked a question, do you usually respond (in words or body movement, or both)?
   D. If you have something important to discuss with your family, how would you approach them?

Space

1. Degree of comfort
   A. Moves when space invaded
   B. Does not move when space invaded
2. Distance in conversations
   A. 0–0.5 m
   B. 0.5 m–1 m
   C. 1 m or more
3. Definition of space
   A. Describe degree of comfort with closeness when talking with or standing near others
   B. How do objects (e.g., furniture) in the environment affect your sense of space?
4. Ask these and similar questions:
   A. When you talk with family members, how close do you stand?
   B. When you communicate with co-workers and other acquaintances, how close do you stand?
   C. If a stranger touches you, how do you react or feel?
   D. If a loved one touches you, how do you react or feel?
   E. Are you comfortable with the distance between us now?

Social Organization

1. Normal state of health
   A. Poor
   B. Fair
   C. Good
   D. Excellent
2. Marital status
3. Number of children
4. Parents living or deceased?
5. Ask these and similar questions:
   A. How do you define social activities?
   B. What are some activities that you enjoy?
   C. What are your hobbies, or what do you do when you have free time?
   D. Do you believe in a Supreme Being?
   E. How do you worship that Supreme Being?
   F. What is your function (what do you do) in your family unit/system?
   G. What is your role in your family unit/system (father, mother, child, adviser)?
   H. When you were a child, what or who influenced you most?
   I. What is/was your relationship with your siblings and parents?
   J. What does work mean to you?
   K. Describe your past, present and future jobs.
   L. What are your political views?
   M. How have your political views influenced your attitude towards health and illness?

Time

1. Orientation to time
   A. Past-oriented
   B. Present-oriented
   C. Future-oriented
2. View of time
   A. Social time
   B. Clock-oriented
3. Physiochemical reaction to time
   A. Sleeps at least 8 hours night
   B. Goes to sleep and wakes on a consistent schedule
   C. Understands the importance of taking medication and other treatments on schedule
4. Ask these and similar questions:
   A. What kind of timepiece do you wear daily?

B. If you have an appointment at 2 p.m., what time is acceptable to arrive?
C. If a nurse tells you that you will receive a medication in "about a half-hour," realistically, how much time will you allow before calling the nurses' station?

Environmental Control

1. Locus-of-control
   A. Internal locus-of-control (believes that the power to effect changes lies within)
   B. External locus-of-control (believes that fate, luck and chance have a great deal to do with how things turn out)
2. Value orientation
   A. Believes in supernatural forces
   B. Relies on magic, witchcraft and prayer to effect change
   C. Does not believe in supernatural forces
   D. Does not rely on magic, witchcraft or prayer to effect change
3. Ask these and similar questions:
   A. How often do you have visitors at your home?
   B. Is it acceptable to you for visitors to drop in unexpectedly?
   C. Name some ways your parents or other persons treated your illnesses when you were a child.
   D. Have you or someone else in your immediate surroundings ever used a home remedy that made you sick?
   E. What home remedies have you used that worked? Will you use them in the future?
   F. What is your definition of good health?
   G. What is your definition of illness or poor health?

Biologic Variations

1. Conduct a complete physical assessment, noting:
   A. Body structure (small, medium or large frame)
   B. Skin colour
   C. Unusual skin discolourations
   D. Hair colour and distribution
   E. Other visible physical characteristics (e.g., keloids, chloasma)
   F. Weight
   G. Height
   H. Check lab work for variances in hemoglobin, hematocrit and sickle phenomena if Black or Mediterranean
2. Ask these and similar questions:
   A. What diseases or illnesses are common in your family?
   B. Describe your family's typical behaviour when a family member is ill.
   C. How do you respond when you are angry?
   D. Who (or what) usually helps you to cope during a difficult time?
   E. What foods do you and your family like to eat?
   F. Have you had any unusual cravings for:
      (1) White or red clay dirt?
      (2) Laundry starch?
   G. When you were a child, what types of foods did you eat?
   H. What foods are family favourites or are considered traditional?

Nursing Assessment

1. Note whether the client has become culturally assimilated or observes own cultural practices.
2. Incorporate data into plan of nuring care:
   A. Encourage the client to discuss cultural differences; people from diverse cultures who hold different world views can enlighten nurses.
   B. Make efforts to accept and understand methods of communication.
   C. Respect the individual's personal need for space.
   D. Respect the rights of clients to honour and worship the Supreme Being of their choice.
   E. Identify a clerical or spiritual person to contact.
   F. Determine whether spiritual practices have implications for health, life and well-being (e.g., Jehovah's Witnesses may refuse blood and blood derivatives; an Orthodox Jew may eat only kosher food high in sodium and may not drink milk when meat is served).
   G. Identify hobbies, especially when devising interventions for a short or extended convalescence or for rehabilitation.
   H. Honour time and value orientations and differences in these areas. Allay anxiety and apprehension if adherence to time is necessary.
   I. Provide privacy according to personal need and health satus of the client (*Note:* the perception of and reaction to pain may be culturally related).
   J. Note cultural health practices:
      (1) Identify and encourage efficacious practices.
      (2) Identify and discourage dysfunctional practices.
      (3) Identify and determine whether neutral practices will have a long-term ill effect.
   K. Note food preferences:
      (1) Make as many adjustments in diet as health status and long-term benefits will allow and that dietary department can provide.
      (2) Note dietary practices that may have serious implications for the client.

SOURCES: Schematic design by Geneva Turner, PhD, CFLE; Joyce Newman Giger, EdD, RN, CS, FAAN; and Susan Wieczorek, MSN, RN. From Bobak & Jensen, 1993.

Components of the Health History

A comprehensive health history describes people's past and present health and illness patterns and records their responses to health problems. It provides a complete picture of the person as a whole and how that individual interacts with the environment. It identifies usual patterns of daily living, strengths and coping capabilities, and what the patient does or does not do to stay healthy (health-promotion and health-protection patterns).

The health history yields information that the nurse uses to plan and modify care that conforms with the patient's preferences and usual patterns of living. The nurse also uses this information to identify opportunities for teaching and for enabling individuals and families to satisfy their needs and to achieve optimum health and wellness.

The health history format provides structure to the data collection process and an organized system for recording the patient's responses. There are a variety of formats for taking health histories; however, they all share a common set of components patterned after the traditional medical model for history taking. These include introductory aspects, chief complaints (concerns), present illness, past history, current health status, family history, psychosocial history and review of symptoms (Bates, 1995). These components are described in Table 16.1.

Nurses have adapted the traditional medical history format to reflect nursing's holistic focus on the human experiences with health, illness and healing. The nursing history formats are often based on nursing models; the components are organized or grouped to ensure that the theoretical concepts central to nursing (person, environment, health and nursing) are incorporated into the data collection. One format used by nurses is the functional health pattern typology developed by Gordon (1982) as a framework for the diagnostic process (see Table 16.2). The basic components of the health history are contained within these categories (see box). These guides provide an outline of the information that is customarily gathered in the health history and are adaptable to any nursing model or format for history-taking.

In practice, you will use the agency form and follow agency protocol for obtaining the health history. The amount of information you need will vary according to the setting, the patient's needs and the purpose of the history-taking interview. For example, you would elicit different information from a person with a chronic health challenge

TABLE 16.1 Traditional health history format

Component	*Description*
Introductory aspects	• Date and time of history • Identifying data: include age, birth date, birthplace, gender, marital status, ethnic origin, religion, occupation • Source of referral, if any, and the purpose • Source of history, e.g., patient, family member, friend, patient's medical record or referral letter • Reliability of source, if relevant, e.g., knowledge, memory, trust, motivation (this is a judgement made at the end of the history-taking interview)
Chief concern	• Identifies, in the patient's own words, the reason for seeking health care
Present illness	• A narrative of the problem for which the patient is seeking health care. It gives a full, clear chronological account of the symptoms and the events related to them • Significant negatives (absence of certain symptoms that will aid in differential diagnosis) are also noted
Past History	• Determines other illnesses experienced in the past, relapses, recurrences and medical interventions
Current health status	• Identifies the patient's present state of health and any environmental conditions, personal habits and health-related measures that may impinge on it (e.g., medication use, allergies, tobacco, alcohol, recreational/street drugs and related substances, diet, screening tests, immunizations, sleep patterns, exercise and leisure activities, environmental hazards and use of safety measures)
Family history	• Used to rule out hereditary/genetic influences; identifies age and health, or age and cause of death, of immediate family (parents, siblings, spouse and children; may also include grandparents or grandchildren)
Psychosocial	• Determines daily lifestyle and usual patterns of living; includes home situation and significant others' daily life, important experiences (e.g., schooling, occupational history, financial circumstances, marriage, retirement), religious beliefs that are relevant to perceptions of health
Review of systems	• Explores symptoms relating to the systems and regions of the body to reveal related or new information the patient may have forgotten to mention when giving the history of the present illness

SOURCE: Bates, 1995.

TABLE 16.2 Typology of 11 functional health patterns

Pattern	Description
Health perception/health management pattern	• Describes patient's perceived pattern of health and well-being and how health is managed
Nutrition/metabolic pattern	• Describes pattern of food and fluid consumption relative to metabolic needs and pattern indicators of local nutrient supply
Elimination pattern	• Describes patterns of excretory function (bowel, bladder, skin)
Activity/exercise pattern	• Describes patterns of exercise, activity, leisure and recreation
Cognitive/perceptual pattern	• Describes sensory-perceptual and cognitive pattern
Sleep/rest pattern	• Describes patterns of sleep, rest and relaxation
Self-perception/self-concept pattern	• Describes self-concept pattern and perception of self (body comfort, body image and feeling state)
Role/relationship pattern	• Describes pattern of role engagement and relationships
Sexuality/reproductive pattern	• Describes patient's satisfaction or dissatisfaction with sexuality pattern; describes reproductive pattern
Coping/stress tolerance pattern	• Describes general coping pattern and its effectiveness in terms of stress tolerance
Value/belief pattern	• Describes values and beliefs (including spiritual pattern, or goals that guide choices or decisions)

SOURCE: Gordon, 1992, p. 81.

receiving home care than from a person with an earache visiting a family practice walk-in clinic, or a person working in a large corporation receiving personal wellness counselling. Three types of health histories may be obtained: complete, interval and focussed.

COMPLETE HEALTH HISTORY A complete health history is taken on the first visit to a health care agency in order to establish a data base when the health professional within the agency will be providing ongoing care (Barkauskas, Stoltenberg-Allen, Bauman & Darling-Fischer, 1994). This can occur in a primary care setting (e.g., family practice clinic, home care or community health agency), or upon admission to a long-term care facility or an acute care hospital. In the hospital setting, data may have already been collected in the medical history. If this is the case, use the information recorded by the physician rather than questioning the patient about the same things again. Collect only the information you need to complete the nursing health history.

Health History Guide Components

Health and illness patterns	• Usual patterns of daily living; habits related to eating, eliminating, activity/exercise, rest/sleep and hygiene • Perceptions of usual patterns of physiologic, psychologic, social and spiritual functioning • Recent changes in patterns of physiologic, psychologic, social and spiritual functioning; includes review of relevant body system(s) • Presenting health problem: chief concern, reason for seeking health care • Medical history • Family history • Concerns and expectations of care: worries/expectations and the care anticipated from health professionals
Health-promotion/-protection patterns	• What the person does or does not do to remain healthy • Health beliefs • Lifestyle/recreation practices • Environmental factors that may affect health (e.g., occupation or role within family; place of work/residence) • Developmental considerations

INTERVAL HEALTH HISTORY An interval health history is obtained periodically to follow up on the status of identified problems or concerns and to update the data base. This occurs in all settings when patients are receiving ongoing or continuous care.

PROBLEM-FOCUSSED HISTORY A problem-focussed history is used for episodic, short-term problems. The data collected are directed to specific problems or need, as opposed to the person's overall health status. For example, the information collected from the person with an earache visiting a walk-in clinic would focus on the ear, the symptoms associated with the earache and relevant body systems, such as the upper respiratory system.

Health History-Taking Throughout the Life Cycle

The health history for pediatric and older adult patients is not unlike that used for an adult. In the following section we will discuss how history taking differs among the various age groups.

INFANTS, CHILDREN AND ADOLESCENTS

The pediatric health history incorporates information pertinent for the age and developmental stage of the child, such as birth history (mother's health during pregnancy, history of birth and the perinatal period), physical growth, developmental milestones, social development, injury prevention and safety, immunizations and nutrition.

The parent is often the primary informant for the pediatric health history; however, it is important to remember that children, too, can provide valuable information. Children tend to be honest, but they can present data from an exaggerated point of view. The reliability of the child's data is likely to increase with advancing age. Parents, then, become the sole informant for infants and toddlers. When interviewing parents, the nurse should keep in mind that they are just as emotionally involved as their child, and particularly in an acute care setting, may be just as anxious. Parents may feel guilt or anger in relation to the reason for the child's admission. These feelings need to be explored during the interview.

The interviewing techniques and communication patterns used to elicit information from the parent are similar to those used in obtaining a health history from an adult. There are specific approaches to be taken with children in obtaining a health history at each developmental stage, and these will be discussed here. Even though many children either cannot or will not participate verbally, it is crucial to remember throughout the interview that all children need to be acknowledged as individuals and made to feel both accepted and important to the interviewer. Just as the behavioural responses for each group are unique, so should be the nursing approaches.

Infants

Little needs to done to involve infants during the interview with their parents. It is best not to attempt to pick up infants or to get too close. Separation anxiety and stranger fear usually peak at around six to nine months of age. Provided infants are content, alert and responsive to their surroundings, periodically turn to them to gain their attention by speaking softly, addressing them by name and, perhaps, capturing their interest with a bright toy. This technique reassures parents that you are both interested in their child and comfortable interacting with him or her. The child also takes pleasure in this stimulation and is more likely to develop a sense of trust in this new environment.

Toddlers

Toddlers may become frightened in a new environment amidst strange noises, people and equipment. They are likely to be subdued, clinging to parents and wary of all strangers. Do not expect most toddlers to volunteer information. As well, do not push to elicit their participation in the interview with parents, for this may only add to feelings of discomfort and mistrust. Maintain a comfortable distance from these children and acknowledge them by name. You can also tell them, in simple terms, that you need to ask their mother or father a few questions and that they can stay with mom or dad. It would be wise to have a variety of interesting toys close by and within the toddlers' view. Their curiosity may get the better of them, and they may feel secure enough to approach the toys and play.

Preschoolers

Preschoolers are usually able to explain their chief concern simply and relatively clearly. Some may require a little time before they feel comfortable enough to offer information. Others may be too shy or even too distressed, and therefore may be unwilling to interact with you. If this is the case, acknowledge their presence and give them time to acquaint themselves with the strange environment. You may need to try different approaches to gain the preschooler's trust. Get down to the child's eye level to minimize feelings of threat. Sometimes conversing by means of a hand puppet, or directing the conversation to an item of importance to the child, may spark the preschooler's participation. If the child remains unresponsive despite your efforts, do not pursue this issue. Continue your interview with the parents without ignoring the child completely. The occasional friendly comment that acknowledges the child as an individual is a useful tactic.

School-Aged Children

School-aged children have much to offer to the health history. It is not unusual for this group to provide even more information than the parents can. Include these children in the history taking from the very start. If the children are actively participating and not in any distress, direct all questions to them that you feel they are capable of answering.

As well, give them a chance to ask questions of you. School-agers need frequent explanations. You may need to explain why certain questions are important and relate these explanations to treatment modalities and subsequent progress.

Adolescents

For the most part, the adolescent can be approached much as the adult patient in obtaining the health history. Although parents often accompany adolescents and may offer important details to the history, older adolescents, in particular, should be treated as the primary informant unless their condition restricts participation. Adolescents need respect and acceptance. Because they may be suspicious of adults, an honest, straightforward approach is essential to gain their trust; you want the adolescent to be totally honest in revealing necessary information to you.

Adolescents should always be asked whether they want their parents present during the interview. If they request to be interviewed alone, the nurse should arrange to speak with the parents afterward. You should emphasize both to the parents and to the adolescent that the information given to you will be kept confidential. This is especially reassuring to the adolescent, and encourages more open dialogue. However, under rare and extenuating circumstances when the information points to a serious and potentially life-threatening situation, the nurse must inform the adolescent beforehand that such information may have to be shared with the parents.

Older Adults

The history format for the older adult is basically the same as for the younger adult. Modifications to the health history may be made if the individual has age-related sensory changes. In addition, because of the aging process and the effects of chronic health problems, older adults may experience a variety of symptoms and require more medications. Therefore, the nurse should focus on current health status rather than on past problems, and should complete a medication history (Ebersole & Hess, 1998).

There are a number of special considerations when taking a health history from an older adult. These are outlined by Staab and Hodges (1996):

1. Conduct the interview in a private, comfortable, well-lit area with a minimum of background noise to compensate for sensory losses of aging. Ensure that lighting is not glaring, and provide a chair with arms.
2. Sit close enough to be seen and heard, but respect the individual's need for personal space.
3. Provide ample time for slower responses; however, take care to limit the interview time in order to reduce fatigue.
4. If the patient has a memory impairment or is anxious or in psychological distress, arrange for a family member to be present to fill in missing or inaccurate information.
5. Be aware that older adults may not report significant symptoms because they may think these are just part of the normal aging process.
6. With regard to the usual patterns of daily living, ask the older adult to tell you how he or she spends the day. This will provide information about lifestyle and life problems, as well as life satisfaction, chief concerns and desire for change.

Symptom Analysis

The review of systems or functional abilities includes a long and specific list of symptoms. The student nurse can refer to specific chapters in this text to determine relevant questions to ask about related physical and psychological needs.

When the history of present problems and the review systems are discussed with the patient, it is important to get a full description of symptoms. Because symptoms are subjective sensations, the thoroughness of a symptom analysis depends on the examiner's ability to elicit accurate information about the patient's perception of the symptom. Descriptions of symptoms should be recorded using the patient's own words. For example, some people who have difficulty breathing may not respond positively when asked if they are "short of breath," but might instead describe their sensation as "tightness in the chest" or state, "I can't catch my breath." A systematic approach to questioning patients about the characteristics of their symptoms might use the following criteria:

- onset
- location
- quality
- quantity
- frequency and duration
- aggravating or alleviating factors
- associated factors
- course (Fuller & Schaller-Ayers, 1994).

Physical Examination

The physical examination is the systematic assessment of a patient's physical and mental status and yields objective data for the patient's data base. Data are objective because the information about the patient is observed, perceived or measured by the examiner through the use of the sense organs or with the aid of an instrument. Typically, the physical examination is performed after the nursing health history; however, subjective data may also be obtained during the course of the examination. The nurse may request more information

Questions the Nurse Might Ask to Analyse Symptoms

Onset	• When did you first experience the symptom (time and date)? • Was it a sudden or gradual onset? • Have you experienced this symptom before now?
Location	• Where do you feel the chest tightness? Does it spread to other parts of your body? • Can you point to where it hurts?
Quality	• Describe the quality of your cough. Is it dry and hacking, or wet and rattling? • Describe the progress of your cough since you first noticed it. Is it better? Worse? Unchanged? • What does it feel like (sound like, look like)? • What has it done to your lifestyle or daily activities? For example, does it keep you awake at night? • How would you describe your breathing difficulty? Is it a feeling of tightness? Of exhaustion? Do you feel you cannot get enough air?
Quantity	• How severe is the cough/chest tightness? (use scale of 1 to 10, with 10 being the worst) • Describe the amount of sputum. What colour is it? Describe the odour.
Frequency and duration	• How often do you get these symptoms? How long do the episodes last? • Are there particular settings or times in the day or night when these symptoms are worse or better?
Aggravating or alleviating factors	• What situations or treatments have been helpful in alleviating the symptoms? • What situations or treatments aggravate the symptoms? • What situations precipitate the tightness in your chest?
Associated factors	• Did you notice any other symptoms with this experience (e.g., pain)?
Course	• Have you noticed a changing pattern in these symptoms over time?

about a particular finding, or the patient may remember something he or she forgot to mention during the interview.

Physical examination involves the use of four sensory techniques: *inspection*, *palpation*, *percussion* and *auscultation*. The nurse should be equipped with all the tools that are necessary for a comprehensive and detailed examination. Use of the visual senses is necessary for inspection, which is facilitated by specific instruments such as the **ophthalmoscope** (for examining the eyes) and the **otoscope** (for examining the ears). The hands and the fingers are the main tools for palpation and percussion. In auscultation, the examiner uses the ears to listen to sounds produced by various organs and tissues, such as the heart, lungs, bowel and blood vessels. This may entail a direct process in which the examiner places his or her ear against the patient's body, or an indirect process, in which an instrument such as a **stethoscope** is used to amplify body sounds. Proficient use of these sensory techniques depends on the human tools of skill, knowledge and interpretation.

Preparation for Physical Examination

The physical assessment should be carried out in an organized fashion to avoid omission of necessary components. The beginning student is advised to develop a sequence for the complete basic physical examination and stay with this sequence until it becomes a habit. This will yield a systematic approach to assessments and avoid the possibility of missing portions of the examination.

Assessment of bodily organs and systems requires specific techniques, which are outlined in the related needs chapters throughout this text. For example, assessment of the lungs and thorax is detailed in Chapter 24.

The physical examination typically follows the health history interview. Following are general guidelines for conducting a health assessment.

1. Observe body movement, gait and general status of patient on entry.
2. Take a health history; conduct a symptom analysis. Observe for state of health, alertness, mood, intelligence.
3. Record vital signs, height and weight.
4. Have the patient change into a gown if needed, and ask him or her to void. If a urine sample is required, the specimen can be collected at this time. Having the patient's bladder empty promotes comfort, particularly during abdominal and pelvic examination.
5. Assemble all needed equipment. To promote efficiency and avoid interruptions, ensure that equipment is in working order before the exam.

6. Provide a warm, comfortable setting. Maintain the patient's privacy and modesty throughout the examination by closing the door or drawing the drapes, and by draping those areas of the body not being examined.
7. Wash your hands in the presence of the patient before and after the examination. This reassures the patient of your concern for his or her safety, as well as the safety of others. Practise universal precautions when coming in contact with any body fluids (blood, mucous membranes, urine, stool discharge, open skin lesions or wound drainage).
8. Explain the purpose of the examination to promote the patient's participation and help reduce anxiety. As you proceed through the exam, briefly explain each step and provide clear instructions so that the patient knows what to expect with each procedure. For example, "I am going to examine your breasts now; can you bring your arm behind your head?"
9. Much of the examination will be conducted with the patient in the sitting or supine position. Some patients, owing to their illness, cannot tolerate holding these positions for long. Monitor the patient's comfort throughout the examination, keeping position changes to a minimum and delaying the most uncomfortable manoeuvres to the last. The examiner performs most of the special manoeuvres from the patient's right side, moving to the foot of the examining table or the other side as needed. (Patients may need to assume particular positions to allow maximum exposure of specific body parts. The rationale for, and the limitations of, particular examination positions are shown in Table 16.5 later in this chapter.)
10. Throughout the examination, the nurse uses the four techniques, described in the following pages, to assess each body region, organ or system. The usual order is inspection, palpation, percussion and auscultation. An exception to this order is in the abdominal exam, when inspection is immediately followed by auscultation and then percussion. Palpation is performed last because it often stimulates peristalsis and alters the auscultatory sounds.
11. Proceed from head to toe, as outlined in Table 16.3, modifying the sequence and selecting tests and manoeuvres according to the patient's age, health status and acuity. For each body region, note the skin's colour, condition and pigmentation.
12. Carefully examine those areas identified in the health history as concerns or potential problems. For example, the patient who reports difficulty breathing will require a thorough examination of the upper airway, lungs and thorax, heart, skin and nails (for cyanosis and clubbing).
13. The physical examination provides a good opportunity to introduce certain topics for health promotion, such as the self-breast examination for women, and the testicular self-examination for men. Health teaching can occur as the examiner assesses these areas; return demonstrations by the patient can then be evaluated.

TABLE 16.3 Outline for head-to-toe physical examination

HEAD

Skin

Inspect the skin overlying the face, neck and ears for:

- colour, areas of pigmentation or depigmentation
- lesions such as rashes, ulcers, scars and tumours

Scalp

Inspect and palpate the scalp and skull from frontal to occipital areas, including the temporal and postauricular areas, for:

- hair distribution, colour, texture and quantity
- contour and size of the head
- areas of tenderness
- size and fullness of the anterior and posterior fontanelles in infants
- head circumference of infants and children up to the age of 2 years

Face

Inspect the palpebral fissures and nasolabial folds for symmetry

Palpate temporal arteries for symmetry and quality

Test the facial cranial nerve (VII) by asking the patient to perform the following motions as you observe for symmetry:

- raise eyebrows and frown
- smile and show teeth
- puff out both cheeks

Test the trigeminal cranial nerve (V) by:

- palpating for symmetrical strength of the masseter and temporal muscles as the patient clenches teeth
- assessing for intactness and bilateral sensation to light touch over the patient's forehead, cheeks and jaw

Ears

Inspect the auricle and mastoid processes bilaterally for:

- horizontal alignment by using an imaginary line from lateral canthus of the eye to the occipital prominence; the helix of the ear is normally above this line
- lesions or disfigurement of the external ear

Palpate the pinna tragus, auricle and mastoid process of each ear for:

- tenderness
- swelling
- nodules

TABLE 16.3 Outline for head-to-toe physical examination *Continued*

Palpate the preauricular and postauricular lymph nodes

Using an otoscope, inspect the auditory canal for:

- presence, amount and characteristics of cerumen (earwax)
- swelling and redness of the canal
- discharge—serous (clear, watery), purulent (yellowish) or sanguineous (bloody)
- colour and intactness of the tympanic membrane
- presence of foreign objects in children's ears

Assess the acoustic cranial nerve (VIII) of each ear using:

- whispered voice test from a distance of 1 m (the average person can hear a normal conversation from a distance of approximately 5 m)
- tuning fork tests such as the Weber test (to assess the lateralization of sound to one ear) and the Rinne test (to compare air conduction with bone conduction of sound)
- Romberg test (to assess the vestibular function of the acoustic cranial nerve)

Eyes

Inspect the eyebrows, eyelids, lashes, conjunctiva, sclera and cornea for:

- symmetry of position and lid closure
- distribution of hair over the brow and lashes
- redness
- swelling
- tearing
- discharge or crusting
- lesions such as a nodule or sty
- colour and clarity of conjunctiva and sclera
- transparency, shine and smoothness of cornea
- presence of foreign bodies
- forward bulging of the eyes (exophthalmus)

Inspect and palpate the lacrimal apparatus by:

- asking the patient to look up and milking the nasolacrimal sac towards lower inner orbital rim; observe for regurgitated discharge

Assess pupillary responses (cranial nerve III) by shining a penlight from the temporal area towards the pupil and observing for:

- size and shape of each pupil (normal pupils are 4–5 mm in diameter; they are round and equal in size)
- direct and consensual reaction to light (normally, pupillary constriction is observed in the eye directly stimulated by the light [direct response] and the opposite pupil constricts simultaneously [consensual response])
- accommodation (pupils dilate when gazing at a distance; they constrict and converge when gazing at the examiner's finger, placed 15 cm from the nose)

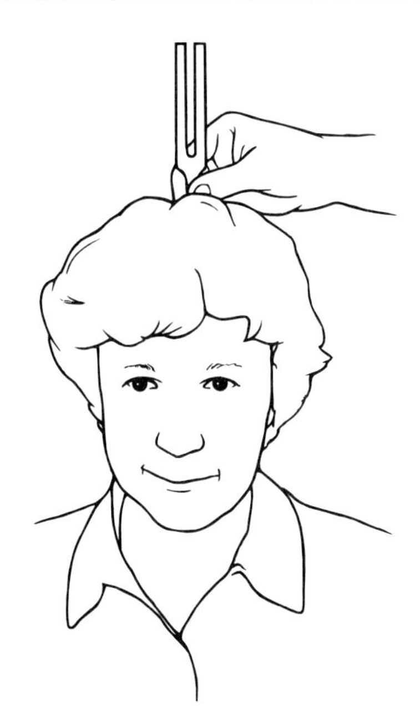

Weber Test

Place the base of a lightly vibrating tuning fork firmly on top of the patient's head or on the midforehead. Ask where the patient hears it: on one or both sides. Normally, the sound is heard in the midline or equally in both ears. If nothing is heard, try again, pressing the fork more firmly on the head.

SOURCE: Bates, 1995, p. 181.

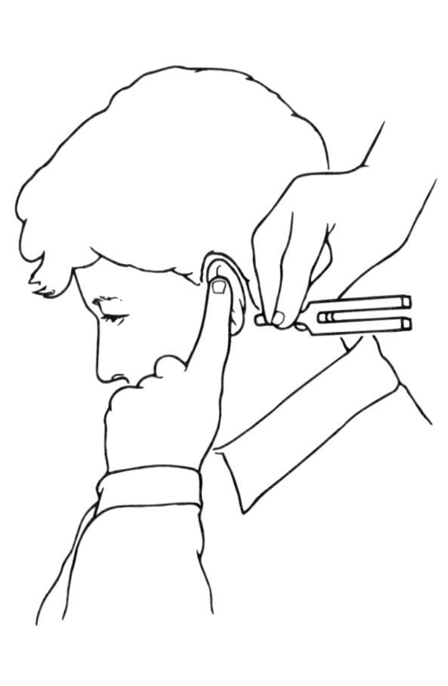

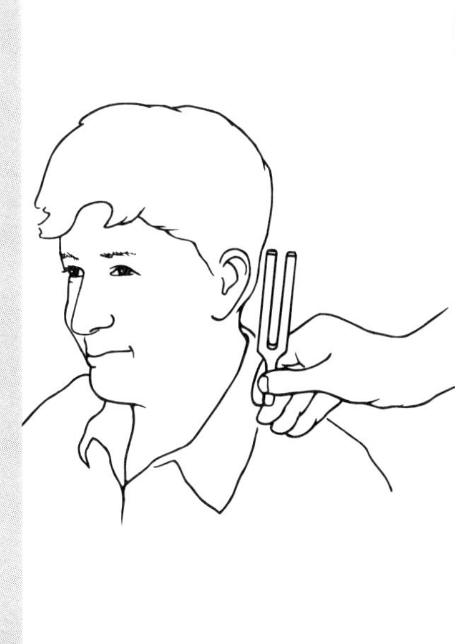

Rinne Test

Place the base of a lightly vibrating tuning fork on the mastoid bone, behind the ear and level with the canal. When the patient can no longer hear the sound, quickly place the fork close to the ear canal and ascertain whether the sound can be heard again. Here the "U" of the fork should face forward, thus maximizing its sound for the patient. Normally the sound is heard longer through air than through bone.

SOURCE: Bates, 1995, p. 182.

TABLE 16.3 Outline for head-to-toe physical examination *Continued*

Visual acuity can be tested using:

- Rosenbaum chart to assess near vision
- Snellen chart to assess distance vision (cranial nerve II)

Peripheral vision is assessed using confrontation, in which the patient's ability to see an object held at an extreme peripheral position is compared with the examiner's vision. Peripheral vision is tested in the nasal, superior, inferior and temporal fields

Extraocular muscle function is tested by:

- observing for symmetry of the corneal light reflex when the examiner shines a penlight onto bridge of the patient's nose (cranial nerves VI and VII)
- observing for nystagmus and strabismus through the six cardinal fields of gaze (cranial nerves III, IV, and VI)

Nose

Inspect and palpate the nose for:

- symmetry
- characteristics and quantity of nasal discharge
- tenderness

Assess patency by asking the patient to occlude one nostril and sniff inward through the opposite side

Inspect the septum and nasal mucosa for:

- intactness of the septum
- septal deviation that occludes air flow
- colour of the mucosa

Assess the olfactory cranial nerve (I) by occluding each nostril in turn, and asking the patient to identify two familiar odours

Inspect and palpate the frontal and maxillary sinuses for:

- redness
- swelling
- tenderness

Mouth and pharynx

Inspect and palpate the tympanomandibular joint for:

- limited opening or locking
- crepitus or clicking
- tenderness or pain

Note breath odour (foul, fruity, alcoholic)

Inspect the lips, buccal mucosa, teeth and gums, and the dorsal and ventral surfaces of the tongue for:

- colour
- moistness of the mucosa
- cracking, bleeding or ulcerations
- lesions
- condition of the teeth (presence of dental caries) and gums (bleeding)
- size, surface characteristics and movement of the tongue

Using a tongue depressor and penlight, inspect the soft and hard palates, tonsils and pharynx for:

- colour and surface characteristics
- lesions
- intactness and symmetry of the palates
- midline position of the uvula when the patient says "ah"
- intactness of the gag reflex (cranial nerves IX and X)

Neck

Inspect the neck for:

- bilateral symmetry of the neck muscles
- midline position of the head
- midline position of the trachea

Test range of motion by observing the patient in the following movements:

- flexion of the head towards the chin
- extension of the head backward
- lateral bending of the head from side to side
- rotation of the head towards the left shoulder and to the right

Test the strength of the neck muscles by adding resistance of your hand against the patient's head as patient repeats the above movements

Test cranial nerve (XI) by observing the patient's ability to shrug shoulders against the resistance of your hands

Inspect and palpate the following lymph nodes for redness, swelling and tenderness:

- occipital
- tonsillar
- submandibular
- submental
- anterior superficial cervical
- posterior cervical
- supraclavicular
- infraclavicular

Inspect the external jugular vein for distention, and the internal jugular vein pulsations

Palpate one carotid artery at a time

Auscultate each carotid artery using the bell of the stethoscope and listen for a bruit (an abnormal finding)

Inspect and palpate the thyroid gland for:

- enlargement
- nodules
- tenderness

THORAX

Lungs

Inspect the anterior and posterior chest wall for:

- contour and shape by comparing anterior–posterior and lateral diameters
- respiratory rate and breathing pattern
- chest deformities
- posture assumed by the patient for breathing
- whether accessory muscles are used for breathing

Inspect the skin, nails and lips for colour

Palpate the trachea for midline position

Palpate the anterior and posterior chest wall for:

- ribcage stability
- bilateral respiratory excursion
- symmetrical tactile fremitus (palpable vibration as the patient says "99")
- note areas of tenderness, asymmetrical excursion and increased or decreased fremitus

TABLE 16.3 Outline for head-to-toe physical examination *Continued*

Percuss over the posterior and lateral chest wall for:

- resonant percussion tones over the lung fields
- areas of hyperresonance or dullness

Auscultate over the following areas using the diaphragm of the stethoscope and comparing from side to side (note quality of breath sounds and their location; presence of adventitious sounds)

- apices of lungs
- intrascapular areas
- lung bases
- lateral chest walls

Breast

Inspect and palpate the breasts, nipples and areola for:

- rashes, dimpling, vascularities
- areas of tenderness
- nodules and masses

Inspect and palpate the axillary nodes for:

- nodules, masses

Heart

Inspect the precordium for:

- visible pulsations
- retractions
- lifts

Palpate for pulsations, heaves or thrills (palpable vibrations) over the following areas of the precordium:

- aortic—over the second intercostal space (ICS) at the right sternal border
- pulmonic—over the second ICS at the left sternal border
- right ventricular—over the third, fourth and fifth ICS at the left sternal border
- mitral—over the fifth ICS at the midclavicular line. This area is also referred to as the apex

Palpate the apex for the point of maximal impulse (PMI), noting the location, amplitude, duration and width of the impulse. Normally, the apical impulse is at the fifth ICS medial to the midclavicular line; it has a small amplitude, brief duration and is 2–3 cm in diameter (Thompson & Wilson, 1996)

Auscultate for heart sounds and murmurs, using the diaphragm and then the bell over the following areas:

- aortic—over the right second interspace at the sternal border
- pulmonic—over the left second interspace at the sternal border
- Erb's point—over the left third interspace at the sternal border
- tricuspid—over the left fourth interspace at the sternal border
- mitral—over the left fifth interspace at the midclavicular line

Auscultate over the mitral area for 60 seconds, using diaphragm of the stethoscope; count the apical pulse rate, assessing rhythm

Abdomen

Inquire about areas of tenderness; examine these areas last

Inspect the abdomen for:

- contour
- surface characteristics, scars, striae, vascularities
- surface movements (visible peristalsis)

Auscultate for bowel sounds, pressing the diaphragm of the stethoscope lightly on the abdomen; listen to the four quadrants

Auscultate with the bell of the stethoscope for:

- arterial bruits (aortic, renal, iliac, femoral)
- venous hum (over the umbilicus)

Percuss the four abdominal quadrants for:

- tympanic tones; note areas of dullness, which may be due to the presence of fluid or a mass
- the gastric bubble of the stomach—an area of increased tympany is normally found over the left lower ribcage
- liver span—the area of liver dullness is located over the right midclavicular line between the fifth ICS and the costal margin
- splenic dullness—a small area of splenic dullness is normally found at the sixth to tenth rib at the left midaxillary line

Palpate the abdomen lightly for:

- muscle tone
- superficial masses
- note areas of tenderness or hypersensitivity
- note areas of muscle rigidity

Palpate the abdomen deeply for:

- deeper masses
- tenderness
- aortic pulsation—located at the epigastrium, and above and slightly to the left of the umbilicus
- umbilical bulges and hernias
- lower liver border and tenderness—palpate under the right costal margin
- lower splenic border and tenderness—palpate under the left anterior costal margin
- lower poles of the right and left kidneys—palpate the right and left posterior costal margins (flanks). When palpable, the kidneys are normally smooth, firm and nontender
- bladder—the nondistended bladder lies below the symphysis pubis and is not palpable

Percuss for kidney tenderness posteriorly at the right and left costovertebral angles

Inspect and palpate the femoral and inguinal areas for:

- enlargement or tenderness of the inguinal lymph nodes
- bulges and hernias over the femoral and scrotal areas
- femoral artery pulsations

Genitalia

Inspect and palpate the external genitalia, perineum and anal area for:

- hair distribution
- skin colour and pigmentation
- swellings, ulcerations and lesions
- discharge from the vagina (female) and the urethral meatus (male and female)
- areas of tenderness or induration

TABLE 16.3 Outline for head-to-toe physical examination *Continued*

SPINE AND EXTREMITIES

Observe the patient's gait for:

- rhythm
- trunk posture and arm swing
- symmetry of stride and arm swing
- note unsteadiness or jerky motions
- note use of assistive devices, such as a cane or walker

Spine

Inspect the spine for:

- alignment and symmetry of shoulders, hips, knees, ankles and feet
- normal curvatures—cervical concave, thoracic convex, lumbar concave
- deformities

Upper and lower extremities

Inspect for:

- skin colour and pigmentation
- edema
- masses
- contractures, deformities
- involuntary movements: tremors, muscle spasms
- symmetry of muscle size (dominant side is usually slightly larger than nondominant side)

Palpate the peripheral pulses bilaterally, comparing their symmetry (see Figure 16.7):

- radial artery—located on the inner aspect of the wrist at the radial or thumb side
- ulnar artery—located opposite the radial artery on the inner aspect of the wrist
- brachial artery—found medial to the biceps tendon at the antecubital fossa
- femoral artery—found midway between the symphysis pubis and the anterior iliac spine, below the inguinal ligament
- popliteal artery—located in the popliteal fossa behind the knee (this pulse is difficult to find)
- posterior tibial artery—found behind and inferior to the medial malleolus on the inner aspect of the ankle
- dorsalis pedis artery—located between the extensor tendons of the first and second toe on the dorsum of the foot

Assess capillary refill by squeezing the fingerpads and the toes until they blanche (with normal capillary refill, original colour returns within 4 seconds)

Palpate the major bones, joints and muscles for:

- symmetry of muscle tone
- heat, edema or tenderness
- crepitus on movement

Assess passive and active range of motion of the major joints and adjoining muscle groups for:

- limitations of movement
- tenderness on movement
- joint instability

Assess the strength of the major muscle groups for:

- full resistance against the examiner's opposing force
- symmetry with the contralateral side

Assess the distal dermatomes of the extremities for sensation to:

- light touch
- heat and cold stimuli
- sharp and dull stimuli

Assess the following deep tendon reflexes:

- biceps
- triceps
- patellar
- Achilles
- Babinski

Assess the patient's general coordination, using one of the following tests:

- finger-to-nose test
- rapid tapping of the thighs with palms up, alternating with palms down
- running heel of one foot down the shin of the opposite leg

Grading Deep Tendon Reflexes

Deep tendon reflexes are graded on a scale of 0 to 4:

0 No response
1+ Diminished (hypoactive)
2+ Normal
3+ Increased (may be interpreted as normal)
4+ Hyperactive (hyperreflexia)

The deep tendon responses and plantar reflexes are commonly recorded on stick figures. The arrow points downward if the plantar response is normal and upward if the response is abnormal.

SOURCE: Fuller & Schaller-Ayers, 1994, p. 351.

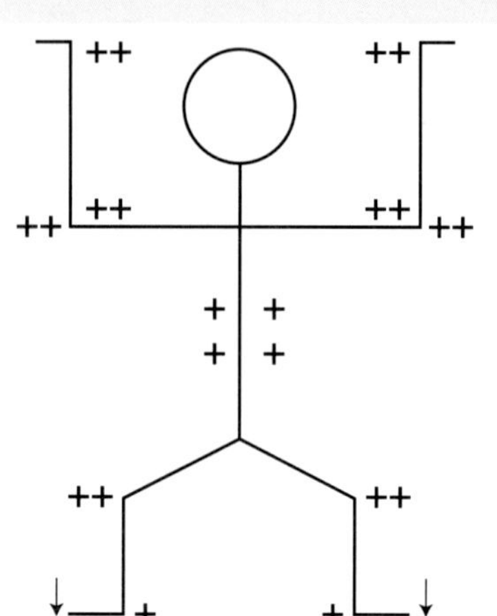

Recording deep tendon reflexes

TABLE 16.3 Outline for head-to-toe physical examination *Continued*

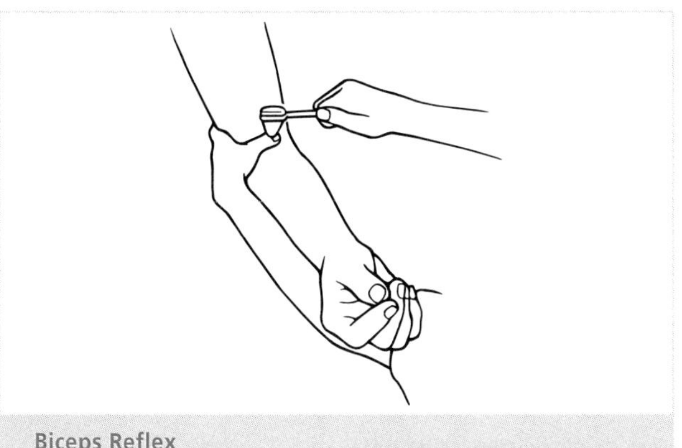

Biceps Reflex
Support the patient's forearm on yours to relax and partially flex the patient's arm. Place your thumb on the biceps tendon and strike a blow on your thumb. You can feel as well as see the normal response, i.e., flexion of the forearm.

SOURCE: Jarvis, 1996, p. 736.

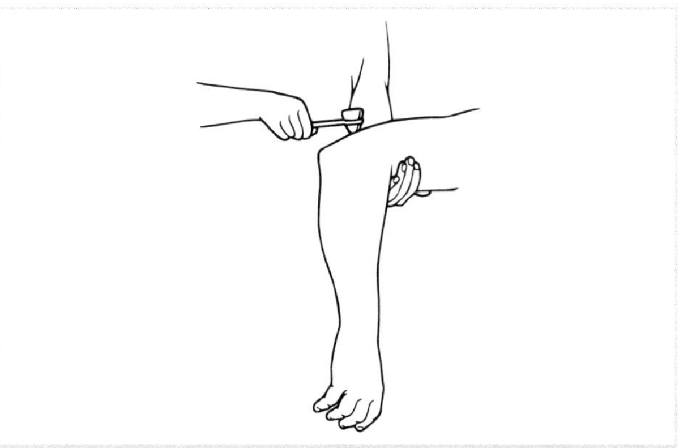

Triceps Reflex
Ask the patient to let the arm "go dead" as you suspend it by holding the upper arm. Strike the triceps tendon directly just above the elbow. The normal response is extension of the forearm.

SOURCE: Jarvis, 1996, p. 736.

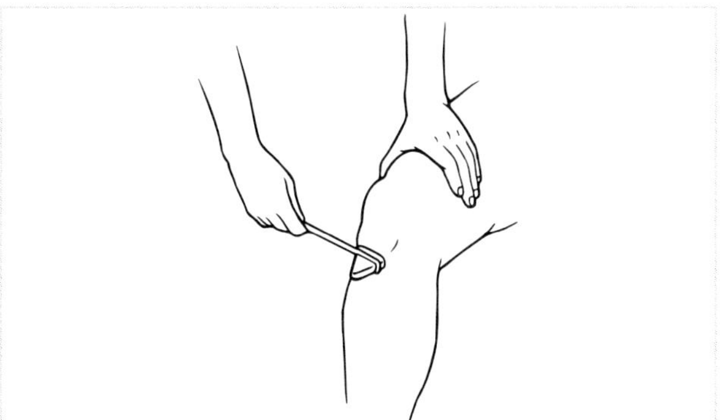

Patellar ("Knee-Jerk") Reflex
Let the patient's lower leg dangle freely to flex the knee and stretch the tendons. Strike the tendon directly just below the patella. Extension of the lower leg is the normal response.

SOURCE: Jarvis, 1996, p. 737.

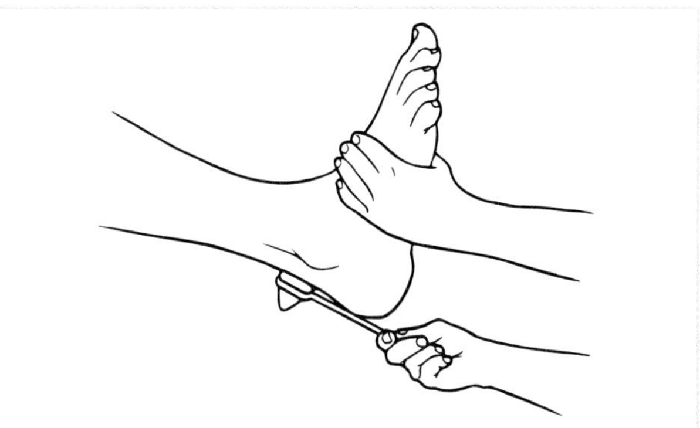

Achilles Reflex
Position the patient in the same manner as you would for testing the patellar reflex. Support the foot in a dorsiflexed position and tap the Achilles tendon above the heel. The normal response is plantar flexion, which may be observed visually or felt by placing your hand against the sole of the foot as the reflex is tested.

SOURCE: Fuller & Schaller-Ayers, 1994, p. 362.

Inspection

Inspection is the most valuable, least mechanical, and most difficult technique to learn. It involves the use of the senses—primarily vision—to assist in making judgements, comparisons and decisions. Because inspection is a highly subjective process, it requires skill, repetition and practice to establish reliable findings for distinguishing among ranges of normal, borderline and abnormal.

One of the criteria of thorough inspection is the conscious systematic use of one's senses. The examiner observes the patient with a critical eye, comparing the left side of the body with the right (to assess symmetry) and noting any variations from normal. As the examiner proceeds from one body system or area to another, he or she inspects the relevant body part for particular observations. For example, when assessing over the precordium, the examiner observes for pulsations and heaves that may indicate an underlying abnormality. Inspection also includes notation of any odours emitted from the skin or body orifices.

Adequate lighting and adequate exposure of the area to be inspected are also essential criteria. Direct lighting allows the examiner to assess colour and texture. Tangential lighting—directing a light at right angles to the area being inspected—is helpful for determining contour and pulsations on the body surface (Thompson & Wilson, 1996).

A diagnostic set that includes an ophthalmoscope, an otoscope and a nasal speculum is necessary to examine the internal eye structures, the inner ear and the internal nose, respectively. An ophthalmoscope and an otoscope are depicted in Figure 16.1. It is important to care for the battery housing of both instruments to ensure complete, dependable service.

Equipment Used in a Physical Examination

Item	Use
Tongue depressor	For examining the pharynx and to stimulate the gag reflex
Ruler	For linear measurements of body parts
Measuring tape	For measuring length and circumferences of body parts
Skin-marking pen	To enable accurate measurement taking
Penlight or flashlight	To aid inspection by illuminating areas and to test pupillary constriction
Thermometer (mercury, tympanic or electronic)	For measuring body temperature
Watch with a second hand or digital display	For counting pulse and respirations
Sphygmomanometer and cuff	For measuring blood pressure
Stethoscope with bell and diaphragm	For listening to sounds arising from the body that are not easily heard with the naked ear
Paper clip and cotton balls	For testing tactile sensory perception
Cotton-tipped applicators	To aid in everting the eyelid in eye examination
Snellen charts	For measuring visual acuity (far or distant vision)
Tuning forks (100–400 Hz and 500–1000 Hz)	For testing sound conduction, auditory nerve function and vibration sensation
Ophthalmoscope	For examining the internal structures of the eye
Otoscope	For examining the external auditory canal and the tympanic membrane
Nasal speculum	For examining the internal surfaces of the nose
Percussion (reflex) hammer	For testing deep tendon reflexes
Vaginal speculum	For examining the vagina and cervix
Water-soluble lubricant	To ease insertion of vaginal speculum into the vagina
Clean gloves	To protect the nurse from infection

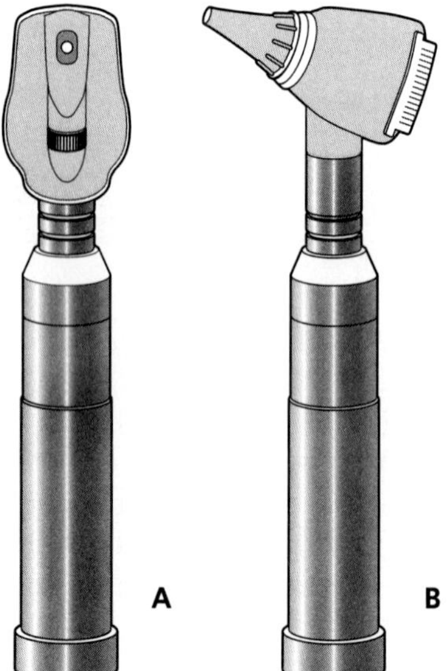

FIGURE 16.1 A. The ophthalmoscope illuminates and magnifies the interior of the eyes, permitting examination of the internal structures.
B. The otoscope illuminates the external ear canal, permitting examination of the canal and the tympanic membrane.

SOURCE: Block & Nolan, 1986, pp. 138, 155.

Palpation

Palpation is the use of touch to detect both superficial and deeper characteristics of the body. It helps to identify areas reported by the patient as being tender. Palpation follows inspection because in many instances it validates visual impressions. It is used to examine all accessible parts of the body. Specific parts of the hand are used to palpate for particular findings. Because the palmar surfaces of the hand and fingers (fingerpads) are more sensitive than the fingertips, they are used to determine position, texture, size and consistency of a mass, fluid and crepitus (air in the subcutaneous tissues) (Thompson & Wilson, 1996). Vibration, as in tactile fremitus, is best assessed with the ulnar surface of the hand (along the side of the little finger), while temperature is assessed with the dorsal surface (the back of the hand). A thorough knowledge of anatomy is essential in differentiating palpation of normal body structure from abnormal. Light and deep palpation yield different types of data.

Light palpation is especially helpful in determining temperature, muscular resistance, superficial organs, masses and abdominal tenderness. It should be done gently to help reassure and relax the patient. Complete relaxation of the patient is essential to good palpation. Deep palpation is used to locate organs, determine their size and consistency, feel masses and check for organ tenderness and muscle rigidity.

PALPATION OF THE ABDOMEN

To relax your patient's muscles:

- warm your hands; ensure your fingernails are short
- instruct the patient to breathe through the mouth
- place a pillow under the head and shoulders.

LIGHT PALPATION Using the palmar surfaces of the fingers of one hand in a gentle, dipping motion, indent the skin 1 cm. Avoid sudden short jabs. Light palpation is used to assess skin, pulsations and tenderness; it always precedes deep palpation. If resistance is present, try to determine whether it is a voluntary or an involuntary spasm.

DEEP PALPATION Place one hand on top of the other and press the palmar surfaces of the bottom hand to indent the patient's skin by 4 cm. The top hand is used to exert downward pressure, while the bottom hand feels the underlying tissues. Another technique, called bimanual palpation, is used to assess deeper organs, such as the kidneys and the uterus. The examiner places one hand anteriorly and the other posteriorly, and brings both hands together to entrap the organ between the fingertips. Deep palpation is considered an advanced skill.

Percussion

Percussion involves striking or tapping the body surface to produce sounds that correlate with the type of underlying tissue density. As the body surface is tapped, it produces a vibration 4–5 cm deep in the body tissues. The subsequent sound produced is a percussion note. The notes vary in quality according to the density of the underlying structures. Percussion is used:

1. to determine the size and borders of certain organs, such as the liver and the spleen
2. to determine the presence of fluid or air in organs, such as the stomach or the lung
3. to detect tenderness over deep organs, such as the kidneys
4. to obtain deep tendon reflexes by stretching specific tendons with a percussion hammer. Both direct and indirect percussion are used in the physical examination. The examiner uses direct percussion over the sinuses to elicit tenderness, while direct fist percussion over the costovertebral angle elicits kidney tenderness. Indirect percussion is used to assess the organs in the thorax and the abdomen.

INDIRECT PERCUSSION

Place the nondominant hand, as illustrated in Figure 16.2A, over the area to be percussed, making sure that only the middle finger (pleximeter) is in contact with the skin surface. Use a quick, sharp but relaxed wrist motion to strike the middle finger of the nondominant hand, at the distal interphalangeal joint, with the middle finger (plexor) of the dominant hand (see Figure 16.2B). Use the tip of this finger rather than the pad. This necessitates short fingernails on the examiner. The two fingers should almost be at right angles. The movement is at the wrist, not in the finger. Percuss two or three times in one location before moving to another. Listen for the percussion tone produced by the tapping.

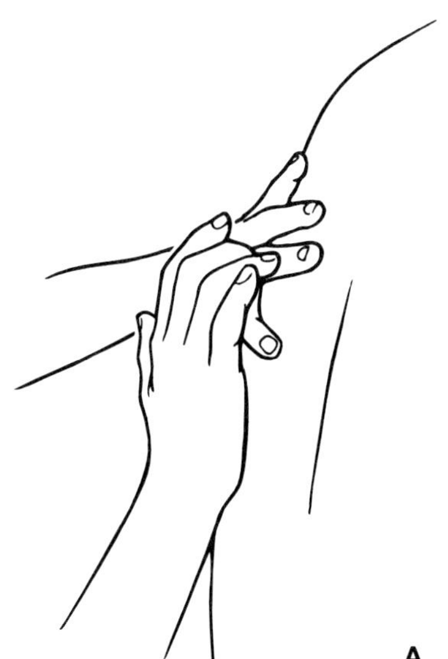

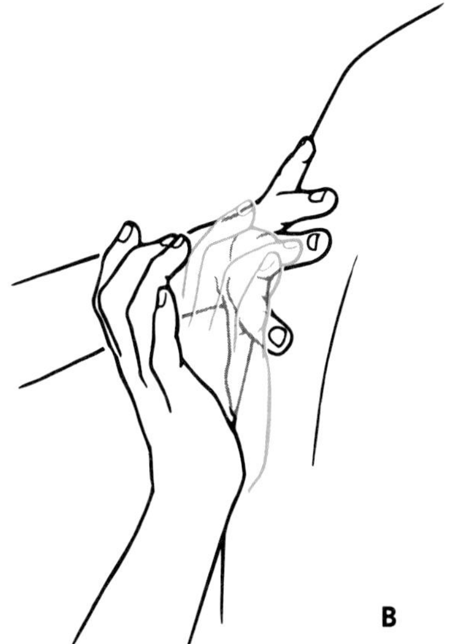

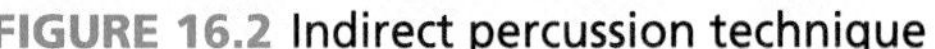

FIGURE 16.2 Indirect percussion technique

SOURCE: Jarvis (1996).

FIVE PERCUSSION NOTES The percussion technique can invoke five percussion notes or sounds. Each sound has its own intensity, pitch, duration and quality. Table 16.4 differentiates the five percussion sounds. The principle of percussion can be understood by remembering that the more solid a structure, the fewer the vibrations produced and the softer and quieter the sound. For example, the solid thigh vibrates very little, hence you hear a flat sound. The liver vibrates slightly more, thus a dull sound is heard. The air-filled lung vibrates even more, creating a resonant sound. The stomach filled with an air bubble vibrates considerably, hence the tympanic or musical sound heard. Normal percussion sounds are resonant over the lungs, tympanic over the abdomen and dull over the liver and viscera. Abnormal percussion notes are flatness and hyperresonance. Percussion will not produce vibrations in structures more than 4–5 cm deep or less than 4–5 cm in size.

Auscultation

Auscultation is similar to percussion in that it involves the evaluation of body sounds. It differs, however, in that the examiner listens for sounds produced by the body arising from the heart, lungs and abdomen, and not for those that are produced exogenously (outside the body). The main instrument used for auscultation is the stethoscope (see Figure 16.3).

The stethoscope can yield valuable information only if it meets certain criteria and is utilized properly. The following points should be followed to promote optimum sound transmission:

1. the *eartips* must fit the external auditory meatus snugly yet comfortably while occluding it. Clean these often, as they become occluded with wax
2. the *binaural curvature* is directed anteriorly towards the nose when the eartips are in the ears
3. the *tubing* should be 30–38 cm long and 3 mm in diameter to decrease sound distortion
4. the correct chest piece must be used. The chest piece has two components. The *diaphragm*, which is flat and broad, transmits high-pitched sounds, such as breath, bowel and heart sounds. It should be held firmly against the skin. The *bell*, which is dome-shaped, transmits low-pitched sounds, such as extra heart sounds, bruit or murmurs. It should be held very lightly against the skin.

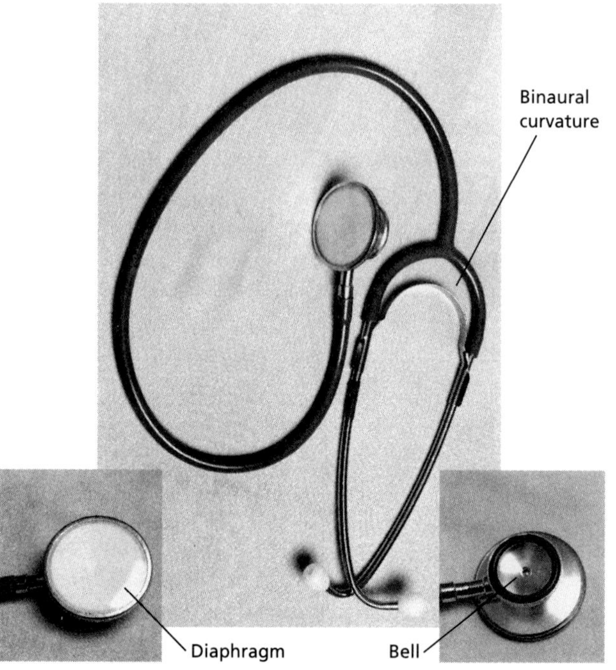

FIGURE 16.3 Stethoscope

Be sure the tubing at the junction of the diaphragm or bell is turned in the correct direction to allow sound to be transmitted to your ears. It is a good idea to insert the eartips and tap the side (bell or diaphragm) you want to use to check for patency. It is not uncommon to hear accidental sounds while auscultating. Three causes of accidental sounds while auscultating are: movement of the tubing against the skin; breathing heavily on tubing, which produces a roaring sound; and friction of the stethoscope on hairs. The nurse should eliminate all extraneous noises, such as television,

TABLE 16.4 Five percussion sounds

SOUND	*INTENSITY*	*PITCH*	*DURATION*	*QUALITY*	*EXAMPLE*
Resonance	loud	low	long	hollow	normal lung
Dullness	medium	medium	medium	thud-like	liver, spleen
Tympani musical	loud	high	medium	drum-like	gastric air bubble, puffed-out cheek, abdomen
Flatness	soft	high	short	quiet, dull	thigh, muscle, bone
Hyperresonance	very loud	lower	longer	booming	emphysematous lung

SOURCE: Thompson & Wilson, 1996.

voices and equipment sounds prior to auscultation. Be sure the stethoscope head is warm before placing it on the patient. Shivering can cause fine muscular contractions that will interfere with normal sounds.

When using the diaphragm, stabilize it between the index and middle fingers, and hold it firmly against the patient's skin. When using the bell, place it lightly over the skin surface, applying just enough pressure to produce an air seal with its full rim (Bates, 1995). The auscultation technique requires the examiner to isolate specific sounds, identify their location and, when appropriate, compare sounds from side to side. Auscultatory sounds are described according to their quality (e.g., crackle, wheeze); loudness (e.g., soft, medium, loud); duration (e.g., during inspiration); and location (e.g., over the lung bases). Normal lung, heart and bowel sounds are described in detail in their respective chapters. Practice, knowledge and concentration are required to develop skill in using the stethoscope.

ASSISTING WITH A PHYSICAL EXAMINATION

The responsibilities of the assisting nurse usually involve gathering the necessary equipment and supplies, preparing the examining room or patient's unit and helping both the examiner and the patient with the examination. Most patients want some explanation about the examination—what is to be done and why. The patient will need to undress fully or partially and may need help in putting on the gown provided; the gown may be removed during parts of the examination. It is important to ensure the patient's privacy and also to make sure that he or she is not cold. If the patient lies on a bed for the examination, a light blanket may be used. During the examination the nurse is usually responsible for draping the patient as appropriate for comfort and modesty, and helping the patient, as needed, to assume the best position to facilitate the examination.

The nurse does not always stay throughout the entire physical examination, although many agencies today, and also many physicians, request that a female nurse be present during the examination if the patient is female and the examiner male. The reason for this is twofold: it contributes to the psychological comfort of the patient and also provides legal protection for the examiner. The nurse should also consider the patient's age, mental alertness, balance and cooperativeness in judging whether to stay with the patient throughout the examination.

Table 16.5 shows the various positions for physical examination. If the patient is ambulatory, a general inspection is often done with the patient standing; that is, one assesses posture and general appearance and notices abnormalities. Alternatively, it is done with the patient lying in a **supine position** (on the back). Most examiners prefer to have the patient sitting up for examination of the head and neck and the chest and lungs (back and front). The supine position is the usual choice for examination of the breasts, heart and abdomen. The examiner may also look at the extremities when the patient is lying down but will often want to do a further examination with the patient sitting and, also, standing. For examination of the rectum, a male patient may be asked to bend over the examining table. For a patient on bed rest, or a female patient, Sims' position or a knee-chest position may be used. **Sims' position** is also known as the semi-prone or three-quarter prone position. It is a position that is frequently used for people who are unconscious, and is described in detail in Chapter 26.

In the **knee-chest position**, the patient kneels with the buttocks upward. It is important that the patient who assumes this position be adequately draped. Many health agencies have special rectal drapes that completely cover the buttocks of a patient except for a circular cutout over the anus. The patient will generally need additional covering for the shoulders and a pillow for the head.

If the health agency does not have special drapes, the nurse can improvise with a cotton drawsheet. The drawsheet is placed across the patient so that the lower edge just covers the buttocks. The corners are tucked around the medial aspect of the patient's thighs. By raising the fold of the sheet, the examiner may expose the anal area.

During this procedure, the examiner needs a rectal glove, lubricant and kidney basin. The examiner inserts a lubricated gloved finger into the patient's rectum, palpating for abnormalities such as hemorrhoids and fissures.

The **lithotomy position** is used chiefly for examinations and operations involving the reproductive and urinary tracts for both genders. In this position the patient lies on the back with a small pillow for the head. The patient's hips are flexed and slightly abducted, and the knees are also flexed. The patient needs support for the feet to maintain this position for more than a few minutes. The stirrups provide a means for supporting the feet.

Because this position is embarrassing for most people, it is important that adequate drapes be provided. One way of draping is to place a drawsheet across the patient so that the lower border is 10 cm below the symphysis pubis. Then each of the lower corners of the drawsheet is brought to the medial aspect of the patient's thighs and tucked around the patient's legs. When the upper fold of the drawsheet is lifted, the patient's perineum is exposed. The nurse should also provide the patient with a covering for the upper part of the body. Another method is to place a bath blanket diagonally over the patient. The opposite corners (at each side of the patient) are wrapped around the legs and anchored at the feet. The lower corner can be drawn back and tucked under the top layer of the bath blanket to expose the perineum.

For a vaginal examination the examiner requires gloves, lubricant, a vaginal speculum, a kidney basin and a good light. This equipment is sterilized after use in order to prevent the transmission of infection. The physician may also require a cytobrush, spatula, fixitive and a microscopic slide

TABLE 16.5 Positions for examination

Position	Areas Assessed	Rationale	Limitations
Sitting	Head and neck, back, posterior thorax and lungs, anterior thorax and lungs, breasts, axillae, heart, vital signs, upper extremities	Sitting upright provides full expansion of lungs and provides better visualization of symmetry of upper body parts	Physically weakened client may be unable to sit. Examiner should use supine position with head of bed elevated instead
Supine	Head and neck, anterior thorax and lungs, breasts, axillae, heart, abdomen, extremities, pulses	This is the most normally relaxed position. It provides easy access to pulse sites	If client becomes short of breath easily, examiner may need to raise head of bed
Lithotomy*	Female genitalia and genital tract	This position provides maximal exposure of genitalia and facilitates insertion of vaginal speculum	Lithotomy position is embarrassing and uncomfortable, so examiner minimizes time that client spends in it. Client is kept well draped
Sims'	Rectum and vagina	Flexion of hip and knee improves exposure of rectal area	Joint deformities may hinder client's ability to bend hip and knee
Knee-chest*	Rectum	This position provides maximal exposure of rectal area	This position is embarrassing and uncomfortable

*Clients [patients] with arthritis or other joint deformities may be unable to assume this position.

SOURCE: Adapted from Potter & Perry, 1995.

in order to take a sample of the cervical secretions, which are then sent to the laboratory for examination for abnormal cells. This is called a Papanicolaou smear (Pap test).

Assessing Functional Abilities

Nutritional Status

In assessing an individual's nutritional status, the nurse may have information about height, usual weight, and present weight from the nursing health history. It is customary practice in most health agencies to take height and weight measurements for all newly admitted patients, and this is usually a nursing responsibility. Many agencies use a combination height and weight measuring scale. Patients are asked to remove their shoes and to stand on the scales. It is a good hygienic measure to use a fresh paper towel on the scales for each patient. The nurse usually measures the height first (with the patient's back to the measuring scale), and then weight. If the patient is too ill, the height and weight measurements might not be taken on admission. A portable scale that can be wheeled to the bedside is used if it is important to monitor the weight of a patient confined to bed. Height and weight may be compared with the average for the patient's age, gender, and type of body frame to aid in assessment of his or her nutritional status. Tables showing desirable weights for individuals of different ages are included in Chapter 20. In addition to noting patients' height and weight, the nurse also observes their general appearance—do they look *obese*, *plump*, *average* in build, *thin*, or *emaciated?*

The health history includes questions to elicit information about patients' nutritional status. What are their usual eating habits? Do they usually have a small, average or big appetite? The nurse inquires about special diets patients have been following, as well as any dietary restrictions they observe for cultural or religious reasons or because of allergies. Observations can be made regarding the

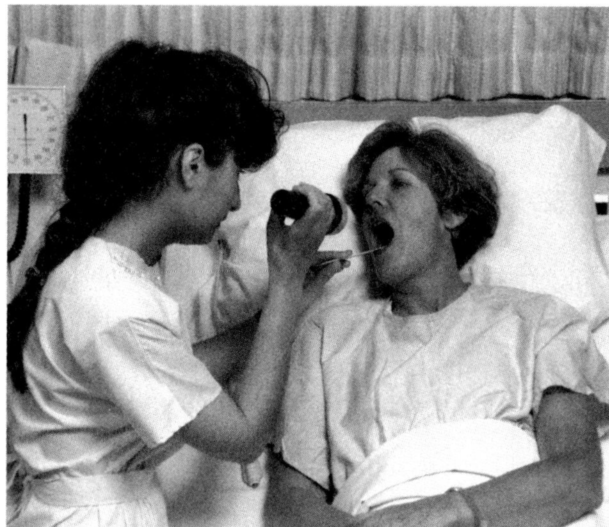

The nurse examines the condition of the patient's mouth and throat.

individual's present response to food and eating. Normally people enjoy food, although they do not always eat enough of the proper nutrients.

The nurse notes the amount of food or fluids that the individual takes. Abnormalities that should be noted in the person's ability to eat or in response to food include: *nausea* (a queasy feeling in the stomach); *anorexia* (loss of appetite); refusal to eat; *dysphasia* (difficulty in swallowing); *distention* (enlargement of the abdomen due to internal pressure of gas or liquid); *dysguesia* (distorted tastes); or *emesis* (the vomiting of contents of the gastrointestinal tract through the mouth). Vomiting is always an abnormal condition. The nurse should make observations about the *amount* (it should be measured or approximated) and the *contents* of the emesis. Common terms used to describe the latter include: *bloody* (containing red blood); *coffee grounds* (dark brown-to-black particles of old blood); *undigested food* (recognizable particles of food); and *bile* (a thick, viscid fluid varying in colour from yellow to brown or green, and having a bitter taste).

Elimination Status

Data about an individual's elimination patterns are usually included in the health history. When inquiring about an individual's current elimination status, the nurse takes note of bowel and urinary status.

BOWEL STATUS

Significant information about current bowel status includes the date and time of the individual's last bowel movement, the colour of the stools and the frequency of bowel movements. Normal stool is brown, soft and formed. Abnormal findings should be noted, such as *clay-coloured* stools or *tarry* stools (black or blackish-brown, viscous semiliquid or liquid stools).

Common problems with bowel functioning that the individual may report are *diarrhea* (frequent bowel movements; stools of more or less fluid consistency); *constipation* (infrequent passage of feces or difficult defecation; stools are unduly hard and dry); and *flatulence* (gas in the digestive tract). When individuals are unable to control the movement of their bowels, they are said to have *involuntary* bowel movements (incontinence). The term *impacted* bowel refers to a condition in which there is an accumulation of feces in the rectum pressed firmly together so as to be immovable.

URINARY STATUS

Normal urine is clear and straw-coloured. Assessments should include colour, clarity and amount. Common terms used to describe abnormalities are: *cloudy*, *dark orange*, *pink*, *red*, *frothy* or *containing sediment*. Common problems in urinary functioning that the individual may report include: *frequency* (urinating at short intervals); *urgency* (the need to void suddenly, with an inability to retain urine without acute distress); *burning* (a scalding sensation on voiding); and *dribbling* (an intermittent flow of urine). A person is said to be *incontinent* of urine when he or she is unable to control urination. Questions and responses about lower abdominal discomfort, lower back or flank pain should be included in the health history.

Sensory Perception

The abilities to see, hear, feel, taste and smell are vitally important in coping with the daily activities of living. In making observations relating to an individual's sensory perception, the nurse is concerned with the integrity of the anatomical structures needed for functioning in these areas: eyes, ears, nose, mouth, throat, and skin, as well as any disturbances in the functioning of these structures. Deviations from the individual's normal abilities, as indicated in the baseline data, should be noted for all sensory areas.

VISION

In assessing current visual status, the nurse makes observations about the condition of the eyes, eyelids and pupils, as well as asking about any visual disturbances the patient may be experiencing. The nurse inquires about itching or burning of the eyes or lids; frequent rubbing of the eyes often indicates this feeling. In addition, the nurse asks the patient about such visual disturbances as *blurring* (seeing objects as vague or lacking in outline) or *diplopia* (double vision, seeing two objects when there is only one). In noting comments about the eyes, the nurse should record which eye is affected—right, left or both.

HEARING

Hearing is one of the senses that becomes less acute as one grows older. Men lose the ability to hear high sounds first (women's voices, for example), whereas women find the low tones more difficult to hear as they grow older. Long-standing deficits in hearing and the use of hearing aids are included in the data collected about an individual. The nurse also asks if the patient has noticed any disturbances in hearing, such as a buzzing or ringing in the ears *(tinnitus)*, or any dizziness or loss of balance.

SMELL

The nose is instrumental not only in the ability to smell; it is also an important part of a person's respiratory system. Common abnormalities include sinus congestion (sensation of pressure or tenderness over the frontal or maxillary sinuses), nasal discharge (secretions from the nose), or bleeding (nosebleed). Disturbances in the sense of smell, such as an absence of this sense, or distorted odours (odours usually considered agreeable are unpleasant, and vice versa), should also be noted.

TASTE

The condition of a person's mouth and throat is important not only to the sense of taste but also to the ability to take food and fluids, thereby affecting nutritional status. Disturbances in taste that the individual may describe include a bad taste in the mouth, an absence of taste or distorted taste (misinterpretation of tastes). Or the patient may report an increased acuteness of this sense or, conversely, decreased ability to distinguish tastes.

TOUCH AND FEELING

Touch and feeling are subjective experiences, and the nurse must rely on the individual's observations regarding deviations from the normal in this sensory area. Disturbances in feeling, such as numbness, prickling or tingling, are most commonly noted in the extremities or in the face. Sometimes there is heightened sensitivity to touch (pressure), heat or cold, or, conversely, decreased sensitivity.

The Skin and Its Appendages

The intact skin provides a protective covering for the body. Normal, healthy skin is clear (free from blemishes), intact (unbroken), warm to the touch and has a characteristic colour, depending on the person's ethnic background and inherited complexion tones. Although each individual's skin colouring varies to a certain extent, the nurse may observe common abnormalities such as *flushing* (redness of the skin, particularly noticeable in the face and neck), *pallor* (lack of colour), *cyanosis* (bluish or greyish cast to the skin, particularly noticeable in the lips, earlobes and nailbeds), and *jaundice* (yellowing of the skin or sclera).

The nurse should also look for blemishes and breaks in the skin. Common blemishes include rashes (eruption of the skin, usually reddish in colour); bruises (superficial discolourations due to hemorrhage into the tissues from ruptured vessels); reddened areas (diffuse red discolouration); *weeping* areas (oozing a watery secretion); dry, itching areas (rough and scaly skin which the individual has a desire to scratch); and *mottled* areas (marked with blotches of different shades of colour). Scabs (crust of a sore, wound, ulcer, or pustule) and *lesions* (moles, blisters, birthmarks) should be noted, as well as scars on the body or incisions from surgical operations. The presence of lumps under the skin (abnormal masses that perform no physiological function) should be noted. Both the location (specific area of the body on which the blemish or lesion appears) and its size should be recorded.

Other observations that the nurse may make about the skin are the presence of excessive perspiration, which may be seen on the forehead, upper lip, palms of the hands and/or soles of the feet, in the axillary area or covering the entire body. If the entire body is bathed with perspiration, the term *diaphoresis* is used. The nurse may also notice abnormalities in the temperature of the skin; for example, it may feel hot or cold to the touch.

Motor Status

A normal individual can sit, stand, walk and perform a great number of movements, provided that the bones and muscles, circulation and nerve supply are intact. Limitations in mobility due to chronic health problems, such as paralysis, weakness or difficulty in movement of one or more limbs (or parts of limbs), should be included in the data collected about the patient.

The nurse inquires about the patient's response to activity. Some common terms that people use to describe abnormal responses to activity are feelings of dizziness (a whirling sensation in the head that gives the affected person a tendency to fall), faintness (a feeling of weakness), fatigue (a feeling of tiredness or weariness) and shortness of breath (slow, rapid respirations on exertion). These observations are predominantly subjective. The nurse must ask if the patient has noticed any of these symptoms in response to normal activities, such as walking and climbing stairs.

The individual's mobility should also be determined. Aids to mobility required at the present time, such as crutches, a cane, a walker, a wheelchair or persons to assist the individual, are noted. If restrictions have been placed on activities because of a current illness (such as bed rest or bathroom privileges only), these are also included.

Nursing observations pertaining to present motor status focus on the integrity and functioning ability of the extremities. Abnormalities to which the nurse should be alert include disturbances in circulation or sensory perception, limitation of movement and abnormal muscular movements.

An important observation the nurse should make relative to circulation is the presence or absence of *distal* (peripheral) *pulses*—that is, whether a pulse can or cannot be obtained by compressing the arteries at the points farthest from the heart in any of the extremities. Other pertinent observations include the presence of swelling (abnormal localized enlargement) or *edema* (an excessive amount of tissue fluid) in any part or all of an extremity. Sensory disturbances that the individual may tell the nurse about include *paresthesia* (abnormal sensation without objective cause, such as numbness, prickling, tingling, or a heightened sensitivity (to pressure, heat or cold) in any part, or all of one or more limbs.

The nurse should also observe the limbs for deficiencies in range of motion of a part or of the whole extremity. Weakness (that is, a lack of strength in any area) should be noted, especially a marked decrease in the ability to grasp an object (weak hand grip).

Abnormal muscular movements include *contractures* (permanent fixation of a muscle due to spasm or paralysis), *tremors* (quivering or involuntary convulsive muscular contraction) and *muscle spasm* (involuntary convulsive muscular contractions). Missing limbs, or parts of a limb, absent as a result of a birth defect, trauma or surgery, should also be noted.

State of Rest and Comfort

The individual's usual patterns of rest and sleep are noted in the nursing health history. Problems such as insomnia or excessive drowsiness should also be noted. The nurse notes the presence of any pain, since it is one of the most common causes of disturbances in rest and sleep. Pain is, of course, a subjective experience, and the nurse must rely on the patient's observations of pain. The exact location of the pain and its nature are recorded. People use a variety of expressions to describe pain. Common terms include sharp (acute or cutting), aching (dull, generalized, persistent), cramplike (severe paroxysmal type), throbbing (pulsating), constant (continuous, unchanging) and intermittent (coming and going at intervals). The nurse also notes whether the pain reacts to therapy—whether the severity or intensity of the pain is, or is not, appreciably alleviated with treatment. Various types of pain scales are used (see Chapter 27).

Reproductive Status

Age, gender and marital status are vital statistics about the individual that are noted in the patient's chart. Other information about reproductive status that is collected in the nursing or medical history of a female patient includes data about menstruation (age of menarche, frequency and duration of menstrual periods, usual amount of flow, any premenstrual symptoms, date of last menstrual period); obstetric issues (number of pregnancies and live births, number of children and their ages; infertility); menopause (when menstrual periods stopped; symptoms of hot flashes, mood swings, vaginal dryness or itching); sexual relations (type and frequency of sexual activity, number of sexual partners; preference for men, women or both; satisfaction with sexual relationship); contraceptive use (type of birth control/protective measures used; satisfaction with method); frequency and result of Papanicolau smears; urinary symptoms (frequency, urgency, pain on urination, incontinence); and vaginal discharge (colour, amount and odour). Common types of discharge include bloody, white or yellow discharges. An intermittent bloody discharge of very light flow is termed *spotting*. Bloody vaginal discharge occurring between menstrual periods is termed *withdrawal bleeding*. If a discharge has a foul odour, this also should be noted.

Health history about the reproductive status of the male patient includes questions about urinary symptoms (frequency, urgency, nocturia, dysuria, hesitancy and straining); past genitourinary problems (infections, testicular or scrotal pain or lumps, penile pain, discharge or lesions); self-examination behaviours; and sexual concerns (relationships and sexually transmitted diseases) (Thompson & Wilson, 1996).

Mental Status

In the patient of "normal" mental status, information about this aspect of health is obtained from the psychosocial component of the history. Additional data are obtained from observations of the patient's appearance and grooming; behaviour (irritability, listlessness, restlessness); orientation (to time, place and person); cognitive abilities (recent and remote memory, abstract reasoning and calculation ability); and emotional status.

Normally, during waking hours, a person is alert and responsive. In appraising the mental status of patients, the nurse should observe their movements. If they are slow or sluggish in moving, or appear to suffer from abnormal drowsiness, they are said to be *lethargic*. If they appear bewildered and perplexed, and/or give inappropriate answers to questions, the term *confused* is commonly used to describe their mental state. *Disoriented* individuals perceive themselves and/or their environment incorrectly in relation to time, place or person. They may not know who they are (or recognize familiar people), where they are or what day it is.

People are said to be *inattentive* when they are unable to focus on an idea or on some aspect of their surroundings or on reality. The term *forgetful* is used when patients have a temporary loss of memory—for example, they cannot remember what you asked them a few minutes ago, or whether they have eaten lunch. When individuals make no response to sensory stimulation (for example, they do not answer or obey simple commands such as, "Please raise your hand," or do not turn their head away from a bright light or react to touch), they are said to be *unresponsive*.

Most people experience a range of emotions in their day-to-day lives. These emotions are communicated to other people both by what the individual says and by his or her actions. In assessing a patient's emotional status, the nurse needs to identify both the individual's feelings as he or she expresses them in words and the person's observable behaviour. These feelings include *depression* (a feeling of sadness or melancholy); *nervousness* (easily excited, irritated, jumpy, uneasy or disturbed); anger (strong feelings of displeasure or antagonism); and fear (unpleasant emotion caused by anticipation or awareness). The patient may claim to want to die, or may have feelings of anxiety concerning possible ill effects from his or her present state of health or from surgery.

Some common nursing descriptions of observable behaviour include: *restless* (continually moving the body or parts of the body); *crying* (weeping or lamenting); *withdrawn* (socially detached and unresponsive); *underactive* (not moving about as much as is desirable); *combative* (physically striking or attempting to strike others); *abusive* (harshly attacking others verbally); and *noisy* (talking loudly, shouting or banging objects).

The "Mini-Mental State" test is a standardized tool used to screen patients for mental status abnormalities (Folstein, Folstein & McHugh, 1975). A sample of this test appears in Table 16.6.

The Glasgow Coma Scale (GCS) is used to assess a patient's level of consciousness using a 15-point scale. This scale assesses for best motor, verbal and eye-opening responses (Thompson & Wilson, 1996; see bottom of Figure 16.8).

Social Status

People normally are gregarious; they enjoy the company of other people. The ability to make contact and to exchange communication with others not only makes life more interesting and enjoyable, but is essential to daily living. People convey messages to others by speaking, by writing and through their behaviour. Deviations from the normal in regard to an individual's social status may be observed through their speech, writing and behaviour.

VERBAL COMMUNICATION

Normally a person has the ability to carry on a conversation with another person and to respond to questions in such a way that the meaning is clear. This, of course, assumes that there are no language barriers. Two common abnormalities of speech that the nurse can identify by listening to a person talking are *stuttering* (stumbling and spasmodic repetition of the same syllable) and *slurring* (sliding or slipping over word sounds that would normally be heard). A person who is unable to make meaning clear (provided everyone is speaking the same language) is said to be *incoherent*. When an individual who previously was able to speak normally is unable to speak at all, the term *aphasia* (or aphasic) is used. *Dysphasia* is a general term used to refer to difficulties in speaking.

In observing an individual's speech, the nurse should note willingness to communicate. He or she may, for example, be *reticent* (inclined to be silent and uncommunicative); *evasive* (avoids answering people directly); or *verbose* (extremely talkative). If the individual is unable to write, this fact should be noted.

SOCIAL RESPONSE

People respond to other people in an infinite variety of ways. Behaviour that is normal for one individual may be abnormal for another. If the individual is ill, however, the nurse should note his or her response to the presence of others.

It is important to note, for example, whether the individual wants to be alone (to have minimal or no contact with anyone) or does not want to be left alone, but desires or needs constant companionship. The nurse should also record his or her observations if the patient becomes upset by contact with family, friends, staff, visitors or roommates.

Vital Signs

Temperature, pulse, blood pressure and respirations have traditionally been referred to as the **vital signs**, or *cardinal signs*, of life. They indicate basic physiological functioning, specifically in the functional areas of temperature status, circulatory status and respiratory status. In making observations about an individual's current functional abilities, the nurse frequently starts with the vital signs.

Determinants of Vital Signs

Age, exercise, hormone levels, circadian rhythms, stress and the environment have an impact on vital signs. In assessing vital signs, it is important to remember that individuals each have their own **circadian (diurnal) rhythm**, or a 24-hour biological "clock," that regulates their daily events. The rhythm is evident in biological functioning such as body temperature, sleep and blood pressure, and the nurse will note differences in the vital signs of patients at different times of the day. For example, a person's temperature is normally lowest in the early morning hours and highest in the late afternoon or early evening. Blood pressure, in most people, is also highest after the day's activities.

Although temperature, pulse, respirations and blood pressure readings vary among and within individuals, there is a range that is generally considered normal for each of these signs. Normal ranges for individuals in different age groups are included in each of the following sections.

Because of the variable nature of vital sign measurements, it is important to establish baseline data for each patient. The patient should be made aware of his or her baseline vital signs and work towards a lifestyle that promotes normal findings. A series of readings, undertaken systematically and consistenly, helps to determine what is normal for a particular individual, to identify deviations from the normal and to pick up trends in the early stages of illness. For example, if a patient's temperature is usually around 36.1° C before breakfast but, one morning, you find it to be 37.5° C and, by noon, it is 37.8° C, you would suspect that the patient is developing a fever, even though all temperature readings fall within the "normal" range.

TABLE 16.6 "Mini-mental state" test, a standardized screening tool of mental status. The maximum score is 30. Depressed patients without dementia usually score between 24 and 30. A score of 20 or less is found in patients with dementia, delirium, schizophrenia or an affective disorder

"MINI-MENTAL STATE"

Patient . . . .
Examiner . . . .
Date . . . .

Maximum Score	Score	
		ORIENTATION
5	( )	What is the (year) (season) (date) (day) (month)?
5	( )	Where are we: (province) (city/town) (hospital) (floor)?
		REGISTRATION
3	( )	Name 3 objects: 1 second to say each. Then ask the patient all 3 after you have said them. Give 1 point for each correct answer. Then repeat them until he learns all 3. Count trials and record. Trials
		ATTENTION AND CALCULATION
5	( )	Serial 7's. 1 point for each correct. Stop after 5 answers. Alternatively spell "world" backwards.
		RECALL
3	( )	Ask for the 3 objects repeated above. Give 1 point for each correct.
		LANGUAGE
9	( )	Name a pencil, and watch. (2 points) Repeat the following: "No ifs, ands or buts." (1 point) Follow a 3-stage command: "Take a paper in your right hand, fold it in half, and put it on the floor." (3 points) Read and obey the following: CLOSE YOUR EYES (1 point) Write a sentence (1 point) Copy design (1 point)
	_____	Total score

ASSESS level of consciousness along a continuum ________________________

Alert Drowsy Stupor Coma

INSTRUCTIONS FOR ADMINISTRATION OF MINI-MENTAL STATE EXAMINATION

ORIENTATION

(1) Ask for the date. Then ask specifically for parts omitted, e.g., "Can you also tell me what season it is?" One point for each correct.

(2) Ask in turn "Can you tell me the name of this hospital?" (province, city, etc.). One point for each correct.

REGISTRATION

Ask the patient if you may test his memory. Then say the name of 3 unrelated objects, clearly and slowly, about one second for each. After you have said 3, ask him to repeat them. The first repetition determines his score (0–3) but keep saying them until he can repeat all 3, up to 6 trials. If he does not eventually learn all 3, recall cannot be meaningfully tested.

ATTENTION AND CALCULATION

Ask the patient to begin with 100 and count backwards by 7. Stop after 5 subtractions (93,86,79,72,65). Score the total number of correct answers.

If the patient cannot or will not perform this task, ask him to spell the word "world" backwards. The score is the number of letters in correct order, e.g., dlrow = 5, dlorw = 3.

RECALL

Ask the patient if he can recall the 3 words you previously asked him to remember. Score 0–3.

LANGUAGE

Naming: Show the patient a wrist watch and ask him what it is. Repeat for pencil. Score 0–2.

Repetition: Ask the patient to repeat the sentence after you. Allow only one trial. Score 0 or 1.

3-Stage command: Give the patient a piece of plain blank paper and repeat the command. Score 1 point for each part correctly executed.

Reading: On a blank piece of paper print the sentence "Close your eyes," in letters large enough for the patient to see clearly. Ask him to read it and do what it says. Score 1 point only if he actually closes his eyes.

Writing: Give the patient a blank piece of paper and ask him to write a sentence for you. Do not dictate a sentence; it is to be written spontaneously. It must contain a subject and verb to be sensible. Correct grammar and punctuation are not necessary.

Copying: On a clean piece of paper, draw intersecting pentagons, each side about 1 in, and ask him to copy it exactly as it is. All 10 angles must be present and 2 must interact to score 1 point. Tremor and rotation are ignored.

Estimate the patient's level of sensorium along a continuum, from alert on the left to coma on the right.

SOURCE: Folstein et al., 1975.

It is important for the nurse to interpret vital signs in relation to other information about a patient. A sudden drop in blood pressure, an increase in pulse rate (or irregularity of rhythm or weakness of the pulse) or a lowered body temperature, with or without rapid and deep respirations, would alert the nurse to a change in status and should be reported promptly to the physician.

Temperature

PHYSIOLOGY

The surface temperature of the body fluctuates with the temperature of the surroundings. In a cool room, for example, exposed skin surfaces soon feel cold and are cold to the touch. On the other hand, the deep body, or core, temperature is precisely regulated and maintained within a very narrow range. Body measurements taken to determine a person's temperature status reflect core temperature. Under normal conditions it does not vary more than a degree or so from the mean, or average, for that person. Variances greater than that usually indicate disturbed functioning of the body's heat-regulating system.

The temperature regulating system is one of the principal homeostatic mechanisms, whereby the internal climate of the body is maintained at an optimal level for functioning. The centre for controlling the internal temperature of the body is located in the hypothalamus, in the lower portion of the brain. In health, this centre maintains a fairly precise balance between heat production and heat loss. Heat is continually being produced in the body as a byproduct of metabolism. It is also constantly being lost through *evaporation* (perspiration from the skin); *radiation* (the transfer of heat in the form of electromagnetic waves), for example, from the body to cooler objects in the environment; *conduction* (the transfer of heat from a warmer to a cooler substance by direct contact), for example, from the body to the surrounding air; and *convection* (movement of air), as currents around the body carry away heat that has been conducted to the air from the body surface. The factors affecting heat production and the processes by which heat is lost from the body are described in more detail in Chapter 25.

DETERMINANTS OF BODY TEMPERATURE

The **body temperature**, as measured by a clinical thermometer, reflects the balance between heat production and heat loss. It usually varies slightly during the course of a 24-hour period in any one individual, being lowest during the early morning hours before a person wakens and highest in the evening. The cycle may be reversed in persons who work at night and sleep during the day. Many people who are ill have an elevated temperature; it is often one of the first observable indications of disturbed body function. In addition, a temperature below normal may indicate ill health. **Pyrexia** and **fever** are two terms used to refer to an elevated temperature. The term **hypothermia** refers to a temperature that is below normal.

Factors other than disease processes can affect body temperature. The activity of the individual can make some difference—the active person usually has a higher temperature than the sedentary person. Exercise can cause a marked, but temporary, elevation in body temperature. Age also affects temperature; for example, infants and older adults often have a body temperature lower than the young adult. Emotions and stress can increase the basal metabolic rate of an individual and thereby elevate temperature. Some medications can cause an elevation of body temperature, referred to as a *drug fever*.

ASSESSING BODY TEMPERATURE

Sites

An estimate of the body's core temperature can be obtained from the mouth, the rectum, the axilla (armpit) or the ear. The usual route used in everyday clinical practice is by mouth (*per os*) or PO. The small blood vessels on the underside of the tongue are supplied with blood by branches of the external carotid artery that are close to the bifurcation with the internal carotid artery (Sunderland, 1996). When a thermometer is placed in the posterior pocket under the tongue, and the mouth is closed, it is possible to obtain a reasonably accurate estimate of the body's internal temperature. The normal body temperature, when taken orally, ranges from 35.8° C to 37.3° C (Thompson & Wilson, 1996). The oral method of temperature assessment is the most convenient for patients who are awake, alert and can follow directions. It is unsafe for young children and for adults who are disoriented, confused, unconscious or experiencing seizures. Accurate readings require that smoking or ingestion of hot or cold foods or fluids be withheld for 20–30 minutes prior to measurement.

An axillary temperature, taken by placing a thermometer under the arm is a safe method of temperature-taking because it is noninvasive. Major arteries situated near the area provide accurate readings, providing the thermometer is kept in place long enough. The axilla is the site of choice for taking temperatures in newborns and preschoolers, but it can be used for people of all ages and conditions. It is an appropriate alternative for patients with conditions of the mouth that contraindicate use of an oral thermometer, such as infections or oral surgery. Axillary temperatures measure approximately 0.5° C lower than oral temperatures; however, readings may vary considerably. A drawback of this site is that it takes 6–10 minutes to register a temperature and therefore its use requires valuable nursing time in order to obtain an accurate reading.

The rectal site is used for adults when it is considered either unsafe or inaccurate to take the temperature by mouth, as when a patient is unconscious, disoriented or irrational. Rectal temperatures should not be taken as standard practice in newborns and infants (because of the danger of damage to the rectal mucosa) and in preschoolers (because of the fear of intrusive procedures). When a rectal temperature is necessary, care must be taken to prevent rectal trauma and fear in the child (Pillitteri, 1995). On average, rectal temperatures are approximately 0.5° C higher than core body temperatures. The rectal method should not be used for people with diseases of the rectum, those with diarrhea or those who have had rectal surgery.

The ear, specifically the tympanic membrane, is an excellent site for taking core temperature. True core temperature exists within and near the hypothalamus, which holds the central thermoregulators. The ear is an ideal site for temperature assessment because it lies close to the hypothalamus and receives its blood supply from branches of the external carotid artery. The tympanic membrane is even more desirable because it shares its blood supply with the hypothalamus, from the anterior cerebral artery, a branch of the internal carotid (Sunderland, 1996).

Temperature measurements are made from the tympanic membrane. This site may be used for all patients, regardless of age or condition. Ear thermometry is noninvasive and causes little discomfort. Temperature assessment is quick, taking up to 15 seconds or less. Its major disadvantage is that improper technique can give inconsistent and inaccurate readings. For instance, nurses may think that they are taking a tympanic membrane temperature but, because of improper placement of the probe, they may in fact be reading the temperature of the ear canal.

The ear canal, like the oral cavity, is subject to variant effects. For instance, a higher reading would be obtained if the temperature were taken in the ear the patient has just slept on, or lower if taken in the outside ear and a fan were blowing overhead. The presence of excess earwax may also affect reading. Nurses must be cautious when using ear thermometry. First, they should know how the thermometer works. That is, does the device use a scanning or shutter method to sense the infrared heat rays? Is the thermometer designed to read tympanic membrane or ear canal temperature? Second, they must use a consistent technique, which ensures that the ear canal is straightened and the probe sensor is placed far enough in the ear canal to exclude the outer ear. In a tympanic temperature, this would mean making sure that the probe sensor is pointing at the tympanic membrane. The techniques for taking temperatures from the various sites are outlined in Procedure 16.1.

Preparing the Patient

Inform the patient that his or her temperature will be taken and explain the method that will be used. The patient needs to know what is expected in order to be able to participate in the procedure. If an oral temperature is to be taken, find out if the patient has been smoking, or has just had a hot or cold drink. If so, wait about 20–30 minutes before measuring the temperature.

Assembling Equipment

Several types of thermometers are available for measuring body temperature. These are the glass mercury thermometer, the electronic predictive thermometer and the infrared ear thermometer. Disposable thermometers and commercially marketed temperature-sensitive tapes are also available. These are particularly useful in the home (and in some health agencies) for infants and small children and for patients in isolation. The tape is usually applied to the child's abdomen and will change colour if the temperature is above or below normal. If deviations are noted, the temperature should be taken with a standard thermometer to obtain a more accurate measurement.

THE GLASS MERCURY THERMOMETER The mercury thermometer is an elongated glass tube (called the *stem*) calibrated in degrees Celsius (centigrade) or degrees Fahrenheit. Within the tube is a column of mercury, which expands or contracts in response to the heat of the body. The scale on the Celsius thermometer generally starts at about 34° C and terminates at 42.4° C. As depicted in Figure 16.4, each long line represents 0.5°; each short line represents 0.1°. The Celsius scale is the only one used in health care agencies; however, the Fahrenheit scale may still be found in some Canadian homes. The formulas for converting centigrade and Fahrenheit scales are given in the box below.

Centigrade and Fahrenheit Conversion Formulas

To convert Fahrenheit to centigrade:

$$C = (F - 32) \times 5/9$$

To convert centigrade to Fahrenheit:

$$F = (C \times 9/5) + 32$$

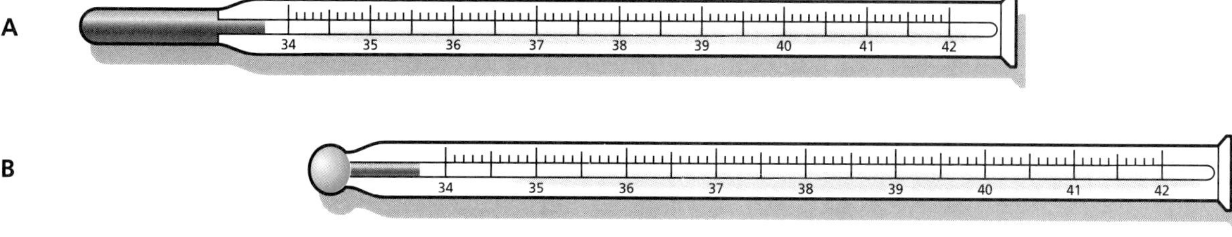

FIGURE 16.4 Glass mercury thermometers. A. Oral thermometer B. Rectal thermometer

The contact surface of a thermometer, called the *bulb*, differs depending on whether it is for oral (and axillary) or rectal use (see Figure 16.4). The oral mercury thermometer has a long, thin bulb that provides a substantial surface for contact with blood vessels under the tongue or in the axilla. The bulb of a rectal thermometer is short and blunt (pear-shaped), its purpose being to prevent injury to rectal tissue on insertion. Rectal and oral thermometers are sometimes differentiated by the colour of the bulb. Oral bulbs are often silver in colour and rectal bulbs are blue.

The glass mercury thermometer is usually kept in a small vial containing a disinfectant. Various kinds of disinfectants are used to soak the thermometers, for example, synthetic phenols or isopropyl alcohol (70%). Because thermometers are soaked in a disinfectant when not in use, they need to be rinsed with cool water and wiped with a tissue before use. Clean thermometers are wiped from the bulb towards the fingers. This prevents the spread of microorganisms from dirtier to cleaner areas.

ELECTRONIC THERMOMETER Electronic thermometers are widely used today. With these, it is possible to get an accurate temperature reading in a few seconds and to monitor temperature over a period of time. An electronic thermometer consists of a heat-sensitive probe that is inserted into the body site, a digital display unit and a connecting cord (see Figure 16.5). It can be set to work in two modes: predictive and monitor mode. In the *predictive* mode, a heat sensor (thermistor) in the probe detects heat from the site through a change in its characteristics with regard to temperature. This change is transmitted to a computer chip in the unit, where a temperature reading is computed and displayed. Using a mathematical formula, the unit electronically calculates an equilibrium temperature. For example, from the initial rate of change in probe characteristics, it predicts what an oral temperature would be if the probe were kept in the sublingual pocket for an optimal period of time. Oral and rectal temperatures are obtained with the thermometer in the predictive mode. The circuitry of electronic thermometers in predictive mode temperature calculations is designed to account for the characteristics of the oral and rectal mucosa. Axillary temperatures, on the other hand, should be taken in monitor mode. The axilla does not have the same characteristics as the mouth and rectum. Therefore, the predictive mode for axillary temperature will not yield accurate readings.

The thermometer is set in *monitor* mode for axillary temperatures or when a continuous reading is needed. This might happen in an emergency unit, for instance, when a person is admitted in a state of hypothermia and the physician orders a continuous rectal temperature. In monitor mode, the thermometer provides a display of the temperature it is actually sensing; there is no predictive computation in between. Simply stated, the predictive mode computes the temperature based on a sampling and the monitor mode provides a direct temperature readout. There is a switch on the back of the unit for selecting the mode.

Most electronic thermometers have a different probe for the oral/axillary sites and for the rectal site. Oral/axillary probes are blue, while rectal probes are red. The probe is capped with a disposable plastic cover every time a temperature is taken and, therefore, does not require cleaning. However, because the unit is battery-powered, it should be promptly put back on its charging unit after use.

INFRARED EAR THERMOMETER The infrared (IR) ear thermometer is the latest development in temperature assessment instruments. It consists of a hand-held device with a sensor probe, similar to an otoscope, which is placed in the external opening of the ear canal (see Figure 16.6). The sensor measures the invisible heat rays emitted by the tympanic membrane and surrounding ear canal tissue. These infrared heat rays travel in a straight line from the source and are absorbed into the thermopile sensor in the thermometer.

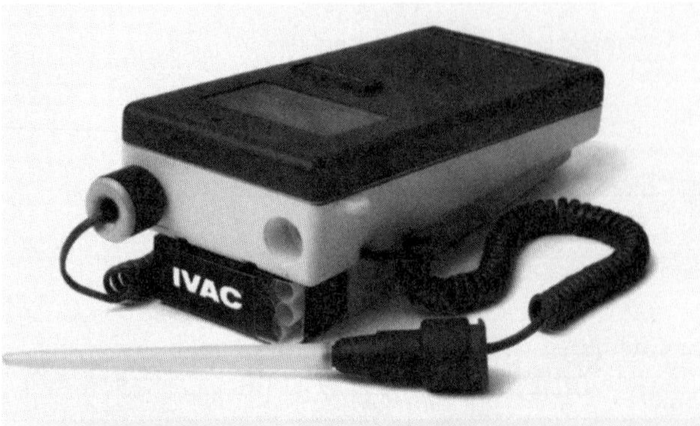

FIGURE 16.5 Electronic thermometer and probe covers

SOURCE: Courtesy of the IVAC Corporation, San Diego, CA.

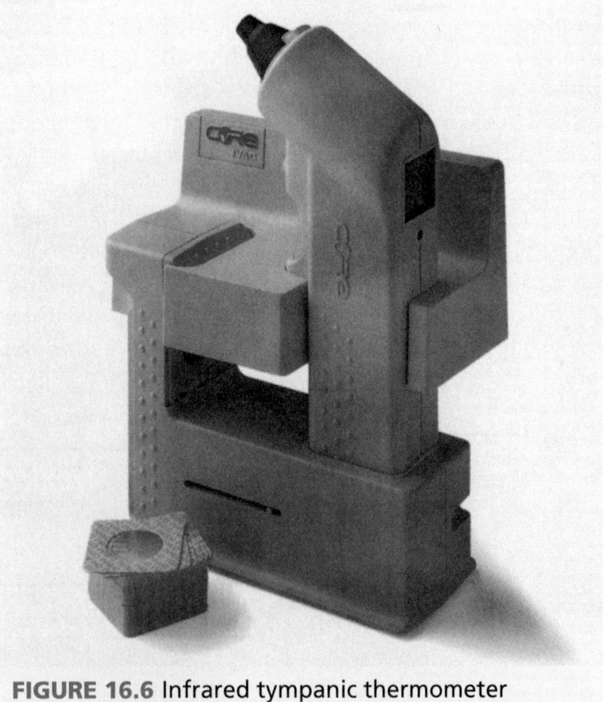

FIGURE 16.6 Infrared tympanic thermometer

SOURCE: Courtesy of the IVAC Corporation, San Diego, CA.

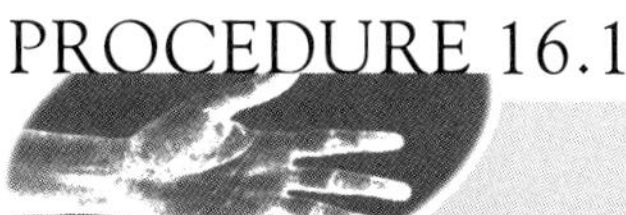

PROCEDURE 16.1 Measuring Body Temperature

Action	*Rationale*
1. Wash hands.	Prevents the spread of microorganisms.
2. Gather appropriate equipment:	Facilitates efficiency and economy of time.
• Glass thermometer, tissue, lubricant for rectal thermometer	
• Electronic thermometer, blue probe for oral/axillary method, red for rectal method, probe cover, lubricant	
• Tympanic thermometer, probe cover	
• Clean gloves as necessary.	When using glass thermometers, gloves should be used if there is visible blood in the patient's oral secretions or in the feces. The risk of transmission of non–blood-borne pathogens, such as pulmonary tuberculosis, infectious diarrhea and hepatitis A, can be reduced by wearing gloves.
3. Prepare the patient.	Promotes well-being and facilitates patient participation in care.
4. Ready the thermometer:	
Glass: Hold the stem horizontally at eye level and rotate it until the scale becomes visible.	Brings the temperature scale into view.
Read the mercury level. If it is above the 34° mark, grasp the stem between the thumb and forefinger and, with a snapping wrist motion, shake down the mercury.	Ensures the thermometer reading is below body temperature. Brisk shaking downward lowers the mercury level.
Electronic: Slide a probe cover on the probe until it locks in place.	Prevents the transmission of microorganisms from patient to patient.
Infrared ear: Apply a probe cover on the probe as directed by the manufacturer.	
5. Take the patient's temperature.	
Oral Method: Glass Thermometer	
• Place the bulb of the thermometer in the right or left posterior sublingual pocket under the base of the tongue.	Heat from the superficial blood vessels in the sublingual pocket warms the thermometer, which registers a temperature reading.

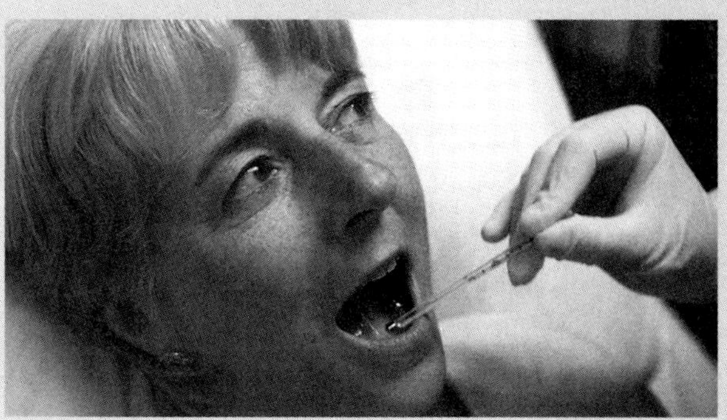

• Instruct the patient to hold the thermometer between closed lips and to avoid biting it.	Maintains proper position and ensures accurate measurement. Prevents trauma and mercury poisoning should the thermometer break.
• Leave the thermometer in place for 3 min. If the temperature is borderline or elevated above normal, leave it in place for 5 minutes.	Optimum placement times ensures accuracy.

Continued on the next page

PROCEDURE 16.1 *continued*

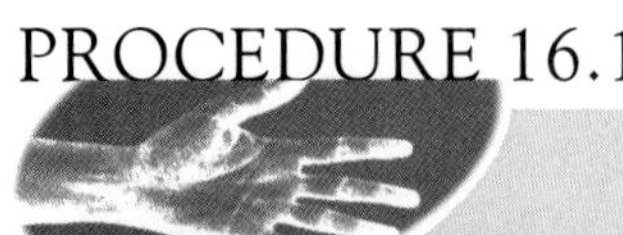

Action	Rationale
• Remove the thermometer and wipe it from the fingers towards the bulb, using a twisting motion.	Prevents the spread of microorganisms from dirtier to cleaner area. A twisting motion facilitates mechanical removal of mucus and secretions.
• Read the temperature.	
Oral Method: Electronic Thermometer	
• Place the probe in the right or left posterior sublingual pocket under the base of the tongue.	As for oral glass thermometer.
• Instruct the patient to keep the mouth closed.	
• Hold the probe in place until a signal is heard and a temperature reading appears on the digital display. Note the temperature.	Ensures accurate reading.
• Remove the probe from the patient's mouth. Eject the cover into a wastebasket.	
Rectal Method: Glass Thermometer	
• Draw curtains and help the patient assume Sims' position (side-lying position with the upper leg flexed). Drape with bed linens.	Makes the rectal area accessible for the procedure. Provides privacy and reduces embarrassment.
• Apply clean gloves.	Protects the nurse from contamination with patient's body substances.
• Lubricate the bulb of the thermometer.	Facilitates insertion and reduces irritation or injury to the rectal mucosa.
• Ask the patient to take a deep breath and then breathe out slowly.	Helps to relax the patient.
• Using the nondominant hand, lift the upper buttock, and with the dominant hand, insert the thermometer about 3.5 cm for adults, or not more than 1.25 cm for infants and 2.5 cm for young children.	Exposes the anal opening. Ensures sufficient contact with blood vessels in the rectal wall.
• Hold the thermometer in place for 2–3 minutes.	Ensures adequate contact time to register an accurate temperature.
• Remove the thermometer and wipe off lubricant and fecal material.	Facilitates reading the thermometer.
• Read the temperature.	
Rectal Method: Electronic Thermometer	
• Prepare and position the patient as when using the glass thermometer.	
• Lubricate the probe cover	Facilitates insertion and reduces irritation or injury to the rectal mucosa.
• Ask the patient to take a deep breath and then to breathe out slowly.	Helps to relax the patient.
• Using the nondominant hand, lift the upper buttock, and with the dominant hand, insert the probe about 7.5 cm for an adult.	Exposes the anal opening. Ensures sufficient contact with blood vessels in the rectal wall.
• Hold the probe in place until a signal is heard and a temperature reading appears on the digital display. Note the temperature.	Ensures accurate reading.
• Remove the probe and eject the cover into a wastebasket.	

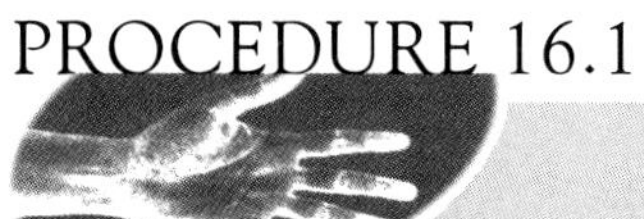

PROCEDURE 16.1 *continued*

Action	Rationale
Axillary Method: Glass Thermometer	
• Pull curtains; remove gown from the arm and dry the axilla, if moist.	Provides privacy and exposes the axilla. Moisture conducts heat.
• Place the bulb of the thermometer in the centre of the axilla, lower the arm over the thermometer, and position the arm across the patient's chest.	Maintains proper contact of the thermometer against blood vessels in the axilla.
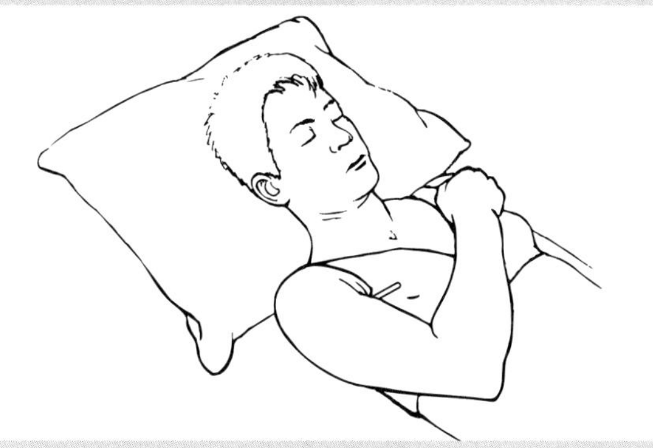	
• Keep the thermometer in place for 5–10 minutes. If the patient is alert, ask him or her to hold the thermometer in place. If the patient is not alert or is confused, hold the thermometer in position.	Ensures sufficient time to register an accurate temperature reading.
• Remove the thermometer; wipe it with tissue. Read the temperature.	
Axillary Method: Electronic Thermometer	
• Pull curtains; remove gown from the arm and shoulder. Dry the axilla, if moist.	Provides privacy and exposes the axilla. Moisture conducts heat.
• Put the thermometer in monitor mode according to the manufacturer's instructions.	
• Place the probe in the centre of the axilla, lower the arm over the thermometer, and position the arm across the patient's chest.	Maintains proper contact of thermometer against blood vessels in the axilla.
• Hold the probe in place for 5–10 minutes. Note the temperature reading appearing on the digital display.	Ensures accurate reading.
• Remove the probe from the patient's axilla. Eject the cover into a wastebasket.	
Ear Thermometry	
• Apply the disposable cover to the thermometer.	
• Hold the thermometer in the right hand to take the temperature in the right ear and in the left hand to take the temperature in the left ear.	Avoids crossing over of the hands; dexterity and accuracy in positioning the probe are promoted.
For adults:	
• Grasp the pinna firmly at the midpoint, then pull up and back.	Straightens the ear canal.
For children up to 3 years of age:	
• Grasp the lower portion of the pinna, pull it down and slightly back.	
• Insert the covered probe completely into the ear canal, pointing the tip midway between the eyebrow and the ears on the opposite side. Make sure the probe seals the ear canal from ambient air.	Ensures that the beam of infrared light points on the tympanic membrane. Prevents inaccurate readings due to environmental conditions.

Continued on the next page

PROCEDURE 16.1 *continued*

Action	*Rationale*
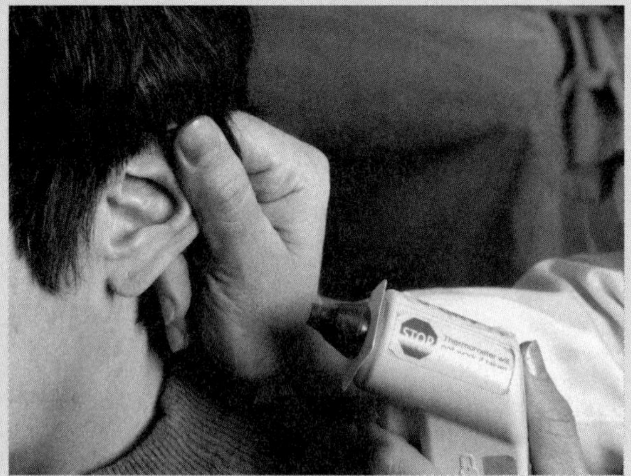	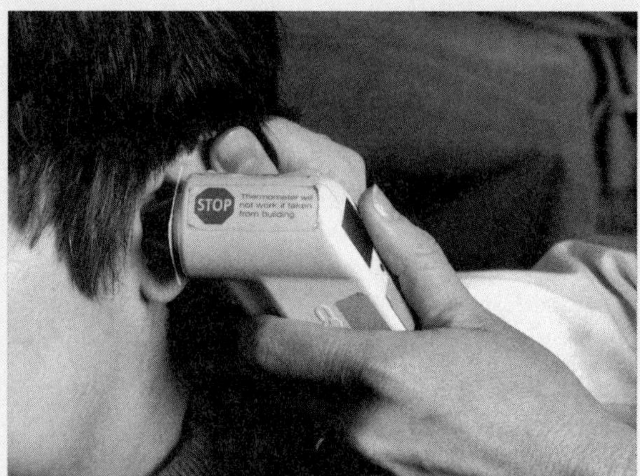
• **Shutter design:** Hold the thermometer in place until a reading is displayed.	
• **Scanning design:** Gently wiggle the probe in the ear until a reading is displayed.	Scans the tympanic membrane using a gentle side-to-side motion.
• Note the temperature and discard the probe cover.	
• If repeating the measurement, wait 10–20 seconds between readings.	
6. Leave the patient comfortable.	Promotes patient well-being.
7. Return electronic and infrared ear thermometers to their charging units.	Maintains battery charge.
Wash glass thermometers in cold soapy water. Rinse in cold water, dry, and return them to their storage container.	Maintains cleanliness and prevents the transmission of microorganisms. Any protein left on the thermometer will interfere with disinfection.
8. Document the temperature and the site on the patient's graphic flowsheet (Figure 16.8) according to agency guidelines. Note only trends of temperature elevations or subnormal temperatures.	Provides a data base for ongoing evaluation of patient status.
9. Report consistent temperature elevations or subnormal temperatures immediately to the physician. Document the patient's temperature in the nurses' notes and that the patient's physician was notified.	Subnormal temperatures and temperature elevations may require treatment. Fulfills requirements for nurse accountability and facilitates continuity of care.

Most IR thermometers have a thermistor, which measures the temperature of the probe itself. These readings are converted into an electrical impulse and are sent to a computer, which interprets the information and displays a reading on a screen. Some IR thermometers may be programmed to make a second conversion and display the readings in equivalent oral, rectal or core readings. This practice is less common now as practitioners become more familiar with the technology. As well, there is some indication that this second conversion results in reduced accuracy of the reading (Terndrup, 1992).

Most IR thermometers on the market use a shutter design, much like a camera, that opens when the examiner presses a button. The infrared heat sensed by the unit in that split second is used by a computer in the thermometer to predict the temperature. It is essential that the tympanic membrane is in the "picture"; otherwise, the reading may be falsely low.

In another design, a series of measurements is taken while the probe is gently moved from side to side in the ear. This is called *scanning*. The maximum temperature observed in the scan is interpreted by the unit to be the tympanic membrane temperature. There are no computer conversions in this design. The highest temperature sensed is displayed, so, again, the tympanic membrane must be scanned to ensure tympanic membrane assessment.

RESEARCH to practice

Henker, R., & Coyne, C. (1995). Comparison of peripheral temperature measurements with core temperature. *AACN Clinical Issues, 6*(1), 21–30.

The purpose of this study was to identify accurate methods of measuring peripheral body temperature that closely reflected core body temperature. A sample of 24 stable postoperative cardiac patients were recruited. Peripheral temperatures were measured using infrared, glass, chemical and electronic thermometers. Infrared measured aural temperature; glass, electronic and chemical measured both oral and axillary temperatures. Glass and electronic thermometers were also used to measure rectal temperatures.

All temperatures were measured between 08:30 and 20:30 hours. Data were collected over a five-month period. Each subject had temperature measured over a 20- to 25-minute period; both peripheral and core temperatures were collected during this time. Because pulmonary artery temperature is an accurate measurement of core body temperature, all peripheral temperatures were measured in relation to this indicator.

The authors found that the aural site was not an effective measure of core body temperature. The oral site using a chemical thermometer was acceptable for screening patients, but this method lacked accuracy in determining a diagnosis and appropriate treatment. Finally, the findings revealed that the electronic thermometer used in the oral or axillary sites was acceptable for diagnostic and treatment purposes. The rectal site using an electronic thermometer had a high correlation with core body temperature. However, the authors do not recommend this method owing to possible cross-contamination and patient discomfort.

Although this design tends to result in more accurate readings, the scanning process is less comfortable for the patient than the simple shutter process.

The effectiveness of IR tympanic thermometry is based on the premise that the probe sensor is aimed at the tympanic membrane (Baird, White & Basinger, 1992). If the tympanic membrane is not included in the "picture" or scan, the reading obtained will reflect the temperature of the ear canal rather than the tympanic membrane. The design of the probe in shutter models has a wide field of view and will "see" the tympanic membrane and surrounding ear canal. Even when properly positioned, the resulting reading is an average of what is in its field of view. For that reason, these thermometers are called infrared ear thermometers rather than tympanic thermometers.

The scanning thermometers tend to have a smaller field of view and are more likely to capture the true tympanic membrane temperature. The probe tips are currently designed for the adult ear canal. This fact should be kept in mind when using IR thermometry with neonates, infants and children under three years of age. At this time, there is only one scanning-type IR thermometer on the market with a probe suitable for neonates and infants (Ototemo Pedi-Q). Ear thermometry is new; as with any new technology, we can expect more growth and change before an efficient and effective thermometer is developed. Like electronic thermometers, the ear probe is capped with a disposable cover for each use and is stored in a charging unit when not in use.

Pulse

PHYSIOLOGY

When the left ventricle of the heart contracts, a wave of blood surges through the systemic arteries. This wave of blood, called a **pulse**, can be palpated at various sites on the body where an artery crosses over a bony prominence.

At rest the heart is required to pump only four to six litres of blood per minute. This volume is increased as much as five times during exercise. Normally each ventricle pumps 70 mL of blood with each contraction, although wide variations in the amount are compatible with life. This volume of output is reflected in the rate, rhythm, strength (volume) and tension (elasticity) of the pulsations that can be felt. The *rate* of the pulse is the number of ventricular contractions or heartbeats per minute.

DETERMINANTS OF PULSE RATE

Deviations from the normal **pulse rate** are frequently seen in illness. Many medications affect the pulse rate; a number of factors other than disease processes and medications may also affect it. Pulse rate varies according to age, gender, size and physical and emotional activity. The pulse rate decreases as a child grows and continues to decrease until old age. Men generally have a slower pulse rate than women. The rate of cardiac contractions increases during exercise and when a person is experiencing strong emotions, such as anxiety, fear or anger. The normal range and average of pulse rates for human beings at various ages are shown in Table 16.7.

ASSESSING PULSE RATES

Pulse rates are assessed by palpation of selected sites located in the periphery of the body (for example, the wrist, neck or foot) and by auscultation of the apical pulse located over the heart. These are called the peripheral pulses and the apical pulse, respectively.

ASSESSING A PERIPHERAL PULSE

When taking a peripheral pulse, the nurse notes rate, rhythm, strength (volume) and tension (elasticity). If the

TABLE 16.7 Normal pulse rates for specific ages

AGE	NORMAL RANGE	AVERAGE
Newborn	90–190	140
1–6 months	80–180	130
6–12 months	75–155	115
1–2 years	70–150	110
2–6 years	68–138	103
6–10 years	65–125	95
10–14 years	55–115	85
14–18 years	65–105	75
Adults	70–100	74
Aging	70–100	74

SOURCES: Bates, 1995; Jarvis, 1996.

pulse rate is greatly accelerated (for example, over 100 beats per minute), the condition is referred to as **tachycardia**. A very slow pulse rate (under 60 beats per minute in adults) is called **bradycardia**.

Pulse rhythm refers to the pattern of the beats. In health the rhythm is regular; that is, the time between beats is essentially the same. The pulse is considered irregular when the beats follow each other at irregular intervals.

The *strength*, or amplitude, of a pulse wave (the **pulse volume**) reflects the volume of blood pushed against the wall of the artery in the ventricular contraction. A weak pulse lacks a feeling of fullness and a definite beat; it may feel thready. When a pulse cannot be felt or heard, it is said to be *imperceptible*. A bounding pulse is one in which the volume reaches a higher level than normal, then disappears quickly. A scale for describing pulse volume is given in the box below.

Pulse tension (elasticity) refers to the compressibility of the arterial wall. If the pulse is obliterated by slight pressure, it is a pulse of low tension. A pulse that is obliterated only by relatively great pressure is a pulse of high tension.

Scale for Describing Pulse Volume

Scale	Description
0	Absent, not palpable
+1	Thready, weak, difficult to palpate, easily obliterated with pressure
+2	Normal, easily palpated, may be obliterated by strong pressure
+3	Strong, forceful, not easily obliterated by pressure
+4	Bounding, difficult to obliterate

SOURCE: Berger & Williams, 1992.

To assess a person's pulse, the examiner places the second, third and fourth fingers lightly on the skin at a location where an artery passes over underlying bone. The thumb is not used because the examiner might feel the pulsations of the radial artery of his or her own thumb. Usually, counting the rate for 30 seconds and then multiplying by two gives an accurate record of beats per minute. Some people prefer to count the rate for 15 seconds and multiply by four. If the pulse is irregular in any way, it is counted apically for a full minute.

LOCATING PERIPHERAL PULSE SITES There are numerous sites on the body from which a pulse may be obtained (see Figure 16.7). When a person is lying on the back, one can normally observe pulsations from the carotid artery and, also, from the jugular vein. The carotid pulse shows as a brisk, localized throbbing; the jugular pulse is slow and undulating. In emergencies, the **carotid pulse** is convenient for assessing cardiac functioning. Care must be taken, though, to make sure that one does not inadvertently cut off, or seriously slow down, carotid circulation. Palpation should be done in the lower third of the neck, to avoid undue pressure on the carotid sinus, which is located just above the bifurcation of the artery into its external and internal branches. Excessive pressure on the artery is to be avoided, and only one carotid artery should be palpated at a time.

In nonemergency situations, the peripheral pulses located in the extremities are commonly used for assessment of a person's circulatory status. Of these, the radial and the brachial pulses are the ones most frequently used by nurses. The radial site is used to assess the pulse, and the brachial site is used in taking the blood pressure. Other peripheral sites may be used for pulse assessment if the radial pulse is obscured, or if there is a need to test the circulation of blood to a specific area. The temporal, femoral and dorsalis pedis pulses are three that are used most often.

The **radial pulse** is located on the inner aspect of the wrist on the thumb side where the radial artery passes over the radius. With slight pressure, the artery may be held against the radius so that the pulsations of blood may be felt. The **brachial pulse** is located on the ventral surface of the arm, at the antecubital fossa, where the brachial artery passes over the ulna. The **temporal pulse** is felt lateral to the eyebrow, where the temporal artery passes over the temporal bone. The **femoral pulse** may be felt below the inguinal ligament in the groin, where the femoral artery passes over the pelvic bone. The **dorsalis pedis pulse** (usually taken to assess circulation in the foot) can be felt on the dorsum of the foot in a line between the first and second toes, just above the longitudinal arch.

Other peripheral pulses that are sometimes used include the **ulnar**, which is on the opposite side of the wrist to the radial, the **posterior tibialis**, on the inner aspect of the ankle and the **popliteal pulse**, which can be felt on the inner aspect of the back of the knee. The technique for assessing a peripheral pulse is detailed in Procedure 16.2.

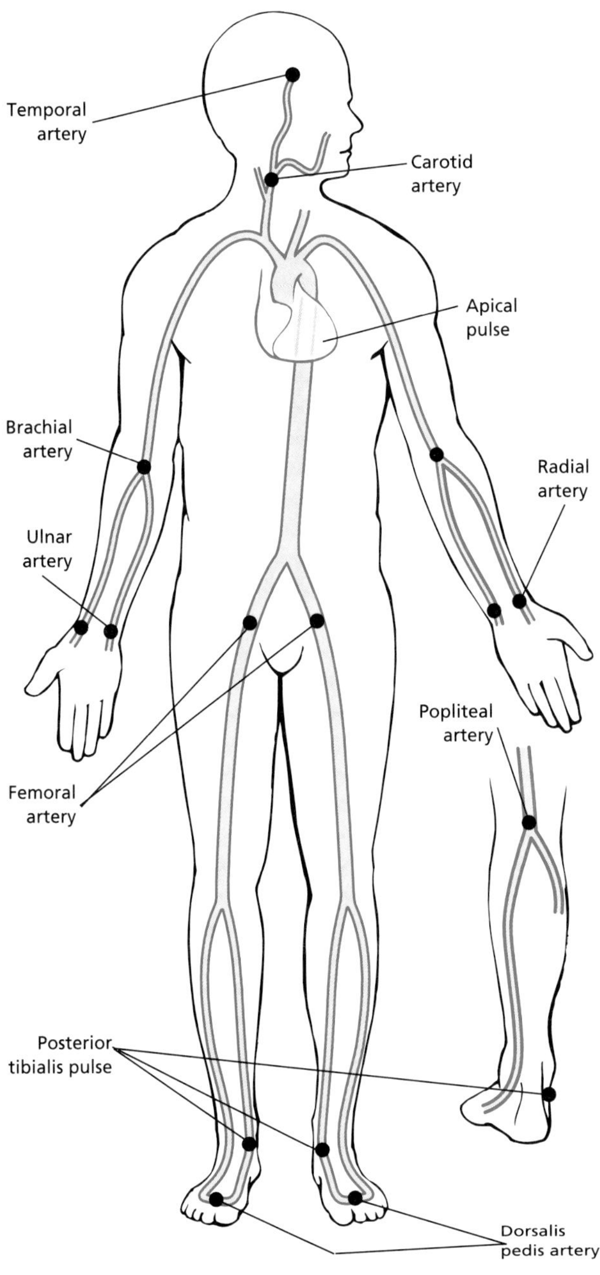

FIGURE 16.7 Peripheral pulse sites

Assessing an Apical Pulse

It is often necessary to assess the heartbeat by listening to the heart sounds rather than palpating a peripheral pulse. The **apical pulse** is the beat of the heart auscultated at its apex. The apex is considered to be the **point of maximal impulse (PMI),** also called the apical impulse. In normal adults, the apical impulse is located in the fifth intercostal space, 7–9 cm to the left of the midsternal line, just below the left nipple. It is located lower, and more laterally, in adults with chronic cardiac problems. In children under seven years of age, the apical impulse is located at the fourth intercostal space, lateral to the midclavicular line. By listening with a stethoscope in this area, the nurse can usually hear the apical pulse.

To determine the apical pulse, the bell of the stethoscope is placed over the apex of the heart and the beats are counted for a full minute. A heartbeat is heard as "lub-dub." The "lub" represents the closure of the atrioventricular or tricuspid and mitral valves (S_1 sound); it occurs at the onset of systole (the contraction of the heart). The "dub" represents the closure of the semilunar (aortic and pulmonic) valves (S_2 sound) at the end of systole. The rhythm of the heartbeat can also be assessed by noting the interval between beats. Procedure 16.2 outlines how to take an apical pulse.

Assessing an Apical-Radial Pulse

In health, the apical and radial pulse rates are the same, but in illness they sometimes differ, as when some apical beats are not transmitted to the radial artery. An *apical-radial* pulse is taken when it is necessary to determine whether such a difference exists. Two nurses are needed for this technique. One nurse counts the patient's radial pulse at the same time that the second nurse counts the apical beats of the heart. Both nurses must use the same watch. Each pulse is counted for a full minute. The difference between the apical rate and the radial rate is termed the *pulse deficit*.

Preparing the Patient

Inform the patient of the procedure and tell him or her what to do to facilitate accurate assessment of the pulse. Generally, the patient should lie or sit quietly for a few minutes before the pulse is counted. Exercise, a change in activity or posture, or anxiety can accelerate the pulse rate to the extent that it does not reflect the normal rate at rest.

Assembling Equipment

The nurse will need a watch with a second hand or a digital watch that displays seconds to count the pulse rate. A stethoscope is needed if an apical pulse is being taken.

Respirations

PHYSIOLOGY

Respiration is a term used to refer to both the movement of air from outside the body to the gas exchange units of the lungs, and the exchange of these gases across the alveolar membranes to the blood and cells. The former is technically called *external* respiration, the latter *internal* (or *tissue*) respiration. When we are assessing respiration as one of the vital signs of body functioning, it is the external process we are measuring.

External respiration, or breathing, involves two principal movements: **inspiration** (inhalation), the act of breathing in, and **expiration** (exhalation), the act of breathing out. Breathing is carried out by the diaphragm and the external intercostal muscles. The process is controlled primarily by the respiratory centre in the medulla oblongata. This centre

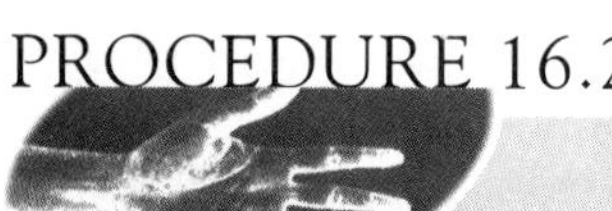

PROCEDURE 16.2 Assessing Peripheral and Apical Pulses

Action	*Rationale*
1. Wash hands.	Prevents the spread of microorganisms.
2. Gather equipment: • Watch with a second hand or digital display • Stethoscope if needed	Facilitates efficiency and economy of time.
3. Prepare the patient.	
4. Take the patient's pulse.	Promotes well-being and facilitates patient participation in care.
Peripheral Sites:	
• If taking a radial pulse, have the patient in a sitting or lying position with the arm resting at his or her side or across the abdomen or chest. The wrist should be slightly extended with the palm facing downward.	Promotes comfort for the patient and convenience for the nurse. Exposes the artery for palpation.
• Place the first, second and third fingertips lightly on the skin along the artery at the selected site.	Sensitivity of fingertips to touch permits palpation of pulsations.
• Feel for pulsation; assess the rhythm and the volume by noting the pattern and strength of the beats.	
• If the pulse is regular, count the beats for 15 seconds or 30 seconds and multiply by 4 or 2, respectively.	Determines the rate of beats per minute.
• If the pulse is irregular, count the beats for one full minute. Note if the irregularity occurs randomly or in a pattern. If the radial pulse rate is irregular, take an apical pulse.	Provides more accurate assessment of rate, rhythm and volume.
Apical Pulse:	
• Pull curtains and assist the patient into a supine position with head elevated or a sitting position. Expose the left side of the chest.	Provides privacy and facilitates access to the point of maximal impulse (PMI).
• Warm the bell or diaphragm of the stethoscope by holding it in the palm of the hand.	Prevents variations in the pulse from the patient's being startled by a cold stethoscope.
• Place the bell or diaphragm of the stethoscope over the fifth intercostal space, medial to the midclavicular line.	Positions the instrument over apex and the PMI.

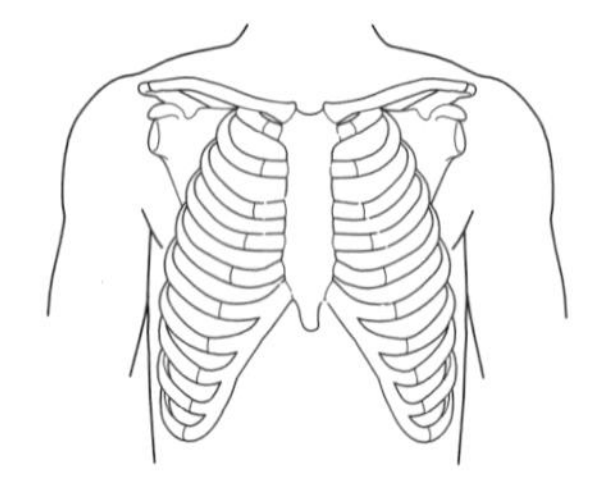

• Listen for normal S_1 ("lub") and S_2 ("dub") sounds and note their strength and regularity. In an adult, count the heartbeats for one full minute.	Ensures accurate measurement of rate. Reasons for taking apical pulse (e.g., digoxin medication, cardiac condition) require it to be taken for a full minute.
5. Leave the patient comfortable.	Promotes patient well-being.
6. Document the pulse rate on the patient's graphic flowsheet (see Figure 16.8) according to agency guidelines. In the nurses' note, record changes in rhythm, volume and tension of peripheral pulses and changes in rhythm and strength of apical pulses.	Provides a data base for ongoing evaluation of patient status.

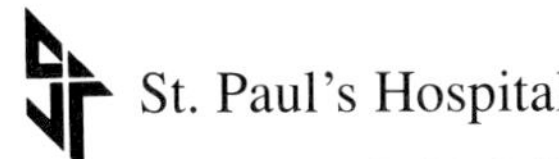

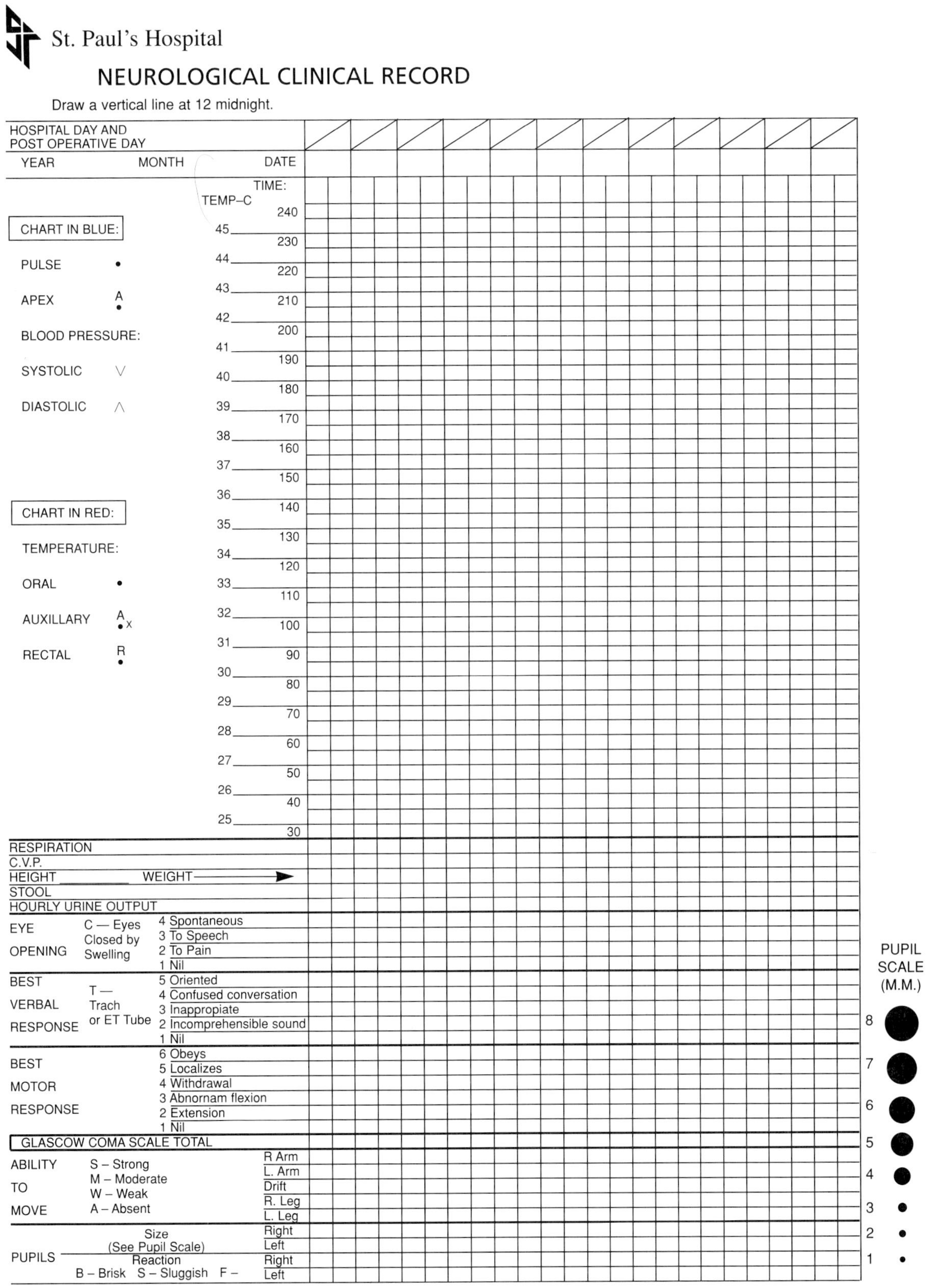

NEUROLOGICAL CLINICAL RECORD

Draw a vertical line at 12 midnight.

HOSPITAL DAY AND POST OPERATIVE DAY

YEAR MONTH DATE

TIME:

	TEMP–C	
CHART IN BLUE:		240
	45	230
PULSE •	44	220
APEX A•	43	210
	42	200
BLOOD PRESSURE:	41	190
SYSTOLIC V	40	180
DIASTOLIC Λ	39	170
	38	160
	37	150
	36	140
CHART IN RED:	35	130
TEMPERATURE:	34	120
ORAL •	33	110
AUXILLARY A•x	32	100
RECTAL R•	31	90
	30	80
	29	70
	28	60
	27	50
	26	40
	25	30

RESPIRATION

C.V.P.

HEIGHT ______ WEIGHT →

STOOL

HOURLY URINE OUTPUT

EYE OPENING	C — Eyes Closed by Swelling	4 Spontaneous
		3 To Speech
		2 To Pain
		1 Nil
BEST VERBAL RESPONSE	T — Trach or ET Tube	5 Oriented
		4 Confused conversation
		3 Inappropiate
		2 Incomprehensible sound
		1 Nil
BEST MOTOR RESPONSE		6 Obeys
		5 Localizes
		4 Withdrawal
		3 Abnornam flexion
		2 Extension
		1 Nil
GLASCOW COMA SCALE TOTAL		
ABILITY TO MOVE	S – Strong M – Moderate W – Weak A – Absent	R Arm
		L. Arm
		Drift
		R. Leg
		L. Leg
PUPILS	Size (See Pupil Scale)	Right
		Left
	Reaction B – Brisk S – Sluggish F –	Right
		Left

PUPIL SCALE (M.M.)

8 ●
7 ●
6 ●
5 ●
4 ●
3 •
2 •
1 •

FIGURE 16.8 Example of a graphic flowsheet for temperature, pulse, respiration and blood pressure. Note the symbols used to identify the methods of assessing temperature and pulse rates. Other agencies may use different symbols. This flowsheet also incorporates the Glasgow Coma Scale.

SOURCE: St. Paul's Hospital, Vancouver, British Columbia.

is influenced by several factors, including chemical changes in the blood (e.g., a high carbon dioxide level, which stimulates respiration), extreme alterations in blood pressure (e.g., severely elevated blood pressure, which inhibits respirations) and stimuli arising from the muscles (e.g., exercise, which increases respiration). A more detailed discussion of the factors affecting respiration will be found in Chapter 24.

Respirations controlled in this manner are automatic. Their rate and depth are regulated within a range that meets the metabolic needs of the body for oxygen. Any activity that necessitates increased oxygen supply will result in more rapid and usually deeper respirations. However, the rate and depth of respirations are to a certain extent under voluntary control. A person can take deep breaths or shallow breaths, or breathe more quickly or slowly, within the limitations imposed by the body's needs for oxygen.

ASSESSING RESPIRATIONS

Respirations are assessed for rate, depth, rhythm and character, or sounds of breathing. The accessory muscles involved in breathing are also examined.

The **respiratory rate** is the number of breathing cycles per minute. An inhalation and an exhalation make up one cycle. Normal respiratory rates vary with age. The average rate for adults is 14–20 per minute (Bates, 1995). For newborns at rest it is 30–60 per minute, slowing to 20–40 at one year. The average respiratory rate for children is 20–30 per minute at two years, slowing down gradually to 17–22 at 10 years. By 20 years of age, the average respiratory rate declines to 15–20 per minute (Pillitteri, 1995). An abnormal increase in the respiratory rate is called **tachypnea** *(polypnea)*; and an abnormal decrease is technically referred to as **bradypnea**. Normal breathing, which is effortless, regular and noiseless (quiet), is called **eupnea**. An absence of breathing is termed **apnea**.

The **respiratory depth** refers to the amount of air inhaled and exhaled with each breath movement. It is observed by watching the chest movements. Normal respirations result in deep and even movements of the chest. In shallow respirations, the rise and fall of the chest and abdomen are minimal. If the respirations are shallow and rapid, the person may report being *short of breath*. The terms *Kussmaul breathing* or *air hunger* are frequently used to describe respirations that are abnormally deep, sighing and accompanied by an increased respiratory rate.

The **respiratory rhythm** refers to the regularity of inhalation and exhalation cycles. Normal respirations follow one another evenly, with little variation in the length of the pauses between inspiration and expiration. *Symmetry* refers to the synchronous movements of each side of the chest. *Asymmetrical* breathing may be observed in some patients with multiple rib fractures, pneumonia or pneumothorax (air in the pleural space).

The **respiratory character** refers to digressions from normal, effortless breathing. **Dyspnea**, which refers to difficult or laboured breathing, for example, involves active participation of accessory inspiratory and expiratory muscles. In normal breathing the principal muscles concerned are the diaphragm and, to a lesser extent, the external and internal intercostal muscles. If, for any reason, respiration becomes difficult, all the muscles attached to the thoracic cage are brought into play. These include the major and minor pectoral muscles, the sternomastoid, the scalene, and the subclavius. Difficulty in breathing accompanied by whistling sounds is called *wheezing*. Laboured breathing accompanied by high-pitched crowing sounds is called *stridor*. On auscultation with a stethoscope, fine sounds that resemble hair being rubbed between fingers is called *crackles*. *Pleural rub* (pleural friction rub) is a creaking sound produced when roughened pleural surfaces grate against each other. These are called *adventitious* lung sounds (Bates, 1995).

When assessing respirations, the nurse counts the rate, watches the chest movements and listens for the character of breath sounds. Women breathe thoracically, while men and young children breathe diaphragmatically, moving the abdomen during respiration. Respirations must be assessed unobtrusively, because people usually find it difficult to maintain their normal breathing pattern when they are aware their respirations are being observed. Thus, respirations are often assessed after taking the pulse, while the nurse has his or her fingers on the wrist. Procedure 16.3 outlines how to assess respirations.

Preparing the Patient

For the reason described above, the patient is not informed that his or her respirations will be assessed. However, if the nurse observes factors in the patient that have altered their normal pattern, for instance, signs of anxiety, distress, pain, exercise, crying or coughing, assessment should be deferred until the patient is in a resting state.

Blood Pressure

PHYSIOLOGY

Blood pressure refers to the pressure of the blood within the arteries of the body. When the left ventricle of the heart contracts, blood is forced out into the aorta and travels through the large arteries to the smaller arteries, arterioles and capillaries. The pulsations extend from the heart through the arteries and disappear in the arterioles. The **systolic pressure** reflects the force exerted against the arterial wall as the left ventricle contracts and pumps blood into the aorta. It is the maximum pressure that is exerted on the vessel wall. The **diastolic pressure** reflects the arterial pressure during ventricular relaxation, when the heart is filling. It is the minimum pressure in the arteries. Blood pressure is measured in millimetres of mercury (mm Hg) and the values are separated by a slash. For example, the blood pressure in a young adult might be 120/80, signifying a systolic pressure of 120 and a diastolic pressure of 80. The difference between the systolic and diastolic pressure is the **pulse pressure**.

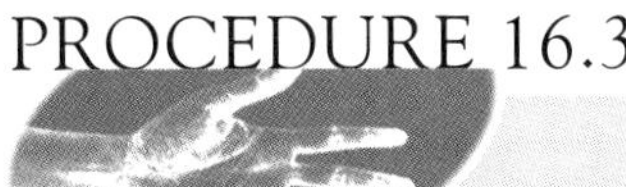

PROCEDURE 16.3 Assessing Respirations

Action	*Rationale*
1. Wash hands.	Prevents the spread of microorganisms.
2. Gather equipment: • Watch with a second hand or digital display	Facilitates efficiency and economy of time.
3. Take the patient's respirations:	
• Place arm across abdomen of lower chest as if to assess pulse.	Allows for inconspicuous assessment of respirations.
• Observe and/or feel the rise and fall of the chest, noting the rhythm. • If respiratory cycles are regular, count for 30 seconds and multiply by 2.	Allows for feeling rise and fall of abdomen as well as visualizing chest movements (respirations are too slow to count accurately in 15 seconds; this is appropriate for counting a regular pulse rate only).
• Count cycles for one full minute if they are irregular, if the patient is younger than two years or if respiratory rate is less than 12 or more than 20.	Accounts for variations in respiratory rate and pattern. Ensures accurate assessment in unusual rates.
4. Document the respiratory rate on the graphic flowsheet (see Figure 16.8) according to agency guidelines. Record changes in rhythm, depth and character in the nurses' notes.	Provides a data base for ongoing evaluation of patient status.

Blood pressure is determined by cardiac output and peripheral vascular resistance. The **cardiac output** is the amount of blood ejected from the heart with the force of each ventricular contraction. The force of the contractions depends on the pumping action of the heart. The greater the strength of the pumping action, the more blood is ejected with each contraction. The amount of cardiac output is also affected by the total volume of blood circulating in the body. A decrease in blood volume, such as occurs in hemorrhaging, will result in less cardiac output, hence a lowered blood pressure.

Peripheral vascular resistance is "the resistance to blood flow primarily caused by friction with the vascular walls" (Martini, 1989, p. 913). Normally, the pressure in the large blood vessels is high, and the pressure in the smaller vessels (the arterioles and capillaries) is low. Blood, as any other liquid, tends to flow from areas of high pressure to areas of low pressure. Peripheral resistance is created by the size of the lumen (the inner channel) of arterioles and capillaries and by the elasticity of vessel walls. Peripheral resistance increases as the size of the lumen decreases, assuming the blood volume remains constant. Thus, the smaller the lumen, the higher the blood pressure. Factors that decrease the lumen of the blood vessels affect the smaller vessels proportionately more than the larger ones, and increase the amount of pressure required to pump the blood through them. Any constriction of the vessels, as when deposits occur on the lining of the vessels, increases the peripheral resistance and, therefore, the blood pressure.

The elasticity of the muscular walls of the blood vessels contributes to vascular resistance and the maintenance of blood pressure. Elasticity refers to compliance, or the ability of the vessel wall to expand or contract in response to the pressure of blood exerted upon it. For instance, arteries normally expand during systole and contract somewhat during diastole to maintain a relatively constant blood pressure. When blood vessels lose their elasticity, as happens with aging, for example, blood pressure goes up.

Blood pressure is also affected by the viscosity (thickness) of the blood, which depends on the number of red blood cells and on the amount of plasma protein it contains. Blood pressure increases as the blood flowing through the vessels becomes thicker. Viscosity may be altered by disturbances of fluid balance.

DETERMINANTS OF BLOOD PRESSURE

A number of variables affect arterial blood pressure. At the outset, normal blood pressure increases with age. At birth, blood pressure averages 80/46 and gradually rises to 130/85 by young adulthood. As a person grows older, blood vessels become less compliant and the systolic blood pressure continues to rise. Women under 50 years of age tend to have lower blood pressures than do males of the same age. The upper limits of normal blood pressures (over the brachial artery) for individuals of different ages are listed in the box on the following page.

An individual's blood pressure varies from hour to hour and from day to day. It falls during sleep and is highest late in the day or early in the evening. Pain; stress; ingestion of caffeine, nicotine or excessive licorice; and activity and exercise cause blood pressure to rise. It may be strikingly

Normal Blood Pressure for Age

Age	Systolic (mm Hg)	Diastolic (mm Hg)
Newborn	78±19	54±16
1 year	91±19	54±17
3 years	91±19	56±16
6 years	96±19	57±17
10 years	102±19	62±16
13 years	109±19	64±18
16 years	112±19	67±18
Adult	100–139	60–89
Adult > 60 years	Maximum 159	60–89

SOURCES: Haynes et al., 1993; Wong, 1995.

elevated by strong emotions, such as fear and anger (Haynes, et al., 1993). Position also affects blood pressure. When a person is lying down, blood pressure is lower than when sitting or standing. Also, the pressure may differ in the two arms of the same patient. Therefore, before taking the blood pressure, the nurse should check (a) the patient's baseline value, (b) the time of day, (c) the arm used and (d) the position the patient was in for the previous reading.

MEASURING BLOOD PRESSURE

Blood pressure is measured indirectly by auscultation. The technique requires a sphygmomanometer and a stethoscope. A **sphygmomanometer** consists of an inflatable cuff, an inflation bulb with a release valve, and a mercury manometer or an aneroid pressure gauge. The mercury manometer is considered to be more accurate than the aneroid pressure gauge, which requires regular calibration (Bailey, Knaus & Bauer, 1991). The most common site used is the upper arm. It is sometimes necessary to take a blood pressure reading on the thigh, such as when assessing blood pressure in children and adolescents with congenital heart anomalies, and in clinical situations where the arms cannot be used. In these cases, the same principles are followed as when taking blood pressure on the arm, auscultating over the popliteal artery instead of the brachial artery. Normally, systolic blood pressure in the leg is 10–40 mm higher than in the arm; diastolic pressures are the same in both the arms and the legs (Thompson & Wilson, 1996).

In the auscultatory method, the examiner listens, with a stethoscope, for a series of sounds created as blood flows through an artery after it has been occluded with a cuff and then the cuff pressure gradually released. At the same time, the blood pressure registers on the manometer. The patterns of sounds the examiner hears are called Korotkoff sounds; they are depicted in Figure 16.9.

The systolic blood pressure is the point on the manometer when the first clear tapping sound is heard (phase 1 Korotkoff). As the cuff pressure is gradually decreased, the artery fills, and swishing or blowing sounds are heard that

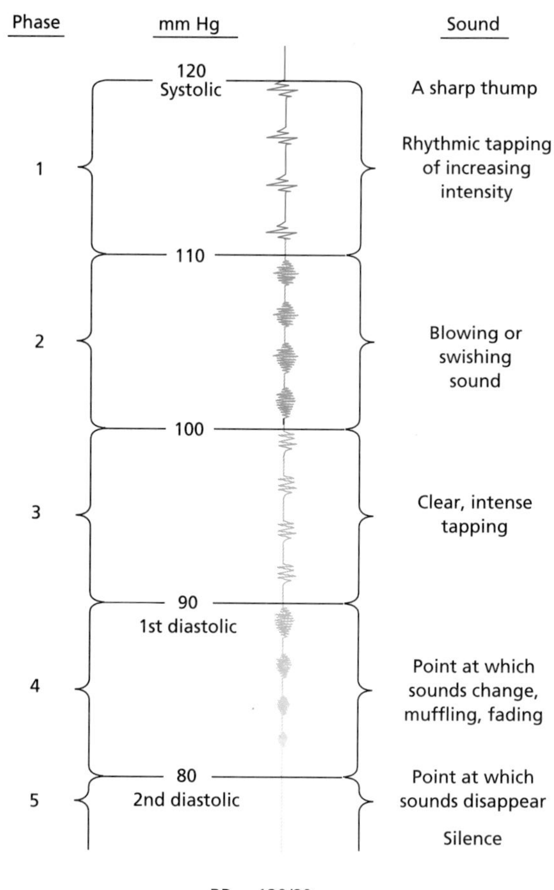

FIGURE 16.9 Phases of the Korotkoff sounds

correspond with phase 2 Korotkoff sounds. Phase 3 sounds are heard as crisp, intense tapping. Further deflation of the cuff will produce soft, muffled, blowing sounds that distinctly fade. The point at which this change in sound is heard is phase 4, sometimes referred to as the first diastolic pressure in patients in whom Korotkoff sounds persist as cuff pressure approaches 0 mm Hg (Haynes et al., 1993). Phase 5, the point at which Korotkoff sounds disappear, is known as the second diastolic pressure. The Canadian Hypertension Society recommends that phase 1 Korotkoff sounds be recorded as the systolic pressure, and phase 5 as the diastolic pressure. For patients in whom Korotkoff sounds persist to 0 mm Hg, phase 4 sounds are recorded as the diastolic pressure (Haynes et al., 1993).

Accurate blood pressure readings require a standardized method and proper technique. The Canadian Hypertension Society recommends the following guidelines for accurate measurement of blood pressure:

1. The patient should refrain from smoking or drinking hot or cold liquids for 30 minutes prior to measurement. There should be no talking during the procedure. The arm should be exposed and free from constrictive sleeves. The patient's legs should not be crossed.

2. Use a mercury or an aneroid manometer. If using a mercury manometer, position it so that the mercury column is at eye level.
3. Select a cuff width size that is approximately 40 per-cent of the arm circumference. Obese individuals may require a thigh cuff, whereas very thin patients may require a child-size cuff.

Adult arm (cm)	Cuff bladder size (cm)
< 33	12 x 33
33–41	15 x 33
> 41	18 x 36

4. Place the cuff so that the lower edge is 3 cm above the elbow crease and the bladder is centred over the brachial artery.
5. The bell of the stethoscope is preferred for auscultating Korotkoff sounds.
6. Venous congestion can result from leaving a partially inflated cuff in place for too long. Venous congestion alters the sounds, making them difficult to hear. To avoid venous congestion, allow one minute to lapse between readings. To correct venous congestion, deflate the cuff, raise the patient's arm over head and "milk" the forearm. Inflate the cuff while the arm is raised, quickly return it to the original position and take the reading.
7. Patients with irregular heartbeats may require additional readings. The average systolic and diastolic pressures are estimated and recorded with the pulse rate and heart rhythm.
8. Blood pressure should be measured at least once in both arms. Where there is a difference in pressures between arms, the higher pressure is recorded. Record the arm used and the patient's position—supine, sitting or standing (Haynes et al., 1993).

Procedure 16.4 outlines the technique for measuring blood pressure by auscultation.

Preparing the Patient

The nurse informs the patient that blood pressure will be taken. The size of the patient's upper arm should be looked at to determine the size of blood pressure cuff that will be necessary (see item 3, above).

Assembling Equipment

There are three basic types of sphygmomanometers for measuring the blood pressure: mercury, aneroid and electronic (see Figures 16.10 and 16.11). The electronic unit is discussed later. The mercury manometer uses liquid mercury within a glass tube calibrated in millimetres. The blood pressure is indicated by the level of the meniscus, or the concave surface of mercury as it descends in the tube. The mercury must be read at eye level; otherwise the value may be distorted. The aneroid gauge is a circular dial calibrated in millimetres and a needle that registers blood pressure as it descends the calibrations on the dial.

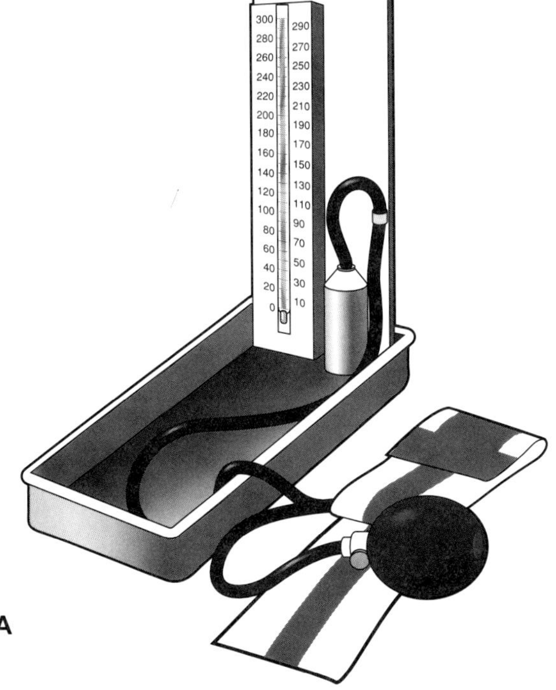

A

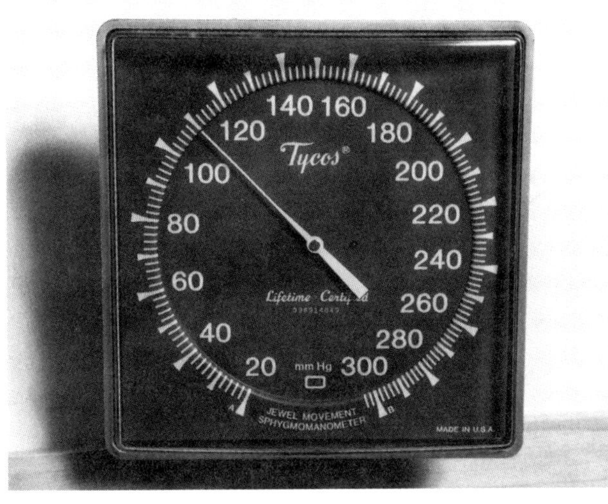

B

FIGURE 16.10 A. Mercury sphygmomanometer B. Aneroid sphygmomanometer mounted on a wall

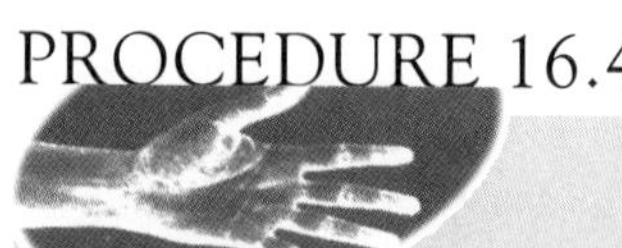

PROCEDURE 16.4

Measuring Blood Pressure

Action	Rationale
1. Wash hands.	Prevents the spread of microorganisms.
2. Prepare the patient.	Promotes well-being and facilitates patient participation in care.
3. Gather equipment: • Sphygmomanometer • Stethoscope	Facilitates efficiency and economy of time.
4. Help the patient assume a lying or sitting position, with the arm supported at heart level, and the palm turned up.	If the arm is above heart level, readings can be falsely low; if it is below heart level, readings can be falsely high.
5. Position the sphygmomanometer so that it is at eye level and in direct view; check that the mercury manometer or aneroid gauge is at zero.	Readies the equipment for accurate reading.
6. Expose the upper arm and palpate brachial pulse.	Locates the artery for placement of the cuff.
7. Fold the cuff's bladder in half. Position the cuff so that the centre of the bladder lies directly over the brachial artery and the lower border about 3 cm above the antecubital space. Then wrap the cuff snugly and evenly around the upper arm.	Finds the cuff's true centre. Promotes the most accurate blood pressure reading. A loose and unevenly placed cuff may cause a false reading.

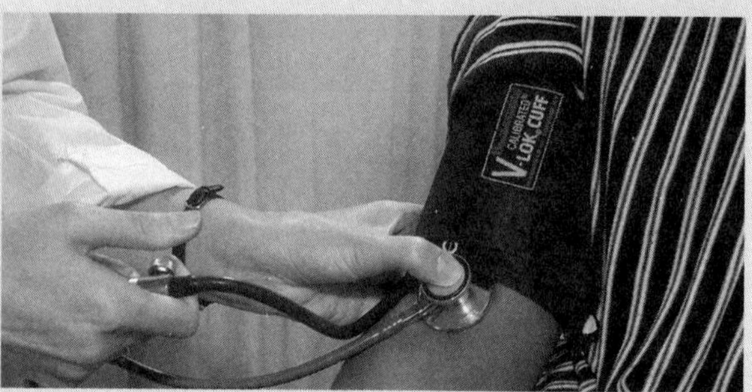

Action	Rationale
8. Palpate the brachial or radial artery with fingertips, close the valve of the inflation bulb and inflate the cuff until the pulse disappears. Note the point on the manometer or gauge where the pulse disappears. Deflate the cuff and wait 30 seconds.	Avoids misinterpreting an auscultatory gap and recording a falsely low systolic or a falsely high diastolic pressure. Allows the blood to circulate through the arm before continuing.
9. Place the stethoscope eartips in the ears and the bell or diaphragm over the brachial artery.	
Inflate the cuff rapidly until the mercury manometer registers 30 mm Hg above the point at which the pulse disappeared.	Ensures ample time to hear the systolic pressure accurately. Excludes the possibility of an auscultatory gap.
10. Carefully open the valve and slowly release the air at a rate of 2–3 mm Hg per beat. While releasing the air, watch the mercury manometer and listen for the Korotkoff sounds.	
Note the point at which the first clear sound is heard.	Indicates the systolic pressure (phase 1 Korotkoff).
Continue to deflate the cuff, noting the point at which the first muffled sound appears and finally, the point at which the last sound is heard.	Indicates the first diastolic pressure (phase 4 Korotkoff). Indicates the second diastolic pressure (phase 5 Korotkoff).
11. Rapidly deflate the cuff. If the reading must be repeated, wait at least one minute.	Re-establishes blood circulation through the veins.
12. Remove the cuff and return it to storage. Assist the patient to a comfortable position.	Promotes well-being.
13. Document the blood pressure on the graphic flowsheet (Figure 16.8) according to agency guidelines. In the nurses' notes, record variations in heart rhythm, pulse rate, position or extremity used.	Provides a data base for ongoing evaluation of patient status and promotes continuity of care.

The blood pressure cuff consists of an inflatable rubber bladder that is covered with self-securing fabric. A tube connects the cuff to the manometer; another connects it to the inflation bulb. The cuffs come in various sizes to fit infants, children and adults; sizes for the thigh as well as the arm are available. Using a cuff that is too small will yield a false high reading because it is not big enough to compress the artery adequately. A cuff that is too big, on the other hand, will give a false low reading. Thus, for a very obese patient, it may be necessary to use a thigh cuff rather than an adult arm-size cuff.

The equipment should be checked before use to ensure proper functioning. The release valve on the inflation bulb should open and close freely. The cuff must be free of residual air, and the manometer or gauge must register zero.

MEASURING BLOOD PRESSURE WITH AN AUTOMATED ELECTRONIC SPHYGMOMANOMETER

Electronic sphygmomanometers that give a digital readout of the blood pressure are available (see Figure 16.11). A cuff with a built-in pressure transducer is placed on the upper arm as is done with the ordinary sphygmomanometer. The machine is then turned on. A flashing light or a beeping sound indicates that systolic and diastolic pressures have registered. These machines may also be set to take blood pressure measurements at precise intervals. Some instruments are designed to provide a print-out of the blood pressures so that they can be examined and recorded appropriately.

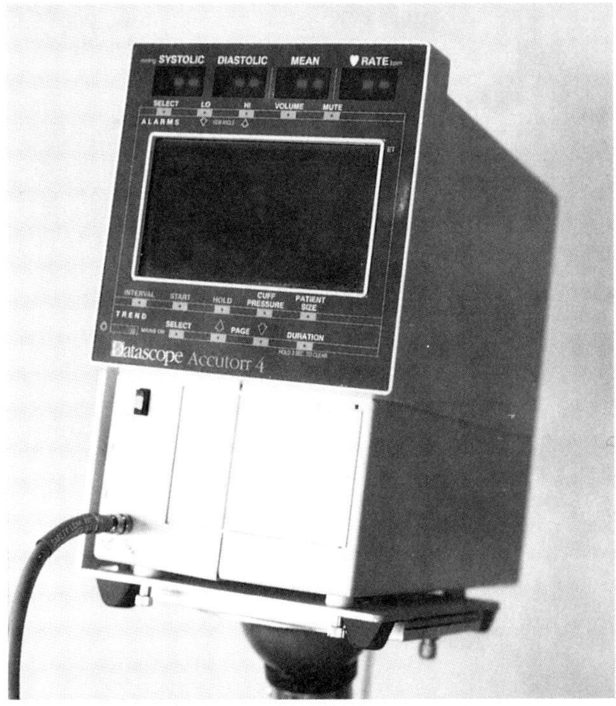

FIGURE 16.11 Electronic unit for measuring vital signs. It includes a sphygmomanometer, thermometer and pulse meter

SOURCE: St. Paul's Hospital, Vancouver, B.C.

Measuring Blood Pressure to Detect Postural Hypotension

Some patients, most commonly the elderly, experience postural hypotension, also called **orthostatic hypotension**. This condition occurs secondary to dehydration, prolonged bed rest, or as a side effect of medications (particularly antihypertensives). These patients often report light-headedness when arising from bed and, consequently, are at high risk for falls. For these patients, blood pressure measurements to detect postural hypotension are conducted.

1. With the patient supine for 5 minutes, measure blood pressure in both arms.
2. Assist the patient to a standing position. Wait approximately 1–5 minutes and repeat blood pressure measurements in both arms.
3. Most patients with postural hypotension will show a drop of 20 mm Hg in their systolic pressure within 2 minutes of standing up.

SOURCE: Goroll, May & Mulley, 1995.

Electronic, automated sphygmomanometers have been accepted as labour-saving devices in many institutions. In patients with normal blood pressures, readings using these automated devices have been found to correlate closely with blood pressure measurements using the auscultatory method. However, among non-normotensive patients, the automated devices tend to overestimate or underestimate blood pressures (Rutten, Ilsley, Skowronski & Runciman, 1986). Therefore, in situations where blood pressure measurements using the automated devices are inconsistent or questionable, the auscultatory method should be used. In clinical situations where a high degree of accuracy is required (such as for drug titration in critically ill patients), the direct method of measurement (by cannulation of an artery) is recommended (Henneman & Henneman, 1989).

Examinations and Diagnostic Tests

A comprehensive health assessment often includes a large number of tests and examinations that may be performed by many other health professionals. The first step in the assessment is usually a complete physical examination, performed by a physician or by a nurse practitioner. In conjunction with the examination, laboratory tests are usually ordered, and x-rays and other special examinations may be scheduled. The gamut of specialized tests and procedures used in the detection of illness today includes not only the standard x-ray but also its sophisticated offspring, the computerized axial tomography (CAT) scan, as well as the

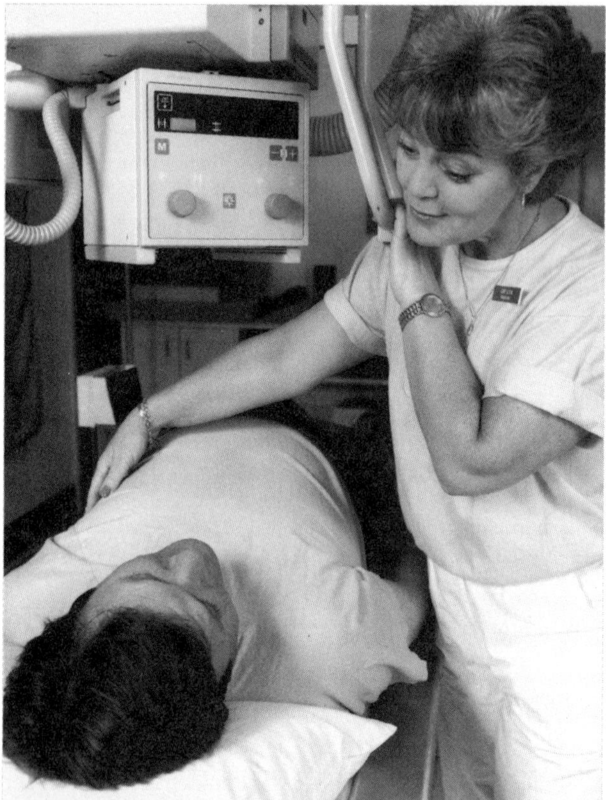

Diagnostic testing is part of a comprehensive health assessment.

ultrasonic scan, nuclear medicine studies, electrodiagnostic studies, magnetic resonance imagery (MRI), cardiopulmonary laboratory examinations and tissue biopsies. The neuropsychiatric field also has a number of specialized tests to help in assessing an individual's mental status.

Examinations and diagnostic tests create a good deal of anxiety in many people. Of primary importance to anyone undergoing them is what the results will mean in terms of prognosis (medical opinion of the final outcome of a health problem) and treatment. Some of the questions that run through a person's mind are: Will the results indicate that I have an incurable disease? Will I be disabled? Will I need to undergo surgery? These questions often preoccupy even the person who is just going to have a routine chest x-ray or blood test. Patients also want to know the reasons for the tests and when they will be able to have the results.

Under present rules of ethical practice, the nurse does not give the patient the results of examinations or tests. This is the responsibility of the attending physician or nurse practitioner. However, the nurse can provide the patient with information about the tests and with emotional support before, during and after many procedures. This is done by confirming and explaining what the physician has said about the "whys" of the test or examination and by giving the patient pertinent information. Nurses explain how the procedure is to be carried out, in terms the patient can understand, and they answer questions to the best of their ability.

The patient often wishes to help in the procedure, and the nurse can assist by explaining what he or she can do before, during and after the test to facilitate the examination. The nurse can also communicate to the patient an understanding of his or her anxiety and need to have confidence in the measures that are being taken for the patient's care. If the nurse feels that the patient does not understand what is being done, he or she has an important responsibility as a patient advocate to communicate this to the physician. The nurse also has an important coordinating function in regard to diagnostic tests and examinations. This may include assisting in the scheduling of tests, carrying out some of the procedures and assisting other members of the health team.

Laboratory Tests

In conjunction with a physical examination, various laboratory tests are usually ordered. These generally include blood tests and a urinalysis in the initial assessment of an individual's health status, or a periodic health checkup. In the blood work, the tests commonly ordered include a complete blood count (CBC). This includes a white blood cell count (WBC) and differential, hematocrit (Hct), a red blood cell count (RBC), platelet examination and a hemoglobin (Hgb) estimate. In many places where laboratory data systems are computerized, it is now common practice to order a battery of tests, instead of ordering them singly. Analyses on one sample of blood can provide an assessment of nutritional status, liver and kidney function, lipid profile, thyroid function and tissue injury. In a routine urinalysis, the urine is tested for pH, specific gravity, albumin and sugar, and a microscopic examination is done. If abnormalities are found in the blood tests or urinalysis, further laboratory investigation or other special tests are undertaken.

Nursing Functions for Specimen Collection

1. Explain the procedure and gain the patient's participation.
2. Collect the right amount of specimen at the correct time.
3. Place the specimen in the correct container.
4. Label the container accurately (this usually includes the patient's full name and identification number, the date, the physician's name and, in a hospital, the number of the nursing unit) and place it in a plastic bag.
5. Complete the laboratory requisition or enter data into the computer (this specifies what tests are to be carried out and gives pertinent data about the patient).
6. Place the specimen in the appropriate place for pick up (e.g., some must be refrigerated, others not).
7. Record anything unusual about the appearance of the specimen.

Frequently, the nurse is responsible for collecting specimens from patients. These may include specimens of blood, urine, sputum and drainage from wounds. For these tests, patients usually need explanations as to what they can do to help. Most patients like to be able to assist, and often the success of a test depends upon the patient's willingness to provide a specimen or perform some activity at a particular time.

Various specimens are sent for microbiological examination in the laboratory. Specimens of a patient's secretions, excretions and any exudates are frequently examined in order to isolate and identify an infecting organism. A **secretion** is a product produced by a gland (e.g., bile); an **excretion** is a substance excreted or discharged by the body (e.g., urine). An **exudate** is an inflammatory fluid, such as pus, that is discharged from an infected area of the body.

For most specimens, a sterile container is required, and precautions must be taken to avoid contaminating the specimen with organisms in the environment. A smear or culture may be needed. If a specimen is required for a smear, clean (preferably new) slides and a sterile, cotton-tipped applicator are needed. The specimen is gathered with the applicator, which is rolled over the centre of the slide. The smear is covered with another glass slide. The slides are appropriately labelled and sent to the laboratory.

For cultures, the specimen is placed in a sterile container. Urine, stool, blood, ascitic fluid and other excretions are usually put in a sterile container. For cultures of specimens of wound discharge, many agencies furnish sterile test tubes that are equipped with sterile applicators suspended from the cork that seals the tube. When the cork is removed the applicator is removed with it. The applicator tip is wiped over the area of discharge and then returned carefully to the sterile tube. Sputum specimens are collected in wide-necked sterile containers. Sputum is ideally collected early in the morning, when the patient is most able to cough up sputum from the lungs. Some specific tests require multiple specimen collection (e.g., otology and tuberculosis).

When stools are sent for culture, it is seldom necessary to send the entire specimen. Normally a sterile applicator dipped in the feces is sufficient. If the feces are to be examined for amebae, the specimen is sent to the laboratory while it is warm and it is examined within 30 minutes after it is obtained. Only a small quantity (approximately 3 mL) of feces is needed for this examination.

It may be necessary to test a culture for differentiation and sensitivity. *Differentiation* is accomplished by means of Gram's stain, which divides bacteria into two classes: gram-negative organisms stain red; gram-positive organisms stain purple. *Sensitivity* refers to the effect of specific antibiotics upon bacteria. The organisms are streaked on nutrient plates, various antibiotics are then added to the plates and the plates are placed in an incubator. The areas where the growth of the bacteria is inhibited indicate the particular antibiotics to which the bacteria are sensitive.

UNDERSTANDING LAB RESULTS

The purpose of laboratory and diagnostic tests is fourfold: (a) to provide baseline data to which future tests are compared, (b) to confirm or rule out the presence of a physiological disorder, (c) to screen for disorders that require further investigation and (d) to evaluate the effect of medications and treatments. The nurse is often the first health care provider to receive reports of these tests and, thus, is responsible for understanding the results and communicating them to the physician. This requires knowledge of human physiology, and an understanding of the relationship of the tests to pathophysiology and the significance of abnormal results on nursing care and medical management. To acquire the necessary knowledge base, the reader is encouraged to refer to textbooks on pathophysiology and laboratory and diagnostic testing listed at the end of this chapter. The purpose of this section is to introduce the basic concepts in understanding laboratory and diagnostic results.

Laboratory test results are interpreted according to reference values that are specific to a given laboratory and its procedures. Because there will be slight variation in reference values from one laboratory to another, test results should be read according to the reference values listed for the laboratory at which the sample was processed. In most laboratory reports, the normal ranges of reference values are listed beside the test results. Upon receipt of a laboratory report, the nurse compares the patient's values to the normal range. Values that fall outside the range are considered significant and should be reported to the physician. It is important to know that the normal range of laboratory values is influenced by age and gender. For example, compare the normal range for serum sodium in the following groups (Treseler, 1995):

Adult	(136–145 mmol/L)
Infant	(139–146 mmol/L)
Older male adult	(134–147 mmol/L)
Older female adult	(135–145 mmol/L)

Efforts have been made to standardize the units of measurement used in reporting laboratory values to a common language worldwide. While some institutions continue to use conventional units of measure (e.g., milliequivalents, or mEq), others are changing to SI units (*Le Système internationale d'unités*), which express laboratory values in molecular units, international units or decimal fractions. Thus, to interpret laboratory reports accurately, it is important to know what unit of measure is used; it may be necessary to convert values from one system of measure to another.

For example, a diabetic patient using a home glucose monitoring unit reports his blood glucose level to be 140 mg/dL (conventional units). Your institution uses SI units, in which the normal reference values for blood glucose are 3.85–6.05 mmol/L. To interpret this patient's blood glucose

Common Terminology Used in Laboratory Studies

Some common terms the nurse will need to be familiar with when reading laboratory reports are listed below (Treseler, 1995).

Blood chemistry screen. An analysis of the major chemical constituents of the blood. These constituents include serum sodium, chloride, potassium, glucose, creatinine, urea nitrogen, uric acid, total protein, bilirubin, cholesterol and enzymes.

Complete blood count. An analysis of the cellular components of blood. Included in this test are the determination of: red blood cell count (RBC), hemoglobin (Hgb), hematocrit (Hct), white cell count (WBC), white cell differentiation (differential) and platelet count.

Immunoassay. The study of antigen–antibody reactions in the blood, and the quantification of antigens or antibodies.

Osmolality. The number of dissolved solute particles in a solution. Serum osmolality is the number of dissolved particles per unit of water in the serum.

Osmolarity. The concentration of a solution. It is measured in osmoles of solute per litre of solution.

Plasma. The fluid portion of blood.

Serum. The fluid portion of blood from which fibrinogen has been separated.

Urinalysis. The systematic study of the physical, chemical and microscopic properties of urine. Tests in this study include gross examination, specific gravity, pH, glucose, protein, ketone bodies, occult blood and bilirubin.

value, it will need to be converted to SI units, using the appropriate conversion factor (i.e., multiply by 0.055). This patient's blood glucose value is equivalent to 7.7 mmol/L, which is above the normal range. The normal ranges of common laboratory values in conventional and international (SI) units.

X-Rays

Radiation is a highly publicized and emotionally charged word these days, and many people are afraid that having any kind of x-ray will harm them. Excessive radiation is most certainly dangerous, and special precautions are taken to ensure that people who work in x-ray departments or in places where radiation therapy is used (such as a cancer clinic) are not exposed to excessive amounts. Radiation exposures are cumulative. The amount a person receives during a single diagnostic test is minimal. A person does not receive enough radiation to destroy tissue unless this is being done therapeutically, for example, in treatment of a tumour.

Every precaution should be taken to minimize unnecessary radiation exposure. The potential hazard of radiation exposure is greatest on tissues of the developing fetus. Women of childbearing age should have x-rays scheduled only up to 14 days after the first day of their menstrual period. Pregnant women should avoid all x-ray exposure (Treseler, 1995). Nurses who are pregnant should wear protective gear, such as lead aprons, when assisting with x-ray procedures.

Today, x-rays are used in diagnosis and therapy on virtually every system of the body. In diagnosis, their purpose is to assist in the visualization of internal structures of the body, so that pictures of these structures can be put on film. X-rays, which are also called *roentgen rays*, are electromagnetic radiations, or energy waves, of short wavelength.

When x-rays are passed through the body, denser structures, such as bone tissue, absorb more of the rays and, hence, register heavier shadows on the photographic film. Less dense structures, such as soft organs (e.g., the stomach), permit the rays to pass through them more easily. These structures register lighter shadows on the film. It is the contrast between light and dark shadows (because of the differing density of tissues and, hence, the differing amount of rays they absorb) that enables the person reading the x-ray to find abnormalities.

In order to visualize softer structures within the body, such as the gastrointestinal tract, a substance (called a contrast medium) is often used to make the structures radiopaque so that they will show on photographic film. The contrast media usually used are either metallic salts or gases. Barium sulfate, for example, is the contrast medium used for the gastrointestinal tract. If the upper part of the tract (the esophagus, stomach and duodenum) is to be visualized, the patient drinks the barium solution. To allow visualization of the lower part (colon and rectum), the barium is given as an enema. Organic soluble iodides are used to visualize the gallbladder, urinary tract and blood vessels.

The ordinary diagnostic x-ray is like a still photograph and provides a permanent record. However, sometimes it is desirable to observe body organs or systems in motion, for example, the filling and emptying of the stomach. *Fluoroscopy* is used to capture movement. In this procedure, x-rays are passed through the body and images of the moving internal structures are projected onto a fluorescent screen. A contrast medium may be used to aid in the assessment.

The CAT scan (also known as CT and CAT) is another form of x-ray. The initials stand for *computerized axial tomography*. In this procedure, x-rays are passed through the body in the region of the structure to be scanned. A 180° sweep of the structure, at three or four different planes, is used. The x-rays are fed into a computer, which records the *absorption potential* of different tissues at varying planes within the structure. The computer prints out a visual representation of these. Photographs are also taken of the image on the screen. Usually these are in black and white, although colour photography is also possible.

Nuclear Medicine Studies

Radioactive isotopes, which are also known as *radionuclides* or *radiopharmaceuticals*, are another form of radiation that is used in both diagnosis and treatment. These substances give off radioactivity in known, predictable quantities as they decay, and they can thus be traced in the body by a monitor that picks up radioactivity. Certain radioactive substances have a particular affinity for specific parts of the body; for example, radioactive iodine taken orally (usually given in a drink) will find its way to the thyroid gland, where it tends to accumulate. Given in large doses, it will destroy tissue in much the same way as radiation therapy using x-rays does. In smaller doses (called tracer doses) it can be used to identify abnormalities in the thyroid gland. The radioactivity given off by the iodine as it decays can be picked up by a scanner (much like a Geiger counter) and the emissions transformed into electrical impulses, which can then be counted. A camera, called a gamma camera, may be used to take photographs of the accumulation and distribution of the radioactive iodine in the body. It is possible, using radioactive substances, to detect abnormalities or malignant tumours in such tissues as the brain, bone, lungs, liver, kidneys, spleen, pericardium and thyroid.

Electrodiagnosis

Various organs of the body, including the heart, brain, stomach, muscles and skin, constantly emit electrical impulses as they function. These impulses can be picked up on a machine and transformed (transduced) into a set of tracings that provides a graphic representation of the impulses. The tracings are then "read," or interpreted, by an expert to assess the functioning of the particular organ. In this way, graphic representations can be made of the electrical impulses emitted by the heart (*electrocardiogram*, also called an ECG or EKG), brain (*electroencephalogram*, or EEG) and muscles (*electromyogram*, or EMG).

Ultrasonic Scan

Auscultation, the listening for sounds within the body, is one of the basic methods of observation we discussed at the beginning of this chapter. The *ultrasonic (US) scan* is a diagnostic tool that utilizes this basic methodology. Sound waves of too high a frequency to be heard by the human ear are directed at the organ or structure of the body that is to be assessed. The vibrations that come back are transformed (transduced) into tracings, called *oscilloscope tracings*, which can be read to detect pathological changes in body tissues. Ultrasonic scans are commonly used to assess fetal development.

Ultrasound is also used to guide invasive procedures such as biopsies, aspirations and centesis. Doppler ultrasound yields information about blood flow velocity and direction of flow; this procedure is used in the assessment of arterial, venous and cardiac disease. The noninvasive nature of ultrasound, its portability to the patient's bedside and the absence of risks to the patient make this technology the preferred diagnostic test in some situations.

Magnetic Resonance Imaging

Magnetic resonance imaging (MRI) is a noninvasive imaging process that is based on the magnetic behaviour of hydrogen nuclei in biological tissues. MRI uses safe magnetic-field radio waves and computer technology to visualize internal organs and soft tissue (Treseler, 1995). Of all the imaging modalities, MRI yields the most complete and detailed image of certain body areas. Because it does not use ionizing radiation or contrast medium, there is no risk of tissue damage from serial studies, or of hypersensitivity reactions. MRI is used to detect hemorrhage, edema, infarcts, tumours and a variety of disorders of the central nervous system. It provides clear images of soft tissues and structures such as muscles, fat, bone and internal organs.

Most ferromagnetic objects become airborne projectiles when exposed to a strong magnetic field. Thus, a contraindication to MRI is the presence of ferrous metallic implants in the patient, such as an inner-ear implant, cardiac pacemaker, cardiac defibrillator, blood-vessel surgical clips, drug infusion pumps and ferrous foreign bodies. Prior to an MRI scan, patients and families are carefully instructed to leave all metal objects (keys, jewellery, pins, watches, coins) and clothing with metal (bras, belts and zippers) outside the scanning room (Treseler, 1995). Some patients become claustrophobic when enclosed within the bore of the scanner. Measures that help alleviate claustrophobia include providing the patient with a mirror so that he or she can see outside the imager, encouraging the patient to keep both eyes closed and to use visualization and, in severe cases, providing sedation prior to the procedure. Depending on the number of images, the procedure may take up to an hour or longer. MRI is an expensive procedure and is not available in many rural areas.

Tissue Biopsies

It is sometimes important to examine a sample of living tissue from a particular structure of the body. Usually this is done to look for either abnormal cells that may indicate the presence of a tumour or structural changes indicative of an infectious process. The procedure for obtaining a specimen of tissue from the body is called a **biopsy**. The specimen is sent to pathology for microscopic examination. There are three ways that a tissue biopsy may be obtained: (a) by use of a needle for puncture or aspiration, (b) by endoscopy and (c) by surgical excision.

Guidelines for Assisting with Tests and Examinations

Before the procedure:

1. Prepare the patient
   - Explain the procedure—what exactly is to be done, how long it will take, why it is being done and what sensations to expect—in terms the patient can understand
   - Explain how the patient can help with the examination
   - Provide the patient with a gown and assist him or her in getting into it, if necessary
   - Provide privacy for the patient to dress and undress and to wait for the examination
   - Help the patient to assume the position required for the examination
   - Drape the patient for comfort and to facilitate the examination
2. Practise body substance precautions
3. Prepare the equipment
   - Obtain all the equipment needed for the examination
   - Maintain the sterility of the equipment before and during the examination, as necessary
   - Obtain the containers needed for specimens and label these with the patient's name, the examiner's name and the date
4. Prepare the examining room
   - Close the windows and eliminate drafts
   - Ensure privacy
   - Place equipment so that it is convenient for the examiner
   - Provide a chair for the examiner when this is indicated

During the procedure:

1. Provide emotional support for the patient
2. Provide physical support as needed, for example, when the patient must keep very still in one position
3. Assist the examiner with equipment as necessary
4. Observe the patient for reactions to the examination

After the procedure:

1. Carry out measures for the patient's comfort, for example, cleaning lubricant off the skin or drying areas that may have been dampened
2. Observe the patient closely for any untoward reactions
3. Send labelled specimens to the laboratory
4. Clean and dispose of equipment as necessary
5. Enter details of the examination on the patient's record, such as date, time, exactly what was done and for what purpose specimens were sent to the laboratory

A sample of bone marrow may be obtained by inserting a hollow needle through the surface tissue of the body and into the marrow cavity of a bone. A small amount of the marrow is aspirated to obtain the specimen. The iliac crest is the most common site for this procedure, although the sternum, the posterior superior ilium and the spine are also used.

Endoscopy is the examination of body cavities and openings through the use of specially designed instruments that enable the examiner to observe tissues more clearly. The instruments are called scopes and usually come equipped with a small light at the inserting end and, often, a small mirror to make visualization easier. If a tissue sample is wanted, a narrow instrument is inserted through the scope to pick up cells for the biopsy.

For obtaining a sample of tissues that are imbedded in a body structure—for example, from a lump in the breast—it may be necessary to use surgical excision to get specimen cells for laboratory examination.

Cardiopulmonary Laboratory Tests

Many tests and examinations have been developed to aid in the assessment of functioning of the heart and lungs—so many that there are now specialized laboratories devoted to this diagnostic area. The electrocardiogram mentioned above is a procedure commonly ordered as part of a complete physical examination for all patients with a known cardiac history or if requested by the physician. In addition, various x-ray techniques may be used to visualize the size, positioning and functioning of the heart, lungs and blood vessels. A number of specialized tests may also be done, such as the stress tolerance test and treadmill test that assess cardiac functioning, and the pulmonary function tests that measure lung volumes, capacities and flow rates. We will be discussing the more commonly used diagnostic tests for cardiopulmonary functioning in Chapter 24.

Tests of Mental Status

In some cases, particularly when it is considered important to establish a psychiatric diagnosis, specialized psychological tests may be used. These include the objective tests, such as the intelligence tests with which most of us are familiar, the vocational interest and aptitude tests and the personality tests (for example, the Minnesota Multiphasic Personality Inventory). These may be supplemented by projective tests, such as Draw-a-Person, the Rorschach inkblot test or the Thematic Apperception Test. The latter two call for the individual to interpret different shapes of inkblots and pictures of people in different situations, respectively. The projective tests are said to reflect a person's fantasies and modes of adaptation. They are always administered and evaluated by a skilled psychologist or psychiatrist.

Nursing Responsibilities Pertaining to Laboratory Testing and Diagnostic Procedures

1. Know the facts about the test:
   - Is this an invasive or noninvasive procedure?
   - What type of sample is needed, and how is it collected?
   - Is the patient required to fast, restrict fluids or force fluids prior to the test?
   - Will a contrast be used? Is the patient allergic to this substance?
   - How long is the procedure?
   - Is sedation required?
   - Is a consent form required? All invasive procedures require a signed and witnessed consent form. Consent forms should be obtained after the patient has received all explanations and before any sedatives are administered.
2. Provide an accurate and simple explanation of the procedure to the patient. Recognize and alleviate psychological concerns by correcting misconceptions and providing emotional support.
3. Review current and previous test results. Trends and changes in test results help determine the plan of care for the patient.
4. Be aware of contraindications for specific contrast media and common complications of the procedure. Conditions in which the use of iodine contrast media is contraindicated include iodine or shellfish allergy, pregnancy, asthma, chronic obstructive pulmonary disease, renal failure, long-term steroid use, multiple myeloma, pheochromocytoma and syphilis. Barium enemas are contraindicated when ulcerative colitis or bowel perforation is suspected. Common complications after invasive procedures include infection, bleeding, perforation of organs and respiratory difficulties.
5. Be aware of postprocedural care:
   - Monitor vital signs closely after diagnostic procedures.
   - Observe the patient for signs of reaction to the contrast media and for signs of shock or infection. Institute methods to flush the contrast media from the patient's body. These may include increasing oral fluids, providing laxatives and avoiding medications that interfere with elimination.
6. Record in the patient's chart the following information:
   - specific preparation of the patient for the procedure
   - medications, treatments and fluid intake taken before and after the test
   - time when the procedure started or specimen was collected and time of completion
   - all nursing interventions made during the diagnostic testing
   - any adverse reactions or complications
   - postprocedural care and monitoring, including follow-up instructions to the patient
   - refusal by the patient to undergo a diagnostic test and the reason for refusal.
7. Be aware of legal and ethical implications related to reporting of test results. Confidentiality of information should be maintained. Some infectious diseases are mandated to be reported to the appropriate centre for disease control.

SOURCE: Fischbach, 1995.

IN REVIEW

- Health assessment involves the collection of subjective and objective data to develop a comprehensive base on which to make informed judgements and decisions about patient care.
- A comprehensive health assessment often includes diagnostic tests and examinations performed by other health professionals. The nurse can alleviate anxiety by providing information and support before, during and after many of these diagnostic tests.
- Data are collected through:
  - interviewing
  - health history
  - physical examination.
- Physical examination of the patient is a systematic assessment using the following techniques:
  - inspection (observation)
  - palpation (touch)
  - percussion (tapping)
  - auscultation (listening).

  Knowledge, practice and experience are necessary to develop skill in using these examination techniques.
- Physical assessments should be carried out in an organized manner to avoid omissions. There are several frameworks that assist the nurse, such as systems, needs or health patterns. These frameworks are often used in a head-to-toe format.
- Vital signs (temperature, pulse, respiration, heart rate and blood pressure) provide an indication of basic physiological functioning.

  Temperature can be obtained from the following sites by electronic tympanic or mercury thermometer:
  - mouth
  - rectum
  - axilla
  - ear.

- Pulses are either peripheral or arterial, and may be palpated or auscultated. They are assessed for rate, rhythm, strength and elasticity. Apical pulse is the beat of the heart auscultated at its apex. Pulse rate varies with:
  - age
  - gender
  - physical build
  - physical and emotional activity
  - medication
  - illness.
- Respirations involve both external and internal movements. External respiration (inhalation and expiration) is controlled by the respiratory centre in the medulla oblongata. Respirations are usually assessed for depth, rhythm, rate and character. Respirations should be measured without the patient's awareness, as changes are automatic but can also be voluntary.
- Blood pressure is the force with which blood flows in the arteries. Blood pressure is determined by cardiac output and peripheral vascular resistance. It is affected by:
  - age
  - gender
  - stress
  - activity
  - positioning
  - illness.

Critical Thinking Activities

In consultation with your teacher, select a patient who has recently been admitted to your agency.

1. Review the patient's data base, paying particular attention to the nursing health history and the physician's medical history and progress notes.
2. Undertake a clinical assessment of the patient's functional abilities, including:
   - temperature, pulse and respirations
   - blood pressure
   - nutritional status
   - elimination status (bowel status, urinary status)
   - sensory perception (vision, hearing, smell, taste and touch)
   - motor status
   - state of rest and comfort
   - reproductive status
   - mental status
   - emotional status
   - social status (verbal communication and social response).
3. Identify deviations from the normal that you observed in the patient's functional abilities.
4. What is the significance of these deviations in terms of planning nursing care for this patient?
5. What diagnostic tests and examinations have been ordered for this patient? Was a complete physical examination done? What laboratory tests were ordered? Roentgenography? Other? Why were they ordered? Review the laboratory reports, taking note of reference values, the units used for reporting and any deviations from normal. What are the implications of these deviations in terms of nursing care?

KEY TERMS

ophthalmoscope p. 373
otoscope p. 373
stethoscope p. 373
inspection p. 379
palpation p. 380
percussion p. 381
auscultation p. 382
supine position p. 383
Sims' position p. 383
knee-chest position p. 383
lithotomy position p. 383
vital signs p. 388
circadian (diurnal) rhythm p. 388
body temperature p. 390
pyrexia p. 390
fever p. 390
hypothermia p. 390
pulse p. 397
pulse rate p. 397
tachycardia p. 398
bradycardia p. 398
pulse rhythm p. 398
pulse volume p. 398
pulse tension p. 398
carotid pulse p. 398
radial pulse p. 398
brachial pulse p. 398
temporal pulse p. 398
femoral pulse p. 398
dorsalis pedis pulse p. 398
ulnar pulse p. 398
posterior tibialis pulse p. 398
popliteal pulse p. 398
apical pulse p. 399
point of maximal impulse (PMI) p. 399
external respiration p. 399
inspiration p. 399
expiration p. 399
respiratory rate p. 402
tachypnea p. 402
bradypnea p. 402
eupnea p. 402
apnea p. 402
respiratory depth p. 402
respiratory rhythm p. 402
respiratory character p. 402
dyspnea p. 402
blood pressure p. 402
systolic pressure p. 402
diastolic pressure p. 402
pulse pressure p. 402
cardiac output p. 403
peripheral vascular resistance p. 403
sphygmomanometer p. 404
orthostatic hypotension p. 407
secretion p. 409
excretion p. 409
exudate p. 409
biopsy p. 411

References

BAILEY, R., KNAUS, V., & BAUER, J. (1991). Aneroid sphygmomanometer: An assessment of accuracy at a university hospital and clinics. *Archives of Internal Medicine, 151*, 1409–1412.

BAIRD, S.C., WHITE, N.E., & BASINGER, M. (1992, August). Can you rely on tympanic thermometers? *RN, 55* (8), 48–51.

BARKAUSKAS, V.H., STOLTENBERG-ALLEN, K., BAUMAN, L.C., DARLING-FISCHER, C. (1994). *Health and physical assessment.* St. Louis: Mosby.

BATES, B. (1995). *A guide to physical examination and history taking.* (6th ed.). Philadelphia: Lippincott.

BERGER, K.J., & WILLIAMS, M.B. (1992). *Fundamentals of nursing: Collaborating for optimal health.* Norwalk, CT: Appleton & Lange.

BLOCK, G.J., & NOLAN, J.W. (1986). *Health assessment for professional nursing.* (2nd ed., p. 155). Norwalk, CT: Appleton-Century-Crofts.

BOBAK, I.M., & JENSEN, M.D. (1993). *Maternity and gynecologic care.* (5th ed.). St. Louis: Mosby.

EBEROLE, P., & HESS, P. (1998). Toward health aging. *Human Needs and Nursing Response.* (5th ed.) St. Louis: Mosby.

FISCHBACH, F. (1995). *Quick reference to common laboratory and diagnostic tests.* Philadelphia: Lippincott.

FOLSTEIN, M.F., FOLSTEIN, F.E., & McHUGH, P.R. (1975). Mini-mental state: A practical method for grading the cognitive state of patients for the clinician. *Journal of Psychiatric Research, 12*, 189.

FULLER, J., & SCHALLER-AYES, J. (1994). Health assessment: A nursing approach. (2nd ed.). Philadelphia: Lippincott.

GORDON, M. (1982). *Nursing diagnosis: Process and application.* New York: McGraw-Hill.

GOROLL, A., MAY, L., & MULLEY, A. (1995). *Primary care medicine.* (3rd ed.). Philadelphia: Lippincott.

HAYNES, R.B., LACOURCIERE, Y., RABKIN, S.W., LEENEN, F.H.H., LOGAN, A.G., WRIGHT, N., & EVANS, C.E. (1993). Report of the Canadian Hypertension Society Consensus Conference: 2. Diagnosis of hypertension in adults. *Canadian Medical Association Journal, 149*(4), 409–418.

HENKER, R., & COYNE, C. (1995). Comparison of peripheral temperature measurements with core temperature. *AACN Clinical Issues, 6*(1), 21–30.

HENNEMAN, E.A., & HENNEMAN, P.L. (1989). Intricacies of blood pressure measurement: Reexamining the rituals. *Heart and Lung, 18*(3), 263–273.

JARVIS, C. (1996). *Physical examination and health assessment.* (2nd ed.). Philadelphia: Saunders.

MARTINI, F. (1989). *Fundamentals of anatomy and physiology.* Englewood Cliffs, NJ: Prentice Hall.

PILLITTERI, A. (1995). *Maternal and child health nursing: Care of the childbearing and childrearing family.* (2nd ed.). Philadelphia: Lippincott.

POTTER, P.A., & PERRY, A.G. (1995). *Basic nursing: Theory and practice.* (3rd ed.). St. Louis: Mosby.

RUTTEN, A., ILSLEY, A., SKOWRONSKI, G., & RUNCIMAN, W. (1986). A comparative study of the measurement of mean arterial blood pressure using automatic oscillometer, arterial cannulation and auscultation. *Anaesthesia and Intensive Care, 14*(1), 58–65.

STAAB, A.S., & HODGES, L.C. (1996). *Essentials of gerontological nursing: Adaptations to the aging process.* Philadelphia: Lippincott.

SUNDERLAND, P.M. (1996). In S.E. Huether & K L. McCance (Eds.), *Understanding pathophysiology* (chap. 11, Structure and function of the neurological system). St. Louis: Mosby.

TERNDRUP, T. (1992). An appraisal of temperature assessment by infrared emission detection thermometry. *Annals of American Medicine, 21*, 1483–1492.

THOMPSON, J., & WILSON, S. (1996). *Health assessment for nursing practice.* St. Louis: Mosby.

TRESELER, K.M. (1995). *Clinical laboratory and diagnostic tests.* (3rd ed.). Norwalk, CT: Appleton & Lange.

WONG, D.L. (1995). *Whaley & Wong's nursing care of infants and children* (5th ed.). St. Louis: Mosby.

Additional Readings

ATTREE, M., BUTTON, D., & COOKE, H. (1994). Student's evaluation of the process of conducting a patient assessment. *Nurse Education Today, 14*(5), 372–379.

BILLINGS, P.C. (1996). *Instant nursing assessment: Paediatric.* Albany, NY: Delmar.

FIRTH, P., & WATANABE, S.J. (1996). *Instant nursing assessment: Women's health.* Albany, NY: Delmar.

GRIMES, J., & BURNS, E. (1996). *Health assessment in nursing practice.* (4th ed.). Boston: Little, Brown.

HANSON, C. (1996). *Instant nursing assessment: Gerontologic.* Albany, NY: Delmar.

HEATH, H. (1995). Health assessment of people over 75. *Nursing Standard, 9*(37), 30–37.

HYER, K. (1996). Home safety assessment. *Home Health Focus, 2*(9), 70–71.

JAFFE, M. (1997). *Home health nursing: Assessment and care planning.* (3rd ed.). St. Louis: Mosby.

LEININGER, M. (1995). *Transcultural nursing: Concepts, theories, research and practices.* (2nd ed.). New York: Wiley.

LINDELL, D.F. (1997). Community assessment for the home healthcare nurse. *Home Health Care Nurse, 15*(9), 618–628.

MABBETT, P.(1996) *Instant nursing assessment: Mental health.* Albany, NY: Delmar.

NARAYAN, M.C. (1997a). Cultural assessment in home healthcare. *Home Healthcare Nurse, 15*(10), 663–670.

NARAYAN, M.C. (1997b). Environmental assessment. *Home Healthcare Nurse, 15*(11), 799–805.

NEAL, L. (1997). Is anybody home? Basic neurologic assessment of the home care client. *Home Healthcare Nurse, 15*(3), 156–169.

NOWAZEK, V., & NEELEY, M.A. (1996). Health assessment of the older patient. *Critical Care Nursing Quarterly, 19*(2), 1–6.

O'HANLON-NICHOLS, T. (1998). Gastrointestinal system. *American Journal of Nursing, 98*(4), 48–53.

QUIRK, M.E., & CASEY, L. (1995). Primary care for women: The art of interviewing. *Journal of Nurse Midwifery, 40*(2), 97–103.

TRIPP-REIMER, T., BRINK, P., & SAUNDERS J. (1984). Cultural assessment: Content and process. *Nursing Outlook, 32*(2), 78–82.

Chapter 17

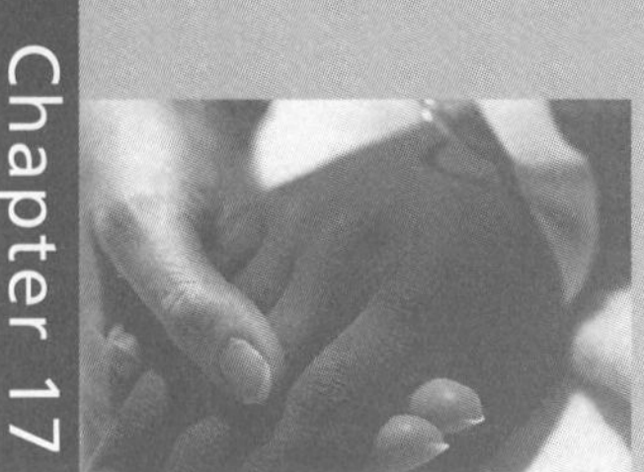

Communication Skills

OUTLINE

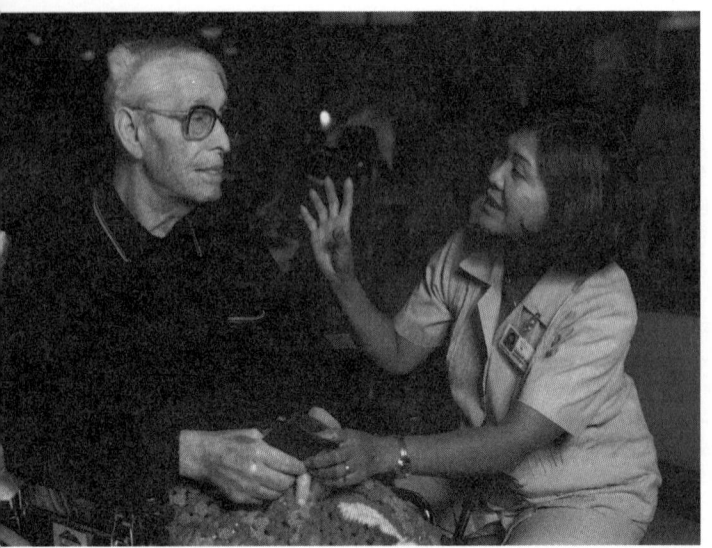

Central Questions

1. What are the five basic characteristics of a helping relationship?
2. What are the three major phases of the nurse–patient relationship?
3. What are the main aspects of the process of contracting with a patient?
4. What is the SMCR model of the communication process?
5. Which factors can interfere with elements of the communication process? Give examples.
6. What factors should the nurse consider when conveying a message?
7. How must characteristics of language be considered by the nurse in communicating with patients?
8. How do people communicate nonverbally? Give examples.
9. What are some of the ways of fostering an open climate for nurse–patient communication?
10. What role does the interview play in nurse–patient communication?
11. How are various media used for information exchange between members of the health team?
12. What are the most significant factors in care for the caregiver?

Introduction

The fundamental core of nursing is the relationship that is established between the nurse and the patient. This is a professional relationship, based on trust and mutual respect. Individuals who come to a health agency are there because they need help with some aspect of their health; nurses and other health professionals are there to provide that help. The relationship that develops between the nurse and the patient is **collaborative**—nurse and patient work together to promote the patient's optimal level of health. In order to develop relationships whereby nurses can help patients, nurses must develop skills in communicating, since, without communication, relationships are not possible.

Communication is the process by which people exchange thoughts, feelings and ideas. It is a tool that provides a means for one person to understand another, to accept and be accepted, to convey and receive information, to give and accept directions and to teach and learn. Communication is always a two-way process. The nurse communicates with the patient and the patient with the nurse. The nurse also communicates with patients' families and friends, with visitors to the agency, with other members of the health team and other personnel and with a host of other people during the course of a day. Nurses should, therefore, understand the process of communication. Like any other nursing skill, good communication requires theoretical knowledge, a positive attitude towards the value of communication and ongoing, self-reflective practice (Balzer-Reiley, 1996).

This chapter will examine the basics of clear communication, focussing on various aspects of the nurse–patient relationship as well as the nurse–colleague relationship.

The Nurse–Patient Relationship

Nursing is one of the helping professions. Nurses help people to promote and maintain optimal health, to protect them from disease, to restore health following an episode of illness and to cope with the exigencies of chronic or terminal illness. The relationship that is established between nurse and patient is a *helping relationship*. This relationship is the basis of nursing practice, and it is woven into the fabric of every interaction that occurs between nurse and patient. In the health field, the helping relationship is often referred to as a **therapeutic relationship**, because it is a key element enabling the health professional to administer care to the patient.

Characteristics

Several characteristics of the helping, or therapeutic, relationship have been identified by different authors (Adler, Rosenfeld & Towne, 1995; Montgomery, 1993; Northouse & Northouse, 1997). One essential element is **empathy**, which is often defined as the ability to imagine oneself in another person's place and to recognize and understand the other's feelings from his or her unique point of view. From a caring perspective, empathy is seen as **receptivity**, the willingness to enter into the perspective of another. This does not mean that the nurse loses his or her sense of self and does not exercise healthy boundaries. Rather, it underscores that empathy is distinct from simply feeling sympathy for another's pain or situation.

Empathy arises when the nurse is receptive to being in a relationship with the patient. When your patient ceases to be "the patient" and becomes a person to whom you are relating, you, the nurse, enter into that person's experience at some level. If you remain receptive, you may understand what he or she is going through. To confirm that you are getting the message, you might ask clarifying questions, for example, "I'm wondering if you are feeling frustrated with having more tests today, Mr. Yuen," or, "How are you feeling now that you've talked to your surgeon?" Questions that invite a response beyond a simple "yes" or "no" create opportunities to share, facilitate a deeper relationship and, as a result, promote empathy (Hills, Chisamore & Lindsey, 1990).

Another element essential to the therapeutic relationship is mutual **respect**. Demonstrating respect means treating the patient as a person, not a case, a bed number, a diagnosis or a list of tasks to be accomplished. Recognizing the uniqueness of each person is necessary to establishing a

A Few Simple Ways to Demonstrate Respect to Patients:

- Address them by the name and title by which they wish to be called.
- Preserve dignity during intimate procedures such as bed baths by drawing curtains and avoiding unnecessary exposure of their bodies.
- Maintain confidentiality by not discussing patients in public areas.
- Say *please* and *thank you* when asking a patient to perform a task, for example, deep breathing and coughing, or when assisting the patient to turn over in bed.
- Ask permission before touching a patient or performing a procedure.
- Acknowledge visiting family members when you enter the room.
- Ask permission before sitting down to speak with a patient.
- Introduce yourself by name and title.
- Inform patients of treatments and explain your actions during them.

caring relationship; respecting the individual and his or her right to make decisions is essential, but not always easy—for example, when a patient refuses a medication or other treatment. Sensitivity to cultural and social courtesies is another sign of respect. While nurses are not expected to know the nuances of every culture or tradition, the attitude of respectful caring can cross both cultural and language barriers. Simple actions and common courtesies speak volumes.

Nurses need to have the respect of patients if the relationships are to be effective—that is, if nursing interventions are to be related to positive patient outcomes. Your nursing education qualifies you to help others with regard to health problems; these qualifications in themselves engender respect from others who have not had this professional training. Competence in carrying out nursing interventions, whether teaching preoperative exercises, putting on a dressing or taking a blood pressure, reinforces the inherent respect for the professional felt by the lay person. The confidence of the patient in the nurse is promoted by the demonstration of self-respect by the nurse. Self-respect is evidenced by such things as personal grooming, good posture, confident tone of voice and deliberative, well-planned actions.

Both empathy and mutual respect contribute to fostering a **climate of trust**, which is a very basic element in the helping relationship. Patients must be able to trust nurses as people who are concerned first and foremost with patient welfare. Before they discuss personal matters or express their feelings, patients must feel that the nurse will not betray their confidence. Once sure of the nurse's competence, patients are able to trust that complex, invasive measures can be carried out safely. As the patient develops trust in the nurse, the nurse is able to assess the patient's readiness to accept responsibility in regard to personal health care. Trust usually develops slowly as rapport is built. Rapport can be facilitated by attention to small details such as remembering to make the phone call a patient asked you to make and reporting back to the patient, by being honest and giving only reliable information, and, again, by demonstrating competent nursing care.

Genuineness, or **authenticity**, is another characteristic of the helping relationship that creates a climate of trust. Spontaneity of response, **self-disclosure**, and a lack of defensiveness on the nurse's part all contribute to authenticity. The nurse's willingness to disclose opinions and feelings will model, for the patient, the ability to express private concerns and anxieties. The nurse may disclose similar feelings, such as grief that he or she may have experienced in the past over the death of a family member, but care must be taken not to burden the patient with the nurse's personal problems. It should be remembered that the purpose of self-disclosure is limited to promoting the development of a therapeutic relationship whereby the patient understands that the nurse is a human being who has a sincere interest in the patient's welfare. The patient's concerns are always the focus of the relationship.

Once the patient's concerns have been established, the nurse uses **specificity** to clarify the exact nature of the patient's problem; ambiguity and vagueness are replaced by clarity as the nurse constantly communicates an understanding of the patient's concerns and seeks to validate that this understanding is accurate. As problems are accurately identified, appropriate interventions can be initiated.

Using open-ended questions to elicit more information can produce surprising results. Patients can surprise themselves by recognizing the answer to their difficulty while responding to a nurse's question; nurses can surprise themselves by recognizing that what they thought was the problem was really not a problem to the patient at all. Clarification and specificity are keys to good communication.

Open-Ended Questions

Asking open-ended questions of the patient can improve communication and help the nurse to understand the patient's perception of the problem.

Open-ended questions are phrased in such a way as to encourage more than a yes-or-no response. Examples include:

- What do you see as the main difficulty you are facing?
- What is concerning you?
- What can you tell me about this situation?
- How would you describe how you're feeling?
- What has this hospitalization been like for you?
- What brings on these feelings?
- What do you fear most about this?
- What else can you tell me?
- What have you tried so far?
- When do you feel most anxious/angry/fearful?
- What has helped in the past?
- How would you like to see this changed?
- What will you do the next time you feel this way?

SOURCES: Hills et al., 1990; Northouse & Northouse, 1997.

Handling Conflict

Mutual respect is imperative to any caring relationship (Wright & Leahy, 1994). Patients, family members or colleagues who threaten nurses or use verbal or other abuse towards them must be dealt with in a manner respectful to all parties. All agencies should have policies in place protecting all persons from sexual harassment and abuse of any kind, and nurses should be aware of them. Procedures and protocols that offer clear direction in dealing with emotionally unstable or violent patients and other individuals must be followed to protect all persons involved. As well, nurses, who deal daily with emotionally distraught or overstressed persons, need to be aware of ways to de-escalate a highly charged encounter or confrontation. Part of this expertise consists of recognizing when a situation has the potential to spiral beyond the capabilities of one person and to call for help promptly. Asking for help when you judge it to be necessary is a sign of respecting yourself.

Empathy within a caring relationship can help to de-escalate a potentially disruptive confrontation. Understanding and recognizing the feelings that underlie a patient's aggressive behaviour can alert the nurse at a point at which de-escalation is possible. Such feelings may include anxiety, fear, frustration, isolation, overwhelming grief and powerlessness (Hills et al., 1990; Northouse & Northouse, 1997). We all experience these feelings at times; however, when coupled with situational stresses such as language or cultural barriers, prolonged illness, hospitalization, pain, mental illness or cognitive dysfunction, addiction withdrawal or prolonged lack of personal space, people may become overwhelmed and act aggressively. Usually, such patients have a history of violence, or may exhibit signs of growing emotional turmoil. Such behaviours as handwringing, pacing, fist-clenching, darting eyes, inability to sit or stand still, speech that is becoming louder or faster, refusal to listen or respond, and finally, threatening speech and gestures, are clear indicators that violence may be imminent (Irwin & Simons, 1994).

A simple rule is helpful in handling conflict: *If the nurse feels disrespected it is always time to act, always with the goal of re-establishing mutual respect.* Sometimes, at an early stage when anxiety or moderate frustration is the underlying emotion, the nurse's action may consist of simply offering support by listening and encouraging the patient to talk about his or her feelings. If the underlying problem is a feeling of isolation due to a language barrier or aphasia, a translator, alphabet board or other means of communication must be established. Many small acts of aggression by the elderly, such as hitting or pinching their caregivers, result from their decreased ability to communicate needs or to hear and understand what the caregiver is saying or doing (Hills et al., 1990).

At a moderate stage when frustration is moving towards anger, a supportive stance that offers alternatives to the patient may work (Northouse & Northouse, 1997). For example, a patient may be extremely anxious while going through alcohol withdrawal for reasons not directly related to the primary diagnosis—perhaps he or she is a smoker, and smoking privileges are curtailed in the hospital. A supportive stance would invite this disclosure. Alternative coping strategies might include encouraging the patient to arrange for a friend or volunteer to take him or her outside the hospital for regular smoking breaks, or offering nicotine gum or a patch upon the advice of the physician. This is the critical stage when the nurse must feel able to call upon colleagues for support if needed.

When a patient or other person loses control and becomes aggressive to the point of potential or actual violence, it is frightening for all parties involved: the aggressor, caregivers, other patients, visitors and bystanders. Such a situation requires a prompt response that mobilizes health professionals to take charge by following agency protocol. For many agencies, a "code white" is a call for help that results in a nonthreatening show of force that can effectively re-establish mutual respect by setting secure limits to aggressive behaviour. Sometimes outside law enforcement may be called, if the situation warrants this extreme measure. The message needs to be clear: all voices have the right to be heard; all persons, including health professionals, have the right to be treated with respect.

Phases of the Nurse-Patient Relationship

Studies of the nurse–patient relationship have identified three major phases. There is first of all an introductory, or *orientation*, phase, when nurse and patient get to know and trust each other, then a *working phase* and, finally, a *termination phase*. Some authors subdivide these phases, and some identify more than three, but since the components coincide, we will discuss them under the three major headings (Peplau, 1991, 1992; Forchuk & Brown, 1989; Forchuk, 1992).

ORIENTATION PHASE

The time it takes for nurse and patient to get to know and begin to trust each other is referred to as the **orientation phase**. Under normal circumstances, they start off as strangers. The nurse, however, usually has the advantage of having some information about the patient before the initial meeting. If a nurse is assigned a patient in the clinical area, for example, relevant information can be obtained from the patient's chart. The nurse will also be able to obtain a verbal report from the charge nurse (or the primary nurse) before meeting the patient.

The nurse takes the initiative in the relationship that is being established. It is up to the nurse to set the tone for the encounter (or series of encounters). Both nurse and patient are identified by name, and roles are clarified during this introductory, or orientation, phase. Both parties come with preconceived ideas about the nature of the relationship. The patient may hold certain beliefs about hospitals and nurses, and comments about the agency or hospital may have been offered by friends or relatives. Experiences with the health care system will influence expectations of the care to be received.

The nurse comes to the encounter with expectations formed by previous clinical experiences and by the knowledge attained during education. Nurses should be sensitive to the possibility that expectations may not coincide. It is imperative that, during this orientation phase, expectations about the nature of the working relationship be clarified between the two parties. The patient, for example, may expect the nurse to do everything while he or she simply lies in bed getting better. The nurse, on the other hand, may believe in promoting as much self-care as the patient can manage. The importance of exploring the patient's expectations and resolving differences between the nurse and the patient was discussed in Chapter 14.

An orientation to the nursing unit or health agency is usually part of the introductory phase. It is important that the patient be introduced to people who will be participating in his or her care and that the nurse's roles be explained. Taking the nursing history is often a part of this phase and is sometimes the first opportunity the nurse has to get to know the patient. During this phase of the relationship there may be some testing, as both parties attempt to develop trust while exploring the possibilities and limitations of the relationship.

WORKING PHASE

The **working phase** of the nurse–patient relationship begins when the nurse has gathered data and is beginning to draw up a tentative plan of care in collaboration with the patient. Increased emphasis on accountability and responsibility for both providers and consumers of health services has led to the premise that both are equal partners in the process of health care. It is this premise that guides the nurse in the working phase. The nurse and the patient share in developing mutually agreeable goals, and both have a definite role to play in achieving these. There is a division of responsibility, and it is important to clarify at the beginning of the working phase who will be responsible for which aspects of care.

Patient Contracting

One structured type of communication between the nurse and patient is the patient contract. A **patient–nurse contract** "is an agreement between the patient and the nurse that outlines roles and responsibilities for each member of the therapeutic relationship" (Balzer-Reiley, 1996, p. 52).

The contract may simply be a verbal agreement, for example, "I will teach you how to do the deep-breathing exercises before surgery, but I would like you to consider doing them four times a day on your own." Or, the contract may be a written statement that is signed by all parties concerned (a family member or significant other may also be involved, and there may be more than one nurse or other health care provider in the development of the contract).

Herje (1980) specified several characteristics central to an effective patient contract. The contract must be:

1. realistic (are the goals specified attainable for the patient?)
2. measurable/capable of being evaluated (are the goals concrete? can progress be evaluated?)
3. positive (what goals would the patient like to attain? what existing patient strengths can be built on?)
4. time-dated (when can the contract be started? how much progress is expected in a given time frame?)
5. written (have the patient and nurse both signed and retained a copy of the written contract?)
6. rewardable (is the desired patient behaviour rewardable? is the reinforcement desirable to the patient?).

Hayes and Davis (1980) have identified five steps in the process of contracting, and these provide good guidelines:

1. identification of the problem/priority ranking
   (patient and nurse discuss the patient's perception of his or her health and create a problem list that is prioritized)
2. contract development
   (includes the behaviour that is expected from the patient and what reinforcement the patient will receive in return for this behaviour)
3. contract implementation
   (patient and nurse attempt to perform the goals/behaviours that were specified in the contract)
4. contract evaluation
   (together, the patient and nurse periodically evaluate the contract's success to assess whether the stipulated goals are being attained; the contract may have to be periodically re-evaluated, depending on patient progress)
5. contract termination
   (it is useful to include a predetermined termination date in the contract).

Hayes and Davis (1980) stress the importance of making the contract very specific to ensure that the terms of the agreement are clearly understood by all concerned. It should contain not only specific daily activities but also the variables of the activity. For instance, in the verbal contract described above, the nurse would specify the number of times the patient would be helped with deep-breathing exercises and the times of the day the patient should practise alone before surgery. More than one nurse is often involved in the patient's care; they would all need to agree to the arrangements if the contract is to be fulfilled. The patient's primary physician should also be involved in the contract design. Depending on the nature of the activity, the physician's orders may need to be included, and the contract must be consistent with the overall plan of care for the patient.

Nurses have an important motivating role during the working phase of the nurse–patient relationship, in addition to their responsibilities in carrying out specific nursing care measures. Nurses encourage patients to take increasing responsibility for their own care (to the extent that they are able) and help the patient work towards the goals that they have established together. A review of the progress made each day and honest praise for accomplishment of the various tasks help to keep the patient motivated. Family and friends can also provide support in motivating the patient to work towards the established goals.

TERMINATION PHASE

The nurse–patient relationship terminates when the patient is discharged from the agency or the nurse leaves for another assignment, or for any other reason ceases to provide care for the patient. Sometimes the relationship is of short duration, as when the nurse has had the responsibility of caring for the patient for one shift only. For the nurse working in an acute care setting, the relationships are usually short, extending over a few days or a few weeks. In long-term care facilities, in which the patients are often residents, the nurse may work with one group of residents for several months. The community health nurse may have people he or she works with over a period of years. Whatever the length of the relationship, there is an inevitable sense of loss when it is terminated. This feeling is more acute, of course, the longer the relationship has continued.

It is helpful during this **termination phase** to review with the patient the progress that has been made in achieving previously established goals. When the relationship has been of longer duration, feelings of loss can be mediated by drawing the patient's attention to the goals that have been met. In this way the patient is able to accept more readily that the nurse's care is no longer needed. When patients have been adequately prepared for the termination of the relationship, a sense of mutual satisfaction may exist between the patient and the nurse. Sometimes, it is necessary to hand over the care of a patient to another person. In these situations it is always helpful to introduce the patient to the new caregiver. If the patient is to be transferred to another agency, he or she needs to be prepared for the transfer. Reviewing progress to date and giving the patient information about the new agency will help to make the transfer easier. If the patient is being moved from an acute care hospital to an extended care unit, for example, fears and concerns should be fully explored. Knowing where the agency is located, the type of accommodation and the care provided will be greatly appreciated by the patient. If a member of the family can visit the facility and describe in detail to the patient what can be expected, the transfer will be facilitated.

The Process of Communication

Communication involves both the sending and the receiving of a message. If the message is not received, no communication has taken place.

Because communication is such an essential component of most work, as well as a basic social process, it has received a great deal of study. Numerous models have been developed to illustrate the process. The Source, Message, Channel, Receiver (SMCR) model (Rogers & Rogers, 1976) illustrates the process simply, contains all the basic elements and is easily understood (see Figure 17.1).

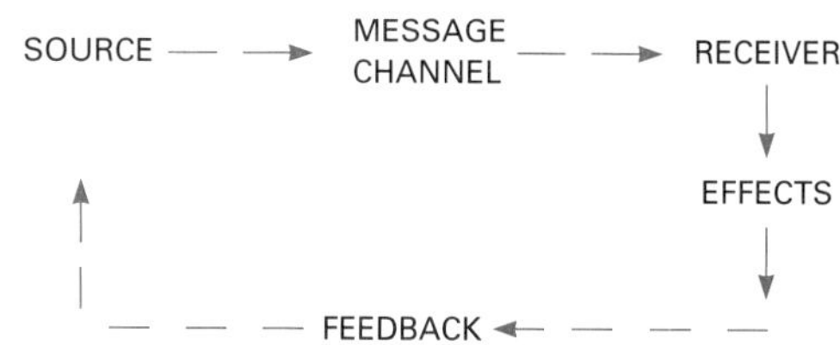

FIGURE 17.1 The SMCR model of communication

SOURCE: Rogers & Rogers, 1976.

The essential elements in the communication process are:

1. a **source** (sender)—someone who sends a message to another person
2. a **message**—the thought, feeling or idea that the sender wishes to convey
3. a **channel**—the means by which the message is conveyed
4. a **receiver**—the person for whom the message is intended.

Let us consider an example. The nurse in a doctor's office wishes Ms. Lim to go into the examining room and tells her so. The *source* is the nurse. The *message* is "Please go to the examining room." The *channel* is the spoken word. The intended *receiver* of the message is Ms. Lim. The desired effect on the receiver is that she get up from the chair and proceed to the examining room. If she does, the nurse will know that she received the message. If she does not, the nurse will assume that the message was not received. The *effects* on the receiver provide the sender with **feedback**, since they enable the person who has sent the message to know if it was received or not. If it was not, communication has not taken place and the sender should try again.

The SMCR is one of many sender–receiver models of communication. A more recently proposed model illuminates the difference that occurs when empathy within a caring relationship is the cornerstone of communication (Montgomery, 1993). This model conveys the importance of the merger that occurs when empathy develops (see Figure 17.2). "Relational communication tells us that messages have both a relational and a content dimension; that one cannot not communicate" (Montgomery, 1993, p. 20). We know this by experience: a look may convey all that is needed from a mother to her child; in a similar way, even a stranger who passes us in the street may send us a message of cordiality, disdain or danger by body language. Somehow, the significance or insignificance of relationship and attitude is sent regardless of words; however, like any message, the relational, or nonverbal, message may or may not be received or interpreted correctly.

The importance of the relational aspect to communication cannot be overstated. Nurses are in a position of implied power over patients who are ill, weak or unable to

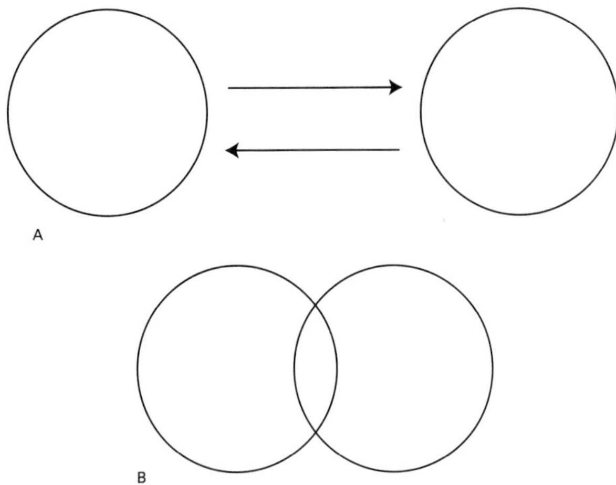

FIGURE 17.2 A. Sender–receiver model of communication B. Merger that occurs with empathy

SOURCE: Montgomery, 1993, p. 24.

express themselves. The nonverbal relational message they inadvertently send may either support or bolster that power structure or help in levelling the playing field. Empathy, an attitude of receptivity and warmth towards the other, can help reduce the sense of powerlessness and helplessness that patients often feel while undergoing care.

The SMART (Zilm, 1998), another model of communication, adds the affective element of tone to the SMCR model. The elements of SMART include:

- Source
- Message
- Audience
- Route
- Tone.

Factors Affecting Communication

Effective communication means that the message the sender intended to convey reached the intended receiver, was received and was interpreted correctly, and that the receiver was able to respond in some meaningful way to indicate that the message was received. Difficulties can occur anywhere along the way in the communication process.

The Source (Sender)

The sender may have trouble putting the message into a form that can be communicated. This is called coding the message. Some people are very skilled at translating their messages into drawing, painting or music. Most of us, however, communicate with words, both spoken and written, and with nonverbal behaviour, such as facial expressions, gestures, body postures and touch. We can communicate some ideas quite eloquently using nonverbal means but, in order to convey most messages, we need to be able to attach symbolic meanings—in the form of words—to those messages. People must also be able to arrange these symbols (words or signs) to form messages that can be understood by others, and they must be able to send these messages clearly.

Consider the person who is in a foreign country, for example, and is unable to speak the language. Getting along is possible to a certain extent by pointing and using gestures but, when it comes to asking directions or ordering a meal, it may be difficult to get the meaning across without the use of words. It is at this stage that difficulties will be encountered. Likewise, a person who has suffered brain damage and is unable to speak, or cannot convert thoughts into verbal expression that can be understood by others, will also have trouble coding messages intelligibly. A person having difficulty making vocal sounds will experience problems communicating and must depend on written forms of communication, gestures or other nonverbal expressions to get messages across.

An individual's physical well-being and emotional state also affect the ability to communicate. A person who is ill may find trying to communicate too much of an effort, or thought processes may not function well enough to enable a coherent message to be put together. A person's emotional state can make communication easier, may hinder self-expression or may prevent communication completely. When a person is at ease emotionally and feels comfortable with another person, it is usually much easier to communicate. Nervousness and anxiety often interfere with the ability to put together a clear message and send it. The nervous applicant at a job interview, for example, frequently finds it difficult to say the right thing in the way it should be said.

Many different emotions can affect the sender's ability to communicate. A person can be so overwhelmed with happiness that the appropriate words cannot be found for

Top Ten Ways to Halt Communication

Are you guilty of any of the following?

1. make demands rather than requests
2. aim to please others rather than tell the truth
3. take everything personally
4. do not consider anyone else's point of view
5. are unassertive
6. assume no one wants to hear what you have to say
7. assume everyone is hanging on your every word
8. react defensively to perceived criticism
9. never make eye contact with anyone
10. never, ever listen.

SOURCE: Grensing-Pophal, 1997.

When You Do Not Speak the Same Language ...

Imagine yourself all alone in a foreign country where no one speaks your language. Now imagine yourself ill and in need of nursing care. How will you communicate your needs to those around you? How will you know if they care about you or if they understand the problem?

Many people face this situation every day. You will nurse many patients who speak a different language and who do not understand the words you speak. All agencies should have access to translators so that consent can be ethically obtained. However, what about daily nursing care?

- It is helpful to compile a list of simple phrases in the patient's language, with a translation to which the patient can point to make his or her needs known. The translator or a family member can help with this.
- Pictures also can be of great help in clarifying needs. Pain and anxiety scales can be effective in spite of language barriers, if graphics such as colours and facial expressions are part of the scale.
- Nonverbal communication in the form of simple, respectful courtesy goes a long way towards establishing a caring relationship and, thus, empathy.
- Sometimes a smile and a supportive touch transcend the greatest of language barriers.

self-expression. Extreme anger and fear can similarly impair communication. But, on the other hand, a clenched fist, pounding on a table, or the slamming of a door can convey anger as eloquently as words can. All these emotions can influence the communication by affecting (positively or negatively) the effectiveness of the source.

The Message

The message itself may not be clear. Sometimes two conflicting messages are being sent simultaneously. For example, a nurse may say to a patient, "I am glad that you came, even if it is late," but the impatient tapping of a foot, or the surreptitious glances at a watch, may convey an entirely different meaning to the patient. Noise or other distractions can also interfere with message exchange.

In order to convey the meaning intended by the sender, the message must be sent in a form the receiver can understand. If Ms. Lim does not speak English, the communication process breaks down unless the nurse is able to put the message into a language the individual does understand, or can convey the intent of the message by nonverbal means. Even with someone who speaks the same language as the nurse, the terminology must be at a level that the person can understand, or again the message will be unclear. If the intent of the message is not completely and explicitly stated— for example, if directions on how to get to the examining room are not included with the request to go there—the message is not complete.

The Channel

The channel chosen for sending a message must be appropriate. There are three main channels by which we communicate with other people: oral (speech), written and nonverbal communication.

For oral communication, we have a number of tools at our disposal: talking directly with a person in a face-to-face meeting, recording messages on tape (audio or video), telephoning or communicating by radio or television. All are media for the spoken word. There are also many forms of written communication: notes, letters, interoffice memos, records and forms, e-mail, faxes, newspapers, books and magazines all convey messages in written form.

Messages are also conveyed nonverbally. It has often been said that a person communicates true feelings more in actions and mannerisms than in words. A whole area of study in recent years has been on "body language"—that is, the interpretation of messages people send through facial expressions, gestures, postures and ways of walking.

Other nonverbal forms of communication include the various sign languages (the most common being American Sign Language, or ASL) used by the deaf community. Sign languages can range from simple gestures to forms similar to ASL. These more complex forms are highly developed languages in which body language combines with a complex system of gestures to communicate messages.

Pictures and diagrams are often useful as an adjunct to, or in place of, words—for example, the use of diagrams, slides, videos and films in educational programs. It is possible to learn to make a bed by listening to a description and reading the directions, but it is much easier to learn by watching a demonstration or a video, or by following an illustrated manual.

The medium chosen must be appropriate for the message and must make the intent of the message clear to the intended receiver. Touch can sometimes convey more empathic understanding than words to someone who has suffered a loss. Direct face-to-face talking is often a more effective means of communication than telephoning or writing a message. On the other hand, some people have difficulty expressing themselves orally and can put their thoughts and feelings down on paper more easily. When there is a long list of instructions for someone to follow, the written channel (supplemented with oral clarification as needed) is more appropriate.

The Receiver

Problems in communication can also occur at the receiving end of the process. The message may reach someone other than the intended receiver. If Ms. Lim is the intended receiver but Mrs. Armani gets up and moves in the direction of the examining room while Ms. Lim continues to sit in her chair, the nurse knows that the wrong person received the message. An individual who is hard of hearing may have difficulty receiving spoken messages. A person who cannot read or write is unable to receive communications sent in written form. The intended receiver must not only receive the message but also be able to interpret it.

Many physical and psychosocial factors can affect a person's ability to understand communications. Age, for example, must be taken into consideration. Children often will not understand messages that are directed to them by an adult. Their language skills have not developed sufficiently for them to be able to symbolize in the same terms as the adult, nor has their intellectual development reached a level where they can comprehend the idea the adult is trying to convey. The integrity of the anatomical structures and physiological processes involved in interpreting messages must also be intact. When mental faculties have been impaired by brain damage, by alterations in the level of consciousness, the ability to receive and interpret messages is decreased.

Emotional state may also interfere with both the ability to receive messages and the ability to interpret them. The frightened individual attends only to those messages that concern the object causing fear. Other messages may not be received or may be misinterpreted. The patient who is afraid that an injection will be painful may perceive the nurse's smile as threatening rather than reassuring.

It has often been said that people hear only what they want to hear. Receiving and interpreting messages is an active process. A woman who is told that she has inoperable cancer may not hear the message because she has "tuned out." Nurses and other health professionals may have difficulties processing the significance of messages being given by their patients for a number of reasons: environmental distractions, multiple demands, cultural differences, personality issues and lack of skill or attentiveness in decoding messages.

Age-Related Considerations in Communication

Respecting the uniqueness of individuals and listening to their concerns means the nurse will recognize the developmental context of the patient. For instance, the concerns of an adolescent will differ vastly from the concerns of a toddler or a middle-aged adult.

Other than the obvious vocabulary choices you would make, what would facilitate communication with a preschooler, given what you know about Erikson's psychosocial developmental stage of initiative versus guilt? Recalling that preschoolers love to master new skills and frequently ask "Why?" can help the nurse to formulate the interview to meet the child's needs and to truly hear the child.

Like any age group, the elderly require a unique approach to communication. It is important to address the elderly by their title and last name until they tell you otherwise. Many seniors have cognitive, visual and hearing impairments; these limitations must be taken into consideration when communicating with this age group. Nurses must speak slowly and clearly, and allow time for patients to respond. Keep interaction short and free of distractions. Repetition may be necessary. If a patient wears glasses or uses a hearing aid, these must be in place.

Families, as well, have stages of life. The nurse, when communicating with a young family with an infant and toddler, will be hearing different needs as well as experiencing different barriers to communication. For example, what difficulties might you perceive when interviewing a family with a newborn? Two barriers to communication might be fatigue and anxiety related to lifestyle adjustment.

SOURCES: Irwin & Simons, 1994; Wright & Leahy, 1994; Sieh & Brentin, 1997.

Communicating with Aphasic Patients

Patients who are unable to speak offer a special challenge to nurses. However, depending on what underlying condition is causing the aphasia, there are numerous devices that the patient can use, from simple alphabet boards to sophisticated computer programs. Patients on ventilators often can use a pad of paper and pen to communicate.

Patience is the key to good communication with persons whose speech is dysfunctional. The nurse must be willing to learn from the individual how he or she communicates.

Compared with the relative speed of speech, communication using a message board or other device may be slow and prone to misunderstanding. However, the rewards of working through such difficulties are great, and good nursing care depends on establishing communication.

SOURCE: Mann & Lane, 1991.

The Nurse as Sender in the Communication Process

There is an old rhyme that says, "I have six honest servants who taught me all I know. Their names are *Who* and *What* and *When*, and *Where* and *Why* and *How*." In thinking about communication and how to get a message conveyed to an intended receiver so that the message is correctly interpreted, the nurse may find it helpful to ask the six questions contained in the rhyme. We will start with the *what*, since the first thing the nurse must do is to get the message clear in his or her own mind before deciding how to send it.

- What is to be communicated?

  Is it directions, such as how to get somewhere or how to do something?

  Is it information, such as what is going to happen in the x-ray department or for a series of tests?

  Is it an attitude, such as a feeling of warmth and acceptance?
- Who is the intended receiver?

  Do I know much about the patient as an individual?

  Do I know anything about the patient's background?

  What is likely to be the patient's point of view?
- Why is this message to be communicated?

  Does the patient need to know something in order to become oriented to the agency?

  Does the patient need help to overcome the fear of surgery?

  Does the patient need this message for safety? To increase independence?
- How should it be communicated?

  Should I speak with the patient, should I give information (or directions) in writing, or would nonverbal communication be best for this particular message?
- Where should the communication take place?

  In the patient's room, in the nursing station, in a classroom outside the nursing unit, in the patient's home?
- When should it be communicated?

  Is the person receptive to the message?

  Does he or she need the message now?

  Should it be delayed?

  Should others, such as family members, be present?

The nurse will probably think of many more questions that could be asked but, if the six basic ones are remembered, it will help to keep in mind some of the fundamental elements of the communication process when the nurse is the sender.

Verbal Communication

In sending messages, either in speech or in writing, the language level chosen for the message should be simple and clear. Some people have a tendency to overcommunicate. The message gets lost somewhere among the explanations, embellishment, or extra verbiage that the sender feels should be included. Some people undercommunicate, so that the message is incomplete and the receiver has to ask for further clarification. If a person has something important to communicate, the message should be sent in the simplest language and with as few words as possible (but as many as necessary to get the meaning across), if the individual wants to be certain the message will be interpreted correctly.

Factors Affecting Communication

- growth and development
- perceptions
- values/beliefs
- emotions
- culture
- gender
- level of education
- roles and relationships
- environment
- space and territory
- language
- self-concept.

SOURCES: Balzer-Reiley, 1996; Sieh & Brentin, 1997.

The choice of words is another important consideration. Although many people in our health-oriented society are quite knowledgeable about health matters, such as the causes and treatment of illness, they often do not understand the technical terms that health professionals use. Each line of work has its own **jargon**—that is, technical terms that are used in that particular field but are not in common use outside it.

The terminology that nurses learn in order to be able to communicate effectively with other health professionals is often not understood by patients. Effective communication with others depends on the use of common terminology. It is important that nurses talk to patients in terms that they can understand. The nurse must assess the patient's language level and use appropriate words to express meaning clearly. For example, a nurse might ask a public health inspector or a medical officer of health, "What measures are taken for vector control?" and expect a satisfactory answer. If an average homeowner were asked the same question, he or she probably would not know what the nurse was talking about. On the other hand, if the nurse were to say, "Do you have screens on the doors and windows to keep out insects?" the person would be able to understand the question more clearly.

Health professionals commonly use technical terms to refer to vital bodily functions. The words *void* and *defecate*, for example, are used for urination and bowel elimination, but terms such as *pass water*, *pee* and *bowel movement* are probably more readily understood by most people. In working with children it is important to find out the particular terms for bodily functions that they have been taught.

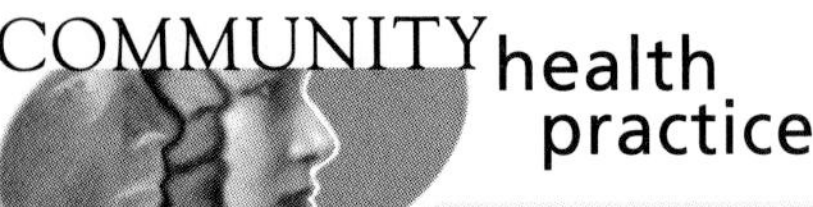

Preschoolers and Communication

Below are some typical difficulties for preschoolers in learning to speak and communicate with others. If the child:

- has difficulty understanding and using language
- has difficulty hearing
- has an unusual voice (nasal, raspy or scratchy)
- seems reluctant to converse with others
- is easily embarrassed or frustrated when talking
- repeats words or sounds
- has difficulty making himself or herself understood

it may be helpful to have a referral to a speech language pathologist. Information can be obtained from your local health unit.

SOURCE: Vancouver Health Department, 1994, 1995.

In verbal communication, the message must be given at an appropriate speed in order to avoid misinterpretation. Timing is also essential for effective communication; for example, it may be difficult for a patient to attend to discharge teaching when he or she is in pain. Humour can be an effective coping strategy for relieving stress, anxiety and pain. While nurses may use humour as a nursing intervention, inappropriate use can create a negative atmosphere, in which the patient may feel belittled or misunderstood. Because humour is culturally defined, nurses must be sensitive to how patients and family members express humour (Balzer-Reiley, 1996).

Inclusive language is also an important tool for good communication in a pluralistic society. Inclusive language seeks not to exclude certain persons or groups from the message being communicated and is a sign of respect to all. Many groups continue to feel marginalized or stereotyped in mainstream Canadian society, particularly women, children, people of colour, the poor, persons with mental illness and persons who are disabled. In speech and writing, nurses should use language that is both clear and inclusive: for example, "humankind," "manufactured" and "sporting" are preferable to "mankind," "man-made," and "sportsmanlike." Avoid outdated suffixes conventionally used to distinguish men's work from women's work (e.g., waitress, actress) or language that identifies only one gender (e.g., chairman, policeman). Be sensitive to current usage of language describing persons with disabilities. These words change frequently as disparaging associations develop and new terms are introduced to maintain respect linguistically. A good rule in speaking or writing is to focus on the person rather than on the externals surrounding him or her (Griffith, 1997; Status of Disabled Persons Secretariat & Department of the Secretary of State of Canada, 1991).

Nonverbal Communication

Feelings and attitudes are conveyed not only in the words a person says, but also in nonverbal behaviour. Nurses should be aware that their facial expression, tone of voice, gestures and posture all convey in subtle ways their regard and feeling for another person. At the same time, the nurse should be aware that clues about the patient's feelings, attitudes and physical condition can be picked up through observations of nonverbal behaviour.

Nurses should be aware that their verbal and nonverbal communication may be incongruent. For example, a nurse might indicate verbally to a patient that she has time to discuss his or her questions, yet her body language (e.g., glancing at her wristwatch, pacing) may convey to the patient that she does not have time. Patients can also demonstrate incongruent communication behaviours. For example, a patient might state that she is not upset, yet her nonverbal behaviour (e.g., reddened eyes) indicates that she has been crying.

Nonverbal signals convey 55% of your message. Voice tone conveys another 38%. Your words carry only 7% of your message.

SOURCE: Robinson, 1997.

FACIAL EXPRESSION Facial expression is perhaps the most common way in which feelings are expressed by people nonverbally. One conveys feelings of happiness, fear, surprise, anger, disgust (contempt) and sadness by using facial muscles. Facial expressions speak a universal language. In cross-cultural experiments, psychologists have found remarkable agreement in people from different countries in interpreting emotions expressed in photographs (see Figure 17.3). Both literate and nonliterate cultures have been tested, with remarkably similar results (Ekman, Friesen, O'Sullivan & Chan, 1987; Matsumoto, 1992).

Human beings can use the muscles around the eyes and mouth to express feelings. Actors on the stage are aware of the impact of facial expression and learn to control their muscles to such an extent that the audience is able to tell, merely by looking at their faces, the emotions they wish to convey. Perhaps the nurse does not need as much skill in facial expression manipulation as the actor, but nurses do need to be able to control nonverbal expressions of dislike, hostility and disgust. This requires examination of personal motivations and feelings.

POSTURE Body posture is also a means of communicating. An erect, upright posture usually indicates a feeling of self-

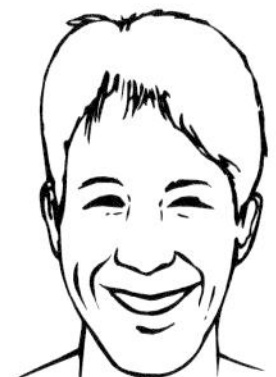 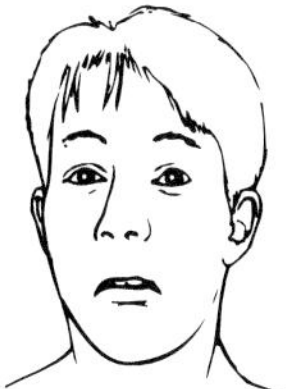 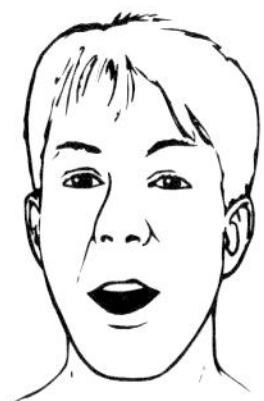 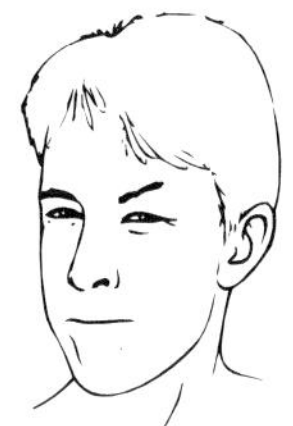 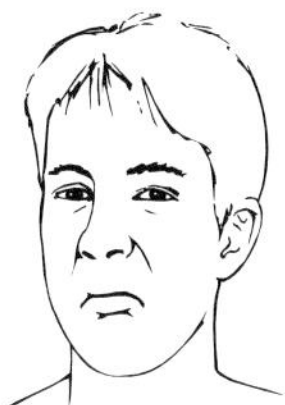 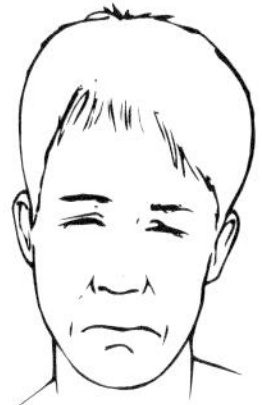

	Happiness	Fear	Surprise	Anger	Disgust Contempt	Sadness
Japan	87	71	87	63	82	74
Brazil	97	77	82	82	86	82
Chile	90	78	88	76	85	90
Argentina	94	68	93	72	79	85
United States	97	88	91	69	82	73

FIGURE 17.3 Judgements of emotion in five literate cultures

SOURCE: Ekman, 1975, p. 36.

esteem and inner poise. Sadness, depression or a low regard for oneself usually makes a person stoop or slouch. It is not uncommon, for example, to see a severely depressed person sitting slumped in a chair or shuffling along with head down and shoulders rounded.

GROOMING Grooming also conveys meaning. A neat, well-groomed look indicates pride in appearance. The attitude of the patient towards grooming often indicates his or her state of well-being. Very ill people often do not have the strength or the desire to keep up their grooming. The request of a patient for a mirror has often been noted as an indication that he or she is feeling better.

GESTURES People are often unaware of the gestures they use, but gestures play an important role in conveying thoughts and feelings. A welcoming gesture as you ask a person to sit down helps to put the patient at ease. A hurried manner with quick gestures on the part of the nurse evokes a feeling that the nurse does not have much time and, as a result, the patient becomes reluctant to ask questions or to confide fears and worries. The patient's gestures are equally important. Lowered eyes or an averted glance usually indicate a wish to avoid communication on a topic. A person who sits with folded arms, occupying as little space as possible, is often tense.

NURSES at work ICU Nurse

Phil, a critical care nurse in the intensive care unit (ICU), reflects about his experience relating with a ventilated patient who has amyotrophic lateral sclerosis (ALS):

When you work with patients on ventilators who are seriously ill and are often surrounded by equipment, it is easy to forget the most important thing in nursing: that you are caring for a person, not operating technology. One patient I had taught me a lot about how important it is to work out a means of communication, no matter how busy you are.

Laura was a 40-year-old woman with amyotrophic lateral sclerosis, a degenerative disease affecting motor neurons. She was unable to use her hands even to point. Her speech was also affected and, now that she was ventilated, she was unable to form words at all. All Laura could do was blink. However, Laura, her family and the occupational therapist devised an alphabet board that was simple and effective.

The board consisted of three rows of letters: A through I, J through R, and S through Z. The rows were numbered one to three. When Laura wanted to tell us something, or to respond to our questions, she would stare at us and blink deliberately. We would begin by asking her, 'Which row? One? Two? Three?' When we hit on the right row of letters, Laura would blink twice. Then, we would read out the letters in that row: 'A, B, C ... ' Laura would again blink twice when we got to the first letter of the first word in the sentence.

For example, if Laura wanted us to turn on her radio, she would blink twice for row two, and twice again for the letter 'R.' As we got to know Laura's likes and dislikes, and learned to use the alphabet board effectively, our communication with Laura improved.

The greatest memory I have of Laura is her radiant smile whenever we hung in there with her and worked out a complicated message.

— Fay Lapka, RN

INTONATION A wide variety of subtle meanings are conveyed by the tone of one's voice. There is an adage that it is not so much what you say as how you say it. Small children, in particular, respond much more to the tone of a person's voice than to the actual words. Adult patients, however, are also sensitive to coldness or warmth as conveyed in the tone of the nurse's voice.

Tone of voice often indicates an individual's feelings of well-being. A person who is ill usually speaks more slowly and in a lower tone than usual. With excitement, the voice often rises and is more highly pitched. Various feelings may be expressed simply by changing the intonation of one's voice as, for example, in saying "Good morning." People are seldom aware of how their voice sounds to others. Listening to a tape recording of one's voice is often useful in helping to hear oneself as others do.

TOUCH Touch can also convey the nurse's thoughts and feelings to patients. Research has revealed that when one individual touches another in a nonobtrusive manner, positive reactions generally occur, even between strangers (Crusco & Wetzel, 1984).

Creating a Climate for Open Communication

In order to foster an atmosphere of openness in which the patient feels free to communicate, the nurse must convey a feeling of warmth and acceptance.

Warmth implies a genuine liking for people. Acceptance involves the ability to understand another person's point of view and to respect the right of each individual to be different. Acceptance means being nonjudgemental. This is not an easy task. We all have conscious and unconscious attitudes, biases and prejudices that reflect our social background and our learning and life experiences. We all tend to evaluate other people and events from our own personal perspective.

As a helping professional, the nurse must learn to understand patients in the light of their backgrounds and experiences. Learning to be nonjudgemental is a conscious undertaking for most people. It is helpful for the nurse first to become aware of personal attitudes and to understand how they were acquired. Attitudes, biases and prejudices are all learned. They can all, therefore, be unlearned, or at least modified by additional learning and life experiences. Taking courses in psychology can help a nurse to gain an increased understanding of self and also greater insight into individual differences and the factors motivating behaviour. Courses in sociology and anthropology help in developing an appreciation of cultural and social influences on behaviour. Working with people from other cultures and from different social backgrounds, and getting to know them as individuals, also helps to change attitudes previously held, consciously or unconsciously.

Giving Information

Communication is always a two-way process and, in order to keep the communication channels open, both the nurse and the patient must contribute. The nurse is an important source of information for the patient, as we have noted. The nurse should always answer the patient's questions, both those that have been verbalized and also, where possible, the unspoken ones. Answers should be specific, with as much information as can be provided and in terms that the patient can readily understand. The patient, for example, may say to the nurse, "Dr. Leroux said he was sending in a referral for a neurologist to investigate this ringing in the ears I've been having. What, exactly, did he mean?" The nurse might answer, "He has asked Dr. Mei to come in and check you over. He thinks the problem may be related to the nerves that are involved in hearing. Dr. Mei is one of our specialists in this field. She will probably be in to see you later this morning." Or, the patient may say, "I hear they are going to operate on me tomorrow. I wish I knew what time." The nurse might say, "I have just seen the schedule for tomorrow's surgery. Your operation is at eight o'clock in the morning" or, "I don't know just yet. They make up the schedule in the afternoon and we usually have it by three o'clock. As soon as it comes, I will let you know."

Learning to Listen

In any nurse–patient communication, the patient's problems, interests, feelings and activities are the primary focus. In order to help the patient, the nurse must learn to **listen**. Most people

What Nonlistening Habits Do You Have?

What are you really doing when you look as though you're listening? Are you a ...

- Mind reader: Asking yourself, "What is this person really saying?"
- Rehearser: Practising what you'll say next.
- Filterer: A selective listener, tuning out what you don't want to hear.
- Dreamer: Not "there" at all.
- Identifier: "I know what you mean," is your favourite reply. You hear only what you've experienced.
- Assessor: Critically appraising the speaker rather than listening to the message.
- Derailer: Interrupting or changing the subject too soon tells the speaker you're not really interested.
- Discounter: Saying something quickly, like, "That's nothing to worry about!" belittles the speaker.
- Placater: Avoiding conflict by agreeing with everything said is not respectful to yourself or to the speaker.

SOURCE: "Why We Don't Hear Others," (n.d.) p.1.

will communicate quite readily if they have an attentive listener who is not going to impose personal values on them, nor proffer unwanted advice. The techniques of being a good listener can be learned. Although most beginners tend to feel a little self-conscious using the techniques described, they soon become a natural way of responding.

One of the first things to learn is to listen attentively. To patients this conveys that someone is interested and is willing to devote time and energy to hearing what they have to say.

POSTURE The nurse's posture is important in conveying to the patient that he or she is listening attentively. Much nurse–patient communication occurs during the process of giving care, and the nurse, particularly in a hospital setting, is usually standing. For an interview (such as taking the nursing history), a discussion of problems the patient has, negotiating a contract or the like, it is always better if the nurse can sit and talk with the patient. Sitting down to talk implies a more relaxed and less hurried manner than standing. Getting out from behind a desk and sitting in a comfortable chair (with the patient also in a comfortable chair) helps to create a more relaxed atmosphere for both the nurse and the patient in a community health setting. Sitting at the same level also helps to convey that you and the patient are equal partners in this relationship. When nurse and patient are on the same level, good eye contact can be maintained. It should be remembered, however, that in some cultures, it is considered disrespectful to look another person directly in the eyes.

The nurse should sit facing the patient directly—this helps to indicate a willingness to listen. Neither arms nor legs should be crossed, as these actions tend to portray a defensive posture. Openness is fostered by a nondefensive posture. It helps for the nurse to lean slightly forward, towards the patient, when talking. Most people do this automatically in conversational situations.

PERSONAL SPACE The distance between the nurse and patient is also important. Each of us likes to have a certain amount of space around us. It is a natural protective instinct, and we feel threatened when other people intrude upon it. If you are in a crowded elevator, for example, and a number of people get off at one floor, you will almost automatically move to put more space between you and the next person. The amount of room a person likes as **personal space** varies, depending on personal idiosyncrasies, on cultural norms, on how a person feels at the time and on the intimacy of the situation. Some people prefer not to be touched (except in intimate family situations) because they feel that their personal space is being violated. Other people use demonstrative affectionate gestures, like hugging, even among people they do not know very well. Some people, when they are ill, do not want anyone near them, while others are comforted by the presence of others.

Studies have been done on the distances most commonly maintained in various types of social interaction. A knowledge of these ranges is useful for nurses in judging the space to keep between themselves and patients in various situations, so that both parties feel comfortable.

For *intimate interaction*, 7.5–45 cm is the average range. This distance is used for confidential information—a whisper can be heard at this distance by most people. It is also used in nonverbal communication, such as putting an arm around the shoulder to comfort someone or cuddling an infant. For *personal interaction*, when you are discussing personal matters, the range is approximately 0.4–1.2 m. At this distance, a soft voice can be heard by the person with normal hearing but people at a farther distance cannot overhear the conversation. This is the distance to maintain when you are discussing personal matters with the patient. You should be near enough to shake hands or touch the patient's shoulder.

Distances from 1.2–3.7 m are used for most *social interactions* (as in small group discussions). The normal speaking voice is used, but it is important to remember that it can be heard by others within the range. This distance is suited to discussions on nonpersonal matters. In *public interactions*, such as teaching in a classroom or giving a talk to a fairly large group of people (more than 10 to 12), the distance may be beyond 4 m. One has to be careful in these situations to speak in a loud, clear voice and to enunciate words clearly. About 6 to 7.5 m is usually as far as the average person can project the voice indoors without the use of a microphone, although some people may be able to do so up to 30 m outdoors (Smith & Cantrell, 1988).

Many of the measures nurses use in caring for patients necessitate being in the intimate range of interaction. People often feel uncomfortable at this distance with someone they do not know well, and they may react with a reflex withdrawal. The nurse should, whenever possible, alert the patient beforehand as to what he or she is going to do, so that the patient isn't alarmed by sudden actions at close range.

Listening attentively is an active process. The patient must have the nurse's undivided attention. Some people feel that the nurse should not take notes when talking to a patient to obtain information; others, however, feel that taking notes does not hinder the communication process. Certainly, if a lot of information is needed from the patient, it is difficult to remember everything that has been said without the benefit of notes. In fact, some patients may feel better listened to, knowing someone is caring enough to take down their words carefully. Again, patients are individuals with unique thoughts and beliefs. A simple statement of courtesy, such as, "Ms. Mauro, I want to make sure I hear you correctly; do you mind if I take some notes during our interview?" will demonstrate the intent of your action: to hear the patient's concerns fully and truly.

RESPONSES THAT HELP

MINIMAL RESPONDERS Sometimes just a word or a nod of the head is sufficient to give the patient the feeling that the nurse is interested in what is being said and would like the patient to continue. Words or utterances such as "Mmm," "Yes" or "I understand" have been termed **minimal responders** and are frequently used to reassure the patient of attentiveness.

SILENCE Sometimes it is best not to say anything, particularly if the nurse feels that the patient has something to add to an earlier statement. Most of us feel uncomfortable when conversation lapses and, if a pause lasts too long, we want to rush in to fill the space. Often, however, people need to think about what they are going to say and, given a little time, will continue with their train of thought. On the other hand, the person may decide that he or she does not want to pursue the matter any further and will introduce a new topic. The nurse should not press, nor give the appearance of prying into the patient's private affairs. Some people just do not like to talk about personal matters, and the nurse should respect their wishes in this regard. Sometimes, just sitting quietly with the patient or walking together down the corridor is enough to convey that the nurse understands the patient's feelings.

TOUCH Touch is a very important form of nonverbal communication for nurses. We use our hands in so many of our nursing measures. Touching a patient's hand or shoulder or holding a sobbing child can convey empathy and attentiveness. There is often no need for words. Touch is something that has to be used with discretion because, as we have already mentioned, some people find touch uncomfortable and disrespectful.

REFLECTING FEELINGS Another way of indicating interest and attention is through the reflection of feelings the patient has expressed. People sometimes express their feelings directly in words, for example, "I was so angry that I ..." Sometimes a description of actions allows the nurse to identify the feelings behind the actions. For instance, if a patient says, "I banged on the door," he or she is obviously expressing feelings of frustration and probably hostility towards whomever was on the other side of the door.

The nurse may also pick up clues about the patient's feelings from nonverbal behaviour, as discussed earlier in this chapter. The nurse might respond in words that acknowledge the feelings, for example, "I understand that you were angry [or annoyed, or hurt]" or "I can see that this bothers you." Although it can be useful to use the patient's own words in response, it is more important to reflect his or her feelings. Repeating the individual's words can sometimes make the nurse's response sound mechanical, as if parroting a learned response.

REPEATING KEY WORDS OR PHRASES At times, though, it is helpful to repeat key words or phrases that the patient has used, particularly if a number of thoughts have been expressed at one time. To use an example, a person might say, "Nothing seems to have gone right since I had that operation a year ago. I can't seem to work the way I used to. I haven't been able to go to the club either and I miss that. The club members are a very nice group of people." Here it might be useful for the nurse to pick up the key phrase "since I had that operation a year ago," rather than responding to the specific mention of the club. The nurse could then explore how things have changed for the patient rather than becoming sidetracked on a discussion of the various club members. Repeating a key word or phrase helps to keep the conversation focussed on important issues rather than irrelevant items.

USING OPEN-ENDED QUESTIONS OR STATEMENTS If the nurse wishes to obtain more information about a specific point, it is often helpful to repeat a part of a question or statement that gives the patient an opportunity to say more. The nurse might say, "You said that you had an operation a year ago; perhaps you could tell me more about it." Or, the nurse might simply ask, "You had an operation a year ago?" Sometimes the nurse can use an open-ended statement or question, such as "You were going to say ..." or "Would you like to tell me more about it?" to elicit more information.

ASKING FOR CLARIFICATION Sometimes it is difficult to identify feelings or to understand the meaning of a person's words. The nurse might sometimes need to ask for clarification. Phrases such as "you mean that you were angry?" or "am I right in thinking that you felt guilty [or depressed, or sad]?" are examples of responses the nurse could make to verify impressions. Asking for clarification also helps to indicate to the patient that the nurse is trying to understand his or her point of view.

EXPLORING ALTERNATIVES Sometimes the nurse can help patients explore possibilities for resolving problems that they have identified. An awareness of factors in the situation that the patient may not be aware of can be useful when selecting strategies to enable the patient to work through problems to create solutions. The nurse should be careful, however, not to give personal opinions on what the patient should do, but rather to enable consideration of all factors and possible alternatives in the situation.

RESPONSES THAT HINDER

DISMISSIVE REASSURANCE Responses that hinder the flow of conversation can be made if the nurse does not think about the impact of his or her words. One of the most common ways of cutting off communication is the use of dismissive reassurance. Nurses want to make the patient feel better and, therefore, often say things such as "don't worry, everything is going to be all right," "everybody feels like that," or "we haven't lost a patient yet." Comments such as these may be said with the intention of reassurance, but they may convey to the patient that the nurse is minimizing their problem.

SOCIAL CLICHÉS Closely allied to dismissive reassurance as hindering responses are the social clichés that seem to come almost automatically to our lips when we are not thinking about what we are saying. Expressions such as "you'll feel better after a good night's sleep," "your doctor knows what is best for you," and "everything will work out in time" are examples of common clichés, that is, pat answers that are trite and have lost their meaning through overuse. They tend to convey to the patient that the nurse isn't really listening.

HOSTILITY People who are anxious frequently react with anger and hostility to those around them. Nurses and other health professionals often bear the brunt of this anger from patients and their families, and it can be difficult not to be hostile in return. A hostile response made by a nurse, such as "you shouldn't say things like that," can humiliate the patient and, most certainly, will hinder the progress of the nurse–patient relationship. A statement along the lines of "this experience must be terribly difficult for you" can enable the patient to express anxiety directly. In turn the nurse will be able to offer support in an effective manner.

IMPOSING VALUES The nurse should be careful not to impose personal values on the patient. "It was wrong of you to do that," or "if I were you, I would have done this or that," are examples of evaluative responses that are best avoided, since they neither support the self-esteem of the patient nor facilitate effective problem solving.

GIVING ADVICE Giving advice implies to patients that the nurse knows better than they do what they should do. If your advice is being requested on matters pertaining to the patient's health, this is an area in which you are expected to have more knowledge, and advice may be appropriate. Advising people on the conduct of personal matters other than health is generally not acceptable. For example, statements such as "I would tell your sister to stop bothering you," or "If I were you, I'd sell the house and move to a condominium" are likely to cut off communication. Most people don't want advice, unless they specifically ask for it. Even if a patient asks for your opinion, it is wise to refrain from giving advice in areas in which you are not an acknowledged expert. Even when it is a matter of health, it is preferable to help patients to explore alternatives, so they can make their own decisions, rather than giving cut-and-dried answers.

PROBING We have already mentioned that the nurse should avoid probing into a patient's private life. Exceptions to this rule exist in the area of psychiatric and mental health nursing. In this area the patient will often expect and accept that feelings about personal matters will be explored. Questions such as "why do you feel this way?" or statements such as "tell me more about your relationship with your sister" tend to be probing unless the patient's specific problem necessitates exploration of this nature. Often, the patient may not know the answer, or may resent the intrusion. Patients can be placed in uncomfortable positions when they are asked to explain their actions. Silence can often be used with an attentive manner to enable patients to explore their feelings, without causing them to feel as if their privacy has been invaded.

BELITTLING Belittling the feelings or actions of another person engenders resentment and diminishes self-esteem. Saying things such as "other people don't seem to feel this way" conveys to patients that there must be something wrong with them to be reacting in this fashion. Telling patients about other people's accomplishments (or problems that are greater than theirs) makes them feel small and insignificant. If a postpartum patient says, "My stitches hurt" and the nurse answers, "You have to expect a little pain. My sister told me she couldn't sit down for a week after she had her baby," the patient is not likely to confide further in the nurse.

REJECTION The nurse can cut off communication, consciously or unconsciously, by rejecting the patient's feelings, thoughts or actions. Statements such as "you shouldn't feel like that," "I don't want to hear about it" or "how could anyone do that?" give the impression that the patient's thoughts, feelings or actions are unworthy. The patient is likely, then, to avoid talking further about that subject, and may be hesitant to bring up other matters. Rejection can also be communicated by nonverbal means. Turning away from a person, averting the eyes and subconsciously backing away can all indicate rejection.

A CASE IN POINT

The following example shows how the nurse can affect the patient's well-being through communication.

Mr. Antonio Niccolini is a 64-year-old widower who was admitted to the hospital suffering from difficulty in breathing and pain in his chest, left arm and back. Mr. Niccolini emigrated from Italy 50 years ago and, although he is fluent in English, he can still communicate in Italian. He lives with his daughter and son-in-law and their four teenage children in a predominantly Italian neighbourhood. He is a baker, head of the family business, which he runs with his three sons, who live in the same neighbourhood. Mr. Niccolini's working day is usually from 04:00 to 18:00 hours, six days a week. He smokes about a pack of cigarettes a day. He enjoys food and is consequently overweight. He drinks what he considers a moderate amount of wine every day. He has never been hospitalized before and appears very anxious about being separated from his family.

Mr. Niccolini is sitting up in bed playing solitaire and muttering to himself when the nurse walks in.

N.: Good morning, Mr. Niccolini. How are you feeling this morning?

Mr. N.: What's good about it? I feel fine. Why can't I go home? I just sit here all day. Why can't I have a cigarette and some decent food? How can you expect me to eat these meals? Now, what I would like is a good steak, some decent bread and a little wine. I can't even taste the food you give me here.

N.: You seem to be upset this morning, Mr. Niccolini.

(reflecting feeling)

You say you want to go home?

(picking up key words)

Mr. N.: Yes, I want to go home. Nobody's doing anything for me here. They just take my temperature and my blood pressure now and then, and expect me to lie around like this. I have better things to do with my time.

N.: You feel you have a lot to do.

(reflecting feeling and asking for clarification)

Mr. N.: Yes, like who's looking after the bakery, for example? They need me there.

N.: Do your sons work in the bakery with you?

(asking for clarification)

Mr. N.: Yes, yes, my sons. But they all have their own jobs to do—who's going to make the bread? I always make it myself every morning. They need me.

N.: I'm sure they do need you, Mr. Niccolini. Is someone making the bread now while you are in the hospital?

(accepting the patient's feelings and helping him to explore the situation)

Mr. N.: Yes, my oldest boy. But he has his jobs to do too. And who will mind the counter when everyone is busy?

N.: You mind the counter as well as make the bread?

(picking up key phrase)

Mr. N.: My daughter does most of the time, but I help out when things get busy. Luigi comes in and helps on the weekends.

N.: Luigi?

(asking for clarification)

Mr. N.: He's my oldest grandson. He seems to like the bakery or maybe he just likes the money he earns.

N.: Could Luigi come in and help after school?

(helping the patient to explore solutions)

Mr. N.: That might be an idea. Luigi is 17 now and should be taking more responsibility. I'll call my daughter and see about it.

When the nurse comes back a little later, Mr. Niccolini seems a little more cheerful.

N.: Well, Mr. Niccolini, you look as if you are feeling a little bit better now. Did that conversation with your daughter help?

(showing interest in the patient)

Mr. N.: Yes, it did, but I just remembered something.

N.: What's that, Mr. Niccolini?

(encouraging the patient to elaborate)

Mr. N.: I'm supposed to give a speech at the bakers' association meeting next week. I've never missed a meeting. I guess that's how I became president. Now I won't be able to go on the day I'm supposed to give my speech.

N.: Do the members of the association know you are in the hospital?

(picking up key words and helping patient to explore the situation)

Mr. N.: No. But my sons will tell them at the meeting tonight. Two meetings in a row I'm going to miss.

N.: Would you like to talk with one of the other members? The vice-president, perhaps?

(helping patient to explore the possibilities to resolve problem)

Mr. N.: Yes, I would, but not until tomorrow. Otherwise, they might decide to let someone else give my speech, and I want to give it myself later on, when I'm out of hospital.

Interviewing

The interview is a basic tool of communication that is used a great deal by health professionals, although its use is not, of course, limited to the health field. Most nursing students will have had experience with interviews. If you have applied for a summer or full-time job, for example, you have probably had an interview with your prospective employer.

In the health field, the interview is used for a number of different purposes. Nurses, in their practice, may use interviewing for gathering information or for verifying it, for assessing the results of nursing care, in counselling people about health matters, in planning care with patients and as a therapeutic tool.

When planning an interview, the nurse should take into account not only its purpose, but also the time and the setting. The nurse should be familiar with some of the basic techniques of interviewing, such as those used in beginning and ending an interview, and in eliciting specific information. As with other skills, interviewing requires practice. Many textbooks and articles have been written on interviewing, and the nurse will probably want to supplement the introductory material presented here with additional readings from the list of references suggested at the end of the chapter.

Setting the Time and Place for the Interview

An adequate amount of time should be set aside; how long is considered adequate will depend on the purpose and nature of the interview. Judgement must be exercised about both the length of time allotted for the interview and the time at which it takes place. If a patient is seriously ill, or has just been admitted to the hospital and is having numerous tests and examinations, it may be best to delay an interview until an appropriate time. Also, if the patient appears to be fatigued, it is wise to terminate an interview and complete the session at another time. Interviews should be scheduled for a time when both the patient and the nurse are free from other commitments. They should not conflict with appointments the patient has for x-rays, laboratory tests, treatments or visiting hours. Nor should the nurse feel hurried or rushed because of other commitments. In short, the nurse should strive to create a relaxed, unhurried atmosphere.

It is always best to have a quiet and private room in which to conduct an interview. This is not always possible in our busy and often crowded health agencies. It is important, though, that the person being interviewed has the undivided attention of the nurse and that confidentiality is being respected. A corner of a lounge or office can be used, or the curtains can be pulled around the bed if the patient is in the hospital and not in a private room.

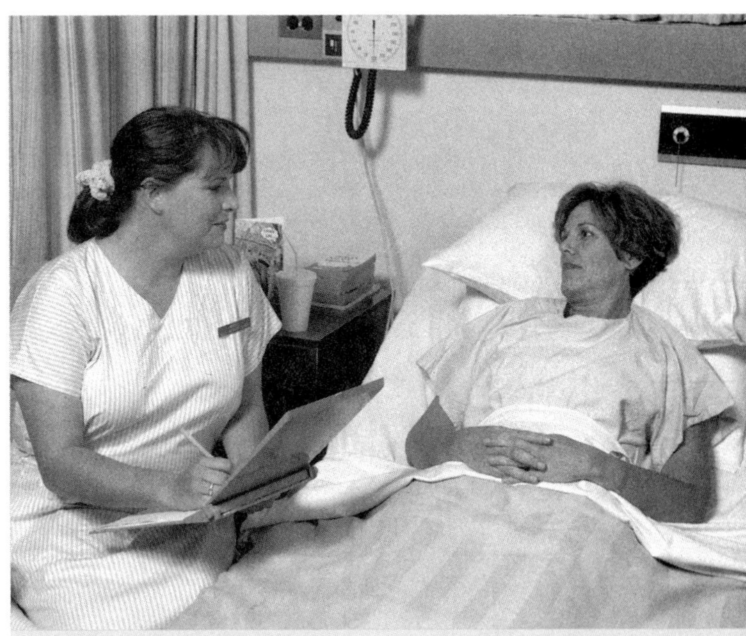

Nurses may use interviews for a number of different purposes in a variety of situations.

Beginning an Interview

An interview is essentially a conversation between two people. Often, when the patient has just been admitted to the agency, it is a conversation between two strangers. The nurse, as the interviewer, has a responsibility to put the other person at ease. For the beginning student, who may be a bit apprehensive about interviewing someone, it is helpful to remember that the patient, too, is probably anxious. Most people who seek the help of health professionals are either ill or in some way concerned about their health. Even those who are well and attending a health maintenance clinic usually have some minor worries. It helps if the nurse observes the common courtesies of greeting people—by name, with a smile or a handshake, by offering a seat (in an ambulatory setting) or asking permission to sit down and talk (if the patient is in an inpatient facility). The nurse should also introduce him- or herself by name. These courtesies convey a feeling of respect for the person who is being interviewed and help to put him or her at ease.

The nurse should also state the purpose of the interview and the approximate amount of time it will take. This information helps to set the climate for the interview. A patient will feel more comfortable knowing what to expect and what the purpose of the interview is. The nurse might say, in an initial assessment interview, for example, that the purpose is to learn something about the patient so that care can be planned to suit individual needs and preferences.

Eliciting Specific Information

Although the nurse often has specific information to obtain from the patient during the interview, it should not be conducted as a strict, one-way question-and-answer session. It may be a structured interview in the sense that the nurse controls and directs the conversation, as when gathering information in the assessment interview, but the patient should feel free to discuss feelings and concerns. Most people will give all the information needed, and more, if an open climate is created.

When there is specific information that the nurse wants to obtain, some direct questions will have to be asked. In such cases it is probably a good idea to start with immediate concerns, that is, the patient's feelings and perceptions about the subject of the interview, without interjecting too many questions in the beginning. If the nurse does not allow the patient to speak freely, important factors may be missed.

It is usually considered most useful, in asking questions, to start with the general and then proceed to specific details. People usually respond much better to impersonal questions at first. The nurse should leave the more personal ones until the patient has had a chance to get to know the nurse a little during the course of the interview. In this age of information, most people are used to filling in forms and answering questions about their name, age, education and place of employment. These are considered relatively impersonal items. An individual's likes, dislikes and feelings are more personal. If the specific information to be elicited requires asking such questions, these should be left until after the general questions have been answered.

Ending an Interview

When the purpose of the interview has been accomplished, the nurse should take some time to ask if the patient has any questions, or if there are other things that he or she is concerned about that were not discussed. Patients often feel reluctant to take up a busy nurse's time. Taking a few minutes to listen to patient concerns often saves the nurse

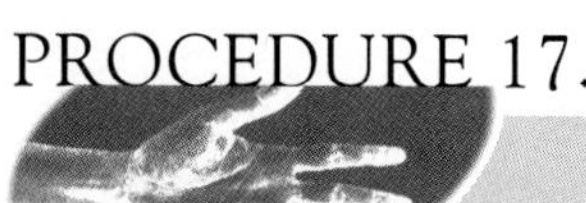

PROCEDURE 17.1 Admission to a Health Care Facility

Action	Rationale
1. Prepare the area and gather equipment required for assessment, e.g., sphygmomanometer, stethoscope, thermometer.	Facilitates efficiency and economy of time.
2. Receive the patient in a welcoming manner. Introduce self to patient and accompanying family or friend. If applicable, introduce to roommates.	Establishes rapport; addresses sensitive emotions and expectations.
3. Assess familiarity to hospital and orientation needs, e.g., any previous experience. If required, provide information pamphlets and orientation to:	
• hospital routines and policies, e.g., mealtimes, visiting hours, smoking restrictions, cellular phone use, bringing appliances into hospital	Promotes safety.
• unit layout, cafeteria location for visitors, lounge, chaplain, use of television and telephones.	Facilitates adjustment.
4. Introduce patient to the individual bed unit, e.g., explain and demonstrate as needed operation of the bed, side rails, bedside stand, overbed table, lights and call bell.	Allays anxiety.
5. Draw bed curtains and allow time for the patient to undress, if indicated.	Providing privacy shows respect.
6. Ask patient if he/she wishes the person who has accompanied him/her to stay during history taking.	Establishes trust and shows respect.
7. Complete required forms according to policies: detailed nursing history, and valuables record.	Provides basis for continuity and supportive care. Prevents loss; provides security of belongings.
8. Take the patient's vital signs, height and weight; do appropriate health assessments; note allergies. Document according to hospital policies.	Establishes areas for ongoing assessment and evaluation of the patient's status; promotes safety.
9. Begin gathering information required for discharge planning; document in patient's chart.	Initiates planning for discharge; promotes awareness of discharge concerns.
10. Explain routine tests, if applicable.	Decreases anxiety; provides opportunity to clarify information.
11. Provide opportunities throughout admission process for questions.	Promotes patient participation in decision making.
12. Address special wishes, leave patient comfortable.	Allows time for rest and promotes well-being.
13. Communicate as necessary with other health professionals and departments relevant information of the patient's admission, e.g., dietitian, social worker, chaplain. Document.	Provides continuity of care.

time in the long run, since patients are less apt to make frequent requests later if they have been reassured that the nurse is concerned about them.

In terminating an interview, it is again important to observe social courtesies. Thanking patients for their time, saying that you will see them again and assuring them that they can call on you if they are concerned about anything, are all ways of conveying that they are worthy of respect (Braverman, 1990; Justice, 1986; Cameron, 1982; Haselfeld, 1990).

Admission and Discharge

Admission and discharge from a health care facility, as we have discussed in Chapter 9, can be stressful and anxiety-producing events for some patients and family members. Using effective therapeutic communication will create a warm, caring introduction, establish a positive initial impression and decrease anxiety.

Exchanging information and coordinating care during the initial interaction and throughout the patient's stay

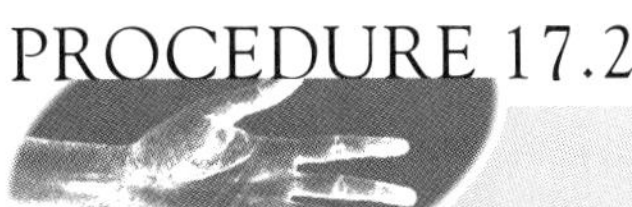

PROCEDURE 17.2 Discharge from a Health Care Facility

Action	Rationale
1. Perform ongoing assessments of patient's post-hospitalization and referral needs throughout his or her stay.	Helps with planning and coordinating of other health services. Ensures a smooth transition to home or other health care facility.
2. Review assessment and mutual goals by involving patient, family and multidisciplinary team.	Identifies needs, safety risks, environmental limitations and need for home or other facility. Promotes patient participation in planning for discharge and maintenance of health and healing.
3. Check physician's orders for discharge, medications, treatments, special appliances, referral and appointments.	Meets facility's requirements for physician's authorization for discharge. Communicates activity restrictions to promote healing.
4. Plan and provide discharge teaching for continued health care at home or transfer to another health care facility regarding: • treatments and medical attention • coordination with other health professionals.	Provides appropriate referrals to other health professionals in the community. Provides continuity of medications and treatments. Provides appropriate information and meets support needs as required.
5. Meet patient's and family's need for information and explanation with pamphlet and ongoing teaching; provide opportunity to ask questions.	Allows for learning and clarification; relieves anxiety.
6. Determine transportation arrangements. If patient is being transferred to another health care facility or unit, ensure appropriate paperwork is completed prior to departure.	Ensures appropriate means of transport according to patient's health status. Ensures continuity of care.
7. Follow health care facility's policies and procedures in returning all valuables, and obtain signature on completed forms as required.	Prevents loss and ensures return of belongings. Fulfills legal responsibility.
8. Assist patient to appropriate transport method for discharge, e.g., wheelchair or stretcher.	Provides safe discharge from unit.
9. Follow facility's policies regarding escorting patient to entrance/unit within agency or transferring to vehicle.	Ensures safe exit and ends liability for facility.
10. Upon return to unit, complete charting and discharge summary according to policies. Notify appropriate departments about the patient's transfer or discharge as necessary, e.g., dietary, pharmacy, housekeeping. Prepare unit for new admission.	Promotes effective communication between and among departments.

makes for a successful transition to home or another health agency. Flexibility in these processes is encouraged to meet the patient's and family needs (see Procedures 17.1 and 17.2).

Communicating with Other Members of the Health Team

Nurses seldom work in isolation. Even in a remote nursing station where the nurse may be the sole provider of health care for a community, there is almost always telephone or, at least, radio contact with a base hospital where communication with other members of the health team is possible. More usually, the nurse is employed in a busy, urban health agency with many nurses and a variety of other health professionals. Irrespective of the setting, nurses, by virtue of their roles, must be excellent communicators.

Communication with other members of the health team is an important part of the nurse's work. It is essential for facilitating the process of patient care. Information gathered by all team members provides the basis for planning comprehensive care for the patient. Sharing information helps to avoid duplication of effort in gathering data and also enables each team member to benefit from the information others have collected. Communication is also essential in the planning of patient care; it ensures that everyone shares the same goals for the patient and that care is coordinated and people are not working at cross-purposes.

The actual implementation of health care today is also very much a team effort. The provision of comprehensive care requires the skills and talents of many different disciplines. The physician and the nurse have always worked closely together in many aspects of patient care and continue to do so. With the number of specialized workers in the health field today, it is more than ever essential that all coordinate their efforts in caring for patients. There must be adequate, effective communication channels for the achievement of this coordination.

Communication between members of the health team takes place in many ways. A great deal of information is exchanged informally, through face-to-face meetings and telephone conversations. But there are also more formal channels, both oral and written, that help to facilitate the exchange of information.

The patient's record is one very important tool that helps to keep all team members up to date on the latest information about a patient and the most recent developments regarding the patient's progress. (Patient records will be discussed in detail in Chapter 19.) Other common communication media that the nurse will use frequently are reports, both oral and written, Kardex, consultations, conferences, referrals and patient rounds.

Owing to recent health care restructuring, "floating" and the delegation of nursing tasks are becoming more prevalent. With this in mind, it is essential that nurses possess strong communication skills. For example, when floating to an unfamiliar unit, the nurse must be able to access information quickly. What are unit routines? Who has first call? When is it appropriate to call the physician? Likewise, with delegation, it is important for nurses to be aware of the scope of practice of other health professionals (Sieh & Brentin, 1997).

REPORTS

Reporting information to other members of the health team is essential if they are to be briefed on events that have taken place (or are likely to take place), be told of developments that have occurred in regard to patients' progress and be alerted to things to watch for in the care of specific patients. Reports may be given either orally or in writing. At the end of each shift, members of the nursing team usually report orally to the oncoming staff on the progress of each patient, including treatments or other activities that are still in progress. The nurse may, for example, say that Dr. X will be phoning Mr. Smith's medication orders this evening, or that the admitting department has called to say that the unit will be receiving a new patient.

Many agencies are now using tape recorders to make the change-of-shift report less cumbersome. Each nurse who has been responsible for the care of a group of patients can dictate the report about those patients. Nurses coming on duty then need to receive only a brief report from the charge nurse going off duty and can obtain direct information about

Confused about End-of-Shift Reporting?

Here's a checklist:

- patient's name, age, room number and primary diagnosis
- any nursing care needed in the next 2–3 hours, e.g.:
  - dressing changes
  - vital signs
  - pain medication due
  - IV therapy start
  - preprocedural checklist
  - specimen collection
- any change in the patient's condition and what you did about it, e.g.:
  - blood pressure 200/140 at 19:00; physician notified
  - red itchy rash following IV antibiotics; diphenhydramine (Benadryl) administered as ordered
- other needs as they arise, e.g.:
  - family interactions
  - learning needs and progress
  - discharge plans
  - interdisciplinary interventions.

Advantages and Disadvantages of Reporting Methods

Method	Advantage	Disadvantage
Oral	• access to in-depth information • ability to interact with outgoing staff	• time-consuming • patients unattended
Taped	• effective use of time • ability to reaccess information	• inability to clarify information
Written	• effective use of time; data can be recorded throughout shift	• illegible writing
Patient rounds	• ability to interact with patient • ability to review aspects of care	• privacy concerns

SOURCE: Sieh & Brentin, 1997.

each patient from the tape-recorded report. The charge nurse reports to the nurse manager about the patients on the unit. A transfer report is given when a patient moves from one unit to another. This may done over the phone or in person.

In addition to patient care reports, most health agencies have a large number of other reports and forms that nurses use. These vary from agency to agency, and nurses must familiarize themselves with those used in the agency in which they are working. There are usually forms for requesting laboratory, x-ray and other types of diagnostic tests, forms for recording the administration of narcotics and other controlled drugs (a count has to be kept of these), forms for ordering drugs and other supplies. Recent transition to electronic documentation has eliminated the need for many of these forms. The accident (incident) report, which is completed whenever an unusual occurrence takes place, will be reviewed in Chapter 30.

Consultations

Often nurses feel the need to consult with other health professionals about the care of patients. If there is a clinical nurse specialist available, the nurse may want to consult with him or her about the patient's plan of care, or about unusual problems the patient has.

Physicians consult with other physicians; they frequently call in specialists to see patients and give opinions regarding diagnostic or therapeutic measures. The nurse will note on the patient's record the requests for specialist consultations and the specialist's report.

Conferences

Nurses and other members of the health team meet routinely in a team conference to exchange information about their patients and to review and revise their care plans. Until very recently, team conferences have been used most frequently in rehabilitation settings, in community health agencies, in psychiatric settings and in agencies providing long-term care. Health care reform has required acute settings to engage in more team conferences.

Referrals

Referrals are basically of two types: those requesting the services of another department within an agency in the care of a patient, and those referring a patient to another agency for care. In a community health agency or the outpatient department of a hospital, patients are frequently referred from one service to another for specialized care. A patient might be referred to the dental or eye clinic, for example, or to the nutritionist or social worker from a generalized service. In a hospital setting, a referral for specialized services might be made to departments such as social services, physiotherapy or respiratory therapy.

Patients may also be referred from one agency to another. A community agency might refer an individual to a hospital for inpatient care (the patient would be admitted under the care of the attending physician), or a hospital might refer a patient to the community. If a patient is being discharged from hospital and requires home care services, a referral would be made to the appropriate agency. Referrals

NURSES at work: Clear Communication

Fatima, a new graduate working as a casual RN on a busy medical ward, recalls the first time she had to telephone a patient's physician to inform her of an assessment:

It was my first night working on my own. I received a report on a new patient who had been admitted late that afternoon with abdominal ascites and was in for tests. She had undergone a procedure to drain fluid from her abdomen, and the fear was that she had advanced liver cancer.

The nurse reporting off shift had written that the patient had not been able to urinate. When I went in to assess the patient I asked her if she had been up to the toilet, but she said no, and told me she was in too much pain.

I administered the analgesic ordered for her and asked her to ring the bell for assistance to use the commode. I noted that her IV was running at 150 mL/h, which was a lot of fluid to go in and not come out. I listened to her chest, which was clear, but couldn't palpate her bladder because her abdomen was so distended.

After assessing the rest of my patients I returned to reassess her and learned she still hadn't any urge to urinate. This time when I listened to her chest I picked up crackles in her lower lobes. I knew she was in danger of fluid overload due to urinary retention, and I knew she needed medical intervention. However, I didn't have all that much faith in my nursing judgement yet!

I went to an experienced colleague and told him of my findings and my concerns. He reassured me that my judgement was on track, so, with a pounding heart, I grabbed the chart and called the physician. I don't even remember what I said, but I guess I got the gist of it across, because she immediately ordered a urinary catheter to be inserted, a diuretic to be given and the IV fluid rate to be cut in half.

Since that night, I've had many telephone conversations with many physicians, and I've learned to keep my communication simple and concise, but with all relevant information: my assessment, including baseline vital signs; my nursing interventions; medications administered; laboratory results. I always keep the chart in front of me, so I can give additional information if required and check for allergies if a new medication is ordered. I learned that my voice is as imperative to the well-being of my patient as are my clinical nursing skills.

— *Fay Lapka, RN*

may be made by a community health nurse (or a school nurse) for individuals to receive care from any number of agencies in the community.

A referral system promotes continuity of care. It is essential that the agency to which the patient is being referred have sufficient information to ensure that continuity. Most agencies have referral forms on which summary information about a patient is written; it is often the nurse who is responsible for completing these forms, although policies vary. In a hospital, the patient's record would be available to the member of the department being called in to see a patient.

Patient Rounds

Another means of communicating information about patients is through multidisciplinary patient rounds. We have already mentioned one type, where nurses make the rounds on a nursing unit during the change-of-shift report. The nurse usually makes rounds with the physician when visiting patients on a hospital nursing unit. A considerable amount of information is exchanged at this time, as opinions are shared regarding the patient's progress and plans are discussed for care. Teaching rounds are also made for the benefit of students; both medical and nursing schools use patient rounds as learning experiences for students.

Care for the Caregiver

Nursing can be an extremely fulfilling and rewarding profession; it can also take its toll in stress. Nurses hear and vicariously experience many stories that are painful, grief-filled and traumatic. How nurses, as individuals, learn to communicate their needs and "talk out" these stories rather than carry them around can spell the difference between burnout and health. Nurses benefit by sharing their stories with one another, or with a trusted friend, family member or counsellor. Support in the workplace—both informal and formal—has recently been recognized as a crucial aspect of employee health (Balzer-Reiley, 1996; Phillips & Benner, 1994).

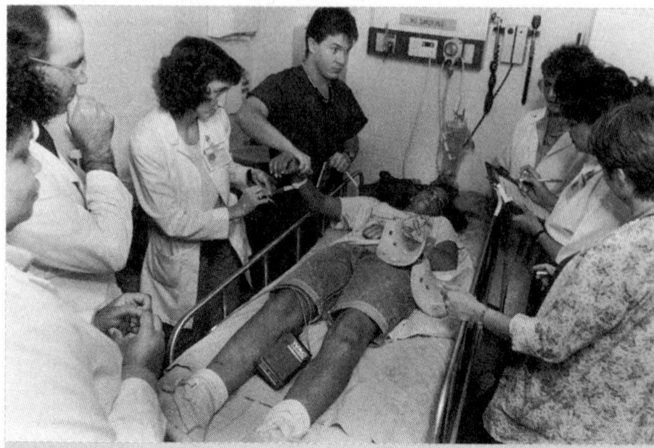

A multidisciplinary team prepares to make rounds on a nursing unit.

Luci, an emergency nurse, tells of her need to "vent" after a trauma case:

> *I really enjoy being a nurse in the ER, but I couldn't keep working there if it weren't for my colleague and friend, Doug. Doug is an ER nurse as well, but at another hospital. Doug and I talk regularly on the phone, especially after either of us has had a tough shift. One night the paramedics brought in this young woman who had been assaulted. She was a mass of bruises and lacerations and shivering in shock. But the picture that stays with me is of her fingernails. Obviously, she was accustomed to keeping her nails long and manicured, with the latest nail-polish colour. Well, her nails were broken off and bent, and some of her nailbeds were bleeding; she had fought off her attacker with the only weapon she had. Although I've seen trauma many times, for some reason, that picture—this patient—stayed with me. It wasn't until I talked it out with Doug that I was able to sleep the next day. I don't know what I'd do without being able to vent to a caring colleague like Doug.*

While informal supports such as this are beneficial, many health facilities have recognized the need for a formally structured care for the caregiver program. Typical components can include staff support groups facilitated by external professional counsellors, occupational health services, referral to community resources through an Employee Assistance Program, customized benefits packages, flexible scheduling and paid leave (Geraci, Flannery, Filman, Durkee, & Lambert, 1997). While employers can make these supports available, the ultimate success of a care for the caregiver program depends on "staff members' willingness and ability to recognize stressful situations, to use the resources available to them and to take care of themselves" (Geraci et al., p. 103).

Factors That Impair Communication in the Clinical Setting

Verbal

- lack of interaction with staff/instructor
- inability to inform staff of their scope of practice
- inability to seek assistance/supervision
- inability to ask for ongoing evaluation
- discussion of patients' care in unsuitable locations
- verbal defensiveness when receiving feedback

Nonverbal

- inappropriate dress code
- inappropriate body language
- lack of initiative
- lack of confidence

SOURCE: Sieh & Brentin, 1997.

IN REVIEW

- The nurse–patient relationship is the core of nursing, often referred to as the therapeutic relationship. Based on shared trust, mutual respect and collaboration, this relationship includes elements of:
  - empathy
  - respect
  - authenticity (genuineness)
  - self-disclosure
  - warmth.
- The nurse–patient relationship has three phases:
  - orientation
  - working
  - termination.
- The process of communication involves four basic elements:
  - source (sender)
  - message
  - channel
  - receiver.
- Many factors can hinder or enhance communication, including:
  - culture
  - gender
  - nonverbal/verbal factors
  - timing
  - space
  - values (judgements)
  - environment
  - individual growth and development.
- Nurses can cultivate a climate for open communication by:
  - conveying a feeling of warmth and acceptance
  - having a genuine liking for people
  - employing a nonjudgemental approach
  - listening attentively.
- To foster communication, the nurse uses many communication techniques, including:
  - minimal responders
  - open-ended rather than closed-ended questions
  - silence
  - reflecting patients' feelings back to them
  - requesting clarification
  - exploring alternatives with patients and families.
- The primary purpose of a patient interview is to collect and validate information.
- The nurse communicates with other health professionals formally and informally, by means of:
  - patient records or Kardex files
  - reports (oral, taped and written)
  - consultation/conferences, referrals
  - interdisciplinary/multidisciplinary patient rounds.
- Because nursing is a stressful profession, supportive networks are needed both in and out of the workplace. Care for the caregiver programs is an important means of maintaining employee health.

Critical Thinking Activities

1. With the help of your instructor, select a patient from the clinical area in which you are working. Arrange a time to visit the patient, and, using the agency's form, take a nursing health history. Use the techniques outlined in the "Learning to Listen" section of this chapter to find out about the patient as a person.
   a. Write a short narrative report describing the patient as a person.
   b. List the techniques you found helpful in establishing a climate that encouraged the patient to communicate freely.
   c. Did the patient request information from you? If so, what information? How did you handle the request? What information did you volunteer?
   d. What listening techniques did you use to facilitate conversation between you and the patient?
   e. How did you terminate the interview?

KEY TERMS

collaborative p. 417
therapeutic relationship p. 417
empathy p. 417
receptivity p. 417
respect p. 417
climate of trust p. 418
genuineness p. 418
authenticity p. 418
self-disclosure p. 418
specificity p. 418
orientation phase p. 419
working phase p. 420
patient–nurse contract p. 420
termination phase p. 421
source p. 421
message p. 421
channel p. 421
receiver p. 421
feedback p. 421
jargon p. 425
warmth p. 428
listen p. 428
personal space p. 429
minimal responders p. 430

References

ADLER, R.B., ROSENFELD, L.B., & TOWNE, N. (1995). *Interplay: The process of interpersonal communication.* (5th ed.). Fort Worth, TX: Harcourt Brace Jovanovich.

BALZER-REILEY, J.W. (1996). *Communications in nursing.* (3rd ed.). St. Louis: Mosby.

BRAVERMAN, B.G. (1990). Eliciting assessment data from the patient who is difficult to interview. *Nursing Clinics of North America, 25,* 743–750.

CAMERON, J.E. (1982). "Giant leap forward" begins with the nurse interview. *Australian Nurses Journal, 12,* 47–48.

CRUSCO, A.H., & WETZEL, C.G. (1984). The Midas touch: The effects of interpersonal touch on restaurant tipping. *Personality and Social Psychology Bulletin, 10,* 512–517.

EKMAN, P. (1975, September). Face muscles talk every language. *Psychology Today, 9,* 35.

EKMAN, P., FRIESEN, W., O'SULLIVAN, M., & CHAN, A. (1987). Universal and cultural differences in the judgments of facial expressions. *Journal of Personality and Social Psychology, 53,* 712–717.

FORCHUK, C. (1992). The orientation phase of the nurse–patient relationship: How long does it take? *Perspectives in Psychiatric Care, 28,* 7–10.

FORCHUK, C., & BROWN, B. (1989). Establishing a nurse–patient relationship. *Journal of Psychosocial Nursing and Mental Health Services, 27,* 30–34.

GERACI, F., FLANNERY, J.S., FILMAN, J., DURKEE, L., & LAMBERT, A. (1997). Care for the caregiver. In *Casey House Hospice: A Model for Collaborative Care* (pp. 99–103). Toronto: Casey House Hospice.

GRENSING-POPHAL, L. (1997, October). Eight signs of poor communication. *Nursing 97* (27), 64.

GRIFFITH, J. (1997). *Eliminating generic-male language: Political statement or just good writing?* Unpublished work, Oak Ridge, TN: Roane State Community College.

HASELFELD, D. (1990). Patient assessment: Conducting an effective interview. *AORN Journal, 52,* 555–557.

HAYES, W.S., & DAVIS, L. (1980). What is a health care contract? *Health Values, 4*(2), 82–89.

HERJE, P.A. (1980, February). Hows and whys of patient contracting. *Nursing Educator,* 30–34.

HILLS, M., CHISAMORE, M., & LINDSEY, L. (1990). *On delivering care: An interpersonal workbook for nurses.* Victoria, BC: University of Victoria.

IRWIN, D.B., & SIMONS, J.A. (1994). *Lifespan developmental psychology.* Dubuque, IO: WCB Brown & Benchmark Publications.

JUSTICE, L.A. (1986). Skill sharpening methods in conducting patient interviews. *Today's OR Nurse, 8,* 32–35.

MANN, W.C., & LANE, J.P. (1991). *Assistive technology for persons with disabilities: The role of occupational therapy.* Rockville, MD: American Occupational Therapy Association.

MATSUMOTO, D. (1992). American–Japanese cultural differences in the recognition of universal facial expressions. *Journal of Cross-Cultural Psychology, 23,* 72–84.

MONTGOMERY, C.L. (1993). *Healing through communication: The practice of caring.* Newbury Park, CA: Sage.

NORTHOUSE, L.L., & NORTHOUSE, P.G. (1997). *Health communication strategies for health professionals.* (3rd ed.). Norwalk, CT: Appleton & Lange.

PEPLAU, H.E. (1991) *Interpersonal relations in nursing: A conceptual frame of reference for psychodynamic nursing.* New York: Springer.

PEPLAU, H.E. (1992). Interpersonal relations: A theoretical framework for application in nursing practice. *Nursing Science Quarterly, 5,* 13–18.

PHILLIPS, S., & BENNER, P. (1994). *Crises of care: Affirming and restoring caring practices in the helping profession.* Washington, DC: Georgetown University Press.

ROBINSON, M. (1997). Egos and eggshells. Greensboro, NC: Stanton & Harper.

ROGERS, E.M., & ROGERS, A. (1976). *Communication in organizations.* New York: The Free Press.

SIEH, A., & BRENTIN, L.K. (1997). *The nurse communicates.* Philadelphia: W.B. Saunders.

SMITH, B.J., & CANTRELL, P.J. (1988). Distance in nurse–patient encounters. *Journal of Psychosocial Nursing, 26,* 22–26.

STATUS OF DISABLED PERSONS SECRETARIAT & DEPARTMENT OF THE SECRETARY OF STATE OF CANADA. (1991). *A way with words: Guidelines and appropriate terminology for the portrayal of persons with disabilities.* Ottawa: Author.

WHY WE DON'T HEAR OTHERS. (n.d.) *Communication Briefings, 16*(4), 1.

WRIGHT, L.M., & LEAHY, M. (1994). *Nurses and families: A guide to family assessment and intervention.* (2nd ed.). Philadelphia: F.A. Davis.

VANCOUVER HEALTH DEPARTMENT. (1994). *Speech language pathology: When do you refer your preschooler?* [Pamphlet]. Vancouver: Author. (Catalogue no. HED595-94/12)

VANCOUVER HEALTH DEPARTMENT. (1995). *What if my child is having trouble speaking or learning to communicate with others?* [Pamphlet]. Vancouver: Author. (Catalogue no. HED504-95/04)

ZILM, G. (1998). *The SMART Way: An introduction to writing for nurses.* Toronto: Harcourt Brace Canada.

Additional Readings

ALFARO-LEFEVRE, R. (1998). *Applying nursing process: A step-by-step guide.* (4th ed.). Philadelphia: Lippincott.

COMMUNICATING WITH VENTILATED PATIENTS. (1997, August). *Nursing 97, 27,* 54.

HANLON, J.M. (1996). Teaching effective communication skills. *Nursing Management, 27*(4), 48B, 48D.

LOVERIDGE, C.E. (1996) Communicating, co-ordinating and collaborating through diversity. *Advanced Practice Nursing Quarterly, 2*(2), 75–78.

McLEOD, R.P. (1996). Your next patient does not speak English: Translation and interpretation in today's office. *Advanced Practice Nursing Quarterly, 2*(2), 10–14.

McLEOD, R.P., & BENTLEY, P.C. (1996). Understanding deafness as a culture with a unique language and not a disability. *Advanced Practice Nursing Quarterly, 2*(2), 50–58.

PRATT, J.R. (1996). Communicating with your subordinates: How? How much? *Home Health Care Management and Practice, 8*(5), 73–75.

SCHULTES, L.S. (1997). Humour with hospice clients: You're putting me on! *Home Healthcare Nurse, 15*(8), 561–566.

STUART, G.W., & LARAIA, M.T. (1998). *Stuart & Sundeen's principles and practices of psychiatric nursing.* (6th ed.). St. Louis: Mosby.

WOLFE, E. (1995, February 3). Mental health matters: Coping with caregiving. *Stratford (ON) Beacon Herald.*

Chapter 18

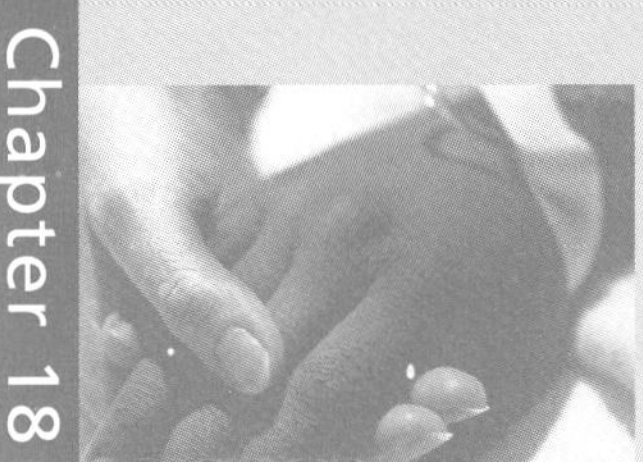

OUTLINE

Teaching and Learning Skills

Central Questions

1. Why is teaching such an important part of the nursing role?
2. How do we learn?
3. Why are teaching and learning considered reciprocal processes?
4. What factors need to be taken into consideration in helping people to learn?
5. What are the three main domains of learning?
6. What teaching strategies are most suitable for learning tasks in each domain?
7. How do you assess a person's learning needs?
8. Are there specific nursing diagnoses related to learning needs?
9. How do you plan, organize and implement a teaching–learning program?
10. How would you assess the success of the program?
11. How can you evaluate your teaching skills?
12. How can you get maximum benefit from your clinical learning experiences?

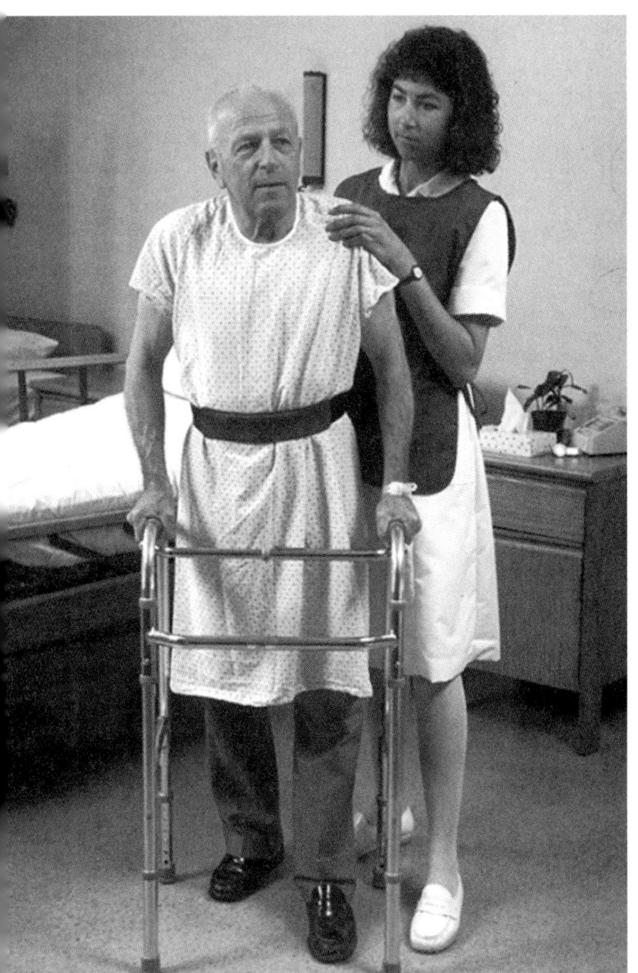

Introduction

Patient education is built on nurse–patient relationships that foster growth through respecting one another, caring, and working together. Patient education is the most powerful tool health professionals have to assure safer discharges from our care and to transfer power to the patient and the family.

Rankin and Stallings, 1990, p. 23

An integral component of nursing care is helping individuals and families learn what they need to know to promote, protect, maintain and restore health. Teaching is a part of the nurse's role through all stages of the life span and in all phases of the health continuum. In Chapter 5, teaching–coaching was identified as one of the major domains of nursing practice. Nurses play a key role in teaching and are regarded by the public as being knowledgeable about health. As people assume increasing responsibility for their own health, they need to gain the knowledge and skills that will enable them to meet their health needs competently and with confidence. As the provinces—and Canada as a whole—adjust to a restructured health care system, patient and public health education has increased in importance. The role of the individual as a health care consumer has changed. Accepting responsibility for preventive health care will bring the patient in contact with the nurse in a teaching relationship. Today, health professionals recognize the importance of sharing their knowledge and skills so that individuals and families can make informed health care decisions. Teaching should be incorporated into the nursing care of every health care consumer.

Health disciplines employ similar terminology with regard to the teaching–learning process. **Health education** is described by Coutts and Hardy (1985) as "a planned process aimed at helping individuals and communities achieve and maintain a level of health which is appropriate for them" (p. 14). **Client education** "is the use of the educational process for individuals who are partners in the health-education effort. The learner and teacher mutually identify the subject matter to be taught and then decide how the educational process will be carried out. Client education often implies an increasingly autonomous and self-directed role for the learner" (Boyd, Graham, Gleit & Whitman, 1998, p. 15). **Patient education** "is the use of the educational process for individuals, their families and other significant persons when dependent upon the health-care system for diagnosis, treatment or rehabilitation" (Boyd et al., 1998, p. 15). Table 18.1 compares the elements of patient education and health education.

In order to incorporate teaching into nursing care, nurses require an understanding of the teaching-learning process as well as the factors that influence an individual's ability to learn. These topics are covered in the first section of this chapter. The next section discusses the assessment of learning needs and the development, implementation and evaluation of teaching sessions. The final section of the chapter describes ways in which teaching–learning is viewed within nursing education.

TABLE 18.1 Comparison of patient education and health education

FOCUS	PATIENT EDUCATION	HEALTH EDUCATION
Philosophy	Patient use of information and skills for whatever purpose is desired	Behavioural change for health promotion and compliance with medical regimen
Unit of service	Individuals, families and other groups	Specific populations
Delivery system	Part of clinical care by all direct care providers in any setting	Campaigns that include mass media and work through community institutions
Content	Patient experiences, coping, helping patient develop self-management skills, decisional support	Risk factors, health behaviours
Theory base	Direction from field's theory of practice, learning and instructional theory	Behavioural science, epidemiology
Ethical concerns	Scientific stability and cultural bias of what patients are asked to learn; subtle manipulation possible in provider–patient relationship; inadvertent side effects (e.g., loss of self-confidence)	Scientific stability and cultural bias of what patients are asked to learn; manipulation by government, under which many programs are carried out; inadvertent side effects such as "blaming the victim"
Literature	Integration of literature of disease entity or health problem	Public health literature and certain specialized health education journals
Challenges	Reliable delivery system, including outcome measurement	Accessing very powerful provider–patient relationship

SOURCE: Redman, 1997, p. 4.

The Teaching–Learning Process

Learning is a lifelong process. We are constantly learning as we gain information, develop skills, acquire attitudes and apply these in adjusting to new situations. While theorists disagree about the precise definition of learning, they agree that to learn is to change, and that experience is the course of learning (Whitman, Graham, Gleit & Boyd, 1992). **Learning** is defined as "a change in the individual caused by the person's interaction with the environment" (Whitman et al., 1992, p. 52). Table 18.2 compares the learner characteristics of children and adults.

Teaching and learning are a collaborative process. The teacher's role is to assist learners to acquire the knowledge, skill and attitudes they need in order to learn. **Teaching** is an interactive process that facilitates learning. It is not just a matter of imparting information, of giving someone the ability to do something or of changing people's opinions or feelings. The behavioural changes must take place in the learner. The teacher can only guide and direct the learning process, so that it takes place more easily and more effectively (Benoliel & Soule, 1988; Benner, 1984).

Learning can take place either informally, through the ordinary activities of living, or formally, through a series of selected experiences designed to achieve specific goals. In the home, parents usually teach children basic hygiene measures, such as washing hands before meals and using facial tissues. Other sources—such as books, newspapers, magazines, television shows and the Internet—contribute to informal learning.

In informal teaching, there is no structured plan. Teaching occurs when a learning need becomes apparent. The majority of patient education is informal in nature. For example, during morning care, a patient may ask the nurse the purpose of taking a particular medication. The nurse can explain the need for the medication at this time.

There are situations where more structured health teaching is required. Because individuals are taking greater responsibility in health promotion, there has been a growing demand for planned programs. Wellness programs, for example, have developed in community centres as well as in corporations, industrial plants and other places of business as a cornerstone of occupational health. The promotion and protection of health are the primary focus of such programs. Many hospitals and long-term care and community agencies have separate patient education departments whose role is to provide resources to nurses. Other examples of formal, structured programs within a hospital or in the community include the Healthy Heart Program, and New Beginnings (for new mothers).

The Phenomenon of Learning

Theories have been postulated by numerous educators over the past century to explain the phenomenon of learning. Most theories have been based on studies that have measured the ease with which learning takes place (how much was learned? how long did it take?), the extent of learning retention (how much was retained? for how long?) and observations of changes in the thinking patterns of children as they develop. You are probably familiar with many of these learning theories from your introductory courses in psychology. Among the schools of thought that have influenced North American education are:

1. **The behaviourist school.** Proponents of this school believe that all learning is manifested in observable changes in behaviour and that learning can be controlled by manipulating factors in the environment.

TABLE 18.2 Comparison of learner characteristics between children and adults

CHARACTERISTICS	CHILDREN	ADULTS
Readiness to learn	Based primarily on biological development	Determined by life tasks, roles and immediate problems
Application of learning	Postponed application; subject-centred	Immediate application related to relevant problems
Orientation to learning	Dependent; other-directed	Independent; self-directed
Value of experiences	Experiences seen as external events	Experiences are internalized: they provide a foundation for further learning and may contribute resistance to change
Rate of learning	Quickly master isolated facts and concepts	Resistant to learning nonrelevant material; the aging process increases the time needed to complete some learning tasks
Barriers to learning	Few competing responsibilities for learning time; accustomed to formal learning through school experiences	Family, work or community responsibilities may compete for learning time and energy; anxieties about self-image as a learner may threaten

SOURCE: Boyd et al., 1998, p. 149.

Also known as operant conditioning, this stimulus–response–reinforcement model has been used in numerous behaviour modification programs to help people substitute desirable behaviours for undesirable ones.

2. **The cognitive school**. Believers in the cognitive model think that learning is not necessarily always observable; it is an intellectual process using cognitive skills. Learning, according to the cognitive theorists, can be thought of as information processing. Programmed learning texts and computer learning packages are based on this model of learning.
3. **The humanist school**. Humanists believe that learning is more than a mechanistic exercise; meaningful learning must involve the whole person including both the intellect and the emotions (Yelon & Weinstein, 1977).

As we noted in Chapter 1, there has been a growing disenchantment with science and a return to humanism and spirituality in many fields of endeavour. In education, the scientific, technological view of learning as operant conditioning or as information processing is giving way to the humanistic approach. One of the main proponents of this approach is Carl Rogers, a humanist whose work has influenced many nurse theorists. Rogers (cited in Knowles, 1990) believed that it is impossible to teach another person directly: one can only facilitate the learning.

The trend to humanism in education is in line with the broadened definition of health we discussed in Chapter 2, as a "resource for everyday living, encompassing social and personal resources, as well as physical capabilities." The humanist school of thought in education views the learner as a whole person and is concerned more with the overall growth of the individual in both cognitive and affective areas than with the content of what is taught per se. The role of the teacher has shifted, too, from that of instructor to that of facilitator (Yelon & Weinstein, 1977), in much the same way that the role of the nurse has shifted from care-provider to collaborator with the individual.

The fact that humanism has become the dominant philosophy in education does not negate the work by people of other schools of thought who have contributed greatly to our knowledge of the process of learning. In the process of teaching, most of us use concepts derived from behavioural theory, from cognitive theory and from humanist theory. Everyone does better when efforts are rewarded—when there is reinforcement of learning. This would happen, for example, when content and presentation are structured (as the cognitive theorists recommend) and we apply the humanist principles of respect for the total person (Yelon & Weinstein, 1977). Goodwin Watson developed a list of "what we know about learning" that incorporates findings from the research of educators from different schools of thought. Malcolm Knowles (1990), one of the leading figures in adult education, suggests that Watson's list could serve as "guidelines for the facilitation of learning."

Guidelines for the Facilitation of Teaching–Learning

Teaching

1. know the learner's capacities
2. motivate the learner
3. provide for learning activity
4. reinforce progress
5. give feedback
6. plan the teaching
7. check the teaching image
8. practise recognizing the teachable moment
9. facilitate discovery learning
10. encourage self-evaluation
11. be realistic.

Learning

1. may be conscious or unconscious
2. occurs when the individual is able to learn (based on language skills, developmental stage, absence of pain/denial)
3. occurs when the individual is willing to learn (based on level of anxiety, satisfaction with care, meaningful content)
4. occurs when material aids are actively used
5. is emotional as well as intellectual
6. is sometimes painful
7. arises out of experience.

SOURCE: Coutts & Hardy, 1985.

A number of factors affect the reciprocal process of teaching and learning. The most important variables in this process are the domains of learning, the characteristics of the learner, the characteristics of the teacher, teaching styles and the environment in which teaching–learning takes place.

Domains of Learning

There are three basic domains of learning: the **cognitive domain** (storage, recall, process of thinking), the **psychomotor domain** (skill acquisition) and the **affective domain** (attitudes, values, beliefs and feelings) (Babcock & Miller, 1994).

In teaching patients and their families, the nurse's primary role is to assist patients to use their knowledge and skill in day-to-day living. This involves the integration and application of knowledge, skills and attitudes—in other words, all three domains of learning. For example, a person may learn about nutrients and calories (cognitive domain) and develop skill in planning meals (psychomotor domain). However, unless a change of behaviour takes place—that is, the person begins to eat more nutritiously—learning will not have occurred (affective domain).

In any teaching situation, all three domains may be involved, or only one. Often, nurses need to teach patients and their families, addressing all three domains. Therefore, understanding the three domains of learning assists the nurse in developing an effective teaching plan.

Foundation Stones of Modern Adult Learning Theory

- Adults are motivated to learn as they experience needs and interests that learning will satisfy; therefore, these are the appropriate starting points for organizing adult learning activities.
- Adults' orientation to learning is life-centred; therefore, the appropriate units for organizing adult learning are life situations, not subjects.
- Experience is the richest resource for adults' learning; therefore, the core methodology of adult education is the analysis of experience.
- Adults have a deep need to be self-directed; therefore, the role of the teacher is to engage in a process of mutual enquiry with them rather than to transmit his or her knowledge to them and then evaluate their conformity to it.

SOURCE: Knowles, 1978, p. 31.

Characteristics of the Learner

"The chief factor that influences the nurse's teaching is the nature of the learner, the physical and emotional state, the age, social and cultural background, education and experience, the voluntary nature of the patient's relationship to the nurse as teacher" (Pohl, 1981, p. 53). In developing an educational program, the nurse must know something about the learner or learners.

Learning Levels of the Three Domains of Learning

Cognitive Learning Levels

- knowledge: facts, concepts
- comprehension: understanding
- application: using knowledge
- analysis: seeing relationships among ideas
- synthesis: forming new patterns of thought, ideas
- evaluation: critiquing value of ideas.

Affective Learning Levels

- receiving: awareness
- responding: willingness
- valuing: commitment
- organization: discussion
- characterization: living the beliefs, values.

Psychomotor Learning Levels

- perception: receiving sensory signals and translating
- set: motivation
- guided response: limitation, trial and error
- mechanism: learned response
- complex overt response: smooth response
- adaptation: altering response
- origination: innovation with response.

SOURCES: Bloom, 1956; Coutts & Hardy, 1985.

AGE

Age is a factor that affects both teaching and learning. Young children do not think in abstract terms. They need the concrete—something they can see, do, feel, touch, taste or smell, or something they have experienced. They usually have fertile imaginations, but their imagery is based on past experience. If imaginary situations are used in teaching, then, they need to be based on experiences familiar to the child, such as going to the store, playing with friends or helping parents (Rankin & Stallings, 1996; Redman, 1997).

Adults are usually more goal-oriented in their learning than children are and more selective in what they learn (Cantor, 1992). With adult learners, it is well to remember Malcolm Knowles's (1978) "foundation stones of modern adult learning theory," shown in the box above.

COMMUNICATION SKILLS

Teaching patients is essentially a communication process, with the interaction between nurse and patient at its core (Rorden, 1987). The individual's ability to communicate needs to be taken into account when planning patient teaching. For example, both hearing and vision become less acute with advancing age. If you are teaching a group of older adults, you will probably find that you have to talk a little louder than you normally would, enunciate your words more clearly and perhaps provide written material in larger print.

Lack of a common language can be a considerable barrier to teaching and learning. If the patient speaks only a language that is foreign to you, you can use nonverbal communication to a certain extent—gestures, pantomiming, diagrams or printed material in the patient's language. When there are complicated instructions, or complex materials to be learned, an interpreter is needed. Often, a family member or friend accompanying the patient can help. Many agencies whose patients include people of different ethnic origins have staff members who speak one or more of the languages commonly used by patients and are often called upon to assist in interpreting. Many agencies also have phrase books in different languages for use in departments such as Emergency and a wide range of teaching materials that have been translated into the languages used by different community ethnic groups. The Canadian Translators and Interpreters Council is also a good resource. Each provincial branch maintains a directory of qualified translators and interpreters for its jurisdiction.

Even when you share a common language, the nurse must use words that are understandable to the patient. Education does not guarantee familiarity with medical terminology, and dealing with those in stress may require

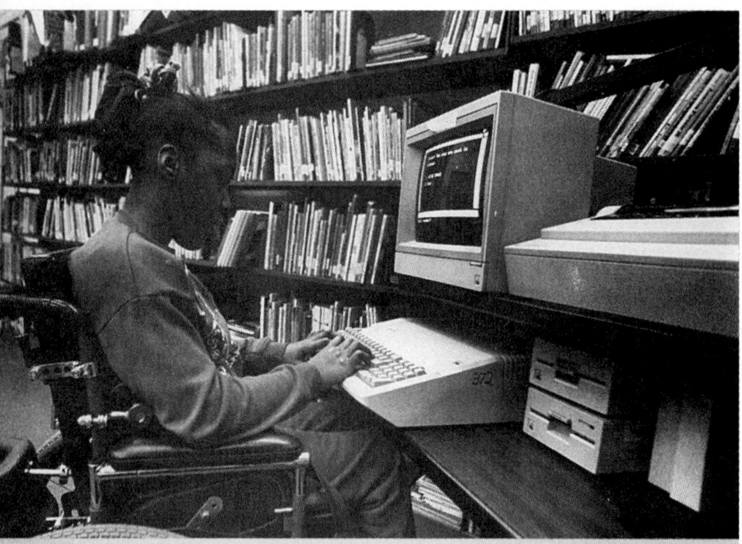

The library is a learning resource for patients and their families as well as for health professionals.

explanation in plain language and repetition of important points. Conversely, the nurse should never make the mistake of "talking down" to people.

Finally, communication cannot occur if body language is incongruent with the verbal message. For example, although a patient indicates verbally that she understands the content that has been reviewed, her facial expression may lead the nurse to believe that the patient does not fully comprehend. (See Chapter 17 for a discussion of communication skills.)

CULTURAL BACKGROUND

As we discussed in Chapter 12, the cultural background of the patient is another factor to be considered. It is important to assess the individual's subjective beliefs and perceptions as well as looking at more objective characteristics of the learner (Rorden, 1987). Customs and mores vary from one ethnic group to another and within ethnic groups, from one part of the country to another and from one socioeconomic group to another.

In one particular instance, new mothers in a hospital in northern India scoffed at a nurse's demonstration of bathing a baby. When asked why they laughed, they said they could bathe six babies in the time it took the nurse to bathe one. On further questioning, they said they would not use a basin, soap and a washcloth as the nurse did. They would sit on the mud floor of their one-room home in the village and, holding the baby between their ankles with one hand, pour water from a jug over him or her with the other, letting the water flow off the baby into an open drain in the floor. The nurse did a little research with a community health nurse and, in the next round of classes, demonstrated a safer method for the procedure the mothers had described. The nurse also showed them the basin method while sitting on a mat on the floor. This time the teaching was accepted with no scoffing. In this case, the nurse was from the same geographic region as the mothers, but from a different socioeconomic group.

STATE OF HEALTH

In health teaching, the state of the patient's health must be considered. Teaching sessions for ill patients need to be short and gauged to the patient's ability to participate. Ideally, deep-breathing exercises should be taught preoperatively, when patients are feeling well, rather than postoperatively, when they may be in considerable pain.

People today are often knowledgeable about health matters. Health information is more readily available today. A patient may, in fact, know much more than the nurse about his or her particular health problem. It is important to find out what patients already know and want to know about their health status to determine the base of experience on which new learning can be built. However, the nurse should never assume that patients know everything about their health problems.

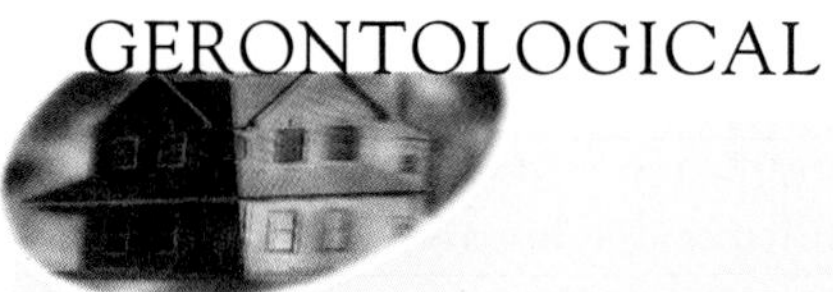

GERONTOLOGICAL

Implications for Teaching–Learning in the older adult

- speak clearly
- present content at an appropriate pace
- foster self-pacing
- teach when patient is alert and rested
- allow adequate response time
- provide opportunities for repetition, recall
- present small amounts of information in short, frequent learning sessions
- eliminate all distracting sounds and sights
- establish attainable short-term goals
- encourage participation in planning and decision making
- apply content to current situation
- integrate new patterns with established ones.

SOURCE: Boyd et al., 1998.

MOTIVATION

The individual's motivation for learning is also an important characteristic of the learner. **Motivation** can be characterized as an individual's willingness and effort to learn (Redman, 1997). Motivation may be either intrinsic or extrinsic. Intrinsic factors include an individual's "anxiety level ... success in past educational settings, and ... openness to

Implications for Teaching–Learning in School-Age Children

- use known terms, age-appropriate diagrams/models
- plan lessons of 15–20 minute duration
- provide explanations
- allow learners to make decisions
- allow time for learners to sort out new terms and concepts
- assign simple psychomotor tasks
- reinforce learning with praise
- consider group learning opportunities
- allow privacy
- allow learners control by inviting their help in planning lessons.

SOURCE: Boyd et al., 1998.

learning. Extrinsic factors include the environment for learning, the pleasure of acquiring new knowledge, and the type of interaction in the process" (Rankin & Stallings, 1996, p. 300). The nurse's ability to recognize what motivates individuals (i.e., their readiness to learn) is important. The nurse can identify factors affecting an individual's motivation during the assessment phase of the teaching–learning process.

Characteristics of the Teacher

The teacher is a key figure in the process of teaching and learning. We can all think of memorable teachers who influenced us, from whom we feel we learned the most and, with their guidance, learned most easily.

KNOWLEDGE OF SUBJECT MATTER

A good knowledge of the subject matter is basic (Cantor, 1992). If you are going to help a group of overweight individuals—or even one individual—to learn how to control their diet to lose weight, you will need to have a good knowledge of foods and the nutrients they contain, as well as their caloric content. You should be familiar with the Canada Food Guide put out by the federal government. It is also helpful to have guides for estimating the number of calories expended during various types of activity, such as swimming, jogging, bicycling, resting and various types of housework.

You, as a knowledgeable health professional, are a resource for the group you are teaching, and you will want to be prepared to answer their questions and have materials available for them. It is a good idea, when you are planning a teaching session, to think of questions people might ask. If, during the actual session, you find you do not have the answer to someone's question, don't be afraid to say, "I don't know, but I will see what I can do to find the answer to your question next session." Or, you might give patients references so they can explore a particular issue further on their own. Even the best of teachers are not expected to have all the answers.

When teaching skills, you must be sure of your mastery of these before you attempt to teach someone else. It is always helpful to practise the skill beforehand, even if you think you know it well, just to refresh your memory.

STRATEGIES AND NEEDS ASSESSMENT

Knowledge of the subject matter is not enough to guarantee effective teaching. The teacher also has to have skill in using teaching strategies to communicate the material effectively. In the next section of the chapter we will discuss strategies commonly used in teaching patients. A knowledge of the various methods that can be used will help you to select the one best suited to meet a particular patient's needs. Skill in using the different strategies will come with practice, as is true of any other skill. A wide range of teaching aids, including models, charts, diagrams and audio- and videotapes on a wide variety of health topics, is available to help you in your teaching. You will need to become skilled in handling the various types of audio-visual equipment to use them successfully.

The teacher must also have skill in assessing the learner's needs and in planning and organizing the material to be taught. In thinking about teaching, the fundamental questions are: What is the patient going to have to do? What does the patient therefore need to learn? We will discuss these questions in detail later in this chapter.

PLANNING AND ORGANIZATION

When the material to be learned has been identified, the teacher needs planning and organizing skills. The following are some questions to ask yourself when you are planning and organizing a teaching session:

- can the material all be taught in one session, or are several sessions needed?
- how much material should be included?
- what should be presented first?
- are there things that need to be taught before something new can be learned?
- where should the teaching be done?
- do I need to prepare the venue beforehand?
- what materials do I need?
- are there teaching aids I can use?

Teaching Styles

The style a teacher uses—the way of conducting classes and guiding other learning experiences—reflects the teacher's leadership role with the learner. At one end of the continuum is the **autocratic** style, in which all decisions are made by the teacher, and there is little or no opportunity for the learner to have a voice in the goals to be achieved or in the nature of the learning experience, or to take any responsibility for its direction. An example of an autocratic style of teaching is the nurse who tells the patient, "these are the things you need to know," and proceeds to give a non-stop talk about the patient's medical condition. This type of teaching gives the impression that nurses know better than the patient what the patient needs to know.

At the other end of the continuum is the **laissez-faire** style of teaching, in which decisions about what is to be learned and how it is to be learned are left entirely up to the learners. While this style may be effective with a group of well-motivated and well-educated adults, it is all too easy for a group to be sidetracked and to deviate from its original goals.

The middle style on the continuum is the **democratic** style, in which the learner participates in establishing goals, assumes some responsibility for the conduct of the learning session and feels free to participate in decisions regarding the direction of the experience. Humanists believe that this style is most effective in facilitating learning (Yelon & Weinstein, 1977).

However, it is important to remember that the styles represent a continuum; teachers may display varying degrees of these styles, and learners will respond better to some styles than to others according to their own background and preferences. While it can be difficult to develop a style that pleases all learners, it is usually wise to strive for a middle-of-the-road, democratic approach to teaching learners.

The Environment

Another important factor that affects teaching and learning is the **environment**. "The external environment can enhance and encourage learning but it cannot create or force learning to occur" (Draves, cited in Boyd et al., 1998 p. 101). The environment can be broken into three components: physical, psychosocial and related variables.

The physical environment includes heat, light, sound, space, colour, time of day and length of teaching activity. For example, the nurse should find a quiet, private location for teaching. The room should be brightly lit with little glare. Furniture should be comfortable and arranged in a manner conducive to interaction. Because the venue may need to be prepared ahead of time, it is always a good idea to check that everything that will be needed (blackboard, flip-chart, audio-visual aids) is there in the room. It is important to check that there are enough chairs and a place to put notes, materials and equipment. Equipment, such as a slide projector or VCR, should be checked to make sure it is in working order. Replacement light bulbs and batteries should be easily accessible. Whenever possible, it is helpful to go through an entire session as a "dry run," either alone or with another person. Educational materials must be replaced and updated as needed.

Early discharge from hospital may allow for only one teaching session by the nurse. Thus, the psychosocial environment is an important variable in the process of teaching and learning. Knowles (1980) describes four basic characteristics of a learning environment: (a) respect for personality, (b) freedom of expression and availability, (c) participation in decision making and (d) mutuality of responsibility in planning and setting goals and in evaluating activities.

Related variables include education of nurses about the teaching–learning process, the value nurses place on teaching within the health care setting, money available for health prevention and promotion and the political climate. The quality and quantity of health education is greatly affected by the learning environment (Boyd et al., 1998).

Teachers need good interpersonal skills to be able to foster a climate that is conducive to learning. People cannot learn easily if they feel threatened (Waines, 1993). Many patients view the nurse as an authority figure, and it is important to dispel any threat the patient may feel. In this regard, the material in Chapter 17, on creating an open climate for communication, is relevant in the process of teaching and learning.

In teaching, both on a one-to-one basis and in groups, it is important to have an atmosphere in which each person feels free to participate and the communication channels remain open. When you are teaching a group of patients, you will find that there is interaction not only between you as teacher and the learners but also among the learners. People feel more comfortable in a group when they know who the other members are and why they are there. It is helpful at the beginning of a teaching session to have participants introduce themselves and, perhaps, tell a little about their background and why they are attending the program.

The authority inherent in the nurse's role is made less threatening if the nurse sits as a member of the group, rather than standing at the front of the room behind a lectern. A more relaxed, informal atmosphere is promoted if everyone

Coutts and Hardy (1985) view teaching and learning as interconnected and interrelated, and dependent on the following factors:

Environment
Space, noise, furniture, time, material resources, support from the system, ethos, expectations.

Learner
Motivation, capacity, energy, culture, age, intelligence, skill, emotional and physical state, values, experience, type of learning, previous experience, learning style.

Teacher
Motivation, capacity, energy, aptitude, knowledge, beliefs, values, communication skills, selection of methods and materials, teaching style, theoretical perspective.

SOURCE: Coutts & Hardy, 1985, p. 49.

Cultural Implications for Teaching–Learning

- become familiar with your own cultural heritage
- be aware of the cultural background of each patient
- identify adaptations to cultural norms
- confirm patient preferences
- base patient teaching on cultural analysis
- recognize and respect patients' health care beliefs
- learn about communities' cultural norms and customs
- identify perceptions of health, illness and wellness
- develop culturally relevant educational programs
- utilize patients' traditional health beliefs and practices in educational design
- foster community and family support.

SOURCE: Price & Cordell, 1994.

can sit around a table. In many situations, however, this is not feasible. If the group is large, or if you need to use aids such as flip-charts or a blackboard, you should stand where everyone can see you and you can see everyone in the class. It is important that both you and the learners feel comfortable and at ease, and that everyone is within sight and hearing range.

BARRIERS TO LEARNING

In considering the factors that affect teaching and learning, the teacher must remember that many of these factors can also be barriers to learning. A person under extreme physical or emotional stress has a reduced attention span and capacity to learn (Anderson, 1990). The nurse may also impose barriers to patient learning—for example, by inappropriately assessing readiness to learn, planning and presenting content in a hurried fashion or failing to provide feedback and evaluation. Rankin and Stallings (1996) cite a number of questions that may be asked to identify common barriers to learning in the practice setting:

- how do physical limitations of the patient and environment affect patient education?
- what are the effects of pain, illness and fatigue on patient education?
- what is the relationship between anxiety and learning? (pp. 320–321)

NURSES at work — Enterostomal Therapist

I am an enterostomal therapist in a regional hospital in northern British Columbia. I have had formal post-basic education in the management of "ostomies," wounds (including pressure sores and leg ulcers) and incontinence.

This morning I visited patients on the surgical ward who have undergone ostomy surgery. One of the patients, Mrs. Gopal, is recovering from colostomy surgery for a ruptured bowel, caused by an acute inflammatory condition of the colon. She had never heard of a colostomy before her surgery and feels overwhelmed by the thought of wearing a pouch. Her ostomy is temporary but she is concerned about how she will manage pouch care because she has limited hand dexterity due to arthritis. I discussed the nature of the surgery and the results with Mrs. Gopal, and I think she has a better understanding of her condition and the reasons for surgery. I also left some of our patient teaching pamphlets with her and arranged to have a member of the United Ostomy Association visit to give her some moral support and help her with the day-to-day concerns of living with a colostomy.

This afternoon, I will see patients in the Ostomy Outpatient Clinic. Mr. Kucera, I know, is slated for surgery and is coming in for his preoperative assessment. He has had Crohn's disease (a chronic inflammatory condition of the small intestine) for 10 years and has had two bowel resections. He still has extensive Crohn's disease in the anal canal. He is exhausted with pain and has elected to have a permanent ileostomy. During the preoperative session I have with him, I will:

- assess the level of his understanding about the surgery, based on what his physician has told him
- use some simple diagrams to show him the structure of the gastrointestinal tract, the section that will be involved in the surgery and the alteration that will be done
- describe in simple terms the stoma, the output and appliance management
- reassure Mr. Kucera that he can resume his activities of daily living after surgery; he does not have to give up his favourite sports of fishing, hunting and curling. Mr. Kucera has discussed with his surgeon possible sexual implications of the surgery
- discuss dietary implications with him and give him a patient teaching handout on this topic
- give Mr. Kucera a list of local ostomy supply retailers and discuss with him the procedure for obtaining financial assistance for these supplies if he should need it
- provide him with a contact number for the United Ostomy Association.

It is also my responsibility to mark the stoma site with indelible pen in the right lower quadrant of the abdomen, below the belt line and within the patient's range of vision. After I have done this, I will tell Mr. Kucera that I will see him in the hospital after his surgery. There, my role will be to promote Mr. Kucera's independence in ostomy self-care so that he can successfully return to the community.

Another part of my role as an enterostomal therapy nurse is to act as a resource consultant to the United Ostomy Association and to other hospitals and agencies in northern British Columbia.

— Lenore Du Gas, RN, BSN, ET
Prince George Regional Hospital

Incorporating Teaching in Nursing Care

People who seek the help of health professionals have learning needs. Teaching–learning interventions should therefore be incorporated into all nursing care. In this section of the chapter, we review the steps of the nursing process that the nurse would carry out in meeting teaching and learning needs in a specific situation: that of surgical patients with a colostomy or ileostomy (the opening of some portion of the colon or ileum to the outer surface of the abdominal wall; the opening is called the stoma). "The teaching process can be seen as a parallel to the nursing process in that each has an assessment, diagnosis, goals, intervention, and evaluation phase" (Redman, 1997, p. 5). Table 18.3 shows the relationship of the teaching process to the nursing process.

Assessment of Learning Needs

In assessing learning needs, the nurse's basic question is what does the patient need (or want) to be able to know or do? It is important to clarify your perception of needs in relation to the perception of the individual who is to do the learning, to be sure that you, as teacher, and the patient, as learner, are both headed in the same direction. The two patients described in the box entitled Nurses at Work would appear to have similar needs. Both need to learn more about their condition, the type of surgery they have had or are going to have, and how to care for themselves at home. The nurse would verify with the patients that these are indeed the things they want to learn. Some health agencies have developed a questionnaire that is given to patients to identify their particular learning needs. A sample questionnaire is shown in Figure 18.1.

In addition to knowing exactly what the patients' learning needs are, it is important to assess the factors that may affect their learning. You will want to assess the level of their knowledge about their condition or disease and past experience in promoting and protecting their health. It is helpful to know how strong their motivation is to learn (why do they want to learn this?). Also helpful is information about age, educational level and ethnic and/or religious background. Ability to communicate is also important; you will want to know if patients speak English (or French) fluently enough to participate in discussions. An interpreter can be available to assist with the teaching process. It is useful to know something about lifestyle, particular strengths, likes and dislikes in regard to learning methods.

Please check as many of the items as you like. Thank you for helping us to help you.

I would like to know more about:

_____ the nature of my medical condition and its causes
_____ the reasons for the surgery
_____ what was done during the surgery
_____ what will my abdomen look like after it has healed
_____ pouch care
_____ care of the skin around the opening
_____ diet considerations
_____ daily living with an ostomy
_____ what to do if something unusual happens

Other things I would like to know:

____
____
____
____
____
____
____

FIGURE 18.1 Questionnaire on learning needs for a patient with a colostomy or ileostomy

SOURCE: Adapted from Haggard, 1989, p. 33.

TABLE 18.3 Relationship of teaching process to nursing process

ASSESSMENT	DIAGNOSIS	GOALS	INTERVENTION	EVALUATION
Nursing process				
General screening questions to detect patient's need to learn	One of problem statements may be a need to learn or a nursing diagnosis	Learning goals are a subject of goals	Teaching intervention may be delivered with other intervention	Evaluating whether nursing care outcome was met
Teaching process				
Refined assessment and readiness to learn	Learning diagnosis	Setting of learning goals	Teaching	Evaluating learning

SOURCE: Redman, 1997, p. 5.

Guidelines for Assessing a Patient's Learning Needs

- What does the patient perceive as the learning need(s)?
- What is the patient's attitude towards health professionals (previous experience)?
- What is the patient's motivation for learning?
- What does the patient know about the disease or condition?
- How old is the patient (developmental tasks)?
- What is the patient's sensory condition: touch, sight, smell, taste, hearing?
- What is the patient's state of health (physical, psychological, signs & symptoms)?
- What is the patient's level of education (literacy)?
- What is the patient's cultural background (beliefs and values: ethnic origin, language(s) spoken, religion practised)?

Nursing Diagnoses and Learning Needs

According to Jenny (1987), *knowledge deficit* is not a nursing diagnosis since it "does not represent a human response, alteration, or pattern of dysfunction but rather a related factor" (p. 184). Individual (or family) teaching, then, is a part of nursing interventions for all nursing diagnoses. For example, if the nursing diagnosis for an individual is *Sleep Pattern Disturbance*, teaching interventions would be indicated to help the person to re-establish a normal sleep pattern. If a lack of knowledge is the principal cause of a diagnosis, the diagnosis might be stated as *Anxiety related to insufficient knowledge of preoperative routines*. Other examples might be *Risk for Infection related to lack of knowledge of safety precautions in handling contaminated equipment* or *Ineffective Management of Therapeutic Regimen due to lack of knowledge regarding medications ordered by physician*. With Mrs. Gopal (from the Nurses at Work box), possible diagnoses might be:

> *Risk of Ineffective Management of Therapeutic Regimen, related to insufficient knowledge of ostomy care*
>
> *Anxiety related to concern over managing ostomy care at home*
>
> *Self-Concept Disturbance related to sudden change in body structure following surgery* (Carpenito, 1997).

With Mr. Kucera, we might add:

> *Anxiety related to possible lifestyle disturbance as a result of surgery*.

Once the diagnoses have been established, they need to be placed in order of priority. What is most important to be achieved first? In this case, the diagnoses are probably in the correct order unless Mrs. Gopal's anxiety was too overwhelming and needed to be dealt with first.

Once the nurse has identified the nature of the learning needs, verified these with the individual and developed diagnostic statements, the next step is to develop expected outcomes (goals or objectives). For example:

> *Mrs. Gopal will independently demonstrate skill in changing the ostomy appliance before she is discharged from the hospital.*
>
> *Mr. Kucera will state less anxiety related to managing ostomy care at home before he leaves the hospital.*

When you have identified the expected (short- and long-term) outcomes, you will want to analyse the learning tasks involved in achieving them. These include the knowledge, skills and attitudes the learner needs to gain. The questions in this case are: What does the person need to know in order to manage ostomy care effectively at home? to reduce anxiety? to restore a healthy self-concept? What does the patient need to be able to do? What skills need to be learned? Are there attitudinal components that need to be considered? In your written plan, it is helpful to list the learning needs under the headings of knowledge, skills and attitudes, so that you do not overlook any in planning your teaching.

Developing a Teaching Plan

Once learning needs have been identified, the next step is to develop a **teaching plan**. A teaching plan includes content to be taught and strategies to be implemented. The learning needs should be organized into logical groups and arranged in sequential order to enhance learning. It is beneficial to start a teaching session with content that the patient already knows, as this will decrease anxiety. A further strategy when organizing content is to move from simple to complex or from concrete to abstract ideas. In the Nurses at Work vignette, an example of simple cognitive content would be Mr. Kucera's understanding of his planned surgery. More complex cognitive content would be his understanding of gastrointestinal pathophysiology. Learning to change an ostomy appliance requires gaining psychomotor skills. Learning to live with an ostomy is abstract content explored within the affective domain.

The next step is to identify suitable learning experiences so that the patient can achieve the desired outcomes. Appropriate strategies need to be selected. It is also a good idea at this stage to identify teaching aids that could be helpful. One-on-one discussion strategy, with the use of aids such as diagrams of the structure of the gastrointestinal tract, could foster learning in the case of Mr. Kucera.

The teaching plan may be brief, including simply the expected outcomes and the method to be used in teaching. It may also include the content in brief or key points.

Many agencies have developed teaching plans for patients with specific problems. Figure 18.2 is an example

British Columbia's **Children's Hospital** Patient Teaching Flowsheet: **Cardiac Surgery** **Preoperative Teaching** Page 1	Addressograph
Teaching Aids Key Title	

Key	Title	Key	Title
1	3G Orientation Checklist	5	Autologous Blood Transfusion Program
2	In the Vicinity of Children's Hospital	6	Computer Aided Instruction
3	Your Heart Matters	7	The Pre-Admission Clinic
4	Heart Defect Specific Pamphlet	8	Instructions for Patients Preparing For Surgery (PAC)

Req'd Yes/No	Objective	Key	Date & Sign when teaching done	Comments & Concerns (Indicate further teaching required, referrals, notes on chart)
	1. (a) Familiarize family with: • Cardiac services (e.g., clinics, 3G, ICU, Catheterization Lab). • Roles of health professionals • Parent services available at BCCH and its vicinity (b) Are there other services you might need?	1 2		
	2. (a) What is your understanding of your child's heart defect and how it will be repaired or managed surgically? • Review normal heart. • Review heart defect. • Review surgical repair.	3 pg 16-19 4,6		

	3. (a) Do you have any questions related to blood transfusions often required during heart surgery?
	(Find out if child is a candidate for this.)
	• Risk of blood transfusion.
	• Reason for blood transfusion.
	  • Small children
	  • Complex surgery
	• Benefits of using own blood
	• Eligibility
	• Process for autologous donation.
	• Preparing your child
	• Description of procedure.
	• Complications to watch for
		5		

	4. (a) What is your child's/family most pressing concern related to having cardiac surgery and/or being in the hospital? (b) Let's review what will happen during your hospital stay. PARENTS—Preparation: • Pre-Admission Clinic visit: • Pre-op prep at home • Family plan for hospitalization. Surgery: • DCS → OR → ICU/PACU → Rm 9 → Ward → Home. • Surgical experience. • ICU experience: Tour (if applicable) • Waiting areas and activities	7 8 9 10 11		

FIGURE 18.2 Patient teaching flowsheet

SOURCE: The British Columbia Children's Hospital, Vancouver, B.C.

British Columbia's **Children's Hospital** Patient Teaching Flowsheet: **Cardiac Surgery** **Preoperative Teaching** Page 2	Addressograph
Teaching Aids Key Title	

9 Yes, You Can Help	12 Video: Understanding Your Child's Heart Surgery (Open)
10 ICU Booklet	13 Teen Video—Straight Talk About Surgery
11 What To Do While You Wait	14 Tell Me About My Operation

Req'd Yes/No	Objective	Key	Date & Sign when teaching done	Comments & Concerns (Indicate further teaching required, referrals, notes on chart)
	• What to expect when they first see their child: In ICU: **Appearance:** Pale color, puffy, asleep and sedated for comfort, cool to touch, no clothes on. Equipment: Ventilator and ETT, CVCs and ART lines, catheter, warmers, temperature probes. In general: Cardiac monitor and leads, chest tubes, IVs, incisions, sedated and medicated for pain. **Recovery:** • Physiotherapy: • Mobilization and holding/carrying child. • DB and C, bubble blowing. • Spirometry. • Diet: When child can drink then eat. Breastfeed. • Resuming ADLs: Bathing, school, play. CHILD (Adapt to child's level of understanding). Involve Child Life Specialist when available. • Discuss anticipated course through hospital stay. • General points about their heart condition and how it will be fixed. • Events on the day of surgery. • Child will go to sleep in OR and wake up in either ICU or PACU. • Where parents will be waiting and when they will visit. Emphasize they will be sleepy and comfortable and that their favourite toy or object can be with them. • Talk about the equipment, what it looks like and how it feels (talk about the equipment the child will have), ETT - can't talk, feel like you have to cough when it is suctioned, chest tube, ECG leads to heart monitor, catheter, IVs in wrist and neck. • Turning and bubble blowing or using an incentive spirometer. • When the child will start getting up and start to drink and eat. **5. What other questions or concerns do you have about the surgery or hospitalization?**	12 3 pg 24-25 13 14		

FIGURE 18.2 *(continued)*

SOURCE: The British Columbia Children's Hospital, Vancouver, B.C.

of a patient teaching flowsheet used in one hospital. Flowsheets help to ensure that all material that people need to learn is covered. On the flowsheet various health professionals may be indicated as responsible for teaching, with the physician or RN explaining the nature of the medical condition, its causes and the aims of treatment. The registered nurse is responsible for the remainder of the teaching. Note also the stated objectives (which have been abbreviated for the written teaching plan), the grouping of learning tasks and the sequence of content indicated. Teaching aids are listed at the beginning of the plan and referred to by number in the plan.

All teachers develop their own style of lesson plan. The important thing to remember is that the plan is to help the teacher to keep in mind the expected outcomes and to serve as a reminder of what needs to be covered (Carpenito, 1997; Redman, 1997; Rankin & Stallings, 1996; Rorden, 1987).

Teaching–Learning Strategies for Different Learning Tasks

Various teaching–learning strategies are particularly suitable for each type of learning task.

STRATEGIES FOR ACQUIRING KNOWLEDGE

A newcomer in the field of patient education that is proving to be very useful in helping people to acquire knowledge is the interactive computer program, which may well revolutionize patient teaching. It is used extensively, for example, in patient teaching at the British Columbia Children's Hospital. Families can gain confidence in decision making, through having the opportunity to consider various alternative courses of action.

In keeping with the philosophy of the learner as an active participant in identifying learning needs and seeking the information needed to meet these needs, the hospital has established a Family Resource library. Learning resources have been developed by staff and materials collected from other sources for use by patients and their families.

The library holdings include reference books, articles and other written materials on various health problems and other relevant subjects, as well as videotapes that can be borrowed for in-agency or home use. A major part of the holdings is a collection of interactive computer programs. Discharge planning is facilitated because families can go to the library and use the computer programs to learn about the care the child requires at home, the danger signals they need to be alert to and other matters about which they would like more information. Printouts can be made from the computer for people to peruse at their leisure and to keep as reference material. Other pamphlets and written material are also available for patients and their families in a number of different languages (British Columbia Children's Hospital, 1994).

Written materials are available from your local health department and other agencies concerned with specific health problems, for example, the Arthritis Society and the Lung Association. There are pamphlets on smoking, nutrition, exercise, hypertension, heart disease and a great many other topics that will be useful in teaching patients. The community health agency has developed patient teaching handouts that are pertinent to the health needs of the area. Handouts are very useful to supplement teaching by other means. They can be taken home and kept at the bedside, to be read and reviewed at leisure, or referred to at a later date. Some samples are shown in Figure 18.3.

Interactive computer programs and written materials may be used separately or in conjunction with other forms of teaching. For example, information may be presented in the form of a lecture or short talk, or during the course of a conversation. Conversation is suitable when you are dealing with one patient, or a very small group. For most groups, a lecture or talk is usually more appropriate. However, a straight **lecture**, or uninterrupted talk, does not involve much activity on the part of the learner except through the sense of hearing, and it depends on the learner's ability to listen. If you are giving a talk, it is wise to remember that the attention span of the average healthy adult is only about 20 minutes. It is less for children and for the elderly, and usually less for those who are ill. In order to ensure that this span will not be exceeded, one should vary the strategies used in teaching, and intersperse lecturing with other strategies.

Discussion, which involves participation on the part of the patient, facilitates the retention of learning. Some structure to the session, that is, someone guiding and directing, is needed for it to be effective. A list with key questions can assist in moving the discussion forward. The combination of a short talk followed by discussion is often a good way of structuring a teaching session.

Many nurses use the strategy of **one-on-one discussion** in order to share knowledge and to help patients learn. It can be used at the patient's bedside, in a health clinic or during a home visit. In this approach, the nurse directly relays content and engages the patient in informal discussion. An advantage of this strategy is that it provides a safe environment for sharing confidential information. One-on-one discussion allows for individualized teaching (Rankin & Stallings, 1996).

Audio-visual materials are also useful aids to teaching. Illustrating a talk with diagrams or pictures on a blackboard or flip-chart will often help to get points across that are difficult to grasp through words alone. Models are also useful supplements for teaching. There are various anatomical models available; for example, the heart model is used in

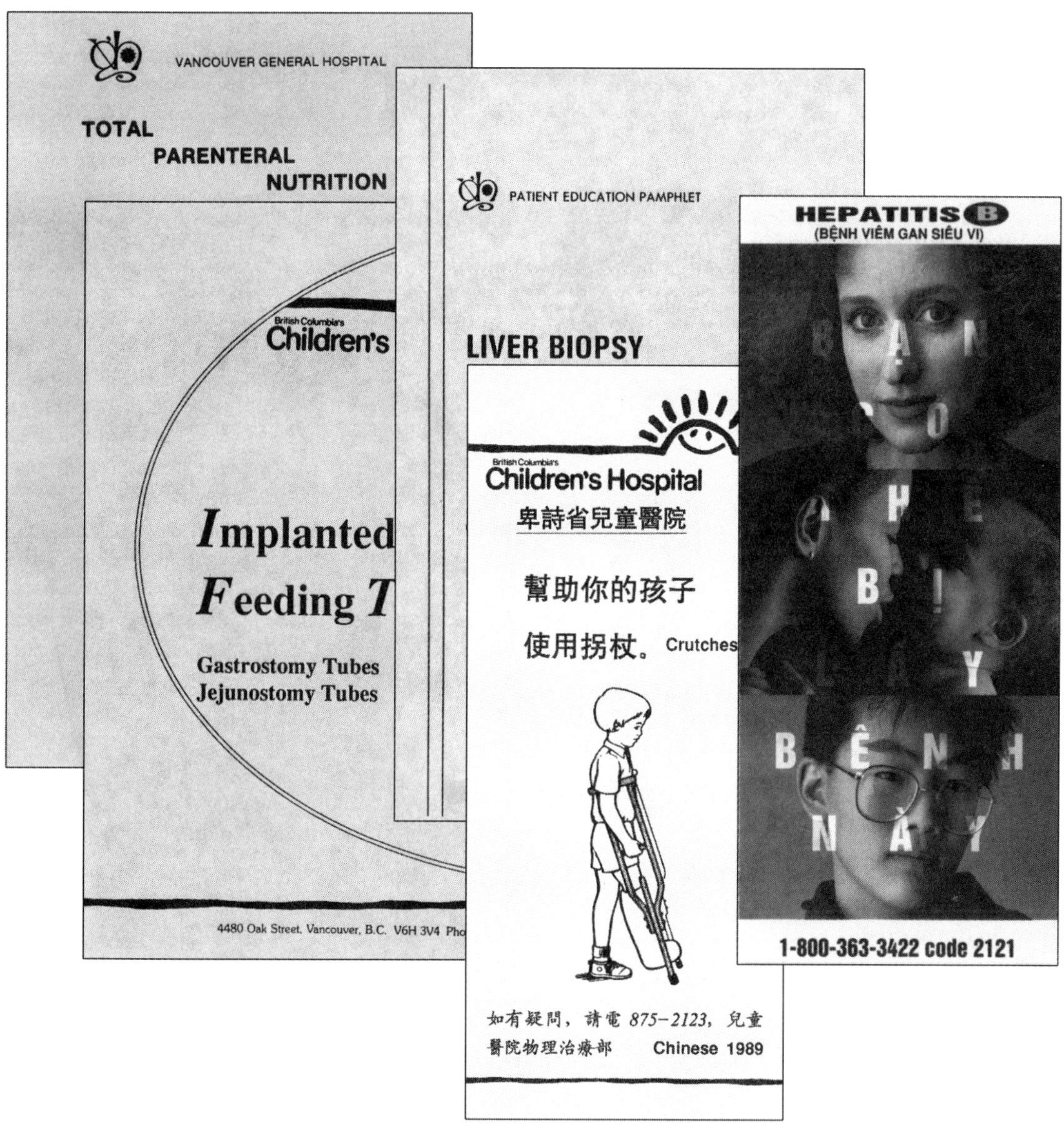

FIGURE 18.3 Sample patient teaching materials

SOURCES: The Vancouver Hospital and Health Sciences Centre; the British Columbia Children's Hospital; the Canadian Liver Foundation.

the Healthy Heart Program as a visual aid to discuss the anatomy and function of the heart.

Many slides, audio- and videotapes about common health problems have been developed to help in teaching patients. When using audio-visual aids in teaching, it is a good idea to review these ahead of time, in order to assess their suitability and relevance to the class and to become familiar with the content. The actual presentation should be introduced with an explanation of the purpose of viewing the slide or video and the points to watch for during the presentation. Opportunity should be provided for discussion during or after the presentation to clarify a point or to emphasize basic concepts.

Storytelling is a useful strategy for presenting information to children. Given the nature of children's imaginations, situations used in the story should be based on things familiar to the child. A number of illustrated children's books are on the market to help children prepare for a hospital experience. Cartoons and comic strips have been developed to help children learn about health topics such as nutrition, brushing their teeth and other hygiene measures.

STRATEGIES FOR DEVELOPING MOTOR SKILLS

Complex movements, such as those needed in skill development, involve the establishment of a series of connections in the neural pathways between the brain and the muscles. Patients learning to give themselves an injection

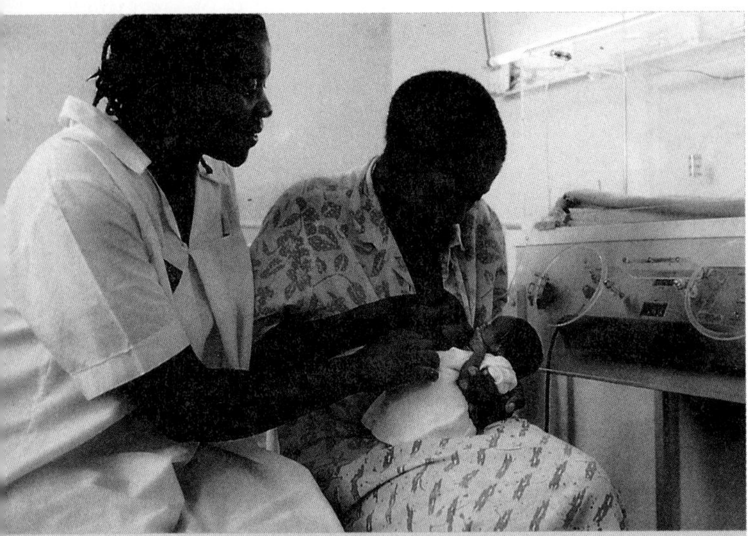
Nurse assisting a new mother to breastfeed.

of insulin have to go through the motions of assembling the equipment, disinfecting the top of the insulin container, drawing up the correct amount, selecting an injection site, cleansing it and giving themselves the injection. A complicated series of sequenced movements is involved in the skill.

In demonstrating a specific skill, the nurse should, wherever possible, use the type of equipment the patient will be using at home.

In giving a **demonstration**, the nurse should first explain what is going to be done and why it is to be done in this way—for example, basic hygiene principles such as washing hands before drawing up insulin. The nurse should always be sure that the learner can see exactly what he or she is doing. For example, the learner should be able to see the numbers on the syringe when learning to draw up insulin. An overview of the procedure is given first; then the procedure is broken down into steps. Key points are stressed while the nurse is demonstrating. The material that is being taught can often be related to something that is familiar to the patient, so that the learning can be transferred from the familiar to a new area.

The patient should have an opportunity to perform the procedure in a **return demonstration** soon after the nurse has demonstrated it—preferably immediately afterward. It is helpful to guide and direct patients through the various steps when they are returning your demonstration, so that they perform the steps correctly and in the right sequence. Initially, accuracy is more important than speed. Efficiency and speed will come with practice. Sufficient practice sessions should be arranged so that the patient (and sometimes family members) feels confident prior to performing the skill independently.

Audio-visual materials can be used advantageously in teaching many skills. A short videotape can help the learner to visualize the procedure and can often be used as a substitute for a demonstration. A written outline of the procedure, with diagrams illustrating key points, is also helpful, particularly if there are several steps involved.

STRATEGIES FOR ATTITUDINAL CHANGES

Learning experiences to help people change their attitude about something are, perhaps, the most difficult to structure. Attitudes often develop over a long period of time; many we acquire almost subconsciously. A person's attitude towards the importance of having regular meals, for example, is usually acquired in the home through early childhood experience.

Attitudes can be changed through a variety of teaching strategies. Over the past few years intensive educational programs, such as ParticipAction, have changed Canadians' attitude towards exercising. We have also changed our attitude towards seat belt use, which today is mandatory. The strategies used to bring about this change have included a massive communication campaign that has used radio and television programs, newspaper articles and a wide distribution of pamphlets to the Canadian public.

Attitudes towards the material to be learned will affect whether or not patients actually put their learning into practice. Patients have to recognize the need to take their medications on time, and appreciate the effect of skipping a dose, if they are to maintain a regular schedule. If the material learned does not seem important or relevant, they are not likely to apply it.

Often, attitudinal changes come about with increased knowledge. A hypertensive individual who understands the effects of obesity on blood pressure will be more likely to recognize the importance of losing weight by participating in a weight-reduction program. An awareness of the potential problems of high blood pressure, such as heart disease, stroke or kidney failure, will help individuals to realize the importance of maintaining their lifestyle change.

In helping people to change their attitude and apply their knowledge and skills, it is important to remember two of the basic guidelines for the facilitation of learning:

- to be meaningful, learning must be in response to what the learner perceives as needed
- learning is made easier when learners achieve a reward as a result of their behaviour.

In changing attitudes, as well as in helping people to acquire knowledge and develop motor skills, it is important to know something about the patients' needs and priorities. What values are important to them? What are the achievements that give them satisfaction? What do they find rewarding? (Cantor, 1992).

The Application of Learning

The nurse's primary concern is that patients apply the knowledge and use the skills they have learned. Having the information, and being able to perform the skills, is not enough; they must apply these. To learn to apply their knowledge and skills, learners must be actively involved. Some teaching strategies are particularly useful in helping people to apply their learning.

PROBLEM SOLVING

The **problem-solving** (or **discovery**) method has been suggested by educators as very appropriate for learning to apply knowledge. This method is useful in teaching patients. The steps in problem solving include:

1. perceiving a learning need
2. exploring possible solutions
3. selecting one solution to be tried
4. putting the solution into action
5. evaluating the results of this action, reconsidering and possibly trying other solutions.

The nurse's role in problem solving is that of supportive assistant. The nurse helps the patient to identify the learning need, gather information and assess the relative merits of various alternative courses of action. The nurse may help the individual (or family) to select and try one course of action, and assist in evaluating it.

For example, an elderly man who has been hospitalized for a kidney condition has been told by his physician that he should stay on a salt-free diet. The dietitian has given this patient information regarding foods that are low in salt, and he appears to accept the idea of salt substitutes to flavour his food. He seems worried about being able to stay on the diet at home. The nurse may help him to identify the problem. The man and his wife live alone; the wife does the cooking. He is afraid that cooking his meals without salt will mean extra work for her.

The nurse helps him to work through possible solutions. Has he talked to his wife about his concerns? As she does the cooking, she should be consulted in solving the problem. Together the patient and his wife might examine possible solutions. The patient's food could be cooked separately, in which case there would be two meals to prepare and two sets of pots and pans to wash. Or, food for both could be cooked together without salt, and the patient's wife could add salt to hers later. Many people find food tasteless when salt is not added during the cooking, and the wife may not like her food cooked this way. Both alternatives should be explored and a decision reached. The couple may decide to try cooking meals for both together without salt. If this solution does not work, then they can try the alternative.

There are many examples that could be cited of situations in which problem solving seems the logical method for helping patients to understand their disease processes and make realistic plans to care for themselves. The patient's family needs to be included, since many problems related to health and illness involve adjustments in family living.

CASE STUDY

This is another method often used in helping people to apply knowledge. The **case study** includes a description of a person with the same problem the patient has, and a series of questions or points to consider in a discussion. Potential real-life situations may be described and the patients asked to tell what they would do. The use of an imaginary person is helpful because it is less threatening to the individual concerned. It is a strategy that is often useful in helping to bring about attitudinal changes. People often feel freer to express their feelings and opinions about an imaginary person than about themselves.

ROLE-PLAY

Role-play is another useful strategy in helping people to apply knowledge and skills. Again, an imaginary situation is used. People in a weight-reduction program, for example, might be asked to think of going to the market and selecting foods for themselves and their families. The situation might then be acted out by participants—or they might actually go to the market. This strategy is helpful in encouraging people to express feelings and attitudes or to work through difficult situations. It is most effective when it is relatively unstructured and the participants are permitted to develop the situation as they go along. Not everyone feels comfortable with role-play, however, and it is time-consuming.

Children usually love role-playing, and this is a strategy that can be used very effectively with them. It is a good way to help them acquire new information, with the nurse in the role of teacher, storekeeper, TV character or other suitable figure. Role-playing can also be used for demonstrations, return demonstrations and practice sessions in learning new skills. It can be very effective in helping children and adults put into practice material they have learned in a simulated situation that is close to real life (Redman, 1997).

BEHAVIOUR MODIFICATION

Behaviour modification is a strategy that is frequently used in helping people substitute healthy habits (or behaviours) for unhealthy ones. In order to do this effectively, the desirable behaviour has to be learned first. The behaviour modification technique is used in many programs designed to help people to stop smoking or to stop overeating.

Methods used for helping people to stop smoking include substituting a new habit, such as walking around the block, instead of their usual coffee and cigarette after dinner. In one "last resort" method, smokers are encouraged to smoke continuously for a period of time until they get to the point where they cannot stand the sight or smell of cigarettes. Pleasure in smoking is replaced by distaste. Behaviour modification has also been used in some instances in treating alcoholism. The technique involves substituting an unpleasant response to alcohol consumption for the pleasurable effect it had for the individual.

Behaviour modification is based on rewarding the desirable behaviour and extinguishing the undesirable through a lack of reinforcement. The child is rewarded for good behaviour with praise, stars on a chart or other suitable tangible rewards. The undesirable behaviour is ignored and is extinguished because it is not reinforced (Redman, 1997). Sometimes an aversive response to the undesirable behaviour, such as separating the child from a group of children temporarily when the child is disrupting it, may be used in combination with rewards for good behaviour.

Implementing the Teaching Plan

Much teaching in the community is done in the patient's home or wherever the individual feels most comfortable. Some may take place in a classroom in the local community centre, or in the health room at a school. With patients coming into a hospital and those who are already inpatients, teaching will be in a class or conference room, an office or at the patient's bedside. It is important, when discussing personal matters, to ensure privacy for the individual; if the patient is not in a private room, it might be a good idea to take him or her to a conference room or lounge on the unit, or to draw the curtains around the bed.

All teaching, if it is to be worthwhile, takes time. Some of the nurse's teaching may be done informally, during the process of talking with the patient, but when specific material is to be taught, a definite plan should be developed and sufficient time allocated for carrying it out. A time that is suitable for both the learner and the nurse—when neither feels rushed and the learner is not overly tired—should be selected. The choice of time varies, depending upon the learner's activities and the nurse's schedule. In an ambulatory care setting, there may be definite times allocated when classes are scheduled for people with common concerns—for example, the diabetic clinic. There may also be regularly scheduled classes in an inpatient facility to accommodate people with similar problems. For example, preoperative videos can be used for demonstrating deep-breathing and coughing exercises.

Often, however, the teaching needs to be done on an individual basis. In inpatient facilities, the period in the morning after treatment and care have been completed, or the early afternoon, are often good times for teaching. For the sick, teaching periods are kept relatively short because most people, during illness, have a decreased attention span, and the nurse must be careful not to try to cover too much in any one session.

Whenever possible, one nurse should initiate and carry through the teaching plan. Patients usually prefer to have the same person teaching them, and the nurse can develop a more effective relationship with the patient and provide continuity by carrying through the complete teaching plan. If this is not feasible, however, a team approach, in which each nurse is responsible for one aspect of teaching, can be used quite effectively.

In conducting a teaching session, whether for one person or a group, it is important that the learners are clear on the expected outcomes. These should be reviewed at the beginning of the session. The session should then proceed logically from one point to the next. The learners should understand one step, or point, before the nurse moves on to the next. Evaluation techniques, such as feedback, are useful in making the decision whether to go on with the next point.

Asking learners to restate in their own words what they have just heard is another useful technique. It is always a good idea to watch for signs of lack of interest or irritability

RESEARCH to practice

Snowdon, A.W., & Kane, D.J. (1995). Parental needs following the discharge of a hospitalized child. *Pediatric Nursing, 21*(5), 425–428.

Previous research has addressed parents' needs only during their child's hospitalization. However, few studies have examined parents' needs posthospitalization. The purpose of this study was to identify the needs of parents after their child had been discharged. The authors used an exploratory, descriptive approach and recruited 16 families from a large acute care general hospital. Each family was visited on two separate occasions in their home.

The questions the authors used to collect data were focussed on exploring parents' needs following discharge and their perceptions of the effectiveness of a discharge home follow-up program. The analysis of the findings revealed that parents expressed needs that fell into two broad categories: the need for detailed information about their child, and the need for support with the multiple stressors they faced related to the hospitalization. The authors recommended further research to determine whether these parental needs developed because the parents did not receive adequate information during the hospitalization, because they had difficulty expressing their needs or because the stressful nature of the hospital environment was a barrier to their learning during the discharge teaching session.

Parents reported high levels of satisfaction with the discharge home follow-up program. The authors perceived that the individualized nature of the visits greatly influenced the parents' favourable responses. In addition, they relate that the home environment was more conducive to learning than the hospital.

The most helpful aspect of the visit was that the information focussed not only on the child's illness but also on preventing its recurrence. Interestingly, two families reported that the visits allowed them an opportunity to ask questions to which health professionals within the hospital had no time to respond. All the families recommended the program's continuance.

that may indicate that learners are not ready to go on to new material. At the end of the session, the learners should be left with a clear idea of the main points of the teaching session.

Evaluating the Learning That Has Taken Place

Evaluation is the assessment of how well the learner has achieved the expected outcomes (goals). If the expected outcomes have been stated specifically in terms of what the learner is expected to be able to do at the end of the teaching session, the task of evaluating the effectiveness of the learning is relatively simple. For example, one goal mentioned in the Nurses at Work box for Mrs. Gopal is that she indepedently demonstrate skill in changing the ostomy appliance. The extent of Mrs. Gopal's learning would be evaluated through the nurse's observations of her actually changing her appliance.

Methods of evaluating learning will vary with each of the learning needs. If the need has been one of acquiring information—for example, learning more about action to take if there are untoward complications when the patient returns home—questioning the patient is a good method of finding out the extent of knowledge. Can the patient list the complications? Does he or she understand their significance? Does the patient know what to do about them?

The acquisition of skills can be assessed by observing the ability to carry out the specific procedures, as we noted above. Some other questions might be: Does Mrs. Gopal use good skin care techniques around the stoma? Does she know how to prepare the equipment to change the appliance, handle it and maintain good technique while doing so? Questioning the patient while she is performing the procedure helps to ascertain whether she understands the principles involved.

In assessing attitudes, it is important to look not only at whether a person applies knowledge and skills, but also at the way they apply them. For example, is the patient careful to maintain good technique in handling the ostomy appliance? Attitudes can also be assessed through talking with the patient. For example, if Mr. Kucera tells the nurse that he is less anxious about how he is going to manage on his own, then the teaching can be considered successful.

Owing to the recent trend towards early discharge, it is often difficult to observe the ongoing integration of knowledge. Therefore, a follow-up appointment by a community health nurse, or a visit to the local outpatient clinic, is essential to assess how well Mrs. Gopal and Mr. Kucera continue to manage and integrate ostomy care into their day-to-day living.

Evaluating Teaching

The questions shown in the box on the next page can be used to help evaluate how well a teaching session with one patient or a group of patients was conducted. As a nursing student, you can apply these questions to your own teaching sessions. The questions are organized under headings that correspond to the skills of the teacher that affect teaching and learning (these were discussed earlier, although not in this order).

Documenting Patient Teaching

In patient teaching, it is essential that all members of the health team are familiar with the teaching plan. The communication tools used by nurses for patient teaching include the patient's chart, nursing care plans and forms that have been designed specifically for patient teaching, such as the patient teaching flowsheet shown in Figure 18.2. It can be a good idea to have a copy of the teaching plan in the patient's room and one at the nursing station to ensure that everyone is aware of the plan (Haggard, 1989; Rankin & Stallings, 1996).

The teaching that is done needs to be recorded on the patient's chart. In some agencies, the patient teaching flowsheet becomes a part of the permanent record. In others, both the teaching plan and the individual's response to it are included on the patient's chart.

Teaching–Learning in Nursing Education

The final section of this chapter explores ways in which the teaching–learning process is viewed within basic nursing education. During your educational program, you will acquire considerable knowledge through the classes you attend, the reading you do, the projects you undertake and your experience in clinical practice. You will also develop a repertoire of nursing skills. In the course of your program, you will probably change your attitude about a good many things. During your clinical experience you will learn to apply your knowledge and skills and put the attitudes you have acquired into practice in the real-life situations that constitute nursing.

In recent years, there has been a shift in thinking towards a new caring paradigm within nursing curricula. "In nursing, our perspectives have shifted from an emphasis on medicine back to nursing, from knowledge to understanding, from hierarchical relationships to partnerships, and from control to emancipation" (Molzahn, 1996, p. 13). The introduction of innovative teaching strategies emphasizes acquiring not only knowledge, skills and attitudes, but also mastery of the process of learning. This change suggests that the roles of both the teacher and the learner have changed. The role of student nurse has moved from passive recipient of information to active participant; the role of the nurse educator has shifted from manager of instruction to facilitator of learning. Knowles (1980) believes that students who assume a greater role in the teaching-learning process create for themselves a sense of ownership, increased feelings of satisfaction and stimulated levels of interest and motivation.

Guide for Evaluation of Your Teaching

Planning Skills

1. Did you have a written plan?
2. Was input obtained from patients regarding the planning?
3. Did you state the objectives for the session clearly and specifically, in behavioural terms?
4. Were the objectives attainable in the time available for the session?
5. Was the content relevant to the patients' needs?
6. Was the content appropriate considering what the patients already knew or were able to do?
7. Did you include appropriate material and strategies?

Organizing Skills

1. Were the time and place for the teaching adequate? Appropriate?
2. Did you make sure the place for teaching was ready?
3. Did you have all your equipment and supplies ready before the session?
4. Did you make sure that all participants had a clear, unobstructed view of equipment and materials used?
5. Did you make the objectives clear to participants at the beginning of the session?
6. Did you develop the lesson logically and sequentially?
7. Did you stop to see if the participants understood and were clear on one point before you proceeded to the next?
8. Did you emphasize key points in your conclusion?
9. At the end of the session, did the participants have a clear understanding of what it was all about?

Skill in Using Teaching Strategies

1. Do you feel the strategies you used were effective in gaining and holding the attention of participants?
2. Do you feel the strategies were appropriate for the content of the session?
3. Were a variety of strategies used?
4. Did you use teaching aids effectively (blackboard, diagrams, audio-visuals)?
5. Was the language you used clear and precise? Was it appropriate for the participants?
6. Did you explain technical terms?
7. Did you project your voice clearly so that everyone could hear you?
8. Do you think the participants found the session interesting?
9. Were the patients attentive?
10. Did the patients participate in the session?
11. Did you use appropriate techniques to evaluate the extent of the patients' learning?

Mastery of Subject Matter

1. Was subject matter correct in terms of current theory and practice?
2. Did you explain basic concepts clearly and simply?
3. Did you explain to the patients how this session related to the total program? How it was related to their needs?
4. Did you use approved technique in demonstrating a skill?
5. Do you feel you answered the patients' questions appropriately?

In recent years the work of Benner (1984) has gained considerable acceptance in nursing education. Barnum claims that "clinical learning is a dialogue between principles and practices. To truly grasp a principle, to learn it functionally, requires many practical experiences in which the principle is embedded" (cited in Benner, Tanner & Chesla, 1996, p. viii). This **situation-based interpretive approach** applies a model of skill acquisition developed by Dreyfus and Dreyfus. These authors believe that nurses learn the practice of nursing by passing through five levels (cited in Benner, 1984):

1. novice
2. advanced beginner
3. competent
4. proficient
5. expert.

According to Benner (1984), there are three aspects of change in skilled performance:

One is a movement from reliance on abstract principles to the use of past concrete experience as paradigms. The second is a change in the learner's perception of the demand situation, in which the situation is seen less and less as a compilation of equally relevant bits, and more and more as a complete whole in which only certain parts are relevant. The third is a passage from detached observer to involved performer. The performer no longer stands outside the situation but is now engaged in the situation.

(Benner, 1984, p. 13)

Using Benner's approach, learners enter a new clinical situation as novices, with little understanding of the contextual meaning other than that acquired from theory. Expert learners, on the other hand, perceive situations holistically and reflect critically with confidence and accuracy. Their knowledge base involves drawing from theory and understanding of self, as well as exposure to a rich, complex practice environment. To understand the behaviour, it is important to look at the bigger picture in which it is found. For example, giving a bed bath to a severely ill patient may be seen as a comfort measure. However, offering a bed bath to a soon-to-be-discharged patient may be seen as fostering dependence.

Student nurses are being encouraged to develop skills in critical and reflective thinking. Lindsey (1996) claims that "critical thinking, based on nursing theory and practice, is deliberate, intentional learning" (p. 11). Central to critical thinking is the concept of praxis. **Praxis** is a reciprocal process of reflection and action that produces opportunities for transformation and emancipation. Thus, learning is embedded within the context of the situation and is acquired through reflective practice (Schon, 1987a). The purpose of **reflective practice** is to enable student nurses to access, understand and learn through their lived experiences.

Reflection on experience needs to be guided to fulfill learning potential. Reflective journal writing is one strategy to enhance learning. The intent of "journalling" is to encourage self-reflection and enhance critical thinking skills. It also promotes a learner-centred dialogue between learner and facilitator and can provide insight into one's own learning (Schon, 1987b). To be a successful nurse today, you must be able to reflect on your nursing practice (Heinrich, 1992). The Registered Nurses Association of British Columbia (RNABC) and the Ontario College of Nurses have mandated, as part of continuing competency for registration, that nurses continue to self-evaluate their practice. Other strategies to facilitate reflection are discussion, questioning, storytelling, narratives, critical incidents and paradigm cases (Molzahn, 1996).

A final teaching strategy that nurse educators use to promote learning is the case study approach, described earlier in the chapter. Case studies form an essential component of the learning process of the novice nurse. For example, under the guidance of the facilitator, a student nurse can explore the meaning within the situation's parameters as well as within the student's own perceptual framework of values (personal meanings). The student is then guided to apply the theory in an appropriate manner relevant to the situation's context.

IN REVIEW

- A primary responsibility of nurses is to help patients, family and the community meet their learning needs, i.e.:
  - health education
  - patient education.

  Thus, nurses require an understanding of the teaching–learning process.
- Three major schools of thought have influenced our thinking with regard to teaching–learning:
  - behaviourist school (operant conditioning)
  - cognitive school (information processing)
  - humanist school (holistic approach).
- Currently, the dominant philosophy of educators is based on the humanist school of thought, in which:
  - the teacher is viewed as a facilitator rather than an instructor
  - the learner is viewed as an active (rather than a passive) participant in the process.
- There are three domains of learning, each involving different strategies:
  - cognitive (storage, recall, process of thinking)
  - psychomotor (skill acquisition)
  - affective (attitudes, values, beliefs, feelings).
- Teaching styles vary on a continuum from laissez-faire (least rigid) to autocratic (most rigid). A democratic (middle-of-the-road) approach is recommended for patient teaching. Teaching strategies must meet a patient's learning style.
- Characteristics of the learner include:
  - age
  - ability to communicate
  - cultural background
  - state of health
  - motivation.
- Characteristics of the teacher include:
  - knowledge of subject matter
  - appropriate use of teaching strategies
  - skill in assessing patient learning style
  - planning and organizing teaching activities.
- Creating an environment conducive to learning is another important factor in teaching.
- The phases of the nursing process parallel those of the teaching-learning process:
  - assessment (an initial assessment should identify learning needs and factors that may affect learning)
  - diagnosis (a learning diagnosis is identified)
  - planning (a teaching plan should be based on the identified learning diagnosis and specific goals/outcome criteria)
  - implementation (the teaching plan is carried out)
  - evaluation (based on two major components, i.e., patient learning and teaching session).
- Documentation is essential in order to communicate to other health professionals that teaching–learning has taken place.

- Nursing education has incorporated several ways of enhancing student learning:
    - reflective practice
    - situation-based interpretive approach
    - caring curriculum.

Critical Thinking Activities

1. Lee, who is eight years old, has an infected cut on his thigh. He is at home where he is being looked after by his grandmother, since both his mother and his father work outside the home. As the community health nurse in the area, you have been asked to visit the home and teach Lee's grandmother how to apply hot compresses to the cut. Lee's grandmother is Chinese and speaks only a few words of English.
    a. What factors would you consider before initiating any teaching?
    b. What strategies would be best to use for teaching Lee's grandmother?
    c. What factors might inhibit learning?
    d. What aids could you use to facilitate learning?
    e. In developing a teaching plan, what specific outcomes would you anticipate?
    f. How would you evaluate what Lee and his grandmother have learned?

KEY TERMS

health education p. 442
client education p. 442
patient education p. 442
learning p. 443
teaching p. 443
behaviourist school p. 443
cognitive school p. 444
humanist school p. 444
cognitive domain p. 444
psychomotor domain p. 444
affective domain p. 444
motivation p. 446
autocratic p. 447
laissez-faire p. 448
democratic p. 448
environment p. 448
teaching plan p. 451
lecture p. 454
discussion p. 454
one-on-one discussion p. 454
storytelling p. 455
demonstration p. 456
return demonstration p. 456
problem solving (discovery) p. 457
case study p. 457
role-play p. 457
behaviour modification p. 457
situation-based interpretative approach p. 460
praxis p. 461
reflective practice p. 461

References

ANDERSON, C. (1990). *Patient teaching and communicating in an information age.* Albany, New York: Delmar.

BABCOCK, D., & MILLER, N. (1994). *Client education: Theory and practice.* St. Louis: Mosby.

BENNER, P. (1984). *From novice to expert: Excellence and power in clinical nursing practice.* Menlo Park, CA: Addison-Wesley.

BENNER, P., TANNER, C.A., & CHESLA, C.A. (1996). *Expertise in nursing practice: Caring, clinical judgment and ethics.* New York: Springer.

BENOLIEL, J.Q., & SOULE, E.S. (1988). Some reflections on learning and teaching. *Journal of Nursing Education, 27*(8), 340–341.

BLOOM, B.S. (1956). *Taxonomy of education objectives. Handbook I: Cognitive domain.* New York: Longman Green.

BOYD, M.D., GRAHAM, B.A., GLEIT, C.J., & WHITMAN, N.I. (1998). *Health teaching in nursing practice: A professional model.* (3rd ed.). Stamford, CT: Appleton & Lange.

BRITISH COLUMBIA CHILDREN'S HOSPITAL. (1994). Discussions with Director of Patient Education.

CANTOR, J.A. (1992). *Delivering instruction to adult learners.* Toronto: Wall & Emerson.

CARPENITO, L.J. (1993). *Nursing diagnosis: Application to clinical practice.* (5th ed.). Philadelphia: Lippincott.

COUTTS, L.C., & HARDY, L.K. (1985). *Teaching for health: The nurse as health educator.* New York: Churchill Livingstone.

HAGGARD, A. (1989). *Handbook of patient education* (p. 33). Rockville, MD: Aspen.

HEINRICH, K.T. (1992). The intimate dialogue: Journal writing by students. *Nurse Educator, 17*(6), 17–21.

JENNY, J. (1987). Knowledge deficit: Not a nursing diagnosis. *Image, 19*(4), 184–185.

KNOWLES, M. (1978). *The adult learner: A neglected species.* (2nd ed.). Houston: Gulf.

KNOWLES, M.S. (1980). *The modern practice of adult education: From pedagogy to androgogy.* Chicago: Follett.

KNOWLES, M. (1990). *The adult learner: A neglected species.* (4th ed.). Houston: Gulf.

LINDSEY, E. (1996). *Collaborative nursing program in British Columbia. Collaborative curriculum guide.* Victoria, BC: University of Victoria.

MOLZAHN, A.E. (1996). Changing to a caring paradigm for teaching and learning. *American Nephrology Nurses Association Journal, 23*(1), 13–18.

POHL, M.L. (1981). *The teaching function of the nursing practitioner* (4th ed.). Dubuque, IA: Wm. C. Brown.

PRICE, J.L., & CORDELL, B. (1994). Cultural diversity and patient teaching. *Journal of Continuing Education in Nursing, 25*(4), 163–166.

RANKIN, S., & STALLINGS, K. (1990). *Patient education: Issues, principles, practices.* (2nd ed.). Philadelphia: Lippincott.

RANKIN, S., & STALLINGS, K. (1996). *Patient education: Issues, principles, practices.* (3rd ed.). Philadelphia: Lippincott.

REDMAN, B. (1997). *The process of patient education.* (8th ed.). St. Louis: Mosby.

RORDEN, J.W. (1987). *Nurses as health teachers: A practical guide.* Philadelphia: Saunders.

SCHON, D. (1987a). *Educating the reflective practitioner.* San Francisco: Jossey-Bass.

SCHON, D. (1987b). The intimate dialogue: Journal writing by students. *Nurse Educator, 17*(6), 17–21.

SNOWDON, A.W., & KANE, D.J. (1995). Parental needs following the discharge of a hospitalized child. *Pediatric Nursing, 21*(5), 425–428.

WAINES, R. (1993, February). AIDS education from a front line worker's perspective. *Canadian Journal of Public Health*, 31–33.

WHITMAN, N., GRAHAM, B., GLEIT, C., & BOYD, M. (1992). *Teaching in nursing practice: A professional model.* (2nd ed.). Norwalk, CT: Appleton & Lange.

YELON, S.L. & WEINSTEIN, G.W. (1977). *The teacher's world: Psychology in the classroom.* New York: McGraw-Hill.

Additional Readings

ATKINS, S., & MURPHY, K. (1993). Reflection: A review of the literature. *Journal of Advanced Nursing, 18*, 1188–1192.

BECHTAL, G.A. (1995). Enhancing functional health patterns among homebound elderly clients' caregivers. *Journal of Nursing Science, 1/2*, 33–39.

COVEY, S.R. (1990). *The seven habits of highly effective people.* New York: Simon & Schuster.

DUFFY, B. (1997). Using a creative teaching process with adult patients. *Home Healthcare Nurse, 15*(2), 102–108.

DU GAS, B.W. (1983). *Introduction to patient care: A comprehensive approach to nursing*. Philadelphia: Saunders.

GOTTLIEB, L., & ROWAT, K. (1987). The McGill model of nursing: A practice-derived model. *Advances in Nursing Science, 9*(4), 51–61.

GREENBURG, J. (1995). *Health education: Learner-centered instruction strategies.* (3rd ed.). Dubuque, IA: Brown & Benchmark.

JOHNS, C. (1995). Framing learning through reflection within Carpers. Fundamental ways of knowing in nursing. *Journal of Advanced Nursing, 22*, 321-329.

JOHNS, C. (1996). Visualizing and realizing caring in practice through guided reflection. *Journal of Advanced Nursing, 24*, 1135–1143.

KATZ, J.R. (1997). Back to basics: Proving effective patient teaching. *American Journal of Nursing, 97*(5), 33–36.

MOORE, P.A. (1996). Decision-making in professional practice. *British Journal of Nursing, 5*(10), 635–640.

PATERSON, B.L. (1995). Developing and maintaining reflection in clinical journals. *Nurse Educator Today, 15*, 211–220.

PEARSON, M., & WESSMAN, J. (1996). Gerogogy in patient education. *Home Healthcare Nurse, 14*(8), 631–636.

SARNA, L., & GANLEY, B.J.A. (1995). A survey of lung cancer patient education materials. *Oncology Nursing Forum, 23*(3), 422–423.

SELEY, J.J. (1994). 10 strategies for successful patient teaching. *American Journal of Nursing, 94*(1), 63–65.

THEIS, S., & JOHNSON, J.H. (1995). Strategies for teaching patients: A meta-analysis. *Clinical Nurse Specialist, 9*(2), 100–105, 120.

Chapter 19

Information Management

OUTLINE

Central Questions

1. Why is documentation of nursing care important?
2. What information is kept on the patient's record?
3. What is a nursing audit?
4. What are the advantages and disadvantages of:
   - narrative charting?
   - the problem-oriented medical record?
   - PIE charting?
   - focus charting?
   - charting by exception?
   - electronic documentation?
5. How are flowsheets used?
6. What standards have been established regarding the documentation of nursing care?
7. What information is considered essential for nurses to document on patient records?
8. What basic guidelines should be kept in mind when documenting nursing care?

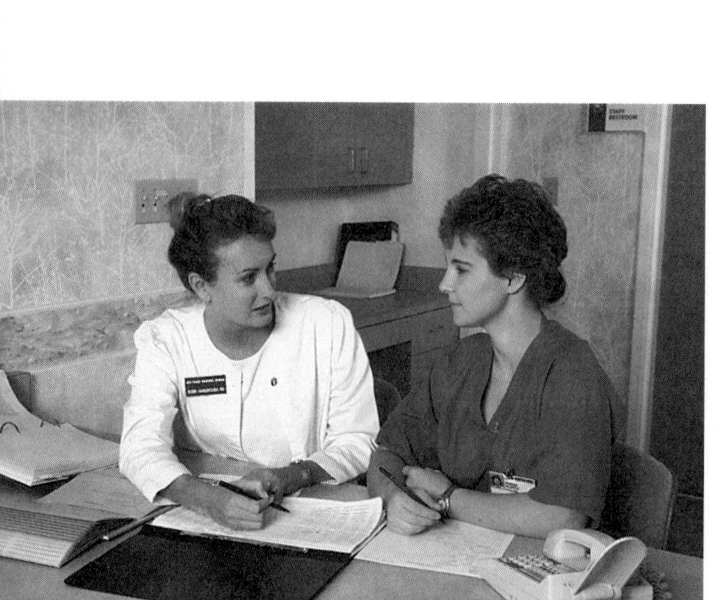

Introduction

... It has been realized that with so many people becoming involved in the care and treatment of patients, it is essential to have an efficient and sophisticated means of communicating information among them.

Rozovsky, 1994, p. 82

Documentation is the communication in writing of essential facts in order to maintain a continuous history of events over a period of time. **Reporting** is the communication of information to another individual (or group of individuals) and may be either written or oral. Giving and receiving reports were examined in Chapter 17. A number of different records and report forms are kept by various health agencies, and the nurse will find that these vary from one agency to another. All types of health agencies maintain patient records or charts. The form of the record usually depends on the type of agency. Hospitals use one type of record, community health agencies another and extended care institutions yet another.

No matter what form of charting is used in the agency in which you work, a knowledge of basic standards in nursing documentation is imperative. In this chapter, we present the basic elements of nursing documentation of patient care. Professional nurses should be able to adapt these elements to fulfill their responsibilities in whatever agency they may be employed.

Purpose of Documentation or Charting

Documentation, or charting, in the patient record serves a number of functions. It provides a means of communication among health professionals and a legal record of patient care. In addition, the record is used for education and research, and for the **nursing audit**—the evaluation of the quality of nursing care.

COMMUNICATION

The documentation on the **patient record** serves as a means of communication among health professionals. It is an account of the patient's history, present health status, treatment and response to treatment. "Since the provider of care has a duty to the [patient] to provide the care in a reasonable and prudent manner and to take reasonable steps to minimize reasonably foreseeable risks, communication of information becomes an integral part of that duty" (Rozovsky & Rozovsky, 1984, p. 6).

The nursing care provided should be reflected by documentation of the nursing process, including assessment, nursing diagnosis, planning, implementation and evaluation. Through documentation of the care plan and the patient's response to care, continuity of care is established and maintained.

LEGAL AND PROFESSIONAL STANDARDS

Nurses are responsible and accountable for their actions. Thus, they can be held legally answerable for these actions. Because the patient's record is recognized as a legal document, accurate record keeping becomes a professional responsibility. In a majority of malpractice suits involving patient care, the patient record serves as documentary evidence and is an invaluable account of actions concerning the issue in question (Iyer & Camp, 1995).

In 1970 the Supreme Court of Canada ruled that:

Hospital records, including nurses' notes made contemporaneously, by someone having the personal knowledge of the matters being recorded and under a duty of care to make the entry or record should be received as prima facie proof of the facts stated therein.

(*Ares v. Venner*, 1970; RNABC, 1996, p. 5)

As a legal record, the chart is the property of the agency or the medical professional responsible for a patient's care. However, a patient has the right to access the information on the chart (RNABC, 1992). To access the record, a patient can submit a written or verbal request. Each agency has its own procedures that a health professional can follow when this situation occurs.

EDUCATION AND RESEARCH

The patient record is used by all disciplines in teaching rounds, for conferences and for study purposes. Trends in specific disease entities identified from chart reviews provide information for the treatment of the individual patient.

When patient records are used for education or research purposes, it is essential to ensure the confidentiality of these records, and it may be necessary to obtain patients' consent (Sanchez-Sweatman, 1997). The fourth value in the CNA *Code of Ethics for Nursing* states: "Nurses safeguard the trust of clients (patients) that information learned in the context of a professional relationship is shared outside the health care team only with the client's (patient's) permission or as legally required" (CNA, 1997, p. 15). Furthermore, the Ontario Guidelines for Professional Behaviour read that patients must be informed that other health professionals will have access to the information in their record.

AUDIT

An audit is a methodical review of the medical record for the purposes of collecting data. The nursing audit consists of a review of patient records to evaluate the quality of nursing care as documented in the record. The nurse must remember that if the care has not been documented, it is assumed that the care has not been given. The audit may be retrospective (that is, a review of the care received by patients who have been discharged), or concurrent (an evaluation of care that is currently being given).

The process of care, as documented in the record, is compared with standards for nursing care as determined by members of the nursing profession. Criteria for evaluation are established through such aspects of care as the data base, the identification of problems, the expected outcomes of care, the selection of nursing interventions and the degree to which the plan of care was carried out as evidenced by the nurses' notations on the patient's record.

A nursing audit may be undertaken to evaluate either the quality of care given by individual nurses or the quality of care provided by an entire agency. In either case, it is the individual patient records that are reviewed. A nursing audit committee within the agency is responsible for determining the standards of care to be met. If the agency's quality of nursing care is being evaluated, an outside committee is established. Representatives on this committee might include members of the provincial nurses' association, nurses from an accrediting agency and, possibly, nurses employed by a government agency. Because an audit is done by members of the same professional group, it is often referred to as *peer review*.

Forms of Charting

Many forms of charting are currently in use in Canadian health agencies. The following is a brief overview of six charting systems. Table 19.1 (page 471) compares their advantages and disadvantages.

NARRATIVE

Narrative charting (also known as *source-oriented medical recording*) is the most traditional approach to documentation. The progress notes are written in simple paragraph form and in chronological order as patient issues are presented. There is little structure to these notes unless documentation guidelines and standards have been established by the health care agency. In some agencies, all disciplines document in the same progress note. This allows for concentration of patient information in one area. However, in agencies where each discipline has its own progress note, information about the same patient problem could be scattered throughout the record. Narrative notes tend to be lengthy and cluttered with accounts of routine care and assessment (RNABC, 1996; Iyer & Camp, 1995).

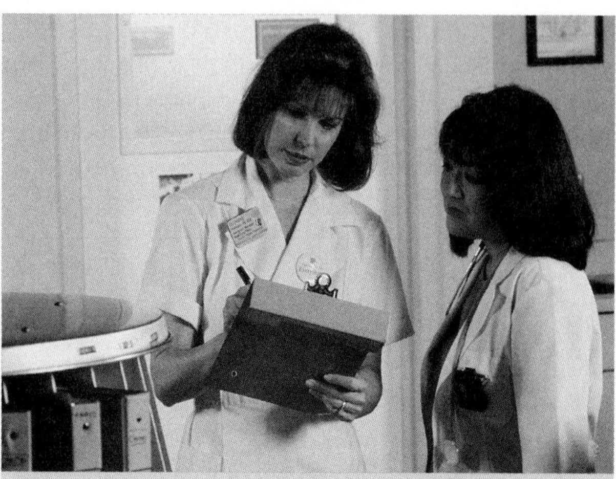

The documentation of patient care is an important nursing responsibility.

With the use of flowsheets, the documentation of routine care and treatments is removed from the narrative note. The purpose of the **flowsheet** is to show in graphic form interventions or observations in respect to one particular problem. Flowsheets are usually developed for use for a designated period of time. They may cover a week or a 24-hour period. The vital signs record used in most hospitals is an example of a flowsheet that is used to record temperature, pulse, respiration and other vital signs for a week at a time. When it is necessary to monitor vital signs more frequently than every four hours, as allowed for on the usual vital signs record, a seperate flowsheet may be used. The minute-to-minute monitoring of vital signs of patients in the intensive care unit of a hospital would be charted in this way.

This leaves a more pure narrative that refers to significant findings and specific patient problems. Flowsheets were developed originally by nurses in intensive care units but are also used in other units for the following reasons:

- to save time
- to document routine care
- to prevent duplication in charting
- to ensure a systematic assessment and
- to provide the greatest amount of patient information in one area of the record.

Flowsheets can be used with other forms of charting as well as with narrative charting (see Figure 19.1).

A narrative note, combined with flowsheet documentation, should provide the information needed for all disciplines to make informed patient care or treatment decisions (Iyer & Camp, 1995). An example of a narrative note follows:

> *Feb. 6, '99, 19:30: Pt complaining of lower abdominal pain in area of abdominal incision; also has sense of "fullness" and a need to void. Scant, old, dried, dark brown drainage noted on abdominal dressing. Wound is clean, no fresh drainage noted. Fresh dressing applied. Urinary catheter tubing repositioned; clear yellow drainage in tubing and bag. Pt instructed re: urinary catheter and its purpose; reassured that voiding on her own not necessary. Medicated for pain with morphine per MD's order. Repositioned to R side.*
>
> — Jane Doe, RN
>
> *Feb. 6, '99, 20:00: Pt indicates she is more comfortable; able to do coughing and deep-breathing exercises with nurse's encouragement; cough is nonproductive. Turned to L side. No further comments re: urge to void. Catheter continues to drain well.*
>
> — Jane Doe, RN

VANCOUVER GENERAL HOSPITAL
BRITISH COLUMBIA'S HEALTH CENTRE

ACTIVITIES OF DAILY LIVING FLOWSHEET

B = Breakfast 2P = 2 person assist SM = Small
L = Lunch 1P = 1 person assist M = Moderate
D = Dinner L = Large

T = Total W = Well NN = See Nurses's Notes
P = Partial I = Intermittent Blank space = not applicable
S = Self Pr = Poor

DATE NURSING UNIT

MR., MISS, MRS., MS. UNIT NUMBER

SURNAME GIVEN NAME

DOCTOR (PLEASE BLOCK CAPITALS)

SEX AGE

	Day														
	Month ______ Year ______ Time														
DIET	No nursing observation/intervention required ✓														
	Diet Change / Time														
	Tolerated ✓ / Amount Taken % B														
	L														
	D														
	Snack														
	Assistance T, P, S,														
HYGIENE	No nursing observation/intervention required ✓														
	Tub/Shower T, P, S														
	Sink/Basin T, P, S														
	Bedbath T, P, S														
	Mouthcare T, P, S														
	Pericare T, P, S														
ACTIVITY	No nursing observation/intervention required ✓														
	Assistance & # (T, 2P, 1P, S) / Last Time Walking														
	BRP														
	Chair														
	Dangle														
	Bedrest ✓														
	Sleep W, I, Pr,														
ELIMINATION	No nursing observation/intervention required ✓														
	Bowel Movements														
	Loose SM, M, L														
	Soft SM, M, L														
	Hard SM, M, L														
	Absent ✓														
	INITIAL														

FIGURE 19.1 Activities of daily living flowsheet

SOURCE: Vancouver General Hospital and Health Sciences Centre, Vancouver, B.C.

PROBLEM-ORIENTED MEDICAL RECORD (POMR)

In the **problem-oriented medical record (POMR)** all patient data are organized according to patient problems. A problem list is established and members of all disciplines are involved in documenting issues concerning problems relevant to their disciplines. The POMR has five components: data base, problem list, initial plan/orders, progress notes and discharge summary (Iyer & Camp, 1995).

The **data base** includes the physician history and physical exam and the nursing history and functional health pattern assessment. The **problem list** is multidisciplinary and generated from the data base. Updates occur as problems are solved and/or new problems develop. A **plan of care** is developed from the problem list. The medical plan of care is documented in the **progress notes**; the nursing care plan is usually in a separate format that includes the nursing diagnoses, expected outcomes and interventions. Progress notes are recorded by all disciplines on the same sheet and are numbered to correspond with the problem from the problem list. Information is organized in the **SOAPIE format**, an acronym for:

S = Subjective data (what the patient tells you)
O = Objective data (what the clinician observes)
A = Assessment (nursing, medical diagnoses)
P = Plan (plan of action based on above information)
I = Interventions (actual interventions implemented)
E = Evaluation (patient's response to plan and changes needed).

Discharge summary concludes the POMR, which includes a discussion of each problem and its outcome. For unresolved problems, a SOAPIE is written. This summary fosters communication among agencies and health professionals.

The POMR system was seen as a great improvement over traditional patient records when it was introduced two decades ago. It focussed on patient problems with a format that could be used by all disciplines and in all types of agencies. It was felt that the use of the POMR would foster collaboration among all members of the health team since all plans would be recorded on the same form. It was felt that it would also help to bring about greater uniformity in recording in different agencies.

However, the SOAPIE format can be redundant with plan and interventions noted both on the care plan and in the progress notes. If flowsheets are included, charting duplication occurs. Because each problem requires an entry, problems tend to overlap, causing repetition. A final potential drawback is that integration with other disciplines may cause resistance from individual clinicians (Iyer & Camp, 1995). The SOAPIE format is illustrated in Figure 19.2.

PIE CHARTING

PIE charting (problems, interventions and evaluation of nursing care) was developed to simplify documentation by eliminating the traditional care plan and incorporating it into the daily documentation. It is a problem-oriented approach similar to SOAPIE charting. However, PIE charting was developed from the nursing process, whereas SOAPIE charting originated from the medical model. The system consists of a 24-hour, daily assessment flowsheet. The nurse initials the portions specific to the patient. Deviations from the normal are flagged with an asterisk; the deviation is then described in the progress notes. Each problem, using the NANDA (North American Nursing Diagnosis Association) list, is labelled with a P and numbered (P#__). The intervention is labelled IP#__ (the number corresponds to the previously identified problem number). The problem is then evaluated each shift and labelled EP#___ (Iyer & Camp, 1995). An example of PIE charting is given in Figure 19.3.

The overall planning component of the nursing process may not be addressed in PIE charting. The nurse will need to ensure that patient outcomes are considered, probably through the addition of standardized or individualized care plans.

FOCUS CHARTING

Focus charting is a type of charting that can be used as an alternative to the more traditional narrative nurses' notes. It provides more specificity than the narrative notes and records nursing concerns rather than the medically oriented problems listed on the POMR.

In **focus charting**, the nurse identifies a patient *concern* rather than a problem. The nurse focusses on a behaviour, a change, an event or a nursing diagnosis. The progress notes are organized into three columns: the date and time in one, the focus in another and the patient care note in the last. The patient care note is further organized into three sections: data (subjective or objective), action (nursing interventions) and response (patient's response to interventions). Assessment forms and flowsheets, developed by the individual agency, support and are necessary to focus charting (Iyer & Camp, 1995; RNABC, 1996). Figure 19.4 shows a focus progress note. Chart audits of focus charting have revealed that nurses tend to revert to narrative charting, because they have some difficulty documenting the correct information under the appropriate focus charting sections (Iyer & Camp, 1995).

CHARTING BY EXCEPTION (CBE)

The **charting by exception (CBE)** system documents only significant findings or exceptions to the norm. There are several components to this system:

- flowsheets—nursing/physician order flowsheet, graphic record, teaching record and discharge note
- standards of practice—a checkmark indicates that previously developed standards of care have been met
- nursing data base (history and physical)
- nursing diagnosis-based care plans
- SOAPIE progress notes (data, action, response)

Problem List:

1. Postoperative pain
2. Bladder discomfort

Date/Time	***Problem***	***Progress Notes***
Feb. 6, '99 19:00	Abd pain postop or #1	S: "I'm having pain in my stomach." O: Pt is 4 h postop abd hysterectomy. Last med for pain 3 h ago in the PACU. Pt lying on her back, tense posture, guarding abd. On scale of 1–10, rates pain at 6. Scant old, dried, dk. brown drainage on abdominal dressing. Wound is clean, no fresh drainage noted. Fresh dressing applied. A: Alteration in comfort: acute pain secondary to surgical trauma today. P: Medicate pt according to MD's orders. Instruct pt to request pain med before pain is severe. Check pt. in 30–45 min to assess for relief. — Jane Doe, RN
	Bladder discomfort or # 2	S: "Please bring me a bedpan. My bladder feels full and I want to use the bedpan." O: Pt has indwelling foley cath; cath draining freely of clear, yellow drainage. A: Knowledge deficit: unaware of cath placement. Urinary Elimination, Alteration in patterns related to foley cath placement. P: Reposition foley cath. Assess for relief of discomfort in 45 min. Instruct pt re: foley cath placement. I: Foley cath repositioned to promote optimum drainage. Pt. instructed that foley cath placed during surgery, would remain in place through the night, and that cath is positioned in bladder allowing continuous drainage and negating need for pt to void on her own. Pt remembers now preop instruction re: cath insertion. — Jane Doe, RN
Feb. 6, '99 19:15	Abd pain postop or #1	I: Pt medicated with morphine re: MD order. Pt positioned on R side. Pt instructed to put on call light if pain continues or when relief begins to wear off. — Jane Doe, RN
Feb. 6, '99 19:45		E: Pt indicates she is more comfortable; rates pain at 2. Pt able to do coughing and deep-breathing exercises with nurse's encouragement. Repositioned on L side.
	Bladder discomfort or #2	E. Cath continues to drain well. Pt has no further complaints of discomfort. — Jane Doe, RN

FIGURE 19.2 SOAPIE format for documentation

Date	*Time*	*Progress Notes*
Feb. 6, '99	19:00	P#1 Alteration in comfort: acute pain secondary to surgical trauma today. P#2 Knowledge deficit: unaware of urinary cath placement during surgery. Wants to void. — Jane Doe, RN
Feb. 6, '99	19:15	IP#1 Pt medicated for pain. Instructed to call RN if pain persists or as relief wears off. Call light within reach. Abd wound assessed. Scant sanguinous, dry drainage on dressing. New dressing applied. Pt positioned on R side. IP#2 Pt instructed re: foley catheter placement during surgery. Pt also instructed re purpose of catheter and position in bladder. Catheter tubing repositioned to encourage optimum drainage. — Jane Doe, RN
Feb. 6, '99	19:45	EP#1 Pt indicates she is more comfortable. Able to do coughing & deep-breathing exercises with Nurse's encouragement. Pt repositioned on L side. EP#2 No further comments re: need to void. Catheter draining. — Jane Doe, RN

FIGURE 19.3 PIE charting

Date	*Time*	*Focus*	*Progress Notes*
Feb. 6, '99	19:00	Alteration in comfort: acute pain secondary to surg. trauma today.	D: Complaining of pain in abd. Lying on back. A: Abd incision site assessed: site clean; scant sanguinous, dry drainage on dressing. New dressing applied.
		Knowledge deficit: Unaware of urinary catheter placement.	D: Wants to void. A: Pt instructed re: urinary catheter placement during surgery, that catheter will remain in place through the night, that catheter is positioned in bladder allowing continuous drainage and negating need to void. Catheter repositioned to promote optimum drainage. — Jane Doe, RN
Feb. 6, '99	19:15		A: Pt medicated with morphine per MD orders. instructed to call RN if pain persists or as relief wears off. Call light placed within reach. — Jane Doe, RN
Feb. 6, '99	19:45		R: Pt indicates she is more comfortable. Able to do coughing and deep-breathing exercises. Catheter. draining appropriately. No further comments re: need to void. States she now remembers pre-op instruction re: catheter placement. — Jane Doe, RN

FIGURE 19.4 Focus progress note

- accessibility of forms—all flowsheets are kept at the patient's bedside, negating the need for transcription of data (Burke & Murphy, 1995).

As with conceptual models, an agency may use a combination of different forms of charting. Figure 19.5 is an example of a flowsheet that combines the use of focus and CBE charting systems.

Educating staff to document only the abnormal findings has proven difficult. Charting by exception was pilot-tested at St. Luke's Hospital in Milwaukee, Wisconsin, under a grant from the Aurora Health Centre. The purpose of the project was to teach nurses to document selectively in order to reduce the amount of time spent on charting. The project was successful in reducing charting time. However, educating staff to document only the abnormal findings proved difficult because nurses have traditionally been taught to record all pertinent observations (both normal and abnormal) about a patient. Some nurses were concerned about checking standard care boxes on a flowsheet instead of writing a narrative note because they were unsure of their accountability when they made such an entry. For these reasons, orientation to CBE involves a major educational effort (Iyer & Camp, 1995).

Murphy and Burke (1995) and the Registered Nurses Association of British Columbia (1997) maintain that CBE is a complete charting system. However, it changes the traditional philosophy of "*if it was not documented, it was not done*" *to* "*all standards of care have been met unless documented otherwise*." At present, there is no case law on CBE. In 1993 an Alberta case, *Wenden v. Trikhas*, accepted that "standard procedure in the hospital, and indeed, the acceptable procedure, is to make nurses' notes at various intervals when there is something worthwhile to say and not necessarily more frequently. This case may help recognize that if CBE is used, and if evidence can be offered that care was given and noted according to this format, then it would be admissible as evidence" (RNABC, 1997, p. 2). To meet legal documentation standards, the CBE system includes "established agency documentation policies and procedures, individual care plans, care protocols and flow sheets" (RNABC, 1996, p. 6).

ELECTRONIC DOCUMENTATION

Increasingly, health facilities are using computerized systems to document patient care. Nursing use of technology in health care agencies varies from very limited use to complete documentation through computers. Electronic systems designed to support the management of patient care are commonly referred to as **patient care information systems (PCISs)** and are a major component of the health care organization's information system. In hospitals, the PCIS is part of the larger hospital information system (HIS). With regionalization initiatives in the Canadian health care system underway, the conceptualization of the HIS has broadened to include continuing care facilities, community health care providers and physicians' offices, as well as acute care hospitals.

Information can be accessed by authorized health professionals in multiple locations within the system including the bedside, community clinics and the physician's office. Documentation of care is entered at each patient entry point in the system, thus creating a continuous electronic health record—from crib to grave. The use of a PCIS for patient documentation is of great benefit to obtain more timely, reliable and complete patient documentation.

TABLE 19.1 Advantages and disadvantages of various forms of charting

SYSTEM	ADVANTAGES	DISADVANTAGES
Narrative	• familiar to nurses • quick/easy to document • quick/easy to document in emergencies	• time-consuming • lacks structure • task-oriented
POMR	• problem list is easily accessible to follow progress • directs care on problems • fosters collaboration	• difficult to maintain list • creates lack of confidence in assessment skills • duplication may occur
PIE	• reduces documentation time	• eliminates planning step of nursing process • no separate care plan
Focus	• gives structure to progress notes • information easily located	• can become narrative in nature • requires change in thinking
CBE	• patterns in pt status easily identified • current data readily accessible • eliminates repetitive charting of routine care	• duplication may occur • requires change in thinking • requires ongoing educational support • legal basis is questionable

SOURCES: Eggland & Heinemann, 1994; Iyer & Camp, 1995.

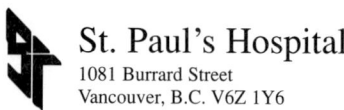

St. Paul's Hospital
1081 Burrard Street
Vancouver, B.C. V6Z 1Y6

NURSING ASSESSMENT AND INTERVENTION FLOWSHEET

NURSING PHYSUICAL ASSESSMENT PARAMETERS:
FUNCIONAL HEALTH PATTERNS

NUTRITION/METABOLIC PATTERN
Tolerates prescribed diet without nausea and/or vomiting. Swallowing without coughing or choking on liquids or solids. No evidence of rash. Skin color within patient's norm. Skin warm and intact. Mucous membranes moist. Wound/incisional Assessment: No evidence of redness, increased tissue temperature, tenderness in surrounding tissue. Sutures/staples/steri-strips intact. Incisional edges well approximated. No drainage present.

YEAR: ________________ MONTH: ________________

ELIMINATION
Abdomen soft. Bowel sounds present on auscultation. No pain with palpation. Having bowel movements within own normal pattern. Able to void with no oliguria, polyuria, dysuria, dribbling, distention, burning or incontinence. Urine clear and yellow to amber. Genital area shows no evidence of edema, bruising or abnormal bleeding. Foley patent if present.

ACTIVITY/EXERCISE PATTERN
Independently ambulates, transfers from bed to chair or stands without pain, dyspnea or fatigue. Active range of motion of all extremities with symmetry of strength. No swelling or tenderness in joints. No muscular weakness. Regular apical/radical pulse. Peripheral pulses palpable. No edema. No calf tenderness. If monitored, patient is in normal sinus rhythm. Affected extremity is pink, warm and movable within patient's average range of motion. Sensation intact without numbness or paresthesia. Respirations 10-20/min at rest, quiet and regular. Breath sounds clear and audible both lung fields and auscultation. Sputum absent or clear. Nail beds and mucous membranes pink.

COGNITIVE/PERCEPTUAL PATTERN
Alert and oriented to person, place and time. Behaviour appropriate to situation. Memory intact. Pupils equal and reactive to light. Verbalization clear and understandable. Patient experiences no pain or current level of pain is no greater than the patients' acceptable level of pain.

Key: ✓ = Normal findings   * = Significant findings   ➜ = Significant findings remain unchanged   D/C = Discontinued   C = See patient chart

DATE IDENTIFIED	NO.	FOCUS ASSESSMENT/INTERVENTION	DATE / TIME											
	1													
	2													
	3													
	4													
	5													
	6													
	7													
	8													
	9													
	10													
	11													
	12													
	13													
	14													
	15													
	16													
	17													
		NURSE'S INITIALS												

FIGURE 19.5 Nursing assessment and intervention flowsheet

SOURCE: St. Paul's Hospital, Vancouver, British Columbia.

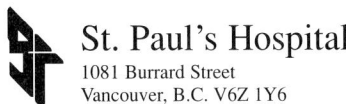

DEPARTMENT OF NURSING
SIGNIFICANT FINDINGS

DATE	TIME	FOCUS	SIGNIFICANT FINDINGS D = Data A = Action R = Response / Evaluation	INITIALS

FIGURE 19.5 *(Continued)*

SOURCE: St. Paul's Hospital, Vancouver, British Columbia.

PCIS Process

Patient data are collected and retrieved using a variety of different methods in a PCIS. These include keyboards, light pens, touch screens, bar code readers, a point-and-click mouse, handwriting or voice recognition. Data are entered and retrieved on a terminal or workstation and by hand-held or palm-top devices. Patient information is stored in the computer (on-line) and can be printed and placed on the patient chart (hard copy). The approach varies between agencies, depending on the type of PCIS they are using and the extent of the health record that is stored electronically. Figure 19.6 illustrates a computer screen in a PCIS.

The components of most PCISs include: order entry and results reporting, medication administration recording, care planning and charting. Ideally, these components are designed for multidisciplinary use and integrated across the functions. For example, order entry is used by physicians to enter diagnostic and treatment orders and by nurses to enter nursing orders. When the charting function is used, information that was entered into the orders and care planning functions prompts the nurse on required charting. The patient information stored in the data base is then available for review, analysis and reporting on a patient-specific or patient-group basis. Ideally, the care-planning and documentation functions support the determination of patient acuity and the calculation of prospective and retrospective nursing workload. All PCISs have the ability to produce many different types of reports that can be used by nurse care providers, nurse educators, nurse administrators and nurse researchers.

Information can be sent and received between the PCIS and other systems in the hospital information system (HIS) via electronic interfaces. For example, orders for lab tests are communicated immediately and directly to the lab system; when the test results are obtained, the data are sent immediately from the lab system to the PCIS. In addition, the PCIS can automatically capture data recorded by other equipment, such as intravenous infusion pumps, analgesia pumps, heart monitoring devices, and thermometers.

The PCIS supports the immediate capture of data, thus eliminating the need for paper notes, duplicate recording and transcription of information. Once data are entered into the system they can be displayed wherever appropriate. For instance, allergy information may be displayed on different screens and/or reports as well as communicated to other systems that require it, such as the one used by the pharmacy.

Uses of the PCIS

The PCIS provides a variety of options to review patient information for health professionals. Some screens show summary information with the ability to "scroll up or down" to details as required. Data such as results and vital signs can be viewed in columnar or graphical formats. Care

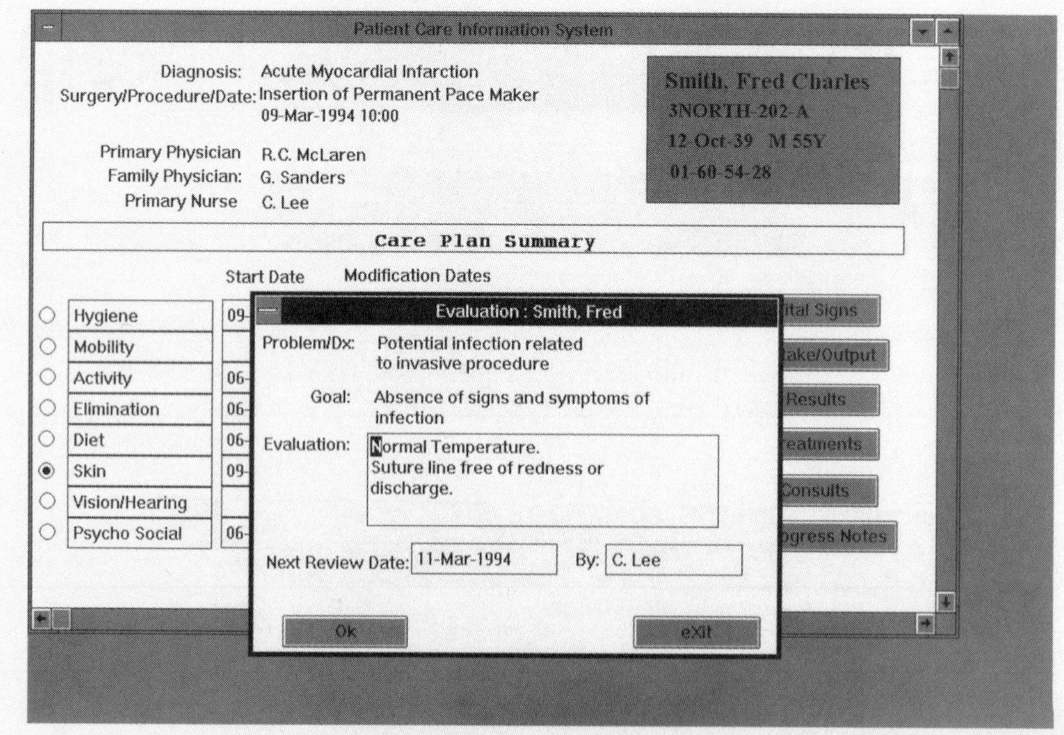

FIGURE 19.6 Patient (client) care information system (PCIS). This is a simulation of a computer screen in a PCIS. In this screen, the nurse is able to view a current summary of the patient's care plan and chart the patient's response to a specific intervention. The nurse could also "click" the buttons on the right or left sides of the screen to access other sections of the care plan or the chart.

SOURCE: Diagram developed by Susan Ball, Christina Beckett and Pat Jesselon.

providers can also control the information display in terms of picking exactly what they want to see at any given time. For example, the nurse may want to view certain lab results and medication records simultaneously, and in another case may wish to see care plan interventions that have an impending review date. Access to information may be from points where patient care is provided such as the bedside, in clinics and in diagnostic or treatment areas, as well as locations remote from the point of care, such as the physician's office or public health unit.

The PCIS supports the nursing process by storing large amounts of data for a variety of purposes and linking related information. Standards of care and individualized care plans are retained in the system. As orders are entered, results reported and care documented, the care plan is automatically updated to reflect the new information. Interventions are automatically added or suggested as the care plan is created and the patient assessment is charted.

Quality Assurance programs are supported by the PCIS through the use of "rules" that can be incorporated into the program to prompt the nurse to provide additional information in specific situations. For example, if a patient's vital signs exceed the normal ranges, the system prompts the nurse to increase the frequency of vital signs monitoring. Teaching materials can be printed for patients from the PCIS. As well, diagnostic procedure preparation information for nurses can also be made available on-line. Many PCISs include access to data bases, such as CINAHL (on-line journal search) and Micromedex (pharmaceutical and trauma data base). Some health care agencies have all their manuals on-line, as part of their PCIS.

In response to tightened health care funding and increased public accountability, a shift is occurring that combines clinical guidelines and standards of care into critical paths. Critical paths are built around **case-mix groups (CMGs)**—called diagnosis-related groups (DRGs) in the United States. The **critical path** outlines the care to be provided patients for each day (or at more frequent intervals) of their stay in hospital by all physicians, nurses and other allied health professionals. Care is recorded against this critical path in much the same way as was indicated in the section on charting by exception. Administrators can review the care delivered and determine when, where, and why variances from expected paths occurred. This allows them to better monitor budgets and care delivery, physician practices, resource utilization (patient costing) and outcomes of care delivered.

Discharge planning is facilitated by the PCIS automatically or, with little additional effort, by including information already in the system in a patient's discharge plan. Referrals to community agencies are now handled electronically in many cases, and community caregivers access the PCIS to view relevant clinical information on-line.

An example of a critical pathway documentation is illustrated in Figure 19.7.

Concerns About the PCIS

The issues of privacy, confidentiality and security of electronically stored patient information are paramount. Nurses must continue to be patient advocates in this area. They must ensure the integrity and security of patient information held in computer information systems to the same degree they do paper charting. All agencies with computerized systems have policies and procedures to ensure the security of patient records. Most PCISs have elaborate and sophisticated security systems within the software, which can restrict access to patient information on a need-to-know basis.

In summary, the PCIS is a valuable information tool to support the provision of patient care. Many of the features of computerized documentation can significantly enhance the quality and timeliness of patient information, thus allowing care providers to enhance the quality of care delivered. PCIS features provide such advantages as:

- reducing the number of phone calls to various hospital departments and physicians
- eliminating duplicate recording of information in multiple locations
- ensuring that patient documentation is more thorough, relevant and complete
- facilitating the development and updating of patient care and discharge plans
- significantly reducing medication errors, order entry errors and charting omissions
- eliminating errors resulting from misinterpretation of illegible writing
- providing accurate and current patient acuity and workload information
- giving immediate access to pertinent patient information by multiple care providers at multiple locations
- creating faster turnaround time between information collection and retrieval
- developing a data base to support nursing administration, research and education
- reducing the risk of record tampering
- allowing graphical display of data
- categorizing according to standards of care.

There are also disadvantages to computer documentation. These include:

- costly initial investment
- insufficient terminals or space at nursing stations
- downtime (due to routine service or failure), which is disruptive and frustrating
- reluctance of some nurses to give up the old system
- slowing of system during peak usage periods
- loss of essential patient information if system crashes
- possible dependency on computerized information; reluctance to question errors

THE SIMON FRASER HEALTH REGION

☐ Royal Columbian Hospital
☐ Eagle Ridge Hospital
☐ Ridge Meadows Hospital

O.R. Day (After Surgery)

SHIFT:		SHIFT	
Care Category	Date:	Care Category	
Clinical Measurement	☐☐☐ VS q6h ☐☐☐ I&O _ _ _ VS stable _ _ _ Fluid balance maintained	Hygiene	☐☐☐ Mouthcare ☐ HS care: Comp/part ☐☐☐ Skin care
Medications	☐☐☐ Pain medication (PCA, IM, epidural) ☐☐☐ Antiemetic prn _ _ _ Nausea controlled	Activity/ Mobility	☐☐☐ Bedrest ☐☐☐ Lockout knee control on ☐☐☐ Bedpan/Urinal ☐ Slept: well, on/off, poorly _ _ _ Turn q3h with assistance
Procedures/ Treatments/ Assessments	☐☐☐ 0_2 Mask/Nasal prongs ☐☐☐ 0_2 Sat prn ☐☐☐ I.S. 10 x h while awake ☐☐☐ NVC as per standard ☐☐☐ Foley catheter ☐☐☐ IV fluids ☐☐☐ IV replacements for wound drain x 12 h prn _ _ _ Skin pressure point clear qh8 _ _ _ States pain at tolerable level q2h x 24 h _ _ _ Dressing dry & intact	Patient/ Family Education	☐☐☐ Instruct re: hip precautions ☐☐☐ Instruct re: I.S. ☐☐☐ Reinforce PCA pain scale
Diet	☐☐☐ NPO ☐☐☐ Bowel sounds assessed	Physio	
		Progress	_ _ _ Maintained on pathway
Initials		Initials	
Symbol key:	☐ = Interventions _ = Expected outcomes ✓ in ☐ or _ Interventions done or outcome as expected	O in ☐ or _ The item was not pertinent to the shift. * in ☐ or _ Interventions was not done or outcomes as expected	

FIGURE 19.7 Clinical pathway: Total hip replacement

SOURCE: Simon Fraser Health Region, British Columbia.

HOUR	MEDICATIONS	TREATMENT & NOTES

FIGURE 19.7 *(Continued)*

SOURCE: Simon Fraser Health Region, British Columbia.

- fewer interactions with other health professionals
- risk of reduced patient–nurse interaction
- fear of staff reductions
- staff resistance to technology
- patient reluctance to disclose fully because they fear data can be accessed by all employees of the agency
- possible inaccurate dissemination of information
- limited standardized terminology in computer programs (Eggland & Heinemann, 1994; Iyer & Camp, 1995; Meyer, 1992).

The legal issue of confidentiality has raised a number of concerns with the use of PCISs. For example, nurses should not reveal their passwords to others, access sensitive information relating to patients other than their own or leave the terminal unattended. To monitor potential abuses of information access, all computer transactions are recorded (Iyer & Camp ,1995).

Several trends in computerization that may modify the documentation process include:

1. development of standing orders that are built into the hospital system
2. automation of critical pathways
3. voice-activated programs for quick documentation in busy settings
4. linking of hospital computer networks with personal home computers
5. graphical interface of patient data (Iyer & Camp, 1995, p. 259).

NURSING INFORMATICS

Graves and Corcoran (1987) define **nursing informatics** "as [a] combination of computer science, information science and nursing science designed to assist in the management and processing of nursing data, information and knowledge to support or enhance the practice of nursing and the delivery of nursing care" (p. 227). Hannah (1985) also describes nursing informatics as any use of information technology in relation to any nursing function that is carried out by nurses.

Because we work in a rapidly changing technological environment, all health professionals must keep current with the latest information in order to maintain standards of practice. The Alberta Association of Registered Nurses (1985) claims that the introduction of computer technology will greatly influence nursing. Informatics is just one method that helps nurses access and process widespread information quickly and maintain a currency of nursing knowledge. Many associations, organizations and schools of nursing have also added to the wealth of knowledge available on the Internet by developing their own websites. The Canadian Nurses Association's home page is located at http://www.cna-nurses.ca/. Individuals who browse their web pages can find a variety of information, including dates of upcoming conferences, journal abstracts and courses offered.

Now recognized as a legitimate area of study and practice in nursing, nursing informatics is being integrated into nursing curricula to enhance student learning. Students use the Internet to access an abundance of information to complete assignments, to offer information to patients and their families and to e-mail their teachers and peers. Students can even maintain dialogue with other students around the world. The Canadian Nursing Students' Association has a website (http://www.cnsa.ca/) to facilitate just such communication.

FACSIMILE (FAX) TRANSMISSIONS

Fax transmissions are another electronic means of expediting communication. "Since a fax is an exact copy of the original documentation, it is [an] acceptable form to communicate information between health care providers and to authorize interdependent functions, such as physician orders" (College of Nurses of Ontario, 1996, p. 21). Faxed information must be kept confidential. Guidelines to maintain the security of patient information have been developed—for example, placing fax machines in nonpublic areas, controlling information sent by fax, and authorizing staff-only use of fax (Peck, 1995).

DOCUMENTATION FOR SELF-EMPLOYED NURSES

Nurses who work in private practice are required to use some type of documentation system. Essential documentation will vary according to the kind of service offered by the nurse. Usually, the forms are straightforward and continue to focus on assessments, plans, actions and the patient's responses (RNABC, 1996).

Standards for Documentation

Standards for charting have been developed to ensure that essential information is consistently documented. All health care agencies have their own standards regarding the content to be included in documenting patient care. The health professional must be oriented to the standards of charting in the agency and must chart according to the system that is in place. However, professional nurses can develop their own standards and adjust these to correspond to whatever area they work in.

General charting standards have been established by professional nursing organizations. It is important for the health professional to become familiar with the general standards of the nursing profession. Nurses will also find it helpful to have access to specific standards of the area or specialty in which they work. From standards that have been formally developed, one usually finds specific references to documentation expectations. Following are some examples of charting standards.

CANADIAN NURSES ASSOCIATION Standards II.1: Nurses are required to collect data in accordance with their conception of the patient (CNA, 1987, p. 4).

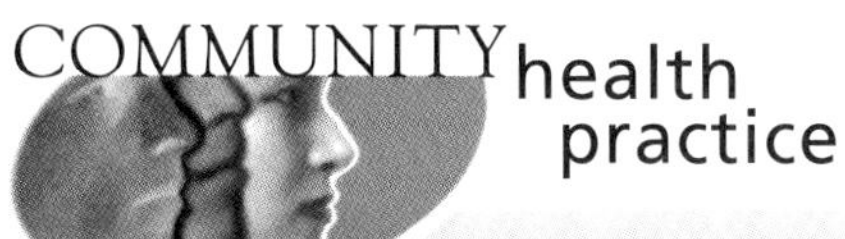

COMMUNITY health practice

Home Care and Long-Term Care Documentation

Documentation in the home and in long-term care settings is as fundamental as in the hospital. Health professionals working in all these settings follow charting standards developed by their respective agencies that help them identify and record patient concerns, the interventions taken and patient response to these interventions. The rationale for charting in the home care setting is to ensure continuity of care, as many individuals will be offering care to the patient in his or her own home (Iyer & Camp, 1995).

In addition to progress notes, a patient record in a home care setting may include an account of conference notes and telephone calls. With long-term care documentation, family concerns and education may also be recorded in the patient record. The frequency of long-term documentation, in contrast to that in the hospital or in the home care setting, varies from agency to agency and depends on the patient's health status. For example, a nurse may be required to complete nurses' notes on a daily basis soon after a patient's admission and then only once a week or once a month thereafter (Iyer & Camp, 1995).

COLLEGE OF NURSES OF ONTARIO 1. Framework for documenting: Documentation needs to provide a clear picture of the needs or goals of the patient, the actions of the nurse and the outcomes. Nurses need to document the care or service provided to individuals, to groups and to communities (College of Nurses of Ontario, 1996, pp. 7–8).

BRITISH COLUMBIA RESIDENTIAL CARE SERVICES/FACILITIES (CONTINUING CARE DIVISION) Standard 4.1, Resident Care Services: Individualized Care Planning: There shall be a current, individualized, written plan of care developed and implemented for each resident (Government of British Columbia, 1992, p. xviii).

Essential Documentation

Following is a description of essential documentation that should be carried out in accordance with charting standards.

1. An admission note will be written at the time of admission on the approved form by the nurse admitting the patient. The admission note will include date and time of admission, mode of transportation and person accompanying the patient. The note will also include the reason for admission as stated by the patient, if appropriate, and a brief description of the patient's presenting signs and symptoms. Allergies, medications the patient is currently taking and assistive devices (such as dentures and eyeglasses) will be noted. The nurse will document the patient's perception of reason for admission, past health problems and problems or concerns in need of immediate attention.

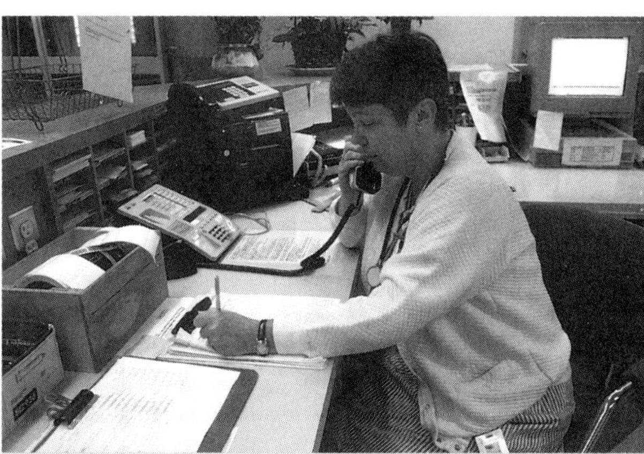

A nurse documenting a telephone order from a physician.

2. An assessment by functional health patterns and an initial care plan will be written for each patient within 24 hours of admission. Each agency usually has developed its own nursing assessment form. In some agencies, a discharge planning form is often part of the patient record and is initiated on admission.
3. A progress note will be written at least once a shift, and as often as the patient's condition warrants, by the nurse caring for the patient. Progress notes will reflect continued assessment of patient condition, planning, mutual goal setting, interventions and patient outcome evaluation. Patient response to nursing interventions for resolution of nursing diagnoses or collaborative problems will be the focus. Patient teaching and patient response to that teaching are also written in the progress notes.
4. Nursing activities generated by the medical plan of care and patient response to those interventions (for example, medications, treatments) will be recorded on the approved forms.
5. A transfer note will be written when a patient is transferred from one unit to another. The note will include date and time of transfer, unit of acceptance and mode of transport and status of current patient problems. The nurse accepting the patient will write a note to include date and time at which the patient is received and a statement of the patient's condition. A notation is made when a patient leaves and returns from a procedure that necessitates a consent and/or premedication (for example, the operating room). Date, time of transfer and mode of transport, scheduled procedure and patient's condition, including response to medications, are all included.

RESEARCH to practice

Adam, L., Traschel, L.C.E., & Love, S. (1994). Interdisciplinary documentation: The challenge of developing a common data base. *Canadian Journal of Rehabilitation, 7*(4), 267–272.

Clinical information on patients at the Glenrose Rehabilitation Hospital in Edmonton had been recorded by different health professionals as separate entries within the patient's chart. The authors undertook the task of developing a system that would integrate all clinical assessment data, from all health professionals involved, into a common data base.

Initially, excessive and duplicative documentation was noted. Following this preliminary review, a set of principles and categories of information were established in order to develop the common data base that all health professionals could use to record their assessment findings. A pilot site was then chosen, guidelines to assist staff were created and documentation was initiated using the common data base. This common data base was used only with new patients. Eighteen patients were assessed over a four-month period.

While the project was underway, evaluation tools for a chart audit and for staff satisfaction were being developed. Health records technicians carried out the audit, which indicated that use of the common data base resulted in substantial reduction in duplication and increased integration of information. Yet, the results also indicated confusion with regard to referrals: it was difficult to ascertain if these were actually made.

The staff were then surveyed regarding their satisfaction with the common data base. Twenty-six staff of 30 responded. Using a Likert rating scale, the results indicated a moderate to strong agreement level. In addition, there was an increase in collaborative planning among staff. While the authors recommend further improvement to the common data base, other staff were interested in testing it on their units.

6. A discharge note is written upon discharge. It includes patient condition, person accompanying the patient, mode of transportation, prescriptions and follow-up appointments.
7. The nurse must check the agency's policy for verbal/telephone orders. Only registered nurses can take verbal/telephone orders, signing their name and indicating the physician responsible for giving the order. To ensure accuracy, the nurse should repeat the order back to the physician before writing it on the patient's record. In addition, the nurse must document VO (verbal order) or TO (telephone order), as well as the date and time the order was taken and transcribed. For example:

   Feb. 6, '99, 19:00: Gravol 50 mg q4h IM prn; TO Dr. Gomes/Jane Doe, RN.

   The physician then signs the verbal/telephone order within a specified time according to agency policy. Verbal/telephone orders have the potential for creating errors.

Charting Guidelines

Entries are written in black or blue ink and signed with full name and registration status. In some agencies, student nurse notes are countersigned by a registered nurse. Each note must be dated with the exact (24-hour clock) time. If initials are used on a flowsheet, the nurse's full signature with initials should appear somewhere on the flowsheet.

Errors in documentation are corrected by putting a single line through the incorrect information, writing "error" above it and initialling it. No correction fluid or erasures are permitted.

Legal Requirements for Charting

- sign every entry
- write the complete date/time of each entry
- avoid spaces
- read previous entries prior to documenting care given
- write neatly, concisely and legibly
- use proper spelling and grammar
- use authorized abbreviations; avoid using medical terms inappropriately
- be precise in documenting information reported to physician
- use graphic record to record vital signs
- chart promptly after delivery of care
- avoid block charting
- do not tamper with records; avoid erasures, back-dating or additions to previous entries
- correctly identify late entries
- chart only the care given or supervised
- document exact quotes
- document in black or blue ink only
- use 24-hour clock
- ensure patient's name is addressographed on each form
- transcribe orders with precision
- avoid using nursing notes to criticize other health professionals
- eliminate bias from written notes
- never leave a terminal unattended after you have logged on
- do not access patient information without a purpose
- do not share access passwords

SOURCES: Eggland & Heinemann, 1994; Smith & Duell, 1996; Iyer & Camp, 1995.

Chart entries must be made in chronological order. Nothing should be written between the lines. Out-of-order notes (recorded in the progress notes by another person before the nurse has had a chance to write) should be written after the last charted note. The words "out-of-order entry" should precede the note. The time the entry is made and the time the care was given must be recorded. Late-entry notes (notes made after the fact) are written after the last charted note and are preceded by "late-entry note." Lines should not be left blank. If a blank line is present, a line should be drawn through it to prevent someone from inserting a note (RNABC, 1996). Only the abbreviations used by the agency in which you are working should be used. Commonly used medical abbreviations are listed in all medical dictionaries. Most agencies have selected one set of abbreviations for use in all departments.

Notes and entries must be made promptly. If the nurse must document the care given by someone else (for example, a nurse's aide or family member), the name and status of the individual involved must be recorded (RNABC, 1992). Notes should be concise, without repetition and free of jargon; writing must be legible and words spelled correctly. Generalizations should be avoided.

IN REVIEW

- The principal purposes of the patient record are:
  - to maintain a legal document
  - to provide a channel of communication among health professionals
  - to serve as a tool for research and education
  - to assess quality of care.
- Health professionals have an ethical responsibility to maintain the confidentiality of patient records.
- Patient records are the property of the agency. However, patients have a legal right to access the information on record.
- Several systems of documentation are used in Canadian health agencies, including:
  - narrative
  - focus
  - POMR
  - CBE
  - PIE
  - electronic

  Each system has advantages and disadvantages.
- Canadian health agencies follow general standards regarding content to be included in the patient record. Essential nursing documentation includes:
  - admission note
  - initial assessment and care plan
  - progress notes (record of nursing interventions, patient response, ongoing assessments)
  - transfer/discharge notes.
- There are basic guidelines that must be adhered to regardless of the agency's system of documentation. These include:
  - mandatory full signature and registration status
  - entries recorded in black or blue ink only with date and time
  - entries in chronological order
  - no spaces or lines left blank in the record
  - concise entries free of jargon or repetition.
- Computerized information systems have assisted nurses in documenting patient information. Nursing informatics and the Internet have helped nurses to access, process and share information quickly and to maintain currency of nursing knowledge.

Critical Thinking Activities

1. Mrs. Rose Wong is a patient who has undergone abdominal surgery. She has been on the nursing unit three days postoperatively. Her orders from the physician include dressing changes once a day as necessary and Demerol, 50–100 mg intramuscularly (IM) or Tylenol #3, every four hours (q4h), as needed (prn) for pain.

   Her dressing is soaked through with reddish-brown fluid and she complains of pain. As her nurse, you give her 50 mg of Demerol and change her dressing. The following questions should be answered and recorded using each of the different charting methods (narrative nurses' notes, a problem-oriented medical record, PIE documentation, focus charting, charting by exception and electronic documentation):

   a. Where should you look for Mrs. Wong's orders?

   b. Give a sample of the charting for Demerol, including what should be recorded about the patient.

KEY TERMS

documentation p. 465
reporting p. 465
nursing audit p. 465
patient record p. 465
narrative charting p. 466
flowsheet p. 466
problem-oriented medical record (POMR) p. 468
data base p. 468
problem list p. 468
plan of care p. 468
progress notes p. 468
SOAPIE format p. 468
discharge summary p. 468
PIE charting p. 468
focus charting p. 468
charting by exception (CBE) p. 468
PCIS (patient care information system) p. 471
case-mix groups (CMGs) p. 475
critical path p. 475
nursing informatics p. 478

c. What should be included in recording the dressing change? Give an example.

d. Where are these data recorded?

e. How would a change in the physician's orders be indicated to nursing personnel? A change in nursing orders?

References

ADAM, L., TRASCHEL, L.C.E., & LOVE, S. (1994). Interdisciplinary documentation: The challenge of developing a common data base. *Canadian Journal of Rehabilitation, 7*(4), 267–272.

ALBERTA ASSOCIATION OF REGISTERED NURSES (AARN). (1985). *Computers in nursing*. Edmonton: Author.

BURKE, L.J., & MURPHY, J. (1995). *Charting by exception applications: Making it work in clinical settings.* Albany, NY: Delmar.

CANADIAN NURSES ASSOCIATION (CNA). (1987). *A definition of nursing practice standards for nursing practice*. Ottawa: Author.

CANADIAN NURSES ASSOCIATION (CNA). (1997). *Code of ethics for nursing*. Ottawa: Author.

COLLEGE OF NURSES OF ONTARIO. (1996). *Nursing documentation standards*. Toronto: Author.

EGGLAND, E.T., & HEINEMANN, D.S. (1994). *Nursing documentation: Charting, recording and reporting.* Philadelphia: Lippincott.

GOVERNMENT OF BRITISH COLUMBIA. (1992). *Standards for residential care services (facilities)*. Victoria: B.C. Ministry of Health & Ministry Responsible for Seniors, Continuing Care Division.

GRAVES, J., & CORCORAN, S. (1987). The study of nursing informatics. *Image, 21*(4), 227–231.

HANNAH, K. (1985). Current trends in nursing informatics: Implication for curriculum planning. In Hannah, K., Guillemin, E., & Conklin, D. (Eds.), *Nursing uses of computer and information science* (pp. 181–187). Amsterdam: North Holland.

IYER, P.W., & CAMP, N.H. (1995). *Nursing documentation: A nursing process approach*. St. Louis: Mosby.

MEYER, C. (1992). Bedside computer charting: Inching toward tomorrow. *American Journal of Nursing, 92*(4), 38–44.

PECK, S. (1995). *Review of the storage and disposal of health care records*. Victoria: B.C. Ministry of Health & Ministry Responsible for Seniors.

REGISTERED NURSES' ASSOCIATION OF BRITISH COLUMBIA (RNABC). (1992). *Nurse to nurse information for nurses. Charting: A review of nursing documentation*. Victoria: Author.

REGISTERED NURSES ASSOCIATION OF BRITISH COLUMBIA (RNABC). (1996). *Nursing documentation.* (Rev. ed.). Vancouver: Author.

REGISTERED NURSES ASSOCIATION OF BRITISH COLUMBIA (RNABC). (1997). *Charting by exception: Nurse to nurse.* Vancouver: Author.

ROZOVSKY, L. (1994). *The Canadian patient's book of rights. A consumer's guide to Canadian health law*. Toronto: Doubleday.

ROZOVSKY, L., & ROZOVSKY, F. (1984). *The Canadian law of patient records*. Toronto: Butterworths.

SANCHEZ-SWEATMAN, L. (1997). Nurses, computers and confidentiality. *Canadian Nurse, 93*(7), 47–48.

SMITH, S.F., & DUELL, D.J. (1996). *Clinical nursing skills.* (4th ed.). Stamford, CT: Appleton & Lange.

Additional Readings

AMERICAN NURSES ASSOCIATION. (1995). *Standards of practice for nursing informatics*. Washington, DC: Author.

BALL, M.J., HANNAH, K.J., NEWBOLD, S.K., & DOUGLAS, J.V. (Eds.). (1995). *Nursing informatics: Where caring and technology meet.* (2nd ed.). New York: Springer-Verlag.

BRASSARD, Y. (1992). *Learning to chart.* Sherbrooke, QC: Loze-Dion.

CALFEE, B.E. (1996). Charting tips: Documenting an AMA discharge. *Nursing 96, 26*(10), 17.

CANADIAN INSTITUTE FOR HEALTH INFORMATION. (1995). *Health data sharing in Canada: A resource guide*. Ottawa: Author.

EGGLAND, E.T. (1996). Charting tips: Making the transition to home health care charting. *Nursing 96, 26*(3), 16.

GEE, P.M. (1997a). The Internet: A home care nursing clinical resource. Part I. *Home Healthcare Nurse, 15*(2), 115–121.

GEE, P.M. (1997b). The Internet: A home care nursing clinical resource. Part II. *Home Healthcare Nurse, 15*(3), 175–180.

GOVERNMENT OF BRITISH COLUMBIA. (1996). *Health information management project. Phase 2—final report.* Victoria: B.C. Ministry of Health and Ministry Responsible for Seniors.

GRANE, N.B. (1996). Charting tips: Comments that should stay "off the record." *Nursing 96, 26*(1), 17.

HAWLEY, P. & DESBOROUGH, K. (1998). The computer as tutor: Interactive learning that builds confidence. *Canadian Nurse, 94*(4), 31–35.

HEBDA, T., CZAR, P., & MASCOVA, C. (1998). *Handbook of information for Nurses and Health care professionals.* Menlo Park, CA: Addison Wesely Longman

HENRY, S.B. (1995). Nursing informatics: A state of the science. *Journal of Advanced Nursing, 22*, 1182–1192.

HUTCHINSON, D. (1997, January). A nurse's guide to the Internet. *RN*, 46–51.

INDIAN & NORTHERN HEALTH SERVICES DIRECTORATE, NURSING DIVISION. (1994). *Standards for documentation by nursing personnel.* Ottawa: Author.

JOHNSON, D., & MARTIN, K. (1996). Preparing for electronic documentation. *Nursing Management, 27*(7), 43–44.

KREMSDORF, R. (1996). Is computerization keeping up with patient-focused care? *Seminars for Nurse Managers, 4*(1), 65–71.

KROTHE, J.S., PAPPAS, V.C., & ADAIR, L.P. (1996). Nursing students' use of a collaborative computer technology to create family and community assessment instrument. *Computers in Nursing, 14*(2), 101–107.

LANGE, L.L. (1997). Informatics nurse specialist: Roles in health care organizations. *Nursing Administration Quarterly, 21*(3), 1–10.

LYBECKER, C.J. (1997). A nurse explores the Internet. *American Journal of Nursing, 97*(6), 42–50.

MARRELLI, T.M., & HARPER, D.S. (1996). *Nursing documentation handbook.* (2nd ed.). St. Louis: Mosby Year Book.

MERKOURIS, A.V. (1995). Computer-based documentation and bedside terminals. *Journal of Nursing Management, 3*(2), 81–85.

NAGLE, L.M., & RYAN, S.A. (1996). The superhighway to nursing science and practice. *Holistic Nurse Practitioner, 11*(1), 25–30.

NETTINA, S.M. (1996). *The Lippincott manual of nursing practice.* (6th ed.). Philadelphia: Lippincott.

SHELEST, K. (1997). Nursing and the Net. *Nursing BC, 29*(2), 15.

SIMPSON, R.L. (1995). Getting wired for success. *Nursing Administration Quarterly, 19*(4), 89–91.

TURLEY, J.P. (1996). Toward a model for nursing informatics. *Journal of Nursing Scholarship, 28*(4), 309–313.

WARNER, I. (1996). Introduction to telehealth home care. *Home Healthcare Nurse, 14*(10), 790–796.

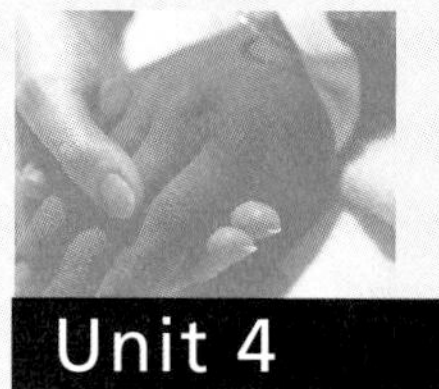

Unit 4

Physiological Needs

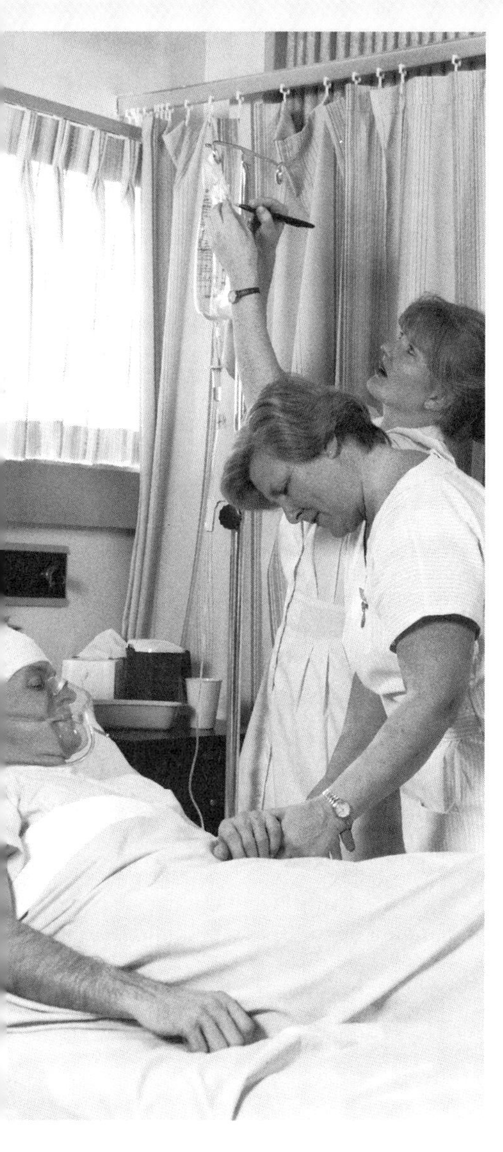

Chapter 20

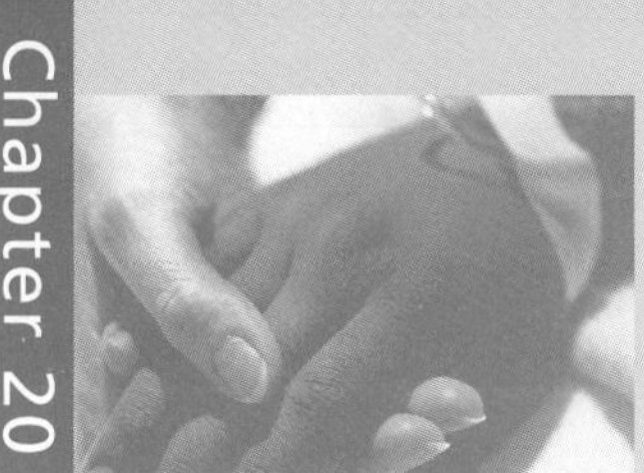

Nutritional Needs

OUTLINE

Introduction

Nutritional Needs in Health

Nutritional Needs Throughout the Life Cycle

Determinants of Nutritional Status

Nutritional Needs in Illness

Common Problems

Assessing Nutritional Status

Diagnosing Nutritional Problems

Planning Nutritional Interventions

Implementing Nutritional Interventions

Evaluating Nutritional Interventions

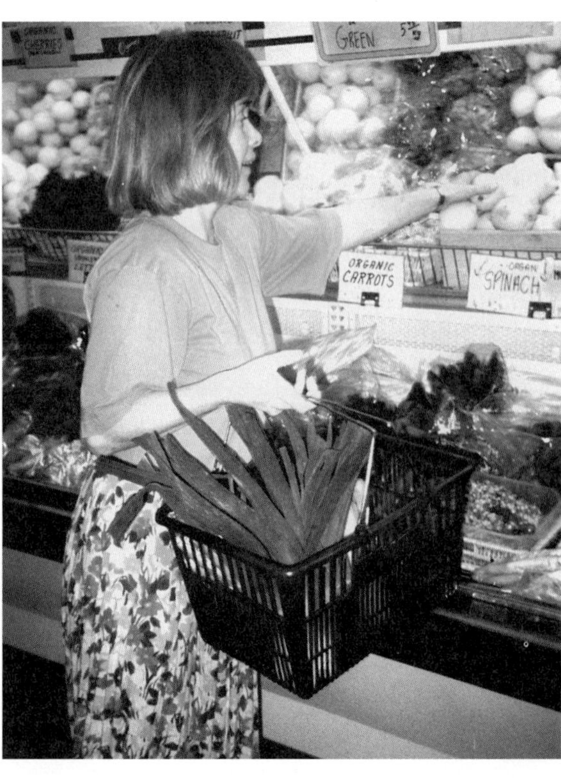

Central Questions

1. What is the role of food in meeting basic human needs?
2. What are the processes involved in the digestion, absorption, and metabolism of carbohydrates, proteins and fats?
3. What are the functions of vitamins and minerals in the body?
4. What are the nutrient and energy requirements of healthy people?
5. How do nutritional needs vary throughout the life cycle?
6. What are the main determinants of nutritional status?
7. How do nutritional needs change in illness?
8. What are some common nutritional problems?
9. What basic principles would the nurse apply in assisting individuals to meet nutritional needs?
10. How does the nurse assess an individual's nutritional status?
11. What are the common nursing diagnostic statements for individuals with nutritional problems?
12. How would the nurse develop a plan of care for individuals with nutritional problems?
13. What strategies might the nurse implement in helping individuals, families or groups to promote optimum nutritional status and protect nutritional functioning?
14. What health-restoring and supporting strategies might the nurse implement in the care of individuals with nutritional problems?
15. How would the nurse evaluate the individual's response to nursing interventions?

Introduction

The term *nutrition* is derived from the Latin root *nutr-*, which means to *nurture* or *nourish* (Williams, 1997). Nutrition is concerned with the foods people eat and how the body uses these foods to sustain life. Food and the partaking of meals also have a significance in human society that goes beyond the provision of nourishment for the body. In addition to fulfilling a basic physiological need, food may also help to satisfy one or more of an individual's many other needs. It has long been recognized, for example, that food is closely related to feelings of security. This security comes not merely from the presence or absence of food in sufficient quantity to satisfy hunger, but from the availability of specific foods. For many people, milk is a basic security food; for others, it may be meat, potatoes, rice or some other familiar food. When people are ill, it is sometimes necessary to deprive them of certain foods. Individuals may feel threatened if foods that hold strong security meanings for them are absent from their diet. By the same token, a person's emotional health, especially in the stress of illness, may be "enhanced by significant 'comfort foods' that hold special meaning for the person and help to heal both the body and the spirit" (Williams, 1989, p. 12).

Food is often used to promote a feeling of social acceptance. Sitting down to eat with another person conveys to the person that he or she is considered an equal. Offering someone a cup of tea or coffee—the "ritual of hospitality"—can do much to foster an atmosphere of warmth and friendliness that is often difficult to attain in other ways.

Some people use foods for their prestige value and to enhance feelings of self-esteem. In many cultures, bread is a prestige food. For many years, steak and roast beef were considered prestige foods in North America. Now that the world has become a "global village," more people have been introduced to foods from other countries, and therefore more exotic fare has become prestige food. Food may also be used to express creativity. Many people enjoy using their creative talents to prepare gourmet meals to please their families and friends.

The sharing of food in one form or another plays an important role in many religious ceremonies. In the Christian ceremony of Communion, for example, food has great significance: the bread symbolizes the flesh of Christ, and the wine, Christ's blood. In Judaism and Islam, the preparation of food is in itself a ritual. There are also many food taboos associated with specific doctrines of religions. The devout Muslim will not eat pork, nor the Hindu, beef. (See Chapter 12 for a detailed discussion of the cultural and religious significance of food.)

Mealtime, in many parts of the world, is a significant aspect of family life. In many cultures, eating is considered a private affair, to be shared and enjoyed only with one's family or intimate friends. Meals often play an impotant role in reaffirming solidarity within the family group. The traditional gathering of a family for Thanksgiving or Christmas dinner serves to strengthen ties within the extended family unit. Meals may provide a time when family roles are defined and clarified.

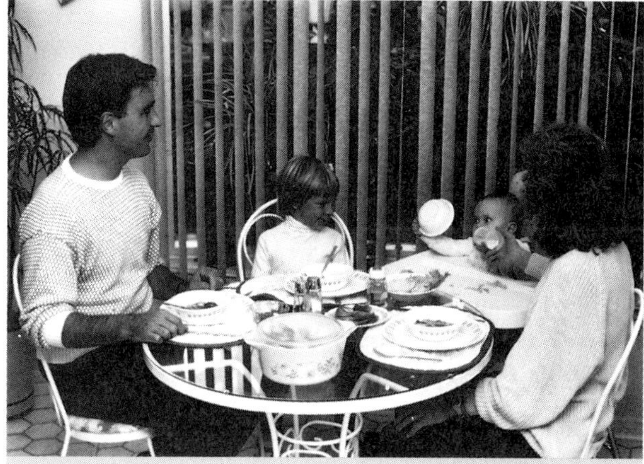

Being together for meals can help strengthen family ties.

In addition, mealtime is often considered a pleasant time—a period of relaxation, when one can enjoy the company of others and engage in social conversation. Health agencies today are doing much to make mealtimes more pleasant for patients. Food is arranged attractively on trays; there is usually a menu from which patients may select the foods that they like; and many hospitals now have small dining areas next to the nursing units, where patients who are able may gather to eat their meals.

Thus, nutrition is vital to all aspects of health. As well as having psychological, social, cultural and spiritual significance in a person's daily life, food is essential for physical health and well-being. Because all cells in the body require adequate nourishment for optimal functioning, all systems of the body many be affected by nutritional problems. When a person is ill, nutrition and diet therapy are primary factors in restoring health. A person's state of health may be restored without medicine, but the body cannot heal without proper nutrition (Poleman & Peckenpaugh, 1991). Whether well or ill, people may need assistance to maintain an adequate nutritional state, to achieve an even better state, or to correct an imbalance. The responsibility for assisting individuals to meet their nutritional needs rests with the physician, dietitian and nurse. This chapter is intended to provide the nurse with basic knowledge of nutrition and diet therapy which will enable him or her to do the following:

1. assess the nutritional needs of individuals in health and illness
2. assist individuals in maintaining adequate nutrition and hydration during illness
3. provide restorative care to individuals experiencing nutritional problems
4. assist individuals in promoting optimal nutritional health for themselves and their families.

Nutritional Needs in Health

A person cannot exist for long without taking some form of nourishment. Food is the fuel that provides the energy for human metabolism. In order for people to function at their optimal level, they must consume adequate amounts of foods containing the essential nutrients for human life. A **nutrient** is defined as any "chemical substance supplied by food that the body needs for growth, repair and general functioning" (Eschelman, 1996, p. 18). The amount of nutrients required varies from one individual to another, depending on age, gender, current physical status, lifestyle, physical environment, medical status and medications. The essential nutrients are carbohydrates, proteins, fats, vitamins, minerals, trace elements and water. Before discussing these important nutrients, we will review the physiological and biochemical processes involved in nutrition—digestion, absorption and metabolism.

Digestion, Absorption and Metabolism

The food we eat is of no benefit unless it is in a form the cells of our body can use. To be usable, the nutrients that are taken into the body, normally via the gastrointestinal tract, must be digested and then absorbed into the blood stream for delivery to the cells. Metabolism, which refers to the chemical processes that sustain life and health, takes place in the cells. Figure 20.1 depicts the organs of the digestive system and summarizes their functions in digestion and absorption.

DIGESTION

Digestion is the process by which complex food forms are changed into simpler, soluble chemical parts so that they can be absorbed into the circulation for use by the body. Two simultaneous activities are involved in digestion—one is mechanical, the other chemical (Dudek, 1997).

Mechanical or physical digestion pertains to the neuromuscular activities that break down food into smaller particles, mix them with digestive juices and propel the contents through the digestive tract so that chemical digestion and absorption can take place. The rhythmic, wavelike muscular contractions that move food down the gastrointestinal tract are called **peristalsis** (Dudek, 1997).

Chemical digestion is carried out by the actions of several gastrointestinal secretions, for example, salivary enzymes and gastric, pancreatic and biliary secretions. Specific enzymes in digestive juices break down food nutrients, namely carbohydrates, fats and proteins, into simple, soluble forms that can be absorbed. The chemical breakdown of nutrients occurs through the process of **hydrolysis**. Under the actions of digestive enzymes, nutrients are split into simpler elements by the addition of water to molecules. Carbohydrates are converted to simple sugars (glucose, fructose and galactose), fats to fatty acids and glycerol, and proteins to amino acids (Dudek, 1997).

Enzymes have specific actions that occur under relatively specific conditions. For example, *pepsin*, which begins the breakdown of complex proteins in the stomach, is activated by hydrochloric acid. *Trypsin*, on the other hand, which acts on proteins in the small intestine, functions best in an alkaline medium. Thus, *hydrochloric acid* is secreted

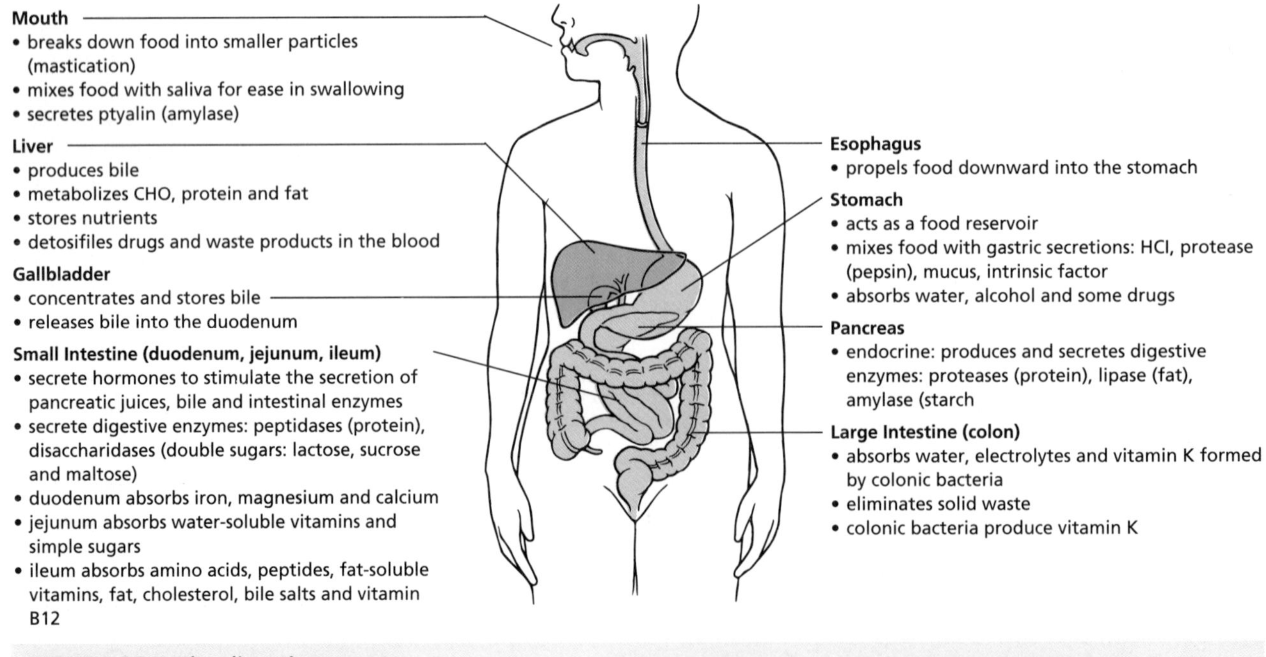

Mouth
• breaks down food into smaller particles (mastication)
• mixes food with saliva for ease in swallowing
• secretes ptyalin (amylase)
Liver
• produces bile
• metabolizes CHO, protein and fat
• stores nutrients
• detosifiles drugs and waste products in the blood
Gallbladder
• concentrates and stores bile
• releases bile into the duodenum
Small Intestine (duodenum, jejunum, ileum)
• secrete hormones to stimulate the secretion of pancreatic juices, bile and intestinal enzymes
• secrete digestive enzymes: peptidases (protein), disaccharidases (double sugars: lactose, sucrose and maltose)
• duodenum absorbs iron, magnesium and calcium
• jejunum absorbs water-soluble vitamins and simple sugars
• ileum absorbs amino acids, peptides, fat-soluble vitamins, fat, cholesterol, bile salts and vitamin B12
Esophagus
• propels food downward into the stomach
Stomach
• acts as a food reservoir
• mixes food with gastric secretions: HCl, protease (pepsin), mucus, intrinsic factor
• absorbs water, alcohol and some drugs
Pancreas
• endocrine: produces and secretes digestive enzymes: proteases (protein), lipase (fat), amylase (starch
Large Intestine (colon)
• absorbs water, electrolytes and vitamin K formed by colonic bacteria
• eliminates solid waste
• colonic bacteria produce vitamin K

FIGURE 20.1 The digestive system

SOURCE: Dudek, 1997, p. 170.

in the stomach and *buffer ions* (bicarbonate) are secreted in the pancreatic and intestinal juices to maintain the proper pH environment for the specific enzymes. Large amounts of *mucous* are secreted by the mouth, stomach and small intestine to lubricate and protect the lining of the entire gastrointestinal tract during its digestive activities. Other substances, such as bile from the liver and certain hormones, also aid in digestion. The secretions of the gastrointestinal tract are influenced and controlled by a number of factors, including hormones, nerves, food passage, sensory stimuli and emotions (Dudek, 1997). These factors are summarized in Figure 20.2.

ABSORPTION

Absorption is the process whereby soluble nutrients pass through the intestinal wall into the blood or lymphatic circulation. Nutrients are mostly absorbed in the small intestine. The extremely large surface area of the small intestine and its unique absorptive inner lining facilitate the process. The mucosal surface of the small intestine has a multitude of folds, called **mucosal folds**. Within these folds are tiny, finger-like projections called **villi**. Each villus contains vascular capillaries and a lacteal (a lymphatic vessel) to receive the absorbed nutrients. The surface of a villus consists of numerous absorptive cells which are capped by smaller projections referred to as *microvilli*. The villi trap the nutrient particles, which are then taken in by the absorptive cells. The mucosal folds, villi and microvilli together increase the inner surface area of the small intestine about 600 times beyond that of the outer serosa (Dudek, 1997).

Nutrients in the form of simple sugars, some fatty acids, amino acids, minerals and water-soluble vitamins enter the blood stream through capillary beds that lead to the portal vein. The absorbed nutrients pass through the portal vein and into the liver, where they are processed before reaching the general circulation. Other fatty acids, certain fat molecules and fat-soluble vitamins enter the lymphatic circulation via the lacteals. Water and electrolytes (sodium and potassium) are absorbed from the large intestine (Dudek, 1997).

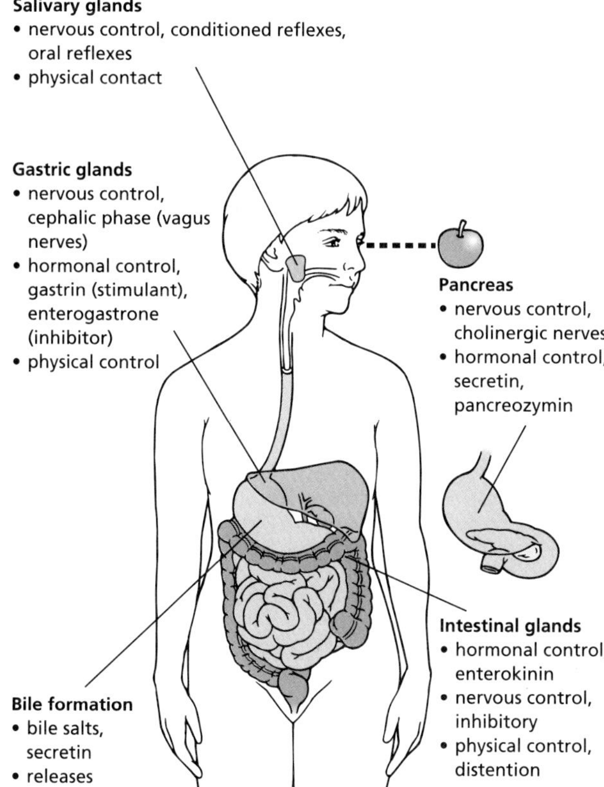

FIGURE 20.2 Factors influencing secretions of the gastro intestinal tract

SOURCE: Williams, 1995a, p. 167.

METABOLISM

Metabolism "refers to how the body obtains and uses energy from the energy-yielding nutrients after they are absorbed—glucose from carbohydrate digestion, glycerol and fatty acids from fat digestion and amino acids from protein digestion" (Dudek, 1997, p. 176). Metabolism is a continuous process that includes two basic metabolic activities: catabolism and anabolism. In **catabolism**, compounds are broken down or oxidized for energy. In **anabolism**, this energy is used in the synthesis of enzymes and proteins needed by the body cells. The restructuring of amino acids to form protein elements of the body is a particularly important part of anabolism (Dudek, 1997).

ESSENTIAL NUTRIENTS

Carbohydrates

As the name implies, **carbohydrates** are organic compounds that contain the elements of carbon, hydrogen and oxygen in varying combinations. For the most part, they are starches and sugars produced in green plants through the process of photosynthesis. Some carbohydrates, such as lactose, come from milk produced by animals. The primary function of carbohydrates is to supply a source of energy for the body and to spare body protein stores. Because of their availability and ease of production, carbohydrates are the most common nutrients in the diets of a vast majority of people throughout the world (Eschelman, 1996).

There are many forms of carbohydrates with varying degrees of complexity. The simple forms are called simple sugars and the more complex forms are called complex carbohydrates and dietary fibre. *Simple sugars* include monosaccharides (meaning one molecule or unit) and disaccharides (meaning two monosaccharides combined). The most common monosaccharides are glucose, fructose and galactose. Glucose and fructose occur naturally in fruits, honey and some vegetables. Galactose does not exist free in nature; it is found only in mammary glands. It occurs in the body as a by-product of lactose metabolism since it is attached to glucose in sugars that are found in milk (Dudek, 1997).

Glucose is the major monosaccharide in the body. It is the end-product of all carbohydrate digestion and the form that is absorbed into the blood. Because it is the major sugar found in the blood stream, glucose is also referred to as *blood sugar* or *dextrose*. In intravenous fluid therapy, dextrose is used as the carbohydrate fuel source. Sucrose, maltose and lactose are the most common disaccharides found in foods. Sucrose, or common table sugar, is the most common dietary disaccharide. Lactose is the sugar found in milk products. Maltose, like galactose, does not exist free in nature. It is found in malt and malt products and, as such, is not a significant source of dietary carbohydrate. Maltose plays an important role in nutrition as an intermediate product formed when starch is changed to sugar during digestion.

Complex carbohydrates, or *polysaccharides*, are composed of many monosaccharide units, mainly glucose. They include starch, glycogen, dextrin and dietary fibre. Dietary sources of complex carbohydrates are commonly known as *starches*. The major foods containing starch are grain products such as wheat and rice, legumes such as beans and peas and potatoes and other vegetables. *Glycogen* is a form of animal starch that is stored in liver and muscle tissues. It is extremely important in energy metabolism as a source of glucose needed to maintain normal blood sugar levels during periods of fasting, such as when a person sleeps or must have nothing by mouth (NPO, or *nil per os*), and during high-intensity and high-endurance exercise. *Dextrin* is an intermediate polysaccharide formed from the breakdown of starch in the body.

Dietary fibre refers to the nondigestible residues of plant foods such as cellulose and pectin. Some fibres, such as cellulose, are water-insoluble. Their presence in the bowel adds bulk which stimulates peristalsis. Water-soluble fibres, such as pectins and gums, absorb and hold water in the intestine which further increases bulk and softens the stool, easing elimination. Dietary fibre has received a lot of attention lately, as scientists have discovered that "there is considerable epidemiological evidence and some experimental evidence that increased fibre intake may help reduce the incidence rates of colon cancer and other intestinal disorders. In addition, some studies have also reported reduced cholesterol levels in the blood following a diet high in soluble fibres" (Williams, 1993, p. 100).

Dietary carbohydrates, with the exception of fibre, are easily digested and eventually converted to glucose, which is easily absorbed into the blood stream. The digestion and metabolism of carbohydrates are illustrated in Figure 20.3. Several things can happen to blood glucose. It may be metabolized directly by tissues (for instance, the brain and nervous system) for energy, or it may be stored in the liver or muscles as glycogen. When glycogen stores are maximized, excess glucose is converted to fat and stored in adipose tissue (Dudek, 1997).

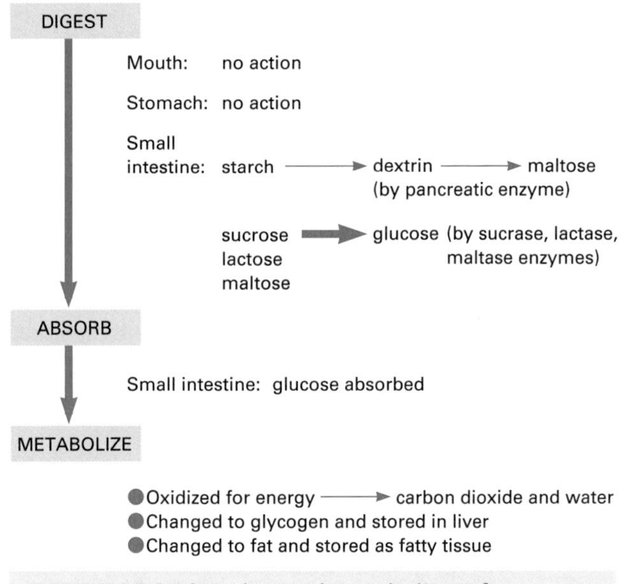

FIGURE 20.3 Digestion and metabolism of carbohydrates

SOURCE: Poleman & Peckenpaugh, 1991, p. 70.

Fats

Fats, or *lipids*, are compounds that are insoluble in water. They too are composed of carbon, hydrogen and oxygen, but in different ratios than in carbohydrates. They function primarily as a source of heat and energy to the body, and because they contain less oxygen, they release their energy more quickly and in greater quantity than do carbohydrates. Moreover, they furnish essential fatty acids for the body, spare the burning of protein for energy, promote absorption of fat-soluble vitamins, insulate vital organs and are required for hormone synthesis and maintenance of cell membranes. Fats add flavour to foods and enhance satiety (the satisfied feeling of fullness) after eating by slowing the digestive process, thereby retarding the development of hunger (Eschelman, 1996). Fats are found naturally in animals and in plant seeds. The most common sources of fats in our diet are butter, margarine, nuts, eggs and oils used for cooking and in salad dressings. Meats and milk products provide variable amounts of dietary fat.

There are two important lipids in human nutrition: triglycerides and cholesterol. **Triglycerides** are compounds made up of three fatty acids to one glycerol base. Glycerol is a sugar alcohol that is similar to carbohydrate. Fatty acids are chains of carbon atoms linked to hydrogen atoms. When all the carbon atoms are linked to hydrogen atoms, the fatty acid is said to be **saturated**. In other words, it cannot take up any more hydrogen atoms. Saturated fatty acids come primarily from animal food sources. They usually remain solid at room temperature, for example, butter or the fat that often surrounds meat (Eschelman, 1996).

Fatty acids that come from plant sources are called **unsaturated** because not all of their carbon atoms are attached to hydrogen atoms, but are linked to each other by double bonds. This makes them capable of absorbing more hydrogen. Unsaturated fatty acids are classified as monounsaturated or polyunsaturated fatty acids, depending on the

```
    H  H  H  H  OH                 H  H  H  H  H  H  OH
    |  |  |  |  |                  |  |  |  |  |  |  |
R—C—C—C—C—C=O              R—C—C=C—C—C=C—C=O
    |  |  |  |                     |        |
    H  H  H  H                     H        H
```

A. Saturated fatty acid B. Unsaturated fatty acid

FIGURE 20.4 (A) Saturated fatty acid (B) Unsaturated fatty acid

number of carbon–carbon double bonds they contain (see Figure 20.4). *Monounsaturated fatty acids* contain one carbon–carbon double bond, which makes them capable of absorbing two or more hydrogen atoms. Olive and canola oils are sources of monounsaturated fatty acids. Fatty acids that contain two or more carbon–carbon double bonds are called *polyunsaturated fatty acids*. They can absorb four or more hydrogen atoms. Soybean, corn and most other vegetable oils contain a good percentage of polyunsaturated fatty acids. Unsaturated fats are usually liquid at room temperature. They can be converted from liquid to solid states by the addition of hydrogen to some of the unfilled bonds (hydrogenation). The conversion of canola and corn oils into margarine is one example (Eschelman, 1996).

There are three fatty acids essential to human health that are not synthesized by the body and must be obtained from food. These essential fatty acids, found in vegetable oils, are linoleic acid, linolenic acid and arachidonic acid. Essential fatty acids help to maintain skin and cell membrane integrity and lower serum cholesterol levels (Dudek, 1997).

Phospholipids are compounds that contain a glycerol molecule, two fatty acids and a phosphate group, to which the choline molecule is attached to complete the chain. Phospholipids act as the structural lipids found in cell membranes and myelin sheaths (Dudek, 1997). They are naturally found in most food; because they can be soluble in water and fat, they are used as emulsifiers. Lecithin is an example of a phospholipid. "They are precursors of prostaglandins, a group of fatty-acid derivatives with hormone-like actions, that perform the following functions: help regulate blood pressure, assist with nerve impulse transmissions, regulate gastric secretions and muscular contractions of the gastrointestinal tract, stimulate uterine contractions, induce labour and inhibit lipid catabolism" (Dudek, 1997, p. 69).

Cholesterol is a fat-like substance (sterol) that is necessary for the production of hormones such as estrogen and testosterone and the formation of bile (a principal emulsifier in fat digestion). It is also an essential component in the formation of cell membranes. Some cholesterol may be obtained from animal foods (for example, egg yolk); however, most of it is manufactured in the liver from fatty acids and products derived from carbohydrates and protein. Epidemiological studies have associated excessive intake of saturated fats and cholesterol with heart disease and certain types of cancer. However, valid cause-and-effect relationships have not been established through experimental research (Health & Welfare Canada, 1990; Dudek, 1997).

Figure 20.5 illustrates the digestive breakdown, ab-

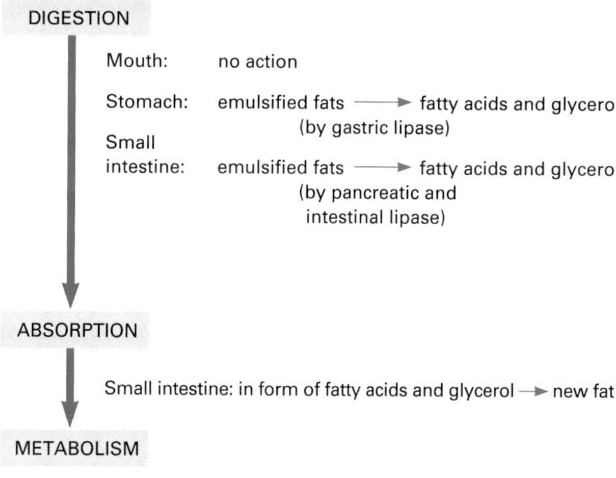

FIGURE 20.5 Digestion, absorption and metabolism of fats

SOURCE: Poleman & Peckenpaugh, 1991, p. 91.

sorption and metabolism of dietary fats. Fats are mostly digested in the small intestine by pancreatic and intestinal juices after emulsification by bile and bile salts. They are changed to fatty acids and glycerol and absorbed from the small intestine. They may then be oxidized for energy, stored as fatty tissue or combined with phosphorous to form phospholids (Dudek, 1997).

Proteins

Like carbohydrates and fats, **proteins** are composed of carbon, hydrogen and oxygen, but with the added element of nitrogen. These four elements are combined to form **amino acids**, the specific compounds (or building blocks) that are then linked together to make protein. The nitrogen component of an amino acid is responsible for a protein's unique function in the human body—the building and repair of tissues. It is also essential for the production of body compounds such as digestive enzymes, hormones and glandular secretions; the formation of hemoglobin, antibodies and other blood proteins; and the regulation of water balance, nitrogen balance and nutrient transport. It can also be used as a source of energy. Protein is found in nature in animals and plants. The most common dietary sources are dairy products, meat, fish, poultry, eggs, legumes (such as peas and beans), nuts and seeds.

There are 22 amino acids that are known to be necessary for the building and repair of body tissues and for life-sustaining physiological processes. Most amino acids can be synthesized within the body, but there are nine that cannot be manufactured in the body and must be acquired from dietary sources. These are called essential amino acids. They are isoleucine, leucine, lysine, methionine, phenylalanine, threonine, tryptophan, valine and histidine (for children).

The amino acids formed in the body are termed nonessential amino acids. It must be stressed, however, that all 22 amino acids are necessary and must be present concurrently for the optimal maintenance of body growth, repair and function. Additionally, amino acids are not stored by the body as are carbohydrates. Thus, the body requires a constant supply of protein food to meet ongoing needs (Dudek, 1997; Eschelman, 1996).

Foods that contain all the essential amino acids in amounts and proportions for proper use in the body are termed **complete proteins**. In order to ensure a balanced supply of amino acids, a diet should include proper amounts of complete proteins or adequate combinations of **incomplete proteins** (deficient in one or more essential amino acids). As a general rule, animal sources of protein are complete proteins. Most vegetable and plant sources are incomplete proteins and, therefore, do not meet the total protein needs of the body unless they are combined to form a complete protein. This poses a challenge to people who choose to avoid animal sources of protein in their diets. They must plan their diets to ensure the proper combinations of vegetable and plant sources of protein needed to supply an adequate balance of all the essential amino acids. For instance, legumes (kidney beans, soybeans, garden peas, black-eyed peas, lentils and lima beans), when combined with grains (wheat, barley) in a meal, provide a complete protein. This balance of intake is of extreme importance in strict vegetarian, or vegan, diets, in which all foods of animal origin are avoided (Dudek, 1997; Eschelman, 1996).

The digestion, absorption and metabolism of proteins are depicted in Figure 20.6. After digestion, amino acids are absorbed and used for synthesis of body tissues and protein substances. Excess protein may be stripped of nitrogen and converted to glucose. Waste products are excreted in the urine.

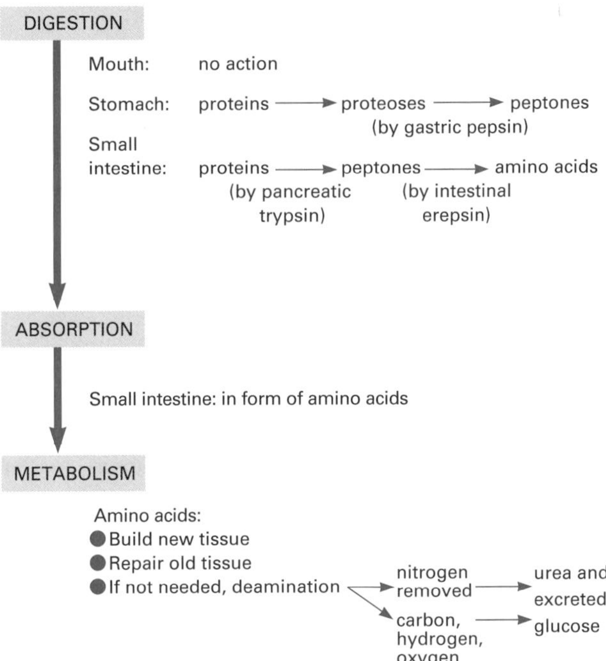

FIGURE 20.6 Digestion, absorption and metabolism of proteins

SOURCE: Poleman & Peckenpaugh, 1991, p. 81.

Vitamins

Vitamins are a natural component of most foods. They are necessary for promoting and regulating chemical processes that convert food into energy, build and repair tissues and protect cells. Vitamins are designated as A, B complex, C, D, E and K, and are classified into two main groups—the fat-soluble and the water-soluble vitamins. *The fat-soluble vitamins* (A, D, E and K) are transported throughout the body in fats. The *water-soluble vitamins*—the B complex (including folic acid, biotin and pantothenic acid) and C—use water as their vehicle. For this reason, foods containing these vitamins are most effective when eaten raw, since cooking tends to remove the vitamins. Some vitamins may be synthesized in the body, such as vitamin A from beta-carotene, vitamin D from the action of sunlight on the skin, activities of vitamin D in the kidney, and vitamin K from the action of bacteria in the bowel (Eschelman, 1996; Dudek, 1997). However, most vitamins must be supplied from food.

A summary of the major vitamins—their functions, some food sources and primary symptoms of deficiency—is provided in Table 20.1. Some vitamins, such as the B vitamins, serve as coenzymes in chemical reactions. **Coenzymes** are essential elements needed for the activation or control of enzyme activity, which regulates physiological processes in the body such as digestion, energy production and carbohydrate, fat and protein metabolism (Eschelman, 1996). Other vitamins, such as C, E and beta-carotene (a precursor to vitamin A), function as antioxidants. Antioxidants are agents that help to prevent DNA alteration caused by electron-seeking (oxidizing) substances. The antioxidants interfere with this oxidative process by donating electrons. Vitamin E also delays or prevents the destruction of cell membranes by protecting polyunsaturated fatty acids from oxidizing compounds. Vitamin D has been found to act as a hormone (Eschelman, 1996).

Minerals

Minerals are necessary to the body in the building and maintenance of bones, teeth and the various body systems. The main essential minerals are considered to be calcium, iron, phosphorus, magnesium, potassium and sodium. Other minerals, called trace minerals, are equally essential, but are needed in much smaller amounts. Some of these other minerals required by the body are copper, iodine, manganese, zinc, selenium and fluorine.

Calcium is important for the proper formation of teeth and bones, for muscle tone and nerve transmissions and for

TABLE 20.1 Essential vitamins

Fat-soluble Vitamins

VITAMIN	FUNCTIONS	RESULTS OF DEFICIENCY	FOOD SOURCES
A (retinol); provitamin A (carotene)	Vision cycle—adaption to light and dark; tissue growth, especially skin and mucous membranes; toxic in large amounts	Night blindness, xerophthalmia, susceptibility to epithelial infection, changes in skin and membranes	Retinol (animal foods): liver, egg yolk, cream, butter or fortified margarine, fortified milk; carotene (plant foods): green and yellow vegetables, fruits
D (cholecalciferol)	Absorption of calcium and phosphorus, calcification of bones; toxic in large amounts	Rickets, faulty bone growth	Fortified or irradiated milk, fish oils
E (tocopherol)	Antioxidant—protection of materials that oxidize easily; normal growth	Breakdown of red blood cells, anemia	Vegetable oils, vegetable greens, milk, eggs, meat, cereals
K (phylloquinone)	Normal blood clotting Bone development	Bleeding tendencies, hemorrhagic disease Poor bone growth	Green leafy vegetables, milk and dairy products, meats, eggs, cereals, fruits, vegetables

Water-soluble Vitamins

VITAMIN	FUNCTIONS	RESULTS OF DEFICIENCY	FOOD SOURCES
B-complex vitamins:			
Thiamine (B_1)	Normal growth; coenzyme in carbohydrate metabolism; normal function of heart, nerves and muscle	Beriberi; GI: loss of appetite, gastric distress, indigestion, deficient hydrochloric acid; CNS: fatigue, nerve damage, paralysis; CV: heart failure, edema of legs especially	Pork, beef, liver, whole or enriched grains, legumes
Riboflavin (B_2)	Normal growth and vigour; coenzyme in protein and energy metabolism	Ariboflavinosis; wound aggravation, cracks at corners of mouth, swollen red tongue, eye irritation, skin eruptions	Milk, meats, enriched cereals, green vegetables
Niacin (precursor: tryptophan)	Coenzyme in energy production; normal growth, health of skin, normal activity of stomach, intestines and nervous system	Pellagra; weakness, lack of energy, loss of appetite; skin: scaly dermatitis; CNS: neuritis, confusion	Meat, peanuts, legumes, enriched grains
Pyridoxine (B_6)	Coenzyme in amino acid metabolism: protein synthesis, heme formation, brain activity; carrier for amino acid absorption	Anemia; CNS: hyperirritability, convulsions, neuritis	Grains, seeds; liver and kidney, other meats; milk, eggs, vegetables
Pantothenic acid	Coenzyme in formation of coenzyme A: fat, cholesterol, and heme formation and amino acid activation	Unlikely because of widespread occurrence	Meats, cereals, legumes, milk, vegetables, fruits
Biotin	Coenzyme A partner; synthesis of fatty acids, amino acids, purines	Natural deficiency unknown	Liver, egg yolk, soy flour, cereals (except bound form in wheat), tomatoes, yeast
Folic acid	Part of DNA, growth and development of red blood cells	Certain type of anemia: megaloblastic (large, immature red blood cells)	Liver, green leafy vegetables, legumes, yeast

continued on next page

TABLE 20.1 *Continued*

Water-soluble Vitamins (continued)

VITAMIN	FUNCTIONS	RESULTS OF DEFICIENCY	FOOD SOURCES
Cobalamin (B_{12})	Coenzyme in synthesis of heme for hemoglobin, normal red blood cell formation	Pernicious anemia (B_{12} is necessary extrinsic factor that combines with intrinsic factor of gastric secretions for absorption)	Liver, kidney, lean meats, milk, eggs, cheese
Vitamin C (ascorbic acid)	Intercellular cement substance; firm capillary walls and collagen formation Helps prepare iron for absorption and release to tissues for red blood cell formation	Scurvy Sore gums Hemorrhages, especially around bones and joints Tendency to bruise easily Stress reactions Impaired wound healing, tissue formation Anemia	Citrus fruits, tomatoes, cabbage, leafy vegetables, potatoes, strawberries, melons, chili peppers, broccoli, chard, turnip greens, green peppers, other green and yellow vegetables

SOURCE: Williams, 1995a, pp. 88, 91, 105–106.

the coagulation of blood. The main sources of calcium in most diets are milk and other dairy products, but calcium is also found in dark-green leafy vegetables, fish with edible bones, eggs, meat and cereals.

Phosphorus aids in the formation and strenghtening of bones and is necessary for energy production (ATP formation), calcium metabolism and muscle function. It can be obtained from dairy products, meat, fish, poultry, nuts, whole grains and legumes.

Magnesium is an important factor in the regulation of the body's temperature, nerve conduction and muscle contractions. Common dietary sources of magnesium are green leafy vegetables, nuts, whole grains and beans.

Iron is important for building hemoglobin in red blood cells and for preventing nutritional anemia. The best sources are liver, red meats and egg yolk, but it is also found in lentils, green leafy vegetables, whole grain and enriched cereals, flours, bread and pastas. Vitamin C-enriched foods enhance iron absorption if taken concurrently (Eschelman, 1996; Dudek, 1997).

Sodium and potassium are discussed in more detail in Chapter 23.

Water

Water is the single most important nutrient in the human body. It is a component of most foods, both liquid and solid. Water is a vehicle of absorption for most nutrients in the body and is present in all body excretions and secretions. Approximately 60 to 70 percent of the adult body is composed of water. Because of its importance in the regulation and maintenance of all body tissues and processes, water is discussed in more detail in Chapter 23 (Dudek, 1997).

Energy Requirements

Dietary requirements are generally considered in terms of both specific nutrients and energy requirements. The body's needs for energy and the energy value of foods are usually expressed in calories (a term taken from the physical sciences), which measure heat. A **calorie** is the amount of heat required to raise the temperature of one gram of water by one degree Celsius. A kilocalorie (kcal) is used in nutrition to indicate that it represents 1000 of the calories used in the physical sciences. As such, a **kilocalorie** is the amount of heat needed to raise the temperature of one kilogram of water by one degree Celsius. The energy value of food is also expressed in kilojoules (kJ), such that one kilocalorie is equal to 4.184 kJ. The energy values of the principal foods are 4 kcal per gram (17 kJ) of carbohydrate, 9 kcal/g (38 kJ) of fat and 4 cal/g (17 kJ) of protein (Eschelman, 1996).

ENERGY USE BY THE BODY

The body uses energy for three basic purposes. These are:

- basal metabolism
- physical activity
- the thermic effect of food.

In addition, there may be a small energy expenditure when a person is cold and the body produces heat through shivering (Dudek, 1997). Growing children and pregnant women also require extra energy for the synthesis of new tissue.

Basal Metabolism

The **basal metabolic rate (BMR)** represents the minimum energy requirements of the body when the individual is awake and at digestive physical and emotional rest (Williams, 1997). It is the amount needed for the internal work of the body, which includes maintaining heartbeat, circulation, respiration, temperature and muscle tone. A measurement of BMR, conducted in a laboratory or hospital setting, is required to get an accurate BMR value for an individual. However, a less accurate estimate (resting energy expenditure, REE) can be obtained by multiplying one's weight in kilograms by 0.9 (calories) for a woman and 1.0 (calories) for a man and then by 24 (number of hours in a day) (Dudek, 1997).

A person's basal metabolic rate is influenced primarily by body composition and lean body mass. Lean body mass consists of muscles, bones and body organs such as the heart, liver and kidneys; it represents the body weight minus fat. Generally, the higher a person's lean body mass, the higher the BMR. The influence of lean body mass on metabolism is the result of higher metabolic activity in tissues such as muscles and the liver. Other factors, such as surface area, gender and age, determine basal metabolism only as they relate to the lean body mass (Williams, 1997). These factors are outlined in the box in the next column.

Physical Activity Needs

To the basal metabolic requirements are added the energy needs for work, movement and exercise. It is primarily the work of body muscles that demands the energy. Mental activity consumes very little extra energy, because the brain is always active and is therefore accounted for in the basal metabolic rate. However, emotional states may increase energy needs as a result of restlessness, agitated activity or muscle tension. Also, catabolic illness and increased temperature can significantly increase energy requirements.

Energy expenditure for physical activity varies widely among individuals. The amount of energy used depends upon the vigour with which the person works and the amount of time per day he or she spends at the activities. People who play a leisurely game of tennis for an hour two or three times a week would not have energy expenditures per hour as great as the professional who puts full effort into every point. There is also a wide variety of energy expenditure involved in the specific jobs that might be found in any given line of work. Table 20.2 presents the expenditures in various types of work and recreation.

Thermic Effect of Food

When food is taken into the body, the body uses energy to digest, absorb, transport and further process the nutrients. This overall stimulating effect of food is called **dietary thermogenesis** (Williams, 1997) and accounts for about 10 percent of the body's total energy needs in adults (Eschelman, 1996; Williams, 1995a). For example, in a person whose daily caloric requirement is 2400 kcal, about 240 kcal would be needed for the thermogenic effect of food.

Factors That Determine Basal Metabolic Rate

Factor	Influence on BMR
Lean body mass	The greater the body mass, the higher the BMR.
Body surface	The greater the area, the greater the heat loss.
Gender	Males average higher energy rates because of greater lean body mass.
Age	BMR rises during the first five years of life, levels off, rises again just before and during puberty, and then declines with advancing age in adults.
Body temperature	Fever increases BMR.
Thyroid hormone activity	Higher levels increase metabolic rate.
Nutritional state	Eating less slows metabolic rate.
Pregnancy and lactation	Metabolic rate increases.
Caffeine and tobacco use	Metabolic rate increases.

SOURCES: Dudek, 1997; Eschelman, 1996.

DAILY ENERGY REQUIREMENTS

The body's energy requirements vary considerably from one individual to another, depending principally on body composition (lean body mass and body fat), age, gender, the kind and amount of daily activity and any superimposed health problem. Thus, there is no fixed level of energy intake that is required by all individuals of the same age, gender and size. Rather, there is a wide range of energy intakes that can be considered adequate, depending on the level of activity performed, on what is considered desirable in the individual's society, and on the person's degree of adaptation to environmental stresses, such as changes in temperature or food intake, and emotional tension (Health & Welfare Canada, 1990). Table 20.3 outlines estimates of average energy requirements according to age, gender and physical activity. These estimates are based on average desirable weights for each age and gender category.

MALNUTRITION

On a global basis, the most common problems associated with nutrition throughout the world are malnutrition, starvation and obesity. Although malnutrition is more prevalent in developing countries, it is also of great concern to health professionals in developed countries.

Malnutrition is "a state of impaired health due to undernutrition, overnutrition, an imbalance of nutrients or ... the body's inability to use the nutrients ingested"

TABLE 20.2 Energy expenditure per hour during various activities*

LIGHT ACTIVITIES (120–150 kcal/h)	LIGHT TO MODERATE ACTIVITIES (150–300 kcal/h)	MODERATE ACTIVITIES (300–400 kcal/h)	HEAVY ACTIVITIES (420–600 kcal/h)
Personal care	**Domestic work**	**Yard work**	**Yard work**
Dressing	Ironing	Digging	Chopping wood
Shaving	Making beds	Mowing lawn (not motorized)	Digging holes
Washing	Sweeping floor	Pulling weeds	Shovelling snow
Sitting	Washing clothes	**Walking**	**Walking**
Peeling potatoes	**Yard work**	5.5–6.5 km/h on level surface	8 km/h
Playing cards	Light gardening	Up and down small hills	Up stairs
Playing piano	Mowing lawn (power mower)	**Recreation**	Up hills
Rocking	**Light work**	Badminton	Climbing
Sewing	Auto repair	Ballet exercises	**Recreation**
Typing	Painting	Calisthenics	Bicycling 17–19 km/h or up and down hills
Writing	Shoe repair	Canoeing 6.5 km/h	Cross-country skiing
Standing or slowly moving around	Store clerk	Dancing (ballroom, square)	Jogging 8 km/h
Recreation	Washing car	Golf (no cart)	Tennis (singles)
Billiards	**Walking**	Ping-pong	Waterskiing
	3.5–4.5 km/h on level surface or down stairs	Tennis (doubles)	
	Recreation	Volleyball	
	Archery		
	Bicycling 8.5 km/h on level surface		
	Bowling		
	Canoeing 4.5 km/h		

*Energy expenditure depends on the physical fitness (that is, amount of lean body mass) of the individual and continuity of exercise. Note that some of these activities can be used as aerobic activities to promote cardiovascular fitness.

SOURCE: Wiliams, 1997, p. 133.

TABLE 20.3 Daily energy requirements according to age, gender and activity (kcal/day)[a]

	19–24 Years		*25–49 Years*		*50–74 Years*		*75 Years+*	
	M	F	M	F	M	F	M	F
Weight (kg)	69	58	67	58	65	56	64	54
BMR	1735	1349	1654	1337	1472	1237	1351	1163
Light activity[b]	2700 (39/kg)	2100 (36/kg)	2600 (38/kg)	2100 (36/kg)	2300 (35/kg)	1900 (34/kg)	2100 (33/kg)	1800 (34/kg)
Moderate activity[c]	3100 (45/kg)	2200 (38/kg)	2900 (44/kg)	2200 (38/kg)	2600 (40/kg)	2000 (36/kg)	2400 (37.5/kg)	1900 (35/kg)
Heavy activity[d]	3600 (53/kg)	2500 (42/kg)	3500 (52/kg)	2400 (42/kg)	3100 (48/kg)	2300 (40/kg)	2800 (44/kg)	2100 (39/kg)

a. 1 kcal is equivalent to 4.184 kJ.

b. Calculated on the basis of average expenditure = 1.55 BMR for men and 1.56 BMR for women.

c. Calculated on the basis of average expenditure = 1.78 BMR for men and 1.64 BMR for women.

d. Calculated on the basis of average expenditure = 2.10 BMR for men and 1.82 BMR for women.

SOURCE: Health & Welfare Canada, 1990, p. 24.

(Eschelman, 1996, p. 18). Malnutrition can manifest as obesity, anemia or wasting. It can also be associated with diseases, for example, heart disease, hypertension, stroke, diabetes and dental or periodontal disease. Young children, adolescents, young pregnant women, the poor, persons with disabilities and people over 65 years of age are the most vulnerable to malnutrition.

There are many causes of malnutrition. In developing nations, the climate and terrain may be such that those crops that do grow well are neither sufficient in quantity nor nutritionally adequate for the resident population. Overpopulation is often a concomitant factor in such cases. If little land is available for agriculture, many foods will have to be imported and will, therefore, be costly, so that only the very rich can afford to eat well. Indeed, the situation in some countries is so extreme that many people starve to death. The United States and Canada, with other countries and international organizations (such as UNESCO, UNICEF and WHO), participate in food distribution programs to countries in need and provide agricultural specialists to advise on food cultivation and processing.

Recommended Nutrient Requirements

Recommended daily requirements of specific nutrients have been established in Canada, as in many other countries. International standards have been issued by the United Nations Food and Agriculture Organization and the World Health Organization (FAO/WHO). Food guides have also been developed to help people select foods that will ensure an adequate supply of essential nutrients in their daily diets. These are discussed later in the chapter.

The latest edition of national nutrition guidelines for Canadians was completed in 1990 by the Scientific Review Committee Report entitled *Nutrition Recommendations*, made to the Minister of National Health and Welfare. The purpose of these guidelines is to aid in the selection of a dietary pattern that will supply adequate amounts of essential nutrients to promote and maintain health and reduce the risk of nutrition-related diseases (Health & Welfare Canada, 1989). *Nutrition Recommendations for Canadians* is summarized in the box. A summary of recommended daily intakes of nutrients is presented in Tables 20.4 and 20.5. (At time of writing, revisions to the above tables were in progress.)

Nutrition Recommendations for Canadians

- The Canadian diet should provide energy consistent with the maintenance of body weight within the recommended range.
- The Canadian diet should include essential nutrients in amounts recommended.
- The Canadian diet should include no more than 30% of energy as fat (33 g/1000 kcal) and no more than 10% as saturated fat (11 g/1000 kcal).
- The Canadian diet should provide 55% of energy as carbohydrate (138 g/1000 kcal) from a variety of sources.
- The sodium content of the Canadian diet should be reduced.
- The Canadian diet should include no more than 5% of total energy as alcohol, or two drinks daily, whichever is less.
- The Canadian diet should contain no more caffeine than the equivalent of four regular cups of coffee per day.
- Community water supplies containing less than 1 mg fluorine per litre should be fluoridated to that level.

SOURCE: Health & Welfare Canada, 1990.

Nutritional Needs Throughout the Life Cycle

Major factors affecting nutritional needs throughout the life cycle were included in the discussion of needs requiring particular attention at each stage of the life cycle (Chapter 8). In this section, we will discuss how changes in growth and development affect specific nutrient requirements in each age group.

THE PREGNANT WOMAN AND THE FETUS

Although a good pregnancy outcome cannot be guaranteed by diet alone, proper nutrition does significantly influence the health of the mother and her fetus. The developing fetus is totally dependent on the mother for nourishment. Inadequate nutrition can seriously impair fetal growth and can result in low birth weight, growth retardation, congenital defects and neonatal mortality. Malnutrition in the first few weeks of pregnancy (two to eight weeks), when organs and structures are developing, may cause irreversible abnormalities. Growth retardation is the effect of nutritional deprivation later in pregnancy, once organ formation is complete (Eschelman, 1996; Weigley, Mueller & Robinson, 1997).

In order to ensure that the nutritional needs of the fetus are met, the mother must maintain a well-balanced diet with the addition of extra nutrients. In particular, more carbohydrates are needed for maternal and fetal energy, protein for fetal tissue development and growth, and calcium for mineralization of the fetal skeleton. As well, increased amounts of folic acid (folacin) and iron are essential for red cell formation required to ensure adequate hemoglobin levels in both mother and fetus. Maternal demands rise

TABLE 20.4 Summary of recommended nutrient intakes based on age and body weight expressed as daily rates

Age	Gender	Weight kg	Protein g	Vit. A RE[a]	Vit. D µg	Vit. E mg	Vit. C mg
Months							
0–4	Both	6.0	12[b]	400	10	3	20
5–12	Both	9.0	12	400	10	3	20
Years							
1	Both	11	13	400	10	3	20
2–3	Both	14	16	400	5	4	20
4–6	Both	18	19	500	5	5	25
7–9	M	25	26	700	2.5	7	25
	F	25	26	700	2.5	6	25
10–12	M	34	34	800	2.5	8	25
	F	36	36	800	2.5	7	25
13–15	M	50	49	900	2.5	9	30[e]
	F	48	46	800	2.5	7	30[e]
16–18	M	62	58	1000	2.5	10	40[e]
	F	53	47	800	2.5	7	30[e]
19–24	M	71	61	1000	2.5	10	40[e]
	F	58	50	800	2.5	7	30[e]
25–49	M	74	64	1000	2.5	9	40[e]
	F	59	51	800	2.5	6	30[e]
50–74	M	73	63	1000	5	7	40[e]
	F	63	54	800	5	6	30[e]
75+	M	69	59	1000	5	6	40[e]
	F	64	55	800	5	5	30[e]
Pregnancy (additional)							
1st Trimester			5	0	2.5	2	0
2nd Trimester			15	0	2.5	2	10
3rd Trimester			24	0	2.5	2	10
Lactation (additional)			20	400	2.5	3	25

a. Retinal equivalents
b. Protein is assumed to be from breast milk and must be adjusted for infant formula
c. Infant formula with high phosphorus should contain 375 mg calcium
d. Breast milk is assumed to be the source of the mineral
e. Smokers should increase Vitamin C by 50%

SOURCE: Health & Welfare Canada, 1990, p. 204.

TABLE 20.4 *Continued*

Folate μg	*Vit. B_{12} μg*	*Calcium mg*	*Phosphorus mg*	*Magnesium mg*	*Iron mg*	*Iodine μg*	*Zinc mg*
25	0.3	250[c]	150	20	0.3[d]	30	2[d]
40	0.4	400	200	32	7	40	3
40	0.5	500	300	40	6	55	4
50	0.6	550	350	50	6	65	4
70	0.8	600	400	65	8	85	5
90	1.0	700	500	100	8	110	7
90	1.0	700	500	100	8	95	7
120	1.0	900	700	130	8	125	9
130	1.0	1100	800	135	8	110	9
175	1.0	1100	900	185	10	160	12
170	1.0	1000	850	180	13	160	9
220	1.0	900	1000	230	10	160	12
190	1.0	700	850	200	12	160	9
220	1.0	800	1000	240	9	160	12
180	1.0	700	850	200	13	160	9
230	1.0	800	1000	250	9	160	12
185	1.0	700	850	200	13	160	9
230	1.0	800	1000	250	9	160	12
195	1.0	800	850	210	8	160	9
215	1.0	800	1000	230	9	160	12
200	1.0	800	850	210	8	160	9
200	0.2	500	200	15	0	25	6
200	0.2	500	200	45	5	25	6
200	0.2	500	200	45	10	25	6
100	0.2	500	200	65	0	50	6

TABLE 20.5 Summary of recommended nutrient intakes based on energy expressed as daily rates

Age	*Gender*	*Energy kcal*	*Thiamin mg*	*Riboflavin mg*	*Niacin NE*[b]	*N-3 PUFA*[a] *g*	*N-6 PUFA g*
Months							
0–4	Both	600	0.3	0.3	4	0.5	3
5–12	Both	900	0.4	0.5	7	0.5	3
Years							
1	Both	1100	0.5	0.6	8	0.6	4
2–3	Both	1300	0.6	0.7	9	0.7	4
4–6	Both	1800	0.7	0.9	13	1.0	6
7–9	M	2200	0.9	1.1	16	1.2	7
	F	1900	0.8	1.0	14	1.0	6
10–12	M	2500	1.0	1.3	18	1.4	8
	F	2200	0.9	1.1	16	1.2	7
13–15	M	2800	1.1	1.4	20	1.5	9
	F	2200	0.9	1.1	16	1.2	7
16–18	M	3200	1.3	1.6	23	1.8	11
	F	2100	0.8	1.1	15	1.2	7
19–24	M	3000	1.2	1.5	22	1.6	10
	F	2100	0.8	1.1	15	1.2	7
25–49	M	2700	1.1	1.4	19	1.5	9
	F	1900	0.8[c]	1.0[c]	14[c]	1.1[c]	7[c]
50–74	M	2300	0.9	1.2	16	1.3	8
	F	1800	0.8[c]	1.0[c]	14[c]	1.1[c]	7[c]
75+	M	2000	0.8	1.0	14	1.1	7
	F[d]	1700	0.8[c]	1.0[c]	14[c]	1.1[c]	7[c]
Pregnancy (additional)							
1st Trimester		100	0.1	0.1	1	0.05	0.3
2nd Trimester		300	0.1	0.3	2	0.16	0.9
3rd Trimester		300	0.1	0.3	2	0.16	0.9
Lactation (additional)		450	0.2	0.4	3	0.25	1.5

a. PUFA, polyunsaturated fatty acids
b. Niacin equivalents
c. Level below which intake should not fall
d. Assumes moderate physical activity

SOURCE: Health & Welfare Canada, 1990, p. 203.

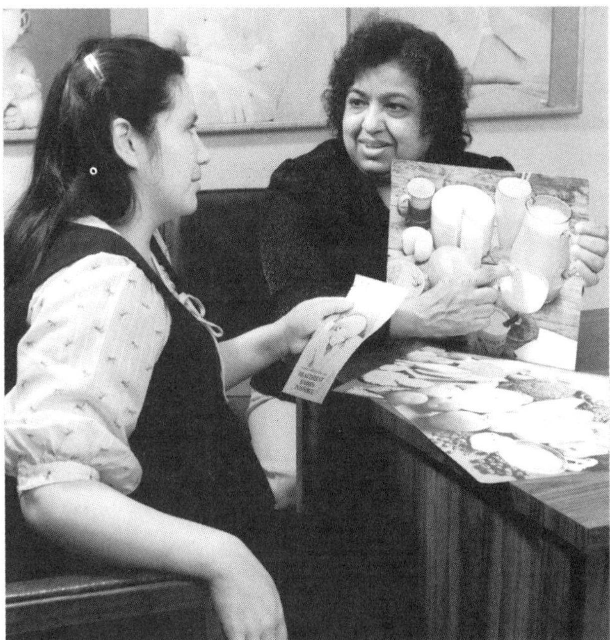

A community health nurse provides counselling for a pregnant woman.

in response to the need for greater red cell production owing to the increased blood volume during pregnancy. In addition to needing iron for building red blood cells and hemoglobin, the fetus also stores iron in the liver to sustain him or her through the first three months of life when intake from milk is low. The recommended nutrient intakes for pregnant women are included at the end of Tables 20.4 and 20.5.

THE BREASTFEEDING MOTHER AND THE INFANT

The woman who is breastfeeding her infant has higher requirements for most nutrients, including energy, proteins, minerals and vitamins, than the expectant mother. These nutrients are needed to cover the demands made on the mother's body for the production of milk as well as the nutrients secreted in the milk that provide nourishment to the infant.

The diet recommended for lactating mothers is essentially the same as for pregnant women and should include plentiful supplies of milk and alternative calcium and protein sources. The nursing mother needs ample fluids to provide the water content of breast milk; two to three litres daily are suggested (Pillitteri, 1995).

The normal newborn generally loses five percent of his or her birth weight during the first two to three days of life, owing to adjustments in total body water. With adequate nutrition (120 kcal/kg/day), the normal healthy infant should gain one kilogram per month from one to three months of age, 500 g per month from three to six months of age and 250 g per month from six to twelve months of age (Townsend, 1994). Adequate nutrition during infancy is important for optimal growth and development of body tissues. Fatty acids are necesary for neurological growth and development.

The gastrointestinal tract of infants is relatively immature. Breast milk, which is the baby's natural food, provides the most easily digested source of nourishment. Breast milk is also the most complete food, needing to be supplemented by only vitamin D for the first few months. However, many babies have been raised to healthy adulthood on goat's milk and formulas made from other substances (soy beans, for example). The formula used must be tailored to the needs of each individual infant (Wong, 1995).

It is now generally recommended that solid foods not be introduced until six months of age. More rapidly growing infants may, however, need solids after four months. Until that time the tongue extrudes, which makes swallowing food difficult. It is also believed that exposure to certain foods (especially those high in protein) in early infancy may lead to food allergies later in life. Solids should be introduced gradually, with one new food at a time, in soft or pureed form (Delmar, 1997).

During the first year of life, the infant's rate of growth and development is quite remarkable. It slows down during the second year, however, and parents may notice that the one-year-old's appetite is not as great as it was. However, loss of appetite is normal in the typical one-year-old. During the second year of life, the child moves from breast- or bottle feeding and soft food supplements, to drinking from a cup and eating table foods (Wong, 1995).

THE CHILD

In the toddler and preschool years the child's physical skills related to eating develop rapidly. A summary of their skills from approximately three months to 12 years is outlined in Table 20.6. Children need the same types of foods as adults, with quantities adjusted to meet their smaller size (these were shown in Tables 20.4 and 20.5). Because their independence is also rapidly developing, small children much prefer foods that they can manage themselves, usually foods that can be eaten with the fingers. Good eating habits can be established at this time, with a pattern of regular meals and a sufficient but not excessive intake of nutritious food (Townsend, 1994).

Malnutrition in childhood results in growth failures and renders the child more susceptible to infections. In addition, iron-deficiency anemia can occur (Eschelman, 1996).

Excess intake of vitamins, in particular vitamins A and D, has become a common problem, presumably because many mothers mistakenly believe that their children can only benefit from consuming large amounts of vitamins. A good diet can provide all the minerals and vitamins that children require. Physicians and baby clinics may recommend supplements in special situations, such as when children are going through a growth spurt, when their appetite is poor during illness, when the child does not like

TABLE 20.6 Development of physical skills related to eating

Age	*Physical Skill*
0–6 months	• sucking, rooting, swallowing reflexes are present and disappear between 3–5 months • head and neck control develops • can transfer food to back of mouth for swallowing • begins sitting up at 6 months
6–12 months	• brings hand to mouth • grasps and reaches for objects • begins feeding self finger foods • at 7 months, begins drinking from cup (holding with two hands) but continues to suck; at about 12 months drinks without sucking • begins chewing; is more refined by the age of 12 months • sits alone • pincer grasp is well developed between 9–12 months
1–6 years	• growth rate decreases, thus appetite may become irregular • biting, chewing and swallowing continue to mature so child can eat greater variety of textures/foods • self-feeds by end of second year • can hold cup with one hand by age of 2 years • begins seeking independently by age of 15 months; "food jags" are normal • muscle mass and bone density increase with adequate protein and calcium • verbalizes dislikes and likes • between 3–5 years, inappropriate food attitudes may develop • food choices influenced by others
6–12 years	• digestive system matures • can handle larger meals • develops regular patterns of meals • period of slow, continuous growth • strong influences outside home • if inappropriate food habits were established they may continue, e.g., skipping breakfast

SOURCES: Dudek, 1997; Eschelman, 1996.

(or cannot tolerate) certain foods or when some foods are unavailable or too expensive, for example, out-of-season fresh fruits and vegetables (Dudek, 1997).

School-age children's rates of growth are slower than they were in infancy or will be again in adolescence. However, it is critically important that their nutritional needs be met to promote optimal growth and development. A nutritious breakfast that includes a good source of protein is particularly important for the school-age child to ensure good work performance and good concentration in the late morning hours. Teachers of special education classes for children with emotional problems have found that the most troublesome youngsters are those who come to school without eating breakfast (Pollitt, 1995).

School-age children are also developing their social skills and enjoying inviting another child home to share meals with them. At this age children also begin to enjoy experimenting with different food tastes and adding to the variety of foods they will eat, although they still prefer plain foods and those they can eat with their fingers.

Among the common deficiencies of childhood, iron deficiency is the most prevalent, and lack of calcium and vitamins C and D are also a problem in many children's diets. Socioeconomic factors play a large part in the dietary sufficiency of children, with those from higher-income families generally having a more adequate intake of essential nutrients, and those with the least income and education having the most problems. Obesity is fairly common in all racial groups, and among rich and poor, during the preadolescent stage. It is often caused by poor eating habits such as eating too many non-nutritious snacks and overeating, particularly rich, high-fat foods. There is, however, some feeling now that heredity is a factor in obesity (Dudek, 1997).

THE ADOLESCENT

During adolescence, both boys and girls undergo growth spurts during which their nutritional needs are greatly increased. They still require the same essential nutrients as adults, with increased quantities of those particularly required for growth. They especially need larger quantities of items from the milk food group. Parents may be amazed at [illegible]

[illegible] often begin to make decisions about the foods they eat. Peer pressure is a very strong influence, and diet fads may be taken up by a group (or sometimes just one adolescent) who may become vegetarian, or adopt a diet that contains only organically grown foodstuffs.

Obesity is a major health problem in this age group. Obese adolescents, as a general rule, tend to be less active physically than those of normal weight, and this seems to be especially true of girls. Some adolescents, particularly girls, develop an obsession with being thin, and a condition known as *anorexia nervosa* (a psychological loss of appetite and self-starvation due to an emotional disturbance in body image and a fear of becoming fat) has become a serious problem in this age group. It may be caused by other problems such as anxiety or depression (which may, or may not, be related to obesity). If unchecked, anorexia nervosa can lead to abnormal water and temperature regulation and deranged hormonal changes. If the anorexia is severe, the adolescent can literally starve herself to death.

Bulimia nervosa is another psychologically influenced eating disorder that may occur during the late teen years; it can continue into the mid-thirties. It is characterized by repeated incidents of binge-eating followed by self-induced vomiting or by purging with the use of laxatives, diuretics and excessive exercising (Eschelman, 1996).

Adolescent girls are particularly vulnerable to *iron-deficiency anemia*, as the monthly loss of blood begins to occur with puberty. Adolescents, both boys and girls, experience a rise in gastric acidity, which is felt to be caused by hormonal changes. They are also prone to abdominal pains of vague origin. It is not wise, however, to ascribe them always to "growing pains." Persistent or severe abdominal pain should always be investigated (Dudek, 1997; Townsend, 1994).

THE ADULT

Growth continues into the early years of young adulthood, although not at so rapid a rate as during adolescence. The young adult needs a good supply of proteins, minerals and vitamins, although not in such large quantities as adolescents. This is the age when good eating habits need to be strengthened to maintain health and to prevent illness in the future. Young adulthood is often a turning point, when individuals are setting up housekeeping away from parental influences. They are on their own to make decisions regarding the foods they will or will not eat, and to establish their own eating habits. Many young adults, because of pressures of work or other commitments, slip into poor dietary habits that will affect their future health. Good nutritional counselling is an important measure in helping young adults protect themselves against problems such as obesity, heart attacks and hypertension in their middle and later years.

Caloric needs usually decline, as does the need for extra supplies of protein when people reach full adulthood, but vitamin and mineral requirements do not. A large number of Canadians are overweight, presumably because they eat [illegible] much and are sedentary (Health & Welfare Canada, 1990). Anemia, due to inadequate intake of iron, is a common problem in women.

During the middle years there is usually a gradual slowing of activity, and individuals require fewer calories than they did in their young adult days. Often, people tend to eat the same amounts, and obesity becomes a major problem. As a person gets older, there is a decrease in digestive enzymes, and heartburn (dyspepsia) is a common problem among middle-aged and older adults. If good oral hygiene has not been practised, problems with teeth and gums may develop and lead to poor nutrition. With the aging process, there is a loss of skeletal calcium (a condition known as *osteoporosis*), and a good intake of calcium and vitamins is required. Women are particularly prone to this problem after menopause because of changes in hormonal secretions (Lutz & Przytulski, 1997).

OLDER ADULTS

The nutritional needs of older adults are the same as those of other adults, although they require fewer calories because of lessened activity and decreased muscle mass. Their nutritional problems usually stem from lack of adequate intake. Older adults may have deficiencies of calories, proteins, vitamins and minerals in their diet. Calcium (for the reason noted above) is particularly important. A lack of vitamin D leads to a condition called *osteomalacia* (softening of the bones). Vitamin D-fortified milk and margarines help to combat this problem.

The failure of many older adults to eat an adequate diet may be due to a number of factors including a lack of money for food; out-of-date nutrition information; physical handicaps that make shopping or cooking difficult; feelings of loneliness, rejection or apathy; and physical changes such as a loss of appetite, poorly fitting dentures and troubles with constipation. Good nutrition counselling is very important. Older adults can be helped to get the most out of their food dollar and to prepare nutritious meals simply. They should be encouraged to share meals with friends and to engage in activities that stimulate the appetite, such as walking in the fresh air or mild exercise. The development of Meals-on-Wheels programs has been a boon for the homebound elderly and for those who find preparing a substantial meal difficult. Volunteers who have participated in these programs often remark that the friendly visit of the person delivering the meal seems to mean as much to the individual as the food (Eschelman, 1996; Dudek, 1997).

Table 20.7 lists typical physiological changes that may affect nutritional needs associated with the aging process.

GERONTOLOGICAL

TABLE 20.7 Nutrition and the aging process

CHANGES IN PHYSIOLOGY AND FUNCTION	NUTRITIONAL IMPLICATIONS
RENAL CHANGES	
Decreased ability to excrete nitrogen and other metabolic wastes related to: • decreased capillary blood flow • decreased glomerular filtration rate (GFR) • inability to regenerate nephrons	If renal failure develops, protein, sodium and other nutrients may need to be restricted in the diet
Urinary incontinence may develop related to impaired bladder sphincter function	The elderly may voluntarily restrict fluid intake to cope with incontinence
SENSORY LOSSES	
Gradual progressive sensory losses may be related to impaired nerve cell function	
Hearing loss begins around age 30	Socialized eating may be difficult or intimidating; lack of socialization can significantly impair appetite and intake in the elderly
Loss of visual acuity, visual accommodation, ability to see in low light, ability to distinguish colour intensities; decrease in depth perception begins at age 50	Food purchasing and preparation may be impaired
Sensory losses can cause decreased salivation, gastric secretion, pancreatic enzyme secretion, and pancreatic hormone secretion, which could alter nutrient utilization	
As many as 50% of the elderly experience major olfactory impairment Loss of taste begins between 50 and 55 years of age and may be related to: • a decrease in the number of taste buds and papilla; sweet and salty tastes are lost first, followed by bitter and sour • oral infections, poor hygiene, decreased flow of saliva	Studies show that the elderly have elevated odour thresholds, lower perceived odour intensities, lower ability to identify odours and olfactory food flavours, and inability to detect spice in a food. Changes in olfaction cause food to be less flavourful and less enjoyable. Many elderly subsequently change their eating habits; elderly women may compensate by eating more, especially more fat and sugar
Decreased sensation of thirst, which may be due to changes in the thirst centre in the hypothalamus	The elderly are prone to dehydration
CHANGE IN INCOME RELATED TO RETIREMENT	
More than 50% of the elderly population are estimated to be economically deprived; as many as 40% have annual incomes under $6000	The first items sacrificed when food budget is limited are milk and meats, which are rich sources of calcium, protein, zinc, iron and B vitamins The lower the income, the less likely an adequate and varied diet will be consumed
CHANGES IN HEALTH	
Degenerative diseases like diabetes, atherosclerosis, hypertension and cancer are more common among the elderly, as are disabling disorders like bone fractures, arthritis and strokes	May affect nutrient requirements, intake, digestion, absorption, metabolism and excretion Disabling disorders may impair food purchasing, preparation or eating
BODY COMPOSITION AND ENERGY EXPENDITURE	
Energy expenditure decreases related to the following: • decrease in REE of about 20% from age 20 to 90 • decrease in physical activity related to retirement or physical impairments (cardiovascular or pulmonary disorders, arthritis, bone fracture, poor vision)	Calorie requirements decrease in response to the decrease in REE, decrease in physical activity and change in body composition. Studies show that people tend to eat less as they get older
Changes in body composition: • loss of lean body mass; muscle mass is replaced by fat and connective tissue • increase in adipose tissue, which requires fewer calories to be maintained than muscle tissue	Loss of muscle mass → loss of muscle strength → loss of range of motion and mobility → impaired ability to purchase, prepare and eat food

TABLE 20.7 *Continued*

CHANGES IN PHYSIOLOGY AND FUNCTION	NUTRITIONAL IMPLICATIONS
ORAL AND GI CHANGES	
Difficulty chewing related to loss of teeth and periodontal [illegible] osteoporosis	If intake is limited to soft, easy-to-chew foods, some essential [illegible]
Decreased saliva occurs in 20% of elderly as a side effect of some diseases and medications	People with dry mouth may have difficulty wearing dentures and may have altered taste and difficulty eating
Constipation is 5 to 6 times more frequent in the elderly than in younger adults, and may be related to the following: • decreased peristalsis related to loss of abdominal muscle tone • inadequate fluid and fibre intake • secondary to drug therapy; antihypertensives, diuretics, sedatives, laxative dependence • decrease in physical activity	40% to 50% of the elderly reportedly use laxatives. A high-fibre diet with an adequate fluid intake can help relieve constipation
Digestive disorders may develop related to the following: • decreased secretion of hydrochloric acid (stomach) and digestive enzymes (pancreatic and intestinal) • decreased GI motility • decreased organ function	Diet modification may be necessary if food intolerances or impaired nutrient absorption develops
Nutrient absorption may decrease because of decreased mucosal mass and decreased blood flow to and from the mucosal villi	
METABOLIC CHANGES	
Altered glucose tolerance. The underlying reason is unclear; may be due to a decrease in insulin secretion or a decrease in tissue sensitivity to insulin	Nutritional implications are not clear
CNS CHANGES	
Tremors, slowed reaction time, short-term memory deficits, personality changes and depression may be related to a decrease in the number of brain cells or the decrease in blood flow to the brain and nervous system. Between 1% and 6% of people over 65 have severe dementia; another 2% to 15% have mild dementia	Food purchasing, preparation and eating may all be impaired
Reliance on drugs. The elderly, who comprise 11% of the population, account for approximately 25% of all drugs used. Compared to younger adults, the elderly are more likely to use drugs, to use a combination of drugs and to take drugs over a longer period of time	Drugs may affect nutritional status by altering appetite, the ability to taste and smell, or the digestion, absorption, metabolism and excretion of nutrients. Likewise, food intake can increase or decrease the effectiveness of some drugs by altering the rate of absorption. If a large percentage of a fixed income is spent on medication, less money is available for food
Alcohol abuse. Some segments of the elderly population may rely on alcohol to relieve boredom, loneliness, depression or pain	Alcohol abuse may cause nutrient deficiencies, particularly of folic acid and thiamine, by altering: • food intake through a decrease in appetite, food buget or alertness • nutrient digestion, absorption, metabolism and excretion
PSYCHOSOCIAL CHANGES	
Social isolation related to: • death of spouse; death of friends • living alone • impaired mobility	The elderly frequently complain that they do not like to cook for one person or eat alone, either at home or in a restaurant. Studies indicate that elderly living alone do not make poorer food choices than those living with a spouse, but they do eat fewer calories
Poor self-esteem related to: • change in body image • lack of productivity • feelings of aimlessness	Poor self-esteem may lead to lack of interest in eating
Institutionalized	Generally, elderly who are institutionalized are more likely to have an inadequate diet than those living independently 30% to 50% of elderly in nursing home residences are estimated to be underweight; up to 50% may exhibit clinical signs of protein-calorie malnutrition

SOURCE: Dudek, 1997, pp. 351–363.

Determinants of Nutritional Status

A person's nutritional status reflects the balance that is maintained between the body's requirements for nutrients, energy and the actual intake of food. It depends on three major factors:

1. the requirements of the individual for nutrients and energy
2. the intake of food
3. the efficiency of bodily processes for absorbing, storing, utilizing and excreting nutrients.

Nutrient and energy requirements in health throughout the life cycle have been discussed in the previous section. Here, we will focus on food intake and health status factors.

Intake

If people eat more food than the body requires, or, conversely, they do not eat enough to meet their energy and nutritional requirements, problems develop. A number of factors—socioeconomic, physical, psychological, and cultural and religious—affect food intake.

SOCIOECONOMIC FACTORS

An analysis of apparent nutrient intake patterns of Canadians by Campbell and Horton (1991), using Statistics Canada's Family Food Expenditure Survey of 1984, revealed the influence of income, family composition and education on nutrient intake. Although the majority of apparent intake patterns were found to be adequate, there were differences in apparent intake of calories, proteins, fats, carbohydrates and a number of vitamins and minerals among households with differing sociodemographic characteristics. The apparent intake for all nutrients increased with income. Households in the lowest economic decile consumed fewer calories than did those in the highest decile. Interestingly, however, the proportion of calories from carbohydrates and fats did not change with income. Canadians consume an average of 40 percent of their calories from fat and 47 percent from carbohydrates. The difference in calories did, however, mean that people in the lowest income decile had apparent protein intakes below the recommended nutrient intakes (RNI) for Canadians. With respect to essential vitamins and minerals, diets were found to be most inadequate in folate, thiamin, iron, calcium and riboflavin for all income groups. However, the proportions of diets with inadequate amounts of these nutrients decreased with increasing income.

Family composition, the presence of a spouse and work status of the wife were found to make a difference in the adequacy of nutrient intake. Dietary patterns in senior households were higher for all nutrients and significantly so for all but folate. "Single-parent households with children had markedly greater proportions of diets apparently inadequate than those with two parents" (Campbell & Horton, p. 376). As well, "households where the wife worked outside the home had lower apparent intakes (especially when the wife worked full time outside the home), and had a greater likelihood of dietary inadequacy" (p. 377). The limited amount of time these individuals have for shopping and food preparation may be the critical limiting factor.

Levels of education of the head of the household beyond high school were found to be important over and above income-related effects. "Higher levels of education were associated with lower intakes of fats and higher levels of Vitamin C, folate and calcium" (Campbell & Horton, 1991 p. 379). This finding supports the importance of knowledge in promoting proper nutrition and suggests that educational programs must reach those with less education.

In countries where food is abundant, many people suffer from excessive caloric intake, resulting in obesity. Intake of other required nutrients may be inadequate despite this excessive intake of food. Contrary to popular belief, people do not necessarily choose naturally the foods their bodies need. In fact, most people choose their foods according to cost and preparation time. The convenience foods, which are relatively expensive, are highly processed and take little or no preparation. They are also usually high in carbohydrates and fats and are low in protein. Foods rich in carbohydrates occur abundantly in nature and therefore are usually inexpensive in comparison with protein-rich food. With the escalating cost of living, the average person is likely to eat more rice and potatoes and less meat, and more canned fruits and vegetables.

PHYSICAL FACTORS

Among the physical factors affecting food intake, the condition of a person's teeth, gums and the mucous membranes of the oral cavity may affect nutritional status. A person with no teeth or with poorly fitting dentures, or one whose mouth is in poor condition, will have difficulty in biting or chewing food effectively. Other physical factors to be considered are the person's general state of health and specific health problems they may have (these are discussed in more detail in subsequent sections). There are also biological variations in the ability to tolerate certain foods. Many people have allergies to specific foods, for example, milk, chocolate, shellfish, nuts and berries.

The need for milk and milk products to provide sources of protein and calcium is not the same for people in all racial groups. Adults in many racial and ethnic groups suffer from lactose intolerance—the inability to tolerate milk. The problem is caused by the absence of lactase, the enzyme that digests milk sugar (lactose). Without this enzyme, lactose in milk ferments in the gastrointestinal tract, and the individual may complain of diarrhea, bloating and discomfort due to the formation of gas. It is felt that one reason for the deficiency may be the dropping of milk from the diet after childhood in many cultures. In addition, acute illness or diseases of the small bowel can decrease an individual's ability to digest lactose, either temporarily or permanently. It has been estimated that between 50 and 75 percent of African Americans, Asians, Inuit and American

75 percent of adults of European descent (Eschelman, 1996). However, even though some groups experience more lactose intolerance than others, almost anyone is prone to it. "Probably 70 percent of adults worldwide experience a large decrease in their abilities to synthesize lactase as they age. This loss of lactase activity is not due to disease; it happens naturally" (Wardlaw, Insel & Seyler, 1992, p. 141). To improve nutrition for these people, sharp cheese (aged over 60 days), yogurt and tofu (soy bean curd) may be used, since the lactose in these foods has been converted to lactic acid, which can be digested. In addition, an individual can use milk in which the lactose has been converted into simpler, easily digested sugars (Lactaid, Lacteeze), take lactose tablets or add lactase drops to ordinary milk to aid in digestion. It is important to note that a milk allergy is not the same as lactose intolerance (an allergy is a reaction to milk protein).

PSYCHOLOGICAL FACTORS

A person's emotional status will also affect his or her intake of food. We have already mentioned this point in connection with anxiety, such as "knots" and "butterflies" in the stomach and pre-examination nausea or vomiting. In one psychiatric hospital setting, dietetic staff observed interesting correlations between food intake and the general anxiety level of both patients and staff. When they were upset by changes in their environment, such as staff changes, hospital policy changes and holidays, the consumption of such "security foods" as bread and milk went up, as did the amount of food left on plates. When things settled down, eating patterns returned to normal (Weigley, Mueller & Robinson, 1997).

Some people use food as a source of comfort and security; they may eat excessively because of their anxieties or because of a lack of fulfillment of the basic needs of love and belonging. Other emotions besides anxiety will also affect people's appetites and, hence, their intake of food. The depressed patient does not want to eat; the happy individual does, unless he or she is too excited by happiness to eat. The attractiveness of a meal and the environment in which it is served also contribute to a person's enjoyment of food and encouragement to eat (Eschelman, 1996).

A substance dependency, whether on alcohol, medications or tobacco, strongly influences an individual's eating habits. For example, household money may be spent on maintaining the dependency rather than on the purchase of nutritious foods. Further, many substances physiologically depress the appetite or alter the senses of taste and smell, thus putting people at risk for nutritional deficiencies (Eschelman, 1996; Dudek, 1997).

CULTURAL AND RELIGIOUS FACTORS

As we noted at the beginning of this chapter (and in Chapter 12), cultural, moral and religious values play a con-

cultures and among different religious groups. They also vary from one family to the next, and from individual to individual.

Among cultural groups, food habits usually have their origins in the types of foods available in the part of the world in which the group originated. Potatoes are plentiful in many parts of North America; hence, they form a staple of the diet in many homes. In many countries, rice is the staple and forms part of the culture. When people from one culture move to another part of the world, they usually carry their food habits with them. In Canada, where people from all over the world have settled, it is important for the nurse to be aware of the cultural food heritage of patients and of their religious backgrounds, since many religions have specific food-related rules.

Vegetarianism

Many people are vegetarian because of religious beliefs or personal preference (it is not unusual in an East Indian household, for example, to find both vegetarian and nonvegetarian family members). Orthodox Hindus subscribe to the doctrine of *ahimsa*, which means "not killing." Many other religious groups also espouse vegetarianism. The largest group in North America are members of the Seventh Day Adventist Church. People may become vegetarians for moral reasons (not wanting to kill animals for food), for health reasons (to reduce saturated fat and cholesterol or because of declining tolerance of meat with advancing age), for environmental reasons (deforestation to create cattle grazing lands) or simply for personal preference. The most common nutritional problems among vegetarians include deficiencies of iron, zinc, vitamin B_{12}, calcium and vitamin D. However, it is possible to have a vegetarian diet that fulfills, or even exceeds, recommended nutrient requirements, provided that foods are selected very carefully.

Other Dietary Restrictions

Various cultural groups have other dietary restrictions. Fasting occurs among various religious faiths. Many religious groups—for example, people of the Islamic, Jewish and Seventh Day Adventist religions—do not eat pork. Nonvegetarian Hindus and Sikhs will usually not eat beef or veal because of the sacredness of the animal from which these meats come. Because the cow is sacred in India to both Hindus and Sikhs, cow's milk and products made from cattle are not consumed by these people (milk from the water buffalo is used instead in India). It is important in caring for people to find out the particular foods they do eat, as well as those they do not.

Food preparation is also a concern for some groups. For people of some religious faiths, the preparation of food is a ritual. Orthodox members of the Jewish religion will eat only foods that are *kosher*, that is, prepared according to prescribed ritual. Many Islamic people will eat meat only if the animal has been ritually slaughtered. Kosher meat may, however, be acceptable.

Besides following formal restrictions, many people limit their diets to food prepared in styles customary to their own culture. In most Asian countries, meat, poultry and fish are usually cut up into small pieces and cooked with vegetables. A large steak or piece of chicken or fish may not be acceptable to the Asian patient. Many people from other cultures are used to foods that have been highly spiced, such as Indian curries, hot Mexican chilies and Korean kimchee (fermented cabbage). People from these cultures often find the typical North American diet very bland and unappetizing. They usually like to add a spicy sauce to most foods to improve the flavour.

HEALTH PROBLEMS

Health problems also affect a person's intake of adequate nourishment. In addition to allergies and poor digestion, most physical and emotional problems affect food intake in some way, often by bringing on anorexia or nausea and vomiting. Some medications can have side effects (such as anorexia and nausea) that affect a person's nutritional intake; medications can also alter requirements for certain nutrients.

People who are ill face an increased risk for malnutrition. Many common diagnostic tests and treatments interrupt normal dietary patterns, and as a result ill people may not have a sufficient intake of essential nutrients and energy-giving foods. Meals may be withheld for tests that are ordered, the patient may be allowed nothing by mouth and be maintained on low-calorie infusions, or a nutritionally inadequate diet may be required as part of the treatment. The term *hospital malnutrition* has been applied to this increasingly prevalent problem. The nurse working in an acute care facility needs to be aware of the need for a careful assessment of patients so that remedial measures can be instituted promptly.

Efficiency of the Body in Processing Food

Any factor that interferes with the body's ability to retain, absorb, store, utilize or excrete nutrients will adversely affect a person's nutritional status. Disease processes, congenital problems or injury to any part of the gastrointestinal system may therefore result in nutritional problems. Probably the most common type of illness affecting the gastrointestinal tract is infection, especially gastroenteritis, which is a major cause of death in many developing countries and a very common cause of illness in Canada.

Illnesses involving parts of the body other than the gastrointestinal tract may also cause disturbances in the processing of food, as well as altering the body's needs for energy and for specific nutrients. This aspect of nutrition will be discussed in further detail.

Nutritional Needs in Illness

Food as a source of nourishment is particularly important for those who are ill. It is not uncommon for those who are ill to have some disturbances in gastrointestinal functioning. They may lose their appetite or be unable to tolerate food and fluids, or there may be a problem in the digestion of food or in the absorption of nutrients from the gastrointestinal tract. Whatever the problem, the ill person's nutritional needs are usually different from those of the healthy individual. Lack of exercise because of illness may decrease the body's need for energy-giving foods but, at the same time, there is a greater need for tissue-building nutrients.

In the well person, the processes of anabolism and catabolism are normally equal. In the ill, particularly those who are incapacitated, the catabolic activities are increased, leading to breakdown of cellular materials and subsequent deficiency of protein. Additional protein foods are important for almost all ill people. There are, of course, some conditions in which a high-protein diet is contraindicated, but the foregoing statement is a good general rule. For example, the patient who has suffered a cerebral vascular accident (stroke) may have altered nutritional needs as a result of difficulties with chewing and swallowing.

There are certain conditions in which metabolic activity is increased, as in patients with fever or certain cancers, and in these cases there is a need for additional energy-giving foods as well as proteins.

In many disease conditions, the patient may be unable to tolerate food or fluids, or may lose these through vomiting, diarrhea or other losses. When food is not available as a source of energy, the body can draw on stored resources. Liver and muscle glycogen, the stored form of carbohydrates, is the most readily available source of stored energy. Through the process of **glycogenolysis**, glycogen is converted to glucose and made available to the body. These sources, however, are able to satisfy basal kilocalorie demands for only a few hours and are readily used up if not replenished by the intake of food. If starvation continues for more than 24 hours and glycogen stores are depleted, the body begins to convert protein into glucose through the process of **gluconeogenesis**. The amino acids that make up protein break down and release nitrogen into the urine in the form of urea and ammonia. As well, in an effort to conserve protein, fatty acids are mobilized from the body's *adipose* (fatty) tissue and are used as fuel to meet energy requirements. Fatty acids break down to ketone bodies, leading to **ketosis**—an abnormal accumulation of ketones in the body resulting from a deficiency or inadequate utilization of carbohydrates. Without an adequate supply of calories from food, the body's nutrient stores are used up quickly and, over time, a state of protein–calorie malnutrition results. In these cases, the replacement of lost fluids and nutrients is an im-

These cases require special adaptation of the diet.

TYPES OF DIET FOR THE ILL

As a part of the patient's therapeutic regimen, food is usually prescribed in the form of a diet. There are many kinds of diets. For example, the average patient is on a *regular* (also called *full* or *general) diet.* This diet includes practically all foods people normally eat that are easy to digest and simply prepared. Generally, fried and highly seasoned foods are not served to patients because of the difficulty some people have in digesting them.

A *minced* or *pureed diet* is indicated for people who have difficulty chewing food. A *clear liquid diet* permits water, tea with lemon, coffee, juices, clear bouillon, carbonated beverages and clear gelatin desserts. A *full liquid diet* is free of irritating condiments and cellulose. Often included in a full liquid diet are all the foods on a clear liquid diet plus such others as strained soups, simple puddings or custards, refined cooked cereals and milk.

Therapeutic diets are special diets designed for the needs of the individual patient and vary greatly in their composition and purpose. The amount and kind of nutrients may be varied or certain non-nutritive compounds eliminated as, for example, in fibre-modified diets and various postoperative diets. There are also diets that restrict the amount of sodium, potassium, sugar or protein. There are high-calorie diets and low-calorie diets, high-protein diets and low-protein diets. There are also diets that control the quantity and type of fats. Each therapeutic diet is ordered by the physician to meet the patient's specific needs. The quantity of each kind of food is calculated by the dietitian or nutritionist, and each meal contains the prescribed amounts of specific foods.

Regardless of the kind of diet, it is important that patients understand why they are served certain foods. A patient's acceptance of the specified food as part of the prescribed therapy, and of his or her commitment to following the diet, will be enhanced if the benefits or reasons for it have been fully explained.

Common Problems

Indigestion, Anorexia, Nausea and Vomiting

Among the most common eating-related problems nurses will encounter in patients in their day to day practice are indigestion, anorexia, nausea and vomiting. Indigestion is often the first indication that something is wrong with gastrointestinal functioning. The inability to take in food and fluids, or the body's rejection of them, poses a serious threat to homeostasis and involves all areas of functioning of the human

[illegible] often, distressing accompaniments of the aging process.

Gastroenteritis, which is a common cause of anorexia, diarrhea, nausea and vomiting, still remains one of the most common types of short-term illness in North America. It is very common in infants and small children; it is also distressing for many international travellers, whose gastrointestinal tracts are exposed to foods and fluids that are not a part of their normal diet. In addition, anorexia, diarrhea, nausea and vomiting frequently accompany so many health problems that the nurse should be acquainted with the physiological mechanisms involved in these disturbances, and be able to take appropriate action to assist patients.

PHYSIOLOGICAL CONSIDERATIONS

Indigestion is characterized by pain and distress in the epigastric region. It may be accompanied by other symptoms, such as eructation (burping) or flatulence (the excessive formation of gases in the stomach or intestine; *flatus* is the term used for gas expelled through the anus). Many pregnant women and older adults complain of heartburn, which is characterized by a burning pain located behind the sternum. It is caused by regurgitation of acid contents of the stomach into the esophagus, the burning sensation being due to irritation of the mucous membrane lining the esophagus.

Anorexia means loss of appetite, or lack of desire for food, and it involves the subjective perception of a distaste for food. The individual often expresses this by saying, "I don't feel like eating." Anorexia may precede nausea. In **nausea**, not only is there a distaste for food but the mere thought of food becomes repellent. In addition, the individual usually complains of an uncomfortable sensation in the region of the stomach. **Vomiting**, the forceful ejection of the stomach's contents, is usually preceded by nausea. Although anorexia, nausea and vomiting are considered by many to be sequential stages of the same physical phenomenon, any one of the three may occur by itself in the absence of the other two (Williams, 1995b; Dudek, 1997).

Appetite is the pleasant sensation of a desire for food. Although appetite and hunger frequently occur together, they are not the same. **Hunger** is an uncomfortable sensation that indicates a physiological need for nourishment, whereas appetite is a learned response. As such, appetite is closely related to cultural and social values. To a large extent, one's appetite is conditioned by previous experiences with food. A number of different stimuli will arouse the appetite. These include olfactory stimuli, such as the pleasant odour of something cooking, visual stimuli, such as an attractively served meal; auditory stimuli, including the clatter of pots and pans in the kitchen as dinner is being prepared; or gustatory stimuli, as when one tastes a sample of food and finds it aggreeable, and when the appetite is whetted for more (Weigley et al., 1997).

When people lose their appetite, specific visceral changes occur. There is usually hypofunctioning of the stomach; gastric tone is lessened and the secretion of hydrochloric acid is decreased. These same physiological findings have been observed in individuals suffering from nausea, except that in the case of the nauseated person, they are more pronounced. In nausea, there is a relaxation of the walls of the stomach, and gastric secretions and muscular contractions cease. Because of this relaxation, the stomach is usually situated lower in the abdominal cavity than it normally is. At the same time as the muscles of the stomach are in a relaxed state, the muscular wall of the intestine shows increased contractility and contents from the duodenum may be regurgitated back into the stomach. *Retching*—an unproductive attempt at vomiting—may occur several times before vomiting actually takes place.

The act of vomiting involves a sequence of events that culminates in the forceful ejection of the stomach's contents. Initially there is a relaxation of the upper portion of the stomach, including the cardiac sphincter. This is followed by strong contractile waves in the lower portion of the stomach, which effectively close the pyloric sphincter and prevent the stomach contents from passing into the duodenum. Subsequently, the diaphragm and the abdominal muscles contract. The strong contractions of these muscles during the act of vomiting account for the feeling of "soreness" that many people experience as an after effect of vomiting. With the simultaneous contraction of the diaphragm and the abdominal muscles, intra-abdominal pressure is greatly increased and the stomach is literally squeezed between the two sets of muscles. The contents in the relaxed upper portion of the stomach are then forced upward through the esophagus and out through the mouth. Normally, the glottis is closed and respirations cease during the act of vomiting in order to prevent the vomitus from being aspirated (entering the lungs).

In *projectile vomiting*, the impulse to vomit is very sudden, occurring with little or no warning (that is, with no symptoms of nausea beforehand). Moreover, the ejection of the stomach's contents is more forceful than in ordinary vomiting. This type of vomiting is often seen in infants with disorders of the gastrointestinal tract and in patients with head injuries.

Prolonged vomiting in children is more serious than in adults because of the relatively greater loss of fluids and electrolytes in proportion to body weight.

COMMON CAUSES OF INDIGESTION, ANOREXIA, NAUSEA AND VOMITING

Indigestion is caused by the body's inability to process the foods that are taken into it. It may result from a diminishing ability to chew food properly. Or, it may result from putting too great a load on the system by overeating, by eating too quickly or by eating highly spiced foods or foods that are foreign to the gastrointestinal tract. Foods that contain a lot of fat or are cooked in fats or oils are particularly troublesome to many people, as are gas-forming foods (lettuce, cabbage and beans) and milk for those unable to tolerate it. Smoking may also be a factor because it stimulates the secretion of acid gastric juices in the stomach. There is increased risk of reflux in people with hiatus hernias or where there is a problem with the gastroesophageal sphincter.

The primary centre controlling vomiting is located in the medulla oblongata. It is thought that stimulation of this centre may give rise to anorexia, nausea or vomiting, depending on the degree or intensity of the stimulus. Thus, a person who does not feel like eating may become nauseated at the sight of food and may vomit if he or she tries to eat. However, vomiting is not always preceded by nausea, and it is believed, therefore, that only certain areas in the vomiting centre are directly involved with nausea. The vomiting centre may be stimulated by a number of factors, including chemical stimuli (drugs and other toxic substances), impulses from the cerebral cortex (strong emotions) and impulses arising from receptors in the viscera (internal factors). Vomiting may also occur in medical conditions where there is delayed gastric emptying or when there is a gastrointestinal obstruction.

Drugs and Other Toxic Substances

Two of the most common causes of nausea and vomiting that the nurse may see in community practice and in emergency units are food and drug poisonings. Toddlers and small children are particularly vulnerable to both because they will often eat or drink food that is left on a counter or table, or ingest household products (such as bleach or insecticides) or medications, if these are within reach.

A number of different chemical agents may give rise to anorexia, nausea and vomiting, for example, digitalis (frequently used in the treatment of people with heart conditions); a number of the narcotics, such as morphine; and many drugs used as anesthetics. When giving a patient any medication, it is important to note whether nausea and vomiting are listed as possible side effects of the drug and, if so, to watch for these symptoms in the patient. Other toxic substances that are circulating in the blood stream, such as bacterial toxins in infections or in food poisoning, may also stimulate the vomiting centre.

Food Poisoning

Every year, a number of deaths from food poisoning receive a great deal of publicity, but countless more cases occur, many of them unreported. Food poisoning is always a potential problem at large gatherings, such as picnics, where food may be held for long periods of time at temperatures conducive to the growth of bacteria.

If food poisoning is suspected, it is important to find out what the person has eaten and also whether any other person who ate the same food is affected as well. The symptoms of food poisoning usually occur within one to five

develop abruptly and may include nausea, vomiting, abdominal cramps and diarrhea. Most cases of food poisoning last no more than five to six hours, or 24 hours at the most. They will usually subside on their own as the body rids itself of the offending substance. The individual should be watched for signs of shock and for the development of neurological symptoms that occur with certain types of food poisoning, including botulism and shellfish and mushroom poisoning. Shock may be caused by excessive fluid loss (from vomiting and diarrhea), by bacterial toxins or by an allergic reaction to the food ingested.

Botulism (caused the the *Clostridium botulinum* organism) is the most serious food poisoning because it can be fatal. Although cases receive a great deal of publicity, its occurrence is relatively rare. The most frequent cause is improperly home-preserved vegetables, although preserved fruits, fish and meat products may also be sources of botulism.

The botulism organism releases gas as it grows and is sometimes evidenced by a bulging can or lid of a jar. The symptoms of botulism usually develop 4–36 hours after the food has been eaten, but may be delayed up to four days. The early symptoms are similar to those of other food poisonings, with the addition of weakness, dizziness, visual disturbances and dryness of the mouth and throat. Often the person will complain of headache. Other neurological symptoms, such as paralysis, limitation of eye movements, dilated pupils, decreased tendon reflexes and impaired speech, often follow. When botulism is fatal, the cause of death is usually respiratory paralysis. If botulism is suspected, the person should be referred for emergency medical treatment immediately.

Shellfish poisoning can also cause neurological symptoms, through the transmission of toxins from the plankton on which shellfish feed. Particularly dangerous are shellfish harvested during "red tide." Fortunately, the mortality rate is not as high as with botulism. The symptoms may develop as soon as 20 minutes after eating, with *parasthesia* (abnormal sensations such as prickling or tingling) of the hands and mouth, weakness of the arms and legs and a feeling of floating. The person may also notice *ataxia* (a failure of muscle coordination), headache and vomiting. Respiratory or *bulbar paralysis* (due to effects of the toxin on motor centres in the medulla oblongata) may ensue. Prompt medical attention is important. No specific treatment is known as yet; the measures used are those for respiratory paralysis. If the person survives the first 12 hours, he or she is likely to recover.

Another common type of food poisoning, particularly in the spring, late summer and early fall, is that caused by certain wild varieties of mushrooms. In mushroom poisoning, the individual usually has an acute attack of nausea, vomiting and diarrhea starting about two to three hours after eating. Hallucinations and intoxication reactions may follow. Some varieties of mushrooms are more poisonous than others and may lead to kidney and renal failure. It is im-

catch, how many and where. If possible, the nurse should get a sample of the mushrooms or save any **emesis** (vomited contents) for analysis. The patient should be hospitalized so that he or she can be watched for delayed reactions. Often, the stomach is washed out, and a strong laxative is given to speed the mushrooms through the gastrointestinal tract (Dudek, 1997; Escheman, 1996; Williams, 1997).

Other common types of food-borne bacteria include *Salmonella* species and *Escherichia coli*, most commonly from undercooked poultry, meat, eggs, fruits and vegetables and unpasteurized milk. These microorganisms can be transmitted from handling food without proper hand washing. Early symptoms include diarrhea, nausea, vomiting, fever and abdominal cramps. If stool is bloody (as with *E. coli* infection), prompt medical attention is imperative as renal failure may result. One particular strain of *E. coli* (0157:H7) can be fatal. The best means to decrease transmission of these bacteria is to follow simple food safety principles, such as cooking meats and eggs thoroughly, washing fruit and vegetables well and washing utensils and surfaces after use (Dudek, 1997; Eschelman, 1996).

Table 20.8 lists examples of bacterial food-borne disease.

Psychosocial Stressors

Indigestion may be caused or aggravated by psychosocial factors. A meal that is taken when a person is under stress, for example, is not easily digested. When people are angry or worried about something, they may feel that their stomach is "tied up in knots"; excessive acid secretion may ensue, and they may also suffer from excessive gas formation and resultant distention in the stomach and intestines.

Stressful situations may give rise to anorexia, diarrhea, or vomiting. The event or situation need not necessarily be unpleassant. An individual may be "too excited to eat." Infants and toddlers will often vomit if overstimulated, particularly after a meal. Older children, too, may become nauseated or vomit if excited or fearful. However, it is in connection with unpleasantly stressful situations that the symptoms of anorexia, diarrhea, nausea and vomiting are most often noted. Worry over a pending examination, pain, anxiety and fear may all give rise to these symptoms. Similarly, other psychic factors such as the sight of something particularly abhorrent, unpleasant odours or even extremely loud noise can also take away one's appetite, make one feel nauseated or cause vomiting.

Internal Factors

The parts of the body containing receptors that initiate vomiting are the stomach, duodenum, uterus, kidneys, heart, pharynx and semi-circular canals of the ear. The stimuli that

TABLE 20.8 Selected examples of bacterial food-borne disease

FOOD-BORNE DISEASE	CAUSATIVE ORGANISMS (GENUS AND SPECIES)	FOOD SOURCE	SYMPTOMS AND COURSE
Bacterial food infections			
Escherichia coli O157:H7 infection	*Escherichia* *E. coli* O157:H7	Undercooked meat, mainly ground beef	Severe cramps, nausea, vomiting; bloody and nonbloody diarrhea; acute renal failure. Appears 1–8 days after eating, typically lasts 3–4 days; sometimes fatal
Salmonellosis	*Salmonella* *S. typhi* *S. paratyphi*	Milk, custards, egg dishes, salad dressings, sandwich fillings, polluted shellfish	Mild to severe diarrhea, cramps, vomiting. Appears 12–24 h or more after eating; lasts 1–7 days
Shigellosis	*Shigella* *S. dysenteriae*	Milk and milk products, seafood, salads	Mild diarrhea to fatal dysentery (especially in young children). Appears 7–36 h after eating; lasts 3–14 days
Listeriosis	*Listeria* *L. monocytogenes*	Soft cheese, poultry, seafood, raw milk, meat products (paté)	Severe diarrhea, fever, headache, pneumonia, meningitis, endocarditis. Symptoms begin after 3–21 days
Bacterial food poisoning			
Staphylococcal	*Staphylococcus* *S. aureus*	Custards, cream fillings, processed meats, ham, cheese, ice cream, potato salad, sauces, casseroles	Severe abdominal pain, cramps, vomiting, diarrhea, perspiration, headache, fever, prostration. Appears suddenly 1–6 h after eating; symptoms subside generally within 24 h
Clostridial Perfringens enteritis	*Clostridium* *C. perfringens*	Cooked meats, meat dishes held at warm or room temperature	Mild diarrhea, vomiting. Appears 8–24 h after eating; lasts a day or less
Botulism	*C. botulinum*	Improperly home-canned foods; smoked and salted fish, ham, sausage, shell-fish	Symptoms range from mild discomfort to death within 24 h; initial nausea, vomiting, weakness, dizziness, progressing to motor and sometimes fatal breathing paralysis

SOURCE: Williams, 1997, p. 289.

give rise to anorexia, nausea and vomiting include irritation of the receptors, for example, the tickling of the back of the throat to induce vomiting; the eating of irritating foods; stretching of the organ, as occurs when a child stretches his stomach by overeating and promptly vomits; or pressure on the receptors. Irritation of the gastrointestinal tract by infectious, chemical or mechanical agents, and distention of (or trauma to) other viscera, also affect the vomiting centre.

A disturbance in motion, as one experiences with the rolling motion of a ship at sea or with any rapid change in direction of the body, stimulates receptors in the labyrinth of the ear. These receptors send out impulses that are carried by the vestibular nerve to the cerebellum, and then to the vomiting centre in the medulla.

Indigestion is often caused by problems in the gastrointestinal tract, where a disturbance in structure or functioning, inflammation or new growths (such as tumours), either in the tract itself or in its accessory organs, may interfere with the body's ability to process and utilize food. In older persons particularly, chewing may be difficult if the person gradually loses teeth or if ill-fitting dentures prevent proper mastication. The motility of the gastrointestinal tract also lessens with age—food is not processed as quickly (Dudek, 1997).

Assessing Nutritional Status

In order to assess a patient's nutritional status, the nurse needs information about all factors that affect that person's state of nutrition. The parameters of data collection include a nutritional history and physical examination, anthropometric measurements (size, weight and body proportions) and laboratory tests. Information about the patient's disease process is furnished by the medical history. Medical management and special diet orders will be found in the patient's chart.

Nursing Health History

A nutritional history is taken as part of the health history. The nurse obtains data such as age and stage of development, gender, height, usual weight and present weight. Usual habits with regard to daily activities and current activity level, usual dietary pattern and any recent deviations from it, and present status with regard to food and fluid intake are explored. Information is gathered about the patient's (and/or family's) socioeconomic status and lifestyle. The person's general physical condition, emotional status and any possible health problems that could cause alterations in nutritional needs or interfere with digestive processes are determined. The person's religious affiliation, ethnic ori- [illegible]

nurse should obtain information about her menstrual history and determine if she is pregnant or a nursing mother.

Indigestion, diarrhea, anorexia and nausea are subjective feelings; hence, their identification is highly dependent on the individual's ability to express discomfort. The person who has indigestion may report pain in the epigastric region. The nurse should identify the location of the pain, its nature, its intensity, when it occurs and its frequency. Is it related to eating certain foods? Is it relieved by any particular measures? Often the patient claims to have "a little indigestion" or "heartburn." The patient may report a "burning" feeling or a bloated feeling in the abdomen, "gas in the stomach," or flatulence.

Patients with anorexia may say that they are not hungry or that they "just don't feel like eating." The nauseated person may complain simply of "feeling sick" or may specifically locate the sensation of nausea in the epigastric region. An uncomfortable feeling in this area is usually accompanied by other symptoms of a distressing nature. Frequently there is increased perspiration and greatly increased salivation. Patients may state that their mouths are full of saliva. Some people feel faint, and some report vertigo (dizziness) or tingling sensations in the fingers or toes. After vomiting, a person often complains of soreness in the stomach area.

The nursing history provides an essential base for identifying nutritional problems and planning individualized care. An evaluation of the patient's (and family's) health-promoting and health-protecting pattern aids in identifying potential problems and opportunities for teaching. A guide for obtaining a nutritional health history follows.

Measurements

An important parameter of a person's nutritional status is weight. Being underweight or overweight is considered a risk factor in many diseases, such as hypertension, cardiovascular disease, diabetes and some cancers. It is believed that every individual has a *desirable weight* for optimal health and fitness and that this weight can be estimated on the basis of certain measurements and by comparing these measurements to selected standards.

A person's weight depends on his or her height, frame size and body composition. Measurements of the size and proportions of the body are called **anthropometric measurements**. These include height and weight, circumferences of various body parts and measurements of skinfold (fatfold) thickness. The measurements are used to estimate the patient's body frame, body mass index and the amount of subcutaneous fat, all of which are needed to determine whether a person's weight is desirable or whether he or she is underweight or overweight. Body mass index calculations can also be helpful in determining a person's risk for nutrition-related health problems such as diabetes, hypertension and cardiovascular disease.

FOR HEIGHT

Tables of desirable weights for height, such as those used by the Metropolitan Life Insurance Company (1983 revision), provide a general guide for establishing a person's desirable weight or determining whether someone is over- or underweight. These tables have recently been criticized as a standard of measure because they are based on weights associated with the lowest mortality rate in insured people and, therefore, do not apply to the entire population. In addition, they provide no information on the distribution of body fat or degree of obesity and they fail to account for the usual weight changes associated with aging. Therefore, these tables should be used only as general guidelines in the evaluation of relative weights and should be used in conjunction with other indices (BCDNA, 1992). The 1983 Metropolitan Life Insurance values of desirable weights for height for adults are found in Table 20.9.

FRAME SIZE

Body weight is influenced by frame size or body build. Understandably, a person with a large frame size will weigh more than a person of the same height but with a smaller body build. Body frame is usually divided into three categories—small, medium and large. One can assess the general type of body frame by looking at the person. However, a more accurate measure of a person's frame size may be determined by calculating the ratio of the individual's height to wrist circumference and then comparing that value to standard values for the different frame sizes. The wrist is measured at its smallest circumference (see Figure 20.7) and a height to wrist circumference ratio is computed as follows:

$$\textit{Ratio} = \textit{height (cm)} \div \textit{wrist circumference (cm)}$$

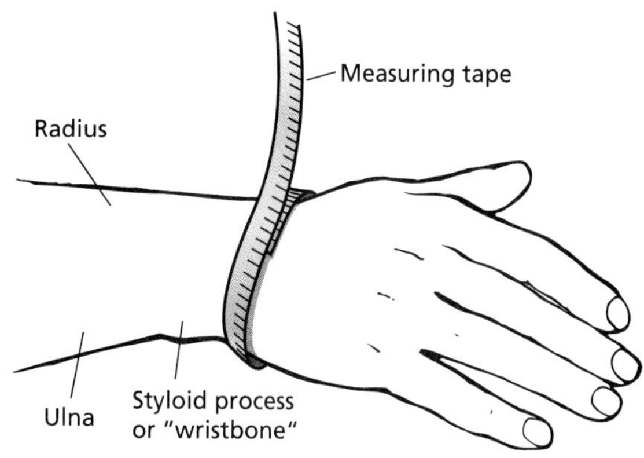

FIGURE 20.7 Measuring wrist circumference: Place the tape around the smallest circumference distal to the styloid process.

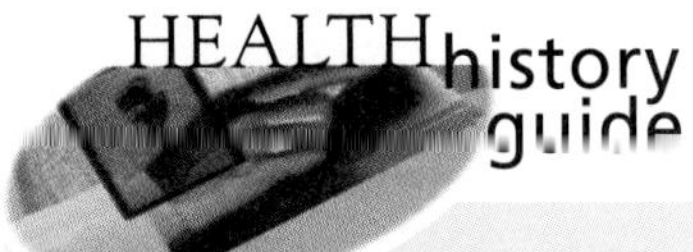

Nutrition

HEALTH AND ILLNESS PATTERNS

USUAL DIETARY PATTERN AND EATING HABITS

- Are you on a special diet? If so, what kind? Do you understand the purpose for it? Do you adhere to it? If not, why?
- What is your basic eating pattern?* Number of meals per day? Snacks? Typical times?
- Do you eat regularly? Do you skip meals? If so, how often?
- Do you often eat when you are not hungry? If so, for what reason? Stress? Anger? Nervousness? Boredom? Habit?
- What foods do you usually eat?* Milk and milk products? Meats and alternatives? Grains? Fruits and vegetables? How much of each in a typical day?
- Do you drink fluids with meals? Between meals? If so, what type? How much?
- Do you have any cultural, religious or moral beliefs and values that influence your eating pattern and food preferences? If so, what are they?
- What foods do you especially like? Dislike?
- Are there certain foods you avoid because they cause unpleasant reactions such as headache, gas, indigestion, diarrhea or constipation?
- Do you have any food allergies? If so, what are they?
- Do you use vitamin and mineral supplements? If so, what kinds? How often? How much?
- What is your usual height and weight?
- Do you need help with your meals? If so, what kind of help?
- In your opinion, are you eating a well-balanced diet? An unbalanced diet? Would you like help to plan a well-balanced diet?

RECENT CHANGES IN DIETARY PATTERN AND EATING HABITS

- Have there been any recent changes in your usual food intake and eating habits? Have you noticed that you are eating and drinking more or less than usual? Do you know the cause of these changes? If so, what is it?
- Have you noticed a change in your weight? Loss or gain? How much over the past week? Past month?
- Have you had a recent illness that affected your food intake and eating habits?
- Have you experienced loss of appetite, diarrhea, nausea, vomiting or abdominal pain?
- Has there been a change in your activity patterns? Why?
- Have you noticed unusual fatigue, tiredness, muscle weakness or recurrent fever lately?

PRESENTING HEALTH PROBLEM

- Describe the symptoms you are experiencing now. (Use questioning techniques as necessary to explore symptoms.)
- When did the symptoms begin?
- Are the symptoms related to a specific cause, such as eating habits, particular foods, medications, personal lifestyle and stressful situations?
- What remedies have you tried for the symptoms? What were the results?
- Do you or does anyone in your family have a history of acute or chronic diseases, surgery or weight problems? For example, obesity, eating disorders, diabetes mellitus, heart disease, cancer, ulcers, gallstones, intestinal disorders?
- Are you taking any prescriptions or over-the-counter (OTC) medications? If so, which drugs and what dosages?

HEALTH PROMOTION AND HEALTH PROTECTION PATTERNS

- Do you drink products containing caffeine (coffee, tea, cola), salt or sugar? If so, how much and how often?
- Do you use OTCs or prescribed medications or street drugs?
- Do you drink alcohol? If so, how much? How often?
- Do you smoke? If so, how much? For how many years?
- Do you have an active or sedentary lifestyle? What are your usual daily activities? Work-related? Recreation-related? Do you exercise regularly? If so, what kind? How often? How long?
- How do you care for your teeth and gums?
- Are you aware of Canada's Food Guide? Do you try to follow it?

* An effective method of obtaining information about nutritional patterns and eating habits is the 24-hour dietary recall. This may be obtained by interview or by asking the patient to prepare a written record of all foods and fluids taken in the previous day or on a typical day. Some agencies also use a self-administered questionnaire.

TABLE 20.9 1983 Metropolitan Life Insurance values for desirable weights for height for adults

Males

7A. Desirable Weight (kg)

HEIGHT cm	SMALL FRAME	MEDIUM FRAME	LARGE FRAME
158	58.3–61.0	59.6–64.2	62.8–68.3
159	58.6–61.3	59.9–64.5	63.1–68.8
160	59.0–61.7	60.3–64.9	63.5–69.4
161	59.3–62.0	60.6–65.2	63.8–69.9
162	59.7–62.4	61.0–65.6	64.2–70.5
163	60.0–62.7	61.3–66.0	64.5–71.1
164	60.4–63.1	61.7–66.5	64.9–71.8
165	60.8–63.5	62.1–67.0	65.3–72.5
166	61.1–63.8	62.4–67.5	65.6–73.2
167	61.5–64.2	62.8–68.2	66.0–74.0
168	61.8–64.6	63.2–68.7	66.4–74.7
169	62.2–65.2	63.8–69.3	67.0–75.4
170	62.5–65.7	64.3–69.8	67.5–76.1
171	62.9–66.2	64.9–70.3	68.0–76.2
172	63.2–66.7	65.4–70.8	68.7–77.5
173	63.6–67.3	65.9–71.4	69.1–78.2
174	63.9–67.8	66.4–71.9	69.5–78.9
175	64.3–68.3	66.9–72.4	70.1–79.5
176	64.7–68.9	67.5–73.0	70.7–80.3
177	65.0–69.5	68.1–73.5	71.3–81.0
178	65.4–70.0	69.6–74.0	71.9–81.2
179	65.7–70.5	69.2–74.6	72.3–82.5
180	66.1–71.1	69.7–75.1	72.8–83.3
181	66.6–71.6	70.2–75.8	73.4–84.0
182	67.1–72.1	70.7–76.5	73.9–84.7
183	67.7–72.7	71.3–77.2	74.5–85.4
184	68.2–73.4	71.8–77.9	75.2–86.1
185	68.7–74.1	72.4–78.6	75.9–86.3
186	69.2–74.8	73.0–79.3	76.6–87.6
187	69.8–75.5	73.7–80.0	77.3–88.5
188	70.3–76.2	74.4–80.7	78.0–89.4
189	70.9–76.9	74.9–81.5	78.7–90.3
190	71.4–77.6	75.4–82.2	79.4–91.2
191	72.1–78.4	76.1–83.0	80.3–92.1
192	72.8–79.1	76.8–83.9	81.2–93.0
193	73.5–79.8	77.6–84.8	82.1–93.9

SOURCE: Ontario Dietetic Association and the Ontario Hospital Association, 1989.

TABLE 20.9 *Continued*

Females			
7A. Desirable Weight (kg)			
HEIGHT cm	SMALL FRAME	MEDIUM FRAME	LARGE FRAME
148	46.4–50.6	49.6–55.1	53.7–59.8
149	46.6–51.0	50.0–55.5	54.1–60.3
150	46.7–51.3	50.3–55.9	54.4–60.9
151	46.9–51.7	50.7–56.4	54.8–61.4
152	47.1–52.1	51.1–57.0	55.2–61.9
153	47.4–52.5	51.5–57.5	55.6–62.4
154	47.8–53.0	51.9–58.0	56.2–63.0
155	48.1–53.6	52.2–58.6	56.8–63.6
156	48.5–54.1	52.7–59.1	57.3–64.1
157	48.8–54.6	53.2–59.6	57.8–64.6
158	49.3–55.2	53.8–60.2	58.4–65.3
159	49.8–55.7	54.3–60.7	58.9–66.0
160	50.3–55.2	54.9–61.2	59.4–66.7
161	50.8–56.7	55.4–61.7	59.9–67.4
162	51.4–57.3	55.9–62.3	60.5–68.1
163	51.9–57.8	56.4–63.3	61.0–68.8
164	52.5–58.4	57.0–63.4	61.5–69.5
165	53.0–58.9	57.5–63.9	62.0–70.2
166	53.6–59.5	58.1–64.5	62.6–70.9
167	54.1–60.0	58.7–65.0	63.2–71.7
168	54.6–60.5	59.2–65.5	63.7–72.4
169	55.2–61.1	59.7–65.1	64.3–73.1
170	55.7–61.6	60.2–66.6	64.8–73.8
171	56.2–62.1	60.7–67.1	65.3–74.5
172	56.8–62.6	61.0–67.6	65.8–75.2
173	57.3–63.2	67.8–68.2	66.4–75.9
174	57.8–63.7	62.3–68.7	66.9–76.4
175	58.3–64.2	62.8–69.2	67.4–76.9
176	58.9–64.8	63.4–69.8	68.0–77.5
177	59.5–65.4	64.0–70.4	68.5–78.1
178	60.0–65.9	64.5–70.9	69.0–78.6
179	60.5–66.4	65.1–71.4	69.5–79.1
180	61.0–66.9	65.6–71.9	70.1–79.5
181	61.6–67.5	66.1–72.5	70.7–80.2
182	62.1–68.0	66.6–73.0	71.2–80.7

TABLE 20.10 Frame size according to height–wrist circumference ratio

Small	>10.4	>10.9
Medium	10.4–9.6	10.9–9.9
Large	<9.6	<9.9

SOURCE: BCDNA, 1992, p. 80.

The patient's frame size is established by comparing the patient's ratio value to standard values, as outlined in Table 20.10.

BODY MASS INDEX (BMI)

The body mass index is a measure of a person's weight in relation to height. It is computed by dividing the weight (in kilograms) by the height (in metres) squared. Thus:

$$BMI = weight\ (kg) \div height\ (m)^2$$

Because the body mass index was found to correlate best with the risk for diseases, an Expert Group on Weight Standards for Health and Welfare Canada recommended the use of BMI as a measure of body weight (1988a). "The BMI provides an estimate of healthy weights and identifies individuals at risk for complications associated with being overweight or underweight" (BCDNA, 1992). Its use is limited to men and nonpregnant, nonlactating women between 20 and 65 years of age. In addition, BMI does not account for weight differences due to frame size or fat distribution. Thus, an assessment of fat distribution is recommended for assessing body weight (BCDNA, 1992).

Measuring the head circumference of children less than two years of age can also be used to reflect the effects of nutrition on brain growth. To measure, place the tape just above the child's eyebrow (middle of the forehead), above the ears and around the bony structure at the back of the child's head (Eschelman, 1996). Usually, this measurement is primarily used to determine non-nutritional health problems (hydrocephaly); it is not used frequently as a nutritional screening device (Dudek, 1997).

Standards for Interpreting Body Mass Index

• BMI <20	May be associated with health problems for some people
• BMI 20–25	Healthy weight for most people
• BMI 25–27	May lead to health problems in some people
• BMI >27	Increased risk for developing health problems

SOURCE: Health & Welfare Canada, 1988b.

FAT DISTRIBUTION

An indirect estimate of the body's fat deposits can be obtained by measuring the thickness of skin folds using calipers. This is referred to as a *fatfold* or *skinfold* test. The measurement is usually taken from the back of the arm—the triceps's skinfold thickness (see Figure 20.8). The fat under the skin in this region, and in other regions such as the back, represents about helf the body's total fat tissue; in most people, it is roughly proportional to total body fat. The fatfold test can yield reliable information, provided it is done by trained professionals using reliable calipers. Interobserver error can be high; thus, it is best if this test is done each time by the same health professional to minimize the possibility of error. Skinfold thickness measurements must be interpreted with caution. Their main use is in monitoring body composition and fat deposits over a long period of time (Dudek, 1997). "Depletion of stores can reflect chronic inadequate intake and, therefore, these measurements provide an estimate of the duration and severity of inadequate intake" (BCDNA, 1992, p. 76).

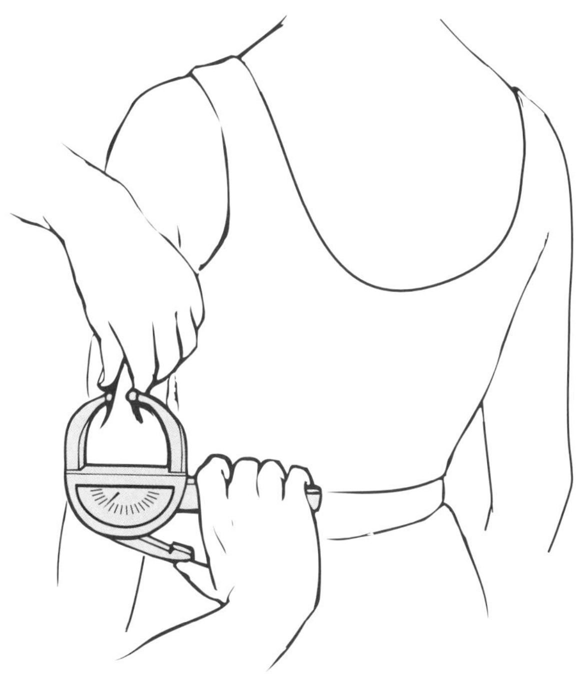

FIGURE 20.8 Measuring triceps skinfold thickness

Physical Assessment

There are many outward signs of both good nutrition and malnutrition that are readily observable to the trained eye. Characteristics that the nurse can observe in people with good nutrition and those with poor nutrition (a comparison) are shown in Table 20.11. Particularly important aspects to note are the eyes, the mouth (especially the teeth and mucous membranes), the skin and its underlying fat and muscle tissues and the limbs. The general appearance, the pace and vigour with which people carry out activities, and general emotional tone should be noted. Do they look overweight or underweight? Do they look emaciated? Do they appear listless and apathetic or do they tackle things with enthusiasm? Are they good-natured, irritable or depressed?

In severe cases of malnutrition, the heartbeat may be accelerated and its rhythm altered. The blood pressure may be elevated and individuals may find it difficult to sit or stand erect. The lips and tongue may be red and swollen; the gums may be spongy and may bleed easily; and the nails may become spoon-shaped, brittle and ridged. The face may look drawn, with hollow cheeks and dark circles under the eyes and on the cheeks. The parotid glands and the thyroid glands often become swollen. The person may become confused, and may have a burning or tingling sensation in the hands and feet. Muscles may appear wasted and the joints sore and swollen (Dudek, 1997).

The person who has indigestion is usually obviously uncomfortable, as is the one who is nauseated. A nauseated person, or one about to vomit, usually shows pallor and increased perspiration. Beads of perspiration may be evident on the forehead or upper lip. Pulse and respiratory rates taken at this time may be markedly increased. The pulse rate may increase at first, but usually then drops to below normal. Blood pressure usually drops as well.

Vomiting should be assessed in terms of both the nature of the vomiting and the characteristics of the vomitus (material vomited). In relation to vomiting, the nurse should determine its type—that is, whether it is projectile or regurgitated (ordinary vomiting); whether it is preceded by

TABLE 20.11 Clinical signs of nutritional status

Features	*Good*	*Poor*
General appearance	Alert, responsive	Listless, apathetic, cachexic
Hair	Shiny, lustrous, healthy scalp	Stringy, dull, brittle, depigmented
Neck glands	No enlargement	Thyroid enlarged
Skin, face, neck	Smooth, slightly moist, good colour, reddish-pink mucous membranes	Greasy, discoloured, scaly
Eyes	Bright, clear, no fatigue circles	Dryness, signs of infection, increased vascularity, glassiness, thickened conjunctivae, fatigue circles
Lips	Good colour, moist	Dry, scaly, swollen, angular lesions (stomatitis)
Tongue	Good pink colour, surface papillae present, no lesions	Papillary atrophy, smooth appearance, swollen, red, beefy (glossitis)
Gums	Good pink colour, no swelling or bleeding, firm	Marginal redness or swelling, receding, spongy
Teeth	Straight, no crowding, well-shaped jaw, clean, no discoloration	Unfilled cavities, absent teeth, worn surface, mottled, malpositioned
Skin, general	Smooth, slightly moist, good colour	Rough, dry, scaly, pale, pigmented, irritated; petechiae, bruises
Abdomen	Flat	Swollen
Legs, feet	No tenderness, weakness, swelling, good colour	Edema, tender calf, tingling, weakness
Skeleton	No malformations	Bowlegs, knock-knees, chest deformity at diaphragm, beaded ribs, prominent scapulas
Weight	Normal for height, age, body build	Overweight or underweight
Posture	Erect, arms and legs straight, abdomen in, chest out	Sagging shoulders, sunken chest, humped back
Muscles	Well-developed, firm	Flaccid, poor tone, undeveloped, tender
Nervous control	Good attention span for age, does not cry easily, not irritable or restless	Inattentive, irritable
Gastrointestinal function	Good appetite and digestion, normal, regular elimination	Anorexia, indigestion, constipation or diarrhea
General vitality	Endurance, energetic, sleeps well at night, vigorous	Easily fatigued, no energy, falls asleep in school, looks tired, apathetic

SOURCE: Williams, 1997, p. 7.

feelings of nausea; its frequency; and its occurrence in relation to intake of food, the administration of drugs and the individual's emotional state. Characteristics of the vom-

(watery, liquid or solid), the presence of undigested food, blood or other foreign substances; and odour.

Gastrointestinal disturbances quickly result in deterioration of the patient's nutritional status. Food and fluids, especially the chloride ions, are lost as a result of vomiting of gastric juices. Prolonged deficiency in nourishment and in fluid intake results in malnutrition and dehydration; dehydration, in turn, can cause constipation. The patient can be expected to be constipated because of the fluid withdrawn from the feces in an effort by the body to compensate for lowered fluid intake or excessive fluid loss. There will probably also be a decrease in the amount of urine excreted, and the urine will be more concentrated.

A person who suffers from anorexia or nausea over a period of time will lose weight and, in addition to showing signs of dehydration and malnutrition, will become weak and listless owing to inadequate intake of nutrients. The individual who has experienced prolonged vomiting will show more pronounced effects due not only to lack of intake but also to the loss of food and fluids through vomiting. This individual may show a marked weight loss and rapidly progressive signs of weakness and prostration, as well as signs of fluid and electrolyte imbalance (see Chapter 23).

Diagnostic Tests

BLOOD TESTS

Blood tests for hemoglobin and hematocrit indicate iron as well as protein deficiencies. Laboratory tests that reflect protein adequacy include total protein and serum albumin, prealbumin and transferrin (total iron-binding capacity). A total lymphocyte count (TLC) is taken to assess the person's immune status. Because the TLC is depressed when nutrient deficiency problems exist, the TLC can be used as a gauge of nutritional status. Blood levels of sodium and potassium, of glucose, and of cholesterol and triglyceride are used to assess electrolyte balance, carbohydrate metabolism, and lipid metabolism, respectively (Dudek, 1997).

However, blood proteins are not necessarily a reliable indicator of nutritional status in certain health problems. For example, people who have renal or liver disease or sepsis, or who suffer from trauma, can have abnormal blood protein counts that are affected by the health problem and not their nutritional status. TLC can also be affected by immunosuppressive medications (e.g., chemotherapy) and health problems (e.g., AIDS).

BLOOD GLUCOSE TESTING

Blood glucose testing, when done by the nurse or the patient, offers a precise method of monitoring blood glucose levels. Several makes and models of blood glucose monitors exist in the marketplace. The meters are small and easy to carry around, relatively inexpensive and simple to operate.

All diabetic patients, whether they are insulin-

monitoring to keep their diabetes under control. Blood glucose monitoring is essential in several circumstances, such as diabetes in pregnancy, when erratic blood glucose levels exist or when hypoglycemia unawareness occurs after a long history of diabetes (Kestel, 1993). Regular testing reveals blood glucose patterns that can be used to modify diet and medications in order to keep diabetes under control and prevent diabetic complications.

Most models of blood glucose monitors operate on similar principles, using electronic sensors that measure electrical potential caused by the reaction of glucose with the reagents on the electrode strip. The measurement range of the meters is usually between 1.1–33.3 mmol/L (20–600 mg/dL). Patients whose testing results show glucose levels below 2.8 mmol/L or above 13.9 mmol/L are recommended to contact their physician or other health professional.

Because of fast-paced technological developments in blood glucose meters, close attention to individual differences and changes in monitoring technique are necessary. Most models use capillary blood specimens from finger-stick blood samples and have common steps in the testing procedure (see Procedure 20.6).

URINE TESTS

A 24-hour sample of urine may be ordered for creatinine levels to assess protein metabolism. Creatinine is a by-product of muscle metabolism and is used as an indicator of muscle protein breakdown, renal function and malnutrition. Similarly, a 24-hour urinary urea nitrogen test is used to determine protein catabolism and nitrogen balance. Urea is formed in the liver as a by-product of protein metabolism. It is excreted from the body through the kidneys; thus, levels in the urine can be used to evaluate protein (nitrogen) balance in the body. When protein intake equals protein output, the body is in a state of nitrogen equilibrium. Often, during illness or starvation, the body loses more protein than it takes in. The body is then in a state of negative nitrogen balance. In practice, the assessment of nitrogen balance requires a battery of tests, which you will learn more about in your advanced-level courses (Chernecky & Berger, 1997).

Diagnosing Nutritional Problems

Nutritional problems that fall within the domain of independent nursing intervention are generally diagnosed as *Altered Nutrition*. In cases where the intake of nutrients is actually or potentially insufficient to meet metabolic demands, the nursing diagnosis is stated as *Altered Nutrition: Less than Body Requirements*. This can include any number of situations in which the person can ingest food but the quantity and/or quality of intake is inadequate. For example, people who eat less than required amounts of food because of anorexia, nausea, fatigue, pain, chewing or swallowing difficulties, inadequate family budgets for procuring food, personal lifestyles and food habits, or lack of knowledge of required nutrient intake may experience, or be at risk for, insufficient intake. Furthermore, because metabolic needs increase during illness, trauma and healing, a person who is ill faces the risk of inadequate intake even when eating patterns remain unchanged. For example, someone who sustained a back injury in a skiing accident might notice a loss in weight even if food and fluid intake is not affected during the course of healing. Defining characteristics of insufficient nutrient intake might include reported or observed food intake below daily nutrient requirements, weight loss, BMI below 20, presence of hypermetabolic disease states (such as fever, trauma, infection, cancer), decreased energy level and muscular weakness and tenderness.

The diagnostic statement, *Altered Nutrition: Less than Body Requirements* should not be used for patients who are NPO (taking nothing per mouth) or unable to ingest food, because there are no interventions nurses can prescribe to improve the nutritional status of these patients. Instead, the nursing diagnoses should focus on the resulting problems that nurses can treat, such as *Altered Comfort* or *Altered Oral Mucous Membrane Integrity*. In addition, potential problems that may result from the patient's NPO status and the medical treatment regimen, which nurses have a collaborative responsibility to monitor, manage and minimize, should be stated as collaborative problems. For example, a person who is NPO might be at risk for hypoglycemia and negative nitrogen balance.

Altered Nutrition: More than Body Requirements is the diagnosis used for individuals who are experiencing, or are at risk of experiencing, weight gain because their food intake is greater than their metabolic needs. This diagnosis might apply to patients who gain (or are at risk for gaining) weight because of their sedentary lifestyle, changes in taste or smell or medications, such as corticosteroids (Carpenito, 1997). Carpenito advises that the nurse should be careful using this diagnostic statement with patients who are overweight or obese because of the multiplicity of factors usually involved in obesity. Furthermore, a successful weight loss program includes more than limiting food intake; behaviour modification and lifestyle changes are also necessary. Thus, a better diagnosis would be *Altered Health Maintenance related to intake in excess of metabolic requirements* (1997).

Some examples of nursing diagnoses for patients with nutritional problems are:

- *Altered Nutrition: Less than Body Requirements related to chewing difficulty secondary to wired jaw.*
- *Altered Nutrition: Less than Body Requirements related to difficulty procuring food secondary to lack of transportation to supermarket.*
- *Risk for Altered Nutrition: Less than Body Requirements related to anorexia secondary to pain and chemotherapy.*
- *PC: Hypoglycemia.*

Planning Nutritional Interventions

A plan of care for people with nutritional problems is based on the nursing diagnoses and focusses on maintaining adequate nutrition and hydration during illness, restoring satisfactory nutritional status if nutritional balance has been disturbed and promoting optimal nutrition in daily living.

As we discussed previously, dietary habits and food intake are greatly influenced by personal preferences and lifestyle practices, cultural and religious beliefs and practices, psychological and emotional factors and socioeconomic determinants. A plan of care must take these factors into consideration and must involve the patient (and family, as necessary). The patient's participation is mandatory when setting goals and planning strategies to change dietary habits and food intake. Unless the goals reflect outcomes that the patient is willing or able to achieve, the plan of care will likely be ineffective. Goals and expected outcomes should be stated as short-term steps towards long-term achievement. For example, a long-term goal of reducing weight by 25 kg in 12 weeks may be overwhelming to the patient, whereas a short-term goal of reducing weight by one kilogram per week may be easier to deal with.

Examples of goals or expected outcomes pertaining to nutritional problems include:

- The patient will show adequate nutrition by eating all foods on the meal tray.
- The patient will list high-fibre foods and the amounts he or she will add to the daily diet.
- The patient will describe how to select restaurant foods to avoid high-fat and high-salt intake.
- The patient (family) will explain how he or she will buy and prepare nutritious meals and snacks according to Canada's Food Guide.

Implementing Nutritional Interventions

Health-Promoting Strategies

Proper intake of food is essential for optimal health. "Eating the right kinds and amounts of food and following good dietary habits throughout one's entire life means a healthier body and mind, greater vitality, greater resistance to disease, efficiency, happiness, and longevity" (Poleman & Peckenpaugh, 1991, p. 9). Inadequate food intake and poor eating habits can affect one's immune system and physical fitness (e.g., decrease strength and endurance) (Williams, 1992) and interfere with the capacity to think, work and cope with the stresses of everyday living. N

1. by encouraging and helping people to examine lifestyle factors and personal, cultural and religious values and practices that affect their dietary patterns and eating habits
2. by providing information that will enable individuals, families and groups to determine whether their usual patterns and habits need changing
3. by teaching healthy eating and other health practices, such as regular exercise and dental care, that are intended to promote optimal nutrition and wellness.

Table 20.12 identifies dietary problems and interventions specific to the elderly patient. The section that follows describes health-promoting strategies for the general population.

PROMOTING HEALTHY FOOD INTAKE

The wise selection of foods can significantly affect an in

supply the amounts of essential nutrients that are needed to sustain life and health. In addition, while epidemiological and experimental studies linking nutrition and disease have not been conclusive, available evidence suggests that a diet containing the recommended essential nutrients has the potential for reducing the risk of chronic diseases such as cardiovascular diseases, diabetes and cancer.

Guidelines for Healthier Nutrition

A resource used by nurses, nutritionists and physicians in teaching and counselling individuals, families and groups about nutrition is *Canada's Food Guide to Healthy Eating*. Issued by Health Canada, the *Food Guide* is based on daily nutritional recommendations. It specifies amounts to be included in a daily diet from each of four basic food groups:

TABLE 20.12 Dietary intervention for eating problems of the elderly

PROBLEM	RATIONALE	DIETARY INTERVENTIONS
Difficulty chewing	Missing or decayed teeth Periodontal disease Missing or ill-fitting dentures	Provide liquid, semi-solid, mashed or chopped foods as tolerated. Progress to liquid diet as soon as possible
Difficulty swallowing	Paralysis related to stroke Parkinson's disease	Thickened and gelled liquids are usually better tolerated than thin liquids. Baby food can be used as a nutritious thickener Avoid overuse of pureed foods because of the negative connotations associated with it
Lack of appetite	Depression Acute or chronic disease Loss of sense of smell and taste Side effect of medication Loneliness Early satiety	Offer small, frequent meals Solicit food preferences Allow plenty of time to eat Because appetite is usually greatest in the morning, emphasize a nutritious breakfast Encourage group eating
Impaired ability to feed self	Poor vision Arthritis of the hands; stroke	Describe the meal and how it is arranged on the plate Assist the patient by opening packages of bread and crackers, buttering bread and vegetables, cutting meat and opening milk cartons Assess the patient's ability to grasp utensils and guide food to the mouth. Refer the patient to an occupational therapist to evaluate the need for assistive devices or retraining
Loss of taste and smell	Normal aging Endocrine disorders secondary to drug therapy Certain nutrient deficiencies (zinc, vitamin B_{12}, niacin)	Add commercial flavours to foods to intensify smell Add texture, when possible (e.g., crunchiness, chewiness) Appearance of food becomes more important Sour/bitter fruits and vegetables are the foods most likely to be avoided; encourage the intake of other types/forms of fruits and vegetables acceptable to the individual

SOURCE: Dudek, 1997, p. 367.

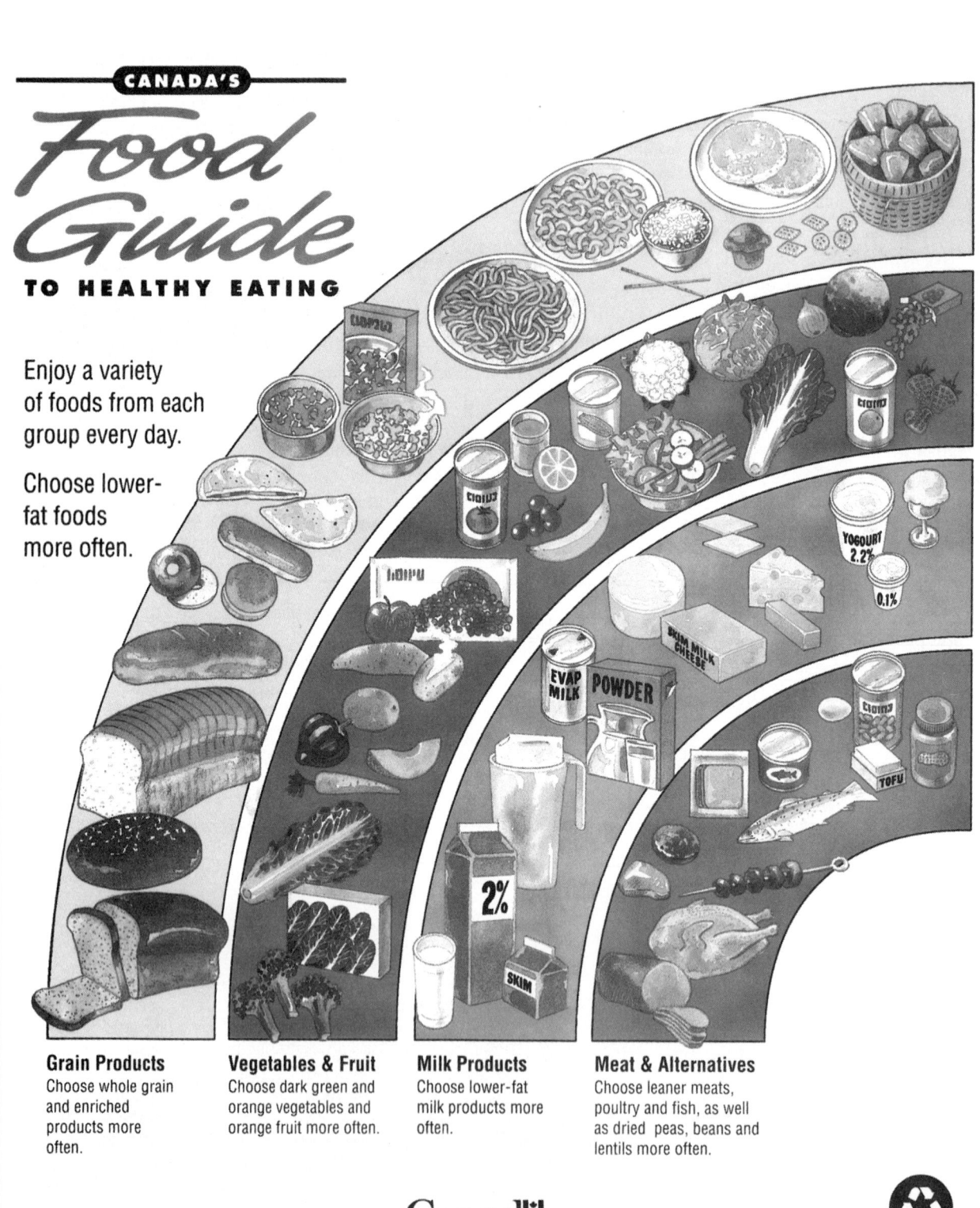

FIGURE 20.9 *Canada's Food Guide to Healthy Eating*

SOURCE: Health Canada, 1992.

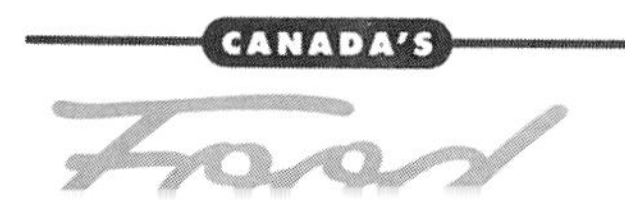

Guide
TO HEALTHY EATING
FOR PEOPLE FOUR YEARS AND OVER

Different People Need Different Amounts of Food

The amount of food you need every day from the 4 food groups and other [illegible] gives a lower and higher number of servings for each food group. For example, young children can choose the lower number of servings, while male teenagers can go to the higher number. Most other people can choose servings somewhere in between.

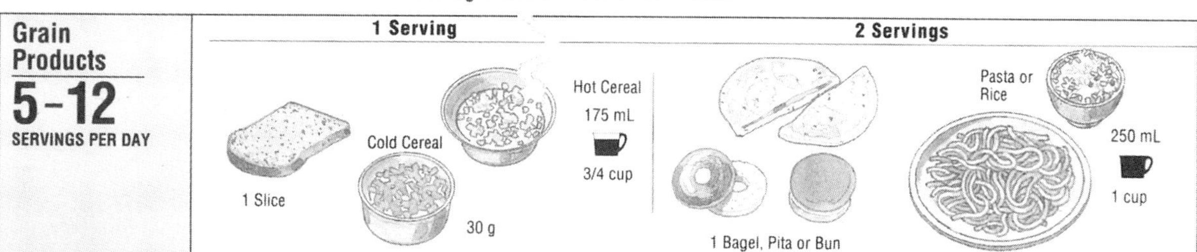

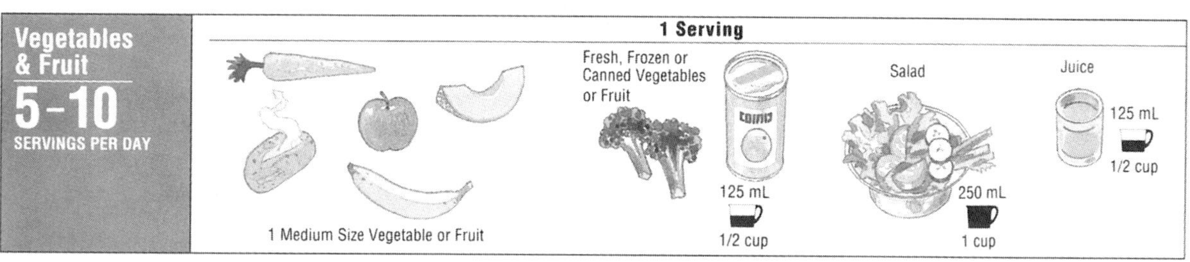

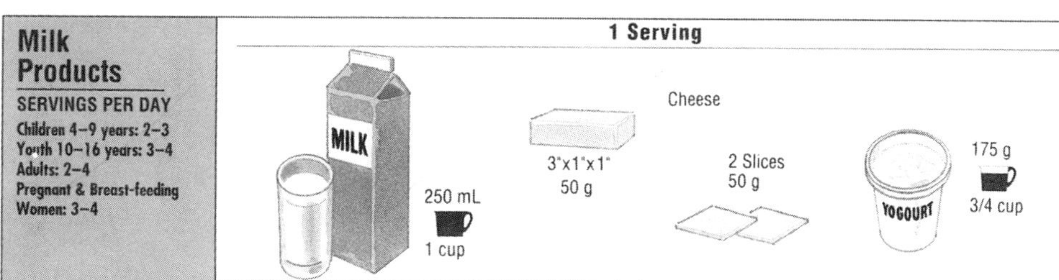

Other Foods

Taste and enjoyment can also come from other foods and beverages that are not part of the 4 food groups. Some of these foods are higher in fat or Calories, so use these foods in moderation.

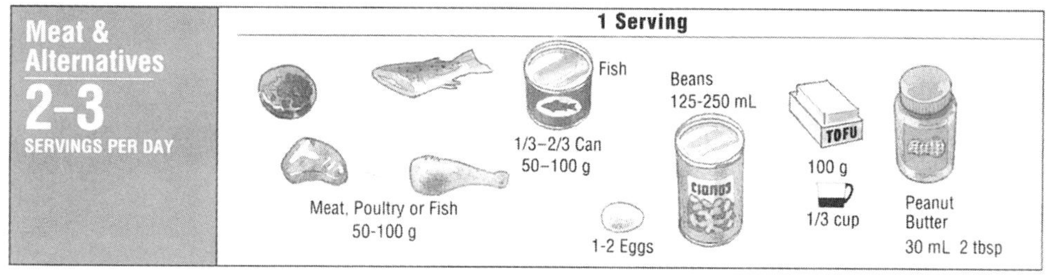

Enjoy eating well, being active and feeling good about yourself. That's VITALIT*É*

ISBN 0-662-19648-1

Reprinted 1994

FIGURE 20.9 *Canada's Food Guide to Healthy Eating (continued)*

SOURCE: Health Canada, 1992.

grain products, vegetables and fruit, milk products, and meat and alternatives. It also includes guidelines for intake of other foods, such as fats and oils, sugars, beverages, herbs, spices, alcohol and caffeine, as well as vitamin and mineral supplements. *Canada's Food Guide to Healthy Eating* is outlined in Figure 20.9. The key nutrients in the *Food Guide* are listed in Figure 20.10. In addition to the *Food Guide*, there are a number of other guidelines that individuals and families may use to make food choices for healthier nutrition. These are outlined in the box, Promoting Healthy Nutrition.

The Vegetarian Diet

Vegetarian diets exclude or limit the intake of meat, poultry and fish and, in some instances, eggs and dairy products. There are four basic types of vegetarian diets:

1. *lacto-ovo-vegetarian*, which avoids meat, fish and poultry but allows eggs and dairy products
2. *lacto-vegetarian*, which avoids meat, poultry, fish and eggs, but allows dairy products
3. *ovo-vegetarian*, which avoids meat, poultry, fish and dairy products, but includes eggs
4. *vegan*, also referred to as strict vegetarian, which avoids all foods of animal origin, including dairy products and eggs.

In practice, there are many individual variations of vegetarian diets. For example, some people call themselves vegetarians because they exclude only red meat, such as beef and pork, from their diet. Others allow only poultry and fish, while excluding all other animal products including milk and eggs.

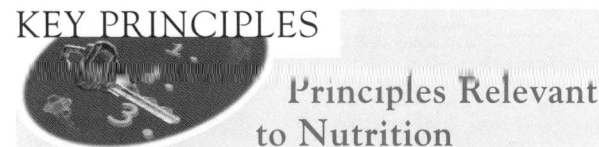

KEY PRINCIPLES

Principles Relevant to Nutrition

1. Adequate intake of essential nutrients and energy-giving foods is required for optimal health.
2. An individual's nutritional status is determined by the adequacy of the specific nutrients and energy-giving foods taken into the body, absorbed and utilized.
3. Nutritional needs depend on an individual's age, gender, body composition, amount and type of daily activity, endocrine secretion and health status.
4. Nutritional needs are usually altered in illness.
5. Food has psychological meaning for people.
6. Food habits are learned.
7. Food habits are related to cultural, religious and moral beliefs.

Acceptable sources of protein include milk and dairy products (if eaten) and meat alternatives. Soybeans, nuts, seeds and whole grains (and foods made from these) are an important source of dietary protein. To ensure an adequate intake of iron, the use of eggs (if permitted), fruits and vegetables containing iron, and whole grain and enriched cereals should be encouraged. To increase the vitamin D content of vegetarian diets, eggs and vitamin D-fortified milk and margarine, or a regular inake of vitamin tablets, may be suggested. Children and expectant and lactating mothers are particularly vulnerable to nutritional disorders because of their additional nutrient needs. Besides the problems

Each food group is essential. That's because it provides its own set of nutrients.

Grain Products	+	Vegetables & Fruit	+	Milk Products	+	Meat & Alternatives	=	The Food Guide
protein				protein		protein		protein
				fat		fat		fat
carbohydrate		carbohydrate						carbohydrate
fibre		fibre						fibre
thiamin		thiamin				thiamin		thiamin
riboflavin				riboflavin		riboflavin		riboflavin
niacin						niacin		niacin
folacin		folacin				folacin		folacin
				vitamin B_{12}		vitamin B_{12}		vitamin B_{12}
		vitamin C						vitamin C
		vitamin A		vitamin A				vitamin A
				vitamin D				vitamin D
				calcium				calcium
iron		iron				iron		iron
zinc				zinc		zinc		zinc
magnesium		magnesium		magnesium		magnesium		magnesium

FIGURE 20.10 Key nutrients in *Canada's Guide to Healthy Eating*

SOURCE: Health & Welfare Canada, 1992, p. 5.

Promoting Healthy Nutrition

- Eat a variety of foods from the four food groups. Eating a [illegible] of all essential nutrients.
- Eat foods rich in calcium and iron (especially important for women and children). For calcium choose skim or low-fat milk and dairy products; dark-green leafy vegetables such as spinach and broccoli; dried peas and beans; cauliflower; fish with bones, such as canned salmon. For iron choose lean meats, shellefish, dried peas and beans; dark-green leafy vegetables, such as spinach and broccoli; and dried fruits, such as raisins, apricots, dates.
- Eat moderate amounts of protein, balancing intake of plant and animal sources. Choose leaner meats, poultry and fish, as well as dried peas, beans and lentils.
- Eat more complex carbohydrates, fibre and natural sugars. Choose whole grain and enriched products, legumes (peas and beans) and fruits and vegetables. Choose dark-green and orange vegetables and orange fruits (high sources of vitamin A, vitamin C and folacin). As well, choose cruciferous vegetables, such as cabbage, brussels sprouts, broccoli and cauliflower, since they appear to provide protection against lung, stomach, colon and rectal cancer.
- Choose lower-fat foods more often since diets high in fat have been associated with heart disease and certain types of cancer.
- Eat less meat with high fat content. Avoid hot dogs, processed luncheon meats, sausage and bacon.
- Use skim, partly skim and [illegible]
- Avoid butter, margarine or rich sauces on vegetables.
- Limit consumption of fast and deep-fried foods.
- Eat more fish, and select meat, poultry or fish that is baked, broiled or microwaved.
- Use less dressing on salads or use lower-fat dressings.
- Limit snacks such as chips and chocolate bars.
- Limit intake of salt and sodium.
- Avoid highly salted foods.
- When shopping check labels; select unsalted foods or foods low in salt or sodium.
- Use less salt at the table.
- Taste foods before adding salt.
- Use herbs, spices and lemon juice instead of salt in cooking.
- Avoid taking dietary supplements in excess of the daily recommended nutrient intakes (RNI).
- Eat fresh, natural foods as much as possible and avoid foods with questionable additives such as dyes, saccharin, sodium nitrate and sulfites.
- Use alcohol and caffeine in moderation. For adults, this means no more than one alcoholic drink a day and no more than 7 drinks a week. Limit caffeine intake from all sources to no more than the equivalent of 4 cups of coffee a day.

SOURCES: Health & Welfare Canada, 1990, 1992; Williams, 1995a.

mentioned above, they may also have a deficiency of calcium if milk and milk products are not included in the diet. It is often necessary to use calcium tablets as a supplement (Barker, 1996; Dudek, 1997).

Extra-firm tofu (made with calcium) and tahini (sesame butter) can also provide some calcium to the diet. Vitamin B_{12} is found in animal foods; thus, supplements may be required in vegan diets. Some special nutritional yeasts grown on a vitamin B_{12}-enriched medium can also provide some vitamin B_{12} to the diet.

When foods are selected carefully, vegetarian diets are healthy and nutritionally adequate. If they are not properly planned, the person may suffer from nutritional deficiencies of protein, iron, calcium and riboflavin. A vital concern for people on a vegan diet is that they obtain the right amounts of protein and supplemental vitamin B_{12}. You will recall from our previous discussion that plant products provide incomplete proteins. While certain vegetable products, such as grains (wheat, rice and corn), legumes (fruit or pod of vegetables including soybeans, peas, beans, lentils) and nuts and seeds, are good sources of protein, they lack one or more essential amino acids in sufficient quantity. If eaten individually, they are not generally adequate in maintaining proper nutrition. However, if eaten in proper combinations or complementary patterns, they can supply all the amino acids essential to life. In what is termed *protein complementation*, a vegetable food low in a particular amino acid is eaten with a food high in that particular amino acid to provide the equivalent of a complete protein. For example, grains complemented by nuts or seeds, such as noodles with sesame seeds, will provide a complete protein. It is important to note that complementary patterns of amino acids are not necessary within each meal, but should be included within the intake for a given day (BCDNA, 1992). A vegetarian food guide is shown in Table 20.13.

CHANGING DIETARY PATTERNS

It is sometimes necessary for people to change dietary patterns and food habits because of illness. They may be told by a physician that they can no longer use salt to flavour their food, or they may have to give up eating a favourite dish. Patients may be put on low-fat diets, or any one of a number of special diets. In these situations, people react differently. Some accept the restrictions of a special diet fairly easily; others are less amenable to change.

TABLE 20.13 Vegetarian food guide

A variety of foods from each of the following groups should be eaten daily:

Breads and Cereals: 6 servings daily

Whole grain products are recommended

Examples of one serving:

- Bread, 1 slice
- Bagel, 1/2
- Bannock, 60 g (2 oz)
- Cereal, ready-to-eat, 200 mL (3/4 cup)
- Cereal, cooked, 125 mL (1/2 cup)
- Chapati or roti, 1
- Crackers, 4–6
- Hamburger or hot dog bun, 1/2
- Muffin, 1 small or 1/2 large
- Pancake or waffle, 1
- Pita bread, 1/2
- Popcorn, 375 mL (1 1/2 cups)
- Rice, cooked, 125 mL (1/2 cup)
- Roll, 1 small
- Rye cracker, 2
- Spaghetti, macaroni or other pasta, cooked, 125 mL (1/2 cup)
- Tortilla, 1

Vegetables and Fruits: 6 servings daily

Include 1–2 servings of dark-green vegetables daily and at least one other vegetable

Examples of one serving:

- Vegetable or fruit, fresh, frozen or canned, 125 mL (1/2 cup)
- Vegetable or fruit juice, 125 mL (1/2 cup)
- Medium-sized potato, carrot, tomato, apple, banana, orange or peach, 1
- Small fruit, apricot or plum, 2

Iron and Protein Foods: 2 servings daily

Eat these plant sources of iron at the same meal with a vitamin C source (a vegetable or fruit) to increase iron absorption

Examples of one serving:

- Legumes, cooked, 250 mL (1 cup)
- Firm tofu, 125 mL (1/2 cup)
- Nuts or seeds, 125 mL (1/2 cup)
- Nut or seed butter, 75 mL (1/3 cup)
- Soy yogurt (cultured soy), 125 mL (1/2 cup)
- Soybean milk, 500 mL (2 cups)

In addition, for ovo-vegetarian diets:

- Eggs, 2

Calcium Foods: 6 servings daily

Each serving provides approximately 100 mg calcium. Some foods can be counted as fruit and vegetable servings *as well as* calcium food servings (for example, dark-green leafy vegetables and broccoli).

Some foods can be counted as iron and protein foods *as well as* calcium foods (for example, moderately firm and firm tofu that is made with calcium; legumes; nuts and seeds)

The serving sizes for some foods are small when counted as calcium servings. Soy milk does not serve as a calcium source.

Examples of one serving:

- Firm tofu made with calcium, 50 mL (1/4 cup)
- Legumes, cooked, 250 mL (1 cup)
- Unhulled sesame seeds or butter, 15 mL (1 tbsp)
- Sesame tahini, 30 mL (2 tbsp)
- Almonds, 30 g (1 oz)
- Seaweeds (hijiki, kelp, wakame), dried, 4–7 g
- Dark-green vegetables (beet greens, bok choy, broccoli, collards, kale, mustard greens, okra, turnip greens), cooked, 125 mL (1/2 cup)

In addition, for lacto-vegetarian diets:

- Milk, 75 mL (1/3 cup)
- Yogurt, 75 mL (1/3 cup)
- Cheddar cheeses, 14 g (1/2 oz)

Also include

For vitamin B_{12}:

5 mL (1 tsp) nutritional yeast grown on a vitamin B_{12}-enriched medium

For vitamin D:

15 mL (3 tsp) vitamin D-fortified margarine

For additional energy:

Add energy-rich foods such as nuts, seeds, nut and seed butters, and oils. Servings of breads, cereals, legumes, fruits and vegetables may also be increased.

SOURCE: BCDNA, 1992, p. 17.

One of the most common reasons a person fails to adhere to a diet is lack of understanding of why it is necessary. Another underlying cause may be fear resulting from the loss of a familiar food. The person who has been used to eating pasta daily, and for whom this represents a basic security food, will likely find it difficult to eliminate or limit this food from the diet. An individual may rebel against being told what to eat or may resent the loss of personal choice in the matter. When helping people to change their dietary patterns, the nurse may find it best to work within the framework of their existing food habits, and to suggest modifications wherever possible rather than a complete change in eating habits.

For example, an elderly person's protein intake may be increased by the addition of cheese to his or her usual lunch of tea and toast. Supplementing a familiar diet of beans and

Complementary Plant Protein

Combination	Examples
	Whole grain crackers and lentil or split pea soup
	Brown rice and tofu
	Cornmeal tortillas and vegetarian chili beans
	Chapatis and dahl
	Falafel (pita bread and garbanzo beans)
	Peanut butter sandwich
	Pita bread and humus
	Toast and scrambled tofu
	Muffins and soy milk
	Cereal with soy milk or tofu yogurt
	Bun with tofu patty
Grains plus nuts or seeds	Whole grain bread and nut butter
	Whole grain bread and tahini (sesame butter)
	Granola or muesli with nuts
	Noodles with sesame seeds

SOURCE: BCDNA, 1992, p. 15.

rice with the addition of meat and milk may be accepted more readily by a Latin American family than the suggestion of a completely different way of eating.

TRAY SERVICE

The dietary department of a health agency should maintain good standards for tray service, as follows:

1. The tray should be large enough to hold the dishes and utensils needed for the patient's meal and, at the same time, small enough to fit on the patient's overbed or bedside table.
2. Food must be served at the proper temperature; that is, hot food should not be allowed to cool and cold food should not be allowed to become warm.
3. Food should always be covered when it is being carried to the patient's bedside. Covering food helps not only to maintain the proper temperature but also to prevent drying out, which affects the flavour, texture and appearance of food.
4. Food should be served as attractively as possible, in arranged portions, with garnishes to give colour appeal. Small portions are more stimulating to the appetite than large portions.
5. Napkins, dishes, utensils and the tray itself should be clean.
6. The arrangement on the tray should be neat and organized. Any spilled food should be replaced.
7. The patient should always get the right tray with the right diet. Each tray has a card with the patient's name, bed number and type of diet. If the nurse has any doubts as to the correctness of a patient's tray, he or she should check the diet orders before the patient is served.

FEEDING THE PATIENT

If it is necessary for the nurse to feed the patient, a few simple rules will enhance comfort:

1. Offer bedpan or urinal before serving the meal.
2. Whenever possible, use the utensils the patient would normally use for the food being served.
3. Never hurry the patient. Sit down to feed him or her whenever possible.
4. Offer the patient small rather than large bites of food.
5. Offer the food in the order that the patient prefers.
6. Note whether any food or liquid is hot and, if it is, warn the patient to take only small portions or sips.
7. Provide a straw or drinking cup if possible—these will often help a patient to take liquids.
8. If the patient can hold bread or toast, let the patient do so.
9. Be careful not to spill food. Wipe the patient's mouth and chin whenever necessary. Always protect the patient with a napkin.

After the patient has finished the meal, remove the tray promptly. Never hurry patients with their meals. If a patient's fluid intake is to be recorded, the amounts should be noted on the fluid balance sheet. Food and fluids consumed should be entered by the nurse on a food record/calorie count sheet if intakes are questionable; the dietitian may then assess the patient's nutritional status using these data. The nurse should be familiar with the amount of fluid contained in the commonly used containers. Many agencies have printed materials defining volumes of specified cups, bowls and containers.

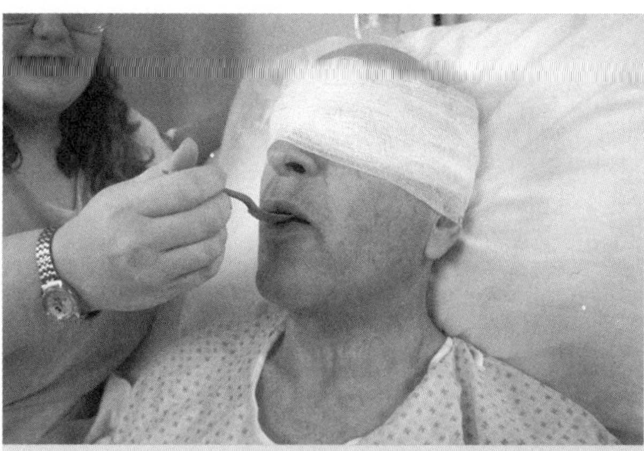

A family member assisting a loved one with lunch.

Patients should be provided with facilities for washing hands and brushing teeth before and after meals. This offers a good opportunity for the nurse to teach oral hygiene and the correct method for brushing teeth.

Health-Protecting Strategies

In caring for people with nutritional problems, nurses implement health-protecting strategies to prevent or minimize indigestion, anorexia, nausea and vomiting and to ensure safety, comfort and hygiene for patients who are unable to swallow, who are experiencing anorexia and nausea or who are vomiting. Nurses can also help protect individuals and families from food poisoning by providing information and instruction on preventive measures in the home.

PREVENTING INDIGESTION, ANOREXIA, NAUSEA AND VOMITING

Indigestion

There are a number of things people can do to prevent indigestion:

1. Eat small meals rather than large ones. Dividing the total daily food intake into five small meals—breakfast, lunch, a mid-afternoon snack (the British afternoon tea), a light supper and a snack before bedtime—is often helpful for older people. Children, with their smaller stomach capacities, often do better with smaller meals and snacks at mid-morning and mid-afternoon and before bedtime than with three large meals. Pregnant women also benefit from having smaller, more frequent meals, because the growing fetus presses on the abdominal organs and can effectively lessen stomach capacity and appetite, and increase reflux and heartburn.
2. Avoid coffee, tea, cola and other drinks containing caffeine.
3. Avoid fried foods and those high in fat content.
4. Avoid highly spiced foods.
5. Avoid any other foods that give indigestion.
6. Take some mild exercise, such as walking, after meals, or before meals to stimulate appetite.

Anorexia, Nausea and Vomiting

The prevention of anorexia, nausea and vomiting always involves a consideration of both the patient and the environment. Nursing measures that are effective in preventing these problems are often specific to the causes that have been discussed. The nurse can often help the patient to identify situations and stimuli that are causing the problem, and then help to modify or eliminate these. Frequently the patient is aware of events or subjective experiences, such as pain, that cause anorexia, nausea and vomiting.

Safety, Comfort and Hygiene Measures

In caring for seriously ill patients, who may not be fully conscious, the nurse should make sure that they are able to swallow before attempting to give them fluids or food. In assessing the swallowing reflex, the presence of the gag reflex should be established first. A standard method of testing for the gag reflex is to touch the back of the throat with a tongue depressor. If the gag reflex is present, the person may be given small sips of water first, while the nurse watches for swallowing movements in the neck. A gag reflex does not always indicate the ability to swallow safely. Patients should be able to follow commands when asked to swallow or should have a strong cough reflex. Signs that a person may have problems with swallowing include lack of gag reflex, drooling, inability to follow commands and pocketing of food. If these signs are present, an occupational therapist should be consulted to assess the patient's ability to swallow.

With most patients who are anorectic or nauseated, the immediate problem is usually to prevent aggravation of the symptoms. The nauseated individual usually feels better lying down in a cool and quiet room with adequate ventilation. If this is not possible, the person should be encouraged to sit quietly and take a few deep breaths. This helps to relax the diaphragm. Measures to take the person's mind off his or her gastrointestinal problems may also help.

PREVENT FOOD POISONING

The prevention of food poisoning involves teaching people about selecting, preparing and storing foodstuffs and cooked foods to prevent unsafe quantities of disease-carrying bacteria (or their toxins) from being consumed. Specifically, people should do the following:

1. Buy from reputable dealers. Patronize only clean stores.
2. Keep hot foods hot (60°C or higher) and cold foods cold (4°C or lower).

3. After marketing, place frozen foods in the freezer compartment of the refrigerator or in a deep-freeze until ready for use.

are actually thawed. Frozen foods that have been completely thawed or have been held at refrigerator temperature for more than one or two days should not be refrozen.

5. Heat precooked frozen foods, such as TV dinners and meat pies, for the time and temperature recommended on the labels. Read the labels.
6. Refrigerate leftovers from prepared dishes within an hour and keep refrigerated until re-serving or re-heating. Store leftover poultry and stuffing separately.
7. After preparing foods containing eggs, meat, milk, gravy, or salads with dressing, such as sandwiches or picnic or buffet dishes, serve them within two hours or refrigerate.
8. If canning foods at home:
   a) always follow professional directions carefully
   b) never can non-acid foods such as meat, fish, meat–vegetable mixtures, soups or non-acid vegetables (beans, peas, asparagus, corn) unless a properly attended pressure-cooker is used.
9. Do not taste foods from bulging or leaking cans, or cans whose contents spurt out or are bubbly, off-colour or off-odour.
10. Do not eat foods that have an "off" flavour.
11. Keep everything in the kitchen clean.
12. Avoid cross-contamination between raw and cooked food by using separate chopping boards and utensils.
13. Always wash your hands before, during and after food preparation. (Eschelman, 1996)

Health-Restoring Strategies

Helping a person to restore hydration and nutritional status is an important nursing function. Some strategies are implemented as independent nursing measures, while others are performed in collaboration with the physician and dietitian. This section will focus on measures to stimulate appetite and relieve nausea and vomiting, on how to insert and manage transnasal tubes and on how to provide enteral and total parenteral nutrition.

RELIEVING NAUSEA AND VOMITING

Antiemetic drugs are often given as prescribed by the physician to control nausea and vomiting. However, there are a number of nonpharmacologic measures that may also be effective and should be attempted. Weak tea, flattened carbonated beverages (such as ginger ale) or Gatorade are frequently tolerated much better than other fluids when the stomach is upset. Dry crackers and toast may help as well. When people have difficulty retaining fluids, offering

to achieve adequate fluid intake. Small amounts taken regularly are more likely to be retained than a large volume taken all at once. Patients must be monitored carefully and, if signs of dehydration become evident, the physician should be notified. When dehydration becomes severe, intravenous fluid therapy will be necessary to restore fluid balance. The nursing responsibilities regarding intravenous therapy are outlined in Chapter 23.

Patients who have been vomiting are usually permitted only clear fluids until vomiting subsides. When other fluids are introduced into the patient's diet, those that are high in carbohydrate and protein are preferable because of the body's need for energy and tissue-building nutrients. For infants and small children, half-strength apple juice (diluted with water) is often easily tolerated. High-carbohydrate fluids containing necessary electrolytes, such as Lytren or Pedialyte, are also available on the market specifically for infants and small children. Lytren also comes in a grape flavour that makes it more palatable and easier for children to ingest.

The patient who is vomiting needs prompt attention, directed first of all at making sure that the patient does not aspirate the vomitus. A person who is lying down and starts to vomit should be helped to a sitting position if this is possible and not contraindicated. Otherwise, the head should be turned to the side and the person positioned so that the vomitus will drain from the mouth. It is particularly important to watch helpless patients, such as those who are unconscious, semi-conscious or paralyzed, to make sure that the airway is not blocked. Other priorities in nursing care of the vomiting patient are to relieve the symptom and to provide comfort and support to the patient.

The nurse can assist the vomiting patient by holding a curved basin (emesis basin) under the chin to catch the vomitus, and supporting the head and shoulders. The nurse should provide tissues and help to wipe the patient's mouth. Vomiting is an unpleasant experience. Not only is it physically distressing but there is a loss of control and dignity, which most people find embarrassing. The nurse can do much to reassure the patient by a calm acceptance of the situation and empathetic yet efficient care. Curtains can be quickly drawn around the patient's bed, or the door of the room closed, to ensure privacy.

After the patient has stopped vomiting, mouth care and a hand and face wash will promote comfort. Any linen that has been soiled should be changed promptly. The room should be aired and the patient allowed to rest. If the patient is unable to tolerate food or fluids, frequent mouth care is essential.

An environment that is clean and pleasant will help to stimulate the appetite and prevent nausea and vomiting. If the patient eats while in bed, the nurse can provide a clean table that is free of equipment. The emesis basin should be kept out of sight. If the patient feels more secure with it nearby, it can be kept within easy reach.

Unpleasant odours, sights and sounds are noxious stimuli that may contribute to anorexia, nausea or vomiting. To dissipate unpleasant odours, a well-ventilated room is important, and the use of deodorants may be necessary at times. Vomitus is always removed immediately, and treatment trays are covered and placed as inconspicuously as possible. Personal cleanliness is particularly important in the case of the person who has anorexia or a tendency to become nauseated. Other preventive measures include those described in the section earlier in this chapter on provision of nourishment for the sick.

Collaborative measures to prevent nausea and vomiting involve the use of antiemetic drugs. Antiemetic drugs have a specific action on the vomiting centre, and they may be given 20–30 minutes before mealtimes or otherwise as ordered. Many people who are susceptible to motion sickness travel much more comfortably if they take an antiemetic shortly before embarking on a plane trip or other journey. These drugs usually produce some drowsiness as a side effect.

GASTROINTESTINAL INTUBATION

Many patients with gastrointestinal problems require gastrointestinal intubation. Intubation refers to the placement of a tube into the stomach or intestine through the mouth (orogastric) or transnasally (nasogastric or nasointestinal) or through an artificial opening made in the abdominal wall to the stomach (gastrostomy) or jejunum (jejunostomy). The transnasal route is preferred over the mouth for gastric and intestinal intubation because it evades the gag reflex at the base of the oropharynx and is more comfortable on a long-term basis. Orogastric tubes are often used in premature infants whose gag reflect is nonfunctional.

Tubes are inserted into the digestive tract for a number of reasons. They are commonly used to prevent distention following surgery or intestinal blockage by removing fluids and gas from the intestinal cavity (gastric decompression) and to provide nutrition to individuals who are not able to ingest foods orally but retain adequate bowel function (enteral nutrition). Nurses are responsible for inserting some tubes and managing associated patient care, such as irrigating decompression tubes, administering tube feedings, monitoring patient status, providing patient comfort and removing nasogastric tubes (Dudek, 1997).

INSERTING A FEEDING TUBE

Feeding tubes are used to provide enteral nutrition. The procedure is performed only with a physician's order. Extra care must be taken during the procedure to avoid trauma to the nasal passages and the esophagus, and to ensure correct placement of the tube. Because of the proximity of the esophagus to the trachea, the tube can easily enter the lungs and result in severe complications. Procedure 20.1 outlines the steps for inserting a nasogastric and nasointestinal feeding tube.

Purposes of Gastrointestinal Intubation

Decompression	To establish a means of draining the stomach by suction following surgery or blockage of the intestinal tract.
Nutrition	To establish a route for feeding the patient who is unable to take nourishment by mouth but whose digestive functions are intact.
Lavage	To aspirate or wash out the stomach contents, for example when a person has taken poisonous materials or an overdose of medication.
Diagnostic	To aspirate contents for laboratory analysis.

Preparing the Patient

Before inserting a feeding tube, explain the procedure to the patient. Not only do most patients want to know how they can help, but explanations frequently allay fear and anxiety. The passage of a tube is not painful but it is uncomfortable. The patient may feel some irritation as the tube is passed through the nose, and may gag or shed tears. Explain that mouth-breathing, panting and swallowing will alleviate some of the discomfort and make it easier to advance the tube. Inform the patient that he or she will be instructed to sip some water as the tube is passed down. Establish a hand signal that will permit the patient to alert the nurse of the need to pause during the procedure.

Assembling Equipment

The nurse must know the purpose of intubation in order to select the appropriate feeding tube. Usually the physician will order the size tube to be inserted. In some cases of enteral nutrition, the size tube is recommended by the manufacturer of the solution (formula) to be administered. Nasal tubes differ in size, length and composition. The size, or outside diameter, of a tube is gauged by use of the French scale and is indicated with a number followed by the symbol *Fr*. Each number on the French scale is approximately equal to 0.33 mm. The larger the number, the larger the diameter of the tube. *Small-bore* tubes are less than 12 Fr in diameter; these are preferred for enteral feeding. Nasogastric tubes are usually shorter than nasointestinal feeding tubes since they terminate in the stomach. Nasointestinal feeding tubes vary in length. Many are designed so that they can be placed in the duodenum or jejunum. Enteral feedings are generally administered into the stomach. In some institutions, patients who are at risk for pulmonary aspirations—for instance, those with altered pharyngeal reflexes or those who are unconscious—are fed into the upper small intestine (Metheney, 1988). However, a recent study indicated that

PROCEDURE 20.1

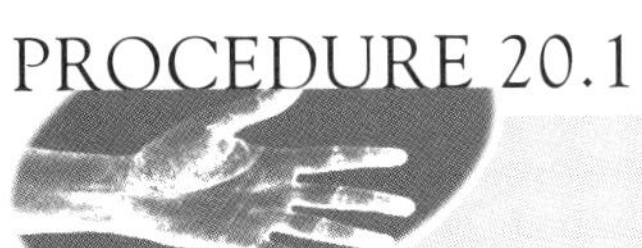

Inserting a Nasogastric and Nasointestinal Feeding Tube

Action	Rationale
1. Prepare the patient for what to expect and what he or she can do to aid in the procedure.	Reduces anxiety and enables patient participation. Insertion is easier if the patient is relaxed.
2. Gather: • NG tube or feeding tube • water-soluble lubricant • 50 mL catheter-tip syringe • glass of water with a straw • waterproof pad or towel • emesis basin • hypoallergenic adhesive tape 2.5 cm wide • clean gloves • penlight • elastic band and safety pin • pH test strip • goggles, if required.	Facilitates efficiency and economy of time. Provides protection from exposure to body fluids if gagging or coughing occurs.
3. Wash hands thoroughly.	Limits the spread of microorganisms.
4. Help the patient into a sitting position unless contraindicated. Cover the patient with a waterproof pad or towel and place the emesis basin, some tissues and the glass of water with a straw on the bedside table in easy reach. Have the patient remove dentures if they don't fit well.	Facilitates passage of the tube by the pull of gravity. Stimulation of the throat may cause gagging and vomiting. Passage of the tube also causes lacrimation. Readies the water for later use. Prevents choking on the dentures if they should become dislodged.
5. If the nurse is right-handed, stand at the patient's right side; if left-handed, stand at the left side.	Facilitates ease of insertion and prevents unnecessary strain on the nurse's body.
6. Apply gloves. Ask the patient to blow nose. Then ask the patient to breathe while alternately blocking each nostril. Using the penlight, examine the patient's nostrils for deformities or obstructions.	Clears the nostrils and determines which side has better air flow. Using the nostril that is larger and has better air flow will facilitate easier passage of the tube.
7. Measure the length of tube to be inserted by holding the distal end of the tube at the tip of the patient's nose, and then extending the tube to the earlobe and down to the xiphoid process. Mark the distance with a piece of adhesive tape.	Approximates the distance from the nose to the gastric cavity, thereby ensuring that the distal end of the tube reaches the stomach.

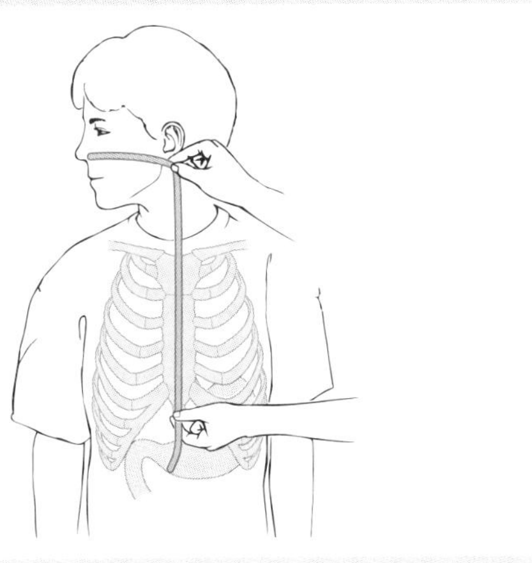

Continued on the next page

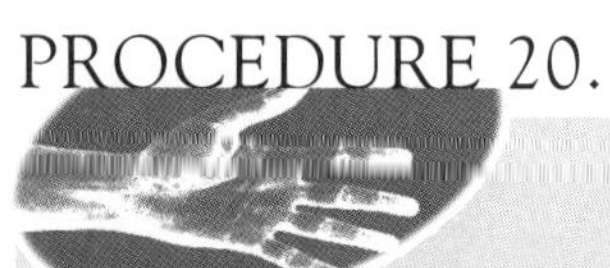

PROCEDURE 20.1 *continued*

Action	Rationale
8. Prepare a feeding tube according to the manufacturer's directions.	Manufacturers differ in the treatment of tubes. Some require the insertion of the wire guide; in others the guides are preinserted but a specified amount of water must be instilled into the tube to activate self-lubricating coating, which eases removal of the guide. Be sure the guide is properly secured in the tube.
9. Lubricate the first 12–15 cm of the tube with water-soluble jelly. If using a self-lubricating tube, immerse the tip in water. **Do not** use mineral oil or petroleum jelly.	Reduces mucosal irritation and facilitates passage of the tube. Some tubes are coated with a water-activated lubricant. Avoids respiratory complications should the tube enter the trachea, since oil-based lubricants do not dissolve as water-soluble preparations do.
10. Have the patient hyperextend his or her neck. Hold the tube with its natural curve pointing downward. Carefully insert the tube into the nostril, directing it downward towards the back of the throat. Advance the tube along the floor of the nostril into the nasopharynx.	Decreases the curvature of the nasopharyngeal junction. Follows the natural contour of the nasal passage and avoids injury to the turbinates (projections) along the lateral wall.

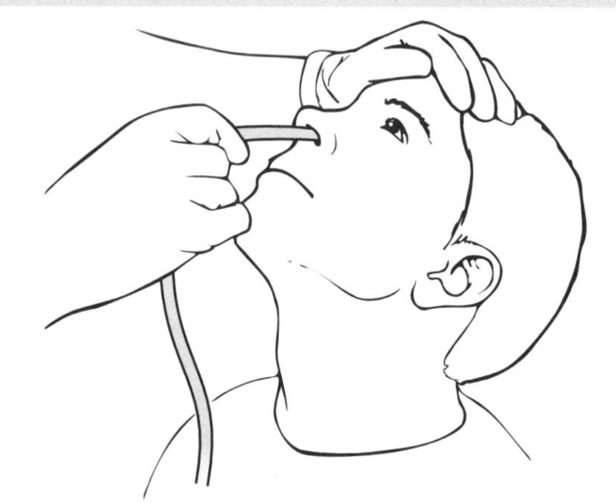

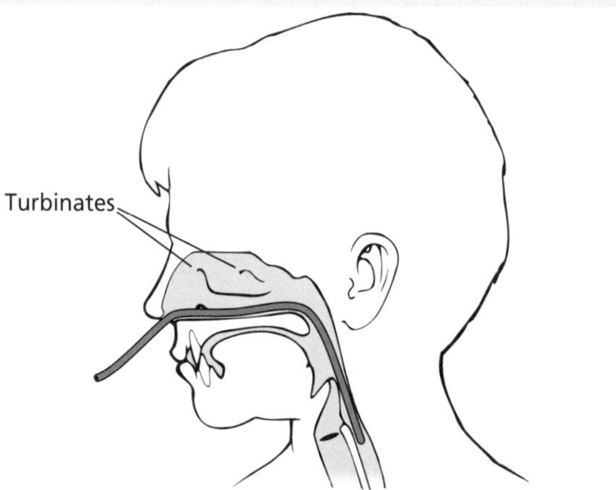

Action	Rationale
11. Slight pressure may be needed to advance the tube. If resistance is met, withdraw the tube a bit, rotate it and readvance it to the nasopharynx. **Do not** force the tube against resistance. If the obstruction persists, withdraw the tube, relubricate it, and try the other nostril.	Alters the direction of the tube, which may better follow the curvature of the nasal canal. Avoids the risk of trauma.
12. When the tube reaches the nasopharynx, resistance will be felt. Ask the patient to lower his or her head slightly.	Closes the trachea and opens the esophagus.
13. Unless contraindicated, hand the patient the glass of water and instruct him or her to sip and swallow, while slowly advancing the tube. Do not push the tube faster than the patient can swallow.	Swallowing closes the epiglottis and aids passage of the tube. May cause the tube to kink at the epiglottis and come out the mouth.
14. Watch the patient carefully as the tube is being advanced. If gagging occurs, instruct the patient to pant and swallow. If gagging continues, check the oropharynx. If the tube is coiled in the throat, withdraw it until it is straightened and continue the procedure.	Suppresses the gag reflex. Determines whether the tube has coiled in the throat.
If respiratory distress occurs (e.g., patient coughs, gasps for air, becomes cyanotic) immediately withdraw the tube back into the nasopharynx. Give the patient a few moments to readjust breathing pattern, then continue the procedure.	Indicates the tube has entered the trachea and is obstructing breathing.

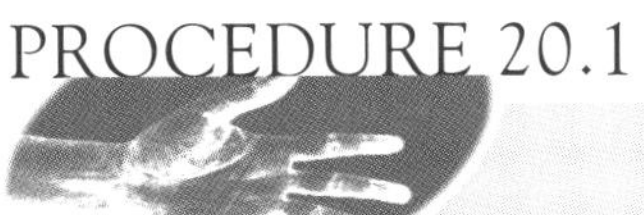

PROCEDURE 20.1 *continued*

Action	Rationale
15. Should the guide of a small feeding tube slip out during insertion, **do not** reinsert it while the tube is in the patient. Instead, withdraw the entire tube, explain to the patient what has happened, and reinsert the guide, making sure it correctly joins to the weighted tip and that all necessary connections are secure. Then, relubricate and reinsert the tube.	Prevents potential trauma to surrounding tissue should the guide puncture the tubing as it is being pushed back into the tube.
16. Once the tube is inserted to the premeasured position, tape it lightly to the nose.	Prevents displacement while proper placement is confirmed.
17. Confirm proper tube placement.	
a) Aspirate stomach contents and measure the acidity with pH test strip.	Provides a reliable indication of proper placement. The mean pH of gastric aspirate is 3.02, compared with 6.57 for intestinal and 7 or more for lung aspirates.
b) Obtain an x-ray.	Confirms placement of the tube. (The tube cannot be aspirated because the lumen is occluded by the guide.)
18. Once placement of a feeding tube is confirmed, remove the guide according to the manufacturer's directions. Store it in a place designated by agency policy (e.g., taped to the head of the patient's bed).	Keeps the guide available for use in case the tube is accidentaly removed and must be reinserted. (These tubes are expensive.)
19. Secure the tube with hypoallergenic tape as in Figure 20.11. Loop a rubber band around the tube and fasten it to the patient's gown using a safety pin.	Prevents pressure against the nostrils causing irritation and excoriation; reduces the risk of displacement and promotes comfort.
20. Connect the tube to the feeding apparatus as ordered.	Initiates treatment as ordered.
21. Discard supplies and wash hands.	Maintains cleanliness and safety in the workplace.
22. Document the procedure: note the type and size of tube, the means by which placement was confirmed and how the patient responded.	Fulfills requirement for nurse accountability. Promotes continuity of care.

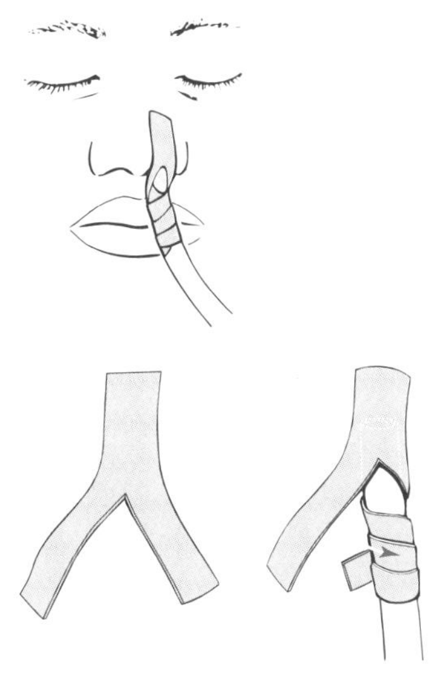
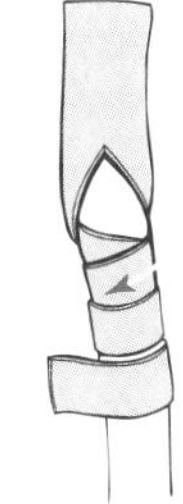
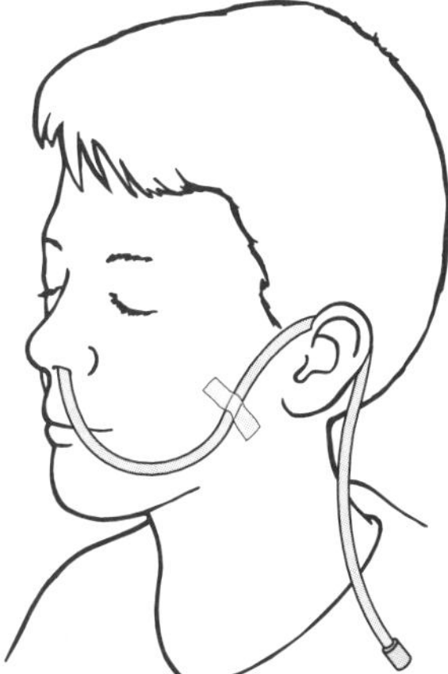
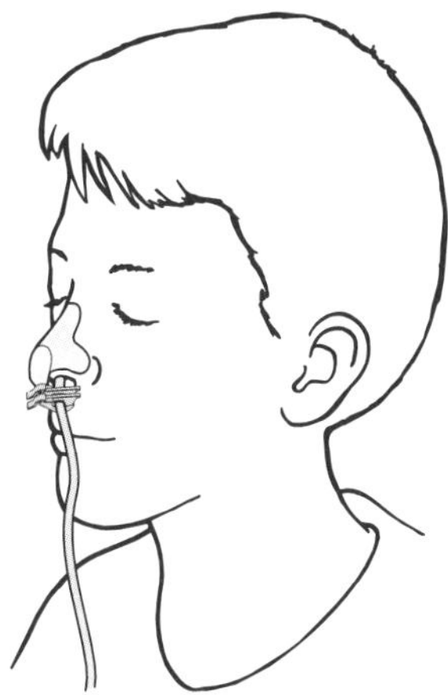

FIGURE 20.11 Nasogastric tube anchoring devices

SOURCES: Flynn & Hackel, 1990, p. 575; Hollister Incorporated.

these complications did not decrease with postpyloric feedings (Strong et al., cited in Davis & Sherer, 1994).

Transnasal feeding tubes are made of soft silicone rubber or polyurethane, which reduce oropharyngeal irritation, cause less trauma to the tracheoesophageal wall and increase patient comfort and tolerance. Because of their flexibility and softness, these tubes are weighted with tungsten and contain a wire guide or stylet that facilitates their passage through the nose and esophagus into the stomach or upper intestine. The guide is removed once the feeding tube placement has been confirmed by x-ray. The weight also helps to keep the tube in its proper place once inserted. Polyvinyl chloride feeding tubes have a radiopaque strip or marker at the distal end, which allows visualization of the tube's placement on x-ray.

INSERTING A NASOGASTRIC DECOMPRESSION TUBE

Nurses may insert nasogastric tubes for abdominal decompression. The procedure is performed once a physician's order is obtained. Large-sized tubes are referred to as *large-bore* and are usually used for gastric decompression. They are usually 12 Fr or larger in diameter. Two basic types of tubes are used for gastric decompression: the single-lumen Levin tube and the double-lumen sump tube (Salem sump tube). The Levin tube is a straight non-vented tube with holes near the tip. It is used less commonly nowadays because it does not have the venting capability of the Salem sump tube. The Levin tube works effectively as long as flow is maintained and the tube openings do not adhere to the gastric mucosa. If flow stops and the tube adheres to the stomach lining, a vacuum forms, producing suction levels that can cause trauma to the mucosa. The Salem sump tube overcomes this problem by providing a constant flow of atmospheric air through a venting lumen which prevents the tube from adhering to the stomach lining. The blue "pigtail" on the Salem sump tube connects the venting lumen to the outside air. Both types of tubes are made of stiff polyvinyl chloride, which can cause erosion of the nose and oropharynx, along with other discomforts such as difficulty swallowing. They should not be used for enteral nutrition.

Inserting a nasogastric tube for decompression is similar to the steps outlined in Procedure 20.1, with the following additions:

- In step 2, you also want to gather a stethoscope.
- In step 12, suggest that the patient swallow to aid in the tube insertion. Sips of water assist the patient to swallow, pushing the tube past the oropharynx.
- In step 18, you can gently aspirate stomach returns and measure the acidity with a pH test strip to confirm accurate tube placement. Another way of ensuring tube placement is to inject 10–20 mL of air with a 50-mL catheter-tip syringe while auscultating over the epigastric area with a stethoscope. A whooshing or gurgling sound indicates that the tube is in the stomach.

PROVIDING NASOGASTRIC SUCTION AND TUBE CARE

Gastric decompression refers to the drainage of fluid and gaseous contents from the stomach by use of negative pressure or suction. It is indicated as a measure to prevent or relieve distention and vomiting following surgery with general anesthesia and to remove the stomach contents of patients who have gastrointestinal obstructions. A large-bore NG tube, commonly the Salem sump or the Levin tube, is used for gastric decompression. The external end of the tube is connected to a suction device which drains and collects the gastric contents. Effective decompression depends on equipment that functions properly and an NG tube that is patent and placed correctly in the stomach. Thus, care involves monitoring the equipment for proper functioning as well as ensuring patency and correct placement of the tube. Patency is maintained by irrigating the tube at regular intervals to keep it free of blockage from accumulated secretions.

Nurses must be aware that the constant presence of the large, inflexible tube in the nasopharynx is a source of discomfort and potential trauma to the patient. Prolonged pressure from the tube on the mucous membrane lining of the nose can cause irritation and painful excoriation. Because one of the nostrils is occluded by the tube, the patient tends to breathe more through the mouth. This, combined with the lessened flow of saliva (due to NPO), leads to a dry mouth and throat. Special care is needed to prevent local excoriation and discomfort in the nose and to keep the lips and mucous membranes moist and clean. To ease irritation by the tube on the patient's throat, the patient is often allowed to have throat lozenges or to chew gum. Techniques for establishing and maintaining gastric suction, for irrigating the NG tube and for providing hygiene and comfort to the nose and mouth are detailed in Procedure 20.2.

Since gastric suction returns are an important part of the patient's fluid output, the amount of drainage is measured and the clarity, colour and consistency of the drainage are noted. Large amounts of drainage are often replaced by intravenous therapy. These observations are reported on the patient's chart. Any untoward changes in the patient's suction returns, such as bright red returns, or in the patient's condition, such as an accelerated pulse, are reported to the physician.

Preparing the Patient

The techniques for managing suction, maintaining tube patency and providing hygiene to the nose and mouth are painless. Telling patients what to expect and how they can help will enable them to participate in the procedure.

Assembling Equipment

Decompression is established by connecting the NG tube to a suction device. There are a variety of suction devices available. Some are wall-mounted units that generate continuous or intermittent negative suction; others are portable

PROCEDURE 20.2

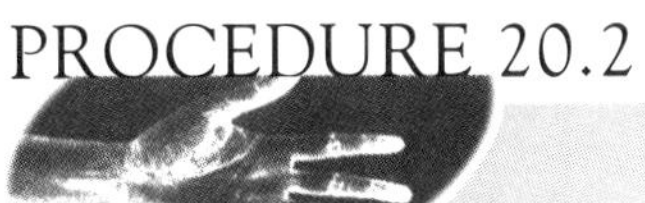

Providing Nasogastric Suction and Tube Care

Action	Rationale
A. ESTABLISHING GASTRIC SUCTION	
1. Check the physician's order for type and amount of suction.	Ensures accuracy and reduces the risk of error.
2. Prepare the patient.	Promotes the patient's well-being and enables participation in care.
3. Gather: • suction device • connecting tubing • connector, if one is not supplied with NG tube.	Facilitates efficiency and economy of time.
4. Wash hands thoroughly.	Limits the spread of microorganisms.
5. At the bedside, set up the suction device according to agency protocol. Attach the connecting tubing to the suction container. Check that all connections are tight. Turn on a portable machine to check that it is working. A continuously flashing red light indicates proper functioning. To check a wall unit, squeeze the connecting tubing, turn on the regulator and watch the gauge for movement of the dial.	Prepares the device for effective functioning.
6. Set the type and amount of suction. **Single-lumen Levin:** Set the suction on "intermittent" and "low." **Salem sump tube:** Set the suction on "continuous" and "low" unless otherwise ordered.	Reduces mucosal trauma should the tube adhere to the stomach lining. Air vent prevents suction pressures that would traumatize tissue.
7. Attach the NG tube to the connecting tubing using a connector and turn the suction on. With a Salem sump, connect the primary (larger) lumen to the suction device.	
8. Check for proper functioning of the system:	
a) Gastric contents in the tubing are moving towards the collecting container.	Indicates that suction is effective and that tube is patent.
b) Red light on a portable unit is continuously flashing.	Indicates machine is working.
c) There is no leakage of air or fluid at connection points and no fluid leakage from the blue venting (pigtail) of a Salem sump.	Indicates that connections are tight and that the tubing and collection container are placed correctly.
d) For intermittent suction, the portable suction pump turns on and off in cycles lasting several seconds. Or, the pressure gauge of a wall suction moves up and down at regular intervals.	Indicates effective suction.
9. Anchor the tubing to the patient's gown. Keep a Salem sump pigtail higher than the level of the stomach.	Promotes effective suction and prevents reflux of gastric contents through a Salem sump pigtail. Negative pressure decreases when tubing lies below the collection container because the suction device must work against the force of gravity to draw fluids from the stomach. When the pigtail is placed below the level of the stomach, the venting mechanism, aided by the pull of gravity, acts like a siphon, drawing gastric contents into its lumen.

Continued on the next page

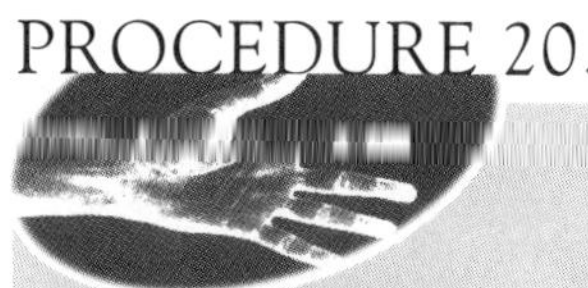

PROCEDURE 20.2 *continued*

Action	*Rationale*
B. MAINTAINING GASTRIC SUCTION	
1. Monitor the patient and the suction system regularly.	
Patient: Note abdominal distention, stated discomfort, nausea and feeling of fullness in stomach. Assess bowel sounds and look for electrolyte imbalances if gastric output is excessive.	Indicates tube blockage or ineffective system function. Bowel sounds indicate gastric function. Electrolytes are lost in gastric drainage.
System: Review step 8 in A. Also, inspect the tubing for kinks or blockages.	As above.
Drainage: Note the amount, colour, consistency and odour. Normal secretions may appear colourless or yellow-green if bile is present and have a mucoid consistency. Note a coffee-ground colour and consistency. Test for pH and blood according to agency protocol.	Provides data for ongoing assessment of patient status and evaluation of care. May indicate bleeding.
2. Irrigate the NG tube at regular intervals according to the physician's order, agency protocol or as necessary (if a blockage occurs). Section C on the next page details the procedure.	Prevents or corrects tube blockage.
3. If available, insert the blue end of an anti-reflux valve into the pigtail of a Salem sump.	Prevents soiling of patient's gown and bed linen from inadvertent reflux through the venting lumen.

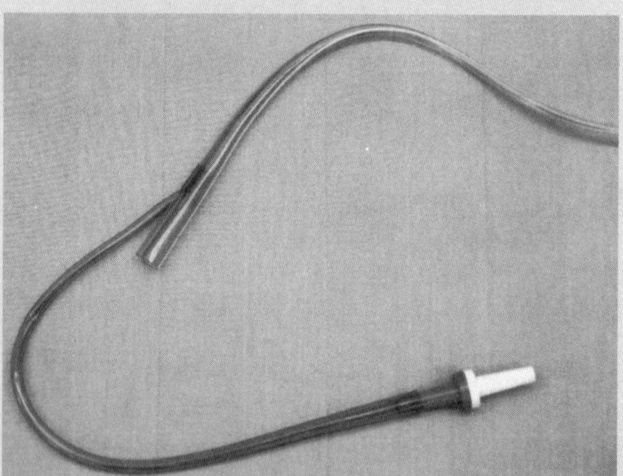

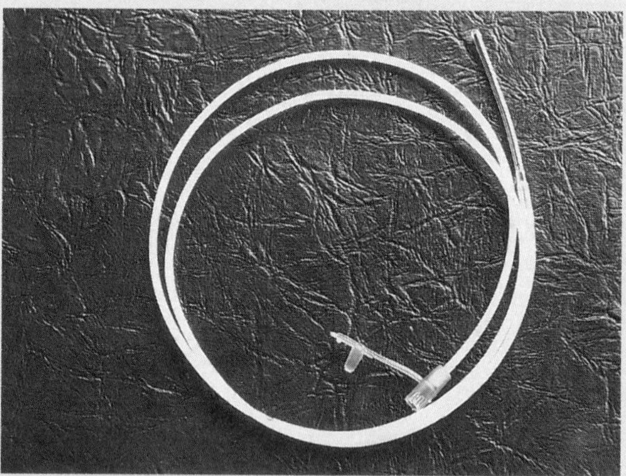

4. To ambulate the patient, turn off the suction. Disconnect the NG tube from the suction source. If using an anti-reflux valve on a Salem sump pigtail, close the primary lumen by inserting the white end of the antireflux valve into it.	Prevents gastric contents from draining from the tube when the patient is ambulating.
5. Empty and measure gastric drainage from the collection container when the container is three-quarters full or at least q12h. Disconnect the tube from the suction device as in B, step 4, above. Remove the container from the suction unit. Inspect the drainage; measure and discard. Rinse the container with warm water. Replace the container and re-establish suction. Record the amount of drainage on the fluid balance sheet (see Chapter 23 and the characteristics of drainage in the nurses' notes).	Maintains cleanliness and provides data for assessment and evaluation of care. A full collection container may reduce the effectiveness of suction.

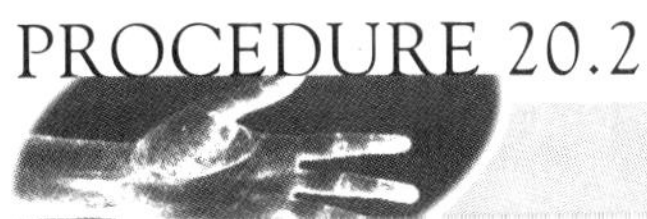

PROCEDURE 20.2 *continued*

Action	Rationale
C. IRRIGATING THE NG TUBE	
1. Check the physician's order or agency protocol for the frequency, type and amount of irrigant.	Promotes accuracy and avoids risk of error.
2. Gather: • irrigation set • irrigating solution • waterproof pad • clean gloves.	NG irrigation is a clean procedure. Thus, to conserve equipment and supplies, the materials are kept at the bedside and reused.
3. Place a waterproof pad on the bed under the NG tube–tubing connection.	Prevents soiling bed linen.
4. Apply gloves and check tube placement.	Prevents accidental instillation of irrigant into lungs.
5. Draw up 30–50 mL of irrigant, or amount as ordered, into the syringe.	
6. Disconnect the NG tube from the connector and attach the catheter-tip syringe. Instill the irrigant gently and slowly. **Do not** force solution.	The mucosal lining of the stomach is easily damaged. Excessive suction may cause trauma.
7. Gently aspirate the solution. If fluid returns freely, re-establish gastric suction. Check the system for proper functioning as in A, step 8.	Prevents excessive pressure on a suture line or gastric mucosa.
8. If there is no gastric return, repeat the irrigation and aspirate. If no fluid returns, inject 20–30 mL of air and aspirate, reposition the patient, or reposition the tube slightly. If using a Salem sump, instill 10–20 mL of air into the venting lumen (blue pigtail).	Injecting air or altering the position of the patient and the tube may shift the tube away from the stomach wall and, thereby, promote drainage. Maintains and verifies patency of the venting lumen.
If there is still no fluid returns, set the suction on "low" and notify the physician.	Normal gastrointestinal functioning has returned.
D. PROVIDING PATIENT COMFORT AND HYGIENE	
1. Provide mouth care at least q4h or as needed (see Procedure 31.1, Chapter 31).	Promotes comfort and prevents dryness of mucous membranes and lips.
2. Clean the nose and remove secretions with moistened cotton-tip applicators as necessary. Apply water-soluble lubricant to inside of nares.	Prevents irritation from dried secretions. Soothes the tissues and provides a cushion against friction caused by movement of the tube.
3. Remove tape anchoring the tube if it loosens. While holding the tube in place, wash the skin and remove adhesive residue from the skin with a solvent. Slightly reposition the tube and retape as in Figure 20.11.	Skin oils cause the tape to loosen and may produce a gummy residue that is not water-soluble. Changes the point of contact in the nose and throat, thereby reducing the risk of irritation and excoriation.
E. DOCUMENTATION	
1. Document the procedures in the nurses' notes per agency protocol. Record nursing assessments, date and time suction was established, suction pressure and any equipment malfunctions. Note tube placement, any blockages, irrigations and gastric return characteristics. Record hygiene and comfort measures as well as the patient's physical and emotional responses to NG intubation and continuing suction. On the fluid balance sheet, record the amounts of drainage.	Fulfills requirements for nurse accountability and promotes continuity of care.

machines that create an intermittent negative pressure by use of an electric pump. Figure 20.12 presents examples of two common types of suction units. The type and amount of suction to be maintained are dictated by the physician's order and the type of NG tube in place. When a single-lumen Levin tube is used, the suction is usually set at "intermittent low" to avoid the risk of mucosal trauma, as discussed previously. A continuous high or low setting may be ordered for the double-lumen Salem sump. For wall-mounted suction devices, a high setting is established by adjusting the regulator between 80–120 mm Hg; a low setting means 40–80 mm Hg. Connecting tubing and a connector will be needed to attach the NG tube to the suction apparatus. Some tubes, for example, the Salem sump, come packaged with a connector. If available in the agency, an anti-reflux valve can also be used on the blue venting lumen (pigtail) to prevent spills and soiling of bed linen due to reflux of gastric contents (see Procedure 20.2–B, step 3).

Nasogastric tubes are usually irrigated with normal saline. Water should not be used as an irrigant because it may cause electrolyte imbalances (Earnest, 1993; Lee, Barrett & Ignatavicius, 1996). Disposable irrigating sets are available that contain a basin and a 50 mL catheter tip syringe; some may also contain a waterproof pad. Since NG tube irrigation is a clean procedure, the irrigation set is kept at the bedside and reused. The set is changed every 24 hours.

PROVIDING ENTERAL NUTRITION

Enteral nutrition is the provision of nourishment in liquid form directly into the stomach or upper intestine through a feeding tube. The tube may be inserted nasally, surgically or percutaneously through an incision in the abdominal wall. A tube surgically inserted into the stomach is called a *gastrostomy*; one inserted into the small intestine is a *jejunostomy*. Enteral nutrition is indicated for persons who are unable or unwilling to take food but who retain at least some gastrointestinal function. Those unable to take food may include, for instance, a person with impaired swallowing because of cancer or neuromuscular dysfunction, or one with oral or esophageal trauma or obstruction. An example of a patient who is unwilling to take food orally is someone with anorexia nervosa. Gastric and intestinal feedings are also given to unconscious patients and to intubated and ventilated patients.

Tube feedings can be given for an indefinite period of time provided an appropriate formula and volume of formula are given. A registered dietitian can assess the patient's nutrient requirements. The nasogastric route is most commonly used for short-term feeding. It is not recommended for long-term use because the presence of the tube interferes with the functioning of the lower esophageal sphincter—reflux esophagitis, regurgitation and aspiration are high risks, particularly in unconscious patients. Similarly, a nasointestinal tube inserted into the duodenum or jejunum does not eliminate the risk of regurgitation and aspiration, but the risk is decreased. Furthermore, the need for radiographic verification of placement and the ease of displacement from coughing, sneezing or vomiting, or more commonly, from confused patients pulling them out, make nasogastric and nasointestinal tubes less desirable for long-term use. Thus, permanent feeding tubes, percutaneously inserted through a surgical gastrostomy or jejunostomy, are indicated for long-term feedings (Davis & Sherer, 1994). Patients may be sent home with feeding tubes in place after they or their family caregivers have been provided with education for home management.

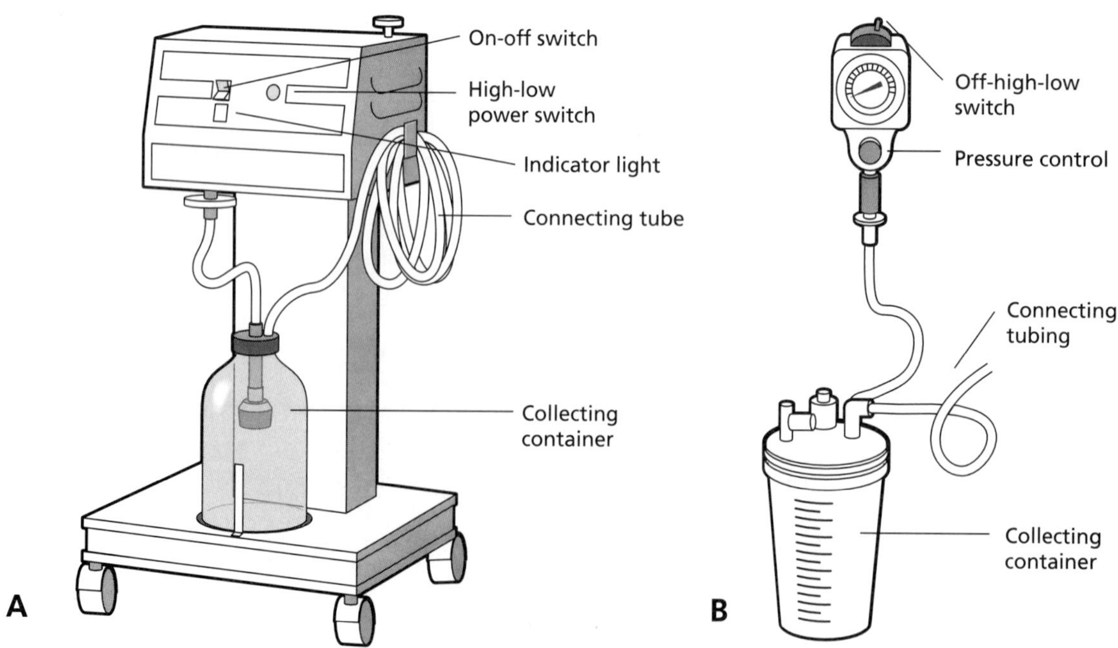

FIGURE 20.12 Gastric suction units. A. Portable suction machine B. Wall-mounted unit

Enteral feedings are given on an intermittent schedule (for example, every four hours) or by a continuous low infusion over a 24-hour period. Cyclic nocturnal feedings

ings, as well as the rate of continuous feedings, are ordered by the physician in collaboration with the dietitian. The dietitian monitors the patient's weight, tolerance to tube feeding, electrolyte balance and hydration status to avoid electrolyte and fluid imbalances and to ensure the nutritional adequacy of the feedings. In addition to administering the tube feedings, the nurse monitors the patient for common problems and provides protective or therapeutic measures as necessary—some independent and some collaborative. Table 20.14 lists the advantages and disadvantages of various feeding routes, while Table 20.15 shows common problems associated with tube feedings, as well as the possible causes and preventive or treatment measures.

Procedures 20.3 and 20.4 outline the steps for administering enteral feedings via the nasogastric, nasointestinal, gastrostomy and jejunostomy routes. Finally, the steps for moving a nasogastric tube are outlined in Procedure 20.5.

Preparing the Patient

As for all procedures, explain to the person what is to be done. A tube feeding is not painful, but the patient may expect a feel

comforts such as nausea, vomiting, cramps, bloating or diarrhea must be reported. Intermittent feedings generally take about 45–60 minutes; volumes should not exceed 350–500 mL per feeding. A continuous feeding is administered with a pump, and it carries on day and night. The feeding will be stopped periodically so that assessments can be made and the tube flushed. Generally, feeding tubes are flushed q4h for continuous feeds and before and after each intermittent feed. Feeding tubes are also flushed before and after the administration of any medications through the feeding tube. This procedure is outlined in Chapter 34. The patient does not have to remain in bed because of the feeding. He or she may be up in a wheelchair or walking around as the condition permits. Before preparing the feeding, the nurse assesses the patient for abdominal distention and bowel sounds. Feedings are withheld if bowel sounds are absent or if the abdomen is distended.

TABLE 20.14 Advantages and disadvantages of various feeding routes

ROUTE	INDICATIONS	ADVANTAGES	DISADVANTAGES
Nasogastric (NG)	Short-term feeding (less than 6 weeks) with functional GI tract	Uses stomach as reservoir Can use intermittent feedings "Dumping syndrome" less likely than with NI feedings	Contraindicated for clients at high risk for aspiration Not appropriate for long-term use Unaesthetic for client
Nasointestinal (NI)	Short-term feeding for clients with normal digeston and absorption	Less risk of aspiration; especially important for clients with impaired gag or cough reflex, decreased consciousness, who are ventilator-dependent or who have a history of aspiration pneumonia	Increased risk of "dumping syndrome" Not appropriate for intermittent or bolus feedings Not appropriate for long-term use Unaesthetic for client
Gastrostomy	For long-term use in clients with a functional GI tract Frequently used for clients with impaired ability to swallow	Same advantages as NG, but more comfortable and aesthetic for client Confirmation of tube placement easier Cannot be misplaced into trachea	PEG (percutaneous endoscopic gastrostomy) insertion contraindicated for clients who cannot have an endoscopy Risk of aspiration pneumonia in clients with gastroesophageal reflux Risk of wound cellulitis
Jejunostomy	For long-term use in clients at high risk for aspiration pneumonia and for clients with altered GI integrity above the jejunum For short-term use after GI surgery	Low risk of aspiration No risk of misplacing tube into the trachea More comfortable and aesthetic for clients than transnasal tubes Can be used immediately after GI surgery	Small-diameter tubes become clogged easily Peritonitis can occur from tube dislodgement Cannot be used for intermittent or bolus feedings

SOURCE: Dudek, 1997, p. 439.

TABLE 20.15 Common problems associated with tube feedings

PROBLEM	POSSIBLE CAUSE	PREVENTION/TREATMENT
Nausea, vomiting; abdominal distention, cramping	• Administration rate too rapid • Delayed gastric emptying • Ileal or GI obstruction • Intolerance of concentration or volume of feeding	• Avoid bolus feedings; administer by slow, continuous drip • Decrease rate, then gradually increase as tolerated
	• Lactose intolerance • Bacterial contamination • Improper position of pt during feeding	• Use lactose-free formulas • Ensure clean technique • Elevate head of bed 30–45° during feeding and 30 minutes after • Position pt on right side to facilitate gastric emptying • Consider gut motility-enhancing medications or placing tube postpylorically
Diarrhea	• Intolerance to hypertonic formula	• Decrease rate, then gradually increase it as tolerated
	• Rapid administration of formula	• Administer via slow, continuous drip
	• Bacterial contamination/ infection	• Ask MD to order stool cultures, treat infection medically • Refrigerate open containers of formula • Use medical sepsis when handling formula and equipment • Change bag and tubing per agency protocol; rinse equipment with each use
	• Drug therapy • Lactose intolerance • Maldigestion/malabsorption • Impaction with overflow incontinence	• Consult with MD and increase rate as tolerated • Use lactose-free formula • Consider use of elemental formula • Disimpact and prevent constipation
Clogged feeding tube	• Medications not adequately flushed through tubing	• Use liquid forms of drugs if possible • Crush tablets finely, mix with water • Flush tube with water before and after medications
	• Tube inadequately flushed (e.g., with pop or juice)	• Flush per agency protocol or with pancreatic enzyme per MD's order • Avoid flushing with beverages as sugars can crystallize and increase bacterial growth
Dehydration	• Diarrhea • Insufficient fluid intake	• See above • Calculate fluid needs; administer supplementary fluids (via increased flush) prn • Monitor urine output, serum electrolytes, urea and creatinine
	• Osmotic diuresis related to high carbohydrate concentration • Glucose intolerance	• See hyperglycemia
	• Vomiting or other fluid losses	• Replace fluids; control loss
Hyperglycemia	• High carbohydrate concentration • Glucose intolerance secondary to diabetes or catabolic stress	• Assess blood/urine glucose; change to lower-carbohydrate formula or slow rate of administration • MD may consider giving insulin
Aspiration	• Delivery rate too rapid • Improper tube placement • Improper positioning of pt • Gastric retention	• Decrease rate or volume • Check tube placement prior to feeding per agency protocol • Elevate head of bed 30–45° during feeding and 30 minutes after • Hold feeding until gastric residual is <100 mL • Alert MD • Consider GI motility medications, feeding into small bowel instead of stomach or permanent tube

SOURCES: Berger & Williams, 1992, p. 1113; BCDNA, 1992, pp. 128–131.

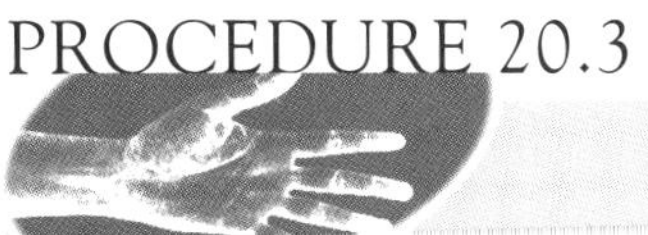

PROCEDURE 20.3

Administering Enteral Feedings through Nasogastric and Nasointestinal Tubes

Action	Rationale
1. Check the physician's order for frequency, type, amount and rate of infusion.	Ensures accuracy and reduces the risk of error.
2. Prepare the patient. Auscultate for bowel sounds and observe for distention. Withhold feeding if bowel sounds are absent and/or distention is present. Report to physician.	Promotes the patient's well-being and enables participation in care. Bowel sounds indicate gastrointestinal function. Abdominal distention may indicate delayed gastric emptying and increases the risk of regurgitation and pulmonary aspiration.
3. Gather: • prescribed formula • tube feeding administration set • adapter (if one not supplied) • feeding pump as necessary • large catheter-tip syringe • IV pole • basin • 10 x 10 cm gauze pad and elastic band (optional).	Facilitates efficiency and economy of time.
4. Wash hands thoroughly.	Limits the spread of microorganisms.
5. At the bedside, set up the feeding. Clamp the tubing on the administration set and pour the formula into the bag. Hang the feeding set on the IV pole. Open the clamp and slowly run formula through the tubing (referred to as priming the tubing). Close the clamp. For a **continuous** feed, attach the tubing to the pump according to the manufacturer's directions. Set the infusion rate.	Prepares the equipment for the feeding. Prevents infusion of air, which may cause discomfort.
6. Help the patient into a semi- or high Fowler's sitting position.	Aids gastric emptying, prevents regurgitation and reduces risk of pulmonary aspiration.
7. Attach the syringe to the feeding tube and **gently** aspirate contents.	Excessive or vigorous suction will collapse small-bore tubes.
a) Check the pH as in Procedure 20.1, step 17a).	Confirms correct placement of tube.
b) **Intermittent feeding:** Measure the amount of gastric residual and reinstill. If gastric residual is more than amount specified (by physician or agency protocol), withhold the feeding.	Prevents overfilling, which can lead to vomiting and aspiration. Residuals contain gastric secretions; returning residuals prevents electrolyte imbalance.
c) **Continuous feeding:** Measure after a 4-h volume has been infused and reinstill.	
d) If placement of the feeding tube is in doubt, obtain x-ray confirmation.	The small-bore feeding tubes are prone to displacement even if they are weighted. Coughing, sneezing, retching or vomiting, for example, can displace a gastric tube into the esophagus or the lungs.
8. Administer the feeding. **Intermittent:** Connect the feeding tube to the administration tubing. Slowly open the roller clamp and adjust the rate of infusion, allowing the formula to infuse over 45–60 minutes. Ensure that the formula container is about one metre above the patient's head. Generally, no more than 350–500 mL of formula should be administered at each feed.	A large volume introduced into the stomach quickly can cause diarrhea, nausea, cramping and vomiting. Flow depends on the force of gravity.
Continuous: Connect the feeding tube to the administration tubing. Open the roller clamp and start the feeding pump. Check the infusion rate.	A slow, continuous rate of infusion is better tolerated and reduces the likelihood of diarrhea, nausea, vomiting and aspiration. Promotes safety and accuracy of infusion.

Continued on the next page

PROCEDURE 20.3 *continued*

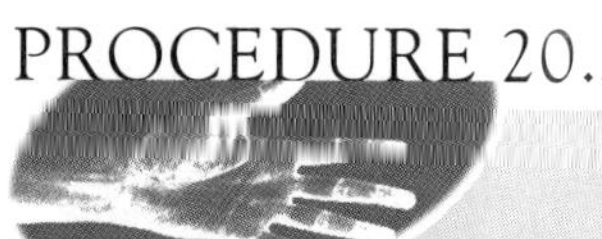

Action	Rationale
9. Intermittent feeding:	
a) Monitor the feeding.	
b) When the infusion is finished, flush the feeding tube per agency protocol or physician's order.	Helps to prevent clogging of the tube and decreases the risk of bacterial growth.
c) Pinch the tube while disconnecting it from the administration set. Then insert a catheter plug.	Prevents air from entering the stomach and gastric contents from draining out.
d) Flush the bag and tubing with warm water. Hang it upside down to drain and dry. Store it for reuse. Replace the set per agency protocol.	Removes residual formula, thereby reducing the risk of bacterial growth.
10. Continuous feeding:	
a) Monitor the patient and the feeding every hour. Check the flow rate and assess for diarrhea, abdominal distention, nausea and cramping. Precise rates of flow are crucial for tolerance of the formula.	Indicates the patient's tolerance of the feeding. The rate of infusion is generally set to lessen complications such as diarrhea and abdominal cramping. An antidiarrheal, such as diphenoxylate (Lomotil), may also be ordered to control diarrhea, if stool cultures are negative and no other cause for diarrhea is identified.
b) Interrupt the feeding q4h or as ordered.	
1) Flush the feeding tube per agency protocol or physician's order.	Prevents clogging of the tubes.
2) Rinse the set with warm water before adding new formula.	Prevents buildup of residue, which may invite bacterial growth.
3) Administer supplemental water if ordered.	Patient may require water to prevent dehydration.
4) Replace the feeding set per agency protocol.	
11. Leave the patient comfortable. Ask him or her to stay in a sitting position for at least 30 minutes or raise head of bed to 30–45°.	Facilitates gastric emptying.
12. Document the feedings. Note the frequency, type, amount and rate of infusion. Include patient responses and associated assessments. Enter volume of feedings and water delivered on the fluid balance sheet.	Fulfills requirement for nurse accountability and promotes continuity of care.

PROCEDURE 20.4 Administering Gastrostomy or Jejunostomy Tube Feedings

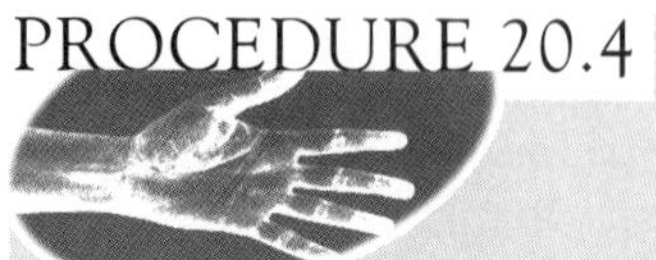

Action	Rationale
1. Follow steps 1 to 6 of Procedure 20.3.	
2. Flush the tube per agency protocol or physician's order.	Establishes patency of the tube.
3. Administer the feeding as in Procedure 20.3, steps 8–11.	
4. Provide care to the gastrostomy or jejunostomy site according to the physician's order or agency protocol. Use principles of wound care outlined in Chapter 33.	Leakage of gastric or jejunal contents can cause irritation and skin breakdown.
5. Document as in Procedure 20.3.	

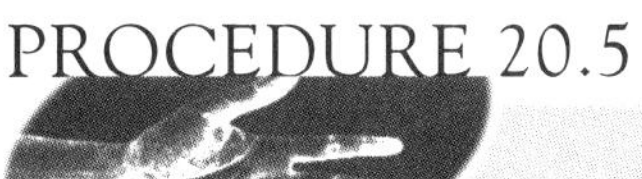

PROCEDURE 20.5 Removing a Nasogastric Tube

Action	*Rationale*
1. Check the physician's order to remove the tube.	Ensures accuracy and reduces the risk of error.
2. Prepare the patient: a) Some irritation of the nose and throat may occur and the eyes may water as the tube is removed. b) Breathing out as the tube is removed will reduce irritation and ease removal.	Promotes well-being and enables patient participation in the procedure.
3. Gather: • waterproof pad • clean gloves • moisture-proof bag • tissues.	Facilitates efficiency and economy of time.
4. Help the patient into a sitting position if able. Place the pad over the patient's chest. Give the patient some tissues.	Protects patient's gown from secretions and drainage in tube.
5. Disconnect the tube from the suction device or feeding pump, detach the tubing from the patient's gown and remove the tape anchoring the tube. Apply clean gloves.	Prepares tube for removal. Protects the nurse from contact with patient's secretions.
6. Instruct the patient to take a deep breath and blow out. Pinch the tube and withdraw it smoothly and rapidly as the patient exhales.	Creates a distraction for the patient and relaxes the pharynx, which eases removal, decreases irritation and prevents aspiration.
7. Wrap the tube in the waterproof pad, remove gloves and place in moisture-proof bag.	Maintains cleanliness and prevents transfer of micro-organisms to environment.
8. Provide mouth care and hygiene as needed (see Chapter 31).	Promotes patient comfort.
9. Provide fluids as ordered. Instruct the patient to sip fluids at first and gradually increase intake.	Rapid, large intake of fluid may cause nausea and vomiting, especially if the patient was NPO and receiving gastric suction.
10. Measure drainage in collecting container if gastric suction was used. Dispose of equipment and discard supplies according to agency policy. Wash hands.	Maintains cleanliness and safety in the workplace.
11. Document the procedure and the patient's response. Record the amount of drainage in suction container on the fluid balance sheet.	Fulfills legal requirements for nurse accountability and promotes continuity of care.

Enteral Formula

Enteral formulas consist of commercially prepared solutions containing carbohydrates, fat, protein, vitamins, minerals and other nutrients. There are numerous commercial formulas on the market made to suite the differing clinical needs and to permit feeding with small-bore tubes (see Table 20.16). The formulas vary in their composition of carbohydrates, fats, proteins and residues and in their osmolality (the osmotic pressure of a solution that results from the concentration of particles in a given volume of fluid). It is the responsibility of the dietitian to determine the formula most suited to the patient's needs.

If a person's gastrointestinal tract is functioning normally (allowing for the digestion and absorption of nutrients), a polymeric or meal replacement formula made from intact nutrient sources may be prescribed. If a person's gastrointestinal tract is not fully functional, an elemental formula made from predigested nutrients may be administered. Elemental formulas require minimal digestion because basic nutrients are ready to absorb and do not overly stimulate the pancreatic, biliary and intestinal secretions (Davis & Sherer, 1994). They are absorbed readily from the upper intestinal tract. Modular nutrient units consist of one essential nutrient—either protein, carbohydrate or fat. Modular units may be mixed together or added to a basic formula to meet the specific needs of patients. There are also formulas designed for special problems and specific disease states, such as a hepatic formula especially planned for the decreased functional abilities of the liver.

TABLE 20.16 Classification of enteral formulas

Type	*Commercial Preparations*
Monomeric	
Hydrolyzed protein formula	Vital HN (Abbott) Criticare HN (Mead Johnson) Reabilan (Elan Pharmaceutical) Peptamen (Clintec) Vivonex T.E.N. (Sandoz)
Polymeric	
Lactose-free	Nutren 1.0 (Clintec) Osmolite (Abbott) Attain (Sherwood Medical) Isocal (Mead Johnson) Ensure (Abbott)
Protein with fibre	Nutren 1.0 with fibre (Clintec) Sustacal (Mead Johnson) Ensure (Abbott) Fiberlan (Elan Pharmaceutical) Profiber (Sherwood Medical) Jevity (Abbott) Fibersource (Sandoz)
High-nitrogen	Isocal HN (Mead Johnson) Ensure HN (Abbott) Osmolite HN (Abbott) Promote (Abbott) Isotein HN (Sandoz)
Modular	
Carbohydrate	Moducal (Mead Johnson) Polycose (Abbott) Sumacal (Sherwood Medical)
Protein	Casec (Mead Johnson) Promod (Abbott) Nutrisource (Sandoz)
Fat	M.C.T. Oil (Mead Johnson) Nutrisource Lipid (Sandoz) Microlipid (Sherwood Medical)

SOURCES: Dudek, 1997; Eschelman, 1996.

Formulas are provided in ready-to-use or powdered forms. Powdered preparations are reconstituted with water or milk according to manufacturer's directions. Once opened or mixed, formulas must be refrigerated to avoid bacterial contamination. Unused quantities must be discarded after 24 hours. Expiry dates on commercial formulas must be checked; outdated formulas are discarded.

Cans and bottles must be shaken well to mix the contents thoroughly. Refrigerated solutions should be allowed to reach room temperature prior to administration. This decreases the risk of gastrointestinal intolerance.

Assembling Equipment

There are many types of tube feeding equipment. Feeding sets are available that consist of a plastic bag attached to tubing complete with a drip chamber and a roller clamp for regulating the rate of infusion and an adapter to connect the tubing to the feeding tube. A feeding pump or infusion controller is used for all continuous feeds and, in some agencies, for selected intermittent feedings that require careful control of the infusion rate. A feeding set and an enteral feeding pump are illustrated in Figure 20.13. When a continuous feeding is set up, a four-hour supply of formula should be hung to limit the chance for bacterial growth. A 50- or 60-mL catheter-tip syringe will also be necessary for checking tube placement, measuring gastric residuals (amounts of feeding remaining in the stomach) and flushing the tube after the feeding. Tubes are flushed with tap water or normal saline, as ordered by the physician.

TOTAL PARENTERAL NUTRITION

When the body is unable to absorb nutrients through its digestive tract, a person's nutritional status can be improved and maintained over extended periods solely through intravenous feeding. This method of providing nutrients directly into the blood stream is called total parenteral nutrition (TPN).

COMMUNITY health practice: Enteral Nutrition

If a patient has a functioning gastrointestinal (GI) tract but is unable to ingest oral nutrition, then enteral feeding is the preferred route. Enteral nutrition is less expensive than parenteral nutrition, and provides more calories per volume. Many patients receive enteral nutrition in the home environment; therefore, it is important for home care nurses to be skilled in the guidelines, maintenance and troubleshooting strategies needed in caring for such patients.

Choice of feeding device must be considered by the home care nurse, patient and family. Equipment must be easy to use within the home setting. The home care nurse must ensure that the patient and family are able to deal with problems in relation to the feeding tube and equipment.

Complications associated with feeding tubes include clogging, dislodgement, diarrhea, nausea and aspiration. Two reasons that a feeding tube might clog are inadequate flushing and improper administration of medications via the feeding tube. The patient and family must be taught the importance of maintaining a functioning feeding tube. If a feeding tube becomes clogged, flushing with warm water may be helpful. If the tube cannot be unclogged, then it must be replaced.

Patient and family are taught how to administer medications properly through the feeding tube. The liquid form of medications should be used, if possible. Medications that can be crushed should be pulverized with a mortar and pestle and then dissolved in warm water before administration.

Home care patients also need instruction regarding formula types, feeding routines and equipment. Feedings in the home setting vary based on the patient's needs and lifestyle. Continuous assessment by the home care nurse is essential to evaluate how the patient and family are coping in relation to tube feedings. The nurse's ongoing teaching and monitoring are fundamental in preventing or managing circumstances that may lead to further hospitalization.

SOURCE: Loan, Kearney, Magnuson & Williams, 1997.

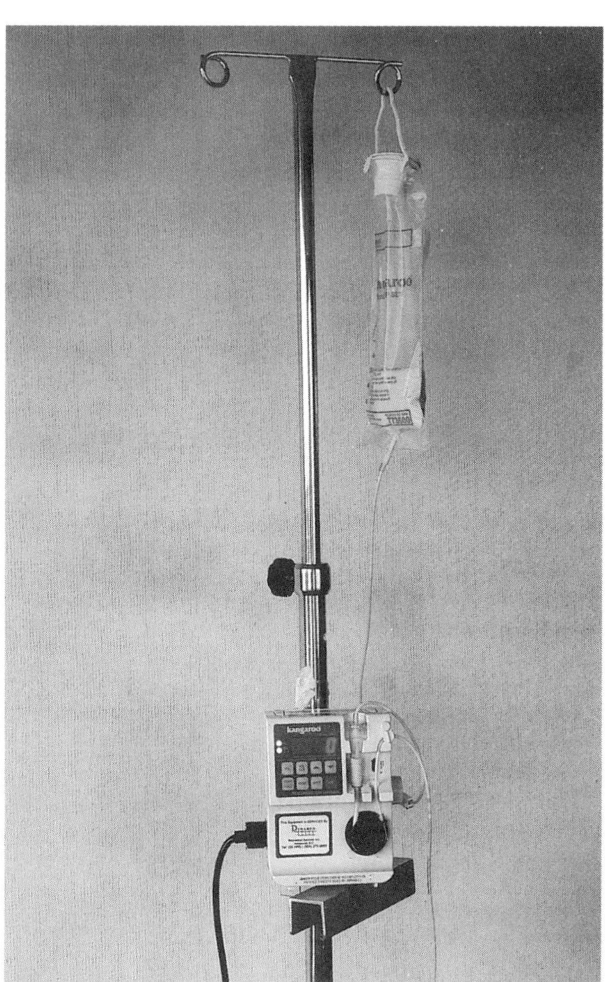

FIGURE 20.13 Feeding set attached to an enteral feeding pump

In a healthy individual, the function of protein is to support the growth and maintenance of body tissues. Adequate protein function is reflected as a state of nitrogen equilibrium. In illness, protein breakdown (catabolism) can exceed protein synthesis (anabolism) and is reflected as a negative nitrogen balance (more nitrogen loss than intake). The goal of TPN is to maintain a state of positive nitrogen balance in an effort to counter catabolic deterioration.

There are three basic indications for use of TPN:

1. **Unavailability of the digestive tract.** If the gastrointestinal tract has been rendered totally unavailable for use, an alternative method of nutrition is an obvious necessity. This may include, for example, conditions in which feeding by means of the gastrointestinal tract is impossible, hazardous or inadequate (as for major abdominal injury, obstruction, fistula, massive small bowel resection) or conditions in which the bowel must rest (such as severe pancreatitis, inflammatory bowel disease or hyperemesis gravidarum, or when the patient has been NPO for more than five to seven days).
2. **Malnutrition.** In the presence of malnutrition, the chances of successful medical intervention are greatly diminished. Patients with conditions such as chronic vomiting, diarrhea or malabsorption states, and poor pre- or postoperative nutritional status, benefit from the nutrient support provided by TPN.
3. **Degree of hypermetabolism or catabolism.** In the presence of severe illness, increased nutritional requirements can place extensive demands on the body's reserves, for example, in people with sepsis or

burns, those with extensive trauma or surgery and those with malignant diseases requiring radiation and/or chemotherapy (Dudek, 1997).

Nutritional Assessment

Prior to the initiation of TPN, it is important to gather a broad assessment of the individual's nutritional and metabolic status to provide a baseline by which to measure progress. Then, at regular intervals throughout TPN therapy, certain tests are repeated to measure the patient's response to therapy. These assessments are presented in the box below.

Administering Parenteral Nutrition

The administration of parenteral nutrition can be approached in two ways: peripheral parenteral nutrition (PPN) and total parenteral nutrition (TPN). The advantages of peripheral parenteral nutrition are the ease of access to the peripheral veins and the much lower rate of infection and catheter-related complications. However, PPN is also subject to complications. For instance, phlebitis and thrombus occur with the administration of hyperosmolar solutions (those containing increased concentration of particles per kilogram of solution) into peripheral veins owing to the slower flow rates within these vessels. As well, peripheral vein access is prone to problems of infiltration. PPN is therefore limited to short-term administration as a supplement (carbohydrates, amino acid solutions and lipid emulsions) for patients who are able to consume some oral nutrients or as a means of providing total parenteral nutrition on a very short-term basis (Eschelman, 1996; Dudek, 1997).

Administration of TPN therapy requires a large central vein such as the subclavian vein. TPN solutions contain 15–35 percent dextrose in addition to amino acids, vitamins, minerals, trace elements and electrolytes. The brisk blood

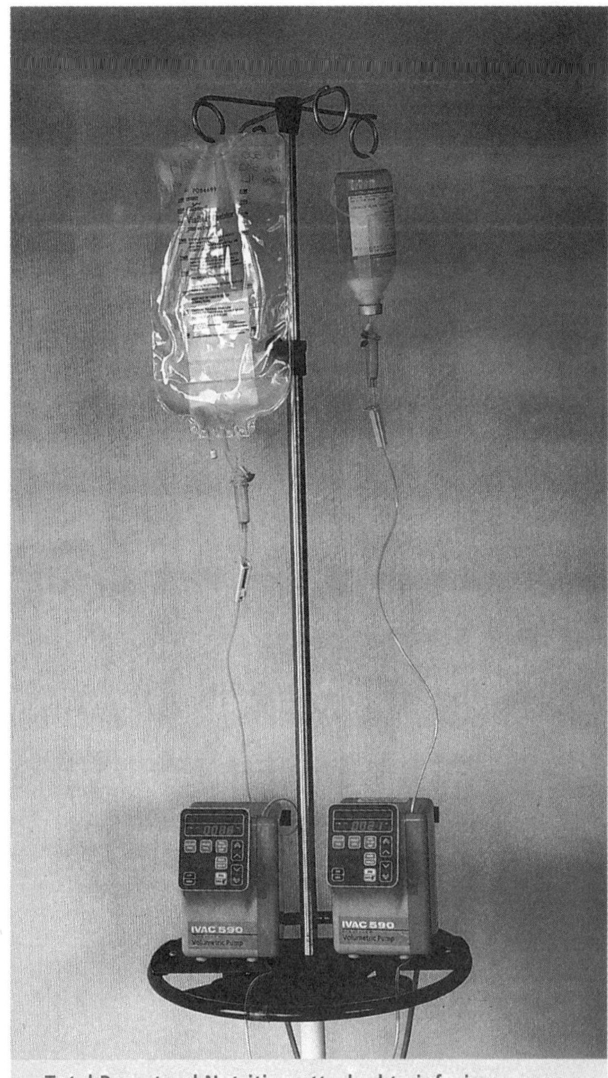

Total Parenteral Nutrition attached to infusion pumps.

Assessment of an Individual During TPN Therapy

1. **Protein status:** To establish the body's need for protein intake, an assessment of the individual's nitrogen balance is essential. Nitrogen balance is determined from 24-hour urine specimens. Protein status is also determined on measurements of lean body mass, body fat stores, skeletal muscle mass, immune function and the patient's medical health problems. A dietitian can make an estimate of the patient's protein requirement.
2. **Possible sources of infection:** The high concentrations of dextrose solutions used in TPN and the person's compromised immune status pose a serious risk for infection. Any existing infection must be cultured and treated prior to initiation of therapy. Patients must be monitored carefully throughout therapy for signs of infection.
3. **Liver function:** Laboratory tests include total protein, albumin, AST (aspartate amino transferase), alkaline phosphatase, LDH (lactic acid dehydrogenase) and bilirubin.
4. **Kidney function:** Laboratory tests include BUN (blood urea nitrogen), serum creatinine and 24-hour urine collection for Na, K and urea. Fluid intake and output records are important to assess renal function and over- or underhydration.
5. **Biochemistry evaluation:** Studies include electrolytes and fasting glucose. Capillary blood glucose levels can also be done to evaluate glucose. A person with TPN is usually monitored four times a day during initial treatment, then twice a day until TPN has been discontinued.
6. **Hematology evaluation:** Studies include CBC and differential.
7. **Fluid balance:** Intake and output should be monitored and recorded to ensure proper hydration with TPN.

RESEARCH to practice

Metheney, N., Reed, L., Berglund, B. & Wehrle, M.A. (1994). Visual characteristics of aspirates from feeding tubes as a method for predicting tube location. *Nursing Research, 43*(5), 282–287.

Nurses are accountable for confirming feeding tube placement upon initial insertion, prior to each intermittent feeding and at least once per shift after continuous feedings are initiated. The literature reveals that visual inspection of aspirates from the feeding tube is highly recommended as a method of assessing tube placement.

The purpose of this study was not only to describe the visual characteristics of aspirates from the tubes but also to determine the extent to which these characteristics can be used to determine feeding tube position. A sample of 880 feeding tube aspirates were classified as being either clear, cloudy or having one of six colours. It was determined that gastric aspirates were mostly cloudy and either green, tan or off-white, bloody or brown, or colourless. Intestinal fluids were clear and yellow to bile-coloured. Pleural fluids and tracheobronchial secretions aspirated from feeding tubes (initial insertion was inadvertently positioned in the respiratory tract) were pale yellow and serous, or tan or off-white and mucous. The respiratory aspirates often contained blood; thus, it was difficult to determine accurate characteristics of respiratory fluids.

One hundred six photos of samples of aspirates—50 gastric, 50 intestinal, four tracheobronchial and two pleural—were then taken, recorded and coded. In addition, a sample of 30 registered nurses who were accustomed to examining feeding tube aspirates were selected from three acute care adult facilities. They were then shown the photographs to determine whether they could predict the feeding tube's location on the basis of visual characteristics depicted in these photographs.

The findings of the study revealed that the nurses were able to identify locations, in particular the gastric and intestinal placements, from the photographs (81% for gastric and 64% for intestinal). After reading a list of suggested characteristics for each location, the ability of the nurse rater rose significantly (91% for gastric and 72% for intestinal). However, the nurses were unable to identify respiratory aspirates accurately, even after reading a list of suggested characteristics.

Implications for practice that can be drawn from this study include that while aspirates from feeding tubes can be distinguished from either the gastric or the intestinal area, they are of little value in ruling out respiratory placement. The authors highly recommend that nurses practise this visual method in combination with testing the aspirate's pH. Aside from an x-ray, these two measurements can best help the nurse predict feeding tube location.

flow through the large central veins allows for rapid dilution of these hypertonic solutions. While the administration of TPN via central lines provides the secure access essential for long-term therapy, it is not without complications (in Chapter 23 we discuss the care for patients with central venous lines). The nurse needs to be aware of potential complications arising from the infusion of the TPN solution, primarily sepsis and metabolic disturbances, namely hyperglycemia (the most common), rebound hypoglycemia, osmotic diuresis, fluid excess or deficit, and electrolyte imbalances. A plan of care that focusses on monitoring for complications and implementing health-protecting strategies is critical in TPN therapy. As with all care, the plan should be made in collaboration with the patient. The nurse should assess the patient's learning needs and provide instruction and information accordingly. Patients should be advised, when possible, to watch for potential complications with their therapy and to notify their nurse.

SEPSIS Patients receiving TPN therapy are in an already compromised state, and their ability to fight infection is limited. The amino acid–dextrose solution is a potential growth medium for yeast organisms, and bacteria thrive in lipid solutions. The nurse needs to be aware of signs and symptoms that would indicate the presence of any superimposed infection. The nurse should monitor for local (erythema, tenderness and drainage at insertion site) and systemic (sudden glycosuria in a previously glucose-tolerant patient as the body mobilizes extra glucose to fight the infection, fever, chills, nausea and vomiting and hypotension) signs of infection. Other nursing interventions should include monitoring vital signs, and daily assessment of capillary blood glucose levels and of urine for ketones. If drainage was present at the site of insertion, a swab would be taken for culture and sensitivity.

HYPERGLYCEMIA Monitor the patient for signs and symptoms such as glycosuria, polyuria, increased thirst, weakness, nausea and vomiting, flushed skin, acetone breath and abdominal pain. The TPN solution should be initiated gradually to allow the patient time to adapt to the increased glucose concentration. Use of an infusion pump will ensure the infusion at the prescribed rate (+ or – 10 percent; *do not* play "catch up"). Insulin may be administered or added to the solution for individuals with persistent hyperglycemia. The patient is also monitored for signs of fluid volume deficit.

HYPOGLYCEMIA TPN therapy should be discontinued gradually in order to prevent hypoglycemia. If concentrated dextrose solutions are discontinued suddenly, an imbalance between pancreatic insulin production and available glucose will occur, resulting in hypoglycemia (unless the patient is eating when TPN is discontinued). The patient is monitored

PROCEDURE 20.6

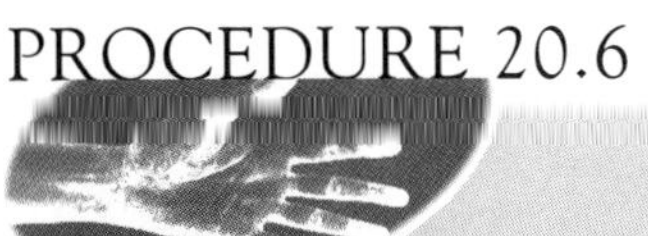

Blood Glucose Monitoring

Action	*Rationale*
1. Gather equipment: • antiseptic swab and cotton ball (optional) • sterile lancet or lancing device • glucose testing meter • glucose test strips that match the meter; calibration test strip • clean gloves.	Ensures efficiency and economy of time.
2. Wash hands and maintain medical and surgical asepsis.	Reduces transmission of microorganisms.
3. Assess patient's understanding of procedure and purpose; explain procedure.	Allays anxiety and enhances emotional well-being.
4. Have patient wash hands thoroughly with soap and warm water.	Prevents infection.
5. Check: equipment and supplies; battery of meter; expiry date of glucose test strips; code numbers of calibration strips and meter performance with test solution on glucose test strip.	Ensures accuracy of test results.
6. Calibrate meter to glucose test strip according to institutional policies and manufacturer's instructions (e.g., inserting calibration or code strip into the slot and matching the number).	Checks the performance of the meter and ensures the accuracy of the results according to each new carton of glucose test strips.
7. Insert test strip into the meter according to manufacturer's instructions.	Ensures that the strip is inserted at the correct time.
8. Don clean gloves.	Reduces transmission of microorganisms.
9. Obtain a blood sample, usually a capillary blood sample with a lancet and finger-stick: • Select the puncture site (sides of the fingertips; sites are usually rotated if tested often).	Avoids areas of bruising and lesions; selects areas with few nerve endings and calluses.
• Clean the puncture site by washing with soap and warm water (some agencies may prefer use of an alcohol swab to clean puncture site; check policy).	Reduces transfer of microorganisms. Warm water enhances flow of blood to the fingers. If alcohol used, ensure puncture is thoroughly dry; ensures alcohol in the sample does not alter test results.
• Prepare the sterile lancet, or load and cock the lancet device.	Enables a simple and safe method for obtaining blood sample with correct depth of penetration. Amount of pressure and position of lancet device against the finger determines depth of puncture.
• Gently position the lancet device on the selected puncture site and prick the finger. • Form a drop of blood on the fingertip by stroking from wrist to palm to finger, avoiding squeezing around the puncture site.	Squeezing the puncture site makes the stick more painful, and tissue serum may interfere with test results.
10. Apply the drop of blood to the target area of the test strip by various methods according to product instructions. Most product monographs do not mention wiping the first drop of blood away and then using the second drop of blood.	Some references suggest this, because the first drop contains more serum. Check agency policy.
11. Insert test strip into the meter.	Ensures that the strip is inserted at the correct time.
12. The meter will indicate when the result is ready and display the result in the window (20–60 seconds).	
13. Remove the test strip; discard strip and lancet in a safe manner. Wash hands.	Prevents spread of microorganisms.
14. Record and report the results.	Documents testing and response to therapy, communicates findings to other members of the health care team and provides indication for initiating or altering treatment.

for diaphoresis, tachycardia, confusion, tremors, anxiety and altered levels of consciousness. If any of these symp- [illegible] doctor's order) is given to maintain glucose level.

OSMOTIC DIURESIS Hyperglycemia increases serum osmolarity, which causes fluid to shift from the intracellular compartment into the plasma, where it is subsequently lost in the urine. A sudden increase in urinary output and signs of dehydration (dry mucous membranes, reduced skin turgor) may indicate osmotic diuresis. Nursing interventions include notifying the physician and infusing additional fluids and electrolytes as prescribed. The TPN nutrient prescription may need to adjusted by the physician. Insulin may need to be considered as a medical intervention.

FLUID EXCESS Fluid excess results from an infusion that is too rapid, from electrolyte imbalances, or from malnutrition and decreased serum albumin, which promotes fluid retention. The patient is monitored for edema (facial, sacral or peripheral), rapid weight gain, pulmonary edema and ascites. Daily weights are taken, and intake and output levels are maintained to monitor fluid excess. The use of an infusion pump for administering solutions should help to prevent this complication. If fluid excess occurs, the rate of infusion is decreased as ordered by the physician and/or the TPN prescription is changed.

FLUID DEFICIT An inadequate rate of infusion, hyperglycemia, electrolyte imbalance, diarrhea and fluid loss from other sites (for example, fistula, NG suction, drains) result in fluid deficit. The patient is monitored for signs of dehydration and imbalances between intake and output. Nursing interventions include increasing the rate of the infusion or changing the composition of the infusion per the doctor's order.

ELECTROLYTE IMBALANCE The composition of the TPN solution is based on each patient's individual requirements. Throughout the course of therapy, alterations may need to be made to adjust to changes in the patient's response to therapy. The nurse should monitor the patient for signs of hypokalemia (such as lethargy, muscle cramps, nausea and vomiting, arrhythmias, glycosuria), hypocalcemia (abdominal muscle cramps, tetany, tingling of fingers and toes, circumoral tingling, positive Chvostek's and Trousseau's signs and convulsions), hypophosphatemia (progressive weakness of muscles in extremeties, pain in long bones) and hypomagnesemia (anorexia, nausea, vomiting, irritability, depression, tremor, tetany, hyperreflexia and paresthesia). Hypomagnesemia is often co-existent with hypocalcemia and hypokalemia. Electrolyte imbalances are further discussed in Chapter 23. Nurses should be aware of the need for blood work to be done daily or several times weekly. They should monitor the results and notify the physician of any abnormalities (Metheney, 1996).

Evaluating Nutritional Interventions

The patient goals, or expected outcomes, provide directions for nursing care. An example of a patient goal for a man who is reluctant to eat might be "eats all his meals each day." Evaluation of the goals depends on the outcome criteria set by the nurse and the patient cooperatively. These should be specifically stated. Some questions for the nurse to keep in mind when evaluating nutritional interventions are:

1. Is the individual eating meals? Has he or she adopted better eating habits, including an adequate, nutritious diet?
2. If on a special diet, is the person adhering to it? If in hospital, does the person select foods that are compatible with his or her prescribed diet from the diet menu?
3. Have the symptoms of digestive disorders been alleviated? That is, has vomiting stopped? Is nausea less troublesome? Is the patient beginning to regain appetite? Is the patient free from indigestion?
4. Is the patient comfortable?
5. Is the patient able to retain fluids for gradually extended periods of time?
6. Is the patient able to take and retain adequate food and fluids for his or her nutritional needs?
7. Do results of laboratory tests reflect adequate nutrition?

The nurse also observes the patient to assess nutritional status and the progress made towards achieving the goals. Comparison of the nurse's observations of the patient with the characteristics of good nutrition and poor nutrition (see Table 20.11) are helpful in this regard. The registered dietitian can provide a more detailed assessment and specific nutritional recommendations for the individual patient's specific health problems and needs. Thus, it is important to consult and collaborate with this member of the health team when caring for individuals with nutritional problems.

IN REVIEW

- Food is vital to all aspects of health. Physiologically, the body needs a constant supply of nutrients to sustain life. Food provides the fuel for:
  - metabolism
  - growth, maintenance and repair of tissues
  - synthesis of enzymes and hormones
  - regulating all body processes.

- Food plays a significant role in psychological, social, cultural and spiritual health. It is used to:
  - promote feelings of security and comfort
  - foster social acceptance and prestige
  - maintain traditional customs and religious ceremonies
  - promote family solidarity and relaxation.
- Metabolism refers to all physical and chemical changes that nutrients undergo after being absorbed from the gastrointestinal tract and their use by body cells. Nutrients are ingested, digested and absorbed into the blood stream for delivery to the cells. They can be:
  - oxidized for energy (catabolism)
  - used in the synthesis of hormones, enzymes and proteins (anabolism).

  Excess nutrients can be stored in the body.
- Essential nutrients include carbohydrates, fats, proteins, vitamins, minerals and water.
- Carbohydrates are starches and sugars, and are used primarily for energy. Carbohydrates:
  - vary in complexity (from simple to complex and fibre)
  - can be converted to glucose (except for fibre)
  - can be converted into fat and stored in adipose tissue or excreted in urine.

  Glucose is metabolized for energy and can be stored in the liver or muscles as glycogen.
- Fats are compounds that are insoluble in water. They function as a source of heat and energy. In addition, fats:
  - provide essential fatty acids to the body
  - spare the burning of proteins for energy
  - promote the absorption of fat-soluble vitamins
  - insulate vital organs
  - help in hormone synthesis
  - add flavour to foods and enhance satiety.
- Proteins are nutrients made up of amino acids. They provide a major source of building material for maintenance and repair of tissues. Of the 22 amino acids needed by the body, nine are considered essential and are supplied by food; the others (non-essential amino acids) are synthesized in the body. In addition, proteins:
  - are either complete or incomplete (depending on amino acid content)
  - are necessary in the formation of hormones, enzymes, antibodies and blood proteins
  - regulate water balance, nitrogen balance and nutrient transport
  - may be used for energy.
- Vitamins are necessary constituents in the chemical processes involved in converting food to energy, building and repairing tissues and protecting cells.
- Minerals function in the building and maintenance of bones, teeth and various body systems.
- Water is essential for the transportation of all nutrients and excretion of body wastes.
- The body uses energy for basal metabolism, physical activity and the thermic effect of food. Daily energy requirements vary greatly, depending on:
  - lean body mass
  - body fat
  - age and gender
  - physical activity
  - health problems and medications
  - stress and anxiety.
- Nutritional guidelines have been established to help Canadians choose foods that will ensure an adequate supply of daily essential nutrients.
- Nutritional needs vary considerably during the life cycle. For example, a woman's nutrient requirements increase during pregnancy and lactation.
- Infants' nutrient requirements change in accordance with their growth and the maturation of the gastrointestinal and neuromuscular systems. Growth:
  - is rapid during the first year of life
  - slows in the second year.
- Children need the same types of foods as adults, but the quantities vary according to their growth and energy requirements. It is important to establish good eating habits during the toddler and preschool years.
- Adolescents' nutritional needs increase greatly as they undergo growth spurts.
- The need for calories and protein usually declines as people reach full adulthood. With aging comes a gradual slowing down of metabolic activity, and the need for calories decreases further.
- The nutritional problems of older adults often stem from inadequate intake. Factors that contribute to inadequate intake include:
  - insufficient funds
  - lack of information
  - physical inability to shop for and prepare food
  - loneliness, depression
  - loss of appetite.
- During illness, demands for energy and proteins may increase. If patients are unable to tolerate food, the body's stored sources of energy may be used up quickly.

- A person's nutritional status reflects the balance between the body's requirements for nutrients and energy and the intake of food. Factors that affect food [illegible]
    - socioeconomic status
    - family composition
    - level of education
    - physical and psychological health problems
    - culture and religion.
- The nurse's role in helping people with nutritional problems includes:
    - comprehensive assessments (including the nursing health history, physical examination, anthropometric measurements and interpretation of laboratory results)
    - identification of problems and development and implementation of a plan of care (including participation from patient and family to ensure successful outcomes)
    - promotion of optimal nutrition (by encouraging patients and families to examine their dietary patterns and then helping individuals to change these patterns)
    - provision of educational information on healthy eating (including therapeutic diets designed to prevent and treat anorexia, indigestion, nausea and vomiting, food poisoning)
    - restoration of patients' hydration and nutritional status (via such measures as enteral feeding and total parenteral nutrition)
    - monitoring of patients' nutritional status and risk for potential complications
    - implementation of preventive and therapeutic measures if complications arise
    - collaboration with other members of the health care team (e.g., physician, physiotherapist, registered dietitian, speech pathologist).

Critical Thinking Activities

1. Record all the food and beverages you consume in a typical day (24-hour period). Compare your intake with *Canada's Food Guide for Healthy Eating*.
    a) What is healthy about your diet? What is not?
    b) What changes should you make to eat a more nutritious diet?
2. Select an ethnic or religious diet and identify the characteristics and main dishes. Examine the diet in terms of the four food groups.
    a) [illegible]
    b) How could the diet be improved?
3. Janice, age 7 years, has iron-deficiency anemia. In an interview, her mother tells you that the family is vegetarian and that Janice has a very poor appetite.
    a) What questions are important in a nutritional assessment for Janice?
    b) Plan a strategy for counselling the mother about nutrition.
    c) What advice could you give the mother to help increase Janice's appetite?
4. You are a home care nurse assigned to a 71-year-old woman who speaks little English. She is in need of teaching to improve her eating habits. What are some of the things you could implement in an attempt to change her food habits?
5. Susan Schwartz, aged 20, works at a day care centre and lives with five other people on a communal farm at the edge of town. Susan has not been feeling well for the past few days. She was admitted to hospital this morning suffering from severe abdominal pains, vomiting and bloody diarrhea. She looks thin and pale, and she has a fever. Susan weighs 43.1 kg. She is 157 cm tall. Her wrist measurement is 15.24 cm. Laboratory test results show that her blood levels of hemoglobin, hematocrit and serum protein are below normal. The physician establishes a medical diagnosis of regional enteritis (Crohn's disease) and prescribed TPN.
    a) What are some of the factors contributing to Susan's nutritional problem?
    b) What assumptions might you make about actual or potential problems for Susan?
    c) What assessments would you make regarding Susan's nutritional status?
    d) What signs and symptoms of malnourishment might you observe in Susan?
    e) How much is she below the average weight for her height and body frame?
    f) What should be monitored while Susan is receiving TPN?
    g) What specific nursing interventions would you consider in Susan's care?
    h) How would you evaluate the effectiveness of these interventions?

KEY TERMS

nutrient p. 486
digestion p. 486
peristalsis p. 486
hydrolysis p. 486
absorption p. 487
mucosal folds p. 487
villi p. 487
metabolism p. 487
catabolism p. 487
anabolism p. 487
carbohydrates p. 487
fats p. 488
triglycerides p. 488
saturated p. 488
unsaturated p. 488
phospholipids p. 489
cholesterol p. 489
proteins p. 489
amino acids p. 489
complete proteins p. 490
incomplete proteins p. 490
coenzymes p. 490
calcium p. 490
phosphorus p. 492
magnesium p. 492
iron p. 492
calorie p. 492
kilocalorie p. 492
basal metabolic rate (BMR) p. 492
dietary thermogenesis p. 493
malnutrition p. 493
glycogenolysis p. 506
gluconeogenesis p. 506
ketosis p. 506
anorexia p. 507
nausea p. 507
vomiting p. 507
appetite p. 507
hunger p. 507
emesis p. 509
anthropometric measurements p. 511

References

BARKER, H.M. (1996). *Nutrition and dietetics for health care.* (9th ed.). New York: Churchill Livingstone.

BERGER, K.J., & WILLIAMS, M.B. (1992). *Fundamentals of Nursing & Collaborating for Optimal Health.* Norwalk, CT: Appleton & Lange.

BRITISH COLUMBIA DIETITIANS' & NUTRITIONISTS' ASSOCIATION (BCDNA). (1992). *Manual of nutritional care.* (4th ed.). Vancouver: Author.

CAMPBELL, C.C., & HORTON, S.E. (1991). Apparent nutrient intakes of Canadians: Continuing nutritional challenges for public health professionals. *Canadian Journal of Public Health, 82,* 374–480.

CARPENITO, L.J. (1997). *Nursing diagnosis: Application to clinical practice* (7th ed.). Philadelphia: Lippincott.

CHERNECKY, C.C., & BERGER, B.J. (1997). *Laboratory tests and diagnostic procedures.* (2nd ed.). Philadelphia: Saunders.

DAVIS, J.R., & SHERER, K. (1994). *Applied nutrition and diet therapy for nurses.* Philadelphia: Saunders.

DELMAR PUBLISHERS. (1997). *Delmar's textbook of basic pediatric nursing.* New York: Author.

DUDEK, S.G. (1997). *Nutrition handbook for nursing practice.* (4th ed.). Philadelphia: Lippincott.

EARNEST, V.V. (1993). *Clinical skills in nursing practice* (2nd ed.). Philadelphia: Lippincott.

ESCHELMAN, M. (1996). *Introductory nutrition and nutrition therapy.* (3rd ed.). Philadelphia: Lippincott.

FLYNN, J.M., & HACKEL, R. (1990) *Technological Foundations in Nursing.* Norwalk, CT: Appleton & Lange.

HEALTH & WELFARE CANADA. (1988a). *Canadian guidelines for healthy weights.* Report of an expert group convened by Health Promotion Directorate, Health Services and Promotion Branch. Ottawa: Author.

HEALTH & WELFARE CANADA (Health Services & Promotion Branch). (1988b). *Promoting healthy weights: A discussion paper.* Ottawa: Author.

HEALTH & WELFARE CANADA. (1989). *Nutrition recommendations: A call for action.* Ottawa: Minister of Supply & Services. (Catalogue no. H39–162/1990E)

HEALTH & WELFARE CANADA. (1990). *Nutrition recommendations: The report of the Scientific Review Committee.* Ottawa: Minister of Supply & Services. (Catalogue no. H49–41/1990E)

HEALTH CANADA. (1992). *Canada's food guide to healthy eating.* Ottawa: Minister of Supply & Services. (Catalogue no. H39–252/1992E)

KESTEL, F. (1993). Using blood glucose meters: What you and your patient need to know. Part 1. *Nursing, 23,* 3, 34-41.

LEE, C.A., BARRETT, C.A., & IGNATAVICIUS, D.D. (1996). *Fluids and electrolytes: A practical approach.* (4th ed.). Philadelphia: F.A. Davis.

LOAN, T., KEARNEY, P., MAGNUSON, B., & WILLIAMS, S. (1997). Enteral feeding in the home in environment. *Home Healthcare Nurse,* 15(8), 531–538.

LUTZ, C.A., & PRZYTULSKI, K.R. (1997). *Nutrition and diet therapy.* (2nd ed.). Philadelphia: F.A. Davis.

METHENEY, N. (1988). Measures to test placement of nasogastric and nasointestinal feeding tubes: A review. *Nursing Research, 37,* 324–329.

METHENEY, N.M. (1996). *Fluid and electrolyte balance: Nursing considerations.* (3rd ed.). Philadelphia. Lippincott.

METHENEY, N., REED, L., BERGLUND, B., & WEHRLE, M.A. (1994). Visual characteristics of aspirates from feeding tubes as a method for predicting tube location. *Nursing Research, 43*(5), 282–287.

ONTARIO DIETETIC ASSOCIATION & THE ONTARIO HOSPITAL ASSOCIATION. (1989). *Nutrition care manual.* (6th ed.) Ontario: Author.

PILLITTERI, A. (1995). *Maternal and child health nursing: Care of the childbearing and childrearing family.* (2nd ed.). Philadelphia: Lippincott.

POLEMAN, C.M., & PECKENPAUGH, N.J. (1991). *Nutrition: Essentials and diet therapy.* (6th ed.). Philadelphia: Saunders.

POLLITT, E. (1995). Does breakfast make a difference in school? *Journal of American Diet Association, 95*(10), 1134–1139.

TOWNSEND, C.E. (1994). *Nutrition and diet therapy.* (6th ed.). New York: Delmar Publishers.

WARDLAW, G.M., INSEL, P.M., & SEYLER, M.F. (1992). *Contemporary nutrition: Issues and insights.* St. Louis: Mosby.

WEIGLEY, E.S., MUELLER, D.H., & ROBINSON, C.H. (1997). *Robinson's basic nutrition and diet therapy.* Toronto: Prentice Hall.

WILLIAMS, M.H. (1992). *Nutrition for fitness and sport.* (3rd ed.). Dubuque, IA: W.M.C. Brown.

WILLIAMS, M.W. (1993). *Lifetime: Fitness and wellness.* (3rd ed.). Madison, WI: Brown & Benchmark.

WILLIAMS, S.R. (1989). *Nutrition and diet therapy.* (6th ed.). St. Louis: Mosby.

WILLIAMS, S.R. (1995a). *Basic nutrition and diet therapy.* (10th ed.). St. Louis: Mosby.

WILLIAMS, S.R. (1995b). *Diet therapy.* Toronto: Mosby.

WILLIAMS, S.R. (1997). *Nutrition and diet therapy.* (8th ed.). St. Louis: Mosby.

WONG, D.L. (1995). *Whaley and Wong's nursing care of infants and children.* (5th ed.). St. Louis: Mosby.

Additional Readings

ANEIROS, S., & ROLLINS, H. (1996). Home enteral tube feeding. *Community*

BAYER, INC. (1995). *The improved Glucometer Elite Blood Glucose Meter.* [Product monograph.]

CATO, Y. (1997). Intradialytic parenteral nutrition therapy for the malnourished hemodialysis patient. *Journal of Intravenous Nursing, 20*(3), 130–135.

DAVIDHIZAR, R., & DUNN, C. (1996). Malnutrition in the elderly. *Home Healthcare Nurse, 14*(12), 948–956.

DIMAND, R.J., VEERMAN-WAUTERS, G., & BRANER, D.A.V. (1997). Techniques, materials and devices. Bedside placement of pH-guided transpyloric small bowel feeding tubes in critically ill infants and small children. *Journal of Parenteral and Enteral Nutrition, 21*(2), 112–114.

FORLOINES-LYNN, S. (1996). How to smooth the way for cyclic tube feedings. *Nursing 96, 26*(3), 57–60.

GOODWIN, R.S. (1996). Prevention of aspiration pneumonia: A research-based protocol. *Dimensions of Critical Care, 15*(2), 58–71.

HOLMES, S. (1993). Force of habit, culture and religion help form our eating habits. *Nursing Times, 89*(35), 48–50.

LAMMON, C., FOOTE, A., LELI, P., INGLE, J., & ADAMS, M. (1995). *Clinical nursing skills.* Philadelphia: Saunders.

LIFESCAN CANADA LIMITED. (no date). One-Touch Profile and Surestep System. [Product monograph.]

LUTZ, B.H. (1996). Client challenge. Total parenteral nutrition in the older adult. *Home Healthcare Nurse, 14*(2), 123–125.

MEDISENSE CANADA INC. (1995). *The revolutionary new Precision Q.I.D. System.* [Product monograph.]

MEHLER, P.S., & WEINER, K.A. (1995). Treatment of anorexia nervosa with total parenteral nutrition. *Nutrition in Clinical Practice, 10*(5), 183–197.

METHENEY, N., REED, L., WIERSEMA, L., McSWEENEY, M., WEHRLE, M.A.,

ing tube placement: An updated nursing [illegible]

METHENEY, N.A., SMITH, L., WEHRLE, M.A., WIERSEMA, L., & CLARK, J. (1998, January). pH, color and feeding tubes. *RN*, 25–27.

MILES INC. (1992). *Glucolet 2: Automatic lancing device for use in obtaining blood for blood glucose testing.* [Product monograph.]

PENDLEBURY, J. (1997). Skills update: Feeding by PEG. *Community Nurse, 3*(4), 11–12.

ROLLINS, C.J. (1997). Total nutrient admixtures: Stability issues and their impact on nursing practice. *Journal of Intravenous Nursing, 20*(6), 299–304.

SHAPIRO, T., MINARD, G., & KUDSK, K.A. (1997). Transgastric jejunal feeding tubes in critically ill patients. *Nutrition in Clinical Practice, 12*(4), 164–167.

SHILS, M.E., OLSON, J.A., & SHIKES, M. (1994). *Modern nutrition in health and disease.* (8th ed.). Philadelphia: Lea & Febriger.

SPIKER, C.A., HINTHORN, D.R., & PINGLETON, S.K. (1996). Intermittent enteral feeding in mechanically ventilated patients: The effect on gastric pH and gastric cultures. *Chest: The Cardiopulmonary Journal, 110*(1), 243–248.

VIALL, C. (1996). When your patient has an NG tube, what's the most important thing? Location, location, location. *Nursing, 26*(9), 43–45.

WHITNEY, E.N., CATALDO, C.R., DEBRUYNE, L.K., & ROLFES, S.R. (1996). *Nutrition for health and health care.* New York: West.

WILSON, J.M. (1996). Nutritional assessment and its application. *Journal of Intravenous Nursing, 19*(6), 303–314.

Chapter 21

Urinary Elimination Needs

OUTLINE

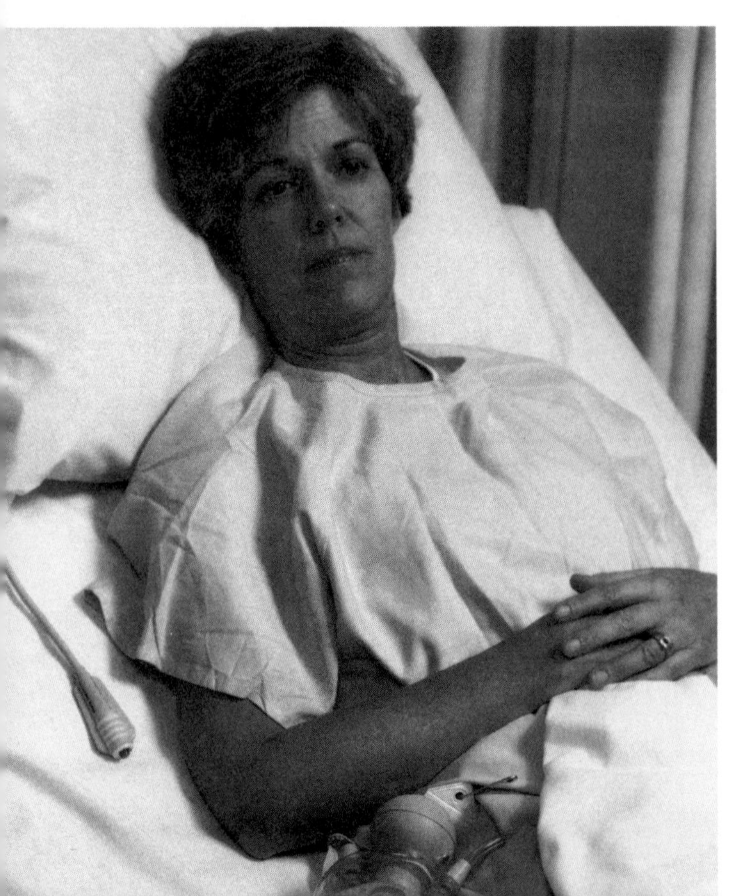

Central Questions

1. In what way is adequate urinary elimination important to health and well-being?
2. What are the structures and functions involved in urinary elimination?
3. How does normal urinary functioning vary throughout the life cycle?
4. What are the main determinants of urinary functioning?
5. What are some common urinary elimination problems?
6. What basic principles would the nurse apply when assisting individuals to meet their urinary elimination needs?
7. How does the nurse assess an individual's urinary elimination status?
8. What are the common nursing diagnostic statements for individuals with urinary elimination problems?
9. How would the nurse develop a plan of care for individuals with urinary elimination problems?
10. What strategies might the nurse implement in helping individuals, families or groups to promote optimal urinary functioning and prevent potential urinary problems?
11. What health-restoring and supportive strategies might the nurse implement when caring for individuals with urinary elimination problems?
12. How would the nurse evaluate the individual's response to nursing interventions?

Introduction

[illegible]
rid itself of wastes. There are four principal [illegible] the removal of wastes: from the urinary tract as urine, from the gastrointestinal tract as feces, through the skin as perspiration and through the lungs as expired air. Each mechanism has its specific function in clearing the body of wastes that result from the processing of nutrients and their subsequent utilization in cells.

The focus of this chapter is on urinary elimination, which primarily functions in removing nitrogenous waste products of cellular metabolism and in regulating fluid and electrolyte balance. Both functions are essential to the maintenance of chemical homeostasis of the blood. When urinary elimination is impaired, all body systems may be affected and the individual may become acutely ill.

In addition, the act of voiding is an important area of independent functioning. Control over voiding is learned early in childhood, and actual or potential loss of independence in this vital function constitutes a serious threat to an individual's social and emotional well-being. Such a loss can lead to fear of a return to the dependent state of infancy, as well as feelings of reduced self-esteem.

This chapter provides the basis for understanding urinary elimination, common urinary problems and their management of these problems. The assessment of urinary elimination and measures by which nurses can promote patients' optimal urinary health, the maintenance or restoration of their usual patterns of functioning when urinary dysfunction has occurred, are also outlined.

Anatomy and Physiology of Urinary Elimination

Normally, the urinary tract consists of two kidneys, two ureters, a bladder and a urethra (see Figure 21.1). The elimination of urine from the body depends on effective functioning of these structures.

KIDNEYS

The kidneys are paired, bean-shaped organs situated in the back of the abdominal cavity, behind the peritoneum and just below the diaphragm, one on either side of the spinal column at the level of the 12th thoracic and third lumbar vertebrae. The right kidney sits lower than the left owing to the position of the liver. In the adult each kidney weighs about 117–170 g and is 10–12 cm long and approximately 5–6 cm wide (Porth, 1998). The kidneys are attached to the dorsal wall by connective tissue and an extensive cushion of fat. They primarily function to control the composition and volume of body fluids, including blood, and to excrete excess fluids, electrolytes, nitrogenous wastes, toxic substances and drugs. These functions are accomplished through the complex processes of filtration, selective reabsorption and secretion in which essential elements needed by the body are retained and waste products are removed in the form of urine.

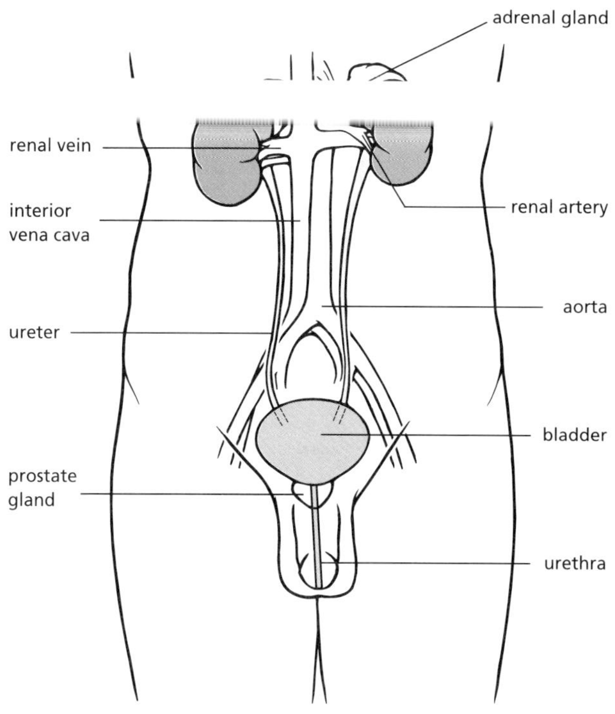

FIGURE 21.1 The urinary system

SOURCE: Porth, 1998, p. 568.

The functional unit of the kidney is the **nephron** (see Figure 21.2). Each kidney contains about one million nephrons. Urine is formed in the nephrons through the processes of filtration, reabsorption and secretion. A single nephron consists of a **glomerulus** (a cluster of capillaries), which filters fluid from the blood, and a tubular component, in which the glomerular filtrate is transformed into urine. The renal tubule begins as a sac (Bowman's capsule) that encases the capillary cluster. It winds through the kidney tissue and opens into a collecting tubule. Each collecting tubule joins other collecting tubules at a collecting duct. The collecting duct carries urine to the pelvis of each kidney.

Blood is brought to the kidneys by way of the renal arteries. About 20 to 25 percent of the resting cardiac output (approximately 1200 mL/min) passes through the kidneys. As the blood circulates through the kidneys, water-soluble waste products and excess water are filtered into the renal tubules. The nephrons process this filtrate by reabsorbing the essential constituents back into the blood stream, ignoring the unwanted constituents and secreting other constituents (hydrogen ions, potassium ions, ammonia) to the filtrate. Waste products are concentrated in the tubule, converting the filtrate into urine (Porth, 1998).

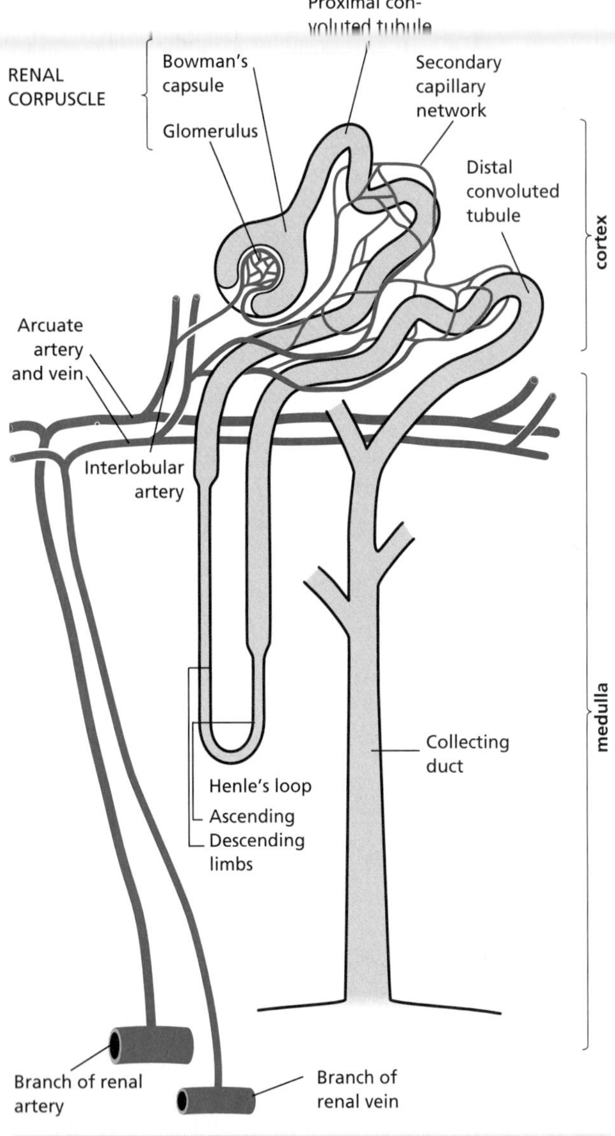

FIGURE 21.2 Cross-section of the kidney, illustrating a nephron

URETERS

Urine produced in the nephron empties into the pelvis of the kidney. From the kidney, urine is transported at a rate of one to five millilitres per minute by means of peristalsis along long muscular tubes called the **ureters** to the urinary bladder. The ureters enter the bladder at an oblique angle; the entrances are covered by a fold of mucous membrane, so that urine is not forced back up the ureters when pressure exists within the bladder.

BLADDER

The **urinary bladder** is a distensible muscular sac that lies on the pelvic floor behind the symphysis pubis. The bladder wall contains three layers of smooth muscle and a special mucosal lining (transitional epithelium) that allow the bladder to collapse when empty and then expand as it fills with urine. Normally, the bladder holds about 300–500 mL of urine, but it is capable of holding more than double that amount. The smooth muscle layers form the *detrusor muscle* of the bladder. Contraction of this muscle compresses the bladder and expels urine into the urethra. At the base of the bladder, where it joins the urethra, smooth muscle fibres form the involuntary *internal sphincter*, which controls the release of urine from the bladder. The bladder wall contains sensory receptors, which respond to distention from the accumulation of urine and relay information to the central nervous system, activating the mechanism for urination. The bladder is innervated by the autonomic nervous system. Sympathetic impulses cause relaxation of the detrusor muscle and contraction of the internal sphincter, thus inhibiting urination. Parasympathetic impulses, on the other hand, cause contraction of the detrusor muscle and relaxation of the internal sphincter, which activate urination.

URETHRA

The **urethra** is a short, muscular tube that carries urine from the bladder to outside of the body. The female urethra is approximately three to five centimetres long and opens just above the vagina. The urethra of the male serves both the urinary and reproductive systems. It is about 20 cm long from its origin in the bladder to its external opening in the glans penis. Three distinct regions can be identified in the male urethra: the prostatic urethra, the membranous urethra (where the external sphincter is located) and the penile urethra. In both males and females, the urethra contains a circular band of skeletal muscle that forms the *external sphincter*. This sphincter is under voluntary control; thus, the individual is able to exert control over the act of voiding. **Meatus** is the term used for the external opening of the urethra in both men and women.

The entire urinary tract is lined with a continuous layer of mucous membrane that stretches from the meatus to the pelvis of the kidney. The mucous membrane of the bladder has a phagocytic ability which, combined with the unidirectional flow of urine, guards against ascending infections of the urinary tract (Porth, 1998).

MICTURITION

Micturition refers to the act of emptying the bladder. Two terms more frequently used for this act are *voiding* and *urination*. When a sufficient amount of urine accumulates in the bladder (200–300 mL for most people), stretch receptors are stimulated. These receptors relay information via the pelvic nerve to the micturition reflex centre in the sacral (S2 through S4) region of the spinal cord and to the voluntary control centre in the cerebral cortex. The pelvic nerves also carry parasympathetic motor impulses to the detrusor muscle in the bladder wall and to the internal sphincter.

At the same time that the sensation of the need to void is perceived in the brain, impulses sent to the spinal cord activate the micturition reflex. This reflex produces parasympathetic stimulation, which causes contraction of the bladder muscle and relaxation of the internal sphincter. If [illegible] sphincter, micturition will ensue. If the individual does not cooperate voluntarily, the internal sphincter will remain closed and the bladder wall will gradually relax. As the bladder continues to fill, however, the micturition reflex returns with a more powerful urge to void. Voluntary control of micturition is a learned response that involves the development of an inhibitory mechanism within the cerebral cortex and the maturation of various portions of the spinal cord. Voluntary control of micturition is usually developed by three or four years of age (Wong, 1995).

Urinary Functioning in Health

The average adult usually excretes 1000–1500 mL of urine in a 24-hour period. The total volume varies with the amount of fluid intake, as well as with the amount of fluids lost through other routes, such as perspiration, vomiting or diarrhea.

The number of times a person voids during the day and the amount eliminated each time is highly individual. It is dependent, among other things, upon such factors as early childhood training, habitual response to the urge to urinate, amount of fluids consumed and the capacity of the bladder. Most people void first thing in the morning, possibly four to six times throughout the day and again before retiring. Owing to hormonal influences, the volume of urine produced at night is usually less than half that produced during the day. Therefore, it is not usually necessary to void during the night, unless the individual has consumed a large amount of fluids prior to bedtime.

Normal urine is clear and straw-coloured or light amber in appearance. Darker-coloured urine generally indicates increased concentration. Usually, the first urine voided in the morning is more concentrated than that excreted at other times of the day. Freshly voided urine is generally slightly acidic with a faint odour. When urine is left standing, it develops a stronger odour; it becomes alkaline (owing to the disintegration of its constituents) and a cloudy sediment develops (Huether, 1996).

Urinary Functioning Throughout the Life Cycle

INFANCY

Most newborns void within the first 24 hours of life. The first voiding is usually cloudy and may be pinkish due to uric acid crystals and mucous. Babies who do not void within this time are examined for problems such as obstruction in the urinary tract, urethral stenosis or absence of kidneys or ureters. Because their glomerular filtration rate (GFR) is [illegible] and regulate body fluid composition. The GFR reaches 30 percent of adult values within the first two days of extrauterine life and gradually attains full adult value by the age of two years (Kenner & MacLaren, 1993). Urine is usually dilute and odourless, and voiding may occur frequently. The frequency of voiding decreases gradually during infancy, although this is highly dependent on the amount of fluids consumed and on the surrounding temperature. The infant's body temperature is more readily affected by environmental temperatures than is an adult's, and more fluids are needed for internal processes when body temperature is high.

CHILDHOOD

By early childhood, the specific gravity and other urine findings are similar to those in adults. Children usually have to void more frequently than do adults, owing to the smaller size of their bladders. The urge to void is usually more intensely felt in children, although in many instances it is ignored if they are busy, resulting in a race to the bathroom. The neurophysiological pathways necessary for voluntary control of the bladder mature later than do those for bowel control. Most children become physiologically ready for voluntary bladder control by the age of two to three years. In general, readiness can be assessed by children's ability to hold their urine for one to two hours, communicate their need to void and hold their urine until seated on the toilet. As well, willingness to participate in the process must be considered. Children sometimes learn faster if they have a slightly older sibling whose activities they like to imitate. Night-time control is sometimes accomplished at the same time as the child learns to stay dry during the day. However, control at night occurs later in some children. Most children have achieved night-time control by the age of three to four years.

The school-aged child has generally mastered bladder control. It is not uncommon, however, for accidents still to occur, particularly if the child is under stress or gets too busy, especially with outdoor activities, to get to a bathroom in time. As growth continues, the bladder also grows and its capacity increases. Urinary elimination usually settles into an adult pattern well before adolescence and, unless problems develop, the pattern continues through adulthood, with variations as noted below.

PREGNANCY

Pregnant women usually experience the need to void more often and with greater urgency, particularly during the early and late stages of pregnancy. There is a dilation of the urinary system, partly due to pressure on the bladder by the enlarging uterus, but there is also a relaxation of smooth muscle due to

GERONTOLOGICAL

Effects of Aging on the Urinary System

Kidneys become smaller	Decreased renal function
Decrease in number of nephrons	
Decreased ability to concentrate urine	Decreased ability to excrete waste products
Decreased metabolic and regulatory functions	Risk of medication toxicity
	Urinary tract infections
Bladder becomes funnel-shaped	Decreased capacity
Increased irritability of bladder wall	Increased urgency to void

hormonal changes. This dilation may lead to stasis or slowing down of urine flow, with resultant increased vulnerability to urinary tract infections (Pillitteri, 1995).

ADULTHOOD

Many women in the middle years of adulthood experience difficulty in retaining urine within the bladder as the muscles of the pelvic floor, weakened by childbirth, begin to lose their tone. A small amount of urine may leak from the bladder if the woman laughs heartily, coughs or sneezes. This is known as stress incontinence (Porth, 1998). Men also may experience some age-related changes in their urinary pattern. As the male ages, there is a likelihood that the **prostate gland** (located below the bladder neck, surrounding the urethra) will become enlarged, resulting in such difficulties as increased frequency and nocturia (excessive urination at night). As both men and women age, they may experience a generalized loss of muscle tone, decreased bladder capacity, incomplete bladder emptying and increased residual urine. The lessened efficiency of the kidneys, coupled with delayed sensation to void, contributes to the need to void more frequently and with increased feelings of urgency (Porth, 1998).

Determinants of Urinary Functioning

A number of factors may affect the volume of urinary output and the pattern of voiding, as well as the characteristics of the urine excreted. These factors should be taken into consideration in the nurse's assessment of an individual's urinary elimination status.

INDIVIDUAL DIFFERENCES

In addition to those changes in urinary function that occur throughout the life cycle, there are also inborn differences in anatomical structure and physiological functioning. Some people have a larger bladder capacity than others or a seemingly more efficient urinary system. They may not need to void as often as others. Early childhood training also plays its part in an individual's response to the urge to urinate. Since voiding is under voluntary control, people may alter their voiding patterns in response to situational factors such as the availability of toilet facilities, mealtimes and the pressures of work.

FLUID AND FOOD INTAKE

One of the kidney's functions is to remove excess water from the body; therefore, both fluid intake and the amount of fluids lost through other routes will affect the volume and frequency of urinary output.

When large amounts of liquids are consumed, the kidneys will excrete more urine. Conversely, when fluid intake is decreased or the body is dehydrated, the kidneys will retain fluid, resulting in decreased amounts of concentrated urine.

Urine output is influenced by fluids and foods that contain alcohol and caffeine. Alcohol and caffeine inhibit the release of the antidiuretic hormone (ADH) which, in turn, inhibits the reabsorption of water from the renal tubules, causing a diuretic effect. Cola, cocoa, coffee and tea all have a diuretic effect on the kidney. Fruits and vegetables that have a high water content—for example, celery—may also increase urine output. Conversely, foods that are high in sodium, such as processed cheese and meats, may cause water reabsorption and decreased urine production. Certain foods may also affect the acidity of urine. For example, vegetarian diets may cause alkaline urine (Porth, 1998).

PSYCHOLOGICAL STATES

Psychological factors such as stress, anxiety and pain may also cause urinary disturbances. Anxiety, for example, often stimulates the urge to void more frequently. Strong fear may cause a person to void involuntarily, and pain may inhibit voiding.

DISEASE AND ILLNESS

Urinary elimination patterns are often altered by disease, illness states and associated medical treatments. Infection is one of the most common causes of urinary disturbances. The urinary tract is lined with a continuous mucous membrane; therefore, an infection that begins in one part of the system can progress rapidly to all parts of the urinary [illegible] of urinary tract infection (UTI). The proximity of the openings of the gastrointestinal and urinary tracts contributes to this transfer (Huether, 1996).

In infants and children, UTIs are treated vigorously to prevent possible spread to the kidneys. UTIs continue to be a problem in adolescence and young adulthood, especially in women, suggesting that anatomic and hormonal changes associated with puberty may contribute to their incidence. Frequency of occurrence is thought to increase with sexual activity. A bladder infection sometimes called "honeymoon cystitis," identified as an irritation of the urethral mucosa, often occurs after sexual activity in susceptible young women. Using a spermicide and diaphragm increases the risk. A nonpharmacological means of decreasing the risk for infection is to increase fluid intake prior to intercourse and to void soon after intercourse. This approach eliminates organisms from the bladder (Porth, 1998). The shortness of the urethra and proximity of the meatus to the vagina and rectum in women makes them particularly prone to infections.

Stasis of urine in the bladder, as a result of retention, is another factor predisposing people to infections, as well as to the formation of bladder stones. In hospitalized patients, UTIs are most commonly associated with invasive diagnostic and therapeutic procedures of the urinary tract.

Obstructions may be either congenital or acquired, and occur in almost any part of the urinary tract. Most commonly, they are seen in the pelvis of the kidney, the ureter and the prostatic section of the male urethra. Blockage of the urinary tract, whether by malignancy, stones or stricture, hinders the excretion of urine.

Congenital structural anomalies may cause blockage of the urinary tract or give rise to other functional problems. Many congenital problems are discovered in infancy and early childhood and are surgically corrected at that time. Some anomalies, however, may go undetected until later in life or not at all. An individual with a solitary kidney, for example, may not discover this fact until an x-ray of the abdomen is taken during examination for reasons other than urinary tract dysfunction.

Generalized trauma to the body, such as hemorrhage, burns, shock or systemic infection, can also affect the kidneys. In severe dehydration, for example, there is a depletion in the amount of fluid within the body, which can severely disturb kidney function to the point of failure.

Interference with or injury to the nervous supply of the bladder and urethra can interfere with normal urinary function. Drugs that depress the central nervous system can cause loss of voluntary control over micturition as can damage to the spinal cord, to the pathways that transmit impulses from the spinal cord to the brain, or to the brain itself.

Common Problems

[illegible] sulting from impairment of elimination of waste products from the body.

Localized Problems

URINARY INCONTINENCE **Urinary incontinence**, or the inability to control voiding voluntarily, may result from infection, damage to the nerve supply of the bladder, lesions of the spinal cord or brain, or cerebral clouding of the aged. Urinary incontinence sometimes occurs temporarily after an operation. **Stress incontinence**, the excretion of small amounts of urine involuntarily with exertions such as coughing or laughing, occurs in many middle-aged women.

The inability to control urination is often very demoralizing, and individuals feel embarrassed when it happens. Incontinence may also result in irritation of the skin in the perineal area.

DYSURIA The term **dysuria** refers to difficult, painful voiding. It is generally associated with urinary tract infections as well as a number of other pathophysiological conditions, such as blockage, trauma or muscular abnormalities of the bladder or urethra. In men, hypertrophy of the prostate gland, which surrounds the urethra, is a common cause of dysuria. Dysuria may also be caused by the excretion of more highly concentrated urine than normal.

FREQUENCY **Frequency**, or voiding more often than usual, may simply result from an increased intake of fluids. Anxiety can stimulate voiding and cause distressing frequency, at times with loss of control. However, frequency, particularly combined with urgency, is also commonly seen in individuals with infections of the urinary tract.

URGENCY The need to void in a hurry is known as **urgency**. Its most common cause is urinary tract infection, although it may also be due to the same causes that produce frequency.

NOCTURIA **Nocturia** is the need to get up during the night to void. While nocturia may simply be the result of drinking a large amount of fluids prior to bedtime, particularly those containing caffeine or alcohol, it may also be a symptom of urinary dysfunction. Nocturia should not be confused with **enuresis** (the involuntary loss of urine, or bedwetting), the causes of which can range from psychosomatic sources to actual physical impairment.

POLYURIA The passage of increased amounts of urine is called **polyuria** or **diuresis**. Excessive fluid intake, particularly fluids containing alcohol and caffeine, and disease states such as diabetes mellitus and diabetes insipidus, are among the common causes. Polyuria can also be caused by the use of **diuretics**, drugs given to increase urine output in people who suffer from hypertension and fluid retention.

URINARY RETENTION **Urinary retention** refers to the inability to pass urine despite bladder distention. It is generally the result of an obstruction to the flow of urine. Anesthetics and certain drugs, such as opiates and anticholinergics, may also cause urinary retention. Occasionally an individual will void small amounts of urine, which minimally relieves feelings of pressure within the bladder but does not empty the bladder completely. This residual urine predisposes the individual to bladder infection (**cystitis**).

OLIGURIA AND ANURIA **Oliguria** is the term used for urine production that is less than 30 mL/h. **Renal anuria** is the cessation of urine production and clinically means a urine output of less than 100 mL/day. It usually indicates serious kidney impairment and, if prolonged, will result in the buildup of toxic substances within the body and, perhaps, death. Kidney disease, heart failure, severe dehydration and shock may cause oliguria and anuria.

HEMATURIA The term **hematuria** is used to indicate blood in the urine. Blood in the urine can be microscopic or gross (obvious to the naked eye), and the cause may be benign or pathological. Hematuria may be related to neoplasms of the kidney or bladder and should be carefully investigated.

HESITANCY The term **hesitancy** refers to difficulty initiating urination. This problem is often seen in men with prostate enlargement. Other conditions in which hesitancy is common include anxiety, urethral edema and after removal of a urinary catheter.

Generalized Problems

The impairment of renal function can result in generalized problems affecting most systems of the body. A reduction in the ability of the kidney to excrete the nonprotein nitrogenous waste products of metabolism results in an accumulation of these wastes within the blood. This condition is called **uremia**. It may result from infection, trauma or chronic renal disease.

Impairment in renal functioning has several effects on the body in addition to oliguria and anuria. Fluid retention results in the formation of edema (accumulation of fluid in the tissues) and possible development of hypertension. Retention of the acidic products of metabolism causes disturbance of the acid–base balance, leading to development of metabolic acidosis. Potassium (normally excreted by the kidney) is retained, which may result in neuromuscular irritability and cardiac dysrhythmias. There are significant changes in blood chemistry. The blood urea nitrogen (BUN) and creatinine levels rise. The extent of the increase in blood levels of these substances provides an indication of the severity of the kidney impairment.

In an attempt to rid itself of wastes normally excreted in the urine, the body will use other methods, which lead to additional problems. Perspiration is increased, and deposits of salts may accumulate on the patient's skin *(urea frost)*. The skin becomes pale and powdery, and the patient may have problems such as itching (*pruritus*). An offensive odour develops on the skin due to the urea deposits. When metabolic acidosis occurs, the lungs compensate through changes in respiration. Respirations become rapid and deep (*Kussmaul's respirations*) in an attempt to increase the excretion of carbon dioxide. Occasionally the individual's breath has the odour of urine.

Medications That Produce Urine Colour Change

Blue or green
triamterene (Dyrenium)
methylene blue
amitriptyline (Elavil)

Yellow-orange
sulfasalazine (Azulfidine)
multivitamins
diuretics

Orange-red
rifampin (Rifadin)
phenazopyridine HC1 (Pyridium)
warfarin sodium (Coumadin)

Pink-red
chlorpromazine (Thorazine)
other phenothiazines
phenolphthalein (Ex-Lax)
phenytoin (Dilantin)

Brown-black
nitrofurantoin (Furadantin)
methyldopa (Aldomet)
metronidazole (Flagyl)

Urinary Diversions

When the urinary bladder is removed because of trauma, disease or congenital anomalies, a new route for urinary elimination must be created. An artificial opening or **stoma** is made to divert urine from the kidneys to the abdominal wall. This opening is called a urinary ostomy or **urostomy**. There are a variety of urinary diversion procedures; however, the most common are the ileal conduit and the continent urostomy. The **ileal conduit** consists of a reservoir, constructed from a portion of the ileum, and a stoma (see Figure 21.3A). The ureters are attached to the reservoir. Urine drains continuously from the ileal conduit; thus, it is an *incontinent* diversion. The individual must wear an external collection bag or appliance to collect the urine.

The **continent urostomy** is a type of ileal conduit that functions similarly to a real bladder. In addition to the formation of an internal pouch, two nipple valves are constructed by intussuscepting sections of bowel. One valve

RESEARCH to practice

Jackson, B., & Hicks, L.E. (1997). Effect of cranberry juice on urinary pH in older adults. *Home Healthcare Nurse, 15*(3), 199–202.

Research suggests that consumption of cranberry juice may be helpful in preventing urinary tract infections. However, much of the research has focussed on the consumption of large amounts of concentrated cranberry juice in well individuals. Although urinary tract infections are a frequent cause of illness and hospitalization, little research has been conducted in this population group.

Twenty-one men aged 65 and older, who resided in one unit of a veterans' nursing home, were deemed eligible for this study. All subjects had a history of UTIs or were at risk for UTIs. Most subjects were Caucasian, with a mean age of 73. Urine specimens were collected by voiding or via external urinary devices.

Study design was a double crossover in which the subjects served as their own controls. There were three phases to the procedure: four weeks with no cranberry juice, four weeks with cranberry juice and four weeks again with no consumption of cranberry juice. During the four weeks of cranberry juice consumption, each subject ingested two packaged servings (118.3 mL each) of 25 percent cranberry juice at each meal. A first-voided morning specimen was obtained for 12 specimens from each subject. Specimens obtained from a urinary device were done within one hour of the subject's voiding. The pH was measured immediately by a Corning 106 pH meter, which has an accuracy of +0.01 pH units, and recordings were made to the nearest 10th unit. Calibration of the pH meter was checked at the beginning and once during the duration of the study.

The three analyses yielded no statistical significance. However, urinary pH during the juice consumption period was lower than during the nonjuice periods.

This study supports other research findings that cranberry juice does decrease urinary pH, although it is unclear what level of urinary acidity is needed to affect the frequency of UTIs in the elderly. Based on the findings of this study and others, the consumption of cranberry juice is an intervention that may be used to decrease the risk of UTIs in the elderly.

(inlet valve) prevents urine from flowing back into the ureters, thus reducing the risk of ascending infection. The second valve (outlet valve) prevents urine from flowing from the stoma, thus maintaining continence. Urine is stored in the pouch until it is emptied by means of a catheter passed through the stoma. An external collection appliance is not necessary. Two common types of continent urostomies are the Kock's pouch and the Indiana pouch. In a Kock's pouch, both reservoir and stoma are created from ileum. In an Indiana pouch, the stoma is made from ileum and a larger reservoir is constructed from ileum, ascending colon and cecum (see Figure 21.3B).

Living with a urostomy is a lifelong challenge. Individuals must deal with alterations in body image and learn to manage a stoma. Those with incontinent diversions have to care for an external appliance, and those with continent diversions have to pass a catheter regularly to drain the internal pouch. Nurses in the community and in inpatient facilities may need to assist people with urinary diversions to meet their elimination needs.

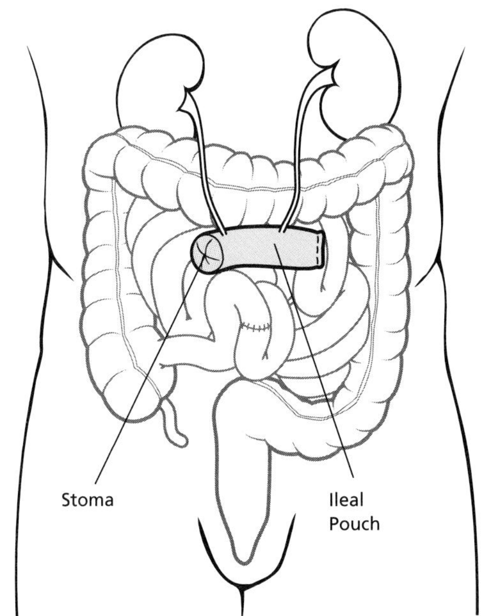

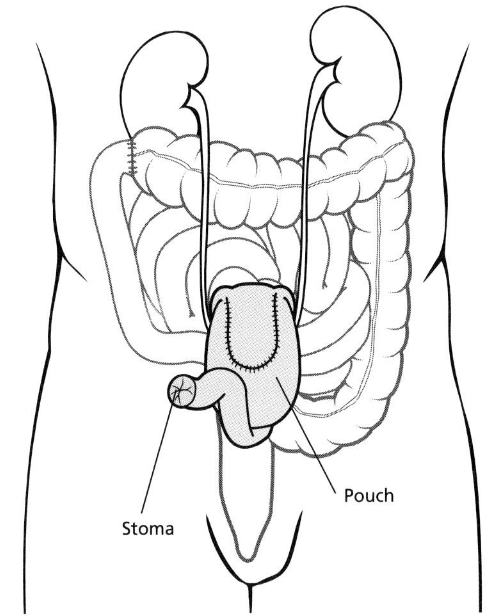

FIGURE 21.3 A. Ileal conduit or Kock's pouch B. Indiana pouch

Assessing Urinary Elimination Needs

The assessment of an individual's urinary status involves the collection of data from all sources. The nursing health history and physical assessment provide the basis for planning individualized care. Information about the nature of the patient's health problem, past and current medical history, and the physician's diagnostic and therapeutic plans of care for the patient will be found in the medical record. Data from diagnostic tests or examinations such as blood work, urinalysis, x-rays, scans, biopsies or cystoscopy will add valuable information to the data base.

The Nursing Health History

In taking a nursing health history pertaining to urinary elimination the nurse questions patients (or a family member) about their usual patterns of voiding, their ability to toilet themselves, urinary control and any aids required in elimination (urinals, bedpans, commodes). The nurse asks about recent changes in patterns of elimination and the nature, onset and severity of symptoms. The presence of urinary diversions and, if these are present, the patient's usual routines, are determined at this time. Factors that may influence the elimination pattern are also considered. This includes, for example, the patient's age, usual food and fluid intake and any disturbances currently being experienced (such as nausea and vomiting).

In many cultures, the subject of elimination is surrounded by social taboos. Once toilet trained, children are taught that this is not a topic for general conversation. The act of urinary elimination usually takes place in private. Further, the intimate anatomical relationship between the urinary and the reproductive tracts contributes to making urinary functioning a sensitive topic. As a result, individuals often have difficulty in discussing urinary functions and any related problems. The nurse can set the patient at ease with a sensitive but matter-of-fact approach. A private, quiet area for discussion may minimize feelings of embarrassment. A guide for obtaining a urinary elimination health history follows.

Physical Assessment

The nurse uses physical assessment skills to obtain objective data. Observation of the characteristics of the patient's urine (colour, odour, consistency, amount and the presence of abnormal constituents) should be compared against normal values. Careful notation of the patient's fluid intake and output should be related to observations of the patient's voiding pattern and the characteristics of the urine.

Examination of the patient's abdomen may reveal kidney tenderness, bladder distention or the presence of a urinary ostomy. For this, the patient is placed in the dorsal recumbent position and draped appropriately. The nurse begins by inspecting the abdomen for skin colour, contour, symmetry and the presence of scars or urinary stomas. Light palpation or percussion over the costovertebral angle (where the 12th rib joins the spine) or flank region may reveal kidney tenderness. Palpation just above the symphysis pubis can determine the presence of bladder distention. If the bladder is distended, the nurse will feel a firm roundness, and the patient may express the desire to void when pressure is applied. As well, percussion with the fingers over this area will cause a dull sound when the bladder is full.

In addition, the nurse should be alert to manifestations of localized and generalized problems in relation to urinary dysfunction, as described in the preceding section. Assessment and recording of pertinent observations is a primary responsibility of the nurse in caring for patients with urinary tract dysfunction. The early detection of edema, changes in skin pigmentation and signs of central nervous system or neuromuscular dysfunction can contribute to the plan of care for the patient.

Measurements

Exact measurement of fluid intake and output is necessary in monitoring patients with urinary dysfunction. Detailed guidelines for measuring fluid intake and output will be found in Chapter 23. Measurements are recorded in millilitres and documented on a fluid balance record on the patient's chart. In extreme cases, it may also be necessary to record the amount of fluid ingested as a part of the patient's food, and the amount lost in perspiration and feces.

For accurate measurement of fluids, the nurse should drain larger collecting containers into a smaller, calibrated container. Placement of this smaller container at eye level on a flat surface allows the nurse to gauge the contents accurately against the calibration. Care must be taken at all times when handling urine and other body fluids. Gloves must be worn and care taken to avoid splashing.

Diagnostic Tests

In order to diagnose and evaluate urinary function, patients may undergo a variety of tests and examinations. These include urine tests such as urinalysis, dipstick examination and culture and sensitivity, as well as diagnostic procedures such as cystoscopy and x-ray examination.

URINE TESTS

URINALYSIS The routine **urinalysis** is probably the most common test available. For this examination, a sterile specimen of urine is not required. The patient is asked to void into a clean container, bedpan or urinal. A small amount of urine (5–10 mL is considered sufficient) is then transferred into a clean test tube, labelled and sent to the laboratory with its accompanying requisition. Some hospitals no longer have hard-copy requisitions, as all lab requests are done using computerized information management systems. Normal urinalysis values are outlined in Table 21.1.

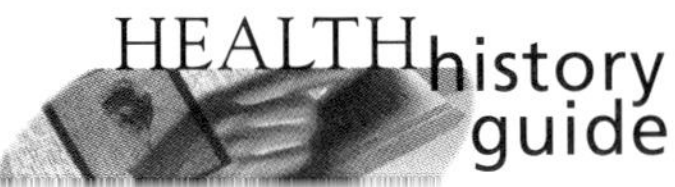

Urinary Elimination

Health and Illness Patterns

Usual Pattern of Urinary Elimination

- How often do you urinate? How many times in a day?
- Describe the usual amount, colour and odour of your urine.
- Do you often awaken in the night to void? How many times a night?
- Do you have any difficulties with toiletting? If so, describe them.
- What assistance will you require while in hospital? Assistance walking to the bathroom? Commode? Bedpan? Urinal?

For patients with urinary diversions:

- What type of urostomy do you have?
- What is your usual urostomy routine?
- Have you had any problems with your urostomy, e.g., skin irritation?
- What assistance will you need managing your urostomy?

For patients with long-term catheters:

- What is your usual catheter routine?
- Do you have any problems with your catheter?
- What assistance will you need managing your catheter?

Recent Changes in Pattern of Urinary Elimination

- Have you noticed any change in your normal pattern of elimination or urine characteristics? If so, describe the changes.
- Have there been any recent changes in your life that may be affecting your normal pattern? Recent illness? Medication use? Surgery? Stressful events?

Presenting Health Problem

- Describe the symptoms you are experiencing now. Frequent small amounts of urine? Large amounts of urine? Urgency? Painful voiding? Bleeding? Dribbling of urine? Passing urine when you cough, sneeze or laugh? Trouble starting or maintaining a urinary stream? Post-void dribbling? The need to strain for urination? Bladder fullness awareness? Childhood enuresis? Ability to defer voiding?
- How long have you had these symptoms?
- What remedies have you tried, if any, for the symptoms? What were the results?
- Do you have a history of acute or chronic conditions that might disrupt urinary elimination? For example, heart disease, high blood pressure, diabetes, multiple sclerosis?
- Have you had urinary tract problems in the past? Infections? Kidney stones? Surgery to the urinary or reproductive tracts?
- Are you taking any medications (prescription and over-the-counter) that could affect urinary function, for example, diuretics, antihistamines, anticholinergics, antihypertensives? Dosage of medications?

Health Promotion and Protection Patterns

- How much and what types of fluid do you drink in a day?
- Do you drink alcohol and products containing caffeine? How much and how often?
- Do you smoke? If so, how much and for how many years?

TABLE 21.1 Normal urinalysis values

General Characteristics and Measurements	*Chemical Determinations*	*Microscopic Examination of Sediment*
Appearance: clear to faintly hazy	Glucose: negative	Casts: moderate clear protein casts
Specific gravity: 1.003–1.030	Ketones: negative	Red blood cells: ≤ 3 cells/HPF
pH: 4.5–8.0	Blood: negative	Crystals: small amount
Colour: yellow	Protein: negative	White blood cells: ≤ 4 cells/HPF
Odour: faint	Bilirubin: negative	Epithelial cells: ≤ 10 cells/HPF
	Urobilinogen: negative or 0.1–1.0 Ehrlich U/dL	Bacteria/fungi: none or < 1000/mL
	Nitrate for bacteria: negative	Parasites: none
	Albumin: negative	

HPF = high-power field

SOURCE: Chernecky & Berger, 1997, p. 148.

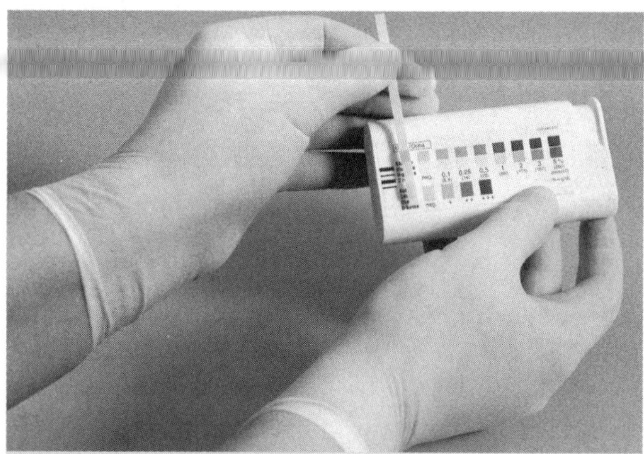

A dipstick is dipped in urine and then held against a colour chart to obtain test results.

DIPSTICK EXAMINATIONS In some cases, the nurse may be asked to perform a test on urine by means of a dipstick. This procedure provides a quick method of determining such aspects as pH, sugar, protein, ketones and the presence of blood in urine. Dipsticks or reagent strips are impregnated with chemicals that react with specific substances in the urine, producing colour changes. Results are obtained by matching colour changes on the dipstick to colour charts usually on the container. A dipstick test is performed on a clean, fresh urine specimen. The tip of the reagent stick is placed into the specimen and, after a specified period of time, the colour changes are compared with the colour chart.

URINE CULTURES Normally, urine is sterile; it does, however, provide an excellent growth medium for those bacteria that invade the urinary tract. Urine samples are cultured to determine the presence of pathogenic organisms. Whenever possible, specimens for culture should be obtained from the first urine voided in the morning, as bacterial counts will be highest at that time. A clean voided midstream specimen of three to five millilitres is generally sufficient; however, specimens may also be collected by catheterization or from an indwelling catheter. Owing to the risk of introducing bacteria into the urinary tract, collection of urine for culture by catheterization should be avoided if at all possible (Chernecky & Berger, 1997).

To obtain a midstream specimen from a male patient, it is necessary to cleanse the urinary meatus with an antiseptic solution. The patient next voids some urine (which is discarded), stops the stream and then voids into a sterile container. Obtaining a midstream specimen from a female patient is somewhat more difficult. The labia and vestibule should be thoroughly cleansed with soap and water or antiseptic solution. If soap is used, it must be rinsed off thoroughly. Holding the labia apart, the patient then voids. The first part of the stream is discarded, the midstream specimen is caught in a sterile container and the remainder of the urine is discarded. The specimen should be sent to the laboratory for immediate processing; otherwise it must be stored at 4°C until processing is possible.

When possible, most patients prefer to do this procedure themselves. A thorough explanation of the procedure will ensure proper collection of the specimen. The nurse can assist in collecting the midstream specimen by positioning the patient on a bedpan or the bedside commode. In this instance, the nurse dons clean gloves, cleanses the patient as above and collects the middle of the stream as the patient voids.

24-HOUR SPECIMENS For some tests a 24-hour sample of urine is required. The first urine voided in the morning is usually discarded and collection begins with the next voiding. All urine voided during the subsequent 24 hours is collected, including the first urine of the following morning. The urine is collected in one large, clean container. Urine must be stored according to agency protocol for the test being performed. Occasionally, this requires that the urine be kept refrigerated. For catheterized patients, keep the drainage bag on ice and empty it into the refrigerated container every hour. With proper preparation, ambulatory patients are often responsible for collecting their own urine. If necessary, a sign may be posted above the patient's bed or in the bathroom as a reminder to staff, family and the patient that a 24-hour urine collection is in progress.

BLOOD STUDIES

Blood tests can provide valuable information about the kidneys' ability to filter, absorb and excrete needed substances. The kidneys also have a role in regulating the composition and volume of body fluids. Some blood chemistry values increase in renal failure, while others decrease (see Table 21.2).

SERUM CREATININE Serum creatinine levels reflect the glomerular filtration rate (GFR) of the kidneys. Creatinine is a catabolic by-product of creatine, which is necessary for skeletal muscle contraction. Creatinine is excreted via the kidneys; therefore, an increase in this level indicates decreased renal function. Creatinine is not affected by dietary or fluid intake, and thus is a more specific measure of renal function. As a rule, a normal serum creatinine level

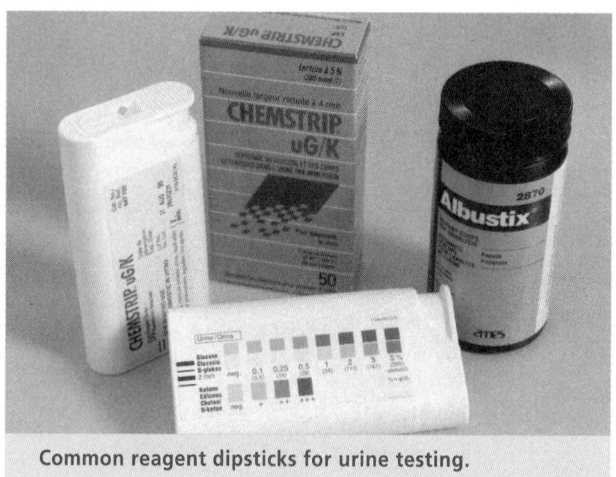

Common reagent dipsticks for urine testing.

indicates normal kidney function. An increase in serum creatinine indicates a loss of nephrons. A serum creatinine level three times the normal value indicates a 75 percent loss

800μmol/L (10 mg/dL) or greater indicate renal function loss of up to 90 percent.

BLOOD UREA NITROGEN (BUN) Urea formed in the liver is the end-product of protein metabolism and is excreted by the kidneys. Urea is normally filtered through the renal glomeruli, but unlike creatinine, it is affected by protein intake, hepatic function and dehydration. Therefore, this value must be evaluated carefully. A rise in BUN will be seen when the glomerular filtration rate drops below 40–60 percent.

BUN is less specific than creatinine for renal insufficiency. However, the BUN-creatinine ratio can provide important diagnostic information. The ratio is normally 10:1. Elevations in the BUN value indicate prerenal causes, such as gastrointestinal bleeding or congestive heart failure, which result in increased values for BUN but not for creatinine (Porth, 1998).

DIAGNOSTIC PROCEDURES

There are many examinations of the urinary tract that facilitate diagnosis of urinary tract dysfunction. A **cystoscopy** is the examination of a patient's bladder with a lighted instrument inserted through the urethra. The physician can visualize the interior of the bladder, obtain a biopsy specimen and perform therapeutic treatments. This procedure is done under a local or general anesthetic in the operating room or in day surgery. The *intravenous* **pyelogram** (IVP) and *retrograde pyelogram* are radiological procedures that outline the pelvis, calices, ureters and urinary bladder by means of a contrast medium. Patients may also undergo more definitive radiological testing, such as ultrasonography and computerized tomography (CT) scanning (Chernecky & Berger, 1997). These procedures are described in Chapter 16.

TABLE 21.2 Normal blood chemistry values

Test	*Normal Values* SI UNITS (CONVENTIONAL UNITS)
Blood urea nitrogen	1.8–7.1 mmol/L (5–20 mg/dL)
Creatinine	53–106 μmol/L (0.6–1.2 mg/dL)
Sodium	136–145 mmol/L (136–145 mEq/L)
Chloride	96–107 mmol/L (97–107 mEq/L)
Potassium	3.5–5.3 mmol/L (3.5–5.3 mEq/L)
Carbon dioxide (CO_2)	20–30 mmol/L (22–30mEq/L)
Calcium	2.15–2.5 mmol/L (8.6–10.0 mg/dL)
Phosphorus	0.87–1.45 mmol/L (2.7–4.5 mg/dL)
Uric acid	143–414 μmol/L (2.4–7.0 mg/dL)
pH	7.35–7.45

SOURCE: Chernecky & Berger, 1997.

The nurse is responsible for preparing the patient for any diagnostic procedure. This can involve physical preparation of the patient, such as evacuation of the bowels. It also

nation of the procedure to be performed and administration of any preprocedure medication. Patient anxiety is thus diminished and patient participation throughout the procedure is achieved.

Diagnosing Urinary Elimination Problems

Urinary elimination problems that can be treated by independent nursing intervention may be generally stated as: *Altered Pattern of Urinary Elimination*. According to Carpenito, this diagnostic statement is too broad for use in clinical practice and should be applied when the etiologic or contributing factors for incontinence have not been identified (1997). When the etiology of incontinence is known, the diagnostic statement should identify the specific nature of the problem. For example, in a woman who has recently had a baby and is now experiencing leakage of small amounts of urine whenever she sneezes, coughs or laughs, the nursing diagnosis would be: *Stress Incontinence related to weakened pelvic floor muscles secondary to childbirth*. NANDA categorizes the types of incontinence as functional, reflex, stress, total and urge incontinence:

- *Functional incontinence*: The state in which an individual experiences difficulty or inability to reach the toilet in time due to urgency, environmental barriers, decreased attention to the urge to void or physical limitations. Example: An elderly person who cannot get to the bathroom in time because of side rails on the bed or because the bathroom is too far away.
- *Reflex incontinence*: The state in which an individual experiences an involuntary loss of urine caused by damage to the spinal cord between the cortical and sacral (S2, S3, S4) bladder centres. Example: A person with a spinal cord injury who has lost voluntary control of micturition.
- *Stress incontinence*: The state in which an individual experiences an immediate involuntary loss of urine upon an increase in intra-abdominal pressure. Example: As above.
- *Total incontinence*: The state in which an individual experiences continuous, unpredictable loss of urine. Example: A confused individual who is not aware of the urge to void.
- *Urge incontinence*: The state in which an individual experiences involuntary loss of urine associated with a strong, sudden desire to void. Example: A person who experiences urgency with incontinence following a cystoscopy (Carpenito, 1997).

Urinary Retention is a diagnostic label used to identify problems in which the individual experiences inability to void, followed by involuntary voiding. Bladder distention will be present and the individual may dribble or void small, frequent amounts and may verbalize the feeling that the bladder is not empty after voiding. This problem occurs frequently following surgery due to the effect of anesthesia or surgical manipulation of tissues proximal to the bladder, as, for example, in prostate surgery. It may also result from drug therapy with antihistamines such as cyclizine (used for motion sickness), adrenergics (sympathetic stimulants) such as epinephrine or isoproterenol or anticholinergics (parasympathetic depressants) such as atropine or propantheline.

Problems with urinary elimination often cause difficulties in other areas of functioning. For example, urinary incontinence may lead to impaired skin integrity. Urinary incontinence may also cause disturbance in self-esteem. A perceived loss of independence and control over the act of micturition may be demoralizing to the individual and, in addition, may lead to ineffective individual coping capacity. Individuals with urinary ostomy diversions may experience a body image disturbance and will initially have a knowledge deficit in self-management of the urinary diversion ostomy. Following are examples of common nursing diagnoses pertaining to urinary elimination problems:

- *Altered Pattern of Urinary Elimination related to unknown etiology as evidenced by incontinence.*
- *Functional Incontinence related to avoidance of the urge to void and mobility deficit secondary to arthritis.*
- *Risk for Urinary Retention related to spinal anesthesia and bladder trauma secondary to pelvic surgery.*
- *Low Self-Esteem related to incontinence.*

Planning Urinary Elimination Interventions

A plan of care for individuals with urinary elimination problems is based on the nursing diagnoses and takes into account each person's elimination patterns and toiletting practices. Patient goals focus on understanding normal urinary elimination, maintaining or restoring normal urinary elimination patterns, preventing associated problems such as skin breakdown and infection and promoting healthy urinary functioning in daily living. Specific goals or expected outcomes are established for each nursing diagnosis. Some examples of expected outcomes include:

- The patient will explain the cause of incontinence and the measures to promote continence.
- The patient will remain continent during the night.
- The patient will remain free of infection from the indwelling catheter.
- The patient will describe the exercises to strengthen pelvic floor muscles.
- The patient will demonstrate self-care for an indwelling catheter.

The successful achievement of patient goals depends on the patient's state of health, his or her ability to participate in care, and the resources available to the patient. Regaining continence, for example, is a learning process that requires maximum participation of the individual and full support of the family and all health professionals. The process takes time—often weeks and even months—and frustration from lapses of incontinence is not unusual. Goals should be stated as short-term steps towards long-term achievement. They should be set mutually with the patient (and family) and reflect levels of performance the patient is realistically capable of achieving. Learning begins in hospital but continues once the person is at home. Thus, planning should also include referrals to appropriate home care services.

Implementing Urinary Elimination Interventions

Health-Promoting Strategies

The urinary tract provides an effective mechanism for eliminating nitrogenous wastes of cellular metabolism and maintaining fluid, electrolyte and acid–base balance in the body. Adequate fluid intake, emptying the bladder when the urge arises, proper hygiene and strong perineal muscle tone will foster healthy urinary functioning in daily living. Nurses can help individuals promote optimal urinary elimination by providing information and encouraging them to examine their urinary patterns and toiletting practices.

Urinary incontinence and retention are symptoms that, with appropriate intervention by a health professional, should improve. Treatment options can be pharmacological, behavioural and/or surgical. In this section we will discuss behavioural management.

DETERMINING TRANSIENT OR PERSISTENT INCONTINENCE

It must be determined whether the urinary incontinence is transient or persistent. Transient incontinence is reversible and can be identified using the acronym DIAPPERS (delirium; infection; atrophic urethritis/vaginitis; psychological [depression]; pharmaceutical [drug side effect]; endocrine; restricted mobility; stool impaction). Management of these factors should potentially reverse the patient's symptoms.

Types of Incontinence

- stress (urethral sphincter incompetence)
- urge (detrusor instability)
- reflex, overflow or functional.

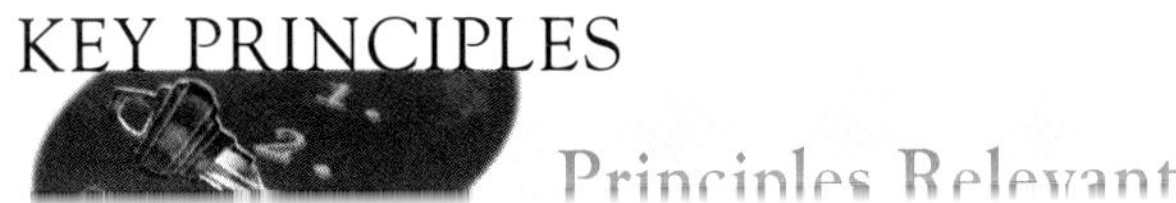

Principles Relevant to Urinary Elimination

1. Most of the nitrogenous wastes of cellular metabolism are eliminated by the kidneys.
2. The kidneys play an important role in maintaining the fluid and electrolyte balance of the body.
3. The suppression of urine formation in the kidneys threatens the life of an individual.
4. The kidneys normally mature to full functioning ability by two years of age.
5. The necessary neuromuscular structures for voluntary control of voiding are not usually sufficiently developed until the age of two to three years.
6. Loss of voluntary control over voiding can be a serious threat to an individual's self-esteem.
7. The average adult voids 1000–1500 mL of urine in a 24-hour period; the average school-age child voids up to 1000 mL in 24 hours.
8. Awareness of the need to void normally occurs in the adult when the bladder contains 200–300 mL of urine.
9. The lining of the urinary tract consists of a continuous layer of mucous membrane.
10. The intimate anatomical relationship between the urinary and reproductive tracts makes urinary functioning a sensitive topic for most people.
11. The location of the urinary meatus in proximity to the anus and to the external sex organs makes the urinary tract vulnerable to infection from these sources.
12. Urinary output of less than 30 mL/h (720 mL in a 24-hour period) is considered inadequate for adults.

Evaluation Techniques

MANUAL PELVIC MUSCLE ASSESSMENT The pelvic floor musculature can be evaluated by manual assessment of the vagina or rectum, by perineometer or by using the functional stop test. A specially trained health professional can determine the pelvic floor contraction strength by inserting a gloved index finger into the patient's vagina or rectum and asking the patient to contract the pelvic floor musculature around the finger. The assessor then categorizes what is felt using the Laycock (1989) scale: 0 = nil contraction, 1 = flicker, 2 = weak, 3 = moderate, 4 = good, 5 = strong. Also needed is the measurement of duration of contraction in seconds. For example, a grading of 2–7 would indicate a grade 2 (weak) squeeze held for seven seconds. Repetitions of contraction are also noted.

PERINEOMETER The perineometer is a pressure-sensing device that is inserted into the vagina to provide numeric dial readings of pelvic floor contractions. The readings can be influenced by changes in the patient's position and intra-abdominal pressure, so reliability is somewhat uncertain.

Causes of Persistent Urinary Incontinence

[illegible] multiple infections or surgeries

2. prolapse of the bladder or uterus due to damage of supporting structures or associated with uterine descent
3. atrophy associated with reduced estrogen and aging, which attacks the elastic and adhesive factors of the urethral wall
4. obstruction of the urethra, e.g., prostate enlargement
5. irritability and hypersensitivity of the bladder
6. musculoskeletal weakness of the pelvic floor structures. This can be the result of trauma to the muscles, nerve supply or adjacent tissues, e.g., difficult or multiple childbirths; fatigue or stretching from overuse, such as repeated coughing, straining at stool due to constipation or heavy lifting; functional underuse, e.g., in the elderly or the disabled
7. psychological problems, e.g., depression, anxiety
8. neuromuscular conditions that interfere with sensory and motor impulses involved in voluntary control of voiding, e.g., Parkinson's disease, multiple sclerosis
9. medical conditions such as diabetes or cerebral vascular accidents
10. trauma to the body involving or affecting the micturition process, e.g., falls or motor vehicle accidents.

FUNCTIONAL MIDSTREAM STOP ASSESSMENT A functional midstream stop test of the pelvic floor musculature is a means by which patients themselves can determine and approximate muscle grade strength of the pelvic floor musculature. This is an evaluation tool only; it should not be performed as an exercise because of the possibility of disturbing the normal micturition reflexes. This test should be done only twice a month. The patient sits on a toilet and, after urinating for five seconds, attempts to stop the flow of urine. The urine flow is graded as follows:

- grade 0 = unable to deflect or slow the urine flow
- grade 1 = partial deflection of the urine flow that cannot be maintained
- grade 2 = maintenance of a deflection of urine flow
- grade 3 = ability to stop the urine flow completely.

CONTINENCE DIARY

After the history and assessment, a treatment program in conjunction with pelvic floor re-education is determined. A well-documented continence diary should be kept for a few days. This allows for interpretation of a regular pattern in the patient's environment. The patient will usually record the fluid input and output; the number of voids and accidents, and the occasion of accidents; and the minimum and maximum time between voids. Over time, the results of the initial and subsequent diaries can be compared to ascertain progress.

DIETARY MANAGEMENT

Since limiting fluid intake as a means of controlling incontinence is common, the nurse should explain the body's physiological requirements for fluids. With less fluid intake, the more highly concentrated urine may irritate the detrusor (bladder), necessitating more frequent voiding. Concentrated urine can encourage bacterial growth, resulting in cystitis. The provision of fluids at regular intervals helps to ensure adequate intake of 1500–2000 mL/day. If the patient is not drinking the required fluid intake, fluids should be introduced gradually over a period of days to avoid overloading the urinary system. Caffeinated and decaffeinated beverages, alcohol and acidic juices and fruits act as irritants or stimulants to the smooth muscle of the bladder and are therefore discouraged. Water and nonacidic fruit juices are recommended.

PELVIC FLOOR STRENGTHENING EXERCISES

The pelvic floor consists of the visceral pelvic fascia and pelvic diaphragm, the urogenital anal triangles with superficial and deep genital muscles, and the urethral and anal sphincters. The pelvic floor can be divided into three levels. The multilayered pelvic floor structure spans from the pubic bone to the coccyx. Supportive ligaments and endopelvic tissue from the urethra, bladder, vagina, uterus, fallopian tubes, ovaries, rectum and colon attach to the pelvic bones to add stability.

Both muscle fibre types are found in the pelvic floor muscles. *Slow-twitch muscle fibres* maintain tone and support to the pelvic organs. *Fast-twitch muscle fibres* enable the urethral sphincters to close quickly. The ability of the pelvic floor to resist sudden rises in intra-abdominal pressure is critical in preventing incontinence. Suppressing the urge to void depends particularly on the reflex control of the pelvic floor.

Pelvic floor exercises, also called **Kegel exercises**, are beneficial for strengthening perineal muscle tone (especially the pubococcygeal muscle) and preventing stress urinary incontinence in both men and women. These exercises consist of repetitive contraction and relaxation of the perineal muscles. The individual is instructed to squeeze the perineal muscles as if trying to stop the flow of urine and tighten the muscles around the anus, then hold to the count of five and release. The person will feel the pelvic floor rise during tightening of the muscles. At least five contraction–relaxation cycles should be performed during a set, and the sets repeated several times a day. Pelvic floor exercises can be performed while lying down, sitting or standing, anywhere and anytime during the day. Procedures 21.1 and 21.2 describe two approaches to teaching pelvic floor exercises.

Protection

When undertaking a continence program that includes pelvic floor strengthening exercises, some protection against incontinence may be necessary. Protection pads made for incontinence are constructed to absorb urine and are more absorbent compared with pads made to absorb blood (which is more viscous). There is a wide variety of incontinence pads—either disposable or made of washable material—for children and adults of both genders. As patients' incontinence improves, they are encouraged to reduce the thickness of the pad and the amount of wearing time. Do not discourage the use of adequate protection.

SKIN CARE AND ODOUR CONCERNS The perineal skin should be washed with warm water or an incontinence cleanser daily. Incontinence cleansers require no subsequent rinsing, which enables their use in home, hospital, office or while travelling. Some products cleanse, moisturize and protect all in one step. The skin should be kept as dry as possible; therefore, the pad or protective undergarment should be changed after every incontinent episode and the skin cleansed.

BIOFEEDBACK

A treatment program that combines pelvic floor exercises and biofeedback is effective in reducing incontinence. Either external patch electrodes or anal and vaginal sensors are used to provide immediate feedback regarding muscle performance. Another patch electrode over the abdominal muscles will give feedback regarding their auxiliary use when a pelvic floor contraction is performed. The goal is to isolate the pelvic floor contractions and eliminate any abdominal activity.

Health-Protecting Strategies

Maintenance of adequate urinary elimination is important to physiological functioning. When people are ill or in hospital their voiding habits may be disrupted and they may need assistance maintaining normal patterns.

MAINTAINING NORMAL URINARY ELIMINATION

The best way to maintain normal urinary patterns is to void at regular times and when the urge is felt. Adequate fluid intake helps to maintain regularity. Patients who are ambulatory can generally attend to their elimination needs by using bathroom facilities. This is most desirable both physiologically and psychologically—psychologically, because the patient can void in private and physiologically, because the patient can assume the natural positions for micturition. For women, voiding is facilitated in a sitting or squatting position. Men void more effectively in the standing position. If they cannot ambulate to the bathroom, women may find it easier to void using a bedside commode rather than a bedpan. Male patients find it easier to stand at the side of the

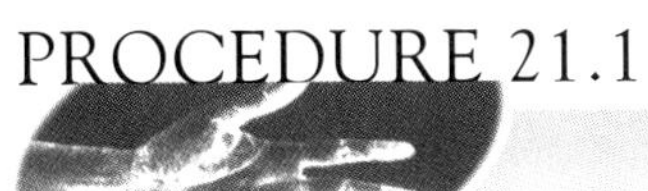

PROCEDURE 21.1 Teaching Pelvic Floor Exercises

Action	Rationale
1. Assess patient's readiness to learn and prepare the patient for teaching.	Reduces anxiety, enables patient participation and increases effectiveness of learning.
2. Provide privacy.	Decreases anxiety and embarrassment; attends to modesty and sexuality issues.
3. Begin by having patient lying supine in a comfortable position with knees bent and apart, feet flat on the surface.	Promotes identification of the correct muscles. Once the muscles have been located, the exercises can be done anywhere and at any time (sitting, lying, standing).
4. Identify the pelvic floor muscles by performing a vaginal/rectal examination and requesting the patient squeeze a gloved, lubricated finger. (The patient can also do a self-examination.)	Promotes awareness of when correct muscles are contracted and discourages contractions of auxiliary substitution of muscles such as abdominal, gluteal or hip adductor muscles.
5. Give verbal instructions to breathe in and out a few times to relax, then have patient contract the pelvic floor muscles by lifting or drawing up and in from the anal sphincter (the back passage), and then forward in the perineum to the urethra (the front passage). Ask the patient to squeeze the muscles as though to stop the flow of urine.	Relaxation prevents breath-holding. Exercising the correct muscles increases muscle strength and coordination, assists in controlling urinary continence and promotes sexual functioning.
6. Inform the patient that both prolonged-hold and quick-contraction exercises should be included.	Strengthens slow-twitch muscle fibres.
a) for the long-duration exercise, have the patient contract for 5–10 seconds, then relax completely and breathe normally for 10 seconds. Repeat 5–10 times, progressing to 15 times. Rest for 1 minute before doing the following "quick" exercise set.	Pelvic floor muscles fatigue easily. Complete relaxation of the pelvic floor is required for normal urination.
b) for strengthening the rapid-response muscles, have the patient contract the muscles for 1 second and relax completely for 1 second. Repeat this cycle 5–10 times, followed by a 10-second rest. Repeat 5–10 times, progressing to 15 times.	Strengthens fast-twitch muscle fibres. Progression should be gradual over several weeks or months.
7. Emphasize importance of performing both these exercises 4–6 times a day.	Success of the Kegel exercises depends on proper technique and adherence to a regular exercise program.

— Based on exercises prepared by Jackie Wells, Physiotherapist, Continence Clinic, Vancouver General Hospital

bed when using a urinal. When patients need assistance with urinary elimination, prompt attention to their call for help is essential to avoid delaying the micturition reflex. In addition, teaching and encouraging patients to perform Kegel exercises will promote bladder emptying.

ASSISTING THE PATIENT WITH A BEDPAN OR URINAL

Patients who are confined to bed must use the bedpan or the urinal for elimination. Female patients use the bedpan for both urination and defecation; the male patient needs the bedpan for defecation and the urinal for voiding. Having to use these utensils is embarrassing for many people. Thus, the nurse must ensure the patient's privacy, avoid unnecessary exposure of body parts and make the procedure as safe and as comfortable as possible for the patient, both physically and psychologically.

To ensure privacy, the curtains are drawn around the patient's unit, or the door of a private room closed. The nurse assesses the patient's need for assistance. If the patient can use the bedpan or urinal independently, the nurse ensures that these utensils and the call bell are within easy reach. The patient who needs help is assisted onto the bedpan as described in Chapter 22. Assisting the male patient with a urinal will be described later in this section. The nurse remains available just outside the patient's unit or room to provide help as necessary.

Generally, men do not require cleansing following urination, other than provision of the means for washing their hands (although Hindus, Sikhs and Muslims customarily wash their genitals, preferably with running water).

PROCEDURE 21.2 Teaching the Use of Vaginal Cones

Some women may use vaginal cones to strengthen the muscles of the pelvic floor. Vaginal cones consist of five to nine equal-sized cones that weigh 10–100 g. One cone at a time is used. They facilitate the correct pelvic muscle contraction in order to retain the vaginal cone. As the pelvic musculature increases in strength, the incontinence decreases.

Action	Rationale
1. Assess the pelvic muscles for suitability of using pelvic cones.	Prevents purchase of the cones by women who have very weak pelvic muscles or overstretched vaginas, and who cannot retain even the lightest cones.
2. Insert one cone into the vagina, beginning with the heaviest weight that can be retained for one minute while walking around.	Facilitates choice of the correct weight cone for pelvic muscle contraction that will retain the cone.
3. Gradually increase the time period of cone retention to 15 min. Do not extend time period beyond 15 min.	Indicates strengthening of the pelvic musculature. Avoids the development of chronic muscle-holding patterns.
4. When the cone does not slip during the 15 min, the patient chooses the next heaviest cone.	Progressively strengthens the pelvic floor muscles.
5. Repeat these exercises twice a day.	Ensures success of these exercises with adherence to a regular exercise program.

Female patients may require assistance in cleansing the perineal area following urination.

As in all other contact with patients, the nurse must remember to use body substance precautions (these are described in detail in Chapter 32). Hands must be washed before and after assisting patients, and clean gloves worn when handling urine and feces or when providing perineal care following urination.

The nurse assesses the amount and characteristics of the urine prior to disposal in the toilet or hopper. Cleaning of the bedpan is outlined in Chapter 32. If the patient requires intake and output measurements, the amount is documented on the patient's record.

In most institutions, separate bedpans and urinals are available for each patient. These are usually stored in the bedside locker. Once the patient is discharged from the hospital, these utensils are returned to the central supply department for sterilization.

USING A URINAL The male urinal is designed to fit over the patient's penis so that urine can be excreted without spillage. It has a handle for convenience (specially designed urinals are available for patients who have the use of only one hand) and is usually flat on either one side or the bottom so that it can be set down after use without spilling the contents. Some agencies provide a bag for storing the urinal at the patient's bedside.

The patient can use a urinal in the supine position, the lateral position (either side) or Fowler's position, or when standing at the side of the bed. Most patients prefer to use the urinal without help. If help is needed, however, the nurse separates the patient's legs sufficiently to allow placement of the urinal between them. Then, holding the urinal with one hand, the nurse inserts the penis into the urinal far enough to prevent urine from spilling onto the bedclothes or the patient's skin. If necessary, the nurse holds the urinal in place until the patient has finished voiding.

Although not common, urinals for use by female patients are available. These are similar in design to the male urinal, but with a long, wide top, shaped like a spout (Figure 21.4).

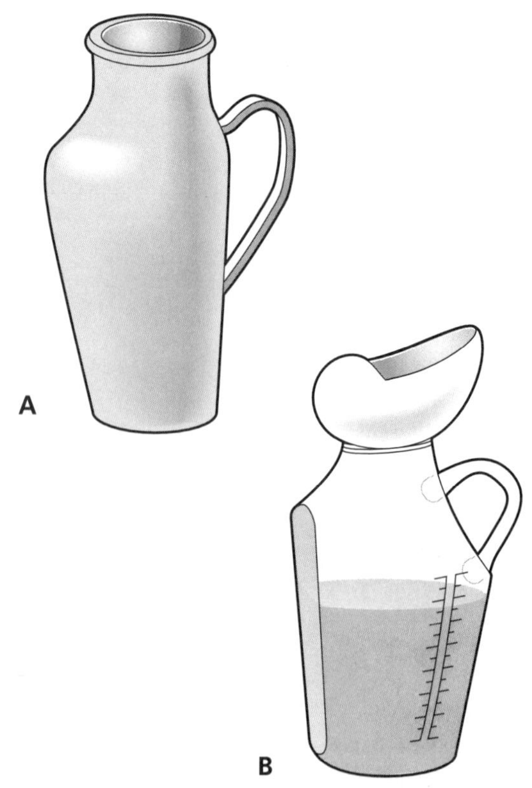

FIGURE 21.4 A. Male urinal. B. Female urinal

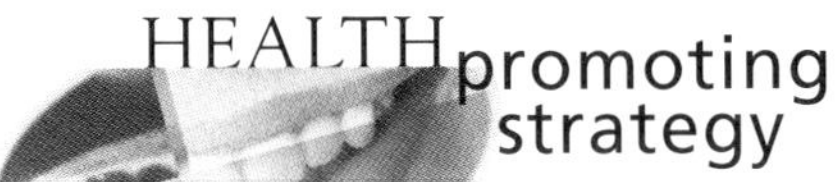

Promoting Healthy Urinary Elimination

Ignoring the urge to void will lead to urinary stasis and bladder distention, which may cause infection and, in older persons, may lead to urgency and possibly incontinence.

- Drink about two litres of fluid daily.
- Limit foods containing sodium, caffeine and alcohol.
- Wash hands before and after urinating.
- Practise pelvic floor strengthening exercises (Kegel exercises) regularly.

For people who tend to wake up in the night to void:

- Limit intake of fluids in the evening.
- Limit foods containing caffeine and alcohol.
- Void before retiring.

For women:

- Wipe the perineum from front to back. This prevents the transfer of organisms from the anus to the urethra.
- Void soon after intercourse. This helps to flush organisms from the urinary meatus and reduces opportunities for bacterial growth.

In order to use the urinal, the patient stands at the side of the bed, sits on the edge of the bed or sits in bed. If necessary, the urinal may also be used in the side-lying position. To use the urinal correctly, the spout must be positioned towards the rectum and must be in contact with the patient's skin. Otherwise, urine will leak out.

Health-Restoring Strategies

Restorative care for urinary elimination problems includes measures to re-establish normal voiding patterns (bladder retraining programs) and facilitate bladder emptying. The choice of bladder retraining program will be determined by a person's physical and cognitive ability, as well as by an assessment of the urinary diary to establish the pattern of voiding. Ensure that the patient is not hampered by concerns over activities of daily living (ADL) such as dexterity or inability to remove clothing quickly, or environmental issues such as proximity to the bathroom, commode or urinal. Physical capabilities must be assessed regarding general health. The patient's ambulatory status and transfer ability must also be determined. There are different types of bladder management procedures, ranging from scheduled voiding to deferment techniques. Measures to stimulate or defer micturition, urinary catheterization, indwelling catheter care, bladder irrigation, external drainage (condom catheter) and urostomy care will be outlined here.

RETRAINING FOR BLADDER CONTROL (SCHEDULED URINATION)

Individuals with urinary dysfunction may experience urinary retention or incontinence. For instance, a patient who has had a catheter in place over a period of time may experience a phase of urinary incontinence before regaining bladder control. Neuromuscular conditions that interfere with sensory and motor impulses involved in voluntary control of voiding, psychological changes (such as anxiety, fear or disorientation) and the use of medications affecting urine output can also result in urinary incontinence.

Incontinence can affect all age groups; however, older individuals are more likely to experience this problem. Urinary incontinence can cause psychological and physiological problems for individuals and their families. People with urinary incontinence may suffer lowered self-esteem, depression and apathy, all of which can lead to a pattern of social isolation (MacLeod & MacTavish, 1988). Nurses can help patients to train their bladders to function at regular and predictable times. To achieve success, the patient must be willing and physically able to undertake a training program.

A program to re-establish bladder control begins with an assessment of the patient's normal pattern of voiding and usual times for toiletting. A program is then established to comply with these usual habits. It is important that all nursing and support personnel adhere to the planned schedule for the patient. Consistency is the key to an effective retraining program.

All measures for promoting normal urinary elimination are used in a bladder retraining program. Individuals who require toiletting assistance should not be kept waiting or be allowed to become incontinent because their call for assistance has been ignored. If incontinence does occur, bed linen should be changed at once, thus preventing skin irritation and promoting psychological well-being.

In a bladder retraining program it is essential that the micturition reflex be activated at regular intervals. Therefore, an adequate intake of fluids is necessary so that sufficient urine is produced to distend the bladder and stimulate the micturition reflex. Withholding fluids in a mistaken attempt to control incontinence can lead to fluid and electrolyte imbalances, as well as constipation and cystitis. The provision of fluids at regular intervals helps to ensure an adequate intake; that is, under normal circumstances, a minimum of 2000 mL/day, although 3000 mL or more is preferred if tolerated by the patient. Patients are encouraged to avoid caffeine-containing beverages, which stimulate the urge to void. Water, milk and fruit juices are recommended (Dudek, 1997).

Bladder retraining is a learned behaviour. Achievement of continence can take from six weeks to several months. Patients require both physical and psychosocial support during a bladder retraining program. Dependence on others and the lack of control over a basic function such as voiding can be very distressing. It is important that the health professional have a good working relationship with the patient, as this will help to lessen any anxiety the patient may experience. A sensitive, caring approach and patience are required of the nurse in helping people with urinary problems. Every effort should be made to provide only positive reinforcement during the program. The individual can be very sensitive to signs of displeasure on the part of staff.

In some patients, however, voluntary bladder control cannot be achieved. For these people, the plan of care may include a schedule of regular toiletting (using the toilet, commode chair, urinal or bedpan) and the use of absorbent pads or waterproof garments. The male patient may benefit from the use of an external urine-collecting device such as a condom catheter. As a last resort, intervention may involve the long-term use of an indwelling catheter.

DEFERMENT

The strategy of deferment involves deliberately delaying urination in patients who have a pattern of frequent, low-volume voidings. The nurse can review the urinary diary with the patient to confirm recordings of larger voiding volumes, which would indicate that the bladder has the physical capacity of storing these volumes. The nurse can then reinforce the teaching that voiding more than five to eight times daily is unnecessary, even though the patient may feel the urge.

When the patient verbalizes the urge to void, briefly instruct him or her to stop the activity of the moment and perform a series of quick pelvic floor contractions. Doing these rapid contractions elicits an effective reflex arc to inhibit the bladder from contracting. Gradually, the patient practices deferment of urination in five-minute increments until the desired goal is reached. It is normal to urinate every three to four hours; a guideline for the maximum period between voidings is five hours. Patients with cystitis should not defer urination.

PELVIC BRACING

Pelvic floor bracing, also known as counterbracing, is a method used to gain control over events that cause incontinent episodes. These events increase intra-abdominal pressure, causing physical stress to the bladder. Stresses include coughing, sneezing, lifting, laughing or nose-blowing. The patient is advised to contract the pelvic floor hard before and during the event, and to relax when the event is over.

FACILITATING MICTURITION

There are a number of measures the nurse can implement to stimulate micturition in patients who are having difficulty in initiating voiding. These include:

1. providing privacy and helping the patient to assume a natural position for voiding
2. providing a commode or, preferably, assisting the patient to the bathroom if this is possible (male patients frequently find it easier to void when standing rather than sitting or lying down)
3. running water within the patient's hearing
4. providing warm water in which patients may dangle their fingers
5. pouring warm water over the perineum (the water must be measured if the patient requires intake and output measurements.)
6. gently stroking the inner thighs or applying pressure over the symphysis pubis
7. providing relief of pain.

The application of warmth to the bladder and perineal areas helps to relax the muscles used in voiding and therefore facilitates this process. If possible, having the patient sit in a sitz-bath or bathtub with warm water is also very helpful. When conservative measures have been unsuccessful in stimulating micturition and the patient is very uncomfortable, a urinary catheterization may be ordered.

URINARY CATHETERIZATION

Catheterization of the urinary bladder is the introduction of a narrow tube, called a catheter, through the urethra into the bladder. It provides a means of emptying the bladder for individuals unable to control micturition and those with urinary obstructions. It is inserted prior to operative procedures in which there is a high risk of bladder trauma or urinary complications. It is also used as a means of monitoring urinary output when frequent, accurate measurements are essential to the patient's care. The insertion of a urinary catheter carries a high risk of nosocomial infections. If at all possible, catheterization should be avoided. However, when it is required, careful attention to meticulous aseptic technique is absolutely essential during every phase of catheter care from insertion to removal. Surgical aseptic technique is described in Chapter 32. The steps for inserting a catheter in a female and a male patient are outlined in Procedures 21.3 and 21.4, respectively.

Preparing the Patient

Before carrying out a catheterization, the nurse explains the procedure and the reasons for it to the patient. It is important to emphasize that insertion of a catheter should not be a painful experience; however, a sensation of pressure may be felt as the catheter is inserted. The patient will be asked to assume a dorsal recumbent or lithotomy position during the procedure. A side-lying or Sims' position may also be used for a female patient who cannot abduct her legs at the hip joint. Drapes will be used to minimize exposure. Every effort should be made to alleviate anxiety and put the patient at ease. Catheter insertion is easier for the nurse, and discomfort is minimized, when the patient is relaxed.

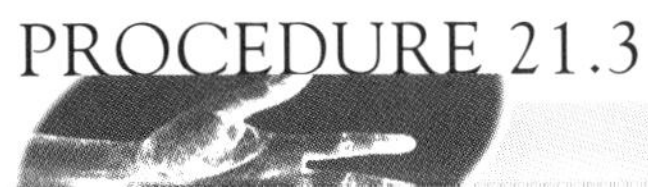

PROCEDURE 21.3 Inserting a Straight or Indwelling Catheter in a Female Patient

Action	*Rationale*
1. Prepare the patient.	Reduces anxiety and enables patient participation.
2. Wash hands thoroughly for 1 min with antiseptic agent.	Prepares for sterile technique and use of sterile gloves (see Chapter 32).
3. Gather: • catheter kit • two catheters, size and type as appropriate • extra pair of sterile gloves • light • urine collection bag with tubing • tape, elastic band and safety pin • moisture-proof bag • waterproof protective pad • bath blanket (optional).	Facilitates efficiency and economy of time.
4. Ensure adequate lighting. If necessary, enlist the aid of an assistant to hold a flashlight.	Facilitates visualization of the urinary meatus.
5. Close the door (if private room) and pull bed curtains.	Provides privacy and may lessen feelings of embarrassment.
6. Don clean gloves.	Prevents exposure to body fluids.
7. Place a protective pad under the patient and position her.	Prevents soiling of bed linen. Enables access to urinary meatus.
• Assist the patient to a dorsal recumbent position. Knees should be flexed and thighs externally rotated. Pillows can be used to support the knees and to elevate the buttocks.	Reduces muscle tension and promotes comfort.
• If the patient is unable to lie supine or abduct the thighs, assist her to a side-lying position with the upper leg flexed at the hip and knee. Position the buttocks close to the edge of the bed.	Promotes comfort and, for some women, lessens feelings of exposure.

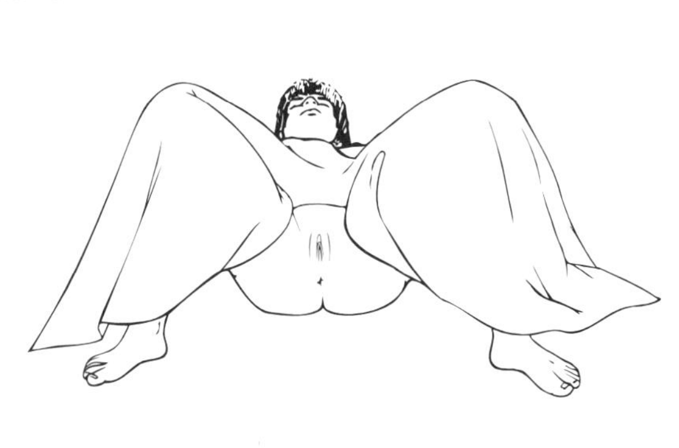

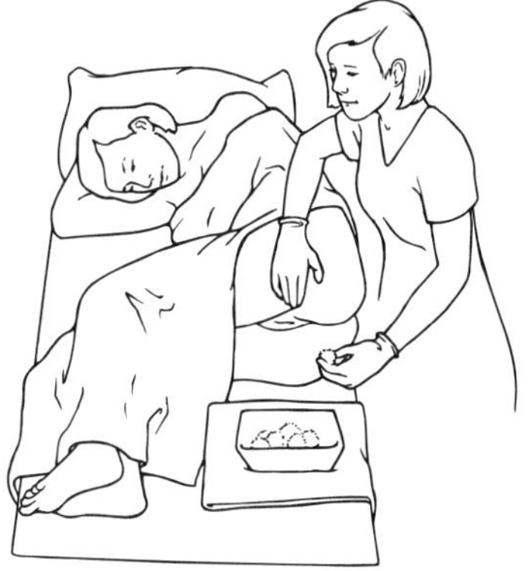

8. Drape the patient. Cover her upper body with a bath blanket; pull the gown up over her hips. Cover her legs and feet with the bed sheet.	Lessens feelings of exposure and keeps the patient warm.

Continued on the next page

PROCEDURE 21.3 *continued*

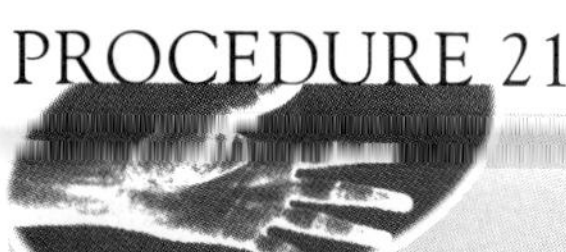

Action	*Rationale*
9. If not done by the patient, wash the genital area with warm soap and water. Rinse well and dry. Discard gloves and wash hands again.	Reduces microorganisms near the urethral meatus and enables the nurse to see the meatus in women with increased vaginal secretions.
10. If inserting an indwelling catheter, attach the urine drainage set to the bed according to the manufacturer's specifications. Leave the cover on the connector end of the tubing.	Prepares equipment for connection to the catheter after insertion. Maintains sterility.
11. Attach the moisture-proof bag to the side of bed, placing it to ensure minimal reaching over the sterile field.	Provides a receptacle for wrappings and used equipment. Prevents spread of microorganisms.
12. Position the light to illuminate the perineal area.	Provides sufficient light to view the urinary meatus.
13. Set up a sterile field on the over-bed table using the inner wrapper of the catheterization kit (see Procedure 32.4). Open catheter package, if not included in kit, and add to sterile field.	Allows for easy access to equipment. Aseptic technique prevents contamination of sterile supplies by micro-organisms.
14. Don sterile gloves (see Procedure 32.3).	Allows the nurse to handle sterile equipment without contamination.
15. Organize the equipment on the sterile field.	Readies equipment for the insertion while both gloves are sterile.
• If the catheter is indwelling, attach the prefilled syringe to the valve of the balloon lumen and inject the fluid until the balloon inflates. Then withdraw all fluid from the balloon and leave the syringe attached to the valve port.	Tests for intactness of the catheter balloon and allows replacement of faulty equipment.
• Open and add cleansing solution to cotton balls.	Cleanses the urinary meatus and reduces the possibility of introducing microorganisms into the bladder.
• Separate cotton balls with forceps.	Promotes easy manipulation.
• Open the specimen container if a specimen is to be obtained.	
• Lubricate 2.5–5 cm of the catheter tip and place in collecting basin.	Aids in catheter insertion and reduces trauma to the tissues.
16. Drape the patient.	
• Pick up the plain drape and open it away from any unsterile surfaces. Wrap the drape around gloved hands and place it between the patient's legs at the edge of the perineum, without allowing the gloves to come in contact with the patient's skin.	Provides a sterile surface close to the perineal area. Protects the hands from contact with unsterile surfaces and maintains sterility of work area.
• Open the fenestrated drape in the same manner and wrap it around gloved hands. Place the drape over the patient's perineal area, taking care not to touch any unsterile surfaces.	

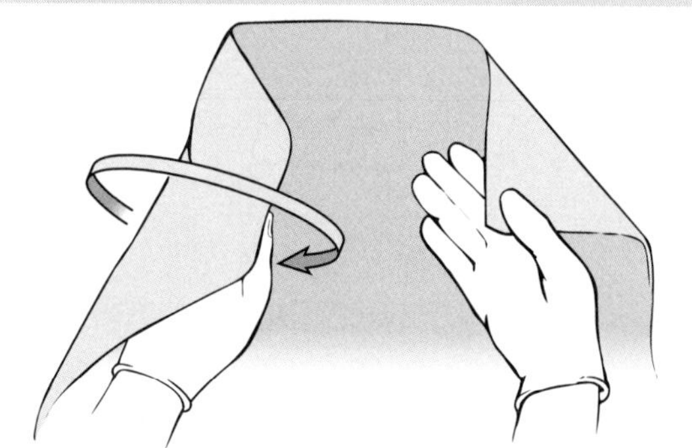

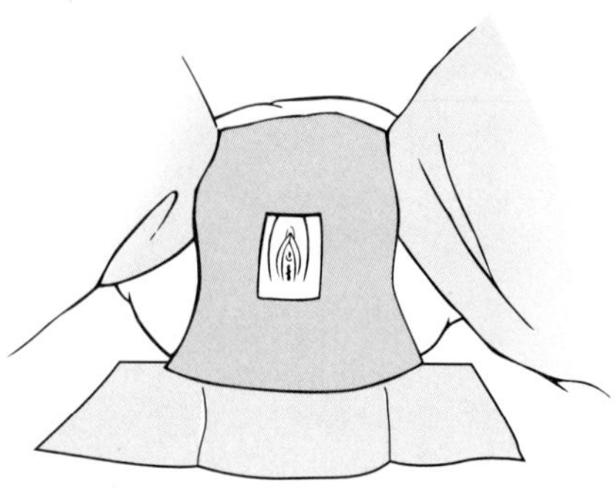

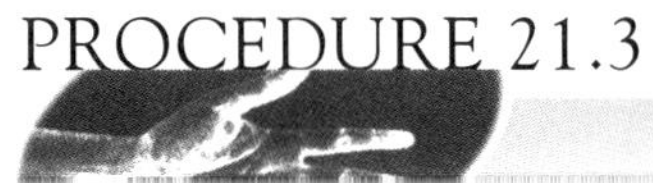

PROCEDURE 21.3 *continued*

Action	*Rationale*
17. Place the sterile collecting basin containing the necessary supplies on the drape between the patient's thighs.	Maintains asepsis and allows access to supplies during the procedure.
18. Using the nondominant hand, gently open the labia to expose the urethral meatus. Keep the labia separated and maintain this hand position throughout the procedure.	Allows the nurse to see the meatus and prevents contamination of the area around the meatus as well as the catheter. *This hand is no longer sterile and cannot be used to touch sterile items.*

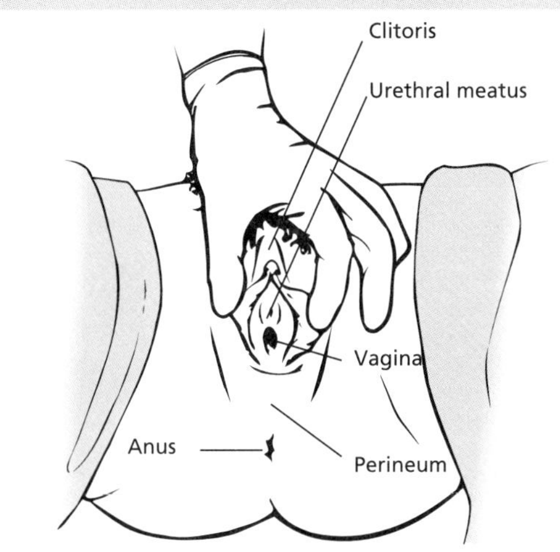

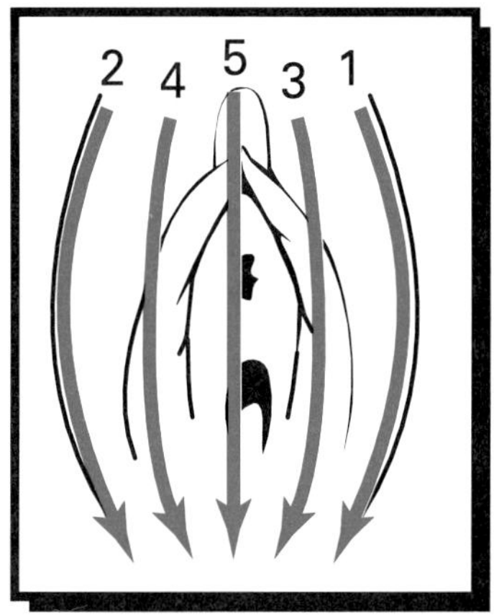

Action	*Rationale*
19. Using forceps to hold the cotton balls, cleanse between the labial folds and over the urinary meatus. Use each swab just once and discard after use. Clean from the cleanest area (near the symphysis pubis) towards the most contaminated area (near the rectum). A minimum of five cotton balls is needed.	Prevents the spread of microorganisms from dirtier to cleaner areas. Cleaning over the urinary meatus last helps to prevent the introduction of microorganisms into the bladder during insertion of the catheter.
20. Pick up the lubricated catheter approximately 4–7 cm from the tip and ensure the distal end is in the collecting basin. Ask the patient to bear down as if to void or to take a deep breath. Insert the catheter gently into the urethra to a distance of 4–6 cm or until urine begins to flow. If inserting an indwelling catheter, advance catheter a further 1–2.5 cm. Do not force the catheter if any resistance is felt.	Facilitates control of catheter. Prevents drainage onto the bed when the catheter is inserted. Allows the sphincter to relax, making passage of the catheter easier. The female urethra is about 3–4 cm in length. Ensures placement of the catheter and allows inflation of the balloon without traumatizing urethral mucosa. Prevents dislodgement.
21. **Straight catheter:** Hold the catheter in place with thumb and forefinger of the nondominant hand until the bladder empties. Collect a specimen if required.	
Indwelling catheter: Hold the catheter in place with thumb and forefinger of the nondominant hand. Gently inflate the balloon according to the manufacturer's directions, while watching for any signs of patient discomfort. Detach the syringe without allowing any of the fluid to flow back into the syringe. Gently tug on the catheter (before detaching the syringe). Collect a specimen if required.	Prevents dislodgement. Holds the catheter in place in the bladder. If the balloon is not fully inflated, the catheter may slip out of the bladder.

Continued on the next page

PROCEDURE 21.3 *continued*

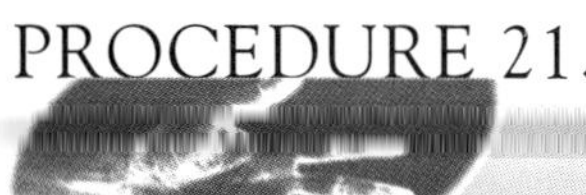

Action	Rationale
22. **Straight catheter:** Once the urine has stopped flowing, the catheter is pinched and withdrawn slowly.	
Indwelling catheter: Attach the catheter to the urinary drainage system and secure the tubing to the patient's thigh using tape or commercial tube holder (Cath-Secure®). Anchor the tubing to the patient's gown using a safety pin and elastic band.	Establishes a closed urinary drainage system. Prevents trauma to the urethral meatus during movement.

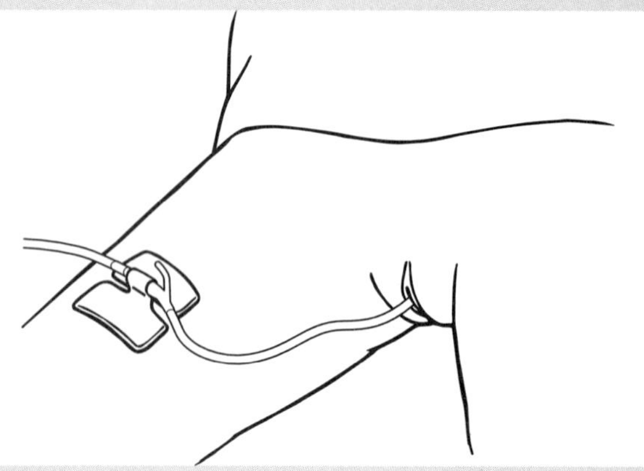

Action	Rationale
23. Dry the perineal area and assist the patient to assume a comfortable position.	Promotes patient comfort and well-being.
24. Discard used equipment per agency protocol. Send the specimen to the laboratory and wash hands.	Maintains cleanliness and safety in the workplace.
25. Measure amount of urine in collecting basin and discard.	Provides assessment data.
26. Document the procedure on the patient's record. Include the size and type of catheter used, a description of the urine obtained (amount, colour, clarity and odour), the patient's tolerance of the procedure, and that a specimen was obtained.	Fulfills legal requirements for nurse accountability and promotes continuity of care.

PROCEDURE 21.4 Inserting a Straight or Indwelling Catheter in a Male Patient

Action	Rationale
1. Follow steps 1 to 6 of Procedure 21.3.	
2. Assist the patient to a supine position with thighs slightly abducted.	Prevents tensing of abdominal and pelvic muscles.
3. Follow steps 8 to 14 of Procedure 21.3.	
4. Organize the equipment on the sterile field.	Readies equipment for the insertion while both gloves are sterile.
• If the catheter is indwelling, attach the prefilled syringe to the valve of the balloon lumen and inject the fluid until the balloon inflates. Then withdraw all fluid from the balloon and leave the syringe attached to the valve port.	Tests for intactness of the catheter balloon and allows replacement of faulty equipment.

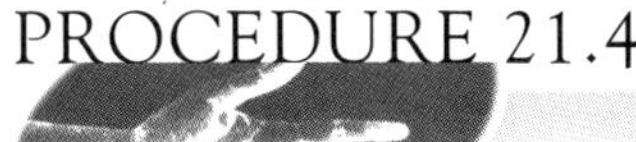

PROCEDURE 21.4 continued

Action	Rationale
• Open and add cleansing solution to cotton balls.	Cleanses the urinary meatus and reduces the possibility of introducing microorganisms into the bladder.
• Separate cotton balls with forceps.	Promotes easy manipulation.
• Open the specimen container if a specimen is to be obtained.	
• Lubricate the catheter generously for a length of 16.5–18.5 cm and place in collecting basin.	Aids in catheter insertion and reduces trauma to the tissues.
5. Drape patient.	
• Pick up the plain drape and open it away from any unsterile surfaces. Wrap the drape around gloved hands and place it over the patient's thighs below the penis.	Provides for a sterile surface close to the perineal area. Protects gloves from contact with unsterile surfaces and maintains sterility of the work area.
• Open the fenestrated drape in the same manner and wrap it around gloved hands. Place the opening of drape over the patient's penis.	
6. Place the sterile collecting basin containing the necessary supplies on the drape between patient's thighs.	Maintains asepsis and allows access to supplies during procedure.
7. Pull penis up at a 90° angle.	Straightens urethra.
8. If the patient is not circumcised and the foreskin is not already retracted, gently retract it. With the nondominant hand, grasp the penis just below the glans. Keep the hand in this position throughout the procedure.	If the foreskin is released, the area becomes contaminated and cleansing has to be repeated. *This hand is no longer sterile and cannot be used to touch sterile items.*
9. Using forceps to hold the cotton balls, cleanse the tip of the penis, using a circular motion. Proceed outward from meatus to the base of the glans. Repeat the procedure at least three times, using a clean cotton ball each time. A final cotton ball may be held for a few moments over the urinary meatus.	Reduces the number of microorganisms in the area of the meatus. Cleansing from an area of least contamination to an area of greater contamination helps to prevent the spread of microorganisms. Cleansing over the urinary meatus last helps to prevent the introduction of microorganisms into the bladder during insertion of the catheter.

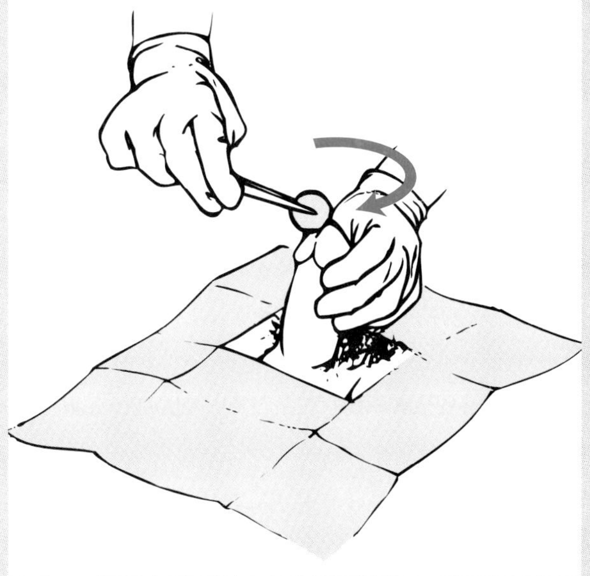

Continued on the next page

PROCEDURE 21.4 *continued*

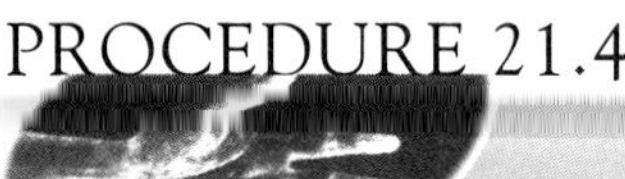

Action	*Rationale*
10. Ensure the penis is at a 90° angle to the patient's body and apply slight traction. Pick up the lubricated catheter approximately 5–6 cm from the tip and ensure the distal end is in the collecting basin. Ask the patient to bear down as if to void and insert the catheter gently into the urethra. Advance the catheter up to the bifurcation or until urine begins to flow. It is not unusual to feel some resistance when the catheter reaches the area of the external sphincter. The nurse may also keep a gentle forward pressure on the catheter while the patient takes a few deep breaths.	Straightens the downward curvature of the prepubic urethra. Facilitates control of the catheter. The male urethra is approximately 20 cm in length. Ensures that the balloon is in the bladder and not in the urethra. Permits the sphincter to relax, allowing the catheter to pass more readily.
11. Lower penis to a 45° angle after catheter is inserted about halfway.	Places penis in position for urine to be released into collecting basin.
12. If inserting an indwelling catheter, advance 1–2.5 cm more. Do not force the catheter if any significant resistance is felt.	Ensures placement of the catheter and allows inflation of the balloon without traumatizing urethral mucosa.
Gently tug on the catheter.	Checks that balloon is inflated.
13. Follow steps 22 to 26 of Procedure 23.1. Before leaving the patient who is uncircumcised, ensure that his foreskin has been pulled forward over the glans.	If the foreskin is left retracted, circulation of blood to the glans can be impeded.

In most cases, the patient should be encouraged to wash the perineal area thoroughly with warm, soapy water immediately prior to the procedure. If the patient is unable to do this independently, the nurse can carry out this function. While washing the patient, the nurse can identify the urinary meatus in the female and retract the foreskin in the uncircumcised male. This also expedites the cleaning process during the catheterization.

Assembling Equipment

There are many types of catheters available, and the choice of the catheter is determined by the reason for the catheterization. A straight, single-lumen catheter is used to collect a sterile specimen, measure a residual urine (amount of urine left in the bladder after voiding) or intermittently drain the bladder. If the catheter is to remain in place for a period of time, an indwelling or retention catheter (often called a Foley catheter) is used.

Retention catheters are kept in place by a balloon which is inflated once the catheter has been inserted. Most common balloon sizes are 5–10 mL. Retention catheters have two or three lumens. In the double-lumen catheter, one lumen is connected to the balloon that holds the catheter in place, while the second lumen drains the urine from the bladder. The triple-lumen catheter has an additional lumen that is used for instilling solution during bladder irrigation. Figure 21.5 provides an illustration of the types of catheters.

In most institutions, sterile, prepackaged catheterization sets are available for catheter insertion. Each kit contains a pair of sterile gloves, sterile drapes, one of which is fenestrated (has an opening in the middle), cleansing solution, lubricant, cotton balls, a specimen container, forceps, a prefilled syringe and a basin to collect urine. Some kits may contain a standard-size catheter, and all kits can be used for both male and female patients. The kits are discarded after use. Catheters are graded in size according to the French scale; 14 Fr and 16 Fr catheters are commonly used for the catheterization of the adult patient. The larger the number, the larger the lumen of the catheter. Smaller-lumen catheters are generally not necessary, and the smaller lumen results in increased length of time required to empty the bladder. However, if there is any chance of injury to the urethral mucosa, or if the patient experiences discomfort during the procedure, smaller-sized catheters can be used. It is always wise to take an extra catheter and an extra pair of sterile gloves along in case of contamination during the procedure.

When an indwelling catheter is being inserted, a urine drainage bag and tubing will also be needed (Figure 21.6). The tubing connects the catheter to the collecting bag, forming a closed drainage system that should not be entered unless absolutely necessary. The drainage bag and tubing are sterile and must be attached to the catheter using aseptic technique to prevent the introduction of micro-organisms into the system.

In order to see the urinary meatus and prevent contamination of the catheter as it is inserted, the nurse requires

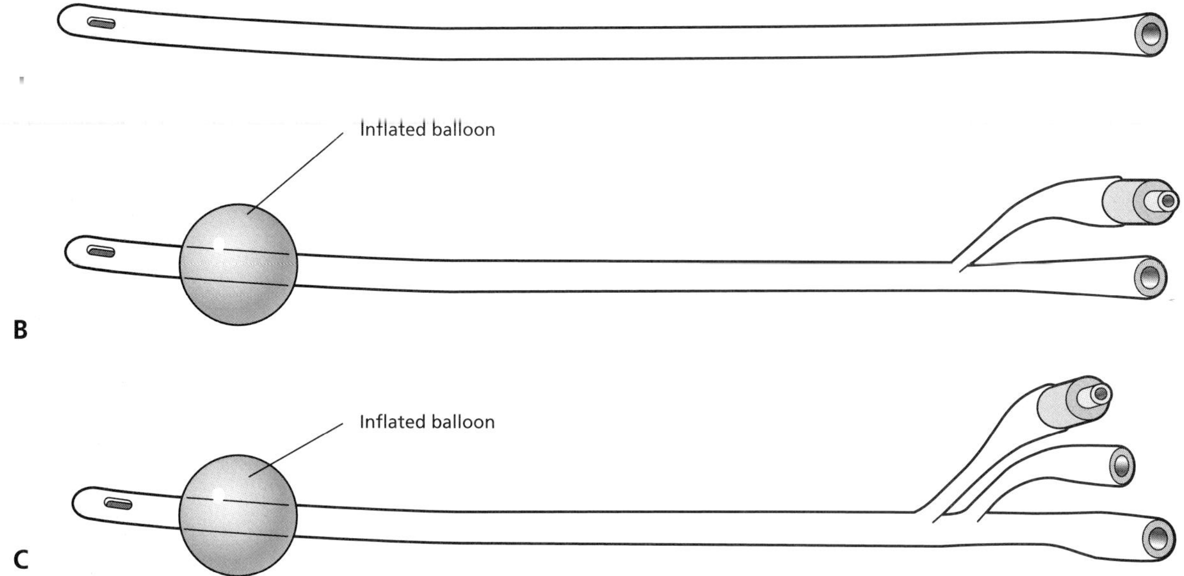

FIGURE 21.5 A. Straight catheter B. Double-lumen indwelling catheter C. Triple-lumen indwelling catheter

a good light source. Either an extension lamp or an extendible goose-neck lamp can be used to illuminate the perineal area. If necessary, the nurse can enlist the aid of an assistant with a flashlight.

PROVIDING INDWELLING CATHETER CARE

Care for the patient with an indwelling catheter primarily includes monitoring for problems, preventing infection and maintaining unobstructed flow of urine through the drainage system. Many patients can participate in the care of their catheter once they know how the system functions and what care is required.

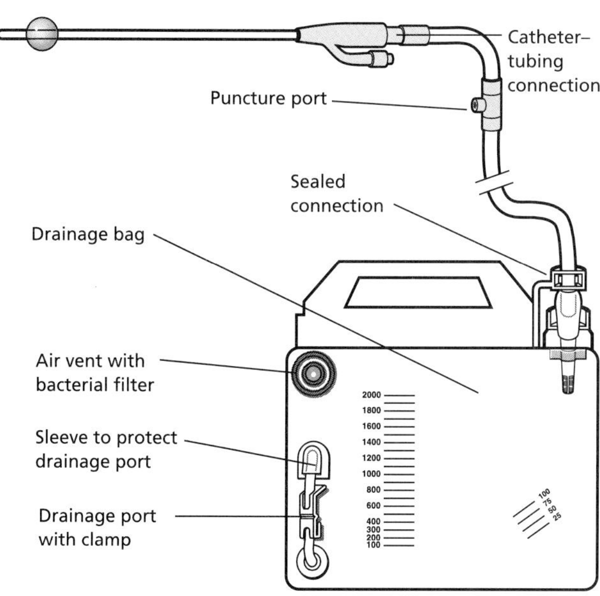

FIGURE 21.6 Urinary drainage system

Immediately after a catheter insertion, some patients may experience irritation of the urethral mucosa. The nurse can reassure the patient that such discomfort is usually of short duration. The patient is encouraged to drink adequate fluids (3000 mL/day if the patient's condition permits) to aid the urinary tract in flushing out unwanted microorganisms and to keep the tubing free of sediment.

Hand-washing and basic hygiene are essential for preventing infection. Hands must be washed before and after caring for a patient with an indwelling catheter. In addition, gloves should be worn to protect the nurse from exposure to blood and body substances. Patients should have perineal care administered at least twice a day to remove secretions and encrustations on the catheter which may cause infection (perineal care is outlined in Chapter 31). Tub baths or showers should be taken as the patient's condition permits.

The correct positioning and maintenance of the urinary drainage system is an essential aspect of care. Urine drains from the bladder into the drainage bag by the force of gravity. The bag must be kept lower than the level of the patient's bladder for urine to drain freely. When the drainage bag is positioned higher than the bladder, urine will flow back into the bladder (backflow), bringing with it unwanted microorganisms. If the catheter bag is positioned above the level of the bladder (for example, for a tub bath), the tubing must be clamped to prevent urine backflow. The tubing should not loop below the receptacle because a kink may form, occluding the lumen. The tubing should be kept secured, with excess loops coiled on the bed, allowing the urine to drain into the drainage bag in a straight drop from the bed. Care must be taken to ensure that tubing does not become trapped under the patient's leg, causing occlusion of the lumen.

When a continuous drainage system is in place, the drainage bag should be emptied as it fills or at regular intervals. The amount, colour, clarity and odour of the urine are noted at that time. Urometers are often used when the measurement of hourly urine outputs is required. The meters are rigid plastic containers attached to a drainage bag and are calibrated to measure small amounts (300 mL or less) of urine (see Figure 21.7).

A closed drainage system should never be opened to measure urine or to obtain a specimen. Doing so would allow bacteria to enter the system and cause infection. The drainage bag is emptied through a drainage port at the bottom of the bag into a graduated container. This provides a means of measuring the amount of urine and then disposing of it, usually into a hopper in the dirty utility room (the technique for obtaining a urine specimen from an indwelling catheter is outlined in Procedure 21.5). If it is necessary for the catheter to be disconnected from the tubing for a period of time, for example, during a bladder irrigation, it is important that the sterility of both the catheter and the tubing be maintained. Small disposable devices are available that provide a sterile cover for the tubing and a plug for the catheter.

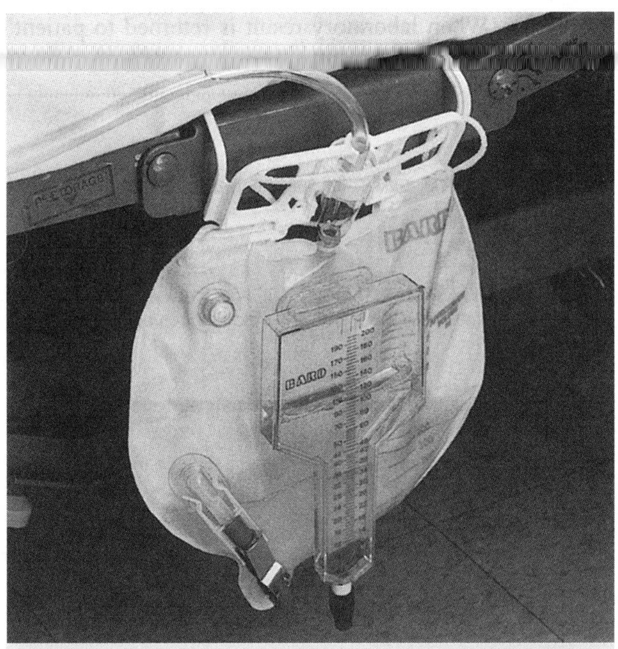

FIGURE 21.7 Urinary drainage bag with urometer attached

PROCEDURE 21.5 Obtaining a Urine Sample from an Indwelling Catheter

Action	*Rationale*
1. Wash hands and gather: • alcohol swab • sterile 5 mL syringe with 23- or 25-gauge needle attached • sterile container for specimen • clamp • clean gloves.	Reduces transfer of microorganisms and facilitates efficiency and economy of time.
2. Tell the patient what you are going to do.	Promotes patient well-being and participation in care.
3. Check that the drainage tube has urine in it. If necessary, apply a clamp to the tubing below the puncture port and wait (usually 10–20 min) until urine collects in the tubing.	
4. Cleanse the puncture port with an alcohol swab.	Prevents contamination of the specimen and introduction of surface microorganisms into the system.
5. Insert the needle into the port and withdraw the sample of urine. Usually 3–5 mL of urine provides a sufficient sample. If used, be sure that the clamp is removed from the tubing.	
6. Put the specimen into the sterile container. Dispose of syringe into a sharps container, remove gloves and wash hands.	Ensures safe handling of used equipment.
7. Send the specimen to the laboratory.	
8. Document the procedure. Record the time that the specimen has been sent to the laboratory.	Fulfills requirement for nurse accountability.

Note: Urine collected for culture and sensitivity needs to be clean and as recently produced as possible; therefore, it is never obtained from the urine in the collecting bag.

Patients with indwelling catheters are not confined to bed. In fact, such patients should be up and about as much as possible. The benefits of remaining as well being are [illegible] receptacles designed to hold the drainage bag, which the patient then can carry, much like a shopping bag. Ambulatory patients may also use drainage bags that strap to the leg. These leg bags are equipped with a drainage port that can be opened to drain the urine into the toilet or other receptacle as the bag fills. Leg bags are easily concealed under clothing and allow patients to participate in public without the embarrassment of displaying a catheter.

On occasion, it is necessary to change a retention or indwelling catheter. This is usually done according to the physician's order or agency protocol. Owing to the risk of introducing microorganisms into the patient's bladder, catheters are never changed without good reason. Any obstruction to urine flow that is not cleared by irrigation would indicate a need for catheter replacement. Other signs that a catheter may need changing are insufficient urine in [illegible] and abdominal distention just above the symphysis pubis. When a catheter is changed, the catheter *in situ* is removed as outlined in Procedure 21.6, perineal care is completed and a new catheter is inserted as outlined in Procedure 21.3 or 21.4.

REMOVING AN INDWELLING CATHETER

Following the doctor's order for removal of an indwelling catheter, the nurse first needs to assess the patient's understanding of the procedure to be performed. If an explanation is appropriate, the reason for the removal and the procedure is explained. If this is a first-time experience for the patient,

PROCEDURE 21.6

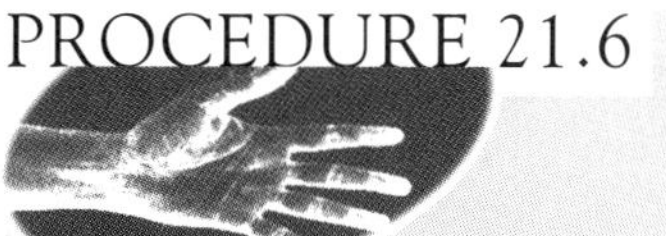

Removing an Indwelling Catheter

Action	*Rationale*
1. Wash hands and gather: • clean gloves • 10-cc syringe (without needle) • moisture-proof bag • waterproof protective pad • graduated container.	Prevents the transfer of microorganisms and facilitates efficiency and economy of time.
2. Assist the patient to a dorsal recumbent position, with legs slightly apart. Place the protective pad under the patient's buttocks.	Promotes patient comfort. Protects bed linens.
3. Apply clean gloves.	Protects the nurse from exposure to body secretions.
4. Empty the urinary drainage bag into the graduated container and measure the output.	Readies the bag for removal.
5. Remove the tape securing the tubing to the patient's thigh.	Readies the tube for removal.
6. Insert the tip of the syringe into the valve of the balloon lumen and withdraw the fluid until negative pressure is felt.	Readies the catheter for removal.
7. Ask the patient to take several deep breaths and then, while the patient is relaxed, wrap the catheter in a protective pad and gently withdraw it from the urethra. Observe the patient for signs of discomfort. If discomfort occurs, stop the procedure and again attempt to withdraw fluid from balloon port.	Promotes relaxation. If the balloon has not been emptied completely, the patient may experience discomfort.
8. Place used equipment into the moisture-proof bag, remove gloves and discard appropriately. Wash hands.	Promotes cleanliness and safety in the workplace.
9. Ask the patient to perform (or, if necessary, help the patient to perform) perineal care.	Cleanses area of any spilled urine.
10. Document the procedure. Record the time, patient tolerance and any teaching done.	Fulfills requirements for nurse accountability and promotes continuity of care.

Note: In some agencies, a routine sample of urine for culture and sensitivity is obtained prior to removal of the catheter.

Patient Teaching for Indwelling Catheter Care

1. It is common to feel the need to void while the catheter is in place.
2. Increased amounts of fluid (approximately 3000 mL/day) are needed to flush the bladder and keep the tubing free of sediment.
3. Move freely in bed and, if allowed, be up and about with catheter in place.
4. Avoid lying on the catheter tubing.
5. Keep the drainage bag below the level of the bladder.
6. If able, wash the perineal area (and the urinary meatus, for male patients) and catheter with soap and water at least twice daily. If unable, this will be done by the nurse. When taking tub baths or showers, clamp the tubing if the drainage bag must be suspended above the level of the bladder.
7. Watch for and report untoward signs such as strong odours, burning sensations or discharge at the meatus.

he or she will likely be concerned about pain on withdrawal of the catheter. The nurse can assure the patient that at most there may be a slight burning sensation. This will be more pronounced for the male than for the female patient. Prior to the procedure, thorough cleansing of the perineal area must be performed. Most patients will prefer to do this independently; however, on occasion it will be the responsibility of the nurse. This is a good time for the nurse to assess the size of the balloon holding the catheter in place so that the appropriate size syringe can be collected later. The technique for removing an indwelling catheter is detailed in Procedure 21.6. Once the catheter is removed, the nurse discusses measures to promote return of the patient's normal urinary elimination pattern. These are summarized in the box below.

Patient Teaching Following Removal of an Indwelling Catheter

1. Void into a urinal or bedpan until otherwise directed so that output can be measured.
2. Continue increased fluid intake.
3. A burning sensation during the first couple of voidings is a normal occurrence.
4. Report any untoward signs such as continued burning on voiding, bleeding, unusual odour or indications of fever.

BLADDER IRRIGATION

A bladder irrigation is performed to maintain or restore patency of a catheter when drainage is obstructed with blood or sediment. It is also done to flush a bladder or instill medications. For example, the physician may order an irrigation to flush the bladder for extensive bleeding with clots in a patient with cancer, or to instill an antibiotic agent in a patient with an infection. If the patient does not have an indwelling catheter in place, one has to be inserted first.

Bladder irrigations are performed with a physician's order. They may be carried out on an intermittent or continuous basis. There are two methods for bladder irrigation: open and closed. The *open method* is used for intermittent irrigation when the patient has a double-lumen indwelling catheter in place. It involves separating the catheter from the drainage tubing and flushing the catheter with a syringe. The *closed method* uses a triple-lumen catheter. The irrigating solution (irrigant) is instilled through the third (irrigating) lumen while the return solution is drained through the catheter drainage system (see Figure 21.8). This method permits frequent intermittent or continuous irrigation without disruption of the sterile drainage system. The steps for performing a bladder irrigation using the open method are outlined in Procedure 21.7. The closed method for continuous bladder irrigation is detailed in Procedure 21.8. Meticulous aseptic technique is required throughout the procedure.

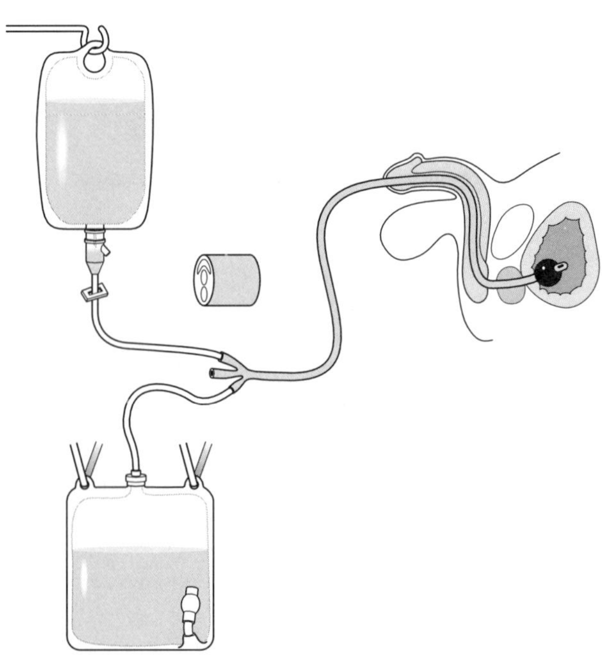

FIGURE 21.8 Continuous bladder irrigation using a closed system via a triple-lumen catheter

PROCEDURE 21.7 Open Bladder Irrigation

Action	*Rationale*
1. Prepare the patient.	Promotes patient well-being and enables participation in care.
2. Wash hands thoroughly.	Prevents the spread of microorganisms.
3. Gather: • disposable irrigation kit • sterile irrigation solution • Toomey syringe (optional) • sterile gloves • sterile tip to protect end of drainage tubing • waterproof protective pad • bath blanket (optional) • sterile alcohol swab.	Facilitates efficiency and economy of time.
4. Close the door to the room and pull bed curtains.	Promotes privacy.
5. Help the patient into a dorsal recumbent position, with legs slightly separated. Pull down the bed covers to expose the catheter where it joins the drainage tubing and place a protective pad under the patient's buttocks. Cover the patient's upper body with a bath blanket.	Promotes patient comfort, facilitates access to the catheter and aids flow of irrigant into the bladder. Protects bed linen from soiling. Provides warmth.
6. Open the irrigation kit on the over-bed table, creating a sterile field. Add solution and sterile alcohol swab.	Maintains sterility of equipment.
7. Put on sterile gloves.	Maintains asepsis and protects the nurse from exposure to body substances.
8. Place the sterile drape between the patient's thighs, under the catheter–tubing junction, and put the irrigating equipment on it.	Creates a sterile field. Readies equipment for the procedure.
9. Disconnect the catheter from the tubing, place a sterile cap over the end of the drainage tube and secure it to the bed linen. Position the end of the catheter in the collecting basin, holding the catheter about 2.5 cm from its open end. Cleanse the end of the catheter with an alcohol swab.	Keeps the end of the drainage tube sterile. Protects the bed linen from spillage of urine. Prevents entry of microorganisms into the system.
10. Aspirate 30–50 mL of irrigant into the syringe.	Prepares the syringe for irrigation and ensures a record of the amount of irrigant instilled.
11. Insert the syringe into the catheter lumen, compress the bulb and gently instill the solution.	Minimizes the potential for discomfort and damage to delicate bladder tissues.
12. Keeping the bulb of the syringe compressed, remove the syringe from the catheter and allow the solution to drain by gravity into the collecting basin. If there is no fluid return, gently aspirate solution from the bladder. Repeat the procedure as indicated by the effect of irrigation or per physician's order.	Repetition may be required to dislodge obstructions and establish urine flow.
13. Reattach the catheter to the drainage tube, ensuring that the ends remain sterile. Secure the catheter to patient's thigh.	Re-establishes closed drainage system.
14. Remove gloves and assist the patient into a comfortable position.	Promotes patient well-being.
15. Discard equipment and wash hands.	Promotes cleanliness and safety.
16. Document the procedure. Note how the patient tolerated the procedure as well as the characteristics and amount of drainage obtained.	Fulfills requirements for nurse accountability.

PROCEDURE 21.8 Continuous Bladder Irrigation

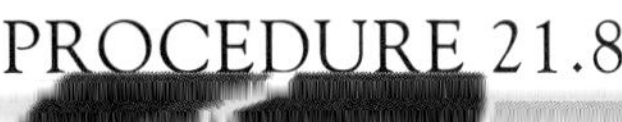

Action	Rationale
1. Prepare the patient.	Promotes patient well-being and enables participation in care.
2. Wash hands thoroughly.	Prevents the spread of microorganisms.
3. Gather: • sterile irrigation solution • irrigation administration set • IV pole • waterproof protective pad • clean gloves • alcohol swab • moisture-proof bag.	Facilitates efficiency and economy of time.
4. Prepare the irrigant. • Remove the solution bag from its outer wrapper and hang it on the IV pole. • Attach and prime the tubing as in Procedure 21.3, maintaining sterility of equipment.	Readies equipment.
5. Close the door to the room or pull bed curtains. Put on gloves, expose the catheter and place a protective pad under the catheter where it joins the drainage tubing.	Promotes privacy. Gloves protect the nurse from exposure to body substances. Protects bed linen.
6. Cleanse the irrigation lumen of the catheter with an alcohol swab.	Reduces the risk of introducing microorganisms into the system.
7. Connect the tubing to the irrigation lumen.	
8. Slowly open the roller clamp and establish flow of irrigant. Adjust the flow rate according to the amount ordered over time or by the character of the irrigation returns.	Provides for continuous flushing of the bladder. The amount is regulated to irrigate the bladder without distending it.
9. Remove gloves and leave the patient in a comfortable position. Discard unnecessary equipment and wash hands.	Promotes cleanliness and safety.
10. Monitor the patient and the irrigation regularly. It will be necessary to empty the bag more frequently.	Promotes safety and establishes need for care. For patients with hematuria and clot formation that blocks bladder drainage, the rate of the irrigation may have to be changed frequently. This does not require a specific physician's order, but changes in the character of returns must be recorded.
11. Document the procedure. Note the time irrigation was established, the type of solution used, changes in the character of urinary returns and the patient's tolerance of the procedure. In some agencies, the amount of fluid instilled into the bladder is subtracted from the amount of returns obtained, giving a record of urinary output.	Fulfills requirements for nurse accountability and facilitates continuity of care.

Preparing the Patient

Explain the procedure to the patient. Patients may experience a feeling of fullness in the bladder. They should inform the nurse of any discomfort.

Assembling Equipment

Normal saline is most commonly used for bladder irrigations. Irrigating solutions (irrigants) are administered at room temperature. Disposable irrigation kits are available for open bladder irrigations. A kit includes a container for the irrigating solution, a receptacle for the irrigation return (outflow) and an Asepto syringe. An Asepto syringe is a large bulb-type syringe with a tip that fits into the urinary catheter (see Figure 21.9). In cases where there are large blood clots occluding urinary drainage, the nurse might choose to use a 50- to 60-mL piston-type syringe, called a Toomey syringe, which permits greater forward pressure and return suction than does the Asepto syringe.

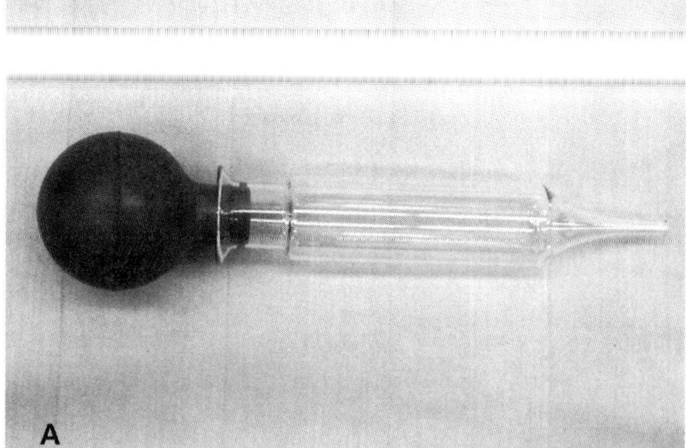

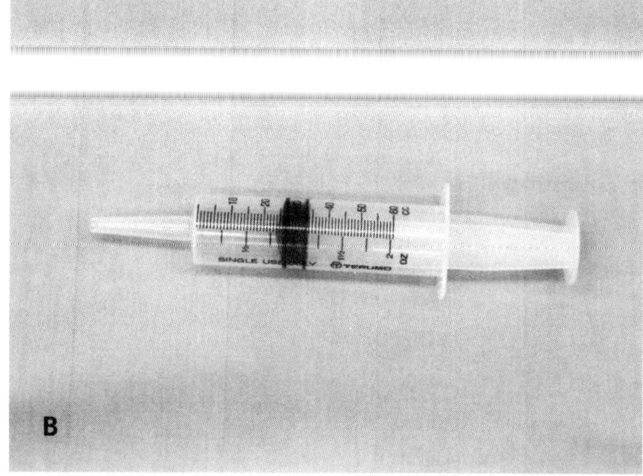

FIGURE 21.9 A. Asepto syringe B. Toomey syringe

A continuous bladder irrigation is set up much like an intravenous infusion (see Procedure 23.1 in Chapter 23). Sterile irrigating solution is usually supplied in three-litre bags of normal saline. The irrigation administration set consists of straight or Y-type tubing which connects to the solution container(s), a roller clamp for adjusting the rate of irrigant entering the bladder, and an adapter end that attaches to the catheter. The Y-type tubing is used when it is necessary to hang two solution bags at once. The solution container is suspended on an IV pole and the tubing is primed in the same manner as intravenous tubing.

EXTERNAL URINARY DRAINAGE

Alternative methods are sometimes used instead of a retention catheter for individuals who are unable to control urination. For women, protective pants made of a non-absorbent plastic or rubberized material are worn over an absorbent pad. An external urinary appliance, called a condom catheter, is often used by men. This appliance consists of a latex condom with a short tube which can be connected to a drainage bag. Known by various names, such as urosheath, Texas condom or condom catheter, it provides a convenient method of collecting urine from patients who are incontinent and reduces the risk of infection from an indwelling catheter. The psychological benefit of being able to empty the bladder in a more "normal" fashion cannot be overemphasized. The condom is disposable, relatively inexpensive and easily applied, all of which make frequent changes possible. It comes with a self-adhesive or Velcro tape which is used to secure the condom in position at the base of the penis (see Figure 21.10). The technique for applying a condom drainage device in outlined in Procedure 21.9.

CARE FOR A CONDOM DRAINAGE DEVICE Once condom drainage has been established, it is important to assess the patient from time to time to ensure that the condom has not become twisted at the point where it joins the drainage tubing and that the tubing has not become kinked, thus blocking drainage. Removal and reapplication of the condom device is dependent upon the integrity of the skin on the patient's penis and the patient's ability to be continent for any length of time.

UROSTOMY CARE

Individuals with urostomies generally have achieved a measure of independence in dealing with their unique method of urinary elimination. When they are ill or hospitalized they may need assistance in carrying out their usual routines.

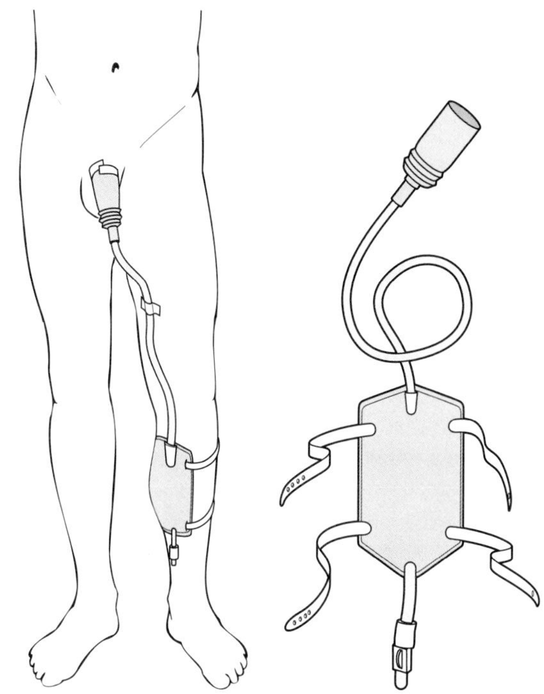

FIGURE 21.10 An external urinary appliance. The urine is collected in a bag that can be attached to the calf or thigh.

PROCEDURE 21.9 Applying a Condom Drainage Device

Action	Rationale
1. Explain the procedure to the patient.	Promotes well-being and enables participation in care.
2. Wash hands and gather: • basin with warm water, soap, washcloth and towel • condom catheter with Velcro or adhesive strap • urinary drainage tube and collecting bag or urinary leg bag and straps • clean gloves • bath blanket.	Lessens transfer of microorganisms and promotes efficiency and economy of time.
3. Close the door to the room or draw bed curtains. Assist the patient into a dorsal recumbent position, cover him with a bath blanket and expose the genitals.	Promotes privacy and lessens feelings of embarrassment. Keeps the patient warm.
4. Apply gloves and thoroughly wash and dry the penis and perineal area.	Removes urine and other secretions that may be harmful to skin integrity.
5a. Unroll the condom over the the penis so that the narrow tube opening at the end is over the urinary meatus. Leave approximately 2.5–5 cm space between the end of the penis and the end of the condom.	Permits proper application of condom. Decreases the chance of skin irritation and allows urine to drain more freely.
b. To apply a self-adhering condom: Place the condom catheter funnel over the tip of the penis; squeeze the funnel to seal the catheter to the penile tip. Gently pull the catheter to expose the penile shaft. Unroll the condom and squeeze to seal.	

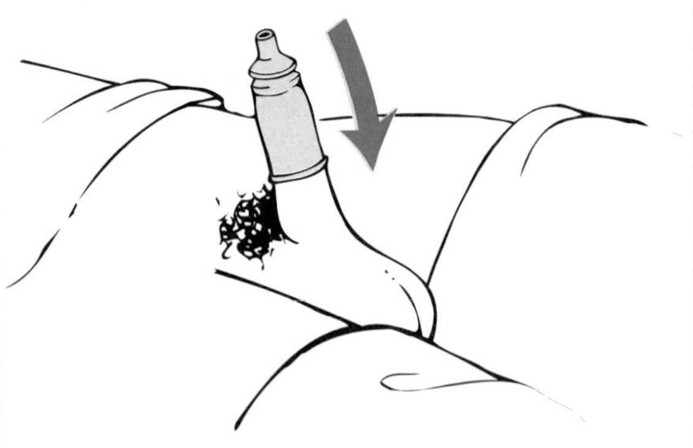

Action	Rationale
6. Wrap the tape or Velcro strap snugly (but not too tightly) over the condom around the shaft of the penis in a spiral; do not encircle the penis or overlap the tape.	Encircling with tape impedes the circulation to the penis and does not allow for expansion in the event of an erection; a spiral allows for expansion.
7. Connect the tube opening of the condom to the urinary drainage set (or leg bag).	Establishes a route for collecting urine.
8. Remove gloves and assist the patient to a position of comfort. Remove used equipment and wash hands.	Promotes patient well-being. Promotes cleanliness and safety in the workplace.
9. Document procedure. Record the patient's response to the procedure. Record urinary drainage as necessary.	Fulfills requirements for nurse accountability and facilitates continuity of care.

The nurse should assess the individual's ability to care for the urostomy independently. As well, the condition of [illegible] agency has access to an enterostomal therapist, the nurse can enlist his or her aid in formulating the most effective plan of care for the patient.

INCONTINENT URINARY DIVERSIONS Individuals with incontinent urinary diversions (for example, an ileal conduit) wear an external collecting appliance. This is a one- or two-piece appliance consisting of a collecting bag with an adhesive wafer that sticks to the skin surrounding the urinary stoma. The appliance can be kept in place for three to seven days, but generally, it is changed twice a week. If it is a two-piece appliance, the collecting bag can be changed more frequently and the wafer can stay in place up to 10 [illegible] through which it is emptied into a toilet or other receptacle. For most individuals, the collecting bag is attached by means of a connector to a closed urinary drainage system (as is used for catheter drainage) for drainage during the night. This reduces the risk of leakage or rupture of the bag and ensures peace of mind while the person sleeps. The technique for changing an external collecting appliance is outlined in Procedure 21.10.

Throughout the procedure, the nurse should observe the condition of the peristomal skin, condition of the stoma

PROCEDURE 21.10 Changing an External Two-Piece Urostomy Appliance

Action	*Rationale*
1. Wash hands and gather: • type and size of appliance used by the patient • clean gloves • waterproof protective pad • basin with warm water, soap, washcloth and towels (or cotton gauze wipes) • urine collection container • scissors • moisture-proof bag.	Reduces the spread of microorganisms. Promotes efficiency and economy of time.
2. Provide for privacy; position the patient and place the protective pad under the patient on stoma side.	Individuals with incontinent diversions have no control over urinary elimination. Protects bed linens.
3. Don clean gloves.	Protects nurse from exposure to body fluids and substances.
4. Position the urine collection container under the valve and open it. Drain any urine collected in the bag into the container. Measure and discard urine.	Provides accurate measurement of urinary output. Allows for appropriate disposal of urine.
5. Prepare the new wafer. If necessary, cut an opening on the wafer large enough to accommodate the size of stoma. Some patients may have a guide to gauge the size of the opening.	Allows the barrier to be fitted over the stoma.

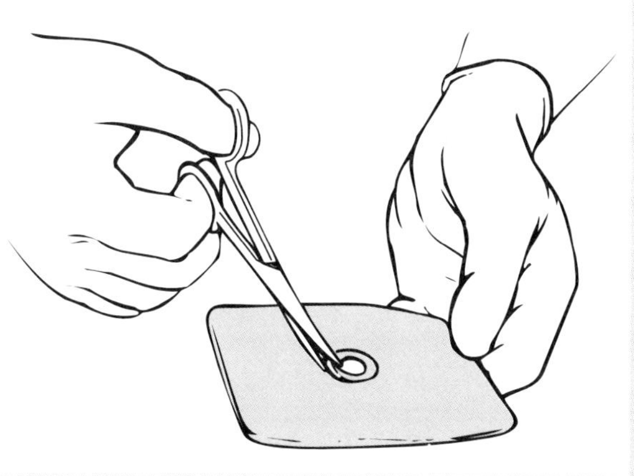

Continued on the next page

PROCEDURE 21.10 *continued*

Action	Rationale
6. Remove the old appliance by carefully lifting one corner of the wafer from the skin using one hand while pressing down with the other. Discard into garbage bag.	Protects the patient's skin from damage. Maintains a clean environment.
7. Gently cleanse area around the stoma with warm soapy water, rinse clean and dry well.	Provides for skin protection from urine. The stoma is fragile and will bleed readily if handled in a rough manner.

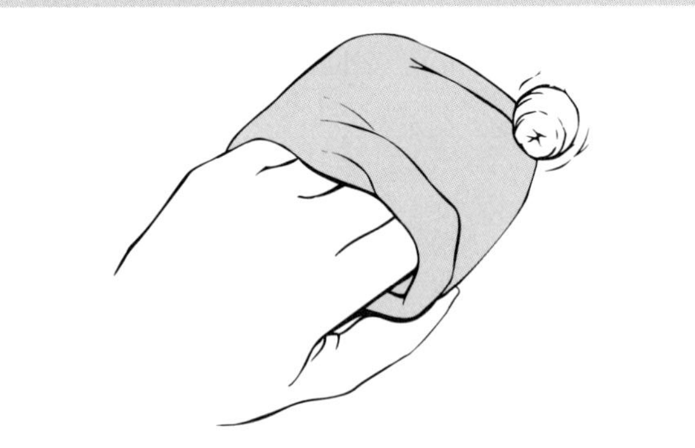

Action	Rationale
8. Apply the new wafer quickly, pressing the wafer firmly to the skin around the stoma.	A urinary stoma drips urine constantly. If the appliance is applied quickly, the skin will remain dry and the wafer will stick.

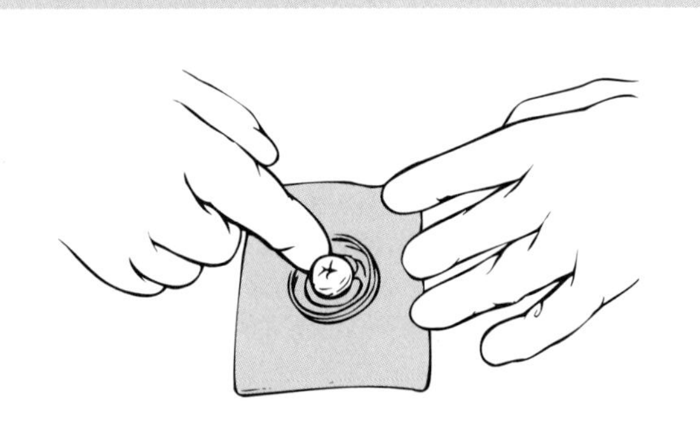

Action	Rationale
9. Attach the collecting bag to the wafer. Ensure that the valve is closed and positioned at the bottom.	Allows for effective drainage and proper filling of collecting bag.

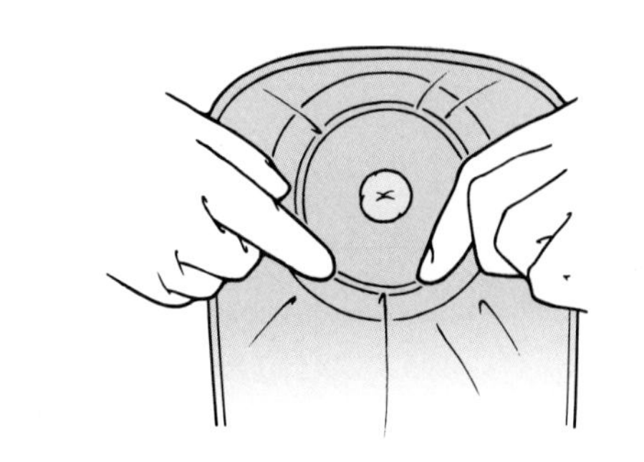

SOURCE: ConvaTec, 1986.

and characteristics of the urine. One of the normal functions of the bowel is to produce mucus to facilitate passage of fecal matter. For individuals with urinary reservoirs cre-

urine to be somewhat cloudy and to contain mucous shreds. However, the nurse must remain alert for any signs of urinary tract dysfunction such as foul-smelling urine, hematuria and increased body temperature.

COLLECTING A SAMPLE OF URINE FROM URINARY DIVERSIONS To collect a urine sample for urinalysis from a patient with a urinary diversion, the nurse first empties the collecting bag, waits for more urine to collect and then takes the sample from the fresh supply. If a urine for culture and sensitivity is required, the nurse will need to remove the collecting bag, insert a sterile, straight catheter into the stoma, position the other end of the catheter into the sterile specimen container and, once the specimen is collected, withdraw the catheter and reapply the collecting bag.

CONTINENT URINARY DIVERSIONS Individuals with continent urinary diversions meet their need for urinary elimination by catheterizing their urinary reservoirs on a regular basis throughout the day. If assistance is required, the nurse needs to know the size of catheter used and the frequency of catheterization.

Causes of Acute Renal Failure

decreased circulating volume
- volume shifts
- decreased cardiac output
- renal vascular obstruction
- decreased peripheral vascular resistance.

Renal failure
- acute tubular necrosis
- trauma
- severe muscle exertion
- certain genetic conditions
- infectious disease
- metabolic disorders
- glomerulonephritis
- vascular lesions.

Postrenal failure
- obstruction
- spinal cord injury
- pelvic trauma.

SOURCE: Black & Matassarin-Jacobs, 1997.

ASSISTING WITH MEASURES TO REDUCE THE WORKLOAD ON THE KIDNEYS

The primary function of the kidneys is to maintain the composition and volume of the body fluids in homeostasis. In cases of renal failure, the kidneys are unable to excrete the waste products of metabolism, chiefly the nitrogenous wastes of cellular metabolism. This may be an acute, potentially reversible state resulting from major trauma, metabolic disturbances or surgery. It may also be a chronic condition requiring long-term management.

Careful monitoring of the patient's fluid intake and output, electrolyte balance and response to therapy and medications can identify those individuals who are at risk for development of acute renal failure. Acute renal failure requires comprehensive medical and nursing intervention.

The nurse can implement various measures to relieve some of the workload on the kidney. The patient is generally prescribed bed rest in an effort to minimize activity and lessen cellular metabolism. Diet therapy for the renal patient is highly individualized. Protein metabolism results in the formation of nitrogenous waste products. Therefore, unless the patient is losing large amounts of protein in the urine (which occurs in some conditions), the patient is placed on a low-protein diet in an attempt to minimize the amounts of nitrogenous wastes produced.

In renal failure, the kidney does not excrete or retain sodium and potassium appropriately. Higher levels of sodium cause fluid retention, while accumulation of potassium can result in serious neuromuscular disturbances. Fluid intake may be restricted in an effort to prevent or lessen edema. Meticulous monitoring of fluid intake and output is critical to the patient's therapeutic management. Patients with renal disorders often suffer from anorexia and may need encouragement to eat their meals. The nurse needs to ensure that the patient is made aware of the importance of adhering to the ordered diet and fluid intake. Many patients are able to keep track of their fluid intake, and gains in their fluid management can often be achieved by encouraging them to participate in their own care.

Edematous tissue is more prone to breakdown than is normal tissue; therefore, if edema is present, the nurse must be alert for any sign of impaired skin integrity. Patients who are confined to bed require particular attention to prevent the development of pressure areas. Fluid tends to collect in the dependent parts of the body, such as the lower limbs and the sacral area in bed patients. These areas particularly should be monitored for signs of impending tissue breakdown, and measures should be taken to prevent this. See Chapter 31.

Meticulous skin care is important in the care of patients with renal impairment, not only as a factor in maintaining skin integrity, but also to cleanse the skin of perspiration and rid the patient of any unpleasant odours arising from the accumulation of nitrogenous wastes being eliminated by this route. Bathing is particularly important for the patient's cleanliness and comfort.

In an effort to compensate for the decreased ability of the kidneys to excrete excess acid, an increased amount of carbonic acid is eliminated through the respiratory tract.

COMMUNITY health practice: Treating Incontinence with Biofeedback

In 1995, Vancouver General Hospital and Health Sciences Centre in Vancouver, British Columbia, established a Physiology Centre to meet the needs of individuals with various physiological disorders. One such disorder is urinary incontinence.

Referrals come directly to the centre from the referring specialist's office. Services provided include diagnostic testing, education, treatment and research. The centre is staffed by two physiotherapists.

The goal of therapy is to assist patients to understand their health problem and to teach effective strategies to cope with the physiological disorder. Prior to their initial assessment at the centre, patients are required to keep a continence diary for seven days, including a list of any medications taken.

Treatment consists of biofeedback, which is covered by the provincial health plan. Biofeedback equipment must to be purchased by the patient prior to the first appointment. Treatment is carried out at home between centre visits.

Measures to facilitate breathing are therefore important. The position of the patient when in bed should be such that maximum expansion of the chest is possible. The room should be well ventilated and an adequate supply of oxygen ensured.

Accumulated nitrogenous wastes may cause disturbances in neuromuscular functioning. Headaches and lethargy are not uncommon and, in severe cases of renal impairment, the patient may become disoriented and subsequently comatose. In these cases, it is especially important to consider the safety needs of the patient. Although the sensorium can remain clear even in patients with considerable kidney damage, the nurse must be alert to any signs of mental confusion. Measures such as side rails to protect the confused patient from injury and the application of mitts to prevent pulling at catheters or other tubing are frequently needed.

Muscle weakness may result from the retention of potassium, and the renal patient is usually easily fatigued. The heart is particularly susceptible to changes in potassium levels. Therefore, the apical heartbeat provides a more accurate assessment of the patient's cardiac status.

At times, if the kidneys have ceased to function adequately or if the kidneys need to be put at complete rest in an effort to promote recovery, the patient will be put on *renal dialysis*. This can be accomplished by means of hemodialysis or peritoneal dialysis.

Hemodialysis removes waste products and excess water by circulating blood from an artery through an external dialyzer (sometimes referred to as an artificial kidney). Waste products are removed by the process of diffusion across a semi-permeable membrane, which mimics the processes of filtration, reabsorption and secretion normally carried out by the kidney. The composition of the *dialysis fluid* on one side of the membrane is the same as the blood, with the exception of urea and other waste products. Thus, movement of the waste products across the membrane occurs by diffusion and filtration. The cleansed blood is then returned to the patient through a vein. Several types of machines for renal dialysis are now available, including units for home use. Some patients require renal dialysis for a short period of time, until recovery from the acute episode has been achieved. However, many individuals with nonfunctioning kidneys and no hope of recovery have been maintained on dialysis over a period of years. For those patients without access to home dialysis, outpatient departments or renal clinics provide dialysis on a scheduled basis, usually three times a week.

In place of hemodialysis, patients may be treated by **peritoneal dialysis**. This technique requires large amounts of *dialyzing fluid* to be instilled into the peritoneal cavity and later removed. Dialysis occurs in this method by the circulation of waste products through the peritoneal capillaries diffusing across the peritoneal membrane into the dialysis fluid. This procedure has been refined to the extent that patients no longer need be hospitalized and are taught to do dialysis at home.

A patient's initial experience of undergoing renal dialysis can be very frightening. Often the individual is very ill, and the exposure to highly technical machinery, the numerous personnel involved and the attendant tests required can provoke anxiety. Many large acute care hospitals are equipped with renal units staffed by specially trained personnel who can provide the thorough explanations required to allay patient anxiety. However, the nurse in the general patient areas or in the community should be aware of patients' (and families') need for continuing encouragement and supportive care. It is important for the nurse to consider the patient's ability to adjust to the effects of renal failure as a chronic condition. Stress, such as that caused by the inability of the individual to work, may be a significant factor to be addressed in the nursing care plan.

Once the condition is stabilized, the patient is usually treated on an outpatient basis. For some, dialysis may be done in the home environment. On occasion, however, these individuals may require hospitalization. Usually all that is required is notifying the renal unit of the patient's admission and noting the scheduled times for dialysis on the patient's Kardex. However, the nurse in the general patient areas should also be aware of the need to assess the patient's access site for dialysis. Normally, a thrill can be felt by palpation over the vascular access site or a bruit can be heard by use of a stethoscope. This would indicate patency of the site

ing that no venipunctures or blood pressures be done on this arm should be posted above the patient's bed.

For the patient receiving peritoneal dialysis, the nurse should assess the peritoneal catheter insertion site. Usually the patient can be provided with the necessary supplies and is able to change the dressing independently. If assistance from the nurse is required, the dressing around the catheter should be changed daily and whenever necessary.

Evaluating Urinary Elimination Interventions

The expected outcomes established in the planning phase of the nursing process provide the basis for evaluating the effectiveness of nursing interventions. Changes in the patient's plan of care are made accordingly. Examples of questions the nurse might ask in evaluating care for urinary elimination problems are given below.

1. Is the patient voiding an adequate amount in relation to fluid intake?
2. Are the laboratory test results showing improvement in the patient's condition?
3. Does the patient maintain voluntary control of micturition?
4. Can the patient state or identify factors that interfere with his or her normal voiding pattern?
5. Can the patient describe measures to promote or maintain normal urinary elimination?
6. Is the patient's skin in good condition?
7. Is the patient comfortable—free from pain, restlessness and anxiety?

IN REVIEW

- The primary functions of urinary elimination are:
  - to remove nitrogenous waste products
  - to regulate fluid and electrolyte balance.

  These functions are essential in the maintenance of homeostasis. When elimination is impaired, the individual may become very ill.
- The urinary tract consists of:
  - two kidneys
  - two ureters
  - one bladder
  - one urethra.
- The functional unit of the kidney is the nephron. Urine is formed in the nephrons through the processes of:
  - [illegible]
  - reabsorption
  - secretion.
- Urine is transported to the urinary bladder by the ureters. The urinary bladder stores urine, and the urethra transports urine from the bladder to the exit point from the body.
- Micturition (urination) may occur both voluntarily and involuntarily.
- Urinary function changes throughout the life cycle and is affected by:
  - individual differences
  - fluid and food intake
  - psychological states such as stress, anxiety and pain
  - disease states and illness
  - associated medical treatment.
- Common urinary problems include localized disturbances such as:
  - incontinence
  - dysuria
  - frequency
  - urgency
  - nocturia
  - polyuria
  - oliguria
  - anuria
  - retention
  - hematuria
  - hesitancy.
- Some medical problems of the urinary tract, such as trauma, congenital anomalies of the bladder and cancer of the bladder, require urinary diversions. In a urinary diversion, urine is eliminated from the body through a urostomy, an artificial opening created to divert urine from the kidneys to the abdominal wall.
- A urinary status assessment includes:
  - nursing health history
  - physical assessment
  - review of laboratory data.
- Nurses are responsible for:
  - collecting urine specimens
  - performing dipstick examinations
  - preparing patients for diagnostic tests and procedures.
- Nursing care (planning and implementation) for individuals with urinary elimination problems is based on the nursing diagnoses and focusses on:
  - promoting optimal urinary elimination
  - maintaining or restoring normal patterns
  - preventing associated problems.

- Common nursing diagnoses for patients with urinary elimination problems include:
  - Incontinence
  - Urinary retention.
- Restorative care includes:
  - measures to re-establish normal voiding patterns (bladder retraining program; e.g., deferment, pelvic bracing, scheduled urination)
  - measures to stimulate micturition
  - urinary catheterization
  - external urinary drainage.
- Individuals with urostomies may need assistance in carrying out their usual routines when they are ill or hospitalized.
- Renal dialysis may be used when the kidneys have ceased to function or need a rest in an effort to promote healing. There are two kinds of dialysis:
  - peritoneal dialysis
  - hemodialysis.

KEY TERMS

nephron p. 553
glomerulus p. 553
ureters p. 554
urinary bladder p. 554
urethra p. 554
meatus p. 554
micturition p. 554
prostate gland p. 556
urinary incontinence p. 557
stress incontinence p. 557
dysuria p. 557
urinary frequency p. 557
urgency p. 557
nocturia p. 557
enuresis p. 557
polyuria p. 557
diuresis p. 557
diuretics p. 557
urinary retention p. 558
cystitis p. 558
oliguria p. 558
renal anuria p. 558
hematuria p. 558
hesitancy p. 558
uremia p. 558
stoma p. 558
urostomy p. 558
ileal conduit p. 558
continent urostomy p. 558
urinalysis p. 560
cystoscopy p. 563
pyelogram p. 563
Kegel exercises p. 566
hemodialysis p. 588
peritoneal dialysis p. 588

Critical Thinking Activities

1. Mrs. Tavares needs an indwelling catheter prior to her surgery tomorrow afternoon. Mrs. Tavares is an intelligent person; she understands the purpose of her surgery, but she has never had a urinary catheterization. The catheter is to be inserted tomorrow morning.

   This afternoon Mrs. Tavares's husband comes to the nursing unit desk greatly disturbed. His wife has told him that she has to have a tube inserted and he does not understand why. In talking with Mr. Tavares, you learn that his mother had a tube inserted and she died two days later.

   a) What factors should you consider in your explanation?
   b) What should you include in your explanation to Mr. Tavares? Why?
   c) What principles would guide you in carrying out a urinary catheterization?
   d) Why is a urinary catheterization a distressing measure?
   e) What nursing interventions would be essential for Mrs. Tavares, as a result of the indwelling catheter?
   f) How can you evaluate the effectiveness of your nursing care after the catheterization?
   g) What problems could Mrs. Tavares encounter following removal of the indwelling catheter?
   h) What would you teach Mrs. Tavares following removal of the indwelling catheter?

2. With the aid of your instructor, arrange to spend a day with an enterostomal therapist in your agency. How does the enterostomal therapist establish a teaching plan for a patient with a urinary diversion? What techniques does he or she use in helping individuals learn how to manage their urostomies?

References

BLACK, J.M., & MATASSARIN-JACOBS, E. (1997). *Medical–surgical nursing: Clinical management for continuity of care.* (5th ed.). Philadelphia: Saunders.

CARPENITO, L.J. (1997). *Nursing diagnosis: Application to clinical practice.* (7th ed.). Philadelphia: Lippincott.

CHERNECKY, C.C., & BERGER, B.J. (1997). Laboratory tests and diagnostic procedures. (2nd ed.). Philadelphia: Saunders.

CONVATEC. (1986). *For a better way of living with a urostomy—every day.* Princeton, NJ: Squibb & Sons, Inc. (Pamphlet 567-042CE)

DUDEK, S.G. (1997). *Nutrition handbook for nursing practice.* (3rd ed.). Philadelphia: Lippincott.

HUETHER, S.E. (1996). Alterations of renal and urinary tract function. In S.E. Huether & K.L. McCance (Eds.), *Understanding pathophysiology.* St. Louis: Mosby.

JACKSON, B., & HICKS, L.A. (1997). Effect of cranberry juice on urinary pH in older adults. *Home Healthcare Nurse, 15*(3), 199–202.

KENNER, C.A., & MacLAREN, A. (1993). *Essentials of maternal and neonatal nursing.* Springhouse, PA: Springhouse.

MacLEOD, F., & MacTAVISH, M. (1988). Adult incontinence. *Canadian Nurse, 84*(8), 45–47.

PILLITTERI, A. (1995). *Maternal and child health nursing: Care of the childbearing and childcaring family* (2nd ed.). Philadelphia: Lippincott.

PORTH, C.M. (1998). *Pathophysiology concepts of altered health status.* (5th ed.). Philadelphia: Lippincott.

WONG, D.L. (1995). *Whaley & Wong's nursing care of infants and children.*

Additional Readings

ALLEN, P. (1992). Nursing care: Kock pouch continent urinary diversion—the Hamilton experience. *Canadian Association for Enterostomal Therapy, 11*(4), 17–19.

AVORN, J., MONANE, M., GURWITZ, J., GLYNN, R., CHOODNOVSKY, I., & LIPSILZ, L. (1994). Reduction of bacteriuria and pyuria after ingestion of cranberry juice. *Journal of the American Medical Association, 271*(March 9), 751–754.

CONNOR, P.A. (1996). Nurses' knowledge, attitudes, and practices in managing urinary incontinence in the acute care setting. *MedSurg Nursing, 5*(2), 87–92.

FASING, S. (1996). Assessment and treatment of urinary incontinence in the hospitalized adult. *Journal of Wound, Ostomy & Continence Nursing, 23*(5), 269–272.

GALLO, M.L., HANCOCK, R., & DAVILA, W. (1997). Clinical experience with a balloon-tipped urethral insert for stress urinary incontinence. *Journal of Wound, Ostomy & Continence Nursing, 24*(1), 51–57.

GRAY, M. (1996). A traumatic urethral catheterization of children. *Pediatric Nursing, 22*(4), 306–310.

KOHLER-OCKMON, J. (1993). Catheter concerns. *Nursing Times, 89*(2), 34–36.

KURTZ, M.J., VAN ZANDT, D.K., & SAPP, L.R. (1996). A new technique in independent intermittent catheterization: The Mitrofanoff catheterizable channel. *Rehabilitation Nursing, 21*(6), 311–315.

LAW, M.D. (1996). Incontinence management implementing a bowel–bladder management program. *Canadian Nursing Home, 7*(1), 27–29.

MANTLE, F. (1996). Eliminate the problem: Complementary therapies—elimination problems. *Nursing Times, 92*(32), 50–51.

MARCHIONDO, K. (1998). A new look at urinary tract infection. *American*

MILNE, A. (1993). Men only: Male catheterisation procedures. *Nursing Times, 89*(8), 55–58.

MOORE, K. (1992). Indwelling catheters: Problems and management. *Canadian Nurse, 88*(6), 33–35.

NAZARKO, L. (1995). The therapeutic uses of cranberry juice. *Nursing Standard, 9*(34), 33–35.

NESKY, K., & LOEHNER, D. (1994). Urinary diversion with an Indiana pouch. *Nursing 94, 24*(1), 32c–32h.

PALMER, M.H. (1997). Pelvic muscle rehabilitation: Where do we go from here? *Journal of Wound, Ostomy & Continence Nursing, 24*(2), 98–105.

PALMER, M.H., CZARAPATA, B.J.R., WELLS, T.J., & NEWMAN, D.K. (1997). Urinary outcomes in older adults: Research and clinical perspectives. *Urologic Nursing, 17*(1), 2–9.

PEARSON, B. (1993). Liquidate a myth: Reducing liquid intake is not advisable for elderly with urine control problems. *Urologic Nursing, 13*(3), 86–87.

RESNICK, B. (1993). Retraining the bladder after catheterization. *American Journal of Nursing, 93*(11), 43.

SOSA-GUERRERO, S., & GOMEZ, N.J. (1997). Dealing with end-stage renal disease. *American Journal of Nursing, 97*(10), 44–51.

TOOTLA, J., & EASTERLING, A.D. (1992). Current options in bladder cancer management. *RN, 55*(4), 42–49.

WARREN, J.W. (1996). Urethral catheters, condom catheters, and nosocomial urinary tract infections. *Infection Control & Hospital Epidemiology, 17*(4), 212–214.

WOZNIAK-PETROFSKY, J. (1993). Fundamental urodynamics (part 1): Normal bladder function and patient assessment. *Urologic Nursing, 13*(3), 88–92.

Chapter 22

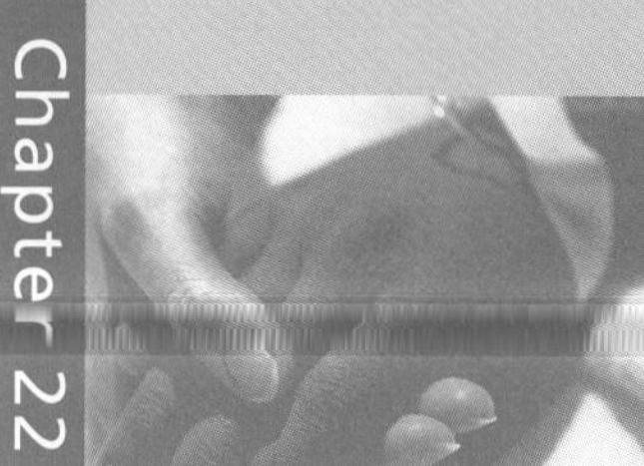

Bowel Elimination Needs

OUTLINE

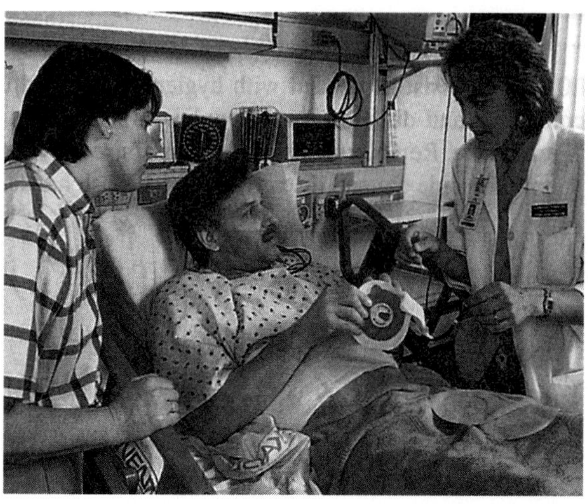

Central Questions

1. In what way is bowel elimination important to health and well-being?
2. What are the structures and functions involved in bowel elimination?
3. How does bowel elimination vary throughout the life cycle?
4. What are the main determinants of bowel functioning?
5. What are some common bowel elimination problems?
6. What basic principles would the nurse apply in assisting individuals to meet bowel elimination needs?
7. How does the nurse assess an individual's bowel elimination status?
8. What are the common nursing diagnostic statements for individuals with bowel elimination problems?
9. How would the nurse develop a plan of care for individuals with bowel elimination problems?
10. What strategies might the nurse implement in helping individuals, families or groups to promote optimal bowel functioning and prevent potential bowel elimination problems?
11. What health-restoring and supportive strategies might the nurse implement in the care of individuals with bowel elimination problems?
12. How would the nurse evaluate the individual's response to nursing interventions?

Introduction

Bowel elimination is the excretion of gastrointestinal waste

an essential part of health. A proper diet, adequate intake of fluids, exercise and regular bowel habits contribute to healthy bowel elimination patterns. Anyone can encounter difficulty maintaining bowel elimination at one time or another. For example, a person may develop mild constipation or diarrhea after eating certain foods or may suffer severe diarrhea from a bout of gastrointestinal flu. Illness, travel, medications, surgery or a change in activity and eating patterns can disrupt normal patterns of elimination.

While most bowel elimination problems are not serious, individuals usually feel uncomfortable and are often distressed. If a disruption in bowel elimination is not restored, the functioning of all other body systems may be affected. For instance, prolonged and severe diarrhea can lead to such problems as nutritional deficits, water and electrolyte imbalances, alterations in comfort and impaired skin integrity. In developing countries, infectious diarrhea is the most significant cause of infant and early childhood mortality. Individuals may need assistance to maintain or promote normal bowel elimination patterns or to restore their usual pattern of elimination when a disturbance has occurred.

This chapter provides basic knowledge of the physiology of bowel elimination, the factors that affect bowel function and common bowel elimination problems. This knowledge will enable the nurse to assess a person's bowel elimination needs and plan individualized care. Also outlined are nursing interventions for helping people to promote normal bowel patterns in daily living; to prevent bowel disruption during illness, diagnostic testing and medical treatment; and to restore bowel function following illness.

Anatomy and Physiology of Bowel Elimination

During digestion, food and fluids taken into the body are mixed and processed, nutrients are selected and absorbed for utilization by body tissues and the waste products of digestion are excreted. The principal structures of the gastrointestinal tract concerned with elimination are the small and large intestine.

The **small intestine** is a narrow muscular tube approximately 2.5 cm in diameter and 7 m in length. It consists of three sections: the **duodenum**, the **jejunum** and the **ileum** (see Figure 22.1). Food in the stomach is propelled into the small intestine by stimulation of the gastrocolic reflex. The duodenum receives food in the form of chyme (viscous, liquid contents of the stomach) from the stomach about half an hour after ingestion. Chyme moves through the small intestine slowly via wave-like contraction and relaxation of smooth muscles (peristalsis). It mixes with digestive enzymes from the gallbladder and pancreas, further breaking down food for digestion. This mixing action is called segmenting. The duodenum is the primary site for iron and calcium

drates; and the ileum absorbs specific vitamins and bile salts (Society of Gastroenterology Nurses & Associates, 1993). By the time chyme reaches the large bowel, it consists mostly of nondigestible substances.

When chyme has moved through the small intestine, the duodenocolic reflex is initiated and pushes the digestive content into the large intestine.

The **large intestine** is larger in diameter (6–7 cm) than the small intestine, but is shorter in length (1.5 m). Divisions of the large intestine include the cecum; the appendix; the ascending, transverse, descending and sigmoid colon; the rectum and the anal canal (see Figure 22.1). The large intestine's primary functions are the absorption of water, electrolytes and remaining nutrients; the synthesis of vitamins; and the storage and elimination of feces (Huether, 1996).

The **cecum** receives unabsorbed chyme from the small intestine and, through peristalsis, moves it forward through the colon. Most absorption of water, nutrients and electrolytes, such as sodium and chloride, occurs in the cecum, ascending and transverse colon. The amount of water that is absorbed depends on the speed of peristaltic action. If propelled too rapidly, the resultant stool will be loose and watery. If peristalsis is too slow, water will continue to be absorbed and the stool will become dry and hard. The synthesis of certain vitamins, including folic acid, riboflavin and vitamin K, occurs in the large bowel aided by the activity of intestinal bacteria. Bacteria are typically found in

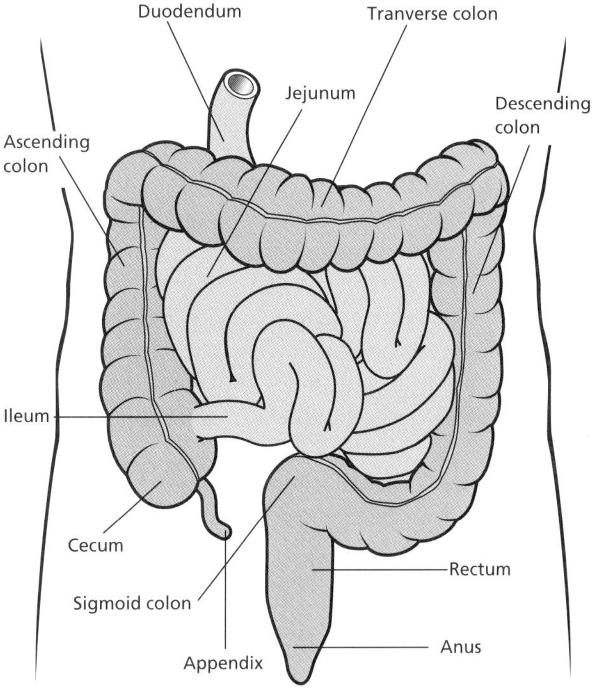

FIGURE 22.1 The small and large intestines

the intestinal cavity and are often referred to as normal intestinal flora. If bowel function is impaired, serious nutritional and electrolyte imbalances can develop.

Finally, the distal colon (descending and sigmoid colon) stores and removes waste products and gas (flatus). To protect itself from injury as the waste moves towards the rectum and becomes drier, the distal colon releases mucus. Waste products are stored in the sigmoid colon and are called **feces**. Normal feces consist of digestive residues and water, with water making up approximately 75 percent of the total. Digestive residues include those from undigested and unabsorbed foods and from digestive secretions. The feces also contain cells and mucous sloughed off the lining of the gastrointestinal tract, as well as bacteria. Added to the resident bacteria are those that have been ingested through food and fluids, from fingers or in swallowed air.

When feces and flatus accumulate in the sigmoid colon, the muscle layers are stimulated to contract. Mass peristaltic movements force the feces into the **rectum**. These movements are strong and occur only a few times a day. The rectum is normally empty of stool. In the adult, the rectum is approximately 12–15 cm in length and 2.5–4 cm in width at the anal opening. The walls of the rectum consist of transverse and vertical folds. The transverse folds assist in keeping the feces in the rectum until defecation (the act of emptying stool from the anus and rectum) is initiated. The vertical folds each contain an artery and veins. Hemorrhoids occur when the veins become engorged owing to pressure from straining during defecation.

The **anal canal** forms approximately the last 2.5 cm of the rectum. Two muscular sphincters control the discharge of feces from the anus. The internal sphincter is composed of smooth muscle and its control is involuntary (i.e., it is controlled by the autonomic nervous system), responding to distention of the rectum; the external sphincter is composed of striated muscle and is under voluntary control (i.e., it is controlled by the cerebral cortex).

The rectal reflex is initiated when the rectum is full. Parasympathetic nerve endings transmit impulses to the brain to initiate the rectal reflex. The internal sphincter of the anus relaxes and the colon contracts. The urge to have a bowel movement is felt. However, the external sphincter can be controlled voluntarily so if the time is not suitable for defecation, the act can be delayed and the urge to defecate will disappear (Porth, 1998).

During the act of defecation, the external sphincter relaxes and a number of accessory muscles are brought into play. Contraction of the muscles of the abdominal wall and fixing of the diaphragm increase pressure within the abdominal cavity, which aids expulsion of feces. Closing of the glottis by holding the breath while bearing down also increases intra-abdominal pressure. This is called the Valsalva manoeuvre. Finally, defecation can be assisted by assuming a sitting or squatting position (Porth, 1998).

Bowel Functioning in Health

Normal stools are brown in colour (due to the presence of urobilinogen), soft and solid in consistency and cylindrical in shape. The amount of fecal matter excreted is highly dependent on the coarseness of the foodstuffs consumed. It may vary from 100–200 g/day, in a person whose diet contains a large proportion of refined food, to 300–400 g/day, in a person who eats a diet high in fibre. The number of bowel movements a person has also varies from one individual to another, with the average being between one or two bowel movements every day to one movement every two to three days. Fecal odour is caused by the by-products of bacterial activity. Flatus (air or gas in the intestine) is formed by bacterial action on the digestive products, diffusion of gas from the blood stream and from swallowing air while eating or talking. It is estimated that 400–700 mL of flatus is produced daily (Guyton, 1996).

Bowel Elimination Throughout the Life Cycle

Bowel elimination patterns are affected by growth and development throughout the life cycle. Knowledge of the variations in bowel function and stool characteristics will assist the nurse in assessing patients and determining their elimination needs.

The first bowel movement of the newborn infant is called **meconium**; it is a greenish-black, tarry substance that is present in the gastrointestinal tract of the full-term fetus. During the first week of life, stools gradually change from greenish-black to yellow. Because the infant's stomach is small and peristalsis is rapid, food moves quickly through the digestive tract. Breast-fed infants may have four to six bowel movements a day, and bottle-fed babies one to three a day. In breast-fed babies the stools are usually looser and lighter yellow in colour and do not have as strong a fecal odour as those of bottle-fed babies. Breast-fed babies also rarely develop constipation, although they may do so when they are weaned, if their fluid intake is not sufficient. With the addition of solids to the diet, the stools become fewer in number, darker brown in colour and firmer in consistency (Wong, 1995).

Infants and young toddlers normally have a bowel movement whenever the rectum is full. The necessary neuromuscular development for voluntary control is usually not present until the age of two to three years (Guyton, 1996). By four years, most children have fairly good control over defecation, although accidents may still happen if the child is in a stressful situation, is too busy to go to the bathroom or has diarrhea.

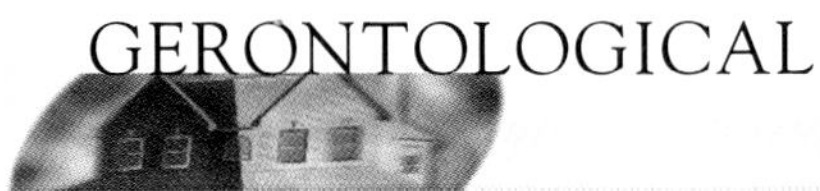

Effects of Aging on Bowel Elimination

Peristalsis is slowed	Constipation
Decreased blood to the intestines	Decreased peristalsis
Gradual loss of anal sphincter control	Fecal incontinence
Slower nerve impulses to the lower bowel	Constipation, impaction
Weakened large intestine musculature	Diverticulosis
Decreased absorption of intestinal mucosa	Protein, mineral, vitamin deficiencies

The elimination patterns of school-age children and adolescents tend to remain fairly constant. However, there is rapid growth of the large intestine during the teenage years and an increase in the amount of food consumed.

Among adults, variations in bowel patterns occur in pregnant women and in older people. During pregnancy, the entire gastrointestinal tract becomes more sluggish owing to the relaxing effect of hormones on smooth muscle. This, combined with the pressure of the growing uterus on the abdominal organs, causes constipation and flatulence. Hemorrhoids also frequently occur in pregnant women and add to the discomfort of bowel elimination (Pillitteri, 1995).

In the older adult, many changes occur that influence elimination. Appetite decreases and the ability to chew food thoroughly may be reduced by the loss of teeth or poorly fitting dentures. Partially chewed food enters the digestive tract and is processed less efficiently because of the decrease in digestive enzyme secretions. Also, peristaltic action slows down and the absorptive ability of the intestinal mucosa changes. There is weakening of the muscle tone in the perineal floor and the anal sphincter, as well as slowing of the rectal reflex nerve impulses. The older adult is more likely to experience constipation and may have difficulty controlling bowel elimination (Black & Matassarin-Jacobs, 1997).

Determinants of Bowel Functioning

In addition to the variations that occur at different stages in the life cycle, many other factors affect bowel functioning. These include health practices such as dietary and fluid intake patterns, personal habits, activity and exercise. Illness, pain, emotions, surgery and anesthesia, and medications also influence bowel elimination.

DIETARY PATTERN AND FLUID INTAKE

The type of food and the amount of fluids a person consumes influence both the nature and frequency of bowel movements. An adequate amount of fibre in the diet is important in providing sufficient bulk to stimulate peristaltic action of the intestines. Fibre is the undigestible residue in food. It absorbs water, which increases stool mass and keeps the stool soft. Raw fruits and vegetables, greens and whole grains contain high amounts of fibre. Natural bran has the highest fibre content of any food and is the most satisfactory bulking agent (Jensen, 1990). People whose diet consists mostly of highly refined foods usually have fewer bowel movements, and their stools are likely to be firmer and darker in colour than those who ensure that they include high-fibre foods in their daily diet.

Certain foods cause flatus in some individuals. Flatus stimulates peristalsis by distending the bowel wall and it can cause abdominal discomfort. Some notoriously gas-forming foods are cabbage, turnips, onions and beans. Fried and spicy foods can cause peristalsis and watery stools. Food-borne infection may also cause gastrointestinal upsets.

An adequate daily intake of water and other fluids (1900–2400 mL) is necessary to maintain the soft consistency of feces (Basch & Jensen, 1991). Reduced fluid intake slows the passage of food through the bowel and makes stool harder. In some individuals, hot liquids stimulate peristalsis and milk causes constipation.

PERSONAL HABITS

Elimination habits affect bowel function. Most people have established a habit of emptying their bowels at a certain time of the day or ingesting certain foods to stimulate peristalsis. A glass of hot water with lemon juice or a cup of coffee before breakfast often promotes regularity. Many people benefit from eating prunes at breakfast or eating a bowl of bran flakes before going to bed at night. Others habitually take laxatives, or use suppositories and enemas to clear their bowels.

Bathroom facilities play an important role in maintaining a regular pattern of elimination. People enjoy the convenience and privacy of their own toilet facilities and are often uncomfortable in situations where bathrooms may be shared, such as the hospital. The odours and sounds associated with using the toilet in a shared environment are often embarrassing and can discourage an individual from heeding the urge to defecate. This can lead to constipation.

ACTIVITY AND EXERCISE

Daily exercise helps to improve muscle tone, stimulate peristaltic action and promote digestion. Inactivity contributes to constipation, and prolonged sitting is conducive to hemorrhoids. People who are bedridden lose tone in their abdominal and pelvic floor muscles very rapidly, and constipation can become a serious problem. Therefore, early ambulation is important after illness or injury to maintain normal bowel function.

MEDICATIONS

Medications may also affect bowel functioning. Laxatives act by softening stool, lubricating stool or stimulating peristalsis. They are a safe aid to defecation if used properly. However, misuse can cause the intestine to lose muscle tone and, over time, the bowel will become less responsive to the medication. Constipation or diarrhea may result from laxative misuse.

Drugs that depress the nervous system lessen the motility of the intestines and have constipating side effects. Narcotic analgesics, such as morphine, and anticholinergics, such as atropine, are examples. Iron preparations cause constipation in many individuals. Antibiotics, on the other hand, may cause diarrhea by changing the normal bacterial flora in the gastrointestinal tract.

ANESTHESIA AND SURGERY

Agents used for general anesthesia impair bowel motility temporarily by blocking the nerve impulses to the intestinal muscles. Peristalsis slows or stops entirely. In addition, surgery that involves direct handling of the intestine stops peristalsis. According to Erwin-Toth and Doughty (1992), it is normal for peristalsis to be affected for a period of 24–48 hours after surgery. This condition is known as paralytic ileus. Further delay in the return of bowel motility occurs if the surgical patient does not ambulate quickly.

PAIN

Defecation is normally painless; however, certain conditions may cause discomfort. These include hemorrhoids, anorectal surgery and perianal skin irritation. People who experience pain on defecation may suppress the urge to defecate, and this results in constipation.

EMOTIONS

The effect of emotions on bowel functioning is not to be underestimated. Stress and anxiety stimulate the parasympathetic nervous system to speed up digestive and peristaltic action so that nutrients may be utilized for defence. Diarrhea and gaseous distention often result. Sadness or depression can have the opposite effect on the digestive tract, as these emotions tend to slow peristalsis.

OTHER ILLNESSES

There are many congenital abnormalities, injuries and disease processes that affect bowel functioning. For example, some infants are born with Hirschprung's disease, a condition in which the intestinal ganglia are absent. This results in failure of the internal sphincter to relax, resulting in severe constipation. Persons with spinal cord injuries may lose control of defecation because of damage to the parasympathetic nerves in the sacral area, which normally transmit the rectal reflex. Incontinence of feces may result. Persons with ulcerative colitis may experience diarrhea as a symptom of the disease.

Common Problems

Because of the multitude of factors that affect bowel function, the nurse is likely to encounter patients with bowel problems in all age groups and practice settings. Common bowel problems include constipation, fecal impaction, diarrhea, incontinence and hemorrhoids.

CONSTIPATION

Constipation refers to the passage of infrequent, hard, dry stools. Feces become hard and dry when peristalsis is slowed or delayed and water content is absorbed.

There are many causes of constipation. The most frequent causes are the self-induced failure to respond to the urge to defecate because of the pressures of time, inconvenient bathrooms or lack of privacy; insufficient dietary fibre and fluid; and lack of daily exercise. Immobility and extended bed rest can contribute to constipation. Constipation can be induced by medications such as opiates, anticholinergics and iron, which slow the motility of the intestine. Strong emotions are believed to be responsible for constipation through the increased production of epinephrine, with resulting inhibition of peristalsis. The physical changes of aging, including decreased peristalsis, weakness in abdominal and pelvic floor muscles and reduced intestinal mucous secretion, make the older adult prone to constipation. Gastrointestinal abnormalities can also cause constipation. These include congenital defects, bowel obstruction from tumours, neurological injury to the spine, and paralytic ileus, to name but a few. Finally, pain from hemorrhoids or anal fissures can contribute to constipation (Jensen, 1990; Porth, 1998).

The person who is constipated usually complains of a "bloated" feeling. This is caused by abdominal distention, which results from the accumulation of gas when waste products remain too long in the gastrointestinal tract. Swallowed air makes up over 75 percent of intestinal gas. Other sources of intestinal gas include the consumption of gas-forming foods and the methane and carbon dioxide produced in the colon by bacterial action on food (Guyton, 1996). If not expelled, the gas can lead to crampy abdominal pain. Headache, anorexia and nausea are additional symptoms that a constipated person may experience. These usually disappear upon defecation and the establishment of a healthier bowel pattern.

KEY PRINCIPLES

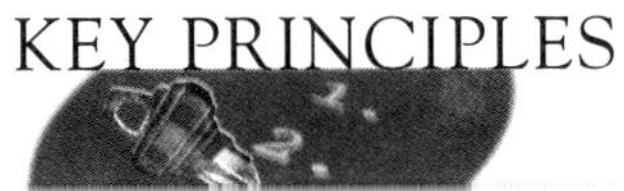

Principles Relevant to Bowel Functioning

1. The function of the bowel is to eliminate the waste products of digestion.
2. Normal bowel elimination is essential to efficient body functioning.
3. The body's fluid and electrolyte balance can be seriously affected by disturbances in bowel functioning.
4. Obstruction of the bowel poses a serious threat to life.
5. The oral intake of food or fluids stimulates a mass peristaltic action in the gastrointestinal tract.
6. The urge to defecate results from stimulation of the rectal reflex by distention of the lower colon and rectum.
7. The act of defecation is normally under voluntary control after the age of two to three years.
8. The necessary neuromuscular structures are not sufficiently developed for voluntary control over bowel elimination until the age of 15 to 18 months.
9. Once achieved, control over defecation is an important area of independent functioning for the individual.
10. The normal pattern of bowel elimination in individuals after infancy varies from one or two bowel movements every day to one bowel movement every two to three days.
11. Patterns of bowel elimination and consistency of feces are highly dependent on an individual's food and fluid intake.
12. Stress, anxiety and other strong emotions may interfere with bowel functioning.

Painful straining in unproductive attempts at defecation is called **tenesmus**. Constipation and tenesmus are serious health hazards and efforts should be made to avoid these, particularly for people who have had recent rectal surgery or who have heart disease, glaucoma or increased intracranial pressure from a head injury.

The full rectum can act as an irritant to the bladder, prompting the urge to void. Continual straining for defecation gradually weakens the pelvic floor, and any increase in abdominal pressure caused by constipation may induce stress incontinence due to sphincter incompetence. The nurse can give advice regarding proper fluid and fibre intake, general exercise and the benefit of maintaining a healthy weight. Individuals should be encouraged to establish a regular bowel routine in a familiar and comfortable environment.

FECAL IMPACTION

Untreated constipation can lead to a large, hardened mass of stool that cannot be expelled. This condition is known as **fecal impaction**. Failure to remove the stool may result in partial or complete obstruction of the bowel. While this may occur in any age group, the condition is most common in the incapacitated elderly. Habitual neglect by children of

Other causes of fecal impaction include dehydration, immobility, medications, neurologic diseases and barium retention. The nurse should be alert to seepage of small amounts of liquid stool from the anus with accompanying symptoms of abdominal distention, cramping and inability to defecate despite the urge. These are indicators of fecal impaction. The seepage, caused by feces higher up in the bowel moving around the mass, can easily be mistaken for a bowel movement, leaving the underlying problem of constipation overlooked.

DIARRHEA

Diarrhea is the frequent discharge of loose, watery stools and has many possible causes. Pre-examination diarrhea, resulting from emotional tension, is a fairly common occurrence among students. Medications, such as antacids, cathartics and antibiotics, may cause diarrhea. Diarrhea may result from dietary indiscretions such as eating coarse foods or an excessive amount of seasonings, alcohol or caffeine. It may occur as an allergic reaction to certain foods. Inflammation of the intestinal mucosa due to pathogenic organisms is a very common cause of diarrhea. Patients with inflammatory bowel diseases such as Crohn's and ulcerative colitis have diarrhea as a symptom of the disease because of anatomical defects in the bowel mucosa that interfere with the absorption of water and nutrients. Surgical operations in which significant portions of the bowel are removed, thus reducing the size of absorptive surface, can also lead to diarrhea.

Patients with diarrhea often complain of generalized abdominal pain. This is usually caused by flatus, which distends the colon. As well, pains of a piercing, gripping nature are not uncommon. They are usually spasmodic in nature and are caused by the strong peristaltic contractions of the intestinal musculature as the waste products are propelled precipitously through the gastrointestinal tract. These pains are frequently accompanied by a feeling of urgency in the need to defecate. Although an increase in the number of stools is not always an indication of diarrhea, it often occurs with diarrhea. The frequency and the irritating nature of diarrheal stools often cause redness and itchiness around the anal area. Care must be taken to cleanse the perineum well after each movement.

If diarrhea is prolonged, fatigue, weakness and general malaise are experienced. In addition, the individual is in danger of fluid and electrolyte imbalance (see Chapter 23). Nausea and vomiting frequently accompany diarrhea and further aggravate the loss of fluids and electrolytes.

INCONTINENCE

Fecal incontinence is lack of control over bowel evacuation that may vary from infrequent, minor soiling to the inability to control stool of normal consistency. The highest incidence is in the older population, most often caused by an detected fecal impaction or simply by degenerative changes in the muscles controlling defecation (Rothenberger & Orrom, 1991). Damage to the muscle or to the innervation of the pelvic floor musculature that affects the puborectalis, or damage to the external anal sphincter, can cause fecal incontinence. Constipation or a history of habitual straining can cause stretching and perineal descent.

Diarrhea is another common cause of incontinence because some individuals cannot control the precipitous delivery of liquid stool to the rectum. Incontinence may also occur as a result of direct injury to the rectal sphincters from childbirth or surgery. Illnesses that impair the neural pathways transmitting impulses from the sacral area to the brain, for example, stroke, spinal cord injury, tumour or multiple sclerosis, can also induce incontinence. Incontinence may also occur in people with mental disorders in which awareness of the need to defecate is altered or awareness of what is socially acceptable behaviour is lost; dementia, confusion or severe depression are some examples (Basch & Jensen, 1991). A sensitive or irritable gastrointestinal tract can be a causative factor for fecal incontinence. Eliminating certain foods and beverages can improve the problem, along with stress management and pelvic floor strengthening.

Fecal incontinence is a distressing problem that can cause great embarrassment and affect self-esteem. Defecation is very much a private matter, so soiling clothes in a social situation can be demoralizing. Fear of having an "accident" can lead to social isolation, which can be particularly harmful to the patient's psychological well-being. Incontinent patients may become extremely anxious and preoccupied with their bowels. The nurse must provide reassurance and support. In many cases, continence can be restored with a good bowel retraining program. This will be discussed in more detail later in the chapter. Scrupulous attention to personal hygiene is necessary, since incontinence can cause severe perianal skin breakdown.

HEMORRHOIDS

Hemorrhoids are swollen veins of the anus or rectum. There are two types: internal or external. Internal hemorrhoids cannot be seen as they develop above the anal sphincter. External hemorrhoids protrude through the anal opening and are visible. Increased pressure on the rectum and anus secondary to straining with constipation, pregnancy, obesity and abdominal tumours are the most common causes of hemorrhoids.

Hemorrhoids can cause bleeding, pain and itchiness. Usually they disappear with conservative treatment, such as warm sitz-baths, preparations containing astringent or anesthetic agents, or a combination of both methods. A common astringent is witch-hazel, supplied in compresses known as Tucks. Anusol or Preparation H are examples of preparations containing astringent and local anesthetic properties. Surgery may be required for unresolved hemorrhoidal pain. Prevention of hemorrhoids can be achieved by proper diet, exercise and the use of stool softeners (Black & Matassarin-Jacobs, 1997).

Bowel Diversions

Some bowel diseases are life-threatening or have such severe symptoms that feces must be diverted from passing through the colon. A temporary or permanent artificial opening from the colon to the surface of the abdomen may be created surgically. The opening is called a **stoma**. An **ileostomy** (see Figure 22.2) is an opening from the ileum of the small intestine to the abdominal wall, whereas a **colostomy** is an opening from the large intestine. A pouch or appliance must be worn over the stoma to collect the stool.

The nature and consistency of the fecal matter that flows from these ostomies are different. Since an ileostomy bypasses the large intestine, fecal discharge or effluent from an ileostomy is frequent and more liquid in consistency. The presence of digestive enzymes in the effluent causes

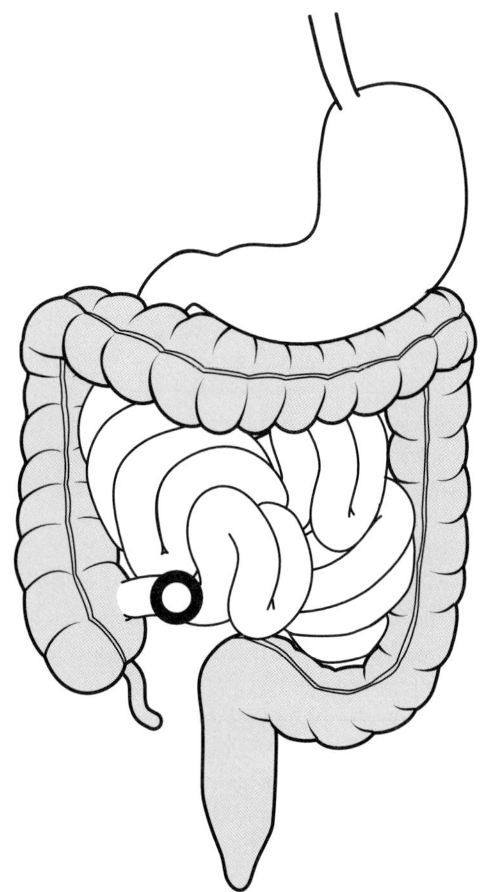

FIGURE 22.2 Ileostomy. The shaded portion, namely the colon and rectum, is usually removed. The surgeon creates a stoma in the lower right-hand quadrant of the abdomen.

irritation to the skin of the abdomen. Feces from a colostomy is generally formed and soft, more like normal stool.

There are three types of colostomies: end, loop and dou-

surgeon creates depends on the patient's medical problem. An *end colostomy* is usually constructed in the treatment of sigmoid or rectal colon cancer. This type of colostomy is usually permanent. The diseased portion of the bowel is removed and the proximal functioning portion is brought to the abdominal wall and sutured in place. Thus, one stoma is created.

A *loop colostomy* is usually created as a medical emergency when the bowel cannot be prepared for surgery, for example, in repairing a gunshot wound to the abdomen or a ruptured diverticulum. This type of colostomy is often performed on the transverse colon and is temporary. In other words, the physician expects to be able to reconnect the bowel at a later date once it has healed. A loop of bowel is pulled up to the surface of the abdomen and a plastic rod is placed under the loop to prevent it from falling back into the abdominal cavity. The loop is sutured to the skin of the abdomen and is opened to create a stoma. This stoma has two openings: a proximal one that emits feces and a distal one that drains mucous. The rod is removed from beneath

A *double-barrelled colostomy* has two separate stomas. Typically a temporary diversion, it is located most often in the descending colon. The affected part of the bowel is excised and both proximal and distal ends of the large intestine are brought to the abdominal surface. As in the loop colostomy, feces drain from the proximal stoma and mucous drains from the distal stoma. The term double-barrelled is sometimes confusing; this procedure is now often referred to as an *end stoma with a mucous fistula*. The mucous fistula is the distal stoma.

A pouch or ostomy appliance must always be worn for continence because the anal sphincter is removed or bypassed in diversional procedures. For ileostomy patients, the pouch must be emptied and cleaned frequently because the stool is so liquid. Management of the appliance for the patient with a colostomy is less concerning, as the stool is

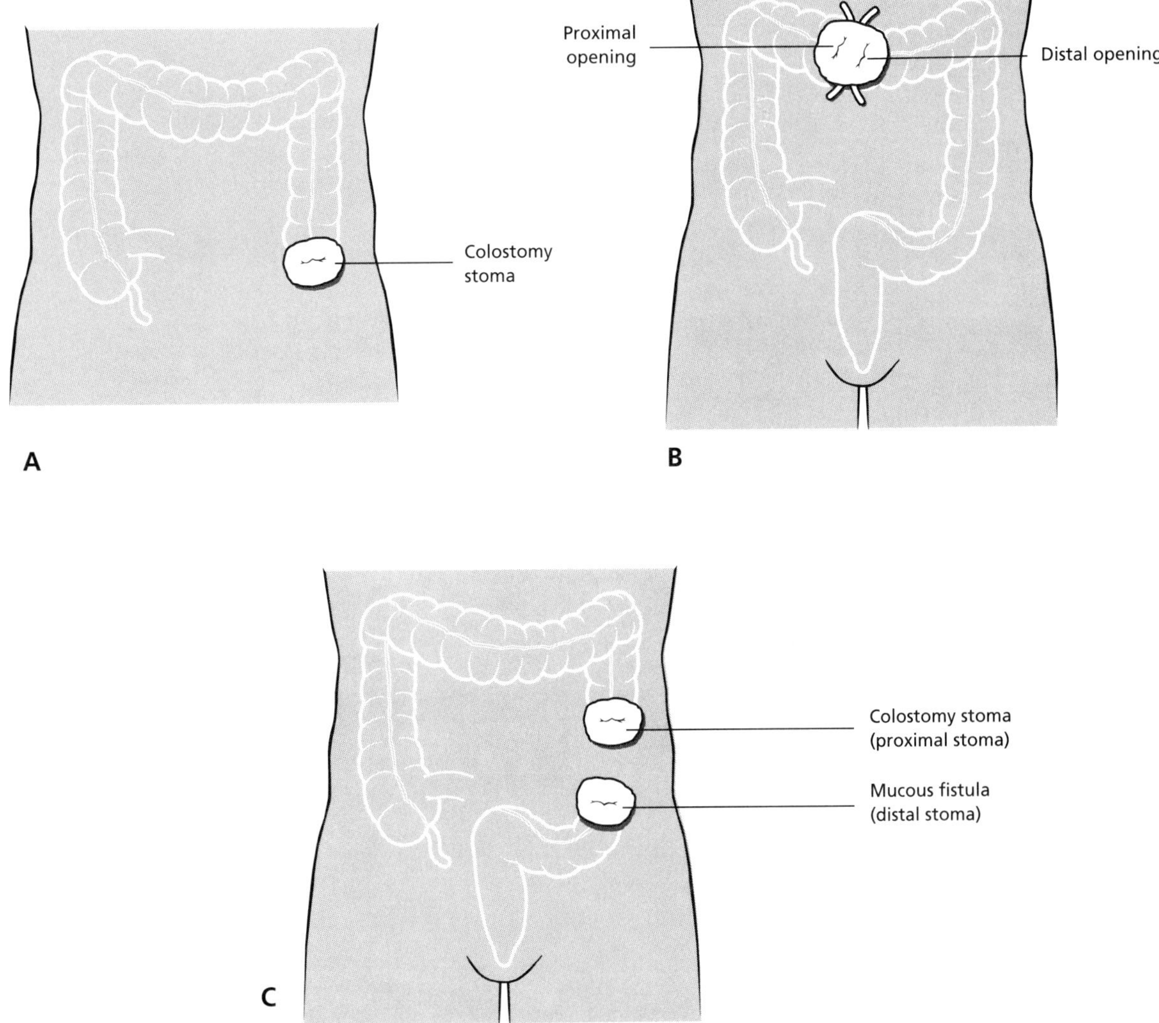

FIGURE 22.3 Types of colostomies. A. End colostomy. B. Loop colostomy. C. Double-barrelled colostomy

more solid and less frequent. Some colostomates can regulate their bowel movements by the food they eat, just as they would do if their bowel were intact. Others establish bowel regularity by irrigating their stoma every morning, although this procedure is not as highly recommended as it once was. Irrigations will be covered later in this chapter.

A great deal of sensitivity is needed by the nurse when caring for the patient with an ileostomy or a colostomy. The operation itself is extensive and the alteration in bowel elimination patterns causes body image changes. Many people are repulsed by a stoma and are overwhelmed by the presence of an appliance and the care it requires. The inability to control defecation and the management of odour, gas and leakage of stool are major concerns for these patients.

CONTINENT OSTOMIES

Certain patients may be candidates for surgical procedures that provide continent ostomies. In a procedure known as the ileorectal anastomosis, the colon is removed and the terminal ileum is anastomosed (i.e., two ends of the bowel are surgically joined) to the remaining rectal stump. The ileal pouch–anal anastomosis (also known as the J pouch or pelvic pouch; see Figure 22.4A) avoids the need for an ostomy. The colon is removed, but the rectal sphincter muscle remains intact. An ileal reservoir is then formed by folding the distal end of the ileum into a J loop, and a side-by-side anastomosis is carried out. The J pouch is then stapled directly to the rectal stump (Pezim, 1993; Hull & Erwin-Toth, 1996). Continence from this procedure should be normal. Average bowel function involves six to eight movements during the day and one at night (Pezim, 1993).

The continent ileostomy or Kock pouch (see Figure 22.4B) is a procedure in which a reservoir is created from a loop of ileum. Stool is stored intra-abdominally and can be drained via a nipple valve constructed from intussuscepted terminal ileum (i.e., one part of the bowel is slipped into another part). The pouch is emptied by the insertion of a wide-bore catheter into a flat stoma on the abdominal wall (Hull & Erwin-Toth, 1996). Today, this procedure is rarely done (Pezim, 1993).

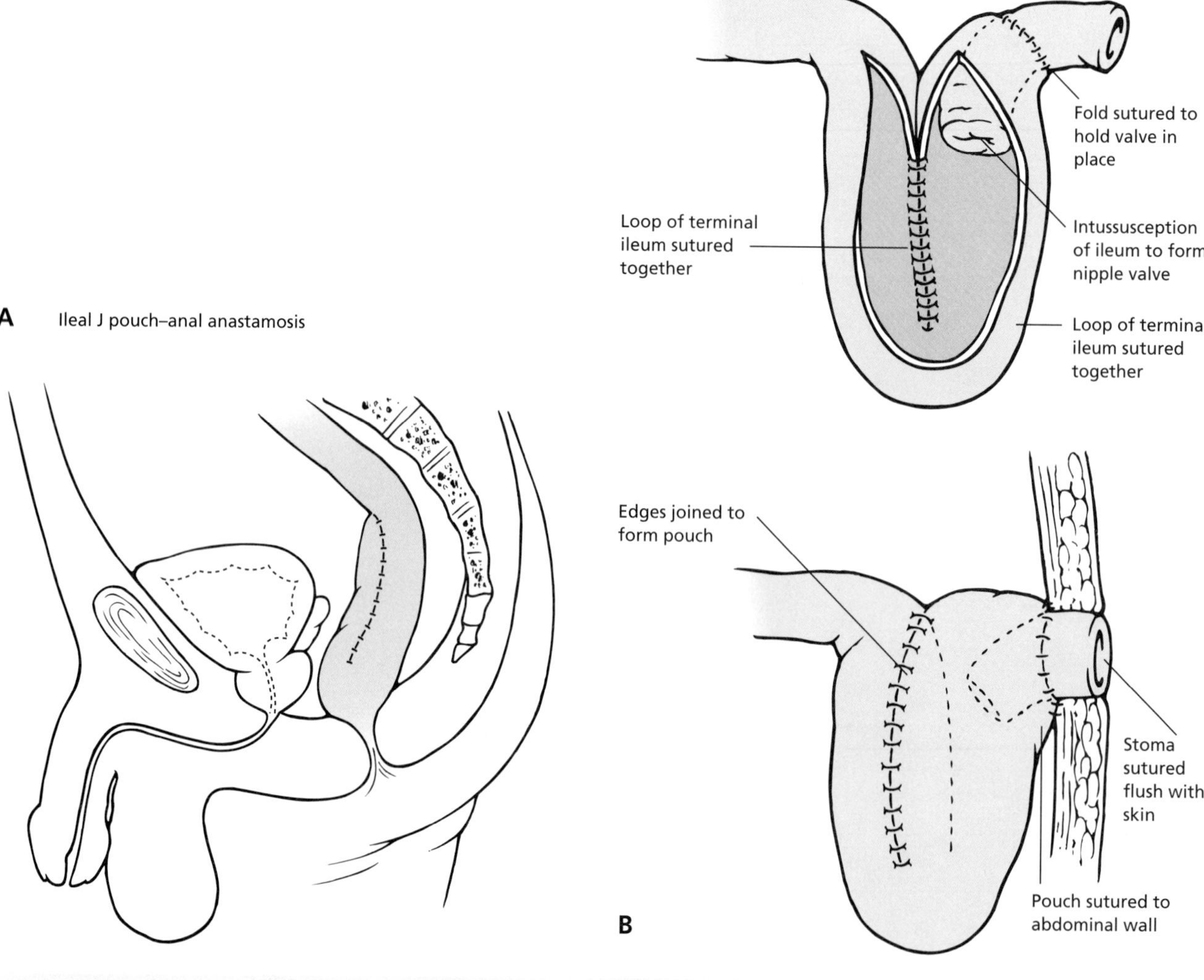

FIGURE 22.4 Continent ostomies

SOURCE: Black & Matassarin-Jacobs, 1997, pp. 1802, 1803.

Assessing Bowel Elimination Needs

To assess bowel elimination status, the nurse needs information about all the factors that affect a patient's bowel functioning. This includes subjective data obtained in a health history and objective data gathered through physical assessment, observation of fecal characteristics and review of diagnostic test results. Information about the patient's illness or any diagnostic or treatment measures that may affect bowel functioning will be found in the chart.

The Nursing Health History

The nursing health history provides the nurse and other members of the health care team with baseline information about the patient's usual bowel habits and patterns of defecation. Because people vary in bowel elimination patterns, it is important to determine what the patient describes as "normal." The nurse can then ascertain whether bowel dysfunction exists, since what the patient considers to be normal may differ from the nurse's knowledge of the parameters of

Knowledge of the normal process and the factors that affect elimination can assist the nurse in structuring the health history. Many people are embarrassed to talk about their bowel functioning. The nurse should take care to ask questions in simple, nontechnical language that allows the patient to provide pertinent information yet maintains feelings of dignity. Privacy during the interview helps to alleviate embarrassment. A guide for taking a health history pertaining to bowel elimination appears below.

Physical Assessment

The physical assessment of bowel elimination status involves an examination of the abdomen, rectum and anus. The skills used for this assessment are inspection, auscultation and light palpation. Palpation is performed

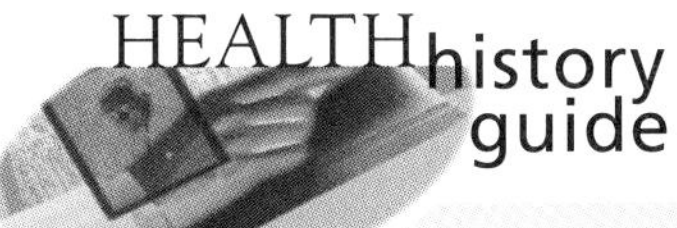

HEALTH history guide

Bowel Elimination

Health and Illness Patterns

Usual Pattern of Bowel Elimination

- How often do you have bowel movements? What time of day?
- Describe a typical stool. Colour? Texture? Shape? Odour?
- Describe your usual routine for bowel elimination.
- Do you use any natural aids for defecation? A glass of warm water? A cup of coffee?
- Do you use any specific foods or fluids, laxatives, suppositories or enemas to aid elimination? If so, what type? How frequently?

For patients with bowel diversions:

- What type of ostomy do you have?
- What is your usual routine?
- Have you had any problems with your ostomy, for example, protrusion, retraction or irritation?
- What assistance will you need in managing your ostomy?

Recent Changes in Pattern of Bowel Elimination

- Have you noticed any change in your normal pattern of elimination or stool characteristics? If so, describe the changes.
- Have there been any recent changes in your life that may be affecting your normal bowel pattern? Recent illness? Surgery? Stressful event? Travel? Change in diet or activity?

Presenting Health Problem

- Describe the symptoms you are experiencing now. Constipation? Diarrhea? Bleeding? Excessive flatulence? Incontinence? Pain in the abdomen or rectum?
- Have you recently had any unintentional weight loss, appetite loss, unexplained fatigue or fever?
- How long have you had these symptoms?
- What remedies have you tried for the symptoms? What were the results?
- Do you have an acute or chronic condition that might be causing your bowel problem? For example, gastroenteritis, inflammatory bowel disease, polyps? Have you had surgery lately?
- Are you taking any medications (prescription and over-the-counter) or treatments for other health problems? If so, what are they? Dosage of medications?
- Has anyone in your family ever had cancer of the colon or rectum, or polyps?
- Do you have any food allergies?

Health Promotion and Protection Patterns

- Do you eat a regular, well-balanced diet high in fibre? Whole grain cereals and breads? Fresh fruit? Raw vegetables such as carrots and celery?
- Are you aware of certain foods that tend to cause bowel problems? If so, do you try to avoid them in your diet?
- How much and what type of fluid do you drink in a day?
- Do you participate in a regular exercise program?
- Do you smoke? If so, how much and for how many years?
- Do you drink products containing caffeine? How much and how often?

last because palpation stimulates peristalsis, which may alter auscultation.

THE ABDOMEN

Prior to beginning the abdominal assessment, the nurse should ensure that the patient has an empty bladder. The patient is then assisted into a supine position with hands by the sides. The abdomen is exposed and the chest and pubic area are appropriately draped. The examiner's hands and the stethoscope should be warmed before touching the patient to prevent muscular contraction, which can alter the findings.

INSPECTION The nurse inspects all four quadrants of the abdomen, noting contour, symmetry, skin colour and appearance, abdominal girth and abdominal movements. The presence of masses, scars or stomas should also be noted. Normally the contour of the abdomen is slightly rounded or flat. A concave abdomen might indicate weight loss; a protuberant abdomen may be caused by intestinal gas, a tumour, hernia or fluid in the peritoneal cavity from cirrhosis of the liver. The abdomen is normally symmetrical; asymmetrical areas may be the result of previous surgery, weak muscles or a mass.

The skin on the healthy abdomen should look smooth and intact, and feel soft and supple. It should be free of abnormal colour, rashes, lesions or scars. For instance, if the individual has liver or biliary tract disease, the abdominal skin may appear jaundiced or yellow. If abdominal distention is severe, the nurse may see tense, glistening skin. In the case of a distended abdomen, the nurse should measure the abdomen's girth daily to determine if the distention is increasing. To measure abdominal girth, a measuring tape is placed around the abdomen at the widest point, usually the umbilicus. For accuracy, measures at this same anatomical site should be taken each day. Finally, the abdomen should be free of observable movements. Visible peristaltic waves may mean impending bowel obstruction.

AUSCULTATION The abdomen is auscultated to evaluate bowel motility via bowel sounds. This is done by placing the diaphragm of the stethoscope over each of the four quadrants, starting with the right lower quadrant (RLQ; see Figure 22.5). The RLQ is the point at which the cecum and ileum join, so if bowel sounds are heard here it may not be necessary to listen further. Proceeding in a clockwise manner, the nurse listens to each quadrant for one full minute. Bowel sounds are caused by air and fluid moving through the intestine and usually occur every 5–15 seconds. They are described as soft, bubbling or gurgling sounds. Hypoactive (infrequent or absent) bowel sounds occur normally after surgery or they may be related to advanced bowel obstruction. Hyperactive bowel sounds may be heard with early intestinal obstruction, diarrhea and hypermotility of the intestine related to hunger.

LIGHT PALPATION Light palpation is used to identify abdominal distention, masses and areas of tenderness. The abdomen is normally soft and nontender. The nurse should ask the patient to identify any tender areas first and should palpate that area last. Usually, the nurse begins at the RLQ

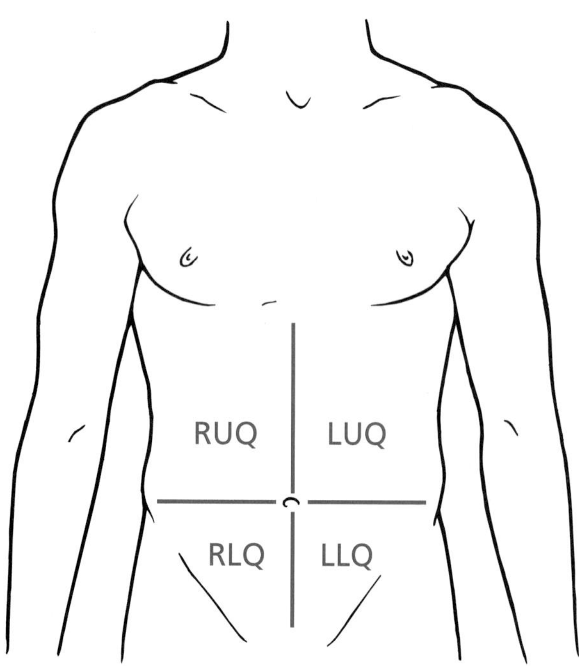

Anatomic Correlates of the Four Quadrants of the Abdomen

Right Upper Quadrant	**Left Upper Quadrant**
Liver and gallbladder	Left lobe of liver
Pylorus	Spleen
Duodenum	Stomach
Head of pancreas	Body of pancreas
Right adrenal gland	Left adrenal gland
Portion of right kidney	Portion of left kidney
Hepatic flexure of colon	Splenic flexure of colon
Portions of ascending and transverse colon	Portions of transverse and descending colon
Right Lower Quadrant	**Left Lower Quadrant**
Lower pole of right kidney	Lower pole of left kidney
Cecum and appendix	Sigmoid colon
Portion of ascending colon	Portion of descending colon
Bladder (if distended)	Bladder (if distended)
Ovary and salpinx	Ovary and salpinx
Uterus (if enlarged)	Uterus (if distended)
Right spermatic cord	Left spermatic cord
Right ureter	Left ureter

FIGURE 22.5 Four quadrants of the abdomen

SOURCE: Thompson & Wilson, 1996, p. 448.

and moves around the abdomen in a clockwise pattern. Using the dominant hand and with fingers close together, [illegible] ing in a dipping, rotating motion. [illegible] hands to the next site. It is important for the individual to breathe slowly during the examination to aid in the relaxation of the abdominal muscles. The nurse must distinguish between voluntary muscle rigidity due to coldness or ticklishness, and involuntary muscle rigidity due to tissue inflammation or injury. Deep palpation of masses or specific body organs is not usually part of the nurse's routine physical abdominal assessment.

THE RECTUM AND ANUS

Usually, a rectal exam is performed only on a person over the age of 40; however, it may be performed on individuals of any age if they have a history of bowel elimination problems. Digital examination of the rectum is not routinely done by the nurse as a component of the physical assessment. However, when fecal impaction is suspected, the nurse may perform a digital rectal exam if institutional policy permits. To examine the anus, the nurse instructs the patient to assume a side-lying position on the bed or examination table with the upper leg flexed towards the chest. Wearing a disposable glove, the nurse gently raises the buttock to view the anus. The anus and surrounding skin are inspected for external hemorrhoids, inflammation, scars, fissures, rectal prolapse or discharge. In addition, the tissue around the anus may be palpated for tenderness or nodules.

The nurse uses the physical findings of the abdominal and rectal assessment to supplement the information collected from the nursing history and records normal and abnormal findings on the patient's chart. The nurse can continue the assessment of bowel elimination by focussing on the characteristics of stool and diagnostic test results.

FECAL CHARACTERISTICS

Assessment of fecal characteristics is the nurse's responsibility. Knowledge of what normal stool is like assists the nurse in determining whether alterations in elimination exist. These characteristics are described in the following box. Stool may also be examined for other constituents, such as fat and pathogenic organisms. Stools that are clay-coloured indicate the absence of bile and the presence of fat. In this case, obstruction in the biliary tract might be suspected.

Diagnostic Tests

Diagnostic examinations of the intestinal tract can reveal helpful information about elimination problems. Common procedures include direct and indirect visualization techniques and laboratory tests of feces. They are usually performed when there are changes in bowel habits, chronic constipation and blood or mucous in the stool (Kee, 1995).

Characteristics of Normal Feces

Consistency	Soft-formed
Shape	Cylindrical
Amount	Adult: 100–400 g/day, depending on coarseness
Frequency	Once or twice a day to 3 times a week
Odour	Pungent
Constituents	Undigested food, bacteria, cells lining the intestinal mucosa, water, fat and bile pigment

VISUALIZATION STUDIES

DIRECT VISUALIZATION TECHNIQUES Direct visualization of the inner cavity of the anal canal, the rectum and the lower colon permits examination of the intestinal mucosa for disease, tumours, fissures or hemorrhoids and allows for the collection of tissue specimens. A tubular instrument or scope with an attached light source is inserted into the anal canal (anoscopy), the rectum (proctoscopy) or the sigmoid colon (sigmoidoscopy) or the colon (colonoscopy).

Prior to the test, the nurse ensures that the patient signs a consent form. An enema or laxative is usually given the evening before the examination and the morning of the test to clear the gastrointestinal tract of fecal material. The patient may be allowed a light breakfast. The nurse should explain that pressure or discomfort may be experienced as the instrument is introduced into the bowel and as air is injected to distend the bowel for better visualization.

For the examination, the patient is asked to assume a knee–chest position, if possible; if not, the Sims' position on the left side may be used. The patient should be draped carefully for comfort, privacy and to reduce embarrassment. Assisting the patient with relaxation breathing techniques, ensuring unnecessary exposure during the procedure and offering reassurance that the discomfort is of short duration are helpful nursing measures during the procedure. The examination usually takes about 30 minutes. After the exam, the nurse observes the patient for rectal bleeding, abdominal pain and fever. The patient is also encouraged to rest for several hours.

INDIRECT VISUALIZATION TECHNIQUES Indirect visualization of the bowel is achieved by x-ray examination and fluoroscopic examination. The small intestine is examined by an upper gastrointestinal (UGI) and small bowel follow-through test (which involves a barium swallow); the lower colon by a barium enema. Both tests use barium, a white, chalky, radiopaque substance, which is usually flavoured to enhance taste and facilitate ingestion. In the UGI series, meglumine diatrizoate (Gastrographin), a water-soluble contrast agent, may also be ingested. The UGI and small bowel follow-through (SBFT) study allow the radiologist to observe for ulcerations of the intestinal mucosa, tumours or diverticula.

Again, the nurse must have the patient sign a consent form. In preparation for the test, the patient must follow a low-residue diet for two days prior to the examination, and an enema and laxative may be ordered the evening before. The patient is permitted nothing by mouth after midnight. In the x-ray department, the patient will be given barium or a Gastrographin drink to swallow and the agent will be observed as it passes through the digestive tract. The patient is positioned supine on a tilting x-ray table that moves to various positions as x-rays are taken. The test can take four to six hours if a bowel series is included. After the examination the patient may resume eating. The patient should be instructed to increase fluid intake, as barium is constipating. The doctor may order a laxative to aid excretion of the barium. Stools are light in colour for up to three days until the barium is expelled.

The barium enema permits observation of the large bowel for abnormalities. Nursing care prior to the procedure is similar to that for the UGI and SBFT series except that a more extensive bowel preparation is required. The patient is restricted to clear fluids the day before the test and permitted nothing by mouth after midnight. A laxative and enemas to clear the bowel are given that same evening. Another enema or a suppository is given the morning of the examination. It is the nurse's responsibility to ensure that the patient's bowel is clear of feces. During the examination, the patient lies on the tilt table and barium is administered slowly via a rectal tube. As different positions are assumed, bowel filling is monitored by spot x-rays. The procedure takes approximately one hour to complete. Posttest observations and instructions to the patient are the same as for the UGI series. Castor oil is often given to the patient for three days after the procedure to clear the bowel of barium.

Laboratory Tests to Assess Gastrointestinal Function

Test	Normal Values SI Units (Conventional Units)
Complete blood count	
Hemoglobin	7.1–9.9 mmol/L (12–15 g/dL) women 8.7–11.2 mmol/L (14–16.5 g/dL) men
Red blood cells	4.5–5 x 10^{12}/L (4.4–5 million/μL) women 4.5–6.2 x 10^{12}/L (4.5–6.2 million/μL) men
Hematocrit	35%–47% women 42%–52% men
Electrolytes	
Sodium	135–145 mmol/L (135–145 mEq/L)
Potassium	3.5–5.0 mmol/L (3.5–5.0 mEq/L)
Calcium	2.12–2.50 mmol/L (8.6–10.0 mg/dL)
Carcinoembryonic antigen (CEA)	<2.5 mg/L (<2.5 ng/mL) nonsmoker <5.0 mg/L (<5.0 ng/mL) smoker
Fecal analysis	
Stool for occult blood	negative
Stool for ova and parasites	negative
Stool cultures	no growth other than normal flora
Stool for lipids	2–6 g/24h (adult, 60 g/day diet)

SOURCE: Chernecky & Berger, 1997.

FECAL EXAMINATIONS

COLLECTION OF STOOL SPECIMENS The collection of stool specimens for laboratory analysis is the responsibility of the nurse. The nurse must know why the stool specimen is required so that an appropriate container is used and the correct method for obtaining the specimen is carried out. For example, some specimen jars have preservative solution in them, whereas others do not. Some tests require a single stool sample; others require a series of timed specimens. Agencies usually have a laboratory resource manual available that details the requirements for specific fecal examinations.

Gloves are always worn when handling stool specimens. A wooden tongue depressor is useful for transferring the stool from the bedpan or other receptacle to the specimen container. Care must be taken not to contaminate the outside of the container. These practices are necessary to lessen the chance of spreading microorganisms, since feces are largely composed of bacteria. The purpose of specimen collection determines the amount of stool needed. Generally about 2.5 cm, or 15–30 mL of liquid stool, is sufficient (Kee, 1995). Specimens must be labelled carefully and sent to the laboratory as quickly as possible along with the appropriate requisitions or computerized labels. If stool specimens are left at room temperature for a period of time, bacteriological changes can occur that can affect the accuracy of the test results.

In most cases, patients can obtain their own specimens. Instructions they will need in order to do this include the following:

- defecate into a special receptacle that fits under the toilet seat or into a clean bedpan or commode
- avoid mixing the stool with urine or blood from menstruation (which may alter test results)
- avoid placing toilet paper in with the stool (which may affect test results)
- alert the nurse as soon after defecation as possible.

TEST FOR OCCULT BLOOD **Occult blood** refers to microscopic amounts of blood in stool that are hidden to the naked eye on gross examination. A simple fecal test can detect occult bleeding in the intestinal tract. It is used as a screening test for colon cancer and in diagnosing conditions known to cause bleeding such as inflammatory bowel disease. The test can be carried out on the ward of an inpatient facility or in the home. There are several test products available; common ones are Hematest and the Hemoccult slide. The testing instructions are given on the product packages and are easy to follow:

Normal Constituents of Feces

	300–400 g, depending on coarseness of diet)
Dry matter	32–64 g/24 h
Water	Approximately 75%
Total fat	< 6.0 g/24 h
Total nitrogen	< 2.0 g/24 h
Urobilinogen	50–300 mg/24 h
Blood	Negative
Ova and parasites	Negative

SOURCE: Springhouse, 1991, p. 437.

- For **Hematest**, apply a thin layer of stool on filter paper, add a tablet to the centre of the specimen and apply two drops of water. Time as directed and note colour changes.
- For a **Hemoccult slide**, apply a thin smear of stool to both boxes of filter paper inside the slide package, add two drops of reagent solution to the paper, and time. Note colour changes.

With both products, a blue colour change indicates a positive test for occult blood. Sometimes blood can be seen on a stool specimen quite easily. This may simply indicate bleeding hemorrhoids. More serious bleeding from the upper gastrointestinal tract usually results in black stools. This is called **melena**.

Diagnosing Bowel Elimination Problems

Problems with bowel elimination that are amenable to nursing intervention include constipation, diarrhea and incontinence. *Constipation* is the diagnosis used for problems in which elimination is infrequent and stools are hard and dry. These problems are often related to inadequate fibre in the diet, inadequate fluid intake, immobility, the use of constipating medications, pain on defecation or a change in routine. When patients pass three or more loose, liquid stools in a day, the diagnosis *Diarrhea* is appropriate. Diarrhea may be caused by stress, the side effect of medications, an allergy, excessive spices in food or inflammation of the bowel. Diagnoses for problems in which people experience involuntary passage of stool because of such factors as fecal impaction, confusion or neuromuscular impairment from stroke or spinal cord injury are stated as *Bowel Incontinence* (Carpenito, 1997).

Bowel elimination disturbances often cause other related problems that require nursing attention. For instance, bowel incontinence or prolonged diarrhea may lead to anal skin breakdown, and fecal seepage from a poorly fitting ileostomy pouch may cause skin breakdown around the stoma. In such cases the diagnosis *(Risk for) Impaired Skin Integrity* would be used. Prolonged diarrhea is a very common cause of fluid volume deficit. When diarrhea is present, the nurse should always consider the diagnosis *Risk for Fluid Volume Deficit* in the plan of care (Carpenito, 1997).

Screening for Colon Cancer

- age >40 years
- previous colon cancer
- high-fat, low-residue diet
- family history of colon cancer
- living in an industrialized urban society.

Early signs
- change in bowel habits
- rectal bleeding.

Screening tests
- to promote early detection, yearly digital rectal exam after age 40
- routine fecal occult blood test and digital rectal exam after age 50
- flexible sigmoidoscopy every 3–5 years for average-risk individuals after age 40
- colonoscopy or barium enema every 2–3 years for higher-risk individuals.

SOURCE: Black & Matassarin-Jacobs, 1997.

People who have difficulty with bowel elimination often experience a disturbance in their body image, self-esteem and coping capacity. Examples of nursing diagnoses for such problems might include: *Body Image Disturbance related to colostomy (or fecal incontinence)*; *Self-Esteem Disturbance related to need for digital removal of stool*; and *Ineffective Individual Coping related to difficulty adapting to ileostomy*. In addition, the diagnosis *Altered Health Maintenance* may be used for patients who need to learn how to live with and care for a bowel diversion, or those who require bowel retraining (Carpenito, 1997).

Following are two examples of nursing diagnoses made from assessment data:

A. Data: Mrs. S, age 83, is bedridden because of arthritis. Her abdomen is distended and her bowel sounds have decreased. She says she feels full and has not eaten much food in the last few days. Her last bowel movement was four days ago.

Nursing Diagnosis:

- *Constipation related to inactivity from disability and insufficient fibre and fluid in the diet.*

B. Data: Mr. B reports having loose, watery brown stools with some blood for the last week. He has crampy abdominal pain when defecating. He is weak and has lost weight. He recently returned from a vacation in Peru, where sanitary conditions were poor. He was not always able to drink bottled water, and he ate some unfamiliar food.

Nursing Diagnosis:

- *Diarrhea related to possible bacterial invasion from contaminated water and food.*

Planning Bowel Elimination Interventions

When planning care for the patient with elimination problems, the nurse includes the patient and family as much as possible. Because bowel habits are learned early in childhood and each individual's pattern of elimination is different, the plan of care must take into account previously established patterns. Previous healthy bowel habits should be maintained, with an emphasis on incorporating new ones. Goals are generally directed towards understanding normal defecation; achieving a regular elimination pattern; understanding the influence of dietary fibre, fluids and exercise on bowel elimination; achieving comfort; and maintaining self-esteem.

Patient goals or expected outcomes are set for specific nursing diagnoses. Following are some examples of expected outcomes for bowel elimination problems:

Constipation:

- The patient will report soft, brown bowel movements every two days.
- The patient will report absence of pain or straining during defecation.
- The patient will verbalize ways to promote regular bowel habits, respond to the urge to defecate when it arises, eat high-fibre foods, increase fluid intake and exercise regularly.
- The patient will describe foods high in fibre.
- The patient will describe the hazards of laxative use and relate intent to avoid their use on a regular basis.

Diarrhea:

- The patient will report no more than two bowel movements per day.
- The patient will defecate brown, solid stool.
- The patient will relate intent to modify known factors that cause diarrhea: avoid intake of spicy foods, participate in relaxation techniques.

Bowel Incontinence:

- The patient will pass a soft, formed stool in the bedpan, in the bathroom or on the commode every second or third day.

Implementing Bowel Elimination Interventions

Health-Promoting Strategies

Bowel elimination is a very basic physiological need. Regular bowel evacuation helps to maintain physiological functioning by eliminating wastes from the body and promotes physical comfort and emotional well-being. Many people experience some degree of disruption in bowel elimination from time to time. Nurses can assist individuals to promote regular bowel evacuation in the course of daily living by providing information and encouraging them to examine their health habits and practices that affect elimination.

RESEARCH to practice

Pieper, B., Mikols, C., & Grant, T.R.D. (1996). Comparing adjustment to an ostomy for three groups. *Journal of Wound, Ostomy & Continence Nursing, 23*(4), 197–204.

The purpose of this study was to explore the psychosocial adjustment of a temporary or permanent ostomy. The initial sample included 64 people who were recruited before they were discharged from hospital (four urban, one rural) and after ostomy teaching.

Forty-seven subjects completed the second interview process. The sample was subdivided into three groups:

- group 1 (n=18)—temporary ostomy due to gunshot injury
- group 2 (n=16)—temporary ostomy due to disease
- group 3 (n=13)—permanent ostomy due to disease.

Each group was interviewed twice, the first time for demographics and consent. Two weeks after discharge, study subjects were contacted and a second interview took place using the Psychosocial Adjustment to Illness Scale (PAIS), Reintegration to Normal Living Index (RNL), Meaning in Life Scale, and Ways of Coping Instrument. Data were collected over a period of two and one-half years.

The results of this study revealed that the three groups did not differ significantly with respect to their score on the PAIS, RNL Index or the Meaning in Life Scale. However, those subjects with a temporary ostomy due to trauma demonstrated higher scores on the Ways of Coping Instrument than the other two groups, although this finding was not statistically significant. Adjustment to the violent act at the same time as the ostomy may account for the difference in scores.

Though the sample size was small, and it was difficult and time-consuming to arrange a second interview, the results of this study suggest further research into individual coping strategies with the incidence of temporary ostomies due to trauma.

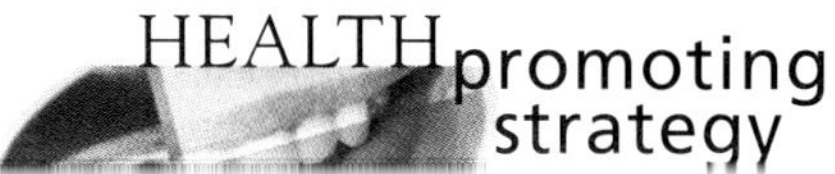

Promoting Healthy Bowel Elimination

- Defecate when the urge arises and take the time to defecate. If needed, establish a routine around the time at which the urge to defecate often occurs. Ignoring the urge to defecate will cause constipation.
- Drink eight to 10 glasses of fluid daily.
- Eat a well-balanced diet including high-fibre foods such as whole wheat cereals, breads and other grain products. Fresh fruits, raw root vegetables and cooked fruits such as apricots and prunes are good sources of fibre.
- Avoid foods that cause troublesome gas distention, cramping or diarrhea—for example, cabbage, turnips, onions, carbonated beverages or fried, spicy foods.
- Participate in a regular exercise program three to four times a week.
- **Female patients:** Always wipe the perineal area from front to back to prevent the introduction of microorganisms from the rectum or vagina into the urinary tract.
- Always wash hands after using the toilet.

The Health Promoting Strategy box gives a summary of guidelines to assist individuals in promoting healthy bowel elimination patterns. The major points are discussed more fully here.

REGULARITY

Regularity of defecation is the key to maintaining healthy bowel habits. To establish regularity, one must defecate when the urge arises and take the time for elimination. People should select a convenient time in the day when they will not be rushed or disrupted by busy or changing work schedules. Since the urge to defecate is usually strongest after breakfast, this is a good time for a bowel elimination routine. Eliminating after breakfast is also beneficial because it allows for the act of defecation in the privacy of one's home. Many people suppress the urge to defecate when they are in a strange environment or when others are present.

DIETARY PATTERN

Normal elimination is influenced by diet. The types of foods and the amount of fluids consumed may impair or promote elimination. Foods high in fibre and a daily fluid intake of 1900–2400 mL are considered sufficient for maintaining soft stool (Basch & Jensen, 1991). Eating a variety of foods containing complex carbohydrates with emphasis on cereals, breads and other whole grain products will ensure adequate fibre in the diet (Health Canada, 1992). Fresh fruits, raw root vegetables such as carrots and celery, and cooked fruits such as apricots and prunes are other good sources of fibre. A regular mealtime schedule will also help to maintain bowel regularity.

Certain foods cause gastrointestinal upsets such as flatulence, distention or cramping in some individuals. For example, cabbage, turnips, onions and beans often cause gas distention; fried, spicy foods tend to cause watery stools. Gum chewing and drinking alcohol and carbonated beverages may contribute to flatulence (BCDNA, 1992). People who experience such upsets should avoid foods and drinks they find troublesome. In some cases, yogurt and buttermilk may reduce flatus (BCDNA, 1992).

EXERCISE

Regular exercise helps to establish a regular bowel pattern and prevent elimination problems. Walking, running, swimming and biking are all excellent exercises for stimulating intestinal motility.

POSITIONING

A squatting or sitting position is the natural one assumed to evacuate the bowels. In this position, it is easier to increase abdominal pressure, which is needed to expel stool. People who have difficulty squatting because of weakness or disability may find regular toilet seats too low. Raised toilet seats can be purchased so that less effort is needed to sit down or stand up from the toilet.

TOILETTING HYGIENE PRACTICES

Everyone should be reminded to wash their hands thoroughly after using the toilet. Female patients should be told of the need to wipe their perineal area from front to back in order to prevent the introduction of microorganisms from the rectum and vagina to the urinary meatus.

Health-Protecting Strategies

Illness and hospitalization often interfere with a person's usual pattern of bowel elimination. Change in food and fluid intake, decreased activity and exercise, medications, diagnostic procedures, surgery, being in a strange environment and lack of privacy all contribute to altered elimination patterns. This section focusses on strategies that a nurse may use in assisting patients to maintain their usual bowel habits, prevent disruptions in bowel functioning and maintain comfort and hygiene.

MAINTAINING USUAL BOWEL ELIMINATION PATTERNS

When people are ill or in hospital (or a long-term care facility), every effort should be made to maintain their usual pattern of functioning. Established routines to aid defecation—for example, drinking hot water at meals—should become part of the individual's plan of care. Sufficient time must be allowed for defecation, and the nurse should ensure that other treatments or nursing activities do not interfere with these routines. In addition, when the patient calls for assistance, the nurse should be prompt in providing help before the urge to defecate passes.

Bowel evacuation is enhanced when people use the natural position for defecation in the privacy of a bathroom. Therefore, unless ambulation is contraindicated, the patient should be assisted to the bathroom or to use the bedside commode (see Figure 22.6). Patients who are restricted to bed will need assistance in using the bedpan. When assisting patients with defecation, the nurse must ensure as much privacy as possible, since the urge to defecate may be suppressed in the presence of others.

Ambulation and exercise are essential for maintaining bowel function and preventing elimination problems such as constipation and fecal impaction. Patients who are ill or who have had surgery are ambulated as early as possible to encourage the return of peristalsis and normal defecation patterns. Bedridden patients can be assisted with exercises to strengthen weak abdominal and pelvic floor muscles. Two simple exercises that will help bowel evacuation are as follows:

- lying supine, pull the abdominal muscles inward, hold for a count of five, and release. Repeat the sequence at least five times, several times a day
- again lying supine, contract the thigh muscle, hold for a count of five, and relax. Repeating the sequence five times, several times a day helps to improve leg strength and thereby facilitate the use of a bedpan.

ASSISTING THE PATIENT WITH A BEDPAN

Patients who are not ambulatory must use a bedpan for elimination. The nurse should do all that is possible to ensure the privacy, safety and comfort of the patient using a bedpan.

There are two types of bedpans: the regular bedpan and the slipper pan (see Figure 22.7). The slipper pan is designed with a low back to facilitate ease of placement for patients who are unable to raise their buttocks or who are restricted from such movements. Bedpans are made of metal or plastic. Metal bedpans can become cold when they are stored; they should be rinsed with warm water and dried before use to lessen the patient's discomfort. Bedpans are usually stored in the patient's bedside table, in an adjoining bathroom or in a clean utility room on the nursing unit. Female patients use the bedpan for feces and urine; male patients use it for feces only.

When assisting a patient with a bedpan, it is important that proper technique is used to avoid muscle strain for both patient and nurse. For patients who can lift their buttocks, the nurse first elevates the head of the bed about 30 degrees to avoid hyperextension of the back. The patient is then asked to bend the knees and push into the mattress with the heels or raise the buttocks. If the patient needs help raising the buttocks, the nurse places a hand under the patient's lower back and rests the elbow on the bed, using the forearm as a lever to help lift the buttocks. The nurse then slides the bedpan under the patient so that the rounded, smooth end is under the buttocks. A slipper pan should be placed with the flat end under the buttocks.

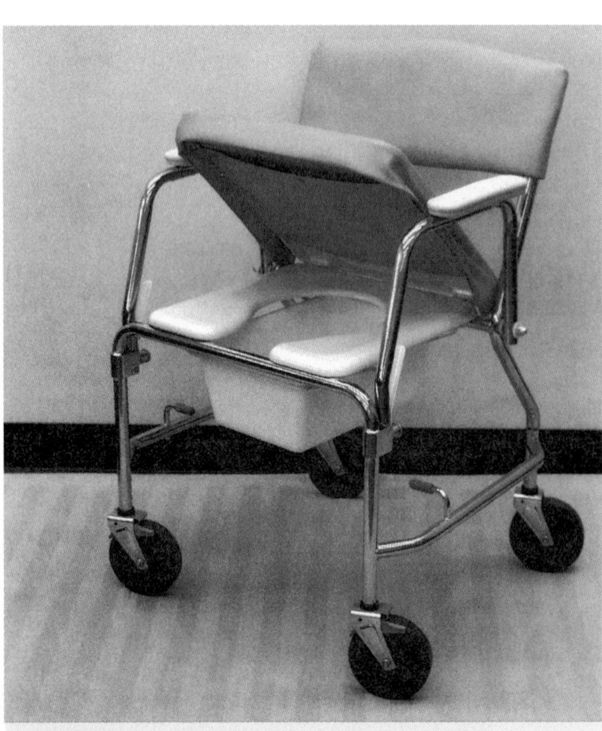

FIGURE 22.6 Bedside commode

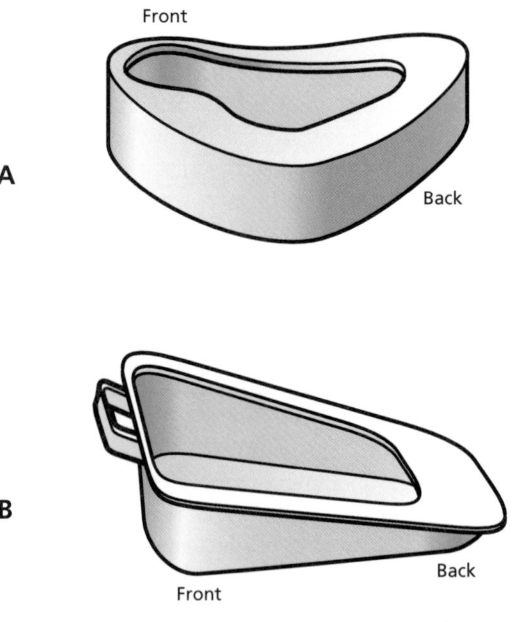

FIGURE 22.7 Bedpans. A. Regular bedpan. B. Slipper bedpan

For the patient who cannot raise the buttocks on and off a bedpan, the bedpan can be given by first placing the bed flat, with the side rail up on the far side of the bed [illegible] backside towards the nurse, and is asked to grasp the side rail. The bedpan is placed in position under the buttocks (see Figure 22.8), and supported there while the patient is rolled to the back-lying position. The head of the bed should then be elevated, if permissible, to bring the patient into a sitting position. Raising or bending the knees may also help support the patient on the pan. The position of the bedpan may need some adjusting for the patient's comfort and to prevent spillage.

The patient's privacy is maintained while on the bedpan. The bed covers are replaced, and the nurse leaves the room unless the patient is weak or requests help. Toilet paper and the call bell are placed within easy reach. The nurse must respond to the call bell as soon as possible to avoid undue discomfort. To remove the pan, the patient should raise the buttocks while the nurse holds the pan steady to avoid spillage when removing it. If the patient cannot raise the buttocks, the nurse can assist the patient to roll off to the side. If assistance is needed cleaning the perineal area, the nurse must wear gloves and wipe from the pubic area back to the anus to reduce the spread of microorganisms. Care to wash and dry the perineal area thoroughly is essential to prevent skin breakdown. The patient should be offered a wet face cloth to wash the hands after defecating.

MAINTAINING COMFORT AND HYGIENE

Meeting the comfort and hygiene needs of patients with elimination problems is very important to their safety and well-being. In the patient with diarrhea, for example, the frequency and enzymatic content of liquid stool, together with [illegible] skin breakdown. The same potential problem exists for the incontinent patient, particularly if the incontinence is frequent and stool remains in contact with the skin for a period of time.

Cleanliness is essential in bowel elimination. The sight and odour of fecal material is unpleasant and the high bacteria count in feces makes them a possible source of contamination. Basic hand-washing prevents the spread of microorganisms. Patients who cannot get to the bathroom for defecation must be provided the opportunity to wash their hands afterwards. The rectal area should be cleaned with soap and water and dried thoroughly after each evacuation. Barrier creams, such as those containing zinc oxide, can be applied to protect the perianal skin from breakdown. Soiled linen should be removed immediately.

After defecation, the environment may require ventilating and freshening to eliminate unpleasant odours. The nurse should take the initiative to use a room deodorizer or open a window, whichever is preferable to the patient.

Health-Restoring Strategies

Measures to restore bowel elimination involve activities related to specific problems. Often, diet alterations are enough to relieve constipation. If not, a laxative, rectal suppository, enema or colonic irrigation may be needed to produce a satisfactory bowel movement. At times, manual extraction of feces is necessary. Diet and medications are also used to bring relief from diarrhea. Individuals with incontinence may require a bowel retraining program, while those with

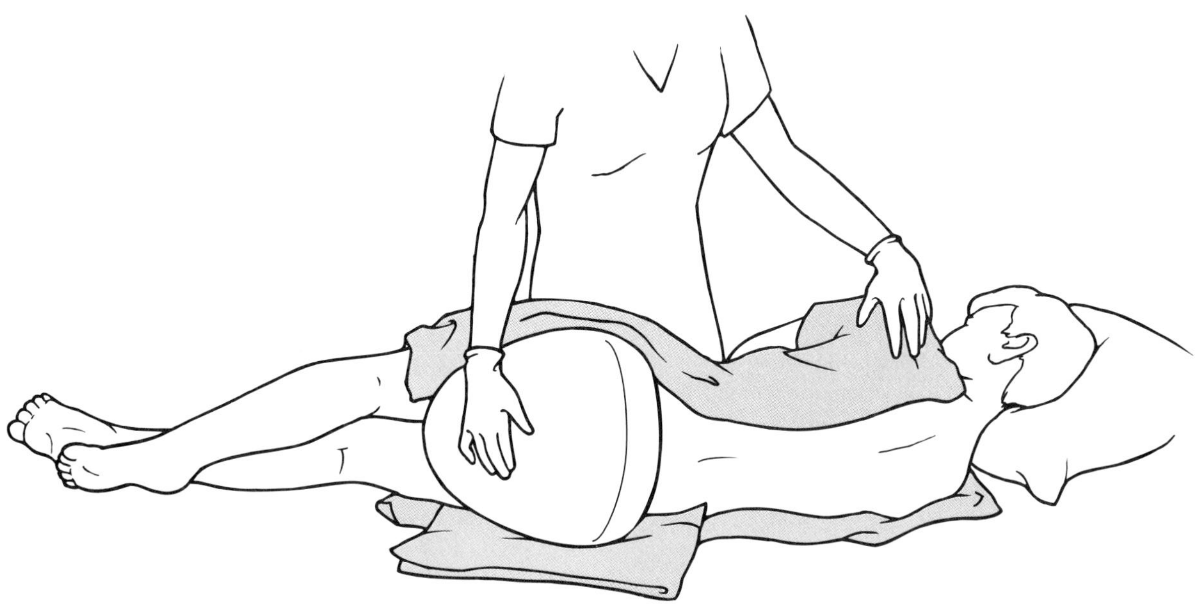

FIGURE 22.8 Assisting the patient onto the bedpan from a side-lying position

bowel diversions may need extensive education in ostomy self care. Some measures, such as diet therapy, may be implemented independently by the nurse; others, such as the use of rectal suppositories and enemas, depend upon the physician's order.

DIET THERAPY

The patient who experiences constipation needs additional high-fibre foods and fluids to activate peristalsis and achieve soft, bulky stools. Bran, fruit and whole grain cereals and breads are excellent high-fibre foods. The usual dose of bran is 15–30 mL daily to establish regularity. Hot liquids stimulate peristalsis, and prune juice has a natural cathartic effect. It is important for people to know that diet is a lifelong measure for healthy bowel patterns and may not provide immediate relief from elimination problems.

When diarrhea is the problem, the patient may try bland foods that are less stimulating to the gastrointestinal tract, such as tea, toast and custards. Foods that are binding, such as rice, cheese, bananas and applesauce, may also be helpful. Extra fluid intake to compensate for fluid lost through the gastrointestinal tract is important. Foods high in potassium, for example, chicken broth, are encouraged because diarrhea can lead to potassium loss. Hot and cold foods should be avoided because they stimulate peristalsis. If the patient cannot tolerate food or fluids, medical help should be sought; hospitalization may be required so that intravenous therapy and potassium replacement can be initiated.

DRUG THERAPY

LAXATIVES AND CATHARTICS **Laxatives** and **cathartics** are agents that promote evacuation of the bowel. "Laxatives promote a soft stool and cathartics result in a soft to watery stool with some cramping" (Kee & Hayes, 1993, p. 440). Some laxatives, such as bisacodyl (Dulcolax), act by increasing intestinal peristalsis while others, such as psyllium hydrophilic mucilloid (Metamucil), act by absorbing water into the intestine and increasing fecal bulk. Still others, including ducosate sodium (Colace), act as emollients that soften stool and decrease straining during defecation. These agents are available in oral and suppository form. How to administer oral medications and suppositories is outlined in Chapter 34.

Laxatives and cathartics are useful on a short-term basis in patients whose activity is restricted and whose food intake is limited. They are also used to evacuate the bowel in preparation for diagnostic tests and abdominal surgery.

Because laxatives are readily available over the counter, many people use them to promote regular bowel function. Long-term use of these agents can lead to fluid and electrolyte imbalances and dependence. The nurse should caution individuals against frequent use of laxatives and cathartics, especially if they are capable of promoting normal bowel function through diet, exercise and regular habits.

Laxatives

Group and Generic Name (Trade Name)

Bulk-forming laxatives
Psyllium hydrophilic colloid (Metamucil, Fiberall)

Surfactants
Docusate sodium (Colace, Disonate)

Lubricants
Mineral oil (Neo-Cultol, Agoral)

Osmotic laxatives
Magnesium hydroxide suspension (Milk of Magnesia)
Sodium phosphate solution (Fleet Phospho-Soda)

Hyperosmotic laxatives
Glycerin (Sani-Supp, Fleet Babylax)

Bowel lavage
Polyethylene glycol solution (CoLyte, GoLYTELY)

Stimulants
Bisacodyl (Dulcolax, Dulcagen)
Phenolphthalein (Ex-Lax, Feen-a-Mint)
Senna (Senexon, Senokot)
Cascara sagrada
Castor oil

Antidiarrheal Drugs

Group and Generic Name (Trade Name)

Opiate antidiarrheal drugs
Diphenoxylate HCl with atropine (Lomotil, Logen)
Paregoric; camphorated opium tincture
Loperamide HCl (Imodium A-D)

Anti-inflammatory antidiarrheal drugs
Bismuth subsalicylate (Pepto-Bismol)

Adsorbent antidiarrheal drugs
Kaolin and pectin (Kaopectate)

Hormonal antisecretory antidiarrheal drugs
Octreotide acetate (Sandostatin)

SOURCE: Pinnell, 1996.

ANTIDIARRHEAL MEDICATIONS **Antidiarrheal agents** are drugs that counteract diarrhea. They act by decreasing intestinal motility or immobilizing toxic substances, for example bacteria, that cause diarrhea. Diphenoxylate (Lomotil) is an example of an opiate-related agent that decreases peristalsis, and kaolin–pectin (Kaopectate) is an adsorbent that binds substances to its surface. It is important to note that antidiarrheal medications do not treat the underlying cause of diarrhea and, therefore, should not be used until the etiology has been identified. Until this is known, nonpharmacologic measures, such as the dietary interventions described above, should be implemented.

ENEMAS

An **enema** is the instillation of fluid into the rectum to [illegible] colon. Enemas act by distending or irritating the bowel or by providing lubrication to make evacuation easier. They are usually administered to relieve constipation, remove fecal impaction, administer medication, cleanse the rectum and colon prior to diagnostic tests or as a safety measure to prevent possible infection in patients who are undergoing surgery. They may also be used to reduce fever or cerebral edema. As with laxative overuse, normal defecation is impaired with frequent use of enemas.

The nurse must check the doctor's order before administering an enema to determine the type and amount of enema and time it is to be given. In some institutions, enemas are given at the nurse's discretion. In this case, it is essential that the nurse be knowledgeable about the types and purposes of enemas so that the enema selected is the best one for the patient's needs and physical condition. Because the bowel contains bacteria, the enema requires clean technique only. The nurse wears gloves to ensure that cross-contamination of microorganisms is prevented. The steps for administering an enema are outlined in Procedure 22.1.

Types of Enemas

There are several different kinds of enemas. These include cleansing, oil retention, carminative and medicated enemas.

CLEANSING ENEMAS **Cleansing enemas** are given chiefly to remove feces from the colon. Preparations commonly used for cleansing enemas include normal saline, tap water, soapsuds and hypertonic solution.

The *normal saline enema* is an isotonic solution given in large volume to distend the bowel and thereby stimulate peristalsis and evacuation. Since normal saline is isotonic—that is, most like the fluid in tissue cells—it minimizes the danger of fluid shifts in the bowel and makes it a very safe solution. For this reason, it is the safest enema for adults with pre-existing fluid and electrolyte imbalances, and for infants and children who tolerate fluid and electrolyte imbalances poorly. A saline enema is prepared by adding 10 mL of salt to 1000 mL of tap water.

The *tap water enema*, on the other hand, is hypotonic. When introduced into the bowel lumen, the difference in osmotic pressure causes the water to move from the bowel lumen into the blood stream. However, before large amounts of water are actually absorbed, the sheer volume stimulates peristalsis and bowel contents are eliminated within minutes. Caution is necessary when administering tap water enemas because the volume of water absorbed can lead to fluid and electrolyte imbalance such as circulatory overload. The nurse is advised to check with the physician or agency policy regarding the number of tap water enemas that can be repeated consecutively.

The *soapsuds enema* acts by irritating the bowel mucosa. Only pure Castile soap should be used since harsh soaps and detergents [illegible] 1000 mL of water or normal saline to make a soapsuds enema.

The *hypertonic enema* is a low-volume, concentrated solution, that pulls fluid from the surrounding tissues into the bowel lumen, thus distending the bowel and promoting defecation. The most commonly used preparation is sodium phosphate (the Fleet Enema). Commercially prepared and disposable, this type of enema is easy to use and comfortable for the patient because of its small volume (100 mL).

OIL RETENTION ENEMA An oil retention enema may be given in cases in which there is severe constipation or the patient has a painful anal condition. The oil not only lubricates the rectal mucosa but also softens the stool, easing its passage. Oil enemas are small-volume (90–120 mL) preparations made with mineral, olive or cottonseed oil. The effectiveness of the oil enema is enhanced if the individual can retain the enema for one to two hours. A cleansing enema may be ordered following an oil retention enema.

CARMINATIVE ENEMA A carminative enema is given to relieve the discomfort from gas distention. These enemas are usually low-volume solutions that help to move gas by stimulating peristalsis. The 1-2-3 enema (30 g magnesium, 60 mL glycerin, 90 mL water) and the Mayo enema (240 mL water, 60 mL brown sugar, 30 mL sodium bicarbonate) are two common examples.

MEDICATED ENEMA A medicated enema is given to administer medications that are absorbed by the rectal mucosa. For example, the antibiotic Neomycin can be administered by enema to cleanse the bowel of microorganisms prior to surgery.

Preparing the Patient

An explanation of the enema procedure for the patient should include the purpose, the position to be assumed (on the left side), breathing instructions to reduce abdominal cramping and the length of time to retain the enema. A feeling of fullness or abdominal cramping may be experienced when the enema is administered. In general, enemas are retained for about 10 minutes, but this depends upon the patient's ability to contract the anal sphincter. In older patients, holding an enema is often problematic, so bed linen should be well protected and a commode readily available at the bedside. If the doctor orders "enemas to clear," the nurse must explain what this means: the enemas are repeated until the results are free of stool. However, it is generally advised that not more than three consecutive enemas be given. The nurse should notify the physician if the third enema fails to produce clear returns.

Assembling Equipment

Disposable, plastic enema kits are available with an attached rectal-tip tubing and sliding clamp. The rectal tip is often

PROCEDURE 22.1 Administering an Enema

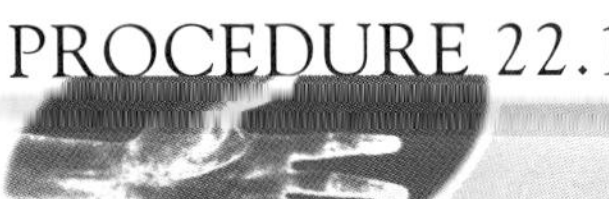

Action	*Rationale*
1. Confirm doctor's order for the type of enema and number to be given.	Prevents error and promotes accuracy.
2. Prepare the patient.	Promotes patient well-being and facilitates participation in care.
3. Gather equipment: • enema kit or reusable container, tubing, rectal tube and clamp; or prepackaged enema • enema solution • water-soluble lubricant • waterproof protective pad • clean gloves • bedpan or commode, if required • toilet tissue • towel and washcloth • paper bag for equipment disposal.	Facilitates efficiency and economy of time.
4. Pull the bed curtains and help the patient into a left-lateral position with the right leg flexed. (This position may be varied according to the patient's condition.) Place a protective pad under the patient's buttocks, then drape the patient appropriately.	Provides privacy. Facilitates the flow of fluid since the rectum and sigmoid colon are on the left side of the body. Flexion of the leg provides access to the anus. Provides warmth and comfort.
5. Apply clean gloves.	Protects the nurse from exposure to blood, body substances and microorganisms.
6. Administer the enema.	
For small-volume prepackaged enemas:	
• Remove the rectal tip covering and inspect for lubricant. Add lubricant if necessary.	Facilitates insertion into the rectum and lessens irritation of the mucous membrane.
• Raise the upper buttock.	Exposes the anus.
• Ask the patient to breathe deeply and insert the rectal nozzle into the anus. Advance the tip 7–10 cm in adults or 5–7.5 cm in children.	Relaxes the internal sphincter and makes insertion easier.
• Squeeze the enema bottle until all the solution has entered the rectum.	
For large-volume enemas:	
• Lubricate the rectal tube if not already lubricated.	As above.
• Insert the rectal tube as above.	
• Hold the tubing in the rectum with one hand.	
• Raise the enema container on the IV pole 30–45 cm above the rectum, measuring the distance from the top of the fluid level. Open the clamp and slowly instill the solution. A litre of solution should take about 10 min, but this can vary depending on the patient's tolerance.	Decreases the force exerted by the solution on the rectal tissue and thereby lessens the risk of injury.
• Allow the solution to infuse slowly. As the fluid level falls, the enema container may be elevated very slowly.	Prevents cramping and pain from rapid distention of the rectum. Maintains the flow rate. Flow slows as the fluid level drops; therefore, the enema container may be raised slightly.
• Instruct the patient to signal if the instillation is painful or if it is becoming difficult to hold the solution. If the patient experiences cramping, lower the enema container or clamp the tubing.	Gives the patient some control over the procedure and directs the nurse's activities. Allows the patient to rest.

PROCEDURE 22.1 *continued*

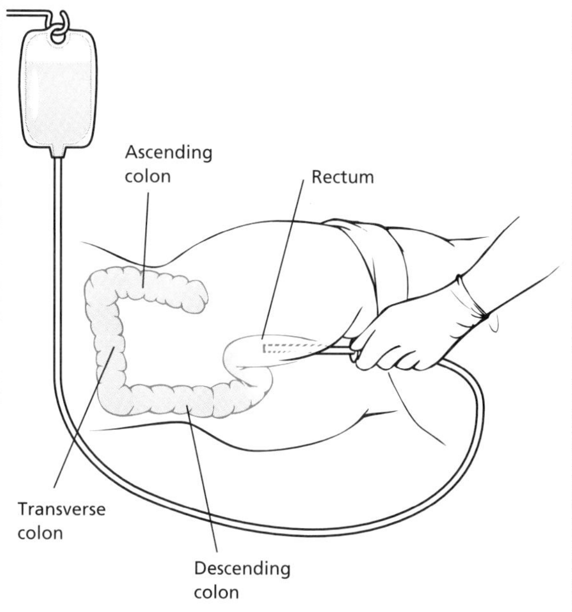

Ascending colon
Rectum
Transverse colon
Descending colon

Action	*Rationale*
Instruct the patient to breathe slowly through the mouth.	Promotes relaxation and enhances tolerance of the solution.
• When all the solution is instilled or the patient is unable to tolerate any more, clamp and remove the tube.	Intolerance is indicated when cramping continues or solution seeps out around the rectal tube.
7. Instruct the patient to remain in the side-lying position and hold the enema for the required time.	Helps to retain the enema.
8. Assist the patient to the bathroom or commode, or with the use of a bedpan.	
9. If the toilet is used, ask the patient not to flush it.	Permits the nurse to observe the enema results.
10. Dispose of equipment according to agency policy. Wash hands.	Maintains cleanliness and safety in the workplace.
11. Record relevant information. Note the type of enema, amount of solution given or tolerated; the amount, colour and consistency of the returns; and relief of gas or abdominal distention.	Fulfills requirements for nurse accountability and facilitates continuity of care.

prelubricated. Reusable equipment may still be used in some agencies. This includes a metal or plastic solution container, tubing, a rubber or plastic rectal tube and a clamp. Rectal tubes come in sizes 12–30 Fr; the sizes of tubes that should be used for the various age groups are listed in Table 22.1. Small-volume enemas, for example Fleet or oil retention, are contained in prepackaged disposable units consisting of a squeezable bottle and a nozzle tip. The nozzle tip is prelubricated and covered with a protective cap. Figure 22.9 illustrates the various types of enema equipment.

Prepackaged, disposable enemas come with their own instructions for use. To prepare enema solutions using a disposable enema kit or reusable equipment, first assemble the equipment and clamp the tubing. Lubricant will be needed for a reusable rectal tube and an IV pole to suspend a soft disposable container. The volume of solution that may be administered varies according to age (see Table 22.1) and should be indicated in the doctor's order. The solutions should be warmed to 40.5°–43.3° C for adults and 37.7°–40.5° C for children (Earnest 1993; Flynn & Hackel, 1990). An enema that is too cold lowers the body temperature and causes cramping; one that is too warm may cause thermal injury. Once the solution is in the container, rid the tubing and rectal tube of air by opening the clamp and

TABLE 22.1 Enema volumes and tube sizes

Age	*Cleansing Volume (mL)*	*Retention Volume (mL)*	*Tube Size (Fr)*
Adult	500–1000	15–200	22–30
School-age/adolescent	350–750	100–150*	18–22
Toddler/preschooler*	250–350	75–150*	14–18
Infant*	Under 250	Under 75*	12

* Should be stipulated in physician's order.

SOURCE: Flynn & Hackel, 1990, p. 620.

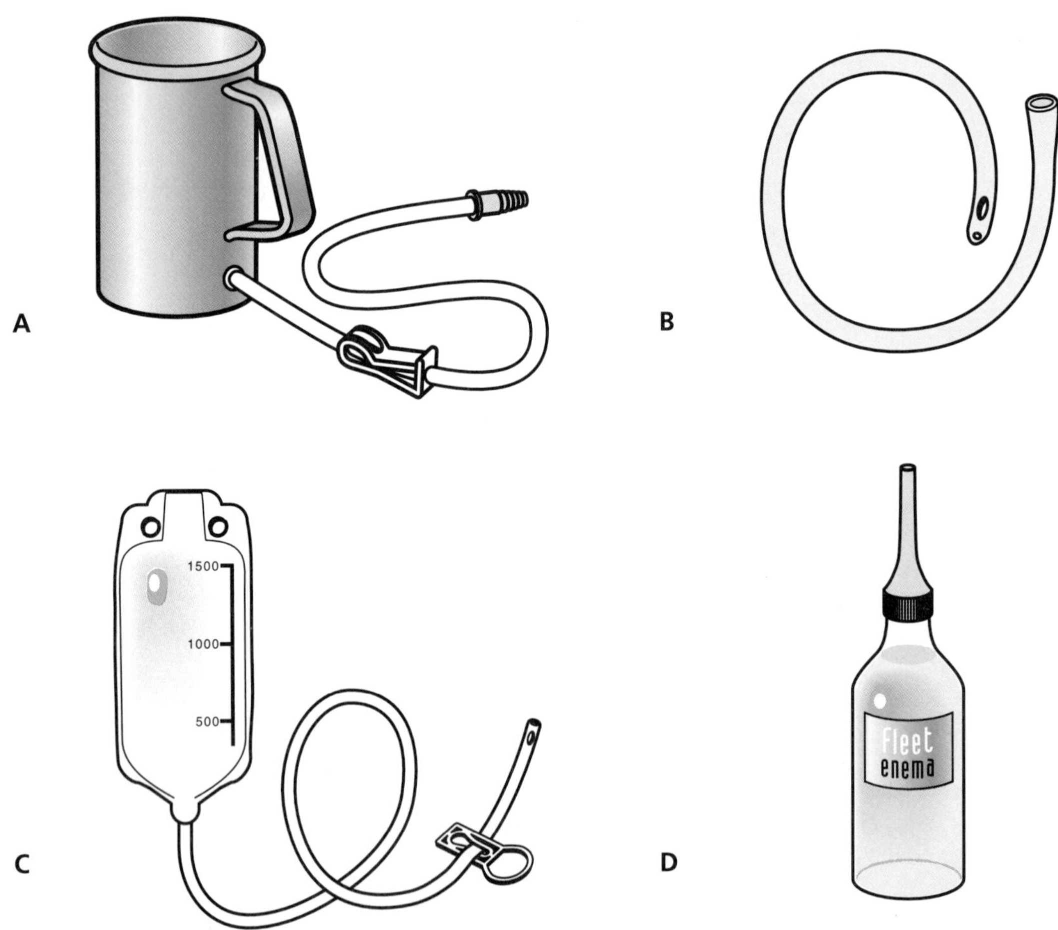

FIGURE 22.9 Enema equipment and supplies. A. Metal reusable container with attached tubing and a clamp. B. Rectal tube. C. Disposable enema kit. D. Prepackaged, disposable enema

SOURCE: Norton & Miller, 1986, p. 610.

running solution through it; then clamp the tubing. If the patient cannot ambulate, a bedpan or commode should be readied.

FECAL DISIMPACTION

If laxatives and enemas administered over a course of days are ineffective in removing feces, a manual extraction of stool from the rectum is necessary. This is done with the finger, and can be painful for the patient. Digital removal of feces can be dangerous for some people because rectal stimulation causes a vagal response which may, in turn, result in a slowing of the heart rate. For this reason, the nurse should check agency policy regarding who can perform a disimpaction.

Digital removal of stool requires a rectal glove, paper bag for glove disposal, lubricant, protective bed covering and a bedpan. Once the procedure has been explained, the nurse proceeds to assist the patient into a lateral position with the knees flexed. Waterproof protective pads are placed under the buttocks, and the bedpan is placed nearby. The [illegible] gently into the rectum. The rectum is massaged along its wall and at the same time the finger works the hard stool mass. The nurse must work the feces down towards the anus and, piece by piece, remove the stool, discarding it into the bedpan. It is important to assess the patient for fatigue, pallor, sweating and pain, and to allow rest periods. After the procedure, the patient should be encouraged to use the toilet, commode or bedpan as rectal stimulation can induce the need to defecate.

Meticulous observation of bowel patterns and fecal characteristics by the nurse is necessary to prevent further impaction. Attention to diet, mobility, bathroom facilities and drug regimens are important aspects of nursing care for the person with fecal impaction.

MANAGING INCONTINENCE

Some people with fecal incontinence, particularly those who have retained some sensory awareness and sphincter control, may be able to achieve normal elimination with a bowel retraining program. A thorough assessment of the cause of the patient's incontinence, physical readiness and ability to gain from bowel training must be completed first. The patient then begins a daily routine using nursing interventions that promote defecation. Patience, consistency and time are necessary for a successful bowel training program. Success may not be achieved for several weeks.

The program usually involves establishing a time for bowel training that fits with the patient's normal elimination pattern or incontinence. The best times are 20–40 minutes after meals, when the gastrocolic reflex is stimulated. Attempts at evacuation are made daily within 15 minutes of the scheduled time. Bulking agents, such as natural bran or Metamucil, are administered daily. As well, hot liquids may be offered each day as a stimulant to defecation 30 minutes before the scheduled time. At the selected time, the patient should be assisted to the bathroom to defecate and given a time limit of 20 minutes. Teaching the patient to lean forward when sitting on the toilet, to bear down and to massage the abdomen are useful measures to aid defecation. Of course, regular meals with adequate amounts of fibre foods and fluids and exercise are important ingredients of a successful bowel retraining program (Basch & Jensen, 1991).

For patients with incontinence related to sensory or motor deficits of the rectum and anus, digital stimulation is a commonly used approach to bowel training. Using a gloved, lubricated finger, the nurse massages the anal wall in a circular motion until the sphincter relaxes. Usually bowel evacuation quickly follows. If not, digital stimulation may be repeated. Again, timing defecation by rectal stimulation after meals, ensuring a sitting position and encouraging abdominal massage help establish a regular defecation pattern.

Other bowel retraining therapies may include sphincter training with biofeedback and pelvic floor exercises. Surgery may be indicated for people with [illegible]

For those with incontinence, a variety of absorbent pads are available, or fecal collection devices can be worn. Prompt disposal of feces, management of odour and skin protection must be provided to restore the comfort and dignity of the patient with incontinence.

OSTOMY CARE

An individual with an ostomy no longer eliminates in the same way as a person with an intact bowel. In most cases, a pouch to collect the feces must be worn on the abdomen at all times. Successful adjustment of the person to the ostomy requires well-planned nursing care. To live independently with an ostomy, the individual must learn about normal stoma characteristics, how to change and empty the pouch and how to care for peristomal skin. In addition, the person needs information about diet and fluid modifications, control of gas and odour and management of many unique health care problems associated with ostomies.

In addition to the practical management of the ostomy, the person must also adjust emotionally to the surgery. Many people find the idea of feces emptying onto the abdomen repugnant and are acutely aware of the reactions of others. They may feel a loss of health and fear that major changes in lifestyle will be necessary. Others may also be coping with a poor prognosis if the ostomy is a palliative measure. It is not unusual for patients and families to go through a period of grieving. It is important for the nurse to communicate understanding of the emotions and reactions of the patient and family. Acceptance and care aimed at protecting the patient's dignity and need for privacy can do much to assist the patient in his or her recovery. Enterostomal therapists are nurses with specialized knowledge and skills in the management of ostomies. Some institutions have enterostomal therapists on staff to assist patients in their recovery and to consult with other nurses in developing and implementing a patient care plan.

Stoma Characteristics

Assessment of the condition of the stoma after surgery is an essential nursing intervention. Stoma characteristics must also be included in the patient's teaching plan and can be addressed preoperatively or in the immediate postoperative phase. Stoma assessment should include location, colour, size and shape, condition of peristomal skin and sutures, stoma bleeding and stoma functioning.

The stoma is normally red or deep pink in colour and appears moist. A pale or dark, bluish-coloured stoma indicates poor circulation and should be brought to the attention of the physician. Loop colostomies are larger in size than end colostomies or ileostomies. Most stomas are round in shape and protrude from the abdomen approximately

1.5–2.5 cm. It generally takes four to eight weeks for a new stoma to shrink to its final size (Erwin-Toth & Doughty, 1992). The peristomal skin (5–13 cm of skin around the stoma) should appear intact and free of redness. The stoma will often bleed when cleaned, as it contains many small blood vessels. When bleeding occurs, the patient should be reassured that this is normal.

Assessment of stoma functioning includes the characteristics of the drainage as well as the presence of flatus. Stoma output from an ileostomy in the first few weeks is likely to be liquid and of high volume—up to 1500 mL/ day (Erwin-Toth & Doughty, 1992). This volume will decrease over time and should thicken slightly. Colostomy drainage, on the other hand, will be like the preoperative bowel pattern in terms of frequency and consistency. Flatus occurs when bowel peristalsis returns after an operation. Large amounts of flatus and noise are commonly experienced by the patient and are usually of concern. It should be explained that flatus can be modified by the diet and that the pouches are odour-proof.

Changing an Ostomy Appliance

In the first few days after surgery, changing an ostomy appliance (also referred to as *pouching the stoma*) is the responsibility of the nurse or enterostomal therapist. During this time the patient is usually emotionally and physically unprepared to learn this skill. Once patient readiness is determined, the instruction process can begin. First the patient is encouraged to watch the nurse change the pouch while explanations are given with each step. Thereafter, the patient takes on more of the pouch changing procedure until the patient can demonstrate the ability to change the pouch independently. Procedure 22.2 outlines the steps in changing an ostomy pouch.

TYPES OF APPLIANCES Many types of ostomy appliances are available. The nurse should be familiar with the available products so that a suitable one can be chosen for the patient. Most have the following common features: a plastic pouch, an adhesive skin barrier and a drainable end. Skin barriers come in various forms: wafers, rings, pastes and powders. They are used to protect the peristomal skin from drainage, build a flat pouching surface on the abdomen or to treat peristomal skin breakdown. Fecal pouches are classified as one-piece or two-piece, disposable or reusable and closed-end or drainable. Figure 22.10 illustrates the ostomy appliance.

In the one-piece system, the pouch is attached to an adhesive barrier or ring, which affixes to the abdomen. The two-piece appliance has a wafer skin barrier with flange separate from the attachable snap-on pouch (see Figure 22.11). The two-piece appliance provides some benefits over the one-piece system, including ease in centring the skin barrier over the stoma, greater visualization of the stoma for assessment and the ability to empty or replace the pouch without disturbing the adhesive wafer. Another advantage of the two-piece system is the type of flange. The floating flange permits the nurse to slide fingers under the flange for pouch application, thereby easing the potential discomfort caused by pressure on the sensitive abdomen of the postsurgical patient.

Another feature of pouches is the size of the stomal opening. Some ringed pouches have this opening already cut in premeasured sizes; others have starter holes. Starter holes are small openings in the centre of the skin barrier that can be cut

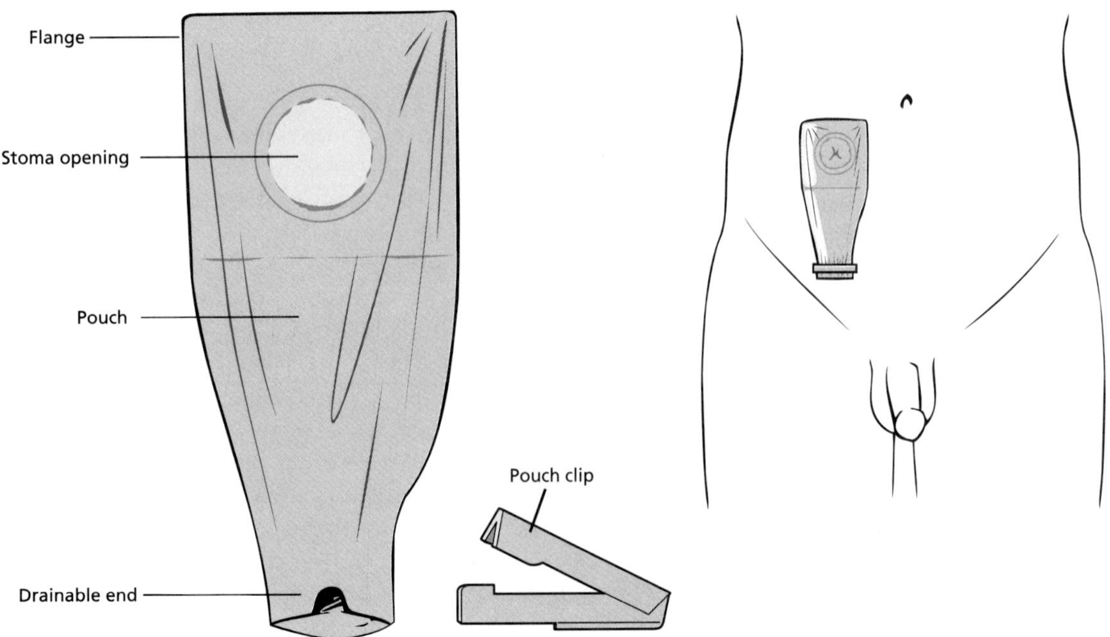

FIGURE 22.10 The ostomy appliance

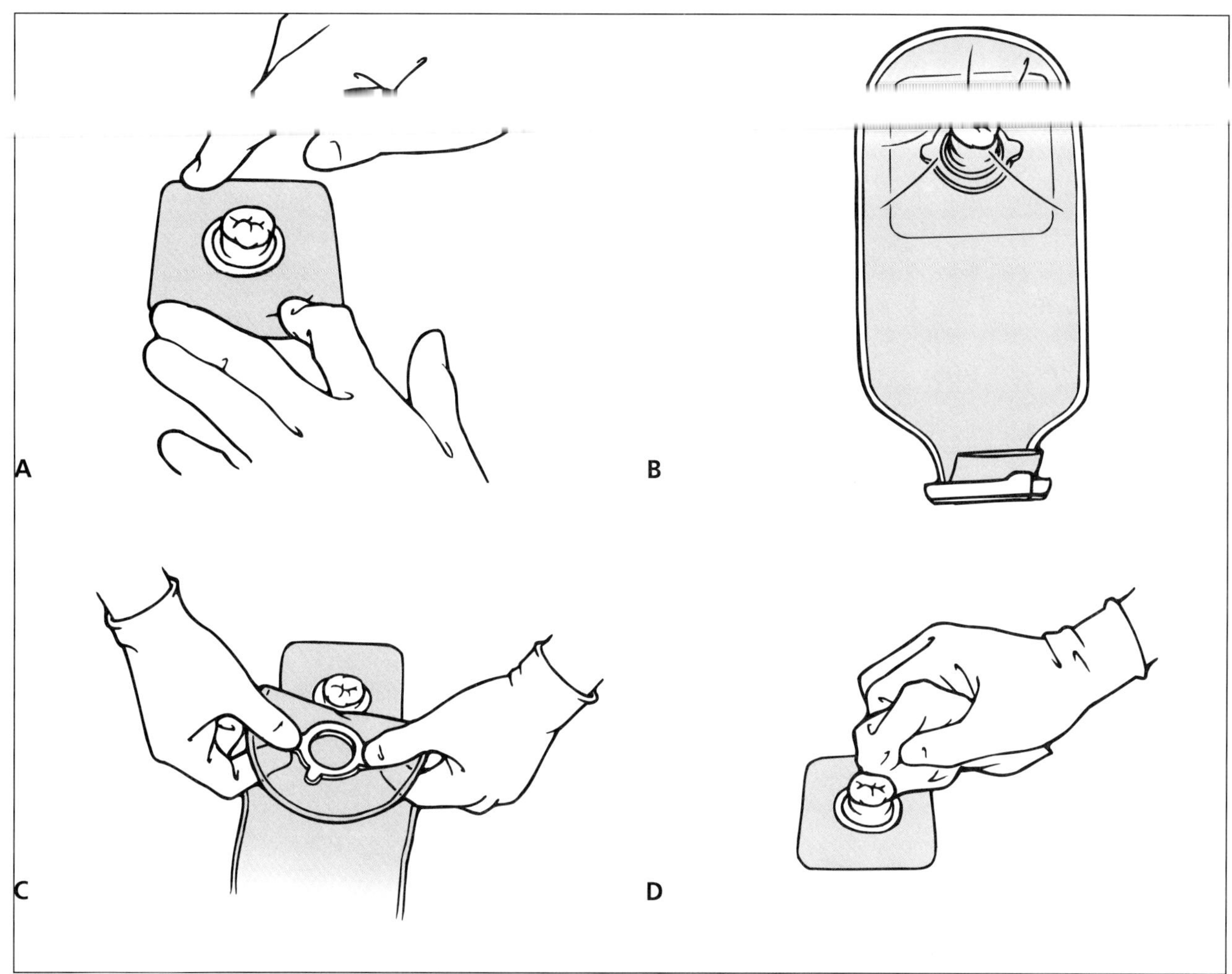

FIGURE 22.11 A two-piece appliance. A. A Stomahesive wafer with flange is applied directly to the peristomal area. B. A pouch is positioned over the stoma and snapped into place. C. and D. The pouch may be removed and the stoma assessed without removing the wafer

SOURCE: Rosdahl, 1995, p. 124.

to fit the exact size and shape of the stoma. While these pouches provide a custom fit, they also demand good eyesight and more dexterity on the part of the patient to apply.

Pouches come in disposable or reusable form. Most agencies stock the disposable pouch. Disposable pouches are made of a lightweight plastic and come in one- or two-piece systems. They are simply discarded after use. The reusable pouch is made of heavier plastic or rubber, comes presized, and in one- or two-piece systems. They may benefit the patient who has a limited budget and needs frequent pouch changes. On the other hand, reusable pouches require more maintenance. The patient must learn how to clean the pouch and how to use and remove the cements that are necessary for adhering the appliance to the skin.

Finally, pouches can be drainable or closed-end. Drainable pouches have an open end that must be closed with a pouch clip until emptying is desired. A closed-end pouch does not permit emptying. It is generally used by colostomates who are well regulated by irrigation.

GUIDING PRINCIPLES FOR POUCHING Protection of the peristomal skin and stoma from damage as a result of effluent or repetitive removal of the appliance serves as the guiding principle for pouching. The degree of skin damage from fecal matter depends on the effluent's enzymatic content, volume and consistency. For example, the effluent from an ileostomy is liquid and high in enzymes. If allowed to pool on the skin, rapid skin breakdown results. Colostomy drainage contains few if any enzymes, and is therefore less corrosive to the skin. The nurse must ensure the appliance is sized snugly to the stoma so that little skin is exposed to the effluent. If the pouch is sized larger than the stoma, a barrier paste must be applied to protect the skin. If leakage occurs around the appliance, it must be changed immediately. Otherwise, disposable ostomy appliances can remain secure for up to seven days. Unnecessary and frequent removal of the pouch can result in skin trauma. Irritated skin requires prompt treatment and more frequent pouch changes so that the appropriate healing products can be applied.

PROCEDURE 22.2 Changing an Ostomy Pouch

Action	Rationale
1. Prepare the patient.	Promotes well-being and enables participation in care.
2. Gather equipment: • flange (if two-piece appliance) • pouch • pouch clip • clean gloves • moisture-proof bag • cleaning materials such as tissues, washcloth, basin of warm water, towel • mild, non-oily, nonperfumed soap, if required • peristomal skin paste or powder, if required • measuring guide and pen • scissors • micropore tape.	Promotes efficiency and economy of time.
3. Provide privacy.	Promotes dignity and comfort.
4. Ideally, the pouch should be changed in the bathroom with the patient sitting or standing. If the patient is unable to ambulate, help him or her into a lying or sitting position in bed.	Lying or standing positions are preferred. In these positions there is less wrinkling of the skin, which makes application of the pouch easier.
5. Apply clean gloves.	Protects the nurse from exposure to blood, body substances and microorganisms.
6. Remove the old appliance.	
• Empty the pouch of drainage and measure.	This prevents spillage during the change.
• Remove the appliance by gently pressing the skin away from the appliance, starting at the top and working towards the bottom.	Minimizes peristomal skin damage and patient discomfort.
• Discard the appliance into the moisture-proof bag.	
7. Prepare the peristomal skin.	
• Remove remaining stool with toilet tissue. Slight stomal bleeding may occur during cleaning and is normal.	
• Clean the skin with warm water and, if required, mild soap or skin cleanser.	Prevents drying or irritation of the skin.
• Dry the skin thoroughly.	Ensures solid bonding of barrier to the skin.
• Remove hair from around the stoma if required using a pair of curved, blunt scissors. An electric or safety razor may be used with caution.	Allowing the hair to grow and then be pulled out during pouch change may cause infection of the hair follicle.
8. Inspect the stoma and skin.	
• Assess the skin for redness, broken areas or rash. Note the condition of peristomal sutures, if applicable.	Provides data for ongoing evaluation of care.
• Note the size, shape and colour of the stoma.	
9. Prepare for pouch application. *For a two-piece pouch system with a wafer skin barrier and flange:*	
• Measure the size of the stoma with the measuring guide. For the first four to eight weeks, the stoma size should be measured with each pouch change.	Ensures a correct fit of the skin barrier. Allows for stomal shrinkage during this time.
• Draw the measured size of the stoma opening on the back of the wafer.	
• Using scissors, cut out the traced pattern.	Makes an opening in the skin barrier.

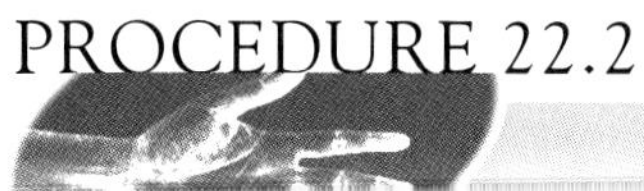

PROCEDURE 22.2 *continued*

Action	*Rationale*
• Remove the paper backing of the skin barrier to expose the adhesive side. Save the paper backing.	Readies the barrier for application. Serves as a template for sizing the skin barrier on the next pouch change.
• Apply a skin barrier paste with the finger immediately adjacent to the stoma, if necessary.	Fills in creases in the skin and provides extra protection from effluent.
• Permit the paste to dry for one minute.	
10. Apply the pouch.	
• Centre the wafer over the stoma and press down. Work in a circular fashion, pressing the skin barrier from the stoma to the outside. Remove any air bubbles.	Ensures a good seal and prevents leakage.
• Snap the pouch onto the flange. Position the end of the pouch towards the feet if the patient is ambulatory or slightly to the side if the patient is not active.	Facilitates emptying.
• Give the pouch a slight tug.	Makes sure it is on.
• Remove any air in the pouch.	
• Secure the end of the pouch with a tail-closure clip. Ensure that the clip snaps into place by giving a slight tug on the closure.	Provides extra reinforcement.
• Apply micropore tape in a window-framing manner around the wafer edges.	Provides extra reinforcement.
11. Attach the belt to the pouch if the patient prefers. Otherwise, the wings to which the belt attaches may be cut off.	Facilitates patient comfort and provides extra security. May be useful for the patient with a large abdomen.
12. Dispose of or clean reusable equipment.	
• Wash reusable pouches with warm water and soap; dry and store.	Promotes cleanliness and prevents the spread of microorganisms.
• Remove and dispose of gloves into the moisture-proof bag and discard into the appropriate garbage receptacle.	
13. Record pertinent information. Note the characteristics of the stoma, the condition of the peristomal skin, the amount and type of drainage, the type and size of appliance used, any significant patient behaviours during the change and any skills learned.	Fulfills requirements for nurse accountability and promotes continuity of care.
14. Modify the teaching and nursing care plan as needed.	Promotes continuity of care.

Assessing the Need for a Pouch Change

The following criteria will assist the nurse in determining when a pouch change is required:

- Note the condition of the existing bag for leakage or meltdown of the skin barrier. Effluent on the skin causes skin irritation. Melting of the skin barrier predisposes the patient to a poor seal and leakage.
- Determine if the patient experiences any discomfort around the stoma. A burning sensation may indicate skin irritation from deterioration of the skin barrier of the pouch.
- Assess the amount of drainage in the pouch. Pouches should be emptied when they are no more than half full, as the weight of the drainage may separate the pouch from the skin.
- Change the pouch if any of the above conditions are seen.

Preparing the Patient

Explain the procedure to the patient and determine, with the patient, an optimum time to change the pouch. It is best to select a time when the ostomy is least likely to function. Avoid meal times and visiting hours. Effluent odour may affect appetite and make an unpleasant environment for guests. The patient's comfort should be ensured before beginning the procedure, since pain will interfere with learning. The patient should observe or participate in the procedure to the extent that he or she is able.

Assembling Equipment

The nurse selects the type of pouch and skin barrier by considering the type of effluent or drainage, stoma size and shape, abdominal contours, visual acuity and manual dexterity of the patient, the patient's preferences in terms of equipment and the cost and availability of supplies. After surgery, as the patient's stoma size decreases, abdominal contours change or activity level improves, pouching needs may require adjustment (Erwin-Toth & Doughty, 1992). When applying a skin barrier, a stoma measuring guide is used to determine the size of the stoma so as to ensure that the hole cut into the skin barrier will fit around the stoma exactly. Tissues, water and a towel will be needed to cleanse the stoma and peristomal skin of effluent or wastes. A mild, non-oily and nonperfumed soap or skin cleanser such as Sween or Bard may also be used if needed, to cleanse the peristomal skin.

POUCH EMPTYING

Most types of pouches are drainable with a pouch clip (tail closure). To empty the pouch, the clip must be removed. Pouch emptying is easiest if the patient can sit on the toilet seat, allowing the fecal effluent to drain into the toilet. At the bedside, a bedpan or other receptacle may be used to collect the output. The patient is taught to cuff the bottom of the pouch after the clip is removed. This helps to keep the end of the pouch clean, which further prevents odour. The cuff also helps to keep the patient's hands clean during the procedure. Squeezing the pouch facilitates emptying, and toilet paper or a damp paper towel is useful in cleaning the bottom of the pouch. The patient may wish to rinse the pouch to remove all the stool, although this is unnecessary as the pouch is odour-proof. A squeeze bottle can be used to direct the water into the pouch, but the patient should be instructed not to be too rigorous with cleaning as the water may disturb the pouch seal. After the pouch is cleaned, the cuff is uncurled and the clip is reapplied.

If the patient is wearing a two-piece pouch system, the pouch may be snapped off and a new one applied. The old one may be rinsed to be used again later. The patient should be taught to empty the pouch when it is no more than half full. The weight of a full pouch risks the integrity of the pouch seal and may cause leakage.

IRRIGATING A COLOSTOMY

The patient with a colostomy may use colonic irrigation as a means of regulating bowel function. However, the individual must understand that irrigation is a management option, and is not essential to maintain healthy bowel patterns. While the choice to irrigate is the individual's, not all people are suitable candidates, and thoughtful assessment and counsel by the nurse is required. For instance, the patient who has a descending or sigmoid colostomy only, who has a history of regular, formed bowel movements and who is capable of learning the procedure is likely a good candidate. Irrigation is ill-advised for the patient with a stoma higher in the intestinal tract, who is very young, has a temporary colostomy, has had pelvis irradiation or has a prolapsed stoma (Erwin-Toth & Doughty, 1992).

Irrigation acts by stimulating the bowel through bowel distention. Routine irrigation trains the bowel to evacuate at the time of irrigation, which is usually performed every second day. The benefit of irrigation is that the patient can avoid wearing the pouch. The disadvantages are that irrigations can take up to an hour to complete and bowel dependency can occur over time. Irrigation does not provide effective bowel regulation at all times; careful attention to diet is also required so that unexpected evacuation is avoided. The technique for performing an ostomy irrigation is outlined in Procedure 22.3. Universal or body substance precautions are necessary when performing this procedure.

Preparing the Patient

At the beginning, the irrigation procedure should be simply explained. The patient needs to understand that the stoma has no sphincter and therefore he or she has no voluntary control over evacuation. The most convenient location for the colostomy irrigation is in the bathroom. The patient can sit on the toilet and the end of the sleeve can be placed directly in the toilet. If the patient is unable to tolerate sitting, the irrigation can be performed in bed. The patient should lie on the side of the colostomy stoma. The end of the sleeve can be closed and drained into a bedpan placed at a lower level when full.

Assembling Equipment

The supplies for the irrigation include an irrigating bag with tubing and a clamp, water-soluble lubricant, a stoma cone and an irrigation sleeve with belt. A stoma cone (see Figure 22.12) is a colon catheter with a seal or cone that prevents backflow of irrigating fluid. A catheter or rectal tube is not recommended for colostomy irrigation, owing to the risk of bowel perforation. Because the stoma does not have nerve endings, the patient cannot report injury. Using a stoma cone reduces the risk that the bowel will be perforated during the procedure. The irrigation sleeve is a disposable, plastic appliance that fits over the stoma to contain the irrigant and evacuated stool as it flows out of the stoma. If a two-piece ostomy appliance is used, the irrigation sleeve will attach to the system.

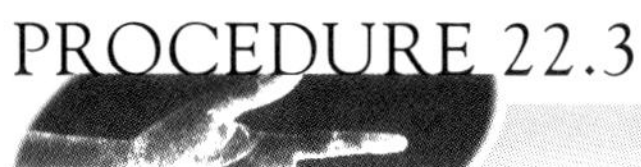

PROCEDURE 22.3 Irrigating a Colostomy

Action	*Rationale*
1. Prepare the patient.	Promotes well-being and enables patient participation.
2. Gather equipment: • irrigation set (solution bag with tubing, clamp; stoma cone; stoma irrigation sleeve with belt) • irrigating solution • clean ostomy appliance • moisture-proof bag • clean gloves • lubricant • IV pole • protective pad • bedpan or commode.	Promotes efficiency and economy of time.
3. Provide privacy.	Promotes patient's dignity and comfort.
4. Assist the patient to a side-lying position if unable to get out of bed, onto a commode at the bedside or to a bathroom toilet. If the procedure is performed in bed, place a protective pad under the stoma and the bedpan on a chair beside the bed. Move the patient's clothing out of the way.	Allows the irrigant to flow into the stoma through the force of gravity. Protects the bed linen from soiling. Exposes the colostomy.
5. Put on clean gloves.	Protects the nurse from contaminants.
6. Attach the irrigation sleeve. A sleeve for a two-piece system will snap onto the flange. A reusable sleeve is belted into place, and a disposable adhesive-backed sleeve sticks to the peristomal skin; both require the removal of the old pouch. Place the sleeve bottom into the toilet, commode or bedpan.	Collects the irrigant and evacuated stool. Directs the returns.
7. Adjust the height of the IV pole so that the solution bag hangs about 30–45 cm above the stoma.	Ensures adequate pressure to allow irrigant to flow into stoma.
8. Administer the irrigation.	
• Lubricate the cone catheter and insert it into the stoma through the top of the sleeve.	Makes insertion easier.
• Hold the cone firmly against the stoma.	Prevents backflow of irrigant.
• Open the clamp and begin the flow of solution. Expect the irrigation to take 10 minutes to infuse. If cramping occurs, stop the flow until it subsides, then resume the flow.	Alleviates discomfort.
• Close the clamp and remove the cone when the solution has been instilled or when the patient senses bowel distention.	
• Expect initial returns to be complete in 15 minutes. Instruct the patient to massage the abdomen. After this, the patient has the option to close the bottom of the bag and move around. Allow about 45 minutes for completion of returns.	Encourages emptying by stimulating peristalsis. Movement stimulates peristalsis.
9. When bowel evacuation is complete, remove and rinse the sleeve.	Maintains cleanliness and prevents transfer of contaminants.
10. Clean the peristomal skin and apply a new pouch.	Promotes skin integrity.
11. Assist the patient to a comfortable position, if required.	
12. Prepare the equipment for repeat use and discard disposable supplies. Remove gloves and wash hands.	Maintains cleanliness and safety in the workplace.
13. Record pertinent information. Note the type and amount of irrigant used, the characteristics of fecal returns, the patient's response and abilities during the procedure.	Fulfills requirements for nurse accountability and promotes continuity of care.

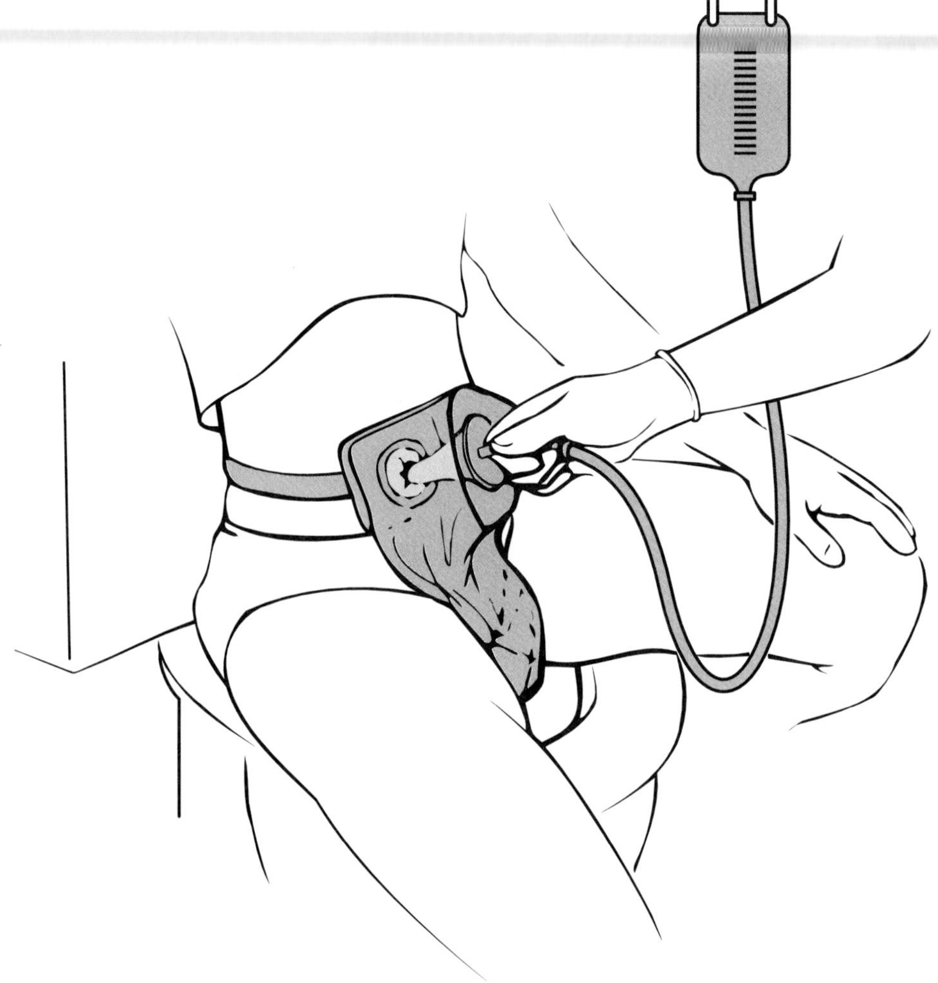

FIGURE 22.12 Colostomy irrigation. The patient sits on the toilet. The irrigating solution is suspended 30–45 cm above the stoma. The plastic irrigation sleeve is applied over the stoma, and the distal end is lowered into the toilet. The stoma cone and colon catheter are inserted through the top of the irrigating sleeve

Tap water is the most commonly used irrigating solution. Patients who are severely debilitated or for whom fluid balance is disrupted may need a saline solution. A normal saline solution may be made by adding 10 mL of salt to 1000 mL of warm water. As with enemas, lukewarm water is most appropriate. Water that is too cold may cause cramping, and water that is too warm may cause mucosal injury and slow the return of feces.

The amount of irrigating solution varies among individuals (500–1500 mL), with 1000 mL generally producing the best results. Too much water can tire the patient and contribute to fluid and electrolyte imbalance. Initially a small amount of solution (500 mL or less) will stimulate the bowel. Pour warm tap water into the irrigation bag to the desired volume. Allow the solution to flow through the tubing to clear the air, then clamp the tubing. Suspend the bag on the IV pole. Attach the cone catheter to the tubing and remove any air. Figure 22.12 illustrates a colostomy irrigation.

PROMOTING OPTIMAL OSTOMY ELIMINATION

Diet management is important for the individual with an ostomy. For most ostomates there are few diet restrictions. Control of odour and gas can be achieved by monitoring the intake of foods that produce gas and may cause odour. The individual may choose to omit these foods, but it should be stressed that the most important odour-control measures are the odour-proof pouch and the practice of keeping the pouch bottom clean and dry. In some cases, buttermilk and yogurt may reduce flatus, and eating parsley, yogurt and buttermilk may also help to reduce odour (BCDNA, 1992). Management of constipation and diarrhea is the same as for the person whose bowel is intact.

The person with an ileostomy must be more cautious about diet because of the location of the ostomy and the nature of the output. Bowel obstruction, for example, is a significant concern. The ileostomate is at risk for food blockage because the ileum, from which the ileostomy is created, has a narrow

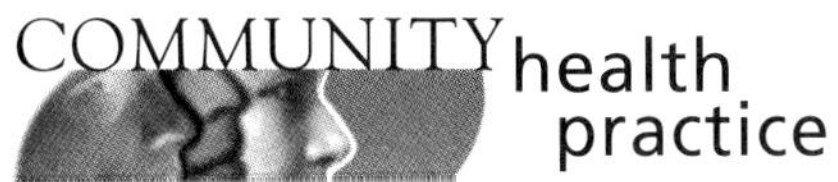

The Crohn's and Colitis Foundation of Canada

The Crohn's and Colitis Foundation of Canada (CCFC) is a nonprofit organization whose purpose is to find a cure for Crohn's disease and ulcerative colitis. Funding is provided for ongoing medical research and educational programs for patients, their families, health professionals and the general public. Educational pamphlets are available free of charge on a variety of topics (e.g., nutrition and diet, sexuality and pregnancy, medication). New pamphlets continue to be produced, such as *The ABCs of IBD for Kids* and *What Parents and Teachers Need to Know about IBD*. Nurses working in the community can obtain these pamphlets by contacting their regional office. Health professionals can support the foundation's mission by becoming a member of the CCFC.

lumen. Further narrowing may occur at the fascia-muscle, or where the intestine comes through the abdominal wall. Consequently, intestinal waste can collect at this point and cause a partial or complete blockage. The nurse describes the types of high-fibre foods that can contribute to blockage and explains preventive measures to the patient: avoid high-fibre foods in the first six to eight weeks after surgery, add high-fibre foods one at a time in small amounts, chew food well and drink plenty of fluid (Erwin-Toth & Doughty, 1992).

The nurse must also inform the patient of the signs and symptoms of bowel obstruction and discuss home management strategies. The signs and symptoms of partial bowel obstruction usually initiate with cramping abdominal pain and diarrhea. Abdominal distention, stomal swelling and nausea may occur, with progression to absence of fecal output as indicative of complete bowel obstruction. To manage these signs and symptoms at home, the patient should sit in a warm bath and massage the abdomen to relax the muscles. Solid food should be avoided and fluids increased. If no stool is passed and vomiting occurs despite these measures, the physician should be contacted.

Gas- and Odour-Producing Foods

Gas-producing foods	Odour-causing foods
broccoli	asparagus
Brussels sprouts	broccoli
cabbage	Brussels sprouts
cauliflower	cabbage
corn	cauliflower
cucumber	cheese
legumes (dried peas, beans and lentils)	eggs
melon	fish
peppers (green and red)	garlic
pickles	legumes (dried peas, beans, lentils)
radishes	onion
sauerkraut	spices
turnip	turnip

SOURCE: BCDNA, 1992, pp. 216, 218.

Evaluating Bowel Elimination Interventions

The effectiveness of nursing care is determined on an ongoing basis by collecting data pertinent to the expected outcomes established by the nurse and patient. Optimally, the desired outcomes might be that the individual will defecate a soft, formed stool every day or every other day; that defecation will be painless; that the patient will demonstrate knowledge of the factors that influence defecation, such as diet and exercise, and apply this knowledge over an extended period of time until the modifications are expressed as a normal pattern of living; that aids to defecation will be used minimally or cautiously to avoid overuse; that the individual with an ostomy will adjust to the ostomy, incorporating it as part of daily life; or that the patient will achieve independence with the technical management of ostomy care and demonstrate an understanding of factors that affect ostomy functioning.

Following is a sample guide for evaluating the effectiveness of interventions to aid bowel elimination:

1. If the patient has been constipated, has the patient had a soft stool and has a regular bowel pattern been re-established?
2. If the patient has had diarrhea, have the stools returned to normal consistency and frequency?
3. If the patient has had abdominal distention, does the abdomen feel soft? Have flatulence and abdominal pain been relieved? Is the patient comfortable and free from distressing symptoms?
4. If the patient has had hemorrhoids, have they disappeared? Has pain on defecation been relieved?
5. Is the patient aware of dietary and fluid needs to ensure adequate fecal elimination? Does the selection of foods and fluid intake indicate this?
6. Is exercise part of the patient's daily routine?
7. Does the patient practise good hygiene? For example, does the patient wash hands after a bowel movement?

IN REVIEW

- Bowel elimination is the excretion of the gastrointestinal waste products of digestion.
- Normal bowel patterns can be disrupted by:
  - some foods
  - gastrointestinal flu
  - illness
  - travel
  - medications
  - surgery
  - change of activity.
- Prolonged diarrhea can lead to imbalances in:
  - nutrition
  - water and electrolytes
  - impaired skin integrity
  - discomfort.
- Principal structures in bowel elimination are the:
  - small intestine (duodenum absorbs iron and calcium; jejunum absorbs fats, proteins and carbohydrates; ileum absorbs some vitamins and bile salts)
  - large intestine (absorbs water, electrolytes and remaining nutrients; synthesizes vitamins; stores and eliminates feces).
- Normal stools are brown, soft, solid and cylindrical in shape.
- Bowel elimination patterns are affected by growth and development. Other factors that affect bowel functioning include:
  - diet
  - fluid intake
  - personal habits
  - activity
  - exercise
  - emotions
  - illness
  - pain
  - anesthesia
  - surgery
  - medications.
- Common bowel problems include:
  - constipation
  - fecal impaction
  - diarrhea
  - incontinence
  - hemorrhoids.
- A bowel diversion is an artificial opening (stoma), created surgically, from the colon to the surface of the abdomen:
  - an ileostomy is created from the ileum
  - a colostomy is created from the colon.

  An ostomy appliance is worn over the stoma to collect stool.
- The continent ostomy provides a reservoir for fecal contents and avoids the need for a stoma pouch.
- Assessment of bowel elimination needs includes:
  - health history
  - objective data
  - physical examination
  - diagnostic tests.
- Common nursing diagnoses of bowel elimination problems include:
  - Constipation
  - Diarrhea
  - Bowel Incontinence.
- Health-promoting strategies for bowel elimination focus on helping individuals who are ill or hospitalized to maintain their normal bowel habits, prevent disruption and maintain comfort and hygiene.
- Measures to restore healthy bowel function include:
  - diet and drug therapy
  - bowel retraining programs.
- Evaluation determines whether the patient's problems have been resolved or a regular elimination pattern has been maintained.

Critical Thinking Activities

1. Mr. S. Norris is a 70-year-old man who has abdominal pain. He has been retired for five years after an active life as a house painter, and he now spends most of his time watching television. Mr. Norris lives alone in a small house just outside the city. He has three grandchildren who live a few kilometres away and he visits them on Sundays.

   Mr. Norris has been increasingly uncomfortable because of constipation during the past few years. He says he never took medicines when he worked but now has to take a laxative every day. Because he does not like to cook, he generally eats frozen TV dinners, sandwiches and cookies, and occasionally eggs. His doctor has referred Mr. Norris to home health care services for assistance in regulating his bowel habits. You have been assigned to his case.

a) What factors should you take into consideration before assisting Mr. Norris?

b) Wh [illegible]

c) For what reasons might Mr. Norris be constipated? What associated problems might he have?

d) What interventions would you think best to try? Outline the expected outcomes of nursing interventions for Mr. Norris.

e) What would you include in your teaching program for this patient? How would you evaluate the effectiveness of your teaching?

f) Mr. Norris's physician has ordered an enema for the patient. How would you explain this measure to him?

g) Describe the best position for the administration of an enema and why it is desirable.

h) What observations should you record regarding the enema?

KEY TERMS

small intestine p. 593	*fecal incontinence p. 597*
duodenum p. 593	*hemorrhoids p. 598*
jejunum p. 593	*stoma p. 598*
ileum p. 593	*ileostomy p. 598*
large intestine p. 593	*colostomy p. 598*
cecum p. 593	*occult blood p. 604*
feces p. 594	*Hematest p. 605*
rectum p. 577	*Hemoccult slide p. 605*
anal canal p. 594	*melena p. 605*
meconium p. 594	*laxatives p. 610*
constipation p. 596	*cathartics p. 610*
tenesmus p. 597	*antidiarrheal agents p. 610*
fecal impaction p. 597	*enema p. 611*
diarrhea p. 597	*cleansing enema p. 611*

References

BASCH, A., & JENSEN, L. (1991). Management of fecal incontinence. In D. Doughty (Ed.), *Urinary and fecal incontinence: Nursing maintenance* (pp. 235–268). St. Louis: Mosby.

BLACK, J.M., & MATASSARIN-JACOBS, E. (1997). *Medical–surgical nursing: Clinical management for continuity of care.* (5th ed.). Philadelphia: Saunders.

BRITISH COLUMBIA DIETITIANS' AND NUTRITIONISTS' ASSOCIATION (BCDNA). (1992). *Manual of nutritional care.* (4th ed.). Vancouver: Author.

CARPENITO, L.J. (1997). *Nursing diagnosis: Application to clinical practice.* (7th ed.). Philadelphia: Lippincott.

CHERNECKY, C.C., & BERGER, B.J. (1997). *Laboratory tests and diagnostic procedures.* (2nd ed.). Philadelphia: Saunders.

EARNEST, V.V. (1993). *Clinical skills in nursing practice.* (2nd ed.). Philadelphia: Lippincott.

ERWIN-TOTH, P., & DOUGHTY, D. (1992). Principles and procedures of stomal management. In B. Hampton & R. Bryant (Eds.), *Ostomies and continent diversions: Nursing management* (pp. 29–103). St. Louis: Mosby.

[illegible] Norwalk, CT: Appleton & Lange.

GUYTON, A. (1996). *Textbook of medical physiology.* (9th ed.). Philadelphia: Saunders.

HEALTH CANADA. (1992). *Canada's food guide to healthy eating.* Ottawa: Minister of Supply & Services.

HUETHER, S.E. (1996). Structure and function of the digestive system. In S.E. Huether & K.L. McCance (Eds.), *Understanding pathophysiology.* St. Louis: Mosby.

HULL, T.L., & ERWIN-TOTH, P. (1996). The pelvic pouch procedure and continent ostomies: Overview and controversies. *Journal of Wound, Ostomy & Continence Nursing, 23*(3), 156–165.

JENSEN, L. (1990). Fecal incontinence. In K. Jeter, N. Faller & C. Norton (Eds.), *Nursing for continence* (pp. 223–240). Philadelphia: Saunders.

KEE, J.L. (1995). *Laboratory and diagnostic tests with nursing implications* (4th ed.). Norwalk, CT: Appleton & Lange.

KEE, J.L., & HAYES, E.R. (1993). *Pharmacology: A nursing process approach.* Philadelphia: Saunders.

NORTON, B.A., & MILLER, A.M. (1986). *Skills for professional nursing practice.* Norwalk, CT: Appleton-Century-Crofts.

PINNELL, N.L. (1996). *Nursing pharmacology.* Philadelphia: Saunders.

PEZIM, M.E. (1993). Inflammatory bowel disease: Surgical aspects. *B.C. Medical Journal, 35*(3), 178–183.

PIEPER, B., MIKOLS, C., & GRANT, T.R.D. (1996). Comparing adjustment to an ostomy for three groups. *Journal of Wound, Ostomy & Continence Nursing, 23*(4), 197–204.

PILLITTERI, A. (1995). *Maternal and child health nursing: Care of the childbearing and childrearing family.* (2nd ed.). Philadelphia: Lippincott.

PORTH, C.M. (1998). *Pathophysiology: Concepts of altered health status.* (5th ed.). Philadelphia: Lippincott.

ROSDAHL, C. (1995). *Textbook of basic nursing.* (6th ed.). Philadelphia: Lippincott.

ROTHENBERGER, D., & ORROM, W. (1991). Anatomy and physiology of defecation. In D. Doughty (Ed.), *Urinary and fecal incontinence: Nursing maintenance.* St. Louis: Mosby.

SOCIETY OF GASTROENTEROLOGY NURSES AND ASSOCIATES. (1993). *Gastroenterology nursing: A core curriculum.* St. Louis: Mosby.

SPRINGHOUSE CORPORATION. (1991). *Diagnostic tests.* Springhouse, PA: Author.

THOMPSON, J., & WILSON, S. (1996). *Health assessment for nursing practice.* St. Louis: Mosby.

WONG, D.L. (1995). *Whaley & Wong's nursing care of infants and children.* (5th ed.). St. Louis: Mosby.

Additional Readings

BENTON, J.M., O'HARA, P.A., CHEN, H., HARPER, D.W., & JOHNSTON, S.F. (1997). Changing bowel hygiene practice successfully: A program to reduce laxative use in a chronic care hospital. *American Journal of Care for the Aging, 18*(1), 12–17.

BENTSEN, D., & BRAUN, J.W. (1996). Controlling fecal incontinence with sensory retraining managed by advanced practice nurses. *Clinical Nurse Specialist, 10*(4), 171–176.

BRADLEY, M., & PUPIALES, M. (1997). Essential elements of ostomy care. *American Journal of Nursing, 97*(7), 38–46.

EPPS, C.K. (1996). The delicate business of ostomy care. *RN, 59*(11), 32–37.

HAUGEN, V. (1997). Perineal skin care for patients with frequent diarrhea or fecal incontinence. *Gastroenterology Nursing, 20*(3), 87–90.

JENSEN, L.L. (1997). Fecal incontinence: Evaluation and treatment. *Journal of Wound, Ostomy & Continence Nursing, 24*(5), 277–282.

LAW, M.D. (1996). Incontinence management. Implementing a bowel–bladder management program. *Canadian Nursing Home, 7*(1), 27–29.

MANWORREN, R.C.B. (1996). Developmental effects on the adolescent of a temporary ileostomy. *Journal of Wound, Ostomy & Continence Nursing, 23*(4), 210–217.

NORTON, C. (1997). Fecal incontinence in adults. 2. Treatment and management. *British Journal of Nursing, 6*(1), 23–26.

PIEPER, B. (1996). Who is being missed in ostomy research. *Journal of Wound, Ostomy & Continence Nursing, 23*(4), 205–209.

ROBERTS, D.J. (1997). The pursuit of colostomy continence. *Journal of Wound, Ostomy & Continence Nursing, 24*(2), 92–97.

SEAMAN, S. (1996). Basic ostomy management: Assessment and pouching. *Home Healthcare Nurse, 14*(5), 334–345.

VAN HORN, C., & BARRETT P. (1997). Pregnancy, delivery, and postpartum experiences of fifty-four women with ostomies. *Journal of Wound, Ostomy & Continence Nursing, 24*(3), 151–162.

ZOUCH, R., & ZAMARRIPA, C. (1997). The significance of culture in the care of the client with an ostomy. *Journal of Wound, Ostomy & Continence Nursing, 24*(5), 270–276.

Chapter

Fluid, Electrolyte and Acid–Base Balance

OUTLINE

Introduction

The Physiology of Fluid, Electrolyte and Acid–Base Balance

Determinants of Fluid, Electrolyte and Acid–Base Balance

Fluid and Electrolyte Needs Throughout the Life Cycle

Common Problems

Assessing Fluid, Electrolyte and Acid–Base Balance

Diagnosing Fluid, Electrolyte and Acid–Base Balance Problems

Planning Fluid, Electrolyte and Acid–Base Balance Interventions

Implementing Fluid, Electrolyte and Acid–Base Balance Interventions

Evaluating Fluid, Electrolyte and Acid–Base Balance Interventions

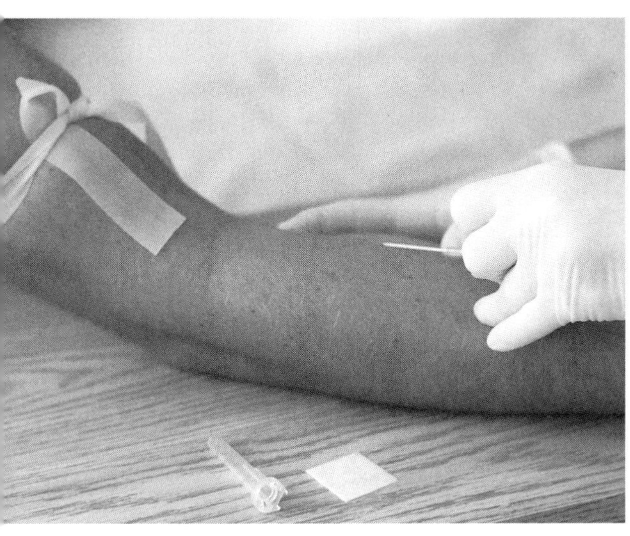

Central Questions

1. In what way is fluid, electrolyte and acid–base balance important to health and well-being?
2. How are water and electrolytes distributed in the body?
3. What mechanisms regulate fluid and electrolyte balance?
4. What are the functions of the major electrolytes?
5. Why is acid–base regulation important?
6. What mechanisms maintain the normal pH range of body fluids?
7. What are the main determinants of fluid, electrolyte and acid–base balance?
8. How does fluid, electrolyte and acid–base balance vary throughout the life cycle?
9. What are the common fluid, electrolyte and acid–base balance problems?
10. What basic principles might the nurse apply in assisting patients in meeting fluid, electrolyte and acid–base balance needs?
11. How does the nurse assess a patient's fluid, electrolyte and acid–base balance status?
13. What are the common nursing diagnostic statements for patients with fluid, electrolyte and acid–base balance problems?
14. How might the nurse develop a plan of care for patients with fluid, electrolyte and acid–base balance problems?
15. What strategies might the nurse implement in helping individuals, families or groups promote optimal fluid, electrolyte and acid–base balance and prevent potential problems?
16. What health-restoring and supportive strategies might the nurse implement in the care of patients with fluid, electrolyte and acid–base balance problems?
17. How might the nurse evaluate the patient's response to nursing interventions?

Introduction

Water has been called the indispensable nutrient. Approximately 60 percent of the total body weight of an average adult is made up of water and its dissolved constituents; 70 to 80 percent of the total body weight of the full-term infant is in a fluid state (see Figure 23.1). The fluid system plays an essential role in the body. Its principal functions are (a) the transportation of nutrients to the cells and the removal of waste products from them, and (b) the maintenance of a stable physical and chemical environment within the body. Important in this latter function are the electrolytes. **Electrolytes** are substances that, when dissolved in solution, split into electrically charged ions of atoms or molecules that conduct an electrical current. Atoms or molecules that carry a positive charge are called **cations**, while those carrying a negative charge are called **anions**—for example, sodium (Na^+) is a cation and chlorine (Cl^-) is an anion. The electrolytes in body fluids are important in the chemical reactions that occur within cells. They help regulate the distribution of water and are vital in the maintenance of acid–base balance. They are also essential in the transmission of electrical energy within the body. Without the calcium ion, for example, muscle contraction could not occur (Lee, Barrett & Ignatavicius, 1996).

Healthy bodies maintain a very precise fluid, electrolyte and acid–base balance. Both the volume and constituents of body fluids vary little from day to day, and they usually return to a state of equilibrium within a few days following any minor disturbance.

Serious fluid and electrolyte imbalance may occur as a result of many health problems. The nature of the imbalance may be either a deficit or an excess. An individual may retain an excess amount of fluid in the tissues, or may lose an inordinate amount of fluids (through persistent vomiting). Whenever fluids are lost or retained in excessive amounts, there is an accompanying loss or retention of electrolytes, so that both fluid and electrolyte balances are disturbed. Disturbances in fluid and electrolytes can cause serious repercussions within the body. Both the transportation and regulatory functions of the fluid system are likely to be affected. The cells may not get enough nourishment, for instance, or there may be an accumulation of waste products owing to inefficient removal. The body's acid–base balance may be upset and temperature regulation impaired. There may also be interference with the transfer of materials across the cell membrane so that a shift occurs in the distribution of fluids and electrolytes. Activities within the body that depend on the transmission of electrical energy, such as muscle contraction and the relay of nerve impulses, may be impaired.

This chapter provides an introduction to the physiology of fluid, electrolyte and acid–base balance in the body, the common imbalances and the management of these problems. Assessment of fluid, electrolyte and acid–base status and nursing interventions to promote, protect and restore fluid, electrolyte and acid–base balance during health and illness are also detailed.

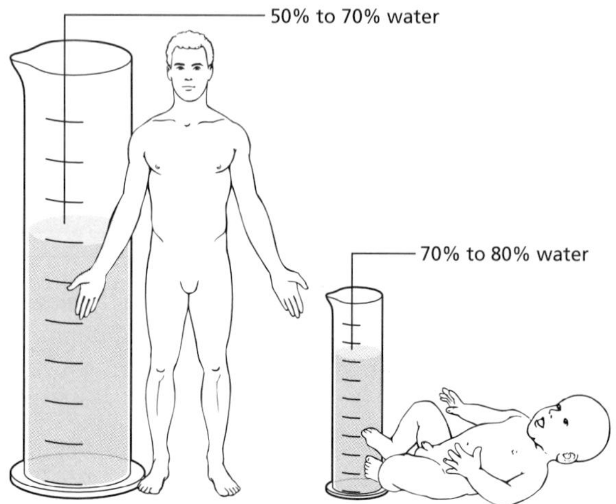

FIGURE 23.1 Percentage of total body weight composed of water and dissolved constituents

The Physiology of Fluid, Electrolyte and Acid–Base Balance

Distribution of Body Fluids

Fluid within the body is generally distributed in two basic compartments. First, body fluids are found within the cells of the body. This type, termed **intracellular fluid** (ICF), accounts for approximately 40 percent of the total body weight. Second, fluid occurs outside the cells of the body; this is **extracellular fluid** (ECF). There are two kinds of extracellular fluid. One is the fluid in the spaces between the cells; called **interstitial fluid** (ISF), this component accounts for about 16 percent of the body weight in an adult. The other component, the plasma or **intravascular fluid,** is the fluid in the blood and lymph vessels; it makes up about four percent of total body weight in an adult. A minor component of ECF is *transcellular fluid*, which includes cerebrospinal, synovial and pleural fluid as well as aqueous humour (Horne, Heitz & Swearingen, 1997). A comparison of the distribution of intracellular and extracellular fluid as related to body weight is depicted in Figure 23.2.

Water, or fluid, from both the ICF and ECF compartments combined is referred to as total body water or fluid. The content of total body water depends on such factors as age, body fat to lean mass ratio, and gender. Infants have proportionately more ECF than adults. Over half of the total body fluid in infants is extracellular as compared to about one-third ECF in adults. Since ECF is more easily lost from the body than is ICF, infants are especially vulnerable to fluid volume deficits (Lee et al., 1996). The infant's percentage of total body fluid gradually decreases over

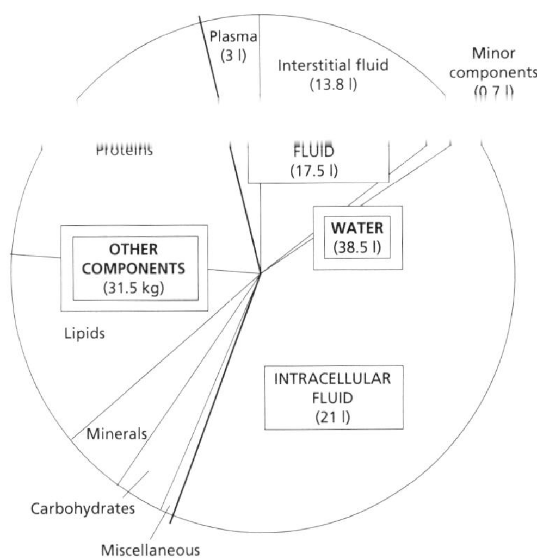

FIGURE 23.2 Distribution of fluid between ICF and ECF in relation to body weight

SOURCE: Martini, 1998, p. 1008.

TABLE 23.1 Approximate values of total body fluids as a percentage of body weight in relation to

Age	*Total Body Fluid* (% Body Weight)
Full-term newborn	70%–80%
1 year	64%
Puberty to 39 years	Men: 60% Women: 52%
40 to 60 years	Men: 55% Women: 47%
More than 60 years	Men: 52% Women: 46%

SOURCE: Metheney, 1996, p. 5.

the first two years, reaching about 64 percent of body weight by one year of age and 60 percent by the end of the second year. However, ECF is proportionately higher (24%) than ICF (36%), and remains so until puberty.

After puberty, the proportions of ECF and ICF reach adult levels but the total body fluid content varies according to body fat and gender. Lean tissue contains more water than adipose tissue. Thus, the leaner the person, the greater the percentage of total body fluid to body weight. Conversely, the more obese the person, the lesser the percentage of body weight that is fluid. Since females have more fat tissue than males, their total body fluid is less than that of males. Correspondingly, as people get older, the percentage of total body fluid to body weight decreases as lean body mass lessens and body fat increases. See Table 23.1 for a comparison of total body fluid in relation to gender and age.

Composition of Body Fluids

Body fluids consist of water and dissolved substances. Water is considered to be the major constituent of the body and the **solvent** in which substances are either dissolved or suspended. Substances that dissolve in a solution are called **solutes**. These include electrolytes, minerals and substances such as glucose, urea and creatinine. The primary solutes in body fluid are the electrolytes.

The principal electrolytes and their concentrations in ECF (plasma) and ICF are given in Table 23.2. As the table shows, the electrolyte composition of ECF and ICF is quite different. The fluid contained within cells is essentially a potassium and phosphate solution, whereas extracellular fluid is high in sodium and chloride.

The electrolyte composition of the two types of extracellular fluid (interstitial and plasma) is essentially the same insofar as principal electrolytes are concerned. The fluid within the blood vessels does, however, contain a much greater concentration of protein than is found in interstitial fluid.

Clinically, plasma is used to measure concentrations of extracellular electrolytes because this component best represents the electrolyte levels in the body as a whole. It is also easily accessible and samples can be obtained with minimal risk and discomfort to the patient. Usually, electrolyte concentrations are measured on serum, the portion of plasma remaining after clotted blood is removed. Thus, the term **serum electrolytes** is used (Lee et al., 1996).

TABLE 23.2 Electrolyte composition in plasma and intracellular fluid

Plasma Electrolytes	mmol/L	*ICF Electrolytes*	mmol/L
Cations:			
Sodium (Na^+)	142	Potassium (K^+)	150
Potassium (K^+)	5	Magnesium (Mg^{2+})	40
Calcium (Ca^{2+})	5	Sodium (Na^+)	10
Magnesium (Mg^{2+})	2		
TOTAL CATIONS	154		200
Anions:			
Chloride (Cl^-)	103	Phosphates &	
Bicarbonate (HCO_3^-)	26	sulfates	150
Phosphate (HPO_4^{2-})	2	Bicarbonate (HCO_3^-)	10
Proteinate	17	Proteinate	40
Sulfate (SO_4^{2-})	1		
Organic acids	5		
TOTAL ANIONS	154		200

Transport of Body Fluids

There is a constant shift or transfer of body fluids and dissolved substances from one compartment to another as nutrients and oxygen are transported to the cells and wastes and manufactured products are removed from cells. This transfer is accomplished by several different means, the four most common being diffusion, osmosis, active transport and filtration (Lee et al., 1996).

Diffusion is the process whereby dissolved particles (ions and molecules) distribute themselves equally within a given space (Horne et al., 1997). Diffusion occurs as a result of the constant motion of molecules. The particles move from an area of higher concentration to an area of lower concentration until equilibrium is reached. In the human body, diffusion usually takes place across a **selectively permeable membrane**. A selectively permeable (or semi-permeable) membrane allows some substances to pass freely through it, but not others. The exchange of oxygen and carbon dioxide both in the lungs (between the alveoli and the blood) and in the tissues (between the cells and the blood) occurs by diffusion across semi-permeable membranes. Electrolytes such as sodium, chloride, potassium and calcium can also diffuse across cell membranes that are permeable to these substances.

Osmosis is the movement of a solvent, such as water, through a selectively permeable membrane. The membrane is freely permeable to water but not to all the solutes. The water passes from the solution with a low solute concentration (more solvent to solute) to the one with a higher solute concentration (less solvent to solute) until the concentrations of solutes in both solutions are equalized.

A common example of osmosis is the movement of water between two salt solutions separated by a semi-permeable membrane. The water goes from the weaker salt solution to the stronger salt solution until both solutions contain the same concentrations of salt. The water is drawn across the membrane by the force of the particles in the more concentrated solution. The force that moves fluid from an area of low solute concentration to an area of high solute concentration is called **osmotic pressure**. The degree of osmotic pressure is dependent on the solute concentration, or the number of osmotically active particles per unit of volume of solvent. The more active the particles are, the greater the osmotic pressure. **Osmolality** is a term used to indicate osmotic pressure. Measured in millimoles, it refers to the number of osmotically active particles per kilogram of water (mmol/kg) (Metheney, 1996).

Some substances dissolved in body fluid—electrolytes, for instance—do not move across membranes as readily as water. Therefore, when it is necessary for the body to transfer electrolytes from within the cells to the extracellular fluid to achieve a balance, an active transport is brought into play. **Active transport** is the movement of solute particles from an area of lower concentration to an area of higher concentration with the use of a carrier molecule. Although the mechanism is not completely understood, it is believed that a substance known as adenosine triphosphate (ATP) is released from the cell. This substance appears to give the electrolytes the energy required to pass through the semi-permeable membrane. The transfer of sodium, potassium and a number of other ions, including amino acids, takes place via this mechanism.

Filtration is the process whereby water and dissolved substances are forced from an area of high pressure to an area of low pressure. In the body, the pressure involved is hydrostatic or fluid pressure. **Hydrostatic pressure** is generated by something pushing against fluid contained within a wall. The pumping action of the heart as it propels blood through the circulatory system creates hydrostatic pressure. Filtration occurs across arterial capillary walls, where water and dissolved nutrients are driven into the tissues. It also occurs in specialized tissues of the kidney in the production of urine.

Fluid and Electrolyte Balance

The mechanisms that maintain fluid and electrolyte balance are closely connected. That is, there are no separate receptors that monitor fluid balance or specific ion concentrations. Instead, fluid and electrolyte adjustments are made in response to osmotic pressure (osmolality) or volume of extracellular fluid. In the healthy adult, body fluid volume remains fairly constant, despite intake variations. This is due to the regulatory mechanisms that balance intake (gains) and output (losses).

FLUID INTAKE AND OUTPUT

People derive fluid and electrolytes from three main sources: the fluid that is ingested in liquid form, the fluid content of the various foods that are eaten, and water that is formed as a by-product of the body's oxidation of foods and body substances. The total adult daily intake of water under normal circumstances is approximately 2100–2900 mL. Water is lost from the body through the skin by perspiration, through the lungs during expiration and from the kidneys in the urine. In addition, a small amount of fluid is excreted in the feces. The total daily loss of water from the body in normal circumstances is approximately 2100–2900 mL, depending largely upon the amount of fluid intake. The average amounts of daily fluid gains and losses are listed in the box on the following page (Horne et al., 1997).

MECHANISMS REGULATING FLUID INTAKE AND OUTPUT

Although individual water molecules move from one fluid compartment to another, the volume of fluid in each compartment remains relatively stable. The main forces at work in holding water within the various compartments of the fluid system of the body (hydrostatic pressure and osmotic pressure) are generated by proteins and electrolytes. In the intravascular compartment (blood vessels) the force is generated largely by the serum albumin; in the interstitial fluid [illegible] Water passes freely through the capillary [illegible] branes, but the protein molecules and the sodium ions do not move as freely. These substances exert an osmotic pressure that tends to hold water in their respective compartments. A patient who has lost a great deal of serum albumin through malnutrition tends to become edematous, as fluid is drawn from the blood plasma into the interstitial spaces. This happens because the osmotic pressure holding the water in the blood vessels has been reduced.

By far the most important regulatory mechanism operating to maintain the body's fluid balance is the kidneys. When the intake of fluid is insufficient or when there is an excessive loss of fluid from the body, the amount of urine that is excreted is decreased. Conversely, when an excess amount of fluid is ingested, urine output increases. This is accomplished through the selective reabsorption of water in the tubules of the kidney.

The kidney also exerts the main control over the sodium and potassium balance of the body through the selective reabsorption of these ions in the tubules. When sodium and potassium levels are low in the body, increasing amounts are reabsorbed into the blood stream. When sodium and potassium levels are high in the body, the excess is excreted in the urine. If there is an acute shortage of sodium in the body, the excretion of this ion through the urine may be cut to almost zero. In the case of potassium, however, there appears to be an obligatory excretion of a certain amount in the urine (Horne et al., 1997). Thus, there is always some potassium in the daily urine output, even though the body reserves may be dangerously low. This factor is taken into account by physicians in planning replacement therapy.

The control of fluid by the kidneys is influenced by two sets of hormones. The *antidiuretic hormone* (ADH), which is produced primarily in the anterior hypothalamus and stored in the posterior pituitary gland, is a major factor in controlling water reabsorption. When the osmotic pressure of the ECF is greater than that of the cells because of insufficient water intake, deprivation of water from other sources or excessive sodium intake, for instance, the secretion of ADH is stimulated. This in turn causes increased reabsorption of water in the kidney tubules and a lessened volume of urinary output. *Aldosterone*, one of several steroid hormones produced in the adrenal cortex, exerts a major influence in promoting the retention of sodium and the excretion of potassium. Aldosterone secretion appears to be stimulated by such factors as lessened sodium intake, an excess of potassium, muscular activity, trauma and emotional tension (Lee et al., 1996).

The gastrointestinal tract also helps to regulate fluid and electrolyte balance. Selective reabsorption of water and solutes takes place principally in the small intestine.

Average Daily Adult Fluid [illegible]

Gains	
Ingested fluids	1000–1500 mL
Ingested foods	900–1000 mL
Metabolic oxidation	200– 400 mL
Total Gains	2100–2900 mL
Losses	
In urine	1000–1500 mL
In feces	100– 200 mL
Through skin	600– 700 mL
Through lungs	400– 500 mL
Total Losses	2100–2900 mL

Although the volume of digestive juices secreted into the intestinal tract each day is considerable (approximately 8200 mL), all but about 100–200 mL of fluid is reabsorbed. Under normal circumstances, only a small amount of the body's daily fluid loss is from the gastrointestinal tract in the feces, and the loss of electrolytes by this route is normally negligible. Both fluid and electrolytes may be lost in considerable quantity, however, in such conditions as vomiting and diarrhea.

Thirst is another of the regulatory mechanisms working to maintain fluid balance. Thirst is the desire for more fluids. It usually indicates a basic physiological need for water, although it may sometimes occur as a result of dryness of the mucous membranes of the mouth and throat from other causes, such as mouth breathing. True thirst, due to a basic lack of water, usually occurs when body cells are dehydrated, extracellular volume is lessened (by hemorrhage) or certain centres in the hypothalamus are stimulated. The thirst mechanism is related to the control of water balance by the antidiuretic hormone (ADH). When the body is suffering from a lack of water, the thirst mechanism operates to increase the desire for intake of water, while ADH acts on the distal convoluted tubules of the kidney to increase reabsorption of water (Woodtli, 1990).

The lungs are also important in the regulation of fluid and electrolyte balance. Ordinarily, the amount of water lost from respiration is quite small. Whenever respirations are increased in rate and depth, however, the amount of water lost via this route is also increased and may become significant. This may occur, for example, with strenuous muscular exercise, in fevers or any condition in which respirations are considerably increased, or when the air that is breathed is very dry. The loss of electrolytes through respiration is normally minimal, although the lungs play an important role in maintaining acid–base balance of the body, as will be discussed later (Metheney, 1996).

Principal Electrolytes

Electrolytes are the primary solutes of body fluid and are necessary for maintaining homeostasis. In this respect they primarily function in three physiological processes: body fluid distribution and osmolality; nerve and muscle irritability and contractility; and acid–base balance. There are many electrolytes in the body; each has its distinct functions and regulating mechanisms. Only the principal cations and anions will be outlined here.

Sodium

Sodium is the major cation within extracellular fluid. In fact, more than 90 percent of osmolality of the ECF comes from sodium salts, namely sodium chloride (NaCl) and sodium bicarbonate ($NaHCO_3$). Because of its abundance in quantity and the fact that it does not move across cell membranes with ease, sodium is largely responsible for maintaining water balance. Indeed, its primary functions are to control the distribution of water throughout the body and to regulate the extracellular fluid volume.

A basic assumption behind sodium's role in water balance is that where sodium goes, water goes with it. If sodium is retained or excreted, water will also be retained or excreted. The regulation of sodium balance is interrelated with the regulation of other electrolytes and with acid–base balance, owing to its ability to combine readily with chloride and bicarbonate. Therefore, sodium imbalances are often accompanied by electrolyte and acid–base disturbances (Lee et al., 1996).

Sodium plays an important role in neuromuscular activity and the transmission of nerve impulses. As part of the cellular sodium–potassium exchange, sodium moves into nerve cells that have been stimulated and generates action potentials. An **action potential** is a change in electrical charge on the cell membrane that activates nerves to transmit impulses to muscles, causing muscles to contract.

The average daily requirement for sodium is two to four grams. Sodium is taken into the body from food and fluid sources. A list of foods rich in sodium is presented in Table 23.3. Sodium ions enter the ECF through the digestive epithelium, mainly in the small intestine, by the processes of diffusion and active transport. The normal serum concentration of sodium is 135–145 mmol/L (Metheney, 1996). The amount that enters the ECF is directly proportional to the amount of sodium in the diet. To maintain a stable extracellular volume, the intake of sodium must equal its output. Sodium balance is regulated within narrow limits by the kidneys, which are influenced primarily by the action of aldosterone, the glomerular filtration rate and the physical condition of the kidneys themselves. Excess sodium is excreted in the urine. Small amounts are also lost through perspiration and feces.

Potassium

Potassium is the main cation of intracellular fluid. About 98 percent of the body's content of potassium lies inside the cells; the remaining two percent is extracellular. It is this two percent of extracellular potassium that represents serum potassium levels. Since it is the major intracellular electrolyte, potassium accounts for a large portion of osmotic pressure within the intracellular fluid compartment and in this way is involved in the distribution of body water.

Potassium is necessary for the transmission of nerve impulses and the contraction of skeletal, smooth and cardiac muscles. Once a nerve impulse has been generated by the influx of sodium ions, potassium shifts out of the cell and in so doing restores the resting state of the cell membrane. Until the neuron is restored to a resting state, it cannot conduct another impulse. In this way potassium regulates the excitability of nerve and muscle cells and controls neuromuscular activity in the body.

Potassium plays a major role in activating specific cellular enzymes necessary for carbohydrate metabolism and it participates in protein synthesis. It is involved in normal kidney function and promotes acid–base balance through its cellular exchange with the hydrogen ion.

The average daily requirement for potassium is three to four grams. Food sources high in potassium are listed in Table 23.3. Virtually all potassium that is ingested is absorbed through the small intestine. The normal serum concentration of potassium is 3.5–5.0 mmol/L. Potassium balance is maintained when the rate of urinary excretion equals the amount absorbed from the digestive tract. Potassium balance in the body is regulated by the kidneys in response to alterations in the potassium ion concentration or pH of the interstitial fluid and through the influence of aldosterone (Metheney, 1996). Small amounts of potassium are eliminated in the feces and through perspiration.

Calcium

Calcium, which is a cation, is the major element involved in maintaining the structure and function of bones and teeth. Only about one percent of the total body calcium is part of extracellular fluid. Of this, over half is bound to proteins such as albumin and globulin or combined with ions such as citrate, sulfate or phosphate. Less than half of the extracellular calcium is freely ionized and available for use in chemical and biological functions in the body. Calcium is needed for the transmission of nerve impulses and for the contraction and relaxation of muscles. It is necessary for maintaining the permeability of cell membranes and is an essential element in blood coagulation.

The average adult requires about 800 mg of calcium daily. Large-bodied people, children and pregnant and lactating women require more. Calcium is primarily absorbed from the small intestine. It is important to note that not all the calcium that is ingested is absorbed. The average adult absorbs 30 to 60 percent of daily ingested calcium; about 15 percent is considered nonabsorbable (Lee et al., 1996). Intestinal absorption is prevented by low vitamin D intake and by binding agents that are present in certain vegetables. Food sources that are high in calcium are listed in Table 23.3.

TABLE 23.3 Functions and Food Sources of Principal Electrolytes

Electrolyte	*Functions*	*Food Source*
Sodium	Regulates body fluid volume Generates and transmits nerve impulses Aids in acid–base balance Involved in enzyme activities	Table salt Baking soda Soy sauce Processed dairy products: cheese, butter, margarine Eggs Processed, canned or smoked meats Celery, spinach Canned vegetables Processed cereals Condiments such as mayonnaise, ketchup, mustard, pickles, salad dressings
Potassium	Helps maintain the intracellular osmotic pressure Regulates body fluids (primarily within the cell) Transmits and conducts nerve impulses Involved in muscle fibre contraction Maintains regular cardiac rhythm Activates cellular enzymes	Fresh apricots, bananas, citrus fruits and juices Dried fruits such as figs, dates, peaches, raisins Avocados, fresh tomato, mushrooms, broccoli, Brussels sprouts, spinach Cooked kidney beans, baked potato Chicken, salmon, sardines, scallops Whole milk, yogurt
Calcium	Forms and maintains healthy bones and teeth Aids in transmission of nerve impulses, muscle contraction, and blood clotting Maintains cell membrane permeability	Milk, cheese, yogurt Green, leafy vegetables such as kale, turnip and mustard greens, broccoli Sardines and salmon Tofu
Magnesium	Aids in transmission of impulses in nerves and muscles Activates enzymes Aids in bone formation	Green vegetables Roasted peanuts Bananas Milk, yogurt Soybeans Grains, bran
Chloride	Transports CO_2 (chloride shift) Maintains osmotic pressure Aids in acid–base balance Component of hydrochloric acid in stomach	Table salt Seafood Meats Eggs Milk
Phosphorus	Provides strength and rigidity to bones and teeth Buffer in acid–base balance Participates in fat, carbohydrate and protein metabolism	Beef, pork, poultry, fish and fish eggs Milk and milk products, especially cheddar cheese Peanuts Cooked dry beans Carbonated beverages Whole grains, fruits and vegetables are fair sources

SOURCES: Dudek, 1997; Metheney, 1996.

The normal serum calcium level is 2.15–2.50 mmol/L (Chernecky & Berger, 1997). This value includes the *ionized*, *complexed* (combined with citrate) and protein-bound calcium. The normal concentration of calcium in plasma is regulated by a fairly complex set of organ and hormonal factors. The primary hormones include parathyroid hormone (PTH), calcitonin (secreted by the thyroid gland) and vitamin D. When plasma levels of ionized calcium drop, PTH is secreted. PTH stimulates the release of calcium from bones and teeth and increases the reabsorption of calcium from the kidney. Calcitonin, on the other hand, has the effect of lowering extracellular calcium concentrations. It decreases plasma calcium levels by inhibiting the release of PTH, facilitating the transfer of calcium from plasma to bone, and increasing renal excretion of calcium. Vitamin D promotes the absorption of calcium from the intestine and assists PTH in the reabsorption of calcium from the bone. The bulk of excess calcium is excreted in the urine. Smaller amounts are also lost in feces, digestive secretions and perspiration.

Magnesium

Magnesium is the second most abundant cation found in intracellular fluid. However, it must be noted that 60 percent of magnesium in the body is located in bone, muscle and soft tissues. In addition, as with calcium, it is only the ionized fraction of serum magnesium that is free for chemical activity and physiological processes.

Magnesium plays a role in neuromuscular activity. It is thought to mediate the release of acetylcholine by motor nerve impulses, creating a sedative effect, and in so doing helps to regulate the transmission of activating impulses in nerves and muscles.

Magnesium is also an important activator of enzymes involved in protein and carbohydrate metabolism. It is necessary for energy production (that is, the formation of ATP) and it works with calcium, phosphorus and vitamin D in the formation of bone. The average daily nutrient requirement for magnesium is 300 mg. The principal sources of dietary magnesium are listed in Table 23.3. The normal serum concentration of magnesium is 0.65–1.25 mmol/L (Chernecky & Berger, 1997). The kidneys play a large role in conserving and excreting magnesium (Lee et al., 1996).

Chloride

Chloride is the principal anion of the ECF. A very small quantity of chloride is present in the ICF, where it plays a significant role in the functioning of specialized cells such as neurons. In the ECF, this electrolyte parallels that of sodium and is generally considered to have a passive relationship with sodium. That is, when serum sodium increases, chloride also increases, and when serum levels of sodium drop, chloride levels also usually drop. Sodium and chloride dissolved in water constitute the saline solution of the ECF compartment; both tend to hold water. Thus, like sodium, chloride functions in maintaining fluid balance and osmotic pressure of the ECF. Chloride also plays a passive role in acid–base balance where the kidneys excrete chloride or bicarbonate ions, and sodium conserves chloride or bicarbonate ions along with it to maintain acid–base balance. In cases where bicarbonate ions are retained, as in metabolic alkalosis, chloride will be excreted while sodium is reabsorbed with bicarbonate. When this happens, chloride losses will not be in proportion to sodium losses, which is a deviation from the parallel, passive nature of chloride's relationship with sodium. Thus, while increases in serum chloride levels follow those of serum sodium, losses in serum sodium and chloride can differ.

Chloride plays a part in the chloride shift, which is the chloride–bicarbonate buffer system that functions to maintain the pH balance of the blood. It is also a necessary component of hydrochloric acid in gastric juice.

The average daily requirement for chloride is three to five grams. Substantial amounts of chloride are found in table salt, dairy products and meats. It is often ingested in combination with sodium or potassium, as a sodium or potassium salt. Normal serum of chloride is concentration 97–107 mmol/L (Chernecky & Berger, 1997). Chloride is absorbed readily from the small intestine along with sodium and potassium. It is chiefly excreted from the body by the kidneys; however, it is also lost in sweat and gastrointestinal secretions.

Bicarbonate

The bicarbonate molecule is the second most abundant anion of extracellular fluid; it is found in intracellular fluid as well. It is an essential component of the bicarbonate–carbonic acid buffer system which functions to maintain normal hydrogen ion concentration and acid–base balance of the body fluids. Bicarbonate differs from the other principal electrolytes in that it is not ingested through food and fluid sources, but is synthesized in the body as the end product of fat metabolism. Base bicarbonate (pertaining to the buffer bicarbonate) is produced when sodium, potassium, calcium or magnesium combines with bicarbonate. Normal serum levels of bicarbonate are 22–26 mmol/L (Chernecky & Berger, 1997). Since it is a principal base buffer within the body, the regulation and excretion of bicarbonate is discussed in the section on acid–base balance (Lee et al., 1996).

Phosphorus and Phosphate

Phosphorus is found in the body in the form of organic and inorganic compounds. Most of it is located in the ICF, mainly as organic phosphate. In fact, 80 percent of the total body phosphorus is comprised of cellular organic phosphate located in bone. Another 10 percent of cellular phosphate is found in muscles and one percent is located in nerve tissues. The remaining nine percent of the total body phosphorus is located in the ECF (Lee et al., 1996).

The phosphate ion is the major intracellular anion. Phosphate plays a role in many body functions. In conjunction with calcium, it provides strength and rigidity to bones and teeth. It acts as a buffer in maintaining acid–base balance [illegible] onism. Phosphate is required for normal nerve and muscle activity, and is important for many cellular activities such as the formation of high energy compounds (for example, ATP), the utilization of B vitamins and the transmission of hereditary traits.

The average daily requirement is 800 mg for phosphorus. Growing children and pregnant and lactating women need more. Dietary sources rich in this electrolyte are listed in Table 23.3. The normal serum phosphorus level is 0.87–1.45 mmol/L (Chernecky & Berger, 1997). Phosphorus is absorbed easily from the small intestine, especially when vitamin D_3 (activated vitamin D) is present. When dietary intake of calcium is excessively high, however, absorption of phosphorus is inhibited. In the presence of too much calcium, phosphorus binds with the calcium, forming insoluble compounds that are excreted in the feces. Phosphorus, like calcium, is regulated by the parathyroid hormone and calcitonin. It is excreted primarily in the urine and is, in fact, the major urine buffer.

Acid–Base Balance

BODY pH BALANCE

Intimately connected with the fluid and electrolyte balance of the body is the maintenance of acid–base (H^+) balance. **Acids** ionize in water and release hydrogen ions (H+). **Bases** combine with the hydrogen ions released by acids to neutralize their effects. Bases make a solution more alkaline. The relative acidity or alkalinity of body fluids is expressed in terms of pH, which refers to the concentration of hydrogen ions in the fluid. The pH is measured on a negative logarthimic scale of 0 to 14. Water, which is considered a neutral substance (being neither acid nor alkaline), has a pH of 7.0. The pH scale is based on a negative logarithm. Acid solutions have a pH lower than 7.0 and alkaline solutions a pH higher than 7.0. Body fluids are not as neutral as water; they tend towards the basic side of the scale (Lee et al., 1996).

When large amounts of fluids are lost or retained in the body, the acid–base balance can swing in the direction of a higher concentration of either acid or base. The term **acidosis** refers to a swing towards the acid side through either a retention of excess acid (H^+ concentration) in the body or a depletion of the body's base reserves. The normally basic state of body fluids becomes more acidic. A pH below 7.35, the lowest point on the normal range for blood, is generally considered to indicate acidosis.

Alkalosis is the opposite of acidosis; there is either a lessening of the acid (H^+ concentration) of body fluids or an excess of base reserves. When the pH of blood exceeds 7.45, the highest point in the normal range, the condition is called alkalosis. When acidosis or alkalosis results from disturbances in metabolism, the term *metabolic acidosis* or *metabolic alkalosis* is used; when it results from disturbed [illegible] *respiratory alkalosis*.

REGULATING MECHANISMS

In order for the body to function normally, the pH of body fluids must be maintained within the normal range, that is, between 7.35 and 7.45. Any deviation from this range poses a threat to homeostasis because changes in hydrogen ion concentration disrupt the stability of cell membranes, alter protein structure and change the activities of important enzymes. The nervous system is particularly sensitive to fluctuations in pH, becoming depressed in acidosis and hyperexcitable in alkalosis. Therefore, the control of pH is essential for normal physiological functioning in the body. The acid–base balance of body fluids is maintained by three mechanisms: buffer systems, respiratory regulation and renal regulation (Metheney, 1996).

BUFFER SYSTEMS The body has a system of *buffers*, which function within the fluid system to correct the tendency towards either acidity or alkalinity. Buffers are pairs of substances consisting of a weak acid and its salt, which act as sponges to absorb extra hydrogen or base ions as required. The principal buffering agents in body fluids are the carbonic acid–bicarbonate system, which operates mainly in the extracellular fluid; the phosphate buffer system, which operates predominantly in the intracellular fluid; and the protein buffer system, which operates in both (proteins can act as acids or bases, as needed). The primary buffer in the body is the bicarbonate–carbonic acid system.

Buffers act immediately to correct changes in the body's pH balance. However, their ability to function on a long-term basis is limited, because as soon as they react, they are used up and eventually have to be replaced. Therefore, the body brings two other mechanisms into play—the *lungs* and the *kidneys* (Horne et al., 1997; Lee et al., 1996).

RESPIRATORY REGULATION The lungs aid in maintaining acid–base balance through their control of carbonic acid. They can eliminate either more or less carbonic acid (in the form of carbon dioxide and water), thus either ridding the body of excess acid or conserving it. When you have engaged in strenuous exercise, for example, you may find that you are breathing more quickly and more deeply than usual, as the body attempts to rid itself of the extra acid from the waste products of muscle cell metabolism.

RENAL REGULATION The kidneys can vary the acidity of the urine in response to the body's need to throw off excess acid or base. They act principally by controlling base bicarbonate. See the box on page 637 on mechanisms for maintaining normal hydrogen ion concentration.

Determinants of Fluid, Electrolyte and Acid–Base Balance

The factors that can disturb the body's fluid and electrolyte balance include insufficient intake, disturbances of gastrointestinal and kidney function, excessive perspiration or evaporation and volume losses.

INSUFFICIENT INTAKE

The sources of water and electrolytes for the body are the food and fluids ingested. Any disturbance in the source of nourishment is reflected in the body. People who do not consume sufficient food and fluids, either because these are not available or because of lifestyle, fad dieting or illness, will usually show a disturbed fluid and electrolyte balance, particularly if the insufficient intake is prolonged (Metheney, 1996).

DISTURBANCES OF GASTROINTESTINAL FUNCTION

A very large volume of fluid in the form of digestive juices is secreted into the gastrointestinal tract each day. Almost all this fluid is reabsorbed during the process of digestion. Interference with the normal processes of secretion and reabsorption can result in serious fluid and electrolyte imbalance. The nature of the imbalance depends to a large extent on the portion of the gastrointestinal tract affected. In order to appreciate the significance of this point, it is helpful to keep in mind the volume, the pH and the electrolyte composition of the various digestive juices (see Table 23.4).

The major components involved in electrolyte and acid–base balance are found in the gastric and intestinal secretions. Gastric juice contains large quantities of hydrochloric acid and a significant amount of sodium. Gastric mucus contains a high proportion of sodium and chloride, small but significant amounts of potassium and a relatively small amount of carbonate. Thus, when fluids are lost from the stomach through vomiting, there may be a significant loss of acid as well. Prolonged vomiting may cause severe sodium depletion and loss of chloride ions. The body's reserves of potassium may also be decreased. Gastric suctioning removes hydrochloric acid, potassium and fluids; gastric washings can severely deplete the store of chloride ions, particularly if these washings are done with water rather than saline. All gastric tube irrigations as well as gastric washings should therefore be done with isotonic saline to prevent the depletion of these electrolytes.

Pancreatic juice, bile and the intestinal secretions are predominantly basic and contain relatively large amounts of carbonate, as well as sodium and chloride. In addition, a portion of the total volume of potassium excreted from the body daily is via feces. Thus, diarrhea generally results in the loss of fluids, and of sodium and chloride ions. Severe diarrhea also depletes the body's potassium levels.

TABLE 23.4 Approximate daily volumes and pH of principal digestive juices

Secretion	*Daily Volume*	*Usual pH*
Saliva	1000 mL	6–7
Gastric juice	2500 mL	1.0–3.5
Small/large bowel fluid	3500 mL	7.5–8.0
Pancreatic juice	1000 mL	8.0–8.3
Bile	1500 mL	7.8

SOURCE: Metheney, 1996.

DISTURBANCES OF KIDNEY FUNCTION

Because the kidney is so intimately connected with the regulation of fluid, electrolyte and acid–base balance, any impairment in renal function may disturb this balance. Damage to the kidney itself may interfere with its ability to reabsorb water and electrolytes in the tubules. An imbalance in the antidiuretic hormone (caused by pituitary gland dysfunction) affects kidney functioning, particularly the reabsorption of water. Similarly, an imbalance in aldosterone (which may result from steroid therapy) affects sodium retention and potassium excretion by the kidneys.

The kidneys are also affected by disturbance in cardiovascular functioning. For example, a poorly functioning heart may cause an insufficient flow of blood through the kidneys to produce an adequate amount of glomerular filtrate. As a result, body tissues may retain fluid. This is evidenced by edema, which frequently accompanies many cardiac conditions.

EXCESSIVE PERSPIRATION OR EVAPORATION

One of the most significant variables in the amount of water lost daily from the body daily is the volume of perspiration. This may range from zero to several litres per day, depending on such factors as the amount of physical activity engaged in, the temperature of the environment and the presence of fever. When there is excessive perspiration, two protective mechanisms are brought into play: thirst, which increases the amount of fluid intake; and adjustment of the water output by the kidneys (Lee et al., 1996).

When fluids are lost through sweating, there is a loss of sodium chloride as well. Hence, people who live in hot climates, and those who must work in temperatures above normal, often find they need more salt in their food to replace that lost through perspiration. As a person becomes acclimatized to higher environmental temperatures, however, the body usually adjusts by lessening the salt content of sweat so that the loss of sodium and chloride ions by this route is minimized.

Mechanisms for Maintaining Normal Hydrogen Ion Concentration

Bicarbonate–carbonic acid (primary buffer system)	Carbonic acid (weak acid) $H_2CO_3 \rightleftharpoons H_2O + CO_2$ Sodium bicarbonate (weak base) $NaHCO_3$
In the presence of a buffer system the pH shifts only slightly	$NaHCO_3 + HCl \rightarrow H_2CO_3 + NaCl$ (strong acid) (weak acid) $H_2CO_3 + NaOH \rightarrow NaHCO_3 + H_2O$ (strong base) (weak base)
The respiratory system	
Acts as a feedback system for controlling hydrogen ion concentration	H^+ concentration increases pH 7.4 → 7 Respirations → rapid and deep More CO_2 exhaled Less CO_2 to combine Therefore, less H_2CO_3
50% to 75% efficient	pH from 7 to 7.2 or 7.3 within minutes or H^+ concentration decreases pH 7.4 → 7.8 Respirations → slow and shallow Less CO_2 exhaled More CO_2 to combine Therefore, more H_2CO_3 pH from 7.8 to 7.6 or 7.7 within minutes
The renal system	
Complex mechanism that continues to act until the pH reaches normal; requires more time	Can excrete more or less H^+ to achieve balance Can excrete more or less bicarbonate to achieve balance

SOURCE: Weldy, 1992, p. 54.

VOLUME LOSSES

Conditions that cause a loss of fluid volume may cause severe disturbances in fluid, electrolyte and acid–base balance. Hemorrhage causes not only a loss of fluid but also a percentage of all the blood elements. The total circulatory volume is decreased and, in a large hemorrhage, the body's adaptive mechanisms may collapse and shock may ensue.

In burns, as well as in some trauma to the body (including surgical trauma), fluid and electrolytes are lost from the general circulation, as these tend to accumulate in the interstitial spaces. Fluids are removed from the plasma, sodium is depleted throughout the body generally and potassium is released in excessive amounts from the damaged cells. Proteins are also depleted. Therefore, there is a need to replace not only fluids but also sodium, potassium and proteins in order to restore a balance.

Fluid and Electrolyte Needs Throughout the Life Cycle

The pregnant woman's circulatory system must take care of the fluid and electrolyte and oxygen needs of the fetus, as well as her own. To cope with these demands, her total blood volume is increased by approximately 50 percent, the production of red blood cells in her body is stepped up by almost one-third, and total cardiac volume is increased by approximately 10 percent. The pregnant woman's heart must also beat faster (her resting pulse rate increases) with the extra demands on her circulatory system. There is also a marked increase in the body's water content. An average of 6.5–7 L is gained, including 3.5 L for the needs of the fetus and the balance for the mother's needs (Metheney, 1996).

Many pregnant women experience fluid retention, which may be caused by such factors as a decrease in blood protein, hypervolemia (in which fluid readily leaves the intravascular spaces to equalize osmotic pressure), an increase in capillary permeability and a tendency to retain sodium. Some edema is common, particularly in the late stages of pregnancy. Some women develop a pregnancy-induced hypertension (a complication that can cause problems for both fetus and mother). This hypertension is related to sodium and water retention (Lee et al., 1996).

As mentioned at the beginning of the chapter, 70 to 80 percent of a newborn's body weight is water. Until around the age of two years, fluids continue to make up a greater proportion of total body weight than they do in older children and in adults. Much of the additional fluid is extracellular and is rapidly lost in the event of illness, a factor that makes the infant very vulnerable to fluid and electrolyte and acid–base imbalances (Metheney, 1996).

The infant also has a high metabolic rate, because of his or her greater proportional body surface area, growth needs and relatively large body organs. The high metabolic rate means that there is more rapid turnover of water in the body of children than in adults, and that children need a larger amount of fluid proportionate to body weight (see Table 23.5). Another factor contributing to the infant's vulnerability to fluid and electrolyte imbalances is the immaturity of the homeostatic mechanisms. For example, the infant's kidneys have a limited ability to concentrate and dilute urine, a mechanism that is important in maintaining fluid balance (Metheney, 1996).

By the time the child is two years of age, fluid volume as a percentage of total body weight, as well as its distribution in the body, is similar to that in an adult. The basal metabolic rate gradually decreases through childhood until maturity, and the water turnover gradually slows down to adult levels. Children, however, continue to need a greater volume of fluids proportionate to body weight than adults do and also lose a proportionately greater volume in urine.

In children there is also a greater exchange of fluids in the gastrointestinal tract than there is in adults. This factor is important because it is through this exchange that water and sodium are absorbed. Thus, problems interfering with the reabsorption of fluids in the gastrointestinal tract can cause major fluid losses in children. Children can become dehydrated quickly with even minor gastrointestinal upsets. Edema is often seen in refugee children who are starving. In this case the fluid flows from the blood vessels into the tissues because lowered levels of plasma protein are insufficient to hold the fluid in the intravascular compartment (Lee et al., 1996).

With adolescence there is a maturing of all body systems, and the homeostatic mechanisms for regulating fluid and electrolyte balance begin to function as they do in adults. In fluid and electrolyte balance, as in so many other aspects of physiological functioning, there is a difference between males and females; women have a tendency to retain fluids during the two or three days immediately prior to the menstrual period. Just before the menstrual period, there is an increase in the level of the hormone progesterone. This hormone is related in chemical composition to aldosterone and has a similar effect in promoting the retention of sodium, which, in turn, leads to the retention of water in the body.

Throughout adulthood, there is a gradual decrease in the functional capacity of the cardiovascular system as blood pressure increases and the individual becomes more vulnerable to cardiovascular diseases. A gradual lessening in

TABLE 23.5 Range of average water requirement of children at different ages under ordinary conditions

Age	*Average Body Weight in kg*	*Total Water Required in 24 hours, mL*	*Water per kg Body Weight in 24 hours, mL*
3 days	3.0	250–300	80–100
10 days	3.2	400–500	125–150
3 months	5.4	750–850	140–160
6 months	7.3	950–1100	130–155
9 months	8.6	1100–1250	125–145
1 year	9.5	1150–1300	120–135
2 years	11.8	1350–1500	115–125
4 years	16.2	1600–1800	100–110
6 years	20.0	1800–2000	90–100
10 years	28.7	2000–2500	70–85
14 years	45.0	2200–2700	50–60
18 years	54.0	2200–2700	40–50

SOURCE: Vaughan, McKay & Behrman, 1992.

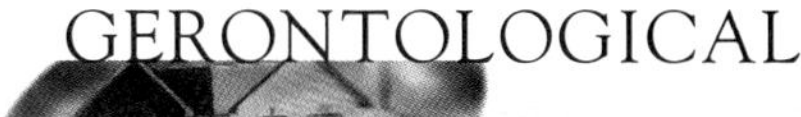

GERONTOLOGICAL

Major Physiologic Changes of Aging That Affect

Change	Consequences
Decreased total body fluid	Prone to dehydration
Dry, inelastic skin	Unreliable as an indicator of fluid status
Diminished thirst mechanism	Decreased fluid intake that can result in dehydration
Decreased glomerular filtration and concentrating capacity	Decreased ability to excrete wastes and regulate water and electrolytes
Atrophy of endocrine glands	Decreased ability to regulate sodium and potassium (adrenal atrophy); decreased ability to respond to fluid and electrolyte changes
Decreased cardiovascular function	Decreased cardiac output Increased peripheral resistance Decreased renal blood flow
Decreased respiratory function	Decreased elasticity of lung tissue Decreased strength of expiratory muscles Decreased partial pressure of oxygen
Diminished gastrointestinal function	Decreased gastric juices Decreased intestinal absorption

SOURCE: Lee, et al., 1996.

efficiency of the fluid and electrolyte regulating mechanisms contributes to making the older adult slower to recover from imbalances than the younger adult.

During menopause many women have a problem with fluid retention. Although a number of theories have been postulated, no single definitive cause has been isolated. Generally it is usually considered to be *idiopathic*, that is, due to no known cause.

In the older adult, the prevalence of hypertension and the incidence of cardiovascular disease increase. The arteries thicken and become less elastic. Many older people have a problem with varicose veins. If the varicosities occur in the deep veins, there will be reduced venous return and edema of the ankles. Older adults have a blunted thirst mechanism that makes it difficult to get them to drink sufficient fluids to meet their bodily needs, particularly when they are ill. It is important to make a point of offering extra fluids between meal times and encouraging them to drink more water, milk and juices (Lee et al., 1996).

Common Problems

Disturbances in fluid, electrolytes and acid–base balance are often not disease entities themselves, but complications of other disorders or trauma. The underlying pathophysiology of many disease processes cause either gains or losses of body water and/or solutes. The resulting fluid, electrolyte and acid–base disturbances can cause many problems to the body's internal environment. As we already discussed, all other systems in the body depend on the effective functioning of the fluid system. It serves not only as the transport mechanism for moving nutrients and removing wastes, but also provides an optimal environment for the efficient functioning of body cells.

Problems caused by fluid, electrolyte and acid–base imbalance often require medical or nursing intervention. The type of problem and the intervention required depend to a large extent on the specific nature of the imbalance and the degree of disturbance. The most common problems that the nurse will encounter are those associated with fluid and electrolyte excesses or deficits, and the accompanying disturbances in acid–base balance.

Fluid Volume Imbalances

FLUID VOLUME DEFICIT

Fluid volume deficit (FVD) is a general term used to designate a condition in which the body or tissues are deprived of water. It may result from a number of causes, such as insufficient intake of fluids, or disease conditions causing excess fluid loss, as outlined in Table 23.6.

There are three types of fluid volume deficit. The first, called **isotonic** (or extracellular) **fluid deficit**, occurs when water and electrolytes are both lost in approximately the same proportions, and the osmolality of the remaining fluids are normal. In this type of disturbance, the loss of fluid comes primarily from the ECF (that is, intravascular fluid and interstitial fluid), leading to hypovolemia (decreased volume of circulating blood) and dehydration. Since there

TABLE 33.6 Fluid volume imbalances

Common Causes	*Signs and Symptoms*
Fluid Volume Deficit	
Insufficient intake Vomiting Diarrhea Gastric suction Fistulas Excessive laxative use or tap water enemas Polyuria Excessive use of diuretics Fever Excessive diaphoresis Muscular exercise Third space fluid shifts Hemorrhage Burns	Thirst (earliest sign) Dry mucous membranes Dry, fissured tongue Decreased skin turgor Weight loss (rapid change) 2% (mild deficit, such as 1 kg in a 50-kg person) 5% (moderate deficit, such as 2.5 kg in a 50-kg person) 8% (severe deficit, such as 4 kg in a 50-kg person) Systolic blood pressure drops 10 mm Hg or more when position changes from supine to standing or sitting Slow filling of peripheral veins Pulse weak and rapid Respirations rapid Temperature subnormal (i.e., 35°–36.7°C) or low-grade elevation (e.g., 37.2°C) unless infection is present Urine output <30 mL/h (in an adult) and concentrated Dizziness, vertigo, syncope Behavioural changes (in severe FVD), e.g., lethargy, irritability, disorientation Laboratory results: Urine specific gravity>1.030 Hematocrit (Hct) is elevated in isotonic and hypotonic dehydration, and decreased in hypovolemia secondary to bleeding Blood urea nitrogen (BUN) and creatinine are decreased
Fluid Volume Excess	
Conditions that cause decreased renal perfusion or blood flow, e.g., renal disease, cardiac insufficiency, cirrhosis Intravascular protein depletion Rapid intravenous infusion of sodium-containing fluids Excessive intake of table salt or other sodium salts Release or administration of aldosterone as occurs with stress or steroid therapy	Pitting edema in upper and lower extremities, periorbital and presacral areas Weight gain (rapid change) 2% (mild excess, such as 1 kg in a 50-kg person) 5% (moderate excess, such as 2.5 kg in a 50-kg person) 8% (severe excess, such as 4 kg in a 50-kg person) Distended neck and peripheral veins Bounding pulse Irritating cough, difficulty in breathing (due to fluid in the lungs) Moist crackles in lungs Laboratory results: BUN, hemoglobin and hematocrit (HCT) decreased (due to hemodilution) Decreased urine output

TABLE 23.6 *continued*

Nursing Interventions

Fluid Volume Deficit

1. Assess the status of FVD:
   - observe signs and symptoms
   - measure and record intake and output from all sources
   - obtain accurate daily weights (1 kg loss in weight represents 1 L of fluid lost)
2. Provide oral fluids if indicated:
   - select fluids containing lost electrolytes and adequate calories
   - establish patient likes and dislikes
   - ensure patient comfort:
     provide frequent mouth care
     choose non-irritating fluids
     give antiemetics as ordered for nausea
3. Fluids may be administered to patients who are unable to eat or drink through tube feedings (i.e., nasogastric, gastrostomy or jejunostomy tubes) as ordered by the physician. Nursing care for tube feedings is discussed in Chapter 20.
4. Fluids will be replaced intravenously if the patient is vomiting, FVD is prolonged or large volumes of fluid are required.
   - Careful monitoring of intake and output and serum electrolytes is necessary for intravenous therapy because the type and amount of fluid prescribed is determined by the type and amount of fluid lost. Nursing interventions for intravenous therapy are discussed later in this chapter.
5. Evaluate the patient's response to fluid therapy. Indicators of effective therapy:
   - increasing urine output (40–60 mL/h)
   - decreasing urine concentration and specific gravity
   - BP returns to normal baseline
   - pulse and respiratory rates return to baseline
   - return to baseline weight
   - return of skin and tongue turgor
   - increasing moisture in skin and mucous membranes
   - improved behaviour and sense of well-being
   - laboratory values return to normal

Fluid Volume Excess

1. Assess the status of FVE:
   - observe signs and symptoms
   - measure and record intake and output
   - obtain accurate daily weights (1 kg gain in weight represents 1 L of fluid)
2. Restrict sodium and fluid intake as ordered.
3. Administer diuretics as ordered.
4. Monitor response to diuretics; observe for potassium depletion and replace as necessary.
5. Regulate intravenous fluids as ordered.
6. If breathing difficulty occurs, position the patient in semi-Fowler's position to facilitate lung expansion.
7. Frequently turn and position the patient on bed rest (edematous tissue is prone to skin breakdown).
8. Provide instruction for self-care:
   - sodium-restricted diet
   - avoidance of OTC drugs containing sodium
   - rest (side-lying positions promote diuresis)
   - monitoring of weight, intake and output, diuretic therapy and potassium replacement
9. Evaluate the patient's response to treatment and care. Indicators of effective care:
   - laboratory values return to normal
   - absence of dependent and pitting edema
   - return to baseline weight
   - pulse returns to baseline
   - clear lungs; easy breathing

SOURCES: Metheney, 1996; Lee et al., 1996; Kee, 1995.

is no change in osmolality, there is very little movement from other compartments. Therefore, loss of fluid from the ICF does not occur.

Extracellular fluid deficit occurs when fluid is lost from the body, as with hemorrhage and diarrhea or when it becomes trapped in a third space. A third space is an area such as a body cavity in which fluid accumulates and cannot be drawn back into the circulatory system. An example of third-space fluid loss is the accumulation of fluid in the bowel due to obstruction. With hemorrhage, in addition to intravascular fluid loss, there is a loss of ICF because the fluid within the red blood cells belongs to the intracellular compartment. Hemorrhage can lead to volume deficit from both the ECF and ICF compartments (Metheney, 1996).

The second type of fluid volume deficit is a **hypotonic dehydration**. In this case, solutes are lost from the ECF without a proportionate loss of water. As a result, the remaining ECF is hypotonic; it has less solute than water. This causes water to move from the extracellular compartment into the cells (ICF) by osmosis until osmotic equilibrium is reached. The ECF volume decreases while the ICF volume increases, and the osmolality of both compartments is lowered. Hypotonic fluid volume deficit can occur after sweating if water is ingested without an adequate intake of salt. It also can occur when diuretic therapy is used in conjunction with a salt-restricted diet. The signs and symptoms (see Table 23.6) tend to be more severe with hypotonic dehydration (Weldy, 1992). In addition, it must be noted that weight loss does not provide a good estimate of hypotonic dehydration because some of the ECF shifts into the ICF compartment, resulting in minimal loss of weight.

Hypertonic dehydration is the third type of fluid volume deficit. It occurs when more water than solute is lost and the remaining body fluids become hypertonic (concentrated). At first the water loss comes from the ECF compartment. This causes water to shift from the ICF compartment until osmotic equilibrium is reached. The end result is that fluid volume is lost from both compartments and the osmolality of both ICF and ECF is increased. Hypertonic dehydration occurs when **insensible water losses** (losses of fluid from the lungs and the skin through respiration and perspiration) are not replaced. This may result from sweating with no intake of water or inability to ingest adequate amounts of water. Since the fluid shifts from the ICF to the ECF compartment, the signs and symptoms of fluid volume deficit are not readily apparent; however, the neurological manifestations (such as confusion and restlessness) become evident (Weldy, 1992).

FLUID VOLUME EXCESS

Fluid volume excess (FVE) is a condition in which excessive fluid is retained in the interstitial fluid space (tissues), causing generalized or localized edema. Fluid is first retained in the peripheral tissues and then in the lungs; in severe cases edema becomes more generalized and fluid passes into body cavities, such as the peritoneal cavity. Fluid volume excess may result from disturbances in kidney function, disturbances in circulatory function (for example, in people with heart conditions), inflammation, increased permeability of the cell membranes or a number of other health problems. This condition is outlined further in Table 23.6.

Electrolyte Imbalances

SODIUM DEFICIT

Sodium deficit is called **hyponatremia**. Specifically, it refers to a condition in which the concentration of sodium in the ECF (serum sodium) is below normal levels, that is, less than 135 mmol/L. It is a hypotonic (hypo-osmolar) state that can result from an excessive loss in sodium without a proportionate loss in water or an excessive gain in water without a proportionate gain in sodium. When there is a deficit in sodium, the extracellular fluid becomes less concentrated; in other words, more dilute. Thus, water is pulled, by osmosis, from the ECF space into the cells, causing an intracellular water excess. While edema is not present *per se*, the tissues swell because of the increased cellular water content. In fact, the signs and symptoms of hyponatremia are probably due to cellular swelling—in particular, the neurological manifestations are the result of cerebral edema (Metheney, 1996).

Hyponatremia can occur alone—that is, a loss of sodium within a normal ECF volume—or it can occur in conjunction with a fluid volume excess or deficit. It is associated with fluid volume excess (edema) in conditions such as congestive heart failure or renal disease, where total body water increases to a greater extent than does sodium. It occurs with hypotonic dehydration when the deficit of sodium is relatively greater than that of total body water; when, for example, a loss of secretions from the gastrointestinal tract is due to vomiting and/or diarrhea.

The treatment for hyponatremia is sodium replacement or restriction of fluid. When the signs and symptoms indicate hyponatremia with a water deficit, treatment is to replace sodium and fluid through oral intake of food and fluids high in sodium or intravenous infusion for those patients unable to eat or drink. Hyponatremia with signs and symptoms of water retention is corrected by restricting fluid intake. The causes, signs and symptoms and nursing interventions for hyponatremia are presented in Table 23.7.

SODIUM EXCESS

Sodium excess, in which the concentration of sodium in the ECF (serum sodium) is above normal levels (more than 145 mmol/L), is called **hypernatremia**. It is a hypertonic (hyperosmolar) state in which there are greater gains in sodium than in water or, conversely, there are greater losses in water than in sodium. Excesses in sodium cause the ECF to become more concentrated and, as a result, water is pulled from the cells by osmosis, causing cellular dehydration.

Consequently, cells shrink and their function is impaired. Indeed, the neurological manifestations of hypernatremia are attributed to cellular dehydration, in particular to the water

As with hyponatremia, hypernatremia can occur in patients whose fluid volume is normal or in those with fluid volume deficits or excesses. People who experience increased insensible water loss, through hyperventilation for instance, can lose water but not sodium, which leads to mild hypernatremia. The amount of water loss, however, is not large enough to deplete the extracellular space; thus the ECF volume remains nearly normal. This type of hypernatremia often goes unnoticed because the body corrects itself by triggering the thirst centre, which induces the person to drink water.

More severe hypernatremia is often associated with hypertonic dehydration, where loss of water exceeds loss of sodium. This can occur with more severe insensible water loss, for instance, from sweating profusely because of high environmental temperature, fever or strenuous muscular exercise. Hypernatremia associated with a volume deficit also occurs in people who are deprived of water because they cannot perceive thirst (for example, unconscious patients or very young children) or because they cannot ingest water (for example, paralyzed individuals). Hypernatremia can also be related to fluid volume excess; for example, when hypertonic saline solutions are administered intravenously there can be a greater gain of sodium in relation to water (Metheney, 1996).

Hypernatremia in conjunction with a water deficit is corrected by replacing water orally or by intravenous infusion of five percent dextrose in water. Sodium excess combined with ECF excess is treated with diuretic drugs, which remove both sodium and water from the body, and by restricting the intake of sodium and fluids. The causes, signs and symptoms and nursing interventions for hypernatremia are outlined in Table 23.7.

POTASSIUM DEFICIT

Potassium deficit, or **hypokalemia**, occurs when the extracellular concentration of potassium is less than 3.5 mmol/L. Hypokalemia is a common condition because the kidneys do not conserve potassium. Even when intake is decreased, the kidneys continue to excrete potassium. In addition to decreased intake, hypokalemia is caused by excessive renal excretion that may result from treatment with potassium-wasting diuretics or steroid hormones, which promote excretion of potassium.

Hypokalemia is also caused by stress and disease of the adrenal cortex, in which excess aldosterone is secreted, since aldosterone causes sodium and water retention and potassium loss from the kidney. Gastrointestinal secretions are rich in potassium. Therefore, fluid loss from the gastrointestinal tract will cause significant loss of potassium and, hence, hypokalemia.

The signs and symptoms of hypokalemia (see Table 23.7) stem primarily from its effect on neuromuscular function. Potassium plays a large role in the transmission and

skeletal, smooth and cardiac muscles. Potassium deficit results in decreased neuromuscular excitability and subsequent diminished muscular contractility, thus muscle weakness.

Early detection and treatment of hypokalemia are important because potassium deficit can be life-threatening. The primary objective in treating hypokalemia is prevention. Patients at risk for hypokalemia require increased potassium through diet and supplements. Individuals who cannot ingest food and fluid receive a maintenance dose of potassium by the intravenous route. Actual potassium losses must be replaced either orally, through liquid or tablet forms, or intravenously, if hypokalemia is severe or oral intake is not possible (Metheney, 1996).

POTASSIUM EXCESS

Extracellular potassium excess or **hyperkalemia** is an increased accumulation of potassium in the blood stream and results when the serum potassium level is above 5.0 mmol/L. Hyperkalemia is not common in people with normal kidney function; however, it can occur in renal dysfunction associated with decreased urinary output. Probably the most common cause of hyperkalemia is excessive or very rapid oral or intravenous fluid intake combined with renal failure.

Like hypokalemia, hyperkalemia affects the excitability of nerve and muscle cell membranes. In the case of potassium excess, the excitability of the cell membrane increases while the resting potential decreases. As a result, the spread of stimuli along nerves and muscle fibres is blocked. Muscle weakness and paralysis follow. The most dangerous effect of hyperkalemia is its influence on the heart. The increased excitability of cell membranes can lead to disturbances in cardiac conduction causing cardiac arrhythmias, bradycardia, heart block and cardiac arrest.

The signs and symptoms of potassium excess are outlined in Table 23.7. It cannot be overemphasized that hyperkalemia is life-threatening; early detection and treatment is imperative. Muscle weakness progressing to flaccid paralysis is the most common sign of hyperkalemia. Paresthesias and tingling sensations are also common. Respiratory paralysis and involvement of the facial muscles are late manifestations.

Prevention is the best treatment of hyperkalemia. For instance, eliminating the use of salt substitutes in a patient taking potassium-sparing diuretics may be required to prevent an accumulation of extracellular potassium. Treatment of hyperkalemia depends on the cause and severity of potassium excess. In mild cases restriction of oral or intravenous potassium may be all that is necessary. For more severe forms and especially when cardiac manifestations are present, treatment may include intravenous administration of

TABLE 33.7 Electrolyte imbalances

Common Causes	*Signs and Symptoms*
Hyponatremia Vomiting Diarrhea Gastric suction Renal disease Potent diuretics Lack of sodium intake Adrenal insufficiency Profuse perspiration followed by a large intake of water Wound drainage and weeping skin lesions Mental confusion Burns Excessive intake of water or electrolyte-free solutions (e.g., 5% dextrose in water)	Headache Faintness Weakness Muscle cramps Anorexia Nausea Vomiting Abdominal cramping Sternal fingerprinting Vertigo Muscle twitching Seizures Coma Serum sodium <135 mmol/L Serum osmolality <285 mmol/kg Urine S.G. <1.003
Hypernatremia Increased insensible loss: Fever High environmental temperature Strenuous exercise Water deprivation Watery diarrhea Renal failure with sodium retention Increased sodium intake: Hypertonic tube feedings without water supplement Excessive ingestion of salt Excessive parenteral infusion of sodium-containing solutions	Mild to moderate: • intense thirst • dry, sticky mucous membranes • swollen, dry tongue • flushed skin • decreased urine output • temperature may rise Severe: • restlessness and agitation • disorientation • hallucinations • lethargy when undisturbed • seizures • coma Serum sodium >145 mmol/L Serum osmolality >293 mmol/kg Urine S.G. >1.035
Hypokalemia Diarrhea Vomiting Gastric suction Potassium-losing diuretics Corticosteroid use Diseases leading to increased adrenal cortical hormone release Metabolic alkalosis Poor intake	Muscle weakness Malaise Decreased muscle tone Hyporeflexia Paresthesias and muscle cramps Hypotension Cardiac arrhythmias due to increased irritability of the heart muscle Anorexia Nausea and vomiting Abdominal distention Decreased peristalsis Polyuria Serum potassium <3.5 mmol/L

TABLE 23.7 *continued*

Nursing Interventions

Hyponatremia

1. Identify patients at risk for hyponatremia, e.g., those with GI fluid losses, diuretic therapy in conjunction with a low-salt diet, or patients with adrenal insufficiency who are exposed to stress such as surgery.
2. Assess the status of hyponatremia.
   - Observe signs and symptoms. Be aware of their significance in the presence of sodium-containing fluid losses, low sodium intake and excessive intake of water and electrolyte-free solutions
   - Measure and record intake and output from all sources
   - Obtain accurate daily weights
3. Administer fluid and foods high in sodium as ordered.
4. Know the sodium content of commonly used parenteral fluids and monitor patients with CV disease for fluid overload (signs of FVE).
5. In cases of severe hyponatremia, hypertonic saline solutions (3% or 5% NaCl) are administered, using extreme caution. These patients are cared for in an ICU where their status and response to therapy can be closely monitored.
6. Evaluate the patient's response to treatment and care. Indicators of effective care:
   - absence of sternal fingerprinting
   - resolution of the gastrointestinal and neurological signs and symptoms
   - return of normal laboratory values

Hypernatremia

1. Identify patients at risk for hypernatremia, e.g., debilitated patients who are not able to perceive or respond to thirst, or stroke patients who are unable to communicate thirst.
2. Assess the status of hypernatremia.
   - Observe signs and symptoms. Be aware of their significance in the presence of risk for water deprivation and insensible water loss, high sodium intake, and excessive intake of salt-containing solutions
   - Observe for fluid volume deficit and excess
   - Measure and record intake and output
   - Obtain accurate daily weights
3. Restrict sodium intake as ordered.
4. Provide fluids at regular intervals to patients who are debilitated or cannot communicate. If intake is inadequate, collaborate with the physician for alternative method of administering fluids.
5. Evaluate the patient's response to treatment and care. Indicators of effective care:
   - absence of thirst
   - moist, shiny mucous membranes
   - normal body temperature
   - resolution of neurological signs and symptoms
   - gradual return of serum sodium to normal value

Hypokalemia

1. Identify patients at risk for hypokalemia, e.g., patients on potent diuretics or corticosteroids, those who are allowed nothing by mouth (NPO) or those who are chronic laxative users.
2. Assess the status of hypokalemia.
   - Observe signs and symptoms
   - Observe for signs of metabolic alkalosis
   - Measure and record intake and output from all sources
   - Check serum potassium reports and notify physician of results
3. Implement preventive care for hypokalemia in patients at risk.
   - Encourage increased intake of potassium, provided there are no dietary restrictions. Patients who use salt substitutes may not need extra potassium because these substances contain significant amounts of potassium.
4. Administer oral potassium supplements as ordered.
5. IV potassium must be administered carefully following strict guidelines because excessive or rapid intake of this mineral can be lethal. Even a transient excess in potassium is dangerous because it can lead to a cardiac arrest.
6. Evaluate the patient's response to treatment and care. Indicators of effective care:
   - resolution of neuromuscular signs and symptoms
   - return of GI function
   - normal pulse rate and rhythm
   - gradual return of serum potassium to normal value

continued on next page

TABLE 33.7 Electrolyte imbalances

Common Causes	*Signs and Symptoms*
Hyperkalemia	
Renal failure with decreased urinary output Excessive or rapid oral or intravenous intake Crush injuries, burns Adrenal insufficiency Respiratory and metabolic acidosis Rapid infusion of old blood (potassium released from deteriorated red blood cells)	Vague muscle weakness Cardiac arrhythmias, tachycardia followed by bradycardia, heart block and cardiac arrest Oliguria or anuria Paresthesias of face, tongue, hands and feet Flaccid paralysis that begins in legs and spreads to trunk and arms; facial and respiratory muscles become involved later Abdominal cramps Nausea and diarrhea Serum potassium >5.0 mmol/L
Hypocalcemia	
Dietary deficiency of calcium or vitamin D Pancreatitis Diarrhea Excessive laxative use Hypoparathyroidism Hyperphosphatemia Renal failure	Numbness and tingling in the fingers, around the mouth, in toes Spasms in the hands, feet and face Hyperactive reflexes Trousseau's sign Chvostek's sign Skeletal muscle cramps Abdominal spasms and cramps Laryngospasm Convulsions Mental changes such as anxiety, confusion, impaired memory Serum calcium <2.15 mmol/L
Hypercalcemia	
Malignant tumours Hyperparathyroidism Hyperthyroidism Excessive vitamin D intake Excessive calcium intake	Muscle weakness Hypotonic muscles Constipation, anorexia, nausea, vomiting Polyuria Thirst Kidney stones Deep bone pain Depression, lethargy Behaviour changes Serium calcium >2.50 mmol/L

TABLE 23.7 *continued*

Nursing Interventions

Hyperkalemia

1. Identify patients at risk for hyperkalemia, e.g., those on potassium-sparing diuretics, potassium supplements or salt substitutes, or those with poor kidney function who are experiencing metabolic acidosis.
2. Assess the status of hyperkalemia.
   - Observe signs and symptoms
   - Observe for signs of metabolic or respiratory acidosis
   - Measure and record intake and output from all sources
   - Check serum potassium reports and notify physician of results
3. Implement preventive care for hyperkalemia in patients at risk.
   - Administer oral and IV potassium safely
   - Administer fresh blood transfusions as ordered
   - Provide self-care teaching. Advise patients to:
     take potassium supplements as prescribed and avoid overuse
     use salt substitutes sparingly if taking diuretics in conjunction with potassium supplements
     avoid potassium-sparing diuretics, potassium supplements or salt substitutes if renal function is impaired
     know the signs and symptoms of hyperkalemia and report any adverse effects immediately
     avoid foods high in potassium if chronically prone to hyperkalemia
4. Implement treatment measures for hyperkalemia as ordered. Use established procedures and guidelines to ensure safety.
5. Evaluate the patient's response to treatment and care. Indicators of effective care:
   - resolution of neuromuscular signs and symptoms
   - GI comfort, absence of diarrhea
   - normal pulse rate and rhythm
   - return of serum potassium to normal value

Hypocalcemia

1. Identify patients at risk for hypocalcemia, e.g., those who have had surgery to thyroid gland or parathyroid glands, patients with malabsorption syndromes or conditions causing increased GI motility with diarrhea.
2. Assess the status of hypocalcemia.
   - Observe signs and symptoms
   - Observe breathing, noting airway status
   - Monitor serum calcium levels for 24–48 hours postoperatively following thyroid surgery or radical neck dissection
   - Observe for prolonged bleeding and clot formation
   - Monitor acid–base status
3. Implement preventive care for hypocalcemia in patients at risk.
   - Institute seizure precaution care
   - Have a tracheotomy tray at the bedside
   - Reduce environmental stimuli
   - Teach individuals with inadequate calcium intake about diets high in calcium or self-administration of calcium supplements as necessary. An adequate intake of vitamin D is necessary to aid intestinal absorption of calcium.
4. Administer oral calcium supplements as ordered.
5. Know parenteral calcium solutions and administer according to established procedure.
6. Evaluate the patient's response to treatment and care. Indicators of effective care:
   - resolution of neuromuscular irritability
   - return of patient's usual pattern of behaviour, mental alertness
   - return of total serum calcium to normal level

Hypercalcemia

1. Identify patients at risk for hypercalcemia, e.g., women with breast cancer or patients using thiazide diuretics.
2. Assess the status of hypercalcemia.
   - Observe signs and symptoms
   - Strain urine to monitor for kidney stones
3. Encourage a fluid intake of 3–4L/day. Unless contraindicated, fluids containing sodium are recommended because sodium enhances calcium excretion.
4. Restrict dietary intake of calcium and vitamin D supplements as ordered. Provide instruction on foods the patient should avoid, i.e., those rich in calcium.

continued on next page

TABLE 23.7 Electrolyte imbalances

Common Causes	*Signs and Symptoms*
Hypomagnesemia	
Prolonged inadequate intake Malnutrition Alcoholism Prolonged IV or TPN without magnesium replacement Nasogastric suction Severe diarrhea Malabsorption syndrome Severe renal disease Diabetic ketoacidosis Hyperaldosteronism Hyperparathyroidism Diuretics Excessive calcium or vitamin D intake	Neuromuscular irritability Increased reflexes Coarse tremors Facial twitching Positive Chvostek's and Trousseau's signs Painful paresthesias of hands and feet Muscle cramps Cardiac tachyarrhythmias Disorientation, confusion Behaviour changes Convulsions Serum magnesium <0.65 mmol/L Signs of hypocalcemia and hypokalemia when hypomagnesemia is severe
Hypermagnesemia	
Renal failure Excessive, prolonged use of magnesium-containing antacids and laxatives Excessive administration of magnesium salts Severe extracellular fluid volume deficit with oliguria	Serum magnesium 1.5-2.5 mmol/L: • hypotension • facial flushing, warmth • diaphoresis Serum magnesium 2.5-3.5 mmol/L: • lethargy, drowsiness • loss of deep tendon reflexes • muscular weakness Serum magnesium 5 mmol/L: • respiratory depression Serum magnesium 6–7.5 mmol/L: • coma Serum magnesium >7.5 mmol/L: • cardiac arrest

TABLE 23.7 *continued*

Nursing interventions

Hypercalcemia, cont'd

5. Ambulate patients as soon as possible. Assist with active and passive exercises for patients on bed rest. Mobility prevents loss of calcium from the bones and promotes the transfer of calcium from the blood stream back into the bones.
6. Implement preventive care for complications in patients with hypercalcemia.
   - Position and transfer patients carefully to prevent pathological fractures
   - Force fluids to dilute the urine and prevent kidney stones. Ensure an intake of fluids that will produce an acid urine, such as cranberry juice and prune juice. An acid urine will increase the solubility of calcium in the urine.
   - Teach patients about and encourage a diet high in bulk to counteract the propensity for constipation
7. Evaluate the patient's response to treatment and care. Indicators of effective care:
   - resolution of neuromuscular weakness and cramps
   - return to normal GI function and comfort
   - absence of pathological fractures or kidney stones
   - return of patient's usual pattern of behaviour, mental alertness
   - return of total serum calcium to normal level

Hypomagnesemia

1. Identify patients at risk for hypomagnesemia, e.g., people who abuse alcohol chronically and do not eat adequately, postoperative patients receiving magnesium-free IV solutions and on NG suction, and people taking calcium and vitamin D supplements.
2. Assess the status of hypomagnesemia.
   - Observe signs and symptoms
   - Monitor vital signs and observe for cardiac arrhythmias
   - Observe breathing, noting airway status (laryngospasm can occur)
3. Implement preventive care for hypomagnesemia in patients at risk.
   - Institute seizure precaution care in severe cases
   - Know the commonly used IV solutions that do not contain magnesium (e.g., D5W, lactated Ringer's solution) and collaborate with physician regarding replacement if necessary
   - Implement safety precautions in patients with behaviour changes
   - Because patients with hypomagnesemia may suffer difficulty with swallowing, check swallowing ability before giving food, fluids or oral medications
4. Teach patients who are able to ingest food and fluid about foods high in magnesium.
5. Administer oral and parenteral magnesium salts as ordered and according to established procedure to ensure safety.
6. Evaluate the patient's response to treatment and care. Indicators of effective care:
   - resolution of neuromuscular irritability
   - normal vital signs and cardiac function
   - return of patient's usual pattern of behaviour, mental alertness
   - return of serum magnesium to normal level

Hypermagnesemia

1. Identify patients at risk for hypermagnesemia, e.g., patients with renal failure who use antacids and laxatives containing magnesium salts or obstetrical patients who are being treated with magnesium sulfate.
2. Assess the status of hypermagnesemia.
   - Observe signs and symptoms
   - Monitor vital signs and observe for hypotension, bradycardia and cardiac arrhythmias
   - Observe breathing, noting shallow respirations with periods of apnea
3. Implement preventive care for hypermagnesemia in patients at risk.
   - Teach patients with poor renal function to avoid antacids and laxatives containing magnesium salts
   - Provide sufficient fluids to ill patients to ensure adequate urinary output. When patients are receiving parenteral magnesium, always have intravenous calcium gluconate available for emergency use.
4. Evaluate the patient's response to treatment and care. Indicators of effective care:
   - resolution of neuromuscular depression
   - normal vital signs and cardiac function
   - return of serum magnesium to normal level

continued on next page

TABLE 23.7 Electrolyte imbalances

Common Causes	Signs and Symptoms
Hypophosphatemia	
Inadequate intake	Anorexia
Malnutrition	Muscle weakness
Vitamin D deficiency	Paresthesias
Hyperparathyroidism	Skeletal muscle pain and aches
Vomiting, chronic diarrhea	Behavioural changes such as apprehension, confusion
Diabetic ketoacidosis	Hemolytic anemia
Glucose administration	Decreased tissue oxygenation
Respiratory alkalosis	Serum phosphorus <0.87 mmol/L
Phosphate-binding antacids	
Thiazide diuretics	
Hyperphosphatemia	
Chronic renal failure	Symptoms of hypocalcemia such as tetany, hyperreflexia, flaccid paralysis, muscular weakness and cramps
Antineoplastic drugs	Symptoms of soft-tissue calcification in such sites as the kidney, joints, cornea and arteries
Excessive use of phosphate-containing laxatives	Serum phosphorus > 1.45 mmol/L
Excessive intake of oral or IV phosphate supplements	
Hypoparathyroidism	

hypertonic glucose and insulin to pull potassium back into the cells. Once the potassium moves back into the cells it is no longer toxic. Calcium gluconate will be given intravenously to stimulate the heart when life-threatening cardiac manifestations are present. Calcium works by antagonizing the effect of excessive potassium on conductivity of cardiac tissue.

Hyperkalemia, particularly when associated with acidosis, may be corrected with intravenous sodium bicarbonate. By buffering the hydrogen ions in the plasma, bicarbonate helps shift potassium back into the cells. Hypertonic glucose and insulin, calcium and sodium bicarbonate are temporary measures for controlling hyperkalemia and are, therefore, used in emergency and transient hyperkalemic states. Acute, nontransient forms of hyperkalemia are treated with cation-exchange resins, such as Kayexalate, that absorb potassium from the intestinal tract; or peritoneal and hemodialysis, which filter potassium along with other waste products from the extracellular fluid.

CALCIUM DEFICIT

Hypocalcemia refers to a deficit in the serum concentration of calcium and is reflected in serum values below 2.15 mmol/L. It is caused by dietary deficiency of calcium or vitamin D, or by diseases that limit intestinal absorption, as in acute pancreatitis or diarrhea. Diseases of the parathyroid gland resulting in an inadequate secretion of parathyroid hormone lead to calcium deficits (Metheney, 1996). Hypocalcemia is also associated with excesses of serum phosphates (hyperphosphatemia) through a mechanism that is not clearly understood, and with renal failure, in which phosphorus is retained while calcium is excreted.

A calcium deficit can also occur when the body is in an alkalotic state, because calcium will not ionize when alkalosis is present. The signs and symptoms of hypocalcemia are related primarily to its effect on neuromuscular irritability. Calcium exerts a sedative effect on the nerve cell membranes. A lack of calcium leads to increased neuromuscular

TABLE 23.7 *continued*

Nursing Interventions

Hypophosphatemia

1. Identify patients at risk for hypophosphatemia, e.g., older, debilitated patients who are being refed after malnourishment; chronic alcoholic patients being treated with IV glucose; or patients in diabetic ketoacidosis being treated with IV glucose and insulin.
2. Assess the status of hypophosphatemia.
   - Observe signs and symptoms
   - Observe urinary output
   - Observe for signs of hypercalcemia (calcium excess is often associated with phosphorus deficit)
3. Implement preventive care for hypophosphatemia in patients at risk.
   - Monitor serum phosphorus values in patients at risk and report to the physician
   - Teach patients about foods high in phosphorus
   - Monitor closely patients taking phosphorus-binding antacids in conjunction with thiazide diuretics or if they have other associated conditions such as hyperparathyroidism or hypercalcemia
4. Administer oral phosphorus as ordered.
5. Evaluate the patient's response to treatment and care. Indicators of effective care:
   - resolution of neuromuscular weakness and pain
   - return of patient's usual pattern of behaviour, mental alertness
   - return of serum phosphorus to normal level

Hyperphosphatemia

1. Identify patients at risk for hyperphosphatemia, e.g., patients with renal insufficiency being treated for peptic ulcer with large quantities of milk or children receiving large quantities of phosphate-containing enema solution.
2. Assess the status of hyperphosphatemia.
   - Observe signs and symptoms
3. Implement preventive care for hyperphosphatemia in patients at risk.
   - Teach patients about the dangers of excessive use of phosphate laxatives and enemas
   - Administer oral and IV supplements cautiously, frequently monitoring serum phosphorus levels
4. Teach patients on a low-phosphorus diet about foods that should be avoided.
5. Evaluate the patient's response to treatment and care. Indicators of effective care:
   - resolution of neuromuscular irritability
   - absence of signs of soft-tissue calcifications
   - return of serum phosphorus to normal level

SOURCES: Metheney, 1996; Lee et al., 1996; Weldy, 1992.

irritability and results in tonic muscle spasms (tetany) and cramps. It decreases the contractility of heart muscle and reduces blood clotting. The signs and symptoms of calcium deficit are listed in Table 23.7. Chronic hypocalcemia is treated with oral calcium supplements. Vitamin D may also be given to enhance absorption from the intestinal tract. Acute hypocalcemia, in which severe tetany or convulsions have set in, is a medical emergency that requires immediate administration of intravenous calcium.

CALCIUM EXCESS

The condition in which there is an excess of extracellular calcium is called **hypercalcemia**. A total serum calcium reading above 2.50 mmol/L indicates hypercalcemia. Extracellular calcium excess is caused by conditions that release calcium from the bones into the extracellular fluid. The most common of these are malignant tumours (cancers) followed by hyperparathyroidism. In hyperparathyroidism, calcium is not only reabsorbed from the bones and teeth but is also absorbed in greater quantities from the intestines and the kidneys.

Excessive intake of calcium and vitamin D can result in hypercalcemia. People who take large doses of pharmacologic vitamin D and people who ingest excessive milk and alkaline antacids, particularly calcium carbonate, may develop hypercalcemia. The signs and symptoms of hypercalcemia (Table 23.7) are related to the increased sedative effect on the nerve cell membranes and the decreased tone of skeletal and smooth muscle. The increased urinary excretion of excess calcium may lead to kidney stones, and the loss of calcium from bones may cause deep bone pain and pathological fractures. Increased serum calcium may also be demonstrated through mental and behavioural changes, notably depression, lethargy and apathy.

Treatment for hypercalcemia must be directed towards the cause, for instance, removal of tumours by surgery, chemotherapy or radiation. However, general measures are also instituted to eliminate serum calcium excesses. A diet low in calcium may be used. Fluids are forced to dilute serum levels and promote diuresis and renal excretion of calcium. Intravenous solutions of normal saline are administered for this purpose as well. Serum calcium concentrations can also be lowered by administering organic phosphorus through oral, nasogastric, enema or intravenous routes.

MAGNESIUM DEFICIT

A magnesium deficit or **hypomagnesemia,** is present when the serum magnesium is less than 0.65 mmol/L. It can occur in conditions that result in an inadequate intake of magnesium, for instance, prolonged malnutrition or starvation associated with alcoholism. Hypomagnesemia is also caused by the administration of magnesium-free intravenous or total parenteral nutrition solutions, particularly when there is no oral intake or when magnesium is also being lost through nasogastric suctioning.

Diseases of the small bowel causing impaired absorption lead to hypomagnesemia, as does hypercalcemia. Calcium and magnesium share a common site for absorption in the distal small bowel. They have a mutually suppressive effect on each other so that excesses in one will inhibit absorption of the other. Thus, excessive calcium intake inhibits magnesium absorption and vice versa. Diuretic therapy and conditions resulting in increased renal excretion and fluid loss, such as renal disease, diabetic ketoacidosis and primary hyperaldosteronism, can also cause magnesium deficits.

The signs and symptoms of hypomagnesemia are primarily associated with its effects on neuromuscular function and on potassium and calcium balance. Since magnesium exerts a sedative effect on the neuromuscular system, deficits in magnesium will lead to hyperactive neuromuscular manifestations. Magnesium facilitates the transport of potassium across cell membranes. When there is a deficit in magnesium the kidneys excrete more potassium; thus a deficit in magnesium leads to a deficit in potassium. With regard to calcium balance, low levels of magnesium inhibit the action of parathyroid hormone causing a hypocalcemia. Mild hypomagnesemia may be treated with diet alone. More severe forms may require oral or parenteral replacement of magnesium salts. See Table 23.7.

MAGNESIUM EXCESS

Hypermagnesemia occurs when the serum concentration of magnesium is above 1.25 mmol/L. The most common cause of magnesium excess is renal failure, in which excretion of the mineral is inadequate. The risk of hypermagnesemia is even greater in these cases if excessive antacids or laxatives containing magnesium salts are being used over prolonged periods of time. Excessive administration of magnesium for other reasons, such as controlling convulsions in pregnancy-induced hypertension, can lead to hypermagnesemia. People suffering from severe extracellular volume depletion with oliguria may also develop a magnesium excess.

The signs and symptoms vary according to serum concentration levels as outlined in Table 23.7. Mild hypermagnesemia is asymptomatic. As the serum levels increase, manifestations beginning with vasodilating effects—hypotension, flushing and diaphoresis—advance to the neuromuscular blocking effects at the myoneural junction—lethargy, drowsiness, hypoactive reflexes, respiratory depression, coma and death. The effects on the heart lead to bradycardia and, eventually, cardiac arrest. Thus, although hypermagnesia is quite rare, when it occurs it can be fatal.

Prevention is the best treatment for hypermagnesemia. Antacids and laxatives containing magnesium should not be given to patients with renal failure or poor urinary output. In milder forms, magnesium excess may be corrected by discontinuing use of magnesium salts. Severe forms with respiratory and cardiac involvement are controlled with intravenous calcium gluconate. Since calcium has a direct antagonistic effect on magnesium, it is an effective temporary measure. Ventilator support may be required. Hemodialysis with a magnesium-free dialysate may also be used.

PHOSPHORUS DEFICIT

A decrease in the serum concentration of inorganic phosphorus is known as **hypophosphatemia**. Concentrations less than 0.87 mmol/L constitute hypophosphatemia. While this serum value generally indicates a deficiency in phosphorus, hypophosphatemia can occur in a wide variety of situations in which the total body stores of phosphate may be normal, increased or decreased.

Hypophosphatemia is associated with low intake, poor absorption from the small bowel (often due to a lack of vitamin D), loss from vomiting and diarrhea and increased renal excretion. Increased renal excretion may be due to hyperparathyroidism (since PTH secretion causes phosphorus excretion) and altered carbohydrate metabolism such as diabetic ketoacidosis (glycosuria and polyuria promote renal excretion while parenteral insulin therapy causes phosphorus to shift into the cells, thus lowering serum phosphorus levels). The intake of nonabsorbable antacids containing aluminum or magnesium hydroxides may also decrease phosphate levels by binding with phosphorus in the bowel and preventing absorption.

The signs and symptoms of hypophosphatemia (Table 23.7) are related to central nervous system (CNS), muscular and hematologic abnormalities. Treatment of phosphorus deficit includes replacement therapy, usually by the oral route, and correction of the underlying pathology.

PHOSPHORUS EXCESS

Hyperphosphatemia is an excess of phosphorus in the ECF and is indicated by serum concentrations above 1.45 mmol/L. The incidence of hyperphosphatemia is relatively rare because normally functioning kidneys excrete excess phosphorus. It is associated with an intake of large amounts

chronic renal insufficiency when the glomerular filtration rate falls below 30 mL/min (Schrier, 1997) and with the administration of antineoplastic agents for cancer, which cause tumour cells to break down and release phosphate into the ECF.

Hypocalcemia usually occurs in conjunction with hyperphosphatemia. While the mechanism by which this occurs is not completely known, it is thought that the increased phosphate concentration stimulates an increase in bone formation, which requires more calcium. The symptoms of hyperphosphatemia are often seen as those of hypocalcemia. Phosphate excess itself causes few symptoms; the most significant is soft tissue calcification, seen most commonly in patients with renal failure. Treatment is directed towards correcting the underlying cause. If excessive intake is the cause, discontinuing dietary ingestion and use of substances containing phosphorus may be all that is necessary. Phosphate-binding antacids may also be used to precipitate and consequently excrete excess phosphate through the gastrointestinal tract.

Acid–Base Imbalances

The acid–base balance of body fluids is kept within a very narrow range by the chemical blood buffers, the lungs and the kidneys. Any condition that interferes with the function of any one of these regulating mechanisms or that either increases or decreases the concentration of hydrogen (acid) or bicarbonate (base) ions will cause an acid–base imbalance in the body. Acidosis will result when there are more hydrogen ions circulating in the blood than there are bicarbonate ions to absorb and buffer them. Alkalosis results when there is too much bicarbonate and not enough acid in the extracellular fluid.

Whenever an acid–base imbalance occurs in the body, a set of processes is put into motion by the lungs and the kidneys to minimize the change in pH and return it to normal. These processes are referred to as *compensation*. Compensation, as it refers to acid–base imbalance, must not be confused with the terms buffering and correcting. **Buffering** is the immediate chemical response to changes in the hydrogen ion concentration of body fluids, whereas **correction** implies the return of all acid–base components to normal.

Compensation is the result of the physiologic mechanisms that attempt to maintain the ratio of one carbonic acid molecule to 20 bicarbonate ions. For example, in compensated respiratory acidosis, the plasma pH values are normal even though carbonic acid is elevated, because the kidneys excrete hydrogen ions and retain bicarbonate ions. When the kidneys are no longer able to help restore balance, the condition is termed *uncompensated*. These compensating mechanisms actually accentuate the abnormal levels of carbon dioxide and bicarbonate in the blood; and they are "expensive" because when compensation occurs,

body function is altered (Metheny, 1996).

There are two primary types of acid–base imbalance: respiratory and metabolic. Each can result in acidosis or alkalosis. These imbalances are depicted in Figure 23.3. The manifestations of acid–base imbalances in the body vary depending on the cause, the amount of cellular injury and the success of the compensatory mechanisms (that is, the retention or release of carbon dioxide by the lungs and the retention or release of bicarbonate or hydrogen ions by the kidneys) that are mobilized to return body pH to normal.

In addition, the signs and symptoms are not always specific to the acid–base imbalance; for instance, in metabolic alkalosis many of the manifestations are attributed to the concomitant deficits in potassium and chloride. Therefore, the best method for assessing and evaluating acid–base status is arterial blood gas analysis. The components of blood gas analysis and their significance in diagnosing acid–base imbalances are presented in Table 23.8. The common types of acid–base imbalance, along with their causes, compensatory mechanisms, signs and symptoms, treatment and nursing interventions, are outlined in Table 23.9.

How to Evaluate Blood Gases

1. Determine whether the pH is acid, alkaline or normal:
   Normal 7.35–7.45
   Acidemia <7.35
   Alkalemia >7.45
2. Determine the cause of the disturbance:
   - Assess pCO_2: is the level acid, base or normal?
   Normal 35–45 mm Hg
   Respiratory acidosis >45 mm Hg
   Respiratory alkalosis <35 mm Hg
   - Assess HCO_3: is the level acid, base or normal?
   Normal 22–26 mmol/L (mEq/L)
   Metabolic acidosis <22 mmol/L (mEq/L)
   Metabolic alkalosis > 26 mmol/L (mEq/L)
3. Identify the primary disturbance:
   - If pH is abnormal, the acid–base component consistent with the pH is the primary disturbance.
   - If pH is normal or near normal, the acid–base component most distant from normal is usually the primary disturbance.
4. Determine presence of compensation:
   - Compensation is present when pCO_2 or HCO_3 is moving in the same direction as the primary disorder.
   - Compensation is absent when one component (pCO_2 or HCO_3) is abnormal and the other normal.

SOURCE: Metheney, 1996; Black & Matassarin-Jacobs, 1997.

Left Side
Related to Respiratory Function

Right Side
Related to Metabolism of the Body

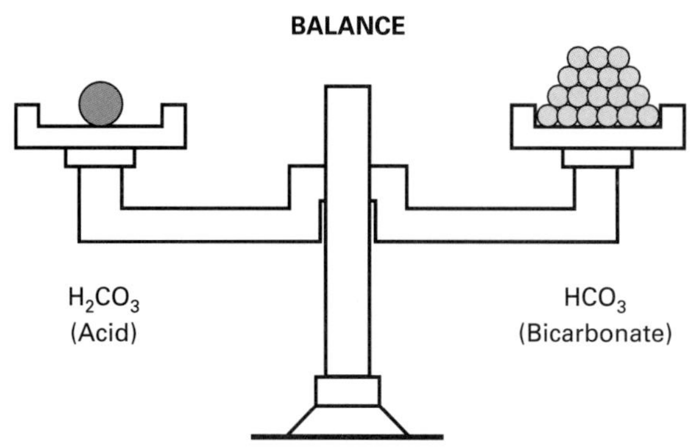

ACIDOSIS

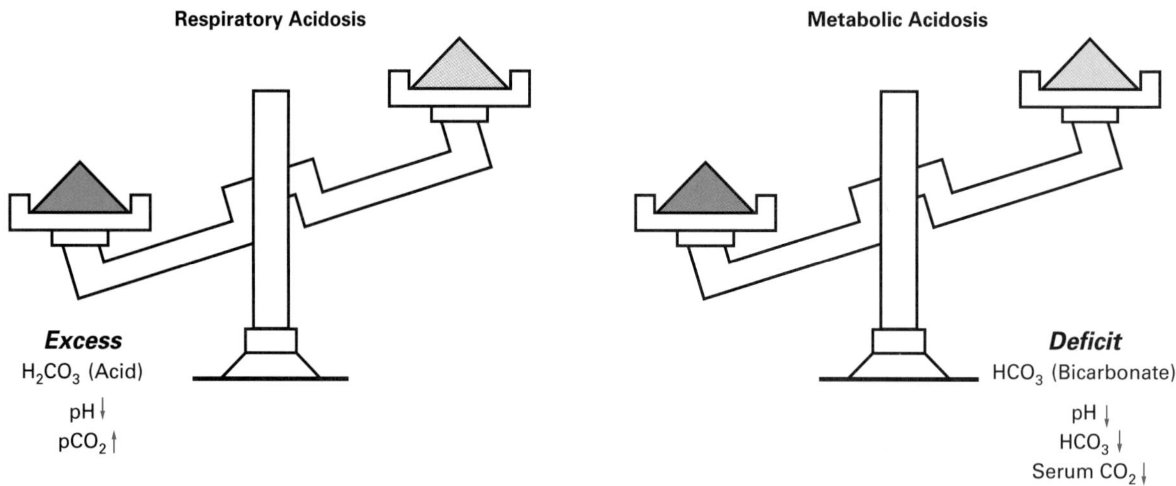

ALKALOSIS

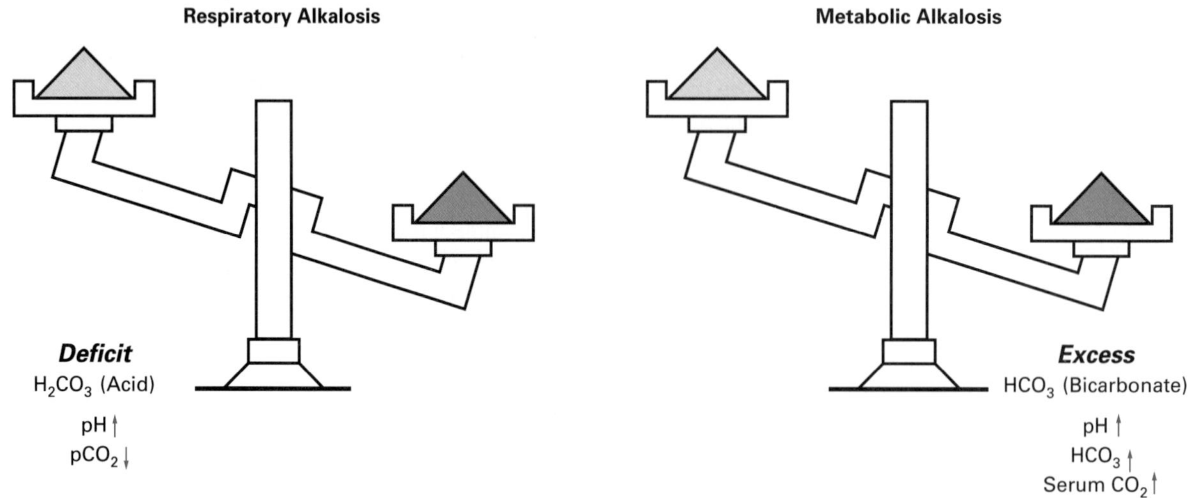

FIGURE 23.3 Acid-base balance and imbalance

SOURCE: Kee, 1986, p. 175.

TABLE 23.8 Arterial blood gases

Term	Normal Value	Definition/Implications
pH	7.35–7.45	Reflects H^+ concentration; acidity increases as H^+ concentration increases (pH value decreases as acidity increases) • pH < 7.35 (acidosis) • pH > 7.45 (alkalosis)
pCO_2	35–45 mm Hg	Partial pressure of CO_2 in arterial blood • When <35 mm Hg, hypocapnia is said to be present (respiratory alkalosis) • When >45 mm Hg, hypercapnia is said to be present (respiratory acidosis)
pO_2	80–100 mm Hg	Partial pressure of O_2 in arterial blood
Standard HCO_3	22–26 mmol/L	HCO_3 concentration in plasma of blood that has been equilibrated at a pCO_2 of 40 mm Hg, and with O_2 to saturate the hemoglobin

SOURCE: Metheney, 1996, p. 161.

RESPIRATORY ACIDOSIS

Respiratory acidosis is caused by conditions that prevent the lungs from exhaling carbon dioxide. Excessive amounts of carbon dioxide are retained in the blood and combine with water to form carbonic acid. The increased carbonic acid causes the blood pH to decrease. The kidneys attempt to compensate for this imbalance by retaining base bicarbonate and eliminating hydrogen ions. However, renal compensation is very slow, taking from a few hours to several days to occur. Therefore, in acute cases, renal compensation may not be effective in shifting the pH back to normal. Very low respiratory rates, as in hypoventilation, or any disease that obstructs the exchange of oxygen and carbon dioxide in the lungs, will result in respiratory acidosis.

RESPIRATORY ALKALOSIS

Respiratory alkalosis occurs when respirations are very rapid. Excessive carbon dioxide is exhaled; as a result, carbonic acid decreases and blood pH rises. Attempting to correct this imbalance, the kidneys save hydrogen ions and excrete bicarbonate ions. Hyperventilation, fever or stimulation of the respiratory centre can cause respiratory alkalosis.

METABOLIC ACIDOSIS

Metabolic acidosis is characterized by a deficit of base bicarbonate (alkali) in the extracellular fluid. It is caused by an excessive loss of bicarbonate from the gastrointestinal tract or the kidneys, or by an excessive accumulation of acids from faulty nutrient metabolism or renal inability to excrete acid products of metabolism. In either case, the ratio of bicarbonate to carbonic acid is decreased, and without enough base the blood pH rises. The lungs try to compensate by getting rid of carbon dioxide; thus, breathing becomes rapid and deep. The kidneys respond by excreting more hydrogen ions and retaining bicarbonate ions; therefore, the urine becomes acidic. Metabolic acidosis is due primarily to altered nutrient metabolism. Some causative conditions include uncontrolled diabetes mellitus, severe diarrhea, excessive exercise, severe infection, starvation and a high-fat diet.

METABOLIC ALKALOSIS

In metabolic alkalosis there is either an excess of base bicarbonate or a loss of hydrogen ions in the blood. Vomiting or gastric suction results in a loss of hydrochloric acid from the stomach. The sodium that is left behind when chloride is lost combines with bicarbonate to form a base bicarbonate excess. Excessive ingestion of bicarbonate-containing antacids (for example, Alka-Seltzer) can cause metabolic alkalosis. In any case, the blood pH is elevated and the lungs retain carbon dioxide, causing slow, shallow breathing. The kidneys also respond by conserving hydrogen ions and excreting bicarbonate; as a result, the urine becomes alkaline.

COMBINED AND MIXED IMBALANCES

Acid–base imbalances can occur as separate entities or as combinations or mixtures of imbalances. That is, a patient can have respiratory acidosis or alkalosis or metabolic acidosis or alkalosis alone, or two of the types can occur at the same time. In *combined acid–base imbalances*, respiratory and metabolic acidosis or respiratory and metabolic alkalosis occur together. For instance, an anxious patient who is hyperventilating and vomiting will experience both respiratory and metabolic alkalosis simultaneously.

Mixed acid–base imbalances occur as respiratory acidosis and metabolic alkalosis or respiratory alkalosis and metabolic acidosis. A common example of the latter mixed imbalance is salicylate (ASA) poisoning. At first, the respiratory centre in the medulla is stimulated, causing hyperventilation and thus respiratory alkalosis. Later, the salicylates cause a metabolic disturbance that leads to an accumulation of acids in the body, resulting in metabolic acidosis.

TABLE 33.[illegible] Acid base imbalances: Causes, compensation, signs and symptoms, treatment and nursing interventions

Causes	*Compensation*	*Signs and Symptoms*
Respiratory Acidosis (Carbonic acid excess) Hypoventilation, e.g., airway obstruction pulmonary edema infection atelectasis paralysis of respiratory muscles overdose of sedatives or anesthetics postoperative pain tight abdominal binders or dressings severe abdominal distention	Kidneys excrete hydrogen ions but the process is slow (takes from a few hours to several days to develop)	Dyspnea Anxiety Disorientation Mental confusion Feeling of fullness in head (due to high pCO_2, which causes cerebral vasodilation and increased blood flow) Dizziness Decreasing level of consciousness Tachycardia Cardiac arrhythmia, e.g., ventricular fibrillation Blood gases: pH <7.35 pCO_2 >45 mm Hg HCO_3 normal or slightly elevated (uncompensated) HCO_3 >33 mmol/L (compensated) Serum K elevated
Respiratory Alkalosis (Carbonic acid deficit) Hyperventilation, e.g., severe anxiety or hysteria (most common) high fever brain lesions involving respiratory centre hypoxemia early salicylate poisoning excessive ventilation with mechanical ventilator	Kidneys excrete bicarbonate but the process is slow	Rapid breathing Signs related to decrease in calcium ionization, e.g., dizziness, numbness and tingling of fingers and toes, circumoral paresthesias tetany Lightheadedness (low pCO_2 causes cerebral vasoconstriction and decreased blood flow) Headache Vertigo Palpitations Blood gases: pH >7.45 pCO_2 <35 mm Hg HCO_3 normal (uncompensated) HCO_3 <22 mmol/L (compensated) Serum K decreased
Metabolic Acidosis (Base bicarbonate deficit) Diabetic ketoacidosis Renal failure (uremic acidosis) Severe diarrhea Excessive exercise (lactic acidosis) Starvation	Lungs "blow off" CO_2, respirations rapid and deep Kidneys excrete hydrogen ion and retain bicarbonate ion	Lethargy Headache Drowsiness Nausea and vomiting Fruity, acetone breath Increased respiratory rate and depth

TABLE 23.9 *continued*

Treatment	Nursing Interventions
Respiratory Acidosis	
Treat underlying cause, e.g., antibiotics for infection Improve ventilation, e.g., • clear airway by suction, postural drainage • deep-breathing exercises • intermittent positive pressure breathing (IPPB) Oxygen therapy for hypoxia Severe cases: • ventilation via endotracheal tube, tracheostomy and mechanical • IV lactate or bicarbonate to help restore balance	Maintain a patent airway: • assist patient to turn and change position frequently • use semi-Fowler's position unless contraindicated • assist patient to deep breathe frequently, cough as necessary • suction nose and throat as necessary Maintain hydration (2–3 L/day), unless contra-indicated to keep secretions thin and facilitate removal Administer O_2 as ordered Monitor the patient's status per signs and symptoms Report signs of difficult breathing promptly, especially respiratory rates of ≤12/min or ≥24/min
Respiratory Alkalosis	
Treat underlying cause, e.g., tranquillizer for hysteria Increase level of CO_2: • rebreathe exhaled air from paper bag or rebreathing mask • voluntary breath-holding • intermittent inhalations of CO_2	Provide reassurance and emotional support to anxious and hysterical patients Teach and encourage slower breathing, breath-holding, or rebreathing techniques
Metabolic Acidosis	
Treat underlying cause, e.g., correct diabetic ketoacidosis with glucose and insulin Replace water, electrolytes, and nutrients	Monitor the patient's status per signs and symptoms Report signs of worsening condition immediately, e.g., restlessness, confusion, Kussmaul's respirations, tetany bradycardia, unconsciousness

continued on next page

TABLE 23.9 Acid–base imbalances: Causes, compensation, signs and symptoms, treatment and nursing interventions

Causes	*Compensation*	*Signs and Symptoms*
Metabolic Acidosis (continued) ***(Base bicarbonate deficit)*** Salicylate poisoning High-fat diet		Kussmaul's breathing (when HCO_3 is very low) Warm, flushed skin Dehydration Restlessness Confusion Unconsciousness Convulsions Blood gases: pH < 7.35 HCO_3 <22 mmol/L pCO_2 <35 mm Hg (compensated) Base excess negative Serum K often elevated
Metabolic Alkalosis ***(Base bicarbonate excess)*** Excessive intake of sodium bicarbonate Excessive vomiting or gastric suction Use of potent diuretics	Lungs retain CO_2, respirations slow and shallow Kidneys retain hydrogen ion, excrete more bicarbonate	Shallow breathing Nausea, vomiting, diarrhea May be signs of hypokalemia May be signs related to decreased calcium ionization, such as muscle cramps, tremors, muscle twitching Irritability Unconsciousness Possible convulsions Blood gases: pH >7.45 HCO_3 >26 mmol/L pCO_2 normal (uncompensated) pCO_2 >45 mm Hg (compensated) Base excess positive Serum K often decreased Serum Cl disproportionately lower than Na

In both the combined and mixed imbalances, the body's compensatory mechanisms are impaired and compensation cannot occur. Medical treatment is necessary to reverse the imbalances and prevent death.

Assessing Fluid, Electrolyte and Acid–Base Balance

In order to assess a patient's fluid, electrolyte and acid–base needs, the nurse has to identify factors in the patient's history which would contribute to health or illness. The nurse should also be alert to signs and symptoms as well as significant laboratory findings in the patient that might be indicative of fluid, electrolyte and acid–base imbalances. In addition, the nurse should know the physician's plan of therapy for the patient and understand the rationale on which this plan is based.

The patient's medical history provides the nurse with information about actual or potential fluid, electrolyte and acid–base problems. The person who has had a history of nausea and vomiting over several days, for example, is likely to show disturbances from the loss of fluids generally, the loss of acid from gastric secretions and possibly a depletion of sodium ions. The patient who is admitted for surgery may develop fluid, electrolyte and acid–base imbalance post-operatively and will need careful observation to detect impending imbalances. The baseline data entered on the patient's record by the physician, other nurses and other health professionals can alert the nurse to the presence of problems.

TABLE 23.9 *continued*

Treatment	Nursing Interventions
Metabolic Acidosis continued	
Alkaline solutions, such as sodium bicarbonate or lactated Ringer's, may be given parenterally	Measure and record intake and output (required for calculating fluid replacement) Administer alkaline solutions according to established procedure to ensure safety Have sodium bicarbonate available for emergency use Implement safety precautions for restless, confused, unconscious or convulsing patients
Metabolic Alkalosis	
Treat underlying cause, e.g., stop use of sodium bicarbonate antacids for relief of indigestion Acidifying solutions, such as ammonium chloride, may be used intravenously or orally Oral or IV sodium chloride is administered Potassium deficits are replaced intravenously or orally	Monitor patient's status per signs and symptoms Report signs of worsening condition immediately, e.g., confusion, irritability, twitching, tremor, unconsciousness, convulsions Measure and record intake and output Monitor potassium, chloride and hydrogen ion losses (necessary to determine replacement) Instruct patients on foods high in potassium Administer oral sodium chloride and potassium supplements as ordered Administer IV sodium chloride and potassium per established procedure to ensure safety Implement safety precautions for confused, agitated, irritable, unconscious or convulsing patients

SOURCES: Metheney, 1996; Lee et al., 1996; Weldy, 1992.

Nursing Health History

The health history for fluid, electrolyte and acid–base balance focusses on obtaining information about the patient's usual patterns of fluid intake and output, determining changes in these patterns and exploring symptoms relating to the presenting health problem. The patient's health-promoting and protecting patterns are also scrutinized to help identify potential problems and opportunities for health teaching.

Measurements

FLUID INTAKE AND OUTPUT

Accurate measurement and recording of fluid intake and output are essential for identifying fluid balance problems and for planning and evaluating patient care. Abnormal gains or losses of fluids are valuable signs of fluid and electrolyte imbalances. Accurate recording of intake and output is especially important for correctly estimating fluid replacement therapy. When patients have existing or potential fluid and electrolyte problems, the nurse should implement fluid intake and output recording as an independent nursing function, even though this may sometimes be ordered by the physician.

All fluids the patient takes into and eliminates out of the body must be measured. Intake consists of fluids given orally, intravenously, interstitially and rectally, as well as fluids administered through tubes (tube feedings) or fluids used for tube irrigations. Fluid output includes urine, emesis and any drainage such as bile and suction returns. Significant amounts of fluid lost in the feces (with diarrhea), from wounds, during hyperventilation or through perspiration are estimated and recorded.

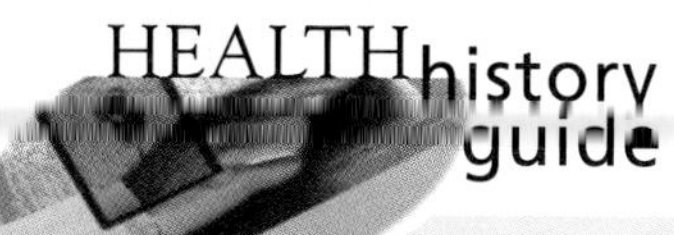

Fluid, Electrolyte and Acid–Base Balance

HEALTH AND ILLNESS PATTERNS

USUAL PATTERN OF FLUID INTAKE AND OUTPUT

- What types of fluid do you usually drink in a day?
- How much water do you drink in a day?
- What foods do you usually eat? (Focus on proteins and foods rich in minerals such as sodium and potassium.)
- What is your usual frequency and amount of urination? How often do you void in a 24-hour period? Is urine concentrated or dilute?

RECENT CHANGES IN PATTERN OF INTAKE AND OUTPUT

- Have there been any recent changes in your usual patterns of intake and output? Have you noticed that you are drinking more or less than usual?
- Have you noticed that you have been voiding more or less often than usual?
- Have you noticed any loss or gain in weight?
- Have you had a recent illness that affected your fluid intake and output?
- Have you experienced nausea, vomiting, diarrhea or excessive perspiration?
- Have you noticed any signs of too much or too little hydration in your body? (Too much—swollen fingers and ankles, difficulty breathing, weight gain. Too little—dry mouth and skin, thirst, concentrated urine.)
- Have you noticed any change in your muscle strength, or signs of muscular irritability, such as tremors or twitching of the muscles?

PRESENTING HEALTH PROBLEM

- Describe the symptoms you are experiencing now. (Use questioning techniques as necessary to explore the symptoms.)
- When did the symptoms begin?
- What remedies have you tried for the symptoms? What were the results?
- Do you have a history of any acute or chronic diseases that might disrupt fluid, electrolyte and acid–base balance? For example, diabetes mellitus, high blood pressure, heart disease, kidney disease?
- Are you taking any medications or treatments that might disrupt fluid, electrolyte and acid–base balance? For example, diuretics, laxatives or enemas, steroids, potassium supplements, tube feedings, total parenteral nutrition, dialysis?
- Have you had any dietary restrictions? If so, what kind? Do you need help to plan a diet to meet these restrictions?

HEALTH PROMOTION AND PROTECTION PATTERNS

- Do you drink products containing caffeine (for example, coffee, tea and cola), salt or sugar? If so, how much and how often?
- Do you drink alcohol? If so, how much and how often?
- Do you exercise regularly? If so, what is the nature of your program? What do you do to maintain hydration during strenuous exercise? What precautions do you take when exercising in hot weather?
- Do you work in a hot, humid environment? Does your work require strenuous activity? For example, using tools in a vigorous way, moving and carrying furniture or engaging in rigorous sporting activity?

Fluid intake and output is recorded on a form commonly referred to as an I&O record or a fluid balance record (see Figure 23.4) that is kept at the bedside or on the patient's chart. In most agencies, printed materials defining volumes of cups, glasses, bowls and containers enable accurate measurement of fluid intake. Graduated containers are also available for measuring output. Patients and their families can help to keep their own records, particularly if they understand the need for documentation and have been taught how to do it. Guidelines for measuring and recording fluid intake and output are outlined in the box on page 662.

The nurse totals the patient's intake and output at the end of each shift and also computes a 24-hour total. Fluid loss should equal fluid intake over a 48- to 72-hour period. The urine output of the average adult is between one and two litres in a 24-hour period. A general rule is that the kidneys produce approximately one millilitre of urine per kilogram of body weight per hour (1 mL/kg/h), regardless of age. Urine output that is less than 30 mL or more than 500 mL per hour is generally abnormal. Abnormalities of either excess or inadequate output must be reported to the patient's physician so that appropriate therapy can be instituted.

DAILY BODY WEIGHT

When patients have fluid and electrolyte disturbances, it is important to measure body weight on a daily basis—rapid changes in fluid volume are reflected in body weight. A loss or gain of one kilogram of body weight is almost equal to the loss or gain of one litre of fluid. To ensure accuracy of measurement, weights should be taken at the same time each day—before breakfast and after voiding. The same scale should be used each time and the patient should wear similar clothing.

LIONS GATE

FLUID BALANCE / IV THERAPY RECORD

INTAKE ☐ OUTPUT ☐

DATE: From 07:00 ____________ to 07:00 ____________

INTAKE										OUTPUT							
INTRAVENOUS							ORAL			URINE			OTHER FLUID LOSS				
													GASRIC			TUBE (Specify)	
START TIME	STOP TIME	SOLUTION VOLUME	RATE	INITIAL	TOTAL IV IN	TOTAL BLOOD IN	TIME	ORAL	TUBE	TIME	VOID	CATH.	EMESIS	N/G	BOWEL		
SUBTOTALS																	
12-H TOTAL:		IN:								OUT:							
START TIME	STOP TIME	SOLUTION VOLUME	RATE	INITIAL	TOTAL IV IN	TOTAL BLOOD IN	TIME	ORAL	TUBE	TIME	VOID	CATH.	EMESIS	N/G	BOWEL		
SUBTOTALS																	
12-H TOTAL:		IN:								OUT:							
24-H TOTAL:		IN:					OUT:						24-H BALANCE + or –				

A601 10M-S-TS
Rev. (03/91)

FIGURE 23.4 Fluid balance record

SOURCE: Lions Gate Hospital, North Vancouver, B.C.

Guidelines for Measuring and Recording Fluid Intake and Output

Establish Intake and Output Protocol

- Post an "Intake and Output" sign on the patient's bed or on the door of the room.
- Place an I&O sheet at the bedside and a fluid balance record on the chart. In some agencies only the fluid balance record is used. It is kept at the bedside and entries are made directly on it, eliminating the need to transfer amounts from one sheet to another at the end of the shift.
- Note fluid intake and output recording on the patient's nursing care plan or Kardex.

Instruct the Patient and/or Family

- Explain why intake and output measurement is necessary.
- If patients are able to participate, explain how to measure and record intake and output:
  - Oral intake may be recorded in millilitres, using the agency list of fluid content in glasses, cups, soup bowls and other containers. Alternatively, the number of glasses, cups, bowls or containers of fluid ingested may be recorded, leaving the computation into millilitres to be done by the nurse.
  - The patient should void into a bedpan, urinal or "hat" that is placed in the toilet, pour the urine into a graduated container, measure the amount and then discard the urine. Demonstrate how to read amounts using the graduated container.
  - Record the time and amounts of intake or output on the I&O sheet.

Measure and Record Intake

- Record the time, amount and type of intake on the I&O sheet.
- Water ingested from the bedside pitcher:
  - Note the amount in the pitcher at the beginning of the shift.
  - Record the amount taken in when the pitcher is refilled or at the end of the shift.
  - Determine the amount of fluid ingested by subtracting the volume remaining in the pitcher from the volume it originally held, that is, the amount at the beginning of the shift or in the refilled pitcher.
- Ice chips:
  - Determine the amount consumed by multiplying the volume of ice by 0.5 (for example, 240 mL of ice equals 120 mL of water).
- Oral fluids taken during or between meals:
  - Record the time and amounts immediately after meals and intakes throughout the day.
  - Indicate the type of liquids ingested (juice, carbonated beverages, coffee, tea, broth, milk, jello, ice cream, sherbet, hot cereals, etc.). Pureed foods are not included.
  - Measure the amount ingested using standard volumes of measurement specified for the agency.
- Enteric fluids or feedings (nasogastric, gastrostomy, jejunostomy):
  - Note the amount in the bag or bottle at the beginning of the shift.
  - Record the type, amount and time when the feeding is completed.
  - For feedings in progress at the end of a shift, measure and record type and amount taken in, and note the amount remaining.
  - Record the time, type and amount of fluid (water or normal saline) used to clear or irrigate the tube that was not withdrawn during the irrigation.
- Parenteral fluids:
  - Record the time, type and amount to be absorbed (TBA) when the bag or bottle is hung or note the amount TBA at the beginning of the shift.
  - Record the time and amount when the bag has infused.
  - Record the time, type and amount of fluid infused with intravenous medications.
  - At the end of the shift, record the time and amount infused and indicate the amount TBA for the next shift.

Measure and Record Output

- Record the time, amount and source of output on the I&O sheet.
- Urine:
  - Measure amount using a graduated container, and record the time and amount following each voiding.
  - For urinary incontinence, estimate the amount or note the amount of clothing or bed linen saturated with urine.
  - For newborn babies or infants, measure output by weighing wet diapers.
  - For indwelling urinary catheters, record the time and amount of urine when the drainage bag is emptied and at the end of the shift. Always empty the drainage bag at the end of the shift, regardless of how full it is. If measuring output hourly, drain the catheter tubing into the collection apparatus before measuring the amount to ensure an accurate measurement.
- Diarrhea, emesis:
  - Measure amounts using a graduated container and record time, type and amount.
  - Estimate amounts that cannot be measured, for example, indicate the area (in cm) of vomitus or liquid stool on clothing or bed linen.
- Drainage tubes (wound drains, chest tubes, nasogastric tubes):
  - At the end of each shift or as frequently as ordered, empty drainage from the collecting container into a measuring device.
  - If the collecting container is graduated, an alternative method is to place a tape on the container and mark the drainage level with the date and time. Determine the amount of drainage by subtracting the previous level from the latest level.
  - Note amount of fluid taken out during tube irrigation if more fluid was withdrawn than was instilled.
- Blood and wound exudate:
  - Describe the amount by measuring the size of the stained area and the thickness of the dressing or by weighing soaked dressings and subtracting the dry weight.
- Perspiration:
  - Describe the amount of clothing or bed linen saturated with sweat.
  - An alternative method is to estimate perspiration as +, ++, +++, or ++++. The value + depicts sweating that is just visible, whereas ++++ depicts extreme sweating.

Total Intake and Output

- At the end of each 8- or 12-h shift, or more frequently if ordered, calculate the total intake and output, and enter these amounts into the appropriate columns of the I&O record.

VITAL SIGNS

Many disturbances in fluid, electrolyte and acid–base balance [illegible] elevated body temperature in a patient who experienced profuse sweating without water replacement may indicate hypernatremia or hypertonic dehydration. Tachycardia is often one of the earliest signs of fluid volume deficit. A full, bounding pulse is commonly associated with fluid volume excess. Deep, rapid respirations may accompany metabolic acidosis as a compensatory mechanism. Blood pressure is a sensitive indicator of hypovolemia. Vital signs are important measures of the occurrence or worsening severity of fluid, electrolyte and acid–base problems and should be monitored carefully.

Physical Assessment

Because many organs and body functions are involved in the maintenance of fluid, electrolyte and acid–base balance, a variety of parameters must be examined. In order to make astute observations, the nurse must have knowledge of the normal characteristics of fluid, electrolyte and acid–base balance, as well as the common defining signs and symptoms of imbalances. The parameters that should be appraised in assessing fluid, electrolyte and acid–base status are outlined here. These have been adapted from Metheney (1996).

SKIN AND TONGUE TURGOR

Skin turgor, which refers to the elasticity of skin, provides an indication of interstitial fluid volume or hydration. It is assessed by pinching a fold of skin on the sternum or forehead, under the clavicle or on the inner aspect of the thigh and then observing how quickly it returns to its normal position. In a well-hydrated person, the skin returns to position immediately. If a fluid volume deficit is present, the pinched skin returns to position slowly and may stay elevated for a few seconds. Skin turgor can vary with age, nutritional state and even complexion and race. It may not be an effective indicator of hydration status in people older than 55 to 60 years because the loss of elasticity associated with aging reduces turgor.

Tongue turgor is an effective indicator of hydration for all age groups, because it does not change with age. The tongue of a hydrated person has one longitudinal furrow. The tongue of a patient with fluid volume deficit will have additional longitudinal furrows and will appear smaller. In a patient with sodium excess, the tongue will look red and swollen.

MOISTURE IN ORAL CAVITY

A dry mouth can be the result of fluid volume deficit or mouth breathing. In fluid volume deficit, all tissues in the oral cavity will be dry. Conversely, if dryness is caused by mouth breathing, the areas where the gums meet the cheek membranes will be moist. Dry, sticky mucous membranes are indicative of hypernatremia.

TEARING AND SALIVATION

Tearing and salivation are reduced in patients with fluid [illegible] may be absent (Metheney, 1996).

APPEARANCE AND TEMPERATURE OF SKIN

The skin takes on a pale appearance and feels cool to the touch in patients with severe fluid volume deficit. This is due to peripheral vasoconstriction that occurs as a compensatory response to hypovolemia. Metabolic acidosis can cause warm, flushed skin due to peripheral vasodilation. Skin temperature is best palpated using the back of the hand or fingers because the skin over these areas is thin, permitting better perception of subtle changes.

FACIAL APPEARANCE

The patient with a severe fluid volume deficit may have a pinched, drawn expression. The eyeballs may appear sunken and feel soft to the touch because the fluid deficit causes decreased intraoccular pressure.

EDEMA

Edema is defined as "an excessive accumulation of interstitial fluid (the body fluid that bathes the cells)" (Metheney, 1996, p. 17). The formation of edema may be localized in one area of the body, such as the swelling in an ankle that sustained trauma, or it may be generalized and spread throughout the body. An accumulation of interstitial fluid predominantly in the lower extremities of ambulatory patients and over the sacral area in bedridden patients is known as *dependent edema*. Edema related to salt retention is described as *pitting* and can be appraised by pressing one's finger into soft tissues over a bony prominence such as the ankle or tibia and then removing it. If pitting edema is present, an indentation will remain (see Figure 23.5).

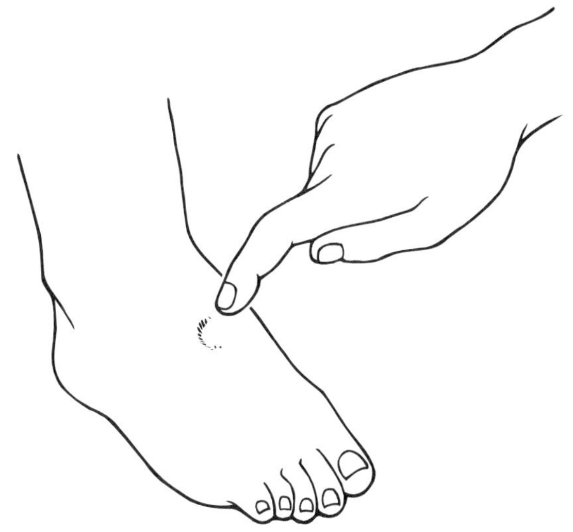

FIGURE 23.5 Pitting edema

Gauging edema by appearance is a subjective measure. Peripheral edema may be described using plus signs to indicate the amount. The value + indicates barely perceptible, ++ and +++ moderate, and ++++ severe edema. A more exact method is to measure the same extremity or body part every day using a metre tape measure. Pitting edema may be described by measuring the degree of pitting (Fuller & Schaller-Ayers, 1994).

NECK AND HAND VEINS

Intravascular fluid volume can be indirectly assessed by observing the filling and emptying of veins in the neck and the hands. Normally, the external jugular veins distend and become visible when a person lies flat in bed or when the head is lower than the heart. The veins should empty easily when the person is brought back to a sitting position. If fluid volume excess is present, the veins may remain distended when the patient's position is changed. In fluid volume deficit, the veins will remain flat even in the supine position, or they will fill slowly.

Normally, the veins on the back of the hand will empty or flatten in three to five minutes when hands are elevated. Likewise, they will fill or expand in three to five minutes when hands are held in a dependent position. Increases or decreases in fluid volume are exhibited by vein-emptying or -filling times that are longer than three to five minutes. A prolonged vein-filling time indicates fluid volume deficit. In fluid volume excess, vein-emptying time is prolonged; the veins will remain distended and clearly visible.

NEUROMUSCULAR IRRITABILITY

Electrolyte changes, in particular changes in levels of calcium, magnesium, potassium and sodium, can cause notable neuromuscular responses. Tests for increased or decreased muscular irritability should be made when imbalances in these electrolytes are suspected.

CHVOSTEK'S SIGN Chvostek's sign is checked by tapping the facial nerve about two centimetres anterior to the earlobe. A positive Chvostek's sign is shown by a unilateral twitching and contraction of the facial muscles—the upper lip, side of the face, nose and eyelid (Figure 23.6A). It is indicative of hypocalcemia and hypomagnesemia.

TROUSSEAU'S SIGN Trousseau's sign can also occur with calcium and magnesium deficits. It is tested by applying a blood pressure cuff on the upper arm and inflating it above systolic pressure for three minutes. A positive response will elicit a carpal spasm (adducted thumb with fingers extended), as shown in Figure 23.6B.

DEEP TENDON REFLEXES Electrolyte and acid–base imbalances can cause hyperactive or diminished reflexes. Deep tendon reflexes often become hyperactive in states of hypocalcemia, hypomagnesemia, hyperkalemia, hypernatremia and alkalosis. Conversely, they are diminished in hypercalcemia, hypermagnesemia, hypokalemia, hyponatremia and acidosis.

OTHER SIGNS

Changes in behaviour, for instance, changes in level of consciousness, restlessness or confusion and varying levels of fatigue, may accompany the signs and symptoms of fluid, electrolyte and acid–base imbalance. Their significance must be considered in the context of the specific imbalances (Metheney, 1996).

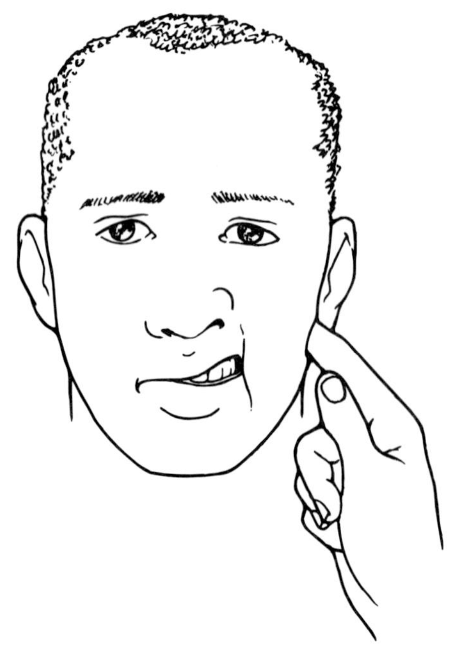

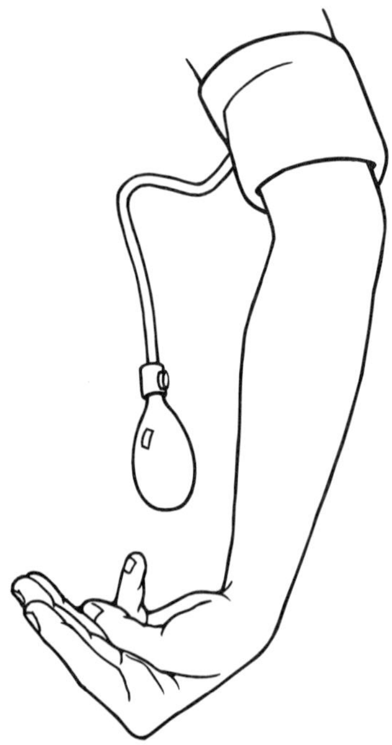

FIGURE 23.6 A. Chvostek's sign. B. Trousseau's sign

TABLE 23.10 Laboratory tests for fluid, electrolyte and acid–base balance

Test	Normal Values	Imbalances Indicated
Serum electrolytes: Measures the concentration of electrolytes in blood serum		
Sodium (Na^+)	135–145 mmol/L (mEq/L)	Hyponatremia and hypernatremia
Potassium (K^+)	3.5–5.0 mmol/L (mEq/L)	Falling trend (0.1–0.2 mmol/day) indicative of a developing deficiency Hypokalemia and hyperkalemia
Calcium (Ca^{2+})	2.15–2.50 mmol/L (mg/dL)	Hypocalcemia and hypercalcemia
Chloride (Cl^-)	97–107 mmol/L (mEq/L)	Hypochloremia and hyperchloremia
Magnesium (Mg^{2+})	0.65–1.25 mmol/L (1.3–2.5 mEq/L)	Hypomagnesemia and hypermagnesemia
Phosphate (PO_4)	0.87–1.45 mmol/L (2.7–4.5 mg/dL)	Hypophosphatemia and hyperphosphatemia
Serum Osmolality: Measures the concentration of dissolved particles (electrolytes, sugar, urea) in the serum	280–300 mOsm/kg H_2O 285–293 mmol/kg H_2O	Elevated levels indicate hemoconcentration, dehydration and hypernatremia Decreased levels indicate hemodilution, overhydration and hyponatremia
Hematocrit (Hct): Measures the red blood cell mass in a volume of whole blood	M 0.42–0.52 (42%–52%) F 0.35–0.47 (35%–47%)	Elevated levels indicate hypovolemia and dehydration
Urine Specific Gravity: Measures the kidney's ability to concentrate urine	1.003–1.035	Low values indicate fluid excess and overhydration. High values indicate fluid deficit and dehydration.
Arterial Blood Gases: Give information on acid–base status and the adequacy of ventilation and oxygen-carbon dioxide exchange	pH: 7.35–7.45 pO_2: >80–100 mm Hg pCO_2: 35–45 mm Hg Bicarbonate: 22–26 mmol/L (mEq/L) Base excess: −3.0–+3.0 mmol/L	A pH <7.35 indicates acidosis; >7.45 alkalosis Elevated pCO_2 indicates respiratory acidosis; decreased pCO_2 indicates respiratory alkalosis Decreased bicarbonate and base excess indicate metabolic acidosis; elevated values indicate metabolic alkalosis

SOURCES: Chernecky & Berger, 1997; Metheney, 1996.

Diagnostic Tests

There is a large number of diagnostic tests for fluid, electrolyte and acid–base disturbances. You will learn about many of them in the more advanced levels of your program. In this section, we will focus on the common laboratory tests performed on blood and urine specimens. These are outlined in Table 23.10.

Diagnosing Fluid, Electrolyte and Acid–Base Balance Problems

Fluid and electrolyte problems that are amenable to nursing therapy are related to deficits or excesses in fluid volume. Fluid volume deficit occurs in situations where oral intake is insufficient or large amounts of fluids are lost from the body. People who feel too ill to eat, who are nauseated, tired, weak or in pain or those who are fasting may experience, or be at risk for, fluid volume deficits as a result of insufficient intake. Similarly, individuals experiencing vomiting, diarrhea, excessive perspiration, gastric suction and wound drainage may develop fluid deficits from abnormal losses. Defining characteristics of fluid volume deficit might include insufficient oral fluid intake, less fluid intake than output, thirst, dry skin with decreased turgor and a decreased volume of concentrated urine.

Problems of fluid volume excess may occur when there is excessive intake of sodium or water, high salt intake, low protein intake or excessive intravenous fluids. Defining characteristics may include peripheral and sacral edema, taut shiny skin, greater intake than output and weight gain. Many problems associated with fluid volume excess, however, are not within the realm of independent nursing intervention and should be viewed as collaborative problems. These might include pulmonary edema, ascites (accumulation of fluid within the abdominal cavity) or massive generalized edema. Electrolyte and acid–base problems should also be regarded as collaborative problems because physicians' orders are necessary for initiation of treatment measures; and many aspects of care, such as initiation and maintenance of intravenous therapy, are directed by agency policy.

Common examples of nursing diagnoses and collaborative problems for fluid, electrolyte and acid–base problems as taken from the list of NANDA diagnoses include:

- *Fluid Volume Deficit related to vomiting, diarrhea and decreased intake.*
- *Risk for Fluid Volume Deficit related to nausea and poor fluid intake.*
- *Fluid Volume Excess related to high salt intake.*
- *PC: electrolyte imbalance.*
- *PC: acidosis (metabolic, respiratory).*
- *PC: alkalosis(metabolic, respiratory).* (Carpenito, 1997)

Planning Fluid, Electrolyte and Acid–Base Balance Interventions

Once diagnosis is complete, the nurse formulates a plan for care. Planning must occur in consultation with the patient, taking into account individual and family beliefs, preferences, lifestyle practices and socioeconomic considerations. In addition to therapeutic interventions for the particular problems, emphasis should be placed on self-care and strategies that enable patients to achieve optimum fluid, electrolyte and acid–base balance in their daily lives.

Goals or expected outcomes direct the selection of nursing interventions. Common expected outcomes related to fluid, electrolyte and acid–base balance might be as follows:

- Patient will maintain a balanced fluid intake and output, averaging 2500 mL/day for 2 days.
- Patient will show signs of hydration.
- Patient will verbalize how to maintain increased fluid intake during strenuous exercise.
- Patient will exhibit arterial blood gases within normal range.

Implementing Fluid, Electrolyte and Acid–Base Balance Interventions

Health-Promoting Strategies

The human body possesses a very effective system for maintaining and regulating fluid, electrolyte and acid–base balance. An adequate fluid intake and a well-balanced diet containing the essential minerals are necessary to maintain optimal fluid, electrolyte and acid–base balance on a day-to-day basis. Difficulties arise when water intake is not adequate or when water losses greatly exceed intake, as can happen during strenuous exercise or manual labour.

Deficiencies or excesses in the intake of minerals may also cause problems. Nurses can help individuals and families maintain optimum fluid, electrolyte and acid–base balance in three basic ways. First, they can encourage and assist individuals and families in exploring lifestyle factors, values and health practices that may affect their fluid, electrolyte and acid–base needs. Second, nurses can provide information that will enable people to decide whether or not they need to change their usual patterns and practices. Third, nurses can provide teaching about healthy living practices aimed at promoting optimum fluid, electrolyte and acid–base balance.

Health-Protecting Strategies

Disturbances in fluid, electrolyte and acid–base balance can have serious effects on body functioning. The nurse must be particularly alert in noting early indications of imbalance. These should be reported promptly so that appropriate therapy can be instituted before the condition becomes too advanced. The consequences of marked imbalances of fluids and the major electrolytes in the body have been documented throughout this chapter. It should be stressed, therefore, that all measures to maintain and restore fluid, electrolyte and acid–base balance are nursing priorities.

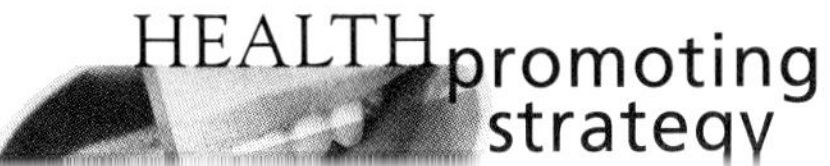

Promoting Healthy Fluid, Electrolyte and

- Drink about two litres of fluid daily
- Eat a well-balanced diet from all four food groups
- Minimize consumption of salt, sugar, caffeine and alcohol
- Keep body weight within normal limits
- Maintain a regular exercise program
- Note early signs of dehydration:
  - Thirst, dry mouth, dry skin, decreased urine output
- Note early signs of fluid retention:
  - Puffy fingers, ankle edema, sharp weight gain
- When undertaking strenuous activity:
  - Wear minimal clothing. Clothes worn should be loose and porous to permit circulation of air and evaporation of heat.
  - Drink fluids frequently. Consume about 240 mL every 25 minutes. Pour water over head and chest to cool down.
- Replenish lost electrolytes. Add extra salt to meals except if high blood pressure is a problem; eat foods high in potassium, such as bananas, dried fruits (figs, peaches) and oranges.
- In hot climates, work or exercise in the morning or evening, if possible, to avoid the heat of the day. Stay in the shade, if possible, to avoid the sun's radiation and wear white clothing to reflect the radiant heat.
- Hyperhydrate if planning to exercise or work in the heat. To do this, drink half to one litre of fluid within an hour of commencing the activity.
- Note signs of heat exhaustion: fatigue, weakness, nausea, cramps and headache. If these should occur, stop exercising, rest in a cool place and drink cool fluids.
- In cold climates, cover head, hands and wrists. Wear several layers of clothing with a windbreaker on the outside. Heat must be allowed to dissipate without getting clothes wet.
- Drink commercial electrolyte products.

Patients with elevated temperatures are especially vulnerable to disturbances in fluid and electrolyte balance. In fever states between 38.3°–39.4° C, an adult's fluid need increases by 500 mL over the basic 24-hour requirement. When body temperatures exceed 39.4° C, an adult requires an additional litre of fluid.

Health-Restoring Strategies

Whenever a disturbance in fluid, electrolyte and acid–base balance occurs, steps must be taken to restore homeostasis. Since the principal sources of fluids and electrolytes are the foods and fluids consumed, adjustments in diet or fluid intake or both may be sufficient to rectify a mild disturbance. In the case of deficiencies of specific electrolytes, supplements may be given in the form of medications. For example, calcium supplements may be ordered for older individuals because they absorb calcium poorly and ingest less in their diets. Often, however, fluid loss is too extensive and the accompanying loss of electrolytes too great to be corrected by oral intake alone; or this method of replacement may be contraindicated. Fluids and electrolytes may then be administered by other routes, namely intravenous infusion, blood transfusion, enteral tube feeding or total parenteral nutrition. The physician orders the route and the type of solutions to be administered based on knowledge of the patient's condition and the particular factors causing the imbalance. Enteral tube feedings and total parenteral nutrition are discussed in Chapter 20.

ORAL FLUID AND ELECTROLYTE THERAPY

Of primary importance in the care of the patient with fluid and electrolyte problems is the maintenance of a therapeutic fluid intake. In many instances the physician orders the exact amount of oral fluid for the patient. Sometimes, however, it is a nursing function to judge the oral needs and prescribe fluid intake. For example, the nurse may determine that a patient with a fever or an infection requires larger amounts of fluid per day.

Generally speaking, patients who are dehydrated or who have lost excessive amounts of fluid should be encouraged to take in extra fluids, unless contraindicated by other conditions. If patients are nauseated or vomiting, for example, it is not reasonable to expect that they will tolerate oral fluids. Patients with kidney or heart conditions may require restriction of their fluid intake. The nurse should be aware of the physician's objectives in medical therapy and never push or force fluids beyond the limit prescribed.

In addition, electrolyte intake may be restricted; for example, the physician might order a salt-free or low-salt diet for the patient. The usual purpose here is to restrict the oral intake of sodium. It is frequently the nurse's responsibility to help patients understand the necessity for the restriction and help them plan meals accordingly. Most people are able to assume responsibility for restricting their diets. Nevertheless, in hospitals it is not unknown for a "helpful" roommate to lend his or her salt to a person on a restricted diet.

INTRAVENOUS THERAPY

Intravenous therapy is the infusion of fluids directly into a vein. It is indicated for patients who cannot ingest fluids or medications orally. Intravenous fluids are delivered into peripheral and central veins. *Peripheral veins* are those found in the hands, arms and feet (scalp veins may be used in infants); these can be accessed by a skilled nurse. Peripheral intravenous access is commonly used for short-term or intermittent therapy, and is common in the hospital and home setting.

Some intravenous therapies are unsuitable for peripheral veins. For example, medications that are irritating or hyperosmotic require the greater blood flow and faster dilution provided by *central veins*. If a patient is medically unstable, or there is a medical emergency, central venous administration is the preferred route. When a patient requires prolonged treatment—for example, total parenteral nutrition (TPN) or hemodialysis—then central access is essential. Catheters for central venous therapy are inserted by the physician with assistance from the nurse.

The decision to administer intravenous fluids rests with the physician. The route of administration, the type and amount of solution, the rate of flow and the duration of infusion is ordered by the doctor according to the patient's age, condition and need for fluid, electrolytes and nutrients. Although nurses may not be required to insert all types of intravenous lines, they are responsible for preparing, maintaining and discontinuing the infusions as well as teaching patients and their families about intravenous therapy and relevant aspects of self-care. Nurses are also responsible for assisting physicians with the insertion of central venous lines.

Types of Intravenous Solutions

The most common intravenous solutions contain sterile water with added nutrients and electrolytes in varying combinations to meet a variety of patient conditions. They are used to supply fluids and calories and to restore electrolyte balance.

Intravenous solutions are classified according to their tonicity or osmotic pressure equivalents to concentrations within cells. A solution that has approximately the same osmolarity as blood plasma is called **isotonic**. One with a lower osmolarity than blood plasma is called **hypotonic** and one with a higher osmolarity is called **hypertonic**. Isotonic solutions produce no change in the osmotic pressure of plasma. They increase circulating fluid volume without altering the interstitial and intracellular compartments. Iostonic solutions are infused to treat hypotension caused by hypovolemia. Hypotonic solutions lower serum osmolarity and cause water to move out of the blood vessels into the interstitial spaces and the cells; they are administered to correct cellular dehydration. When hypertonic solutions are administered, serum osmolarity increases. Fluid is pulled from the cells and interstitial spaces into the blood vessels. Hypertonic solutions are commonly used in postoperative patients to maintain circulating fluid volume and prevent edema (Phillips, 1997).

TABLE 23.11 Common intravenous solutions

Type	*Composition*	*Purpose*
Nutrient Solutions		
Dextrose in water D5W (isotonic) D10W (hypertonic)	Water with carbohydrate	Provides water and calories
Dextrose and saline D5W/0.9 NaCl (hypertonic) D5W/0.45 NaCl (hypertonic)	Water with carbohydrate and NaCl	Provides calories and electrolytes
Electrolyte Solutions		
Saline solution 0.45 NaCl (hypotonic) 0.9 NaCl (isotonic)	NaCl and water	Provides salt and water
Multiple electrolyte solutions Ringer's solution (hypertonic) Lactated Ringer's (RL)(isotonic)	Varying electrolytes: Na, K, Ca, Cl	Maintenance therapy; correct electrolyte and acid–base imbalances
Electrolyte solutions with dextrose D5W/RL (hypertonic)	Electrolytes and dextrose	Provides electrolytes and calories
Blood Volume Expanders		
Serum albumin	Blood components, albumin	Restores normal blood volume
Dextran	Large carbohydrate molecules in water	Temporarily increases blood volume; used to treat shock

Peripheral Intravenous Therapy

When intravenous therapy is ordered, nurses must com- [illegible] doctor's order, prepare the patient, collect and assemble the equipment and solution, perform the **venipuncture** (insert the needle or catheter) and establish the infusion. In some agencies, registered nurses perform venipuncture; in others this is done by a specialized team of nurses, called the IV team. If your agency has an IV team, then the nurse is responsible for calling the team, informing the patient and assembling the equipment for an IV insertion.

PREPARING THE PATIENT It is important to explain the procedure and help the patient relax. Tension and anxiety can cause vasoconstriction, which makes insertion of the catheter or needle more difficult and uncomfortable for the patient. Patients will also feel more relaxed when the nurse is organized. Begin your teaching by asking patients if they have had an IV before. Allow them time to express previous experiences. Try to dispel any misconceptions or apprehensions by providing clear explanations.

Information to give might include why the patient needs intravenous therapy, how the venipuncture will be performed, sensations that might be felt, how long the infusion will last, how the patient can help maintain the infusion, when to call the nurse and any limits the intravenous may put on activity. Explain that slight transient pain may be felt during the insertion of the needle [illegible] vice is in place. Initially, the IV fluid can feel cool but this sensation too subsides in a few minutes. Emphasize that any discomfort or change in the rate of flow should be reported to the nurse. Reassurance that showering and bathing are usually possible is comforting to many patients. If available and if time permits, pamphlets, demonstrations and audiovisual aids may be used to enhance the patient's understanding and comfort. Play therapy is frequently used with children. Encourage patients to ask questions and provide clarification as necessary.

One last detail in preparing the patient for intravenous therapy is to ensure that clothing can be removed over the IV apparatus. Some agencies have special hospital gowns with openings at the shoulder for this purpose.

ASSEMBLING EQUIPMENT The basic equipment for intravenous infusion includes a bag or bottle containing the solution, an intravenous administration set (tubing), a label for the tubing and an IV pole.

Intravenous bags and bottles. Intravenous containers are either plastic bags or glass bottles that are vacuum-sealed (see Figure 23.7). Currently, most solutions come in plastic

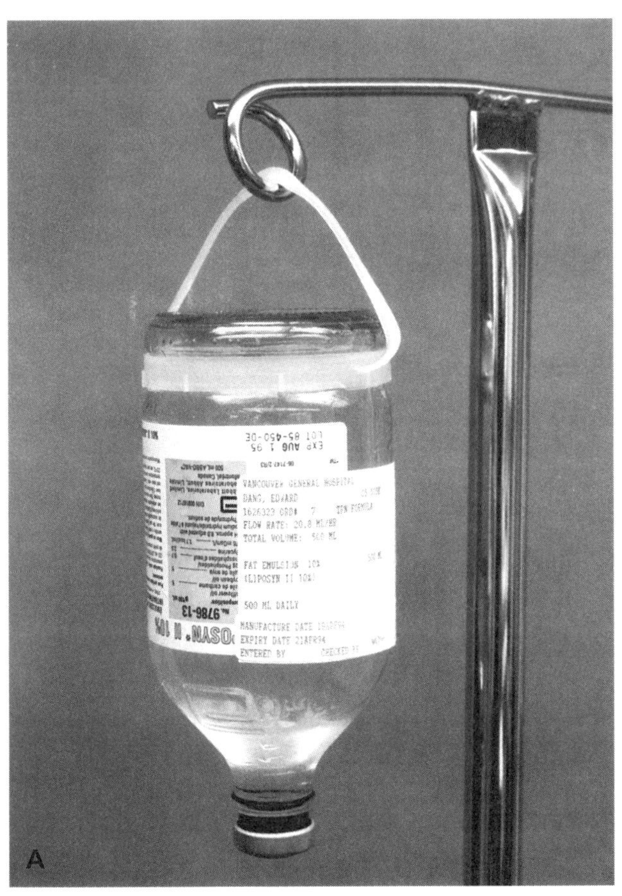

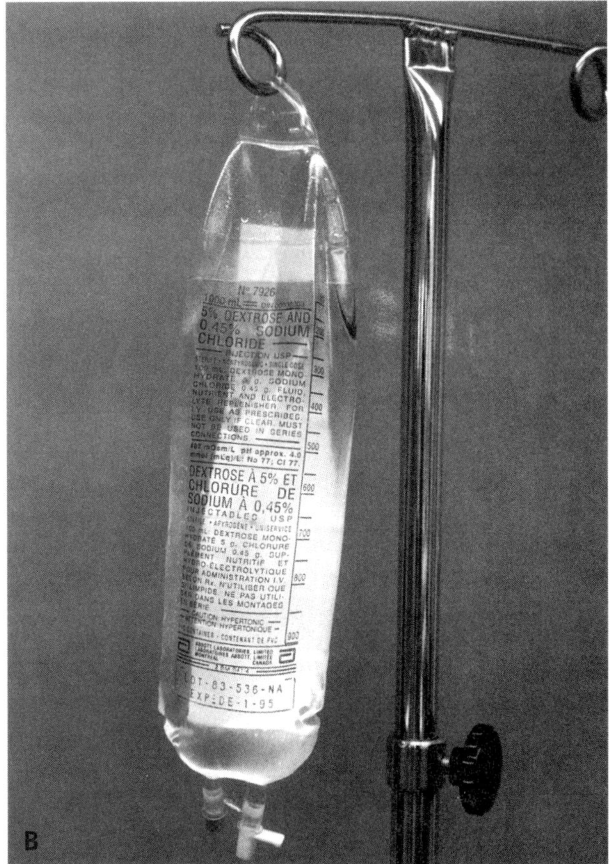

FIGURE 23.7 IV solution containers. A. Glass bottle. B. Plastic bag

bags; however, glass bottles are sometimes necessary for solutions containing substances that are incompatible with plastic, for example, lipid emulsions. Plastic bags are advantageous because they do not require an air vent to enable the flow of solution into the vein. Aided by the pull of gravity and atmospheric pressure, plastic bags simply collapse as solution flows out. Because of their ability to collapse, plastic bags provide a closed system that reduces the possibility of contamination by microorganisms.

Glass bottles, on the other hand, cannot collapse because they are rigid. Therefore, an air vent is needed to draw air into the bottle as fluid flows out. This mechanism is necessary to prevent the creation of a vacuum within the container, which would stop the flow of fluid. The air vent can be a plastic tube placed in the bottle or it can be an attachment on the IV administration set. Because of the air vent, glass containers are open to room air and are thus more likely to become contaminated, posing an increased risk for infection. At the neck end of both plastic and glass containers there is a port or a rubber stopper into which the IV administration set is inserted. Plastic bags also have a resealable port for instilling medication into the bag. Solutions for infusion are commonly supplied in 500- or 1000-mL containers for the adult client.

Intravenous administration set. The IV administration set is a closed system of connective tubing that delivers the solution from the container to the needle or catheter situated in the patient's vein. Figure 23.8 shows the parts of the IV administration set. Commonly referred to as the IV line, the administration set consists of an insertion spike, a drip chamber, tubing, a movable roller or screw clamp, one or more Y-type injection ports, an antireflux or backcheck valve and a needle adapter. Protective caps over the insertion spike and the needle adapter ensure sterility before use.

The *insertion spike* is a sharply pointed plastic cannula that is pushed into the port of the solution container. Below the insertion spike is an enlarged, clear plastic tube called the *drip chamber*. Fluid passes through the spike to the drip chamber through a drip tube in the form of drops. Administration sets are calibrated to deliver a specified number of drops per millilitre of solution. This is called the *drop factor*. The drop factor, indicated as drops per millilitre, is indicated on the package. The drip chamber allows one to observe the drops of solution leaving the container and entering the tubing. The rate of infusion over time can be established by counting the number of drops per minute.

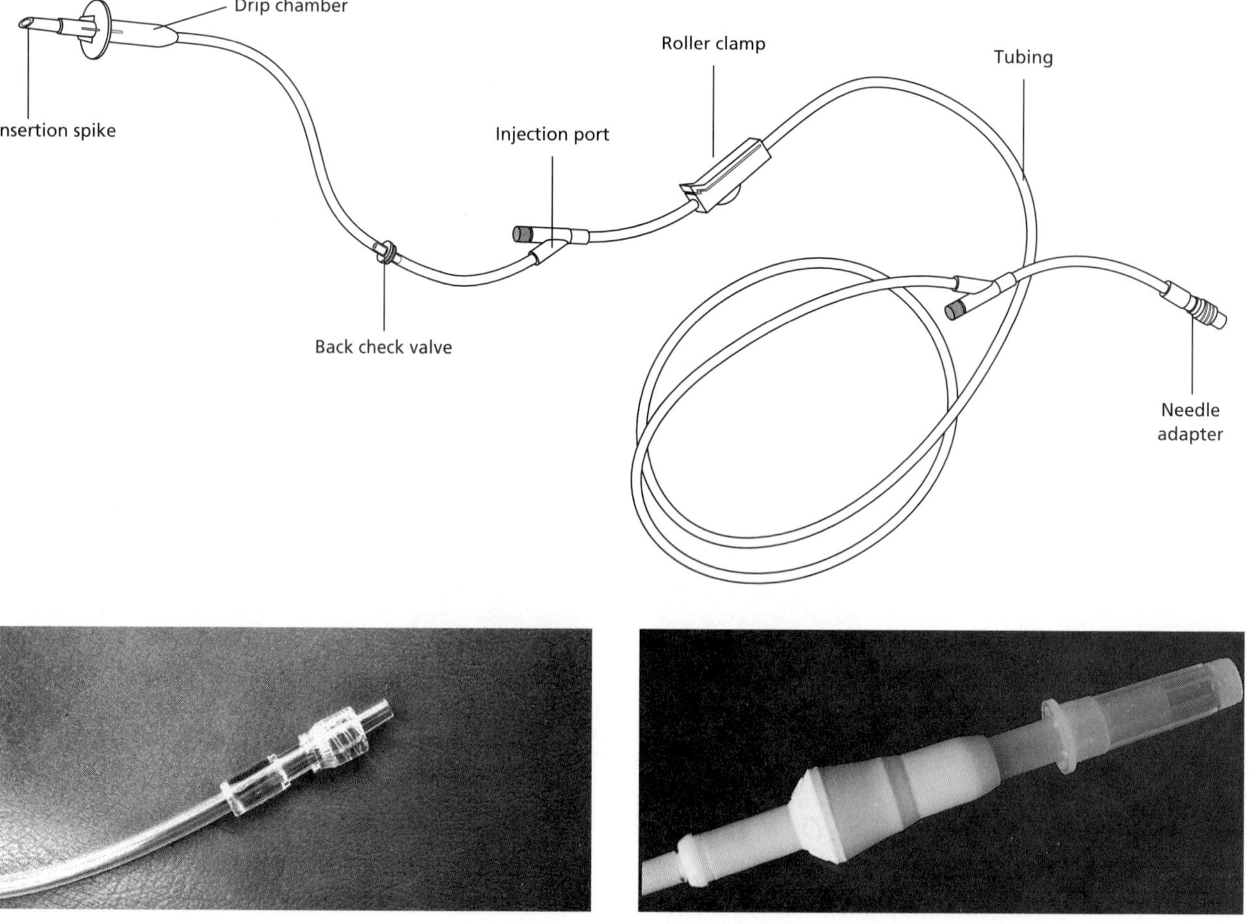

FIGURE 23.8 Parts of the IV administration set: A. Luer lock; B. Flash ball

Situated on the tubing is the *roller clamp*, which is a movable apparatus used to control the rate at which the fluid flows to the patient. [illegible] ous or intermittent infusion of a secondary solution. Many sets also contain *backcheck valves*, which prevent the flow of solution from a secondary line into the main solution. At the end of the tubing is the *needle adapter*, a plastic connector to which the needle or cannula is connected. Many adapters contain a lock apparatus, known as a *Luer lock*, which secures the tubing to the needle or cannula with a twisting motion. Others are slip adapters, which simply fit into the needle or cannula hub by friction. Some administration sets have a resealable injection port, called a *flashball*, between the tubing and the needle adapter. However, this type of tubing is now used less frequently.

There are a number of variations to the basic IV administration set. In most situations that require fluid maintenance or replacement in adult patients, a regular administration set is used. The regular set, called the *macrodrop*, can deliver large quantities of solution at rapid rates because the drops contain a larger volume of solution. On the other hand, where smaller volumes of solution are to be infused, *microdrop* sets are preferred.

Sometimes, particularly when medications are being administered, two solutions may be put up at the same time. This requires a primary administration set with a secondary injection port or a piggyback port and a *secondary set* that connects the second solution to the primary line (this will be discussed in Chapter 34). In some cases, when administering total parenteral nutrition or blood products, for instance, an administration set with a *filter* is required. Other times, such as in the need to deliver very small, precise amounts of fluid to infants, a *volume container device* is attached to the administration set.

In order to assemble the correct administration set, the nurse must know the type of solution that has been ordered, the rate of flow and the type of container that will be used. Many of the variations are built into basic administration sets or they are available as separate devices that can be added as necessary. It is important to note at this point that IV administration sets and related devices vary according to the different manufacturers. To ensure correct use of equipment, nurses should read and follow the manufacturer's instructions carefully. The most common types of IV administration sets and devices are illustrated in Figure 23.9.

Needleless systems. Nurses working with intravenous equipment are at risk for needlestick (sharps) injuries. Needles, including those used for injecting solution into IV tubing, and the IV tubing spike are examples of sharps used in IV therapy. Needlestick injuries have the potential to transmit blood-borne pathogens. Contaminated, as well as clean, needlestick injuries expose health professionals to infection. Nurses are accountable for the safe handling of IV equipment to prevent injury to themselves and other health team members. Some agencies use needleless intravenous devices to protect health care employees. Shields are also [illegible] from splash injuries and skin from the absorption of cytotoxic medications. Examples of needleless devices are illustrated in Figure 23.10.

IV pole. An adjustable rod or pole, called the IV pole, is necessary to hold the IV container above the level of the patient. In order for solution to flow from the container into the patient's vein, the force of gravity is required to overcome venous pressure. This is accomplished by hanging the container on the pole and adjusting the height to approximately one metre above the cannula insertion site. Flow rates can be adjusted by raising or lowering the IV pole. The more distance between the container and the patient, the greater the force of gravity; thus, the faster the solution flows into the vein. IV poles can be attached to the bed or they can hang from the ceiling. They are also mounted on wheels so that patients can get out of bed and ambulate freely (see Procedure 23.1).

PERFORMING THE PERIPHERAL VENIPUNCTURE AND ESTABLISHING THE INFUSION The process of inserting a needle or a catheter into a vein is called venipuncture. This procedure is done to establish intravenous infusion of fluids, to administer medications and to obtain venous blood samples. Agencies have their own guidelines as to who will be responsible for performing venipunctures. In some agencies this is done by registered nurses on the ward after they have successfully completed an in-service education program. In others this task is left to specialized nurses on the IV team. Whether or not you will learn the skill of venipuncture as a student will depend on your school's curriculum. Not all schools regard venipuncture as a skill required for graduation.

While a relatively simple procedure, venipuncture involves a number of tasks that require proper knowledge, skill and dexterity for safe performance. These tasks include selecting an appropriate venipuncture device (needle or catheter) and site for insertion, inserting the device into the patient and establishing the infusion. The procedure, and how it is performed, has great impact on the patient.

Selecting a venipuncture device. Several factors have to be considered in selecting a venipuncture device. The duration and purpose of intravenous therapy; the type of solution; the patient's age, condition of veins and activity level will influence the type of device to be used. A variety of venipuncture devices are available for intravenous therapy. Two of the most common are the over-the-needle catheter and the wing-tipped (butterfly) needle (Phillips, 1997) (see Figure 23.11).

The over-the-needle catheter consists of a plastic tube mounted over a needle, the bevel of which protrudes out of the end of the catheter. The needle functions to stabilize the catheter during insertion and to pierce the skin and vein wall; it is withdrawn once the catheter is inside the

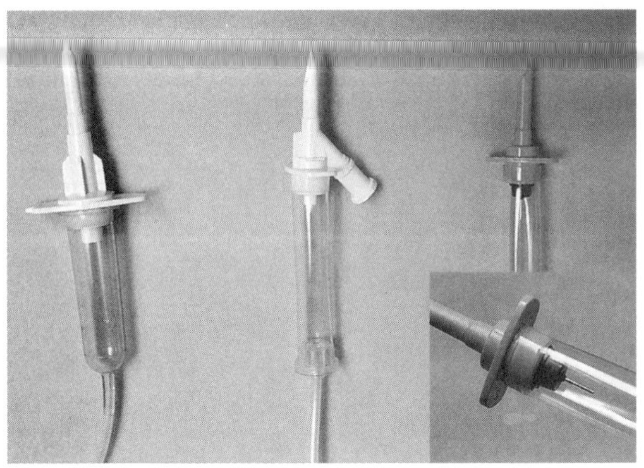

Macrodrop Set

Definition: Refers to the size or diameter of the drip tube that forms the drops entering the drip chamber. The macrodrop delivers 10, 12, 15 or 20 drops per millilitre of solution.

Uses: To deliver large quantities of solution or when rapid infusion is necessary.

Microdrop Set

Definition: The microdrop delivers 50 to 60 drops per millilitre of solution.

Uses: To deliver small quantities of solution or when a very slow, precise rate of infusion is necessary, for example, in infants and small children, or in older patients to prevent circulatory overload.

Nonvented Set

Definition: Refers to tubing without an air vent.

Uses: With plastic bags or vented bottles.

Vented Set

Definition: Refers to tubing that contains an air vent, allowing air to replace solution as it flows out of the bottle. Vented sets usually have filters to remove contaminants from the air before it enters the bottle.

Uses: With nonvented bottles, for example, for albumin and fat emulsions.

In-Line Filter

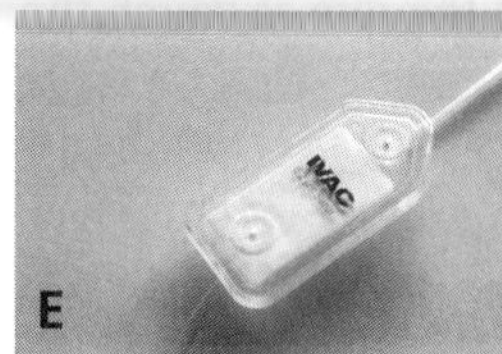

Definition: A filter within the IV line that removes particles and microbes from the solution, helping to decrease the risk of contamination and complications such as infusion phlebitis.

Uses: For total parenteral nutrition for blood products; when administering solutions to immunodeficient patients; or for administering solutions containing several additives.

Add-On Filter (End-Line Filter)

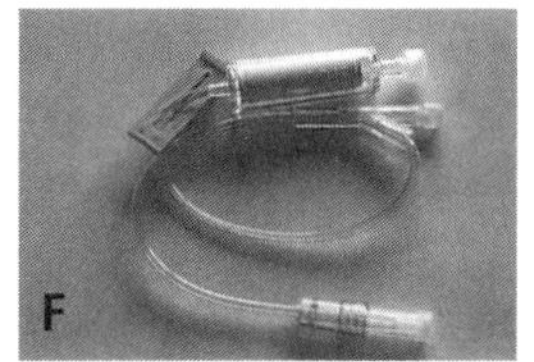

Definition: A filter added on to the tubing serving the same purposes as an in-line filter.

Uses: For total parenteral nutrition and infusion of plasma, blood and blood products.

Volume-Control Container

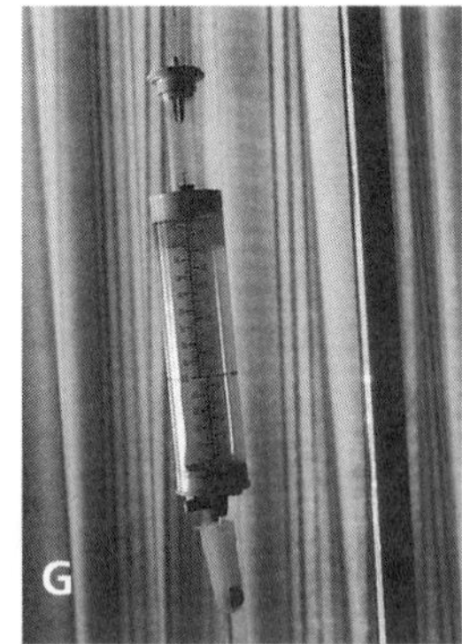

Definition: Small calibrated container situated between the solution container and the drip chamber. Examples: Soluset® and Buretrol®.

Uses: To deliver small volumes of fluids or medications over extended periods. Often used in pediatrics and critical care areas.

Secondary Set

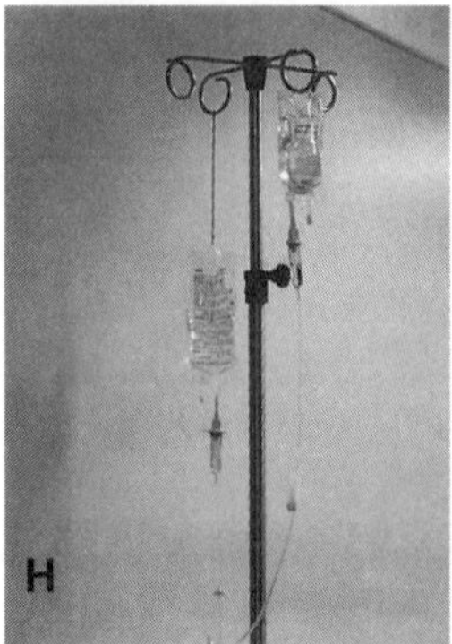

Definition: Tubing that connects a secondary solution to the primary line. This can be a tandem set-up as pictured here, or a piggyback set-up as described in Chapter 34.

Uses: For intermittent or simultaneous infusion of medications with the primary solution.

FIGURE 23.9 Types of administration sets and devices

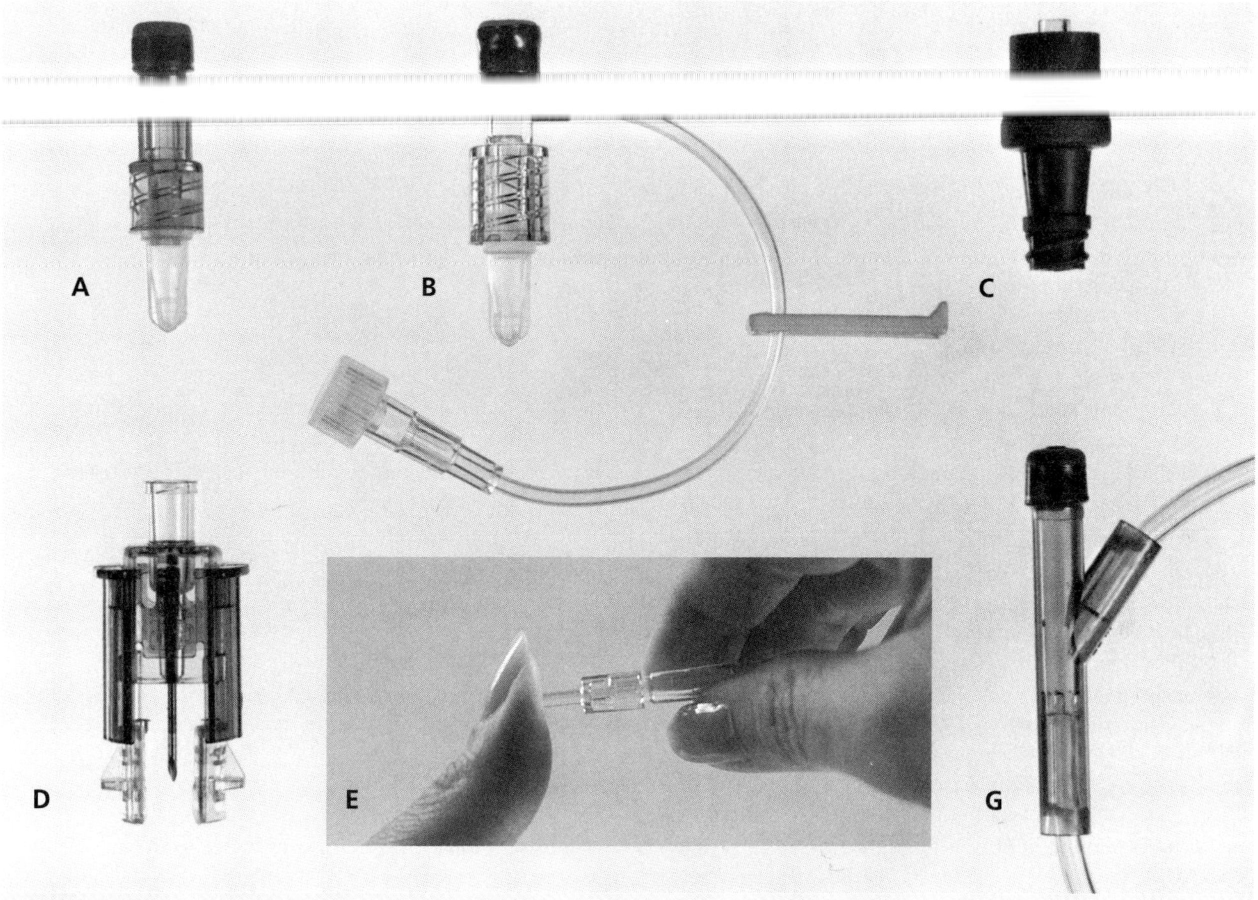

FIGURE 23.10 Needleless intravenous devices. A, B and G are prepierced, self-sealing ports. The blunt cannula in E is inserted into the prepierced port. Use of this system replaces the sharp needle and avoids the risk of injury. C is an adapter that is attached to IV tubing. Secondary IV tubing and syringes can be attached directly to this adapter without a needle. D is a connector used to attach a secondary IV set to a primary line. This adapter shields against injury by having the needle permanently retracted.

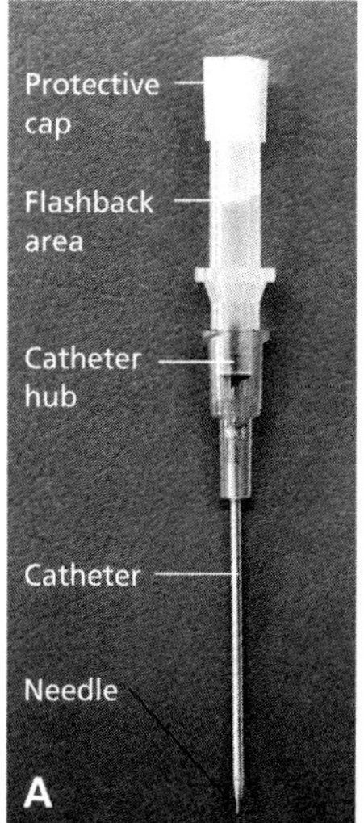

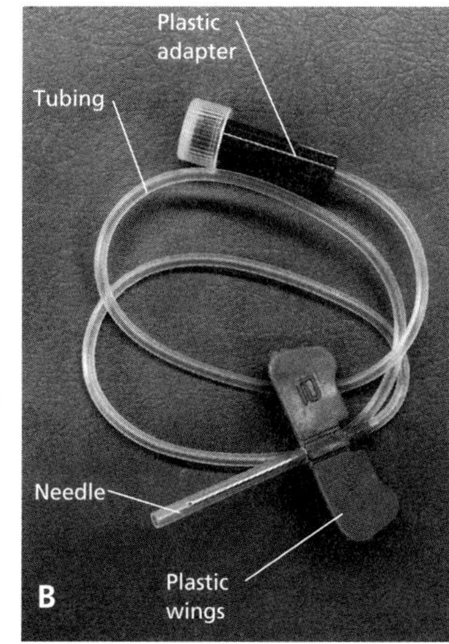

FIGURE 23.11 Common venipuncture devices
A. Over-the-needle catheter. B. Wing-tipped needle

vein. This type of catheter is used for administering all solutions, including blood. It is also used in emergency situations because large volumes of solution can be administered quickly. Since the catheter is a flexible tube, it is less likely to puncture the vein, thus reducing the risk of infiltration. Also, once in place, the catheter is more comfortable and permits the patient to move. One disadvantage is that over-the-needle catheters are more difficult to insert.

The butterfly needle consists of a thin-walled stainless steel stem with plastic flaps attached to the shaft. The flaps are used to hold the needle during insertion. They are flattened and taped to the skin once the needle is inside the vein. The butterfly needle may be chosen for intravenous therapy lasting less than 24 hours and for therapy of any duration in infants, children, older adults or patients with fragile veins. The current design of small, over-the-needle catheters, however, has resulted in a decrease in the use of butterfly needles. As well, butterfly needles can easily dislodge, causing fluid infiltration into tissues.

PROCEDURE 23.1

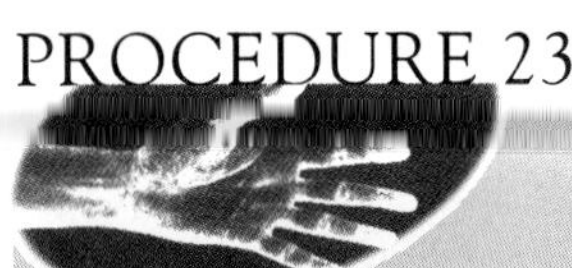

Preparing the Intravenous Infusion

Action	*Rationale*
A. Preparing the Solution Bag	
1. Check physician's order for type of solution and rate of flow.	Ensures accurate delivery and reduces risk of error.
2. Gather equipment: • correct solution • administration set • label for the tubing • IV pole.	Safe, effective infusion depends on correct solution and proper equipment.
3. Wash hands thoroughly and maintain sterile technique throughout the procedure.	Aseptic technique is required to prevent contamination which can lead to local or systemic infection.
4. Inspect the bag for leaks, cracks or tears; the solution for expiry date, clarity and foreign particles; and the tubing for cracks, holes or missing clamps.	Ensures sterility and freshness of solution and sterility of the tubing.
5. Place a bag on a flat surface or hang it on an IV pole; place a bottle upright on a stable surface.	Facilitates ease of inserting spike.
6. Slide the roller clamp below the drip chamber and close the clamp.	Facilitates easy access of clamp and prevents escape of fluid through the tubing.
7. **Bag:** Remove the protective cover from the port by pulling downward, uncap the tubing spike and, while holding the port with one hand, insert the spike with the other hand, using a firm twisting motion. Maintain the sterility of the spike at all times.	Pulling downward quickly removes the cover and maintains sterility of the port. A twisting motion is needed to puncture the seal on the bag.
Nonvented Bottle: Remove the metal cap and inner disk, uncap the spike and push it straight down through the centre of the rubber stopper .	Twisting or angling the spike during insertion can cause pieces of the rubber stopper to break off and fall into the solution.

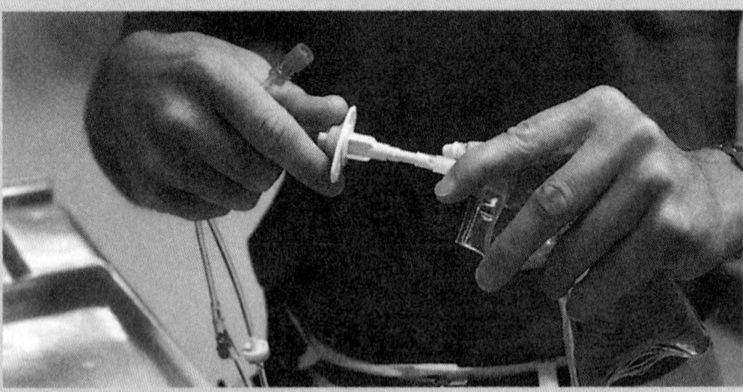

Action	*Rationale*
8. Hang the bag on an IV pole (if not already done) and squeeze the flexible drip chamber until it is half full. Note: Firm drip chambers will fill automatically.	Squeezing the drip chamber pushes air into the bag, causing fluid to flow into the chamber. It also prevents air from moving downward into the tubing. When the chamber is partially filled, drops can be easily seen and counted.

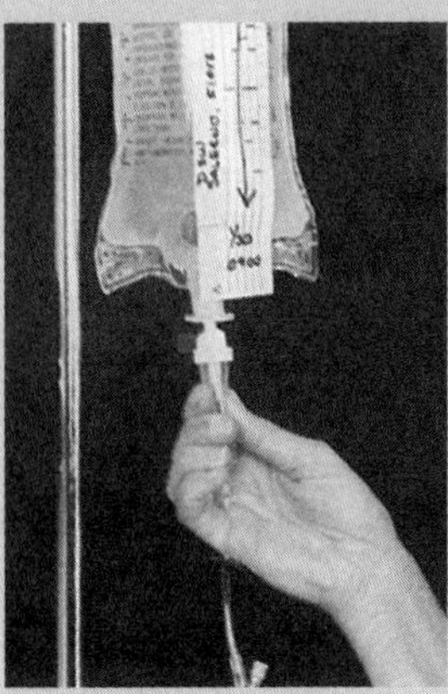

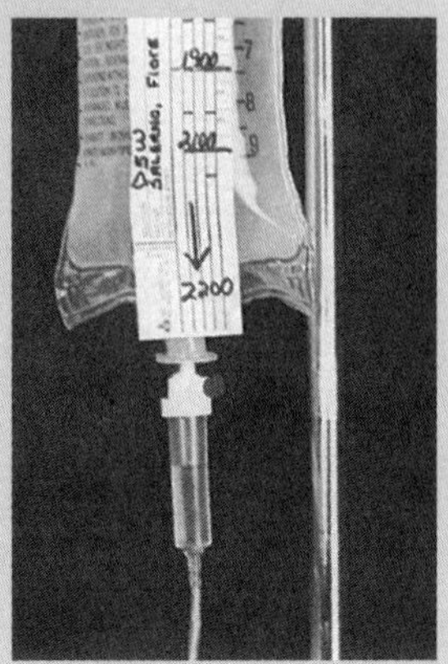

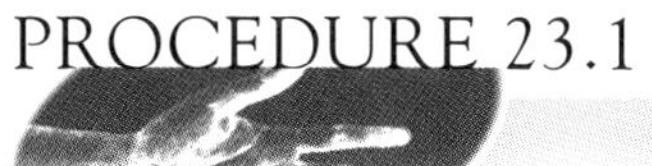

PROCEDURE 23.1 *continued*

Action	*Rationale*
B. Priming the Intravenous Tubing	
1. Hold the capped needle adapter end of the tubing over a sink or clean container. Maintain sterility at all times.	Catches solution. Most protective coverings over the needle adapter permit the flow of solution.
2. Partially open the roller clamp and allow solution to flow slowly through the entire tubing. Invert injection ports and backcheck valve before the solution flows through them.	Forces air out of the tubing, fills ports and backcheck valves with solution and prevents air bubbles. A large collection of air can act as an embolus in the patient's blood stream.
3. Remove air bubbles from the tubing by holding the tubing vertically while lightly tapping the area with fingers. 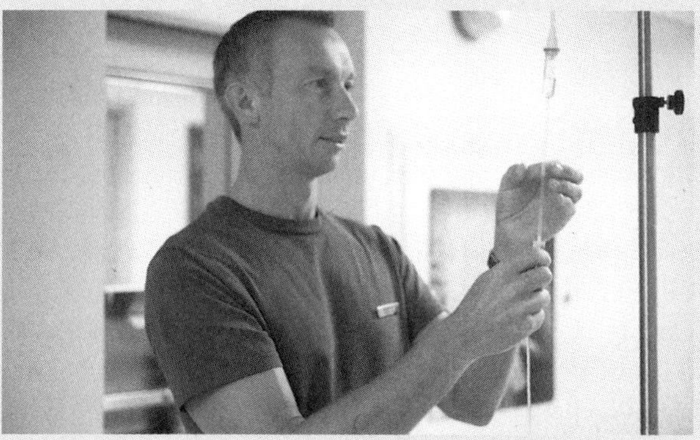	Bubbles will rise.
4. Close the roller clamp.	Prevents contamination of tubing.
5. Loop the tubing over the IV pole or attach it to the roller clamp.	
6. Label the bag and the tubing as required by agency policy.	Labelling the tubing with date and time permits regular replacement according to agency policy.

Catheters and needles vary in length and in the size or diameter of the lumen (the gauge). Lengths vary from 1.5–3 cm; lumen sizes range from 16 to 27 gauge. The gauge number relates inversely to the size of the lumen, so that the smaller the number, the larger the diameter of the lumen. It is generally recommended that the shortest length and the smallest gauge possible of a device used for infusion. Smaller devices cause less trauma to veins and more blood flow around their tips, which results in less risk of clotting.

Choosing the infusion site. The selection of an infusion site is based on a consideration of the duration, type of solution to be infused, patient's age, hand dominance, preference, comfort and need for mobility. It is also important to consider the condition, size and location of the vein. In adults, the superficial veins of the arm or hand can be used for most IV fluids. The most common sites are the basilic or cephalic veins in the arm and the metacarpal or dorsal networks in the hand (see Figure 23.12). The most distal veins in the forearm or hand should be used first. This keeps the more proximal sites (closer to the midline) in good condition for future use. If a vein has been traumatized, sites below the trauma cannot be used until the vein has had a chance to heal.

Sites on the dominant arm or over joints, such as the wrist or elbow, should be avoided because infusions into these areas interfere with the patient's mobility and comfort and can result in phlebitis. In addition, frequent flexion of the joint can alter the rate of flow or cause the device to become dislodged. The insertion of venipuncture devices into the feet should be avoided because circulation to these extremities may be compromised, especially in older patients. The risk of thrombophlebitis is higher with pedal infusions. A limb that suffers circulatory or neurological impairment (for example, the affected arm of a patient with a mastectomy or an arm with an arteriovenous shunt) should not be used for venipuncture. Additionally, an extremity that is edematous, reddened, infected or contused should be avoided. The smallest vein to accommodate the needle or catheter needed for the infusion should be selected. Ideally, the vein should be straight, smooth, firm, resilient and large enough to permit sufficient circulation around

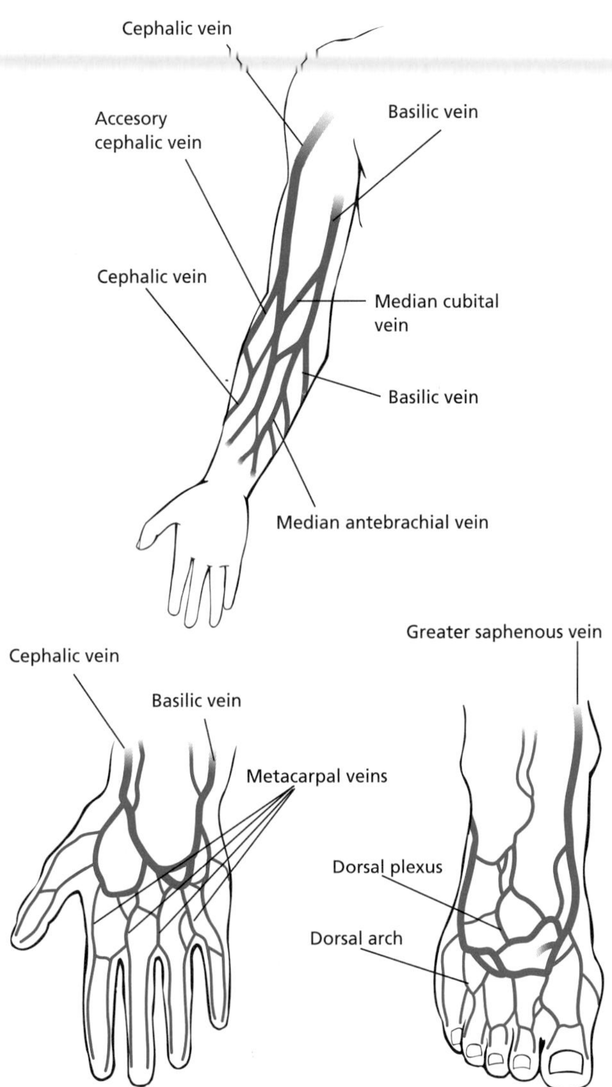

FIGURE 23.12 Peripheral venipuncture sites

the needle or catheter (Phillips, 1997; Weinstein, 1997). Figure 23.13 illustrates the common infusion sites in neonates and infants.

Protection for the nurse. The safe handling of IV equipment is mandatory in order to prevent injury to self and others in the workplace. Body substance precautions must be used when performing a venipuncture and at any time during intravenous therapy where contact with a patient's blood is likely. Body substance precautions warn that blood and body fluids from all patients be treated as potentially infected with viruses such as hepatitis or HIV. If blood is likely to splash, additional protection must be worn, such as a gown, mask or eye goggles. Special attention must be paid to the handling of needles and catheters. Do not bend, break, recap, separate from syringe or in any way manipulate needles or catheters by hand. Place these devices into puncture-resistant containers, called sharps containers, promptly after use.

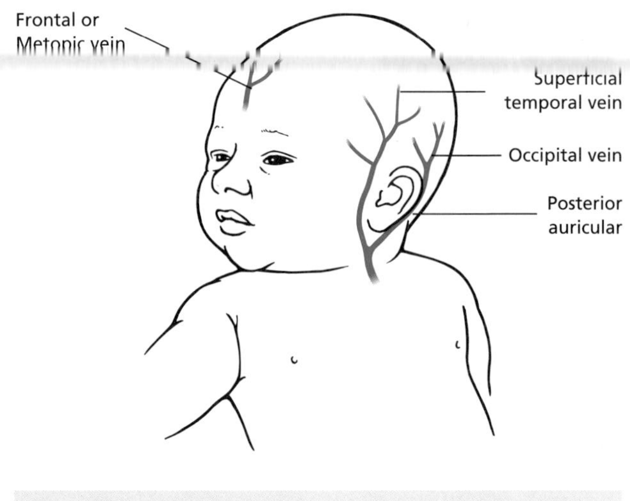

FIGURE 23.13 Sites for scalp vein infusions

Maintaining the Peripheral Infusion

Intravenous therapy carries the risk of many complications. Some of these, such as infiltration and phlebitis, are localized and cause discomfort for the patient. Others, such as fluid overload or sepsis, are systemic and can lead to life-threatening problems. The risk of complications can be reduced through careful assessment and meticulous care. An intravenous infusion must be regulated, assessed and maintained on a regular basis to ensure a constant rate of flow, to identify and correct problems and to reduce the risk of complications. Table 23.12 on page 689 outlines common complications of intravenous therapy.

REGULATING AND MONITORING THE INFUSION RATE OF FLOW The intravenous flow rate is routinely expressed as the total volume of solution to be infused over a specified period of time or as the amount in millilitres per hour (mL/h). For example, the physician's order may be written as *D5W 1 L q8h* or *D5W 125 mL/h* (the latter being far more common). The nurse must ensure that the infusion flows at the specified rate. A rate of flow that is too slow can deprive the patient of needed fluids, electrolytes and nutrients. Conversely, an infusion that is too rapid can cause complications such as circulatory overload. Various devices are used to regulate the rate of infusion. The roller clamp on the IV administration set, which is adjusted manually, is the most basic device used. There are also controllers, flow regulators and infusion pumps that are set to adjust the rate of flow electronically.

When the infusion is regulated with a roller clamp on the IV administration set, the flow rate is measured in drops per minute. In order to calculate the *rate of flow*, also referred to as the *drip rate*, the nurse has to know the amount of solution to be infused, the duration of infusion and the drop factor (the number of drops per millilitre of solution). The most common method of calculating the rate of flow determines first, the number of millilitres per hour (mL/h) and second, the drops per minute (gtt/min).

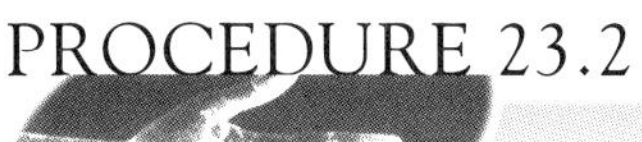

PROCEDURE 23.2 Establishing the Infusion (Peripheral

Action	*Rationale*
1. Gather equipment: • venipuncture device • tourniquet • alcohol or antiseptic swab • gauze sponges, transparent semi-permeable dressing, nonallergenic tape • sharps container, protective underpad, disposable gloves • primed IV solution on IV pole.	Facilitates efficiency and economy of time.
2. Identify the patient.	Avoids error.
3. Prepare the patient for what to expect during each stage of the procedure.	Knowing what to expect reduces anxiety and tension. This enhances the patient's comfort and makes it easier to insert the venipuncture device.
4. Wash hands thoroughly and maintain sterile technique.	Prevents introducing contaminants during preparation.
5. Ready all equipment. Open packages, maintaining aseptic technique. Cut tape and store it on the inside cover of a sterile package.	Facilitates efficiency. Starting an IV infusion is a sterile procedure. Sticking cut tape on hospital surfaces results in the transfer of microorganisms.
6. Place the extremity in a dependent position (below level of heart); apply a tourniquet 15–20 cm above the possible site; ask the patient to clench and unclench the fist. Warm packs can also be applied. Check for a distal pulse. If one is not present, reapply the tourniquet less tightly. Do not use a tourniquet if the veins are fragile or rolling.	These measures distend the vein, making it easier to visualize it and insert the needle or catheter. The tourniquet should be applied tightly enough to dilate the vein but it should not occlude the artery. A palpable radial pulse indicates adequate arterial blood flow. Fragile veins can rupture or "blow" when distended.

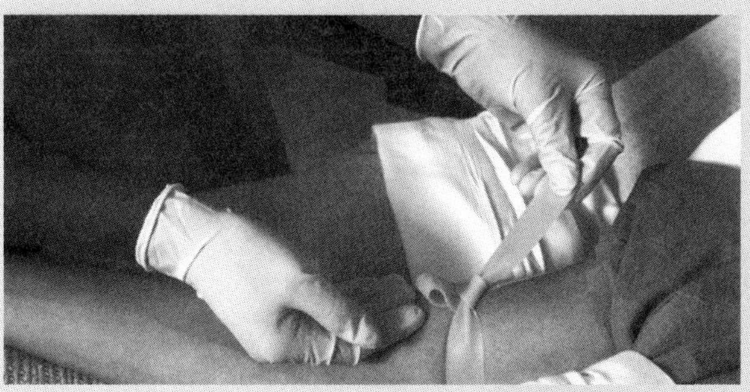

7. Select a venipuncture site by inspecting and palpating the veins. Choose a vein that is visible, feels firm and has a straight section. Avoid areas of flexion. If necessary, clip excessive hair over venipuncture area per agency policy and with permission from the patient.	Makes insertion easier. Prevents the risk of phlebitis. Makes tape removal more comfortable and decreases risk of bacterial contamination.
8. Place a protective pad under the site. Put on gloves and cleanse the site with an antiseptic swab, using a firm, circular motion and working from the centre of the site outward. Let dry.	Protects bed linen if bleeding occurs. Reduces introduction of skin bacteria into the patient's vascular system during the venipuncture.

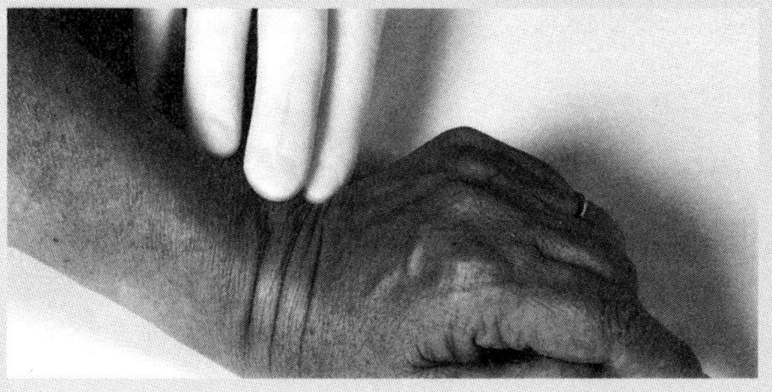

continued on next page

PROCEDURE 23.2 continued

Action	Rationale
9. Using the nondominant hand, hold the extremity so that the thumb is placed below and slightly lateral to the site and the forefinger placed above and lateral to the site. Hold the skin taut by gently pulling downward with the thumb while pushing upward with the forefinger.	Stabilizes the skin and anchors the vein.
10. Insert the needle or the catheter.	
a. Grasp the catheter by the hub, leaving the flashback chamber visible.	Enables the nurse to see the blood return.
b. Holding bevel side up and pointing in the direction of blood flow, pierce the skin at a 30° angle.	Decreases injury to the skin and is more comfortable for the patient.
c. Decrease the angle of the device so that it is almost flush with the skin, then pierce the vein. Watch for a backflow of blood into the needle tubing or the catheter. A sensation of released resistance can sometimes be felt when the device enters the vein.	Reducing the angle of entry decreases the chance of puncturing both walls of the vein. The backflow of blood confirms placement of the device in the vein.
d. Advance the catheter but not the stylet (needle) up to the hub or until resistance is felt, then release the tourniquet.	

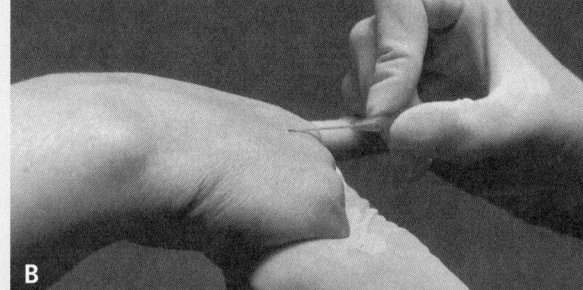

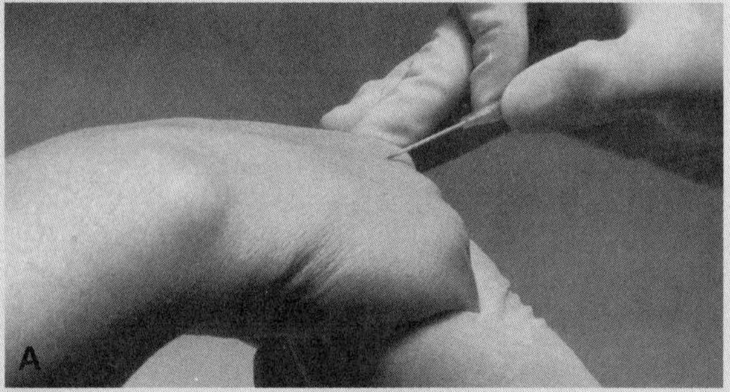

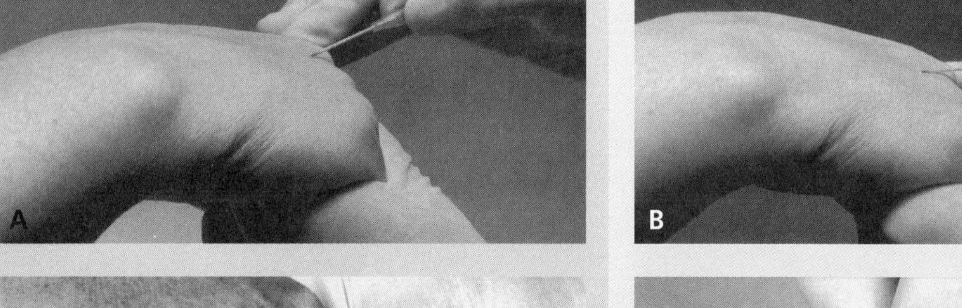

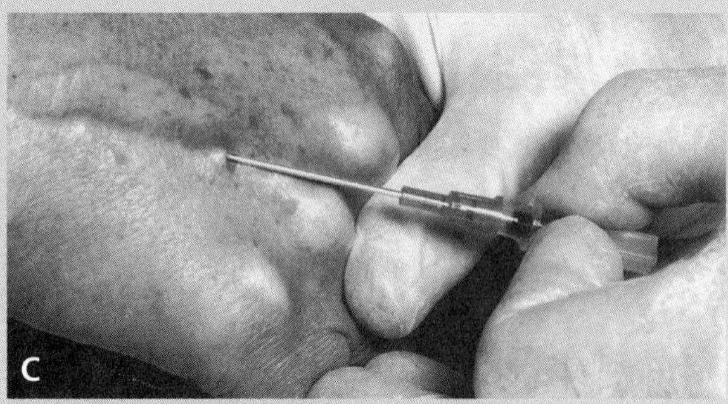

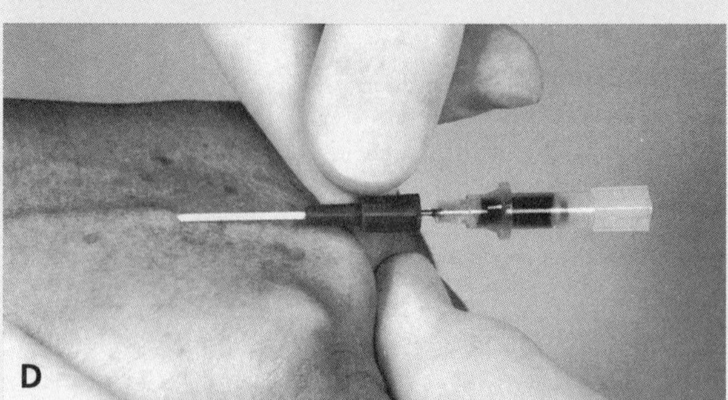

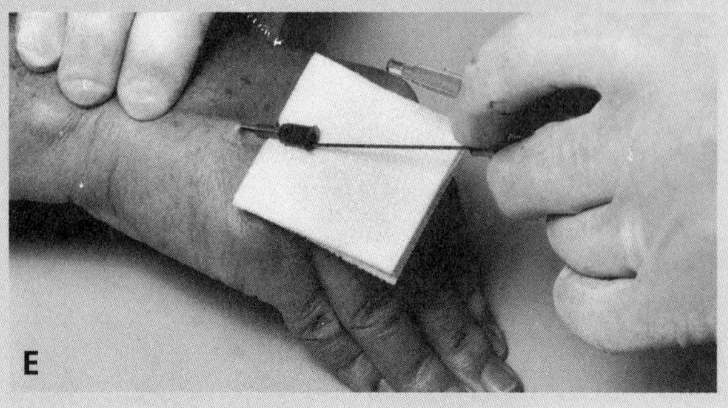

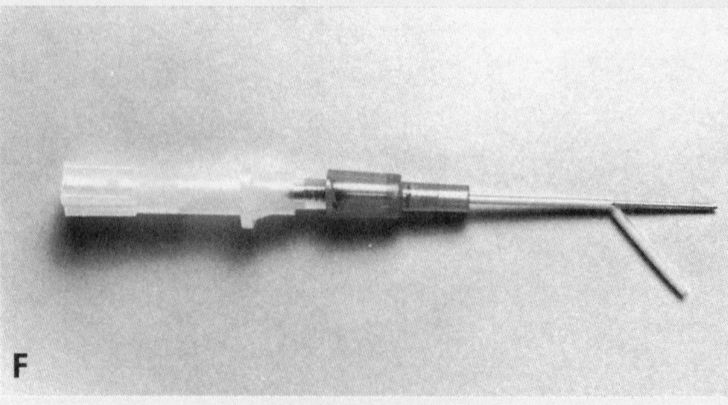

PROCEDURE 23.2 *continued*

Action	*Rationale*
e. Remove the stylet from inside the catheter and discard into a sharps container. Attach the administration set to the catheter and open the roller clamp to start the flow of solution.	
f. **Do not** reinsert the stylet into the catheter at any time.	The needle may sever the catheter and cause it to embolize.
g. If using a needle, advance it into the vein up to the hub. While holding the needle in place with one hand, release the tourniquet with the other, attach the administration set and open the roller clamp to start the flow of solution.	Ensures the device is curently in the vein. The flow of solution is necessary to prevent blood from clotting in the needle.
11. Tape the needle or catheter in place and dress the site using adhesive tape, transparent tape and gauze dressing per agency policy. Secure the device so that the insertion site and the hub–tubing connection is free of tape. See Figure 23.14.	The device must be stabilized to prevent dislodgement. Dressings prevent infection by keeping bacteria from the site. Facilitates inspection of the site and tubing changes later on.
12. Loop the IV tubing on the patient's limb near the venipuncture site and secure with tape.	Prevents the weight of the tubing from pulling on the needle or catheter, thereby dislodging it.
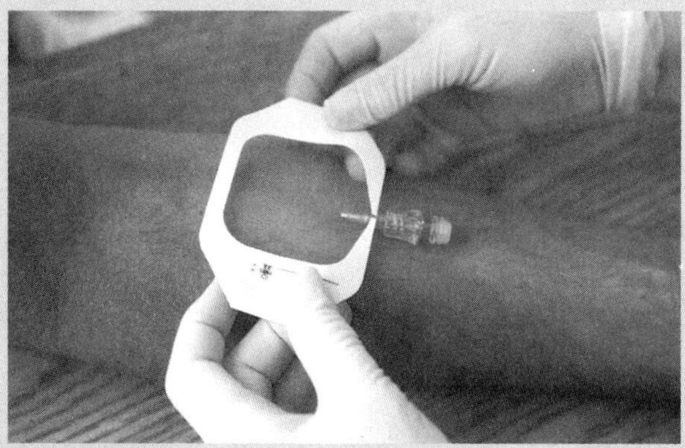	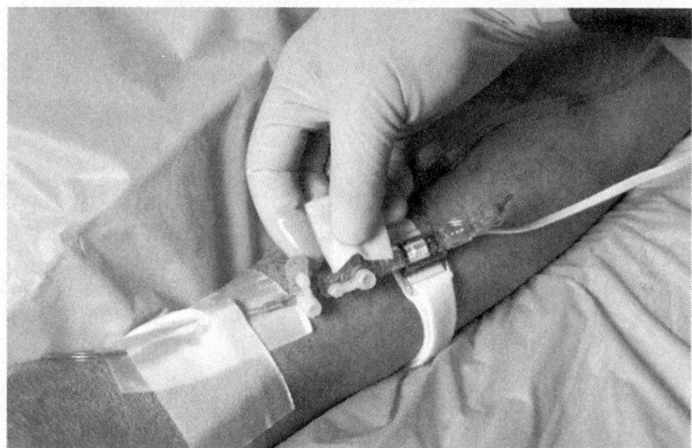
13. Regulate the flow rate as ordered.	Maintains accurate infusion.
14. Remove gloves; wash hands.	
15. Apply an armboard if necessary.	Stabilizes the needle or catheter situated near a joint.
16. Document the procedure noting the time, site, size and type of device, the type of solution and rate of infusion, any problems with the procedure, the patient's response and nursing actions per agency protocol.	Fulfills legal requirements for nurse accountability.

Step 1. $\dfrac{\text{Total volume of solution}}{\text{Number of hours}} = \text{millilitres/hour}$

Step 2. $\dfrac{\text{Number of mL/h} \times \text{drop factor}}{\text{Time in minutes}} = \text{drops/minute}$

Suppose, for example, 1000 mL of solution are to be infused over eight hours. With a drop factor of 10, the drip rate would be calculated as follows:

Step 1. $1000 \div 8 = 125$ mL/h
Step 2. $125 \times 10 \div 60 = 20.8$ or 21 gtt/min

Once the drip rate is determined, the infusion is regulated by adjusting the roller clamp on the administration set and counting drops until the desired rate of flow is achieved. Holding a watch next to the drip chamber expedites the counting of drops. It is recommended that the drops be counted for one minute to account for irregularities in flow (Brown & Mulholland, 1996).

A *time tape* placed on the solution bag is commonly used as a quick guide for monitoring the rate of flow and checking that the correct amount of solution has infused over an hourly period. Commercially prepared time tapes

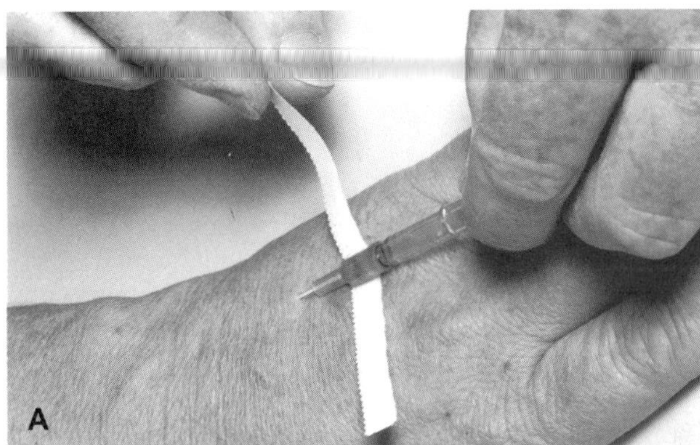

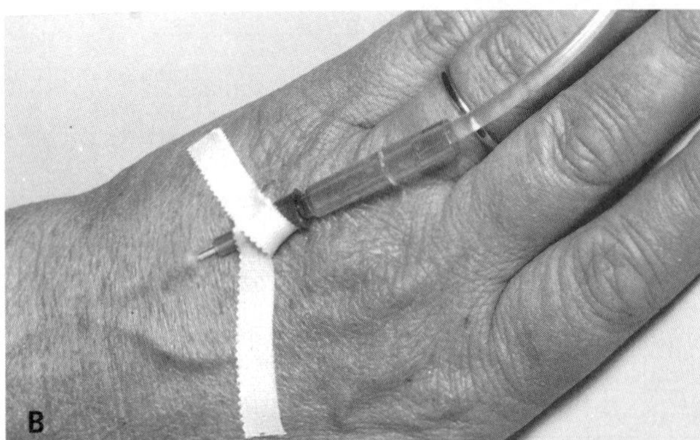

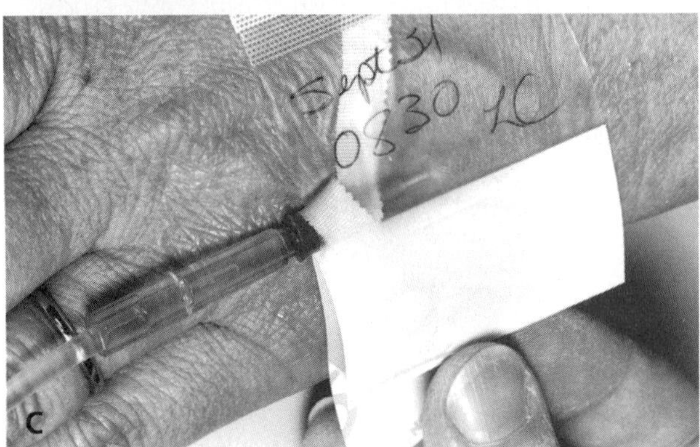

FIGURE 23.14 Securing an infusion needle or catheter with tape and transparent dressing. A. Tape the catheter securely using Chevron technique (or per hospital procedure), pinching tightly to secure the catheter. B. DO NOT apply tape over the sterile entry point. C. Apply a sterile transparent dressing or a sterile Band-Aid. Document with date, time, catheter size and your initials

SOURCE: Chase, 1993.

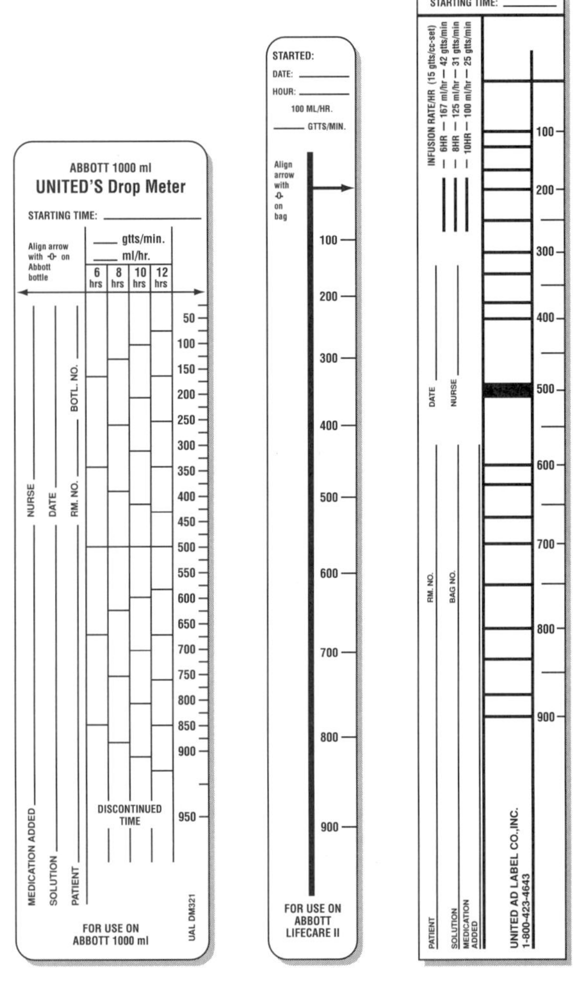

FIGURE 23.15 Time tapes

are available; however, a piece of tape placed vertically on the bag adjacent to the millimetre calibrations is a common alternative. Based on the calculated flow rate, the time tape is marked at intervals showing the expected volume to be infused per hour (see Figure 23.15). The flow rate is monitored by comparing the level of solution in the bag to the expected fluid level on the time tape. Necessary adjustments are made to the flow rate using the roller clamp and validated by counting drops per minute.

One of the biggest challenges in managing intravenous therapy is maintaining a consistent rate of infusion. Several factors alter the flow of solution into the vein, causing the rate to speed up or slow down over time. These include:

1. *The distance of the solution container from the venipuncture site*. The higher the container, the greater the force of gravity overcoming venous pressure; therefore, the more rapidly the solution flows into the vein.
2. *The position of the extremity*. The flow rate may increase or decrease when the limb is moved, flexed, or held above (increases) or below (decreases) the level of the heart.
3. *The patency of the venipuncture site and the tubing*. Taping of the IV site too tightly may restrict flow. An infusion can also slow down if the tubing becomes kinked, crimped, looped, compressed, or if it is allowed to dangle below the insertion site.

4. *The viscosity of the solution.* Thicker fluid such as blood forms fewer and smaller drops than less viscous solutions and, therefore, flows more slowly.
5. [illegible] the flow of solution.
6. *The size of the vein and the venipuncture device.* The smaller the vein and the size of the device, the slower the infusion of solution. Conversely, solution flows more rapidly into large veins when large-gauge venipuncture devices are in place.

Infusions must be monitored frequently in order to ensure consistent flow rates. How often this is done varies according to agency policy, the patient's age and condition, the type of solution and how well it is infusing. Generally, the drip rate is checked and readjusted as necessary at least every hour. Some nurses do this every time they are in the patient's room. If the infusion has been too slow, an increase in the drip rate may be necessary to "catch up," that is, re-establish the infusion at the specified rate. When this happens, the drip rate should not be increased more than 30 percent without consulting the physician first (Krozek, 1993).

Intravenous infusions are also regulated with electric or battery-operated infusion control devices, namely pumps and controllers. These devices maintain flow rates more accurately than the standard gravity flow system. Although infusion pumps and controllers work on different principles, both devices can be used to administer a wide range of fluids, electrolytes, medications and nutrients. Infusion pumps and controllers are used when a precise rate of flow is necessary, for example, in an older patient at risk for developing circulatory overload or when a medication (e.g., heparin), is to be administered (Weinstein, 1997).

An *infusion pump* (Figure 23.16) maintains a preset flow rate by applying variable positive pressure on the fluid or the administration set. Solution [illegible] pressure exerted on the fluid. For example, if flow is restricted because the patient flexes an arm and increases pressure in the vein, the pump responds by increasing pressure on the administration set to overcome the resistance and thereby maintains a constant rate of flow. An *infusion controller* is a device that regulates the rate of flow by using a photoelectric sensor attached to the drip chamber. The sensor recognizes whether the solution is flowing into the drip chamber at the preset flow rate and keeps this rate constant by speeding

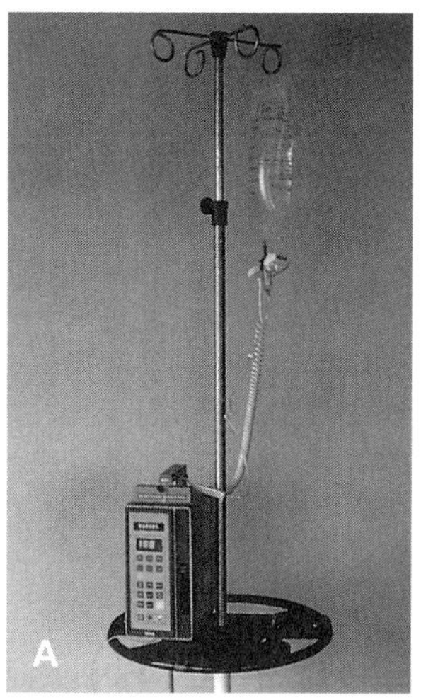

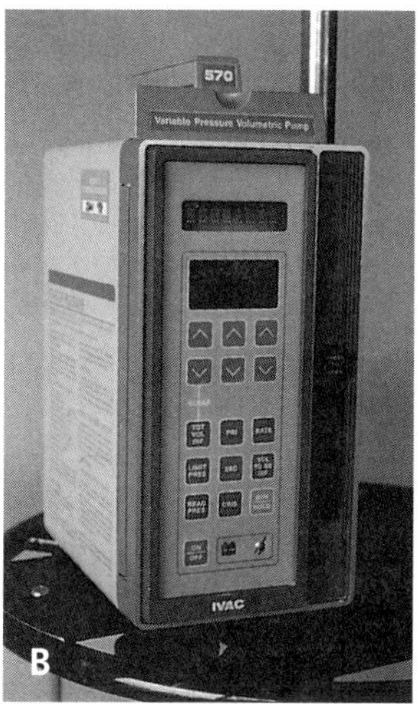

FIGURE 23.16 Infusion control devices. A. Infusion controller with photoelectric sensor on the drip chamber. B. Infusion pump

Peripheral intravenous access sites for pediatric patients*

Preferred sites	Veins
Hand	Digital, metacarpal
Forearm	Supplementary cephalic, basilic, median antebrachial
Antecubital fossa	Median basilic, median cephalic, median cubital
Upper arm (below axilla)	Basilic, cephalic
Foot (before walking age)	Greater saphenous, lesser saphenous
Scalp (before 18 months)	Occipital, frontal, temporal
Lower leg (before walking age)	Greater saphenous, lesser saphenous
Secondary Sites†	**Veins**
Wrist	Superficial veins: infiltration in this area may result in pressure on the radial nerve
Abdomen	Superficial veins: rarely used, usually limited to neonates and chronically hospitalized patients; infiltration may result in damage to abdominal wall
Axilla	Axillary vein: usually limited to neonates; infiltration may cause pressure on structures in chest cavity
Knee	Popliteal vein: usually limited to neonates due to decreased mobility

*Sites listed in order of preference: consider individual characteristics
† Secondary sites should be considered only when preferred sites are not available.

SOURCE: Weinstein, 1997, p. 542.

RESEARCH to practice

Savino, S.R., & Eberhart, T. (1998). A comparison of flow rates between Baxter Continu-Flow and Baxter InterLink Continu-Flow. *Journal of Intravenous Nursing, 21(1)*, 41–44.

The intent of this study was to identify whether Baxter's nonrestrictive tubing delivered IV fluid quicker than its restrictive tubing. A regional oncology centre was the site of this study, which was conducted over a four-day period.

The study was conducted in three phases on separate days. Phase 1 timed separately the flow rate of both systems using a consistent protocol. The distance between the medicine cup and the meniscus of each intravenous bag was 27 in (68.6 cm). The time required for each system to drain 15 mL into a medicine cup was recorded. Phase 2 consisted of two intravenous lines running concurrently using both systems. These lines were placed into separate graduate containers 56 in (142 cm) beneath the meniscus of each intravenous bag. Times were recorded at the start of the infusion and when the first bag emptied. The third and final phase used two separate intravenous lines with separate systems, each having flow-restrictive devices (additional company products) attached to the end of the tubings. The equipment ended in graduate containers 56 in (142 cm) below the meniscus.

The results of this study indicated that the nonrestrictive system took 35 seconds to infuse 15 mL of fluid, whereas the restrictive tubing took 4 minutes, 35 seconds. In phase 2 the 500-mL intravenous bag with nonrestrictive tubing infused in 12 minutes, whereas the restrictive tubing infused only 150 mL in the same time. In phase 3 when flow-restricting devices were used, the nonrestrictive tubing allowed a 500-mL bag to empty more than twice as fast as restrictive tubing.

Different solutions were used in phases 1 and 2 to determine whether they would affect the rate of flow. The results indicated that using different solutions was not a factor in altering the flow rate in either system. An implication for practice is that restrictive tubing has the advantage over nonrestrictive tubing in decreasing accidental infusion of large amounts of intravenous fluid over a short period of time.

up or slowing down the drops of fluid. The controller depends on the force of gravity to propel solution into the vein; therefore, height is an important factor in its effectiveness. To work correctly a controller must be located at least 76 cm above the insertion site.

Infusion devices assist in the safe, accurate infusion of fluids. They also save time because nurses do not have to check and readjust flow rates constantly. Most devices are equipped with alarms that sound if the flow rate is not being maintained or if there are infusion difficulties, such as occlusions or air in the tubing. However, these devices do not always detect inflammation at the venipuncture site or dislodgement of the device, nor do they detect patients' responses to IV therapy. Therefore, it is important to complete the regular assessments required for intravenous infusions. Checks of the pump or controller should also be routinely made to ensure that it is programmed correctly and that it is working properly. A time tape on the solution container is recommended, as a gauge for accuracy (Phillips, 1997).

ASSESSING THE INFUSION Systematic assessment is made of the venipuncture site, the administration set, the accuracy of therapy and the patient's response to therapy. First, the venipuncture site is thoroughly inspected for tenderness, redness, swelling or coolness at or just above the site of insertion. These findings indicate that the needle or catheter may have slipped out of the vein, allowing fluid to flow into the surrounding tissues (infiltration) or that the vein has been irritated by the venipuncture device or solution (phlebitis). When signs of infiltration or phlebitis occur, the infusion should be discontinued and restarted at another location. A warm compress may be applied to the site for patient comfort.

The site is also assessed for leakage or bleeding, which can be caused by a loose connection between the venipuncture device and the tubing, faulty equipment or movement of an improperly secured needle or catheter. A loose connection between the venipuncture device and the tubing is corrected by simply tightening the connection. Faulty equipment must be replaced promptly. When leakage or bleeding occurs from the site because the needle or catheter was not securely taped in place, the site must be cleansed with an antiseptic agent and retaped. The area should be carefully inspected for signs of irritation and infection caused by the movement of the device in the vein and skin. An armboard may be applied to stabilize the insertion site. The site is also checked to ensure that it is free from pressure. Lying on the venipuncture site or keeping the limb tightly flexed increases the blood pressure in the extremity and can cause the infusion to slow or stop completely (Weinstein, 1997).

The venipuncture device is assessed to ensure that it is patent and securely positioned in the vein. There are several ways of doing this. The most common way is to lower the solution container below the insertion site and observe for the passive flow of blood back into the tubing. Patency of the device can also be assessed by inserting a normal saline-filled syringe into the port nearest to the insertion site, and while pinching the tubing, slowly withdrawing some fluid from the tubing and the device. Blood will return if the device is properly situated and in a large enough vein. Lastly, the patency of the venipuncture device can be determined by gently palpating the vein two to three centimetres beyond the end of the device. Palpation will

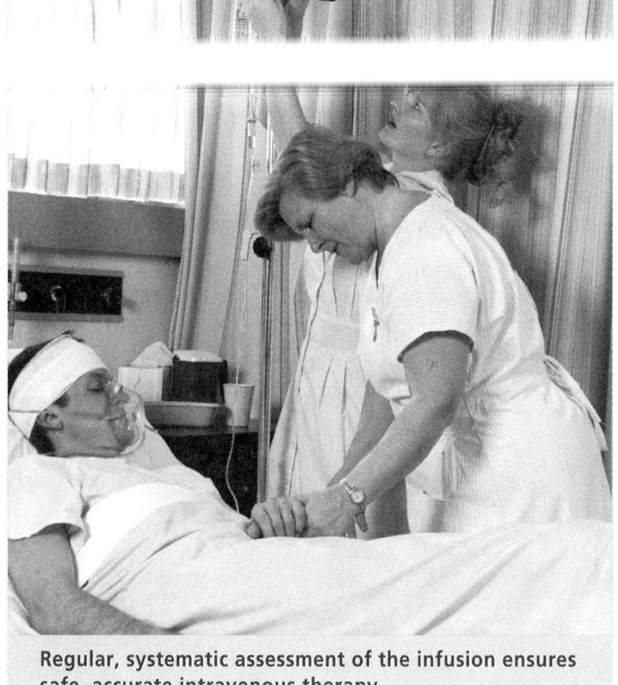

Regular, systematic assessment of the infusion ensures safe, accurate intravenous therapy.

cause a mechanical compression of the vein. If the device is patent, IV flow will slow or stop.

The administration set, namely the tubing, should be assessed for patency. Checks are made to ensure that the tubing is filled with solution and free from air bubbles, particulate matter, kinks, obstructions and disconnections. Inspections are also made to determine that the roller clamp is open at the appropriate rate, the drip chamber is half-full of solution, the spike is securely inserted into the bag and the bag holds enough fluid for the next hour.

It is also important to assess the accuracy of intravenous therapy. At the beginning of each shift, the nurse should check the physician's order for IV therapy and then examine the existing administration set, flow rate, type of solution, amount of solution to be absorbed and the height of the bag. If an electronic infusion device is being used, the flow rate and machine should be checked for proper functioning. Labels on the tubing and the solution should be examined for expiry dates. Necessary changes must be made promptly in order to prevent infection.

Patient response to intravenous therapy is often manifested through the vital signs. An elevated temperature, pulse, respirations or blood pressure may indicate a complication such as infection, pulmonary edema or circulatory overload. Another response is demonstrated by the patient's fluid balance. If IV therapy is effective, urinary output should be proportionate to fluid intake, assuming there are no renal problems. When patients are receiving electrolyte solutions, blood work results should be monitored and the patient examined for untoward effects. For example, when potassium solutions are being infused, laboratory results should be monitored for increased potassium levels and the patient observed for signs of hyperkalemia. High levels of potassium [illegible]

[illegible] tient's emotional response to therapy (Weinstein, 1997).

CARE OF THE INFUSION SITE AND SYSTEM Routine maintenance of a peripheral infusion site and system includes changing solution bags and administration sets, rotating the infusion sites and, in some agencies, changing the IV site dressings. Agencies differ in how frequently administration sets are replaced or IV sites rotated and in the type of dressings that are used. Therefore, agency policies should be followed for all routine maintenance procedures.

IV solutions are ordinarily changed when the bag (or bottle) becomes empty or when the physician writes a new order. Most agencies routinely change the IV every 24–72 hours to prevent contamination. The maximum hang time for IV bags is now 72 hours (increased from 24 hours) with the exception of lipids, blood or blood products (Health Canada, 1997). Lipids should be taken down immediately after completion of the infusion. The maximum hang time for blood products is four hours. In addition, solution containers must be replaced immediately if signs of contamination, such as discoloration, leaks or foreign particles, become evident. Administration sets are generally replaced every 72 hours as a precaution against bacterial growth. These are most simply and efficiently changed when new bags of solution are put up. Sometimes, however, the administration set may have to be changed before the solution bag is empty, for example, if there are leaks, incompatibilities or occlusions in the line, when the tubing becomes contaminated or if a different calibration of tubing (drop factor) is required to facilitate regulation of flow rate.

Venipuncture sites are redressed when they become damp, soiled or loosened. Transparent semi-permeable dressings allow easy assessment of the site; therefore, they are not changed routinely. These dressings provide a warm environment for bacterial growth. There is increased risk of infection if poor sterile technique is used or if drainage is allowed to sit under the dressing. Venipuncture sites should be rotated every 48–72 hours as a precaution against infection and phlebitis. However, this may not be realistic in some cases. For example, frequent changes of venipuncture devices in people who are receiving long-term therapy or in those with poor veins would soon leave few accessible veins. Therefore, in circumstances such as these, the sites are carefully assessed by the nurse and changed only when necessary. When an infusion site is changed, a vein that is proximal to the old site or in the opposite limb should be used in order to promote patient comfort and prevent complications. When rotating an infusion site, the nurse follows the procedure for establishing a peripheral venipuncture (see Procedure 23.2).

Procedures for maintaining the infusion system—that is, changing the solution container, replacing the tubing and redressing the infusion site—are outlined in Procedure 23.3.

PROCEDURE 23.3

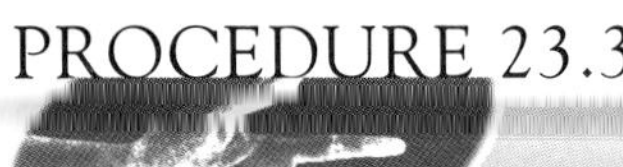

Maintaining the Infusion System

Action	Rationale
A. General Actions	
1. Gather equipment as outlined in each section below.	Ensures efficiency and economy of time.
2. Wash hands thoroughly and maintain sterile technique.	Reduces the risk of contamination during the procedure.
3. Explain the procedure to the patient.	Allays anxiety and enhances emotional well-being.
4. Assess the site and IV system.	Ensures the system is working properly and enables early detection and intervention for complications.
B. Changing the Solution Bag	
1. Collect the prescribed solution, check the bag as outlined in Procedure 23.1 and apply a time tape.	Ensures accurate delivery and reduces the risk of error.
2. At the bedside, hang a bag on the IV pole; place a bottle on the over-bed table.	Readies the equipment for the change-over.
3. Close the roller clamp on the administration set or turn off the infusion control device.	Keeps fluid in the drip chamber and prevents air from entering the tubing.
4. **Bag:** Remove the protective cap from the administration port. **Bottle:** Remove the cap and seal.	Maintains sterility of the port or stopper.
5. Remove the old bag from the IV pole, invert it and remove the spike. Insert the spike into the new bag as in Procedure 23.1. Hang the bag on the IV pole. Maintain sterility of the spike at all times.	Prevents the escape of left-over fluid from the container. Prevents contamination of the solution.
6. Open the roller clamp and adjust the rate of flow, or restart the infusion control device.	Maintains the patency of the system and the desired rate of flow.
7. Discard used equipment.	Maintains cleanliness and safety in workplace.
C. Changing the Solution Bag and the Administration Set	
1. Gather equipment: • administration set • correct IV solution • time tape, label for tubing • sterile gauze sponges, adhesive tape • two pair of clean gloves • hemostat (optional).	Promotes efficiency and economy of time.
2. Prepare the solution bag and prime and label the tubing per Procedure 23.1.	
3. At the bedside hang the new solution bag and primed set on the IV pole and lay the needle adapter end of the tubing near the infusion site. Loosen protective cap on new tubing.	Readies the equipment for the change-over.
4. Put on gloves.	Maintains body substance precautions.
5. Remove tape and dressing from the infusion site to expose the connection, taking care not to displace the needle or catheter. Remove tape anchoring tubing to limb.	Promotes access to the venipuncture device.
6. Place a sterile gauze under the needle or catheter.	Provides a sterile working area and absorbs leakage when the tubing is disconnected.
7. Close the roller clamp of the old tubing.	Avoids undue leakage of solution.

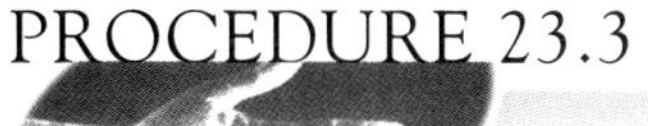

PROCEDURE 23.3 *continued*

Action	*Rationale*
8. Hold the hub of the needle or catheter with the thumb and index finger of the nondominant hand; with the little finger of the same hand, apply pressure to the vein proximal to the needle or catheter. Gently disconnect the old tubing using a twisting, pulling motion.	Using the thumb and index finger ensures the device is kept securely in the vein. The little finger prevents excessive blood loss via the catheter upon disconnection.
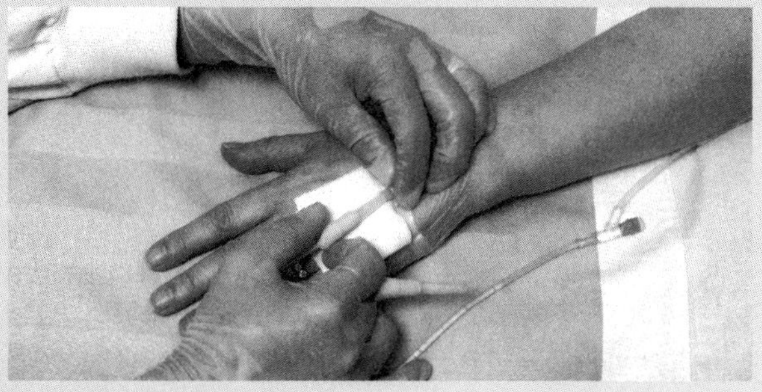	
Option: A hemostat may be used to stabilize the device; however, the hemostat must not be clamped shut on the device, as doing so will crack the hub.	
9. Quickly remove the cap from the new tubing and insert the adapter into the device.	Facilitates exchange with minimal blood loss and minimal risk of infection.
10. Open the roller clamp.	Prevents clotting of the device.
11. Clean the site of any leakage, working from the site outward.	Maintains sterility of the site.
12. If gloves are soiled, remove them and apply new ones.	Prevents contamination of the site.
13. Redress the site as necessary. Loop and tape the new tubing securely onto the patient's limb.	Prevents airborne bacteria from entering the site. Prevents strain on the venipuncture device.
14. Regulate the IV flow rate as prescribed. Label the tubing with date and time.	Maintains accurate infusion. Promotes continuity of care.
15. Discard the used administration set and equipment. Remove gloves and wash hands.	Maintains cleanliness and safety in the workplace.
D. Replacing the Administration Set Only	
1. Gather equipment: • administration set • label for tubing, sterile gauze sponges, antiseptic swab, adhesive tape • two pair of clean gloves • hemostat.	
2. Reduce the infusion rate of flow.	Ensures patency of the venipuncture device and prevents air from entering the tubing.
3. Clamp the port of a bag with a hemostat. Remove the bag or bottle from the IV pole and invert it.	Prevents fluid spilling from the bag.
4. Remove the spike from the bag and keep it upright above the level of the patient's heart. Tape the old spike to the IV pole. Remove the protective cap from the new spike.	Maintains the infusion during the change-over.
5. Insert the new spike into the solution bag, remove hemostat and prime the tubing as in Procedure 23.1.	
6. Put on gloves and continue as in section C, numbers 4 to 15.	

continued on next page

PROCEDURE 23.3 *continued*

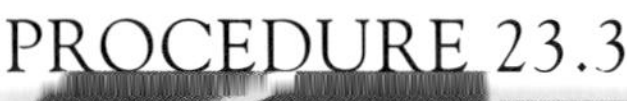

Action	*Rationale*
E. Changing the Site Dressing	
1. Gather equipment: • sterile gauze sponges or transparent semi-permeable dressing, adhesive tape, alcohol swabs • clean gloves.	
2. Put on gloves.	Maintains body substance precautions.
3. Stabilize the venipuncture device with the nondominant hand. Gently remove the old tape and dressing.	Prevents displacement of the device.
4. Clean the insertion site with alcohol, using a circular motion and working from the site outward.	Avoids contaminating the site. An antiseptic solution decreases the risk of infection by reducing the number of microorganisms.
5. Allow the area to dry.	Drying area maximizes effect of antiseptic solution.
6. Retape the device and cover with sterile gauze or transparent semipermeable dressing.	Prevents displacement of the device. Decreases contamination of the site.
7. Remove gloves and wash hands.	Prevents spread of microorganisms.
8. Label the dressing with date.	Promotes continuity of care.
F. Documentation	
Document the procedure in the nurses' notes or fluid balance record per agency protocol. **Changing solution container:** Note the type and amount of solution infused; the time, type and amount of solution added; the flow rate; and the assessment findings. **Changing administration set:** Note the date and time of replacement. **Changing IV site dressing:** Note the date and time the site was redressed. Indicate the cleansing solution used, the type of dressing applied, assessment findings and the patient's response to the procedure.	Maintains a record of intake and fulfills requirements for nurse accountability.

Discontinuing the Peripheral Intravenous Infusion

Intravenous therapy is discontinued when ordered by the physician or when complications such as infiltration or phlebitis develop. An infusion is also discontinued and restarted in another area for routine site rotation. Procedure 23.4 details the nursing actions for discontinuing an infusion.

PREPARING THE PATIENT Before gathering the equipment, the nurse should inform the patient of the procedure. Discontinuing an infusion is usually painless. The dressing and tape are removed from the site, the device is withdrawn slowly and pressure is applied to the site for a few minutes. Pressure is necessary to stop bleeding. A Band-Aid or sterile gauze is placed over the site. It should be kept in place for at least eight hours. Normal activities can be resumed immediately (Phillips, 1997).

Special Considerations for Peripheral Intravenous Therapy

Equipment should be assembled in the utility room and brought to the patient's unit for immediate use. When patients are confused, the roller clamp should be positioned high enough on the tubing so that they cannot reach up and adjust the flow rate. Additionally, restraints may be necessary with confused or aggressive patients to prevent them from pulling out the infusion device.

Some patients may not accept intravenous infusions because of religious beliefs. Jehovah's Witnesses, for instance, will accept blood substitutes but not whole blood. Christian Scientists avoid use of medications or infusions. Patients who choose to refuse intravenous infusions are required to sign a "refusal of treatment" form, which is attached to their record.

The inspection of a site for redness may be difficult to do for dark-skinned patients. In such cases, other techniques, such as palpation of the area for tenderness and warmth, can be used.

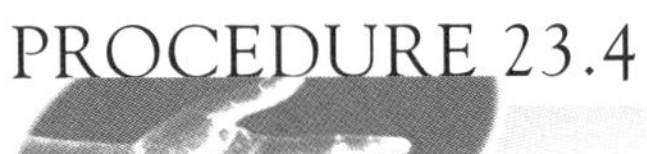

PROCEDURE 23.4 Discontinuing the Peripheral Infusion

Action	Rationale
1. Gather equipment: sterile gauze, Band-Aid, clean gloves.	Ensures efficiency and economy of time.
2. Wash hands thoroughly and maintain sterile technique.	Reduces the risk of contamination during the procedure.
3. Close the roller clamp.	Prevents escape of fluid.
4. Put on gloves.	Maintains body substance precautions.
5. Loosen the tape and dressing by pulling towards the site while applying countertraction to the skin with the nondominant hand.	Countertraction helps to prevent pulling of the skin, thereby lessening patient discomfort.
6. Withdraw the device in line with the vein, using a steady pulling motion. Place gauze over the site and apply gentle pressure with the nondominant hand.	Prevents trauma to the vein and breaking/binding of the device.
7. Apply direct, firm pressure over the site for one or two minutes or until bleeding stops. If the patient is receiving heparin or another anticoagulant, maintain pressure for a longer period and elevate the limb slightly.	Prevents bleeding and hematoma formation.
8. When bleeding has stopped apply a Band-Aid or sterile gauze. Leave in place for at least 8 hours.	Prevents microorganisms from entering the site and slight pressure prevents further oozing.
9. Discard used equipment appropriately. Remove gloves and wash hands.	Ensures cleanliness and safety in the workplace.
10. Document the procedure in the nurses' notes or on the fluid balance record per agency policy. Note date and time; reason for discontinuing infusion; condition and intactness of the device; condition of the infusion site; patient's response; any complications and nursing interventions; and the amount and type of infusion infused.	Fulfills requirements for nurse accountability.

Troubleshooting Peripheral Intravenous Infusion Problems

Begin assessment at the infusion site and work upward to the solution container. Look for obvious problems and then correct them.

Assessment	Intervention
*1. **IV site***	
Check for possible complications: • infiltration • phlebitis • thrombophlebitis • infection.	See Table 23.12 for signs and symptoms and interventions.
*2. **IV device***	
Check for:	
• placement in the vein. Is the device in line with the vein or is it pressed against the vein wall, restricting flow?	If device is pressed against the vein wall, gently pull back on it. Gently rotate an over-the-needle catheter. Never rotate a butterfly, as it will puncture the vein wall. Slightly raise or lower the angle of the device in the vein by adjusting the gauze pad under the hub.
• restriction by tape or pressure from the patient's limb	If device is restricted, retape it or reposition the limb. Apply an armboard if necessary.
• positional flow (rate is affected by joint movement)	Apply a splint or armboard. Instruct the patient to keep the limb below the level of the heart and to avoid direct pressure on the site.

continued on next page

Assessment	Intervention
• patency.	Follow the techniques outlined under "Assessing the Infusion." If the device is patent but the flow is sluggish, pinch and release the tubing near the site several times. This increases the pressure within the tubing, which may clear the device. Do not compress the flashball. Doing so creates pressure, which may rupture the vein. Never irrigate a device without aspirating for blood first. Doing so may dislodge a clot into the blood stream, resulting in an embolism. If the device is obstructed, remove it and relocate the infusion.
3. *Tubing* Check for:	
• kinks, crimps, or pressure (other equipment or patient lying on tubing)	Straighten the tubing or reposition the patient or other equipment.
• sections dangling below the level of the infusion site (prevents gravity from propelling fluid into the patient)	Coil excessive tubing.
• patency and large air bubbles.	If there are large air spaces or if there is precipitate, replace flow and while stretching the tubing downward, tap or flick the tubing with a finger. The air will rise into the drip chamber. Regulate the flow rate. For air low in the tubing, slow the rate of flow. Remove air through the Y-injection port that is below the air space, using a sterile syringe and needle. Regulate the flow rate.
4. *Clamps* Check that all clamps are open.	Open the roller clamp completely, change it to a new position, regulate the flow rate.
5. *Air vent* Check that the air vent is: • present • patent.	Glass containers require air vents. If vent is absent, replace the administration set with one containing an air vent or insert a vent into the rubber stopper. If vent is obstructed, replace administration set or vent.
6. *Filter* Check that the filter is: • present • patent.	Filters are required for solutions with some additives and when administering blood. If obstructed, replace the filter. A blocked filter will interrupt flow.
7. *Drip chamber* Check fluid level (should be able to count drops).	If the drip chamber is full, close the roller clamp, invert the bag and squeeze the drip chamber. The fluid squeezed into the bag will be replaced by air from the bag. Rehang the bag and regulate flow.
8. *Spike* Check placement in port of container.	If the spike is not placed securely into the port, replace the tubing. Do not push the spike into the bag, because it is no longer sterile.
9. *Solution bag* Check:	
• level of fluid	If fluid level is low (50–100 mL), replace the bag.
• temperature of solution	If the solution is cold, which happens when blood is administered, the vein may go into spasm, thereby decreasing flow. Apply a warm compress to the infusion site. Never warm blood unless ordered by the physician.
• height of the bag (should be one metre above the infusion site).	Adjust the height of the IV pole.
10. The system has been systematically assessed; there are no obvious problems, but the infusion has stopped.	Discontinue the infusion and re-establish in another site.

TABLE 23.12 Complications of peripheral intravenous therapy

Complication	Possible Causes	Signs and Symptoms	Interventions
Infiltration: The escape of solution into interstitial tissues	Venipuncture device dislodged from vein Perforated vein wall	Blanching of skin at the site Coolness Swelling at or above the site Feeling of fullness or tightness at the site Pain or burning at the site but may also be painless Infusion continues when the vein is occluded	**Restorative:** Reassure patient there is no permanent harm. Discontinue the infusion. Restart the IV in another site above infiltrated area or preferably in other limb. Apply warm compresses to the site to aid absorption and for comfort. Elevate the limb to encourage venous return. **Protective:** Use an over-the-needle catheter, if possible. Select the most appropriate device. Avoid sites in areas of flexion or excessive movement. Anchor the device securely. Check the infusion frequently. Instruct the patient to report any discomfort or swelling.
Phlebitis: Inflammation of the vein wall	Mechanical trauma during insertion of infusion device or from sliding movement of the device Needle or catheter too large for size of vein Device left in vein too long Infection due to contamination Weakened veins from repeated infusions Chemical irritation from IV solutions, medications, or incompatible additives Infusion rate too rapid	Local tenderness, pain along the vein Redness, warmth, and induration (hardness) along the course of the vein Swelling at or above the site Burning sensation along the vein Slight temperature elevation	**Restorative:** Discontinue the infusion. Apply warm compresses to stimulate circulation and for comfort. Restart the IV in other limb. Report to physician if temperature is elevated. **Protective:** Use the smallest device possible. Use an over-the-needle catheter if possible. Stabilize the device securely to prevent sliding movement. Change the IV site q48–72h. Use intermittent rather than prolonged continuous infusions. Use large veins if infusing irritating solutions. Dilute solutions or additives sufficiently. Infuse solutions at the prescribed rate. Use pumps or controllers for irritating solutions.

continued on next page

TABLE 33.13 continued

Complication	Possible Causes	Signs and Symptoms	Interventions
Thrombophlebitis: A blood clot at the tip of the needle or catheter or along the inner wall of the vein Can be a potential source of bacterial growth	IV inserted in an area of flexion Infusion rate too slow Inflammation leading to damage of the tunica intima (platelets adhere to roughened surface) Incompatible drug additives resulting in obstruction	Tenderness Redness Swollen, hardened vein Slow or stopped infusion	**Restorative:** Discontinue the infusion. Apply warm compresses. Restart the IV in other limb. DO NOT massage or rub the affected limb. Report to physician. Watch for signs of infection. **Protective:** Maintain prescribed rate of flow. Use a microdrop set or an infusion pump or controller for slow infusion rates. Check the infusion frequently. Dilute additives. Check drug incompatibilities carefully.
Infection: Invasion of pathogenic organisms into the body May be local or systemic	Entry of microorganisms during insertion or with breaks in techniques during site care Movement of device allowing organisms into the vein Use of contaminated equipment Leak in the system Opening the system, thus exposing patient to airborne bacteria Patient's own bacteria Device left in vein too long Weakened immune system	Redness, warmth, and swelling at site Tenderness Purulent drainage from site Possible chills, malaise, elevated temperature	**Restorative:** Assess for all possible causes. If local, discontinue the infusion. Send a swab for O&S, if site purulent. Report to physician if temperature elevated. Monitor vital signs. Restart the IV in other limb. **Protective:** Wash hands and use meticulous aseptic technique during all IV procedures. Use sterile equipment. Check equipment for contamination and leaks. Replace contaminated equipment promptly. Change equipment as per agency policy or as recommended by the Health Protection Branch–Health Canada (HPB). Ensure that venipuncture device is securely anchored. Avoid using sites near joints or immobilize the joint with an armboard as necessary.

TABLE 23.12 *continued*

Complication	Possible Causes	Signs and Symptoms	Interventions
Circulatory overload: An increase in circulating fluid volume above normal	Infusion rate overly rapid Excessive volume of infused fluid in patients with impaired cardiac and renal function	Headache Discomfort Flushed skin Engorged neck veins Tachycardia Tachypnea Increased blood pressure Shortness of breath Cough and crackles heard in lung bases on auscultation Cyanosis Chest pain	**Restorative:** Slow the infusion rate and keep the vein open. Place the patient in semi-Fowler's position. Report to physician. Monitor vital signs, intake and output. Administer O_2 as ordered. **Protective:** Maintain prescribed flow rate. Question IV orders that call for excessive amounts of fluids to be infused. Monitor the infusion and patient's response frequently.

Older and very young patients are more susceptible to circulatory overload; therefore, infusion rates must be monitored very carefully. Use of microdrop administration sets or pumps/controllers is recommended for these patients.

Central Venous Therapy

Increasingly, in modern-day health care, patients are receiving intravenous solutions containing medications (anticancer agents) or nutrients (additives in total parental nutrition) that are irritating to small peripheral veins. These solutions, however, are well tolerated by large veins because the high volume of blood flowing through them permits rapid dilution of the irritating substances. In addition, there are many people for whom peripheral intravenous therapy is no longer possible because their veins are inaccessible owing to scarring or sclerosing. Over the last 20 years, three categories of central venous devices have been developed: percutaneous, tunnelled and implanted.

In central venous therapy a large-gauge catheter, made of polyurethane, polyvinylchloride (PVC) or silicone rubber, is inserted into a major vein in the body. The vessels most commonly used are the right and left subclavian veins, the right cephalic vein, the right or left internal and external jugular veins and the femoral vein. A sterile catheter is inserted into a central vein through an incision made in the skin or through a tunnel made in the subcutaneous tissue. The catheter is threaded through the vein until its tip rests in either the superior vena cava, the inferior vena cava or the right atrium of the heart. A central catheter may also be inserted through a peripheral vein and advanced into the central venous circulation. Referred to as a *peripherally inserted central catheter* (PICC), the catheter is usually inserted into the basilic, median cubital veins in the antecubital fossa of the arm and threaded into the axillary vein, the subclavian vein or the superior vena cava.

Figure 23.17 shows several common pathways for central venous catheter insertion. In Canada, some specially trained nurses now insert PICC lines. As the threading of the catheter is done without the benefit of fluoroscopy or direct visualization, the increments on the catheter assist the nurse in determining the length to be inserted in order to reach the superior vena cava.

Midclavicular lines terminate in the subclavian or innominate vein rather than the superior vena cava. Differentiating between the midclavicular and PICC lines is necessary prior to use, as midclavicular lines are used only for administering isotonic fluids and medications. Careful documentation of the catheter tip by the nurse, or the physician inserting the catheter, is necessary for safe practice.

There are several benefits to central venous therapy. As we mentioned above, central venous infusion provides an effective way of administering solutions that must be diluted, such as irritating medications or hypertonic fluids. It allows rapid delivery of large amounts of fluids in emergencies or in cases where peripheral veins have collapsed owing to decreased peripheral circulation. A central venous line also permits monitoring of central venous pressure, which is an indicator of the patient's circulatory functioning, blood volume and pumping efficiency of the heart. By providing long-term venous access, this route eliminates the frequent venipunctures needed to establish peripheral lines or obtain blood samples for diagnostic testing.

Central venous therapy also provides a benefit to patients who require the infusion of two or more solutions

The illustrations below show several common pathways for central venous (CV) catheter insertion. Typically, a CV catheter is inserted into the subclavian vein or the internal jugular vein. The catheter may terminate in the superior vena cava or in the right atrium.

Insertion: Subclavian vein
Termination: Superior vena cava

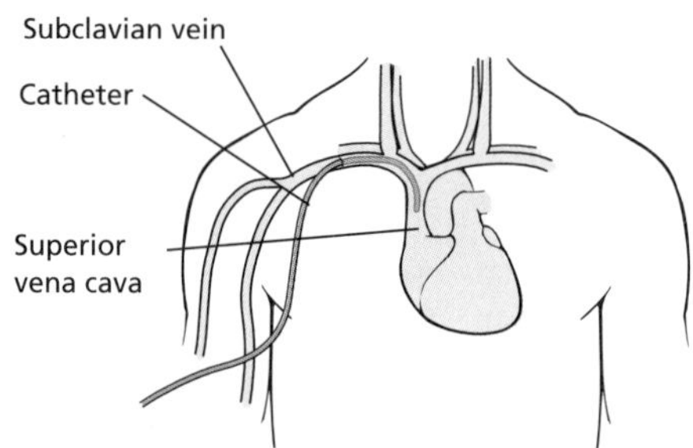

Insertion: Subclavian vein
Termination: Right atrium

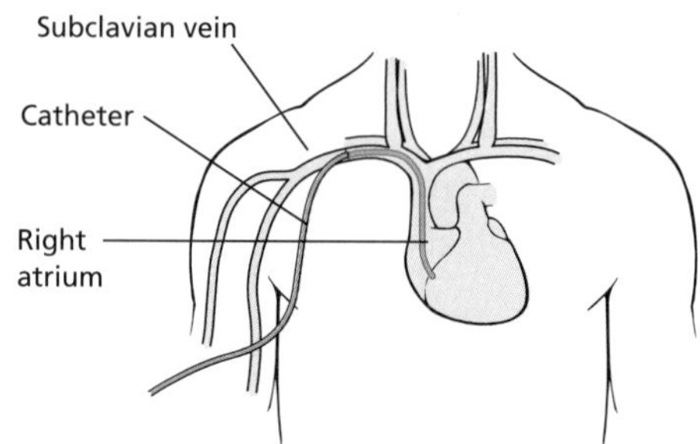

Insertion: Internal jugular vein
Termination: Superior vena cava

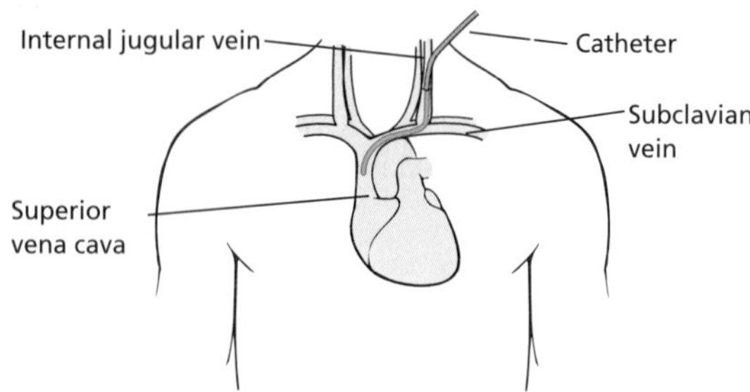

Insertion: Basilic vein (peripheral)
Termination: Superior vena cava

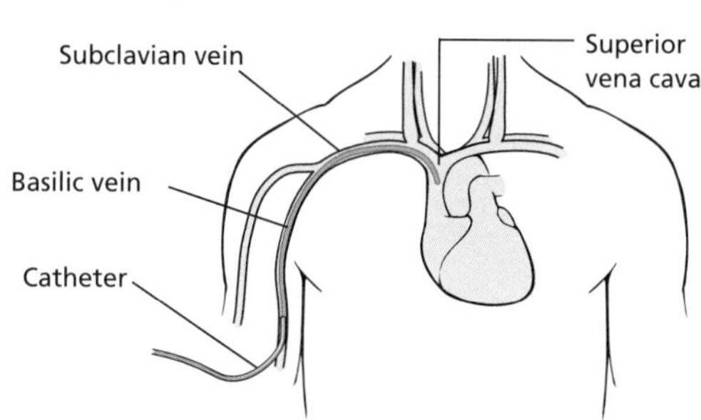

Insertion: Through a subcutaneous tunnel to the subclavian vein (Dacron cuff helps hold catheter in place)
Termination: Superior vena cava

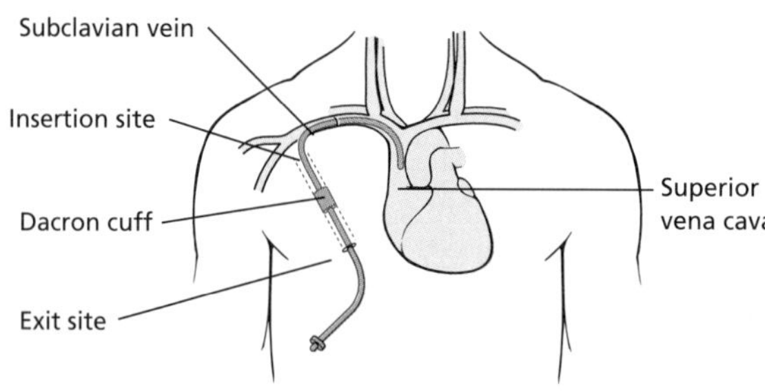

FIGURE 23.17 Central venous catheter pathways

SOURCE: Krozek, 1993, p. 292.

at the same time. For example, a patient with cancer may need to receive analgesics, antibiotics and chemotherapy along with parenteral nutrition. A multilumen catheter in which two or three lumens function separately permits uninterrupted infusion of parenteral nutrition while medications are being administered and also provides a lumen for drawing blood. When used intermittently, the lumens are capped and flushed with a heparin solution to keep them patent (Weinstein, 1997).

Central venous therapy, however, also has a number of disadvantages. More skill and time is required to insert central venous lines: some of the catheters have to be inserted surgically in an operating room or with the assistance of fluoroscopy in the radiology department. Because of the location of the catheters, there is increased risk of life-threatening complications such as pneumothorax, sepsis, thrombus formation and perforation of the vessel. Central venous lines require specialized, meticulous nursing care.

Insertion of a Percutaneous Central Venous Line

Percutaneous central venous catheters are inserted at the bedside using strict aseptic technique. The percutaneously inserted central catheter exits the skin directly over the vein accessed. These catheters are meant for short-term use (days to months) and are the least expensive and most commonly used central venous devices.

[illegible]

stands the purpose and benefits of central venous therapy, the insertion procedure and possible risks involved. In addition, answer any questions or concerns that he or she might have. Tell patients that, for their safety and well-being, it is important that they lie still during the procedure and stay in the position in which they are placed. When the jugular vein is used, a sterile cloth or drape is placed over the head, and the patient may be asked to wear a face mask covering the mouth and nose. Reassure patients that although it may feel dark and warm under the drapes, they will be able to breathe normally, and that the procedure may feel uncomfortable because of positioning and draping. A stinging sensation might be felt at the insertion site when the local anesthetic is given, and the patient may feel pressure when the catheter is inserted. Any pain should be reported to the doctor immediately.

During insertion of the catheter, the patient will be instructed to perform the Valsalva manoeuvre, which prevents air from entering the catheter by raising intrathoracic pressure. It also slows the heart rate, decreases the return of blood to the heart and increases venous pressure. To perform the Valsalva manoeuvre, instruct the patient to take a deep breath, hold it and then bear down for 10 seconds. After this, the patient can exhale and breathe normally.

Once inserted, the catheter will be sutured in place to prevent dislodgement. After the insertion, any feelings of pain or pressure at the site, shortness of breath or light-headedness should be reported to the nurse. The patient should also call the nurse if the dressing becomes wet or loose (Weinstein, 1997).

ASSEMBLING EQUIPMENT Many agencies have specially prepared carts that hold the supplies and equipment for central venous catheter insertions. A typical cart would include:

1. reusable CV catheter insertion bundles or sets containing a sterile gown for the physician, drapes, containers for solutions, forceps and Kelly clamps, a needle driver and gauze sponges
2. disposable CV catheterization kits containing a CV catheter, an inducer needle and vessel dilator, a 5-mL syringe, a scalpel and blade, straight silk suture material, prep sponges and gauze pads
3. dressing trays
4. IV administration sets, extension tubing, vented tubing, pump sets and solutions
5. masks and sterile gloves
6. shave preparation kits and razors
7. local anesthetic solutions and 25-gauge needles
8. skin cleansing solutions such as chlorhexidine, povidone–iodine solution and 70% alcohol
9. [illegible]
10. intermittent injection caps (an IV pole and infusion pump are also needed)
11. Iodium chloride and heparin solution.

The cart is taken to the bedside, where the nurse assists the physician by opening packages and readying the equipment. The choice of catheter type and size depends on the purpose of therapy. For example, a multilumen catheter would be selected for the patient who needs multiple infusions over a short period of time. Catheters vary in length, number of lumens, purposes, duration of use and method of insertion. Table 23.13 illustrates some of the more commonly used central venous catheters. Agency policies vary with respect to priming the administration set.

An extension tubing is attached to the administration set. On this tubing is a *slider clamp* (Figure 23.18), which is used as a safety device to guard against entry of air into the system. It is kept open when an infusion is running but must be closed if an infusion has stopped (see Procedure 23.5).

Surgical Insertion of a Central Venous Line

Tunnelled and implanted central venous catheters are usually surgically inserted in the operating room or with the assistance of fluoroscopy in the radiology department. In a tunnelled central venous catheter, a tunnel is created in the subcutaneous tissue of the chest wall so that the insertion site in the vein is away from the exit site in the skin (Figure 23.17). In the subcutaneous tunnel, the catheter is encircled with a Dacron cuff. Tissue growth into the material of the cuff anchors the catheter and forms a seal against microorganisms (Weinstein, 1997).

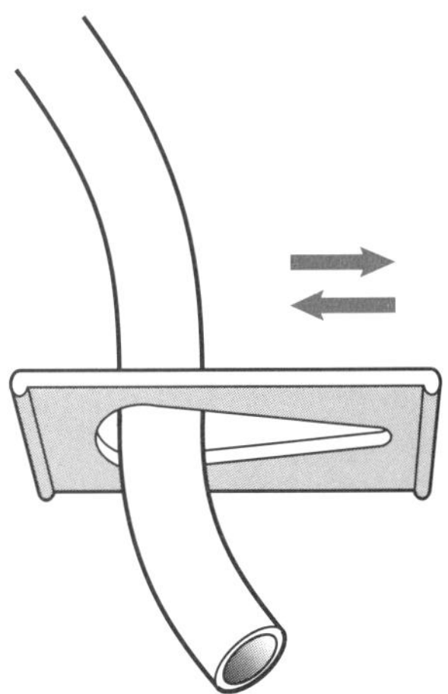

FIGURE 23.18 Slider clamp

TABLE 23.13 Types of central venous lines

Type	*Characteristics*	*Indications for Use*	*Advantages and Disadvantages*	*Nursing Implications*
Percutaneous Single-lumen catheter	• Polyvinylchloride (PVC) or polyurethane • 20 cm long • Lumen gauge varies • Sutured in place	• Short-term CV access • Emergency access • Patient requires one type of infusion solution	**Advantages** • Easy to insert at bedside • Easy to remove **Disadvantages** • Limits infusion to one solution • Short-term therapy • PVC is thrombogenic and irritates inner lumen and vessel	• Minimize patient movement • Assess frequently for signs of infection or clot formation • Smooth-jawed clamp at the bedside at all times • Sterile dressing required
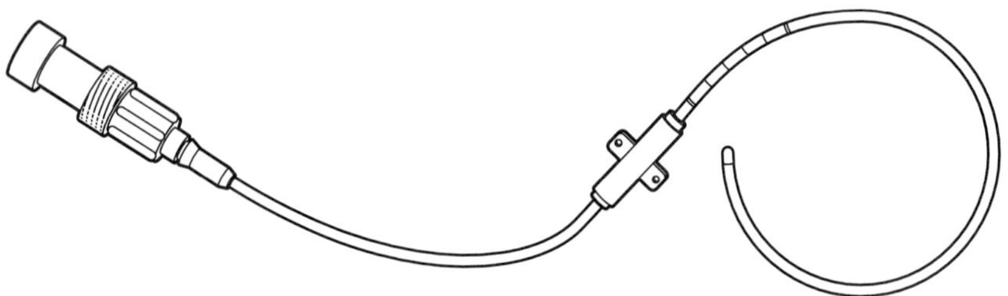				
Percutaneous Multilumen catheter	• PVC or polyurethane • Two or three lumens exiting at 2-cm intervals • Lumen gauges vary • Sutured in place	• Short-term CV access • Patient requires multiple types of infusion solutions	**Advantages** • As for single-lumen catheter • Allows simultaneous infusion of multiple purpose (even incompatible) solutions **Disadvantages** • As for single-lumen catheter	• Know gauge and purpose of each lumen • Use the same lumen for the same purpose • smooth-jawed clamps at the bedside at all times • Sterile dressing required
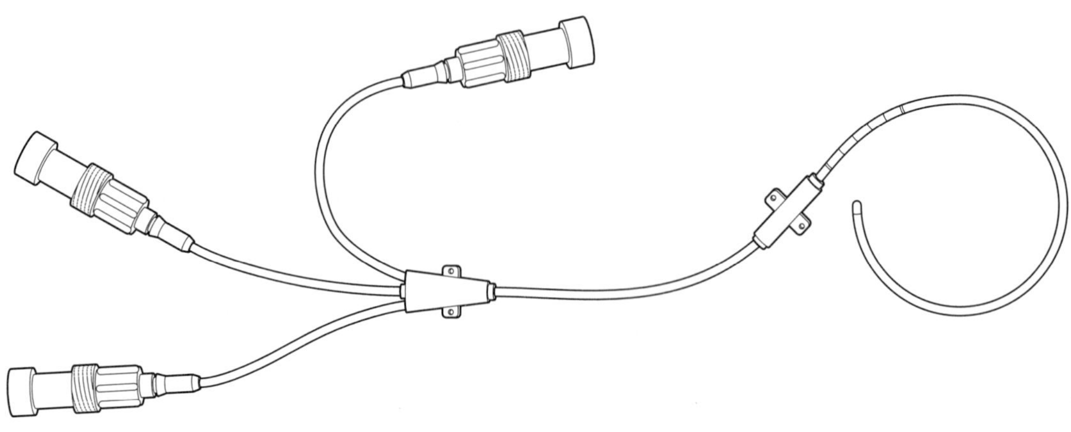				

TABLE 23.13 *continued*

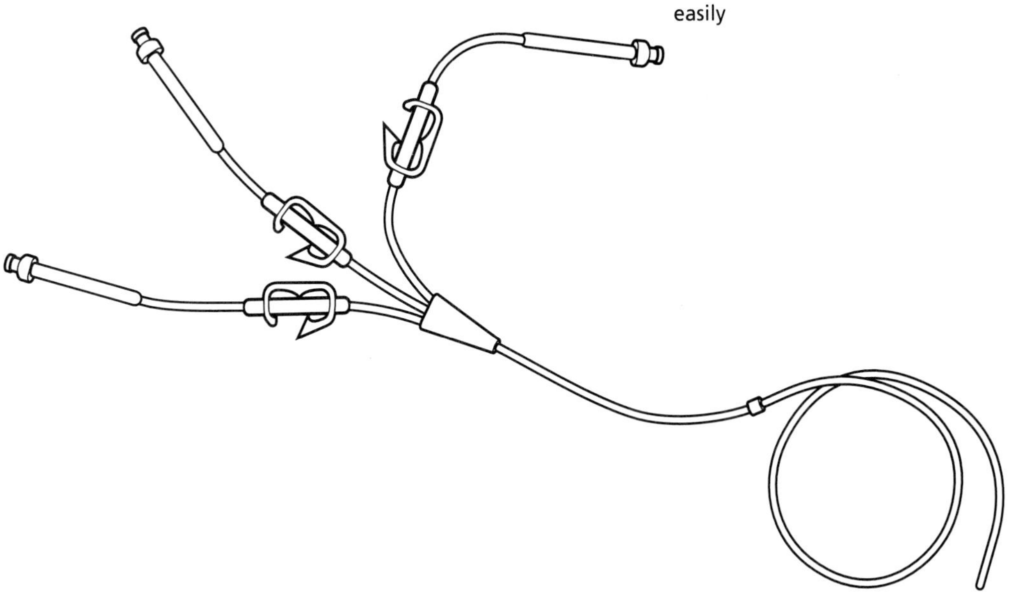

Type	*Characteristics*	*Indications for Use*	*Advantages and Disadvantages*	*Nursing Implications*
Tunnelled Hickman catheter (Broviac, Groshong)	• Silicone rubber • 90 cm long • Dacron cuff • Single- or multilumen	• Long-term CV access • Home therapy	**Advantages** • Less thrombogenic • Dacron cuff prevents excessive motion and migration of bacteria **Disadvantages** • Requires surgical insertion • Requires doctor for removal • Tears and kinks easily	• Sterile dressing required • Handle catheter gently • Observe for kinks or tears • Have repair kit available
Implanted Port-a-Cath/ Bard port	• Silicone rubber catheter combined with a self-sealing rubber disk or septum • Catheter is tunnelled surgically and attached to a port • Port is implanted into a subcutaneous pocket	• Long-term CV access • Home therapy • Intermittent use	• Totally implanted • More discreet • Minimal care when not in use (flush 1x/mo.) • Requires specially designed, noncoring needle to access • Requires surgical insertion, doctor to remove	• Requires training to learn to access port • Sterile dressing required

SOURCE: Krozek, 1993, 294-295.

PROCEDURE 23.5

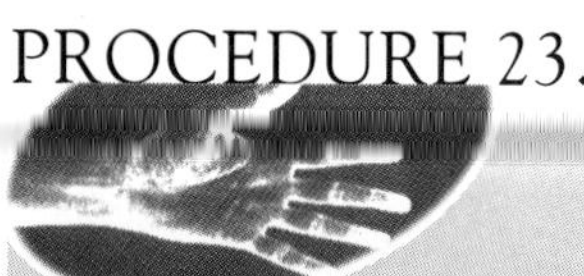

Assisting with a Bedside Central Venous Catheter Insertion

Action	*Rationale*
1. Gather equipment and supplies: • CV catheter insertion set • CV catheterization kit • dressing tray • IV administration set, tubings and solutions per agency policy • masks and sterile gloves • shave preparation kit and razor • skin cleansing solutions, chlorhexidine, povidone–iodine and 70% alcohol • local anesthetic solutions and 25-gauge needle • intermittent injection caps for multilumen catheters, sodium chloride and heparin solution • sterile gauze pads • nonallergenic tape and transparent semi-permeable dressing • IV pole and infusion pump.	Facilitates efficiency and economy of time.
2. Identify the patient.	Avoids error.
3. Prepare the patient for what to expect and provide support during each stage of the procedure.	Helps to reduce anxiety and tension; enhances the patient's well-being and comfort.
4. Apply a mask and wash hands thoroughly.	Prevents introducing contaminants during procedure.
5. Set up a sterile field on the over-bed table and ready the equipment for insertion.	
6. Shave (as necessary) and cleanse the site per agency protocol.	Decreases microorganisms on the skin.
7. When using the subclavian or jugular vein, place the patient in the Trendelenburg position, with a towel between the scapulae.	Dilates the vein and decreases risk of air embolism.
8. Turn the patient's head away from the insertion site.	Makes the site more accessible and prevents possible contamination from airborne bacteria in the patient's breath.
9. After masking, gowning and gloving, the physician will cover the site with sterile drapes.	Creates a sterile field.
10. Assist with injection of local anesthetic as required.	Promotes patient comfort.
11. Support the patient while the catheter is inserted through the skin and threaded through the vein to the vena cava or right atrium.	Promotes physical and emotional well-being.
12. Instruct the patient to perform the Valsalva manoeuvre while the physician attaches the tubing to the catheter hub.	Keeps the vein patent and closes the catheter to air. Because of the forces of fluid flow and pressure changes in the thoracic cavity, a negative pressure develops at the tip of the catheter if it is not filled with fluid or if it is open to air. This negative pressure draws air into the catheter, creating an air embolism. The Valsalva manoeuvre prevents air from being drawn into the catheter by increasing intrathoracic pressure.
13. Set the infusion flow at a keep-the-vein open rate.	Keeps the vein patent. D5W or NS is used until placement of the catheter is confirmed. Infusing an isotonic solution avoids the risk of vessel wall thrombosis.
14. After the catheter is sutured in place, cleanse the insertion site and apply a sterile dressing according to agency protocol.	Stabilizes the catheter and prevents entry of microorganisms.
15. Assist the patient to a comfortable position.	Makes it easier to breathe and decreases the chance of hematoma formation.

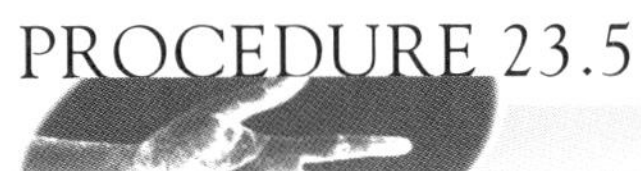

PROCEDURE 23.5 *continued*

Action	Rationale
16. Monitor the patient's response to the catheter insertion. Observe patient's breathing and note any chest pain.	Indicates possible complications of pneumothorax and arrhythmias.
17. Complete requisition for chest x-ray as ordered.	Chest x-ray is needed to ensure correct placement.
18. Document the procedure, noting the date and time of insertion; length, type and location of catheter; name of physician; type of solution and rate of infusion; blood samples drawn; type of dressing applied; condition of the site; and patient's response to the procedure. Once the x-ray has been completed and placement is confirmed, therapy may be initiated.	Fulfills requirements for nurse accountability.

PREOPERATIVE PREPARATION Preoperative care for a patient having a surgical insertion of a central venous catheter is similar to that of any operative procedure. A preoperative checklist is completed and a consent form is signed. As with any invasive procedure, the patient must be informed about and have an understanding of the procedure and the possible risks involved. If a general anesthetic is to be used, the patient may be required to fast after midnight. Frequently, the insertion is completed under local anesthetic, in which case fasting is not required. The morning of the procedure, the patient should have a shower with an antibacterial soap per agency protocol. The anterior chest wall is cleansed thoroughly and the appropriate area is shaved, if necessary.

During the procedure, a small incision is made in the chest wall above the chosen vein and another incision is made between the nipple and the sternum. An instrument is inserted through the subcutaneous tissue to create a tunnel. The catheter is pulled through the tunnel and out the exit incision. The catheter is threaded through the vein under fluoroscopic examination to verify that the tip is positioned correctly in the superior vena cava or the right atrium of the heart. Sutures are used to close the incisions and sterile opaque dressings are applied.

POSTOPERATIVE CARE When the patient returns to the ward the nurse will assess the patient's comfort level, vital signs and dressings per agency postoperative protocol. The patient is asked to stay in bed for a few hours to ensure that there is no bleeding from the sites. The dressing over the insertion sites may be removed after 48 hours. Patients may shower or bathe once the dressings are off, but the incisions must be kept dry for at least seven days. The exit site must be dressed and cared for as long as the catheter remains in place. Surgical placement of a central line is most often done in a day-care setting; thus, discharge instructions must be clear.

Implanted Central Venous Access Device

An implanted vascular access device (IVAD) consists of a small port or reservoir with a self-sealing rubber disc (septum) and a radiopaque silicone catheter (see Figure 23.19). The device is surgically implanted into a subcutaneous pocket adjacent to the central vein (commonly the subclavian or internal jugular) into which the catheter is inserted. A special type of needle, called the Huber point needle, is used to access the catheter. This needle has a curved tip that slices the septum rather than coring it; as a result, the septum reseals itself more effectively. The needle is then taped to the skin and attached to intravenous equipment.

An IVAD is aesthetically more appealing to patients than a central venous catheter because there are no external parts and it allows complete freedom in daily activities when not in use. There is less chance of infection because the catheter does not exit the skin and there are no exposed parts to be subjected to damage or dislodgement.

The purpose and functions of an IVAD are like those of long-term central venous catheters, that is, to deliver intravenous fluids, parenteral nutrition, medications and blood and blood products and to obtain blood samples. IVADs are inserted into patients who require intermittent or continuous venous access for periods of months to years. This includes individuals of any age with terminal illnesses such as cancer, cystic fibrosis and AIDS as well as people with sickle cell anemia, inflammatory bowel disease and congestive heart failure. The IVAD is not recommended for patients with inadequate body tissue (for example, those who are malnourished) to support the device. It is also not recommended for patients who are extremely obese and those who have had mastectomies and radiation to the chest.

Care for an IVAD is the same as for a central venous catheter. Preoperative and postoperative care for implanting an IVAD are like that for a surgical insertion of a central venous catheter. In the first 24 hours postoperative, the

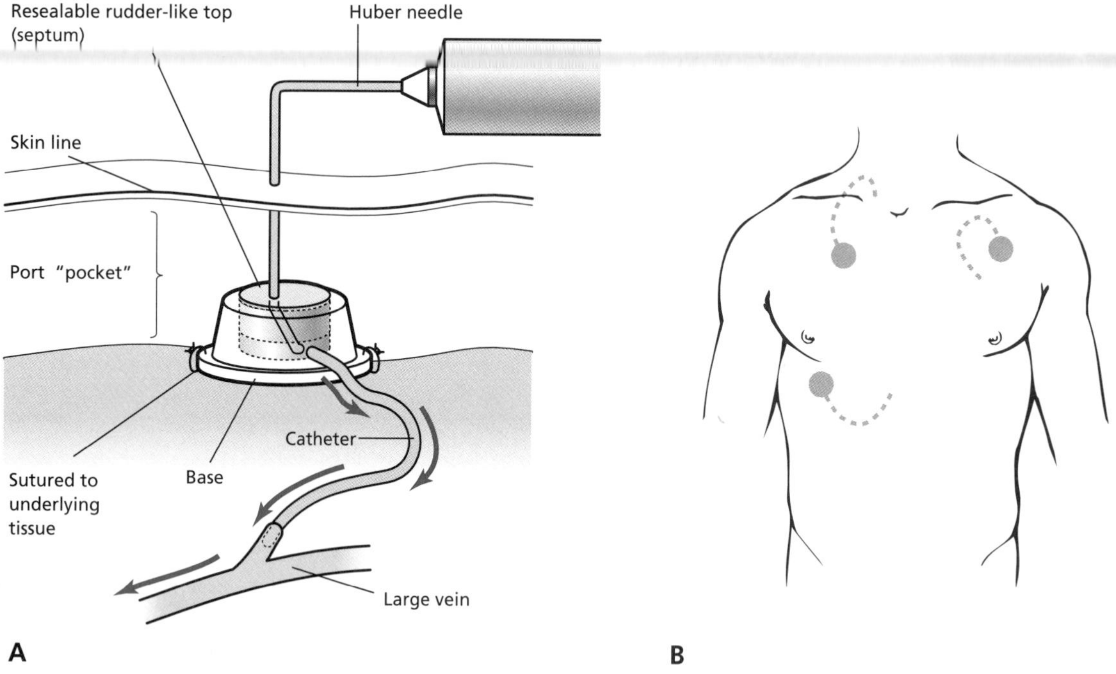

FIGURE 23.19 Implanted vascular access device. A. Port design. B. Common sites

SOURCE: Camp-Sorrell, 1992, p.264 (A only).

head of the patient's bed should be raised 30°–40° to decrease pressure on the area and promote comfort. The tissue surrounding an IVAD is very tender and may be bruised from the creation of the pocket. Patients may require analgesia for the control of discomfort. The pressure dressing over the insertion site is usually removed in 24–48 hours. It is not uncommon to have a scant amount of serosanguineous drainage on the dressing. The site is assessed for tenderness, redness and swelling. After the dressing is removed, the patient may shower or bathe. However, the site should remain dry. The sutures are usually removed seven to 14 days postoperatively.

The care for an accessed IVAD (that is, one being used for intravenous therapy) is similar to the care for a central venous line. In addition to the standard assessment for a central venous catheter, the Huber needle must be checked to ensure that it is firmly secured in the skin at a 90° angle. The covering dressing should be dry and intact. As with central venous lines, the nurse caring for the patient may change solution containers. All other interventions—tubing and injection cap changes as well as flushing and heparinizing the device—are carried out by certified nurses.

Although the incidence is low, the risk of complications with implanted venous access devices is always present. Infection, the most common complication, can be prevented with strict aseptic technique. Thrombosis, occlusions, infiltration and air embolism have occurred occasionally. One unique complication with an IVAD is *Twiddler's syndrome.* In this syndrome the catheter becomes disconnected from the port as a result of frequent manipulation of the device by the patient. The signs and symptoms include tenderness, redness and edema at the insertion site. Should such a disconnection be suspected, the nurse must stop the infusion and notify the physician promptly. Comfort measures such as cold compresses to the site may be implemented. The patient is also prepared for an x-ray.

Implanted venous access devices require minimal care when they are not being used for intravenous therapy. Any type of clothing may be worn, but care should be taken to avoid clothes that rub or apply pressure to the site. Car seat belts, especially shoulder straps, may have to be adjusted. Individuals may bathe, shower or swim as they normally would. There are no restrictions on activities, although aggressive contact sports such as football should be avoided. The patient should manipulate the device as little as possible to decrease the potential for infection and Twiddler's syndrome.

Daily inspection for swelling, redness, tenderness and discharge should be carried out. Any abnormal findings should be reported immediately. IVADs require monthly flushing with normal saline or a heparin solution to maintain their patency. Patients may go to an agency to have the device flushed or they may be taught how to do this procedure at home. The patient should wear a medical alert bracelet or necklace and carry a medical information card stating the type of IVAD that is in place and who should be contacted in case of emergency.

Maintaining a Central Line Infusion

After a central line has been inserted, the primary respon- [illegible] safety and to prevent complications. Each agency has its own specific policies stating who is certified to care for central lines and what care is necessary.

REGULATING THE INFUSION RATE OF FLOW Infusion pumps are recommended for use with central lines to ensure accurate flow and patient safety. The nurse must program the pump correctly and monitor it frequently to ensure proper functioning.

ASSESSING THE INFUSION Frequent, careful and systematic assessments of the central venous line are necessary to ensure safe and accurate infusion. The assessment of a central venous infusion is similar to that of a peripheral intravenous infusion. Beginning at the insertion site, the nurse checks for any tenderness, redness, warmth, swelling or discharge. The catheter is also checked for kinks, obstructions or leakage. The sutures should be clean and should firmly secure the catheter in place. There should be no redness in adjacent tissues. The transparent dressing should be dry and intact; all edges should be well secured to prevent entry of microorganisms. The date and time of last dressing change is noted. In some agencies the external length of the catheter is also noted, so that a measurement can be made to determine whether the catheter may have become displaced.

The administration set is inspected to ensure that all connections are secure. Because accidental disconnections can be life-threatening, a number of steps are taken to ensure patient safety. First, only tubing with Luer-locks and Y-connectors are used in central venous therapy. All tubing connection sites are joined firmly and then Luer-locked. In addition, the connections can be tab-taped with waterproof tape. The tape is tabbed to facilitate ease of removal and to avoid trauma to the connection. The tubing is also pinned onto the patient's gown to prevent pulling at the insertion site. The threads of the locking connectors are inspected daily for wear, tear and cracks. Tubings are checked for kinks, leaks, obstructions, air bubbles or precipitate matter, and the date of the last tubing change is noted. Finally, the safety slider clamp is inspected. The clamp should be open when solution is infusing. However, if the infusion has stopped or the catheter is not in use, the clamp should be closed to prevent air from entering the catheter.

The infusion pump is assessed to make sure the pump is set at the prescribed rate and that it is functioning properly. An inspection is then made of the IV bag, noting the type of solution, the amount and type of additives, the amount infused, the amount remaining and the date and time the solution began.

The patient's response to the infusion is also monitored. The nurse must be especially alert for signs of infection including increased temperature, chills and malaise. It is important to monitor the patient's respiratory status. The pulse or apical beat should be taken to determine arrhythmias, increases in rate or decreases in strength. Finally, the fluid record is examined to determine imbalances in intake

ROUTINE INTERVENTIONS FOR CENTRAL VENOUS LINES In most agencies, routine interventions for central venous lines, with the exception of solution bag changes, are carried out by nurses who are certified. These skills include changing dressings, tubings and intermittent injection caps, as well as flushing and heparinizing the lumens. Central venous dressings are changed every 72 hours or per agency policy. Occlusive dressings must be changed every 48 hours so that the site may be assessed. Administration sets are replaced every 72 hours. Every time a connection in the system is opened, there is a risk that air and microorganisms will enter the catheter. In addition, frequent interruptions of the infusion can cause the formation of clots and occlusions.

When the central venous line or a lumen of a multiple catheter is not kept open with continuous infusion, it may be capped with an intermittent injection cap. An injection cap is a short Luer-lock device placed at the distal end of the line or lumen of the catheter. The cap keeps the line sterile and ready for access when necessary. Central venous catheters must be flushed regularly to keep them patent. Agency policies vary on the flushing procedure, the frequency and the amount and type of flushing solution that is used.

While most of the skills needed for central venous therapy are carried out by specialized nurses, the nurse assigned to care for the patient is responsible for regulating the infusion, making assessments and alerting a certified nurse immediately should problems arise. The nurse caring for the patient (this includes the nursing student) is also required to change the solution bag. In central venous therapy, solution bags are changed the same way as they are for peripheral infusions. Meticulous aseptic technique must be used to prevent the entry of microorganisms into the venous system, and care must be taken to ensure that no air bubbles enter the tubing during a bag change. Should air enter the tubing at this time, the infusion must be changed and the assistance of a certified nurse must be obtained immediately.

Preventing Complications

Complications may occur at any time during central venous therapy. It is essential for nurses to have knowledge of the common complications so that preventive measures are implemented rigorously. Restorative actions must be enacted promptly.

INFECTION The threat of infection is always present; therefore, when providing any care to a central venous catheter, meticulous aseptic technique is mandatory. Once contaminated, the catheter becomes a haven for the growth of microorganisms. Furthermore, bacteria and fungi are readily transported to the heart, the great blood vessels and the cardiac valves.

The chief cause of infection in central venous therapy is a break in sterile technique. Frequent interruptions of the system, wet or soiled dressings that remain in place and contaminated equipment also contribute to infection. The importance of strict, thorough hand-washing as a preventive measure before each procedure cannot be overemphasized. In fact, meticulous hand-washing has been recognized as the most important action against infection.

A number of measures can be implemented to prevent infection in central venous therapy. Ideally, all medications given into central venous catheters should be prepared in the pharmacy department under a laminar flow hood. Blood work, tubing changes, flushings and other procedures should be coordinated to reduce the number of times the system is opened. Intravenous push medications should be avoided, except in emergencies, to decrease the number of times the injection cap is punctured. When the cap is used, a small needle such as a 22-gauge is recommended.

When signs and symptoms of infection such as fever, chills, tenderness along the insertion site or shoulder, redness, swelling or purulent drainage from the site become evident, blood cultures are taken from the central catheter and from peripheral veins. Antibiotic therapy is instituted. If the source of infection is indeed the central venous catheter and the medications are ineffective, the catheter must be removed.

AIR EMBOLISM Although **air embolism**—the presence of a large amount of air in the circulatory system—is a rare complication, its consequences are life-threatening. An air embolism can disrupt the blood supply to parts of the body and cause serious trauma. Death can ensue if the air embolism obstructs the pulmonary circulation. The exact amount of intravenous air that can cause death is not known; therefore, the entry of any amount of air into the venous system should be prevented.

As we discussed earlier, because central veins have a negative venous pressure, air can enter the circulatory system whenever a catheter is open to air or it is not filled with fluid. This can occur when a catheter is inserted or during procedures in which the line is opened, for example, when changing bags, tubings and injection caps. Air can also enter the system when a connection becomes disconnected, a solution bag runs dry or a clamp remains open after a continuous infusion has stopped.

The signs and symptoms of air embolism will depend on the rate and amount of air taken into the venous system. The patient may display a sudden onset of chest pain, difficulty breathing, cyanosis, anxiety and confusion. On examination, the nurse may find an increasing respiratory rate, a rapid, thready pulse and hypotension. The patient may also experience nausea, restlessness, faintness, convulsions, diaphoresis and possibly cardiac arrest.

The entry of air into the patient's venous system is an emergency that must be dealt with immediately. The nurse must remain calm because his or her behaviour will have an impact on the patient's response. The central line must be clamped immediately, using the slider clamp. A padded or smooth-jawed clamp may also be used. The patient is turned onto the left side in a Trendelenburg (head down) position. This position is necessary because it causes air to collect in the apex of the right ventricle, away from the right ventricular outflow tract. This prevents the air from moving through the tricuspid valve, pulmonary artery and on to the lungs (Thelan, Davie & Urden, 1997). The physician must be notified promptly. Oxygen is administered and the patient's vital signs are monitored (Phillips, 1997; Weinstein, 1997).

OCCLUSION AND DISLODGEMENT OF THE CATHETER A central venous catheter can become partially or completely occluded when an infusion flows too slowly or stops for a long period of time, or when it has not been irrigated frequently enough. When an infusion has stopped or is *positional* (will infuse only when the patient assumes a certain position), or will infuse only at a reduced rate, a certified nurse should be notified immediately. Like peripheral infusions, central catheters can become dislodged and cause infiltration. Thrombus formation can occur, but it is rare because rapid blood flow in central veins and the slippery nature of silicone materials in the catheter inhibit clot formation.

BLOOD TRANSFUSION THERAPY

The administration of whole blood or blood components, such as plasma, red blood cells or platelets, into the venous circulation is called a **blood transfusion**. Blood transfusions are given to restore circulating blood volume following hemorrhage, trauma, surgery, shock and burns. Other uses are to correct red blood cell deficiency and improve oxygen-carrying capacity of the blood and to maintain the blood's clotting ability—for example, in patients with bone marrow suppression or hemophilia. While blood transfusion is often a life-sustaining therapy, it is a procedure that is accompanied by the risk of serious and even life-threatening reactions.

One of the major risks associated with blood transfusion occurs because blood is taken from one individual, the **donor**, and infused into another, the **recipient**. After collection, blood is processed and stored under controlled conditions and then infused into a recipient. Known as a **homologous** or **indirect transfusion**, this method carries the potential for incompatibility between the donor's blood and the recipient's blood, and for exposure to blood-borne pathogens such as hepatitis and HIV.

A method that is becoming more popular is the **autologous transfusion**, in which blood is collected from a person, stored and then transfused back into the same person at a later time. This method is safer than the homologous transfusion because it significantly decreases the risk of blood incompatibility and avoids exposure to blood-borne pathogens. Autologous transfusion is discussed later in this chapter (Weinstein, 1997).

BLOOD AND BLOOD COMPONENTS Blood is made up of formed elements and a fluid called plasma. Erythrocytes (red blood cells), leukocytes (white blood cells) and throm- [illegible] plasma contains largely water (serum) and protein (albumin, globulin and fibrinogen), as well as other substances (for example, electrolytes, carbohydrates, lipids and vitamins).

Each component of the blood has its own distinctive function. For example, erythrocytes carry oxygen from the lungs to the cells and carbon dioxide from the cells to the lungs for elimination from the body. Leukocytes guard the body against infection, while thrombocytes aid in blood clotting. The plasma carries the formed elements and other substances. Table 23.14 outlines the most common blood components along with indications for their use in blood transfusion therapy. Whole blood is rarely transfused today [illegible]

BLOOD GROUP AND RH (RHESUS) FACTOR Human blood is classified according to **blood group** (type) and Rh (Rhesus) factor. Successful transfusion therapy depends on blood group and Rh compatibility between recipient and donor blood.

Blood type depends on the presence of specific antigens on the red cell surfaces and corresponding antibodies in the plasma. *Antigens* initiate an immune response and stimulate the formation of *antibodies* to destroy the foreign

TABLE 23.14 Blood and blood components

Type	*Description*	*Uses and Special Considerations*
Whole blood	Contains all blood components	To replace blood loss from hemorrhage, surgical intervention, trauma or extensive burns. Shelf-life of 42 days. Crossmatch is necessary.
Packed red blood cells	Whole blood with 80% of the plasma removed	To restore or maintain O_2-carrying capacity in patients with anemia. To increase red blood cell mass and maintain Hgb levels following surgical blood loss or GI bleeding. Shelf-life of 42 days for stored fresh-packed cells. Frozen cells may be stored for 3 years. Must be used within 24 hours after opening or thawing. Administer within 4 hours of hanging. Crossmatch is necessary.
Platelets	Platelet sediment from platelet-rich blood re-suspended in 30–50 mL plasma	To control or prevent bleeding associated with deficiencies in the number or function of platelets. Can be stored for up to 5 days. Crossmatch is not necessary for red-cell-free products.
Plasma (fresh, fresh-frozen)	Serous component separated from whole blood. Contains clotting factors	To increase clotting factors and plasma protein levels and to expand plasma volume. Fresh plasma must be administered within 6 hours of collection. Fresh-frozen plasma may be stored for 3 months and must be given within 2 hours of thawing. Crossmatch is not necessary.
Cryoprecipitate	Factor VIII (antihemophilic factor) and fibrinogen recovered from frozen plasma	To control bleeding in patients with classical hemophilia or Factor VIII deficiency and to replace fibrinogen. Frozen cryoprecipitate may be stored for 12 months. Must be given within 6 hours of thawing. Crossmatch is not necessary.
Albumin 5% or 25%	Heat treated, chemically processed fraction of pooled plasma	To expand blood volume in patients with hypovolemia, replace plasma albumin and maintain electrolyte balance. May be stored for 3 years at room temperature. Crossmatch is not necessary.

SOURCES: Weinstein, 1997; Phillips, 1997; Earnest, 1993.

invaders. In blood, the antibodies inactivate antigens by agglutination (clumping together of red blood cells) and hemolysis (disintegration of red blood cells with the release of hemoglobin into the plasma). Tests for blood type and compatibility are based on these antigen–antibody reactions.

A person's blood type (A, B, AB or O) is genetically determined by two antigens, A and B, which are present on the surface of the red blood cells. People with A antigens have type-A blood and those with B antigens have type-B blood. Some people have both A and B antigens; their blood group is type-AB. Still others carry neither A nor B antigens on their red cell surfaces. These people have type-O blood.

Correspondingly, plasma contains genetically determined antibodies that act against any A or B antigens that are naturally not present in the blood. For example, type-B blood, which does not normally contain A antigens, has naturally occurring anti-A antibodies present in the serum. Giving type-A blood to a person with type-B blood would result in a blood incompatibility because the anti-A antibodies in the recipient's plasma would act against the A antigen in the donor blood.

Therefore, in homologous transfusion therapy, the blood of the donor must be matched to the blood type of the recipient, since the recipient's plasma contains the incompatible antibodies. Table 23.15 lists ABO compatibilities and incompatibilities. Note that type-O blood has neither A nor B antigens. It, therefore, can be donated to individuals with any of the four blood groups. A person with type-O blood is referred to as a *universal donor*. On the other hand, people with type-AB blood have neither anti-A nor anti-B antibodies in their plasma. These people are called universal recipients because they can receive all blood types.

Another constituent of blood that can cause a hemolytic reaction is the Rh factor. The **Rh factor** is also an inherited antigen, referred to as antigen D, present on the surface of red blood cells. People with antigen D in their blood are classified as Rh positive (Rh+); those without it are Rh negative (Rh–). Unlike the ABO system in which anti-A and anti-B antibodies occur naturally, exposure to the D antigen is necessary for production of Rh antibodies. If a person with Rh negative blood receives Rh positive blood, that person's body will begin to produce anti-D antibodies. These antibodies stay in the system; a subsequent transfusion with Rh positive blood would result in a reaction causing hemolysis and agglutination of red blood cells (Weinstein, 1997).

BLOOD TYPING AND CROSSMATCHING In order to administer blood safely, the recipient's blood must be typed and compared with donor blood to ensure that the two are compatible. The blood test that is done to determine a patient's blood group is called **typing**. **Crossmatching** is a procedure performed to establish compatibility between donor and recipient blood.

ADMINISTERING BLOOD AND BLOOD COMPONENTS Blood transfusions can result in life-threatening complications, the most common resulting from incorrect identification of patients or the administration of incompatible blood (LaRocca & Otto, 1993). When administering blood transfusions, nurses must judiciously follow the agency protocol and guidelines for identifying the patient and blood product, initiating and maintaining the infusion and monitoring the patient for adverse reactions. Procedure 23.6 outlines the nursing actions for administering, maintaining and discontinuing a blood transfusion.

PREPARING THE PATIENT The nurse explains the need for a blood transfusion, the component the patient will be getting and the possibility of adverse reactions. Sometimes patients refuse blood transfusion for religious or personal reasons. When this happens, the patient is asked to sign a "refusal of treatment" form and the physician is notified of the patient's decision. Once verbal agreement for the transfusion is given, the nurse obtains information about allergies and previous experiences with blood transfusions. In addition, the patient is instructed to report chills, nausea, itching, rash, headache, shortness of breath or any other unusual symptoms.

The patient's vital signs are taken within 30 minutes prior to starting the transfusion for later assessment and evaluation. If the patient has a peripheral or central venous line, the nurse should assess the site and the infusion for patency and signs of complications. With peripheral lines, the needle or catheter gauge must be large enough for a blood infusion, that is, at least a 19-gauge butterfly needle and an 18-gauge or 20-gauge catheter. Smaller-gauge needles can cause damage to the red blood cells and significantly

TABLE 23.15 ABO blood compatibilities and incompatibilities

Blood Type	*Antigen*	*Antibody*	*Compatible Donor*	*Incompatible Donor*
A	A	Anti-B	A, O	B, AB
B	B	Anti-A	B, O	A, AB
AB	A, B	None	A, B, AB, O	None
O	None	Anti-A, Anti-B	O	A, B, AB

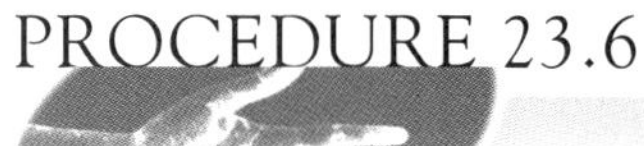

Administering Blood and Blood Components

Action	Rationale
1. Prepare the patient. Assess an existing IV line for patency and note the gauge of the venipuncture device. Take the patient's TPR and BP.	Keeps the patient informed and reduces anxiety. Facilitates decision making and organization of care. Provides baseline values.
2. Gather equipment and supplies: • straight or Y-type blood administration set with filter • primary IV administration set, if using a straight blood set • 500 mL NS solution • supplies for venipuncture if required (see Procedure 23.2). Use an 18- or 20-gauge catheter or larger • alcohol swabs, adhesive tape • clean gloves.	Facilitates efficiency and economy of time.
3. Wash hands.	Reduces risk of contamination.
4. Establish normal saline infusion. **When using a straight blood set with an existing IV:** Replace the solution bag with normal saline. **When using a Y-type blood set with an existing IV:** Don gloves, discontinue the existing solution and tubing and connect the primed Y-type set to the venipuncture device. **When establishing a peripheral line for use of a straight blood set:** Initiate the IV using a primed primary administration set. **When establishing a peripheral line for use of a Y-type administration set:** Initiate the IV using the primed Y-type tubing. Make sure the branch of the tubing that will be attached to the blood bag is clamped off.	Prepares the line and keeps the vein open until the blood transfusion is commenced. Blood and blood components must be commenced within 30 minutes of leaving the refrigerator in the blood bank. Therefore, the infusion should be established before the blood product is obtained from the blood bank.
5. Obtain and, with a second registered nurse, identify the blood product. A. Verify doctor's order. B. Compare the information on the blood bag identification label and recipient identification tag to that on the blood requisition form: • the patient's first and last name, birth date and hospital number • the unit number, the blood group, Rh factor and expiration date. C. Verify that the unit number on the blood identification label is the same as on the recipient identification tag.	Ensures safety. Avoids error and possible reactions.
D. Check the blood for abnormal colour, clumping or bubbles.	Indicates contamination.
E. Enter signatures as indicated on the blood requisition form.	
6. At the bedside, identify the patient. Compare the first and last name, birth date and hospital number on the patient's identification bracelet to that on the recipient identification tag. Blood must NEVER be administered to a patient who is not wearing an identification bracelet.	Ensures that the correct patient will receive the blood product.
7. Gently invert the blood bag several times.	Mixes the plasma and cells.

continued on next page

PROCEDURE 23.6 *continued*

Action	*Rationale*
8. Don clean gloves and prime the blood administration set and start the infusion.	
When using a Y-type set: Insert the spike of the remaining branch into the blood bag and hang the bag on the IV pole. Open the clamp on the tubing that connects the spike to the filter and squeeze the drip chamber until the filter is entirely covered with blood. Clamp the normal saline to begin the infusion of blood.	To function optimally, the filter should be entirely covered with blood.
When using a straight set: Prime the tubing using established procedure. Disconnect the primary tubing with normal saline and connect the blood tubing to the venipuncture device. To begin infusion, open the roller clamp on the blood administration set. Put a sterile cap on the connector end of the primary tubing and attach it to the roller clamp.	Keeps the primary IV line with normal saline ready for hook-up should blood reaction occur.
9. Regulate the infusion rate of flow to no more than 3 mL/min for the first 15 minutes. Remove gloves.	Transfusion reactions of flow frequently occur within the first 15 min.
10. Check vital signs and monitor the patient per agency protocol. Observe for signs of transfusion reaction. See Table 23.16.	Enables early detection of and prompt intervention for transfusion reactions.
11. If signs of reactions appear, stop the blood immediately. Re-establish the primary IV and keep the vein open with normal saline. Take vital signs and notify the doctor.	Minimizes the severity of the reaction.
12. If there are no reactions after 15 minutes, regulate the flow at the prescribed rate. A unit of blood should be infused within four hours. Blood that has not infused within the time allowance must be stopped and returned to the blood bank.	Red blood cells start to deteriorate after 30 minutes out of the refrigerator and lose their effectiveness after two hours. The longer the blood remains at room temperature, the higher the risk of bacterial growth.
13. Document the procedure on the appropriate forms, including date and time infusion commenced, size of needle or catheter, venipuncture site, type of blood component, serial number, sequence number if more than one unit, infusion rate of flow, vital signs, patient responses and any adverse reactions.	Maintains requirements for nurse accountability.
14. Continue to monitor the patient and the infusion according to agency protocol.	Reactions can occur throughout the transfusion.
15. When the infusion is completed, flush the blood tubing with normal saline.	Ensures infusion of the small amounts of blood that remain in the tubing.
16. If the patient is to receive a subsequent unit of blood, keep the vein open with normal saline.	Maintains patency of the IV until the subsequent unit is established.
17. If the transfusion is completed, re-establish an existing IV or discontinue the infusion and document the procedure and time the transfusion was finished.	
18. Return blood bag to the blood bank per agency policy.	
19. Take vital signs and continue to monitor the patient for signs of adverse reactions per agency protocol.	Delayed reactions can occur for two to three hours following an infusion.

What Not to Do When Transfusing Blood

in an unmonitored refrigerator.

- Do not keep blood out of the transfusion service's refrigerator for longer than 30 minutes before starting the transfusion.
- Do not warm blood for transfusion in a microwave oven, in an unmonitored water bath, under running water or in a sink.
- Do not heat blood components to a temperature higher than 38°C.

the appropriate blood filter.

- Do not use the same blood filter longer than four hours.
- Do not transfuse a unit of blood over a period longer than four hours.
- Do not add drugs to blood components or infuse drugs and blood through the same blood administration set.
- Do not use any solution other than 0.9% (normal) saline to prime a blood administration set, to flush the IV line or to dilute the blood product.

SOURCE: NBREP, p. 45.

TABLE 23.16 Common transfusion reactions

Type	*Causes*	*Signs and Symptoms*	*Interventions*
Hemolytic	Antibodies in the recipient's plasma react with antigens in donor blood	Chills, shakiness, flushed skin, fever, nausea, vomiting, headache, backache, dyspnea, cyanosis, chest pain, tachycardia, hypotension, oliguria, flank pain and bleeding abnormalities	Stop the transfusion immediately. Keep the vein open with normal saline. Notify the physician immediately. Return blood bag and administration set to the blood bank along with a sample of patient's blood for repeat typing and crossmatch. Monitor vital signs, intake and output, and observe for signs of bleeding. Administer O_2 and medications as ordered.
Febrile (Bacterial)	Blood contaminated with bacteria	Mild chills, fever, warm flushed skin, headache, malaise, nausea, vomiting, diarrhea Symptoms may be mild to extreme resembling a hemolytic reaction	Stop the transfusion immediately. Keep the vein open with normal saline. Notify the physician immediately. Treat mild symptoms with antipyretics and antihistamines as ordered. Severe cases are cared for like hemolytic reactions.
Allergic	Sensitivity to substances in donor blood	*Mild:* itching, urticaria, mild facial edema, nasal congestion, bronchial wheeze, chills, fever, nausea, vomiting *Severe:* Increasing severity of signs above, tightness in chest, substernal chest pain, difficulty swallowing, progression to shock and death	*Mild:* Slow the infusion. Notify the physician. Administer antihistamines as ordered. *Severe:* Stop the infusion. Keep the vein open with normal saline. Notify the physician immediately. Monitor vital signs. Administer O_2 and medications as ordered.
Hypervolemia (Circulatory overload)	Transfusion too large or too rapid	Dry cough, dyspnea, tightness in chest, pulmonary congestion, distended peripheral and neck veins, full bounding pulse	Stop the transfusion immediately. Keep the vein open with normal saline. Notify the physician immediately. Administer O_2 and medications as ordered.

slow the transfusion. Larger-gauge catheters (16-gauge or 14-gauge) may be necessary in emergencies where blood must infuse rapidly. A smaller-gauge needle (21-gauge or smaller) may be used for children because the rate of infusion is slower owing to the smaller body size and the smaller amount that has to be infused.

When a peripheral line is already in place, the solution that is infusing must be replaced with normal saline. A 0.9% saline solution is preferred in transfusion therapy because it simulates plasma's isotonicity. Other solutions may cause problems. Dextrose solutions, for example, cause hemolysis and clumping of red blood cells while solutions containing calcium, such as Ringer's lactate, cause blood to clot in the bag and tubing.

ASSEMBLING EQUIPMENT The equipment needed for blood transfusion includes a straight or Y-type blood administration set (see Figure 23.20), normal saline solution (500-mL bag) and the blood or blood product. A standard filter is incorporated into all straight and Y-type administration sets to remove small clots, degenerated platelets, leukocytes and large fibrin strands that accumulate during storage. The Y-type set has two branches with spikes; one branch attaches to the blood and the other to the normal saline.

When a straight blood administration set is used, a primary IV line is established using normal saline. If the patient does not have an existing IV line or if the venipuncture device is too small for blood transfusion, equipment is assembled for a peripheral venipuncture using an 18- or 20-gauge catheter. Infusion pumps may be used to administer and regulate the infusion of blood and blood components. Before using a pump, the nurse must check the manufacturer's instructions to make sure it will not cause hemolysis of the red blood cells.

The blood product is obtained from the blood bank according to established agency policy and procedure. Some nurses consider identification of the patient and the proper blood component as the most important measure in transfusion therapy (LaRocca & Otto, 1993). The transfusion process begins with confirmation of the physician's order. The blood is then obtained from the blood bank. The blood bag will have a blood identification label put on by Canadian Blood Services containing donor or unit number, the donor's ABO blood group, Rh factor and the expiration date (Figure 23.21). There will also be a recipient identification tag attached to the bag with a rubber band. This tag is put on by blood bank personnel in the agency. It includes the recipient's name and hospital number, the donor's ABO blood group and Rh factor and the unit number.

All information on the label and tag must be matched and compared with the blood requisition form. If there are any discrepancies in the information, the blood must be returned to the blood bank. As a safeguard, the identification procedure is conducted by two health professionals, first in the blood bank and then at the nursing station. This double-check is documented on the blood requisition form and noted in the patient's chart. In addition, the nurse who administers the blood checks the patient's name, birth date and hospital number against that on the recipient identification tag to ensure the correct patient is receiving the blood. The product's unit number and the time that the transfusion was commenced are entered onto the patient's chart.

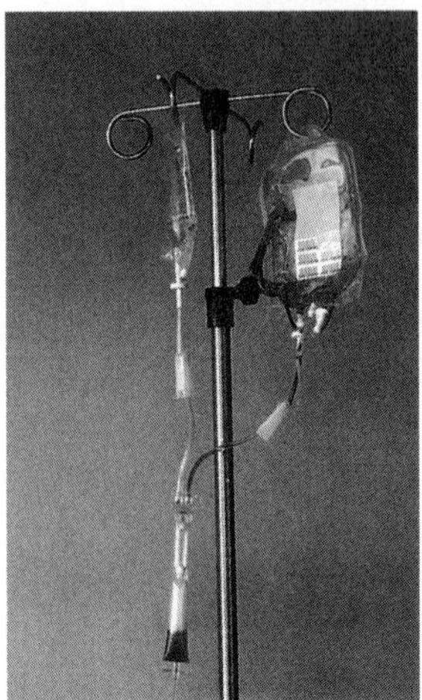

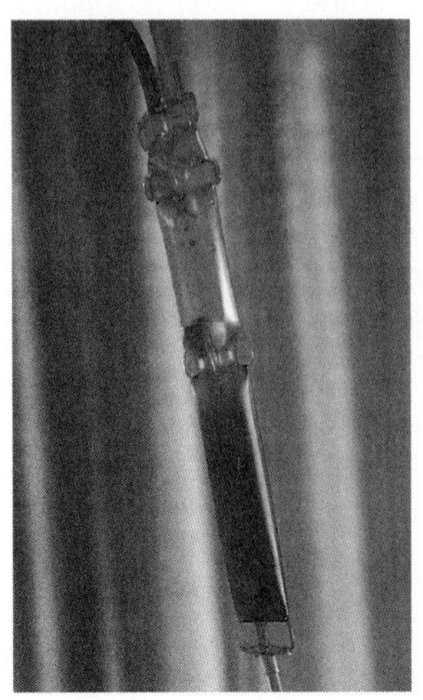

FIGURE 23.20 Y-type blood administration set

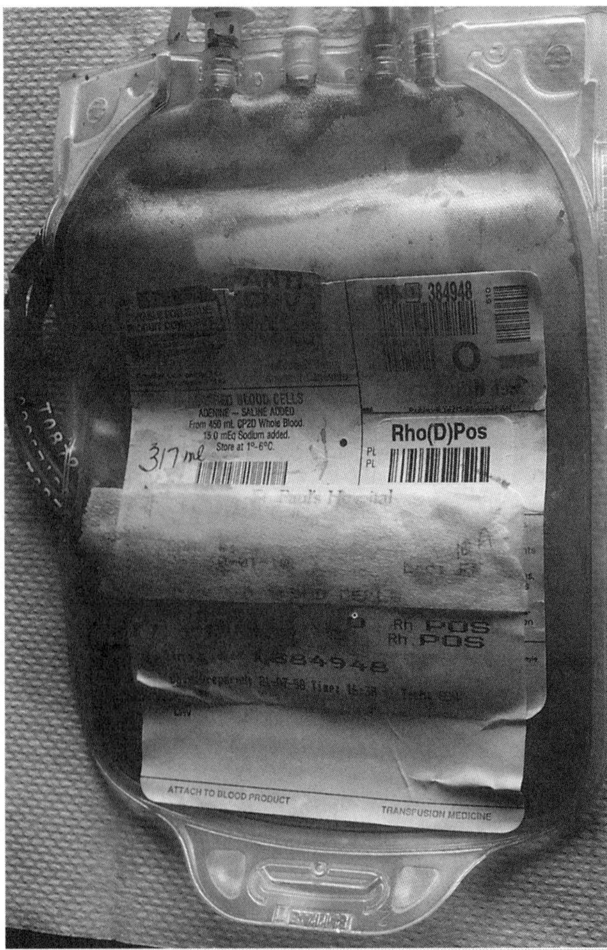

FIGURE 23.21 Blood product label

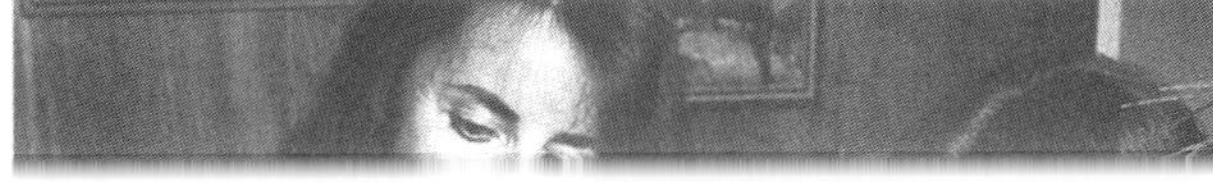

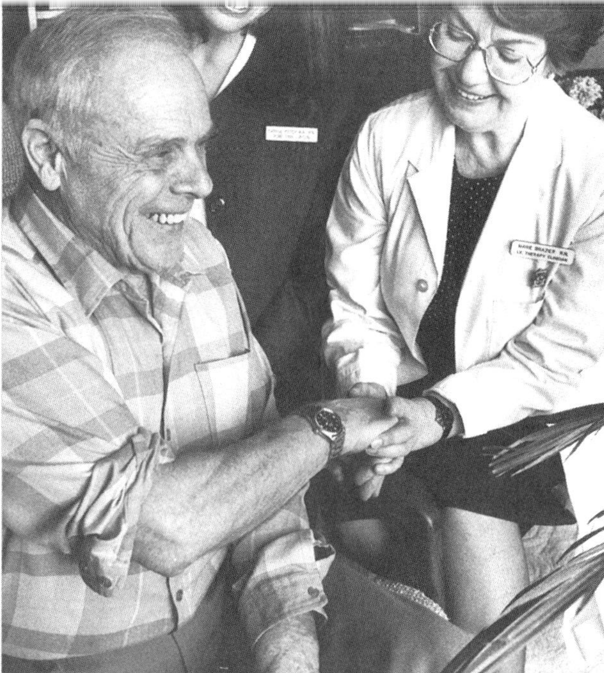

A home IV program allows patients to receive intravenous medications and/or fluids in the comfort and privacy of their home.

Transfusion Reactions

Even when the safety checks have been completed, transfusion reactions can still occur during, immediately after or within 96 hours of a blood transfusion. The primary types of blood reactions are hemolytic, febrile, hypervolemic or allergic. The most serious and potentially dangerous type is the hemolytic reaction, which occurs from incompatibilities between donor and recipient blood. Antibodies in the recipient's plasma react with antigens on the donor's red blood cell surfaces, causing hemolysis and agglutination. Table 23.16 provides an outline of the common transfusion reactions, detailing the causes, signs and symptoms and nursing interventions (Weinstein, 1997).

Autologous Blood Transfusion

An autologous transfusion is the collection and reinfusion of a person's own blood or blood components at a later time. Autologous transfusion is a desirable alternative for individuals whose religious beliefs prohibit homologous blood transfusion and for those concerned about the risk of contracting blood-borne pathogens such as hepatitis and HIV. In addition, receiving one's own blood significantly decreases the risk of febrile, allergic and hemolytic reactions. Another advantage of autologous transfusion is that it reduces the demands for donor blood and, thus, helps to conserve blood supply. However, the risk of bacterial contamination is always present, as is the chance of transfusing the wrong unit of blood into the patient. Therefore, the same [illegible] transfusing homologous blood must be used for autologous transfusion (Phillips, 1997).

Unfortunately, not all patients can qualify for autologous transfusion. Those with malignant cancer, blood clotting disorders or hemolytic conditions involving excessive destruction of red blood cells are not eligible. Patients with active infections are also not eligible for autologous transfusion because the bacteria may proliferate while the blood is stored. Autologous transfusion is most appropriate for healthy patients who are undergoing planned surgery such as a hip replacement. The individual must have a hemoglobin of at least 110 and be free of active infection or enteric contamination. Blood may be collected four to six weeks prior to the surgery. Blood lost during and after surgery or trauma can also be salvaged and reinfused (Drago, 1992).

INTRAVENOUS HOME CARE

One of the trends of the 1990s is the administration of intravenous therapy in the home. Intravenous home care is beneficial for both health care agencies and patients. For the health care system there are reduced costs for care and decreased demands for hospital beds (Coulter, 1997). The benefits for patients are many. Their well-being is enhanced because they feel more comfortable in their own surroundings and they are able to perform many of their normal activities. They feel a sense of control and independence because they are caring for themselves.

The types of intravenous care that are currently undertaken in the home include the administration of fluids and medications such as antibiotics, antifungal agents, analgesics, chemotherapeutic (anticancer) agents and total parenteral nutrition. Some programs also administer blood transfusions in the home. Intravenous therapy may be given via a central venous line or a peripheral line.

Safe and successful home intravenous therapy is dependent on two important factors. The first is a comprehensive assessment of the patient and his or her home environment; the second is thorough patient teaching. Candidates are selected carefully for the program.

Candidates must demonstrate a specific level of self-care and have the cognitive ability to understand the basis of treatment and asepsis, as well as the physical ability and coordination to perform the procedures safely. They must also be able to recognize complications and deal with potential emergencies. Ideally, the candidates must have a caregiver, a relative or a friend in the home who can provide the necessary care for them. The home environment is also evaluated. Obvious essentials such as running hot and cold water, adequate lighting, telephone service and transportation must be present. An area for clean, safe storage of supplies and equipment as well as an area for performing the

COMMUNITY health practice Intravenous Therapies in the Home Care Setting

The administration of intravenous antibiotics and anti-infectives within the home environment is an expanding service within the Canadian health care system. Home care nurses require knowledge about disease states, equipment, peripheral and central intravenous sites and the pharmacology of medications to be administered.

Diagnoses that are treated by home intravenous antibiotics (IVA) include conditions that need long-term therapy or infections that are not easily treated with oral antibiotics—for example, cellulitis, osteomyelitis and wound infections.

Safe administration of antibiotic and anti-infective agents within the home environment requires a detailed past and present medical history, including any allergic reactions. Ongoing assessment by the home care nurse is essential to evaluate therapeutic effectiveness of the medication and the potential for adverse drug interactions, including adverse reactions to the mode of administration. Communication with the multidisciplinary health team is fundamental in providing safe and effective home intravenous therapy.

SOURCE: Barrio, 1998.

procedures must be available. Finally, the accessibility of a hospital or 24-hour health care support service is considered.

Once a candidate is recommended for the program, thorough patient teaching begins. Patients and their caregivers are taught about the following:

- therapy-related procedures
- care of the infusion site
- daily assessments
- restrictions in activities
- troubleshooting problems
- prevention of complications
- when to call for the assistance of a physician or a nurse
- actions to be taken in case of emergencies
- safe methods of discarding used equipment
- where to obtain supplies and equipment
- arrangements for blood sampling or testing.

KEY PRINCIPLES

Principles Relevant to Fluid, Electrolyte and Acid–Base Balance

1. The average adult requires 2100–2900 mL fluid in a 24-hour period.
2. Children require a greater volume of fluids, proportionate to body weight, than adults.
3. Normally, fluid intake is balanced against fluid loss.
4. When fluids are lost or retained in excessive amounts, there is an accompanying loss or gain of electrolytes.
5. The signs and symptoms accompanying electrolyte imbalance vary according to the excess or deficiency of the specific electrolyte.
6. The specific electrolytes lost from the body in any fluid loss depend on the route of the loss.

Patients and their caregivers should feel secure with their knowledge base and the physical skills required before discharge.

INTERSTITIAL INFUSION

Interstitial infusion, *hypodermoclysis* and *subcutaneous infusion* are synonymous terms referring to the administration of large amounts of fluid into subcutaneous tissue. This measure is not used often: it is utilized when a person is unable to take fluids orally, rectally or intravenously. Its purpose is to supply the patient with fluids, electrolytes and occasionally nourishment. Hyaluronidase (Wydase) is often added to the fluid to hasten its absorption. The enzyme breaks down the hyaluronic acid in the connective tissue.

Whether the initiation of an interstitial infusion is the responsibility of the nurse or the physician depends on the policy of the specific agency. The common sites for the administration of an interstitial infusion are just below the scapula, the abdominal wall above the crest of the ilium, the lower aspect of the breast and the anterior aspect of the thigh. The equipment that is used is similar to that used in intravenous infusions. A cysis needle is used. Often, two sites are used simultaneously (Weinstein, 1997).

After the equipment has been set up, the needle is inserted into the skin at a 20° angle. It is then taped in place and the flow of the fluid is adjusted in accordance with the physician's order. The usual rate of flow for an interstitial infusion is 60–120 gtt/min. The rate depends upon the ability of the individual to absorb the fluid. Thin people usually absorb fluid more easily than obese people, because they have fewer fat cells.

The nurse assists the patient in assuming a comfortable position, since this treatment is often lengthy. Observations are indicated to detect untoward signs, particularly those related to circulatory collapse (for example, an accelerated, weak pulse). The patient should be watched for signs of respiratory difficulty that could indicate overhydration, such as dyspnea or moist and noisy breathing.

Sometimes, the infusion is poorly absorbed and the nurse may notice the tissues at the site of the injection are becoming edematous. If untoward symptoms develop, the in- [illegible] promptly.

At the termination of an infusion the needle is removed. A small antiseptic dressing is taped over the wound with slight pressure to prevent leakage of the fluid. The nurse records the time of initiation and termination of the infusion, as well as the type of fluid, the amount of fluid absorbed, the addition of any medications, the rate of flow and the patient's response to the treatment. Again, it is wise to record the site of the infusion so that injection sites can be rotated.

Evaluating Fluid, Electrolyte and Acid–Base Balance Interventions

The evaluation of a care plan for fluid, electrolyte and acid–base balance is based on the expected outcomes or goals outlined in the planning phase of the nursing process. Following is a guide for evaluating the effectiveness of nursing intervention.

1. Is the patient taking adequate food and fluids to meet his or her fluid and electrolyte needs?
2. Is the patient's urine output compatible with fluid intake?
3. If there are restrictions on the patient's fluid or electrolyte intake, are these being followed?
4. If parenteral fluids have been prescribed, have they been given at the correct time? Have sterile precautions been observed in their administration? Is the infusion flowing at the proper rate?
5. Is the patient's skin in good condition? Is the mouth?
6. Do the patient and family have all the information they need to enable them to maintain and restore the patient's fluid, electrolyte and acid–base balance?

IN REVIEW

- The fluid system transports nutrients to the cell, removes waste products and maintains a stable physical and chemical environment in the body.
- Body fluid is made of water (solvent) and dissolved substances (solutes), including:
  - electrolytes
  - minerals
  - glucose
  - urea.
- Water is an indispensable nutrient. Body fluids make up approximately:
  - 60% of the total body weight of an adult
  - [illegible] of the total body weight of a full term infant.
- Body fluids are distributed in the intracellular (ICF) and extracellular (ECF) compartments. The proportion of ICF to ECF varies with age, gender and body fat.
- Solvents and solutes constantly shift from one compartment to another:
  - water moves by osmosis
  - electrolytes move by diffusion and active transport.
- Body fluid and electrolytes are derived from the ingestion of fluids and food and from metabolic oxidation. Electrolytes are lost through urine, expiration and perspiration.
- Fluid and electrolytes balance is regulated by:
  - osmotic pressure
  - kidney function.

  The gastrointestinal tract and thirst also play a role in maintaining balance.
- Fluid and electrolyte needs vary throughout the life cycle:
  - until the age of two, infants are vulnerable to imbalances because their homeostatic mechanisms are immature
  - children become dehydrated quickly and require a greater volume of fluid in proportion to their body weight
  - in adolescence, all body systems mature and the mechanisms regulating fluid and electrolytes begin to function as they do in adults
  - women tend to retain fluid a few days prior to their menstrual cycle, during pregnancy and during menopause
  - in pregnancy, total blood volume is increased by 50%
  - adults experience a gradual inefficiency of regulating fluid and electrolyte balance
  - the elderly are especially vulnerable to imbalances.
- The pH of body fluids is maintained within a narrow range of 7.35–7.45 for normal body function. The body's pH is regulated by three mechanisms:
  - the buffer system (bicarbonate, phosphate and protein)
  - the respiratory regulating system
  - the kidney regulating system,
- The body's acid–base (pH) balance is upset with large losses and gains of fluid or by depletion/excess of essential acid or base reserves. This may result in

alkalosis or acidosis which can be respiratory or metabolic in nature, as confirmed by arterial blood gas (ABG) analysis.

- Fluid and electrolyte imbalances can occur when there is:
  - insufficient intake
  - disturbance in the gastrointestinal tract (e.g., vomiting, diarrhea) or in the kidney
  - excess perspiration and other volume losses from hemorrhage, burns or trauma.

  Severe electrolyte imbalances can be life-threatening and require medical treatment.
- Many imbalances are associated with disease processes that inhibit absorption or excretion of one or more electrolytes.
- Imbalances must be assessed, monitored and documented frequently. A health assessment of a patient's fluid, electrolyte and acid–base balance includes:
  - history of previous imbalances or conditions that precipitate imbalances
  - body weight, physical appearance
  - vital signs
  - inspection of skin/mucous membranes for turgor, moisture, elasticity, temperature
  - fluid intake and output
  - observation for tearing, salivation, perspiration, edema, distended neck veins
  - mental status, neuromuscular irritability
  - laboratory tests.
- Two common nursing diagnoses are:
  - Fluid Volume Deficit
  - Fluid Volume Excess.
- Nursing actions to restore fluid, electrolyte and acid–base balance include:
  - health teaching
  - maintenance of therapeutic fluid intake
  - administration of electrolyte supplements
  - accurate documentation of intake and output
  - measurement of patient's weight, edema, vital signs, mental status
  - awareness of significant laboratory results
  - evaluation of nursing and medical modalities.
- Intravenous (IV) fluids are delivered into peripheral and central veins. Meticulous care and careful assessment are essential throughout IV therapy to prevent complications:
  - strict aseptic technique must be adhered to
  - body substance precautions must be used at all times when handling body fluids.
- Blood transfusion therapy is prescribed to:
  - restore circulating blood volume
  - correct red blood cell deficiency
  - maintain clotting ability.

  While it is often a life-sustaining modality, it is not without risk.
- Strict agency protocol and guidelines must be adhered to during blood transfusion therapy, including:
  - accurate identification of the patient and blood product
  - initiation and maintenance of the infusion
  - monitoring of the patient for transfusion reactions.

Critical Thinking Activity

1. Mr. Miller is admitted to an active treatment hospital in a large city. His diagnosis was tentatively given as dehydration and emaciation. The physician, Dr. Shirley Wong, has ordered food and fluids as tolerated and various laboratory tests. She has also ordered an intravenous of D5W/0.45 NaCl to infuse at 100 mL/h.

   Mr. Miller is 70 years old and lives on Social Security. He has no family and lives alone in a rooming house where he cooks on a small hot plate. A friend accompanied him to the hospital. Mr. Miller is very thin and says he has not eaten well in months. He appears frightened; this is his first admission to hospital.

   a. What is dehydration?
   b. What subjective and objective observations might you anticipate? Why?
   c. What factors should be taken into consideration in explaining the intravenous infusion to Mr. Miller?
   d. The intravenous infusion has been established using a macrodrop administration set with a drop factor of 10. Calculate the intravenous rate of flow in drops/minute.
   e. What observations could you make regarding Mr. Miller's intravenous infusion?
   f. Outline a nursing plan of care for this patient, including nursing diagnoses, expected outcomes and interventions.
   g. How can you evaluate the results of your planned nursing interventions for this patient?

KEY TERMS

cation p. 628
anion p. 628
intracellular fluid p. 628
extracellular fluid p. 628
interstitial fluid p. 628
intravascular fluid p. 628
solvent p. 629
solute p. 629
serum electrolyte p. 629
diffusion p. 630
selectively permeable membrane p. 630
osmosis p. 630
osmotic pressure p. 630
osmolality p. 630
active transport p. 630
filtration p. 630
hydrostatic pressure p. 630
action potential p. 632
acid p. 635
base p. 635
acidosis p. 635
alkalosis p. 635
fluid volume deficit p. 639
isotonic fluid deficit p. 639
hypotonic dehydration p. 642
hypertonic dehydration p. 642
insensible water loss p. 642
fluid volume excess p. 642
hyponatremia p. 642
hypernatremia p. 642
hyperkalemia p. 643
hypocalcemia p. 650
hypercalcemia p. 651
hypomagnesemia p. 652
hypermagnesemia p. 652
hypophosphatemia p. 652
hyperphosphatemia p. 650
buffering p. 653
correction p. 653
compensation p. 653
skin turgor p. 663
edema p. 663
isotonic solution p. 668
hypotonic solution p. 668
hypertonic solution p. 668
venipuncture p. 669
infiltration p. 689
phlebitis p. 689
thrombophlebitis p. 690
infection p. 690
circulatory overload p. 691
air embolism p. 700
blood transfusion p. 700
donor p. 700
recipient p. 700
homologous or indirect transfusion p. 700
autologous transfusion p. 700
blood group p. 701
Rh factor p. 702
typing p. 702
crossmatching p. 702

References

BARRIO, D.J. (1998). Antibiotic and anti-infective agent use and administration in homecare. *Journal of Intravenous Nursing, 21*(1), 50–58.

BLACK, J.M., & MATASSARIN-JACOBS, E. (1997). *Medical–surgical nursing: Clinical management for continuity of care.* (5th ed.). Philadelphia: W.B. Saunders.

BROWN, M., & MULHOLLAND, J.L. (1996). *Drug calculations: Process and problems for clinical practice.* (5th ed.). Toronto: Mosby.

CAMP-SORRELL, D. (1992). Implantable ports: Everything you always wanted to know. *Journal of Intravenous Nursing, 15,* 262.

CARPENITO, L.J. (1997). *Nursing diagnosis: Application to clinical practice,*

CHASE, L. (1993). Venipuncture for initiating peripheral intravenous therapy. *Parenteral therapy manual*. Vancouver: Vancouver General Hospital.

CHERNECKY, C.C., & BERGER, B. (1997). *Laboratory tests and diagnostic procedures.* (2nd ed.). Toronto: W.B. Saunders.

COULTER, K. (1997). Nurses' transition from hospital to home: Bridging the gap. *Journal of Intravenous Nursing, 20*(2), 89–93.

DRAGO, S.S. (1992). Banking on your own blood. *AJN, 92*(3), 61.

DUDEK, S.G. (1997). *Nutrition handbook for nursing practice.* (2nd ed.). Philadelphia: Lippincott-Raven.

EARNEST V.V. (1993). *Clinical skills in nursing practice* (2nd ed.). Philadelphia: Lippincott.

FULLER, J., & SCHALLER-AYERS, J. (1994). *Health assessment: A nursing approach.* (2nd ed.). Philadelphia: Lippincott.

HEALTH CANADA. (1997). *Infection control guidelines for preventing infections associated with indwelling intravascular access devices.* Ottawa: Author.

HORNE, M.M., HEITZ, U.E., & SWEARINGEN, P.L. (1997). *Fluid, electrolyte and acid–base balance.* (3rd ed.). Mosby's Pocket Guide Series. St. Louis: Mosby Year Book.

KEE, J.L. (1986). *Fluids and electrolytes with clinical applications.* (4th ed.). New York: Wiley.

KEE, J.L. (1995). *Fluids and electrolytes with clinical applications.* (5th ed.). New York: Wiley.

KROZEK, C. (1993). Intravascular therapy. In *Nursing procedures: Student version*. Springhouse, PA: Springhouse.

LaROCCA, J.C., & OTTO, S.E. (1993). *Pocket guide to intravenous therapy.* St. Louis: Mosby.

LEE, C.A.B., BARRETT, C.A., & IGNATAVICIUS, D.D. (1996). *Fluid and electrolytes: A practical approach.* (4th ed.). Philadelphia: F.A. Davis.

MARTINI, F. (1998). *Fundamentals of anatomy and physiology.* (4th ed.). Upper Saddle River, NJ: Prentice Hall.

METHENEY, N.M. (1996). *Fluid and electrolyte balance: Nursing considerations.* (3rd ed.). Philadelphia: Lippincott.

NATIONAL BLOOD RESOURCE EDUCATION PROGRAM (NBREP) NURSING EDUCATION WORKING GROUP. (1991). Choosing blood components and equipment. *AJN, 91*(6), 42.

PHILLIPS, L.D. (1997). *Manual of IV therapeutics.* (2nd ed.). Philadelphia: F.A. Davis.

SAVINO, S.R., & EBERHART, T. (1998). A comparison of flow rates between Baxter Continu-Flow and Baxter InterLink Continu-Flow. *Journal of Intravenous Nursing, 21*(1), 41–44.

SCHRIER, R. (1997). *Renal and electrolyte disorders* (rev. ed.). Boston: Little, Brown.

THELAN, L.A. DAVIE, J.K. & URDEN, L.D. (1997). *Textbook of Critical Care Nursing: Diagnosis and Management.* (3rd ed.). St. Louis: Mosby.

VAUGHAN, V.C. III, McKAY, R.J., & BEHRMAN, R.E. (1979). *Nelson textbook of pediatrics.* (11th ed.). Philadelphia: Saunders.

WEINSTEIN, S.M. (1997). *Plumer's principles and practice of intravenous therapy.* (6th ed.). Philadelphia: Lippincott.

WELDY, N.J. (1992). *Body fluids and electrolytes.* St. Louis: Mosby.

WOODTLI, A.O. (1990). Thirst: A critical care nursing challenge. *Dimensions of Critical Care Nursing, 9*(1), 6.

Additional Readings

BRANDT, B., DePALMA, J.M., IRWIN, M., SHOGAN, J., & LUKE, J.F. (1996). Comparison of central venous dressings in bone marrow transplant recipients. *Oncology Nursing Forum, 23*(5), 829–836.

BROWN, L.S., BOGNER, M.S., PARMENTIER, C.M., & TAYLOR, J.B. (1997). Human error and patient-controlled analgesia pumps. *Journal of Intravenous Nursing, 20*(6), 311–316.

CANADIAN INTRAVENOUS NURSES ASSOCIATION. (1996, April). *Intravenous therapy guidelines*. Pembroke, ON: DFR Printing.

CANADIAN RED CROSS SOCIETY. (1993). *Clinical guide to transfusion.* (3rd ed.). Ottawa: Author.

COOK, L.S. (1997). Nonimmune transfusion reactions: When type-and-cross match aren't enough. *Journal of Intravenous Nursing, 20*(1), 15–22.

CROW, S. (1996). Prevention of intravascular infections: Ways and means. *Journal of Intravenous Nursing, 19*(4), 175–181.

DUCK, S. (1997). Neonatal intravenous therapy. *Journal of Intravenous Nursing, 20*(3), 121–127.

FITZPATRICK, L., & FITZPATRICK, T. (1997, August). Blood transfusion: Keeping your patient safe. *Nursing 97*, 34–42.

FLYNN, J.M., & HACKEL, R. (1990). *Technological foundations in nursing.* Norwalk, CT: Appleton & Lange.

HADAWAY, L. (1997). An overview of vascular access devices inserted via the antecubital area. *Canadian Intravenous Nurses Association, 13*(1), 8–15.

KATZ, R.S. (1998). The effects of intravenous solutions on fluid and electrolyte balance. *Journal of Intravenous Nursing, 21*(1), 20–26.

KOKKO, J.P., & TANNEN, R.L. (1996). *Fluid and electrolytes* (pp. 21–127). (3rd ed.). Philadelphia: W.B. Saunders.

MACKLIN, D. (1997). How to manage PICCs. *American Journal of Nursing, 97*(9), 26–33.

OUWENDYK, M., & HELFERTY, N.M. (1996). Central venous catheter management: How to prevent complications. *ANNA Journal, 23*(6), 572–577.

RITTER, H.T.M. (1990). Evaluating and selecting general purpose infusion pumps. *Journal of Intravenous Nursing, 13*, 156.

SITGES-SERRA, A., PI-SUNER, T., GARCES, J.M., & SEGURA, M. (1995). Pathogenesis and prevention of catheter-related septicemia. *American Journal of Infection Control, 23*(5), 310–316.

SPRINGHOUSE CORPORATION. (1996). *Managing IV therapy: A new nursing photobook.* Springhouse, PA: Author.

TERRY, J., BARANOWSKI, R.L., & HEDRICK, C. (1995). *Intravenous therapy: Clinical principles and practice.* Philadelphia: W.B. Saunders.

TRASK, K. (1995). The challenges of teaching universal precautions to multicultural, diverse patients and their family members. *Journal of Intravenous Nursing, 18*(6S) (suppl.), S32-S37.

WEINSTEIN, S.M. (1996). Legal implications/risk management. *Journal of Intravenous Nursing, 19*(3S) (suppl.), S16–S19.

WHITE, V.M. (1997). Emergency! Hyperkalemia. *American Journal of Nursing, 97*(6), 35.

WHITSON, M. (1996). Intravenous therapy in the older adult: Special needs and considerations. *Journal of Intravenous Nursing, 19*(5), 251–255.

WOOD, G.C., BROWN, R.O., & DICKERSON, R.N. (1998). Considerations in the use of lipid-based drug products. *Journal of Intravenous Nursing, 21*(1), 45–49.

Chapter 2

Oxygen Needs

OUTLINE

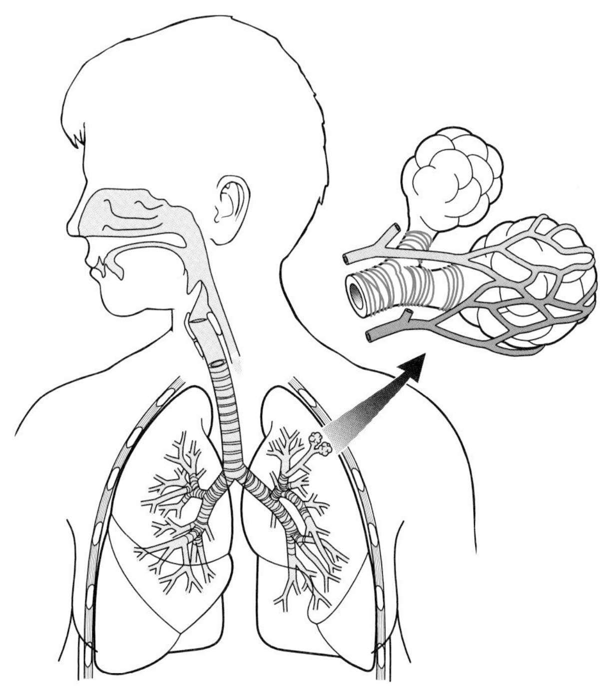

Central Questions

1. In what way is oxygen essential to life?
2. What are the structures and functions of the respiratory and cardiovascular systems?
3. How do the processes of ventilation, diffusion and transportation supply oxygen to body cells?
4. What are the body's lung clearance mechanisms, and how do they function to ensure clean air intake?
5. What are the main determinants of adequate oxygen supply to tissues?
6. How do oxygen needs vary throughout the life cycle?
7. What are the common oxygenation problems?
8. What basic principles does the nurse apply in assisting individuals to meet their nutritional needs?
9. How does the nurse assess an individual's oxygenation status?
10. What are the common nursing diagnostic statements for individuals with oxygenation problems?
11. How might the nurse develop a plan of care for individuals with oxygenation problems?
12. What strategies might the nurse implement in helping individuals, families or groups to promote optimum oxygenation?
13. What health-protecting strategies might the nurse implement to maintain respiratory function, oxygen transport and tissue perfusion in individuals who are ill?
14. What health-restoring and supportive strategies might the nurse implement in the care of individuals with oxygenation problems?
15. How might the nurse evaluate the individual's response to nursing interventions?

Introduction

Oxygen is an essential nutrient for life. Body cells need a continuous supply of oxygen for all metabolic processes and for the production of energy. As the physiologist Haldane noted, "oxygen lack not only stops the motor but wrecks the human machine" (cited in Lacey, 1988, p. 17). Deprived of oxygen, cells malfunction, become damaged and eventually die. Cells of the brain and the heart are particularly sensitive to lack of oxygen. Within only a few minutes of oxygen deprivation, these cells suffer irreversible damage, and death quickly follows.

The supply of oxygen to body cells, referred to as **oxygenation,** is a complex process involving the respiratory and cardiovascular systems. Normally, oxygen is taken into the body by the respiratory system through the air we breathe. It is carried to all body cells within seconds by the cardiovascular system. The cells use the oxygen to produce energy and then release quantities of carbon dioxide, a metabolic waste product. Carbon dioxide is taken up by the blood and carried to the lungs for immediate elimination from the body.

The term **respiration** is used to describe the exchange of oxygen and carbon dioxide between the atmosphere and the cells of the body. The body cannot store oxygen, and excessive amounts of carbon dioxide are poisonous to cells. Therefore, it is essential that both the respiratory and cardiovascular systems are functioning optimally. Problems in either system, or insufficient oxygen in the atmosphere, will interfere with the ability to meet our need for oxygen.

This chapter will provide the nurse with basic knowledge of oxygenation, factors affecting oxygenation and common oxygenation problems. Methods of assessing oxygen health status and measures to protect and restore the health of individuals experiencing problems meeting their oxygen needs are outlined. In addition, ways of assisting people to promote healthy oxygenation in daily living are also presented.

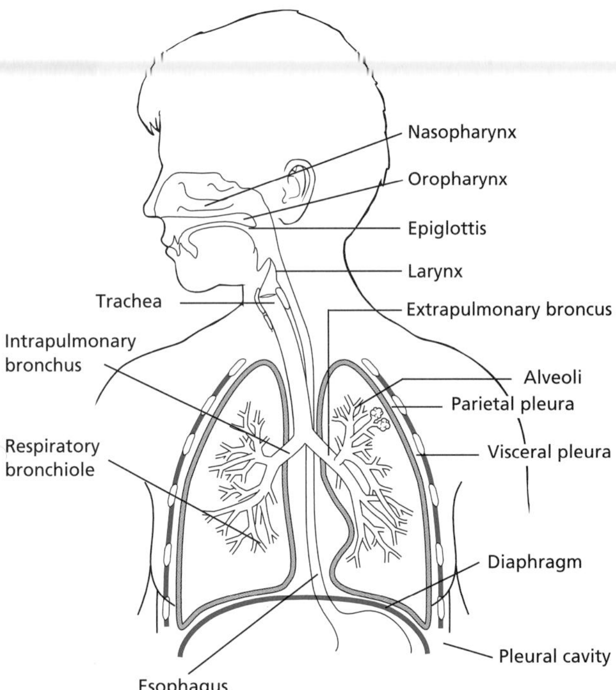

FIGURE 24.1 The respiratory tract

SOURCE: Porth, 1998, p. 476.

Physiology of Oxygenation

The respiratory and cardiovascular systems work together to supply oxygen to the cells and eliminate carbon dioxide from the body. The respiratory system consists of the upper and lower **airways** and the lungs (see Figure 24.1). The upper airways consist of the nose, pharynx, larynx and trachea. Their primary functions are to provide a passageway for air entering and leaving the body and to warm, filter and moisturize it on entry. The lower airways are the two bronchi and their branches, which deliver oxygen to the functional areas of the lungs and return unused air and carbon dioxide to the atmosphere. The lungs are tissues made up of clusters of tiny airways (bronchioles), blood vessels and the alveolar membrane. The exchange of gases occurs in the alveolar sacs of the lungs. The upper and lower airways and the bronchioles are lined with mucous membrane, part of which contains cilia and secretes mucous to trap organisms and other foreign material.

The cardiovascular system includes the heart; the network of arteries, veins and capillaries; and blood. It provides the mechanism for transporting oxygen and carbon dioxide. The heart supplies the force or pumping action that circulates blood throughout the body. Oxygen is carried from the lungs via the arteries to the tissues, and carbon dioxide is carried from the tissues via the veins back to the lungs.

The three major processes involved in oxygenation: ventilation, diffusion and transport.

The heart is a hollow, muscular organ that has four chambers. It lies diagonally in the chest, above the diaphragm and between the lungs. The heart weighs approximately 2.2 kg and is about the size of a fist. The heart wall has three layers: the pericardium (which surrounds the heart), the myocardium (or heart muscle) and the endocardium (the inner lining of the heart muscle). The upper two chambers of the heart are called *atria*; the two lower chambers are the *ventricles*. Each chamber is separated by a cardiac valve. These four valves provide a one-way flow of blood through the heart from the right to left side. Blood is supplied to the heart by the coronary arteries. The heart's conduction system generates the electrical activity needed to initiate and maintain heart rate and rhythm.

The heart has two separate circulatory systems, one providing blood to the lungs (pulmonary system) and the other providing it to the rest of the body (systemic circulation). The right atrium receives venous blood from the superior and inferior venae cavae; the blood then passes

right ventricle receives blood from the right atrium and expels it through the pulmonic valve into the pulmonary artery. The left atrium receives oxygenated blood from the four pulmonary veins and delivers it to the left ventricle through the mitral valve. The left ventricle receives blood from the left atrium and expels it through the aortic valve into the ascending aorta; from there it is distributed to the rest of the body (see Figure 24.2) (McCance, 1996).

Ventilation

Ventilation is the mechanical movement of air in and out of the lungs. It is achieved by a pressure gradient in which gases flow from an area of higher pressure to one of lower pressure. Air is taken into the lungs when the pressure inside the lungs (intrapulmonic) is less than air pressure in the atmosphere. Inhalation ceases when atmospheric and intrapulmonary pressures are equal. When the pressure inside the lungs is greater than atmospheric pressure, air is moved out. Intrapulmonic pressure is generated by changes in the size of the thoracic cavity through the work of breathing.

BREATHING

Breathing has two phases: **inhalation** (inspiration), when air is taken into the lungs, and **exhalation** (expiration), when air is passed out of the lungs. During inhalation, the inspiratory muscles (the diaphragm and the external intercostals) contract, increasing the size of the thoracic cavity. The

outward and the sternum moves outward to lengthen the thorax and expand its lateral and anteroposterior dimensions. The lungs, which adhere to the walls of the thoracic cavity by the attraction of the pleural membranes for each other, expand as the thorax enlarges. Intrapulmonic pressure decreases and air enters the lungs. Air ceases to enter when the intrapulmonic and atmospheric pressures are equal.

Exhalation is a more passive process. The diaphragm relaxes (recoils) and moves upward, the ribs move downward and inward and the sternum moves inward, all of which cause the thoracic cavity to decrease in size. This, combined with the upward push of the abdominal organs against the diaphragm, compresses the lungs and increases intrapulmonic pressure. Air is expelled from the lungs until intrapulmonic and atmospheric pressures are equal. Inhalation normally lasts 1–1.5 seconds and exhalation 2–3 seconds. Figure 24.3 illustrates the mechanics of respiration.

When the effort involved in breathing increases, as, for example, during exercise or with disease, accessory muscles become involved in ventilation. The scalene, sternocleidomastoid and internal intercostal muscles help to increase the size of the thoracic cavity so that more air will enter the lungs. The internal intercostal muscles are activated in forced exhalation to help decrease the size of the rib cage and squeeze air out of the lungs.

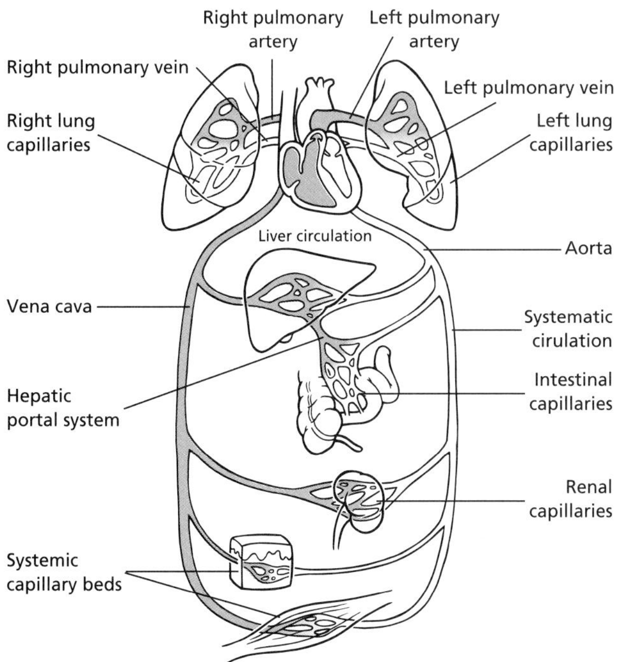

FIGURE 24.2 The cardiovascular system. The right heart chambers propel unoxygenated blood through pulmonary circulation; the left heart propels oxygenated blood through systemic circulation.

SOURCE: McCance, 1996, p. 586.

COMPLIANCE AND RECOIL

Compliance and *recoil* refer to properties of muscles and tissues that allow them to stretch or expand and then to contract or return to their original position. As the ribcage expands and the lungs enlarge during inhalation, the elastic components of the chest wall and the lungs—skeletal muscle fibres, elastin fibres of the lungs, surrounding connective tissues and the parietal pleura—stretch accordingly. When the inspiratory muscles relax, these elastic components are able to contract, thus returning the ribcage and the lungs to their original positions. This phenomenon is called **elastic recoil**. The ease with which the chest wall and the lungs can expand to fill with air and contract to empty the air is called **compliance**. When compliance is low, greater force is needed to fill and empty the lungs. For example, people with emphysema have reduced compliance because they have neither the elasticity to expand the lungs fully, nor the elastic recoil to return them to their normal position on exhalation (Porth, 1998).

PULMONARY VOLUMES AND CAPACITIES

Pulmonary (or respiratory) volumes and capacities represent the amount of air contained within the lungs, the amount of air that moves in and out of the lungs during quiet

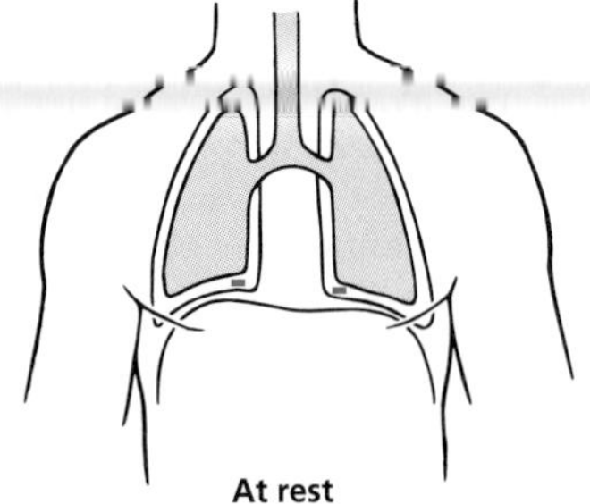

At rest

- Inspiratory muscles relax
- Atmospheric pressure present in tracheobronchial tree
- No air movement

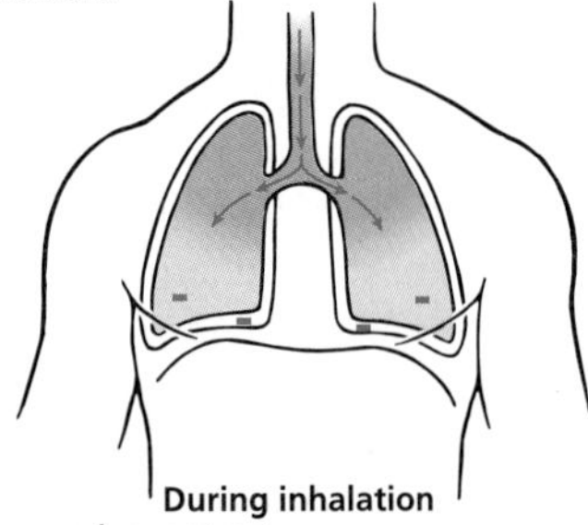

During inhalation

- Inspiratory muscles contract
- Chest expands
- Diaphragm descends
- Negative alveolar pressure present
- Air moves into lungs

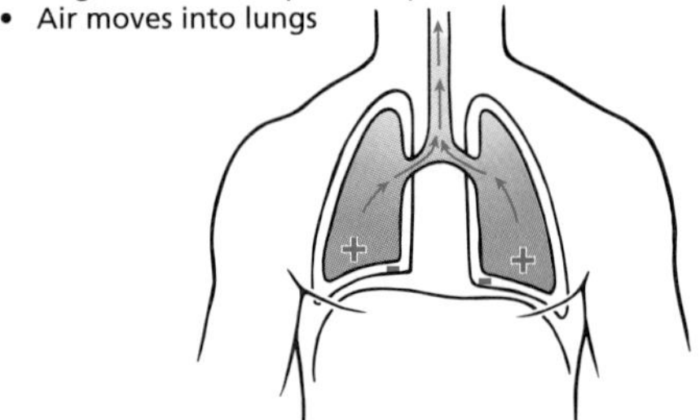

During exhalation

- Inspiratory muscles relax, causing lung recoil
- Diaphragm ascends
- Positive alveolar pressure present
- Air moves out of lungs

Key:
– = negative intrapleural pressure
⊖ = negative alveolar pressure
⊕ = positive alveolar pressure

FIGURE 24.3 The mechanics of respiration

SOURCE: Springhouse, 1983, p. 283.

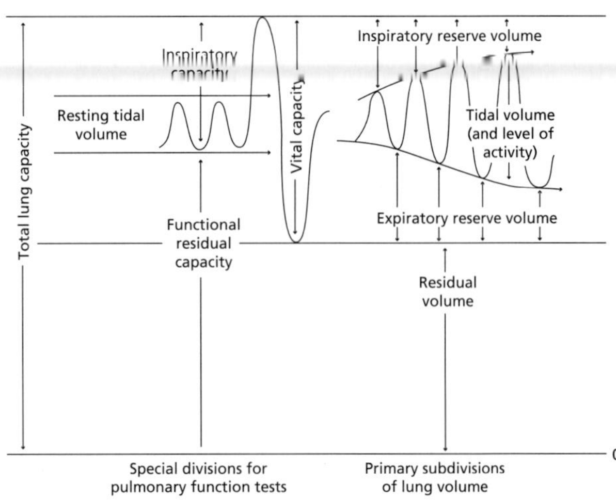

FIGURE 24.4 Respiratory volumes and capacities

SOURCE: Porth, 1998, p. 483.

breathing and the amount that can be moved in and out with forceful breathing. The terms for the various volumes and capacities are described in Table 24.1. Combinations of pulmonary volumes make up the pulmonary capacities. For example, total lung capacity is the sum of the tidal volume, the inspiratory reserve volume, the expiratory reserve volume and the residual volume (Figure 24.4). Pulmonary volumes and capacities vary among individuals depending on such factors as body size and build, gender, age and physical condition (Porth, 1998).

CONTROL MECHANISMS

The principal mechanism controlling respiration includes the medulla and pons, which are the respiratory centre of the brain. The respiratory centre functions as the central control for ventilation. It receives chemical and mechanical impulses from the body, coordinates the information to determine respiratory needs, and forwards nerve impulses to the muscles that control breathing. The nervous system adjusts the rate, depth and pattern of ventilations so that oxygen and carbon dioxide levels remain relatively constant.

Normally, our breathing patterns change without our awareness in response to fluctuations in the chemical composition of blood and body fluids. This involuntary control of respiration is possible because of chemical receptors (chemoreceptors) located in the respiratory centre, aorta and carotid sinuses. These chemoreceptors are groups of nerve cells that sense changes in oxygen, carbon dioxide and hydrogen ion concentrations. Chemoreceptors in the aorta and carotid sinuses are sensitive to concentrations of oxygen and carbon dioxide in arterial blood. Central chemoreceptors respond only to concentrations of carbon dioxide in the cerebral spinal fluid. The chemoreceptors monitoring carbon dioxide levels are sensitive to hydrogen ions released from the dissociation of carbonic acid. Thus, other conditions altering the pH of body fluids can affect respiratory performance (Martini, 1998). Under normal conditions, the level of carbon dioxide in the blood is the primary regulator of ventilation. For most people, an increase in carbon dioxide concentration (hypercapnia) or a decrease in pH causes an immediate increase in respiratory rate.

Mechanical stretch receptors are important in regulating respiratory activity. Stretch receptors located in the visceral pleura around the lungs initiate the Hering-Breuer reflex, which prevents overexpansion of the lungs, particularly during forced ventilations such as those accompanying strenuous exercise. At a specific point in inspiration, these receptors transmit impulses to the respiratory centre, which inhibits inspiration and triggers the expiratory phase of respiration. The reverse takes place during expiration. Other stretch receptors, for example, baroreceptors in the aorta and carotid sinuses, also have an effect on respiration.

TABLE 24.1 Summary of respiratory volumes and capacities

Volume	Symbol	Measurement
Tidal volume (about 500 mL at rest)	TV	Amount of air that moves into and out of the lungs with each breath
Inspiratory reserve volume (about 3000 mL)	IRV	Maximum amount of air that can be inhaled from the point of maximal expiration
Expiratory reserve volume (about 1100 mL)	ERV	Maximum volume of air that can be exhaled from the resting end-expiratory level
Residual volume (about 1200 mL)	RV	Volume of air remaining in the lungs after maximal expiration. This volume cannot be measured with the spirometer; it is measured indirectly using methods such as the helium dilution method, the nitrogen washout technique, or body plethysmography
Functional residual capacity (about 2300 mL)	FRC	Volume of air remaining in the lungs at end-expiration (sum of RV and ERV)
Inspiratory capacity (about 3500 mL)	IC	Sum of IRV and TV
Vital capacity (about 4600 mL)	VC	Maximal amount of air that can be exhaled from the point of maximal inspiration
Total lung capacity (about 5800 mL)	TLC	Total amount of air that the lungs can hold; it is the sum of all the volume components after maximal inspiration. This value is about 20–25% less in females than in males

SOURCE: Porth, 1998, p. 484.

When blood pressure rises, the respiratory rate increases; it decreases when blood pressure falls.

Breathing can be consciously controlled by activating or restricting muscles of the chest and diaphragm. For instance, breathing is controlled while eating, drinking, singing or speaking. We can hold the breath for short periods while swimming under water, or while trying to avoid inhaling noxious fumes in the air. However, we cannot hold the breath to the detriment of our health. When oxygen levels become too low and carbon dioxide levels too high, we lose consciousness. At this point the nervous system regains control, and we begin to breathe again.

Diffusion

Diffusion is the process by which oxygen and carbon dioxide are exchanged between the air and the blood (external respiration) and between the tissue cells and the blood (internal respiration). External respiration takes place in the lungs, specifically, in the alveoli across the alveolar–capillary membrane. The alveolar–capillary membrane is a very thin layer of cells that separates each alveolus from its surrounding capillaries. Each lung contains about 150 million alveoli, and it has been estimated that the total surface for gas exchange provided by the alveoli equals the area of a tennis court (Martini, 1998; Marieb, 1995).

All gases exert pressure. When gases are mixed together, each gas contributes to the total pressure in proportion to its relative amount in the mixture (Dalton's law). The pressure exerted by a single gas in a mixture is called the **partial pressure** and it is indicated by a "p" before the chemical abbreviation for the gas (for example, pO_2, pCO_2). The diffusion of a particular gas from the air into a solution (blood) depends on its partial pressure alone. Thus, the amount of force exerted by oxygen molecules will affect how much oxygen enters the solution, but it will not affect rates of carbon dioxide or nitrogen diffusion. Each gas behaves on its own.

Gases are exchanged in the lungs according to the laws of diffusion. That is, the gases move across a membrane towards the area of lower concentration. On inhalation, oxygen pressure is higher in the alveoli than in the capillary blood; thus, oxygen passes from the alveoli into the blood. The same principle holds true for the passage of carbon dioxide from the blood to the alveoli. The pressure of carbon dioxide is higher in the pulmonary capillaries than in the alveoli; thus carbon dioxide diffuses into the alveoli for excretion.

The rate of gas exchange is influenced by the thickness of the alveolar–capillary membrane and by the size of the gas exchange surface provided by the alveolar walls. In health, diffusion is rapid because the alveolar–capillary membrane is very thin and the alveolar surface is expansive. Conditions that increase the thickness of the membrane or decrease the size of the alveolar surface reduce gas exchange. For example, edema present in lung tissue increases the thickness of the membrane and slows diffusion. Chronic diseases, such as emphysema or silicosis, damage the alveolar epithelium. As a result, less surface area is available for diffusion to take place (Porth, 1998).

Transport

The third process involved in oxygenation is the transport of oxygen and carbon dioxide between the capillaries in the lungs and the cells of the body. This process depends upon an adequate blood volume, an adequate amount of hemoglobin and an effective heart action to pump blood throughout the body.

When oxygen enters the blood it is transported in two forms—a small percentage (about 3%) is dissolved in the plasma and the remaining amount is carried by erythrocytes (red blood cells). Hemoglobin (Hgb) molecules make up the major portion of erythrocyte protein and are responsible for transporting oxygen and carbon dioxide (Black & Matassarin-Jacobs, 1997).

Heme is the oxygen-carrying component of hemoglobin. Heme units hold iron ions, which combine with oxygen to form oxyhemoglobin. The iron–oxygen interaction is such that oxygen can easily separate from hemoglobin, allowing it to leave the blood and enter the body cells. Oxygen that diffuses from the hemoglobin molecules into plasma is carried via interstitial fluid to the cells.

Carbon dioxide, the end product of cellular metabolism, is transported in several forms. About five percent is attached to hemoglobin (carbaminohemoglobin), five percent is dissolved in plasma and the remaining 90 percent is carried in the form of bicarbonate (HCO_3) (Porth, 1998).

Lung Clearance Mechanisms

The body has effective mechanisms for ensuring clean air intake and for removing unwanted debris and contaminants. These include filtration, mucociliary action, coughing and sneezing.

FILTRATION The body's first clearance mechanism is nasal hair. As air is inhaled, large particles such as sand or dust are trapped in the hairs and thus prevented from entering the nasal cavity.

MUCOCILIARY ACTION Mucous-secreting glands and tiny hair-like projections called *cilia* line the respiratory passageways. The mucous traps small particles while cilia move the collected particles towards the pharynx, where it is swallowed. It is estimated that a normal adult swallows about 10 mL of transported mucous daily (Traver, Mitchell & Flodquist-Priestley, 1991).

COUGHING Coughing is a defence mechanism the body uses for clearing the airways of secretions and debris. It is triggered by irritants such as smoke, smog, dust or toxic gases; by the infectious process; or by obstructions in the pharynx, larynx, trachea and bronchi. In the act of coughing, the glottis is forcibly closed while the lungs are relatively full. The abdominal and intercostal muscles contract suddenly, pushing the diaphragm upward and creating pressures that force air from the lower respiratory tract upward against the glottis. The glottis reopens and a blast of air passes upward carrying mucous, foreign particles and irritants out of the respiratory system (Porth, 1998).

SNEEZING A sneeze clears the upper respiratory passages. It is much like a cough except that air is expelled into the nasal cavity instead of the mouth. When someone sneezes, the uvula becomes depressed, closing the oral cavity from the pharynx and directing the air upward through the nose.

Determinants of Oxygenation

Adequate oxygenation of body tissues is affected by many factors, including environment, physiological factors, health status, health practices and lifestyle. Age-related influences on oxygenation are discussed in the next section.

Environment

The presence of atmospheric oxygen in adequate concentrations is vital to optimal respiratory functioning. Normally, the atmosphere supplies all the oxygen an individual requires. At sea level, air contains approximately 21 percent oxygen and 0.04 percent carbon dioxide. These concentrations appear to be the most conducive for normal breathing. At higher altitudes, the situation is different: as altitude increases, atmospheric pressure decreases. The alveolar pressure correspondingly goes down and less oxygen diffuses into the blood. The body responds by increasing the rate and depth of respirations. Visitors to high altitudes may experience fatigue until they become acclimatized to the rarefied atmosphere.

Air pollutants such as smoke, industrial gaseous wastes and automobile exhaust fumes alter the availability of oxygen and have detrimental effects on respiratory functioning. Noxious or toxic gases in the air displace the oxygen normally present and decrease the amount of oxygen available for diffusion.

The respiratory rate is also affected by climate. In hot weather, the peripheral blood vessels dilate. The resistance of blood flow decreases and, consequently, blood pressure drops. The heart responds by increasing cardiac output to maintain blood pressure. With the increase in cardiac output, there is a need for more oxygen. Thus, the rate and depth of respirations increase. In cold weather, blood vessels constrict. Blood pressure increases, cardiac action decreases and the need for oxygen is reduced. As a result, respirations become slower.

Physiological Factors and Health Status

In addition to an adequate supply of oxygen in the atmosphere, our ability to meet our need for oxygen depends on the patency of airways, proper muscular functioning, pulmonary compliance and an adequate mechanism for transporting oxygen and carbon dioxide. Both physiological factors and health status can influence the effectiveness of these processes in oxygenation.

PATENT AIRWAYS In ventilation, oxygen passes through the nose, pharynx, larynx, trachea, bronchi and bronchioles to the alveoli, and then carbon dioxide passes back. Obstructions (partial or complete) in any of the passageways will interfere with the efficiency of ventilation and cause considerable breathing difficulty. Airways can be obstructed by food and fluids. Children often put small objects such as toys and coins into their mouths and subsequently aspirate them. Airway obstruction is always a danger in unconscious individuals, since the tongue can fall back into the oropharynx and block it.

The airway may also be obstructed by excessive or thickened secretions, tumours or tissue growths and edema in the respiratory tract. Diseases such as emphysema, asthma and bronchitis affect ventilation because they obstruct the airway or increase the resistance to the normal flow of air during inhalation and exhalation. Normally, a certain amount of resistance is present in the airways owing to the slight expansion and contraction of the relatively rigid airway structures. When the airways become less elastic because of tissue changes, or obstructed by thickened secretions, the effort involved in breathing increases in an attempt to move air through the narrowed passageways.

Some patients have difficulty clearing secretions for various reasons—because of pain on coughing, unconsciousness or lack of muscle strength. During the aging process, the pressure an individual can achieve during maximum inspiration or expiration decreases, so that the ability to generate the high air flows required for effective coughing is reduced. Also, there is decreased ciliary movement in lower airways, which slows the cough reflex. Whatever the cause, secretions can accumulate and the patient may require assistance for their removal.

MUSCLE FUNCTIONING The condition of the body's musculature affects breathing. If the chest is unable to expand because of trauma or thoracic or abdominal surgery, ventilation will be impaired. Disease processes that weaken or paralyze the muscles that move the ribcage, such as Guillain-Barré syndrome or poliomyelitis, affect the ability to breathe normally.

Continual bed rest and immobility alter ventilation of the lungs. Pressure of the bed against the body limits chest expansion and alveolar ventilations. In the supine or dorsal recumbent position, abdominal organs push against the diaphragm, restricting its movement and thus the movement of air through the lungs. Limited or inadequate chest expansion leads to stasis and pooling of respiratory secretions which harbour microorganisms and may cause infection (hypostatic pneumonia).

PULMONARY COMPLIANCE Lungs that have the elastic properties to expand and recoil with ease during the act of breathing are said to be compliant. Lungs with low compliance (lungs that are stiff) require greater than normal energy expenditure to achieve adequate levels of ventila-

there is less available for other needs, and body functions are compromised. Low or inadequate compliance results from restrictive lung diseases, for example, fibrosis, emphysema, tumour, paralysis, kyphosis, or scoliosis (curvature of the spine).

TRANSPORT OF OXYGEN AND CARBON DIOXIDE Many factors can affect the transport of oxygen and carbon dioxide to and from the cells. There may be an inadequate force from the heart to pump blood through the lungs, or there may be an impediment in the return flow of blood from the lungs to the heart, causing a slowing up (stasis) of blood in the small vessels that surround the alveoli. Such conditions interfere with oxygenation by disturbing the balance of partial pressures of oxygen and carbon dioxide circulating through the lungs.

Similarly, any condition affecting the blood volume and the circulation of blood to the tissues can interfere with the transportation of oxygen from the lungs to the cells. This would include all types of heart diseases, bleeding disorders and arterial or venous disorders, as well as blood dyscrasias. In anemia, for example, the blood lacks adequate hemoglobin to carry oxygen to the cells of the body.

Among the major diseases affecting the cardiovascular system are those that cause the blood vessels to narrow and deteriorate, resulting in inadequate oxygenation and subsequent damage of tissues in vital organs, such as the heart, brain, kidneys or other parts of the body. Most of the damage is caused by three major types of heart disease—atherosclerosis (hardening of the arteries), hypertension (high blood pressure) and congenital defects. These diseases may lead to congestive heart failure, myocardial infarction and cerebral vascular accident (stroke).

Health Practices and Lifestyle

There are many health practices and lifestyle factors that can affect the ability to meet one's oxygen needs. The positive influence of exercise and fitness, as well as the negative effects of cigarette smoking and occupational hazards, will be discussed here.

Exercise increases the efficiency of all body functions and processes. Regular exercise, particularly aerobic exercise, such as sustained speed walking, running or swimming, enhances respiratory and cardiovascular endurance, as well as muscular strength and tone. During exercise, the metabolic rate goes up and demands for oxygen increase. The person breathes more deeply and rapidly to take in extra oxygen, and the heart beats more rapidly and forcefully to supply the needed oxygen to the cells. Over time, the lungs increase their capacity to take up oxygen, the blood increases its capacity to pick up and carry more oxygen, and the heart

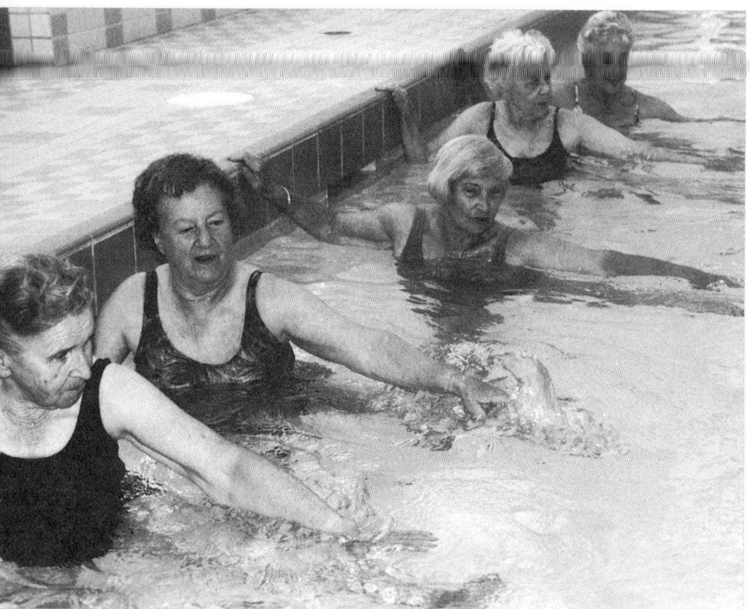

Regular exercise, particularly aerobic exercise such as swimming, enhances respiratory and cardiovascular functioning.

strengthens in its capacity to supply the oxygenated blood to the muscles. Furthermore, the muscles become very effective in using oxygen to generate the energy needed for their activity. The more conditioned the muscles become, the less oxygen they need to accomplish their work. In short, with regular exercise, cardiopulmonary effort and oxygen use in the body become very efficient, bringing significant benefits to health and well-being.

Cigarette smoking is a hazard to health and a major factor associated with lung cancer, chronic obstructive pulmonary disease (COPD) and coronary artery disease (CAD). In the lungs, cigarette smoke induces a variety of inflammatory changes that lead to disease. Small airways become ulcerated, narrowed and fibrosed. Mucous secretion in the bronchi produces sputum and a characteristic smoker's cough. Cilia are damaged and ciliary movement is impaired, thereby interfering with effective ciliary clearance. The alveoli themselves may suffer from inflammation and structural abnormalities that result in disease. While a direct cause-and-effect relationship between smoking and coronary artery disease has not been determined, the relationship is thought to be due to the physiologic effect of nicotine and other chemicals that increase the risk of atherosclerosis. Cigarette smoking "has been shown to cause changes in blood lipid levels, increasing triglycerides and total cholesterol while decreasing high density lipoprotein cholesterol, a lipid profile more prone to atherosclerosis" (Williams, 1993, p. 180).

Not only is smoking detrimental to the health of those who smoke, it is also harmful to those exposed to the passive or sidestream smoke given off by burning cigarettes. Epidemiological studies have found that lung cancer is more prevalent in people exposed to passive smoke than those living in a smoke free environment. Similarly, children of parents who smoke suffer more episodes of respiratory illness such as chronic coughing, bronchitis and laryngitis than do children of nonsmoking parents (Williams, 1993; Ellis & Nowlis, 1994).

Certain occupations expose workers to irritants that may cause lung disease. People working at construction sites, mines, shipyards and chemical plants are exposed to dusts and hazardous materials that pervade the atmosphere, for example, coal dust, asbestos fibres, silica dust or toxic fumes. Irritants infiltrate the lining of the air passageways and lung tissues, causing inflammation and damage. Scar tissue forms, which reduces lung elasticity and restricts air flow along the passageways.

MEDICATIONS

Drugs and anesthetics that act as depressants on the central nervous system decrease the rate and depth of respirations and may, when administered in large dosages, cause respiratory arrest. Morphine and meperidine (Demerol) are common examples of drugs that depress respirations.

Oxygen Needs Throughout the Life Cycle

During pregnancy, the diaphragm is pushed upward as the fetus grows and the uterus expands in the abdominal cavity. The lungs of the mother are gradually squeezed as space in the chest cavity decreases. Pregnant women usually find that they breathe more rapidly than usual and may experience shortness of breath and dyspnea (difficult breathing) after mild exertion (Jarvis, 1996).

The fetus receives its needed oxygen from the mother, the supply being transferred from the mother's circulation to the placenta and, then, via the umbilical cord to the fetus. Readers interested in the fetal circulation and the changes that take place in cardiovascular and pulmonary function after birth are referred to an obstetrical nursing book.

Infants are obligatory nose-breathers during the first year of life. Therefore, congestion in the nasal passages can create problems, especially during feeding. Infants breathe much more rapidly than adults; 30 to 60 breaths per minute is the normal range. The rate remains high through the first months of life, slowing down gradually to about 20 to 40 breaths per minute at 12 months. The higher rate is due to the smaller lung capacity. A normal full-term infant has a total lung capacity of only 300 mL and a tidal volume of 25 mL (Pillitteri, 1995).

Respiratory infections are common in infants and children. Newborns are usually immune, because of antibodies received from the mother, until they are two to three months

GERONTOLOGICAL

Respiratory Changes Associated with Aging

Organ	Change and Rationale	Implication for Health Promotion
Nose	Reduced number and activity of cilia cause reduced bronchoelimination Less effective clearing of respiratory tract predisposes to infections	Avoid smoke-filled environment Wear mask if air pollution exists Avoid allergens Maintain health status and avoid crowds in winter to prevent respiratory infections and pneumonia
Throat	Cough reflex decreased. Sensitivity to stimuli decreased	Teach safety factors, especially when eating (cut food into small portions, chew well, eat slowly)
Trachea	Flexibility is decreased; size of structure is increased	
Ribcage and Respiratory Muscles	Calcification of chest wall causes ribcage to be less mobile Decreased strength of intercostal and other respiratory muscles and diaphragm impairs breathing	Maintain exercise, deep breathing and erect posture to enhance respiratory muscle function
	Osteoporosis of ribs and vertebrae weakens chest wall and respiratory function Calcification of vertebral cartilage and kyphosis stiffen chest wall and impair respiratory movements	Avoid pressure to ribs to prevent rib fracture (e.g., leaning chest on edge of bathtub)
Lungs	Capacity to inhale, hold, and exhale breath decreases wtih age. Vital capacity at 85 is 50–65% of capacity at 30	Encourage deep breathing, full exhalation and erect posture throughout life. Maintain exercise to enhance lung function
	Elastin and collagen changes cause loss of elasticity of lung tissue; lungs remain hyperinflated even on exhalation, and proportion of dead space increases Decreased elasticity and increased size of alveoli. Increased diffusion and surface area across alveolar–capillary membrane	Activity should be adjusted to respiratory efficiency and ventilation–perfusion ratio

SOURCE: Murray & Zentner, 1997, p. 717.

old. During the first two to three years of life, respiratory infection is not uncommon as children gradually build up active immunity to the organisms normally prevalent in their environment. Immunization (which confers passive immunity) to pertussis (whooping cough) is routinely started in infancy to protect the child from this disease.

During childhood, the diameter of the upper respiratory tract is small, and obstruction caused by the accumulation of secretions from infection, allergy or inhalation of a foreign body can be serious. Coins and toys are common sources of obstruction in young children.

With adolescence, there is a rapid increase in lung capacity as the chest expands. Boys show a greater increase than girls; the chest cavity of the male becomes larger and the shoulders broader. Adolescence can be a time of respiratory health risk, as many teens begin smoking, exposing themselves to serious future health problems.

Respiratory infections, in the form of colds, bronchitis and pneumonia, are a common cause of short-term illness in adults. People appear to be most resistant to these infections in the late middle years. However, this is also the time that chronic respiratory ailments become more prevalent. The term *chronic obstructive pulmonary disease* (COPD) is used to refer to a group of disorders associated with chronic obstruction of air flow into and out of the lungs. COPD includes such conditions as emphysema, chronic bronchitis and asthma. These are irreversible conditions commonly associated with cigarette smoking, air pollution and exposure to hazardous substances.

The efficiency of an individual's cardiorespiratory system gradually declines with age. The effects may not be evident at rest but become noticeable when effort is required. Adults who remain physically active, however, maintain higher aerobic capacities than do sedentary individuals. In

RESEARCH to practice

Madge, P., McColl, J., & Paton, J. (1997, March). Impact of a nurse-led home management training programme in children admitted to hospital with acute asthma: A randomized controlled study. *Thorax, 52,* 223–228.

The purpose of this study was to identify whether a nurse-led home education program for parents of children with asthma would decrease the rate of hospital readmissions. The design was a randomized controlled study using four wards of a busy children's teaching hospital in Scotland.

The study group consisted of 201 children who were less than two years of age. Ninety-six were allocated to the nurse-led training program and 105 to usual care. The study nurse, who had specialized asthma training, met with parents for three teaching and discussion sessions of approximately 45 minutes. The study group received discharge education, follow-up and telephone support. The control group received limited advice on discharge.

The results of this study indicated that fewer children with asthma who received the nurse-led education program with follow-up support and education were readmitted to hospital than children who received the usual treatment. However, the groups did not differ significantly on the number of emergency department visits.

the normal aging process, the chest wall stiffens and the lungs lose their elasticity. As a result, the ability to ventilate the lungs slowly decreases. In addition, as people age, their ciliary activity and cough efficiency decrease, making them more vulnerable to respiratory infections. The cardiovascular system also undergoes gradual change during aging. Usually, maximum cardiac output decreases so that by the age of 65 years it is typically 20 to 30 percent less than that of a young adult. In middle age, blood pressure increases, owing to the diminishing elasticity of blood vessel walls, but stabilizes by about the age of 65 years (Ebersole & Hess, 1998; Murray & Zentner, 1997).

Common Problems

Disturbances in oxygenation may cause a number of health problems. These commonly include hypoxemia and hypoxia, dyspnea, cough and chest pain.

HYPOXEMIA AND HYPOXIA **Hypoxemia** refers to a decrease in the oxygen content of the blood and is frequently associated with **hypoxia**, which is an insufficient supply of oxygen to the tissues. The body's responses to hypoxemia and hypoxia depend on how suddenly these states develop. With rapidly developing hypoxia there are changes in CNS functioning because the higher centres are more sensitive to oxygen depletion. The patient may exhibit motor incoordination and impaired judgement; increased (rapid) pulse; rapid, shallow respirations; dyspnea; increased restlessness; and flaring of nares. Patients with long-standing conditions (for example, COPD) may show signs of fatigue, drowsiness, apathy, inattentiveness or delayed reaction time, altered thought process, headache, chest pain, enlarged heart, anorexia, decreased urinary output, weakness of extremity muscles or muscle pain.

DYSPNEA People whose oxygen needs are not being met often experience **dyspnea**, defined as difficult or laboured breathing. An individual with dyspnea may not be able to climb a flight of stairs or walk a block to the corner store without finding it hard to breathe. Often, it is more difficult to breathe when lying flat (orthopnea). Asthmatic patients, those with chronic obstructive lung disorders and those with heart conditions frequently use numerous pillows to raise themselves to a sitting position for more comfortable sleeping. The sitting position promotes maximum expansion of the chest and also prevents the pooling of blood in the large abdominal vessels. Excessive fatigue is commonly experienced, as even normal daily activities can be exhausting to the person who does not have enough oxygen to supply bodily needs.

COUGH Coughing is the body's mechanism for ridding the respiratory tract of irritations and obstructions. It is also a troublesome symptom associated with respiratory disease. The characteristics of the cough and the nature of sputum produced are often indicative of specific diseases. For instance, a harsh productive cough of yellow-green sputum is indicative of bacterial infection. Clear, white sputum can be characteristic of asthma and pink froth sputum indicative of pulmonary edema. A brassy, **nonproductive cough** (a cough without the production of mucous) is associated with pressure on the trachea. **Hemoptysis** is the coughing up of sputum containing varying amounts of blood. It may be associated with cancer of the lung or chronic conditions such as bronchiectasis.

CHEST PAIN Many patients with respiratory problems experience pain in the chest. The pain may or may not be associated with the act of breathing. Pain may be caused by a number of different factors, such as inflammation, the presence of space-occupying lesions or increased muscular activity as the patient works harder to breathe. The presence or absence of chest pain should be noted. A description of the pain (for example, sharp, dull, intermittent or steady) should be reported, as should the location of the pain and its relationship to breathing.

Assessing Oxygen Needs

[illegible] techniques and physical assessment skills, the nurse gathers subjective and objective data about the patient's oxygenation status. In determining oxygen needs and developing a plan of individualized care, the nurse also draws information from the medical history, from laboratory and diagnostic test results and from the physician's plan of care.

Nursing Health History

The health history provides the basis for planning individualized patient care. The nurse gathers information about the patient's usual pattern of oxygenation, including information about home environment, activity level, and whether or not the patient or family members smoke. Recent changes or deviations from the patient's usual breathing pattern, any recent or past related health problems (for example, respiratory and cardiovascular diseases) and symptoms relating to the presenting problem are explored. The patient's family history is also pertinent. Problems such as allergies, asthma, chronic bronchitis or frequent bouts of pneumonia tend to be genetically predisposed. Many people with chronic respiratory problems use oxygen at home (portable units), and they often use humidifiers, nebulizers and other aids. These should be noted on the patient's chart. Finally, the individual's health-promoting and health-protecting patterns are examined to determine opportunities for health teaching.

Patients who are admitted with oxygen problems may be in severe distress. They may be hypoxic, or have difficulty breathing or severe chest pain. They may not have the energy to speak and they may be anxious and confused. A quick visual assessment before undertaking the health history will determine the degree of distress a patient is in. When patients are in distress, the health history interview is deferred until their immediate needs are met and they are more comfortable. The nurse may need to collect data during several visits or allow for periods of rest for patients who become short of breath or experience chest pain during the interview. The history may also be obtained from a family member. A guide for taking an oxygen health history follows.

Measurements

VITAL SIGNS

The assessment of oxygenation status includes measurement of the vital signs—temperature, pulse, respirations and blood pressure. The techniques for obtaining these measurements are described in Chapter 16.

PULSE OXIMETRY

Pulse oximetry is a simple, painless and noninvasive method of measuring a patient's arterial blood oxygen saturation levels. Oxygen saturation ($Sa\ O_2$) is the amount of oxygen being carried by hemoglobin, expressed as a percentage of the maximum oxygen-carrying capacity of the hemoglobin. Measurements are made with an oximeter that uses a light-sensitive probe attached to cutaneous tissue with a pulsating vascular bed, such as the fingertip, ear lobe, toe or bridge of the nose. Oximetry is used in a wide variety of situations to monitor responses to treatment or to observe patients who are at risk for developing hypoxemia. For instance, it may be implemented for patients recovering from anesthesia in the immediate postoperative period. Monitoring can be intermittent or continuous. The steps involved in conducting pulse oximetry are outlined in Procedure 24.1.

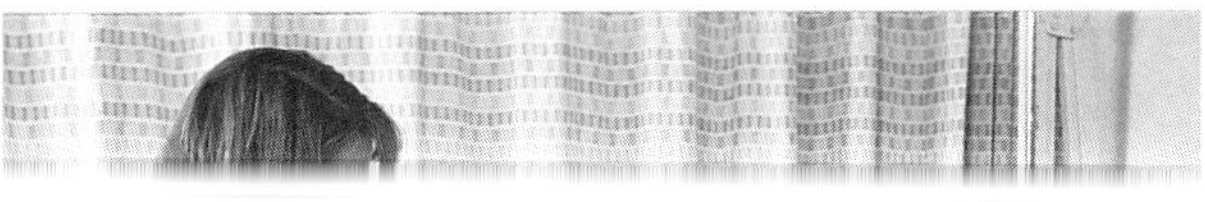

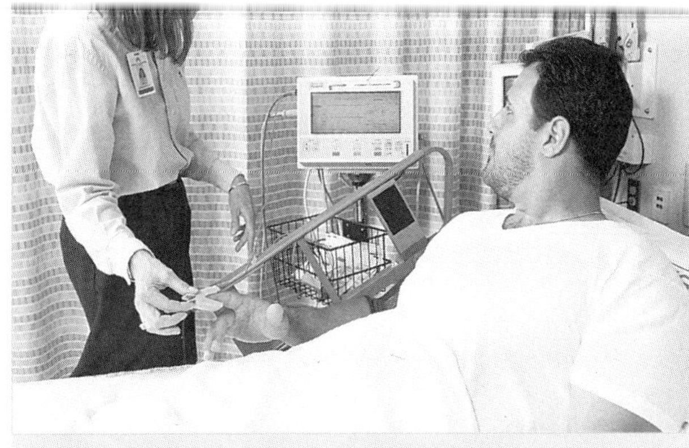

Pulse oximetry carried out by a respiratory therapist.

Preparing the Patient

Explain the purpose and procedure for the test. Pulse oximetry requires little time and is painless.

Assembling Equipment

The pulse oximeter is a small device with a spectrophotometer probe that contains two sensors. One sensor emits red and infrared light beams through the tissues and the other receives wavelengths of light reflected from capillary hemoglobin. Hemoglobin that is saturated (red) absorbs light differently than does hemoglobin that is desaturated (blue) and reflects light in accordance with the amount it absorbs. The probe measures the amount of light reflected from the hemoglobin and sends the information to a computer, which calculates the oxygen saturation and displays the value on a digital screen. The pulse rate is also displayed (Ehrhardt & Graham, 1990).

PEAK FLOW

Peak flow is the measurement of peak expiratory flow rates (PEFRs). Often used with asthmatics, a peak flow meter can be used at the bedside to monitor a patient's respiratory

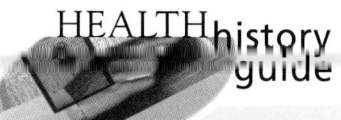

Oxygenation

Health and Illness Patterns

Usual Pattern of Oxygenation

- Describe your usual pattern of breathing. Is it effortless? Difficult?
- Does activity affect your breathing?
- Do you tire easily?
- Does your breathing pattern affect your activities of daily living?
- Do you have allergies in different seasons?
- Do you smoke? If so, what type of tobacco (cigarette, cigar, pipe)? For how many years? How many cigarettes per day?
- Does anyone in your home smoke? Are you exposed to smoke at work?
- Are you exposed to respiratory irritants at home or at work? For example, glue, paints, silica, asbestos, pesticides, grain dust, plants?
- Do you use any aids for breathing such as oxygen, humidifiers or nebulizers?
- Do you routinely use over-the-counter nasal sprays or inhalers?
- How many pillows do you sleep with?

Recent Changes in Pattern of Oxygenation

- Have there been any recent changes in your usual pattern of oxygenation? Shortness of breath? Difficulty breathing? Wheezing? Troublesome cough? Excessive sputum? Fatigue? Chest pain?
- Have you had a recent illness that affected breathing? A cold? Respiratory infection (for example, strep throat, tonsillitis)?
- Any recent injuries to the thoracic cage (ribs), surgeries or other procedures on your chest?
- Have you received any vaccinations against pneumonia or the flu?

Presenting Health Problem

- Describe the symptoms you are experiencing now. Do you have wheezing? Tightness in the chest? Shortness of breath? Do you have a cough? How did it begin (sudden or gradual)? Is it dry or accompanied by sputum? Does it cause fatigue? Does it affect your sleep? Does it occur at a specific time of day?
- Do you have a fever?
- Do you have sputum? If so, describe it. What is the amount? Appearance (clear, mucoid, yellowish, greenish, purulent, blood-tinged, bloody)?
- Do you have pain associated with breathing? If so, describe it. Onset (gradual or sudden)? Intensity? Frequency? Location? Any radiation?
- Do your lips or nail beds turn blue?
- Do you feel dizzy when you change positions?
- Do your shoes or rings feel tight?
- Does your heart sometimes feel as though it is pounding?
- Do you feel tired or fatigued?
- Have you experienced anorexia or weight loss?
- When did the symptoms begin? Duration? Are they constant or intermittent?
- Are the symptoms associated with an activity, time of event or environmental factors? For example, asthma attack brought on by exposure to cats?
- What remedies have you tried for the symptoms? Have you tried sitting up? Sleeping with pillows? Over-the-counter drugs such as decongestants, nasal sprays? What were the results?
- Do you have a history of any acute or chronic diseases that disrupt oxygenation? For example, colds, allergies, asthma, bronchitis, pneumonia, emphysema, high blood pressure, pleurisy, tuberculosis, myocardial infarction, congestive heart failure, anemia?
- Are you taking any medications for respiratory problems, high blood pressure or heart disease? If so, what kind? Dosage? Frequency?
- Have you had rheumatic fever or a heart murmur?
- Has any member of your family had emphysema, asthma, respiratory allergies, tuberculosis, heart disease, high blood pressure, cystic fibrosis or lung cancer?
- Have you had past occupations that exposed you to respiratory irritants?

Health Promotion and Protection Patterns

- Do you drink alcohol? If so, how much and how often?
- Do you exercise regularly? If so, what is the nature of your program?
- Do you own, or are you around, any pets or other animals?
- Are you currently experiencing stress in your life?
- When was your last chest x-ray?
- When was your last tuberculin test?
- Are your immunizations up to date?
- What home remedies do you use for respiratory problems?
- Do you use an air conditioner, air purifier or humidifier in your home?
- If smoking, do you have any feelings about or interest in quitting?
- Would you like to know about ways to protect yourself from respiratory irritants and pollution?

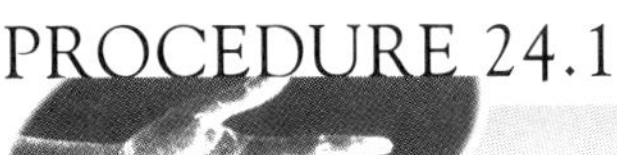

PROCEDURE 24.1 Performing Pulse Oximetry

Action	Rationale
1. Prepare the patient.	Promotes well-being and enables patient participation.
2. Wash hands and gather pulse oximeter and sensor probe.	Reduces transmission of microorganisms.
3. Select a site with adequate peripheral circulation, for example, finger, ear, toe or bridge of nose. If using a finger or toe, check the proximal pulse and capillary refill closest to the site.	Test requires an adequate vascular area for transmission of light.
4. Cleanse the site with water and dry well.	Body oils, artificial nails or nail polish interfere with transmission of light.
5. Attach the probe to the site according to manufacturer's directions.	Incorrect placement gives an inaccurately low reading or no reading at all.
6. Ask the patient to remain still. If the patient is restless, the probe may be lightly taped.	Saturation reading may be inaccurate if circulation is restricted.
7. Turn the machine on.	
8. When the oxygen saturation reading has stabilized, wait 30 seconds and note reading.	Readings can be affected by motion, low perfusion, vasoconstriction, impaired tissue perfusion, intravenous fluids, nail polish and direct excessive lighting.
9. Remove the probe, turn off the machine and clean the probe with alcohol.	Prevents the spread of microorganisms.
10. Indicate if reading was taken on room air or on oxygen (state amount and method).	Provides baseline data.
11. Document the date, time, oxygen saturation, observations and nursing care.	Fulfills requirements for nurse accountability and facilitates interventions.

status and response to bronchodilator treatment. This hand-held device is an important clinical tool for assessment of a patient's respiratory status. Because readings are effort-dependent, variability may occur. A patient should be instructed to breathe in deeply, place the lips tightly on the mouthpiece, and blow out as hard and as fast as possible. Two or three trials may be needed to perfect the technique, with the average peak flow recorded. The nurse should monitor the patient for respiratory fatigue during this procedure and be aware that bronchospasm may occur.

Physical Assessment

Physical assessment of oxygen status involves an examination of the patient's cardiovascular and respiratory functioning. The nurse uses inspection, palpation, auscultation and percussion techniques as outlined in Chapter 16.

Before starting the physical examination it is important to ensure the room is well lit, quiet, warm and private. Natural lighting is necessary to examine subtle colour changes and breathing patterns. Minimal noise facilitates detection of respiratory sounds. Every effort should be made to ensure patient privacy and to prevent interruptions. This enables the patient to relax and helps ensure a comprehensive assessment. Each step of the examination should be carefully explained and clear directions given when needed, for example, "Please breathe in deeply and hold it," so the patient knows what to expect. A calm, matter-of-fact manner can often allay anxiety, even for patients who are in distress.

For examination of the chest and lungs, the patient should wear a gown that can be dropped to the waist. Bras and undershirts should be removed to provide maximum view of the chest. The patient should sit upright, lean slightly forward and have the arms rest comfortably across the lap; shoulders should be brought forward to abduct the scapula so that a greater lung surface can be examined. Assessments should be made in an organized manner. The posterior and lateral aspects of the chest are examined first; then the nurse moves to face the patient for the anterior examination. One side is compared to the other for variations, proceeding from the top downward.

INSPECTION

The nurse begins inspection by exposing the chest and observing the patient's posture and the contour or shape of the thorax. Normally, the transverse diameter should be greater than the anteroposterior (AP) diameter. The normal chest is symmetric with bilateral muscular development, although slightly greater muscle development may be present on the patient's dominant side. The rib cartilages should curve slightly out from the sternum. The spinal processes of C7 and T1 to T7 should be straight, and the scapulae should be symmetrical. The intercostal spaces should be flat or depressed. Normal and abnormal configurations of the thorax are illustrated in Table 24.2.

The patient's respiratory movements and breathing pattern are examined next. At this time, the nurse also listens for audible breath sounds (sounds heard without the use of a stethoscope). During breathing, the chest should expand symmetrically and without obvious use of accessory muscles. There should be no retractions or bulging of the intercostal spaces on inspiration. The normal adult breathing pattern is smooth and regular with 12 to 20 breaths per minute. The ratio of respirations to pulse rate is 1:4. Breathing should be quiet and effortless. Audible breath sounds are usually the result of extra breathing effort combined with obstruction. **Stridor** is a harsh high-pitched "crowing" sound heard on inspiration when there is a narrowing of the upper airway, that is, the larynx or trachea. Infants and young children with croup often manifest stridor. **Stertor** is a snoring sound made when secretions are present in the trachea or large bronchi. **Wheezing** is a high-pitched whistling sound often made on inspiration when the airway is partially obstructed. People with asthma make wheezing sounds. Table 24.3 describes and illustrates normal and abnormal breathing patterns.

Sputum, if produced, must be inspected. Sputum is not saliva. It is a mucous secretion from the lungs, bronchi and trachea composed of mucous, dust particles and microbial debris, saliva, nasal and sinus secretions, normal oral bacteria and epithelial cells. Normal sputum is clear, white and slightly frothy because it contains air bubbles. Abnormal sputum is produced as a pulmonary reaction to any constant recurring irritant, including nasal discharge. The characteristics and amounts of sputum reflect the patient's overall condition and the particular pulmonary dysfunction. In assessing sputum, the nurse notes the amount (in millilitres), consistency (thin, watery, thick, sticky, tenacious, mucoid), odour (musty, foul), colour (clear, cloudy, white, yellow, greenish, pink or rusty) and the presence of blood (hemoptysis).

The colour of skin and mucous membranes is also assessed. The patient's skin colour should be consistent with his or her genetic background. If well oxygenated, the skin, nail beds and mucous membranes should be pink in colour. People with darker skin colour should have rosy undertones. There should be no pallor or cyanosis in highly vascular areas. In light-skinned people, cyanosis can be detected in the lips, nail beds, tip of the nose, top of the ear and underside of the tongue. Colour changes can be more subtle in dark-skinned individuals. A bluish hue in the nail beds, lips

TABLE 24.2 Configurations of the thorax

Normal Adult (for Comparison)

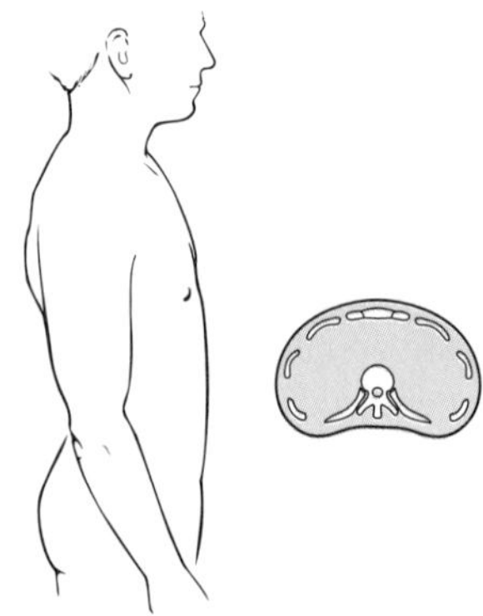

The thorax has an elliptical shape with an anteroposterior: transverse diameter of 1:2 or 5:7

Barrel Chest

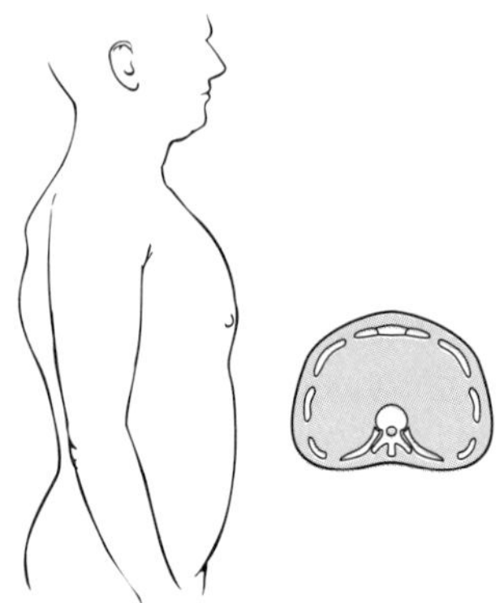

Note that anteroposterior and transverse diameters are equal, and that ribs are horizontal instead of the normal downward slope. This is associated with normal aging and also with chronic emphysema and asthma due to hyperinflation of lungs

TABLE 24.2 *continued*

Pectus Excavatum

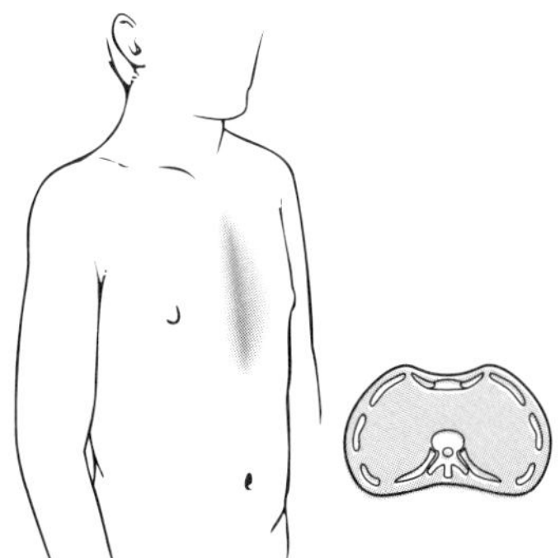

A markedly sunken sternum and adjacent cartilages (also called funnel breast). Depression begins at second intercostal space, becoming depressed most at junction of xiphoid process with body of sternum. More noticeable on inspiration. Congenital, usually not symptomatic. When severe, sternal depression may cause embarrassment and a negative self-concept. Surgery may be indicated for cosmetic purposes

Pectus Carinatum

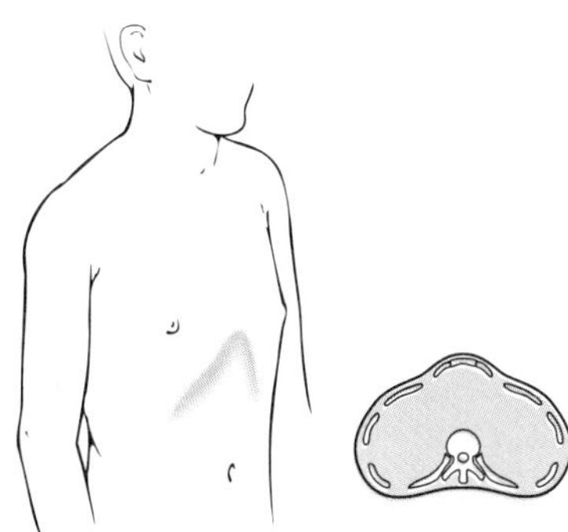

A forward protrusion of the sternum, with ribs sloping back at either side and vertical depressions along costochondral junctions (pigeon breast). Less common than pectus excavatum, this minor deformity requires no treatment. If severe, surgery may be indicated for cosmetic purposes

Scoliosis

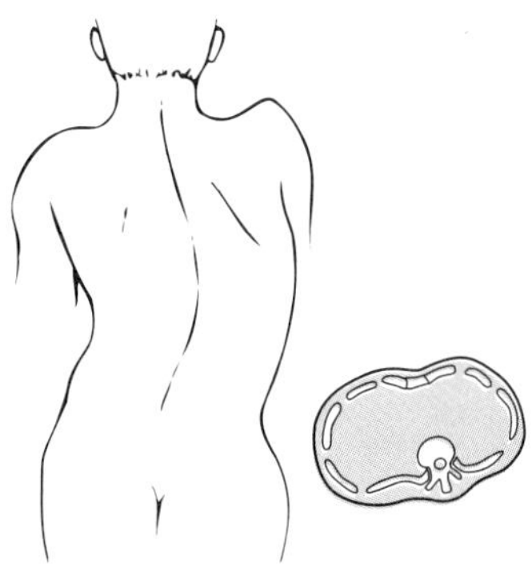

A lateral S-shaped curvature of the thoracic and lumbar spine, usually with involved vertebrae rotation. Note unequal shoulder and scapular height and unequal hip levels, rib interspaces flared on convex site. More prevalent in adolescent age groups, especially girls. Mild deformities are asymptomatic. If severe (> 45°) deviation is present, scoliosis may reduce lung volume; then person is at risk for impaired cardiopulmonary function. Primary impairment is cosmetic deformity, negatively affecting self-image. Refer early for treatment, often surgery

Kyphosis

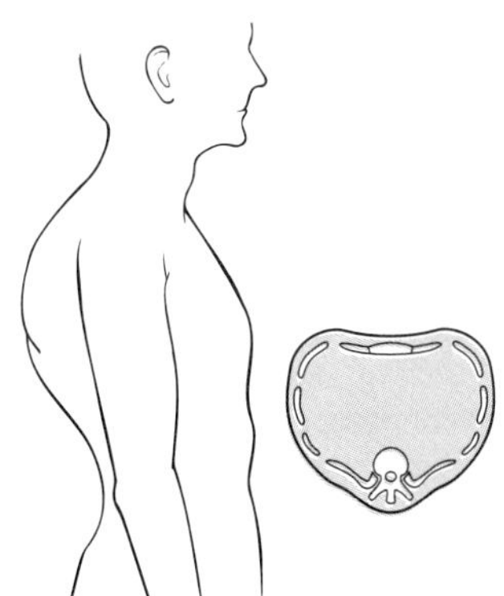

An exaggerated posterior curvature of the thoracic spine (humpback). Mild deformities are asymptomatic. Severe deformities impair cardiopulmonary function. Also associated with aging. Compensation may occur by hyperextension of head to maintain level of vision

SOURCE: Jarvis, 1996, pp. 497–498.

TABLE 24.3 Breathing patterns or rhythms

Normal Adult

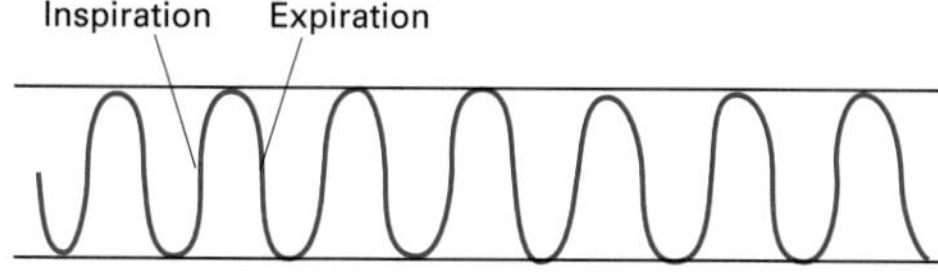

Rate: 10–20 breaths/min
Depth: deep
Pattern: easy, smooth, quiet, even, effortless, occasional sigh, automatic
The ratio of pulse to respirations is constant, about 4:1

Sigh

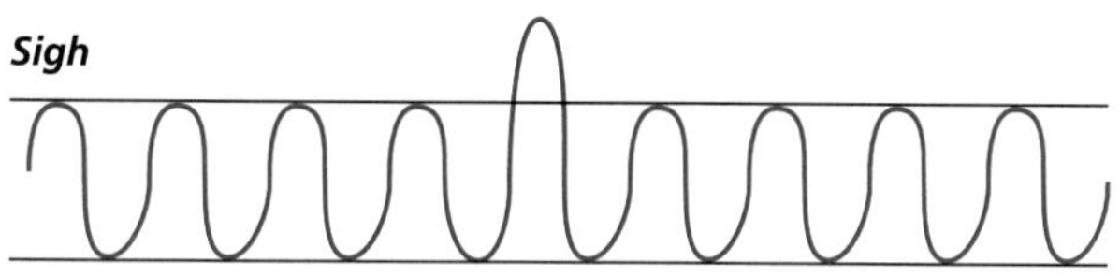

Occasional sighs are normal; their purpose is to expand alveoli. Frequent sighing may indicate emotional dysfunction and may lead to hyperventilation and dizziness

Tachypnea or Polypnea

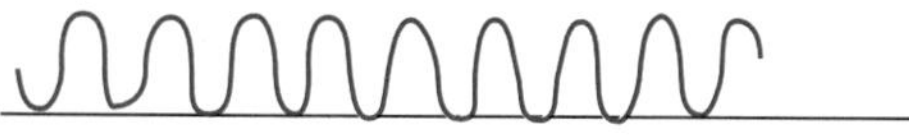

Rapid, shallow breathing
Rate: increased over 24 breaths/min. This is a normal response to fever, fear or exercise. Also occurs with respiratory insufficiency, pneumonia, alkalosis, pleurisy

Bradypnea

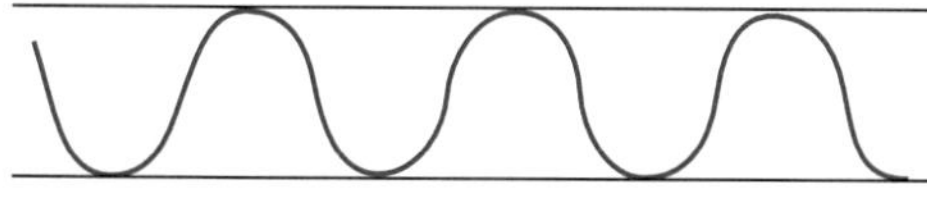

Slow breathing—fewer than 10 breaths/minute
Regular rate
Occurs in protective response to pain, depression of medulla (respiratory centre), increased intracranial pressure, diabetic coma

Hyperventilation (Hyperpnea)

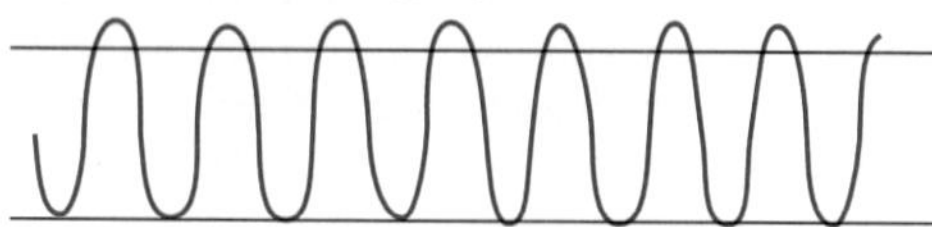

Increase in rate and depth. Normal with extreme exertion, fear or anxiety or when amphetamines are given. Also occurs when blood gas concentrations are altered (either an increase in carbon dioxide or decrease in oxygen). Hyperventilation blows off carbon dioxide, causing a decreased level in the blood (alkalosis).
Amount of air in alveoli exceeds the body's metabolic requirements

Hypoventilation

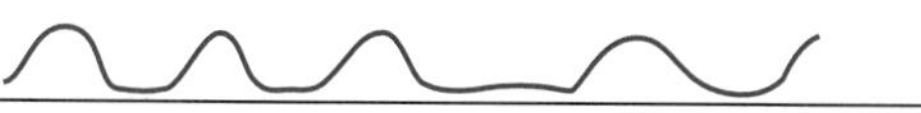

An irregular, shallow, slow pattern of inadequate alveolar ventilation which does not meet the body's requirements. Carbon dioxide is retained in the blood (hypercapnia). May be caused by prolonged bed rest, conscious splinting of the chest to avoid respiratory pain, side effect of some medications. Occurs in respiratory diseases such as pneumonia, asthma, emphysema, airway obstructions

TABLE 24.3 *continued*

Cheyne-Stokes Respiration 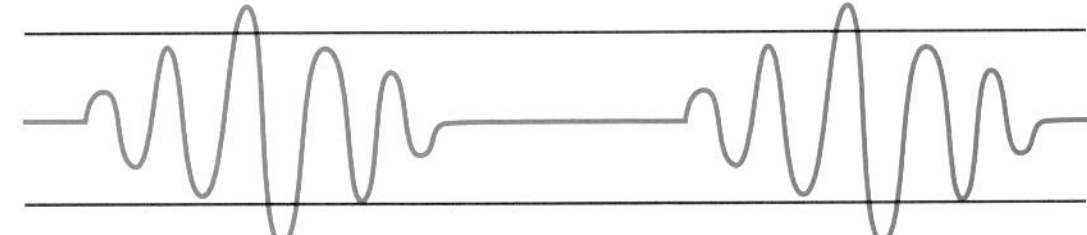	A regular cycle in which there is a gradual increase (wax) followed by a gradual decrease (wane) in the depth of respiration and then a period of apnea (temporary cessation of breathing). Breathing periods last 30–45 seconds with periods of apnea lasting 20 seconds. Most common causes are congestive heart failure, renal failure, increased intracranial pressure or drug overdose. Occurs normally in infants and aging persons during sleep
Ataxic 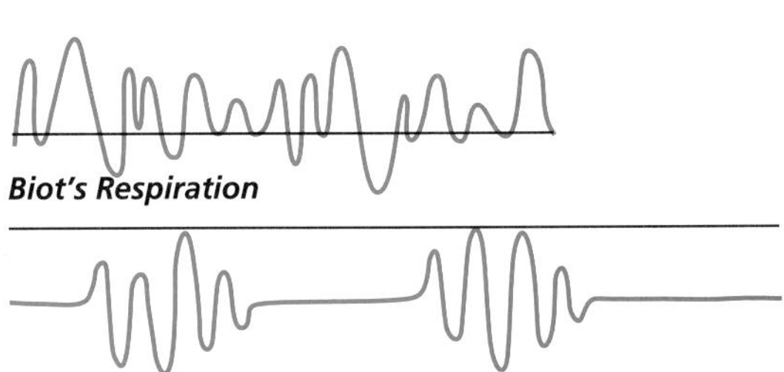	Irregular breathing pattern with both deep and shallow breaths occurring randomly. Seen in patients with lesions of the medulla
Biot's Respiration 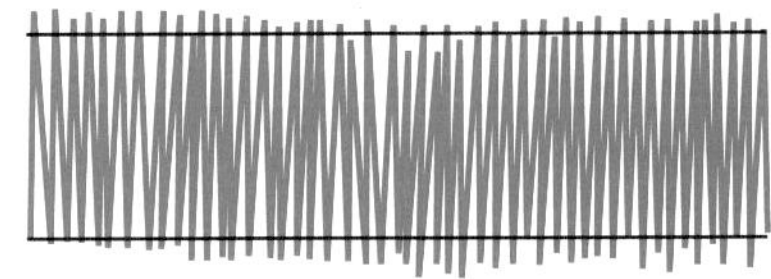	Disorganized pattern of shallow breaths with irregular periods of apnea. The cycle length is variable, lasting anywhere from 10 seconds to 1 minute. Usually seen in patients with CNS disturbances, for example, meningitis, encephalitis, head trauma or brain abscess
Kussmaul's Respiration	Also called air hunger. Characterized by increased rate (greater than 20 breaths/min) and increased depth, that is, deep sighing breaths without pauses, laboured breathing. Body attempts to give off excess hydrogen ions by blowing off carbon dioxide. Seen in patients with metabolic acidosis and renal failure
Chronic Obstructive Breathing 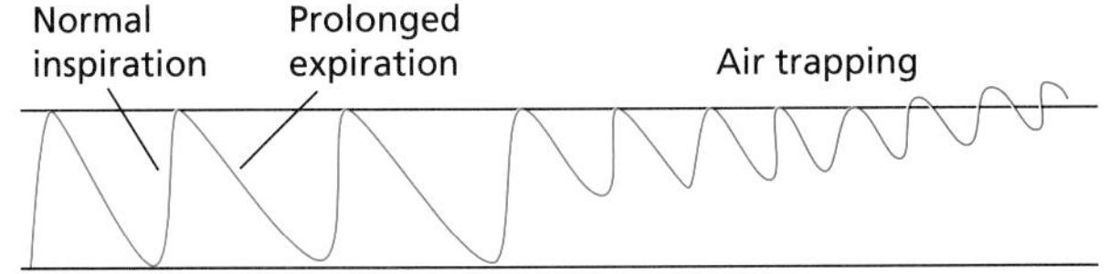	Normal inspiration and prolonged expiration to overcome increased airway resistance. In a person with chronic obstructive lung disease, any situation calling for increased heart rate (exercise) may lead to dyspneic episode (air trapping), because then the person does not have enough time for full expiration

SOURCES: Jarvis, 1996; Thompson & Wilson, 1996.

and gums is normal in people with very dark skin, so the buccal mucosa or conjunctivae are the most reliable areas for detection of cyanosis. The facial skin may also be pale grey in a dark-skinned person with central cyanosis.

The fingers are examined for signs of clubbing. **Clubbing** is an increase in the angle between the base of the nail and fingernail from the normal angle of 160°–180° (Figure 24.5). It is also manifested by an increase in the depth of the nails; they feel bulky and spongy compared to a normal firm nail base. Clubbing is best seen in the fourth and fifth fingers. It indicates signs of lung disease found in patients with chronic hypoxic conditions, for example, cystic fibrosis, chronic lung infections or cancers of the lung (Porth, 1998).

Finally, quickly and gently compress the nail bed between your thumb and index finger. With this compression, the capillary bed is occluded and the nail bed becomes pale. When the nail bed is released, oxygenated blood returns to it. This is known as **capillary refill**. Normal capillary refill occurs within three seconds. A refill time of longer than three seconds indicates an alteration in peripheral blood flow (Black & Matassarin-Jacobs, 1997).

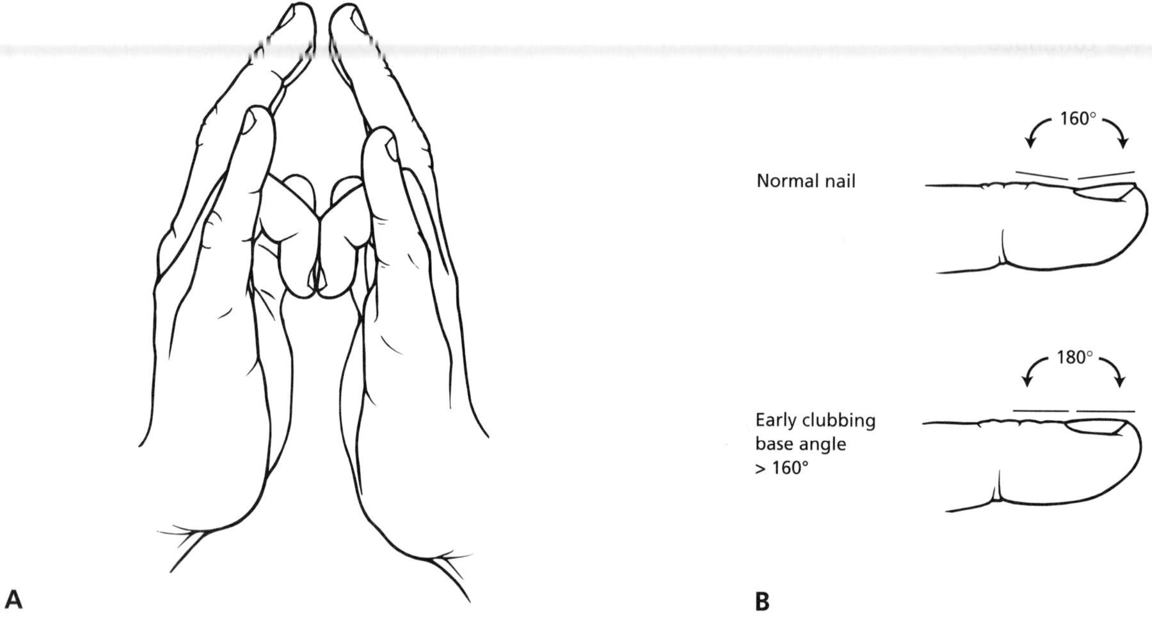

FIGURE 24.5 Clubbing of fingers

SOURCE: A. Black & Matassarin-Jacobs, 1997, p. 1044; B. Porth, 1998, p. 554.

PALPATION

Palpation is performed to evaluate thoracic expansion, spasticity or rigidity, chest symmetry during respiration, areas of sensitivity, masses, edema and depressions, unusual movements with respiration, vibrations or pulsations. Skin temperature, turgor or moisture are also assessed. The nurse's hands should be clean and warm before proceeding with the examination.

Palpation of the Posterior Chest

To palpate the posterior chest, place the hands flat against the chest on the lower third of the ribcage (level of 10th rib), with thumbs pointing towards each other almost touching, and fingers pointing laterally (see Figure 24.6). Ask the patient to inhale deeply. Note the movement of the area between your thumbs. It should move upward and outward equally during inspiration. The space between the thumbs on inspiration is a rough measure of expansion and equality of movement. Normal expansion is two to five centimetres; both sides should move equally.

Next, palpate the chest wall for fremitus. **Fremitus** is a vibration that can be felt on the exterior chest wall when a person speaks. Sounds produced in the larynx are transmitted through patent airways and lung tissue to the chest wall, where they are felt as vibrations. To palpate for fremitus, place the palmar base of the fingers of one hand over the chest wall and ask the patient to say "ninety-nine" or "one, two, three" or "how now, brown cow." These words are effective in examining fremitus because they are resonant and thus produce strong vibrations. Begin at the lung apices and palpate from one side to the other as shown in Figure 24.7. Normally, all people have fremitus. It is loudest at the level of the tracheal bifurcation and should be equal bilaterally. Fremitus is increased in conditions that increase lung density, for example, consolidated lobar pneumonia. It is decreased or absent in airway obstruction or in any condition that blocks the transmission of vibrations, such as emphysema or thickening (fibrosis) of the pleura. Fremitus is assessed on the posterior thorax since there is less muscle tissue and no breast tissue to interfere with the transmission of vibrations (Jarvis, 1996).

Finally, palpate the entire posterior surface, noting the presence and location of tenderness, masses, depressions or unusual movements with respiration. Palpations that produce audible crackling sounds, called *crepitations*, indicate subcutaneous emphysema in which fine beads of air are trapped under the skin. A coarse, crackling sensation may also be felt over the skin surface. This is called *crepitus* (Jarvis, 1996). The skin surface should feel warm, smooth and dry, and have elastic turgor. The spinal processes should be straight and nontender. The ribcage should feel somewhat elastic, but the sternum and xiphoid process should be relatively inflexible.

Palpation of the Anterior Chest

Standing directly in front of the patient, palpate the sternal notch. This aids in identifying the location of the internal organs. Palpate the intercostal spaces, noting the presence, location and characteristics of tender or painful areas or masses. To identify the extent of chest expansion with respirations, place your hands on the patient's lateral ribcage with thumbs placed along the costal margins. The thumbs

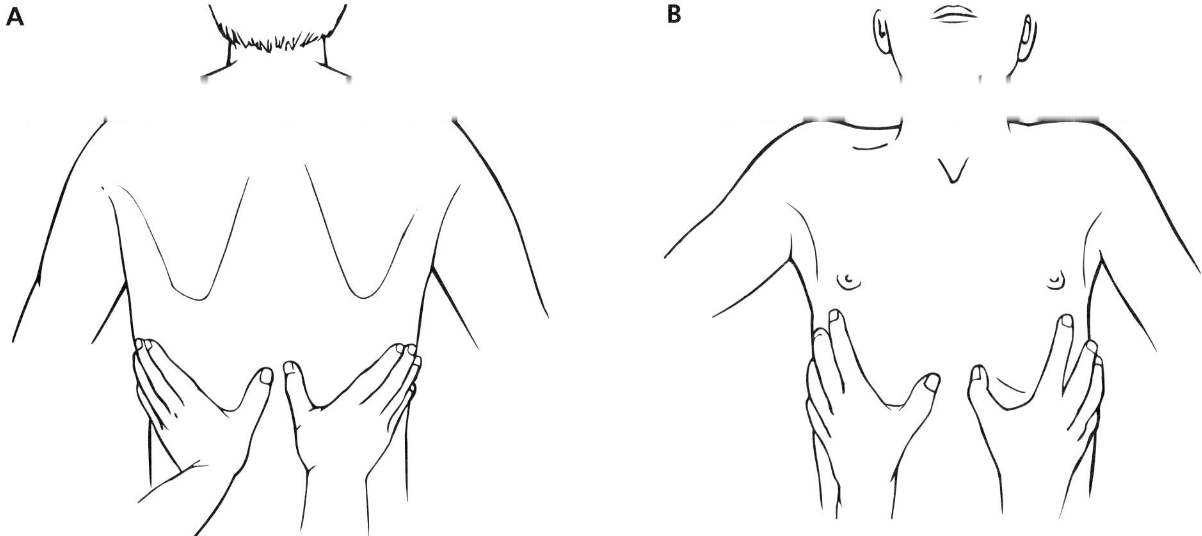

FIGURE 24.6 Palpating the chest for respiratory expansion. A. Posterior. B. Anterior

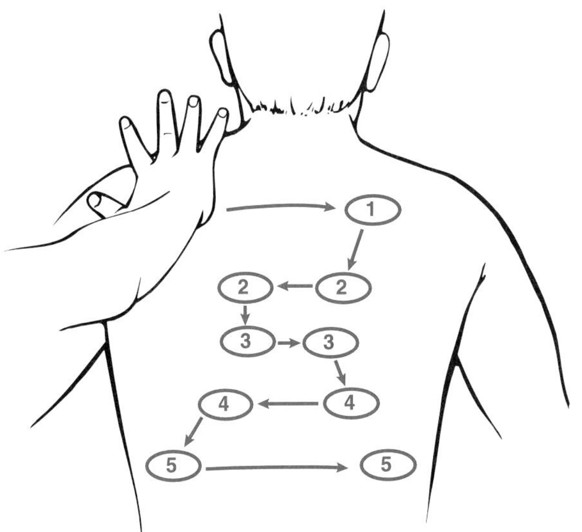

FIGURE 24.7 Palpating fremitus

are placed together (see Figure 24.6). Ask the patient to take a deep breath and, again, note the movement of the areas between the thumbs; this represents the chest expansions. Movement should be symmetrical.

PERCUSSION

Percussion is used in the chest examination to determine the presence of air, fluid or solid material in the underlying lung tissue and to help identify the location and boundaries of underlying organs such as the diaphragm, lungs, heart and liver. Both the posterior and anterior thoracic cage should be percussed. Percussion techniques are discussed in Chapter 16. If the patient is too ill or is unable to sit up, percussion of the posterior thorax is performed with the patient positioned on the side. Start at the top of the shoulder to identify the apices of the lung. Then progress downward and side to side at five- to six-centimetre intervals. Compare the sounds of each area with the sound of the opposite side as percussion proceeds. Normally, the entire thorax to the level of the diaphragm elicits a resonant sound: that is, a loud, hollow, low-pitched sound of long duration. A dull, flat sound is heard over the heart and liver, or in the presence of a mass, pneumonia or atelectasis (Jarvis, 1996).

AUSCULTATION

The nurse listens to the patient's chest using a stethoscope to determine the presence of normal and abnormal breath

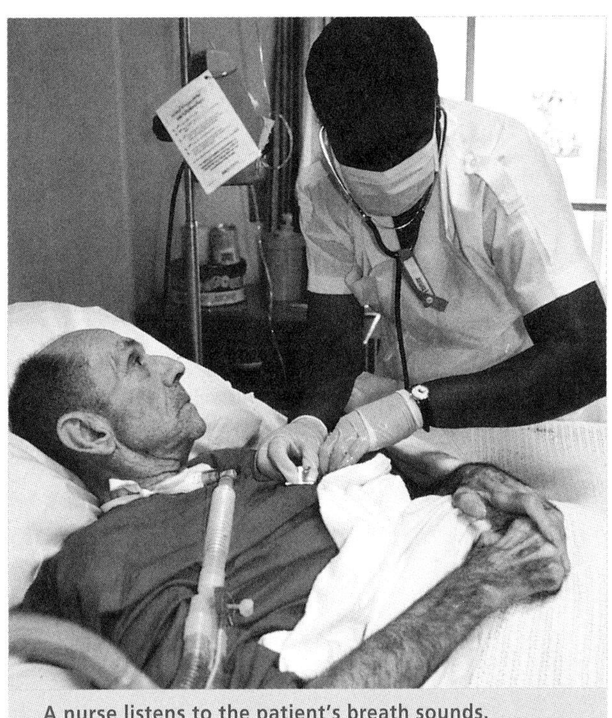

A nurse listens to the patient's breath sounds.

sounds. The breath sounds are created by air passing through the tracheobronchial tree (trachea, bronchi and branching bronchial tubes). Before starting, explain the procedure and ask the patient to take slow, deep breaths through the mouth, a little deeper than normal. Nasal breathing tends to produce false abnormal sounds. Hyperventilations can develop quickly, so the patient should not breathe too fast. If the patient feels light-headed or dizzy, he or she should inform the examiner so that auscultation can be stopped and time allowed for the patient to rest and breathe normally.

The diaphragm of the stethoscope is used to auscultate the chest because it transmits the higher-pitched sounds more common in respirations. Hold the diaphragm firmly on the patient's chest to eliminate outside extraneous sounds. Beginning posteriorly at the apices, proceed downward towards the lung bases at four- to five-centimetre intervals, comparing the right and left sides (see Figure 24.8). Ask the patient to raise his or her arms when auscultating the lateral chest walls.

Take time to evaluate and correlate what is being heard; listen for at least one full respiration in each location and compare sides. The examiner's ear must be trained to differentiate the various sounds. Listen for the pitch (high/low), intensity and duration of breath sounds. These will vary over different parts of the lung. If abnormal breath sounds are heard the nurse should ask the patient to cough and should then auscultate again for at least two breaths to note any change. Note the location of the sound and the phase (inspiration or expiration) in which it occurs.

The characteristics of normal breath sounds are depicted in Table 24.4. Abnormal breath sounds include two categories: (a) absent or diminished sounds and (b) superimposed sounds not normally heard in the lungs. Absent or diminished sounds occur when air does not enter a portion of the lung due to obstruction of the air passages, or from the accumulation of pleural fluids or air between the chest wall and the adjacent lung. Superimposed sounds include **crackles** (formerly called rales), **gurgles** (formerly called rhonchi), **wheezes** and **pleural friction rubs**. These are caused by air colliding with secretions in the tracheobronchial passageways or by the reopening of previously deflated airways. These abnormal breath sounds are described in Table 24.5.

Diagnostic Tests

A number of laboratory and diagnostic tests are used to evaluate oxygenation status. Testing includes blood, sputum and pleural fluid analysis, direct and indirect visualization techniques and pulmonary function studies. Nurses must be knowledgeable about these procedures so that they can prepare patients for these tests and provide post procedure care. The nurse may also assist in some procedures performed at the bedside, such as a thoracentesis.

BLOOD STUDIES

Complete Blood Count (CBC)

A complete blood count is a routine screening test that provides general information about overall state of health and respiratory function. The elements that most directly relate to respiratory status are the red blood cell (RBC) count, hematocrit (Hct), hemoglobin (Hgb) and white blood cell (WBC) count and differential. Table 24.6 outlines the purpose and clinical significance of these tests, along with the normal values of the elements being measured.

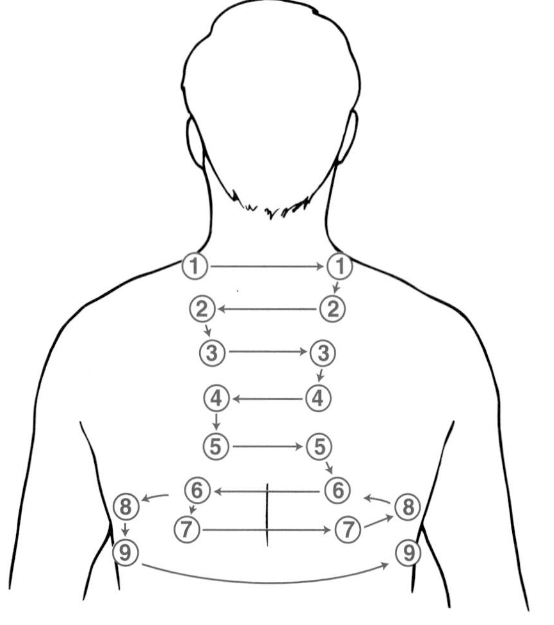

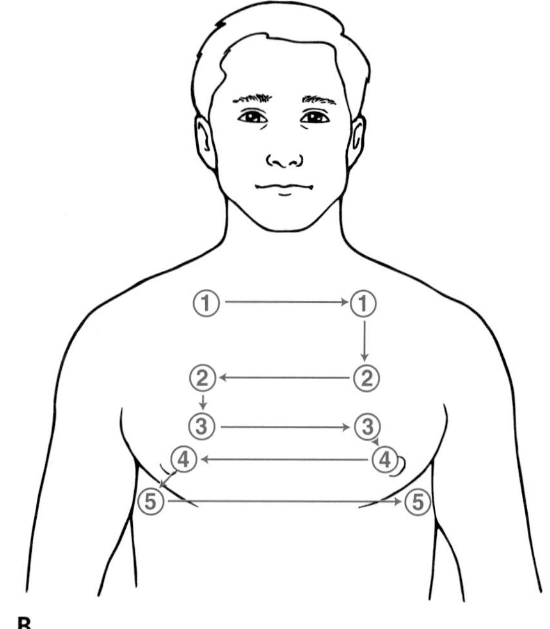

FIGURE 24.8 Locations and sequence for percussing and auscultating the chest. A. Posterior. B. Anterior

TABLE 24.4 Characteristics of normal breath sounds

	Pitch	Amplitude	Duration	Quality	Normal Location
Bronchial (Tracheal)	High	Loud	Inspiration < expiration	Harsh, hollow, tubular	Trachea and larynx
Bronchovesicular	Moderate	Moderate	Inspiration = expiration	Mixed	Over major bronchi where fewer alveoli are located: posterior, between scapulae especially on right; anterior, around upper sternum in first and second intercostal spaces
Vesicular	Low	Soft	Inspiration > expiration	Rustling, like the sound of the wind in the trees	Over peripheral lung fields where air flows through smaller bronchioles and alveoli

SOURCE: Jarvis, 1996, p. 479.

Arterial Blood Gases (ABG)

Arterial blood gas analysis is essential in diagnosing and monitoring patients with respiratory disorders. The tests measure the partial pressures of oxygen and carbon dioxide dissolved in the arterial blood. They also reveal the acid–base status and how well the oxygen is being carried in the blood.

The blood sample is taken by a specially trained nurse, doctor or respiratory therapist. The nurse on the unit provides care before and after the procedure and, in addition, may be asked to assist the health team member who is drawing the sample.

In preparing the patient, the nurse explains the purpose and the procedure for collecting the blood sample. Because the sample is taken from an artery, the procedure may be uncomfortable for a few minutes. In order to obtain the most accurate reading, the patient should rest for 20–30 minutes before the test. Check the physician's order to determine whether the ABG is to be collected while the patient is on or off oxygen. If the patient is receiving oxygen therapy, the rate of flow should not be changed, nor should interventions such as suctioning or positioning be performed for 20 minutes before obtaining the sample unless absolutely necessary.

The sample may be taken from the radial, brachial or femoral arteries. An Allen test should be conducted to assess the circulation to the hand. In the event that the radial artery is damaged during the procedure, this test ensures patency of the collateral ulnar artery. Circulation is assessed by placing one thumb over the patient's ulnar artery and the other thumb over the patient's radial artery. The patient then makes a fist, thereby squeezing the blood from the hand. The nurse then asks the patient to open the hand; the palm should be blanched. When the nurse removes the thumb from the ulnar artery, the circulation should return to the hand within five seconds. This indicates adequate ulnar artery blood flow.

During the procedure, the nurse provides support and reassurance, and helps the patient to maintain proper positioning. Because the pressure from these arteries is quite high, direct pressure must be applied to the site for 5–10 minutes after the needle is withdrawn to prevent hemorrhage. The site is then covered with a firm dressing. The blood sample must be placed in a bag of ice and taken to the lab immediately. Specimens stored at room temperature will yield lower pH and pO_2 levels. Further, if the sample is not analyzed straight away, continuing blood cell

TABLE 24.5 Abnormal breath sounds

Sound	*Characteristics*	*Comments*
***Crackles* (previously called rales)**	Described as fine, medium or coarse discontinuous sounds. Can be heard on inspiration as well as expiration. **Fine**: high-pitched, soft, crackling, short Sounds like several hairs rubbing together between fingertips, air-filled rice breakfast cereal in milk or crinkling of cellophane Crackling, popping sound **Medium**: lower-pitched, moist Sounds like bubbling or a fizzing carbonated drink **Coarse**: low-pitched, loud, short Sounds like bubbling or gurgling, or like opening a Velcro fastener; heard on inspiration; can be cleared only somewhat with a cough.	Produced in the small airways by air passing through fluid or mucous. Can also be found in alveoli Patients with pneumonia, heart failure, asthma, or pulmonary edema may have these sounds
***Gurgles* (previously called rhonchi)**	Continuous sound, coarse Prominent on expiration **Low-pitched:** sounds are sonorous, rumbling and originate in the larger airways **High-pitched**: musical quality, rattling; may be changed or cleared with coughing	Produced by air flowing through large passages narrowed by secretions, mucosal swelling, edema, tumour or obstruction Occurs in patients with lung disease e.g., asthma, emphysema, COPD
Wheeze	High-pitched, continuous More apparent on expiration Sounds like musical whistling, squeaky; may clear somewhat with coughing	Occurs with constriction of large or small airways; in patients with bronchospasms, fluid, mucus, inflammation or obstructive lesion Caused by rapid vibrations of bronchial walls
Pleural Friction Rub	Loud, low-pitched, coarse, dry Jerky sound, rubbing, grating Sounds like two pieces of leather being rubbed together Loudest over lower lateral anterior surface Heard during inspiration and expiration May get louder with coughing Variable duration	May be confined to a small area of the chest Originates in inflamed pleura that has lost its normal lubricating fluid Opposing roughened pleural surfaces rub together during respiration Pain with breathing; patient may splint the chest when breathing

SOURCES: Thompson & Wilson, 1996; Jarvis, 1996; Black & Matassarin-Jacobs, 1997.

metabolism could alter the results of the test. If the patient is receiving oxygen therapy, the laboratory requisition or computer data entry should include the amount and method of oxygen administered over the last 20–30 minutes.

After the sample is drawn, the nurse assesses the patient's vital signs and response to the procedure, and examines the puncture site for bleeding, arterial thrombosis (a common occurrence) and signs of infection or ulnar nerve trauma. Documentation includes the date and time the blood sample was drawn, the puncture site, the name of the health team member who drew the sample, the oxygen concentration and flow rate (if applicable), the patient's response to the test and any relevant observations (for example, patient's vital signs, colour, condition of site). Table 24.7 outlines the purpose and significance of arterial blood gases tests along with normal values.

SPUTUM STUDIES

Sputum analysis is valuable in identifying the cause of pulmonary dysfunction, diagnosing bacterial infections and

TABLE 24.6 Common blood studies for assessing oxygenation

Test	*Normal Values SI Units (Conventional Units)*	*Purpose*	*Clinical Significance*
RBC (erythrocytes)	M: 4.5–6.2 × 10^{12}/L (4.5–6.2 million/mm^3) F: 4.0–5.5 × 10^{12}/L (4.0–5.5 million/mm^3)	Determines oxygen-carrying capacity	Increased in chronic lung disease Decreased in anemia. Results from insufficient dietary intake of iron or folic acid, RBC destruction, blood loss, or bone marrow suppression
Hemoglobin	M: 8.7–11.2 mmol/L (14.0–18.0 g/dL) F: 7.4–9.9 mmol/L (12.0–16.0 g/dL)	Determines amount of Hgb available for combining with oxygen	Same as RBC
Hematocrit	M: 0.40–0.54 (40–54 mL/dL) F: 0.37–0.47 (37–47 mL/dL)	Determines the percentage of RBCs to plasma	Increased in severe dehydration (when blood plasma is lost, concentration of RBCs increases), disease and high altitude Decreased in overhydration, disease and reaction to blood transfusions
WBC	4.5–11.0 × 10^9/L (4500–11 000/mm^3)	Determines immune system response to antigen	Increased in acute bacterial infections, carcinoma, diabetes mellitus, acute hemorrhage Decreased in acute viral infections, bone marrow depletion

SOURCE: Chernecky & Berger, 1997.

TABLE 24.7 Arterial blood gases (ABGs)

Test	*Normal Values*	*Purpose and Significance*
pH	7.35–7.45	Assesses acid–base status. It is the free H+ ion concentration in circulating blood. The pH must remain constant for health Values <7.35 indicates acidosis; >7.45 indicates alkalosis Values <7.2 or >7.6 (panic values) can be life-threatening
pCO_2	34–45 mm Hg	Assesses the amount of carbon dioxide in blood and indicates the effectiveness of alveolar ventilation High values indicate impaired respiratory function, e.g., airway obstruction, lung damage Low values indicate hyperventilation Critical values: <20 or >70
pO_2	75–100 mm Hg	Assesses the amount of oxygen dissolved in plasma and represents the status of alveolar gas exchange with inspired air pO_2 values decrease with age
SaO_2	96–100%	Is the percentage of available Hgb that is saturated with oxygen and available for transport throughout the body
HCO_3	22–26 mmol/L	Bicarbonate is a component of the body's acid–base system that influences pH; tells how the kidneys are able to absorb or excrete bicarbonate ions to maintain normal pH

NOTE: pO_2 and pCO_2 refer to partial pressures of oxygen and carbon dioxide in arterial blood. SaO_2 refers to oxygen saturation of arterial blood.

SOURCE: Chernecky & Berger, 1997.

determining and evaluating treatment regimens. Periodic sputum exams may be necessary for patients receiving antibiotics, steroids and immunosuppressive drugs for prolonged periods, as these agents give rise to opportunistic infections. The most common tests performed on sputum are culture and sensitivity (C&S) to determine the organisms causing bacterial infection and their sensitivities to antibiotics; acid-fast stain (AFB) to detect the acid-fast bacilli when tuberculosis is suspected; and cytology to identify cancer, including the specific cell type.

Because the results of a C&S may take 24–48 hours, a gram stain is performed to determine whether the organisms are gram-negative or gram-positive. The gram stain report is available within a few hours and, therefore, is useful in selecting immediate antibiotic therapy until the C&S results are obtained. C&S and gram-staining examinations require one specimen collected in a sterile container. The specimen should be collected before antibiotic treatment is started. Specimens for AFB are collected in a sterile container for three consecutive mornings. The results are usually available in three to eight weeks. A single specimen is needed for cytology. It is collected in a special container with a fixative solution. The specimen must be sent to the lab promptly to ensure accuracy of the examination.

Collection of Sputum Specimens

Sputum is best collected in the morning because secretions pool in the bronchi during the night and require only a few deep coughs to bring them to the back of the throat. The patient should be supplied with the correct wide-mouthed specimen container and taught how to collect the specimen. If the sight of a specimen is objectionable to the patient or others in the room, the outside of the container may be covered. To produce a suitable specimen, the patient must know the difference between saliva (the clear liquid secreted by the salivary glands in the mouth) and sputum, and that it is necessary to cough to bring up sputum. The patient can be taught how to cough, if necessary. The patient should brush the teeth, clear the throat and rinse the mouth so that saliva and oral debris do not contaminate the specimen. Mouthwash and toothpaste should be avoided because these substances affect the mobility of organisms. The patient then takes a deep breath to full capacity and exhales with an expulsive, deep cough directly into the sterile sputum container without touching the edges. Usually, 5–30 mL of sputum is enough for examination.

Once the specimen is produced, the container is labelled and the specimen sent to the laboratory. If the specimen is a series specimen, the number of the specimen is included on both the requisition (written or computer) and the label. When patients are taking antibiotics, this should also be indicated. In addition, specimens obtained by suctioning should be noted because these commonly appear watery and may resemble saliva. The specimen should be taken to the laboratory immediately, because results are most accurate when analysis is completed within one hour of collection. Some specimens may be refrigerated; consult the laboratory manual for specific directives. Mouthwash or water should be offered to the patient after producing a specimen to remove any unpleasant taste.

The specimen collection is documented in the patient's record. The date and time of collection, number of the specimen if serial, method used to obtain the specimen, how the patient tolerated the procedure, the characteristics of the sputum and its proper delivery to the laboratory are recorded.

THORACENTESIS

Thoracentesis (also called a thoracocentesis) is the aspiration of fluid or air from the pleural cavity (the cavity within the thorax that contains the lungs). It involves the insertion of a needle through the chest wall and into the pleural space to remove fluid for diagnostic or therapeutic purposes or to obtain a needle biopsy of the pleura. Medication can also be instilled into the pleural space.

The procedure is performed at the bedside using sterile technique. The nurse assists by preparing the patient and providing support during the procedure.

Patient preparation includes an explanation of the reasons for the procedure, what is going to happen and how the patient can help. Normally, thoracentesis is not painful; some pressure will be felt when the needle is inserted. A local anesthetic is given to promote comfort. When the needle is inserted, the patient must avoid movement and refrain from talking or coughing to avoid puncturing of the lung. An informed consent is obtained per agency policy, and allergies to local anesthetics are determined. Preprocedure sedation or analgesia may be ordered.

The patient is helped into a comfortable position for the procedure. This may be a sitting position, or a side-lying position with the patient lying on the unaffected side, as illustrated in Figure 24.9, or a side-lying position with the patient lying on the unaffected side. The nurse offers support and reassurance and monitors the patient's response during the procedure. After the needle is withdrawn, pressure and a small sterile dressing are applied to the puncture site. The patient is prescribed bed rest on the unaffected side to permit the pleural site to seal itself and to prevent fluid seepage from gravity or coughing.

Specimens, if any, are sent to the laboratory and a chest x-ray is requisitioned. A chest x-ray is taken to verify the absence of pneumothorax and to evaluate the result of the procedure (if the purpose was to remove excessive fluid or air). Vital signs, including oxygen saturation, are taken and the patient is monitored for signs of respiratory problems (dyspnea, coughing, hemoptysis [blood-tinged sputum], chest pain, wheezing, cyanosis, hypoxia, headache and lightheadedness). An assessment of the puncture site is made for bleeding or seepage of fluid. The documentation of the procedure should include the total amount of fluid withdrawn, the characteristics of the fluid (colour, viscosity), specimens sent, thoracentesis site, response of the patient and whether or not a chest x-ray was taken.

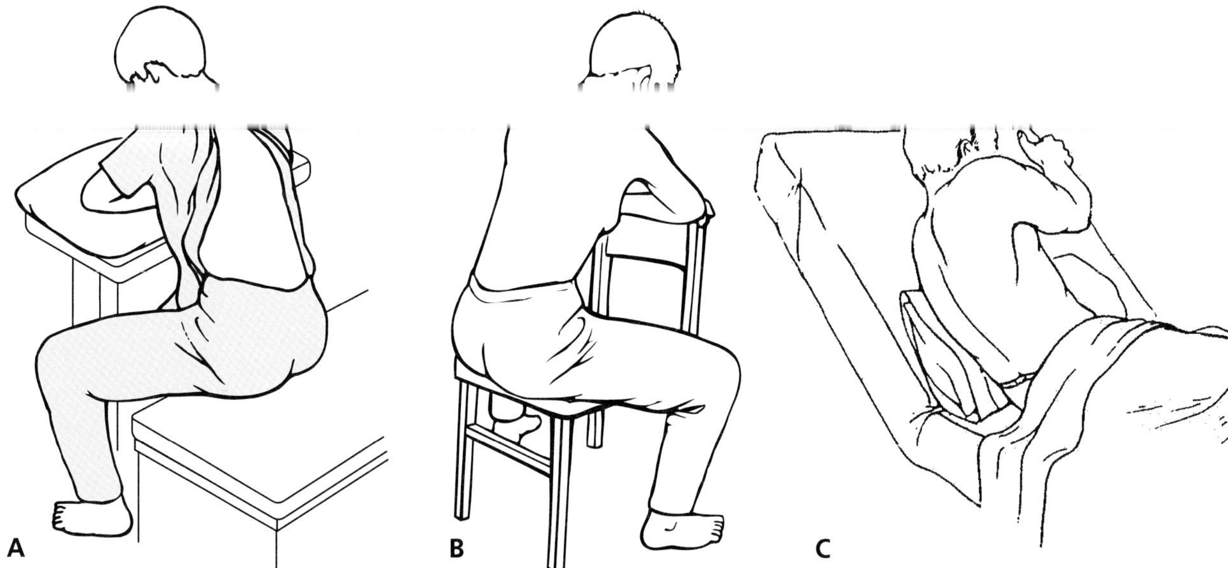

FIGURE 24.9 Positioning the patient for thoracentesis. The nurse assists the patient to one of two positions, and offers comfort and support throughout the procedure. A. Sitting on the edge of the bed with head and arms on and over the bed table. B. Straddling a chair with arms and head resting on the back of the chair. C. Lying on unaffected side with bed elevated 30–40 degrees.

SOURCES: A. Smeltzer & Bare, 1996, p. 457; B. Suddarth, 1991, p. 168; C. Lammon, Foote, Leli, Ingle & Adams, 1995, p. 174.

VISUALIZATION STUDIES

Bronchoscopy

The larynx, trachea and bronchi may be examined with a fibre-optic bronchoscope, a tubular instrument with an attached light source (see Figure 24.10). **Bronchoscopy** permits direct examination of tissues for abscesses, tumours or localized bleeding. It is also used to obtain tissue biopsies, remove foreign objects or mucous plugs and aspirate secretions for laboratory analysis.

An informed consent is obtained prior to the test per agency policy, and allergies to local anesthetics are determined. The purpose and procedure must be carefully explained to the patient to reduce anxiety and correct misinformation. Patient participation during the test is very important. The patient will be asked to assume a sitting or lying position with the neck hyperextended. The throat is sprayed with a local anesthetic to reduce the cough reflex and promote easier passage of the scope. A flexible fibre-optic scope is passed through the mouth or nose into the larynx and trachea. This may create a feeling of being unable to breathe. The patient must be reassured that the airway remains open, and that the procedure will be more comfortable if the patient concentrates on breathing normally. The procedure takes approximately 45–60 minutes. Test results (except secretion analysis) are available within one to two days. The patient may experience hoarseness, a sore throat or blood-tinged sputum after the procedure.

The patient must fast for a minimum of 6–12 hours before the test to prevent aspiration. In some agencies fasting begins at midnight. Contact lenses, eyeglasses and dentures are removed. Loose or capped teeth are noted on the chart. Preprocedure medication is administered as prescribed. This may be atropine (to inhibit vagal stimulation and guard against bradycardia, dysrhythmias and hypotension), a sedative or tranquillizer (to sedate the patient and relieve anxiety) or an analgesic (to promote pain tolerance).

After the procedure the patient is placed in a semi-Fowler's position to prevent aspiration; the patient is permitted to turn from side to side. Vital signs are monitored q15 min or as ordered until stable. The physician is notified immediately if complications develop or the patient's condition deteriorates. An emesis basin is provided and the patient is instructed to spit out saliva rather than swallow it because the anesthetic impairs the protective laryngeal reflex and interferes with correct swallowing. Sputum is observed for bleeding, especially if a biopsy has been taken. Patients who have had a biopsy are instructed to refrain from clearing the throat and coughing so as not to dislodge the clot at the biopsy site and cause bleeding.

The patient is advised to avoid smoking for the rest of the day because smoking irritates the tissues and may cause coughing and clot displacement. Fluids or foods, are restricted until the gag and swallowing reflexes return (approximately two hours). The return of reflexes may be tested by touching the back of the throat with a tongue depressor. The patient is started with ice chips, sips of water and then a normal diet (soft, if throat is sore) within a few hours. Medicated lozenges or warm saline gargles may be provided to ease throat discomfort. Patients are encouraged to avoid straining the voice and, if necessary, an alternative means of communicating may be used such as a magic slate, letter board or pad and pencil.

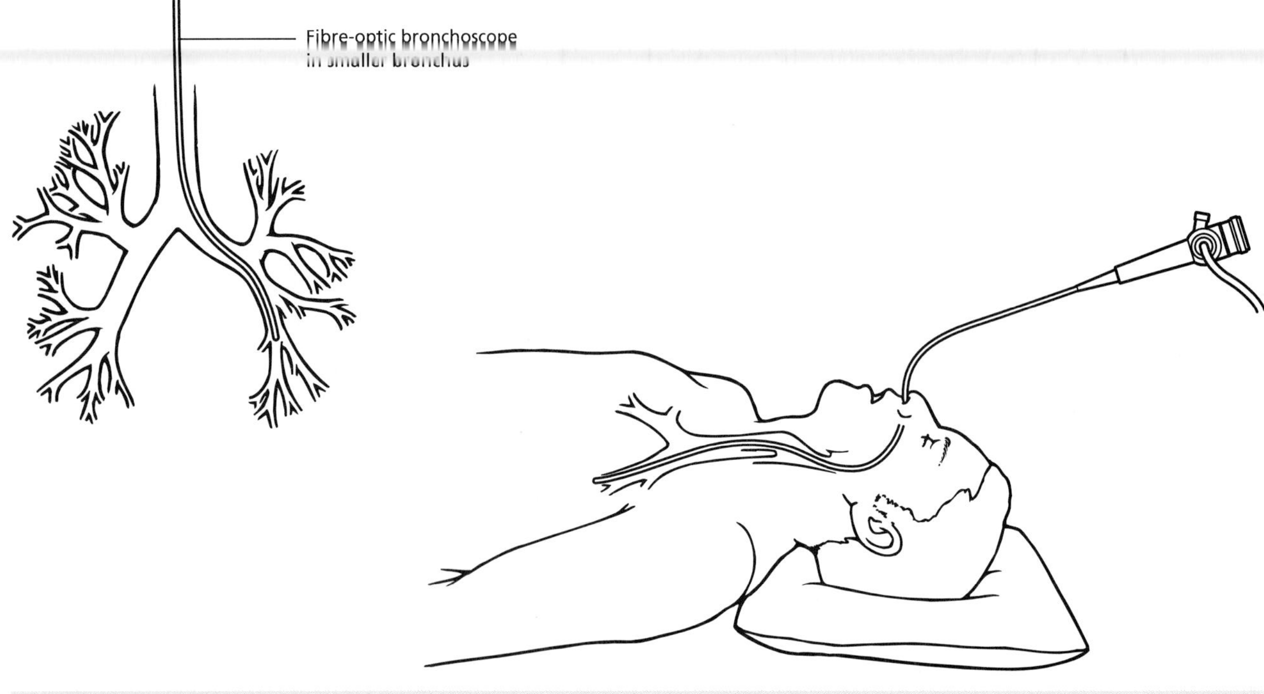

FIGURE 24.10 Fibre-optic bronchoscopy

SOURCE: Smeltzer & Bare, 1996, p. 455.

Indirect Visualization Studies

A number of indirect visualization techniques are used to examine respiratory function. These include the standard chest x-ray, fluoroscopy, computerized tomography (CT scan) and lung scans. X-ray, fluoroscopy and CT scanning are discussed in Chapter 16. Lung scans are performed to assess pulmonary blood flow and ventilatory function when pathology is suspected. Abnormalities such as pulmonary embolism, tumours, lung cancer, bronchitis and emphysema may be detected.

The chest x-ray is a radiographic diagnostic tool used to assess a patient's respiratory status. Since many pulmonary changes do not always show up on imaging, chest x-rays are always assessed in conjunction with clinical findings. Normal anatomical structures are examined first. These include the diaphragm, heart shadow, tracheobronchial tree and lung parenchyma. From this basis abnormalities such as atelectasis, pneumothorax, tumors or infection can be determined.

Usually, two tests are involved in lung scanning: the perfusion scan and the ventilation scan. A perfusion scan is obtained by injecting a radioactive agent labelled with technetium into a peripheral vein. The isotope particles pass through the right side of the heart and are distributed throughout the lungs in proportion to the active blood flow. The radioactive emissions are traced with a scanner and the image is recorded with a camera. Areas in which radioactive uptake is absent or low indicate vascular obstruction or poor perfusion. In the ventilation scan, the patient inhales a radioactive gas (xenon or krypton) through a mask. The gas diffuses through the lung but does not cross the alveolar–capillary membrane (the radioactive particles are too large). Scanning shows the air spaces in the lung and can detect abnormalities in ventilation such as pneumonia, emphysema or infarction.

In preparation for lung scanning, the nurse explains the purpose and procedure of the tests. The tests usually cause minimal discomfort. When the radioactive agent is injected into a vein for the perfusion scan, the patient may feel a flushed sensation or nausea. This is normal and lasts a very short time. The scanning time lasts 20–40 minutes; the patient will be asked to lie very still under the camera so as to ensure the most accurate results. A mask may be placed over the nose and mouth during the test. The patient should breathe normally.

For the ventilation scan the patient will be asked to inhale a gas and hold the breath for a short time. The gas is not harmful and will not cause any distressing symptoms. The scanning process will take approximately five minutes. Both tests are completed in about two hours. The radioactive isotope disintegrates and is excreted within 6–24 hours. It will cause no harm to the patient or visitors. An informed consent is obtained, and any previous reactions to diagnostic dyes or allergic reactions to shellfish or iodine are determined. Jewellery and metal objects are removed so the results of the test will not be distorted. Following the tests, the patient is watched for allergic reactions to the radioactive materials. The patient is encouraged to drink fluids to help flush the contrast materials from the kidneys.

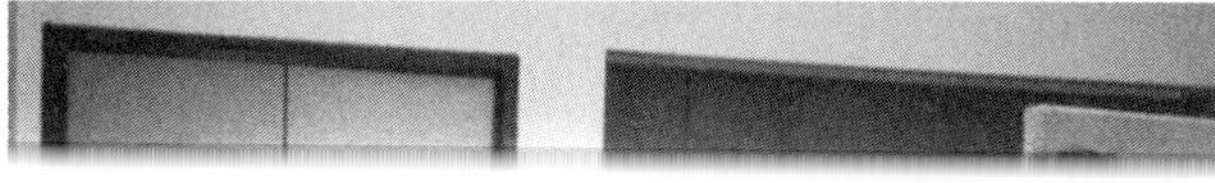

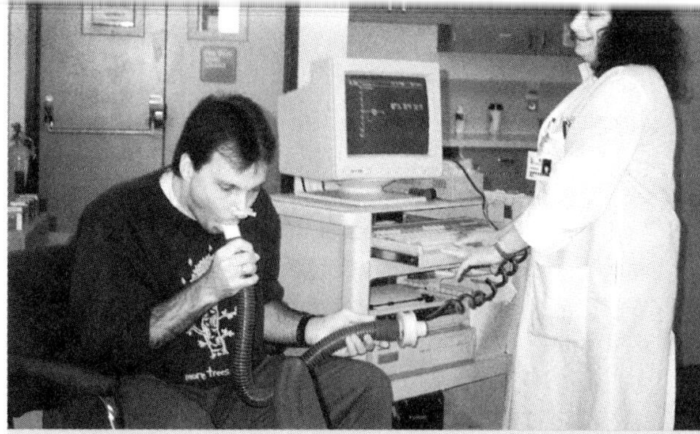

A pulmonary function test underway.

PULMONARY FUNCTION TESTS

Pulmonary function tests (PFTs) are performed to assess lung function and to identify the presence and severity of respiratory disease. A number of tests are carried out because no single measurement provides a complete picture of pulmonary functioning. These include measurements of ventilation function, lung volumes, diffusion capacity and gas exchange.

Pulmonary function tests are usually performed by a respiratory therapist. As with all procedures, the nurse prepares the patient for the testing. The tests are painless but patient participation is essential. Testing involves breathing as deeply as possible and blowing as hard, as fast and as long as possible into a machine. The tests take approximately 20–30 minutes. They are tiring, so resting prior to and following the tests will be helpful. A nose clip is applied for the testing. Patients often report feeling as though they can't catch their breath or that they are "going to suffocate." Reassure the patient that this will not happen but that it is essential to breathe through the mouth. Practising mouth breathing prior to the test helps to alleviate distress. A consent is not required for pulmonary function studies. The patient is advised not to smoke prior to the tests. Eating is permitted, but a heavy meal is discouraged four to six hours before testing to prevent gastric distention, which may alter test results. Dentures can remain in the mouth. The patient is advised to avoid restrictive clothing and to void before performing the tests.

Diagnosing Oxygenation Problems

Actual or potential problems with oxygenation that are treated by independent nursing interventions may relate to respiratory dysfunction itself or to the effects of respiratory dysfunction on other facets of functioning. Alterations in respiratory function may include difficulties with airway clearance and ineffective breathing patterns. When patients cannot cough effectively, the diagnosis *Ineffective Airway Clearance* is useful. This diagnosis applies to cases where a suppressed cough reflex (for example, due to medications or anesthesia), pain, weakness, fatigue or improper positioning interfere with effective coughing. It may also be used for patients who are able to cough but for whom the tenacity of secretions prevents effective airway clearance.

The diagnosis *Ineffective Breathing Patterns* may be used when a patient's breathing pattern fails to provide adequate ventilation. In this situation the patient will be either hyperventilating or hypoventilating. He or she will display changes in the respiratory rate or pattern from the baseline measure, as well as changes in pulse rate and rhythm. According to Carpenito (1997), the diagnosis *Risk for Altered Respiratory Function* may be used to describe potential problems that may affect both the passage of air through the respiratory tract and the exchange of gases between the lungs and the vascular system. She identifies smoking, immobility and environmental allergy as etiologies for this diagnosis. Nursing interventions are directed towards health protective measures, such as teaching deep-breathing exercises and ways to maintain an allergen-free environment and providing education about the effects of smoking on respiratory health.

The diagnoses *Ineffective Airway Clearance* and *Ineffective Breathing Pattern* should be used only when the nurse can initiate treatment measures independently. For instance, in a patient with *Risk for Ineffective Airway Clearance related to postoperative incisional pain*, the nurse may intervene by providing pain relief measures and teaching the patient how to cough effectively. Many oxygenation problems, however, are medical problems for which the nurse collaborates with the physician in monitoring the patient's status and implementing therapeutic interventions. Hypoxemia in a patient with emphysema, impaired gas exchange due to pulmonary embolus or destruction of lung tissue, and decreased tissue perfusion secondary to anemia are but a few examples. These problems are best identified as collaborative problems, in which case the label *potential complication* (PC) is used.

Insufficient oxygenation often interferes with the ability to function effectively in daily living. A major problem is activity intolerance. The diagnostic label *Activity Intolerance* is appropriate for individuals with respiratory and cardiovascular disorders who experience dyspnea or shortness of breath when attempting physical activity. This diagnosis is outlined more fully in Chapter 29. *Anxiety* almost always accompanies breathing difficulty and lack of oxygen. To be unable to breathe normally is a frightening experience. People with chronic respiratory problems may live in constant fear that the next breath will be their last. In addition, the demands of living with a chronic illness often require adjustments in lifestyle and compliance with therapeutic regimens that individuals may find difficult. Diagnoses such as *Alteration in Health Maintenance* and *Ineffective Individual Coping* may be used to describe such problems. Some examples of nursing diagnoses and collaborative problems follow.

- *Ineffective Airway Clearance related to inadequate coughing secondary to chest pain, positioning in bed and thick secretions.*
- *Ineffective Breathing Pattern: hyperventilation related to anxiety and extreme pain.*
- *Risk for Altered Respiratory Function related to immobility.*
- *PC: Hypoxemia.*
- *Altered Health Maintenance related to dyspnea with exertion, confusion and difficulty remembering therapeutic regimen.*

Planning Oxygenation Interventions

A nursing plan of care for individuals with oxygenation problems is based on the established nursing diagnoses and is generally directed towards maintaining and restoring airway patency, pulmonary ventilation and oxygen/carbon dioxide transport; preventing deterioration of respiratory function; and promoting optimal functioning in daily living. Expected outcomes are set and interventions are selected jointly by nurse and patient, to the extent that the condition allows. When patients are very ill, the nurse may collaborate with the patient's family and other health professionals in establishing the plan of care. Care is provided through a multidisciplinary team approach involving nurses, physicians, respiratory therapists and physiotherapists. The nurse must take into account treatments prescribed by the physician as well as interventions implemented by the respiratory therapist and the physiotherapist.

As with all care planning, expected outcomes are developed from the nursing diagnoses and reflect the changes in behaviours or health status anticipated as a result of care. Some expected outcomes might be:

- The patient will show an effective breathing pattern as evidenced by rate, depth and rhythm in normal range.
- The patient will describe the allergens causing asthmatic attacks and the methods of avoiding contact with them.
- The patient will demonstrate correct use of an inhaler.
- The patient will walk to the bathroom and back to bed without dyspnea.

KEY PRINCIPLES

Principles Relevant to Oxygen Needs

1. Oxygen is essential to life.
2. A person can survive only a few minutes without oxygen.
3. An insufficient supply of oxygen impairs functioning of all body systems.
4. Irreparable brain damage may result from prolonged periods of inadequate oxygen.
5. Cells of the cerebral cortex begin to die as soon as they are deprived of oxygen.
6. Air at sea level containing approximately 21% oxygen and 0.04% carbon dioxide is normally adequate to meet human oxygen needs.
7. Carbon dioxide concentrations between 3% and 10% increase the rate and depth of respirations.
8. The body's ability to meet its oxygen needs depends on the adequacy of functioning of the cardiovascular and the respiratory systems.
9. A patent airway is essential to normal respiratory functioning.
10. The respiratory tract is lined with muco749
us-secreting epithelium.
11. Coughing, swallowing and sneezing are mechanisms by which the body attempts to rid itself of foreign materials in the respiratory tract.
12. Difficulty in breathing provokes anxiety.

Implementing Oxygenation Interventions

Health-Promoting Strategies

A constant supply of oxygen to the body is fundamental to life. Most people take oxygenation for granted until they experience a serious problem. There are many ways to preserve and promote optimal oxygenation. Nurses can assist individuals by providing information and encouraging an exploration of lifestyle factors and health practices that may ultimately affect optimal oxygenation.

Health-Protecting Strategies

Patients who are ill, especially those who are immobilized or who have undergone major surgery, often need help in maintaining optimal respiratory function, oxygen transport and tissue perfusion. The nurse assists by implementing measures to enhance these processes and prevent complications.

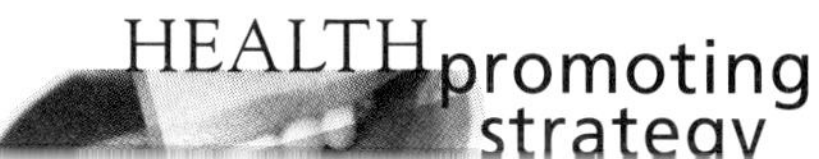

Promoting Healthy Oxygenation

- Engage in a regular exercise program, preferably aerobic, three to four times a week for at least 30 min of continuous activity.
- Eat a nutritious, well-balanced diet, low in fat. Avoid excessive intake of salt and maintain normal body weight.
- If you are a smoker, consider quitting.
- If you are not a smoker, do not start.
- Avoid passive or sidestream smoke.
- Use protective masks, gloves and clothing when exposed to hazardous materials or gases.
- Avoid occupational hazards by adhering to safety regulations of the industry.
- Avoid going outside when the air is severely polluted.
- Support public programs aimed at promoting a pollution-free environment.
- Maintain a pollution-free environment in the home.
- Avoid stagnation of air. Open windows and allow fresh, clean air into the house. Sleep with a window open, but avoid a direct draft.
- Keep dust to a minimum by damp-dusting and vacuuming at least once a week.
- Use an air purifier, if possible, and have carpets cleaned to remove animal hair, dust and smoke.
- Maintain a clean air filter in the furnace.
- Visit the physician regularly for health-screening examinations.

Techniques include positioning to ensure a clear airway and to promote ventilation, breathing exercises to facilitate maximum lung expansion, effective coughing to clear the airway, use of an incentive spirometer to enhance deep breathing and coughing, and leg exercises to strengthen circulation and venous return. Leg exercises are discussed in Chapter 29. Here we will focus on positioning, breathing exercises, effective coughing and use of an incentive spirometer.

POSITIONING

Airway patency and ventilation are affected by body positioning. Patients who are unconscious or partially conscious (for example, those recovering from anesthesia) or those with swallowing difficulty should never be positioned on their back. In the supine position, the lower jaw and tongue fall backward and occlude the airway. Also, secretions pool at the back of the throat, making aspiration likely. These individuals should be placed in a semi-prone position with the lower jaw (mandible) extended forward and upward. This prevents the tongue from falling back and also permits drainage of fluids from the mouth. For the conscious patient, an upright position (Fowler's or semi-Fowler's) is best because the abdominal contents move downward and away from the diaphragm, allowing maximum expansion of the thorax. Expectoration of sputum is also easier in a sitting position. Patients are encouraged and helped to change position (that is, from side to side) frequently while in bed to aid expansion of all lung areas and prevent stasis and pooling of pulmonary secretions.

Individuals experiencing dyspnea will be most comfortable in an orthopneic position, which promotes use of the accessory muscles to help obtain maximum expansion. In this position, the patient sits in bed or on the side of the bed and leans on the over-bed table (raised a suitable height). The patient can also press the lower part of the chest against the table to help in exhalation.

BREATHING EXERCISES

Breathing exercises are performed to improve ventilation and blood oxygenation, decrease the work of breathing by coordinating patterns of respiratory muscle action and relieve anxiety due to dyspnea. Three basic breathing techniques are deep breathing, diaphragmatic or abdominal breathing, and pursed-lip breathing. Procedure 24.2 outlines how to teach these exercises to patients.

DEEP BREATHING Patients who are at risk for respiratory impairment should be taught this technique. This includes people who are immobile, obese, elderly and those receiving medications (narcotics) that depress the rate and depth of respiration. Patients undergoing surgery are taught deep breathing and coughing (discussed later) in the preoperative period. Teaching should begin upon admission, and practice should be encouraged hourly while awake. Even while semiconscious, a person who has been instructed in these techniques will respond to a verbal reminder. Postoperatively, deep breathing helps to clear general anesthetic (which are agents given by inhalation) from the body and hastens recovery, thereby preventing stasis of secretions and the tendency to hypoventilate.

DIAPHRAGMATIC OR ABDOMINAL BREATHING Diaphragmatic breathing uses the diaphragm instead of the accessory muscles to achieve maximum inhalation. During inspiration, the diaphragm moves downward and outward, resulting in an enlargement of the upper abdomen, which allows air to flow in. During exhalation, the abdominal muscles contract, pushing air out. Diaphragmatic breathing helps to expand and ventilate the bases of the lungs. It slows

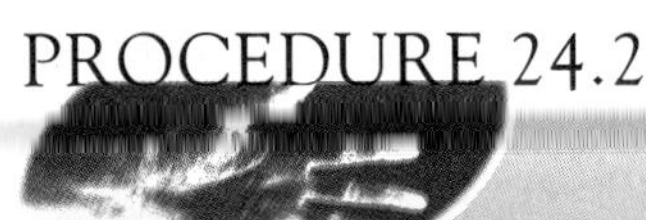

PROCEDURE 24.2 Teaching Breathing Exercises

Action	Rationale
Explain the purpose of the breathing exercise.	Understanding the benefits of the exercise facilitates learning and promotes active participation.
A. Deep Breathing	
1. Assist the patient to a comfortable sitting or Fowler's position. Make sure there are no constricting clothing or restraints.	Permits full chest expansion.
2. Instruct and demonstrate how to:	
• Take a slow, deep breath in through the nose (unless prevented by a nasal condition), raising the ribcage and making the bottom ribs move outward.	Allows maximum inspiration, decreases work of respiration and relaxes the patient.
• Exhale slowly through the mouth.	Facilitates maximum expiration.
3. Repeat the exercise, slowly inhaling and exhaling a few times every hour while awake.	Repetition reinforces learning. Regular deep breathing promotes ventilation and prevents complications.
B. Diaphragmatic or Abdominal Breathing	
1. Assist patient to a comfortable semi-Fowler's or supine position.	Enables full contraction and relaxation of the diaphragm.
2. Instruct and demonstrate how to:	
• Place one hand on the stomach and one on the mid-chest area.	Enables awareness of the diaphragm and its movement in breathing.
• Slowly, take a deep breath in through the nose, letting the lungs fill. The chest should not move.	
• Hold breath for a count of three.	Slows the respiratory rate.
• Purse the lips and slowly exhale, while tightening the abdominal muscles. Press inward and upward on the abdomen with the hand while breathing out.	Increases pressure within the bronchi, minimizing collapse of the small airways and allowing more complete exhalation.
3. Repeat the technique for 1 min or 15 times, with a short rest after each group of five.	Promotes maximum benefit of the exercise without causing undue fatigue.
4. Practise the exercise several times during the day. If you become short of breath, concentrate on breathing slowly and rhythmically.	Regular exercise is needed to improve pulmonary function.
C. Pursed-Lip Breathing	
1. Help the patient to a comfortable upright position.	Decreases pressure of the abdominal organs on the diaphragm, thus creating space for lung expansion.
2. Instruct and demonstrate how to:	
• Inhale slowly through the nose while counting one, two, three or "one one hundred," "two one hundred," "three one hundred."	Facilitates deep inhalation.
• Purse the lips as if about to whistle, or as if blowing through a straw. Then exhale slowly and evenly through the pursed lips for six seconds. The sound made will be like a small soft whistle.	Prevents collapse of the small airways and promotes more complete exhalation. Exhalation takes twice as long because expiratory airflow is slowed due to collapse of airways.
3. Practise the technique eight to ten times per interval, three to four times a day until it becomes automatic. Practise the technique in other positions, for example, lying flat in bed, standing, or walking. While walking, the patient should inhale for two steps and then exhale through pursed lips for the next four steps.	Prepares for use of the exercise in daily living.
4. Document the teaching, patient response and effectiveness of teaching.	Fulfills requirement for nurse accountability and promotes continuity of care.

respirations, opens more alveoli and permits better gas exchange. It also helps to relax the entire body and is, therefore, useful as a sleep aid. This technique is beneficial for

PURSED-LIP BREATHING The goal of pursed-lip breathing is to prolong exhalation by increasing airway pressure and preventing bronchiolar collapse and air trapping. It provides a way of controlling respirations when a patient is experiencing dyspnea or anxiety.

COUGHING

Coughing is used to force collected and consolidated secretions from the lungs and to maintain a clear airway. Postoperatively, patients are often reluctant to cough because of pain. Secretions can pool in the lungs causing airway obstruction, decreased alveolar gas exchange and lung complications such as hypostatic pneumonia. Because deep breathing tends to stimulate the cough reflex, deep breathing and coughing were formerly taught together in preoperative teaching. This is not recommended, however, in current practice. "Routine coughing in the absence of secretions has been found to cause atelectasis and, because of associated pain, to decrease motivation for effective deep breathing" (Berger & Williams, 1992, p. 1261). Thus, postoperative coughing should be done only when secretions are present. The steps for teaching effective coughing are given in Procedure 24.3.

Because incisional pain limits the effectiveness of deep breathing and coughing for the postoperative patient, the nurse also teaches how to splint the incision so that the patient can obtain maximum benefit from the exercises. **Splinting**, which provides support to the incision during coughing, involves applying external pressure against the abdominal muscles. This limits pain and strengthens the force of the muscular contraction. To splint an incision, the patient can put his or her hands across the incisional site with fingers interlaced or place a pillow or bath blanket against the abdomen (Figure 24.11). Splinting can be done

Patients with lung secretions may need to be reminded to cough. Coughing is advised upon awakening, because secretions consolidate through the night, and before meals to aid oxygenation, promote ease of respirations and allow more energy for eating. (In addition, the removal of foul secretions, along with mouth care, may improve the taste of food.)

INCENTIVE SPIROMETRY

Incentive spirometers are used to increase lung functioning and improve pulmonary ventilation. They are effective in counteracting the effects of anesthetic agents and/or hypoventilation, loosening respiratory secretions, facilitating gaseous exchange, preventing atelectasis and expanding collapsed alveoli. Patients prescribed prolonged bed rest and postoperative patients at risk for pulmonary complications (those who have had abdominal or thoracic surgery, older people, those who are obese, smokers and people with decreased ability to cough effectively and expel lung secretions) benefit from incentive spirometry.

The incentive spirometer is designed to increase the depth and duration of lung inflation beyond normal deep breathing in what is called a *sustained maximal inspiration*. The device measures the flow of air through the mouthpiece during inhalation and gives visual feedback to the patient, providing an incentive to improve deep breathing. If spirometry is to be used postoperatively, teaching takes place preoperatively along with deep breathing. Teaching a patient to use an incentive spirometer is outlined in Procedure 24.4. There are two general types of spirometers: the flow-oriented spirometer and the volume-oriented spirometer.

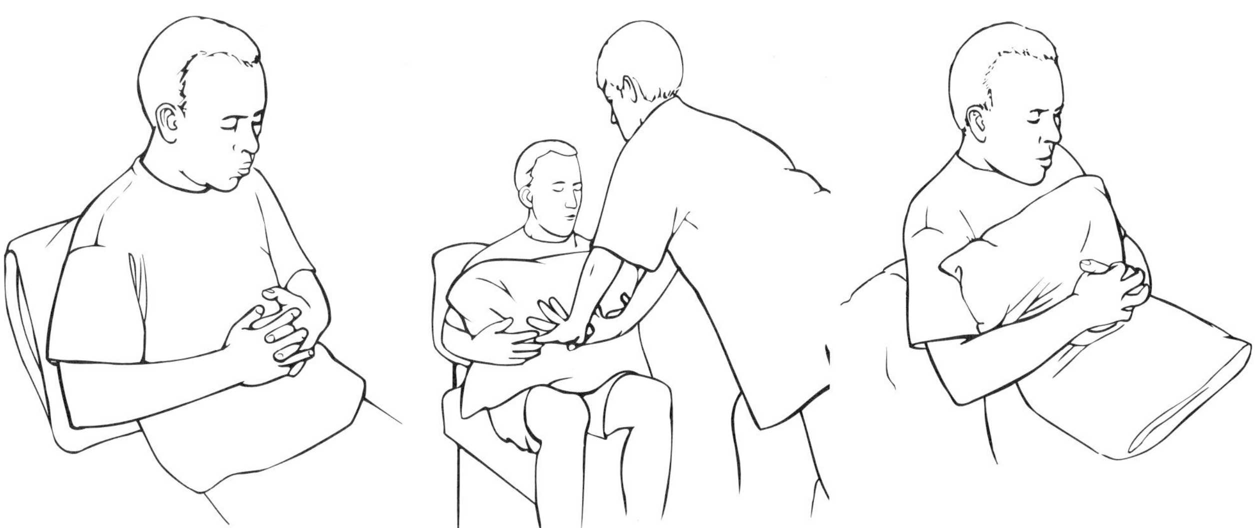

FIGURE 24.11 Splinting incisions to aid effective coughing

PROCEDURE 24.3 Teaching Effective Coughing

Action	*Rationale*
1. Explain the purpose of the breathing exercise.	Understanding the benefits of the exercise facilitates learning and promotes active participation.
2. Auscultate lungs.	Establishes a baseline for evaluating effectiveness of coughing.
3. Help the patient to a comfortable sitting or well-supported Fowler's position.	Aids full expansion of the lungs, permitting maximum ventilation and removal of retained secretions.
4. Provide tissues and/or an emesis basin.	Prepares for collection of secretions.
5. Splint the incision, if necessary.	Decreases pain and promotes lung expansion.
6. Instruct the patient to:	Prevents secretions from being taken deeper into the lungs.
• Take a slow, deep breath and exhale. Repeat two or three times.	Deep inhalations stimulate the cough reflex and build up air within the airways behind the secretions, aiding in moving them upward.
• Lean forward, take another deep breath, hold it for a second; then exhale, with the throat closed, by contracting the diaphragm and abdominal muscles.	Builds up intrathoracic pressure. Maximal air volume combined with pressure creates a bolus of air, which moves secretions.
• Open the mouth and cough forcefully, without inhaling, until nearly out of breath. Expectorate into tissues or basin.	Clears trachea and bronchi and moves secretions out of the smaller airways.
• Pause and breathe normally for 10–15 seconds. Repeat coughing technique until secretions are expectorated.	Relaxes the muscles, provides rest and permits normal ventilation between coughing episodes.
7. Auscultate the lungs.	Evaluates the effectiveness of coughing.
8. Assist the patient with mouth care.	Removes secretions retained in the mouth and refreshes the patient.
9. Encourage fluids, if not contraindicated.	Liquefies secretions, making expectoration easier.
10. Leave the patient in a comfortable position. Encourage rest.	Restores energy used in coughing.
11. With gloves on, dispose of tissues or basin.	Eliminates microorganisms from contaminated secretions; gloves prevent contact with blood and body secretions.
12. Document the procedure, the patient's response, effectiveness of treatment, characteristics of the secretions, chest auscultation findings.	Fulfills requirements for nurse accountability and promotes continuity of care.

FLOW-ORIENTED DEVICE This device consists of one or more clear plastic chambers containing freely movable coloured balls or discs that move up and down as the patient breathes (see Figure 24.12A). It does not measure the specific volume of inhaled air. The patient's task is to elevate the balls and keep them elevated for as long as possible before exhaling. This device is low-cost and disposable, and can be used independently by patients.

VOLUME-ORIENTED DEVICE The volume-oriented device measures the inhalation volume maintained by the patient. It contains pistons or bellows that are raised by inhalation to a predetermined volume (see Figure 24.12B).

Health-Restoring Strategies

Restorative care for individuals experiencing interferences with oxygenation involves a variety of measures to establish airway patency, increase ventilatory efficiency, ensure adequate oxygen intake and decrease bodily needs for oxygen. Nurses work in collaboration with physicians, respiratory therapists and physiotherapists in administering necessary interventions.

MEASURES TO DECREASE DEMANDS FOR OXYGEN

The need for oxygen by the body is related to the rate of metabolism of the tissue cells. Factors affecting metabolic rate include physical activity, disease processes and emotional reactions. Although a certain amount of activity is essential to promote optimum ventilation of the lungs, excessive activity should be avoided. The patient's level of tolerance must be carefully assessed, and care must be taken to avoid overexertion. Patients who experience dyspnea on exertion will need assistance from the nurse in completing

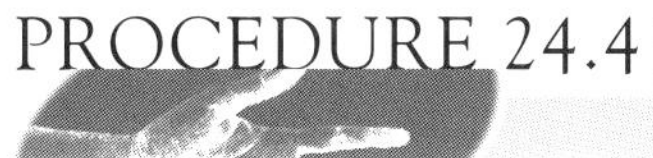

PROCEDURE 24.4 Teaching Use of an Incentive Spirometer

Action	*Rationale*
1. Explain the purpose of the incentive spirometer.	Understanding the benefits of exercise facilitates learning and promotes active participation.
2. Teach the patient how to use the spirometer. For a volume device, set the volume level pointer at a predetermined level.	Enables independent use of the spirometer.
3. Assess the patient's breath sounds and comfort level. Administer pain medication if necessary.	Establishes a baseline for evaluation of treatment. Pain control allows maximum effort and chest expansion.
4. Help the patient into a comfortable sitting or semi-Fowler's position. If the patient can't assume or maintain an upright position, the procedure can be performed in any position as long as the device remains upright.	Promotes optimal lung expansion.
5. Instruct the patient to:	
• Exhale normally.	
• Seal the lips tightly around the mouthpiece.	A weak seal may alter flow or volume readings.
• Hold the spirometer in an upright position.	A tilted flow device requires less effort to raise the ball, and a volume device will not function correctly unless upright.
• Take a slow, deep breath in to elevate the balls or cylinder while watching the balls or gauge rise in the spirometer.	Achieves maximum lung expansion. Indicates when the preset goal is achieved.
• Hold the breath for two seconds initially and increase to six seconds as tolerance increases. Try to keep the balls or cylinder elevated during this time.	Facilitates maximum ventilation of the alveoli.
• Remove the mouthpiece and exhale normally.	Spirometers are not designed for exhalation through the chambers.
• Relax and take several normal breaths before repeating the exercise.	
• Try to cough; splint the incision as necessary.	Deep ventilations may loosen secretions that can be expectorated.
• Repeat the procedure several times (i.e., 10 per hour while awake).	Repetition increases inspiratory volume, maintains alveolar ventilation and prevents atelectasis.
• Avoid exercising at meal times.	Prevents nausea.

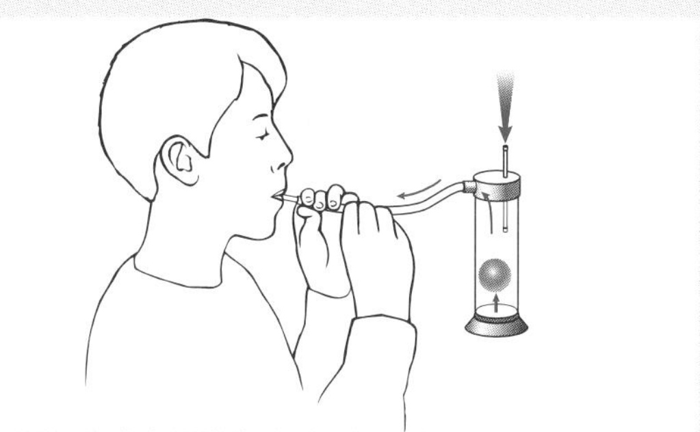

Action	*Rationale*
6. Auscultate the breath sounds.	Determines effectiveness of treatment.
7. Clean the mouthpiece with water and shake dry. Do not immerse the spirometer. Change disposal mouthpieces q24h.	Moisture enhances bacterial growth and impairs effectiveness of the internal filter.
8. Label the spirometer with the patient's name and store at the bedside within easy reach.	Limits transmission of microorganisms and reminds the patient to use it.
9. Document the procedure, type of spirometer, volume or flow levels achieved, number of breaths taken, patient's tolerance and results of auscultation.	Fulfills requirements for nurse accountability and promotes continuity of care.

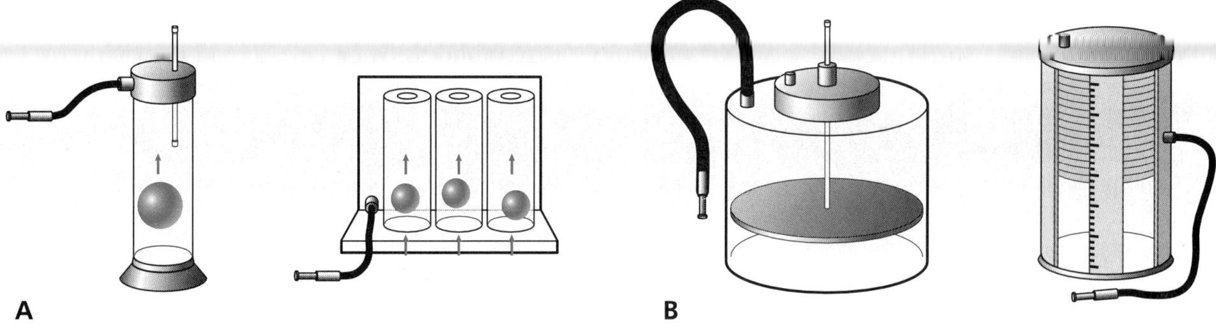

FIGURE 24.12 Incentive spirometers. A. Flow-oriented devices. B. Volume-oriented devices

SOURCE: Traver, Mitchell & Flodquist-Priestly, 1991, p. 112.

activities of daily living until activity tolerance improves. Uninterrupted periods of rest are essential to restore energy and support optimal oxygenation.

Because elevated body temperature increases the basal metabolic rate, oxygen requirements increase accordingly. Patients with oxygenation problems may not be able to meet these extra demands for oxygen. Measures to keep body temperatures within normal limits are essential. Care must be taken to prevent infection; when infections develop the causative organism(s) must be identified and treatment instituted promptly.

Emotional tension is also a factor to be considered in patients with respiratory problems. Anxiety may stimulate the parasympathetic nervous system and result in constriction of the smooth muscles of the bronchioles. The expression of other emotions, such as fear, anger and grief, is also closely related to respiration. Strong emotions initiate responses to prepare the body for action, and respirations become faster and deeper.

The patient's anxiety contributes to respiratory problems, and a vicious cycle may develop. The patient becomes dyspneic; the dyspnea produces anxiety; the anxiety results in more dyspnea. It is essential that this cycle be broken.

Helping to establish the patient's confidence in the care being given is an important factor in alleviating anxiety. Prompt attention to the patient's needs, such as answering the call bell immediately and attending to needs without delay, can often prevent or minimize an attack of dyspnea. It is important in this regard to remember that anxiety is not always expressed openly. Patients may not necessarily say "I am frightened," but often their actions convey this meaning to the observant nurse. The patient may make a seemingly excessive number of requests, or attempt to keep the nurse engaged in conversation. The physical presence of someone competent who can help if needed is reassuring to the patient.

Efficient handling of equipment and skillful execution of procedures contribute to the patient's feeling of security and well-being. The nurse should be familiar with the equipment used in the care of patients with respiratory problems and should feel confident about performing the necessary procedures.

NUTRITION AND FLUID THERAPY

Patients with dyspnea often have little energy for eating and may have difficulty holding the breath while swallowing. In addition, eating large amounts of food creates difficulty in breathing because a full stomach pushes upward on the diaphragm, limiting its movement. A well-balanced diet, taken in small, frequent meals over the day, is recommended. Activities should be scheduled so that meals are eaten one to two hours after treatments or exercises—when respirations are easier, airways are clear and the patient has had some rest.

Adequate hydration is essential for people with respiratory secretions. Water depletion increases the viscosity of secretions and impairs clearance of the lungs. A fluid intake of one to two litres daily is necessary to keep secretions thin and easy to expectorate. People who are mouth-breathers need extra fluids because they are also losing fluids through respiration.

HUMIDITY THERAPY

The provision of air with a high water content is a therapy that has been used for respiratory problems for many generations. Traditionally this has taken the form of steam inhalations, but there are now other devices available for humidification. The purpose of humidity therapy is to provide extra moisture to the mucous membranes lining the respiratory tract. The moisture prevents drying and irritation of the mucous membranes, and helps to dilute thick secretions.

Humidifiers are devices that add moisture to inspired air. Vapour is produced by passing air or oxygen through water in a process called *bubbling*. One of the most common humidifiers in use is the bubble humidifier for humidifying oxygen in oxygen therapy. It consists of a bottle filled with sterile distilled water that is attached to an oxygen source by means of a flow meter. Moisture is picked up as the gas bubbles through the bottle before moving through the

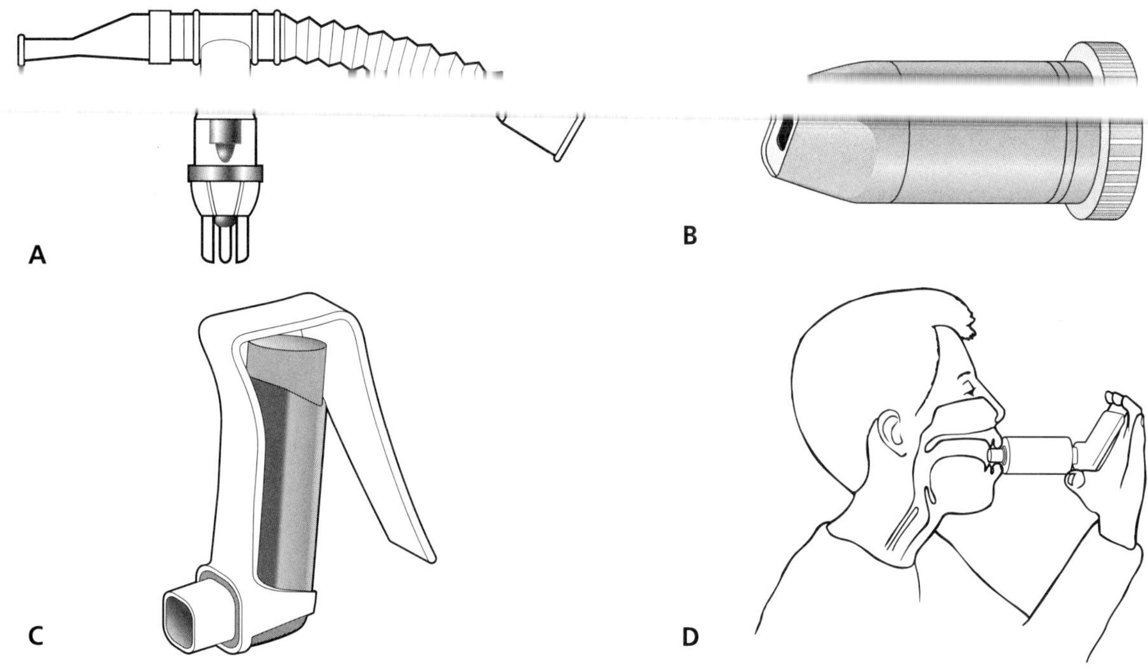

FIGURE 24.13 A. Jet nebulizer. B. Turbuhaler. C. Metred-dose inhaler. D. Spacer

SOURCES: Traver, Mitchell & Flodquist-Priestly, 1991, p. 87; Shapiro, Kacmarek, Cane, Peruzzi & Hauptman, 1991, p. 69.

tubing to the patient. Room humidifiers are also used at the bedside to humidify the atmosphere immediately surrounding the patient.

AEROSOL-NEBULIZATION THERAPY

Aerosol-nebulization therapy involves the delivery of medications into the tracheobronchial tree by inhalation. Medication is *nebulized* (reduced to a fine aerosol spray) and then inhaled deeply into the respiratory tract, where absorption occurs. Nebulized medications avoid the systemic complications associated with parenteral or oral administration. Two commonly used **nebulizers** for medication therapy are the small-volume jet nebulizer and the hand nebulizer (inhaler).

A jet nebulizer is a hand-held device that uses oxygen or air under pressure to create a suspension of microscopic particles in the form of a mist which the patient inhales (see Figure 24.13A). The jet nebulizer utilizes either a mouthpiece or a mask to deliver the prescribed medication. "Approximately 8% to 12% of the aerosol reaches the lower respiratory tract" (Turner, McDonald & Larter, 1994, p. 233).

These inhalers are referred to as either metred-dose inhalers (MDIs), which provide a liquid form of medication, or dry-powder inhalers (DPIs), which provide the powdered form of medication. With the MDI, the canister contains the medication and a gas propellant. When the inhaler is activated by pressing down on the canister, a dose of medication, suspended in the propellent gas, is released from the inhaler. Use of the MDI requires coordination with the inspiratory phase of respiration. "Only 9% to 11% of the aerosol from an MDI reaches the lower respiratory tract" (Turner et al., 1994, p. 232). A *spacer* (Figure 24.13D) may be used with an MDI for patients who have difficulty coordinating delivery with inspiration (young children, the elderly). Also called *chambers* or *extenders*, these devices provide a reservoir to hold the aerosol until the next inspiration. Spacers also facilitate greater absorption of the aerosol in the airways.

DPIs are hand-held nebulizers that are activated with inspiration. They do not contain gas propellants. They are recommended for those patients unable to operate MDIs. Patients use inhalers independently once instructed in the correct technique. Medications commonly delivered by aerosols include bronchodilators, corticosteroids, antibiotics and mucokinetics. Mucokinetics are drugs that alter the consistency and clearance of tracheobronchial secretions. They include diluents (water and saline), mucolytics (which liquefy and loosen thick secretions) and expectorants (which loosen bronchial secretions so they can be removed with coughing).

Preparing the Patient

Prior to initiation of therapy, the patient should be assessed to determine the appropriate device for aerosol nebulization. Successful administration through an MDI, for example, depends upon the patient's ability to coordinate delivery of the medication with the beginning of inspiration. If this is not possible, such as with children or the elderly, an alternative method such as the DPI or jet nebulizer should be employed. The nurse explains the purpose of the therapy and the procedure and places the patient in a comfortable, upright position. Baseline vital signs, including oxygen saturation, should be obtained. Treatment should be given before meals to increase lung ventilation and therefore decrease the fatigue that accompanies eating. The procedure is painless and not tiring; it usually lasts 15–20 minutes. The steps in administering aerosol-nebulization therapies are outlined in Procedure 24.5 and in the Guidelines for Using Inhalers.

Assembling Equipment

A jet nebulizer is a small device that is attached to a gas source. In a hospital, wall oxygen or compressed air is used for this purpose; at home the patient may have an air-powered compressor. The nebulizer has a small reservoir (nebulizer cup) into which the medication and diluent are added. The medication is prepared in a syringe (according to the procedure outlined in Chapter 34) and added to the nebulizer cup. (It is also available in prefilled ampoules.) If necessary, water or saline may also be added to dilute the medication. The nebulizer cup and tubing are changed according to agency policy to maintain cleanliness and prevent respiratory infections.

CHEST PHYSIOTHERAPY

Chest physiotherapy, also referred to as **postural drainage**, is used to loosen and move secretions into the large airways so they can be expectorated with greater ease. It is usually performed by a physiotherapist or respiratory therapist, and in some situations by a specially trained nurse. The procedure uses positioning to aid in drainage of secretions by the flow of gravity, and incorporates deep breathing (see Figure 24.14), coughing, percussion and vibration techniques to mobilize secretions. Percussion is carried out by lightly and rhythmically striking the chest wall with cupped hands (see Figure 24.15A). Vibration is achieved by a rapidly repetitive shaking and a gentle compression of the chest wall during exhalation. Figure 24.15B shows the proper placement of hands for vibration. Effective coughing is necessary to help raise the secretions. It may take several hours following therapy before secretions are expectorated.

Chest physiotherapy is usually performed at least two hours after meals to prevent nausea, and before bed. Bronchodilators are sometimes ordered before the procedure to dilate the bronchial tubes and reduce spasm of the

PROCEDURE 24.5 Administering Nebulization Using a Jet Nebulizer

Action	*Rationale*
1. Prepare the patient.	Promotes patient well-being.
2. Wash hands and gather: • jet nebulizer • air or oxygen flow meter • medication.	Reduces transfer of microorganisms; promotes efficiency and economy of time.
3. Prepare the equipment at the bedside: • Attach the flow meter to the air or oxygen outlet. • Attach the nebulizer to the gas source. • Inject the medication into the medication cup. • Adjust the flow meter to about 6 L/min.	 Usually 5–7 L/min are adequate to create a fine mist.
4. Help the patient to an upright position.	Facilitates maximum chest expansion and aerosol dispersion.
5. Auscultate the chest for breath sounds.	Establishes a baseline for evaluation of care.
6. If patient is using the mouthpiece, instruct to close lips tightly.	Creates a seal. Be careful not to occlude the opening with either the tongue or the teeth.
7. Instruct the patient to breathe in slowly and deeply through the mouth, hold the breath for two to three seconds, and then exhale normally through pursed lips.	Ensures maximum benefit of aerosol therapy.
8. After the treatment, encourage the patient to cough and expectorate the secretions. Provide suction if necessary.	Removes liquefied and loosened secretions.
9. Auscultate the chest.	Determines the effectiveness of treatment.
10. Document the treatment including the date and time, type and amount of medication, breath sounds and patient's response to treatment.	Fulfills requirements for nurse accountability and promotes continuity of care.

Guidelines for Using Inhalers

using the inhaler. *Maximizes inhalation and absorption of the medication.*

- For MDIs, make sure the canister is firmly and fully inserted into the outer shell of the inhaler. *Ensures correct delivery of the prescribed medication.*
- Remove the cap from the mouthpiece. Hold the inhaler in the upright position and shake well five to six times. (Do not shake DPIs.) *Ensures even suspension of the medication.*
- Exhale slowly and fully, then administer the medication using either open- or closed-mouth technique.*

Open-Mouth Technique (used with MDIs):

- Place the mouthpiece 3–5 cm in front of open mouth. Keep the tongue and teeth from blocking the mouthpiece of the inhaler.
- Take a slow, deep inhalation through open mouth while firmly pressing down on the canister.
- Hold breath for 10 seconds or as long as comfortable. *Creates a resistance against airflow from the lungs and increases pressure within the bronchi, forcing full expansion of the airway.*

**Note:* If the patient is unable to use the open-mouth technique with the MDI, the closed-mouth technique may be used. However, inhalation should be slow and deep.

Closed-Mouth Technique (used with DPIs):

- Place the mouthpiece over the tongue and well into mouth. Keep the teeth and tongue from blocking the mouthpiece of the inhaler.
- Close lips tightly around the mouthpiece and breathe in quickly.

slowly and deeply.

- It is not necessary to hold breath after inhalation with DPIs.
- Remove the inhaler from the mouth, purse the lips and breathe out slowly. *Permits greater expansion of the airway.*
- Wait 1–2 min to deliver a second puff (if prescribed).
- Rinse mouth with water after using the inhaler. *Prevents dryness of the mouth and throat and side effects from oropharyngeal deposits.*
- If two inhalers are prescribed, that is, a bronchodilator and a corticosteroid, use the bronchodilator first. This opens the airways and allows the corticosteroid to get into the airways more effectively. It will take a few minutes for the medication to be effective.
- Cough. *Mobilizes secretions.*
- Clean the inhaler once a week. If using an MDI, remove the canister and wash the outer shell in warm soapy water; rinse it well and let it air dry overnight. DPI should be completely dried before use, since moisture will cause the medication powder to clump.

Spacers

- Shake MDI.
- Attach spacer to MDI.
- Depress the MDI once to release the aerosol particles into the spacer.
- Inhale slowly and deeply from the mouthpiece of the spacer.
- Wash frequently in soapy water per manufacturer's instructions.

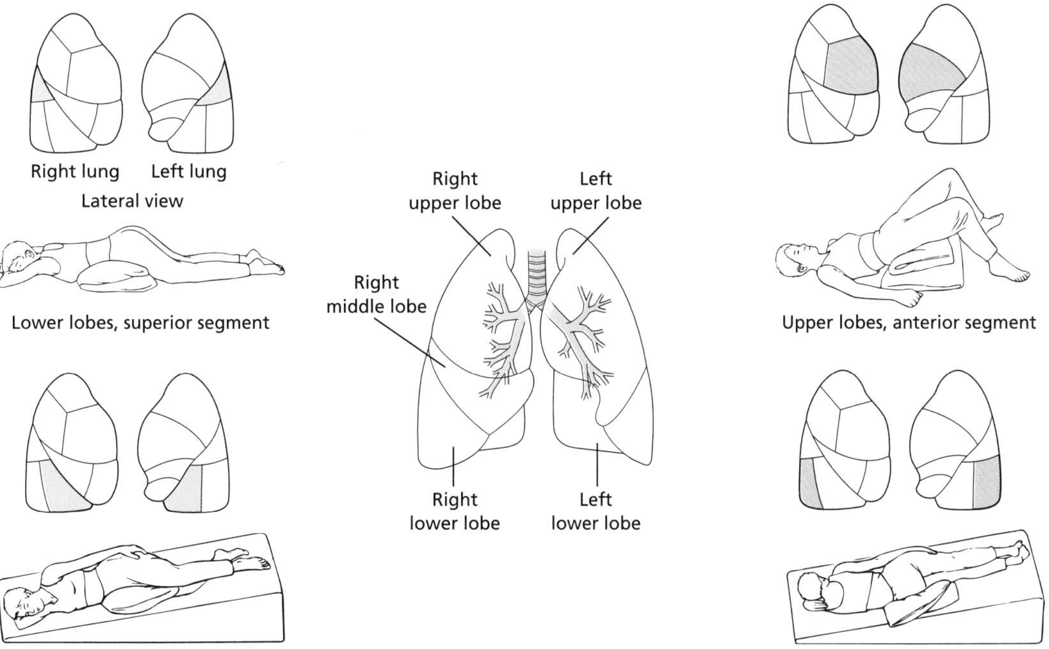

FIGURE 24.14 Postural drainage positions and the areas of the lung drained by each position

SOURCE: Smeltzer & Bare, 1996, p. 549.

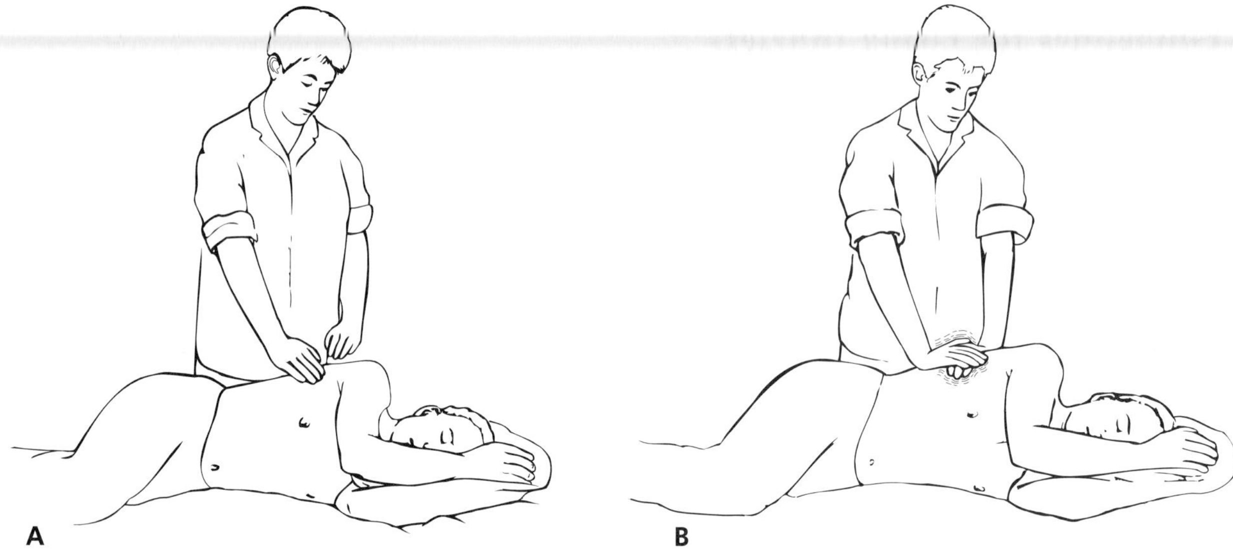

FIGURE 24.15 A. Hand position for cupping. B. Hand position for vibration

bronchial walls. These should be administered 20 minutes prior to the procedure. Chest physiotherapy is very tiring. A rest period beforehand will conserve energy for the procedure and improve the patient's tolerance.

OROPHARYNGEAL AND NASOPHARYNGEAL SUCTIONING

Oropharyngeal and nasopharyngeal suctioning refers to the removal of secretions from the pharynx by means of a catheter inserted through the mouth or nose (as shown in Procedure 24.6). It is used to maintain a patent airway in patients who have difficulty swallowing or expectorating secretions. Suction is provided by a suction machine or wall outlet. Because the suction catheter may inadvertently slip into the lower airway or esophagus, sterile technique (discussed in Chapter 32) is used throughout the procedure. When both nasal and oral suctioning are required at the same time, the nose is suctioned first. This limits the introduction of microorganisms from the mouth to the nasal passages. Normally, the mouth harbours more organisms than does the nose.

The mucous membrane of the respiratory tract can easily be injured during suctioning. Therefore, suctioning should be used only when secretions have accumulated and abnormal breath sounds are audible. These are indicated by noisy, wet respirations or rattling, bubbling breath sounds. Signs of respiratory distress caused by obstruction (restlessness, cyanosis), drooling or the obvious presence of secretions alert the nurse to the need for suctioning.

Preparing the Patient

The patient is reassured that the procedure will make him or her more comfortable by relieving the breathing difficulty. Suctioning of the throat is usually a painless procedure but it can cause the patient to gag, cough or sneeze. If the patient can cough during the procedure, it will facilitate removal of mucous.

Assembling Equipment

Suction is established by a device that creates a negative pressure to draw liquids and solid materials towards the source of pressure (much like a vacuum cleaner). A suction unit consists of a collection container, a regulator with a gauge that registers the degree of negative pressure during suctioning and a control knob for setting the pressure (see Figure 24.16). Tubing connects the suction unit to the catheter. Wall-mounted and portable suction units will be

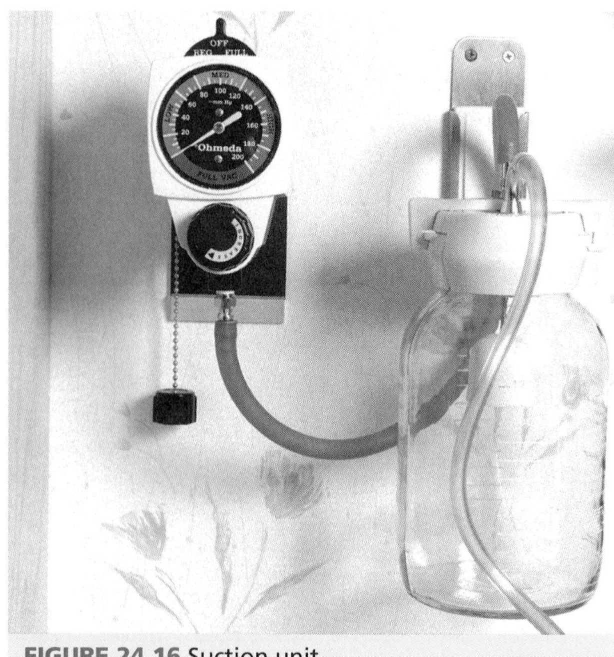

FIGURE 24.16 Suction unit

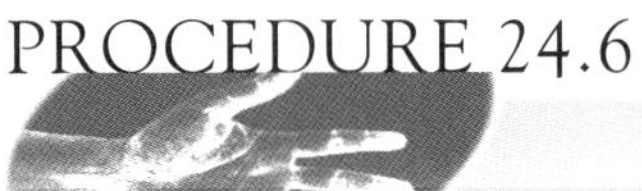

PROCEDURE 24.6 Performing Oropharyngeal and Nasopharyngeal Suctioning

Action	Rationale
1. Prepare the patient.	Reduces anxiety and fear; enables patient participation.
2. Wash hands and gather: • portable or wall suction unit with tubing • sterile suction kit and appropriate-sized catheter, if necessary or • sterile suction catheter • sterile gloves • sterile water or saline • sterile disposable container • towel or waterproof pad • clean glove, if suction kit used.	Reduces transfer of microorganisms and facilitates efficiency and economy of time.
3. Draw the bed curtains.	Promotes privacy.
4. Help the patient to a semi-Fowler's position, if conscious. If patient is unconscious, place him or her in a lateral recumbent position, facing the nurse.	Catheter insertion aided by gravity. Promotes drainage of secretions and lessons the risk of aspiration.
5. Place a towel or waterproof pad across the patient's chest.	Protects patient's clothing from secretions.
6. Turn suction to appropriate pressure. **Wall unit:** Adult: 100–120 mm Hg Child: 80–110 mm Hg Infant: 50–95 mm Hg **Portable:** Adult: 10–15 mm Hg Child: 5–10 mm Hg Infant: 2–5 mm Hg	Negative pressure must be at a safe level to minimize injury to mucosa.
7. Prepare the sterile equipment using sterile technique (see Procedure 32.4). Add sterile saline or water to the container. Open a sterile suction catheter (if appropriate).	Reduces the risk of infection. Patients with pulmonary dysfunction are very vulnerable to infection.
8. Don sterile gloves (Procedure 32.3). Or, apply a clean glove on the nondominant hand and a sterile glove on the dominant hand.	The dominant hand will be used to handle the catheter; it must be kept sterile. The nondominant hand will be used to manipulate unsterile equipment. The glove protects the nurse from contact with body secretions.
9. Using the dominant hand, pick up the catheter and coil it around the hand. Grasp the connecting tube with the nondominant hand and attach the catheter to the tubing.	Prevents inadvertent contamination of the catheter.

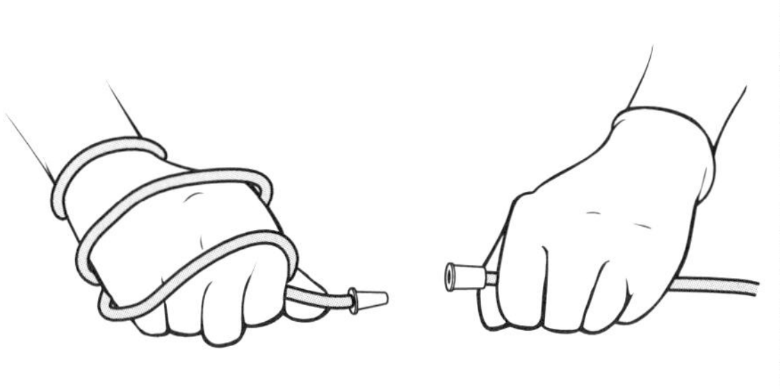

continued on next page

PROCEDURE 24.6 continued

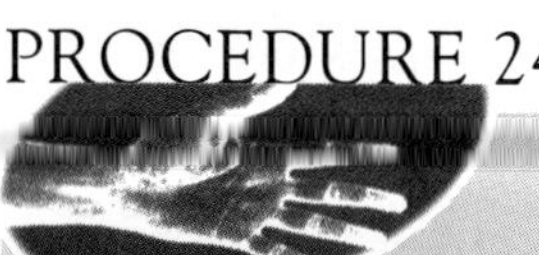

Action	Rationale
10. Moisten the catheter by dipping it into the container of sterile irrigant and occlude the thumb port. Fluid should move through the tube.	Lubricates the lumen of the catheter which aids movement of secretions and checks that equipment is functioning.
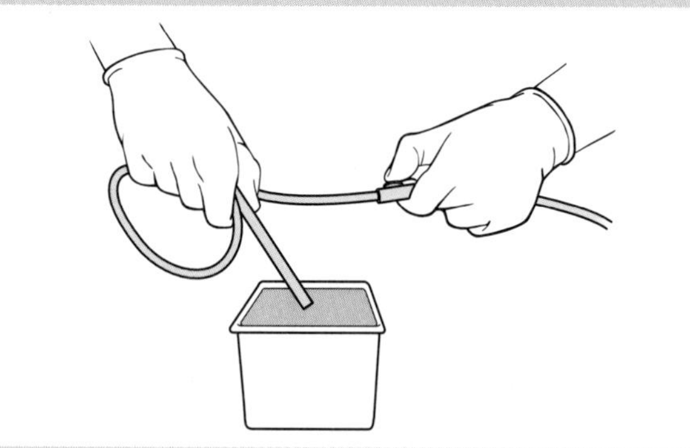	
11. Coil the catheter around the dominant hand so the tip is between the thumb and forefinger.	As in Step 9.
12. Insert the catheter. **Nasopharynegeal suction:** • Estimate the distance from the ear lobe to the patient's nose and hold at that point between thumb and forefinger.	Determines the length of catheter needed to reach the pharynx.
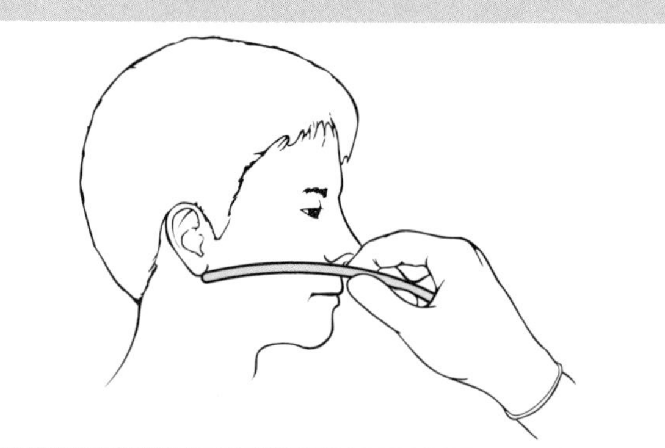	
• With the thumb port open, gently insert the catheter into one nostril as the patient inhales.	Absence of negative pressure lessens injury to the mucosa and reduces oxygen depletion.
• Direct the catheter along the floor of the nasal cavity (medially and inferiorly).	Prevents injury to the nasal turbinates or coiling in the nasal cavity.
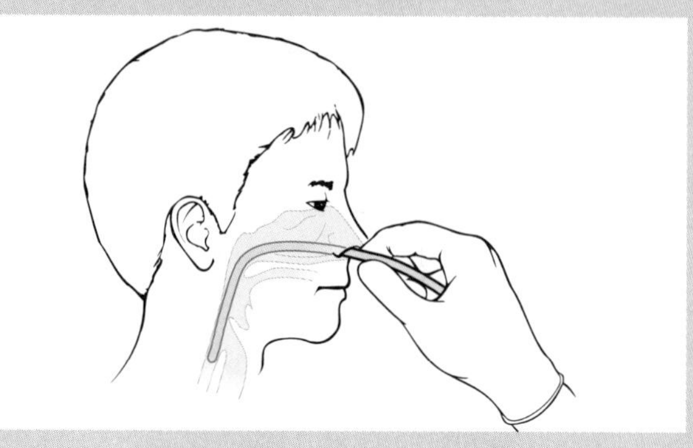	

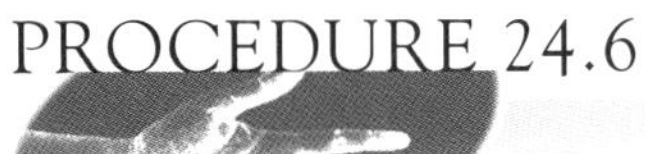

PROCEDURE 24.6 *continued*

Action	Rationale
Oropharyngeal suction: • With the thumb port open, insert the catheter along the side of the mouth towards the oropharynx.	Minimizes gagging.
13. Apply suction by placing the thumb of the nondominant hand over the thumb port for 5–15 seconds at a time. Apply intermittent suction as you rotate and withdraw the catheter.	Reduces mucosal trauma and clears mucous from all the walls of the airway. Limiting suctioning to 15-second intervals reduces the risk of hypoxia.
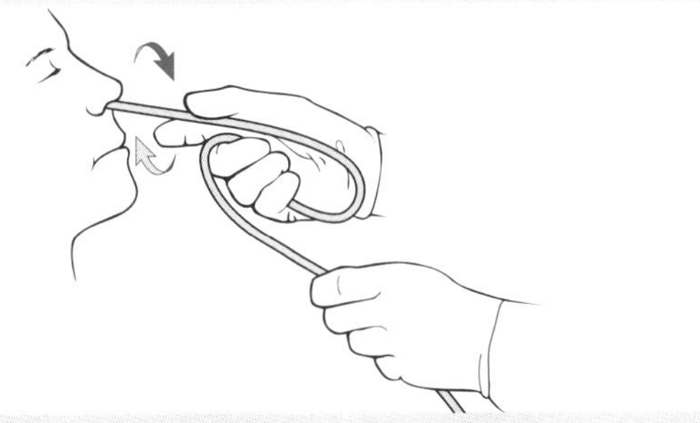	
14. Flush the catheter with sterile irrigant and wipe it with sterile gauze if it is thickly coated with secretions.	Cleans and clears the catheter and lubricates it for the next insertion.
15. Repeat suctioning until the air passage is clear. Allow at least 20–30 seconds of rest between suction passes. Apply oxygen and encourage coughing and deep breathing between suctionings.	Helps to compensate for hypoxia caused by suctioning. Helps to eliminate secretions naturally and reduces the need for further suctioning, or moves the secretions from the trachea and bronchi into the pharynx so they can be removed.
16. If the patient shows signs of increasing hypoxia, the heart rate becomes excessively slow or rapid, or if there are sudden frank bloody secretions, stop suctioning and have someone notify the doctor. Monitor oxygen saturation (via pulse oximetry) throughout procedure.	
17. When suctioning is complete, disconnect the catheter from the tubing, coil the catheter in the palm of the sterile hand and remove the glove so that it turns inside out over the catheter.	Prevents the transfer of microorganisms.
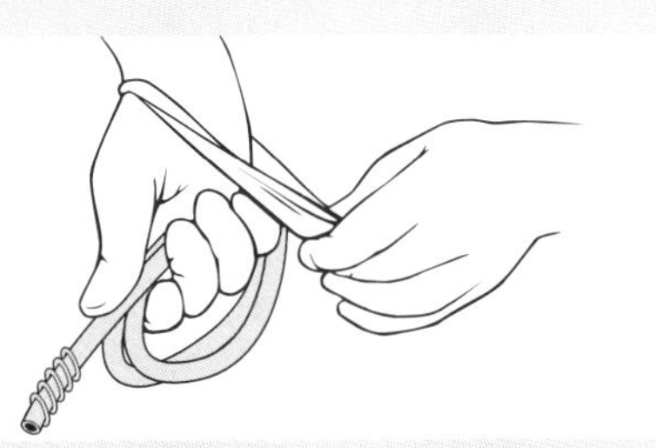	
18. Turn off the suction, dispose of equipment in the proper receptacle and wash hands.	Maintains cleanliness and safety in the workplace.
19. Auscultate the breath sounds, note the patient's colour and respiratory status. Take pulse, respirations and oxygen saturation (pulse oximetry).	Determines effectiveness of suctioning.
20. Assist the patient with oral or nasal hygiene and leave him or her comfortable.	Enhances patient well-being.
21. Document the procedure, including the frequency and method of suctioning, patient's colour, respiratory status and characteristics of secretions.	Fulfills requirements for nurse accountability.

found in agencies. Wall-mounted units are attached to a piped-in source of negative pressure. The negative pressure is measured in millimetres of mercury (mm Hg). In some portable units the negative pressure can be set only as "low," "medium" or "high."

Suction catheters are made of soft plastic material and are available in different sizes ranging from 5 Fr to 18 Fr. (Recall from previous chapters that the smaller the French number, the smaller the diameter of the catheter.) Sizes 12 Fr to 18 Fr are used for adults. The size of catheter selected for a patient should be large enough to remove secretions but not so large as to occlude the airway. Most catheters have a suction control port on the distal end, called a thumb port, which is used to establish suction once the catheter is inserted. This permits insertion of the catheter without causing trauma to tissues along the way.

Sterile suction kits are available that are used once and then discarded. These kits contain a catheter with a thumb port, one or two gloves, water-soluble lubricant and a container for the irrigant. Sterile water or saline is used to flush the catheter during the procedure. If the catheter in the kit is not the correct size for the patient, a separately packaged catheter is obtained. A clean glove will also be necessary when using a suction kit that provides only one glove. When a patient is in distress, the airway must be cleared promptly. For this reason, a suction unit and a supply of necessary equipment are usually kept at the bedside of patients who require suctioning.

SUCTIONING THE OROPHARYNX WITH A TONSILLAR TIP CATHETER The mouth can also be cleared with a *tonsillar* or *Yankauer suction tip*. It is a rigid catheter that can be easily directed to all parts of the mouth. Patients can be taught to use this type of catheter themselves. Once the catheter is connected to the suction source, suction is continuous (the catheter has no suction control mechanism). Clean technique is used with a tonsillar tip device because it is used only to remove secretions from the mouth. The procedure is the same as for oropharyngeal suctioning. All areas of the mouth are cleared: along the top of the tongue, under the tongue and along the sides of the mouth to the pharynx. The catheter is reusable. After use, it is cleaned with water and hydrogen peroxide to remove secretions, rinsed with water and air dried.

CHEST DRAINAGE

Chest tubes are inserted into the intrapleural space to promote evacuation of air and serosanguineous fluid. This re-establishes normal negative pressure, re-expands the lung and prevents mediastinal shift.

A physician usually inserts two chest tubes (either anteriorly or posteriorly) after thoracic surgery, pneumothorax or hemothorax. Chest tubes can be inserted in the operating room, emergency department, treatment room or at bedside. After the tubes are placed and secured, the wounds are sutured, airtight dressings are applied and the tubes are connected to a closed drainage system or a Heimlich valve, which functions like a water seal.

Preparing the Patient

The nurse ensures that the patient understands the reasons and purpose for the chest tube(s) and the risks involved, and answers any questions the patient may have. The patient may be in a sitting position or lying down with the affected side elevated. Sterile drapes are placed around the site. Tell the patient to maintain the position and not to touch the drapes or supplies during the insertion procedure.

Once inserted, the catheter is sutured and air-occlusive dressings are applied. The tubing is attached to the drainage apparatus and the connections securely taped. Instruct the patient to report any pain or shortness of breath following the procedure.

Assembling the Equipment

If the chest tube is to be inserted by the physician outside the operating room, the nurse must obtain the chest tube insertion equipment and supplies. Some agencies have specially prepared carts that contain a local anesthetic, antiseptic solution, chest tube insertion tray, chest drainage system, sterile drapes, gowns and gloves, and various sizes and types of chest catheters. Chest tubes are single-lumen catheters made of silicone or polyvinyl chloride. Drainage tubing connects it to the pleural drainage system.

A drainage system or valve receives fluid and/or allows air to escape the intrapleural space. Drainage systems used in early years consisted of three bottles: the collection bottle, which received the fluid and air from the chest cavity; the water-seal bottle, which acted as a one-way valve; and the suction-control bottle, which regulated a controlled amount of suction to the intrapleural space. Today, a variety of disposable plastic chest drainage systems are commonly used. They often combine the three-bottle system into a single device, which may be a waterless (dry) system or a water-seal (wet) system, or a combination of both (Figure 24.17; see Procedure 24.7).

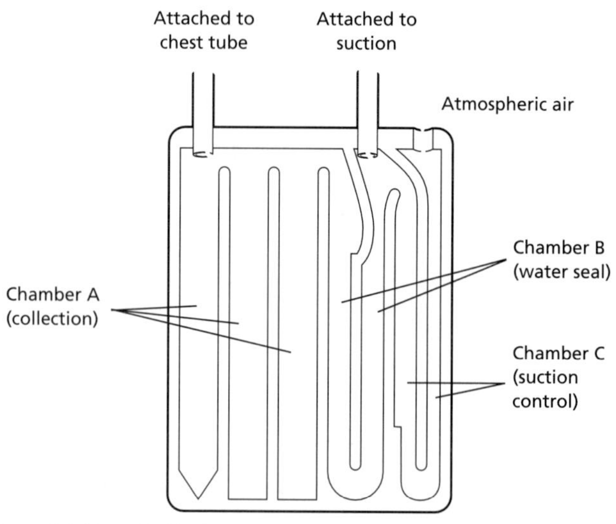

FIGURE 24.17 Water-seal chest drainage system

SOURCE: Timby, 1996, p. 416.

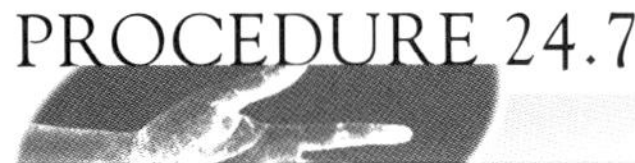

PROCEDURE 24.7 Assisting the Physician with Chest Tube Insertion

Action	Rationale
1. Prepare patient.	Reduces anxiety and fear; enables patient participation.
2. Assess the patient's respiratory and cardiac status.	Provides baseline data.
3. Wash hands and gather equipment and supplies: • chest tube insertion tray • chest tubes of physician's preference • closed drainage system • surgeon's sterile gown and gloves • sterile water • portable or wall suction with connecting tubing • sterile petrolatum gauze • antiseptic solution • local anesthetic • air-occlusive tape • 2 rubber-tipped clamps.	Reduces transfer of microorganisms and facilitates efficiency and economy of time.
4. Draw bed curtains.	Promotes privacy.
5. Prepare the chest drainage system using strict surgical asepsis:	
• With funnel provided, fill water-seal chamber through the short tube to the "fill to here" line or to the 2-cm water level.	Appearance of blue water indicates the water-seal chamber is prepared.
• Fill suction-control chamber with sterile water according to physician's order.	Controls amount of suction applied to the pleural space.
• In a dry unit, test the suction and drainage set by using the dial to obtain a setting according to physician's order.	
• Connect the short section of the suction chamber to the suction source with a connecting tube.	Ensures that the equipment is working properly.
• Keep the tubing clamped until the chest tube is inserted and connected.	Prepares for connection to the chest tube once inserted into the patient.
6. Position patient sitting up or in side-lying position with the affected side up.	Provides physician access to surgical area.
7. Assist physician as required by setting up sterile field and dispensing antiseptics, local anesthetics and supplies.	Facilitates efficiency and economy of time.
8. Support the patient during the procedure (i.e., a local anesthetic is injected; a small incision is made; the chest tube is inserted, sutured and dressed with petroleum gauze and an airtight pressure dressing).	Promotes patient comfort, physical and emotional well-being. Secures chest tube in place and prevents air entry into intrapleural space.
9. Assist with attaching the chest tube to the prepared chest drainage system:	
• Connect the long latex tubing from the collection chamber of the drainage system to the chest tube, maintaining surgical asepsis at the connection.	Provides sterile means of drainage, preventing contamination.

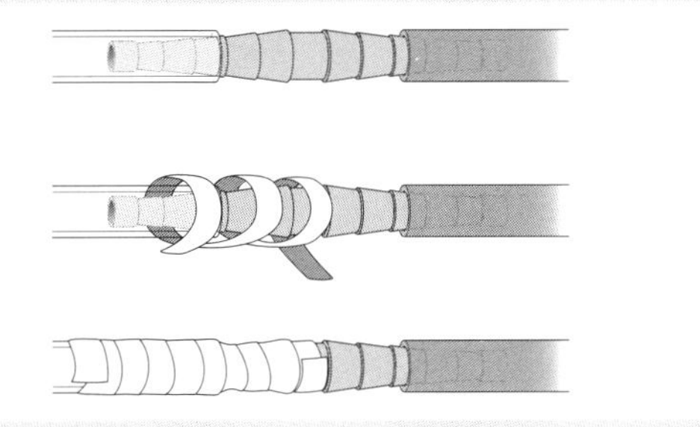

continued on next page

PROCEDURE 24.7 *continued*

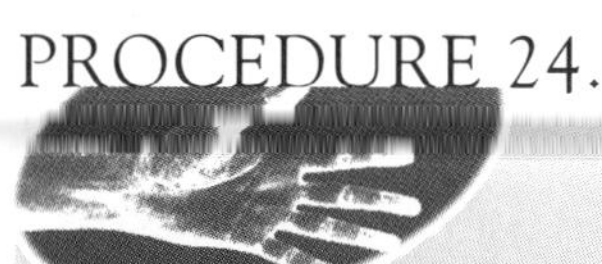

Action	*Rationale*
• Turn on suction until gentle bubbling appears in the suction chamber.	Provides suction to the intrapleural space and promotes evacuation of air and fluid.
• Tape all connections securely with waterproof tape.	Prevents accidental separation of tubing.
• Keep chest drain apparatus below chest level at all times.	Promotes drainage by gravity and prevents reflux or siphoning of fluid back into the pleural space.
10. Turn on the suction. Increase the suction until the orange float or bellows appears in the suction control indicator window in a dry unit. In a wet unit, the water in the suction control chamber bubbles gently but continuously.	Provides adequate amount of suction.
CARE OF THE CHEST TUBE AND PLEURAL DRAINAGE	
A. MAINTAINING THE DRAINAGE SYSTEM	
1. Maintain patency of the chest tube:	
• Keep all tubing straight or loosely coiled without dependent loops, and prevent patient from lying on it.	Kinks or compression of the tubing will occlude the lumen.
• Use chest tube clearance techniques, such as "milking" or "stripping," with caution and according to agency policies.	Briefly increases negative pressure in the tube and dislodges clots; enhances the evacuation of fluid. Excessive negative intrapleural pressure may damage lung tissue. Agency policies may vary.
• Chest drainage apparatus must always be placed below chest level.	Promotes gravity drainage and prevents backflow of drainage into the pleural space.
2. Keep all connections between chest tubes, connecting tube, collection apparatus and suction source tight:	Prevents accidental disconnection and pneumothorax from air leak into the closed system.
• Tape all connections with waterproof tape.	
• Check for the absence of bubbling in the suction control chamber.	Absence of bubbling means that the correct amount of suction is not being maintained.
3. Observe for intermittent bubbling and tidalling in the water-seal chamber.	Indicates pressure changes in the pleural space (rises with inspiration and falls with expiration). Absence of fluctuations may indicate lung re-expansion or blockage in the drainage system. Large amounts of continuous bubbling indicate a drainage system leak.
4. For specimen collection, use a sterile needle and syringe. Swab with alcohol prior to specimen collection. Remove fluid from the specimen collection port on the back of the collection chamber of the drainage system.	Ensures that a fresh specimen is collected.
5. Suction can be disconnected, but do not clamp the tubing.	The drainage system continues to provide water seal and fluid collection.
6. After initial insertion of chest tube, drainage should be recorded per agency policy.	Monitors patient status.
7. Change dressing per agency policy.	
B. REPLACING THE CHEST DRAINAGE SYSTEM	
1. Replace the drainage system when the collection chamber is full (approximately 2500 mL):	Allows for continuity of drainage.
• Set up a new unit.	
• Untape the connection tubing of the old unit.	Provides for a quick change-over.

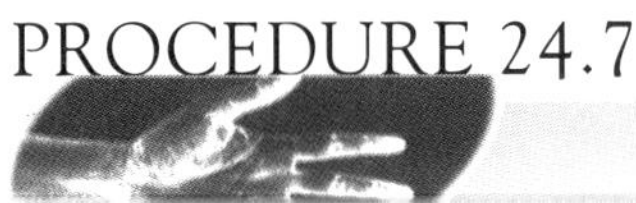

PROCEDURE 24.7 *continued*

Action	*Rationale*
• Change the unit by double-clamping the chest tube about 5 cm (2 in) from the patient (use rubber-shod Kelly clamps and place second clamp about 2.5 cm [1 in] distal to the first clamp).	Prevents air from entering the system and causing a pneumothorax.
• Disconnect old unit and connect quickly to the new unit.	Decreases the possibility of causing a tension pneumothorax.
• Do not leave the chest tube clamped for more than 1 min.	
• Remove the clamps and ask the patient to take a deep breath.	Prevents tension pneumothorax.
• Tape connection securely.	Prevents accidental disconnection.
C. Removal of Chest Tube	
1. The physician orders the chest drain to be discontinued when water-seal fluctuations have ceased for 24 hours, lung auscultation and percussion sounds are normal, drainage is less than 50 mL/day, chest x-ray reveals lung re-expansion, clamping of chest tube produces no changes in vital signs and patient is comfortable.	Indicates lung re-expansion is complete.
2. Assess the need for analgesic and administer as necessary 30 min before removal procedure.	Provides for patient comfort.
3. Wash hands, set up sterile field with air-occlusive pressure dressing and suture scissors.	Prevents transmission of microorganisms.
4. Position patient according to physician's preference, and support patient physically and emotionally.	Facilitates chest tube removal.
5. Ask patient to take a deep breath and hold it while the physician cuts the sutures and pulls the chest tube out. Immediately apply the occlusive pressure dressing.	Prevents air from entering the pleural space through the chest wound.
D. Postprocedure	
1. In addition to monitoring equipment, observe patient status, coughing and deep breathing, chest tube insertion site, chest assessment and vital signs, as necessary.	Ascertains effectiveness of treatments, provides for early identification of complications and gives information for further care.
2. Reposition patient.	Provides comfort.
3. Remove used equipment, applying body substance precautions; dispose appropriately as medical waste.	Prevents transmission of microorganisms.
4. Record and report respiratory status; check chest dressing, amount, colour and type of chest drainage output. Note any complications and nursing actions taken.	Provides information regarding the patient; contributes to record of drainage system operation; documents patient care given. If the drainage rate is greater than 100 mL/h or the rate is increasing, notify the physician.

OXYGEN THERAPY

Oxygen therapy is a method of supplying supplemental oxygen in concentrations greater than that of environmental air. It improves cellular oxygenation, decreases the work of breathing and reduces stress on the heart. In clinical use, oxygen is considered a drug. Therefore, the principles of medication therapy (as discussed in Chapter 34) apply when oxygen is being administered. A physician's order is needed to administer oxygen. The physician specifies the method of oxygen delivery and the rate of flow or the concentration, expressed as a percentage of oxygen in inspired air. Sometimes the physician orders the level of oxygen (hemoglobin) saturation to be maintained, as determined by pulse oximetry. For example, the order might read: *Administer oxygen by nasal cannula and keep* O_2 *saturation at 96%*. In this case the nurse adjusts the flow rate to maintain the necessary oxygen saturation level.

Oxygen must be administered carefully because excessive oxygen is not only harmful, but is also potentially fatal in some people. It can produce toxic effects in the lungs and central nervous system, and cause depression of ventilation. High concentrations of oxygen are especially dangerous in people with chronic hypoxia, for example, a patient with COPD. Such patients become accustomed to abnormally high pCO_2 levels in the blood and, for them, the stimulus to breathe is a lack of oxygen. Administering high levels of oxygen to these patients would take away their respiratory stimulus and they may stop breathing completely. In general, patients with respiratory conditions are given oxygen at the lowest flow rate or concentration that will maintain the arterial oxygen pressure at their normal baseline. This can vary from 75 to 100 mm Hg.

Oxygen is an odourless, colourless and tasteless gas. People may not be aware of its presence. In addition, while oxygen by itself does not burn, it does support combustion. Therefore, safety measures must be taken by everyone, including visitors, when oxygen therapy is in progress. Precautions to be taken during oxygen therapy are outlined in the accompanying box.

In order to administer oxygen safely the nurse must have an understanding of oxygen equipment and know how to use it. Procedure 24.8 outlines the steps involved in setting up oxygen equipment.

Safety Measures During Oxygen Therapy

- Instruct patients and visitors regarding safety precautions.
- Avoid smoking, open flames, matches and lighters. For the confused patient, remove cigarettes and lighters from the bedside.
- Eliminate sparks by ensuring electrical equipment (electric call bells, razors, radios, television sets) is in good working order. Ground electrical equipment.
- Avoid materials that generate static electricity (woollen blankets, synthetic fabrics).
- Avoid volatile, flammable materials, for example, alcohol, petroleum-based lip agents (Vaseline), nail polish remover. Oil can ignite spontaneously in the presence of oxygen. Use water-soluble lubricants.

Assembling Equipment

Therapeutic oxygen is supplied from central storage reservoirs piped to wall outlets or from portable tanks or cylinders. Most hospitals today use a piped-in oxygen system; however, portable units are necessary for transporting patients (for example, to the x-ray department) or in case of emergencies in designated areas. Portable tanks are also used for home care.

Oxygen tanks are steel cylinders containing oxygen under high pressure (Figure 24.18A). A pressure regulator with a pressure-reducing valve is used to control the release of oxygen from the tank. The regulator normally has two gauges: a content gauge and a flow meter. The content gauge, calibrated in pounds per square inch (psi), indicates the amount of oxygen in the tank. A flow meter controls the release of oxygen to the patient. This is measured in litres per minute (L/min). Figure 24.18B shows an oxygen tank with an attached regulator, content gauge and flow meter.

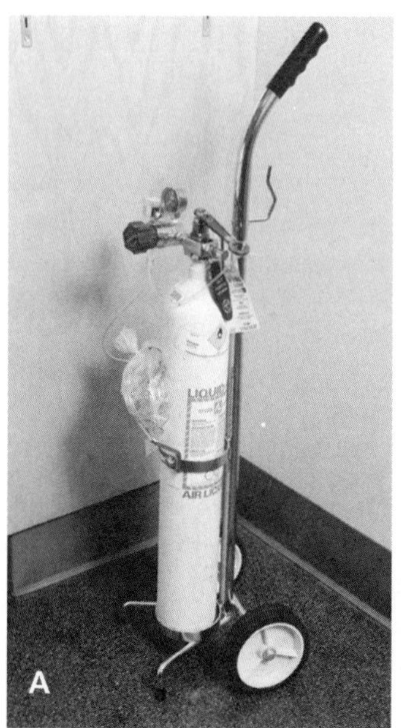

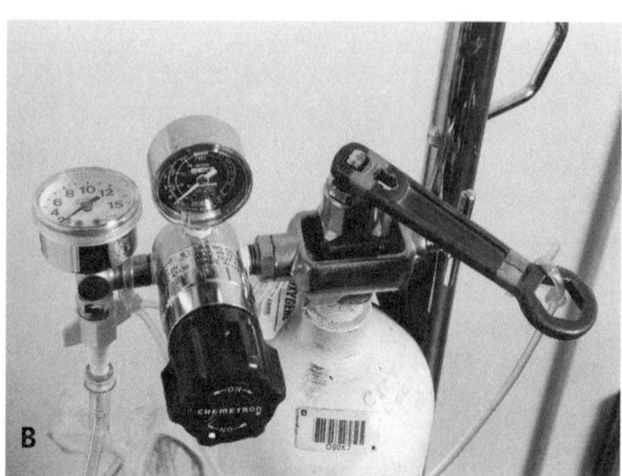

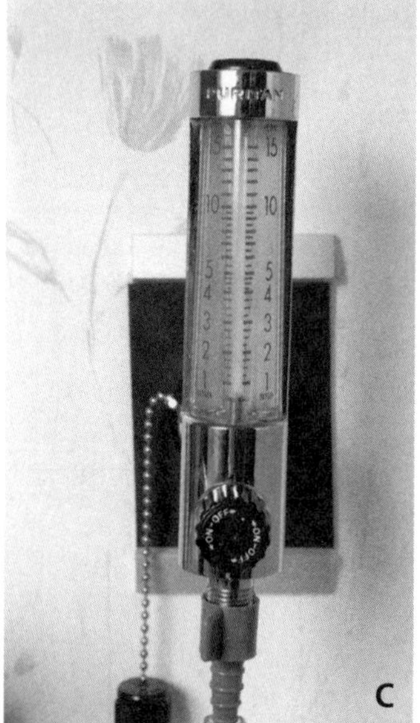

FIGURE 24.18 A. Oxygen tank. B. Close-up of regulator, content gauge and flow meter. C. Flow meter used with a piped-in oxygen source

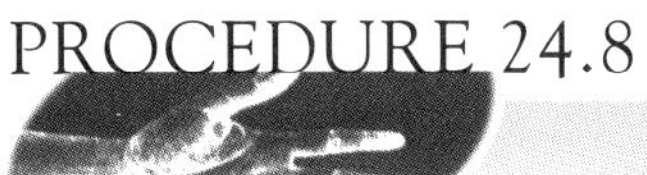

PROCEDURE 24.8

Preparing Oxygen Equipment

Action	*Rationale*
1. Gather equipment: • oxygen flow meter or portable tank and regulator with flow meter • humidifier, as appropriate • oxygen-connecting tubing.	
A. Wall-Outlet System	
1. Make sure the flow meter control is in the off position. Push the flow meter into the wall outlet using firm pressure.	Prevents escape of oxygen when the flow meter is attached to the wall outlet.
2. If appropriate, attach a humidifier to the flow meter. Attach the adapter to the top of the humidifier bottle. Then connect the humidifier to the flow meter and turn the adapter clockwise until it is tight.	Prevents oxygen from leaking around the connection and causing a fire hazard. Indicates that oxygen is flowing freely.
Open the flow meter to establish oxygen flow and look for bubbles in the container. Turn the flow meter off.	
3. Connect one end of the oxygen tubing to the flow meter if a humidifier is not used, or to the outlet port of the humidifier, if used.	Readies the equipment for connection to the oxygen delivery device.
B. Portable Oxygen Tank	
1. If necessary, set up a new cylinder. • Remove the protective cap from the cylinder outlet.	When cylinders drop to about 500 psi, they should be replaced.
• Open the hand wheel at the top of the cylinder slightly by turning it clockwise and then closing it quickly. A loud hissing sound will be made.	Called "cracking the cylinder," this removes dust from the outlet.
• Connect the pressure regulator with flow meter to the cylinder outlet and tighten it with the wrench, supplied with the tank.	Oxygen is stored under pressure. The connections must be tight to ensure safety during use.
2. Open the cylinder valve by slowly turning the hand wheel until it is fully open and then turn it back a quarter turn.	Readies the tank for the flow of oxygen.
3. Follow steps 2 and 3 of section A.	
4. To turn off the flow of oxygen, close the hand wheel by turning it clockwise. Wait until both gauges indicate empty. Then, turn the flow meter control off.	Clears oxygen from the regulator during storage.
5. Store the unit in a safe location away from high traffic areas and heat.	Promotes safety in the environment. Heat causes gases to expand.

The oxygen gauges are generally attached to the tank before it is brought to the patient. In most hospitals, respiratory technologists supply and service the oxygen equipment. Because of the extreme pressure within the cylinder, oxygen tanks must be handled with caution and care. The force of gas escaping from a damaged regulator or outlet could cause the tank to behave like a rocket. Cylinders are held in wheeled carriers or stands and secured with metal straps to prevent them from falling and damaging the regulator and outlet. They should be placed away from high traffic areas and heat registers when in use. Tanks in storage have a protective cap to avoid accidental damage to the cylinder outlet.

Piped-in oxygen is stored in reservoirs under low pressure between 50 and 60 psi. A flow meter is used to regulate the amount of oxygen released from the wall outlet (see Figure 24.18C).

Oxygen is a dry gas (has no moisture content). Continuous administration of oxygen above 4 L/min dries respiratory tissues and mucous secretions, both of which can lead to airway obstruction and risk for infection. Thus, oxygen delivered at high flow rates (>4 L/min) should be humidified. In some agencies, it is standard practice to humidify all oxygen delivered to patients, regardless of the flow rate. The nurse should consult agency policy in this regard. Oxygen is humidified with a humidifier attached to the oxygen flow meter. Prefilled disposable humidifiers are commonly used. Reusable humidifiers are packaged in sterile wrappers and must be filled with sterile distilled water before use. An adapter is needed to connect the humidifier to the flow meter. Adapters may be packaged separately or with the humidifier. Tubing is needed to connect the oxygen source to the delivery device.

Establishing Oxygen Therapy

Oxygen is administered by a delivery device, such as a nasal cannula or a mask, in an amount prescribed by the physician. The amount is ordered as a rate of oxygen flow, indicated in litres per minute, or a concentration, expressed as a percentage of oxygen in inspired air. For example, the physician may order *O_2 per nasal cannula at 4 L/min* or *O_2 by mask at 36%*.

Oxygen delivery devices are categorized as either low-flow or high-flow systems. In a low-flow system, the device delivers a set flow of 100 percent oxygen, which is then mixed with room air as the patient inhales. The amount of room air that is entrained (pulled in and trapped, like air in a vacuum) varies according to the person's rate and depth of respirations and consequently influences the final concentration of oxygen delivered. For instance, when respirations are shallow, little room air is drawn in (entrained) to dilute the supplemental oxygen. Therefore, the percentage of oxygen in the inspired air increases. On the other hand, when a person takes a deep or rapid respiration, more room air is drawn in. As a result, the room air–oxygen mixture is more diluted and the inspired oxygen concentration decreases. "Low flow refers to this variable mixing with room air, not the oxygen flow rate set on the flow meter" (Traver et al., 1991, p. 96). The nasal cannula and simple face mask are the two most common low-flow delivery devices. They are indicated for people who require supplemental oxygen but not in precise concentrations.

High-flow delivery systems are able to control the percentage of oxygen more precisely. This is achieved primarily with masks designed to regulate the amount of room air that is entrained to mix with supplemental oxygen. The mask's ability to deliver a precise percentage of oxygen is not affected by the patient's respiratory pattern, but a properly fitting mask, consistently kept in place, is required. The most common high-flow device in use is the Venturi mask. Table 24.8 outlines the advantages and disadvantages

TABLE 24.8 Oxygen administration devices

Device	*Suggested Flow Rate (L/min)*	*O_2 Percentage Setting*	*Advantages*	*Disadvantages*
Cannula	1–2 3–5 6	23–30 30–40 42	Lightweight, comfortable, inexpensive, continuous use with meals and activity	Nasal mucosal drying, variable FIO_2 (fraction of inspired oxygen)
Catheter	1–6	23–42	Inexpensive	Variable FIO_2, requires frequent change (q8h), gastric distention can occur
Mask, simple	6–8	40–60	Simple to use, inexpensive	Poor fitting, variable FIO_2, must remove to eat
Mask, partial rebreather	8–11	50–75	Moderate O_2 concentration	Warm, poor fitting, must remove to eat
Mask, non-rebreather	12	80–100	High O_2 concentration	Poor fitting
Mask, Venturi	4–6 6–8	24, 26, 28 30, 35, 40	Provides low levels of supplemental O_2 Precise FIO_2, additional humidity available	Must remove to eat
Mask, aerosol	8–10	30–100	Good humidity, accurate FIO_2	Uncomfortable for some
Tracheostomy collar	8–10	30–100	Good humidity, comfortable, fairly accurate FIO_2	
T-piece, Briggs	8–10	30–100	Same as tracheostomy collar	Heavy with tubing
Face tent	8–10	30–100	Good humidity, fairly accurate FIO_2	Bulky and cumbersome

SOURCE: Smeltzer & Bare, 1996, p. 545.

of various oxygen administration devices. The techniques for establishing oxygen therapy by nasal cannula and face mask are outlined in Procedure 24.9.

Preparing the Patient

The administration of oxygen is often a frightening experience for the patient and family. To many people, it denotes a serious illness; some may remember a relative or a friend who died while receiving oxygen. Oxygen is essential to life and to have to depend upon equipment in order to live is in itself anxiety-producing. It is a situation over which patients often have little control and, because they are dependent upon others for the air they breathe, they may feel helpless.

Such fears can often be allayed with knowledge and an opportunity for the patient to become familiar with the equipment. Information about oxygen equipment should be geared to the patient's needs. Some people want to understand in great detail; others are satisfied with a simple explanation. When possible, patients should hold the device, put it on their face and get used to the sensation of wearing it. When patients are well enough to help with the therapy, the nurse can teach them to administer the oxygen themselves and thus help them to feel that they have some control over the situation. The nurse must also review the safety precautions for oxygen therapy and ensure that patients have a good understanding of them.

Assembling the Oxygen Delivery Device

There are many different devices for delivering oxygen. An oxygen hood and oxygen tent (croupette) are used primarily in pediatrics. The nasal cannula, oxygen masks, face tent and croup tent will be described here.

NASAL CANNULA The nasal cannula, also referred to as *nasal prongs*, is the most commonly used aid to breathing. It is an inexpensive, disposable plastic tube with two protruding curved, hollow prongs that fit into the nostrils. The device is secured around the patient's head with an elastic band (see Procedure 24.9). A nasal cannula has several advantages. It is easy to apply, relatively comfortable for the patient and does not cause feelings of claustrophobia, or interfere with eating, talking or coughing. It permits some freedom of movement without interrupting oxygen flow. To use a cannula effectively, the patient must have clear nasal passages and must be alert and able to keep the device in place. Nasal obstruction from a deviated septum, mucosal edema, polyps or excessive secretions, for example, prevents effective use of a cannula, and it can be easily dislodged. Because of the limited area of the nasal cavity to act as a reservoir, the nasal cannula delivers a low range of oxygen concentration. Flow rates of 1–6 L/min are recommended.

SIMPLE FACE MASK The simple face mask is a dome-shaped, clear plastic mask that can be moulded to fit over the nose and mouth (see Procedure 24.9). It has a metal clip that is bent over the bridge of the nose to ensure a snug fit and prevent leakage of oxygen. It is held in place by an elastic strap [illegible]

side of the mask through which room air is taken in and mixed with oxygen, and carbon dioxide is exhaled. A flow rate of at least 5 L/min is necessary to flush exhaled carbon dioxide from the mask. The simple face mask delivers a moderate range of oxygen concentrations at 5–8 L/min. It is indicated when a patient requires an increased delivery of oxygen for a short period, for instance less than 12 hours.

Face masks have several disadvantages. First, they are very uncomfortable to wear. Because of the snug fit, masks are warm and confining, and cause a closed-in feeling. Pressure can also cause irritation of the face, tops of the nose and ears. Masks must be taken off to eat, speak or cough, thus interrupting the continuity of treatment. If the patient is vomiting, there is danger of aspiration because the mask inhibits clearance of the vomitus from around the mouth; the danger increases with unconscious or comatose patients. Close observation is mandatory.

VENTURI MASK The Venturi mask can deliver precise concentrations of oxygen, provided the mask fits snugly and remains in place. The Venturi system (see Figure 24.19) is designed to limit the amount of room air that is blended with a fixed flow of oxygen. The mask has a specific setting for the desired oxygen concentration. Therapeutic oxygen

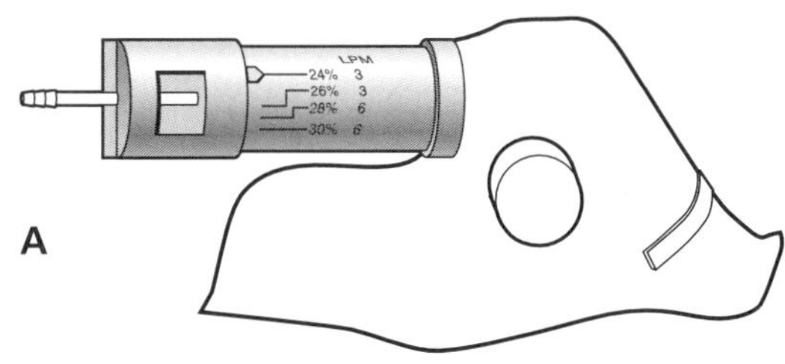

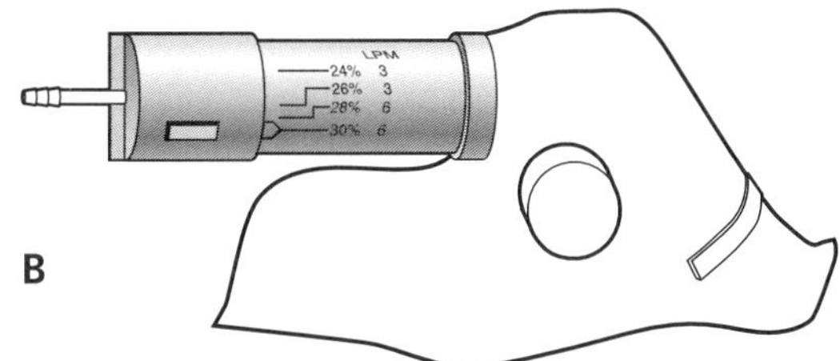

FIGURE 24.19 Venturi mask. Two views of the mask are shown. In A, the mask is set to deliver 24% oxygen; note that the litre flow is indicated as 3 L/min and the entrainment opening is wide. In B, the mask is set to deliver 30% oxygen; the litre flow is now to be set at 6 L/min and the air entrainment opening is much smaller.

SOURCE: Traver, Mitchell & Flodquist-Priestly, 1991, p. 99.

PROCEDURE 24.9

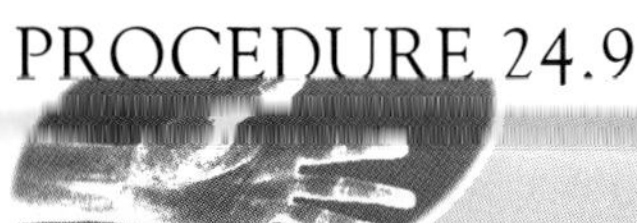

Establishing Oxygen by Nasal Cannula and Face Mask

Action	*Rationale*
1. Check the physician's order for the amount and route of administration.	Protects the patient from injury and promotes accuracy.
2. Prepare the patient. Review safety precautions.	Reduces fear and anxiety; enables patient participation.
3. Gather: • oxygen source • flow meter and tubing • humidifier bottle containing sterile distilled water • oxygen delivery device.	Facilitates efficiency and economy of time.
4. Set up the equipment as in Procedure 24.8 and connect the delivery device. Adjust the flow meter control to the prescribed rate.	
5. Apply the delivery device.	
Nasal Cannula:	
• Position the prongs so they follow the natural curve of the nostril and are directed into the nasal passages. Adjust the strap and tubing according to the type of equipment:	Ensures proper oxygen flow.
a) Slip the elastic band around the patient's head. b) Adjust the tubing around the patient's ears and slide the plastic holder to secure the tubing under the chin.	Secures the cannula in place.
• Ensure that adjustments are not too tight.	Avoids pressure areas and patient discomfort.

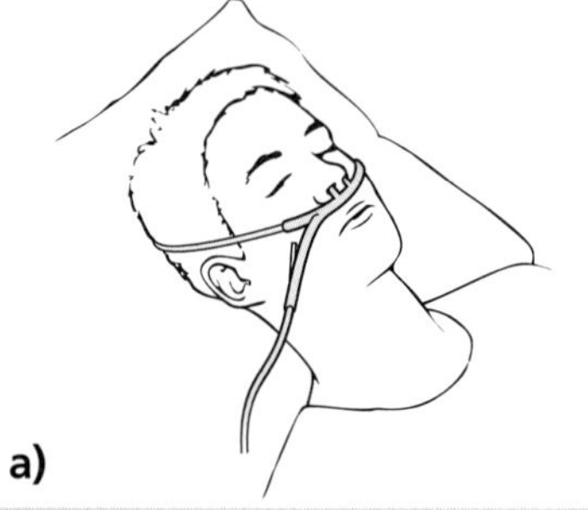

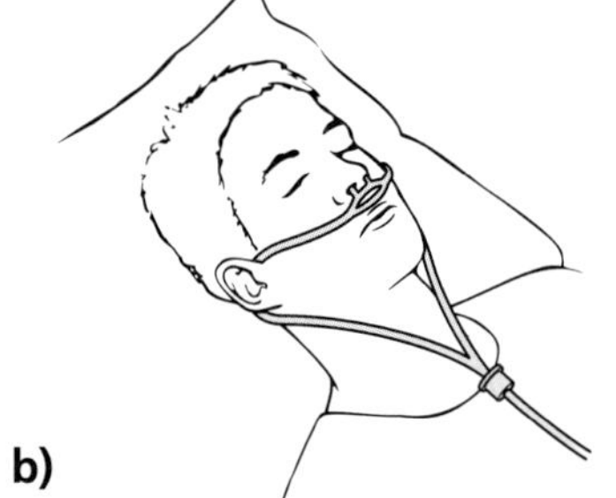

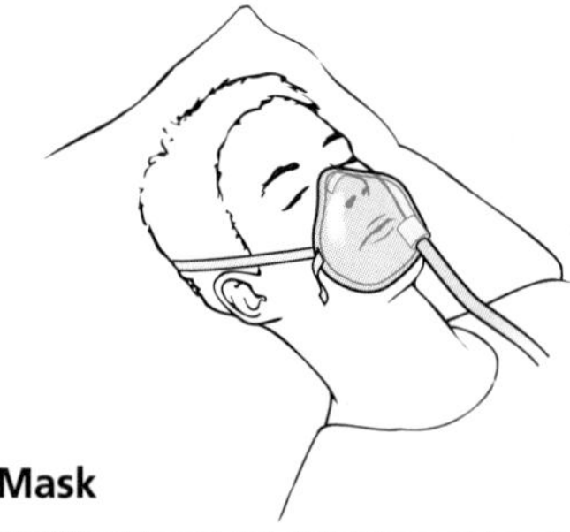

Action	*Rationale*
Simple Mask:	
• Position the mask so that it covers the nose and mouth, and fits the contours of the patient's face.	Ensures maximum benefit from the oxygen being delivered by preventing its escape around the edges of the mask.
• Fasten the elastic strap over the patient's ears and adjust it so the mask fits snugly against the face.	Avoids skin irritation, breakdown or necrosis.
• Mould the nose clip to fit snugly, but avoid excessive pressure.	
Venturi Mask:	
• Adjust the control device on the mask to the prescribed concentration.	Ensures delivery of specified concentration oxygen.
• Apply the mask using the same steps as for the simple mask, above.	The device should be free of blankets or other obstructions.
6. Monitor the patient's status frequently. Note the patient's colour, respiratory status and activity tolerance. Take the pulse,respirations and oxygen saturation (pulse oximetry).	Determines effectiveness of oxygen therapy.
7. Document the procedure. Note the device applied, the flow rate, assessments of the patient's oxygenation and respiratory status and the patient's response to therapy.	Fulfills requirements for nurse accountability.

is delivered at the flow rate (L/min) indicated on the mask, to a small jet (Venturi device) in the centre of a side base

cone through an opening, called an entrainment port, which mixes with the oxygen. The size of the entrainment opening can be adjusted to control the amount of room air entrained and the percentage of oxygen delivered to the patient. The mask also has large vents through which exhaled air can escape.

When using the Venturi mask it is very important to prevent occlusion of the air entrainment ports by bed linen or clothing. If the jets are occluded the efficiency of the Venturi mask is reduced to that of a simple mask, and the concentration of oxygen delivered will vary. The Venturi mask is used for individuals with COPD because it can provide precise low levels of supplemental oxygen, while avoiding the risk of suppressing the hypoxic drive. The disadvantages of using a Venturi mask are the same as for simple masks.

FACE TENT The face tent is an enclosure that covers the lower half of the face and fits snugly under the chin (see Figure 24.20). It is open at the top at about the level of the eyes. It is beneficial for patients who cannot tolerate the simple mask or who have facial burns. A large-bore tubing connection at the base of the shield supplies the oxygen. The concentration of oxygen delivered by a face tent is unpredictable. Therefore, it is often used in conjunction with a Venturi system. When using a face tent, the nurse should frequently inspect the patient's face for dampness, chafing or irritation and provide care as necessary.

CROUP TENT A croup tent (also called a croupette, mist or oxygen tent) is often used as a medical treatment for illnesses such as croup or infections of the epiglottitis, larynx, trachea or bronchi. Although the therapeutic benefits are controversial, the croup tent is still used to help maintain a patent

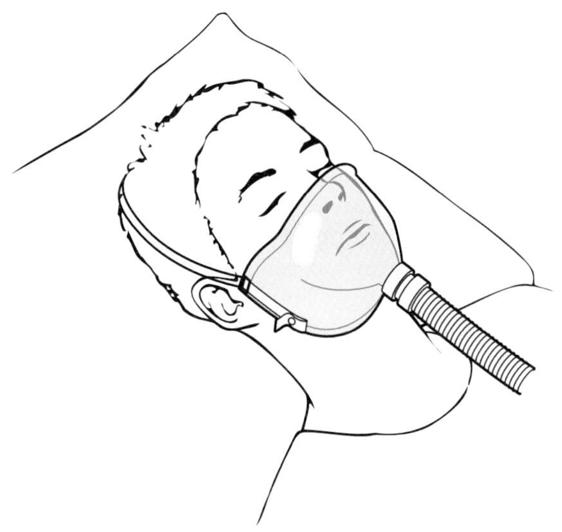

FIGURE 24.20 Face tent

airway. By delivering cool mist and oxygen, it provides an environment that is intended to decrease epiglottal inflam-

respiratory distress. Oxygen may be prescribed by the physician if hypoxia or cyanosis is present (see Procedure 24.10).

MAINTAINING OXYGEN THERAPY

When oxygen is being administered, frequent monitoring of the patient and the equipment is important. The nurse assesses the patient's vital signs, oxygenation status, colour, level of consciousness, activity tolerance and respiratory pattern. Pulse oximetry for oxygen saturation levels may also be taken at specified intervals. In addition, blood gas analysis may be performed. Oxygen therapy is considered completely effective if it improves a patient's oxygen status and acid–base balance. Equipment must be checked at frequent intervals to ensure proper functioning. The nurse notes, for example, the oxygen flow rate, water level in the humidity bottle (if appropriate) and position of the device on the patient's face. If a Venturi mask is in use, the ports are examined for obstructions to ensure delivery of the correct percentage of oxygen.

Therapy will be most effective if the delivery of oxygen is maintained at a constant level. Oxygen flow should be interrupted only to provide necessary care to the face, or the nose in the case of a cannula. Patients who are receiving oxygen via a face mask are provided with nasal prongs for ambulating and eating meals. If the patient is able to sit in a chair or ambulate to the bathroom, tubing long enough to allow these activities will be required. A portable tank may offer the patient more mobility and freedom, if the condition permits. The patient can maintain the health of mucous membranes and keep secretions thin by drinking as much fluid as possible.

Care must be taken to promote patient comfort and protect the skin around the delivery device. With a cannula, the patient's nostrils are inspected q2h for dryness, irritation or bleeding. The nares are cleansed and then lubricated with a water-soluble lubricant as necessary to prevent skin breakdown. Petroleum-based agents, such as Vaseline, should not be used because they can ignite spontaneously in the presence of oxygen. Gauze pads are placed under the tubing around the patient's ears or along the cheekbones, if necessary, to reduce irritation and pressure and prevent skin breakdown. The cannula is removed and cleaned as frequently as recommended by the manufacturer to maintain patency of the openings and, as specified by the agency infection control policy, to limit the spread of microorganisms. The patient with a mask is monitored q2–4h for moisture build-up. The mask is removed temporarily and the skin dried as necessary to prevent skin breakdown.

Oxygen therapy equipment is a potential source of bacterial cross-infection. The delivery devices and tubing must be changed frequently according to manufacturer's recommendations and agency infection control policies to reduce the spread of microorganisms.

PROCEDURE 24.10

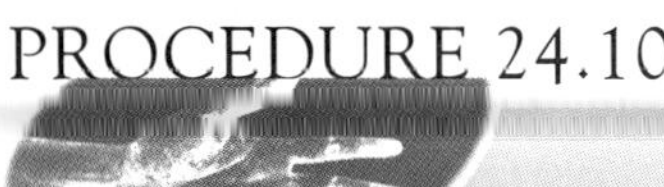

Administering Oxygen with a Croupette, Mist or Oxygen Tent

Action	*Rationale*
1. Prepare the patient; explain procedure, elicit cooperation.	Reduces anxiety in the patient and family and enables participation.
2. Gather equipment: • tent or canopy • humidifier or nebulizer • sterile distilled water • oxygen flow meter, tubing (if ordered by physician) • extra warm clothing (sweater, hat, socks) • non-fire-hazardous, age-appropriate toys.	Facilitates efficiency and economy of time.
3. Set up the equipment:	
• Install the croup tent on the crib so that the complete bed is covered.	Contains humidified air or oxygen concentration inside the tent.
• Fill nebulizer reservoir with sterile water.	Provides humidity, decreases transmission of microorganisms.
• Plug unit into electrical outlet and select "cool" if it is a refrigeration unit, or fill ice reservoir.	Provides means for cooling the air.
• Connect air or oxygen supply hose and adjust gas flow to desired mist output.	Provides flow for mist output and prevents excessive CO_2 concentration.
• Allow 10 min for the tent to cool.	Provides cool environment and oxygen concentration as ordered.
4. Dress the child warmly and check often that the clothes and linen are not damp.	Prevents hypothermia (temperatures inside the tent may be 4°–8°C (6°–15°F) below room temperature.
5. Use various techniques to get the child to remain in the tent; elicit parents' cooperation.	Maintains effectiveness of the treatment.
6. If oxygen is in use, the plastic canopy must be tucked under the mattress on all sides of the crib, or a folded sheet can be used to keep the bottom of the tent tight. Organize nursing care so that repeated opening of the tent is minimal. If humidity alone is used, tight tucking is not necessary.	Keeps the humidity and oxygen inside the tent.
7. Perform frequent assessments:	
• Check for needs and comfort of the patient and parents.	Provides for physical comfort and decreases anxiety level.
• Evaluate respiratory status.	Determines effectiveness of treatment.
• Check operation of the equipment such as water level and ice in the reservoir, and flow of air or oxygen.	Maintains correct functioning of equipment.
• Monitor oxygen concentration if in use, humidity and temperature.	Determines need for adjustments and provides effectiveness of treatment.
• Check that side rails are up at all times.	Promotes safety as the tent will not prevent a child from falling out of the crib.
8. When humidity is used, change equipment and tent per agency policies.	Prevents growth and spread of microorganisms.
9. Record and report assessments, which may include pulse oximetry, respiratory assessments, rate of air flow (and oxygen flow, if oxygen is being administered) and effects of the treatment.	Maintains record of treatment and communicates to other members of the health care team.

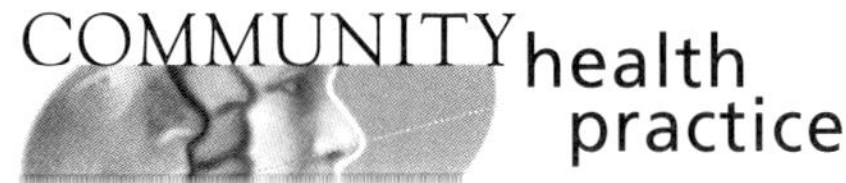

Medigas

Medigas is a national organization that provides home oxygen therapy to individuals. Its services include delivering and maintaining oxygen equipment; educating patients, family members, health professionals and the general public in the proper use of oxygen/nebulizing medications; and giving support to those who use Medigas's service.

The physician writes an order for home oxygen therapy. The agency home care liaison nurse then contacts a respiratory technologist (RT) at Medigas with the details of the patient's therapy and the time of discharge.

A representative from Medigas collects the appropriate equipment and meets the patient at the patient's home. There, the RT sets up the equipment, reviews its safety precautions, demonstrates to the patient and/or family members the correct way to administer the prescribed therapy and evaluates the patient's understanding before leaving. Within 24 to 48 hours, the RT makes a follow-up visit to determine any difficulties or address questions or concerns with oxygen equipment or therapy that the patient or family members may have.

Oxygen Home Care

For some patients, oxygen therapy becomes a lifelong need. Individuals learn to manage oxygen therapy at home as a part of daily living. The doctor determines the choice of delivery system according to the patient's problem. The systems available for home use are oxygen concentrators, compressed oxygen and liquid oxygen in portable devices (see Figure 24.21). These allow the patient the convenience of being able to leave the home while receiving oxygen therapy.

Patients and family members require support and teaching to manage oxygen therapy efficiently and safely. The nurse can help the patient and family by providing information and coordinating the efforts of the health care team. This may include, for instance, the respiratory therapist, the home care nurse and the oxygen supplier in the community.

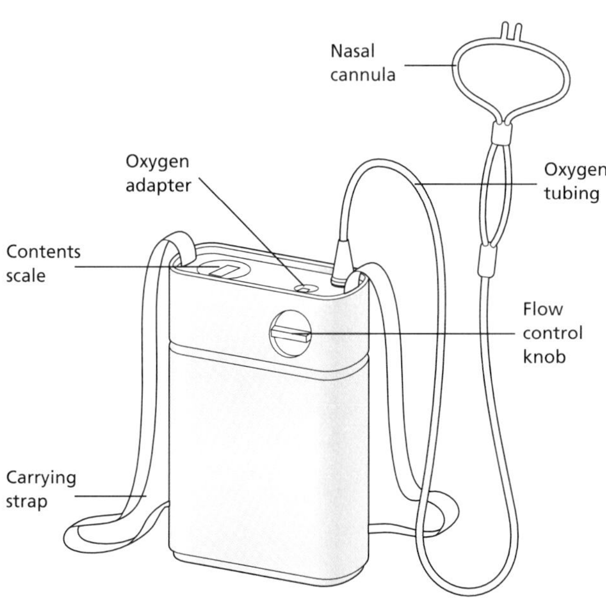

FIGURE 24.21 Liquid oxygen unit

SOURCE: Timby, 1996, p. 407.

The patient and family members are taught the reason for the treatment, the importance of using the oxygen only as prescribed by the doctor, correct administration, safety precautions and maintenance of the equipment. Safety issues are extremely important. Oxygen therapy must be avoided around open flames, for example, lit cigarettes, a gas cooking flame, a fireplace or a wood-burning stove. Tanks or cylinders should be secured on a cart or stand to prevent accidental falls and punctures. Lengthy tubing is useful for mobility, but creates many physical hazards. The patient must be careful to avoid tripping over the tubing or draping it over the cooking stove. Pets or small children must be kept away from tubing so they cannot chew it.

Cleanliness is very important. Oxygen tubing must be cleaned weekly with gentle soap and water to prevent the growth of microorganisms. Extra-long tubing must be replaced monthly. Distilled water used for humidification is always capped and stored in the refrigerator. Hand-held nebulizers (inhalers) should be washed daily in soap and water, rinsed with water, soaked for 20–30 minutes in a 1:1 white vinegar–water solution, rinsed with water and finally air-dried. Commercial respirator cleaning agents may also be used if instructions are followed. Cleaning the inhaler in the top shelf of an automatic dishwasher saves time and the hot water destroys most organisms.

ARTIFICIAL AIRWAYS

An **artificial airway** is a tube inserted into the airway by way of the mouth or nose, or through a surgical opening in the trachea called a *tracheostomy*. It is used to maintain airway patency, to provide a route for administering mechanical ventilation and to facilitate suctioning of secretions. The insertion of a tube is called *intubation*; removing it is *extubation*.

An **oral** (oropharyngeal) **airway** is a curved, plastic device that slides over the tongue to hold it down and forward (see Figure 24.22). Its main purpose is to prevent the tongue from falling back into the pharynx of the unconscious or semiconscious patient. It also facilitates easy removal of secretions. An oral airway is used in emergencies such as

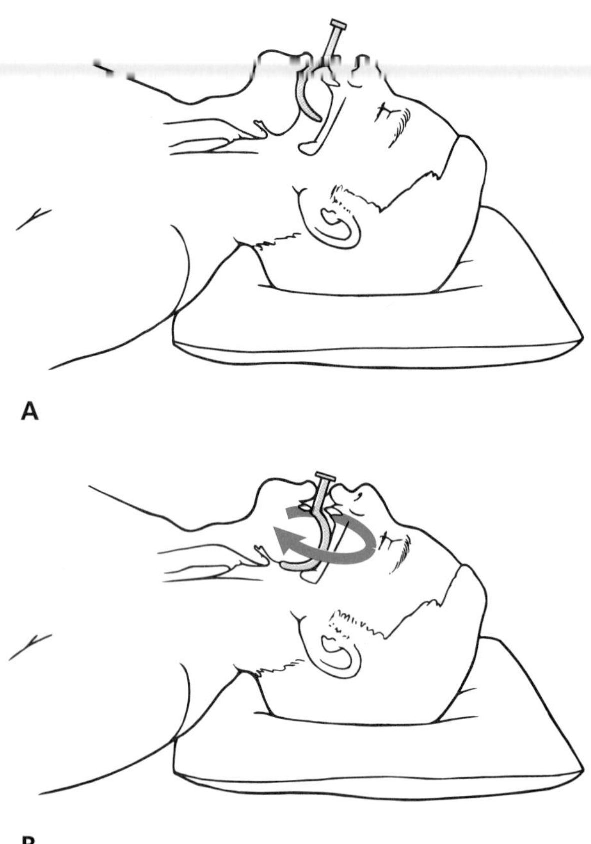

FIGURE 24.22 An oral airway in place. Once the airway is inserted (A), rotate it over and down into the correct position (B)

SOURCE: Lammon et al. 1995, p. 537.

Inserting an Oral Airway

- Select the proper size airway.
- Explain procedure.
- Don clean gloves.
- Suction mouth, if necessary.
- Remove dentures.
- Rinse the airway in cold water. *Lubricant effect aids insertion.*
- Place the patient in a supine position with the neck hyperextended (if not contraindicated). *Prevents the tongue from falling back into the pharynx.*
- Open the mouth and place a tongue blade on the front half of the tongue. *Flattens the tongue and facilitates insertion.*
- With the airway in a horizontal position, insert it into the mouth. Once it reaches the back of the throat, rotate it over and down to the correct position. *Promotes insertion without stimulating the gag reflex.*
- Suction the mouth if needed.
- Position the patient on the side. *Decreases risk of aspirating secretions.*

respiratory or cardiac arrest when bag-mask ventilation (Ambu bag and mask) is employed. The airway facilitates adequate ventilation.

An oral airway is often inserted by the nurse. To be effective, the artificial airway must not be too long and it must be positioned correctly. If an airway is too long or positioned incorrectly, it can stimulate the gag and cough reflexes, causing gagging, vomiting and aspiration. A properly sized airway for a patient is equal in length to the distance from the corner of the patient's mouth to the angle of the jaw below the ear. The steps for inserting an airway are listed in the box above. An airway is *never* inserted if the patient is alert or conscious enough to resist or to push it out. Similarly, an airway is removed as soon as the patient has regained consciousness and the gag and cough reflexes have returned. Keeping airways in conscious patients could stimulate the gag reflex and cause them to aspirate their secretions.

An *endotracheal tube* is passed via the nose or mouth, through the larynx and into the trachea when short-term airway assistance is needed. It is a soft rubber tube used to provide mechanical ventilation in unconscious or semiconscious patients and to administer anesthetic gases to individuals undergoing surgery. Endotracheal tubes also permit the removal of pulmonary secretions and the administration of medications. The procedure is performed by physicians, anesthetists, respiratory therapists and specially trained nurses. Care for a patient with an endotracheal tube requires advanced nursing skills.

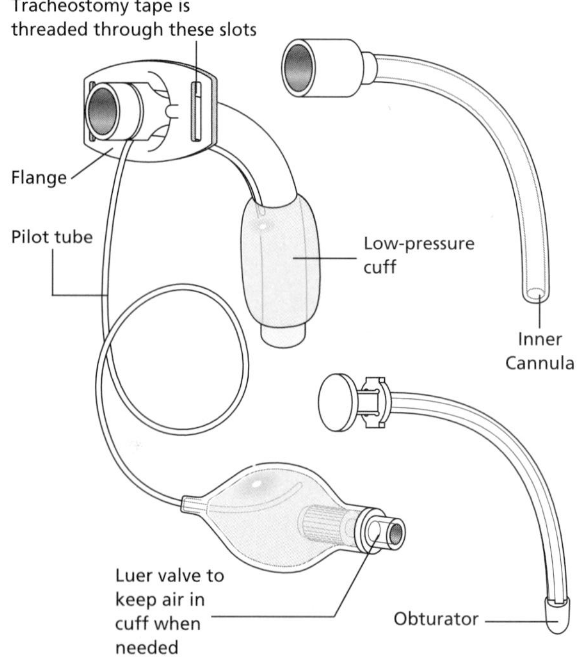

FIGURE 24.23 A tracheostomy tube

SOURCE: Lammon et al., 1995, p. 535.

A *tracheostomy* is a surgical incision creating an external opening into the trachea when an endotrachial intu-

maintains the patency of this opening. Artificial airways are indicated whenever the airway has become, or may become, obstructed. They may be temporary or permanent.

Tracheostomy tubes are constructed from plastic or metal and come in many sizes. The parts may consist of the outer tube with flange, inner cannula and the obturator. Tracheostomy tubes come in different types, such as cuffed or non-cuffed. The cuffed tracheostomy tube has a soft, inflatable cuff that forms an airtight seal between the tube and the trachea, thus preventing aspiration of secretions and air leakage. Various cuffs, such as single low-pressure or double high-pressure and foam, are available for different

Cuffed tubes are essential when the patient needs to be ventilated or when an airtight seal is required between the trachea and the tracheostomy tube. The tube may be fenestrated or unfenestrated. The fenestrated tube allows for speech when the inner cannula is removed and the tracheostomy is capped, enabling air to pass the vocal cords. Figure 24.23 shows the parts of a tracheostomy tube. Procedure 24.11 describes the steps involved in tracheostomy care and suctioning.

PROCEDURE 24.11 Performing Tracheostomy Care and Suctioning

Action	*Rationale*
A. General Actions	
1. Assess respirations and need for tracheostomy care: cuff deflation or inflation, suctioning, tracheostomy tie or dressing change, peristomal care and/or inner cannula cleaning.	Ascertains need for airway clearance by suctioning, cannula cleaning. Determines need for or various aspects of tracheostomy care.
2. Prepare patient; explain procedure. Position appropriately.	Decreases anxiety, promotes cooperation, enhances patient's comfort.
3. Wash hands and gather equipment: • suction equipment • wall or portable suction • connecting tube • tracheostomy suction catheter with suction control valve • body substance precaution attire: mask, gown, clean gloves, sterile gloves, sterile drape, goggles • oxygen source and delivery equipment • resuscitation bag.	Promotes medical and surgical asepsis; provides access to oxygen, if needed.
Note: Have available in immediate vicinity: extra inner cannula, tracheostomy obturator, tracheostomy dilator.	Enables reinsertion of tracheostomy tube in the event of dislodgement. Follow agency policy and/or do not attempt reinsertion of fresh tracheostomy tube within 5–7 days post-op.
a) **Tracheostomy suctioning and inner cannula care:** Suction catheter 12–16 Fr for adults, or less than one-half the diameter of the tracheostomy tube; waterproof disposal bag, 3 sterile solution bowls, sterile normal saline and hydrogen peroxide, cotton-tipped applicators, cleaning brush.	Decreases potential for hypoxia during suctioning. Provides receptacles for soaking and rinsing cannula and for clearing suction tube.
b) **Dressing change and aseptic stoma care:** Solution containers, antiseptic of choice and/or normal saline, tracheostomy tray, dressing tray or cotton-tipped applicators, sterile 4″ x 4″ gauze or prepackaged sterile tracheostomy dressing, sterile gloves.	Woven 4″ x 4″ gauze is folded and not cut for fit around tracheostomy tube, as frayed thread may enter wound or tracheostomy stoma.
c) **Tracheostomy tie change:** Tracheostomy ties; either 24–30 inches (60–76 cm) twill tape and scissors, or prepackaged ties, gloves and hemostat.	Reduces risk of contamination during procedures; facilitates efficiency and economy of time.
4. Don body substance769 precautions attire as appropriate.	Reduces transmission of microorganisms.

continued on next page

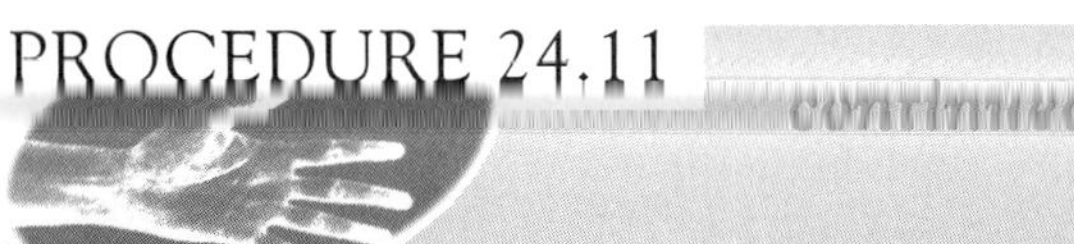

PROCEDURE 24.11 *continued*

Action	*Rationale*
B. Tracheostomy Suctioning and Cleaning of Inner Cannula	
1. Have open sterile field within easy reach. Add sterile brush and pour normal saline and hydrogen peroxide into separate bowls for the cannula cleansing, using surgical asepsis. Pour normal saline into another bowl for clearing the suction catheter.	Decreases contamination of the lower respiratory tract by microorganisms.
2. Open sterile suction catheter package.	
3. Turn suction on and set between 80 and 120 mm Hg.	Higher pressures may cause traumatic injury to the tracheal mucosa.
4. Don clean glove on nondominant hand and sterile glove on dominant hand.	Allows manipulation of sterile catheter with sterile technique. Protects other hand from suction secretions.
5. Control sterile suction catheter with sterile hand and attach connecting tubing with clean gloved hand.	Clean nondominant hand manipulates unsterile supplies.
6. Suction a small amount of saline through the suction catheter.	Checks for proper functioning of the equipment and lubricates catheter with saline.
7. Oxygenate the patient by asking him or her to take a few deep breaths.	Decreases atelectasis and possible hypoxia from the suctioning procedure. An assistant may be required to use the resuscitation bag.
8. Without applying suction, quickly insert suction catheter until resistance is felt; draw back slightly.	Ensures proper depth of insertion; prevents hypoxia and atelectasis through suctioning air from airways during insertion.
9. Encourage the patient to cough. Withdraw and rotate the catheter gently while applying intermittent suction with thumb on vacuum control vent.	Loosens upper airway secretions. Prevents tracheal mucosal trauma.
10. The procedure from insertion to withdrawal of the catheter should not take longer than 10–15 seconds.	Allows reoxygenation and re-expands alveoli between suctioning passes. Longer time increases risk of hypoxemia.
11. Rinse catheter with normal saline between suctioning passes.	Removes secretions from catheter and tubing and lubricates it.
12. Repeat 2–3 times as necessary, while observing patient's respiratory status.	Ensures removal of secretions and determines if more suctioning is necessary.
13. Reapply oxygen or humidification source.	Allows for prescribed oxygenation.
C. Cleaning of Tracheostomy Inner Cannula	
1. Don clean gloves. Unlock inner cannula and remove it in the direction of the curvature. Place the inner cannula into hydrogen peroxide.	The flange of the inner cannula is not sterile. Prevents transmission of microorganisms. Hydrogen peroxide removes secretions.
2. Don sterile gloves and clean the cannula quickly with the brush and hydrogen peroxide.	Removes mucous secretions by oxidation and effervescence.
3. Rinse the cannula thoroughly with sterile normal saline and tap off excess.	Prevents hydrogen peroxide from irritating tissues. Prevents aspiration of saline.
4. Replace cleaned cannula.	
5. Lock the inner cannula in place and check that it is secure.	Ensures that the inner cannula does not come out.
D. Peristomal Care	
1. Don glove (sterile, if fresh tracheostomy) and remove soiled tracheostomy dressing.	Prevents transmission of microorganisms.
2. Use hydrogen peroxide and cotton-tipped applicators or gauze swabs to clean tracheostomy flange and stoma, working outward.	Hydrogen peroxide loosens secretions.

PROCEDURE 24.11 *continued*

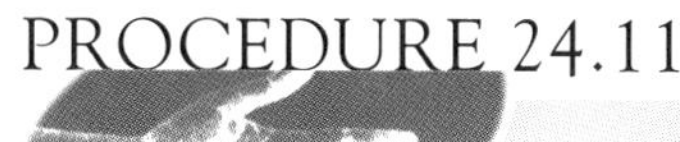

Action	Rationale
3. Using normal saline, rinse hydrogen peroxide from tracheostomy flange and peristomal skin.	Removes hydrogen peroxide, which can damage tissue if left on.
4. Dry the cleansed area.	Prevents maceration of tissue.
E. Changing of Tracheotomy Tie	
1. **Threading the tape:** Thread one end of the precut tie through one side of the tracheostomy flange; pass both ends around the patient's neck, keeping the ties flat. Thread the tape next to the patient's neck through the other flange from underneath. Tie new knot on the opposite side from old knot.	Prevents skin irritation Prevents accidental removal of tracheostomy tie.
2. Check for tautness of ties by slipping one or two fingers under the tie with the neck flexed.	Prevents the tie from becoming too tight when action such as coughing flexes the neck and increases its circumference.
3. Tie the ends with two square knots and tape the knot.	Prevents slippage and untying of knot. Prevents confusion of tracheostomy tie with ties of the patient's gown ties.
4. Cut and remove the soiled tie.	
5. Apply a folded sterile 4" X 4" gauze or prepackaged tracheostomy dressing under the flange. Do not cut gauze dressings.	Prevents aspiration of frayed threads and lint.
F. Postprocedure	
1. Dispose of used suction catheter by enveloping it in the inverted glove. Discard other soiled supplies, solutions and equipment appropriately and wash hands.	Reduces transmission of microorganisms.
2. Replace sterile suction catheter on connecting tube with wrapper left on, or place unopened suction catheter nearby.	Provides immediate access to suction catheter.
3. Assess respiratory and cardiac status.	Evaluates effectiveness of procedure in clearing airways and identifies physiologic effects of suctioning, such as hypoxia, cardiac dysrhythmias and vagal stimulation.
4. Reposition patient.	Promotes breathing and patient comfort.
5. Document procedure.	Communicates care and observations.

EMERGENCY MEASURES

The Heimlich manoeuvre and cardiopulmonary resuscitation (CPR) should be familiar to the reader and thus will not be considered in this text. Nursing students are required to complete a course in basic life support before entering their program of studies and then maintain their skills through yearly recertification. As well, health professionals working in facilities across Canada must maintain certification in basic life support or advanced life support by taking yearly courses set by the Heart and Stroke Foundation of Canada.

In the health care setting, a compressible bag, called an Ambu bag, and a mask are used to assist ventilations in the patient who has suffered a respiratory or cardiac arrest (see Figure 24.24). To use the Ambu bag, position the patient with head tilted back and jaw pulled forward to open the airway. An oral airway is inserted to prevent airway obstruction, which could interfere with adequate ventilation. Connect the Ambu bag to wall oxygen at a rate of 15 L/min. Hold the mask tightly over the patient's nose and mouth with one hand and, with the other hand, squeeze the bag at a rate of approximately 16 to 20 breaths per minute. The bag will inflate automatically; a one-way valve in the mask allows exhaled air to escape. Continue artificial ventilations ("bagging") until spontaneous breathing is established, until another mechanical assistance is established or until death is confirmed by a doctor. Oxygen tubing is attached to the bag to increase the oxygen supply to the patient. Many devices also have an adapter that can be directly connected to a tracheostomy or endotracheal tube for manual ventilations of a patient who is intubated.

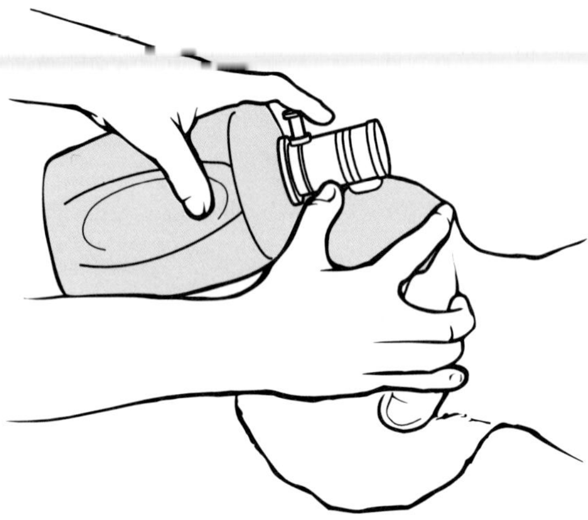

FIGURE 24.24 Using an Ambu bag and mask. Note the basic position of the hands in holding a bag mask in place. A tight seal should be maintained between the mask and the patient's face with one hand while the bag is squeezed with the other hand. The patient's airway must be kept open by keeping the neck extended as shown

Evaluating Oxygenation Interventions

Evaluation of the effectiveness of measures to improve oxygenation is based on the expected outcomes. Following is a list of criteria that the nurse may generally find useful in evaluating care.

1. Is the patient breathing more easily?
2. Has the patient's anxiety been relieved?
3. Is the patient's airway patent?
4. Has ventilatory efficiency been improved?
5. Have distressing symptoms such as coughing been relieved?
6. Has cyanosis been lessened?
7. Is the patient able to bring up sputum sufficiently to clear the bronchial tree?
8. Has activity tolerance increased?
9. Has the patient or the patient's family gained the knowledge and skills necessary to continue treatment at home?

IN REVIEW

- Oxygen is an essential nutrient for life. Without oxygen, cells:
  - malfunction
  - become damaged
  - die.

  Tissues of the brain and heart are particularly sensitive, as they can die within a few minutes of oxygen deprivation.
- Oxygenation is a complex process carried out by the respiratory and cardiovascular systems.
- The upper respiratory tract provides a passageway that:
  - warms
  - filters
  - moisturizes the inhaled air.
- The lower respiratory tract:
  - delivers oxygen to the alveoli
  - returns carbon dioxide to the atmosphere.
- The exchange of oxygen and carbon dioxide between the lungs and the circulation occurs in the alveoli.
- The cardiovascular system includes the heart, blood vessels and blood. It transports oxygen from the lungs to the tissues and carbon dioxide from the tissues back to the lungs.
- The three major processes involved in oxygenation are:
  - ventilation
  - diffusion
  - transportation.
- The body has an effective set of lung clearance mechanisms to ensure the intake of clean air and the removal of harmful debris. These include:
  - filtration
  - mucociliary action
  - sneezing
  - coughing.
- Effective oxygenation depends on:
  - patent airways
  - proper muscle functioning
  - pulmonary compliance
  - adequate oxygen/carbon dioxide transport.
- Health practices, such as regular aerobic exercises and avoidance of exposure to cigarette smoke and hazardous occupational materials, have a positive influence on oxygenation and well-being.
- Assessment of oxygenation status is a critical nursing activity.
- The nursing health history collects subjective data about the individual's:
  - usual pattern of oxygenation
  - smoking history
  - recent changes in pattern of oxygenation
  - symptoms of the presenting health problem
  - recent or past health problems
  - family history.

- The patient's chart supplies the nurse with objective data such as the results from diagnostic tests. Specific respiratory tests include:
  - CBC
  - arterial blood gases (ABGs)
  - sputum studies
  - bronchoscopy
  - lung scans
  - pulmonary function tests (PFTs)
  - chest x-ray.
- A physical assessment includes:
  - inspection of the chest, respiratory movements and breathing patterns
  - inspection of fingers for capillary refill and clubbing
  - measurement of pulse, respiration, blood pressure and oxygen saturation
  - examination of sputum, colour of skin and mucous membranes
  - palpation of the chest for expiratory expansion and fremitus
  - auscultation of the chest for the presence of normal and abnormal breath sounds.
- Once an assessment of the patient's oxygenation status is complete, a nursing diagnosis can be identified along with related interventions. Nursing interventions include:
  - maintaining and restoring airway patency, pulmonary ventilation and oxygen/carbon dioxide transport
  - preventing deterioration of pulmonary function
  - promoting optimal functioning of daily living.
- Health-protecting strategies include positioning, breathing exercises, effective coughing, use of an incentive spirometer and leg exercises.
- Health-restoring strategies establish airway patency, increase ventilatory efficiency, ensure adequate oxygen intake and decrease bodily needs for oxygen. Specific strategies include:
  - assistance with completing activities of daily living
  - uninterrupted rest periods
  - a well-balanced diet in small, frequent meals
  - measures to give emotional support
  - hydration, medications and humidity therapy
  - chest physiotherapy
  - suctioning
  - oral/pharyngeal care
  - chest drainage
  - tracheostomy care
  - oxygen therapy.
- Evaluation of the effectiveness of strategies to improve an individual's oxygenation status is a final step of nursing care.

Critical Thinking Activities

1. Mr. Rowlands is a 38-year-old patient who has been in the hospital for three weeks. His medical diagnosis is acute bronchial asthma. When he was admitted his breathing was dyspneic; he appeared cyanotic, and his respiratory rate varied from 28 to 34 respirations per minute.

   Mr. Rowlands did not want his bed to be flat; he demanded five pillows from the nurse and spent most of his time bent forward in bed. He was thin and appeared anxious. In addition to intravenous corticosteroids and bronchodilators administered by a jet nebulizer, the physician ordered oxygen by nasal cannula. Mr. Rowlands liked to use the oxygen and preferred to turn it on and off himself.

   a. What factors should be taken into consideration in explaining to this patient how to use the oxygen equipment?
   b. By what means can the patient's need for oxygen be assessed?
   c. For what reason might the patient demand five pillows, and why would he like to handle the oxygen himself?
   d. Identify the nursing diagnoses in this situation. Outline expected outcomes and interventions to resolve the identified problems.
   e. How can the effectiveness of these measures be evaluated?
2. With the aid of your instructor, arrange to spend a day with a respiratory therapist in your agency. What types of care does the respiratory therapist provide? In what ways do nurses and respiratory therapists collaborate to provide care in this agency?

KEY TERMS

oxygenation p. 714
respiration p. 714
airway p. 714
inhalation p. 715
exhalation p. 715
elastic recoil p. 715
compliance p. 715
partial pressure p. 717
hypoxemia p. 722
hypoxia p. 722
dyspnea p. 722
nonproductive cough p. 722
hemoptysis p. 722
pulse oximetry p. 723
peak flow p. 723

KEY TERMS

stridor p. 726
stertor p. 726
wheezing p. 726
clubbing p. 729
capillary refill p. 729
fremitus p. 730
crackles p. 732
gurgles p. 732
pleural friction rubs p. 732
wheezes, p. 732
arterial blood gas analysis p. 733
thoracentesis p. 736
bronchoscopy p. 737
pulmonary function tests p. 739
splinting p. 743
incentive spirometer p. 743
humidifier p. 746
nebulizer p. 747
postural drainage p. 748
artificial airway p. 765
oral airway p. 765

References

BERGER, K.J., & WILLIAMS, M.B. (1992). *Fundamentals of nursing: Collaborating for optimal health.* Norwalk, CT: Appleton & Lange.

BLACK, J.M., & MATASSARIN-JACOBS, E. (1997). *Medical–surgical nursing: Clinical management for continuity of care.* (5th ed.). Philadelphia: Saunders.

CARPENITO, L.J. (1997). *Nursing diagnosis: Application to clinical practice.* (7th ed.). Philadelphia: Lippincott.

CHERNECKY, C.C., & BERGER, B.J. (1997). Laboratory tests and diagnostic procedures. (2nd ed.). Toronto: W.B. Saunders.

EBERSOLE, P., & HESS, P. (1998). *Towards healthy aging: Human needs and nursing response.* (5th ed.). St. Louis: Mosby.

EHRHARDT, B.S., & GRAHAM, M. (1990, March). Pulse oximetry: An easy way to check oxygen saturation. *Nursing,* 50–54.

ELLIS, J.R., & NOWLIS, E.A. (1994). *Nursing: A human needs approach.* Philadelphia: Lippincott.

JARVIS, C. (1996). *Physical examination and health assessment.* (2nd ed.). Philadelphia: Saunders.

LACEY, G. (1988). Physiology of oxygenation. *Emergency Prehospital Medicine, 2*(4), 17–22.

LAMMON, C.C., FOOTE, A.W., LELI, P.G., INGLE, J., & ADAMS, M.H. (1995). *Clinical nursing skills.* Philadelphia: Saunders.

MADGE, P., McCOLL, J., & PATON, J. (1997, March). Impact of a nurse-led home management training programme in children admitted to hospital with acute asthma: A randomized controlled study. *Thorax, 52,* 223–228.

MARIEB, E.N. (1995). *Human anatomy and physiology.* (3rd ed.). Redwood City, CA: Benjamin/Cummings.

MARTINI, F. (1998). *Fundamentals of anatomy and physiology.* (4th ed.). Upper Saddle River, NJ: Prentice Hall.

McCANCE, K.L. (1996). Structure and function of the cardiovascular and lymphatic systems. In S.E. Huether & K.L. McCance (Eds.), *Understanding pathophysiology.* St. Louis: Mosby.

MURRAY, R.B., & ZENTNER, J.P. (1997). *Nursing assessment and health promotion: Strategies through the life span.* Norwalk, CT: Appleton & Lange.

PILLITTERI, A. (1995). *Maternal and child health nursing: Care of the childbearing and childrearing family.* (2nd ed.). Philadelphia: Lippincott.

PORTH, C.M. (1998). *Pathophysiology: Concepts of altered states.* (2nd ed.). Philadelphia: Lippincott.

SHAPIRO, B.A., KACMAREK, R.M., CANE, R.D., PERUZZI, W.T., & HAUPTMAN, D. (1991). *Clinical application of respiratory care.* (4th ed.). St. Louis: Mosby.

SMELTZER, S., & BARE, B. (1996). *Brunner and Suddarth's textbook of medical–surgical nursing.* (8th ed.). Philadelphia: Lippincott.

SPRINGHOUSE CORPORATION. (1983). *Nurse's reference library: Assessment.* Springhouse, PA: Author.

SUDDARTH D.S. (1991). *The Lippincott Manual of nursing practice.* (5th ed.). Philadelphia: Lippincott.

THOMPSON, J., & WILSON, S. (1996). *Health assessment for nursing practice.* St. Louis: Mosby.

TIMBY, B.K. (1996). *Fundamental skills and concepts in patient care.* (6th ed.). Philadelphia: Lippincott.

TRAVER, G.A., MITCHELL, J.T., & FLODQUIST-PRIESTLY, G. (1991). *Respiratory care: A clinical approach.* Gaithersburg, MA: Aspen.

TURNER, J., McDONALD, G.J., & LARTER, N.L. (1994). *Handbook of adult and pediatric respiratory homecare.* St. Louis: Mosby.

WILLIAMS, M.W. (1993). *Lifetime: Fitness and wellness.* (3rd ed.). Madison, WI: Brown & Benchmark.

Additional Readings

ACKERMAN, M.H. (1993). The effect of saline lavage prior to suctioning. *American Journal of Critical Care, 2*(4), 326–330.

BOWDEN, V., DICKEY, S., & GREENBERG, C. (1998). *Children and their families: The continuum of care.* Philadelphia: W.B. Saunders.

BURTON, G.C., HODGKIN, J.E., & WARD, J.J. (1997). *Respiratory care: A guide to clinical practice.* (4th ed.). Philadelphia: Lippincott.

CARPENTER, K.D. (1993, August). A comprehensive review of cyanosis. *Critical Care Nurse,* 66–71.

CARROLL, P. (1997, Feb.). Pulse oximety at your fingertips. *RN,* 22–27.

CRAPO, R.O. (1994). Pulmonary function testing. *New England Journal of Medicine, 331*(1), 25–30.

EISENHAUER, B. (1996). Action stat: Dislodged tracheostomy tube. *Nursing, 26*(6), 25.

JESURUM, J. (1997). Tissue oxygenation and routine nursing procedures in critically ill patients. *Journal of Cardiovascular Nursing, 11*(4), 12–30.

KACMAREK, R.M., HESS, D., & STOLLER, J.K. (1993). *Monitoring in respiratory care.* St. Louis: Mosby.

McPHERSON, S.P. (1995). *Respiratory care equipment.* (5th ed.). St. Louis: Mosby.

O'HANLON-NICHOLS, T. (1998). Basic assessment series: The adult pulmonary system. *American Journal of Nursing, 98*(2), 39–45.

PETTINICCHI, T. (1998). Trouble-shooting chest tubes. *Nursing, 28*(3), 58–59.

SMITH, R., FALLENTINE, J., & KESSEL, S. (1995). Underwater chest drainage: Bringing the facts to the surface. *Nursing, 25*(2), 60–63.

STIESMEYER, J.K. (1993, August). A four-step approach to pulmonary assessment. *American Journal of Nursing,* 22–28.

Chapter

Temperature Regulation Needs

OUTLINE

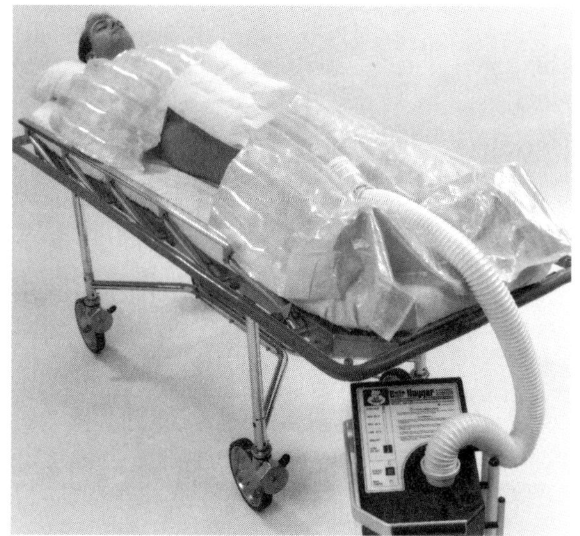

Central Questions

1. What are the heat-regulating mechanisms of humans, and how do these maintain a stable body temperature?
2. What are the main determinants of body temperature regulation?
3. How does temperature regulation vary throughout the life cycle?
4. What are the common problems of altered temperature regulation?
5. How are the temperature regulation needs of patients assessed?
6. What are the common nursing diagnoses for patients with temperature regulation problems?
7. What considerations should be included in the care of patients with altered temperature status?
8. What information might the nurse give to individuals, families or groups in helping them to promote optimum temperature regulation?
9. What health-protecting measures can the nurse implement for a patient with a fever?
10. What health-restoring and supportive strategies can the nurse implement in the care of patients with temperature regulation problems?
11. How is the patient's response to nursing interventions evaluated?
12. What basic principles does the nurse apply when administering heat and cold treatments?
13. What are the therapeutic applications of heat and cold?

Introduction

The surface temperature of the body varies with environmental changes, and humans have had to learn to dress appropriately for protection from both hot tropical sun and cold northern winds. Over the centuries, we have also developed the ability to modify our immediate surroundings to provide a comfortable environmental temperature.

With regard to **core temperature** (or internal temperature), humans are **homeothermic**, or warm-blooded, with inborn mechanisms for maintaining a stable temperature within the body. **Normothermia** for humans means a temperature ranging from 36.6° to 37.5°C (Smeltzer & Bare, 1996).

Heat regulation, or **thermoregulation**, usually refers to core temperature and involves not only those mechanisms concerned with the production of heat within the body, but also those involved in heat dissipation. These bodily mechanisms maintain a precise balance between heat production and heat loss. In this way, internal body temperature is kept within a very narrow range, usually varying less than 0.5°–1°C within a 24-hour period (Cooper, 1969; Ganong, 1997). The heat-regulating system is one of the body's most important homeostatic mechanisms.

Heat Production – Heat Loss = Body Temperature

Every once in a while, imbalances occur with resultant deviations outside the normal range of body temperature. Many people who are ill have an elevated temperature. It is, indeed, one of the cardinal signs of illness, often being one of the first observable indications that there is a disturbance of body function. The maintenance of a higher-than-normal temperature puts considerable stress on the body's adaptive mechanisms and is very debilitating.

The balance also may be upset in the opposite direction. Mild degrees of lowered body temperature (1°–2°C) apparently do not do as much harm to the body as fever does. At lower temperatures, all body processes slow down and when the body warms up, they resume functioning at normal levels. However, *hypothermia* (excessively low body temperatures) both in accidental and clinical situations due, in most cases, to prolonged exposure to cold environmental temperatures continues to be a concern. *Frostbite*, which involves freezing of the skin tissues in one area of the body, such as exposed ear lobes, the tip of the nose, cheeks, fingers or toes, has always been a problem in cold climates. *Chilblains*, a mild form of frostbite, also are a common source of discomfort, particularly to older people who live in cold, damp climates and whose homes are not equipped with central heating.

Pharmacological and nonpharmacological interventions, such as applications of heat and cold, have been used for centuries to treat various disorders of the human body. Both have systemic and localized effects on body tissues and continue to be used frequently in therapy. This chapter describes the mechanisms underlying body temperature regulation and the therapies employed to maintain thermal health.

The Body's Mechanisms For Temperature Regulation

Humans are in a state of thermal health when their core or internal body temperature is about 37°C. Body temperature is a measure of the body's heat; it reflects the ability to maintain a balance between heat gain and loss. Humans produce heat continuously through the process of cellular metabolism. The body heat produced through metabolism must be lost to the environment so that a constant body temperature can be maintained. Heat is lost from the body through a variety of means, as outlined in the accompanying box.

To maintain thermal health, it is necessary to adapt to changing conditions in the surrounding environment and also to internal metabolic processes. Humans have various adaptive mechanisms to promote heat if body temperature falls too low, or to lose excess heat if the temperature goes too high. Figure 25.1 illustrates thermal health and adaptation. According to Erickson (1982), thermal health exists when environmental challenges (ambient and metabolic) are balanced by the individual's adaptive capabilities, which include biological, behavioural and social modes. When environmental demands exceed an individual's adaptive capacities, body temperature rises or falls below normal range, and thermal dysfunction occurs. The goal of nursing is to tip the balance towards thermal reserve and wellness by enhancing the patient's adaptive potentials.

Biological Adaptive Modes

The regulatory mechanisms controlling body temperature are located in the preoptic area of the hypothalamus, which acts as the body's thermostat. Neurons (in the hypothalamus) respond to changes in the temperature of the blood circulating through it by sending impulses either to its anterior heat-losing centre or to its posterior heat-gaining centre. These centres have a reciprocal effect on each other; when one is activated, the other is depressed. Both peripheral (skin) and core temperature receptors play a role in the control of thermoregulation.

It is generally believed that body temperature is regulated around a narrowly defined temperature or *setpoint* (Benzinger, 1969; Bruck, 1983). Although individuals vary somewhat in the temperature at which their body is maintained (Ganong, 1997), temperature homeostasis results in a relatively constant central temperature. When body temperature deviates from the setpoint, the heat-losing or heat-gaining centre is stimulated.

Mechanisms of Body Heat Loss

Conduction: The direct transfer of heat from the body to cooler objects in the immediate environment	Lying on a cold stretcher
Convection: Body heat is transferred to air currents circulating around the body	The cooling effect of a fan
Evaporation: Body heat is used to convert moisture on the surface of the skin to vapour	The effect of sweating
Radiation: The transfer of heat, in the form of electromagnetic waves, from the body to cooler objects in the environment; over half of body heat loss occurs through this process	Lying next to a cold window

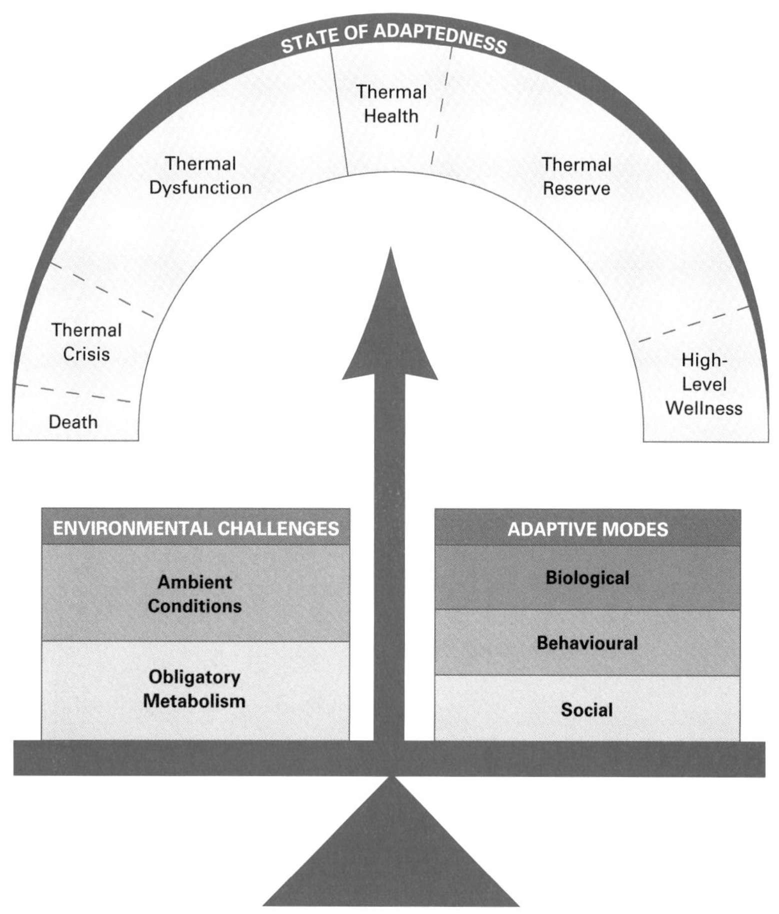

FIGURE 25.1 A model of adaptation to the thermal environment

SOURCE: Erickson, 1982.

When the temperature at the preoptic nucleus drops below the setpoint, the heat-gaining centre is activated. Stimulation of the heat-gaining centre initially increases wakefulness and stimulates muscular activity. If the individual does not engage in some form of exercise in response to this, the body will involuntarily initiate its own muscular activity in the form of shivering. This can produce a considerable amount of heat within the body—as much as 400 percent (Martini, 1998).

At the same time, stimulation of the sympathetic nervous system facilitates the release of both epinephrine and norepinephrine into the blood stream. As a result, glucose stores in the liver are released for energy. Cellular metabolism is accelerated and heat is produced.

Stimulation of the sympathetic nervous system also results in the phenomenon of *piloerection*, in which hairs stand on end. In animals with long hair, this mechanism serves to entrap a layer of warm air next to the skin. In humans, it is usually manifested in the milder reaction of a "goose flesh" appearance of the skin. This mechanism, though not as effective in providing insulation, occurs nonetheless. Cessation of sweating usually occurs as well, to reduce the amount of heat lost through evaporation of water from the body surface.

Concomitantly, vasoconstriction takes place and blood is drawn away from surface vessels to minimize heat lost from conduction, convection and radiation. Individuals become pale and their skin is cold to the touch. They also feel cold.

With prolonged exposure to colder temperatures than normal, the thyroid gland is stimulated to increase production of the hormone thyroxine. This results in an increased metabolic rate and subsequent increased heat production. However, this process is slower, occurring over a period of weeks.

Conversely, stimulation of the heat-losing centre when the temperature setpoint is exceeded has an inhibitory effect on the mechanisms for heat production, and the reverse effects are seen. Muscular activity is decreased and metabolism is slowed; vasodilation occurs, resulting in increased circulation to the skin; and the rate of thyroxine production gradually decreases.

The body also has two mechanisms unique to the facilitation of heat loss; these are panting and sweating. In other animals rapid shallow breathing (panting) increases heat loss by evaporation of moisture from the respiratory tract or tongue. Rapid, deep breathing (hyperventilation) in humans has the same effect. However, the principal mechanism for cooling the human body is by increasing perspiration. This greatly facilitates the loss of heat from the body through the process of evaporation of moisture from the skin. When environmental temperature exceeds body temperature, perspiration is the only mechanism available to humans for heat loss.

Behavioural Adaptive Modes

Our ability to modify the surrounding environment is the most powerful mode of adaptation to extremes in environmental conditions. This behavioural adaptation is motivated by the conscious appraisal of the thermal environment. Thermal comfort is the subjective feeling of satisfaction with the temperature of the surrounding environment. Thermal comfort is said indirectly to reflect the heat balance in the body. It is related to an individual's level of activity and clothing, and to ambient conditions (Worfolk, 1997). Individuals at rest, wearing light clothing, usually feel comfortable in an ambient environment of 24°–25°C and, when unclothed, are comfortable in an environment of about 28°–30°C (Erickson, 1982).

Adaptive behaviours to maintain thermal comfort include altering posture to change the amount of exposed body surface (by curling up or stretching out), ingesting hot or cold foods or beverages, creating a favourable environment by using artificial heating or cooling devices and donning clothing appropriate to the ambient temperature. Clothing, of course, decreases the effects of environmental temperatures on body heat. The insulation of the body by adequate, warm clothing lessens the impact of cold temperatures. In warm climates, cottons are more comfortable to wear because they absorb moisture. Synthetic fibres and wool do not absorb as well; hence, they inhibit the removal of perspiration from the body.

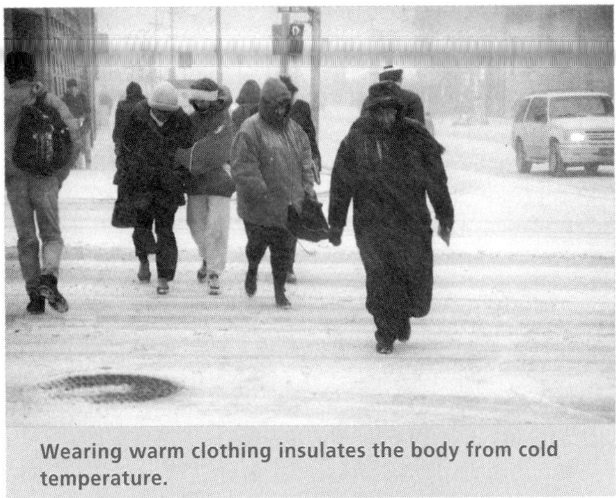

Wearing warm clothing insulates the body from cold temperature.

Several factors influence the ability to adapt behaviour to the environment. Conscious perception and voluntary movement are essential for all behavioural responses (Erickson, 1982; Worfolk, 1997). The unconscious or immobilized patient is therefore at risk for thermal dysfunction. Furthermore, the individual's knowledge of risk factors and available resources will affect behaviour.

Social Adaptation

Individuals with impaired ability to adapt biologically or behaviourally to thermal challenges in their environment can achieve thermal comfort and health through social adaptation. Direct practical assistance through physical care, material resources and education can help individuals to achieve comfort (Erickson, 1982). For example, nurses can provide a warming blanket and warm intravenous solutions to the hypothermic patient.

Determinants of Body Temperature

Body temperature may be affected by a number of factors, including conditions that increase metabolic rate, emotions, body size and mass, illness, medications, health problems and environment.

Conditions That Increase Basal Metabolic Rate

temperature of the body; conversely, a decreased metabolic rate will lower body temperature. In exercise, muscular activity increases body temperature as a result of heat production by body muscles. With heavy muscular exercise rectal temperature may rise as high as 40°C (Guyton, 1996). When body temperature begins to rise, the body's heat-regulating mechanisms start to function. Blood is drawn to the surface for cooling and the person starts to perspire. Usually an elevated temperature due to exercise quickly returns to normal with the cessation of activity.

Disturbances in the production of thyroxine by the thyroid gland also affect body temperature. An excess production of thyroxine (due to hyperthyroidism) increases the basal metabolic rate, thereby stimulating heat production. People with hypothyroidism, on the other hand, are deficient in thyroxine production; they have a lower metabolic rate, and consequently a body temperature that is usually at the low end of the normal range. Persons with thyroid dysfunction usually report an intolerance to hot or cold temperatures (Bates, 1995).

An increase in body temperature itself will stimulate the cells to increase the rate of cellular metabolism and heat production. For each 1°C rise in temperature, the rate of heat production increases 13 percent and the metabolic rate may be 40 times as high as normal (DuBois, 1921). As a result, an increased temperature tends to heighten a fever. A lowered body temperature for a prolonged period has the reverse effect of decreasing metabolism, which, in turn, lessens body temperature still further.

The specific dynamic action of foods also affects body temperature. The body's metabolic rate is stimulated by the intake of food and remains elevated for several hours after a meal. Underfeeding, on the other hand, decreases the metabolic rate, reducing internal heat production. Foods differ in their specific dynamic qualities. Proteins increase metabolic rate (up to 30 percent) more than fats and carbohydrates, and the increase remains high over a longer period of time (3–12 hours after a meal) (Martini, 1998).

There is a circadian rhythm to metabolism and body temperature. In humans, core temperature may fluctuate between 0.2° and 0.5°C over a 24-hour period. It is generally lowest between midnight and 06:00 and peaks between 16:00 and 20:00 (Ludwig-Beymer & Huether, 1996).

Emotions

Strong emotions, such as anger, can raise body temperature because of stimulation of the sympathetic nervous system. It is thought that this may be the result of muscle tensing (Ganong, 1997). "The heat of anger" and "feverish with excitement" are common expressions that represent genuine physical conditions. One notices the relationship between emotional and physical states particularly with children, whose body temperatures are more labile (that is, th [illegible]

Body Size and Mass

Other factors such as body size and mass influence an individual's capacity to maintain thermal health. Subcutaneous fat is an efficient insulator, conducting heat at a slower rate than other tissues (Martini, 1998; Worfolk, 1997). This is how long-distance swimmers (who generally have a thicker layer of adipose tissue) maintain their body temperatures even in relatively cold water. Conversely, those with a thinner layer of subcutaneous tissue are more vulnerable to cold, such as older people. Obese individuals tend to retain heat and have difficulty tolerating hot environmental conditions.

When body surface area is large in proportion to weight, such as in infants, there is less muscle mass to produce metabolic heat. Infants lose heat rapidly and therefore require warmer environments than adults (Pillitteri, 1995).

Illness and Health Problems

Health problems affect the efficiency of the body's temperature-regulating mechanisms. Poor circulation related to cardiac or vascular disease impairs the body's ability to dissipate heat. Disorders that affect the nervous system can interfere with the reflexive responses to changes in body temperature.

Infections, trauma and inflammatory processes induce a series of responses in the body, resulting in fever. Fever is observed in bacterial infection and autoimmune diseases such as Crohn's disease and rheumatoid arthritis; it is sometimes an indicator of silent disease, such as renal carcinoma and Hodgkin's disease (Dinarello, 1996).

Environment

The surrounding environment has a pronounced effect upon body temperature. Permanent changes, such as those encountered when moving to a hot or cold climate, and temporary changes, such as a brief hot spell, affect the body by raising or lowering its temperature. The body's ability to withstand high environmental temperatures depends on the humidity of the atmosphere. When the air is dry and there are sufficient air currents to carry heat away from the body by convection, an individual can stand very high temperatures with little or no increase in body temperature. On the other hand, if the humidity is high, then heat loss through evaporation from the surface of the body is decreased and body temperature begins to rise quickly. This explains why one feels uncomfortable on hot, muggy days.

Similarly, a cold environment decreases body temperature. Cold, damp weather is much more chilling than cold dry weather, and when there is considerable amount of air movement, more heat is carried away from the body. This "wind chill" factor can produce the effect of a temperature much lower than that shown on the outdoor thermometer.

There is a range of ambient temperatures within which normal body temperature is maintained with minimal metabolic work or evaporative losses. This temperature range, called the thermoneutral zone, is between 27° and 33°C for the naked adult (Mitchell & Laburn, 1985).

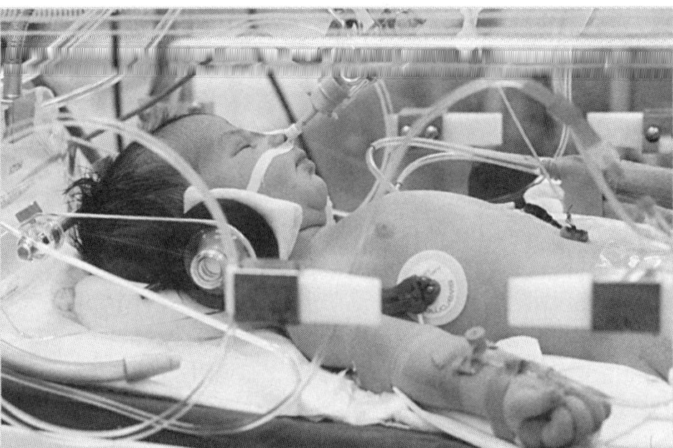
Premature infants are cared for in a unit with a neutral thermal environment.

Temperature Regulation Throughout the Life Cycle

Early in pregnancy, there is a slight rise in the body temperature of most women, which continues until about the fourth month. At about this time, body temperature generally returns to normal levels and stays within the normal range for the remainder of the pregnancy.

Maternal fever in early pregnancy (four to six weeks) can be *teratogenic*, that is, it can cause the development of physical defects in the fetus, particularly in the brain. Pregnant women should take precautions to avoid developing a fever during this time.

Normally the fetus is maintained for nine months in the warm, protected environment of the uterus. Immediately after birth, the newborn's temperature usually falls 2°–3°C because of the evaporation of amniotic fluid from the skin as the infant's total body surface is exposed to the cooler ambient environment (Behrman, Kliegman & Arvin, 1996). Further heat loss is prevented in the birthing room by drying and placing the newborn under radiant heat. The newborn may also be placed on the mother's abdomen. By maintaining skin-to-skin contact, the newborn is kept warm by the mother's body heat. A newborn's temperature is quite unstable because the heat-regulating system is not yet fully developed. Hence, it is important to maintain a stable environmental temperature. A **neutral thermal environment** (32°C) is considered best because it requires minimum oxygen consumption for the infant at rest. This point is particularly important in the care of premature infants, whose heat-regulating mechanisms are even less mature than those of full-term infants.

During the first year of life, infants continue to be highly dependent on environmental temperature to maintain their own internal temperature because of immaturity of the heat-regulating system. The shivering mechanism does not usually begin to function until after the first year. Heat must be produced through the use of specialized adipose tissue known as *brown fat* that can quickly accelerate the infant's metabolic rate (Martini, 1998). This mechanism, although short-lived, plays an important role in temperature maintenance during infancy (McCance & Huether, 1994). The sweat glands, both eccrine and apocrine, are present at birth. The eccrine glands are equivalent in size, structural maturity and position within the dermis in the full-term infant and the adult (Wong, 1995). However, the eccrine sweat glands do not begin to function until after the first month of life, and the apocrine glands remain inactive until puberty (Thompson & Wilson, 1996). Because their body surface area is relatively large, it is important that infants be protected from becoming too cold, or too warm, with changes in the environmental temperature. Appropriate clothing for the climate is essential (warm wool clothing for winter weather and cool cottons for summer or in the tropics).

Infants can develop a high fever rapidly, and this frequently occurs with acute respiratory infections that are common in early childhood. The high fever may produce convulsions—a very frightening experience for the new parents. Another concern is that febrile seizures, as a result of fever, may cause brain damage. Although many children have seizures at relatively low temperatures (38.3°C) on the first day of illness, these seizures do not recur on subsequent days when the fever reaches its peak (Fruthaler, 1985). Unless they are due to brain injury or tumour, seizures accompanying fever rarely result in permanent damage to neurologic tissue (Fruthaler, 1985; Dinarello, 1996).

During childhood, the body temperature averages approximately 37°C. Although a child may run a fever as a result of excitement, fever in children is usually secondary to infection, and is often the first indication of illness. It is not until adolescence that sweating in the axilla occurs; younger children do not have this mechanism to assist in cooling the body.

With the onset of menses, girls experience a cyclical rise and fall of body temperature that continues through the childbearing years. There is a fall in the early morning temperature of most women just after the onset of menstruation. The temperature remains at this lower level until ovulation takes place. With ovulation, an abrupt rise of

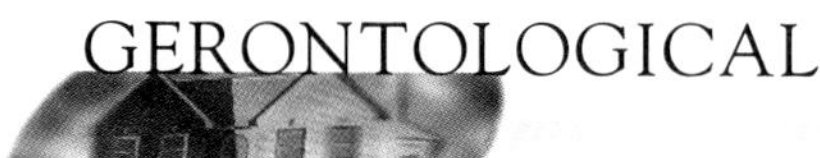

GERONTOLOGICAL

Factors That Influence Temperature

Age-Related Alterations:

- Slowed blood circulation
- Decreased subcutaneous tissue
- Decreased heat-producing activities
- Diminished or absent sweating
- Decreased peripheral sensation
- Desynchronized circadian rhythm
- Decreased kidney function (may increase risk for heat-related dehydration)
- Decreased or no fever response to infection
- Less effective thirst mechanism

Factors That Increase the Risk for Hypothermia:

- Impaired thermal regulation system, i.e.:
  - inefficient vasoconstriction
  - decreased perception of heat and cold
  - lack of stimulus to take action to protect oneself
  - decreased shivering response
  - slowed metabolic rate
- Common health problems associated with hypothermia, e.g.:
  - poor nutrition
  - hypothyroidism
  - immobility
  - diabetes
  - conditions that increase heat loss (burns, open wounds)
  - conditions that alter thermal regulation (stroke, brain tumour, alcoholism)
- Medications:
  - tranquillizers
  - sedatives
  - antidepressants
  - vasodilators
  - morphine
  - polypharmacy (taking several drugs simultaneously)
- Poverty
- Social isolation

SOURCES: Carpenito, 1997; Worfolk, 1997; Ludwig-Beymer & Huether, 1996; Ebersole & Hess, 1998.

0.5°–1.0°C occurs. The body temperature remains at this increased level until the beginning of the next menstrual period. This pattern in body temperature can be used by women to determine ovulation and is therefore helpful in family planning (Pillitteri, 1995).

Women also experience variations of body temperature during menopause. The average woman will go through menopause at the age of 51. For five to 10 years prior to menopause, the ovaries gradually produce less of the hormone estrogen. The most common symptom associated with estrogen loss—affecting approximately 75 percent of Western women—are hot flashes (Carlson, Eisenstadt & Ziporyn, 1996). Fluctuations in estrogen levels during the perimenopausal years cause a downward resetting of the hypothalamic thermoregulating mechanism and peripheral vasodilatation (Shaw, 1997). During a hot flash, the woman suddenly feels warm, her skin becomes visibly reddened and she experiences profuse sweating in the chest, neck and face. Hot flashes are more common at night, often interfering with sleep, and contribute to the problems of insomnia and emotional lability among menopausal women. Interestingly, hot flashes are reported less frequently by women from non-Western cultures. The reason for this cultural difference remains unknown.

To minimize hot flashes, menopausal women are advised to avoid common triggers such as stress, hot weather, warm rooms, hot drinks, alcohol, caffeine and spicy foods (Carlson et al., 1996). Hormonal replacement therapy (HRT) is recommended for the treatment of hot flashes and other symptoms of menopause (American College of Physicians, as cited in Shaw, 1997). Combination therapy using estrogen and progestin is used for the control of hot flashes, as well as for protection from cardiovascular and bone density changes associated with menopause (Shaw, 1997). HRT is not for all women; those at high risk for breast cancer need to discuss the risks and benefits of HRT with their physician. Alternatives to hormonal therapy

Factors That Influence Temperature Regulation in Infants

- Inability to conserve heat owing to large body surface area relative to body mass
- Increased BMR
- Little subcutaneous fat
- Exposure to ambient environmental conditions (e.g., delivery room)
- Presence of non-shivering thermogenesis mechanism
- Tendency to infection due to immature immune system

SOURCES: Thomas, 1995; May & Mahlmeister, 1994.

include medications such as clonidine, bellargal, vitamin B complex, vitamin E and evening primrose oil. Foods containing phytoestrogens such as soybeans, legumes, berries and sunflower seeds help to supplement the body's natural estrogens (Shaw, 1997). Self-care strategies—such as keeping a diary of episodes and triggering agents, and wearing layered cotton garments—are also helpful (Manitoba Health, 1990).

Basal metabolic rate gradually decreases with age, so that older men and women usually have a body temperature lower than that of young adults. The upper limits of normal temperature for the elderly are 37.2°C (oral) and 37.5°C (rectal) (Norman & Yoshikawa, 1996). The presence of fever in the aged person always indicates a serious infection. However, older people tend to have blunted fever responses. Fever should be considered when the older person's body temperature remains elevated at least 1°C over baseline, or if an oral temperature of more than 37.2°C is observed (Norman & Yoshikawa, 1996).

The decreasing efficiency of most body systems that accompanies the aging process also renders the older person more vulnerable to the effects of changing environmental temperatures. Older people often do not cope well with heat. Sweat glands atrophy and circulation becomes sluggish, limiting their ability to dissipate heat through perspiration (Miller, 1995). Hypothermia also can be a problem because the older person tends to be undernourished and has a slower metabolic rate, which limits heat production. The vasoconstrictor response and shivering reflex also become delayed and less effective (McCance & Huether, 1994).

In addition, medications such as diuretics ("water pills") and anticholinergics (used to treat neuromuscular symptoms) inhibit the normal thermoregulatory processes of vasodilation and sweating. The physiological changes associated with aging, combined with underlying disease states and medications, place older people at high risk for heat-related illnesses and hypothermia.

Common Problems

Although normal processes can cause mild fluctuations in body temperature, many illnesses also cause deviations from the normal. Most frequently, the fluctuations are in the direction of an elevated temperature, giving rise to a fever. The most common of these illnesses are infections, diseases of the central nervous system, neoplasms and metabolic disorders. Fluctuations in the opposite direction, resulting in hypothermia (in both accidental and clinical situations), can also create challenges for the health professional.

Fever

Fever is defined as a rectal temperature above 38°C (Lopez, McMillin, Tobias-Merrill & Chop, 1997; Thomas, 1995).

Fever is defined as:

- rectal temperature >38°C
- oral temperature >37.6°C

There are age-related variations to the lower limit of fever. For infants less than three months of age, the lower limit of fever is a rectal temperature above 38°C, whereas older children with rectal temperatures above 38.3° are considered febrile (Thomas, 1995). Older adults, however, are considered febrile when their rectal temperatures are repeatedly above 37.5°C (Norman & Yoshikawa, 1996). The physiological mechanisms responsible for fever are not known for all disease processes. It is generally felt that fever may be caused by abnormalities in the brain itself or by toxic substances that affect the heat-regulating mechanisms.

Infections, trauma and inflammatory processes induce heat-regulating mechanisms to elevate the body temperature, producing fever. Pyrogens, substances that cause fever, are either *exogenous* (derived from outside the body), such as bacterial endotoxins, or *endogenous* (produced by the body in response to exogenous pyrogens), such as cytokines. Once a pyrogenic substance reaches the hypothalamus via the circulatory and lymphatic systems, substances called *prostaglandins* are released. Elevated levels of prostaglandins, particularly PGE-2, cause the temperature-regulatory centre in the anterior hypothalamus to raise its setpoint, resulting in fever (Dinarello, 1996). In addition to pyrogenic causes of fever, a raised hypothalamic setpoint can result from local trauma, hemorrhage, tumour or malfunction of the hypothalamus itself.

There is evidence to suggest that fever caused by pyrogens has some beneficial effects in helping the body to combat infection. It is felt that the fever acts in two ways: (a) it creates an undesirable temperature for the survival of bacteria; and (b) the increased rate of metabolism in the cells increases their production of immune bodies and also their ability to phagocytize foreign bodies, thus impeding bacterial and viral invasion.

Fever frequently accompanies a head injury and is often seen in patients with spinal cord injuries. In the case of head injury, fever is felt to be caused by pressure on, or injury to, the hypothalamus or the tracts leading to and from the heat-regulating centres. In the patient with a spinal cord injury, vasoconstriction, piloerection and sweating mechanisms are impaired below the level of the injury in the spinal cord (Boss, Farley & Mooney, 1996).

Fever may occur postoperatively owing to a number of causes. It may be due to excessive heat production, as in the case of pathogenic infection, or due to inadequate heat elimination as a result of peripheral vasoconstriction. Fever may occur secondary to the surgical stress response, to respiratory atelectasis or to lung congestion.

A term often used synonymously with fever is **pyrexia**. *Hyperpyrexia* designates an abnormally high fever, that is, 41°C or higher (Dinarello, 1996). [illegible]

nervous system, in HIV infection and in drug-induced fevers (Cunha, 1996a; Dinarello, 1996). Although fever is generally considered beneficial, it increases oxygen consumption by as much as 13 percent for every 1°C. Fever can aggravate pre-existing cardiac or pulmonary conditions, and cause delirium in patients with organic brain disease and seizures in those children with propensity to them (Dinarello, 1996). In these situations, aggressive treatment of fever is recommended.

Although prolonged fevers are less common today than in the years before the use of antibiotics, it is worth knowing the terms used for the different patterns of fevers (see box).

A single isolated fever spike is never caused by infection, and is likely due to a blood transfusion or to tissue manipulation during a procedure. On the other hand, hypothermia or subnormal temperature in the presence of an underlying infection is a sign of poor prognosis (Cunha, 1996a). The magnitude of the fever is important for diagnosis. Most fevers of viral or bacterial origin are below 39°C; fevers above 39°C are observed in severe and complicated infections. Furthermore, elevations of body temperature are usually accompanied by a proportionate increase in pulse rate. Febrile patients are usually tachycardic, and the absence of this relative tachycardia is diagnostic of either drug fever or legionnaire's disease (Cunha, 1996a). Fever of unknown origin (FUO) is one in which a temperature elevation above 38.3°C is observed for three weeks or longer, the cause of which is undiagnosed after one week of intensive investigation (Cunha, 1996b). Common causes of FUO are malignancies, connective tissue disorders, abdominal infections and tuberculosis (Cunha, 1996b). The term *fever of unknown origin* is used incorrectly when describing any patient with undiagnosed fever.

Fever patterns will vary

Intermittent Fever: Temperature rises each day but falls to normal sometime during a 24-hour period, most often during early morning hours.

Remittent Fever: Marked variations in temperature occur during a 24-hour period. The lowest reading, however, always remains above the patient's normal level.

Relapsing Fever: Temperature may be normal for one or two days, then elevated for varying periods. Periods of normalcy are interspersed irregularly throughout the course of a relapsing fever.

Hectic or Septic Fever: Intermittent fever with wide fluctuations in daily temperature readings. Temperature may vary as much as 2.2°C within a 24-hour period.

Sustained or Continuous Fever: Temperature remains elevated at essentially the same level over a period of days or weeks.

THE STAGES OF A FEVER

The typical stages of fever occur in response to the physiological processes taking place within the body. There are three distinct stages: (a) the *chill* phase, or period of rising temperature; (b) the *course* of the fever, when the temperature is maintained at an elevated level; and (c) the *termination*, or period when the temperature falls to normal. During the three stages, different sets of mechanisms are operating, giving rise to the signs and symptoms characteristic of each stage.

The Chill Phase

During the onset of a fever, it is thought that there is a resetting of the body's internal "thermostat" or setpoint at a higher level (Guyton, 1996; Martini, 1998). This may be a response to the presence of pyrogenic substances, or to any one of the other causes listed in the section on the etiology of fever. The resetting of the internal thermostat brings the body's heat-producing mechanisms into play as an attempt is made to bring the temperature up to the desired level. Until this level is reached, the patient experiences what is known as a **chill**. Muscular activity, in the form of shivering, is increased, and may vary in severity from merely a feeling of being cold, with slight shivering, to violent muscular contractions (shaking chills).

At the same time as the shivering mechanism is induced, the rate of cellular metabolism increases, and the waste products of metabolism—carbon dioxide and water—are formed in greater quantities. The increased carbon dioxide level in the blood stimulates the respiratory centre, and breathing becomes faster and deeper. This leads to extra fluid loss, and the patient often feels thirsty. Also, as metabolism is accelerated, there is an increased demand by the cells for more oxygen and glucose. The heart beats more rapidly in response to this demand, and the nurse will note that the patient's pulse rate is higher than normal.

Concomitantly, heat-conserving mechanisms are instituted. Vasoconstriction occurs, the patient becomes pale, and the skin is cool to the touch. As a result of feeling cold, the patient may ask for extra blankets. Often, there is a "goose flesh" appearance to the skin as piloerection takes place. Sweating also may cease.

During the chill phase, body temperature rises steadily and may last for a few minutes or as long as an hour. In mild cases of fever, such as one sees with the common cold or in mild cases of influenza, the chill phase is usually brief. It is important that temperature be assessed at the completion of the chill phase in order to determine its upper limit. The chill phase resolves when the new setpoint is reached.

The Course of a Fever

During the second stage, when the fever is "running its course," the temperature has reached the preset level and there is a balance between heat production and heat loss. Because of increased body temperature, there is usually a generalized flushing of the skin, and it feels warm to the touch. The increased metabolic rate required to maintain the elevated temperature puts heightened demands on the body for more oxygen and glucose. The heart and respiratory rates remain high, and water loss through respiration increases the patient's feeling of thirst. The elevated temperature also increases nervous irritability. Headache, photophobia (sensitivity to light) and restlessness or drowsiness (or both) are not uncommon symptoms. An abnormally high fever is often accompanied by a state of mental confusion, which may progress to delirium. Patients may become disoriented as to time and place; they may have hallucinations, or become irrational and combative. Finally, prostration (collapse) may ensue. In young children, a convulsion not infrequently accompanies fever, usually at the outset.

The maintenance of an elevated temperature is very debilitating to the patient. During the first week or so of a fever, there is some destruction of body protein and *albuminuria* (protein in the urine) is usually noted in the laboratory findings (Guyton, 1996). The patient may complain of generalized weakness and not be inclined to much activity. Aching of the muscles and joints is frequently present. In addition to the destruction of tissue protein, it is believed that the parenchyma (the tissue of an organ, not of the supporting or connective tissue) begins to be damaged when body temperature rises above 40°C (Guyton, 1996).

Most authorities concur that children and adults can tolerate temperatures up to 41°C (Fruthaler, 1985; McCance & Huether, 1994). In sustained high fevers above 41.7°C, there may be permanent damage to brain and nervous tissue that does not regenerate (Fruthaler, 1985; McCance & Huether, 1994). The upper limit for survival of vital organs is at a body temperature of 43°C (McCance & Huether, 1994; Mitchell & Laburn, 1985; Porth, 1994).

Febrile patients usually lose weight. Although the increased metabolic rate maintained during the course of a fever increases the body's need for nourishment, most patients have little interest in food. The combination of increased need for food and loss of appetite (anorexia) leads to weight loss.

The temperature does not remain at a constant level but fluctuates during the course of a fever. Thus, periods when body temperature is rising are usually interspersed with periods when it is falling, even though the lowest temperature reached may always be above normal. When the heat-loss centre is stimulated, temperature falls and mechanisms for heat loss dominate. Vasodilation occurs and the skin becomes flushed and warm. **Diaphoresis** (sweating) is usually present to maximize heat loss through evaporation. The body thus loses more fluids, and the possibility of dehydration becomes a problem.

When fever is prolonged, dehydration is more likely to occur. This is due to several factors, including the greater loss of water through increased respiration and the further loss of fluids from sweating during periods when the elevated body temperature is falling. Urine output falls as more than the usual amount of fluid is lost through the skin and lungs. Other evidences of dehydration may be noted. The skin and mucous membranes may appear parched and dry. The patient's lips may become cracked and sore, and lesions may occur at the corners of the mouth. These lesions, often referred to as "fever blisters," may be activated forms of the herpes simplex virus. The nurse may note other signs and symptoms of dehydration, such as those discussed in Chapter 23. It is well to remember that young children in particular become dehydrated very quickly if there is a sustained fever.

The Termination of a Fever

When the cause of the elevated temperature has been removed, for example, when antibiotics have eliminated the cause of infection, the body's thermostat is reset at its original level. The mechanisms for increased heat production cease to operate, and mechanisms for increased heat loss are instituted. The patient's temperature may drop to normal quickly over a period of hours, or gradually over a period of days or weeks.

Other Heat Disturbances

Other disturbances in the body's homeostatic heat balance that require prompt intervention include drug fever, heat cramps, heat exhaustion, heat stroke and malignant hyperthermia.

DRUG FEVER

Drug fever is a febrile response that develops coincidentally with the administration of a drug and disappears with its discontinuation, and for which no other cause can be established (Hanson, 1991). Drug fevers have been attributed to several mechanisms: hypersensitivity reactions, idiosyncratic reactions, pharmacologic actions, drug administration-related reactions and altered thermoregulatory reactions. Hypersensitivity is the most common cause. This allergic response is accompanied by rash, urticaria, serum sickness, eosinophilia and drug-induced systemic lupus erythematosus (Johnson & Cunha, 1996). Idiosyncratic reactions occur in individuals who have a heritable biochemical disorder or enzyme deficiency that influences the body's reactions to some general anesthetics and particular drugs (Hanson, 1991). Many medications cause fever by inducing vasoconstriction, impairing sweating and increasing metabolic rate. Similarly, the pharmacologic effect of some drugs on microorganisms or on malignant cells can elicit a febrile reaction (Johnson

Drug fevers frequently occur after one to two weeks of drug therapy. These patients present with fevers above 39°C, a generalized maculopapular rash and a pulse rate that is inappropriately low relative to the elevated temperature. The drug-induced fever usually resolves within 72 hours of discontinuation of the offending medication (Johnson & Cunha, 1996). A list of medications that have been implicated in drug fevers is provided below.

Drugs Implicated in the Development of Fever

Atropine	Penicillins
Amphotericin	Phenytoin
Bleomycin	Salicylates
Cimetidine	Sulfonamides
Cephalosporins	Streptokinase
Interferon	Vancomycin
Methyldopa	Quinidines

SOURCE: Johnson & Cunha, 1996.

HEAT CRAMPS

Heat cramps may develop in hot climates or hot weather as a result of prolonged, excessive sweating. This depletes the sodium chloride in body fluids and results in the subsequent painful cramping of stressed skeletal muscles. Putting the individual with heat cramps in a cool room and giving fluids with salt added will relieve mild cases (Boyd, 1996). One-half to one teaspoon of salt in a quart of water is generally recommended (Drake & Nettina, 1994). Salt tablets are not recommended because they are absorbed slowly and may result in gastric irritation, vomiting and cerebral edema (Porth, 1998; Barnes & Walker, 1995).

HEAT EXHAUSTION

Also known as *heat prostration*, heat exhaustion may result from lengthy exposure to a hot environment, especially if combined with high humidity. Predominantly associated with either salt depletion or water depletion, this condition may range from fairly mild disorders to more severe forms (Wenger & Hardy, 1990). The individual may experience profuse sweating, nausea and vomiting, culminating in dehydration. The patient usually becomes very pale, and has cold, clammy skin, lowered blood pressure and generalized weakness, impending signs of shock. Core temperature is usually less than 40°C (Khogali, 1997). Generally, moving the patient to cooler and less humid surroundings and giving fluids will relieve this condition. Severe cases may require emergency treatment.

HEAT STROKE

A potentially lethal but preventable condition, heat stroke

primary factor is heat stress such as occurs during a sustained heat wave (Barnes & Walker, 1995). It is most frequently seen in the elderly and is believed to be due to predisposing factors such as atrophy of sweat glands, decreased circulation, underlying disease conditions and the side effects of drug therapy (Worfolk, 1997). Other factors that increase the risk for heat stroke include dehydration, obesity, lack of acclimatization, lack of sleep, chronic illness, alcoholism and restrictive clothing (Khogali & Mustafa, 1984; Mitchell & Laburn, 1985).

Exertional heat stroke, on the other hand, results primarily from metabolic heat production. Consequently, victims of this form of heat stroke tend to be younger and physically fit, such as athletes. In the classic form, sweating is absent, resulting in hot, dry skin. With exertional heat stroke, however, absence of sweating may occur as a late event (Wenger & Hardy, 1990). Heat stroke is further characterized by a very high rectal temperature (above 40.6°C) (Khogali, 1997) and coma (Kohl, 1996).

It is generally accepted that temperatures above 43°C are incompatible with life (McCance & Huether, 1994). The physiological effects of a dangerously high body temperature include damage to the brain and central nervous system tissues, increased blood clotting, metabolic acidosis, tissue hypoxia and severe potassium imbalance that leads to cardiac arrest (Khogali & Mustafa, 1984). Heat stroke requires prompt medical intervention and immediate action to lower the body temperature as quickly as possible (Kellerman & Todd, 1996). Some authorities recommend the optimum rate of cooling to be a decrease of 0.3°C every five minutes (Khogali & Mustafa, 1984).

MALIGNANT HYPERTHERMIA

Malignant **hyperthermia** is a sudden and potentially lethal hypermetabolic crisis state triggered by certain volatile anesthetic or neuromuscular blocking agents in persons genetically prone to this (Simon, 1994). A rapid elevation in temperature at a rate of 1°C every five minutes may result unless appropriate treatment is initiated rapidly. Careful family history assessment preoperatively is necessary to screen patients for this genetic defect.

Hypothermia

On the other side of the temperature spectrum, the most common problem from lack of heat is accidental hypothermia.

Hypothermia is a chilling of the whole body from exposure to cold such that the core temperature drops below 35°C (Britt, Dascombe & Rodriguez, 1991; Dexter, 1990). This state can occur in accidental situations (such as from exposure to cold weather or from immersion in cold water); it can be induced clinically during specific types of surgery (such as in cardiac and neurosurgery); or it can occur as a secondary clinical problem resulting from a predisposing disease condition (such as hypothyroidism, hypoglycemia, alcoholism, hypopituitarism or severe burns) (Dexter, 1990).

Although older patients account for the majority of victims of hypothermia, children and young adults can also be exposed to environmental conditions leading to life-threatening drops in body temperature. Nor does accidental hypothermia occur only in cold, northern climates or in people who have been caught in a snowstorm in the mountains. People vary considerably in their ability to withstand cold temperatures. Persons with darkly pigmented skin, older people and those in poor physical condition are more affected by the cold than others. The amount and type of clothing worn for insulating the body are also important. Multiple layers of lightweight clothing serve to entrap warm air close to the skin and have been found to be more effective for keeping the body warm than fewer layers of bulky, heavy clothing. Water acts as a heat conductor, and damp clothing therefore conducts heat away from the body. The "wind chill" factor, as mentioned earlier, considerably increases the effect of cold environmental temperatures on the body.

Regardless of the underlying cause or the victim's age, treatment of hypothermia takes precedence over any accompanying problems because of the threat to life. In one instance, a two-year-old survived several hours of extreme winter conditions on the Canadian prairies (Roberts, 1994). The body is well preserved at low temperatures because metabolism is suppressed and oxygen stores to the vital tissues are maintained (Cohen & Moelleken, 1996). For this reason, it is generally accepted that even profoundly hypothermic patients should be resuscitated and warmed to normal body temperature regardless of their apparent unresponsiveness on admission to hospital.

If the patient is in the early stages of mild hypothermia (body temperature of 34° to 35°C) (Cohen & Moelleken, 1996), he or she should be protected from the elements and from the cold and possibly wet ground. If possible, wet garments should be removed, the individual should be wrapped in dry clothing and put into a sleeping bag for gradual rewarming. Other acceptable forms of warming the mildly hypothermic patient include direct body contact with a normothermic individual, immersion in a warm bath or consumption of hot liquids.

If the patient has become stuporous or unconscious, it is probable that moderate to severe hypothermia (body temperature lower than 34°C) has occurred (Cohen & Moelleken, 1996). This condition requires prompt medical intervention because of the possibility of lethal complications such as myocardial irritability. It is necessary to transport such a patient to medical facilities where intensive rewarming techniques and monitoring are available. The victim should be placed between blankets and protected from further cold en route. Rewarming measures will vary depending on the severity of the hypothermia. These measures include surface warming (such as the application of external heating measures) or core warming (such as peritoneal dialysis or cardiopulmonary bypass (Garchinsky, Gilmore, MacKay & Ostapowich, 1994). "Afterdrop" (in which body temperature drops at the onset of rewarming) is a major concern, as cold blood from the limbs returning to the core causes a further drop in core temperature (Dexter, 1990).

The basic physiological mechanism operating in hypothermia is a constriction of the blood vessels in the peripheral tissues of the body. With the vasoconstriction, there is decreased flow of blood to the area and consequently decreased supply of oxygen to the tissues. The decreased blood flow results in diminished local sensation (a numbness is perceived) and weakness of the muscles. The skin feels cold and becomes pale. The walls of blood vessels in the area may be directly damaged by the cold, with the result that plasma fluid leaks into interstitial spaces and the area becomes swollen as the blood in the vessels becomes more concentrated and small clots begin to form, giving a typically mottled look to the tissues. Eventually, the clots close the vessel completely and the area becomes avascular (without blood supply). A peripheral pulse can no longer be felt. If there is a quick freezing of the tissues, as sometimes happens to exposed noses, cheeks or ears in very cold climates, the affected part becomes white and shiny, sometimes with a blue tinge.

The skin is the first tissue to be cooled and is the most likely to be damaged. Blood vessels, nerves and muscles are also very vulnerable and easily damaged. Bones, connective tissue and tendons are more resistant to damage from cold exposure. The areas of the body that are most vulnerable to damage from the cold are those that are most exposed, such as the hands, face (especially the cheeks and nose), ears and feet.

In addition to the localized reactions to cold, the patient who has suffered from exposure under conditions of extreme cold may develop cold exhaustion. This usually begins with mild hypothermia, characterized by intense shivering, profound vasoconstriction and accelerated heart rate, all of which help to resist lowering of temperature. Urinary flow is increased (cold diuresis) and the patient will hyperventilate—a reaction that could culminate in dehydration during early hypothermia (Cohen & Moelleken, 1996).

In response to the prolonged cold exposure, physical and mental responses slow down. At a body temperature of 34°C, the patient becomes clumsy and muscle control is impaired as the temperature of the muscles becomes lower. Speech is slurred and the patient becomes amnesic and irrational (Martini, 1998; McCance & Huether, 1994). The thermoregulatory mechanisms of shivering and vasoconstriction are lost when body temperature drops below 33°C (McCance & Huether, 1994). If body temperature drops

fall asleep. Loss of consciousness and cardiac arrest ensue at a body temperature of 28°C. The lowest limit for survival is considered to be a body temperature of 23°C, except in unusual situations.

Assessing Temperature Regulation Needs

Usually the first thing nurses do on admission of patients to a health care agency is take their temperature. Indeed, fever is such a universal sign of illness that it is important to interview and observe all patients for the signs and symptoms of disturbed body temperature. In order to know what to look for and the relevant questions to ask the patient (or family), the nurse needs to understand the mechanism of fever—the types of fever commonly encountered and the stages of fever. The nurse should also understand the effect of cold on body tissues and be able to make pertinent observations. The nursing health history, temperature measurements and observations made during physical assessment of the patient that are recorded on the patient's chart furnish data that aid the nurse in determining patient problems and needs for care.

In addition, the patient's record will provide information about actual or potential problems with temperature regulation. The nurse will want to check for conditions that place the patient at risk for temperature disturbances. These may include:

- open wounds
- recent surgery
- recent invasive diagnostic procedures (colonoscopy, catheterization)
- drug therapy that causes immunosuppression (steroids, chemotherapy)
- malnutrition
- burn injury.

The Nursing Health History

When patients running a fever are admitted to a health agency, it is important to find out how long they have had it, how high the temperature has been and whether they have had any other signs and symptoms of illness. In the case of children, it is particularly important to ask if they have been exposed to a communicable disease, so that they may be isolated to protect other children on the unit. Some agencies have a policy of putting all children with an elevated temperature on isolation precautions for 24 hours to observe them for development of a rash or other indication of one of the childhood diseases.

When a patient is admitted with a cold weather in

cident. How long was the exposure? Under what conditions? What parts of the body are affected? What first aid measures were used before admission? It is also helpful to know how old the patient is, the general physical condition and any existing health problems.

As with all needs, the nurse will also question the patient or family about usual health-promoting and health-protecting patterns to help identify potential problems and opportunities for promoting optimal thermal well-being. A health history guide is on the following page.

Measurements

TEMPERATURE, PULSE AND RESPIRATIONS

Body temperature, taken with a clinical thermometer, is an objective measure of the body's temperature-regulating status. The methods of taking a body temperature are given in Chapter 16. In order to have a baseline on which to judge whether a patient's temperature is above, or below, his or her normal range, it is helpful to take the temperature over a period of several successive days at different times of the day and to plot the readings on a vital signs flowsheet.

Many inpatient agencies have specific policies for the taking of temperatures. Some require that all patients have their temperature taken once, or sometimes twice, a day to screen for fever. If temperature is taken once a day, early evening is usually the best time, since this is the time when temperature is most elevated in many febrile patients. If temperature is taken in the morning, this should be done an hour or so after the patient wakens, when the body temperature is stabilized.

When a patient has a fever, the temperature should be monitored at more frequent intervals. All newly admitted patients have their temperature taken, as do all preoperative and postoperative patients. Postoperatively, the temperature is usually taken every four hours for the first 48 hours. In addition to these general guidelines, when signs and symptoms indicating fever are present, the nurse should monitor the patient's temperature. The temperature should be evaluated in relation to such factors as the patient's usual normal temperature, the time of day, the environmental temperature and the normal physiological processes that may affect body temperature. Pulse and respiratory rates are elevated in hyperthermic disturbances, while in hypothermia these are decreased.

Physical Assessment

The physical examination has a twofold purpose: (a) to assess those sites commonly associated with infection, such

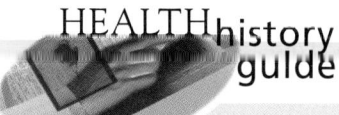

Temperature Regulation

Health and Illness Patterns

Usual Temperature Pattern

- Do you know your normal temperature range? If so, what is it?
- Do you usually feel cold and need an extra sweater or blanket even in warm weather?
- Are you usually too warm when others are comfortable indoors or outdoors?

Recent Changes in Temperature Pattern

- How long have you noticed this occurrence?
- Have you had any accompanying symptoms?

Presenting Health Problem

If admitted with a fever:

- How long have you had this fever?
- How high has the temperature been?
- Describe any symptoms you are experiencing now. Chills? Headache? Fatigue or malaise? Pain or absence of sensation in a body part? Anorexia, nausea, diarrhea, cough, dyspnea, dysuria or vomiting? Thirst?
- Have you done any travelling recently?
- Do you have a history of acute or chronic disease that may cause a fever? Flu? Chronic bronchitis? Bladder infection?
- Have you recently been exposed to anyone with an infection?
- Are you taking any medications at present (including over-the-counter medications)? If so, what?
- Have you had prolonged exposure to excessively hot or cold environmental temperatures?

If admitted with a cold-weather injury:

- What was the nature of your accident?
- How long were you exposed to the cold?
- What parts of your body are affected?
- Were any first aid measures used to treat the injury? If so, what?

Health Promotion and Protection Patterns

- Do you spend a lot of time in a hot environment or in the sun? Examples: Working on road maintenance, at construction sites or in steel mills? Spending time on the beach?
- What precautions do you take in very hot weather or in a hot environment?
- Do you spend a lot of time in a cold, windy environment? Examples: Skiing or working outdoors in the winter?
- What precautions do you take in very cold weather?

as the skin, the ears (particularly in children), the respiratory tract, the gastrointestinal tract and the genitourinary tract; and (b) to assist in the determination of the etiology of the disturbance. The typical manifestations observed in the patient with body temperature disturbances are listed as objective data in the following box.

All patients with body temperature disturbance are observed for changes in their level of consciousness, which can progress from restlessness to drowsiness and, in severe temperature disturbances, to delirium. The skin is observed for colour, warmth and turgor. Mucous membranes are assessed for integrity and moisture. The nurse notes signs of dehydration, which include a rapid and weak pulse, hypotension, decreased skin turgor, a dry and furrowed tongue, absence of tearing or salivation and dark, concentrated urine. Patients who present with hypothermia are assessed for neurological impairment and circulatory and respiratory collapse. Regardless of the type of temperature disturbance, intake and output are monitored carefully, and laboratory values are evaluated for fluid and electrolyte imbalances.

The patient who presents with fever is examined for possible sites of infection. The symptoms reported by the patient during the health history often help to guide the physical assessment.

Diagnosing Temperature Regulation Problems

Clinical problems in temperature regulation amenable to nursing intervention are related to an imbalance between heat losses and heat gains, leading to an excessive rise or fall in core body temperature. Common nursing diagnoses related to temperature regulation are: *Hyperthermia*, *Hypothermia* and *Risk for Altered Body Temperature* (Carpenito, 1997).

Trauma, illness, infection, increased metabolic rate, exposure to a hot environment, inability to perspire, dehydration and the side effects of certain medications on thermoregulatory responses are situations that could lead to increased heat production and a nursing diagnosis of *Hyperthermia*. Along with a body temperature above normal range, the patient who is hyperthermic will exhibit warm,

Subjective and Objective Data in Patients with Disturbances of Body Temperature

SUBJECTIVE DATA	OBJECTIVE DATA
Fever	
Chill Phase	
Feeling of being cold	Skin cool to touch
Intermittent chills	Pale "goose flesh" appearance
Apprehension	Observable shivering or shaking
	Increased pulse rate
	Increased respiratory rate
	Increased body temperature
Course of the Fever	
Feeling of being warm	Skin flushed
Thirst	Hot to touch
Lips sore	Perspiration (may be profuse)
Feeling of generalized weakness	Elevated temperature (may fluctuate)
Headache	Dry mouth and lips
Sensitivity to light	Fever blisters
Aching muscles and joints	Tongue coated, "furry"
Anorexia, nausea, vomiting	Scant urine
	Restlessness, drowsiness
	Lethargy
	With high fever, may show disorientation, delirium, irrational combative behaviour
	Convulsions (in children)
	Loss of weight
	Dehydration
Termination of Fever	
Feels improved	Skin flushed
	Sweating (diaphoresis) often profuse
	Respirations within normal limits
	Pulse within normal limits
	Dropping temperature
	Clearing sensorium
	Gradual return to normal functioning
Hypothermia	
Exposed area feels cold	Skin cold to touch
Diminished local sensation (feeling of numbness)	Pale—becoming white or blue-tinged
	Sometimes mottled appearance of skin
Weakness of muscles	Absence of pulse to affected extremity
Inability to flex joints	Swelling of affected site
Tiredness	Slow, often stumbling movements
	Sometimes irrational behaviour
	Drowsiness
	Respirations slow and shallow
	Pulse rate slow

flushed skin, increased pulse rate (tachycardia) and an increased respiratory rate (tachypnea). This person may report headache and may appear lethargic or restless. Complete blood count results may reveal an elevated white blood cell count, if infection or inflammation is present. An elevated hematocrit and hemoglobin may be suggestive of dehydration.

Hypothermia is the nursing diagnosis applicable to the patient who is exposed to a cold environment for a prolonged period, or whose thermoregulatory responses are affected by alcohol, disease, trauma, medications or anesthetics. Other related factors include aging, inadequate clothing, inactivity, malnutrition and inability or decreased ability to shiver (McFarland & McFarlane, 1997; Dexter, 1990). Defining characteristics of a hypothermic individual may include a reduction in body temperature below normal range; cool, pale, blanched or reddened skin; piloerection; decreased heart rate (bradycardia); decreased respiratory rate (bradypnea); decreased blood pressure (hypotension); and decreased level of consciousness (drowsiness, confusion or coma). Severely hypothermic patients may appear clinically dead with no palpable pulse or respiratory effort (Garchinski et al., 1994).

The nursing diagnosis *Risk for Altered Body Temperature* may be applied to individuals who are identified to be at risk. Risk factors may include extremes in age or weight, exposure to extremes in environmental temperature, inappropriate clothing, infection, disease or trauma affecting temperature regulation, dehydration and intake of alcohol or medications affecting temperature control (McFarland & McFarlane, 1997).

The management of severe hyperthermia and profound hypothermia requires collaboration between nursing and medicine. These and other problems associated with these potentially lethal conditions, such as compartmental syndrome from thermal injury, fluid volume deficit and decreased cardiac output, should be labelled as collaborative problems. Examples of nursing diagnoses and collaborative problems are *Risk for altered body temperature related to surgery and sedation*, *Hyperthermia related to dehydration*, *Hypothermia related to exposure to a cold environment*, *PC: Hyperthermia* and *PC: Compartmental syndrome thermal injury*.

Common expected outcomes of interventions for the patient with a body temperature problem include the following:

- oral temperature will be within normal limits (35.80–37.3°C) (Bates, 1995)
- blood pressure, pulse and respirations will be within the normal limits
- patient's skin will be of normal warmth
- oral mucous membranes will be moist
- patient will be alert and oriented
- patient will verbalize environmental risk factors for hyperthermia or hypothermia
- patient will verbalize necessary behavioural changes to maintain normal body temperature during temperature extremes.

Planning Temperature Regulation Interventions

The plan of care for patients with thermoregulation problems is based on the severity of the problems and on the appropriate treatment modalities to restore body temperature. In cases of fever, nursing interventions are selected to reduce the amount of heat produced within the body, to facilitate the elimination of heat from the body, to minimize the effects of fever on vital bodily functions (circulation, respiration, nutrition and fluid balance) and to collaborate with other health professionals in identifying and eliminating the cause of the fever. For example, collaborative nursing interventions (actions) may include collection of specimens (urine, sputum, wound, blood) to identify a causative organism. Nursing interventions for patients with excessive lowering of surface or core body temperature focus on rewarming the patient, preventing tissue damage and, in severe hypothermia, preventing and treating complications such as acid–base imbalance, fluid and electrolyte imbalance, hypoxemia and cardiac arrhythmias. As with all needs, the plan of care incorporates patient preferences and beliefs, usual lifestyle practices and socioeconomic status. Strategies that enable self-care and achievement of optimal thermal regulation in the course of daily functioning are essential.

In determining priorities for nursing interventions, the nurse must assess the severity of the patient's condition. If the patient's temperature is extremely high (above 40°C) or profoundly low (below 32°C), the situation is considered a medical emergency and requires immediate intervention (McFarland & McFarlane, 1997).

Implementing Temperature Regulation Interventions

Health-Promoting Strategies

Humans are equipped with an efficient heat-regulating mechanism for maintaining a stable body temperature. The body's adaptive mechanisms produce heat when temperature falls and lose excess heat when temperature rises. Thermal dysfunction occurs when environmental challenges (ambient temperature and metabolic processes) exceed the individual's adaptive capacity. People can promote optimal thermal health in the course of daily living by modifying environmental conditions or behaviour to conserve or dissipate body heat.

Health-Protecting Strategies

MANAGING FEVER

The presence of an elevated temperature puts stresses on the body's adaptive mechanisms. Patients are usually uncomfortable; they are losing more than the normal amount of fluids and using more energy than usual to maintain the elevated body temperature. Nursing interventions should be directed towards minimizing these stresses and enhancing the body's coping capabilities.

MAINTAINING REST The patient who has an elevated temperature needs rest. It is essential to minimize the patient's energy requirements. Rest and inactivity decrease the metabolic rate and thereby decrease the amount of heat

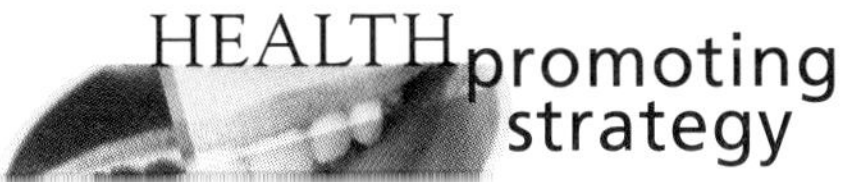

Promoting Healthy Temperature Regulation

- Keep a comfortable temperature in the home. An ambient temperature of 21°–23°C is considered comfortable for day-time; lower levels are recommended for sleeping.
- Avoid extremes of environmental temperature whenever possible.
- In hot climates, stay out of the sun as much as possible. Wear loose, light-weight, and light-coloured clothing to allow air circulation and dissipation of heat. White is best for reflecting radiant heat. Wear a large hat to shade your eyes and deflect the radiant heat from the head and back of the neck.
- In cold climates, wear multiple layers of light-weight clothing to entrap warm air close to the skin. Cover the head, hands and wrists. The head and neck can lose up to 40 percent of body heat (Williams, 1993).
- If planning strenuous work or exercise in hot weather, drink ample fluids within an hour of commencing activity. It takes more energy to work in a hot climate. Pace yourself and work slowly.

produced in the body. Usually, patients are restricted to bed in order to curtail their activities. Physical activity should be kept to a minimum. During the convalescent stage, activity should be gradually increased to prevent tiring the patient.

However, rest involves more than restrictions on physical activity; it also means mental rest. Sometimes the simple act of taking a patient's temperature may cause anxiety. An elevated temperature may result in having surgery postponed, or in delaying a much anticipated return to home and family. Febrile patients need to be assured that all is being done for their welfare. Anticipating the needs of patients helps them to relax. Very often, a simple explanation of procedures and treatments will alleviate many anxieties.

The patient with a fever needs a cool, quiet environment. He or she may be irritable and may be hypersensitive to stimuli. An effort should be made to minimize noise and to provide the opportunity for rest. A cool, comfortable room increases heat elimination and helps the patient to rest more easily. Sometimes a fan is used to increase air circulation in the room and facilitate the removal of heat from the body through conduction and convection. Care should be taken to ensure that the patient does not become chilled. The bedclothes of the patient with a fever should be light and comfortable, since heavy coverings inhibit heat elimination.

MAINTAINING COMFORT AND HYGIENE Good hygiene is important to the patient's health and comfort. Diaphoresis, which frequently accompanies fever, is uncomfortable. Bathing, and a change of gown and bedding, may be required to ensure that the patient remains clean and dry. Because sweat glands are more numerous in the axilla and around the genitalia, these areas need particular care when the patient is bathed. Flannelette sheets, because of their greater absorbency, are often used in place of ordinary cotton ones on the beds of patients who are perspiring profusely.

MAINTAINING HYDRATION The hydration of the febrile patient is of primary importance. Diaphoresis and the loss of additional fluids through increased respirations increase the amount of fluid eliminated from the body, and this fluid needs to be replaced. In addition, during a fever, there is increased production of metabolic waste products, which must be eliminated. The necessity for removing these products from the body, together with any toxic substances that may be present, emphasizes the importance of fluids. If the patient is unable to take fluids orally or in sufficient amounts, parenteral fluids may be ordered. A temperature between 38.3° and 39.4° C increases the 24-hour fluid requirement by a minimum of 500 mL. If the temperature is above 39.4°, this increases the 24-hour fluid requirement by at least 1000 mL (Metheney, 1996).

An accurate record of the patient's fluid intake and output must be maintained. Intake records should include all fluids taken orally and those given parenterally. In computing output, urine should be measured accurately and a note made of the extent of sweating and the loss of any fluids through vomiting or diarrhea. Suction and drain returns should also be included in the output calculations.

The patient should be observed carefully for signs of dehydration. When a patient becomes dehydrated during the course of a fever, the skin often becomes dry and scaly. The application of creams helps to keep the skin in good condition. Dehydration frequently results in cracks in the patient's lips, tongue or mucous membrane lining the mouth. Good oral hygiene is imperative to prevent infection from developing and also to contribute to the patient's comfort. There is a need to cleanse, hydrate and lubricate the mouth and lips.

Frequent intake of fluids helps to maintain hydration of the oral cavity. Rinsing the mouth with water (or mouthwash) and chewing gum also help to preserve hydration. If patients are unable to take fluids orally, rinse the mouth or chew gum, the nurse can help by providing mouth care. Commercially prepared swabs or swabs dipped in mouthwash are used in many agencies.

Lubrication may be accomplished by the application of creams or petrolatum to the lips. Sterile petrolatum should be used because of frequent splits or cracks in the lips due to the fever, which provide a portal of entry for infection.

MAINTAINING NUTRITIONAL STATUS As a result of the body's increased metabolic rate and the increased destruction of tissues that often occur with fever, there is a need for additional proteins and carbohydrates in the diet of the febrile patient. Proteins aid in the formation of body tissue; carbohydrates supply the body with much-needed energy. Frequently these products are supplied in the liquids taken orally or given parenterally. The patient's weight should be checked at frequent intervals. The physician should be kept informed of the patient's nutritional status so that appropriate therapy may be instituted.

An important function of the nurse is the communication of observations to other members of the health team. The nutritional status of the patient with a fever must be carefully monitored and accurately reported and recorded (see Chapter 20).

Health-Restoring Strategies

MEASURES TO REDUCE HEAT PRODUCTION AND FACILITATE HEAT LOSS

Fever is now thought to promote the activity of the body's immune functions and to increase the bactericidal effect of some antimicrobial agents (Klein & Cunha, 1996). Because fever is an important indicator of disease progression, it is not always advisable to suppress or treat it. However, fever may have a deleterious effect on some patients, such as seizure-prone children, the elderly (who are prone to delirium manifestations of the temperature disturbance) and cardiac patients. In situations where it has been deemed necessary to treat fever, a number of measures may be used to bring about a rapid reduction in body temperature. These include the use of antipyretic medications, which have a systemic action, as well as various techniques for surface cooling of the body. Overall, the primary management of fever should be directed at the cause of the disease rather than the fever itself.

Antipyretic and Antibiotic Drug Therapy

Antipyretic drugs, such as acetaminophen, ASA and non-steroidal anti-inflammatory drugs (NSAIDs), are ordered to relieve the discomfort of fever. These drugs work by inhibiting the synthesis of prostaglandins and lowering the hypothalamic setpoint to normal (Klein & Cunha, 1996). In addition, NSAIDs and ASA provide relief of inflammation and pain. ASA has been associated with hepatic, gastrointestinal and kidney toxicity, and Reye's syndrome when given to children with influenza or chicken pox. It is considered to be more toxic than acetaminophen as an antipyretic. Acetaminophen is, therefore, the preferred antipyretic for young children and patients with clotting disorders, gastric ulcers or asthma (Klein & Cunha, 1996). NSAIDs, such as ibuprofen, have also been shown to be clinically effective in reducing fevers greater than 39°C (Murphy, 1992).

Antibiotics are generally prescribed when the causative organism is identified. These agents reduce fever by eliminating the cause of the disease process.

Tepid Sponge Bath

A tepid sponge bath is a temporary measure to lower a patient's temperature. The technique is based on the principle that the body loses heat through the mechanisms of conduction to a cooler substance (in this case the tepid water), evaporation of water from the surface of the body and convection of the heat away from exposed body surfaces during the bathing process.

Although baths were used frequently in the past, controversy exists regarding their usefulness (see Research to Practice), because decreasing the temperature below the setpoint may trigger the shivering response and consequently increase heat production (Friedman & Barton, 1990; Sharber, 1997). The degree of discomfort experienced by the patient, and the nursing time involved in carrying out this procedure, may outweigh the benefits.

Using a Fan

A nursing intervention that is somewhat similar to the tepid sponge bath is the use of a fan to increase heat elimination from the body. The patient is covered only by a sheet and a fan is positioned so that there is constant movement of air over the sheet. This measure promotes evaporation and convection and thereby increases heat loss from the body.

Hypothermia Machines

Many hospitals have a hypothermia machine (cooling blanket) that is used for rapid surface cooling of the body. This machine may be used when it is deemed essential to lower body temperature down quickly (for example, in a case of malignant hyperthermia) or when there has been injury to the heat-regulating centres of the brain and it is necessary to maintain artificial cooling of the body over a prolonged period of time.

This technique uses the mechanisms of radiation and conduction. The patient is placed on or between cooling blankets, which are attached to a refrigerating machine. The blankets contain coils in which a liquid, often water, circulates. The machine is set to operate according to either the desired body temperature or to the desired water blanket temperature. The temperature of the patient is continuously monitored with an attached rectal temperature probe. A considerable amount of heat is lost from the body through direct conduction to the cooling substance and through the radiation of heat waves from the body to the cooler blankets. Because some people shiver in response to the application of the hypothermia blanket, medication is sometimes given

RESEARCH to practice

Kinmouth, A., Fulton, Y. & Cambell, M. J. (1992). Management of feverish children at home. *British Medical Journal, 305,* 1134–1136.

This study compared the acceptability and effects on body temperature between the use of antipyretic agent paracetamol (acetaminophen) or warm sponging to unwrapping and encouraging cool drinks among feverish children at home. The sample comprised 52 children aged from three months to five years with axillary temperatures before treatment ranging between 37.8° and 40°C. The children were randomized within blocks stratified by age into four treatment groups: unwrapping, warm sponging plus unwrapping, paracetamol plus unwrapping, and paracetamol and warm sponging plus unwrapping. The children were treated at home by parents. A research nurse studied each child over four hours after treatment and followed the children until they were well. The nurse advised parents on the treatment measures as follows:

Unwrapping—Dress your child in light clothing (shirt and diaper) in a room warm enough for an adult to feel comfortable naked. Encourage frequent cool drinks.

Warm sponging—In a warm room (as above), sit your child in a tub or basin containing a few centimetres of warm water (at a temperature just below that of your child). Wet the child all over for 10–20 min or as long as the child is comfortable. Do not leave the child unattended. Then unwrap the child (as above).

Paracetamol—Give amounts as prescribed according to age. Then unwrap as above.

Paracetamol and warm sponging—The advice given above was combined.

The response to advice was assessed over four hours. Temperature was measured by continuous logging from an axillary thermometer. Acceptability of treatment to child and parent were scored on Likert scales immediately after treatment and on return to health. The response to treatment advice varied. Unwrapping alone had little effect on temperature. Paracetamol increased the time spent below 37.2°C by 109 min compared with unwrapping. Warm sponging caused the fastest reduction in temperature (and almost half of the children enjoyed warm sponging). Parents, however, were happiest with treatments that included paracetamol. The researchers concluded that giving an antipyretic is more effective and is more acceptable to parents than sponging or unwrapping alone. Warm sponging has an additive effect and reduces fever more quickly than does the antipyretic.

to minimize shivering. Patients receiving hypothermia treatment frequently need a great deal of reassurance and explanation.

THERAPEUTIC MEASURES TO FACILITATE HEAT PRODUCTION AND PROMOTE HEAT GAIN

Patients with lowered body temperature require generalized warmth in order to maintain or regain normal body temperature. In addition to the simple application of additional blankets, particularly flannelette sheets, which help to conserve heat, other measures are available. In some agencies, warming cupboards in which sheets or blankets are heated may be useful, particularly in postanesthetic (recovery room) areas. As a result of cool temperatures in the operating room, patients frequently exit these areas with lowered body temperature.

For patients requiring additional warmth, commercial warming devices are available. One such device (Bair Hugger®) injects warmed air into disposable light-weight plastic/paper blankets. Small openings on the patient side of the blanket allow the air to circulate over the patient. This simple but effective device is user-friendly and is especially useful in the emergency department and postanesthetic areas where patients with varying degrees of hypothermia may be admitted. Temperature settings of low, medium or high may be selected.

Another device, the hyperthermia blanket (warming blanket), may also be used (Figure 25.2). This apparatus is similar to the hypothermia blanket described earlier, with the exception that warmed, instead of cooled, liquid circulates through the coils in the blanket. The hyperthermia machine is particularly useful for patients with extreme hypothermia. Again, rectal temperature is continuously monitored throughout the procedure and the physician orders the desired rectal or blanket temperature to be achieved.

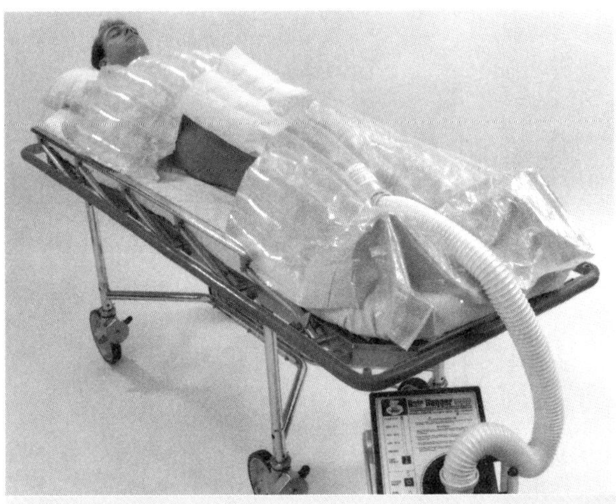

FIGURE 25.2 Warming blanket

SOURCE: Augustine Medical, Inc.

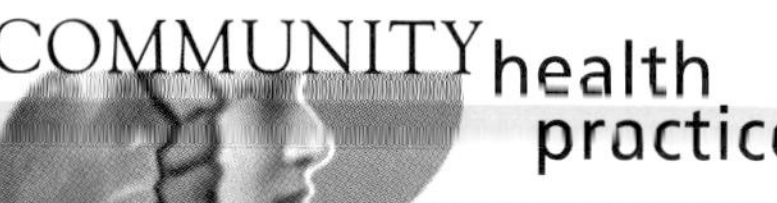

Home Care: Managing Fever in a Child at Home

Fever in children is commonly treated at home by parents who may need guidance and reassurance. Nurses can teach parents how to care for their child during a febrile episode. The following guidelines should be included in parent teaching.

1. Children are considered febrile when their temperature is greater than:
   - 37.3°C (axilla)
   - 37.8°C (oral)
   - 38.3°C (rectal).
2. The child's doctor should be consulted if the febrile child:
   - is under 3 months of age.
   - has persistent diarrhea, vomiting or difficulty breathing
   - is very lethargic or irritable
   - is feeding poorly.
3. The child whose fever persists beyond 24 hours should be brought to the attention of a doctor.

Treatment of fever:

1. Unwrap the child into light clothing (for example, vest and diaper). Keep the room comfortably warm.
2. Give the child acetaminophen or ibuprofen according to instructions on the bottle.
3. Encourage the child to drink plenty of fluids.

SOURCES: Lopez, McMillan, Tobias-Merrill & Chop, 1997; Victoria General Hospital, 1994.

Therapeutic Use of Heat and Cold

Applications of heat and cold as therapeutic measures are well known to most people. Applying a hot water bottle or a heating pad to cold feet is a comfort familiar to many, particularly to those who live in cold climates. The application of ice as a means of stopping nosebleed (epistaxis) is a common therapeutic measure carried out in the home. The student has probably already had firsthand experience with many of these therapeutic measures.

Because perceptions of temperature sensations vary, applications of heat and cold pose hazards to skin integrity. Therefore, they must be carried out with caution. In many agencies, these measures require a written order from a physician. If patient comfort is the sole reason for their use, it is often left to the judgment of the nurse and patient whether and how to apply them. Nurses therefore need a knowledge of the physiological reactions resulting from these measures and of the untoward reactions that may occur. If nurses are ever in doubt about the use of heat or cold, they should consult the physician before applying these measures.

Applications of heat and cold also are used in the course of certain rehabilitation programs. In these instances physical therapists use measures such as paraffin baths and whirlpool baths.

Temperature Sensation

Heat and cold are relative degrees of warmth dependent to some extent upon the perception of the individual. The temperature at the surface of the skin of the torso is generally 33.9°C. Local skin tolerance to cold and heat is thought to range between 4.4° and 43.3°C. Generally, any application that is outside this range can cause tissue damage.

Temperature is perceived in gradations: cold to cool, tepid, indifferent, warm and finally, very hot. Extremes in temperatures, both hot and cold, are perceived as painful. Different areas of the body have varying sensitivity to changes in heat and cold. People perceive temperature more acutely when the temperature of the skin is changing. Eventually the skin's heat and cold receptors that relay sensation become conditioned to the given temperature. That is why a hot bath feels hotter at first than it does after the skin becomes adjusted to it. This mechanism can be dangerous, as it allows people to be burned or frost-bitten without knowing it. For this reason, testing of skin for temperature sensitivity to both extremes of temperature is required prior to treatments to avoid thermal injury.

Types of Applications

Many different types of hot and cold applications can be used as therapeutic measures. Both heat and cold can be applied as dry treatments or as moist treatments, and the source can be varied according to the purpose. Hot and cold applications must be applied with good nursing judgement. Good judgement is based on knowledge of the reasons for the therapeutic heat and cold measures, as well as on the patient's health status.

REASONS FOR THE APPLICATION OF HEAT

Heat is applied to the body for several reasons and can produce a local or a systemic effect. A *local effect* is one that is specific to a defined area of the body, for example, one that relieves a local muscle spasm. A *systemic effect* is one that is reflected in the body as a whole—for example, general warmth felt throughout the body.

The effect of local application of heat involves several responses: peripheral vasodilation, which increases blood supply to the area, and increased cellular metabolism and oxygen demand by the local tissues. The maximum effect of heat is reached after 20 minutes of application. After an

sult in detrimental rather than beneficial effects (Pillitteri, 1995). To avoid this secondary effect, 20–60 minutes should be allowed to elapse between heat treatments.

Heat is known to relieve pain in two ways: by relaxing muscle tone and by increasing blood flow where circulation is poor. Pain caused by the contraction of muscle fibres is relieved when the muscle spasm is reduced by heat. Heat can relieve pain related to ischemia (decreased blood supply) by increasing circulation to an area. Similarly, the pain and swelling caused by increased pressure accompanying the collection of fluid in an area can be reduced by the application of heat. As blood circulation improves, fluid is more easily absorbed from the tissues and, consequently, swelling or edema is reduced. Toxins and waste products are also thought to be causes of discomfort that can be relieved by an increase in blood circulation to the irritated tissues.

Heat helps the healing process by bringing leukocytes and lymph to the area. The suppurative process (pus formation) is increased and wound healing is enhanced. Heat can be applied to improve the oxygenation and nourishment of tissues, thus aiding tissue metabolism and subsequent healing. For example, heat applied to an infected surgical incision not only hastens suppuration but also increases the nourishment of the tissue cells and the healing process.

Another purpose of applying heat locally is to soften exudates. An exudate is a discharge produced by body tissues. Sometimes the discharge from an open wound forms hardened crusts over the area. Hot, moist compresses are often used to soften these crusts so they can be easily removed.

The fact that heat helps to alleviate many types of pain does not mean that it is indicated for all instances of pain. Since heat can hasten the suppuration process, it could aggravate an underlying inflammatory process. In the case of an inflamed appendix, heat applied to the abdomen can cause the appendix to rupture. Although the physician supplies the directions regarding the application of heat, the nurse must always be aware of the purpose of the treatment and alert to possible untoward actions. There is, for instance, always a danger that a burn may result from the local application of heat, or that deeper-lying tissues may be affected and an inflammatory process aggravated. Patients should be encouraged to advise the nurse if the application becomes uncomfortable.

If a systemic effect is desired, a hyperthermia blanket is applied. Patients should be encouraged to advise the nurse if the application becomes uncomfortable.

REASONS FOR THE APPLICATION OF COLD

Cold is applied to the body for both local and systemic effects. The local response to cold includes vasoconstriction and decreased blood flow to the area, decreased cell perfusion and slowed cellular metabolism. Cold can be applied to stop hemorrhage, since it constricts the peripheral arterioles and increases the viscosity of the blood, in addition to contracting the muscles and depressing cardiac action. Ice bags are applied routinely to patients after a tonsillectomy as a prophylactic measure against hemorrhage.

Cold applications slow the suppurative process and the absorption of tissue fluids. Cold applied immediately after an injury such as a sprained ankle helps reduce swelling by decreasing blood flow to area. Once edema has formed, cold prevents its absorption. For this reason, cold application is recommended only within the initial 24 hours after an injury and heat is applied thereafter (Kemp, Pillitteri & Brown, 1989).

Pain can also be relieved through the use of cold applications. Intense cold reduces nerve impulse conduction and decreases the perception of pain. As a result, cold is used as a local anesthetic. There is a danger in the prolonged use of intense cold: it interferes with the supply of oxygen and nourishment to the tissues and may result in tissue death. As with heat, a secondary vasodilation effect occurs after an hour of cold application. The maximum therapeutic effect of cold applications is reached in 20 minutes, and it is recommended that at least 20 minutes be allowed between treatments (Pillitteri, 1995).

For systemic purposes, cold is used to slow the basal metabolic rate. This is indicated in certain kinds of heart surgery, because a low basal metabolic rate results in a lessened demand of the body tissues for oxygen and nourishment, and thus decreases the work of the heart. Cold also slows the blood circulation. For this reason a patient's limb may be packed in ice prior to amputation. The effect of the cold enables the surgeon to control bleeding more easily during the operation.

Guide for Assessing Therapeutic Application of Heat or Cold

1. Does the patient understand the purpose of the treatment?
2. What precautions need to be taken to protect the patient from harm?
3. Is the patient aware of the dangers?
4. Are added safety precautions required because of age, general physical condition, the skin condition or the mental state of the patient?
5. Is the patient able to participate in the treatment? Is this desirable?
6. Are there specific skills that the patient (or family) needs to learn or knowledge that must be gained in order to carry out the treatment at home?
7. Is the patient safe during the application?
8. Is the patient comfortable?
9. Is the hot or cold application producing the desired physiological effect, for example, increased circulation to the part, or relief of pain?
10. Is the patient able to perceive extremes of temperature when tested for sensitivity?

Assessments for Therapeutic Applications of Heat and Cold

Prior to implementing heat and cold treatments, nurses must assess their patients for age and condition of the skin, general physical health, the area of the body that is affected and ability to perceive extremes of temperatures. The choice of the application to be used will depend on its purpose, the duration of the treatment and the availability of equipment.

AGE OF THE PATIENT AND CONDITION OF THE SKIN Infants and older adults tend to have thinner and more fragile skin. Because older adults have decreased perception of pain, and infants are not able to describe these sensations, both groups require special consideration when applying heat and cold treatments.

GENERAL PHYSICAL HEALTH Patients with circulatory problems or heart disease are particularly sensitive to applications of heat and cold (Kemp, Pillitteri & Brown, 1989). Heat applied to a large area of the body draws a significant volume of blood supply to that area and away from other areas. This could result in an inadequate amount of blood within the central circulation and compromise kidney function. Alternatively, cold application to an area with poor circulation could result in cell damage.

People who are sedated (by analgesics, anesthetics or sedatives) and those who have decreased neurological sensation (for example, diabetics, paraplegics) are less able to detect heat or cold. They may sustain tissue injury without realizing its severity.

AREA OF THE BODY AFFECTED Certain body areas, depending on the condition of the skin, are better able to tolerate heat and cold. The hands, for example, can withstand greater warmth or cold than can the abdomen or the neck. Newly formed tissues (such as a fresh surgical incision) are more tender than surrounding tissue. Thus, applications of heat or cold to the new tissue may not be tolerated (Kemp, Pillitteri & Brown, 1989).

KEY PRINCIPLES

Principles Relevant to the Therapeutic Use of Heat and Cold

1. Heat is distributed throughout the body by the circulating blood and by direct conduction throughout the tissues.
2. Heat is lost from the body chiefly through conduction, convection and evaporation at the surface of the skin.
3. The amount of heat that is lost from the body is directly proportionate to the amount of blood that is circulating close to the surface of the skin.
4. The amount of blood that circulates close to the surface of the skin is influenced by the dilatation and constriction of peripheral arterioles.
5. Applications of heat and cold influence the dilatation and constriction of peripheral blood vessels.
6. Moisture conducts heat better than air does.
7. People vary in their ability to tolerate heat and cold applications. People at both extremes of the age spectrum—that is, the very old and the very young—are particularly at risk for tissue damage from heat and cold treatments.
8. The length of time of exposure to extremes in temperature affects the body's tolerance of the temperature.
9. Decreased sensitivity to heat and cold occurs with prolonged applications.
10. Prolonged applications of heat and cold result in secondary (vasoconstriction/vasodilation) effects that may reduce the benefits of the treatment.
11. The maximum therapeutic effect of heat and cold applications is reached after 20 minutes of application.

Local Applications of Heat

Heat can be applied as radiant heat, conductive heat or conversive heat. *Radiant heat* is heat with a wavelength in the infrared portion of the electromagnetic spectrum. A commonly used example is the infrared lamp. *Conductive heat* is heat transferred by direct application, for example, by a hot water bottle or hot compress. Radiant and conductive heat provide heat to the superficial tissues only, penetrating between 2 and 10 mm in depth (Jackins & Jamieson, 1990). *Conversive heat* is heat converted from primary sources of energy, for example, from short-wave or ultrasound wave energy. The application of this latter type of heat is classified as medical diathermy; it is used to provide heat to deep tissues. Use of this type of heat treatment requires consultation with the physical therapist or physician because the increased temperature in the deep tissues may accelerate underlying inflammatory processes, such as cartilage inflammation in arthritis (Burrell, 1992).

Both moist and dry forms of heat can be applied to the skin or mucous membranes. All patients receiving dry and moist heat should be observed closely for any untoward reactions to heat applications, such as a prolonged erythema (redness), blister formation or discomfort.

DRY HEAT APPLICATIONS

The advantages of dry heat applications are that they can be directed to the local site without macerating surrounding tissues, and they help prevent contamination from microorganisms. Dry heat does have disadvantages. These include fluid loss from evaporation at the site and less penetration than moist heat.

Hot Water Bottles

The hot water bottle has long been used as a vehicle for applying dry heat to the body. It is used as both a therapeutic

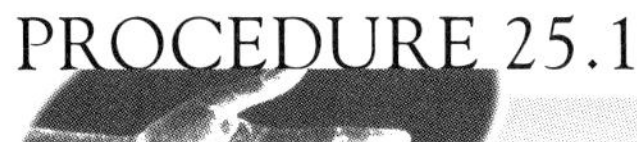

PROCEDURE 25.1 Applying a Hot Water Bottle

Action	*Rationale*
1. Prepare the patient.	Promotes patient well-being.
2. Gather: • hot water bottle • protective cover • thermometer.	Facilitates efficiency and economy of time.
3. Fill the hot water bottle and let it remain full for a few minutes, then empty it.	Allows the rubber to warm.
4. Fill the hot water bottle one-half to two-thirds full, then squeeze the sides together before putting on the top.	Expels air from the remainder of the bottle, making it light and easy to mould to the body.
5. Dry the outside of the hot water bottle, test it for leakage, then place it in its entirety in a cloth cover before taking it to the patient.	The cover slows the transmission of heat, absorbs perspiration and thereby lessens the danger of burning the patient.
6. Place the hot water bottle on the desired area and mould it to the patient's body. If the patient burns easily, place a sheet or blanket between the patient and the bottle.	Facilitates the effectiveness of heat. Protects the patient from thermal injury.
7. Caution the patient against refilling the bottle without checking the temperature.	Protects the patient from thermal injury.
8. Document the procedure and any responses to the treatment.	Fulfills requirements for nurse accountability.
9. When a hot water bottle is not in use, hang it upside-down with the top unscrewed.	This allows the bottle to dry inside and prevents the sides of the bottle from sticking together.

and a comfort measure, although therapeutically its use is being surpassed by the electric heating pad. Some hospitals and other inpatient health agencies have prohibited the use of hot water bottles because of the ever-present danger of burns to patients. Procedure 25.1 outlines how to administer a hot water bottle.

PREPARING THE PATIENT Explain the purpose and duration of the procedure to the patient. Since patients become accustomed to heat after prolonged applications, they should be cautioned not to refill a hot water bottle without checking the temperature. Any pain or discomfort should be reported immediately. The TPR is taken prior to commencing the application as a baseline for evaluating the patient's response to treatment.

ASSEMBLING EQUIPMENT Because the rubber of the hot water bottle readily heats up to the temperature of the inside water, it can cause a burn. Therefore, the water for a hot water bottle must be tested for its exact temperature. Maintaining water temperature between 38° and 43°C is generally considered to be a safe guideline. A temperature at the lowest end of this range is considered safe for children (Wong, 1995) and for adults who are unconscious or debilitated or who have impaired circulation. The water for a hot water bottle can be obtained from the hot water tap; its temperature is checked by the thermometers that most agencies provide for measuring the temperature of unsterile solutions. As a general guide, the temperature of the water should be comfortable when tested on the nurse's inner wrist.

Heating Pads

Electric heating pads and electric blankets are frequently used as a means of providing dry heat. They have the advantages of being light, of being easily moulded to the patient's body and of providing constant heat at a constant temperature. Their disadvantages are related to their cleaning and to the danger of short circuits. Guidelines for applying heating pads are outlined in Procedure 25.2.

PREPARING THE PATIENT Patient preparation is the same as that for applying a hot water bottle. The patient should be cautioned against turning up the temperature setting on the heating pad to avoid the risk of thermal injury.

ASSEMBLING EQUIPMENT There are two basic types of heating pads. The first, called an *electric heating pad*, is a flat waterproof pad made up of a control switch and a coiled element that converts electric current to dry heat. The temperature should be set at the lowest setting unless otherwise prescribed by the physician. High and medium temperature settings place the patient at risk for burn injury; this is of particular concern with children, older people and patients whose perception of pain and warmth may be dulled by analgesics or other medications. The temperature

PROCEDURE 25.2 Applying a Heating Pad

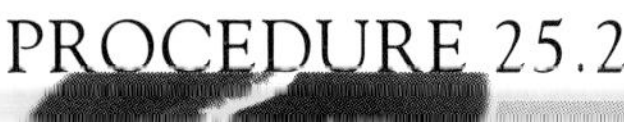

Action	Rationale
1. Prepare the patient.	Promotes the patient's well-being.
2. Gather: • electric heating pad or aquathermia pad and unit • towel or flannel cloth • distilled water for aquathermia unit.	Promotes efficiency and economy of time. Prevents mineral deposits in the unit.
3. Wrap a thin towel or flannel cloth around the heating pad.	Avoids direct contact with the patient's skin. Controls the rate of heat transfer.
4. **Electric heating pad:** Set the temperature at its lowest setting, or as ordered. **Aquathermia pad:** Set the temperature at 40.5°C, or as ordered.	Prevents burn injury.
5. At bedside, plug unit into an electrical outlet and allow pad to warm for a few minutes. Place aquathermia unit on a stable surface and slightly higher than the patient.	Force of gravity assists the flow of water through the pad.
6. Check the temperature of the pad by pressing it against the inner aspect of the forearm.	Alerts the nurse to mechanical dysfunction and prevents accidental burning.
7. Apply the pad to the designated area for 20 minutes.	Ensures patient safety.
8. Monitor the patient for untoward reactions.	
9. Remove the pad after treatment is completed. Store unit as per agency policy.	
10. Document the procedure and any responses to the treatment.	Fulfills requirements for nurse accountability.

control switch should be secured so that is cannot be changed. This can be done by putting adhesive tape on both sides of the control switch, and placing it out of reach of the patient. It is recommended that this be done routinely for children under 12 years of age, and for those patients who may be tempted to increase the temperature setting.

The second type of heating pad is the *aquamatic* or **aquathermia pad**. It is a vinyl pad consisting of channels through which heated water circulates, transmitting dry heat of a constant temperature. The pad is attached to an electrically operated unit that stores, heats and circulates warmed distilled water (see Figure 25.3). Distilled water is used because tap water leaves mineral deposits in the unit. The temperature is preset with a plastic key and is thermostatically controlled. This adds a safety feature in that the temperature setting cannot be changed without the use of a key. Aquathermia pads come in various sizes.

Both types of heating pads are made of a plastic material. If this covering comes in contact with perspiring skin, maceration can occur. Therefore, these electric pads must be covered before use on patients. Towelling further controls the rate of heat transfer (Lehmann & deLateur, 1990).

Chemical Heat Packs

These packs are made of heavy-duty plastic with separate compartments filled with chemicals that produce heat when they react with each other. To activate the chemical reaction, the nurse strikes the pack against the countertop or kneads it between the hands. The temperature of the pack reaches between 40.5° and 46°C and may vary according to the manufacturer (Kemp, Pillitteri & Brown, 1989).

The principles for applying chemical heat packs are similar to those used for a hot water bottle and electric pad.

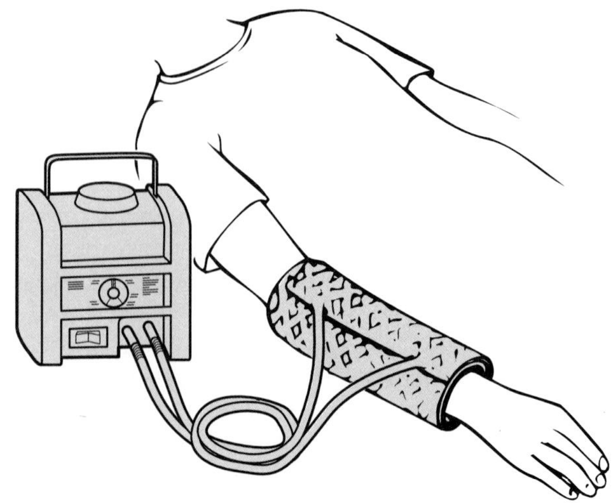

FIGURE 25.3 The aquathermia pad and unit

SOURCE: Norton & Miller, 1989, p. 438.

Specific to heat packs, safety pins should not be used to secure the pack because a puncture could precipitate leakage and a chemical burn.

MOIST HEAT APPLICATIONS

Moist heat applications have the advantage of providing more penetrating warmth than dry heat because moisture is conducive to heat transfer. By the same token, moist heat applications tend to cool more quickly (through evaporation) and they need to be reapplied to maintain the therapeutic effect. Moisture on the skin makes it prone to maceration; nurses must carefully assess the site of application and the surrounding skin for breakdown.

Hot Compresses

Hot compresses are moist applications of sterile or unsterile [illegible] compress is to be applied to an open wound or to an organ such as the eye. Hot compresses are often indicated to hasten the suppurative process and to improve the circulation of blood to the tissues. Normal saline and antiseptic solutions are frequently ordered by the physician. Procedure 25.3 outlines how to apply hot compresses.

PREPARING THE PATIENT Explain the purpose, duration and sensations the patient may feel during the procedure. The compresses will feel warm but should not be painful. Pain should be reported immediately.

PROCEDURE 25.3 Applying Hot Compresses

Action	*Rationale*
1. Prepare the patient.	Promotes patient's well-being.
2. Gather clean or sterile: • basin • tap water or solution • gauze sponges or prepared compresses • forceps • gloves • sterile absorbent pad or towel • plastic wrap • petroleum jelly and applicator • waterproof protective pad • dressing supplies.	Promotes efficiency and economy of time.
3. Expose the area to be treated. Place a waterproof pad under the treatment site.	Protects the bed linen from moisture.
4. Prepare solution and compresses. For a sterile procedure, open a sterile basin, add sterile gauze sponges and pour in hot sterile solution. For an unsterile procedure, add gauze sponges and hot tap water to a clean basin. Test temperature. Have commercially prepared packs in easy reach.	Readies supplies for the procedure. Protects the patient from thermal injury.
5. Using gloves, remove old dressing, if present, and discard. Remove and discard gloves. Apply petroleum jelly to area if necessary. Use sterile gloves or applicator for a sterile procedure.	Acts as a water barrier and protects the skin from maceration.
6. Using clean or sterile technique, wring out excess fluid from the compresses.	Prevents rapid evaporation and cooling of compresses.
7. Apply the gauze to the area. Check for skin reaction. If there is no excessive redness, blistering or pain, mould the compress to the site.	Protects the patient from thermal injury. Moulding the compress facilitates heat retention.
8. Cover the moist dressing with plastic wrap and then a dry towel. For sterile procedures, place a sterile abdominal pad over the compress before applying the plastic wrap. If ordered, apply a hot water bottle or aquathermia pad over the compress. Never use an electric heating pad for this purpose.	Facilitates heat retention by slowing evaporation and the cooling process. Holds the heat of the compress more uniformly. Moisture may cause an electric shock.

continued on next page

PROCEDURE 25.3 *continued*

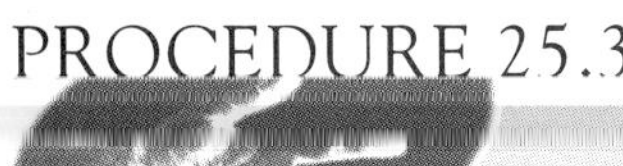

Action	Rationale
9. Leave the compress on for 15–20 min. Monitor the site and the patient's response during the procedure.	Maximum therapeutic effect is reached in this time.
10. Remove the compress, assess the condition of the site and dress it as necessary.	Provides data for evaluating the effectiveness of treatment.
11. Discard supplies and clean and store equipment per agency protocol.	Promotes cleanliness and safety in the workplace.
12. Document the procedure, the condition of the site and the patient's response to treatment.	Fulfills requirements for nurse accountability.

ASSEMBLING EQUIPMENT Hot compresses may be applied by clean or sterile techniques. When clean technique is used, a basin with hot tap water is assembled along with clean forceps, gauze sponges, towels, plastic wrap, dressing supplies and a waterproof protective pad. When the compress is to be applied with sterile technique, the solution, basin, gauze sponges, forceps and dressing supplies must be sterile. Sterile gloves may also be used. Sterile solution is heated by placing the solution container in a sink or large basin of hot water. The temperature of the solution should be 55°C for adults and 40.6°C for children, older people and for eye compresses (Malloch, 1993). The temperature can be tested by pouring a small amount of solution into a container, checking it with a thermometer and then discarding the solution. Clean tap water can be tested directly.

Some agencies use commercially prepared compresses. These eliminate the need for a basin of solution. The compresses (contained in sealed packages) are heated in a special heater and then taken to the bedside. A sterile absorbent pad or towel and plastic wrap are placed over the compress to retain heat and moisture during the procedure. If the patient's skin is prone to maceration, petroleum jelly is applied to the area (sterile jelly is used on the edges of an open wound, if present). Petroleum jelly acts as a water barrier and protects the skin from maceration. It also protects the area from burns because it decreases the rate of heat penetration (Malloch, 1993).

Hot Packs

A hot pack is sometimes referred to as a *hot fomentation* or *foment*. It is a piece of heated moist flannel or similar material that is applied to a patient's skin in order to supply superficial moist heat. It is used for a larger area than the hot compress is. Hot packs are frequently indicated to relieve muscle spasm. They are also applied to hasten the suppurative process and to decrease muscle soreness.

A hot pack can be prepared by boiling or steaming pieces of flannel or by heating commercially prepared packs. If the flannel is boiled it is necessary to wring it out before applying it. There are hot pack machines available that steam the flannel to prepare it for application. Because intense heat can be applied in this manner, there is a danger that the patient may be burned. This danger is minimized if the hot pack is sufficiently dry that water does not drip from it.

The procedure for applying a hot pack is similar to that for a hot compress. The patient is prepared by explaining the procedure. Sometimes petrolatum is applied to the skin beforehand to serve as a protective coating and to slow the transfer of heat. Once the foment has been heated, it is shaken slightly before it is applied. This step distributes the heat evenly, and reduces the danger of burning the patient. The hot foment is covered with an insulating waterproof material and then secured to the patient with a towel or binder. As with hot compresses, a hot water bottle or aquathermia pad may be applied over a hot pack to maintain its heat.

A hot pack usually keeps hot for 10–15 minutes. Once it has cooled it is removed and, if a longer treatment is required, it is replaced with another pack. If the patient does not need another application for some time, the skin is dried.

Erythema (redness) of the skin is expected with the application of hot packs because the heat causes dilatation of the local blood capillaries. If blistering of the skin occurs, it should be reported and the treatment withheld until the physician is consulted.

Hydrotherapy

Hydrotherapy, also known as "tubbing" or "tanking" (from Hubbard tanks), is used in burn therapy for wound cleansing, range of motion exercises and total body bathing. Whirlpool baths are units that are small enough to accommodate a leg or an arm for these same purposes. These units can also serve as a source of heat treatment for patients with traumatic injury or those with stiffness and swelling of joints. Special portable containers, such as arm and foot baths, also are available commercially for use at home. Water agitation in whirlpools and Hubbard tanks is created by air bubbled into the water. This swirling motion stimulates circulation, promotes relaxation and helps to clean wounds. When the body is totally submerged in water, the limbs

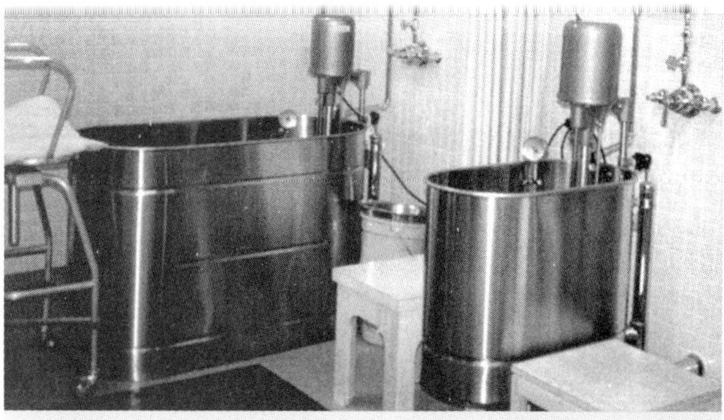

Whirlpool bath.

become weightless, thus facilitating active and passive range of motion exercises. Hydrotherapy is often carried out in the physiotherapy department or in specialized burn units.

Sitz-Baths

The **sitz-bath** is a special bath, the purposes of which are chiefly to provide warmth, to cleanse and to provide comfort to the patient's perineal area. It is often indicated after rectal or perineal surgery and is used routinely after childbirth for promoting perineal healing and comfort. Procedure 25.4 outlines how to administer a sitz-bath.

PREPARING THE PATIENT Explain the purpose and the procedure, as well as sensations the patient may feel. Comfort is an important concern for patients who have experienced perineal trauma. Tell patients that initially they may experience some discomfort because the tissues are tender. However, this should subside within a few minutes. Some patients may require analgesia prior to the procedure. The bath takes about 20 minutes. The patient may want to take some reading material to help pass the time. Because of the localized vasodilation that occurs in response to the heat, dizziness and faintness may occur when getting out of or off the sitz-bath. The patient should be warned about this and instructed to stand up and change position very slowly.

ASSEMBLING EQUIPMENT There are several commercially manufactured sitz-baths available. Some models are portable and disposable (Figure 25.4). These models can fit over toilets, on commode chairs or on beds. There are also comfort seats and inflatable rings that can be placed in bathtubs, as well as separate sitz-bath units. The sitz-bath is generally ordered with saline solution or tap water. The temperature should be 38.9°–40.6°C.

Ultraviolet Lamps

Ultraviolet radiation is used clinically to treat wounds and skin diseases such as psoriasis. The sun is a natural source of ultraviolet light, but artificial sources such as ultraviolet

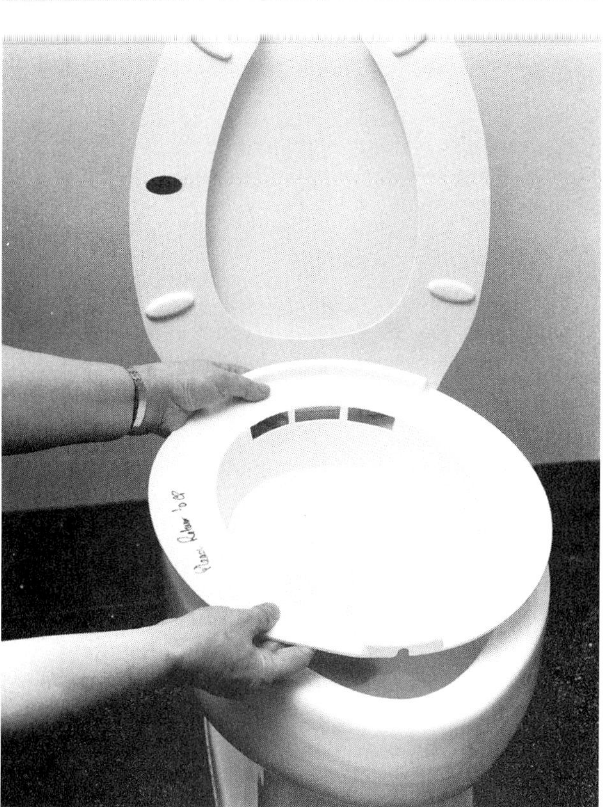

FIGURE 25.4 Portable sitz-bath

lamps and booths are used therapeutically. The hot quartz mercury lamp, the carbon arc lamp and the sun lamp are all used.

Generally, ultraviolet radiation treatment is carried out in a special department, such as the physiotherapy department. The normal skin reaction produces an erythema, tanning and a proliferation of the cells of the epidermis. The physician generally orders ultraviolet treatments every other day for maximum effect. Fair-skinned people are more sensitive to ultraviolet radiation than dark-skinned people. Sulfonamides also increase sensitivity.

Diathermy

Medical diathermy is the provision of heat to the deep tissues of the body by transforming certain kinds of physical energy into heat. It is usually done in a physical therapy department under the direction of a physician.

Various high-frequency currents are used: short-wave, microwave and ultrasound. The treatment is painless; the patient's chief perception is one of warmth. Diathermy is used for much the same reasons as superficial heat is. It is generally not administered to individuals with cardiac pacemakers because the currents may interfere with the function of the pacemaker (Jackins & Jamieson, 1990).

PROCEDURE 25.4 Administering a Sitz-Bath

Action	*Rationale*
1. Prepare the patient.	Promotes patient participation and well-being.
2. Gather: • portable sitz-bath or inflatable ring • towels • bath blanket • patient's clean clothing.	Facilitates efficiency and economy of time.
3. Fill the basin or bathtub with water or ordered solution until it is two-thirds (basin) or one-third (tub) full.	Ensures the perineal area will be adequately immersed.
4. Check the temperature of the water with thermometer or the inner aspect of the wrist.	Protects the patient from thermal injury.
5. **Bathtub:** Place an inflatable ring on tub bottom. **Portable basin:** Place the basin on the toilet or commode.	
6. Assist the patient into a comfortable position in the sitz-bath, ensuring that the perineal area is immersed in water. Provide adequate support with towels, particularly if there is doubt about the patient's ability to tolerate the procedure.	Promotes patient comfort and effectiveness of therapy.
7. Cover the patient with a towel or bath blanket.	Promotes privacy and avoids chilling.
8. Stay with the patient if an analgesia was given; otherwise, show the patient how to use the call bell and assess condition at regular intervals.	Protects the patient from injury. Analgesia may cause light-headedness.
9. After 20 min, assist the patient to get off the sitz-bath or out of the tub. The patient should stand up slowly and hold onto a safety rail if one is available.	Protects the patient from falling.
10. Dry the area and dress the wound as necessary. Assist patient to dress and to return to bed.	
11. Dispose of supplies and clean the sitz-bath per agency protocol.	Ensures safety and cleanliness in the workplace.
12. Document the procedure, the condition of the site and the patient's response to treatment.	Fulfills requirements for nurse accountability.

Local Applications of Cold

Cold applications are available in dry or wet forms. Tissue damage can ensue from intense and prolonged cold applications. Signs of tissue damage include mottling, purplish or bluish colour of the skin surface, blisters and numbness.

DRY COLD APPLICATIONS

The ice bag, ice cap, ice collar and ice pack are commonly used means of applying dry cold to the body. An ice collar is a long, narrow rubber or plastic bag that fits around the neck. Commercial plastic packs that can be frozen and reused are frequently used in lieu of the ice bag. Care should be taken to avoid puncturing these packs because the chemicals in the coolant liquid can cause tissue injury. An ice bag can also be made by filling a disposable glove with crushed ice.

Ice bags are usually made with an opening through which small pieces of ice are inserted. The procedure for applying an ice bag is similar to that for a hot water bottle. Once the ice bag is filled to two-thirds of its capacity, the air is expelled before the top of the ice bag is secured. As with the hot water bottle, the air in the ice bag is removed so that it can be moulded to the patient's body.

Ice applications should never be in direct contact with the skin; a cold injury could result from the intense cold. Therefore, a flannel cover should be put over an ice bag once it is dried. The cover retains cold for more gradual application and it absorbs the water formed by atmospheric condensation. The bag is placed on the area of the body to be cooled.

When an ice bag is in place, it is important to ensure that the pressure of the bag does not cut off circulation. At the first sign of tissue numbness and a mottled bluish appearance, the bag should be removed and the physician notified. These signs could be the result of either the cold or pressure upon the tissues.

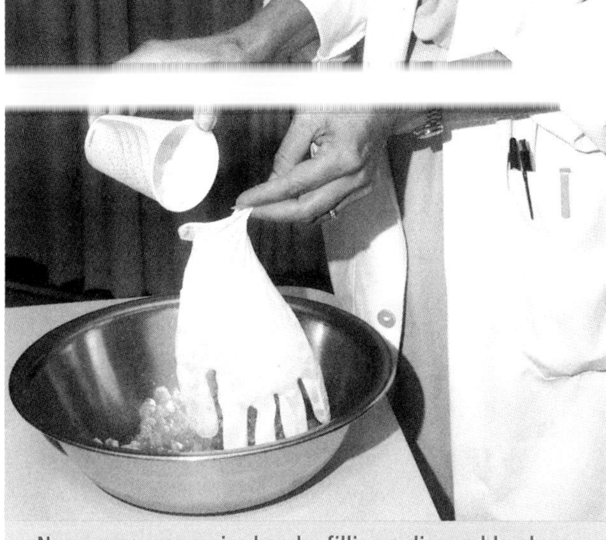

Nurse prepares an ice bag by filling a disposable glove with crushed ice.

Ice bags that are not in use are stored with the tops removed so that the air will dry the inside and prevent the sides from sticking together. An economic alternative to an ice bag, which can be used at home, is a small bag of frozen peas that can be easily moulded and applied. The bag of peas, can be refrozen for future use. It should be labelled "for external use only" since defrosted and refrozen foods should not be eaten.

MOIST COLD APPLICATIONS

Moist cold can be applied by means of ice compresses. These are frequently used to control a nosebleed (epistaxis) or to supply moist cold to the eye.

An ice compress is usually made of gauze or other cloth material. Moistened gauze is cooled over ice chips, wrung out and then applied. The compress is covered with a waterproof pad to keep it cool longer and for patient comfort, as this prevents moisture from dripping on the patient. It is replaced as it becomes warm.

Evaluating Temperature Regulation Interventions

The evaluation of care for patients experiencing disturbances in temperature regulation is based on the expected outcomes for identified problems. The following guidelines may assist the nurse in determining effectiveness of care.

1. Has the patient's temperature come down? gone up? Is it within safe limits?
2. Is the fluid intake adequate for the patient's needs?
3. Is the diet adequate?
4. Is the patient comfortable?
5. Is the patient obtaining sufficient rest?
6. Are the skin and oral cavity in good condition?

IN REVIEW

central body temperature is about 37°C. Temperature is a measure of body heat, reflecting a balance between heat gain and heat loss.

- To maintain a constant body temperature, heat produced by cellular metabolism must be lost to the environment. This is accomplished by the mechanisms:
  - conduction
  - convection
  - evaporation
  - radiation.
- Thermal dysfunction occurs when the body temperature rises or falls outside the narrow range of normal.
- Body temperature is affected by any condition that increases the basal metabolic rate, such as:
  - activity
  - thyroxine production
  - digestion and absorption of food
  - circadian rhythm
  - strong emotions
  - body size and mass
  - external environment (climate)
  - illness and health problems.
- Temperature regulation varies throughout the life cycle.

  Infants and children:
  - at birth, regulating mechanisms are immature
  - high fevers are common in early childhood

  Adolescents:
  - sweating begins
  - young women experience a cyclic rise and fall associated with their menstrual periods

  Women:
  - high fever during pregnancy is teratogenic
  - during menopause, "hot flashes" are experienced by most women

  Older adults:
  - have a lower body temperature
  - are unable to cope with extreme temperature variations.
- Fever is thought to be caused by abnormalities in the brain or by toxic substances that affect the temperature-regulating mechanisms.
- The stages of fever are:
  - chill phase
  - course of the fever
  - termination of the fever.

- Signs and symptoms of fever include:
  - increased cellular metabolism
  - increased bodily demands for fluid, oxygen and glucose
  - increased respiratory and pulse rates.
- As the cause of fever is controlled, the process reverses and mechanisms for heat dissipation are instituted.
- Common health problems associated with thermal dysfunction include:
  - heat cramps
  - heat exhaustion
  - heat stroke
  - malignant hyperthermia
  - hypothermia.
- The nurse's role in caring for an individual with a thermal dysfunction includes:
  - assessing the patient's temperature-regulating status (measuring body temperature; taking a health history; observing for signs of disturbed thermal regulation)
  - identifying nursing diagnoses related to thermal dysfunction
  - planning and implementing nursing interventions (collaborating with other health professionals; educating individuals and families; providing rest, comfort and hygiene measures and adequate fluid; administering antipyretics/antibiotics; administering local and systemic heat/cold therapy)
  - evaluating the effectiveness of planned care.
- Nonpharmacological therapies include:
  - ice pack/hot water bottle
  - cold compress/heat pack
  - cooling/warming blanket
  - cold/hot fluids
  - hydrotherapy/sitz-bath
  - heat lamp.

Critical Thinking Activities

1. Mrs. S. Lopez is a 34-year-old woman who works as an aide in a city hospital. She is married and has a 5-year-old son. Mrs. Lopez was admitted to the hospital with an elevated temperature, intermittent shaking, chills, nausea, vomiting and diarrhea over the past 24 hours. Her temperature at admission was 39.1° C, her pulse 100 and her respirations 24. She has no known allergies. The patient continued to have chills and diarrhea during her first evening in the hospital, and her fever rose to 40° C.

   The doctor left the following orders for Mrs. Lopez:

   - acetaminophen 325 mg, two tablets q4h for temperature greater than 38°C
   - IV D5W at 100 mL/h
   - clear fluids as tolerated
   - stool specimen for C&S.

   a. How can the loss of body heat be facilitated?
   b. What is the action of acetaminophen?
   c. How would you evaluate the effectiveness of the nursing care?
   d. What observations would indicate that the patient is taking insufficient fluid?
   e. Describe an environment that would be therapeutic for this patient.
   f. Why has the doctor requested a stool specimen for culture and sensitivity?
   g. What observations would you include in your assessment of Mrs. Lopez?
   h. What nursing strategies would you employ to promote Mrs. Lopez's comfort and hydration?

2. Mrs. J. Watson has an infected cut on her right hand. She is at home and the physician has ordered hot compresses for her hand. As the home care nurse, you have been asked to assist Mrs. Watson. This patient is 75 years old and has poor blood circulation.

   a. What are the specific problems of this patient in relation to her infected cut?
   b. What factors should you take into consideration in helping to plan this patient's care?
   c. What physiological reactions are to be expected as a result of the hot compresses?
   d. How could the effectiveness of the compresses be evaluated?
   e. What specific precautions should be taken? Why?
   f. Outline the nursing diagnoses, expected outcomes and a plan of care for this patient.

KEY TERMS

core temperature p. 774
homeothermic p. 774
normothermia p. 774
thermoregulation p. 774
neutral thermal environment p. 778
fever p. 780
pyrexia p. 781
chill p. 781
diaphoresis p. 782
hyperthermia p. 783
hypothermia p. 783
aquathermia pad p. 796
hot compress p. 797
hydrotherapy p. 798
sitz-bath p. 799

References

BARNES, S.B., & WALKER, J.S. (1995, June). Summertime emergencies: How to keep the heat from taking its toll. *Consultant*, 803-807, 811–812

ed.). Philadelphia: Lippincott.

BEHRMAN, R., KLIEGMAN, R., & ARVIN, A. (1996). Fever. In A. Arvin (Ed.), *Nelson textbook of paediatrics* (pp. 692–704). (15th ed.). Philadelphia: W.B. Saunders.

BENZINGER, T.H. (1969). Heat regulation: Homeostasis of central temperature in man. *Physiological Review, 49*(4), 671–759.

BOSS, B.J., FARLEY, J.A., & MOONEY, K.H. (1996). Alterations of neurologic function in children. In S.E. Huether & K.L. McCance (Eds.), *Understanding pathophysiology* (chapter 15). St. Louis: Mosby.

BOYD, V. (1996). Dealing with heat stress. *Occupational Health & Safety, 65*(7), 37–39.

BRITT, L.D., DASCOMBE, W.H., & RODRIGUEZ, A. (1991). New horizons in management of hypothermia and frostbite. *Surgical Clinics of North America, 71*(2), 345–356.

BRUCK, K. (1983). Heat balance and the regulation of body temperature. In R.F. Schmidt & G. Thews (Eds.), *Human physiology* (pp. 531–547). Berlin: Springer-Verlag.

BURRELL, L.O. (1992). *Adult nursing in hospital and community settings.* Norwalk, CT: Appleton & Lange.

CARLSON, K., EISENSTADT, S., & ZIPORYN, T. (1996). *The Harvard guide to women's health.* Cambridge, MA: Harvard University Press.

CARPENITO, L.J. (1997). *Nursing diagnosis: Application to clinical practice.* (7th ed.). Philadelphia: Lippincott.

COHEN, R., & MOELLEKEN, B.R.W. (1996). Disorders due to physical agents. In L.M. Tierney, II, S.J. McPhee, & M.A. Papadakis (Eds.), *Current medical diagnosis and treatment* (chapter 37). Stamford, CT: Appleton & Lange.

COOPER, K.E. (1969, June). Regulation of body temperature. *British Journal of Hospital Medicine*, 1065–1067.

CUNHA, B.A. (1996a). The clinical significance of fever patterns. *Infectious Disease Clinics of North America, 10*(1), 33–34.

CUNHA, B.A. (1996b). Fever of unknown origin. *Infectious Disease Clinics of North America, 10*(1), 111–127.

DEXTER, W.W. (1990). Hypothermia: Safe and efficient methods of rewarming the patient. *Postgraduate Medicine, 88*(8), 55–64.

DINARELLO, C.A. (1996). Thermoregulation and the pathogenesis of fever. *Infectious Disease Clinics of North America, 10*(2), 433–449.

DRAKE, D.K., & NETTINA, S.M. (1994). Recognition and management of heat related illness. *Nurse Practitioner, 19*(8), 43–47.

DuBOIS, E.F. (1921). The basal metabolism in fever. *Journal of the American Medical Association, 77*(5), 352–355.

EBERSOLE, P., & HESS, P. (1998). *Towards healthy aging: Human needs and nursing response.* (5th ed.). St. Louis: Mosby.

ERICKSON, R. (1982). A model of adaptation to the thermal environment. *Advances in Nursing Science, 15*(2), 1–12.

FRIEDMAN, A., & BARTON, L. (1990). Efficacy of sponging vs. acetaminophen for reduction of fever. *Pediatric Emergency Care, 6*(1), 6–7.

FRUTHALER, G.J. (1985, November). Fever in children: Phobia vs. facts. *Hospital Practice*, 49–53.

GANONG, W.F. (1997). *Review of medical physiology.* (18th ed.). Norwalk, CT: Appleton & Lange.

GARCHINSKI, L., GILMORE, A., MacKAY, J., & OSTAPOWICH, S. (1994). Miracle child: Resuscitation from profound hypothermia—A case study. *Official Journal of Canadian Association of Critical Care Nurses, 5*(4), 28–29, 32–34.

GUYTON, A.C. (1996). *Textbook of medical physiology.* (9th ed.). Philadelphia: W.B. Saunders.

HANSON, M. (1991). Drug fever. *Postgraduate Medicine, 89*(5), 167–173.

JACKINS, S., & JAMIESON, A. (1990). Use of heat and cold in physical therapy. In J.F. Lehmann (Ed.), *Therapeutic heat and cold.* (4th ed.). Baltimore:

JOHNSON, D., & CUNHA, B. (1996). Drug fever. *Infectious Disease Clinics of North America, 10*(1), 85–91.

KELLERMAN, A.L., & TODD, K.H. (1996). Killing heat. *New England Journal of Medicine, 335*(2), 126–127.

KEMP, B., PILLITTERI, A., & BROWN, P. (1989). *Fundamentals of nursing.* (2nd ed.). Glenview, IL: Scott Foresman.

KHOGALI, M. (1997). Heat illness alert program: Practical implications for management and prevention. *Annals of the New York Academy of Sciences, 813*, 526–533.

KHOGALI, M., & MUSTAFA, M.K.Y. (1984). Physiology of heat stroke: A review. In J.R.S. Hales, (Ed.), *Thermal physiology* (pp. 503–510). New York: Raven.

KINMOUTH, A., FULTON, Y., & CAMPBELL, M.J. (1992). Management of feverish children at home. *British Medical Journal, 305*, 1134–1136.

KLEIN, N. & CUNHA, B. (1996). Treatment of fever. *Infectious Disease Clinics of North America, 10*(1), 211–215.

KOHL, J. (1996). Heat stroke. *American Journal of Nursing, 96*(7), 51.

LEHMANN, J.F., & deLATEUR, B.J. (1990). Therapeutic heat. In J.F. Lehmann (Ed.), *Therapeutic heat and cold.* (4th ed.). Baltimore: Williams & Wilkins.

LOPEZ, J., McMILLIN, K., TOBIAS-MERRILL, E., & CHOP, W. (1997). Managing fever in infants and toddlers. *Postgraduate Medicine, 101*(2), 241–252.

LUDWIG-BEYMER, P., & HUETHER, S.E. (1996). Alterations of neurologic function in children. In S.E. Huether & K.L. McCance (Eds.), *Understanding pathophysiology* (chapter 15). St. Louis: Mosby.

MALLOCH, K. (1993). Physical treatments. In Springhouse Corporation (Ed.), *Nursing procedures: Student version.* Springhouse, PA: Springhouse.

MANITOBA HEALTH. (1990). *Menopause and midlife health for women.* Winnipeg: Author.

MARTINI, F. (1998). *Fundamentals of anatomy and physiology.* (4th ed.). Upper Saddle River, NJ: Prentice Hall.

MAY, K.A., & MAHLMEISTER, L.R. (1994). *Maternal and neonatal nursing: Family-centered care.* (3rd ed.). Philadelphia: Lippincott.

McCANCE, K., & HUETHER, S.E. (1994). *Pathophysiology: The biologic basis for disease in adults and children.* (2nd ed.). St. Louis: Mosby.

McFARLAND, G.K., & McFARLANE, E.A. (1997). *Nursing diagnosis and intervention: Planning for patient care.* (3rd ed.). St. Louis: Mosby.

METHENEY, N.M. (1996). *Fluid and electrolyte balance: Nursing considerations.* (3rd ed.). Philadelphia: Lippincott.

MILLER, C.A. (1995). *Nursing care of older adults.* (2nd ed.). Glenview, IL: Scott Foresman.

MITCHELL, D., & LABURN, H.P. (1985). Pathophysiology of temperature regulation. *The Physiologist, 28*(6), 507–517.

MURPHY, K. (1992). Acetaminophen and ibuprofen: Fever control and overdose. *Pediatric Nursing, 18*(4), 428–432.

NORMAN, D., & YOSHIKAWA, T. (1996). Fever in the elderly. *Infectious Disease Clinics of North America, 10*(1), 93–99.

NORTON, B.A., & MILLER, A.M. (1989). *Skills for professional nursing practice.* Norwalk, CT: Appleton-Century-Crofts.

PILLITTERI, A. (1995). *Maternal and child health: Nursing care of the childbearing and childrearing family.* (2nd ed.). Philadelphia: Lippincott.

PORTH, C. (1998). *Pathophysiology: Concepts of altered health states.* (5th ed.). Philadelphia: Lippincott.

ROBERTS, D. (1994, March 1). Frozen child's revival makes medical history. *The Globe and Mail.*

SHARBER, J. (1997). The efficacy of tepid sponge bathing to reduce fever in young children. *American Journal of Emergency Medicine, 15*(2), 188–192.

SHAW, C.R. (1997). The perimenopausal hot flash: Epidemiology, physiology, and treatment. *Nurse Practitioner, 22*(3), 55–66.

SIMON, H.B. (1994). Hypothermia and heat stroke. *Hospital Practice, 29*(8), 65–68, 73, 78.

SMELTZER, S., & BARE, B. (1996). In *Brunner & Suddarth's textbook of medical–surgical nursing*. (8th ed.). Philadelphia: Lippincott.

THOMAS, D.O. (1995, April). Fever in children: Friend or foe? *RN*, 42–48.

THOMPSON, J., & WILSON, S. (1996). *Health assessment for nursing practice*. St. Louis: Mosby.

VICTORIA GENERAL HOSPITAL. (1994). *Fever in a child* (teaching pamphlet). Winnipeg: Victoria General Hospital Education Department.

WENGER, C.B., & HARDY, J.D. (1990). Temperature regulation and exposure to heat and cold. In J.F. Lehmann (Ed.), *Therapeutic heat and cold*. (4th ed.). Baltimore: Williams & Wilkins.

WILLIAMS, M.H. (1993). *Lifetime: Fitness and wellness*. (3rd ed.). Madison, WI: Brown & Benchmark.

WONG, D.L. (1995). *Whaley & Wong's nursing care of infants and children*. (5th ed.). St. Louis: Mosby.

WORFOLK, J.B. (1997). Keep frail elders warm! *American Journal of Care for the Aging, 18*(1), 7–11.

Additional Readings

BRAUN, S.K., PRESTON, P., & SMITH, R.N. (1998, March). Getting a better read on thermometry. *RN*, 57–60.

ERICKSON, R.S., MEYER, L.T., & WOO, T.M. (1996). Accuracy of chemical dot thermometers in critically ill adults and young children. *Image, 28*(1), 23–33.

HASKELLER, M., BORUTA B., & FRANKEL, H.L. (1997). Hypothermia. *Journal of Advanced Nursing Practice, 8*(1), 368.

HENKER, R., & COYNE, C. (1995). Comparison of peripheral temperature measurements with core temperature. *AACN Clinical Issues, 6*(1), 21–30.

HENKER, R., & ROGERS, S. (1997). Fever. *Journal of Advanced Nursing Practice, 8*(1), 351.

HOLTZCLAW, B.J. (1992). The febrile response in critical care: State of the science. *Heart & Lung, 21*(5), 482–501.

HOLTZCLAW, B.J. (1997). Perioperative problems: Threats to thermal balance in the elderly. *Seminars in Perioperative Nursing, 6*(1), 42–48.

KOHL, J. (1996). Heat Stroke. *American Journal of Nursing, 96*(7), 51.

SHEERAN, M.S. (1996). Thermoregulation in neonates: Obtaining an accurate axillary temperature measurement. *Journal of Neonatal Nursing, 2*(4), 6–9.

WATSON, R. (1998). Controlling body temperature in adults. *Nursing Standard, 12*(20), 49–55.

YOSHIKAWA, T. (1994). Approach to the diagnosis and treatment of the infected older adult. In W.R. Hazzard, E.L. Bierman, J.P. Blass, W.H. Ettinger, II, & J.B. Halter (Eds.), *Principles of geriatric medicine and gerontology* (pp. 1157–1163). (3rd ed.). New York: McGraw-Hill.

Chapter

Rest and Sleep Needs

OUTLINE

Introduction

The Physiology of Sleep and Rest

Determinants of Sleep and Rest

Sleep and Rest Throughout the Life Cycle

Common Problems

Assessing Rest and Sleep Needs

Diagnosing Rest and Sleep Problems

Planning Rest and Sleep Interventions

Implementing Rest and Sleep Interventions

Evaluating Rest and Sleep Interventions

Central Questions

1. How are rest and sleep important to health and well-being?
2. What are the characteristics of the five stages of sleep?
3. How do normal sleep patterns vary throughout the life cycle?
4. What is the relationship between illness and sleep disturbances?
5. What are the main factors that interfere with rest and sleep?
6. What are the common sleep problems?
7. What basic principles does the nurse apply in assisting patients meet their rest and sleep needs?
8. How does the nurse assess rest and sleep needs?
9. What are the common nursing diagnostic statements for patients with rest and sleep problems?
10. What is a sleep plan, and why is it important in patient care?
11. What information might the nurse give to individuals, families or groups in helping them to promote optimum rest and sleep?
12. What health-protecting measures does the nurse implement to maintain normal rest and sleep patterns and to prevent the development of sleep problems in hospitalized patients?
13. What strategies does the nurse implement to restore normal patterns for patients with rest and sleep problems?
14. How does the nurse evaluate the patient's response to nursing interventions?

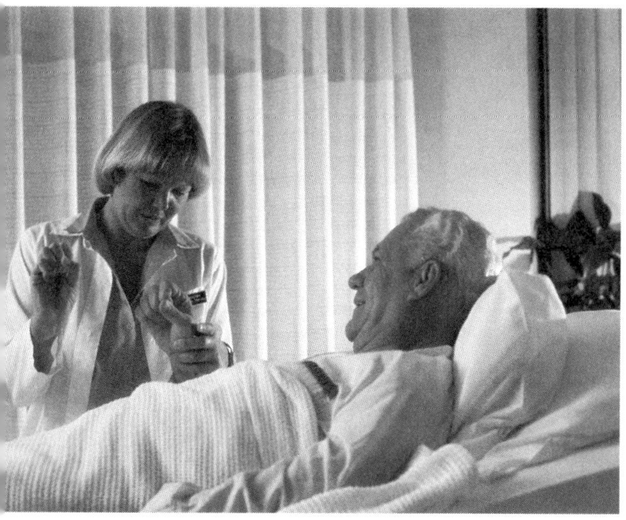

Introduction

O sleep, it is a gentle thing
Belov'd from pole to pole!
To Mary-queen the praise be yeven
She sent the gentle sleep from heaven
That slid into my soul.

— Samuel Taylor Coleridge, 1798

Rest is synonymous with repose or relaxation, and implies freedom from emotional tension and physical discomfort. Rest does not necessarily mean inactivity. People often find a change of activity as relaxing as sitting or lying down to rest. The person who has a sedentary job, for example, may find that physical activity in the form of walking, skating or swimming is relaxing and restful. The person who has been physically active all day may feel rested by watching television, reading, playing cards or just sitting down and talking with family or friends. People who are ill may also find these activities more restful than lying in bed.

Sleep is an essential part of life that takes up approximately one-third of our time. It is a period of decreased mental alertness and physical activity and is part of the normal pattern of daily living. Sleep is a natural process that is both restorative and recuperative, giving body cells a chance to refresh and restore themselves (Du Gas, 1993). Sleep is vital for growth and healing. Drastic changes in sleep and rest patterns disrupt homeostatic balance. The "jet lag" commonly experienced by long-distance travellers is an example of the disturbance in body functioning caused by upsets in our usual pattern of sleep and rest.

The Physiology of Sleep and Rest

Sleep is a cyclical phenomenon affecting all body functions. Stages of sleep have been identified through the use of sophisticated methods of measurement such as the electroencephalogram (EEG). The EEG provides a graphic representation of the electrical waves emanating from the brain. The use of instruments such as the EEG has made possible the identification of the changes occurring in the brain during sleep. Cardiovascular and muscular activity and changes have also been recorded and used to identify the sequence of sleep stages.

Circadian Rhythms

Humans, like plants and animals, possess biological clocks that regulate body functions in regular cyclical fashion. Some cycles, such as the female menstrual cycle, occur monthly; others occur at approximately 24-hour intervals. **Circadian rhythms**, from the Latin words *circa* (about) and *dies* (day), refer to physiologic events that follow a 24-hour cycle. Sleep–wake cycles; changes in body temperature, heart rate and blood pressure; and fluctuations in metabolism and hormonal secretions are influenced by circadian rhythms.

The sleep–wake cycle follows a sequential pattern of awareness (wakefulness) and unawareness (sleep), which constitutes circadian rhythm. These patterns vary among individuals. Some people are early risers, performing their best in the morning. They prefer to go to bed early and sleep throughout the night. Others perform at their best late in the evening and into the night; they prefer to sleep in the morning. Generally, however, "morning is also a time of peak alertness in most people ..." (Dotto, 1990, p. 49). This is because the sleep–wake cycle coincides with other biological rhythms such as body temperature, heart muscle contraction and hormone secretions that decline during sleep and rise during the day. A disruption in the sleep–wake cycle may affect other physiological functions and interfere with general health and well-being.

Stages of Sleep

Normally, the adult sleep cycle recurs every 90 minutes. There are usually four to six 90-minute cycles in a person's sleep time. There are five stages in each 90-minute sleep cycle.

Stage 1 sleep is the lightest and shortest sleep phase. A person is easily aroused from this stage and may be unaware of having been asleep. This is a transitional state during which vital signs begin to slow, muscles become relaxed and body temperature begins to decrease. The EEG reading flattens. A sudden involuntary muscle jerk may be experienced at this point in the cycle.

It is more difficult to wake someone who has entered *Stage 2 sleep*. Some activity appears on the EEG and the individual, although in a more relaxed state, may still be aroused. A person in *Stage 3 sleep* is difficult to rouse. Blood pressure, pulse and body temperature decrease. EEG waves are larger and slower. The individual in *Stage 4 sleep* is completely relaxed and may not move. It is extremely difficult to wake a person in this stage of sleep. It is believed that bedwetting and sleepwalking are most likely to occur at this time, owing to incomplete arousal. During this phase of the sleep cycle there is an increase in the release of hormones regulating growth and promoting tissue healing.

Stage 3 and Stage 4 sleep are commonly referred to as slow-wave sleep (SWS) owing to the large, slow brain waves depicted on EEG tracings. This state is the phase of physically restorative sleep (Dotto, 1990; Edwards & Schuring, 1993; Hayter, 1980).

Upon completion of Stage 4 sleep, the individual retraces the cycle back to Stage 2 and then enters **REM (rapid-eye movement)** sleep (see Figure 26.1). It is during REM sleep that dreaming occurs. Dreams are believed to promote the psychological integration of daily activities. This stage is considered the psychologically restorative stage of sleep (Dotto, 1990; Edwards & Schuring, 1993; Knapp, 1993).

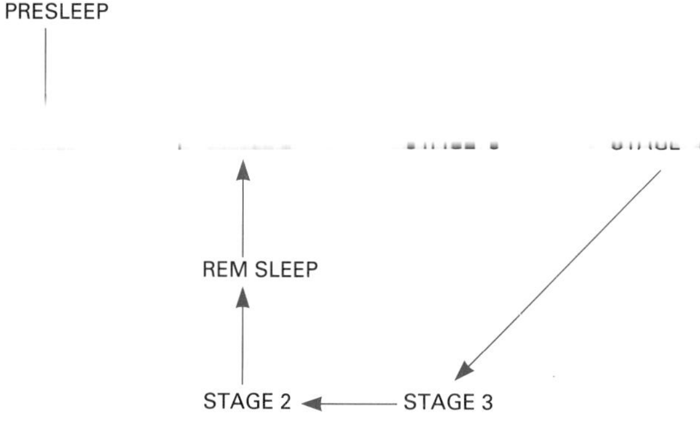

FIGURE 26.1 The adult sleep cycle

During this stage, there is also a great deal of autonomic activity—vital signs fluctuate widely, the eyes move rapidly back and forth and muscular relaxation increases. The EEG reading is similar to that of a person who is awake.

With the completion of the REM stage, approximately 90 minutes after falling asleep, the individual recommences the cycle at Stage 2, proceeds through to Stage 4, returns to Stage 2 and again experiences REM sleep. During the first few hours of sleep, the individual will spend more time in Stage 3 and Stage 4 than in later cycles. The length of the REM stage increases towards morning and may last as long as 60 minutes. Most adults will experience four to six complete sleep cycles during the night. In the final cycle, the individual continues beyond REM to Stage 1, and wakens.

Anytime an individual is awakened, sleep is regained by starting again at Stage 1 and proceeding directly to REM sleep. Consequently, patients disturbed frequently by nursing care may suffer deprivation of the other sleep stages (Dotto, 1990; Hayter, 1980). The importance of REM sleep suggests that dreaming is a very necessary part of our lives.

Sleep Deprivation

Sleep deprivation refers to a decrease in the amount, quality or consistency of sleep. Lack of sleep has a profound effect on an individual's abilities, particularly physical endurance, mental alertness and social relationships. A person deprived of sleep is likely to appear tired, irritable, depressed, anxious or apathetic. Thought processes may be impaired; the ability to concentrate is reduced, forgetfulness occurs and response to stimuli may be inappropriate. Minor troubles may become major problems. Sensory perception may be distorted, causing increased sensitivity to pain. Delusions or hallucinations may occur. When a person experiences gross deprivation of sleep, the body will try to catch up and REM stage sleep may be entered almost immediately. Sleep deprivation is common among hospitalized patients owing to frequent interruptions for assessments and care. Nurses can do much to help patients satisfy their rest and sleep needs by thoughtful planning and implementing of care so as to prevent sleep deprivation.

Determinants of Sleep and Rest

There are a multitude of factors, both physical and psychological, that may affect a person's ability to rest and sleep. Age, personal habits, illness, medications, emotional stress, nutrition and exercise are common determinants. As well, environmental factors and feelings of comfort or discomfort affect one's ability to rest and sleep.

Sleep Habits

Most people have a bed-time ritual that forms part of their sleep habits. For example, many adult Canadians like to watch the late news on television as one of their nightly rituals. For many people, a warm bath or shower is part of their nightly ritual. Each person has particular habits related to going to bed and getting ready for sleep. Most people also have a particular position they find most comfortable for sleeping. Some like to curl up in a ball, some are "tummy" sleepers and others prefer a back-lying position.

Interferences with these bed-time habits are likely to cause disturbances in sleep patterns. In unfamiliar environments people often find it hard to get to sleep the first night or so. A major change in habit can result in stress that disturbs all body functions. Nurses, because they frequently have to work evening or night shifts, often experience disturbances in their normal circadian rhythm. It usually takes a few days to become accustomed to sleeping in the day-time and having one's first meal late in the day. Other people who work shifts report the same problems.

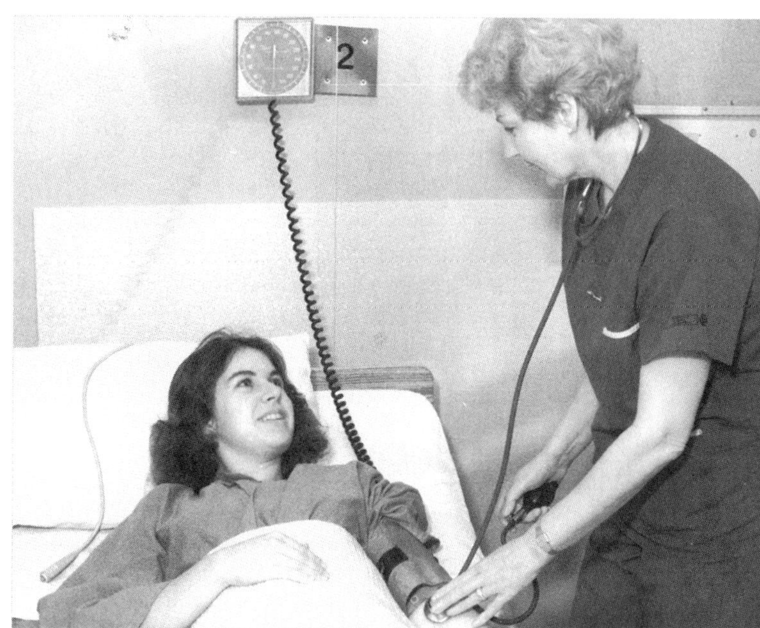

Frequent interruptions for assessments and care can cause sleep deprivation.

Physical Factors

Excessive stimulation will often make it harder for people to get to sleep, unless they are exhausted by the stimulation. A lack of sufficient exercise may be another reason some people find it difficult to sleep; the muscles are not tired enough. A person who is hungry often cannot rest. On the other hand, an excessive intake of food, particularly highly seasoned food that may cause problems in digestion, may also interfere with sleep. A larger than usual amount of fluid intake before retiring usually means having to get up during the night to relieve a distended bladder. Factors that often disturb rest patterns of hospitalized people are medications that must be taken at night and the early morning awakening (often followed by a long delay before breakfast is served) that is still part of the routine in many agencies.

Psychological Factors

Emotional stress and anxiety are common causes of an inability to rest. As a person lies awake and worries, the worries magnify and sleep becomes increasingly elusive. In addition, once sleep comes, the sleep cycle is disturbed. REM sleep, in particular, is decreased, which leads to more stress and anxiety.

Environmental Factors

Excessive sensory stimulation can disturb the comfort, rest and sleep of hospital patients (see Chapter 28). Noise and other disturbances may interrupt the cyclical pattern of a patient's sleep. Other environmental factors that may be a problem include the warm temperatures of most hospital rooms, the hardness of most hospital pillows, lights that are turned (or left) on, the noise of nurses at the nursing station and the sudden stillness after patients have been awakened by some noise.

Discomfort and Illness

Discomfort of any kind interferes with the ability to rest and to sleep. Discomfort may result from myriad psychosocial, spiritual or physical stimuli. A person who is afraid or worried may be as uncomfortable as one who is cold or in pain. Pain is, of course, always a deterrent to rest and sleep. Often, however, it is the minor irritations and discomforts that are most troublesome to patients.

Illness and sleep problems go hand in hand. People who are ill require more sleep because of their need for increased growth hormone to promote tissue repair, and yet this increased need is often thwarted by the fact that illness disturbs the normal rhythm of sleep and wakefulness. Sleep deprivation can itself be a cause of illness.

Medications

Drugs will also distort sleep patterns. The reticular formation in the brain is thought to control sleep. Cerebral depressant drugs that induce sleep work in one or more of several ways. First, they may depress the reticular formation so that it no longer responds to stimuli. Second, they may depress the response of the cerebral cortex to stimuli from the reticular formation. Third, they may cause a specific reduction in the response to stimuli, producing wakefulness (for example, anxiety, depression or pain). Alcohol, for instance, has this effect, as do many of the tranquillizing drugs.

Hypnotics and barbiturates have a tendency to depress REM sleep, resulting in an abnormal sleep cycle. Amphetamines and antidepressant drugs also reduce REM sleep. A patient who is taken off these drugs after having taken them for several days, or who fails to take them, usually has a considerable increase in dream activity, and may be convinced that he or she never slept at all. Barbiturates also depress the parts of the brain that are responsible for inhibitory activity. Hence, they often have an excitatory effect, somewhat like alcohol. Older people are particularly susceptible to this reaction and may become confused and excited instead of going to sleep when they are given barbiturate sedatives.

Sleep and Rest Throughout the Life Cycle

Growth and development are crucial factors in the sleep–wake cycle. Our need for sleep and certain stages of sleep change as we mature. As well, the manner in which we meet our sleep and rest needs alters with maturation.

The developing infant is said to sleep in *utero* or, at least, to have rest periods. Newborns fall into a deep sleep shortly after birth. Most newborns sleep for an average of 16 hours/day, with the longest uninterrupted sleep being a little more than four hours. Approximately half of newborns' sleep corresponds to REM-stage sleep.

The infant quickly proceeds to establish a diurnal pattern and sleep cycle. By about six weeks of age, most infants are sleeping for longer periods during the night than during the day, and by four months most are sleeping through the night, with the longest sleep period averaging around eight-and-a-half hours. The pattern of the sleep cycle in the three-month-old infant begins to resemble that of the adult. Approximately two-thirds of the infant's total sleep is quiet sleep by this time.

Toddlers generally sleep 10–14 hours/day in total, and usually require daily naps until they are approximately three years old. During the toddler stage, bed-time rituals become important. Bed-time rituals such as story time, or engaging in some other quiet activity, help establish good sleep habits. A quiet period and consistent bed-time routines are important for all children. Preschool-age children are often apprehensive about being left in the dark and may need a night light.

Nightmares and bed-wetting (enuresis) are common problems that usually disappear as the child matures. A school-aged child usually sleeps 11–12 hours per night. The amount of

age 12. Teenagers require longer periods of sleep once again, a fact that may be related to their growth needs.

Healthy adults generally sleep six to eight hours a night. During pregnancy, however, women require extra sleep, particularly during the first and third trimesters. Their sleep is frequently interrupted because of the need to void, caused by pressure of the enlarging uterus on the bladder. Additional rest is important throughout pregnancy, and a short nap or rest period during the day is advocated.

As adults mature the amount of sleep required remains the same, though the quality of sleep seems to degenerate. Older adults tend to have difficulty falling asleep and staying asleep. Many older adults experience frequent periods of wakefulness during the night as well as early morning awakenings. Some of the difficulty may be due to aging brain cells and a concomitant decrease in Stage 3 and Stage 4 sleep (Dotto, 1990). Lost night-time sleep results in the need for daily rest periods.

Common Problems

Sleep problems may be divided into two broad categories—*dyssomnias* and *parasomnias*. **Dyssomnias** are characterized by difficulties with the quantity and quality of sleep and include problems such as insomnia (inability to fall asleep or excessive wakefulness), hypersomnia (excessive sleeping, especially during the day) and narcolepsy (sudden, irresistible sleep attacks). **Parasomnias** refer to disruptions of the sleep cycle and include problems such as somnambulism (sleepwalking), enuresis and night terrors (Dotto, 1990). Sleep apnea is a physiological difficulty affecting the sleep–wake cycle that does not fall into either of the principal categories.

Dyssomnias

INSOMNIA

may be described as difficulty falling asleep or staying asleep. Most people, at some time, have problems falling asleep, usually during periods of stress and anxiety. This type of insomnia is termed *situational* or *temporary insomnia* and, over the short term, does not significantly affect waking performance. Individuals who experience *chronic insomnia*, however, often feel continuously fatigued owing to difficulty falling asleep or frequent awakenings. These people may also suffer from depression and anxiety. Their work or school performance may be severely affected. Insomnia is usually treated symptomatically with the use of various relaxation techniques and by encouraging the development of appropriate sleep habits.

HYPERSOMNIA

One explanation for sleeping excessively (**hypersomnia**) is that sleep is being used as a defence mechanism to escape anxieties or frustrations in the fulfillment of basic needs. This, of course, is not always the case; a person who seems to require more than a usual amount of sleep requires referral to a physician for a complete medical examination. Patients exhibiting signs of hypersomnia are generally investigated for possible causes such as insufficient sleep, drugs, tumours or other medical conditions. Often the cause is related to sleep apnea or narcolepsy (Dotto, 1990).

NARCOLEPSY

Narcolepsy is a disorder characterized by brief episodes of sleep that are uncontrollable. The sleep attacks, which may occur frequently, may or may not be preceded by drowsiness. Sleep attacks may last from 30 seconds to 20 minutes. Narcoleptic individuals often have vivid dreams and may be

GERONTOLOGICAL

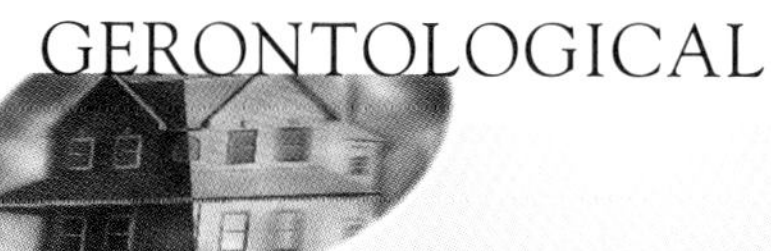

Changes in Sleep Patterns Associated with Aging

Aging brings with it a number of changes in sleep patterns:

- frequent awakenings during the night owing to need to void, arthritic pains, foot and leg cramps
- morning wakening earlier than for younger adults
- more time spent in light sleep, less time in deep sleep (Stages 3 and 4)
- disturbed breathing patterns common
- snoring more frequent, especially among men
- tendency to nap during day
- bad reactions common with medications prescribed for sleep.

IMPLICATIONS FOR NURSING

In addition to the health-promoting strategies suggested for people of all ages to promote healthy rest and sleep, the nurse should encourage the older person to:

- establish a bed-time ritual, such as having a light snack
- try drinking warm milk or a sleep-inducing herbal tea at bed-time
- avoid the use of sleep-inducing medications.

unable to move on waking. They experience hypersomnia during the day and yet during the night often experience insomnia. Many of these people also experience *cataplexy* (profound loss of muscle tone), often brought on by strong emotions (Dotto, 1990; Rogers & Aldrich, 1993). Accidents are more common among narcoleptics than the general population. People with this condition are usually prohibited from working with machinery or at occupations where falling asleep without warning would be a safety hazard. Treatment generally involves taking stimulants and naps.

Parasomnias

SOMNAMBULISM

Somnambulism (sleepwalking) is more common among children than adults. It tends to occur during Stages 3 and 4 of the sleep cycle; hence people who are sleepwalking are usually confused and disoriented. It is not wise to wake them; rather, they should be gently guided back to bed.

NIGHTMARES AND NIGHT TERRORS

While nightmares may occur occasionally among adults, nightmares and night terrors are common sleep problems in children. These disturbances reach their peak in the preschool years. **Nightmares** occur during REM sleep. The child wakes completely following the frightening dream. He or she will be reassured by the presence of someone else and will return to sleep once calm. **Night terrors** often occur during Stage 4 sleep. The child may sit bolt upright in bed, or assume bizarre postures and scream, or cry. The child is terrified. Pulse and respirations are rapid, and diaphoresis occurs. The child is usually disoriented, and may not recognize the person attempting to offer reassurance. It is often difficult to wake the child from this state (Wong, 1995).

ENURESIS

Enuresis, or bed-wetting, generally occurs in Stage 4 sleep and is a common problem in children. Some adults may experience this difficulty as well. It generally occurs more frequently in males and in emotionally disturbed children. Some reports indicate that enuresis is more prevalent among children in low socioeconomic groups. It is believed to be caused in many cases by immaturity of the bladder and many children "grow out of it." Enuresis may, however, be a sign of health problems, and sufferers should be referred for medical attention (Wong, 1995).

Sleep Apnea

Sleep apnea is characterized by "repetitive pauses in breathing lasting from 10 seconds to 2 minutes" during sleep (Dotto, 1990, p. 106). This disorder most commonly occurs in men over the age of 50 and in postmenopausal women. Individuals with this disorder often experience hypersomnia, insomnia and loud snoring. Severe morning headaches, impotence, depression and confusion, day-time lethargy and poor performance are common symptoms. High blood pressure and heartbeat irregularities also occur; these cardiovascular problems usually get progressively worse unless the sleep disorder is treated (Dotto, 1990). These secondary symptoms are the result of periods of decreased blood oxygenation during the night.

The pathology of sleep apnea is classified as obstructive, central or mixed. The most common form, obstructive sleep apnea, is characterized by complete occlusion of the upper airway despite continued respiratory effort by the diaphragm. Loud snoring signals the resumption of breathing. The usual treatment of obstructive sleep apnea is continuous positive airway pressure (CPAP). The patient wears a face mask connected to a device that forces air through the upper airway. The force of the air maintains the airway in an open position. Many patients do not like the device, however, because of the noise it creates. Weight loss can often lessen the severity of sleep apnea and is suggested for many patients. Surgery, specifically a uvulopalatopharyngoplasty (UPP), may be an option for less serious obstructive apnea. In this procedure, the tonsils, uvula and posterior portion of the soft palate are excised and the posterior pharyngeal wall is tightened (Weaver & Millman, 1986).

Central sleep apnea is often associated with infections such as encephalitis or bulbar poliomyelitis. Spinal cord surgery or brainstem infarction may also be causes. These patients do not have the characteristic snoring of obstructive apnea and often require sophisticated ventilatory support. Mixed sleep apnea involves episodes of central apnea (no respiratory effort), followed by obstructive apnea (respiratory effort) and finally by airflow (Weaver & Millman, 1986).

Assessing Rest and Sleep Needs

Making sure that patients are comfortable and that they receive sufficient rest and sleep is an essential nursing responsibility. In order to assess a patient's health status with regard to rest and sleep, the nurse needs information about usual rest and sleep patterns, specific problems the patient may have and the nature of any health problems that may be affecting his or her sleep patterns. Much of this information is collected during the health history; however, focussed enquiries about rest and sleep status are made on a day-to-day basis.

Anxiety is a common cause of sleep and rest problems. Therefore, the nurse needs to be aware of any particular health-related worries the patient has. Knowing the nature of the patient's current health problem and the physician's plan of care—that is, the medications the patient is receiving, the nature of planned diagnostic and therapeutic measures and the results of diagnostic tests—will enhance the nurse's sensitivity to the patient's needs. This information is contained in the patient's chart. It is also helpful to know of any other stresses that may be causing the patient anxiety. Many people are aware of the sources of their anxiety, and when given the opportunity, will make them known. The nurse who takes the time to listen can frequently identify specific sources of worry and discomfort.

Nursing Health History

As we mentioned earlier in the chapter, people vary in their patterns of sleeping and being awake. Still, in hospitals there is a tendency to treat all patients in a similar fashion. Often, it is expected that everyone will go to sleep between 22:00 and 23:00 and sleep until 06:00. This assumption does not respect differences in patients' circadian rhythms, nor does it acknowledge individual habits and preferences. It is essential that nurses identify and note each patient's unique routines and find the measure or combination of measures that will effectively promote comfort, rest and sleep for each individual. Data about a patient's usual rest and sleep pattern and bed-time habits are collected in the nursing health history. This information is also recorded on the Kardex to ensure effective communication among the health team members. In addition, as is the case with other needs, the patient is questioned about recent changes in rest and sleep patterns; if a problem becomes evident, a more detailed exploration of it ensues.

Physical Assessment

People may communicate their inability to sleep to the

dicate sleep disturbances. During the night, nurses make frequent rounds of patients, noting those having difficulty falling asleep or who are wakeful. Nurses on the day shift check the night report to determine how well patients slept. Nurses also observe patients during the day and evening to see if they appear to be getting sufficient rest and sleep.

Both mental and physical relaxation are essential for rest and sleep. In assessing a patient's physical and mental comfort, the nurse must be attentive to both verbal and behavioural cues. The patient who is uncomfortable may appear restless or tense, perspire profusely or lie rigidly in bed. Nurses also need to be aware of any restrictions on the patient's level of activity. Is the patient confined to bed, or restricted to a certain position for therapeutic reasons? Individuals with cardiac or respiratory problems may be most comfortable sleeping with the head of the bed elevated—this is also the best position for them therapeutically. The patient with a fracture may have to lie flat, or have an injured extremity maintained in a specific position. The nature of the

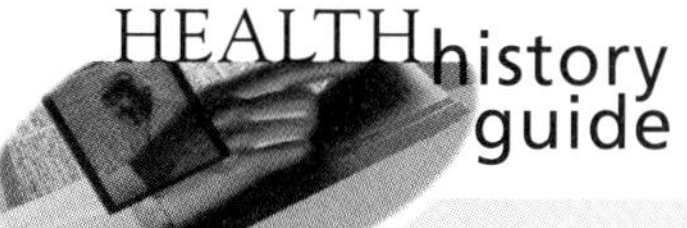

Rest and Sleep

Health and Illness Patterns

Usual Pattern of Rest and Sleep

- What are your usual hours of sleeping (including naps)?
- Describe a typical night's sleep. Do you sleep through? Wake up? If so, how many times a night? Why do you wake up? Thirst? To use the bathroom?
- Describe your usual routine before bedtime. Do you have a snack or warm beverage? What are your hygiene practices? Do you read? Listen to music?
- Do you usually take medicine to help you sleep at night? If so, what?
- What are your usual sleeping habits? Describe the placement and number of pillows. Describe your position. Do you use other aids for sleeping?
- Describe your usual sleep environment. Is your room warm or cool? Is it dark? Quiet or noisy? Do you use a night light?
- Do you feel sufficiently rested in the morning?

Recent Changes in Pattern of Rest and Sleep

- Have there been any recent changes in your pattern of rest and sleep? If so, describe the changes. Do you find you sleep more? Sleep less?
- Are you having difficulty falling asleep? Staying asleep?
- Can you identify any recent changes in your life that may be upsetting your sleep pattern?

Presenting Health Problem

- Describe the difficulty you are having with rest and sleep (falling asleep, staying asleep). Are you sleeping more or less than usual? Snoring?
- Have you been having bad dreams? Nightmares?
- Do you have difficulty waking up in the morning?
- How do you feel when you awaken in the morning? Tired? Depressed? Irritated? Do you often have a headache? How has this sleep difficulty affected your daily functioning? Have you noticed changes in your behaviour? Do you always feel tired? Have trouble concentrating? Feel irritable?
- When did this sleep disturbance begin? What remedies have you tried for the sleep disturbance? What were the results?
- Do you have an acute or chronic condition that may be causing your sleep disturbance? Any medications?
- Do you have a history of long-standing problems with sleeping and resting?

Health Promotion and Protection Patterns

- Do you try to maintain a consistent pattern for sleep and rest?
- Do you exercise regularly? If so, at what time of the day?
- Do you drink products containing caffeine? If so, how much and at what times during the day?
- Do you usually drink alcohol after dinner?

surgical intervention a patient has undergone often determines the position taken in bed. Even an intravenous infusion affects the patient's position in bed.

Diagnosing Rest and Sleep Problems

Problems associated with the quantity and quality of sleep that the nurse can independently treat are labelled *Sleep Pattern Disturbance*. Carpenito defines a *Sleep Pattern Disturbance* as "the state in which the individual experiences or is at risk of experiencing a change in the quantity or quality of [his or her] rest pattern that causes discomfort or interferes with desired life-style" (1997, p. 831). The defining characteristics can include difficulty falling or remaining asleep, fatigue on awakening or during the day, mood alterations and dark circles under the eyes (Carpenito, 1997). It is important to determine the precise etiology of the problem, so that proper interventions can be implemented. For instance, the diagnosis, *Sleep Pattern Disturbance related to hospitalization* does not indicate the treatment measures that should be instituted. However, saying *Sleep Pattern Disturbance related to a noisy environment or a stuffy overheated room* gives direction to the care that may be implemented, in this case eliminating the noise or cooling down and ventilating the room.

Problems with rest and sleep that fall under the diagnosis of *Sleep Pattern Disturbance* must be differentiated from sleep disorders such as narcolepsy or sleep apnea. These are chronic conditions treated by the physician that nurses care for as collaborative functions. Thus, a problem such as sleep apnea is better identified as *Potential Complication: Sleep Apnea* (Carpenito, 1997).

The body needs sufficient rest and sleep for optimal health. A deficit in the quantity and quality of sleep affects daily functioning and causes difficulties in other facets of life. For instance, an individual's performance at work and coping capabilities may be decreased by a prolonged lack of sleep. Thus, the sleep disturbance itself becomes the etiology of other problems. Using the example above, the diagnosis might be stated as *Ineffective Individual Coping related to prolonged lack of sleep*.

Examples of nursing diagnoses and collaborative problems related to rest and sleep are:

- *Sleep Pattern Disturbance related to uncomfortable position and pain associated with fractured elbow*.
- *Sleep Pattern Disturbance related to the changes in usual bed-time routine and noisy hospital environment*.
- *Fatigue related to sleep deprivation*.
- *PC: Dependency on sedatives prescribed for sleep*.

KEY PRINCIPLES

Principles Relevant to Rest and Sleep

1. Definite periods of sleep are an essential component of the circadian rhythm in humans.
2. Adequate amounts of sleep are needed for optimal physical and psychosocial functioning.
3. Growing people require more sleep.
4. Individual needs for sleep vary with age, growth patterns, health status and individual differences.
5. Lack of sufficient sleep impairs physical functioning, mental alertness and social relationships.
6. Individual habits vary with regard to bed-time rituals.
7. Sleep patterns may be disturbed by changes in normal daily living patterns, by social and emotional problems, by physical problems and by minor irritations or discomforts, as well as by pain.
8. Sleep patterns are almost invariably disturbed by illness.

Planning Rest and Sleep Interventions

Interventions to promote rest and sleep are an integral part of nursing care for all patients. Particularly with ill patients, in whom rest and sleep are essential for healing, the nurse must ensure that factors causing the patient discomfort or interfering with rest and sleep are eliminated or, at least, minimized. This aspect of nursing care is considered so important that, in some agencies, the nurses have developed "sleep care plans" for patients (Grant & Klell, 1974).

A specific sleep care plan, or a sleep and rest plan, is helpful in focussing attention on these important aspects of patient care and in facilitating communication about individual needs, preferences and problems with regard to rest and sleep. Sleep care plans ensure that a definite series of nursing activities is planned to help each patient obtain adequate sleep. Interventions that nurses have found helpful for a particular patient are communicated to others so that there is consistency in the approach used by all nursing personnel.

As with all care planning, a sleep and rest plan is based on the patient goals, which are derived from the nursing diagnoses. Examples of patient goals or expected outcomes may include the following:

- The patient will have six hours of uninterrupted sleep.
- The patient will describe factors that prevent or inhibit sleep.
- The patient will report feeling refreshed and energetic after awakening.
- The patient will fall asleep within 15 minutes of using relaxation techniques to induce sleep.

Implementing Rest and Sleep Interventions

Health-Promoting Strategies

People usually fall asleep more easily when their lifestyle permits regular habits for meal times, work or school hours, periods of relaxation and bed-time. Adequate nutrition and exercise are important in promoting restful sleep. Generally it is suggested that strenuous exercise not occur within two hours of bed-time. Restful and relaxing activities should be encouraged prior to sleep. Many find specific relaxation techniques helpful (some of these are discussed in Chapter 36). Tea, coffee and alcohol are best avoided prior to bed-time. A bed-time snack that includes milk is considered by some to be an aid to sleep. Warm milk is particularly effective. Milk contains a potentially sleep-inducing amino acid (L-tryptophan) that is activated when milk is warmed. The development of effective sleep habits needs to begin early in childhood. An especially effective habit is the use of the bedroom for no other activity but sleep.

It is important for individuals who work rotating schedules, such as nurses, to be especially aware of sleep habits. Circadian rhythms may be disturbed and individuals may experience sleep deprivation when continually shifting from a day to a night routine. Shift workers generally require more sleep than usual when they begin working through their usual sleep time. Therefore, it is important to have a quiet, comfortable place to sleep uninterrupted during the day.

Almost everyone has an occasional sleepless night. However, if the sleeplessness continues for more than two or three nights, a physician should be consulted for a thorough investigation of the problem.

Health-Protecting Strategies

Rest and sleep are crucial for restoring health. Yet, many patients in hospital fail to obtain sufficient rest and sleep. There are a number of health-protecting strategies that nurses can implement to foster adequate rest and sleep in [illegible] [illegible] fortable bed and administering a back massage.

PREVENTING SLEEP–WAKE CYCLE DISRUPTION

Normal patterns of daily living, including the sleep–wake cycle, are disrupted during illness. There are a number of measures that can be implemented to avoid or lessen the disruption in a patient's sleep–wake cycle. Diversional activities, if these are not ruled out by health problems, will keep patients from sleeping so much during the day that sleep at night becomes difficult. Morning naps are considered more beneficial than afternoon ones, because they are a continuation of light REM sleep; afternoon sleep is often slow-wave sleep, which can result in the patient's waking up feeling groggy.

Maintaining some of the patient's usual bed-time rituals facilitates a sense of security and promotes rest and sleep. The dietary department needs to be alerted to usual bed-time snacks; if the patient is accustomed to having a bath or shower before retiring, the opportunity to continue this practice will be beneficial to sleep.

Most bed-time rituals involve some type of personal hygiene. In hospital, patients require an opportunity to wash their hands and face and clean their teeth prior to sleep. As well, patients need to be assisted to the bathroom or offered the use of a bedpan or a urinal.

Some people are fond of their own pillow, and may find hospital pillows uncomfortable. Patients may have their own pillow if desired. Familiar objects or routines also help promote a sense of security. A patient may like the pillows arranged in a certain way, the head of the bed elevated to a certain angle, position just so, or a clock turned to facilitate viewing. Small things like these contribute to a patient's effective rest and sleep. The nurse will find that it is worthwhile

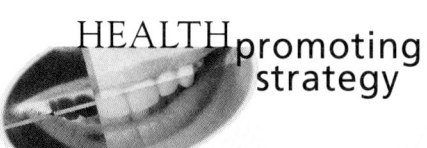

Promoting Healthy Rest and Sleep

1. Get up at the same time of day, every day, regardless of the amount of sleep obtained during the night.
2. Exercise as vigorously as possible in the afternoon or early evening.
3. Reduce caffeine intake.
4. Avoid alcohol after supper.
5. Set aside some quiet time before sleep to relax and unwind.
6. Go to bed only when feeling sleepy.
7. Use the bedroom for sleeping only.
8. Control the sleep environment. Keep the bedroom dark, cool and quiet.
9. If you have difficulty falling asleep, focus on something monotonous. If sleep does not come within a reasonable length of time, get up and do something boring until you feel sleepy. Also, drink a glass of warm milk.

SOURCES: Dotto, 1990; Knapp, 1993; Walgenbach, 1990; Webster & Thompson, 1986.

RESEARCH to practice

Cohen, F.L., Nehring, W.M., & Cloninger, L. (1996). Symptom description and management in narcolepsy. *Holistic Nursing Practitioner, 10*(4), 44–53.

Narcolepsy is a neurological condition described in the literature as chronic and lifelong. It is characterized by excessive day-time sleepiness. Invariably, this results in uncontrollable sleep attacks and cataplexy. Despite the many types of medications that are used to treat narcolepsy, individuals continue to report that control is limited.

The purpose of this study was to explore the individual's experiences living with narcolepsy—the most prevalent symptoms and management strategies employed. One thousand, five hundred individuals were recruited through the American Narcolepsy Association using a random sample design. Each individual received a questionnaire. The questionnaire explored two primary areas: (a) the frequency and severity of narcoleptic symptoms and (b) the pharmacologic and nonpharmacologic strategies in managing the narcoleptic symptoms. The return response rate was 47.4 percent, which consisted of 292 men and 396 women.

The results of the study revealed that the single most frequent symptom was excessive day-time sleepiness (40%), followed by cataplexy (38%) and sleep attacks (19%). The prevailing factor reported for provoking excessive day-time sleepiness or a sleep attack was situations in which the individual had to contend with monotony: driving a car, eating or talking. Individuals reported feeling sleepy at least two to six times a day; time would vary in length. Thus, they perceived themselves as never truly alert.

The most common method of managing symptoms included a combination of medication and other treatment (strict scheduling, naps, exercise, light meals, drinks with caffeine, splashing face with water, avoiding stuffy rooms, pinching self, support of others, alarm clock, chewing gum). In addition, participants described major changes to their personal, professional and social lives.

The authors emphasize that the first step a nurse should take is to comprehend the symptoms associated with narcolepsy and understand that each individual's management style is unique and ongoing. Therefore, nurses can educate people, such as teachers and employers, about this condition and how it is managed. The authors strongly encourage further research, as there is limited information about the effectiveness of some of the nonpharmacologic strategies on large groups of narcoleptics.

to spend a few extra minutes "settling" patients by attending to these small but important details.

Most patients find a back massage soothing and an aid to sleep. For some, relaxation techniques are beneficial. Besides relaxing exercises, a number of techniques for learning to control tension in the muscles and induce relaxation have been developed. The use of progressive relaxation techniques is especially useful with older adults (Johnson, 1993).

When the patient is settled, and all details attended to, the lights are dimmed. Noise is kept to a minimum, and the patient is not disturbed unless absolutely necessary.

MAINTAINING A COMFORTABLE BED

The bed is particularly important to most people who are ill. Much of a patient's comfort depends on the condition of the bed, particularly if he or she is in it for long periods of time. A neat, clean and wrinkle-free bed is necessary for comfort. Often patients who are exacting in regard to their beds and bed units may be clinging to a position from which they can control some aspect of their environment at a time when they believe that many decisions and activities are beyond their control. The ill patient's horizons often narrow, and matters about which he or she normally would have no concern become important.

There are two types of bed making: *occupied* (with the patient in it) and *unoccupied* (with the patient out of it). Whether the nurse makes an occupied or unoccupied bed depends on the patient's condition and the physician's order. An occupied bed is often made as part of the patient's daily hygiene care, after the bath. The nurse should try to schedule the making of an unoccupied bed when the patient is in the bath or shower, taking a walk or off the unit for tests

Infection Control and Bed Making

1. Microorganisms are present on the skin and in the general environment.
2. Some microorganisms are opportunists; that is, they can cause infections when conditions are favourable. For example, a break in the skin or mucous membrane of the patient may become a site of infection.
3. Patients are often less resistant to infections because of the stress resulting from an existing disease process.
4. Microorganisms may be transferred from one person to another or from one place to another by air, by inanimate objects or by direct contact among people. Therefore:
   - avoid holding soiled linen against the uniform
   - never shake linen
   - always wash your hands before going to another patient.
   - never put linen on the floor or on another patient's bed or chair.

Effective Body Mechanics and Bed Making

1. *Maintain good body alignment.* For example, stand facing the direction in which you are working and move so as not to twist your body.
2. *Use the large muscles of the body rather than the small muscles.* For example, flexing the knees and bringing the body to a comfortable working level is preferable to bending at the waist. The former uses the large abdominal and gluteus muscles, whereas the latter puts strain upon the back muscles and shifts the centre of gravity outside the base of support.
3. *Work smoothly and rhythmically.* This is less fatiguing because the muscles are alternately contracted and relaxed.
4. *Push or pull rather than lift* because this requires less effort.
5. *Use your own weight to counteract the weight of an object.* This decreases the effort and strain involved. Shifting your own weight when pulling a mattress requires less effort than pulling the mattress with your arms. In addition, back and arm strain is reduced.

and treatments. Linen is also changed whenever it becomes damp or soiled. Soiled or wet linen predisposes a patient to skin breakdown and infections.

When the bed is made, soiled linen is changed and the bed is aired and remade. Making an occupied bed is similar to making an unoccupied bed, except that in the former case the nurse is also concerned about maintaining the patient's body alignment, safety and comfort. Some patients are unable to assume a supine position because of their condition; for example, they may have difficulty breathing. In such cases, the nurse makes a comfortable, neat bed while the head of the bed is elevated.

When changing bed linen, the nurse must remember that microorganisms are present in the environment and be aware of the methods by which they spread. The use of good body mechanics is also important when making a bed. The principles that underlie body movements in helping the patient to move (see Chapter 29) are equally applicable to bed making. The boxes on the preceding page and above outline principles of infection control and the effective use of body mechanics with respect to bed making.

The method used for stripping and making beds differs among agencies. Basically, however, every health agency wants the end product to be neat, clean, comfortable and durable, and the bed-changing process to be an economical use of time, equipment and the patient's and nurse's energies. Procedure 26.1 details the steps involved in stripping and making an unoccupied or an occupied bed.

Assembling Linen and Equipment

The linen required for the basic hospital bed includes two [illegible] drawsheet (optional), one or two blankets (also optional) and one bedspread.

Cotton drawsheets and rubber catch pads have traditionally been used on the ill person's bed for two reasons: they are easier to change than bottom sheets are, and they protect the mattress. With the availability of plastic-covered mattresses, however, and increasing use of cotton mattress pads (similar to the ones that are commonly used in the home), the routine use of drawsheets, both rubber (or plastic) and cotton, is disappearing. In many agencies the use of drawsheets is now reserved for the beds of patients who need them; they are no longer put on every bed.

When a rubber catch pad is used, it is placed on top of the fitted bottom sheet. The catch pad or drawsheet usually extends from above the patient's waist to the mid-thigh. Thus it can serve to absorb secretions in cases of urinary or fecal incontinence.

The cotton that is used for sheets, pillowcases, drawsheets, or cotton-with-rubber-backing catch pads must be of a heavy weight that wears well in spite of strong pulling and frequent washing. Moreover, because linen is often washed in disinfectant solutions in order to kill microorganisms, a heavy weight is necessary to withstand the laundering.

The bedspreads that are used in hospitals and most other health agencies are frequently made of a loose cotton weave or a mixture of flannel and cotton. The bedspreads should be able to withstand frequent washings without damage or shrinkage. In many hospitals, patients' rooms are warm enough that no blankets are needed. However, blankets are sometimes necessary for warmth. Usually one or two blankets suffice. An extra blanket is sometimes used as a throw blanket over the spread. The extra blanket can be rolled and stored at the foot of the bed, fan-folded down to the bottom of the bed, or put in the patient's closet until it is needed. Blankets should never be used by more than one patient because of the danger of transferring microorganisms from one patient to another. Elderly patients are often more sensitive to the cold than younger patients are and require more covers for warmth.

A complete linen change is not made every day. This is unnecessary and would only serve to increase already costly health care expenditures. It is customary practice to change a pillow slip and the drawsheet or catch pad on a daily basis and other linen only when it becomes soiled. A receptacle is needed for soiled linen. In some agencies hampers are provided that may be taken right into the patient's room. If such a hamper is not available, the corners of the bedspread may be tied to the foot of the bed to collect soiled linen. Clean gloves are necessary if the linen is soiled with body substances and fluids.

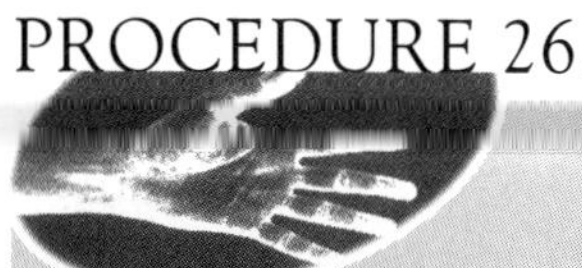

PROCEDURE 26.1 Making an Unoccupied and an Occupied Bed

Action	*Rationale*
A. General Actions	

1. Gather equipment:
• receptacle for soiled linen
• clean linen as needed:
  • top and bottom (fitted) sheet
  • drawsheet/catch pad
  • bedspread
  • blanket
  • pillowcases
• clean gloves as necessary.
	Ensures efficiency and economy of time.

2. Wash hands thoroughly.	Reduces the risk of contamination.
3. Explain procedure to the patient.	Enhances emotional well-being and enables patient participation.
B. Stripping the Bed	
1. Remove equipment from the bed. Detach the call light and garbage bag, and place them on the bedside table.	Provides a clear working space.
2. Lower the head of the bed and raise the bed to a comfortable working height.	Promotes the nurse's use of good body mechanics.
3. Place a chair beside the bed. An over-bed table may be used in place of a chair.	Provides a clean area to place linen.
4. Remove pillowcases and place them in the laundry bag. Place the pillows on the seat of the chair or on top of the table.	Promotes organization of work space.
5. Starting at the head of the bed, loosen the top and bottom sheets from the mattress while walking around the bed.	
6. Remove the blanket by grasping it at the centre and near side and folding it to the bottom of the bed. Pick the blanket up at the centre and lay it, folded in quarters, across the back of the bedside chair. Remove the bedspread and top sheet in the same way, if they are to be reused.	Prevents linen from touching the floor. Folding the linen in such a manner permits efficient replacement on the bed.
7. Linen not to be reused is rolled into itself and discarded into the laundry hamper.	Prevents contact with the nurse's uniform, thereby preventing transmission of microorganisms.
8. If necessary, turn the mattress side to side, or push to the head of the bed.	Adjusting the mattress after bed making loosens the linens.
9. If linens are very soiled, you may want to wear gloves.	
10. Wash hands thoroughly when finished stripping the bed and before putting on the clean linen.	Avoids transferring microorganisms.
C. Making the Unoccupied Bed	
1. Place the bottom sheet on the lower half of the mattress with its centre fold on the centre of the mattress. Align the end of the sheet with the lower edge of the mattress. Open the sheet to the head of the bed. If using a fitted sheet, secure the nearest top and bottom corners. If using a flat sheet, tuck the top under the mattress at the head of the bed and mitre or square the corners on one side (see Figure 26.2 following this procedure). Tuck the sheet in smoothly along the sides so that it is free of wrinkles.	Prevents wrinkles, which are a source of irritation against the patient's skin.
2. Place and tuck in the drawsheet/catch pad.	

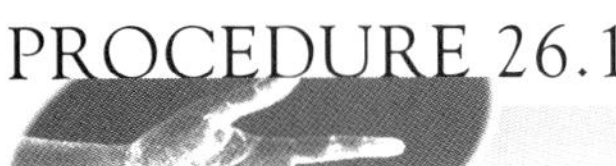

PROCEDURE 26.1 continued

Action	Rationale
3. Place the top sheet on the lower half of the mattress as with the bottom linen. Unfold the sheet towards the top of the bed. Align the top edge of the sheet to the top edge of the mattress. The blankets and bedspread are applied in the same manner but are brought to within about 23 cm of the edge of the mattress. Fold the top sheet down to make a cuff over the blankets and bedspread.	

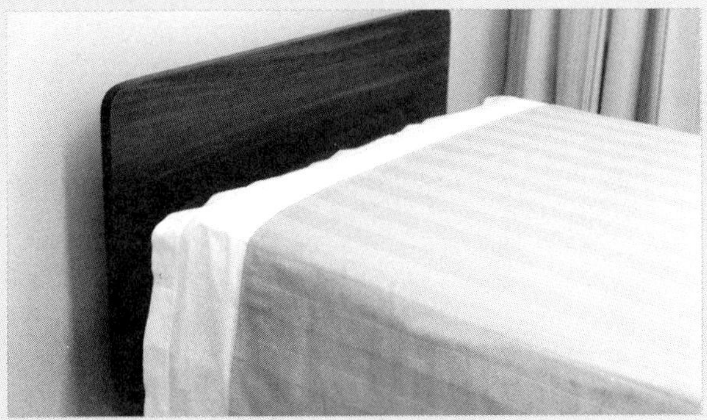

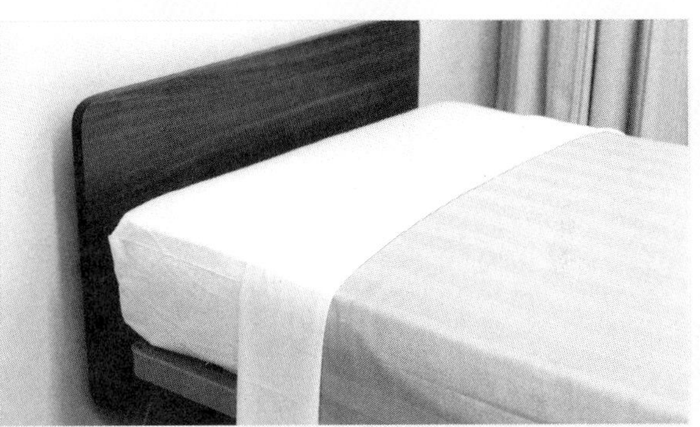

Action	Rationale
4. Tuck the remaining top linen under the mattress and make a modified mitred corner. This is done as in Figure 26.2, except that the top edge is left to hang down at the side of the bed.	

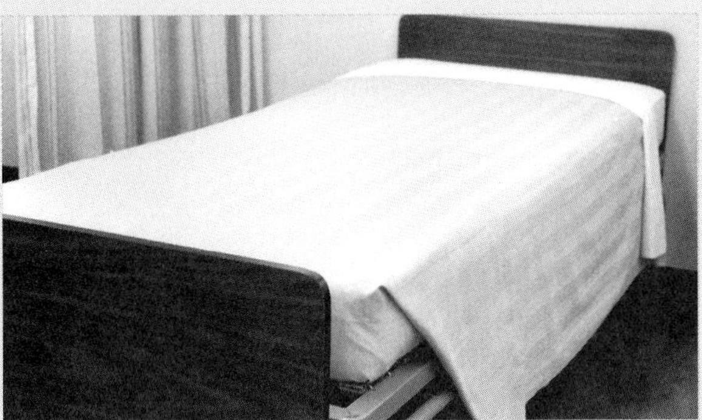

Action	Rationale
5. When the bed has been made completely on one side, make the other side in the same way.	
6. Make a toe pleat in the top covers. To do this, raise the upper sheet and blankets and make a 5-cm vertical fold, perpendicular to the bed. Tuck the linen under the mattress. As an alternative, the top covers may be loosened at the foot of the bed.	Allows room for the patient's feet and prevents pressure that can cause discomfort, skin breakdown and foot drop. Promotes efficiency and economy of time.

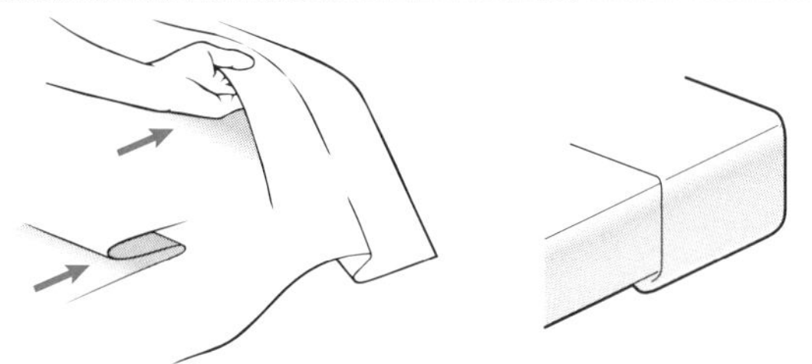

continued on next page

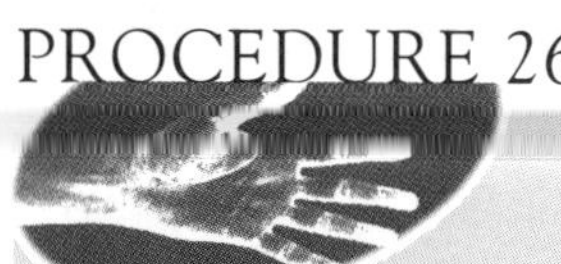

PROCEDURE 26.1 *continued*

Action	*Rationale*
7. To replace a pillowcase, grasp the closed end of the pillowcase in one hand. With the other hand gather up the sides of the pillow case and rest them over the forearm of the hand holding the case. Then, with the hand holding the pillowcase, grasp the pillow and slide the sides of the case over the pillow. Align the corners of the case and the pillow.	

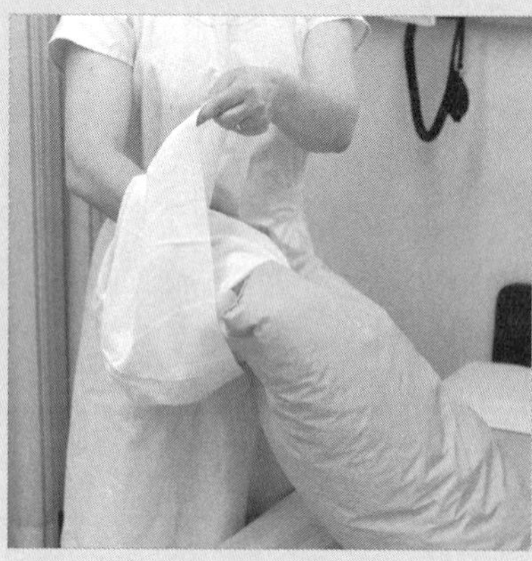

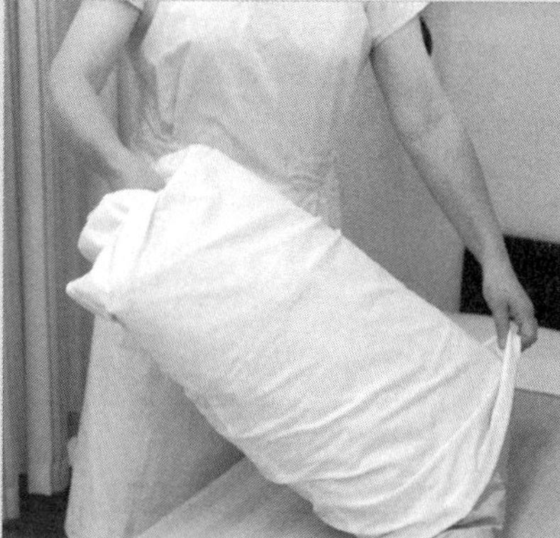

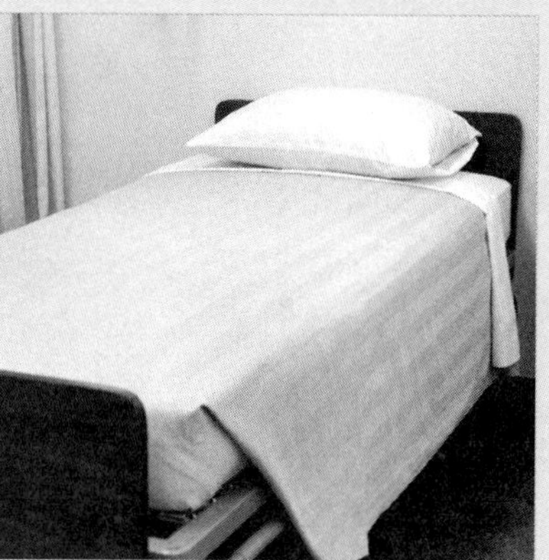

Action	*Rationale*
8. Replace any equipment the patient requires. Attach the call light to the bed, place the bedside chair beside the bed, and place the bedside table within the patient's reach. Remove all unnecessary equipment and place small articles in the bedside table. Ask the patient's permission before discarding any belongings, including flowers.	Promotes patient's well-being, comfort and safety. A neat environment promotes a sense of comfort.
D. Making the Occupied Bed	
1. Check the physician's orders regarding the patient's position and activity.	Ensures safety and avoids errors.
2. Draw privacy curtain around bed.	Maintains privacy, promoting comfort and security.
3. Raise the bed to a comfortable working position. Lower the side rail on the near side and remove the call bell.	Promotes the nurse's use of good body mechanics.
4. When stripping the bed, leave a pillow under the patient's head.	Promotes comfort.
5. Remove the spread and blankets, then place a bath blanket over the top sheet. Remove the top sheet by drawing it down from under the bath blanket. If the patient is to be washed, it is done at this time, before the foundation of the bed is changed.	Prevents the clean sheet from becoming dampened or soiled during the bath.
6. Help the patient move to the far side of the bed. Loosen the foundation on the near side. Fold the linen to be removed into the centre of the bed. Place clean linen on the near side of the bed and tuck it in. Raise the side rail on the near side. Help patient to roll over the folded linen to the near side of the bed.	Promotes patient safety and security.
7. Move to the other side of bed. Lower the side rail. Remove the soiled linen and pull the clean linen tightly across the bed and tuck it in.	

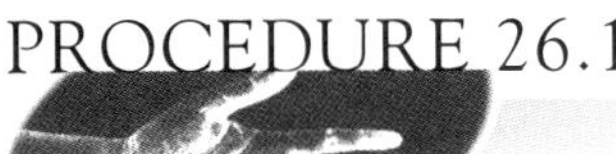

PROCEDURE 26.1 *continued*

Action	Rationale
8. Assist the patient to the centre of the bed and replace the second pillow.	
9. Remove the bath blanket and replace the top covers as for an open bed.	
10. Replace the patient's call bell and lower the bed. Return all equipment to proper position. Tidy the bedside unit.	Promotes patient safety and comfort.

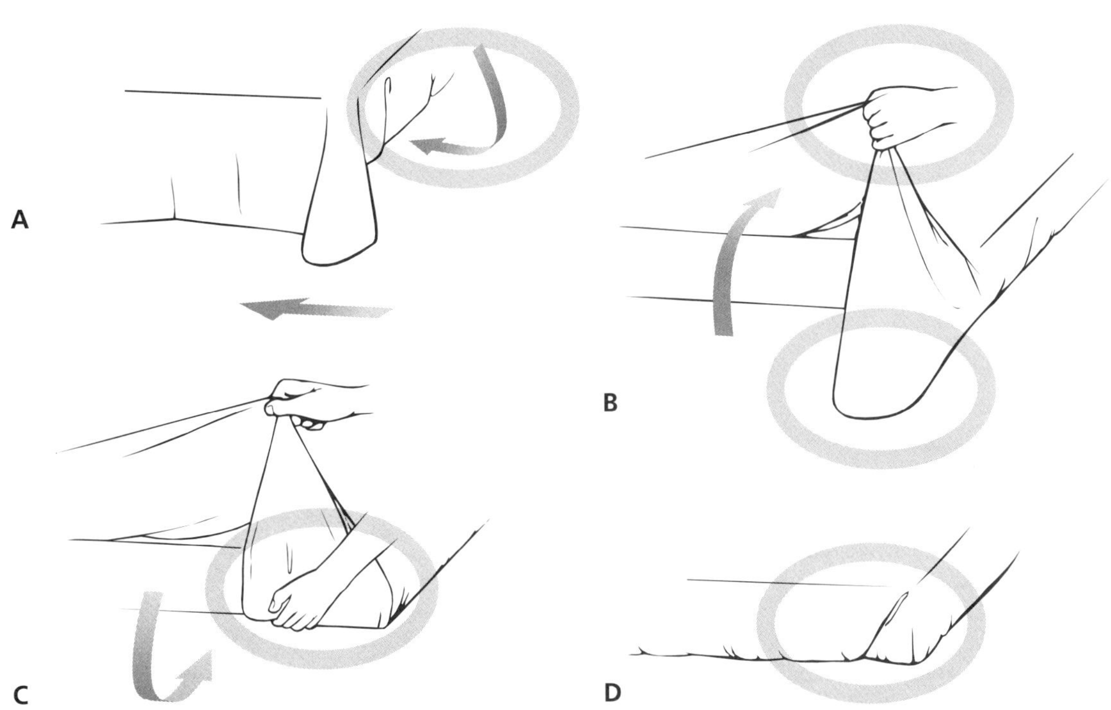

FIGURE 26.2 Mitring a corner. A. To mitre a corner, tuck the bottom edge of the sheet securely under the mattress. B. Lift the side edge of the sheet about 30 cm from the corner, and hold it at a right angle to the mattress. C. Tuck in the part of the sheet that hangs below the mattress. D. Drop the triangular edge down and firmly tuck it under the mattress

ADMINISTERING THE BACK MASSAGE (BACK RUB)

Many patients have trouble sleeping because they feel anxious about being in a hospital. A back massage can be a very effective way of increasing a patient's comfort and alleviating stress, allowing the patient to sleep more soundly.

To administer a massage in preparation for sleeping, after a bath and at other times as indicated, the nurse rubs the patient's back with an emollient lotion or cream. In addition to promoting relaxation, the back rub also increases circulation to the skin, thereby reducing the risk of skin breakdown. The technique of administering the back rub is outlined in Procedure 26.2.

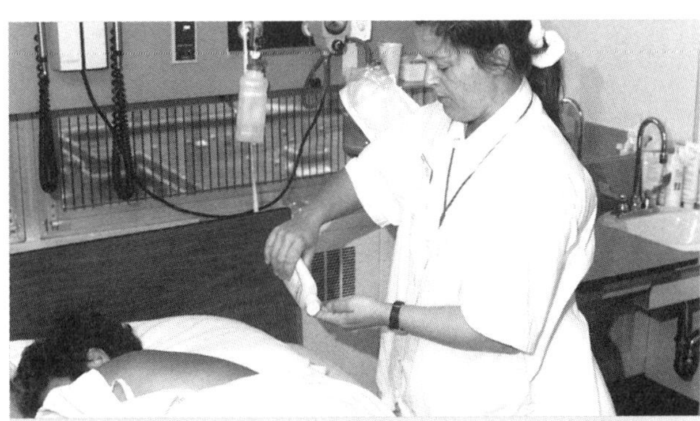

A soothing back rub helps to relax the patient and promotes comfort and rest.

PROCEDURE 26.2 Administering a Back Massage

Action	*Rationale*
1. Wash hands thoroughly.	Reduces the risk of contamination.
2. Explain the procedure to the patient.	Enhances emotional well-being and enables patient participation.
3. Help the patient to lie in the prone or side-lying position.	Permits use of long, firm strokes, which are both soothing to the patient and stimulating to the blood circulation.
4. Expose the patient's back from shoulders to sacrum.	
5. Warm the lotion by holding a small amount in the palms of your hands for a minute. The bottle of solution may also be placed in warm water.	Warm solutions feel more comfortable.
6. Starting at the shoulders and using the palms and fingertips, rub the patient's neck with circular motions extending to the hairline.	Helps to relax the shoulder and neck muscles, which often are tense.

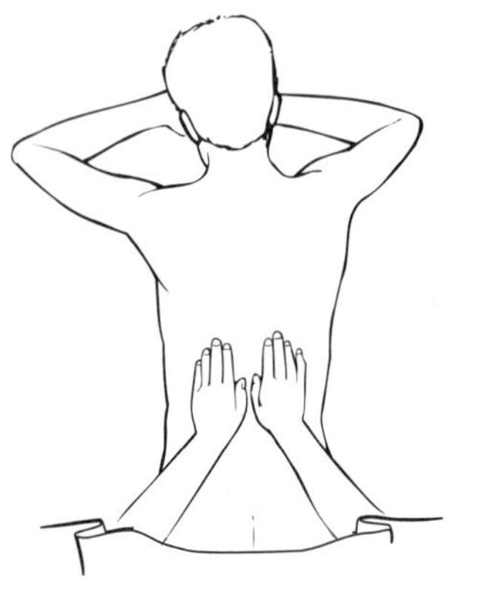

Action	*Rationale*
7. Move the hands to the sacral area and repeat the circular motions with palms and fingertips.	
8. Move to sacrum and rub up the centre of the back to the hairline, using long smooth strokes, then over to the shoulders and down the sides of the back, using broad circular motions.	The circular motions are designed to increase circulation to bony prominences. The pressure of the nurse's motions should be sufficiently firm to stimulate the muscle tissue.
9. Now, move to the lower edge of the patient's buttocks and sacrum, continuing with the broad circular motions.	

Health-Restoring Strategies

THERAPEUTIC BEDS, MATTRESSES AND DEVICES

Mattresses

There are many different kinds of mattresses available for both therapeutic and comfort purposes. The regular hospital mattress is firm and often covered with a plasticized material. Patients allergic to these mattresses have a foam pad placed on top of the usual mattress. This pad also has an advantage in that it places less pressure upon the patient's bony prominences. Because of this it is often used in the prevention and treatment of pressure ulcers for patients who must remain in bed for long periods of time.

Another type of mattress is the alternating pressure mattress. An air pump alternately deflates and inflates areas of the mattress, with the result that there is a continual change in the pressure upon the various parts of the patient's body. These alternations of pressure stimulate circulation to the skin, which facilitates tissue nourishment and waste product removal. This mattress is most effective with only a single layer of linen between the mattress and the patient. Care must be taken not to prick the mattress with safety pins or sharp instruments, or pinch or shut off the tubing to the motor.

There are a variety of other therapeutic mattresses available to assist in making patients feel comfortable. Air-fluidized beds use the flotation principle to provide uniform support to the body. The mattress portion of the bed consists of fine glass beads. Air is blown through these spheres to keep them constantly moving, and the patient experiences a sensation of floating. Other types of mattress available

port surfaces, static air mattresses and water mattresses. Each of these mattresses has specific indications for use, often related to pain management or wound healing. An increased sense of comfort is the outcome experienced by the patient.

It should be noted that the use of these special mattresses is not a substitute for nursing care. Patients continue to require turning, skin care and proper positioning.

The Fracture Board

The **fracture board** (bed board) is placed under the patient's mattress to increase support. It is usually made of wood or Plexiglas. Some fracture boards have hinges so that the head and knee gatches (adjustable joints) of the bed can be used with the board in position. The fracture board is used in situations where patients require additional support, such as following a spinal injury or surgery.

The Bed Cradle

The **bed cradle** is a device used to keep the weight of the top bed covers off the patient. Patients who have burns, uncovered wounds or wet casts often need to keep the top bedclothes away from the injured area. When applying a cradle to the patient's bed it is securely fastened to, or under, the mattress. Some bed cradles are hoop arrangements that extend from one side of the bed to the other; others extend only to the midline of the bed. The cradle is carefully positioned so that the area of the patient's body that is to be free from the weight of the top bed covers is directly under the cradle. The top bedclothes must be pulled up higher than usual to cover the patient's shoulders. Bed cradles are made of metal or plastic.

The Footboard

The **footboard** is placed at the foot of the patient's bed to serve as a support for the feet. Footboards are usually made out of plastic or wood and fit onto the bed frame across the foot of the bed.

Normally the feet of the patient lying in the dorsal position will be bent into plantar flexion (see Chapter 29). In time, if the patient's feet are not exercised or supported, they may become fixed in plantar flexion. This condition, known as *footdrop*, is the result of contractures of the gastrocnemius or soleus muscles and prevents the patient from standing with heels flat on the floor. Footdrop is usually treated by physiotherapy, but sometimes can only be modified by surgery.

The Balkan Frame

The **Balkan frame** is a metal frame that extends lengthwise above the bed, supported at either end by a pole attached to the bed frame (see Figure 26.3). A trapeze may be attached to the frame just above the patient's head as a mobility aid. This simple measure provides patients with the ability to

dependence and ultimately their comfort. The Balkan frame may also be used as an attachment for the pulleys and weights of traction equipment used for patients who have fractures of the lower limbs, particularly the femur.

Specialized Beds

A number of specialized beds have been devised for patients who will be immobilized for long periods of time and for those with specific health problems. Examples include the Stryker frame, the CircOlectric bed, the HighLow Tilt bed, the rocking bed and the chair bed. The use of these beds is generally confined to a specific area, and nurses will be educated about their use when working in the area.

POSITIONING THE PATIENT IN BED

Generally, patients assume the positions that are most comfortable for them. For the patient who is able to move easily and freely in bed without therapeutic considerations, the nurse's chief responsibility in regard to position is comfort. The astute use of pillows and the provision of a firm foundation assist in achieving a comfortable position for the patient.

Patients must sometimes assume positions for therapeutic reasons. Some of the reasons are to maintain good body alignment, to prevent contractures, to promote drainage, to facilitate breathing and to prevent the development of skin breakdown over bony prominences.

The physician may prescribe the appropriate therapeutic position for a patient, but usually the nurse decides which position is best. Intelligent assessment of a patient's problems and a knowledge of anatomy and physiology are important bases for such judgements. Also, the nurse needs to be aware of the variety of positions possible and the supportive measures available to promote comfort in these positions.

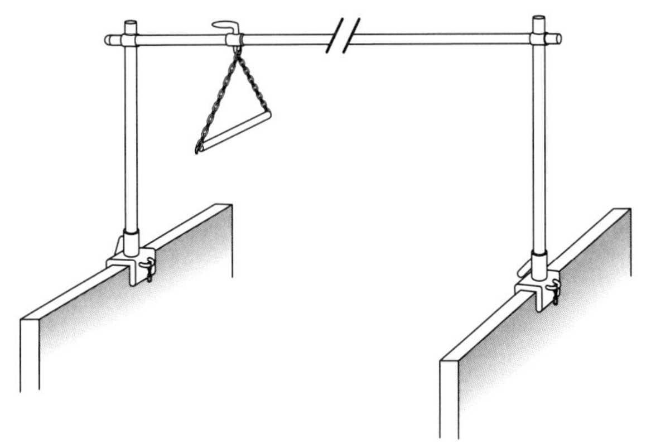

FIGURE 26.3 Balkan frame

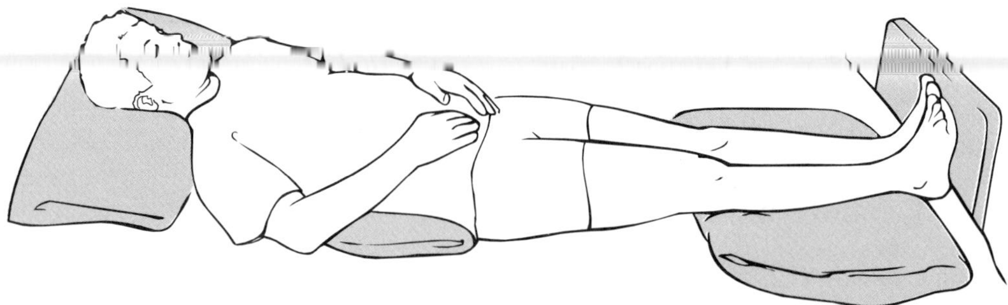

FIGURE 26.4 Dorsal recumbent position

Common Bed Positions

DORSAL RECUMBENT AND SUPINE POSITION In the **dorsal recumbent position** (see Figure 26.4) the patient lies on the back with the head and shoulders slightly elevated. Usually one pillow suffices for this purpose. A small pillow is placed under the lower legs to flex the limbs slightly and prevent hyperextension of the knees. It also keeps the patient's heels off the bed and helps to reduce lumbar lordosis.

The patient who does not have support for the thighs will tend to rotate outward. Two rolled towels or a rolled bath blanket tucked in at the lateral aspects of the thighs under the trochanter of the femur will maintain the patient's legs in alignment. In the dorsal recumbent position, the patient's feet will normally assume a plantar flexion position. Prolonged positioning in plantar flexion, however, can result in footdrop. Preventive measures for this complication include use of the footboard, which helps the patient to maintain the feet in dorsal flexion and removes the weight of the bedclothes from the toes; and use of the heel protector, which supports the foot's position as well as providing protection for the heel. Flexion, extension and circumduction of the patient's ankles help maintain muscle tone and ankle joint mobility.

In some cases, the patient's head and shoulders are not elevated by pillows and rolls. The patient lies on the back with the head and shoulders on the flat surface. This is called the **supine position**. It is frequently prescribed for patients who have had spinal anesthetics. Supports similar to those just described are used when indicated.

PRONE POSITION The **prone position** is one in which the patient lies on the abdomen with the head turned to one side. Many people are relaxed and sleep well in this position; some find it most comfortable to flex their arms over their heads (see Figure 26.5).

Supportive measures for the patient in this position include a small pillow or pad, as needed, under the abdomen at the level of the diaphragm in order to give support to the lumbar curvature and, in the case of the female patient, to take weight off the breasts. A small pillow or towel roll under each shoulder helps to maintain the anatomical position. In addition, a pillow under the lower legs elevates the toes off the bed and permits slight flexion of the knees. Alternatively, the patient can extend the toes over the end of the mattress to take the weight off the toes. Plantar flexion is minimized if the patient's lower legs are also supported. When the patient is in a prone position, there is pressure on the knees. A small pad under the thighs can be used to relieve this pressure. Sheepskin or sponge rubber pads may also be used under the knees.

The patient may want a pillow for his or her head. Unless the physician wishes the patient's head to lie on a flat surface, in order to promote drainage of mucous, for example, a small pillow may be provided to make the patient more comfortable; however, the pillow should not be so thick as to hyperextend the patient's head.

LATERAL (SIDE-LYING) POSITION In the **lateral position**, the patient lies on the side with both arms forward and knees and hips flexed (see Figure 26.6). The upper leg is

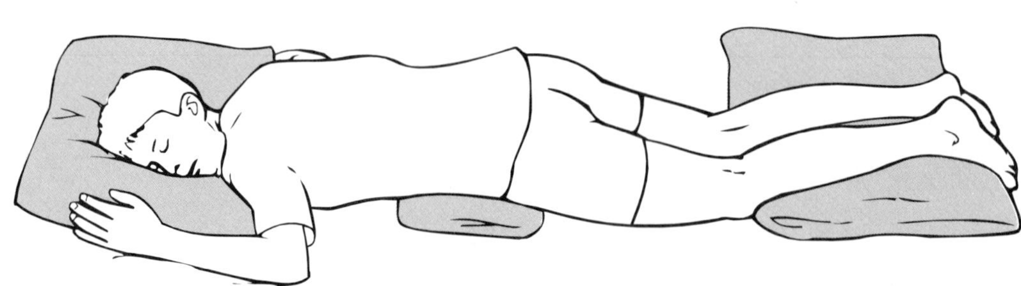

FIGURE 26.5 Prone position

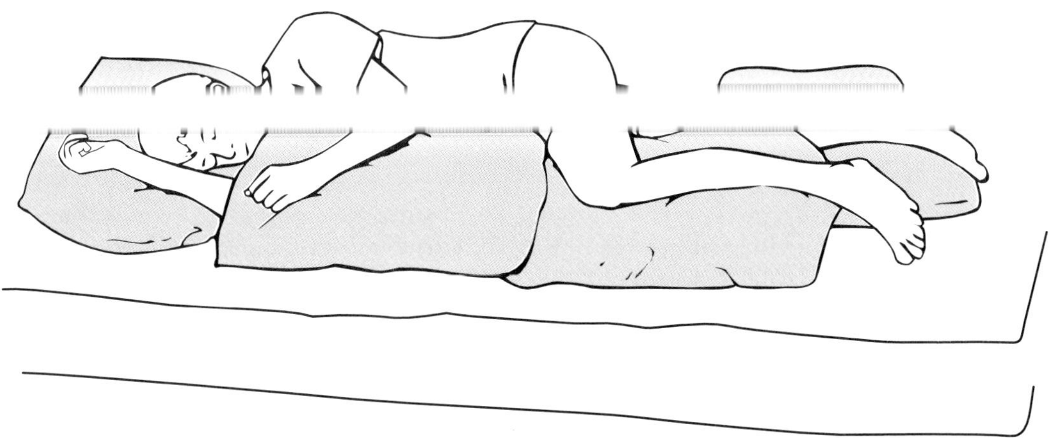

FIGURE 26.6 Lateral (side-lying) position

flexed more than the lower leg. Weight is borne by the lateral aspects of the patient's ilium and by the scapula.

The upper knee and hip should be at the same level; the upper elbow and wrist should be at the same level as the upper shoulder to prevent the limbs from being in a dependent position. The heels and ankles may be protected by using small pads (sheepskin or sponge rubber) to keep them from rubbing against the bedclothes.

If the upper arm falls across the chest, the patient's lung capacity may be restricted; a pillow to support the patient's arm permits greater chest expansion and enables the nurse to observe the character and rate of respirations.

The patient who lies laterally will probably want a pillow for the head. A pillow of proper depth should prevent lateral flexion of the head. Frequently, the patient will also require the support of a pillow placed lengthwise behind the back.

The lateral position is prescribed in situations where it is necessary to take weight off the sacrum of the patient. The patient can also eat more easily in this position than in the supine position. It also facilitates some kinds of drainage. Finally, many people find it a relaxing position.

FOWLER'S POSITION **Fowler's position** is one of the most frequently assumed positions. It is a sitting position in which the patient's head and trunk are raised between 45° and 90° (see Figure 26.7). There are two variations of Fowler's position: the *semi-Fowler's* (or *low Fowler's*) and *high Fowler's* positions. In the semi-Fowler's position the head and trunk are elevated 15° to 45°. This is a comfortable position for the patient who must keep the head and chest slightly elevated. The high Fowler's position refers to the full sitting position, that is, with the head of the bed elevated 90°; the knees may or may not be flexed.

In Fowler's position the patient usually needs at least two pillows for support and comfort. The first pillow is best placed far enough down the patient's back to provide support for the lumbar curvature. A second pillow supports the head and shoulders. An emaciated patient will probably need three pillows. For patients who are very weak, pillows placed laterally will support the arms and help to maintain good body alignment.

Small pillows or a pad under the patient's thighs permits slight flexion of the knees; a footboard permits dorsal flexion and prevents the patient from sliding towards the foot of the bed. Occasionally the knee gatch of the bed is used to support flexion of the knee. If the knee gatch is used, the knees should not be flexed too much because of the danger of putting pressure on the popliteal nerve and major blood vessels that are close to the skin surface in the popliteal area. Prolonged pressure can cause serious interference with both nerve supply and circulation to the lower limbs. Hence, the knee gatch is seldom used for patients now.

In Fowler's position the main weight-bearing areas of the patient are the heels, sacrum and posterior aspects of the ilium. The nurse should pay particular attention to these areas when giving skin care.

Fowler's position is indicated for patients who suffer either cardiac or respiratory distress, since it permits maximal chest expansion. A position somewhat similar to the

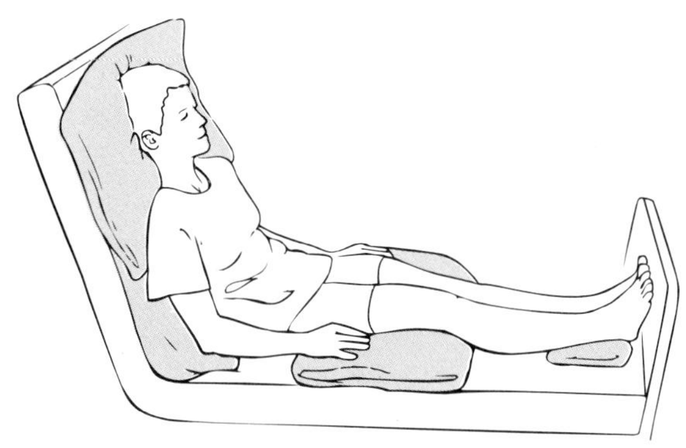

FIGURE 26.7 Fowler's position

high Fowler's is the sitting position in which the patient leans over an over-bed table upon which several pillows have been placed for comfort. Some patients with respiratory problems find this position makes breathing easier. Patients who have difficulty exhaling tend to lean forward to compress the chest for additional force on expiration. The pillows on the over-bed table provide support for the arms and help to maintain the individual in as erect a position as possible to increase total lung capacity.

SIMS' (SEMI-PRONE) POSITION **Sims' position** is similar to the lateral position except that the patient's weight is on the anterior aspects of the shoulder girdle and hip (see Figure 26.8). The patient's lower arm is behind the back, and the upper arm is flexed at the shoulder and elbow. The upper leg is acutely flexed at the hip and knee, and the lower leg is slightly flexed at the hip and knee.

A rolled pillow placed laterally and in front of the patient's abdomen will support the patient in this position. Pillows for the upper arm and upper leg will prevent adduction of these limbs, and a small pillow for the patient's head will prevent lateral flexion. If, however, the patient is unconscious and the nurse wants to promote mucous drainage from the mouth, a pillow under the head is contraindicated.

In Sims' position the patient's feet naturally assume the plantar flexion position. If the patient is to maintain Sims' position for some time, supports should be provided in order that the feet assume the dorsal flexion position. A footboard or sandbag can be used for this purpose.

Sims' position can be established on both the left side and the right side. The patient's position should be changed frequently; if he or she is unable to move unaided, the nurse can help the patient turn every two hours, or more often if needed. When turning the patient who is unconscious, the nurse should be sure that the patient's eyelids are closed to prevent the possibility of the cornea's being scratched by the bedclothes. Good skin care, particularly to the anterior aspects of the patient's ilium and shoulder girdle, is also indicated.

This position is prescribed for patients who are either unconscious or unable to swallow. It permits the free drainage of mucous. Sims' position also allows maximal relaxation and is therefore a comfortable sleeping position for many people.

Positioning the Patient

When patients are confined to bed and cannot move, improper positioning and support of joints can lead to contractures and skin breakdown. Regardless of the position of the patient, certain principles must be applied. The body parts must be properly aligned and the joints adequately supported. The patient's position must be changed frequently. Adequate exercise (to the extent the patient's condition allows), good skin care and supportive measures must always be carried out. A general guide for positioning patients as well as the principles of anatomical position and body alignment are listed in the boxes below. Although there are situations in which positions that do not follow the therapeutically anatomical position fully may be required, the basic principles should be kept in mind and applied insofar as is possible. The steps for helping patients assume the various positions are detailed in Procedure 26.3.

Guide for Positioning Patients

1. Positions that are as close as possible to the basic anatomical position provide good body alignment.
2. Joints should be maintained in a slightly flexed position. Prolonged extension creates undue muscle tension and strain.
3. Positions should be changed at least every two hours. Prolonged pressure on one area may cause the skin to break down, with resultant pressure sores (decubitus ulcers).
4. All patients require daily exercise unless medically contraindicated.
5. When a patient changes position, joints should be manipulated through the full range of motion unless medically contraindicated.

Principles of Anatomical Position

1. Good alignment of all body parts
2. Equal weight distribution of body parts
3. Maximal space in body cavities for internal organs
4. Joints in functional position (for walking, grasping objects, etc.)

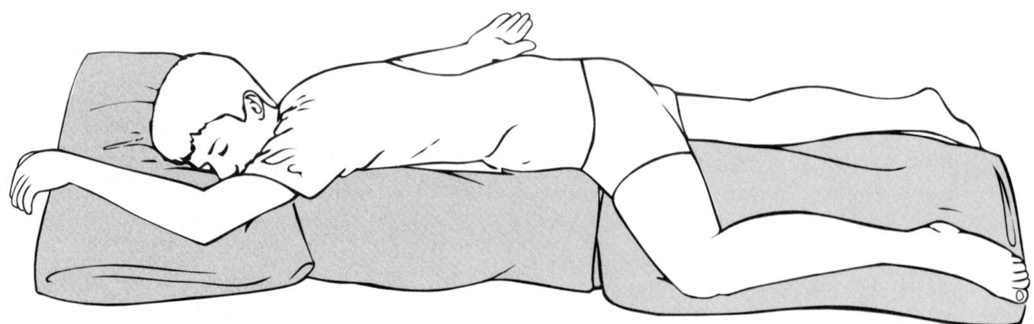

FIGURE 26.8 Sims' position. A small pillow may or may not be placed under the patient's head

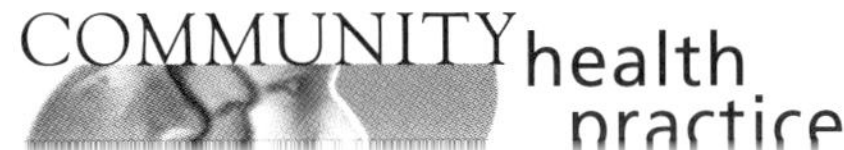

Canadian Red Cross Society

The Canadian Red Cross Society operates a loan service for medical equipment, with depots located in most large communities across the country. Equipment loaned includes hospital-type beds and accessory devices, wheelchairs, walkers, commodes, canes and other items needed for the care of people in the home setting.

Mobility aids are loaned only on referral from a health professional such as a physician, physiotherapist or home care nurse. The service is provided free of charge for a period of up to three months. If the equipment is needed on a permanent basis, the items can be borrowed while arrangements are being made for their purchase.

When patients cannot move, care must be taken to maintain the fingers in a functioning position, that is, with fingers flexed and thumb in opposition. A small hand roll may be placed in the palm of the hand and the fingers curved around it. This is particularly important for unconscious patients and for those who have limited movement in one or both hands. Wristdrop must also be prevented. The hand should never be left in a dependent position. It should be supported so that it is in a straight line with the lower arm.

Assembling Aids for Positioning and Comfort

Pillows are used to maintain proper position and provide support to joints. There are also a number of aids and supportive devices that may be used to ensure comfort and safety.

SHEEPSKIN PADS AND SMALL PILLOWS Sheepskin pads and small pillows serve as supportive devices. Placed under bony prominences, they relieve pressure; placed in the lumbar curve or under a limb, they support or elevate an extremity. Figure 26.9 shows a heel protector that supports the foot in dorsal flexion and protects the skin from friction against the bed linen.

SPONGE PAD A small sponge pad placed in the patient's hand can be used as an exercise aid. It can also be used to prevent flexion of the hand and to separate skin surfaces in conditions of spastic contraction. The size of the pad allows slight flexion of the hand and fingers, with the thumb comfortably placed in its normal anatomical position, that is, in opposition.

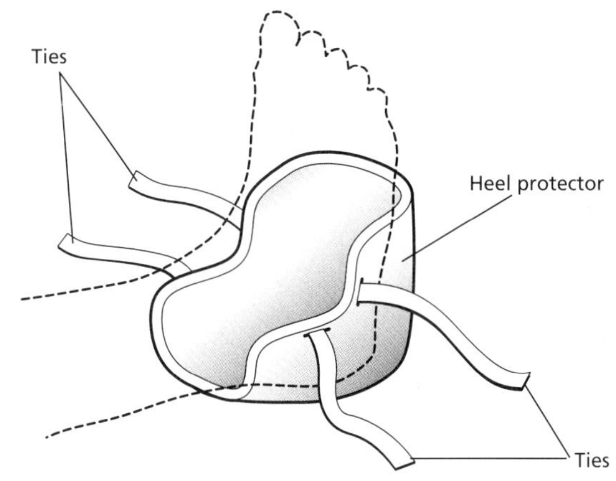

FIGURE 26.9 Heal protector

TROCHANTER ROLLS **Trochanter rolls** are used to prevent external hip rotation. They may be made from bath towels or bath blankets. The towel is folded lengthwise once and then rolled to within 15 cm of one end. The roll may be secured with safety pins fastened between the body and the tail of the roll. To support the patient's thigh and prevent external rotation, the tail of the roll is placed under the patient's thigh, with the safety pins away from the patient. The roll is then firmly secured along the patient's thigh until the patient's toes point directly upward. Figure 26.10 illustrates a trochanter roll.

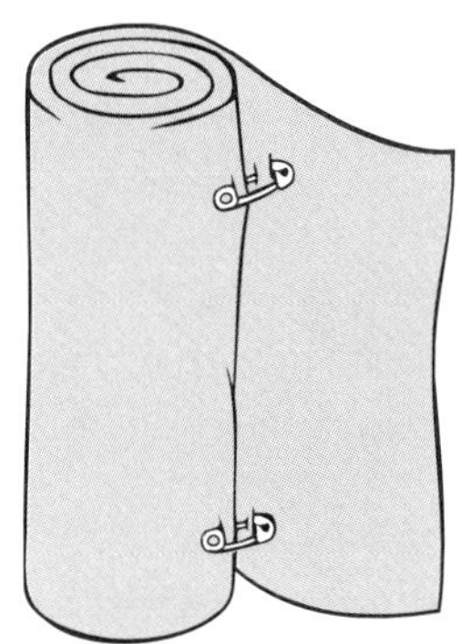

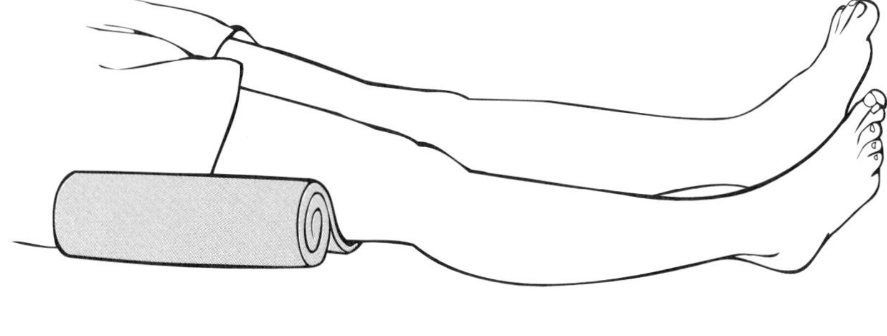

FIGURE 26.10 A trochanter roll can be used to prevent external rotation of the hip. The safety pins used to secure the roll are placed so that they face away from the patient

PROCEDURE 26.3 Positioning Patients

Action	Rationale
A. General Actions	
1. Assess the patient's alignment and comfort level.	Determines equipment that will be needed.
2. Gather equipment and supplies as necessary: • pillows • aids for positioning and comfort • sheepskin pads • sponge pads • heel or elbow protector • trochanter roll • footboard	Ensures efficiency and economy of time.
3. Obtain assistance as necessary.	Ensures safety for patient and nurse.
4. Explain procedure to the patient.	Enhances emotional well-being and, where possible, facilitates patient's participation in care.
5. Wash hands.	Prevents transmission of microorganisms.
6. Provide privacy.	Promotes patient comfort.
B. Dorsal Recumbent Position	
1. Position the patient on the back with one pillow under the head and shoulders.	Prevents hyperextension of the neck.
2. Place a small pillow or folded towel under the lumbar curvature of the back.	Supports the lumbar curvature.
3. Place rolled towels or a rolled bath blanket at the lateral aspects of the thighs.	Supports the thighs, prevents outward rotation and maintains the patient's legs in alignment.
4. Place a small pillow under the lower legs, below the popliteal area.	Slightly flexes the limb and prevents hyperextension of the knees. Placing the pillow below the popliteal area avoids possible interference with circulation to the extremities and injury to the popliteal nerve.
5. Place a footboard at end of the bed.	Helps to maintain the feet in flexion and removes the weight of the bedclothes from the toes.
C. Prone Position	
1. Assist the patient to lie on the abdomen with the head turned to one side. The head may or may not be supported with a small pillow. If a pillow is used, it should not be so thick as to hyperextend the patient's head.	
2. Position a small pillow or pad under the abdomen below the level of the diaphragm.	Provides support to the lumbar curvature and, in the case of the female patient, takes weight off the breasts. A pillow placed at or above the level of the diaphragm will impede respiration.
3. Place a pillow under the patient's lower legs. Alternatively, the patient can extend the toes over the end of the mattress.	Takes the weight off the toes. Lifts the patient's toes off the bed and permits slight flexion of the knees. Plantar flexion is minimized.
D. Lateral (Side-Lying) Position	
1. Position the patient on the side with both arms forward and the knees and hips flexed. The upper leg is flexed more than the lower leg. Weight is borne by the lateral aspects of the patient's ilium and scapula.	
2. Place a pillow under the patient's head.	Maintains alignment of the head to trunk.
3. Place a pillow under the patient's upper arm.	Support of the patient's arm permits greater chest expansion and enables the nurse to observe respirations.

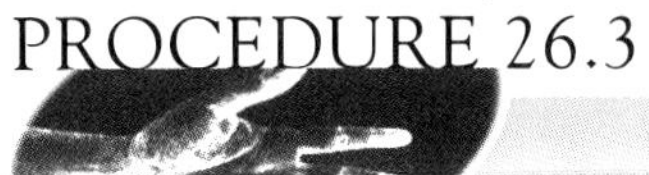

PROCEDURE 26.3 *continued*

Action	*Rationale*
4. Place one or two pillows under the upper leg.	Promotes correct alignment and decreases pressure of top leg resting on bottom leg.
5. Place a pillow lengthwise behind patient's back.	Increases support and promotes sense of comfort.
E. Fowler's Position	
1. Place a pillow behind the patient's back. A second pillow supports the head and shoulders.	Provides support for the lumbar curvature.
2. Place a small pillow or a pad under the patient's thighs.	Permits slight flexion of the knees.
3. Place a footboard at the end of the bed.	Permits dorsal flexion and prevents the patient from sliding towards the foot of the bed.
F. Sims' Position	
1. Position patient laterally but lying partially on abdomen. The lower arm is placed behind the body and the upper arm is flexed at the shoulder and elbow. The upper leg is acutely flexed at the hip and knee, and the lower leg is slightly flexed at the hip and knee.	
2. Place a rolled pillow laterally and in front of the patient's abdomen.	Supports the patient in this position.
3. Place pillows under the patient's upper arm and upper leg.	Prevents adduction of these limbs.
4. Place a small pillow under the patient's head.	Prevents lateral flexion. However, if the patient is unconscious and the nurse wants to promote mucous drainage from the mouth, a pillow under the head is contraindicated.

SANDBAGS Sandbags also serve as a means of providing support to the patient. They are firmer than trochanter rolls and, because of their weight, are less easily moved. For this reason, sandbags are desirable when body alignment must be maintained—for example, in the case of fractures.

Evaluating Rest and Sleep Interventions

All interventions must be evaluated for effectiveness. This is especially important when considering the patient's level of comfort and the quantity and quality of rest and sleep.

When an intervention related to comfort is implemented, the patient's comfort level is assessed every two to four hours. The following questions can help in evaluating the effectiveness of care.

1. Does the patient verbally indicate increased comfort?
2. Does the patient appear more comfortable, that is, more relaxed or less restless?
3. Has the frequency of the patient's requests for analgesics decreased?

Expected outcomes of interventions regarding rest and sleep relate to the amount of rest and undisturbed sleep the patient achieves, as well as the ease with which he or she falls asleep. Questions that may assist evaluation of rest and sleep interventions might include the following.

1. Has the patient been able to fall asleep without difficulty?
2. Has the patient been able to rest quietly?
3. Does the patient feel refreshed following sleep?

Sedatives or hypnotics may be prescribed for patients having difficulty sleeping. These drugs tend to decrease the length of time spent in REM sleep. There is also a rebound effect when these drugs are discontinued. That is, once the drug is discontinued the patient may encounter a significant increase in REM sleep and may experience considerable dreaming and possibly nightmares (Knapp, 1993).

IN REVIEW

- Rest is synonymous with repose or relaxation. It implies freedom from emotional tension and physical discomfort, and does not necessarily mean inactivity.
- Sleep is a normal part of our daily living patterns, taking up approximately one-third of our time. It is essential for growth and healing.
- Sleep is a cyclical phenomenon. The sleep–wake cycle follows a sequential pattern (circadian rhythm) and is intimately involved with other body rhythms. The sleep cycle is usually 90 minutes in adults.
- Each sleep cycle has five stages. It is important to pass through all five stages sequentially to receive full physiological and psychological benefits from sleep.
- Inability to progress through the stages of sleep sequentially (e.g., because of frequent awakenings) may lead to sleep deprivation.
- Sleep deprivation is a decrease in the amount, quality or consistency of sleep. It can have profound adverse effects on physical and psychological functioning if prolonged.
- Factors affecting ability to sleep and rest include:
  - age
  - sleep habits
  - discomfort
  - emotional stress
  - environment
  - illness
  - medications.
- Newborns require the most sleep; one-half of their sleeping time is REM sleep. By four months, the sleep cycle starts to resemble the adult's pattern.
- Children require less sleep than infants. Sleep needs gradually decrease until about the age of 12.
- Adolescents require more sleep than young children, possibly because of growth needs (growth hormone is secreted during sleep).
- Sleep needs remain the same through adulthood, although the quality of sleep deteriorates with age. Older adults may require day-time rest periods to make up for periods of wakefulness and early morning awakenings.
- Common sleep disturbances include:
  - dyssomnias (insomnia, hypersomnia, narcolepsy)
  - parasomnias (sleepwalking, nightmares, night terrors, enuresis).
- Sleep apnea is a physiological difficulty affecting the sleep–wake cycle.
- The nursing health history should include:
  - usual sleep and rest patterns
  - any sleep problems
  - usual bed-time routine
  - present worries or anxieties.
- Nursing diagnoses associated with quantity and quality of sleep include *Sleep Pattern Disturbance*.
- Sleep disorders such as narcolepsy are identified as collaborative problems, for which nurses collaborate with other health professionals in delivering and evaluating care.
- A sleep care plan facilitates communication about:
  - a patient's rest and sleep needs
  - individual preferences and problems
  - a definite series of activities to help each patient obtain adequate sleep.
- Health promotion for individuals, families and groups includes information sharing and teaching.
- Health-protecting interventions include:
  - day-time diversional activities
  - morning naps
  - fostering usual bed-time rituals
  - back massage
  - teaching and encouraging use of relaxation techniques
  - ensuring a quiet environment and a comfortable bed
  - use of therapeutic mattress, fracture board, bed cradle, footboard or Balkan frame for comfort and therapeutic purposes
  - proper patient positioning to promote comfort, relaxation and healing.
- Positioning is used for therapeutic purposes, such as to:
  - maintain good body alignment
  - prevent contractures
  - promote drainage
  - facilitate breathing
  - prevent skin breakdown.
- Common positions a nurse may use for therapeutic purposes include:
  - dorsal recumbent
  - supine
  - prone
  - lateral
  - Fowler's
  - Sims'.

- Equipment that can be used for comfort and proper positioning includes:
  - [illegible]
  - sheepskin or sponge pads
  - rolled towels and sandbags.

Critical Thinking Activities

1. Keep a record of your hours of sleep (including naps) for a typical week. Note factors in your lifestyle that may affect your sleep. Analyse your sleep pattern and determine whether or not it is adequate. If not, what changes should you make to promote optimum rest and sleep?
2. Mrs. R. Rogers is a 56-year-old woman who was admitted to hospital with acute rheumatoid arthritis involving her back, knees and feet. Mrs. Rogers is an obese woman and she finds it difficult to breathe when the head of her bed is flat. She experiences pain in her joints continually. Mrs. Rogers has a limited income and lives by herself in a small apartment. Her husband died four years ago, and her one daughter lives out of town and finds it difficult to visit frequently.

   The physician has ordered a low-calorie diet. Her medications include enteric-coated acetylsalicylic acid (650 mg q.i.d.) and serax (30 mg po. h.s.).

   a. What factors might cause Mrs. Rogers to have problems with regard to comfort, rest and sleep?
   b. How would you assess Mrs. Rogers' present comfort, rest and sleep status?
   c. What objective data (signs) would indicate to you that Mrs. Rogers is uncomfortable or is not resting or sleeping well?
   d. What subjective data (symptoms) of Mrs. Rogers might you note?
   e. What other members of the health team are, or might be, involved in helping Mrs. Rogers? For what purpose?
   f. What positions do you think might be most comfortable for Mrs. Rogers?
   g. What supportive devices might make Mrs. Rogers more comfortable? How should you use them?
   h. Outline a nursing care plan for Mrs. Rogers.

KEY TERMS

rest p. 806

circadian rhythm p. 806

REM (rapid eye movement) p. 806

sleep deprivation p. 807

dyssomnias p. 809

parasomnias p. 809

insomnia p. 809

hypersomnia p. 809

narcolepsy p. 809

somnambulism p. 810

nightmare p. 810

night terror p. 810

enuresis p. 810

fracture board p. 821

bed cradle p. 821

footboard p. 821

Balkan frame p. 821

dorsal recumbent position p. 822

supine position p. 822

prone position p. 822

lateral position p. 822

Fowler's position p. 823

Sims' position p. 824

trochanter roll p. 825

References

CARPENITO, L.J. (1997). *Nursing Diagnosis: Application to clinical practice.* (7th ed.). Philadelphia: Lippincott.

COHEN, F.L., NEHRING, W.M. & CLONINGER, L. (1996). Symptom description and management in narcolepsy. *Holistic Nursing Practitioner, 10*(4), 44–53.

COLERIDGE, S.T. (1798). The rime of the ancient mariner. *Lyrical Ballads.* Bristol, England: Biggs & Cottle.

Du GAS, B.W. (1993) in BECKINGHAM, A.C., & Du GAS, B.W. (1993). *Promoting health aging: A nursing and community perspectcive.* Toronto: Mosby.

DOTTO, L. (1990). *Losing sleep: How your sleeping habits affect your life.* Toronto: Stoddart.

EDWARDS, G.E., & SCHURING, L.M. (1993). Sleep protocol: A research-based practice change. *Critical Care Nurse, 13*(2), 84–88.

GRANT, D.A., & KLELL, C. (1974). For goodness sake, let your patients sleep. *Nursing '74, 4*, 54–57.

HAYTER, J. (1980). The rhythm of sleep. *American Journal of Nursing, 30*(3), 457–461.

JOHNSON, J.E. (1993). Progressive relaxation and the sleep of older men and women. *Journal of Community Health Nursing, 10*(1), 31–38.

KNAPP, M. (1993). Night shift: The restorative sleep specialists. *Journal of Gerontological Nursing, 19*(5), 38–42.

ROGERS, A., & ALDRICH, M.S. (1993). The effect of regularly scheduled naps on sleep attacks and excessive daytime sleepiness associated with narcolepsy. *Nursing Research, 42*(2), 111–117.

WALGENBACH, J.C. (1990). Lullabye and not a good night? *Geriatric Nursing, 11*, 278–279.

WEAVER, R., & MILLMAN, R.P. (1986). Broken sleep. *American Journal of Nursing, 86*(2), 146–150.

WEBSTER, R.A., & THOMPSON, D.R. (1986). Sleep in hospital. *Journal of Advanced Nursing, 11*, 447–457.

WONG, D.L. (1995). *Whaley & Wong's nursing care of infants and children.* (5th ed.). St. Louis: Mosby.

Additional Readings

BARHYTE, D.Y., McCANCE, J., VALENTA, A., Van TATENHOVE, J., WALKER, S., & BETHEA, S. (1995). Selection of a standard hospital mattress: Data-based decision making. *Journal of Wound, Ostomy & Continence Nursing, 22*(6), 267–270.

BLAYLOCK, B. (1995). A study of risk factors in patients placed on specialty beds. *Journal of Wound, Ostomy & Continence Nursing, 22*(6), 263–266.

BOETTGER, J.E. (1997). Effects of a pressure-reduction mattress and staff education on the incidence of nosocomial pressure ulcers. *Journal of Wound, Ostomy & Continence Nursing, 24*(1), 24–25.

CAMERON, B.L. (1993). The nature of comfort to hospitalized medical-surgical patients. *Journal of Advanced Nursing, 18*, 424–436.

CARTY, E.M., BRADLEY, C., & WINSLOW, W. (1996). Women's perceptions of fatigue during pregnancy and postpartum: The impact of length of hospital stay. *Clinical Nursing Research, 5*(1), 67–80.

CHEN, M.F., & WANG, H.H. (1995). Quality of sleep and its related factors among elderly women. *Nursing Research, 3*(4), 323–334.

CLOSS, S.J. (1988). Assessment of sleep in hospitalized patients: A review of methods. *Journal of Advanced Nursing, 13*, 501–510.

COOK, N.F., & BOORE, J.R.P. (1997). Adult/elderly care nursing. Managing patients suffering from acute and chronic fatigue. *British Journal of Nursing, 6*(14), 811–815.

CREIGHTON, C. (1995). Effects of afternoon rest on performance of geriatric patients in a rehabilitation hospital: A pilot study. *American Journal of Occupational Therapy, 49*(8), 775–779.

CURETON-LANE, R.A., & FONTAINE, D.K. (1997). Sleep in the pediatric ICU: An empirical investigation. *American Journal of Critical Care, 6*(1), 56–63.

DAVIS, I., PACK, G., & LOGAN, J. (1997). Promoting patient sleep: A critical but forgotten practice? *Canadian Association of Critical Care Nurses, 8*(1), 12–17.

DIAMOND, W.J. (1997). Reflections on healing. Curing chronic fatigue with homeopathy. *Alternative Medicine Digest, 16*, 72–74, 76.

DONELLY, G.F. (1996). The healing potential of sleep, rest and dreams. *Holistic Nursing Practice, 10*(4), v.

DREHER, H.M. (1996). Beyond the stages of sleep: An emerging nursing model of sleep phases. *Holistic Nursing Practice, 10*(4), 1–11.

EVANS, J.C., & FRENCH, D.G. (1995). Sleep and healing in intensive care settings. *Dimensions of Critical Care Nursing, 14*(4), 189–199.

FULLER, N.S., & MORRISON, R.E. (1998). Chronic fatigue syndrome: Helping patients cope with this enigmatic illness. *Postgraduate Medicine, 103*(1), 175–176, 179–182, 195–197.

GOTTSCHLICH, M.M., JENKINGS, M., MAYES, T., KHOURY, J., KAGAN, R., & WARDEN, G.D. (1997). Lack of effect of sleep on energy expenditure and physiologic measures in critically ill burn patients. *Journal of American Dietetic Association, 97*(2), 131–139.

HOUDE, S.C., & KAMPFE-LEACHER, R. (1997). Chronic fatigue syndrome: An update for clinicians in primary care. *Nurse Practitioner, 22*(7), 30, 35–36, 39–40.

HUDSON, R. (1996). Nursing. The value of lavender for rest and activity in the elderly patient. *Complementary Therapies in Medicine, 4*(1), 52–57.

KOLCABA, K.Y. (1992). Holistic comfort: Operationalizing the construct as a nurse-sensitive outcome. *Advanced Nursing Science, 15*(1), 1–10.

MAHON, N.E. (1995). The contributions of sleep to perceived health status during adolescence. *Public Health Nursing, 12*(2), 127–133.

RICHARDSON, S.J. (1997). Assessment techniques. A comparison of tools for the assessment of sleep pattern disturbance in critically ill adults. *Dimensions of Critical Care Nursing, 16*(5), 226–239.

SIMPSON, T., & LEE, E.R. (1996). Patient guide. Getting a good night's rest. *American Journal of Critical Care, 5*(3), 182–189.

TIESINGA, L.J., DASSEN, T.W.N., & HALFENS, R.J.G. (1996). Fatigue: A summary of the definitions, dimensions and indicators. *Nursing Diagnosis, 7*(2), 51–62.

TORRES, C., HOLDITCH-DAVIS, D., O'HALE, A., & D'AURIA, J. (1997). Effects of standard rest periods on apnea and weight gain in preterm infants. *Journal of Neonatal Nursing, 16*(8), 35–43.

VYHLIDAL, S.K., MOXNESS, D., BOSAK, K.S., Van METER, F.G., & BERGSTROM, N. (1997). Mattress replacement or foam overlay? A prospective study on the incidence of pressure ulcers. *Applied Nursing Research, 10*(3), 111–120.

WAGNER, L.I., & JASON, L.A. (1997). Outcomes of occupational stressors on nurses: Chronic fatigue syndrome-related symptoms. *Nursing Connections, 10*(3), 41–49.

WATSON, S., & WATSON, S. (1997). The effects of massage: An holistic approach to care. *Nursing Standard, 11*(47), 45–47.

ZIMMERMAN, L., NIEVEEN, J., BARNASON, S., & SCHMADERER, M. (1996). The effects of music interventions on postoperative pain and sleep in coronary artery bypass graft (CABG) patients. *Scholarly Inquiry for Nursing Practice, 10*(2), 153–174.

Chapter

OUTLINE

Pain Management

Central Questions

1. How is pain important as a protective mechanism for the body?
2. How do the mechanisms of pain reception, transmission, perception and modulation function in the physiology of pain?
3. What is the gate-control theory of pain?
4. What are the various types of pain stimuli, and how do they cause pain?
5. What are the types of pain and the determinants of the personal experience of pain?
6. How do pain experiences vary throughout the life cycle?
7. How does the nurse assess a patient's pain experience?
8. What are the common nursing diagnostic statements for patients with pain?
9. How can the nurse apply principles relevant to pain and pain management in planning and implementing nursing interventions
   a. to prevent or minimize pain
   b. to help patients cope with their pain
   c. to modify the patient's perception of pain?
10. How does the nurse evaluate the patient's response to nursing interventions?

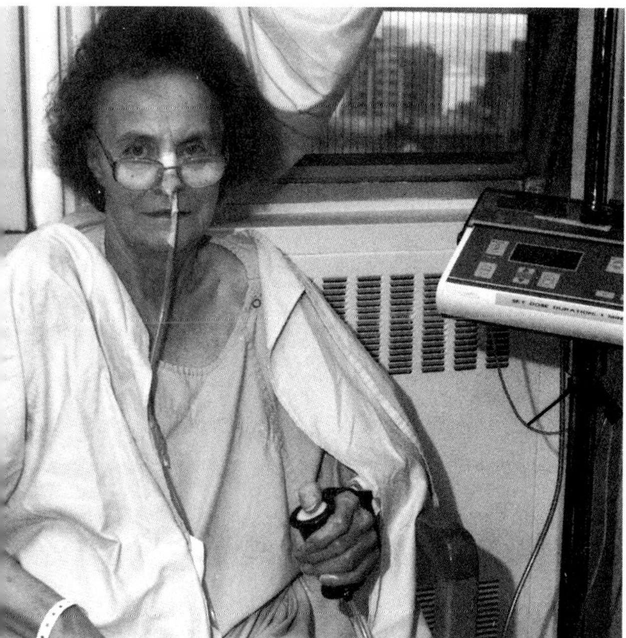

Introduction

We all must die. But if I can save him from days of torture, that is what I feel is my great and ever new privilege. Pain is a more terrible lord of mankind than even death himself.

—Albert Schweitzer, cited in Health & Welfare Canada, 1984

Pain is a multidimensional, universal experience. There are a number of definitions to describe pain. For example, "Pain is an unpleasant sensory and emotional experience associated with potential or impending tissue damage or described in terms of such damage" (International Association for the Study of Pain, cited in Twycross, 1994, p. 32). However it is defined, pain is a phenomenon not yet completely understood. Clinically, it is difficult to measure. Though sophisticated equipment and methods of diagnosis exist for most other disease symptoms, pain measurement remains almost completely subjective. Health professionals rely both on subjective reports and on observable behaviour. The individual experiencing pain is the authority and the only person able to describe the experience. According to McCaffery (1979), pain is "whatever the experiencing person says it is, existing whenever he [she] says it does" (p. 11).

Cassell (1991) describes **suffering** as a state of distress induced by the threat of the loss of intactness or the disintegration of a person from whatever cause. Suffering is linked to issues of meaning and quality of life. It is an all-encompassing hurt that can result from, but is not limited to, physical pain experiences (Mirka, 1996). Pain may be part of suffering, but one can suffer without pain. Therefore, pain and suffering are not the same. Themes associated with suffering include helplessness, social isolation, loss, struggle, threat and spirituality.

Another perspective is the concept of **total pain**. This term was first used by Dame Cicely Saunders in an effort to describe the multidimensional (physical, psychological, social and spiritual) suffering experienced by cancer patients (Twycross, 1994).

In most circumstances, the sensation of pain is due to **noxious** (harmful, injurious) stimuli, and is a protective mechanism that warns the individual of actual or potential damage to body tissues. This type of acute experience is familiar to most people. However, pain can become chronic. Prolonged or intractable pain lasting longer than six months is considered to be chronic pain. We will discuss acute and chronic pain in more detail later in the chapter.

Published research indicates that pain is often undertreated. There are some common misconceptions about pain and pain management that may account for this lack of treatment. Many health professionals are concerned that use of pain medications will promote drug abuse. It is often assumed that individuals with chronic pain grow accustomed to it and therefore require less attention to pain management. Another common misconception is that children may not feel pain, and that if they do, they quickly forget the experience. Older adults are assumed to be less sensitive to pain and therefore do not require pain management. These common fallacies have led to the discomfort and anxiety of many people of all ages.

Pain is a major factor affecting the functional capacity to cope with the activities of daily living. Healing can be interrupted or prolonged if pain is unmanaged. Untreated pain may cause a number of negative responses, including blood pressure, pulse and respiratory changes, as well as anxiety, fear and feelings of helplessness. Therefore, a significant nursing function is assisting patients to achieve relief from pain. Appropriate assessment and analysis of data enable nurses to develop and implement a plan of care that will assist patients to alleviate or manage their pain. In order to do this, nurses must understand the physiology of pain and the interventions available for pain management.

The Physiology of Pain

The experience of pain is a complex process involving both the nervous and the endocrine systems. Though the physiology of pain is not completely understood, the physiological mechanisms of pain may be characterized by four components: reception, transmission, perception and modulation.

Pain Reception

Free sensory nerve endings (**nociceptors**) are responsible for the reception of noxious stimuli and for beginning the transmission of pain impulses along afferent nerve fibres. Nociceptors are not found in all areas of the body. The skin, arterial walls, joints, periosteum and some internal organs such as the gallbladder and bile duct are richly supplied with nociceptors, while other areas, such as the brain and alveoli of the lung, lack these free nerve endings.

It is generally assumed that acute cellular damage stimulates the production of biochemical substances released at the site of injury that enhance pain impulses. These substances include acetylcholine, histamine, prostaglandins, potassium, serotonin and substance P. Not all noxious stimuli generate pain impulses. A stimulus must reach a sufficient level of intensity to create a nerve impulse. The point at which a stimulus reaches sufficient intensity to create a nerve impulse is called the **pain threshold**. This is the point at which the pain is first felt. "Pain threshold varies both between and within ethnic groups even under controlled conditions in the laboratory" (Twycross, 1994, p. 31). "Similar reactions to pain may be employed across cultural groups; they serve different functions and purposes, which are influenced by cultural beliefs and patterns" (Zborowski, cited in Leininger, 1995, p. 267). **Pain tolerance** is the amount of pain an individual is willing to endure. Pain tolerance is influenced by the physical and emotional condition of the individual, as well as cultural conditioning (McCaffery & Beebe, 1989; Bates, Edwards & Anderson, 1993).

Pain Transmission

SPINAL MECHANISM

ways. Once the nociceptor receives a stimulus of sufficient strength, an electrical impulse is generated along peripheral afferent nerve fibres to the spinal cord. Pain impulses are primarily transmitted by two types of peripheral nerve fibres: larger-diameter, myelinated A-delta fibres and smaller, unmyelinated C-fibres.

Myelinated A-delta fibres rapidly transmit impulses. These fibres permit information to be localized and degrees of intensity to be differentiated. The type of impulses transmitted are usually sharp or pricking. Pain transmitted by A-delta fibres generally subsides quickly.

Persistent, diffuse, burning sensations are conducted slowly by unmyelinated or poorly myelinated C-fibres. Approximately two-thirds of the fibres in the peripheral nerves are C-fibres. The abundance of C-fibres permits the transmission of large amounts of information despite slow conduction (Meinhart & McCaffery, 1983).

The difference between the experiences of A-delta and C-fibre pain is easily exemplified. Catching the tip of a finger in a door initially produces sharp, intense and well-localized pain—A-delta pain. Several moments later, aching and diffuse C-fibre pain are experienced.

Both A-delta and C-fibres enter the spinal cord through the dorsal roots of a spinal nerve and terminate in the grey matter (*substantia gelatinosa*) of the dorsal horn. From here the impulses ascend to brain centres including the thalamus, reticular formation, limbic system and somatosensory cortex.

Impulses ascend to the reticular formation and thalamus by neurons that form the anterolateral pathway, which is divided into two divisions: the neospinothalamic and the paleospinothalamic (Figure 27.1). The neospinothalamic tract is composed of A-delta fibres and transmits sharp, stabbing localized pain sensations. It is believed that this tract conveys sensory–discriminative information regarding the location, duration and intensity of pain. Innervation of this tract may also be responsible for initiating autonomic reactions, such as the "fight or flight" response.

The thalamic or paleospinalthalamic tract is composed primarily of C-fibres. This tract conducts impulses slowly and is associated with diffuse, dull, aching sensations associated with chronic and visceral pain. Visceral sensations are also transmitted along this tract. It is further hypothesized that this system affects brain structures that regulate memory and recall, and consequently, influence the emotional component of pain (motivational–affective component).

The thalamus, limbic system and reticular formation are important in the facilitation and inhibition of pain. The thalamus plays an important role in the perception of pain, while the limbic system is involved in the memory of pain. Activity in the reticular formation influences the individual's level of arousal. The reticular formation can facilitate or inhibit the transmission of noxious stimuli by increasing or decreasing attention. Thus, nursing interventions are highly important to prevent pain from occurring, and to treat it promptly when it does arise.

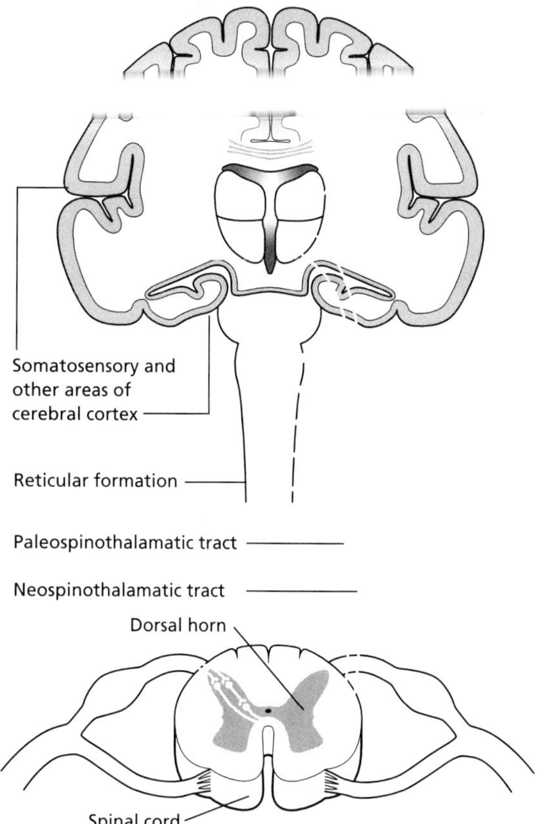

FIGURE 27.1 Neospinothalamic and paleospinothalamic subdivisions of the anterolateral pathway.

Pain Perception

Perception begins the moment an individual experiences pain. The ability to perceive pain depends upon the integrity of the nerve fibres and structures that receive, transmit and interpret pain impulses. Injury to sensory nerves, sensory tracts in the spinal cord, the thalamus or sensory areas in the cerebral cortex will interfere with pain perception. However, the pain after a spinal cord injury may be intractable. This chronic neurogenic pain may be present in as many as 50 percent of those who have suffered a spinal cord injury (Beric, 1997).

Sources of information about another's pain may be verbal or nonverbal. Factors that affect an individual's level of consciousness can pose a challenge for assessing and treating pain. Patients with dementia or those with altered levels of consciousness are unable to express their pain. However, through observation of the similarities that these patients display compared with observations of people who are able to articulate their pain, health professionals tend to agree that practitioners can make inferences pertaining to a patient's pain, even though these observations cannot be verified with the patient (Merskey, 1997).

In some circumstances, individuals become hypersensitive to painful stimuli (hyperalgesic). Unlike other receptors, nociceptors adapt poorly, or not at all, to continuous stimulation. Pain is triggered as the receptors increasingly respond to any type of stimulation. The pain threshold is lowered, and individuals experience increased sensitivity to pain. Indeed, they may continue to experience the sensation of pain long after the initial pain stimulus has stopped.

In contrast, intense pain in one part of the body may raise the pain threshold in other areas. An individual suffering considerable pain from a broken leg may be unaware of pain from an elbow abrasion. This is due to selective perception, whereby the stimulus of greater priority (or intensity) assumes precedence in attention over the less intense, or less significant stimulus.

Areas of the body adjacent to injured areas are usually more sensitive to pain. The skin adjacent to a wound, for example, is generally tender. Damaged tissues also react to additional painful stimuli, even of minimal intensity, more readily than intact tissue. The sensitivity of sunburned skin attests to this phenomenon.

Pain Modulation

Several factors within the central nervous system moderate pain perception. In some instances, the stimulus is of sufficient intensity for a protective response to be initiated in the spinal cord before the impulse reaches the somatosensory cortex and conscious perception. For example, touching a hot stove will generate a reflex action, causing an individual to withdraw the hand immediately.

Pain impulses travelling via the spinothalamic tract, reaching the thalamus and finally the cortex, may also be modified by *endogenous opiates* such as the *enkephalins*, *endorphins* and *dynorphins*. Enkephalin-containing fibres are prevalent throughout the nervous system. Enkephalins produce a weak analgesic effect by binding to opiate receptors on nociceptive fibres and inhibiting the release of excitatory neurotransmitters, such as substance P. This decreases the intensity of the pain impulse being transmitted.

Endorphins are large polypeptides with an opioid-like pharmacological action. Endorphins are believed to be synthesized and stored by the pituitary gland. These molecules, like enkephalins, alter pain impulse transmission by binding to opiate receptor sites throughout the nervous system and inhibiting the release of neurotransmitters. Several endorphins have been isolated; the most powerful is beta-endorphin.

Dynorphins are the most powerful of the identified endogenous opiates. These substances have an analgesic effect 50 times more powerful than beta-endorphin (Meinhart & McCaffery, 1983).

Enkephalins, endorphins and dynorphins are triggered by pain and stress. Stimulation of this internal system of endogenous opiates activates descending nerve fibres that transmit inhibitory impulses to cells in the dorsal horns of the spinal column. The result is an alteration of the intensity of the pain impulse and analgesia. However, the degree, or amount, of pain necessary to trigger the system is unknown.

The phenomenon of *wind-up* continues to be explored in the pain literature. Constant repetition and intensity of C-fibre stimulus can induce this phenomenon, in which the responses of certain dorsal horn neurons increase dramatically even though there is no change in input into the spinal cord. Wind-up increases dorsal horn response by up to 20 times in magnitude, intensity and duration, with the response continuing after the withdrawal of peripheral input. The receptor NMDA (*N*-methyl-D-aspartate) is required for persistent and intense nociceptive activity. This spinal event is imperative to central hyperalgesia, as the NMDA receptor transforms low-level pain activity into high-level activity without change in the input to peripheral nerves (Dickenson, 1990).

Pain Theories

Despite rigorous research, the mechanisms of pain are not completely understood. Several theories of pain, such as the specificity theory, pattern theories and the gate-control theory, have been proposed. The gate-control theory, however, dominates present thinking about pain.

Gate-Control Theory

The gate-control theory proposed by Melzak and Wall (Melzak, 1973) is presently the most popular theory of pain. This theory proposes that a neural mechanism located in the substantia gelatinosa of the spinal cord dorsal horns acts as a gate that controls the flow of pain impulses to higher centres in the brain. Typically, the gate is partially closed. Stimulation of the substantia gelatinosa further closes the gate, thereby blocking the transmission of impulses. Inhibition of the substantia gelatinosa, on the other hand, opens the gate and allows impulses to flow through it. Beyond the gating mechanism are T (transmission) cells. When the degree of stimulation passing through the gate to the T cells reaches a critical (threshold) level, these cells fire, activating areas within the central nervous system that are responsible for pain perception and response.

Activity in both the peripheral and the central nervous systems may alter the position of the gate and either increase or decrease the transmission of pain impulses from the peripheral fibres to the somatosensory cortex and conscious awareness. Pain impulses carried by A-delta and C-fibres enter the spinal column at the level of the dorsal root and terminate in the substantia gelatinosa. Input from A-delta and C-fibres has an inhibiting effect on the gating

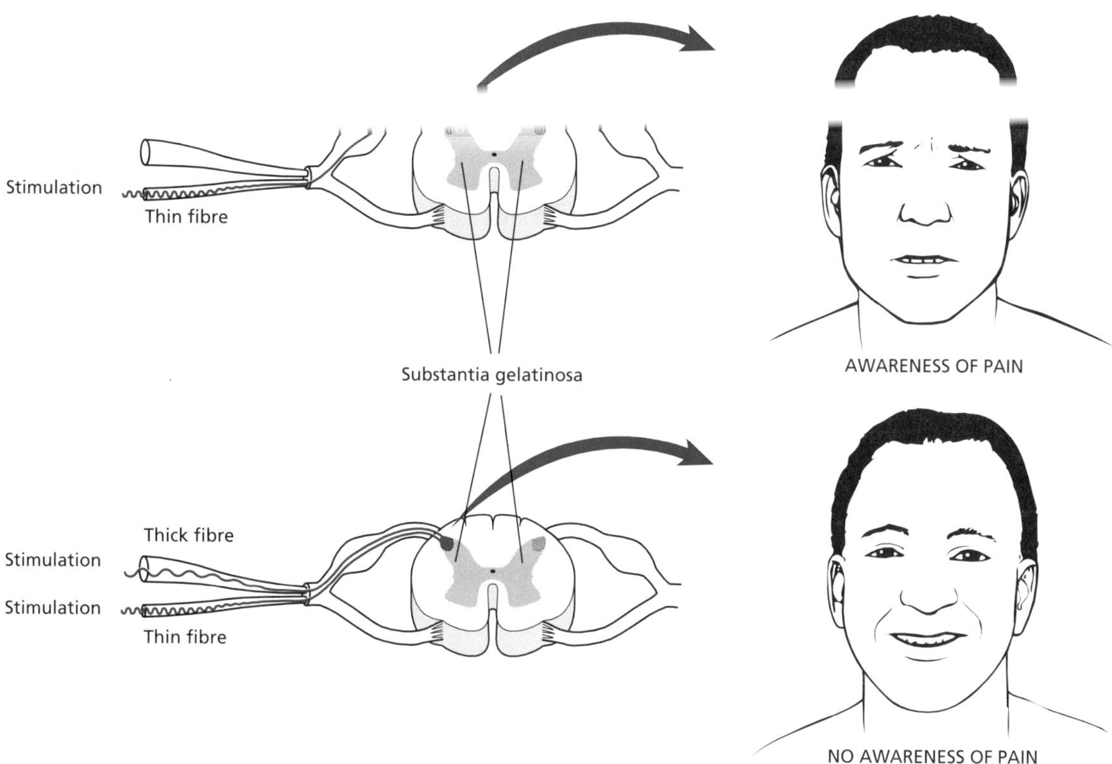

FIGURE 27.2 Stimulation of thick nerve fibres, which may be achieved by nursing measures such as massage, may stimulate the release of endorphins so that pain impulses from thin nerve fibres are blocked in the substantia gelatinosa

mechanism, causing the gate to remain open, or to open further.

Large-diameter A-beta (touch) fibres have been identified. These large afferent fibres also enter the spinal cord at the level of the dorsal root. Stimulation of A-beta fibres opposes the activity of the smaller-diameter fibres, thereby closing the gate and inhibiting the transmission of pain impulses. Stimulation of the A-beta fibres also facilitates the release of enkephalins in the dorsal horn, which further modifies pain impulse transmission along the spinothalamic tracts.

The majority of the larger-diameter A-fibres lie close to the skin surface. Cutaneous stimulation of these fibres by massage, heat, cold or TENS (transcutaneous electrical nerve stimulation) provides effective modalities for decreasing pain impulse transmission and contributing to pain relief.

The gating mechanism is also affected by motivational and cognitive influences from the higher brain centres. These influences, which include such factors as attention, anxiety, expectations, suggestion and memories of previous experiences (including cultural and social background), send messages from the brain that modulate pain impulses travelling upward from peripheral sites. Through a process of input comparison from the sensory systems, the thalamus and the cerebral cortex, the spinal gating mechanism will be closed or opened.

There are a number of pain-relief measures that stimulate the activity of the thalamus and cerebral cortex to close the gating mechanism. These include relaxation strategies, distraction techniques, guided imagery and hypnosis (see Figure 27.2). It is believed that these methods may also activate the endogenous opiate system. The gate-control theory provides plausible explanations for some of the observations about pain, such as why stimulating a painful area—by rubbing it, for example—may result in pain reduction. This theory also recognizes the potency of cognitive activities, such as distraction, in decreasing the perception of pain.

Common Causes of Pain

Pain begins with stimulation of free sensory nerve endings located near the skin surface or within deeper structures. Stimulation of nociceptors may be generated by a number of different stimuli including chemical substances, mechanical trauma and thermal extremes.

Chemical Stimuli

Ischemic pain is an example of the effect of endogenous chemicals. An insufficient blood supply results in tissue death. The decaying cells liberate endogenous chemical substances that irritate the nociceptors and generate pain impulses. Ischemic pain is further intensified by the inability of the blood supply to remove the accumulated metabolic waste products. An example of this pain is the accumulation of lactic acid in the gastrocnemius muscle experienced by runners. When the acidic waste products of cellular metabolism collect, pain results from the irritating effect of these substances on nociceptors.

Mechanical Trauma

Mechanical stimulation usually involves trauma to body tissue, such as spraining an ankle or accidentally hitting the thumb when hammering a nail. The pain felt initially is due to pressure on the free nerve endings.

Pain may also result from overstretching or contraction of tissues. Distention of a hollow organ such as the stomach is an example of overstretching the tissues. An individual who eats a large meal may feel considerable discomfort in the region of the stomach. This feeling of pain is related to two factors: stretched nerve endings in the sensory receptors and occlusion of small blood vessels in the stretched tissue, producing localized ischemia.

Muscle spasm is an example of pain occurring during contraction. Intramuscular blood vessels are compressed, producing localized ischemia. In addition, prolonged muscular contraction increases the cellular metabolic rate, resulting in an accumulation of metabolic waste products, which constricted blood vessels cannot remove. These metabolic waste products are chemically irritating to sensory nerve endings and contribute to the sensation of pain.

Thermal Stimulation

Extreme heat or cold causes pain and damage to body tissues. Pain due to sunburn or a small burn on the tip of the finger is a common experience. The initial burning pain probably results from the intensity of the thermal stimulus. The lingering after-pain is due to the chemical substances released following tissue destruction.

Extreme cold, particularly if there is freezing of body tissues, as in frostbite, causes tissue damage and pain. Cold constricts the blood vessels in the affected tissue and may completely obliterate the blood supply. The pain in a frostbitten nose or finger is most severe when the blood flow is returning and the constricted vessels are being dilated.

The Experience of Pain

The personal experience of pain is mediated by the type of pain perceived and by the influence of a variety of determinants.

Types of Pain

Pain may be divided into two categories: acute and chronic. **Acute pain** is a protective mechanism that warns of potential or actual tissue damage. This type of pain has a rapid onset, varies in intensity and generally lasts less than six months. Acute pain usually has an identifiable pathology, tends to resolve as healing occurs, and is usually responsive to treatment modalities. Pain lasting longer than six months, that may or may not be connected to a pathological process, is **chronic pain**. Chronic pain varies in intensity and requires both pharmacological and nonpharmacological approaches.

Both acute and chronic pain may arise from two sources: somatic and visceral. **Somatic pain** originates from the skin, muscles or joints and may be superficial or deep. *Superficial somatic pain* is usually described as having a sharp, burning or pricking quality. It arises from stimulation of receptors in the skin or the mucous membranes of the body. As a rule, an individual is able to localize surface pain fairly accurately because of the large number of free sensory nerve endings on the surface of the body. *Deep somatic pain* comes from the deeper structures of the body, such as the muscles, tendons, joints and fasciae. Pain originating from these areas is easily localized. It is frequently described as dull, aching, cramping, gnawing or boring. Muscles and tendons are particularly sensitive to pain and may give rise to pain of considerable intensity.

Visceral pain arises from sources in the abdominal cavity or thorax. It is more difficult to localize its source because there are fewer sensory nerve endings in the viscera than in the skin and mucous membranes. Visceral pain is similar to deep somatic pain and frequently includes gripping, cramping, dull aching and burning sensations, as well as a feeling of pressure. In the case of a peptic ulcer, the patient may describe the pain as having a gnawing, burning or sometimes knife-like quality.

Psychogenic pain arises from an emotional or psychological origin. This type of pain has no identified physical cause, yet it is real and is as intense as somatic pain. "Pain is only primarily somatogenic or psychogenic; it is rarely, if ever, purely one type or the other" (Ludwig-Beymer & Huether, 1996, p. 320).

ACUTE PAIN

There are two categories of acute pain: intermittent pain and referred pain. **Intermittent pain** is characterized by exacerbations and remissions of acute episodes of pain. The patient is generally free of pain between these episodes. This pain syndrome is common in conditions such as sickle cell anemia or migraine headaches.

Pain that is felt in one region of the body from a stimulus in another area is called **referred pain**. This type of pain most commonly occurs with visceral pain. It originates in an organ, but the sensation is felt in a somatic area—often, superficial areas in the skin. In referred pain, the afferent fibres carrying impulses from the viscera and those from cutaneous tissues often converge onto the same spinal neuron tract. The brain is unable to distinguish between the two sources of painful stimuli, and the pain sensation is referred to the most superficial structures innervated by the converging neurons (Seeley, Stephens & Tate, 1992). The individual may experience the sensation of pain coming from the skin alone or from both viscera and skin.

The nature of the referred pain is [illegible] curring. For example, a person with myocardial infarction (ischemia of the heart muscle) often describes the pain as constricting, vise-like or compressing, radiating to the left shoulder and down the left arm. Pain may or may not be felt in the region of the heart.

CHRONIC PAIN

Chronic pain is pain that is experienced continuously and is often resistant to relief measures (intractable). It is often described as chronic malignant (cancer) or chronic nonmalignant pain. There is no predictable endpoint in chronic pain. Consequently, people with chronic pain often encounter significant disruption in their personal and professional life. They may become overwhelmed by the pain and lose their ability to cope with the activities of daily living. Feelings of frustration, helplessness and hopelessness in managing the pain frequently lead to anxiety and depression. Behaviour can be adaptive and is focussed on modifying the pain (Ludwig-Beymer & Huether, 1996).

Cancer pain is the pain attributed to advancing disease or clinical treatment. For example, pain may increase in intensity as a tumour grows, pressing on nerves and internal organs. Patients often find it difficult to pinpoint the nature and location of their pain (Twycross, 1994). The concept of total pain, mentioned earlier in this chapter, embraces the pain that patients with cancer may experience.

Phantom limb pain and central pain syndromes are examples of chronic nonmalignant pain. **Phantom limb pain** occurs following amputation of a limb. Individuals with this syndrome usually experience pain prior to the amputation and feel pain as though the affected limb had not been amputated. The pain tends to be severe and may be described as burning, crushing or cramping. Individuals may also feel that the limb is edematous, or lying in a distorted position. Phantom limb pain may be triggered by touch, illness, fatigue or stress (Meinhart & McCaffery, 1983). The physiology of phantom pain is not well understood, but it is suggested that a pattern of impulses may be generated between the brain and the sensory receptors, even though the receptors are not present. Also, the lack of usual neural mediating mechanisms, due to the amputation, tends to result in sensations of increased intensity. Research is currently underway to investigate the role of continuous peripheral input from an area of injury.

Central pain syndromes usually arise from injury to sensory nerves, neural pathways or areas in the brain concerned with pain perception. The pain is severe, occurs spontaneously and is often continuous. It may be described as gnawing, burning or crushing. Trigeminal neuralgia (*tic douloureux*) is an example of a central pain syndrome.

Neuropathic pain can occur from injury to peripheral nerves that have been cut or exposed to chemotherapeu- [illegible] normal impulse firing. Treatment may involve a wide variety of agents such as analgesics, anticonvulsants or antidepressants. Common examples of neuropathic pain are post-herpetic neuralgia, phantom pain and peripheral neuropathy. Neuropathic pain is characterized by descriptions such as burning, tingling or shocking. The patient experiences a delay in onset after the precipitating injury.

Responses to Pain

An individual's response to pain is characterized by physiological and behavioural manifestations. Pain activates both the **sympathetic** and **parasympathetic** divisions of the autonomic nervous system. The physiological manifestations of low- to moderate-intensity acute pain, or superficial pain, are generally the result of sympathetic nervous system stimulation. Commonly referred to as the "fight or flight" reaction, observable signs and symptoms include an elevated blood pressure, pulse and respiratory rate. Pallor, diaphoresis, dilation of the pupils and the bronchial tubes, increased skeletal muscle tension and decreased gastric motility are also evidence of autonomic nervous system response. Restlessness and irritability are frequently observed.

In the experience of severe or deep (visceral) pain, the parasympathetic nervous system is activated and the individual exhibits pallor and a decrease in blood pressure, heart rate and muscle tension. Nausea and vomiting often occur, and the body's defences may collapse. In such an event, there are observable signs of exhaustion and prostration. The patient may appear "as white as a ghost," collapse and loss of consciousness may ensue.

An individual with chronic pain does not usually demonstrate the same overt signs and symptoms of pain. The exact mechanism of the compensatory response of the body to chronic pain is not well understood, but, over time, there is a decrease in the sympathetic nervous system response. As a result, the individual may display fewer physiological and behavioural pain indicators.

Determinants of the Pain Experience

The behavioural responses to pain differ much more widely from one individual to another than do the physiological manifestations. Everyone has observed people who "never flinch," even though the pain they experience is intense. On the other hand, some people react to pain with loud groans, weeping, screaming or attempts to remove themselves from the source of pain. An individual's response to pain is influenced by several factors, such as the individual's physical condition, emotional state and culture (cognitive–evaluative component).

RESEARCH to practice

Riddell, A., & Fitch, M.I. (1997). Patients' knowledge of and attitudes toward the management of cancer pain. *Oncology Nursing Forum, 24*(10), 1775–1784.

The purpose of this study was to explore the knowledge that patients had toward the management and treatment of cancer pain, and to examine from a patient's perspective the factors that contributed to effective and ineffective pain management.

This descriptive correlational study was conducted at a 105-bed ambulatory care setting in a large urban teaching hospital in Canada. The sample comprised 42 patients receiving pain medication for chronic cancer-related pain. Patients in the study completed a modified version of the Patient Pain Questionnaire (PPQ). This tool measures the knowledge, attitudes and experience of patients managing chronic cancer pain. A demographic questionnaire was included, as well as two open-ended questions intended to determine factors that contributed to effective or ineffective relief of cancer pain.

Data were collected during a 30-minute single session with each study participant by the investigator. Study findings indicate that patients lacked knowledge regarding pain management and had concerns (which were often unrealistic) about taking pain medication. Many participants in this study believed that patients were given too much pain medication, that it should be given on an as-needed rather than a regular basis and that medication should be given only when pain is severe.

Study results indicated that many patients were able to identify alternative methods of pain relief. The support of family and friends, and maintaining a positive attitude, were seen as important in the relief of their pain.

Results of this study "emphasize the need for patient education to address patients' misconceptions and concerns about using pain medications and the principles involved in effective pain management" (Riddell & Fitch, 1997, p. 1782). Nurses have a primary role in designing educational strategies for effective cancer pain management.

PHYSICAL CONDITION

When tired or physically weak, people have diminished resistance and control over their reactions. In such circumstances the individual may react to a minimal stimulus with an exaggerated response. Thus, a busy parent attempting to cook dinner and, at the same time, look after small children may find the pain of a slight burn at the stove to be intense.

In cases of extreme exhaustion, an individual's attention span is reduced and sustained concentration on any one stimulus is unlikely. Therefore, an exhausted patient may be unable to focus on the location or intensity of the pain.

EMOTIONAL STATE

The emotional state of the individual also modifies the reaction to pain. Pleasurable emotions tend to nullify pain perception. A contented or happy person often does not feel pain to the same extent as someone who is worried.

Anxiety and fear aggravate pain. All three feelings provoke the same physiological "fight or flight" reaction. If anxiety is relieved, the patient's reaction to pain is lessened. It is suggested that anxiety-relieving measures are associated with the release of endorphins that block or moderate the transmission of pain impulses.

Strong emotional responses to stimuli other than the pain stimulus may block out the awareness of pain. A football player injured during a game may not notice an injury until the game is over. Excitement and the desire to win may be so intense that the sensory impressions of pain from the injury are of less priority and, therefore, are not perceived. A similar explanation may account for the numerous reports of wounded soldiers who stated they did not feel pain despite significant injuries. The overriding fear during battle, and the necessity for self-preservation at all costs, took precedence over impressions from other sensory stimulation; thus, pain perception was inhibited.

CULTURE

Cultural values and beliefs influence perceptions and behavioural responses to painful stimuli. Culture is a complex and multifaceted influence involving ethnicity, age, gender, religion and socioeconomic status. Many sociologists have investigated the differing reactions of various cultural groups to pain.

It is important for nurses to be aware of their own cultural biases with respect to pain. Cultural influences, though subtle, may affect the manner in which a nurse perceives and reacts to another's pain. Nurses who have been raised with the belief that "only babies cry" may find themselves reacting negatively to patients who do not handle their pain in the "approved" manner. Similarly, nurses raised to expect open displays of suffering must not assume that a patient is not in pain simply because he or she does not cry. If nurses realize that their reactions are a reflection of their own social values, which may be different from those of the patient, they will be better able to understand that these feelings should not interfere with judgements about the patient's pain experience (Leininger, 1995). Bates (1987) has proposed a biocultural model of pain perception and response that integrates physiological, psychological and sociocultural influences on pain perception.

The Canadian Pain Society Position Statement on Pain Relief

Almost all acute and cancer pain can be relieved, and many patients with chronic nonmalignant pain can be helped. Patients have the right to the best pain relief possible.

1. Unrelieved acute pain complicates recovery
2. Routine assessment is essential for effective management
3. The best pain management involves patients, families and health professionals.

SOURCE: Canadian Pain Society, 1997.

KEY PRINCIPLES

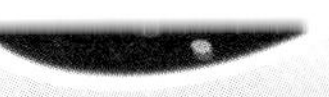

to Pain

1. Pain has a protective function in warning of present or potential damage to body tissues.
2. Pain may be caused by a number of different stimuli.
3. Tissues of the body differ in their sensitivity to painful stimuli.
4. Severe pain can cause collapse of the body's adaptive mechanisms.
5. The ability to perceive pain depends upon integrity of the neural structures that receive, transmit and interpret pain impulses.
6. Pain perception may be altered by physical and emotional factors.
7. Reactions to pain are highly individualized and depend on a number of physical, emotional and cultural factors.

The Pain Experience Throughout the Life Cycle

People of all ages experience pain as a reaction to noxious stimuli. Response to pain and pain tolerance, however, are unique to each individual. As we age, responses and tolerance to pain may change owing to physiological maturity and to the acquisition of a greater number of cognitive responses.

Neonates exhibit a reflex withdrawal response to harmful or potentially harmful stimuli. Other signs of pain include intense crying, restlessness or lethargy. Neonates in pain have also been observed to lie very quietly, as though sleeping. Poor sucking and decreased appetite are further indicators of pain. Infants, like older people, may try to protect the painful area by positioning themselves in a particular way. For example, infants with abdominal pain will draw their legs up to the abdomen.

All children experience pain, but their ability to describe the pain they are experiencing is affected by their limited cognitive understanding, insufficient verbal skills and fear of consequences. Toddlers, in particular, have limited cognitive ability to describe pain. Nurses must rely on behavioural manifestations of pain in these children. Abnormal gait, guarding of a part of the body, persistent crying or consoling behaviours such as rocking or sucking are a few examples of pain manifestations in young children. Older children (those over three years of age) have ample cognitive ability to describe their pain, but they may be reluctant to do so because they fear painful diagnostic or treatment measures. Nurses must be sensitive to the pain management needs of children, who require the same attention to their pain as do adults. With respect to pain-relief measures, children are able to tolerate opioid analgesics and effectively use many behavioural and cognitive strategies for pain relief (McConnan, 1992).

Older adults frequently suffer from chronic illnesses that may cause pain. It is important to note that pain is not a symptom of aging. Some older adults, however, may believe pain to be related to aging, and may hesitate to verbalize what they think is a normal process. Therefore, any statement of pain, or behaviour that may indicate pain, must be investigated.

Older adults often experience sensory-related age changes. Perception and information processing are slower, but the intensity of the pain experience is *not* reduced. Cardiovascular disease, diabetes, arthritis, osteoporosis and cancer are some common pathologies that may cause pain for older adults. The usual presentation of pain in these pathologies may not occur because of age-related physiological changes. For example, in older patients, backache may indicate osteoarthritis of the spine or osteoporosis. It is important to assess the older adult as a unique individual whose pain experience is also unique.

Assessing Pain

Pain is one of the most subjective and distressing of all disease symptoms. Therefore, the primary source of information about pain is always the patient. When patients themselves are unable to provide adequate descriptions of their pain, the family or significant others become essential sources of information. The nurse also makes observations about the patient's physiological and behavioural responses to pain and consults with other members of the health care team for observations they may have made (Romyn, 1992). Figure 27.3 provides an example of a pain assessment tool.

Pain in Infants, Children, Adolescents and the Elderly

	Pain Threshold	Physiologic Manifestations	Behavioural Responses	Nursing Actions
Infants	Lower than adults	• increased P, R, BP • decreased SaO_2 • flushing or pallor • diaphoresis	• changes in facial expression • vertical bulge/furrow in forehead • broadened nose • crying with lowered brows • tightly closed eyes • chin quiver/mouth open and squarish • withdrawal of affected limb • rigidity, flailing • sleep from exhaustion	• hold/cuddle
Children	Lower than adults	• similar to infants • nausea/vomiting	Responses vary.	
			Toddlers: • overactive/restless • cry loudly/grimace • cling to parent • clench teeth/bite lips • rub eyes • show physical aggression	• distraction • diversion • verbalization • holding
			Preschoolers: • fear bodily harm • see procedures as punishment	• allow to act out fear • be present
			School-aged: • passive requests for help • talk about being in pain • fear never being well again	• allow to ask questions • discuss fears
Adolescents	May be similar to adults	• increased P, R, BP • dilated pupils • diaphoresis	• fear of bodily alteration • fear of losing control • verbal comments minimal • perceive that health professionals know when they are in pain • changes in mobility • irritability • quiet, withdrawn, exhausted	• encourage discussion • review how to ask for relief • identify strategies used at home
Elderly	Increased from middle age or may have no change	• Similar to adults	• may be unable to describe • may not use the word "pain" • may perceive pain to be part of aging • perceive that health professionals know they are in pain • perceive that hospitals are for the dying (denial of pain) • wrinkled forehead • tightly closed/widely opened eyes/mouth • pacing, guarding or pulling at body part • sudden change in confusion • fear of addiction	• use family as resource • try other terms • encourage talking • assess facial expressions

SOURCES: McCaffery & Beebe, 1989; Ludwig-Beymer & Huether, 1996; Pasero & McCaffery, 1996; Delmar, 1997.

Nursing Health History

Because pain is highly subjective, most data about a patient's [illegible] [illegible] the standard nursing history form with a special pain assessment tool. When gathering information about an individual's pain experience, the nurse needs to ascertain, whenever possible, the following aspects of the pain:

1. quality
2. location
3. intensity
4. time and duration
5. precipitating factors
6. aggravating factors
7. effect on activities of daily living
8. personal meaning
9. usual coping strategies and pain-relief measures
10. affective responses.

QUALITY Graphic terms are frequently used when describing pain. Patients generally characterize pain in terms of something familiar to them. For example, sharp pain may be compared to the cutting action of a knife. When recording and reporting pain, the nurse should use the patient's exact words, in order to convey an accurate description of his or her perceptions. If the patient is having difficulty describing the pain, it may be necessary to provide some prompting. One way to do this is to ask the patient to describe what would be necessary to make you feel the same pain.

LOCATION The patient is usually able to identify fairly accurately superficial pain and pain originating from bones, muscles and joints. It is more difficult to identify the source of visceral pain. The patient may complain of pain in the general epigastric region, lower abdomen, chest or lower back when a visceral organ is affected. Pain from the viscera may also be referred to a surface area, such as the referral of myocardial pain to the left shoulder.

When assessing the location of pain, the nurse should ask patients to point to the area of discomfort on their own body and also any area where the pain radiates. If patients have difficulty doing this, it sometimes helps to ask them to show you the area of discomfort by pointing to that area on a body chart. This is a useful technique with both adults and children.

INTENSITY The intensity of pain is completely subjective, and it is sometimes difficult for a patient to quantify the severity of the experience. There are many tools available to assist with this area of assessment. The simplest technique is to ask the patient to indicate the severity of the pain numerically on a scale of one to 10: one represents no pain, and 10 indicates the most severe pain. Similar tools may be used with children three years of age and older. These are discussed further in the section on measurement of pain.

For children younger than three years, and for cognitively impaired adults, it is necessary to rely on behavioural cues to determine [illegible] increased irritability may indicate increasing intensity of pain. Often, it is only by 24-hour monitoring of all activities that a picture of the individual's response to pain can be determined.

When the intensity of a patient's pain changes abruptly, it is usually an indication of a change in his or her condition. For example, when an inflamed appendix ruptures, or a peptic ulcer perforates, the patient usually experiences persistent sharp and severe pain, different both in quality and intensity from the pain felt previously.

TIME AND DURATION An accurate description of a patient's pain includes when it begins, how long it lasts and whether it is intermittent or persistent. Does the pain come and go, or does it remain constant? Does the pain become more severe at night? Does it wake the individual? Pain sometimes seems more severe at night, when a person is alone and unoccupied. It is suggested that, in the absence of other people or distracting activities, the patient's full attention becomes focussed on the pain.

PRECIPITATING FACTORS Pain is often precipitated by certain physical or emotional activities. In some cardiac conditions, chest pain may be caused by exertion. Patients with musculoskeletal problems frequently have pain associated with movement of the affected limb. Pain in the gastrointestinal tract may be precipitated by eating certain foods. Pain may also be related to an intolerance to factors in the environment. Noise, for example, may induce a headache. Often, the patient is able to identify the specific factor or factors that cause pain, and these should be recorded and reported, again using the patient's own words. If the patient cannot identify precipitating factors, it is often helpful to ask about activities engaged in prior to noticing the pain. The answer may provide a clue to the precipitating cause. Arguing with a teenager, for example, may raise a parent's blood pressure and precipitate a headache. Similarly, waiting for a job interview may activate stomach ulcers.

AGGRAVATING FACTORS A variety of factors may worsen the patient's pain, for example, secondary symptoms such as nausea, constipation or dyspnea. Patients with peripheral vascular disease or a herniated disk often find their pain increases with the physical exertion of walking. It is important to ask patients about activities that worsen their pain.

EFFECT ON ACTIVITIES OF DAILY LIVING Sometimes pain can be so overriding that it interferes with a patient's ability to carry out daily activities. For example, the pain associated with rheumatoid arthritis may be severe enough to prevent patients from washing, dressing and feeding themselves as well as getting to and from the bathroom. Pain interferes with rest and sleep, decreases appetite and reduces concentration. Severe pain may keep a person away from work or school and curb usual leisure and social activities. Knowing the extent of disruption in daily functioning gives clues about the severity of pain and provides information needed to determine the assistance patients may require in coping with the activities of daily living.

PERSONAL MEANING OF THE PAIN How people interpret their pain depends on its significance to them, their past experiences and on social and cultural influences. Individuals may withstand pain if they identify the painful experience with a positive outcome. For example, a woman giving birth or an individual undergoing cosmetic surgery often tolerate pain. Conversely, pain with no benefit is viewed as a threat to well-being. People with chronic, unabating pain experience fear, anxiety and depression, which further exacerbate the pain experience.

USUAL COPING STRATEGIES AND PAIN-RELIEF MEASURES People in pain often use the same coping strategies they do with any illness. Some people do not allow the pain to disrupt their functioning; they implement pain-relief measures and continue the activity at hand. Other people allow the pain to take precedence over everything else. They stop what they are doing and attempt to relieve the pain. Some people turn to others for help and comfort, perhaps a vestige of a coping strategy learned in childhood. Knowing something about a patient's coping strategies helps the nurse better understand the patient in pain. In addition, identifying pain-relief measures the patient has tried and noting their effectiveness provides valuable information when developing a pain management plan. For example, does rest relieve pain brought on by exertion? Does holding the limb in a certain way prevent pain? Does medication relieve the pain?

AFFECTIVE RESPONSES Many feelings accompany pain, depending on the severity and duration of discomfort and the degree of disruption in a person's life. Feelings of fear, anxiety, depression and exhaustion are common with long-standing pain. Furthermore, individuals may feel powerless to control their pain and consequently lose hope. Expressions like "I can't take this anymore," "I feel like I don't have a life" or "I don't know what else to do" indicate feelings of hopelessness. Information about affective responses to pain are necessary in determining the supportive care patients will need.

A health history guide (see the following guide) for assessing a patient's pain experience is a useful tool. It draws the nurse's attention to the presenting pain pattern as well as the patient's usual health patterns that promote and protect

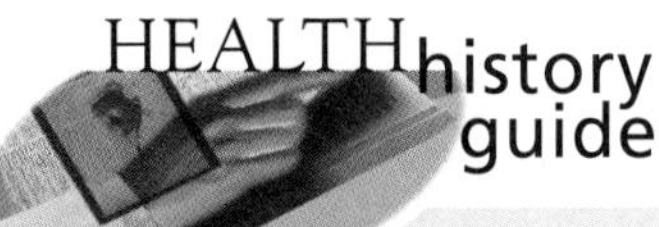

Pain Experience

Presenting Pain Pattern

- Describe the quality of pain you are experiencing. (Is it sharp, burning?)
- Where do you feel the pain?
- Does the pain radiate anywhere? Can you point to the pain on yourself? On this chart?
- On a scale of one to 10, if 10 is the worst pain, how would you rate your pain?
- Have you noticed any patterns to the pain? Is it worse at certain times of the day? In the morning or during the night? Does the pain wake you?
- Do you have a history of any disease that might bring on pain?
- What were you doing when the pain started?
- Does anything bring the pain on?
- Does anything make the pain worse?
- Have you had difficulty with nausea, vomiting, constipation, diarrhea or shortness of breath?
- How does the pain affect your usual daily functioning? Are you able to perform hygiene activities, continue to work (or go to school), exercise, socialize with friends? Are you able to rest?
- What does this pain mean to you? Do you have any fears about the pain?
- How do you usually cope with pain?
- Is there anything that makes the pain better or go away?
- What have you tried to make the pain go away?
- Have you taken any drugs to relieve the pain? If so, have the drugs helped?
- How does the pain make you feel? Anxious? Depressed? Helpless? Hopeless?
- What do you expect from health care professionals in regard to treating the pain?

Health Promotion and Protection Patterns

- What is your usual outlook on life? Optimistic? Positive? Happy? Sad? Depressed? Unhappy?
- Describe your usual mood. Do you tend to be relaxed? Calm? Tense?
- Do you eat a well-balanced diet and avoid foods and beverages that cause gastric upset, abdominal pain or headache?
- Do you keep fit, exercise regularly but avoid excessive, overzealous workouts?
- Do you wear a seat belt when riding in a car?
- Do you practise proper body mechanics when moving or lifting heavy objects?
- Do you practise safety in the workplace?

pain-free, healthy living. The nurse is cautioned, however, to use such a guide in a sensitive manner. For example, if the patient is in severe, acute pain, the nurse would logically

administering pain-relief measures first. Then, when the pain has subsided, a more detailed assessment of the pain experience may continue.

Measurements

PAIN RATING SCALES

Pain rating scales are objective measurement tools used to help patients describe the intensity of their pain. These scales use numbers, words or faces to describe pain of varying intensity. Patients are asked to rate their pain by selecting the word, number or face that describes the intensity of the pain they are feeling. Figure 27.3 gives an example of a word scale. There are similar scales that use numbers instead of words.

A "faces" rating scale is depicted in Figure 27.4a. It consists of a range of faces, from happy to grimacing. Patients point to the face that best represents how they feel. Faces scales are commonly used with children. Another tool used to rate pain intensity is the visual analogue scale (VAS), also depicted in Figure 27.4b. This scale consists of a 10-cm line that represents a continuum of pain intensity. One end of the line represents *no pain* and the other end *unbearable pain*. The patient places a mark on the line that represents the intensity of pain experienced. The distance from the zero point of the line to the patient's mark signifies the intensity of pain. The Hester Poker Chip tool (Figure 27.4c) is often used with children. The number of poker chips indicate the amount of "hurt" the child is experiencing. Pain rating scales provide a valuable tool for evaluating pain-relief measures because the patient's descriptions before and after treatment can be compared. These techniques require that patients be alert and cognitively aware.

Assessing pain in the cognitively impaired elderly patient is complex. Recently, research in this area was conducted at Vancouver General Hospital. Figure 27.5 shows Amy's tool and a flowsheet, which are used to assess pain in cognitively impaired patients or those who are unable to express themselves verbally. This tool consists of verbal, facial, behavioural and physical expression descriptors to help staff assess a patient's pain level. The flowsheet is used for ongoing assessment and monitoring (Galloway & Turner, 1996).

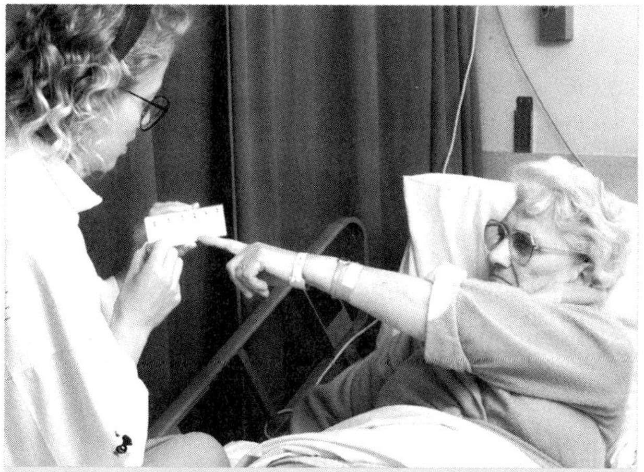

This patient describes the intensity of her pain on a rating scale.

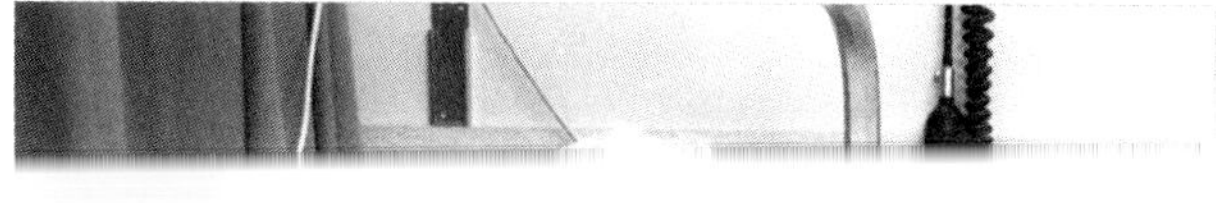

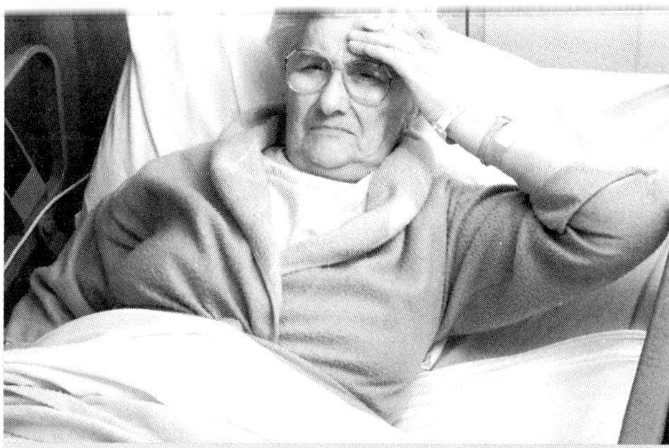

Facial expression and body posture can be behavioural manifestations of pain.

VITAL SIGNS

Pain is accompanied by autonomic nervous system responses that are reflected in the patient's vital signs. Acute or superficial pain of low to moderate intensity will cause stimulation of the sympathetic nervous system, resulting in elevations of heart rate, blood pressure and respirations. Severe visceral pain causes parasympathetic stimulation and a concomitant decrease in blood pressure and heart rate. Patients with chronic pain do not display overt changes in vital signs.

Physical Assessment

When assessing a patient in pain, it is important to supplement information obtained from the patient with observations of physiological and behavioural manifestations of pain. An individual's facial expression, posture and body movement will indicate pain. Patients in pain often appear tense and drawn. In addition, they may assume a particular position to minimize the discomfort. For example, individuals with abdominal pain often draw their knees up and curl into a ball. Patients in severe pain sometimes lie rigidly because the discomfort is intensified by any movement.

Some patients do not like to complain of pain. As a result, they may not verbally acknowledge its existence. Pallor, muscle tension (demonstrated by drawn facial muscles or clenched fists), posture, inactivity and diaphoresis may be the only outward evidence of pain in these individuals.

UNIVERSITY OF OTTAWA SCHOOL OF NURSING FACULTY OF HEALTH SCIENCES

PAIN ASSESSMENT

Name ______________________ Ward ____________ Room ______________

Age __________ Diagnosis ____

Doctor ______________ Nurse assessing ______________ Date ______________

Medications for pain ____

LOCATION

Mark drawings with an X where pain is felt. Indicate sites of pain with an I (internal), E (external) or EI (if both). Use arrow to indicate direction and spread.

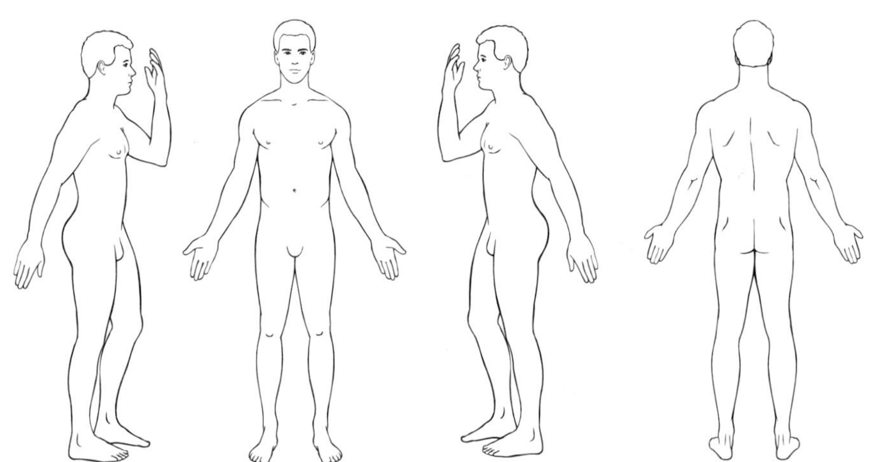

SEVERITY

Rate pain on a 0–5 scale:

0. no pain
1. mild
2. discomforting
3. distressing
4. horrible
5. excruciating

At present ______________________

Worst it gets ______________________

Best it gets ______________________

1 h after meds ______________________

FIGURE 27.3 Pain assessment tool

SOURCE: Logan & Fothergill-Bourbonnais, 1991, pp. 25–26.

QUALITY

____

____

Note nonverbal observations ______________________________

____

TIMING

When did the pain start? ______________________________

How long have you had it? ______________________________

How often does it appear? ______________________________

How long does it last? ______________________________

AGGRAVATING/RELIEVING FACTORS

What brings on the pain? ______________________________

What makes it worse? ______________________________

What makes it better? ______________________________

IMPACT ON PATIENT

Does pain affect your sleep? ______________________________

Does pain affect your mood? ______________________________

How is pain affecting your activities? ______________________________

What is pain preventing you from doing that you would like to do? ______________________________

Describe your food intake (appetite) ______________________________

Are you experiencing other symptoms? ______________________________

PREVIOUS THERAPY (Drugs and other therapies that have helped or failed to relieve pain)

____

FAMILY INFORMATION

Patient's personality/coping prior to cancer ______________________________

____

View on the impact of pain to the patient ______________________________

____

Strengths, weaknesses and dynamics of family ______________________________

____

FIGURE 27.3 *continued*

	Pain Scale/Description	*Instructions*	*Recommended Age*
A	Faces scale (Wong & Baker, 1988). Consists of six cartoon faces ranging from very happy, smiling face for "no pain" to increasingly less happy faces to final sad, tearful face for "worst pain"	Explain to the child that each face is for a person who feels happy because there is no pain (hurt) or sad because there is some or a lot of pain. Face 0 is very happy because there is no hurt. Face 1 hurts just a little bit. Face 2 hurts a little more. Face 3 hurts even more. Face 4 hurts a whole lot, but Face 5 hurts as much as you can imagine, although you don't have to be crying to feel this bad. Ask child to choose face that best describes own pain.	Children as young as 3 years

0 **No Hurt** — ***1*** **Hurts Little Bit** — ***2*** **Hurts Little More** — ***3*** **Hurts Even More** — ***4*** **Hurts Whole Lot** — ***5*** **Hurts Worst**

B	Visual analogue scale Consists of a 10-cm line ranging from "no pain" to "unbearable pain"	Explain to the patient that one end of the line represents "no pain" and the other end represents "unbearable pain"—"the worst pain imaginable." Ask the patient to place a mark on the line that shows the intensity of pain he or she is feeling.	Adults

No Pain ——————————————————— ***Unbearable Pain***

C	Hester poker chip scale. A way to quantify pain by using poker chips to represent pain intensity		Ages 5 and up

1. Say to the child: "I want to talk with you about the hurt you may be having right now.
2. Align the chips horizontally in front of the child on the bedside table, a clipboard, or other firm surface.
3. Tell the child, "These are pieces of hurt." Beginning at the chip nearest the child's left side and ending at the one nearest the right side, point to the chips and say, "This (first chip) is a little bit of hurt and this (fourth chip) is the most hurt you could ever have."

   For a young child or for any child who may not fully comprehend the instructions, clarify by saying, "That means this (one) is just a little hurt, this (two) is a little more hurt, this (three) is more yet, and this (four) is the most hurt you could ever have."
   - Do not give children an option for zero hurt. Research with the Poker Chip Tool has verified that children without pain will so indicate by responses such as, "I don't have any."
4. Ask the child, "How many pieces of hurt do you have right now?"
   - After initial use of the Poker Chip Tool, some children internalize the concept, "pieces of hurt". If a child gives a response such as "I have one right now", before you ask or before you lay out the poker chips, proceed with instructions #5.
5. Record the number of chips on a Pain Flow Sheet.
6. Clarify the child's answer by words such as, "Oh, you have a little hurt? Tell me about the hurt."

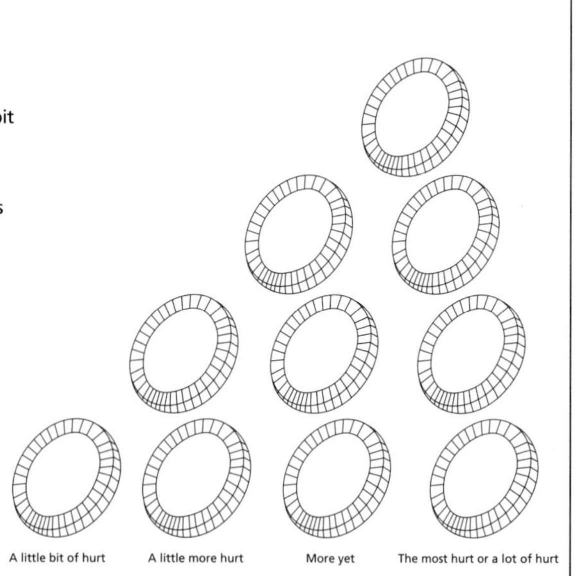

FIGURE 27.4 A. Faces scale. B. Visual analogue scale. C. Hester poker chip tool

SOURCES: A. Wong & Baker, cited in Wong, 1995, p. 1085; **B.** B. Wong, 1995, p. 1086; **C.** Developed in 1975 by Nancy Hester, University of Colorado Health Sciences Center, Denver, CO.

VANCOUVER HOSPITAL & HEALTH SCIENCES CENTRE

PAIN ASSESSMENT

DATE	NURSING UNIT	
MR, MISS, MRS, MS	UNIT NUMBER	
SURNAME	GIVEN NAME	
DOCTOR	(PLEASE USE BLOCK CAPITALS)	
	SEX	AGE

Pain-Associated
Medical Diagnosis:______________________________

Mark, on diagrams below, areas where pain is identified or suspected.

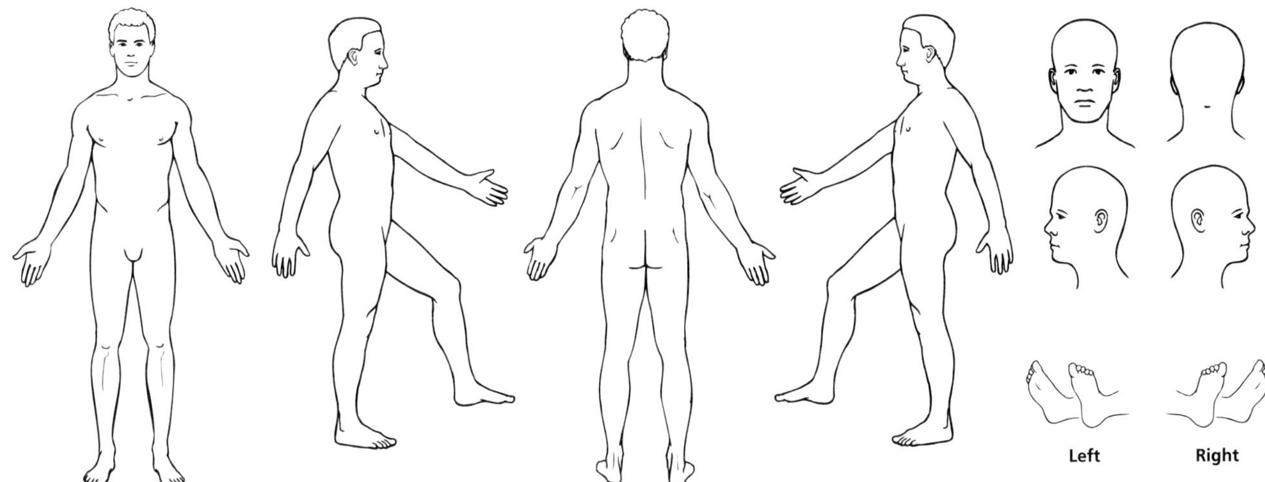

Complete the LOTARP chart below

	A	B	C	D
LOCATION (Mark letter on drawing.) Show radiation				
ONSET (Duration, Variations)				
TYPE (Quality—Use resident's own words)				
AGGRAVATING FACTORS (What causes or increases pain?)				
RELIEVING FACTORS (What relieves the pain?) What has pt/resident done in the past?				
PRECIPITATING FACTORS (What brings the pain on?)				

FIGURE 27.5 Amy's tool and flow sheet

SOURCE: Vancouver Hospital & Health Sciences Centre, 1997.

Verbal Expression	Facial Expression	Behavioural Expression	Physical Expression
Cries with touch	Grimace, such as wincing or painful look	Jumps when you touch a spot	Becomes cold
Hollers	Closes eyes	Increased confusion	Becomes pale
Volume of voice increases or becomes shrill	Winces with touch	Points with hand to spot	Becomes clammy
Becomes very quiet	Pitiful or sad expression	Persistently wears an item, e.g., slippers, hat	Red or swollen body part
Yells or shouts	Worried expression	Doesn't want to eat	Colour changes
Swears, calls names		Forces self back in chair or bed	Vital sign increases, i.e., BP, P, R (acute pain only)
Talks without making sense		Rocking, shaking or tremors	
Grunts		Grumpy	
		Increased movement	
		Limp	
		Withdrawn	
		Agitated, increased movement, anxious, restless	
		Temper tantrum, throws things	
		Pushes away	
		Grabs at you	
		Childlike or baby-like	
		Decreased concentration/not fully there, forgets easily	
		Difficulty settling/sleep disruption	
		Hangs head, withdrawn, depressed or flat	
		Bed seeking, increased sleeping	

If these behaviours are present, consider administering a trial of analgesic for 48 hours and observe behaviour closely.

FIGURE 27.5 *continued*

Other people may respond to pain with restlessness and increased sensitivity to stimuli in the environment, such as noise and bright lights. Some patients may demon-

people or events. They may also exhibit a change in common routines and a decrease in social interactions. When working with individuals in pain, nurses should be aware of these important observations that provide cues in the diagnosis and management of pain. However, it is also important to remember that patients with chronic pain may not present with easily observable, behavioural responses.

INFORMATION FROM OTHER HEALTH CARE TEAM MEMBERS

Pain is frequently the principal symptom that prompts people to seek medical help. A physician may have investigated the nature of the patient's pain, and the nurse can often obtain much information from the patient's physician or from notes made on the patient's chart. Of particular importance are notations regarding factors that precipitate pain, since the nurse may be able to institute measures to eliminate or minimize these factors.

Sharing observations made by all members of the nursing team contributes to the completeness of the patient's pain assessment and intervention plan. All observations should be accurately reported and recorded so that all nursing personnel are aware of measures that prevent, minimize or alleviate the patient's pain, as well as factors that aggravate it.

In addition, other members of the health team, such as the physiotherapist, often contribute information regarding a patient's pain. The physiotherapist usually assists in assessing mobility and functional ability and may be able to provide insight to nursing team members regarding activities and schedules that the patient can tolerate.

The patient's family may also be helpful in establishing the nature of the patient's pain, precipitating factors and effective relief measures. Some people minimize the severity of pain when talking to health professionals, yet may have confided the extent of their discomfort to their spouse. Additionally, a spouse may be aware of the patient's inability to sleep or increased restlessness and irritability. Therefore, it is important to include information given by family members as part of the assessment data.

Diagnosing Pain

Diagnosing pain problems presents a challenge to nurses. Pain may be a response that nurses identify and treat independently (nursing diagnosis) or a problem that nurses treat in collaboration with the physician (collaborative problem). Furthermore, pain may have an etiology stemming from other problems for which nurses prescribe treatment.

The nursing diagnoses as described by NANDA (1994) for patients manifesting pain are *Pain* and *Chronic Pain*. The diagnosis should include an accurate description of the type, intensity and nature of the pain, as well as its cause (if known). These aspects are necessary for planning inter-

on the patient's lifestyle and daily functioning. To identify a specific pain, for example, *Headache*, without a statement of etiology, gives no direction for selecting measures to eliminate the cause of the headache. However, the diagnosis *Headache related to stressful daily living and skipping meals* tells us what interventions are necessary to alleviate the problem.

Chronic or acute pain related to medical conditions that involve nurse-prescribed and physician-prescribed interventions should be stated as collaborative problems. For example, in treating pain related to cancer, the nurse would be responsible for evaluating the pain, administering pain-relief medications, monitoring for adverse reactions to the medications, teaching patients how to self-administer pain-relief measures and assisting them in coping with necessary lifestyle modifications.

Pain is a powerful etiological factor affecting many aspects of a person's life. For example, in a postoperative patient, pain can cause impaired mobility, ineffective breathing patterns, self-care deficits, fear and anxiety, just to name a few responses. Patients with prolonged chronic pain may experience hopelessness, powerlessness, ineffective individual coping or altered health maintenance, all of which may be caused by the pain itself, fear of the consequences of pain or a lack of knowledge of effective relief modalities.

Thus, pain is not a simple problem to diagnose. A correct diagnosis requires complete and accurate information about a patient's pain and the effects of the pain on his or her lifestyle and daily functioning. It requires collaboration with the patient and family as well as other members of the health team.

Examples of nursing diagnoses and collaborative problems related to pain are:

- *Pain in legs related to improper positioning and use of pillows when in bed.*
- *Impaired Mobility related to postoperative incisional pain.*
- *Altered Health Maintenance and Hopelessness related to lack of knowledge of pain-relief measures for arthritis.*
- *PC: Angina secondary to myocardial infarction.*

Planning Pain-Relief Interventions

Nursing actions for patients who are or may be experiencing pain are primarily directed towards protective strategies that assist patients to prevent, minimize and cope with pain. Restorative strategies focus on modifying the perception of pain by decreasing or eliminating painful stimuli. When determining appropriate pain-relief measures, the nurse uses knowledge about the patient's condition and unique reaction to pain.

Common patient goals or outcomes expected from pain-relief interventions might include:

- Patient will describe relief of pain as evidenced by a decreased rating on a pain scale of 0 to 10.
- Patient will perform selected pain-relief measures.
- Patient will show decreased pain as evidenced by walking to the bathroom without guarding incision.

Implementing Pain-Relief Interventions

Health-Promoting Strategies

Because pain is a protective mechanism that alerts us to potential injury or trauma in the body, no one can always be pain-free. However, there are a number of things people can do to maintain most freedom from pain in the course of daily living. For example, we know that fatigue, lack of physical fitness and a poor mental outlook will increase one's perception of pain. We also know that eating certain foods brings on headaches and stomach and bowel ailments in certain people. People can promote a pain-free existence by limiting or avoiding potential sources of pain and by maintaining a healthy lifestyle.

Health-Protecting Strategies

People recover from illness better and faster when their pain is controlled and they are able to get up, move around and perform the activities of daily living. Health-protecting strategies in pain management focus on measures to prevent or minimize pain and to help patients cope with their pain. For example, in some cardiac conditions, chest pain may be caused by exertion. Therefore, the nurse should know how much activity a cardiac patient can tolerate in order to avoid causing undue discomfort. It may be necessary to space nursing interventions to permit the patient to rest between activities. In some cases it may be wise to leave a patient's bath until an hour or so after breakfast, so that he or she may rest after the exertion of eating a meal.

MEASURES TO HELP PATIENTS TOLERATE AND COPE WITH PAIN

One of the most important nursing functions is the provision of psychological support for the patient in pain. Discussing the meaning of pain for the patient is one way to provide support. The nurse may find that it is not really pain that is bothering the patient but something else. The patient may be concerned about the results of surgery or about his or her ability to tolerate pain.

Knowing what to expect in the way of pain often enables a person to cope with an upcoming situation; it also removes the fear of the unknown so that anxiety is lessened. Many diagnostic and therapeutic procedures are uncomfortable or painful. It is wise to explain to the patient exactly what is going to be done, the nature of the pain that may be felt and what the patient can do to assist. Explanation of this sort often helps change the individual's attitude towards the experience.

It is important to be honest with children. Telling them that a procedure is going to hurt a little and what the hurt will be like is preferable to telling them that it will not hurt and then inflicting pain. The latter course of action can destroy a child's sense of trust. A factual explanation of exactly what is going to happen usually eliminates fear and anxiety for both adults and children.

Reassuring patients that pain will not be beyond their level of tolerance is advisable. Assure patients that something will be done to relieve their pain. During a painful procedure, placing a hand on the patient's arm is often considered supportive. Care needs to be taken with touch, however, as some patients dislike it, particularly if they are striving to maintain their independence.

Enabling the patient to retain a measure of control over the situation can also help minimize the reaction to pain. "Tell me when it hurts and we will stop for a minute" is one way of doing this. The nurse can also involve patients in some part of the activity. Holding a piece of the equipment, for example, is an effective way to allow children to feel involved. Distraction can sometimes be used effectively in these situations. The patient is less focussed on pain when concentrating on taking deep breaths.

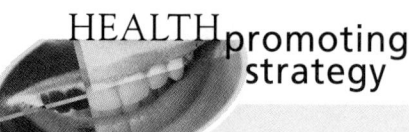

Promoting Pain-Free Health

- Obtain adequate rest and avoid fatigue
- Avoid foods and beverages you associate with pain
- Keep physically fit and in good condition
- Exercise in moderation
- Avoid sporadic episodes of strenuous exercising
- Practise safety in the home and workplace
- Use proper body mechanics for lifting and moving heavy objects
- Wear a car seat belt at all times
- Avoid stress and keep a positive, happy outlook on life.

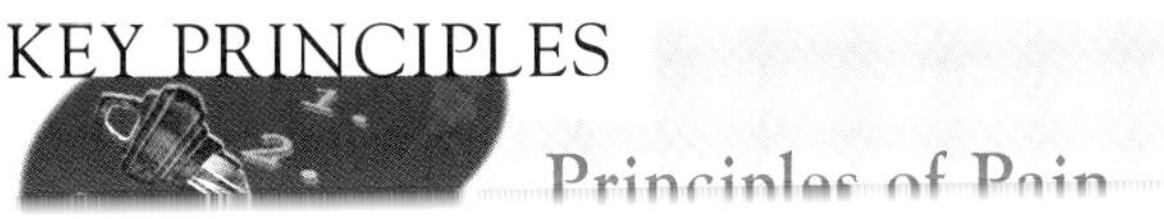

KEY PRINCIPLES

Principles of Pain Management

1. Allow the patient to be in control
2. Involve the whole family
3. Utilize a team approach
4. Use multiple modalities
5. Acknowledge and treat secondary symptoms.

Be sure that the patient is settled comfortably following a painful experience. Evidence of the procedure, such as the dressing tray, should be removed as quickly as possible. Some nurses have found that encouraging the patient to talk about the experience helps put it into perspective.

Health-Restoring Strategies

The management of pain is based on several principles of therapy that guide all health professionals in the development of health-restoring interventions for pain. These principles were formulated in 1984 by the Expert Advisory Committee on the Management of Severe Pain in Cancer Patients, charged with preparing a Monograph on the management of cancer pain to the Minister of National Health and Welfare (1984). Nurses can also use nonpharmacological pain-relief measures as well as pharmacological measures to help patients manage pain.

ALLOW THE PATIENT TO BE IN CONTROL

The foundation of effective pain management is to allow patients to be in control. Participation and commitment to therapeutic regimens increase when patients are involved in discussions regarding treatment options.

Allowing patients to be in control also requires prompt attention to requests for pain relief. Many treatment modalities are more effective when administered before pain intensity peaks. Early intervention, at the beginning of pain, often prevents a serious attack. This is important in conditions such as biliary or renal colic (stones in the bile duct or the ureter of the kidney), in which the pain can reach agonizing proportions.

INVOLVE THE WHOLE FAMILY

When any member of a family experiences pain there is disruption to the usual structure, roles and functions of the family. As well, the meaning and the expression of pain within the family is a significant variable. Therefore, it is important to involve the whole family in the treatment plan. Acute pain is often quickly relieved, allowing family functioning to return to normal. Chronic pain, however, generally has a significant and long-term effect on family behaviours.

It is important that family members be viewed as active participants in the therapeutic process. They often are able to contribute valuable information needed to complete the

often develop unique methods of coping with pain, which, when shared with health professionals, may provide insight into treatment modalities most suited to the patient. It is also important to provide family members with practical advice, aid and emotional support so that they, in turn, can support the family member in pain.

UTILIZE A TEAM APPROACH

Pain, particularly unrelenting chronic pain, is a complex experience that involves physiological and psychosocial

Members of the Pain Team

- patient and family
- family physician
- specialist/internist
- surgeon
- psychiatrist
- psychologist
- acute care nurse
- home care nurse
- palliative care nurse
- social worker
- pharmacist
- chaplain
- physiotherapist
- occupational therapist
- dietitian
- volunteers
- chiropractor
- music therapist
- art therapist
- homeopath
- naturopath

Methods of Pain Relief

Modify the Disease Process:

- chemotherapy
- hormonal therapy
- radiation
- surgery

Modify Pain Perception:

- application of cold/heat
- distraction
- guided imagery/visualization
- hypnosis
- pharmacological treatment
- relaxation techniques
- Therapeutic Touch
- herbal remedies

Interrupt Pain Transmission

- massage
- acupuncture
- acupressure
- TENS (transcutaneous electrical nerve stimulation)
- nerve blocks
- surgery

Secondary Symptoms of Pain

- agitation
- anorexia
- constipation
- contractures
- cough
- dehydration
- despair
- diarrhea
- dyspnea
- edema
- hiccups
- hopelessness
- hunger
- incontinence
- inflammation
- insomnia
- isolation
- muscle spasms
- nausea
- pathological fractures
- pressure sores
- restlessness
- vomiting
- weakness

dimensions. Consequently, pain is best managed by a comprehensive multidisciplinary team of professionals. Health professionals have a responsibility to assess pain routinely, to believe patients' pain reports, to document these and to intervene in order to prevent pain.

Pain teams may function within acute care hospitals, ambulatory care departments or free-standing pain clinics. The team is directed by the needs of the patient in pain, and generally concentrates on long-term methods to relieve pain completely or to control it. Usually, these teams develop individualized programs integrating physical, cognitive and psychosocial strategies for alleviating pain. Working collaboratively, multidisciplinary pain teams ensure practical, integrated and consistent therapy for individuals in pain.

USE MULTIPLE MODALITIES

According to the gate-control theory of pain, there are several points along the nervous system where pain impulses may be modulated: at the peripheral site of the pain; in the spinal cord fibres; in the spinal cord; and in the cerebral cortex. Therefore, effective pain management involves employing a combination of pain-relief measures. These are presented in the box on the preceding page.

ACKNOWLEDGE AND TREAT SECONDARY SYMPTOMS

There are a variety of secondary symptoms that, independently, may cause significant discomfort. When these symptoms are combined with another painful process, patients may have a perception of increased pain.

Control of secondary symptoms can decrease the perception of pain. For example, mint tea can prevent or relieve feelings of nausea. Ensuring that patients are taking sufficient fluids helps prevent the distressing effects of dehydration. The pain caused by a distended bladder and the discomfort of constipation are both preventable by specific nursing techniques (see Chapters 21 and 22). Ensuring that patients obtain sufficient rest and sleep is another important consideration.

MEDICINE MODALITIES

Methods to alter the disease process or interrupt the transmission of the pain impulse tend to involve specialized modalities. These procedures are often performed by specialized practitioners. They include such Modalities as surgery, chemotherapy, radiation and nerve blocks.

Surgery, chemotherapy and radiation therapy are within the realm of the physician. The physician attempts to decrease pain by interfering with the disease process. Surgery may also be performed to interrupt pain impulse transmission. For example, rhizotomy (resection of dorsal nerve root) may be performed to relieve intractable pain. Physicians may also try to interrupt the pain impulse using a nerve block, in which a small amount of anesthetic is injected along the course of the nerve innervating the painful area.

NONPHARMACOLOGIC PAIN-RELIEF MEASURES

The experience of pain can be lessened or relieved by modifying the perception of the pain impulse. Many strategies are available to alter the perception of pain. Nurses may independently implement a variety of noninvasive and nonpharmacologic strategies to assist patients in achieving pain relief. Some of these nursing measures are easily accomplished. For example, changing patients' position to ensure proper body alignment aids in preventing painful contractures and muscle spasms, relieves muscle strain and prevents pressure sores from developing. Consequently, patients may perceive less pain. A back rub often assists patients to relax by easing muscular tension. Removing external sources of irritation, such as loud noises or bright lights, also aids in the elimination of painful stimuli. All the comfort measures identified in Chapter 26 are useful for eliminating sources of pain.

There are many other noninvasive pain management modalities that nurses may independently employ with patients. These include cognitive strategies such as visualization, distraction, hypnosis and many relaxation techniques. According to the gate-control theory, these measures stimulate the activity of the thalamus and cerebral cortex to close the gating mechanism and thereby decrease the perception of pain. Massage, the application of heat or cold and Therapeutic Touch are physical therapies that the nurse may implement. The effective use of modalities such as hypnosis and Therapeutic Touch generally requires the completion of continuing studies in the specific area. These and other alternative therapies are described in Chapter 12.

Application of Heat or Cold

The application of heat or cold to modify the perception of pain is a familiar strategy (see Chapter 25), and may be used with both acute and chronic pain. Muscular aches and pain are often effectively relieved by heat. Heat increases the circulation in the part of the body where it is applied. The increased circulation transports metabolic waste products (a factor in causing muscular pain) away from the painful area. Consequently, a warm bath may help to relieve aching

Cold has the opposite effect—it decreases circulation. In doing so, edema and pressure on sensory nerve endings may be reduced. Ice is frequently used to relieve edema and pain for many joint-related problems. Most athletes and arthritis sufferers are aware of the benefits of ice applied to sore and inflamed joints. Cold may also be used as a local anesthetic agent. The cold numbs the sensory nerve endings, decreasing the transmission of pain impulses. Prior to the administering of an injection, ice may be briefly applied to the site. The patient will experience less puncture pain due to the numbness. This technique is useful both with children and with adults who have difficulty accepting an intramuscular injection.

Distraction

Distraction is a useful tool for helping alleviate both acute and chronic pain. Distraction techniques work equally well with adults and children. The patient's attention is simply diverted away from the sensation of pain towards other thoughts. The number of sensory impressions competing for attention produces a decreased perception of pain. Because the effectiveness of this technique is based on competing sensory impressions, it is important to involve as many of the senses as possible in these strategies. Specific techniques include the following:

1. Encourage the patient to recount a recent exciting or pleasant experience. Narrating the action of a sports event, the plot of a movie or a story may all function as distracters. Encourage the patient to relate information from all the senses: touch, taste, smell, hearing and sight. Children can be encouraged to recite rhymes, or participate in a game. The key component is active participation by the patient.
2. Music is an excellent distracter and relaxant. The type of music selected is crucial to the effectiveness of this method, so the patient should select music based on personal preference. For example, older adults may prefer music from the time when they were growing up, or music that reminds them of a happy time (McCaffery & Beebe, 1989). Encourage active listening. Have the patient close the eyes, concentrate on the music and tap out the rhythm.
3. Participating in rhythmic singing is also an effective distracter. Chants, hymns or simple songs with a strong beat are good to use with both adults and children. Adults are usually more self-conscious than children, however, and often prefer to mouth the words silently. Tapping the foot or fingers for emphasis is an additional distracter that can be used with this technique.
4. Teach the patient rhythmic breathing exercises. The patient may do these exercises with eyes closed, or by focussing intently on an object. Breathing is to be

   patient focusses on the breath and silently repeats "In, 2, 3, 4—Out, 2, 3, 4." Another technique, especially useful with children, is blowing bubbles using, for example, a straw in a glass of water.
5. Humour is also a powerful distracter. Research has shown that humour can reduce muscle tension and stress, and improve an individual's psychological and emotional outlook (Ackerman, Henry, Graham & Coffey, 1993). Patients may choose to watch comedies, read humorous books, make jokes or tell funny stories. Some pediatric units have a mobile humour wagon to bring humour to the patient's bedside. As discussed in Chapter 17, humour is culturally defined and its use as a therapeutic intervention may not always be appropriate.

Visualization

Visualization is a form of distraction that uses images to modify the perception of pain and decrease the intensity of the pain experience. This technique is useful with all age groups; practising it for approximately 20 minutes, two to three times a day, will improve the effectiveness of the images. One common method of visualization is guided imagery.

The following steps provide a guideline for implementing imagery. Until the technique is learned by the patient, it is necessary for the nurse to spend time guiding him or her through the process.

1. Identify the focus of the imagery. The patient needs to be clear about the problem that will be the focus of attention. Is it a headache, stomach pain or a backache?
2. Create a relaxed environment. It is advantageous to darken the room and remove any sources of distraction.
3. Encourage the patient to relax using rhythmic breathing. Spend a few minutes simply relaxing. It is helpful at this point to have the patient visualize a safe and comfortable place.
4. Ask the patient to visualize an image that represents the pain—for example, a tight headband around the forehead for a headache; knotted ropes for muscular pain; a mound of cold, rough cement for back pain. It is important that the image is identified by the patient; rather than suggest images, allow the patient to find an image that represents his or her pain.
5. Have the patient visualize an image that represents relieving the pain: the headband loosening, the ropes untangling, the cement being smoothed out like glass. Once the headband is loose or the ropes are untangled, the patient should focus on this image for a few minutes.

6. Have the patient imagine the positive effects of less pain. The patient visualizes him- or herself as being dynamic, energetic and in good health (Dossey, 1991).

Guided imagery is also an effective technique with children. An imaginary "magic glove" or "magic blanket" may be put in place before a painful procedure such as an intravenous injection (Kachoyeanos & Friedhoff, 1993). The child's perception of pain is lessened by imagining that the magic glove or blanket is protecting him or her during the procedure.

Hypnosis

The clinical application of hypnosis is usually executed by a registered hypnotherapist. This technique works with all age groups. Hypnosis is an altered state of consciousness during which the patient is sensitive to suggestion. Even though the patient may be in a suggestible state, he or she remains in control, and will not perform any action that is incompatible with personal beliefs or values. Many patients with chronic pain use self-hypnosis as one method of achieving pain relief.

A hypnosis-like technique that may be used with some patients is conscious suggestion. This technique involves achieving deep relaxation, and then listening to or giving oneself positive suggestions. When patients are first learning this technique, suggestions may be given by the nurse. Begin by having the patient perform rhythmic breathing. It is helpful for the patient to visualize a safe place at home or in natural surroundings. Allow the patient a few minutes simply to relax; then in a calm, soothing voice, offer the patient positive suggestions of well-being or of decreased sensations of pain.

Massage

Massage has had a long history of use in the treatment of muscular pain. The effect of massage is similar to heat in that circulation and removal of cellular waste products is enhanced. The gate-control theory of pain suggests that massage stimulates the large A-beta and A-delta fibres that cause closure of the gating mechanism to pain impulses.

When it is impossible to reach a painful area—a limb in a cast, for example, or an area covered by a dressing that cannot be removed—the skin in an opposite area can be stimulated (contralateral stimulation). This may provide some relief in the painful area.

Massage is a valuable technique for reducing anxiety and promoting relaxation. The muscular relaxation generated by massage may promote decreased sensations of pain for many hours. This technique is also an excellent modality for promoting family involvement. Family members may actively participate in care by massaging a patient's back, hands or feet unless due to inflammation.

Relaxation Techniques

As we discussed earlier in the chapter, anxiety and fear are contributing factors in pain and may intensify an individual's reaction to it. Successful reduction of anxiety and fear will assist the individual to feel more comfortable and experience a decreased perception of pain. Some techniques that may be used for relaxation include biofeedback, meditation, rhythmic breathing exercises, Therapeutic Touch, acupuncture, acupressure and TENS (transcutaneous electrical nerve stimulation).

BIOFEEDBACK Biofeedback is useful for alleviating chronic pain. Individuals learn to control nonconscious physiological responses, such as blood pressure and muscle tension, through the use of mental images and thought processes. Biofeedback techniques require training with the use of special monitoring equipment that measures nonconscious events and feeds information back to the person in the form of varying tones or meter readings. With practice, people develop mental strategies to control the nonconscious processes enough to promote relaxation and relieve problems such as high blood pressure and tension headaches.

MEDITATION Meditation is a useful relaxation technique for patients with acute or chronic pain. Prior to beginning the meditation, the patient selects a soothing word, such as *relax* or *calm*. The patient begins by performing slow rhythmic breathing and imagining a safe place. He or she may wish to close the eyes or leave them open and focus on an object. With every breath in, the patient silently repeats the word that was chosen. Frequent practice facilitates the effectiveness of this technique.

RHYTHMIC BREATHING EXERCISES Rhythmic breathing, as discussed in the section on distraction, can also be used on its own for relaxation. Slow, deep breathing is a powerful technique for promoting relaxation. Patients can participate in this method of relaxation whenever they are feeling uncomfortable and anxious.

THERAPEUTIC TOUCH Therapeutic Touch (TT) is a method of directing energy through the hands. The technique involves internally centring yourself and consciously focussing on the intent to assist a person in pain. Practitioners assess the patient's energy field by passing their hands over the individual, just above the body. Areas that feel warm or cool, or stimulate pins-and-needles sensations in the practitioner, are areas of energy congestion, blockage or depletion. Through a technique known as *unruffling the field*, the practitioner smoothes the patient's energy field (Brown, 1993; Krieger, 1979).

The technique of unruffling produces a relaxation response and a perception of pain relief. TT has been used effectively with acute and chronic pain. This technique is easy to learn, but requires some continuing education to be completed by the nurse.

ACUPUNCTURE Acupuncture has, for centuries, been used in China for the treatment of various disorders, for the relief of pain and for surgical anesthesia. During the past few years

now being used as an alternative method of treating pain. The acupuncture technique consists of inserting long, fine needles into particular areas of the body. The peripheral needle placement sites are associated with specific internal organs of the body. The disposable sterile needles are inserted with a continuous twirling motion. Additional heat in the area may be generated by applying moxa to the skin or to the needle.

The physiological mechanisms involved in the relief of pain by acupuncture are not fully understood. However, the gate-control theory suggests that stimulation of particular nerves or tissues by acupuncture needles results in increased input to the gate-control mechanism, causing the gate to close and interrupting the pain impulses from selected areas of the body.

ACUPRESSURE Acupressure works on the same principles as acupuncture. However, in this case, pressure is applied to specific peripheral points, without the use of needles. Pressure is applied with the hands, elbows and knees, depending on the point to be stimulated. These techniques may be used effectively for both acute and chronic pain.

TRANSCUTANEOUS ELECTRICAL NERVE STIMULATION (TENS) Transcutaneous electrical nerve stimulation is an effective adjuvant therapy for pain relief that can be used with all age groups. There are two common types of TENS—CTENS (conventional TENS) and ALTENS (acupuncture-like TENS). CTENS interrupts the transmission of pain impulses by stimulating peripheral nerve fibres with low-voltage electrical impulses, causing the gating mechanism to close. It is suggested that stimulation of peripheral fibres by ALTENS initiates the release of endorphins (Finlay, 1992).

Transcutaneous electrical nerve stimulation is usually applied by physiotherapists, but nurses may need to assist patients with therapy during the evening and night. CTENS involves the placement of two to four small electrodes around the painful area. The electrical impulse is adjusted for comfort. Stimulation of the area needs to be strong enough to induce numbness, but not so intense as to induce spasm. The effect of CTENS may decrease over time as peripheral fibres accommodate. The unit may be turned off, or the intensity increased for a few minutes to promote neural excitability (Finlay, 1992).

Acupuncture-like TENS electrodes are positioned over muscle motor points. The objective is to produce nonpainful, rhythmic, muscular contractions. ALTENS treatments are usually administered twice a day for 20–45 minutes (Finlay, 1992).

Most patients are able to monitor TENS independently. Children may require more supervision. Nursing care for individuals using TENS involves assessing the skin for reactions to the conductive jelly or to the electrodes. Dermatitis requires that electrode positions be altered. Patients cannot shower or bathe with the units (Finlay, 1992).

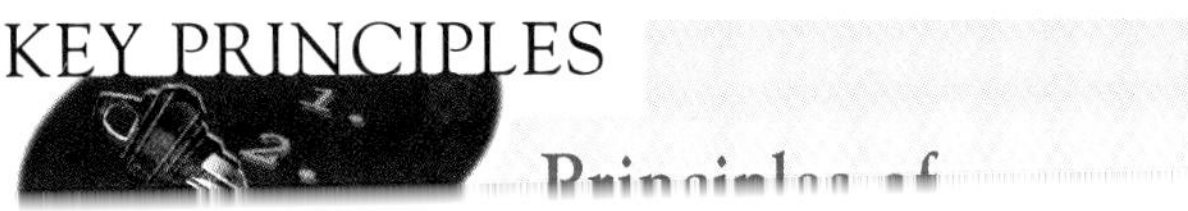

Principles of Analgesic Administration

- Use the oral route whenever possible
- Administer the medication regularly (around the clock)
- Titrate dose individually
- Use adjuvant medications to enhance analgesia
- Treat tolerance appropriately
- Use modalities other than just opioids
- Do not use placebos.

PHARMACOLOGICAL PAIN-RELIEF MEASURES

The administration of medication continues to be a major focus in pain management. There are various categories of drugs available for pain relief, including opioids and agonists/antagonists, which are commonly referred to as narcotic analgesics. Other categories of medication include non-opioid pain relievers, of which ASA and acetaminophen are the most common agents; nonsteroidal anti-inflammatory drugs (NSAIDs); and some tranquillizers. Pain-relief medications are given by oral, transdermal, subcutaneous, intramuscular, intravenous, rectal, epidural and intrathecal routes. The administration of medication and the observation of patients' responses to it are within the purview of the nurse. Nurses need to be aware of the principles that guide decision making regarding analgesic administration.

Nurses have a crucial responsibility in the administration of analgesics. They must understand the actions and effects of the drugs being administered in order to ensure that patients are achieving maximum pain relief. They must also understand how the different routes of delivery may alter or enhance the outcome of medications administered. The timing of administration is very important. Prescriptions may be written for analgesics to be given every four hours or at other specified times (as is frequently the case with patients who have arthritic and rheumatic disorders). In most instances, however, the orders are written *prn* (an abbreviation for *por re nata*, the Latin phrase meaning "as needed"). Nurses must judge the most suitable time of administration and the interval between doses. Medications for pain relief are most effective when given regularly, around the clock, because it is easier to prevent pain than to control it. This is true even for the postoperative patient receiving intramuscular analgesics. The different categories of pharmacological agents used for pain relief are summarized in Table 27.1 and outlined in the text that follows. Table 27.2 lists equivalent

TABLE 27.1 Categories of drugs for pain management

Medication	Action	Uses	Route	Side Effects	Toxic Effects
Opioids	Alter pain perception by binding to opiate receptors within the CNS	Treatment of moderate to severe pain Used for acute and / or chronic pain Primarily used to treat visceral pain	PO SC IM IV *PR *epi *inth *TD *neb	Nausea Vomiting Constipation Pruritis Sedation or drowsiness Hypotension Urinary retention	Respiratory depression (usually relieved with nalaxone)
Agonists/ Antagonists	Produce a narcotic effect, but in the presence of a true narcotic will counteract the effect of the narcotic	Used for patients unable to tolerate true narcotic analgesics	PO IM IV SC nasal spray	Drowsiness Nausea Psychotomimetic effects such as hallucinations or euphoria	
Non-Opioids	Act at the peripheral level by inhibiting the release of prostaglandins Have analgesic, antipyretic and anti-inflammatory effects	Used alone for mild to moderate pain May be used as an adjuvant for severe and persistent pain	PO TD	Hepatotoxicity Gastric irritation ASA use inhibits platelet formation	Tinnitus with ASA Renal failure
NSAIDs	Act at the peripheral level by inhibiting the release of prostaglandins Have a ceiling effect—reach a point where increasing the dose does not have further effect Have analgesic, antipyretic, antiplatelet and anti-inflammatory effects	Used alone for pain due to inflammation May be used as an adjuvant for severe and persistent pain Especially effective for metastatic bone pain	PO IM PR	GI upset and irritation May prolong coagulation time Hepatotoxicity Renal toxicity	GI bleeding

*PR = per rectum
*epi = epidural
*inth = intrathecal
*TD = transdermal
*neb = nebulized

TABLE 27.2 Equianalgesia and opioid dosing

[illegible]	Equal to oral morphine	Equal to IM/IV morphine
Dilaudid (hydromorphone) 1 mg	4 mg	1.3 mg
Codeine 30 mg	4.5 mg	1.5 mg
Darvon (propoxyphene hydrochloride) 65 mg or Darvocet N 50 (propoxyphene napsylate + acetaminophen) or Demerol (meperidine) 50 mg	4.8 mg	1.6 mg
Tylenol no. 3 (30 mg codeine + 300 mg acetaminophen) or Percocet (oxycodone 5 mg + 325 mg acetaminophen) or Percodan (oxcodone 5 mg + 325 mg ASA)	7.2 mg	2.4 mg
Vicodin (hydrocodone 5 mg + 500 mg acetaminophen) or Tylox (oxycodone 5 mg + 500 acetaminophen) or Darvocet N 100 (propoxyphene napsylate 100 mg + 600 mg acetaminophen)	9 mg	3 mg
Methadone (dolophine) 10 mg	15 mg	7.5 mg
Tylenol (acetaminophen) 325 mg ASA 325 mg	2.7 mg	0.9 mg
Tylenol Extra Strength (acetaminophen) 500 mg	4 mg	1.3 mg
Tylenol no. 4 (60 mg codeine + 300 mg acetaminophen)	11.7 mg	3.9 mg
Duragesic patch (transdermal fentanyl) (based on 25-microgram patch applied q 3 days = 50 mg oral morphine q 24 h or divided into 6 doses = 8.3 mg)	8.3 mg	2.77 mg

SOURCE: Ferrell & McCaffery, 1997, p. 211.

dosages for some commonly used analgesics, while Figure 27.6 illustrates the steps in choosing analgesics according to severity of pain.

Opioids

Opioids are drugs that bind to opiate receptors in the central nervous system and inhibit or alter the transmission of pain impulses. Codeine, hydromorphone (Dilaudid), meperidine (Demerol), methadone and morphine are examples of opioids. These medications all produce similar outcomes. All are effective analgesics, and may produce side effects such as sedation, nausea, vomiting and constipation (see the box on the next page on coping with the side effects of opioids). There is also a possibility of toxicity, which usually manifests as respiratory depression. Morphine tends to be the most frequently used of the opioids, likely because it is effective for both acute and chronic pain, and because it can be administered in any form.

While opioids are effective analgesics, there is often reluctance to use these drugs. The concern generally expressed by physicians and nurses relates to addiction and

Indications for Using Opioids

- moderate to severe acute pain
- moderate to severe chronic pain
- when immediate pain relief is required.

WHO (World Health Organization) Analgesic Ladder

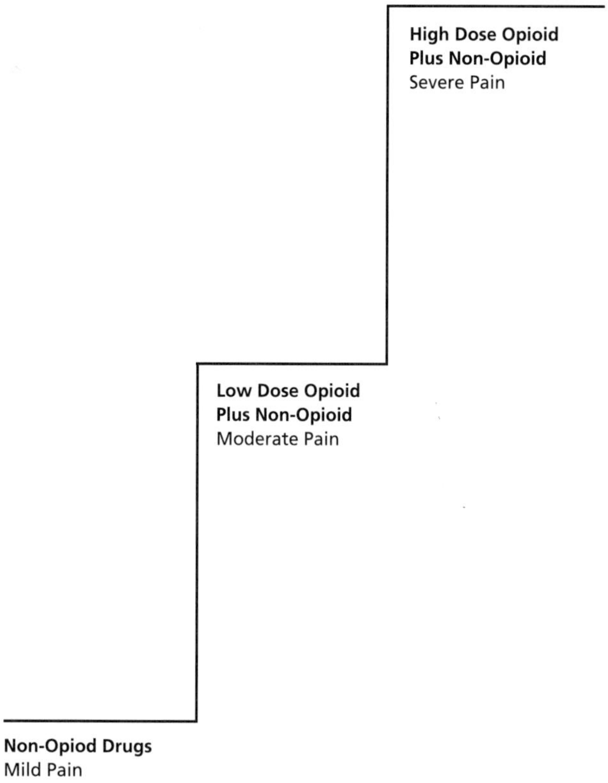

High Dose Opioid Plus Non-Opioid
Severe Pain

Low Dose Opioid Plus Non-Opioid
Moderate Pain

Non-Opiod Drugs
Mild Pain

At any of these levels, analgesic adjuvants may be useful.

FIGURE 27.6 Analgesic steps

SOURCE: World Health Organization, 1990.

Coping with the Side Effects of Opioids*

Constipation:

- Stool softeners are a must with opioid therapy. Patients using opioids tend to become constipated.
- Monitor and record bowel movements.
- Encourage fluids—at least eight glasses of water a day.
- Include high-fibre foods in the diet.

Sedation:

- All patients will experience sedation initially. This is normal, and should decrease in approximately three days.
- If the patient remains persistently sedated, drowsy or confused, the dose may have to be decreased, or another opioid tried.
- Monitor for hypotension.

Nausea and Vomiting:

- This is often the most distressing side effect for patients. If it persists, the opioid may need to be changed. An antiemetic may also be necessary.
- Encourage the patient to avoid foods with strong smells.

*Remember that not only analgesics cause these symptoms. Assess all patients carefully and thoroughly.

toxicity. Physicians are reluctant to prescribe opioids in adequate dosages, and nurses are hesitant to administer these drugs in adequate amounts regularly, fearing that patients will experience toxic reactions or become dependent on the drugs. To use these drugs effectively, then, the health professional must have an understanding of the effects of therapeutic opioid drug use. This understanding begins with knowing the meanings of the terms *addiction*, *dependence*, and *tolerance*.

Addiction refers to the psychological need to use drugs for other than medical reasons. The addicted individual exhibits compulsive drug use and craving for the opioid. **Dependence** is the state in which the individual experiences symptoms of withdrawal, which occur when the drug is abruptly discontinued. Signs of physical withdrawal may include anxiety, irritability, chills, diaphoresis, nausea, vomiting, abdominal cramps and, occasionally, seizures. **Tolerance** occurs when there is a need to increase the dose of the drug in order to achieve the same initial effect. Tolerance does not suggest psychological dependence (McCaffery & Beebe, 1989).

Any individual receiving opioids for an extended period may develop physical dependence and tolerance. However, this does not imply addiction. Behaviours such as clock-watching and frequently requesting medication may be interpreted as addictive behaviours, but it is more likely that such a patient is experiencing inadequate pain relief due to inadequate dosage or frequency. If a patient is experiencing tolerance, he or she may require an increased medication dose in order to maintain an effective state of analgesia. Symptoms of physical withdrawal can be minimized by decreasing the dosage slowly.

Children can safely be administered opioids. Those 12 years of age and older are often able to tolerate an adult dose of medication. Children between the ages of seven and 12 usually require about half an adult dose. Youngsters between the ages of two and six years need about a quarter of an adult dose for effective pain relief. Children younger than two years generally require the medication dosage to be adjusted according to body weight (Pinnell, 1996). Older adults may also safely use opioids, but owing to slower excretion of the drug, they may require a slightly reduced dose.

Agonists/Antagonists

Examples of these drugs include pentazocine (Talwin), buprenorphine (Temalsil) and butorphanol (Stadol). These narcotic analgesics also interact with the opiate receptor sites within the central nervous system to alter the perception of pain. It is important to note that agonists/antagonists,

Rescue Orders

[illegible] injections) requires a rescue order.

- A rescue order is a medication order of the same drug that the patient is receiving.
- The rescue order is used when the patient begins to experience breakthrough pain.

such as pentazocine, will inhibit the effectiveness of pure agonists or opiates, causing ineffective analgesia when simultaneously administered with opioids.

Non-Opioid Pain Relievers

Analgesic–antipyretic medications are the primary non-narcotic pain relievers. These agents block the transmission of pain impulses at the peripheral level, by interfering with the production of prostaglandin. ASA (acetylsalicylic acid) and acetaminophen are used extensively for the relief of mild to moderate pain and are examples of non-opioid analgesics. Non-opioids are often used in conjunction with opioids. Because one group of drugs (opioids) acts on the central nervous system and the other acts peripherally, the combination strikes the pain at two levels. When this type of combination is effective, analgesia is often achieved using less opioid (narcotic).

Nonsteroidal Anti-Inflammatory Drugs (NSAIDs)

Medication in this category acts similarly to non-opioid analgesics. The action occurs peripherally through inhibition of prostaglandin. Generally, the effects of NSAIDs include analgesic, anti-inflammatory, antipyretic and anticoagulant properties. Ibuprofen, indomethacin and naproxen are examples of drugs in this group. While all medication within this classification may have similar properties, not all NSAIDs have the same degree of each property. Consequently, patients may need to try several drugs in this group before finding one that is effective. It may also be necessary to titrate the medication dose for each individual carefully. NSAIDs may be used in conjunction with opioids and antagonists to facilitate analgesia.

METHODS OF MEDICATION ADMINISTRATION

There are numerous methods for administering medications. The preferred route for the administration of analgesic medication is oral. The oral route is considered to be effective and the least invasive of all routes. However, there are a variety of conditions, such as nausea and vomiting or gastrointestinal obstruction, that prevent patients from swallowing or absorbing medication taken orally. The conventional alternative method for the delivery of analgesia is via intramuscular or intravenous routes.

Adjuvant Medications for Pain Relief

These medications are not classified as analgesics. However, they are effective in the relief of secondary symptoms of pain.

Anesthetics, local
Antibiotics
Anticonvulsants
Antidepressants
Antiemetics
Antithermatoids
Benzodiazepines
Corticosteroids
Muscle relaxants

SOURCES: Twycross, 1994; McCaffery & Beebe, 1989.

Intramuscular Injections

The administration of medication via the intramuscular injection is a familiar strategy. It is often used for patients unable to swallow. However, some difficulties do exist with this method. The administration of the medication may create some difficulties. Many patients dislike the puncture pain of injections. In addition, absorption may be erratic, depending on the age and weight of the individual and on previous use of analgesics.

It is difficult to maintain pain control using the intramuscular route. There is frequently a significant lapse of time between the administration of an analgesic and the initial request for it. After the analgesic has been requested, the patient must wait for the nurse to obtain the narcotic keys, sign for the medication and prepare the injection. This time lag increases the patient's anxiety and promotes the development of peaks and troughs. The patient was likely feeling uncomfortable at the time of the initial request; by the time the medication is administered and absorbed, the degree of pain control will probably have decreased significantly. The sudden rise in the blood level of the narcotic analgesic may precipitate observable side effects. Sedation is more likely to occur because of the sudden peak of medication in the patient's system.

Attempts to overcome inadequate pain control with intramuscular injections for both acute and chronic pain have led to the development of innovative methods for delivering analgesics. These include subcutaneous infusions, transdermal patches, and intravenous, epidural and intrathecal medication administration.

Continuous Subcutaneous Infusion (CSCI)

Continuous subcutaneous infusions provide an effective means of achieving pain control for patients who may not be able to tolerate oral analgesics, or for whom oral analgesics are ineffective. However, CSCI is not an acceptable means of analgesic administration for all patients. Patients experiencing pain due to nerve damage, or patients with intermittent acute pain, do not achieve effective analgesia with this method. The other important consideration when selecting patients for this therapy is the amount of subcutaneous tissue. Emaciated patients have too little subcutaneous tissue for satisfactory absorption of the medication.

This therapy does, however, have some significant advantages. The frequency of injections is decreased, and the lightweight portable pumps do not affect mobility. The system is easy to maintain in a home environment. As well, side effects are less frequent and severe because a smaller dose of opioid is administered. This method also avoids the peak and trough levels observed with intramuscular injections (Poniatowski, 1991).

To begin treatment with CSCI, the 24-hour dose is calculated and the correct concentration of narcotic is diluted and added to the pump reservoir. The pump is then programmed to infuse the medication at a rate of 1–2 mL/h. A rate greater than this tends to cause irritation at the site. A 25- or 27-gauge needle is inserted into subcutaneous tissue usually in the anterior chest, abdomen or thighs. The site is covered with a transparent occlusive dressing. The infusion is begun and peak effect is usually achieved within 30–120 minutes (Poniatowski, 1991).

Assessment and evaluation of the effectiveness of this technique proceeds as with any other pain treatment. The site requires routine monitoring every four to six hours for pain, redness, edema and leakage. Sites require changing every three to seven days (Logan & Fothergill-Bourbonnais, 1991). The pump is checked routinely to ensure accurate medication delivery. Evaluation of the effectiveness of treatment occurs by assessing the patient's level of pain and reaction to the opioid being administered. Side effects are noted and treated appropriately.

Patients and families discharged home with this modality require teaching about the type of medication and what to expect regarding side effects. Information about assessing the site and pump is also necessary. As well, the patient and family need to know how to contact resources for problem-solving assistance at any time during a 24-hour period. Patients and families are encouraged to maintain a comfort record so that the effectiveness of the medication dose can be assessed.

Another method of subcutaneous delivery involves inserting a butterfly (needle) for a short duration to administer medications such as morphine. This method accesses the port each time the patient requires an analgesic. The site requires routine monitoring and should be changed per hospital policy. Dressing and site selection are the same as for CSCI.

Transdermal Patches

This is a new route for administration of analgesics. Fentanyl (Duragesic) is available as a patch that is applied to the skin. It takes 8–14 hours for the blood level of the drug to reach a steady state; therefore, this route is not appropriate if an immediate response is desired. Once the drug is discontinued, the nurse and patient should keep in mind that it can take up to 16 hours for the drug to be eliminated from the system.

Intravenous Delivery Systems

Traditionally, the intravenous method of delivering analgesics was reserved for terminally ill patients. Continuous morphine infusions were only for the dying. However, continuous opioid infusions often require as long as 15 hours to reach a therapeutic level of analgesia (Lubenow & Ivankovich, 1991). To combat the ineffectiveness of this route, an innovative intravenous technique known as **patient-controlled analgesia** (PCA) has been developed. This method allows the patient to remain in control of his or her pain-relief needs. Published research indicates that patients on the PCA system use less narcotic and experience fewer side effects than do patients who receive conventional intermittent intramuscular injections of narcotics (Fleming & Coombs, 1992; Ryder, 1991; St. Marie, 1991).

Patient-controlled analgesia is administered intravenously through an indwelling catheter by use of a special electronically controlled infusion pump that contains a timing device. Many of the pumps are small and portable, allowing the patient freedom of movement. The PCA pump permits patients to self-administer, on a demand basis, predetermined doses *(bolus injections)* of narcotic analgesics within prescribed time intervals to maintain a more stable serum level of analgesia.

The nurse programs the pump to deliver the prescribed analgesic dose. When pain is felt, the patient administers a bolus injection, for example, 1–2 mg of morphine sulfate,

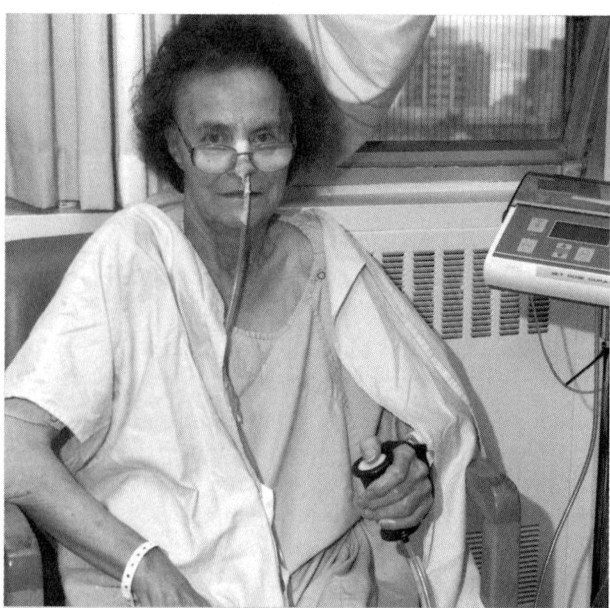

Patient-controlled analgesia allows patients to self-administer doses of analgesia as needed.

Patient-Controlled Analgesia Terms and Definitions

- *Bolus Injection Dose:* A predetermined amount of narcotic delivered when the patient presses the control button.
- *Lockout Interval:* The delay time during which no additional medication can be administered.
- *Basal Rate:* The rate of low-dose continuous infusion.
- *Attempts:* The number of times the patient attempts a bolus injection. The difference between successful attempts and the number of attempts before pain relief is achieved is an indication of pain control. Frequent unsuccessful attempts may indicate that pain is out of control.
- *Loading Dose:* A predetermined amount of narcotic delivered at the beginning of treatment.

into the intravenous catheter by pressing a control button. The timer ensures that repeat doses are administered within a prescribed time interval and prevents the patient from administering a second dose before the first has had time to take effect.

There are two types of PCA administration: low-dose continuous narcotic infusion with bolus injections, or bolus injections only. The continuous narcotic infusion with bolus injections delivers a maintenance dose of narcotic continuously, yet allows patients to self-administer bolus doses as patients feel they are needed. This method is beneficial for postoperative patients. It has "the advantage of maintaining analgesia while a patient is sleeping and minimizes the problem of patients being awakened by sharp, unrelenting pain" (Lubenow & Ivankovich, 1991, p. 38).

There are a number of safety features within the PCA system. The amount of medication that the patient can administer, as prescribed by the physician, is set and locked into the pump controls. All pumps have a "lockout" feature that prevents overdosage. The patient presses the button to administer the medication but the pump will administer only the programmed amount. Once the programmed amount is used up, the patient must wait a set amount of time before the next bolus can be administered. Many pumps have a four-hour maximum that prevents the patient from administering more than a preset total during a four-hour period. Another feature of the PCA system is that the nurse may provide the patient with additional analgesic using the bolus feature. This may be used to assist the patient to achieve pain control.

Effective use of PCA requires that patients be cognitively aware, physically able and psychologically willing to participate in their treatment. This modality is feasible with all age groups, though it is generally suggested that children be at least seven years of age (St. Marie, 1991). PCA is a valuable therapy for patients with acute intermittent pain or constant pain. It may be effectively used for chemically dependent patients, but the amount of medication may have

members and visitors should be instructed not to push the button for the patient.

Patient teaching is critical for PCA users. The patient must understand the reason for the type of medication being administered. All questions need to be honestly answered. A working knowledge of the pump, the control button and safety features is essential. The patient needs to be confident that inadvertent overdosage cannot occur.

Assessment and evaluation of the patient's response to patient-controlled analgesia are crucial for safe care. A flowsheet indicating sedation level, pain control and respiratory rate is usually maintained. If the agency does not use a flowsheet, the nurse enters these assessment parameters in the nurses' notes. Any side effects that are noted are treated and recorded.

Epidural and Intrathecal Medication Administration

Epidural analgesia has become an accepted method of analgesic delivery for postoperative patients. An external catheter with a bacterial filter attached to the distal end is inserted by an anesthesiologist into the potential space between the dura mater and the spinal cord (see Figure 27.7). This space is composed of fat, connective tissue and a network of thin-walled veins (St. Marie, 1991). Opioids, administered by a physician into the epidural space, bind to opiate receptor sites on the dorsal horns of the spinal cord. Generally, patients who receive analgesics in this manner require less opioid and experience fewer side effects (Faut-Callahan, 1991; Paice & Magolan, 1991; Woodin, 1993; McShane, 1992).

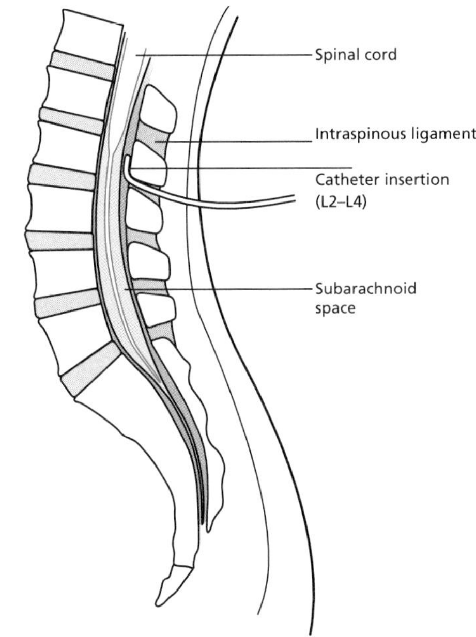

FIGURE 27.7 Epidural analgesia

Safety Measures When Giving Opioids

- Any patient receiving an opioid must have respirations monitored frequently
- A respiratory rate of less than 8/min requires immediate action
  - Notify the physician
  - Be sure that naloxone (Narcan) is available.

The effect of an epidural injection may last from 8 to 24 hours. Patients often experience fewer side effects than they do with IM injections. Consequently, they are able to perform deep-breathing and coughing exercises and to mobilize with ease. There are some disadvantages to this method of medication delivery. The catheter may kink or migrate into the subarachnoid space, resulting in toxic side effects such as respiratory depression.

Opioids are also administered by bolus or pump-controlled continuous infusion. Continuous infusions may be used for postoperative patients with severe pain. In long-term management, a port and catheter may be implanted to decrease the risk of infection.

Nurses caring for patients receiving epidural analgesia must check the insertion site frequently for redness, warmth, edema and leakage. The patient's level of pain is assessed to determine the effectiveness of the analgesic. Agency policy usually dictates the frequency of monitoring neurological vital signs. An increased temperature may indicate the beginning of infection and hypotension may occur due to vasodilation. Patients should be encouraged to move from a lying to a sitting or standing position slowly and with assistance. The effect of the opioid on nerves innervating the bladder may lead to urinary retention. Often, there are predetermined standing orders for common side effects such as nausea, vomiting and pruritis.

Implanted ports are generally used for the administration of **intrathecal analgesia** (medication injected into the subarachnoid space). A small reservoir is implanted and a catheter is tunnelled directly to the intrathecal space (see Figure 27.8). The intrathecal space contains circulating CSF and is located between the subarachnoid and pia membranes (Paice & Magolan, 1991). Accessing the implanted port in home use is often difficult. Because the reservoirs tend to be implanted in the back, the assistance of a willing family member is necessary for the patient to be maintained at home with this treatment.

Intrathecal opioids behave in a manner similar to opioids administered epidurally. The drug binds to opiate receptors and alters the transmission of the pain impulse. However, the dosage is one-tenth that of epidural analgesia. With intrathecal opioids, as with epidural opioids, patients experience fewer side effects. They are, therefore, able to mobilize and perform deep-breathing and coughing exercises.

The monitoring of patients receiving intrathecal opioids is similar to epidural administration. However, temperature must be observed more frequently with these patients, owing to the possibility of developing meningitis.

Evaluating Pain-Relief Interventions

All therapeutic modalities must be evaluated for effectiveness. A key nursing responsibility is to evaluate the effectiveness of any intervention. This is especially important when evaluating pain management regimes. The patient's level of comfort and response require continual monitoring using a flowsheet (see Figure 27.9). Initially, the patient's comfort level is assessed every two to four hours when a new modality, or a change in pain management, is implemented. The following questions suggest some of the ways pain management interventions might be evaluated:

1. Does the patient verbally indicate increased comfort? Has the pain disappeared or lessened in intensity?
2. Does the patient appear more comfortable; that is, is he or she more relaxed or less restless and irritable?
3. Has the patient been able to get to sleep without difficulty, or to rest quietly?
4. Is the patient able to enjoy his or her usual activities?
5. Is the pain more tolerable?

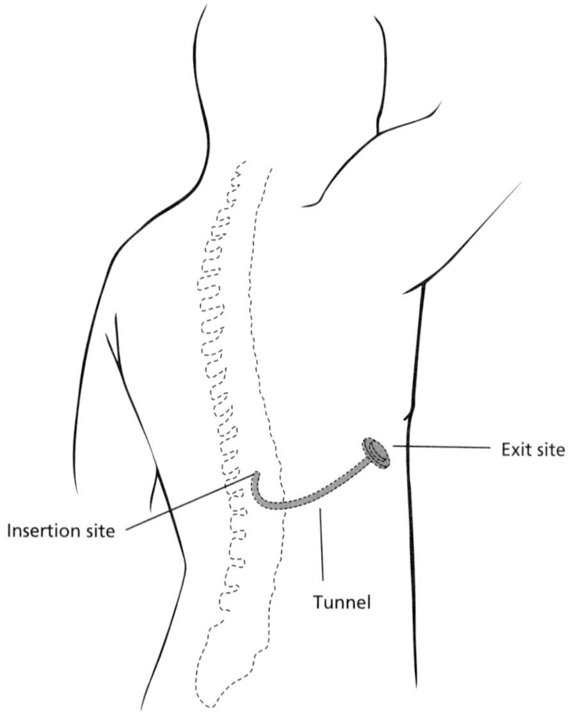

FIGURE 27.8 Implanted port for intrathecal medication

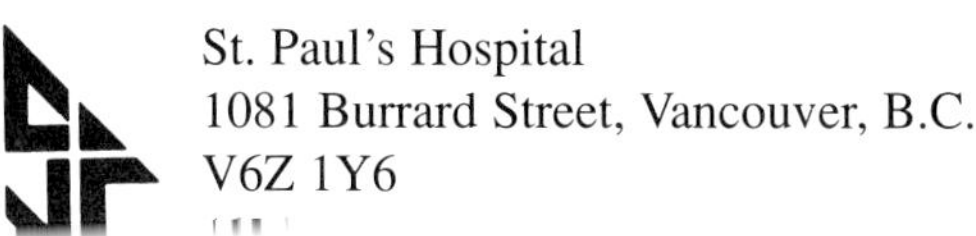
St. Paul's Hospital
1081 Burrard Street, Vancouver, B.C.
V6Z 1Y6

PAIN ASSESSMENT FLOWSHEET

ANAGELSIA SCALE / PAIN SCALE

☐ 0 - 10 ☐ 0 - 5 ☐ COLOUR ☐ FACES ☐ OTHER

PAIN RATING CHART

DATE											
TIME											
PAIN RATING SCALE 10											
9											
8											
7											
6											
5											
4											
3											
2											
1											
0											

*Indicate pain level with an "X" in the appropriate column.
*Notations on medication chart below to correspond with date and time in pain rating chart.

MEDICATION CHART

CONTINUOUS INFUSION											
REGULAR DOSING											
BREAKTHROUGH DOSES/PRN											

*Indicate with a "3" if the patient is continous infusion or regular medication dosing/PRN medication dosing.
*Note times breakthrough doses are given.
*Refer to MAR for type and dose of medication given.

SEDATION SCORE											
SIFE EFFECTS											
RESPIRATIONS											
PAIN LOCATION											

FOR NON-COMMUNICATIVE PATIENT (I.P. CVA PATIENT)

POSSIBLE PAIN											
BEHAVIOURS											
POSSIBLE COMFORT											
BEHAVIOURS											
NURSE'S INITIALS											

NURSE'S SIGNATURE: ____________________

FIGURE 27.9 Pain assessment flowsheet

SOURCE: St. Paul's Hospital, Vancouver, B.C.

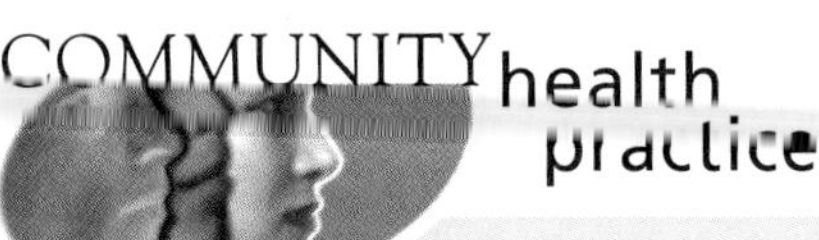

Thoroon Health Centre

The Thorson Health Centre was established by Gordon K. Thorson in 1989. Its main mandate is to help patients take responsibility for their own health and wellness. There is a multidisciplinary team approach at this independent facility. The approach is holistic in nature and its aim is to assess, diagnose and manage acute and chronic pain. The program consists of seven steps:

1. acknowledging pain
2. a desire to change
3. motivation to action
4. seeking professional help
5. understanding the mind–body link
6. taking responsibility for one's own health
7. graduation.

Treatment lasts between one and four months, with an average of one to four visits per week. Medical referral is required, and treatment is covered by the Medical Services Plan of British Columbia. However, there are some services not covered, for example, acupuncture and psychological counselling. These services are often covered under extended employee benefits or third-party insurance.

In 1996, the clinic was officially affiliated with the University of British Columbia's Postgraduate Residency Program.

Barriers to Effective Pain Management

The main barriers to effective nursing management of pain include the attitudes of health professionals; the level of knowledge among professionals, patients and their families; and a lack of support in the working environment of some health care agencies.

ATTITUDES Attitudes of health professionals have not kept pace with advances in knowledge about pain and its management (Weis, et al 1983). Research has shown that nurses underestimate their importance in effective pain control management. Students, from their earliest clinical experiences, should take part in the responsibility for pain control.

KNOWLEDGE Knowledge of all the available methods to relieve the components of pain is important to nursing practice. Nurses need to understand how analgesics work and how to apply this knowledge so that patients gain the maximum relief without unpleasant side effects (Fothergill-Bourbonnais & Wilson Barnett, 1992). In addition, a thorough understanding of different treatment modalities is required to maximize the benefits of pain-relief therapy and for patient and family teaching.

WORKING ENVIRONMENT Application of current pain knowledge and practices is facilitated when the working environment is supportive. A commitment to pain management at all levels of the agency is essential if lasting changes in attitude are to occur (Fothergill-Bourbonnais & Wilson Barnett, 1992).

In an effort to ensure that quality care is provided by the most cost-efficient methods, the Agency for Health Care Policy and Research (AHCPR) in the United States identifies some common health problems for study. Practice guidelines based on scientific evidence were established for acute pain and for cancer pain (see box).

Pain Management: Guidelines for Practice

- Promise patients attentive analgesic care
- Chart and display assessment of pain and relief
- Define pain and relief levels to trigger a review
- Survey patient satisfaction
- Analgesic drug treatment should comply with several basic principles
- Provide access to specialized analgesic technologies
- Provide nonpharmacological interventions
- Monitor the efficacy of pain treatment.

SOURCE: U.S. Department of Health & Human Services, 1992.

Caring for the Surgical Patient

Postoperative pain may be the result of more than just the surgical incision or wound itself. There may also be pain due to the effect of the anesthetic drugs and to the position of the patient during surgery. It is therefore important that all the patient's statements about pain be acknowledged and considered when developing and implementing a pain management plan. Pain may also be the result of misconceptions about the effect and duration of narcotics, tolerance levels and drug addiction. Physicians and nurses concerned about oversedation or respiratory and other complications have been reluctant to administer narcotic analgesics. Consequently, many postoperative patients are undermedicated.

RESEARCH to practice

Puntillo, K., & Weiss, S. J. (1994). Pain: Its mediators and associated morbidity in critically ill cardiovascular surgical patients. *Nursing Research, 43*(1), 31–35.
This study explored the effects of age, gender, personality adjustment and analgesic administration on the extent of pain experienced by patients during the first few days following cardiac and abdominal vascular surgery. It also examined the relationship between pain magnitude and postoperative complications. The sample consisted of 60 cardiac patients (44 male, 16 female) and 14 abdominal vascular patients (13 male, 1 female). The mean age was 64, with a range of 34 to 83. Pain intensity was measured by a 10-cm horizontal numerical rating scale (NRS); sensory and affective pain were measured using word descriptors derived from the McGill Pain Questionnaire–Short Form (MPQ–SF). Personality adjustment was measured by the California Q-Set, a 100-item Q-Sort procedure. The amount of analgesia was computed by summing all dosages of opiates administered by IV and by mouth during the course of the study. Dosages were converted to morphine sulfate equivalents. Once a day, beginning no sooner than 12 hours after admission to the unit and at least two hours after the last opiate administration, patients rated their pain using the NRS and MPQ–SF tools. Sometimes during their recovery a family member or significant other completed the personality Q-Set in order to minimize patients' stress because of the critical nature of their condition.

The study found that pain intensity was moderate and did not diminish over the first few postoperative days; physical sensations and emotional tension associated with pain caused minimal distress. The primary consistent mediator of pain magnitude after surgery was the amount of analgesics received, although small amounts were administered. The findings indicated that the analgesics administered were not effective in reducing pain. The researchers suggest that less conservative use of analgesics may be warranted, as well as increased use of nonpharmacologic interventions. Age and personality adjustment did not influence the extent of pain experienced. However, women and patients having abdominal vascular surgery reported more disturbing physical sensations associated with their pain. Finally, patients with greater pain intensity were found to have a significantly greater incidence of atelectasis (collapse of lung tissue) as a postoperative complication. Sixty-seven percent of patients in this study experienced atelectasis. The implications of this finding cannot be ignored. More aggressive pain reduction strategies are necessary to support patients' abilities to breathe deeply, cough and ambulate. These aggresive measures should minimize the development of atelectasis.

Strategies for alleviating postoperative pain begin preoperatively. Decreasing anxiety can reduce later complications and aid in reducing pain. Informing the patient during the preoperative teaching session about what to expect regarding the surgery and afterward may ease feelings of fear and anxiety. Developing and explaining the plan for pain relief preoperatively will also enable the patient to participate in pain management strategies postoperatively.

When the patient returns from the postanesthetic area, the nurse should complete a thorough assessment. The type of anesthetic the patient received and any analgesics that were administered during the operation or in the postanesthetic room should be noted. Following the initial assessment, the patient should be assessed for pain every two to four hours. During the first 24–48 hours postoperatively it is wise to administer analgesics around the clock.

Postoperative patients in pain tend to guard their surgical area. The resultant muscle tension decreases circulation to the injured area, thereby decreasing the transport of nutrients and waste products to and from the healing area. A patient in pain is generally reluctant to move or ambulate, and respirations also tend to become shallow. Effective analgesia permits the patient to breathe deeply and to relax tense muscles, facilitating circulation and healing and decreasing the possibility of complications. It is helpful to explain this to the patient preoperatively.

It is a good idea to assure the patient that the use of narcotics for 24–48 hours will not encourage addiction. While the administration of analgesics provides the patient with effective pain relief, the need for other comfort measures remains paramount. Nursing actions such as supporting the incision with a pillow during deep-breathing and coughing exercises, ensuring proper positioning, also assist in achieving pain relief.

Other modalities should also be used with surgical patients. Relaxation techniques, imagery and massage may all be effective adjuncts for the surgical patient feeling pain.

Postoperatively, patients often experience muscle pain and backache. Muscle aches—the "hit by a truck" feeling—may be due to the relaxants used during surgery. Some relaxants, such as succinylcholine, cause muscle fasciculations which may leave the patient tired and sore. These aches usually resolve spontaneously, but oral analgesics may also be beneficial (Rowland, 1990).

Many patients experience low back pain postoperatively. Muscle relaxation during anesthesia and the resultant stretching of the ligaments in the lower spine is generally the cause. Patients who received spinal or epidural anesthesia may have a sensation of bruising at the injection site. The application of heat to the lower back provides many patients with comfort for this type of pain (Rowland, 1990).

Caring for the Chemically Dependent Patient

Caring for patients with chemical addictions, whether to alcohol or drugs, is complex and challenging. Misconceptions regarding addiction and tolerance often precipitate inadequate pain management practices for these patients.

Individuals with chemical addictions often have a higher tolerance to opioids and require larger doses of narcotic analgesics to experience pain relief. Consequently, the first challenge is to identify chemically addicted patients so that appropriate analgesic treatment may be instituted. Many times, these patients do not overtly identify their addiction, and the first suspicion of addiction is raised when patient behaviours become a concern. In most instances, the solution is to raise the dose of the prescribed analgesic.

There is, however, often a hesitancy to increase the narcotic dose for chemically dependent patients. There seems to be a fear that increasing the dose will contribute to the addiction. There may also be concerns that the patient is feigning pain to obtain more medication. It is of paramount importance in these situations to remember that pain is a subjective experience. Only the patient truly knows the severity and intensity of the pain. It is the professional responsibility of the nurse to assist the patient to achieve pain relief. If the patient is not genuinely experiencing pain and is attempting to obtain more medication, a firm, consistent plan is required. It is also important to remember that rehabilitation is not possible when the patient is experiencing acute pain. Furthermore, rehabilitation needs to occur in a specialized setting. Acute care units are not organized to provide the intense counselling and physical care required (McCaffery & Vourakis, 1992; Lea, 1992).

Former opioid abusers will often refuse narcotic analgesics for fear of readdiction. These patients must be carefully assessed and counselled. It is best to consider pain and addiction separately, and to use appropriate interventions for each (Gonzales & Coyle, 1992).

Chemically dependent patients deserve the same respect and sensitivity to their needs as other patients. All statements of pain must be assessed and appropriate treatment implemented.

Caring for the Cognitively Impaired Older Adult in Pain

Assessment and evaluation of pain management techniques for the cognitively impaired older adult are often frustrating. Older adults may suffer from a variety of conditions that affect cognition, including aphasia, confusion, dementia, depression, memory loss, chemical and physical restraints and sensory deficits. Unable to articulate the experience of pain, the cognitively impaired older adult often expresses pain behaviourally.

Assessment of these patients must occur over a 24-hour period with input from all health professionals who have contact with them during that time. Expressions such as frowning or widely opening the eyes; aggressive behaviour, such as biting or hitting; rocking movements; sudden onset of confusion; and the guarding of a body part may all be behavioural indicators of pain. Remember that, though this patient may not be able to communicate the experience verbally, the pain experience is as intense as it would be for a younger person. Older adults who suffer from memory loss or certain types of aphasia may be able to communicate the experience if the nurse speaks slowly and uses short sentences or even just a few words. Terms such as *sore* or *hurt*, accompanied by pointing to a body area, may be all that is required to obtain a response (Parke, 1992).

Once pain has been identified for an older adult, it is necessary to implement an appropriate plan of care. Careful documentation of all attempted strategies for pain management and the patient's response is critical. Because the patient cannot verbally indicate the effectiveness, it is necessary to observe for behavioural cues. Watch for evidence of increased relaxation, willingness to participate in daily care and decreased irritability.

IN REVIEW

- Pain is a multidimensional, subjective experience and can only be described by the person experiencing it.
- Pain:
  - is a protective mechanism
  - is often undertreated
  - is viewed through various misconceptions about management
  - interferes with physiological and psychological functioning
  - is influenced by age, gender and culture.
- The physiology of pain is not completely understood. It involves four components:
  - reception
  - transmission
  - perception
  - modulation.
- There are several theories that propose how pain is transmitted and perceived; however, the gate-control theory is the most popular.
- The gating mechanism is opened or closed depending on input from nerve fibres, as well as motivational and cognitive influences from the higher brain centres.
- Pain may be categorized into two broad types:
  - acute pain
  - chronic pain.

  Chronic pain may be further subdivided into malignant and nonmalignant types.

- Pain has three sources:
  - visceral
  - psychogenic.
- The principles of pain management include:
  - allowing the patient to be in control
  - involving the family
  - using a multidisciplinary approach
  - using multiple modalities
  - acknowledging and treating secondary symptoms.
- Some barriers to effective pain management include:
  - attitudes of health professionals
  - lack of knowledge
  - lack of support in the health care environment.
- The primary source of information about pain is the patient. Other health professionals and the patient's family members can also contribute information about the patient's pain.
- Many agencies use a variety of pain assessment tools. The assessment of pain should include:
  - quality
  - location
  - intensity
  - time and duration
  - precipitating and aggravating factors
  - effects on activities of daily living
  - personal meaning of pain
  - usual coping strategies
  - affective responses
  - physical and behavioural manifestations of pain.
- Nursing actions are directed towards the following strategies:
  - protective (measures to prevent, minimize and cope with pain)
  - promotive (measures to avoid sources of pain and to maintain a healthy lifestyle)
  - restorative (measures to help manage pain).
- Pharmacological approaches to pain management include:
  - opioids
  - agonists/antagonists
  - non-opioids
  - NSAIDs
  - adjuvant medications.
- Nonpharmacological approaches to pain management include:
  - distraction
  - visualization
  - hypnosis
  - massage
  - relaxation
  - Therapeutic Touch
  - acupuncture/acupressure
  - transcutaneous electrical nerve stimulation (TENS)
- Evaluation of the effectiveness of any pain management strategy is part of nursing care. Continual monitoring and documenting of the patient's response and comfort level is essential.

Critical Thinking Activities

1. Explore at least three cultural groups with respect to the values and beliefs that influence behavioural responses to pain. What are the similarities and differences among the various groups in their reactions to pain? How do your own values and beliefs about pain compare to those of the cultural groups studied? What have you learned from this exercise that will help you understand the personal experiences of pain and implement individualized pain-relief measures?
2. Mrs. Kovalek is admitted to hospital after an automobile accident in which she has possibly fractured her ribs. Mrs. Kovalek's husband was also injured at the same time, and he is admitted to a nearby nursing unit. He has a fractured pelvis. Mrs. Kovalek is 33 years old, has three small children at home and is in a great deal of pain upon admission. Her orders include meperidine (Demerol) 100 mg IM q4h prn; oxazepam (Serax) 30 mg po qhs; up and about as desired; food and fluids as desired; chest x-ray.
   a. Describe the physiology of this patient's pain.
   b. What factors might enter into this patient's perception of and reaction to pain?
   c. How might this patient describe her pain?
   d. What observations would indicate to the nurse that the patient has pain?
   e. What should the nurse include when recording this patient's pain? Give an example of the recording, including subjective data, objective data and assessment.
   f. What are the goals of nursing care of this patient?

g. What specific measures might help alleviate this person's pain?

h. By what criteria can the nurse evaluate the success of the nursing care?

3. Find out about the services that are available in your community for people who have pain.

KEY TERMS

pain p. 832
suffering p. 832
total pain p. 832
noxious p. 832
nociceptor p. 832
pain threshold p. 832
pain tolerance p. 832
acute pain p. 836
chronic pain p. 836
somatic pain p. 836
visceral pain p. 836
psychogenic pain p. 836
intermittent pain p. 836
referred pain p. 836
cancer pain p. 837
phantom limb pain p. 837
central pain syndrome p. 837
neuropathic pain p. 837
sympathetic nervous system p. 837
parasympathetic nervous system p. 837
addiction p. 858
dependence p. 858
tolerance p. 858
patient-controlled analgesia p. 860
epidural analgesia p. 861
intrathecal analgesia p. 862

References

ACKERMAN, M.H., HENRY, M.B., GRAHAM, K.M. & COFFEY, N. (1993). Humor won, humor too: A model to incorporate humor into the healthcare setting. *Nursing Forum, 28*(4), 9–16.

BATES, M. (1987). Ethnicity and pain: A biocultural model. *Social Science Medicine, 24*, 37–50.

BATES, M.S., EDWARDS, W.T., & ANDERSON, K.O. (1993). Ethnocultural influences of variation in chronic pain perception. *Pain, 52*, 101–111.

BERIC, A. (1997). Post-spinal cord injury pain states. *Pain, 72*, 295–298.

BROWN, J. (1993). When words can't take the pain away. *Nursing BC, 25*(4), 16–19.

THE CANADIAN PAIN SOCIETY. (1997). Statement of pain relief. Ottawa: Author.

CASSELL, E.J. (1991). *The nature of suffering and the goals of medicine.* Oxford: Oxford University Press.

DELMAR PUBLISHING. (1997). *Delmar's textbook of basic paediatric nursing.* Albany, NY: Author.

DICKENSON, A.H. (1990). A cure for wind-up: NMDA receptor antagonists as potential analgesics. *Trends in Pharmaceutical Science, 11*, 307–309.

DOSSEY, B. (1991). Awakening the inner healer. *American Journal of Nursing, 91*(8), 30–34.

FAUT-CALLAHAN, M. (1991). Update on drug interventions. *Nursing Clinics of North America, 26*(2), 463–475.

FERRELL, B.R., & McCAFFERY, M. (1997). Nurses' knowledge about equianalgesia and opioid dosing. *Cancer Nursing, 20*(3), 201–212.

FINLAY, C. (1992). TENS: An adjunct to analgesia. *Canadian Nurse, 88*(8), 24–26.

FLEMING, B.M., & COOMBS, D.W. (1992). A survey of complication documented in a quality-control analysis of patient-controlled analgesia in the postoperative patient. *Journal of Pain and Symptom Management, 7*(8), 463–469.

FOTHERGILL-BOURBONNAIS, F., & WILSON BARNETT, J. (1992). A comparative study of intensive therapy unit and hospice nurses' knowledge of pain management. *Journal of Advanced Nursing, 17*, 362–372.

GALLOWAY, S., & TURNER L. (1996). Pain assessment in the cognitively impaired older adult. Unpublished paper. Vancouver, B.C.

GONZALES, R.G., & COYLE, N., (1992). Treatment of cancer pain in a former opioid abuser: Fears of the patient and staff and their influence on care. *Journal of Pain & Symptom Management, 7*(4), 246–249.

HEALTH & WELFARE CANADA. (1984). *Cancer pain: A monograph on the management of cancer pain.* Ottawa: Minister of Supply & Services (Catalogue No. 1442-25 1984E).

HESTER, N. (1975). University of Colorado Health Sciences Center. Denver, Co.

KACHOYEANOS, M.K., & FRIEDHOFF, M. (1993). Cognitive and behavioural strategies to reduce children's pain. *MCN, 18*, 14–19.

KRIEGER, D. (1979). *The therapeutic touch: How to use your hands to help or heal.* Englewood Cliffs, NJ: Prentice Hall.

LEA, P. (1992). Pain and the chemically dependent patient. *Canadian Nurse, 88*(6), 24–25.

LEININGER, M. (1995). *Transcultural nursing: Concepts, theories, research and practices.* (2nd ed.). New York: McGraw-Hill.

LOGAN, M., & FOTHERGILL-BOURBONNAIS, F. (1991). *Continuous subcutaneous infusion of narcotics: Patient care and family support.* Markham: Knoll Pharmaceuticals Canada.

LUBENOW, T.R., & IVANKOVICH, A.D. (1991). Patient-controlled analgesia for postoperative pain. *Critical Care Nursing Clinics of North America, 3*(1), 35–41.

LUDWIG-BEYMER, P., & HUETHER, S.E. (1996). Pain, temperature, sleep, and sensory function. In S.E. Huether & K.L. McCance (Eds.), *Understanding pathophysiology* (pp. 312–345). St. Louis: Mosby.

McCAFFERY, M. (1979). *Nursing management of the patient with pain.* (2nd ed.). Philadelphia: Lippincott.

McCAFFERY, M., & BEEBE, A. (1989). *Pain: Clinical manual for nursing practice.* St. Louis: Mosby.

McCAFFERY, M., & VOURAKIS, C. (1992). Assessment and relief of pain in chemically dependent patients. *Orthopaedic Nursing, 11*(2), 13–27.

McCONNAN, L. (1992). Measuring a child's pain. *The Canadian Nurse, 88*(6), 20–22.

McSHANE, F.J. (1992). Epidural narcotics: Mechanism of action and nursing implications. *Journal of Post Anaesthesia Nursing, 7*(3), 155–162.

MEINHART, N.T., & McCAFFERY, M. (1983). Pain: A nursing approach to assessment and analysis. Norwalk, CT: Appleton-Century-Crofts.

MELZAK, R. (1973). *The puzzle of pain.* New York: Basic Books.

MERSKEY, H. (1997). Pain, consciousness and behaviour. *Pain Research Management, 2*(2), 118–121.

MIRKA, T. (1996). The pain of suffering. *Canadian Journal of Cardiovascular Nursing, 7*(1), 15–18.

NORTH AMERICAN NURSING DIAGNOSIS ASSOCIATION (NANDA). (1994). *NANDA nursing diagnoses: Definitions and classification 1995–1996.* Philadelphia: Author.

PAICE, J.A., & MAGOLAN, J.M. (1991). Intraspinal drug therapy. *Nursing Clinics of North America, 26*(2), 477–497.

PARKE, B. (1992). Pain in the cognitively impaired elderly. *Canadian Nurse, 88*(7), 17–20.

PASERO, C.L., & McCAFFREY, M. (1996). Managing postoperative pain in the elderly. *American Journal of Nursing,* 96(10), 38–46.

PINNELL, N.L. (1996). *Nursing pharmacology.* Philadelphia: Saunders.

PONIATOWSKI, B.C. (1991). Continuous subcutaneous infusions for pain control. *Journal of Intravenous Nursing, 14*(1), 30–35.

[illegible] *43*(1), 31–35.

RIDDELL, A., & FITCH, M.I. (1997). Patients' knowledge of and attitudes toward the management of cancer pain. *Oncology Nursing Forum, 24*(10), 1775–1784.

ROMYN, D. (1992). Pain management: Know the facts. *Canadian Nurse, 88*(6), 26–27.

ROWLAND, M.A. (1990, May). Myths and facts about postop discomfort. *American Journal of Nursing*, 60–64.

RYDER, E. (1991). All about patient-controlled analgesia. *Journal of Intravenous Nursing, 14*(6), 372–380.

ST. MARIE, B. (1991). Narcotic infusions: A changing scene. *Journal of Intravenous Nursing, 14*(5), 334–343.

SEELEY, R.R., STEPHENS, T.D., & TATE, P. (1992). *Anatomy and physiology.* (2nd ed.). St. Louis: Mosby.

TWYCROSS, R. (1994). *Pain relief in advanced cancer.* London: Churchill-Livingstone.

U.S. DEPARTMENT OF HEALTH & HUMAN SERVICES. Agency for Health Care Policy & Research. (1992). *Acute pain management: Operative or medical procedures and trauma.* Washington, DC: Author.

WEISS, O.F., SRIWATAKANL K., ALLOZA, J.L., WEINTRAUB, M. & LASAGNA, L. (1983). Attitudes of patients, house staff and nurses toward post-operative analgesic care. *Anaesthesia and Analgesia*, 62, 70–74.

WONG, D.L. (1995). Whaley & Wong's nursing care of infants and children. (5th ed.) St. Louis: Mosby.

WOODIN, L.M. (1993). Cutting postop pain. *RN, 56*(8), 26–33.

WORLD HEALTH ORGANIZATION. (1990). Cancer pain relief and palliative care. Report of a WHO Expert Committee. Geneva: WHO Technical Series #804.

Additional Readings

AHMEDZAI, S., & BROOKS, D. (1997). Transdermal fentanyl versus sustained-release oral morphine in cancer pain: Preference, efficacy, and quality of life. *Journal of Pain Symptom Management, 13*, 254–261.

BROWN, L.S., BOLGER, M.S., PARMENTIER, C.M., & TAYLOR, J.B. (1997). Human error and patient-controlled analgesia pumps. *Journal of Intravenous Nursing, 20*(6), 311–316.

CAHILL-WRIGHT, C. (1991). Managing postoperative pain. *Nursing 91, 21*(12), 42–45.

COPP, L.A. (1993). An ethical responsibility for pain management. *Journal of Advanced Nursing, 18*, 1–3.

DALTON, J.A., & McNAULL, F. (1998). A call for standardizing the clinical rating of pain intensity using a 0 to 10 rating scale. *Cancer Nursing, 21*(1), 46–49.

DOLAN, M.B. (1993). Pain empowerment for patients and families. *Caring, 12*(2), 34–37.

DOWEIKO, H.E. (1996). *Concepts of chemical dependency.* (3rd ed.). Pacific Grove, CA: Brooks-Cole.

FERRELL, B.R. (1991). Managing pain with long-acting morphine. *Nursing 91, 21*(10), 34–39.

FERRELL, B.R., NASH, C.C., & WARFIELD, C. (1992). The role of patient-controlled analgesia in the management of cancer pain. *Journal of Pain & Symptom Management, 7*(3), 149–154.

FINLAY, G.A., & MCGRATH, P.J. (1997). Measurement of pain in infants and [illegible]

FULTON, J.S., & JOHNSON, G.B. (1993). Using high-dose morphine to relieve cancer pain. *Nursing 93, 23*(2), 35–39.

HANSON, E.J., & ARNASON, R.C. (1996). Easing the pain of cancer patients at night. *Canadian Nurse, 92*(7), 22–24.

KALSO, E., HEISKANEN, M., RANTIO, M., ROSENBERG, P., & VAINIO, A. (1997). Epidural and subcutaneous morphine in the management of cancer pain: A double-blind cross-over study. *Pain, 67*, 443–449.

KEMP, C. (1996). Managing chronic pain in patients with advanced disease and substance-related disorders. *Home Healthcare Nurse, 14*(4), 255–263.

MALEK, C.J., & OLIVIERI, R.J. (1996). Pain management: Documenting the decision making process. *Nursing Case Management, 1*(2), 64–74.

McCAFFERY, M., & BEEBE, A. (1992). Do you know the value of a nonnarcotic? *Nursing 92, 22*(10), 48–49.

McCAFFERY, M., & FERRELL, B.R. (1994, August). Understanding opioids and addiction. *Nursing 94*, 56–59.

McCAFFERY, M., & FERRELL, B.R. (1995). Nurses' knowledge about cancer pain: A survey of five countries. *Journal of Pain & Symptom Management, 10*(5), 356–369.

McCONNELL, E.A. (1993). Myths and facts about pain in the elderly. *Nursing 93, 23*(6), 83.

McGRATH, P.J., & FINLAY, G.A. (1996). Attitudes and beliefs about medication and pain management in children. *Journal of Palliative Care, 12*(3), 46–50.

PAICE, J.A., & COHEN, F.L. (1997). Validity of a verbally administered numeric rating scale to measure cancer pain intensity. *Cancer Nursing, 20*(2), 88–93.

RIPAMONTI, C., ZECCA, E., & BRUERA, E. (1997). An update on the clinical use of methadone for cancer pain. *Pain, 70*, 109–115.

SAWAKI, Y., PARKER, R.K., & WHITE, P.F. (1992). Patient and nurse evaluation of patient-controlled analgesia delivery systems for postoperative pain management. *Journal of Pain & Symptom Management, 7*(8), 443–453.

SIEPPERT, J.D. (1996). Attitude toward and knowledge of chronic pain: A survey of medical social workers. *Health & Social Work, 21*(2), 122–130.

SIMMONDS, M., WESSEL, J., & SCUDDS, R. (1992). The effect of pain quality on the efficacy of conventional TENS. *Physiotherapy Canada, 44*(3), 35–40.

WALKER, A.C., TAN, L., & GEORGE, S. (1995). Impact of culture on pain management: An Australian nursing perspective. *Holistic Nursing Practice, 9*(2), 48–57.

WALLACE, K.G. (1997). Analysis of recent literature concerning relaxation and imagery: Interventions for cancer pain. *Cancer Nursing, 20*(2), 79–87.

YEAGER, K.A., MIASKOWSKI, C., DIBBLE, S.L., & WALLHAGEN, M. (1995). Difference in pain knowledge and perception of the pain experience between outpatients with cancer and their family caregivers. *Oncology Nursing Forum, 22*, 1235–1241.

ZHUKOVSKY, D.S., GOROWSKI, E., HAUSDORFF, J., NAPOLITANO, B., & LESSER, M. (1995). Unmet analgesic needs in cancer patients. *Journal of Pain & Symptom Management, 10*, 113–119.

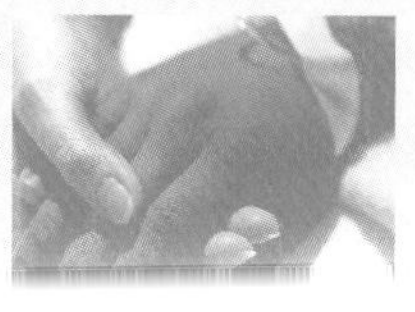

Activity Needs

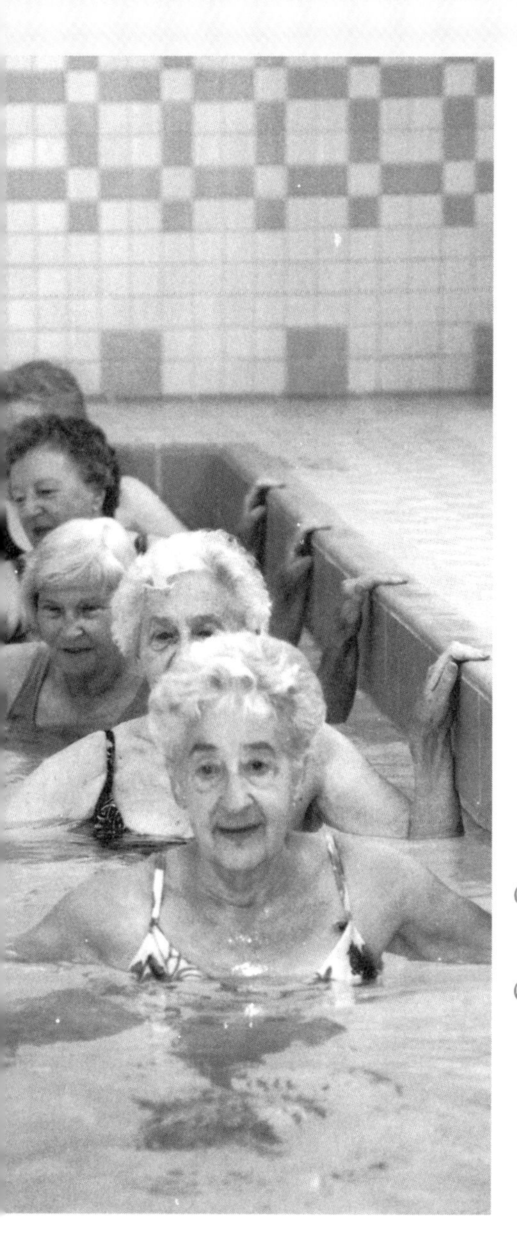

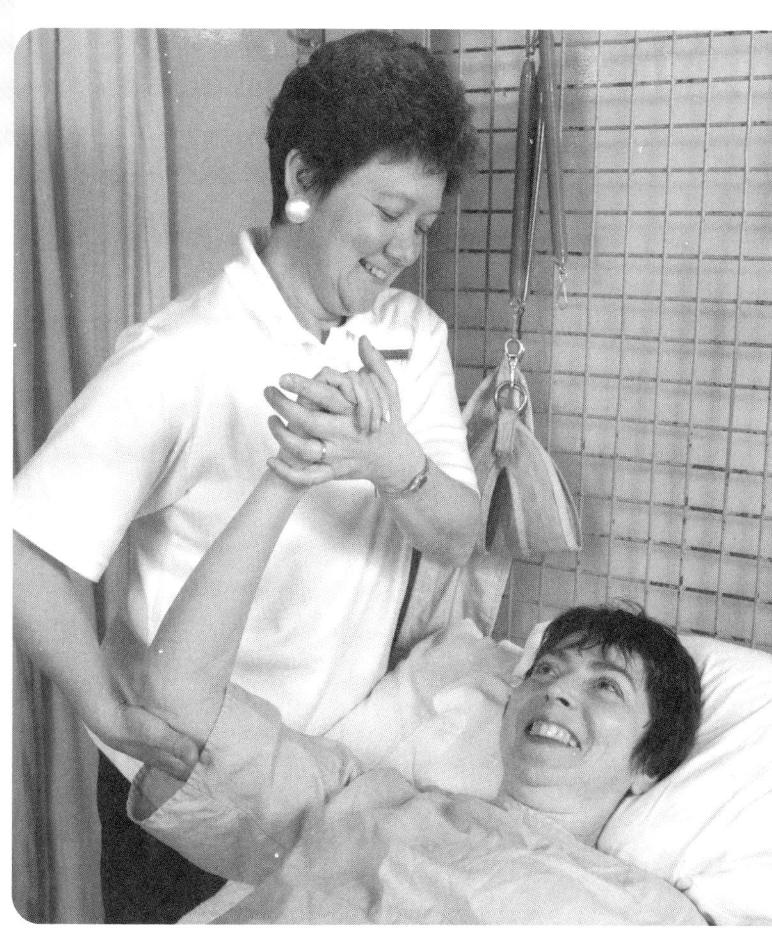

Chapter 28

Cognitive–Perceptual Needs

OUTLINE

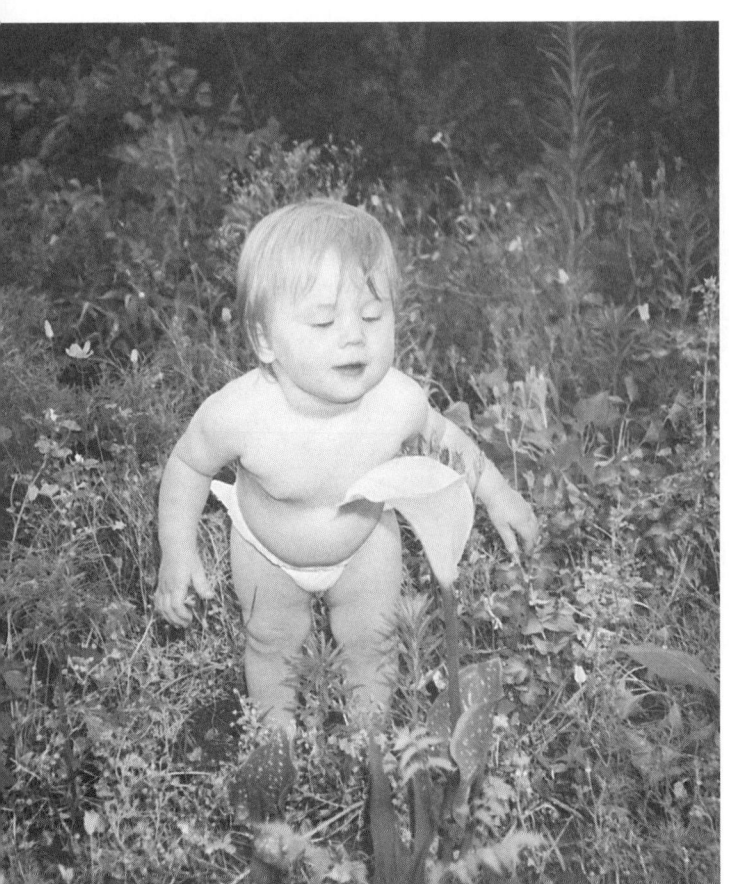

Central Questions

1. In what way is sensory stimulation a basic human need?
2. What is cognition?
3. What are the main determinants of cognitive–perceptual functioning, and how do they affect cognition and sensory perception?
4. How does cognitive–perceptual functioning vary throughout the life cycle?
5. What are some of the common problems in cognitive–perceptual functioning?
6. What basic principles would the nurse apply in assisting individuals to meet their cognitive–perceptual needs?
7. How does the nurse assess the patient's cognitive–perceptual abilities?
8. How would the nurse identify nursing diagnoses pertaining to cognitive–perceptual functioning?
9. How would the nurse develop a plan of care for patients with cognitive–perceptual disturbances and deficits?
10. What strategies might the nurse use to promote and protect the patient's cognitive–perceptual functioning?
11. What strategies would the nurse use to help the patient and family to cope with cognitive impairment, with a partial or complete sensory deficit?
12. How would the nurse evaluate the patient's response to nursing interventions?

Introduction

Sensory stimulation is a basic human need. Psychologists [illegible] quate sensory stimulation to promote the optimal growth and development of children, but only in recent years has the subject received much attention in other areas of the health field, and only recently has its importance to adults been acknowledged.

Sensory stimulation is a vital component of our lives. Our sensory faculties of sight, hearing, smell, taste and touch are the antennae that enable us to pick up signals that give us information about our environment. Without these abilities, we would not know what is going on in the world around us. Nor would we be able to communicate with other people, since communication involves both visual and auditory abilities, as well as the abilities to symbolize, to write and to make sounds.

The human body is often likened to a complex machine, with the brain functioning much as a computer does to receive, process and store data. The human brain, however, can do much more than any machine. Not only does it receive vast amounts of data from a multitude of sources in the external and internal environments; it has the ability to sort, classify, organize and interpret the information it receives. Then, it analyses and interprets the data on the basis of past experience and other sources of information, decides on a course of action and sends messages throughout the body to implement the action (Murray & Zentner, 1997).

Cognitive functioning is the broad term used to encompass these competencies. It includes the ability "to perceive, to think, to solve problems and communicate thoughts and feelings" (Murray & Zentner, 1997, p. 262). If cognitive functioning is impaired, a person's ability to carry out the normal activities of daily living is lessened. One has only to think of the number of motor vehicle accidents in which alcohol is a factor to realize the dangers of impaired cognitive functioning (see Chapter 30).

Receiving and accurately interpreting **sensory input** (stimuli from the external environment) is essential for survival. Losing the use of one of the senses is considered a handicap; it means that one of the antennae is missing and that stimuli must be picked up from other sources to compensate.

The person who is blind, for example, learns to distinguish sound with much more discrimination than does the person whose sense of sight is intact. Such a person also develops the sensitivity of the fingers in learning to read Braille. But he or she may still require the help of another person or of a seeing-eye dog to offer protection from hazards in the environment.

Similarly, the person who is deaf learns to "listen" to other people by reading their lips. People who are deaf may learn to talk in sign language. They also develop their sense of sight more keenly to interpret the meaning of nonverbal communications. Limitations in the ability to communicate, either in speech or in writing, can reduce one's ability to make contact with other human beings and, hence, these limitations cut off a major area of sensory stimuli. If [illegible] sages or depend on nonverbal means of communication.

Appetite is aroused by the sight and smell of food, but it is also dependent on direct stimulation of the taste buds. Thus, if the ability to taste is lost, appetite diminishes, and the nourishment taken in may be insufficient to meet bodily requirements. Loss of the sense of smell lessens the pleasure of many foods, since aroma contributes a great deal to the enjoyment of eating and drinking. In addition, people without the sense of smell may not be able to detect important odours, such as fumes or smoke from a fire, and may have to depend on their senses of sight and hearing to alert them to danger.

The loss of the sense of touch in a part of the body, for example, through the paralysis of an arm or leg as a result of stroke, can also leave an individual vulnerable to danger. He or she will be unable to tell if tissues in the affected extremities are being damaged (by burning from a hot water bottle, for instance). Loss of the sense of touch affects the ability to perceive pain, heat and cold and pressure. It also affects balance, since we use touch to align our bodies with objects or persons in the immediate environment. A person without the sense of touch is cut off from contact with other objects or human beings so far as the affected area is concerned.

We have talked mainly of sensory deficit; but, of course, people can also suffer from too much sensory input. The excessive noise and constant barrage of stimuli from a variety of sources that are a part of contemporary life can overload sensory-receiving mechanisms and result in problems in sensory functioning.

Cognition and Sensory Perception

Cognition means "the mental process characterized by knowing, thinking, learning and judging" (Stuart & Laraia, 1998, p. 857). It involves the organization of thoughts to give meaning to what is perceived. It incorporates reasoning, intuition and memory (Edwards, 1993). We are aware because of the information picked up (perceived) by our senses from stimuli in the external or internal environment. The term used for the apparatus within the body for receiving and interpreting sensations is the **sensorium**. It includes the brain, spinal cord and nervous system.

The perception of sensory stimuli is a complex process that has its origin in the five sense organs: the eyes (visual), the ears (auditory), the skin (**tactile**), the nose (**olfactory**) and the mouth (**gustatory**). Receptors in the sense organs pick up sensory input and send this information along to the brain via channels in the nervous system. The sensory information passes through several levels of increasing complexity in the brain, where it is modified, refined and interpreted. This interpretation depends on a number of factors, including the individual's state of well-being, past experiences with stimuli of this sort and the interrelationship of stimuli coming in from various sources. The result of this process, which takes less than a second to occur, is known as **perception**.

In order to process sensory perception, the brain (in particular, the reticular activating system of the reticular formation) depends on a constant and varied input of stimuli from the environment. If the receptors are not picking up enough stimuli or are getting too much of the same stimuli, **adaptation** occurs, and the brain will no longer perceive the available stimuli. To illustrate this effect, try sitting in a quiet, darkened room and staring at a luminous object. Gradually, the object will seem to disappear until it can no longer be seen. Extreme concentration on any object or person will produce the same effect.

A lack of environmental stimulation will likewise result in a form of sensory adaptation. It is believed that, in such a case, the brain will focus on higher thought processes and disregard the small amount of external stimulation that is available. Either situation—too much of one stimulus or not enough stimuli altogether—results in sensory deprivation.

In addition to the sense organs, which receive information from the outside world, the body also possesses **proprioceptors** (sensory nerve endings), which provide information about movement and the position of the body in space. Proprioceptive senses allow us to move about effectively and to orient ourselves to the environment. **Kinesthesia** is the sense that tells us where our body parts are in relation to one another. Kinesthetic information, which comes primarily from joint receptors, enables smooth, coordinated movement of the body. We would not be able to develop any motor skill, from walking to complex athletic movements, without kinesthetic information. The **vestibular system** in the inner ear is another proprioceptive sense. It conveys information about the position of the body in space and is often thought of as the sense of balance. We are usually not aware of the vestibular sense unless we overstimulate it, by spinning around, for example, until we become dizzy (Bernstein, Roy, Srull & Wickens, 1988).

Determinants of Cognitive–Perceptual Functioning

Two major sets of factors affect both cognitive and sensory functioning: environmental and biological. Environmental determinants involve either inadequate or excessive sensory stimuli in the environment. Besides the physiological changes that occur throughout the life cycle, biological determinants include the impairment of the sensory receptors themselves or the neural structures transmitting sensory impulses, and the impairment of the centres for processing sensory stimuli.

Environmental Factors

INADEQUATE STIMULI

People who have all their mental and sensory abilities intact are just as likely to suffer from a lack of sensory stimuli as are people with impairment of these abilities. The lack of stimulation may come from the physical environment, the psychosocial environment or both. People with limited mobility, such as those confined to a wheelchair or bed or those whose ability to get around is limited in any way, are particularly vulnerable. Their opportunities for varying their surroundings and for meeting and talking with other people are seriously hampered. The potential for inadequate sensory stimulation is therefore greatly increased. People whose work or home environments are monotonous and lacking in stimulation may also suffer from sensory deprivation. The person who works on an assembly line, for example, and has few hobbies or after-work activities, and the parent who stays home day after day with the same monotonous round of housework and who has no interests outside the home, are both likely to suffer from sensory deprivation.

Lack of stimulation is a very common problem in people who are ill, particularly in the hospital setting. Whether at home or in hospital, sick individuals fail to receive adequate sensory input because of monotony from meaningless stimuli or restrictions imposed by therapeutic interventions. Having to remain in the same room, look at the same walls, be exposed to dim lighting and a quiet environment, undergo a repetitive, unchanging routine and have limited contact with others are common examples of factors which lead to sensory deprivation. Disturbances caused by this form of sensory deprivation have been documented on patients in isolation, in intensive care units and in coronary care units, all of whom have minimal contact with the outside world (Halm & Alpen, 1993; MacKellaig, 1986).

EXCESSIVE STIMULI

It is also possible to experience an overload of sensory stimulation. This can occur even in the hospital setting. Although the atmosphere of the hospital is traditionally quiet and conducive to rest, this is not always the case. Many humorous articles have been written by patients about the disturbances in a hospital, but the situation is not always amusing. The patient may be subjected to bright lights or disruptive noises, for example, those produced by a respirator or a renal dialysis (artificial kidney) machine. The patient's rest may be constantly interrupted by members of the health team checking his or her vital signs or those of a roommate. Adequate rest and sleep are important to physical and psychological well-being, as well as to sensory perception; the specific effects of sleep deprivation are discussed more fully in Chapter 26.

IMPAIRMENT OF THE SENSORIUM

The mechanisms within the body for receiving, interpreting and processing sensations must be intact for optimal cognitive functioning. These include the brain, spinal cord, nervous system and other systems that affect these structures, such as the circulatory and endocrine systems. Any clouding of the sensorium (depression of the nervous system) or injury or disease affecting the anatomical structures or physiological processes involved in cognitive functioning will impair competence in this area. Cognitive–perceptual functioning is also affected by psychosocial stressors. People who are anxious may be so distraught that they do not know what they are doing and cannot think clearly. Similarly, people living alone in remote areas may experience disturbances in their thinking processes. The isolated trapper, for example, may suffer from "cabin fever," see polar bears that are not really there or come to believe that his nearest neighbour is plotting to kill him.

The sense organs and their accessory muscles, nerves and blood supply must be intact for optimal sensory stimulation to occur. Disease, injury or a congenital defect can interfere with the ability to receive adequate sensory input. The impairment may be temporary, or it may be permanent. A patient recovering from eye surgery who has both eyes bandaged may be suffering only a temporary loss of vision, but it is nonetheless a very distressing experience. While the patient's eyes are bandaged, he or she must adjust to life as a blind person. The person with a permanent sensory deficit must learn to adapt by making greater use of remaining sensory abilities and learning to live with the deficit.

Sensory impairment may be either partial or total. Partial loss of any of the senses can be almost as disturbing as total impairment. The individual who has some hearing loss often becomes very anxious and frustrated trying to hear what other people are saying. Social relationships may be impaired and sensory stimulation may be lost because of the difficulties in receiving spoken messages.

Distorted sensory perception can be equally distressing and potentially harmful. A person with distorted vision, for example, may stumble and fall while trying to find where to put his or her foot next. If you have ever walked through a "fun house" in an amusement park, you may remember how it feels to have your vision distorted in one of the convex or concave mirrors. This experience helps to give some idea of the feelings of a person with distorted vision.

IMPAIRMENT OF THE CENTRES FOR PROCESSING SENSORY STIMULI

Any factors that impair the functioning of centres in the brain that refine, modify and interpret sensory input interfere with sensory abilities. Diseases or injury affecting mental processes or causing damage to the brain may cause disturbances in sensory functioning. Fever, for example, often distorts sensory perception—a very high fever may cause hallucinations. **Hallucinations** (false perceptions unrelated to reality) may be visual or auditory. Other senses, such as smell and touch, may also be involved, and sometimes several sensations may be experienced at the same time. When this occurs, the feeling that this is real, and not a hallucination, may be overpowering (Gregory, 1997).

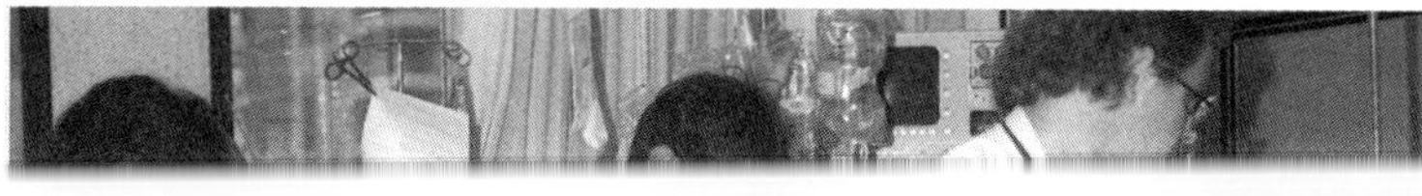

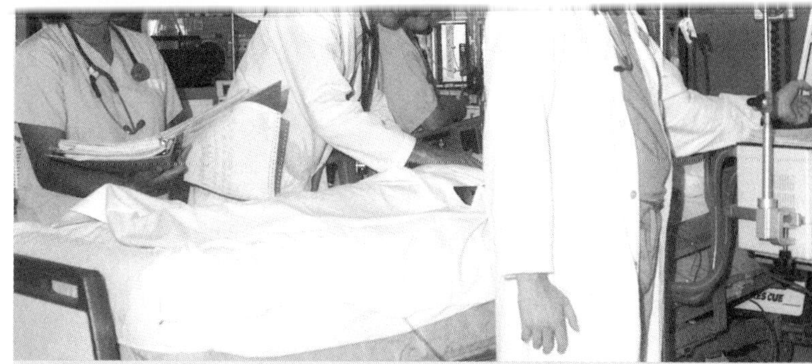

Sensory overload is possible in the hospital, especially in an intensive care unit.

A stroke (cerebrovascular accident) is a common cause of temporary or permanent impairment to brain tissues that interferes with sensory functioning. Paralysis and interference with speech and hearing often result from a stroke. Because the speech area in the brain is located in the dominant hemisphere, a stroke affecting this side of the brain may cause difficulties in speaking or **aphasia** (the loss of the ability to speak; patients with **expressive aphasia** know what to say, but cannot verbalize their thoughts). Patients with **receptive aphasia** cannot understand what is being said. In patients with existing heart problems, general circulation is impaired and there may be interference with the blood supply to the brain. These patients may also experience disturbances in sensory functioning because of inadequate oxygenation of brain tissues.

One's level of consciousness affects both the ability to receive sensory input and the ability to process it. The ability to receive sensory stimuli and the complicated mechanisms in the brain that process the input function at less than optimal efficiency when the level of consciousness is decreased.

Drugs that depress the central nervous system can decrease sensory functioning, since this system carries information from the sensory receptors and processes it. Many drugs are known to cause distortions in sensory perception. Hallucinogenic drugs, such as marijuana and LSD, cause hallucinations. Other drugs commonly used in the treatment of illness may have side effects that cause disturbances in sensory functioning, such as blurring of vision, ringing in the ears or distorted taste. When caring for patients receiving any type of medication therapy, the nurse should be aware of potential side effects and be alert for their appearance in the patient.

Emotional state can also affect sensory abilities. When people are happy they tend to see everything in a different light than when they are worried or depressed. Depressed people, on the other hand, may be unaware of things in their immediate environment—their eyes just do not see them.

Cognitive–Perceptual Functioning Throughout the Life Cycle

During normal growth, human cognition develops in systematic patterns. As we discussed in Chapter 8, Piaget divided cognitive development into four periods: sensorimotor (from birth to two years), preoperational (from two to seven years), concrete operational (from seven to 11 years) and formal operational (11 to 16 years). Piaget believed that a person reaches his or her highest level of cognitive development by the end of adolescence. However, it is now felt that full mental capacity is not reached until about the age of 25.

Newborn babies possess amazing sensory capabilities. Even before birth, sensory antennae are beginning to function. The fetus responds to sound starting in the fifth month of gestation (Caplan & Caplan, 1979). At birth, most of the essential sensory organs are fairly well developed and ready to function. From birth, infants are very sensitive to touch and pressure. Newborn babies will respond to cutaneous stimulation (soothing touch) with quiet, relaxed behaviour and they will withdraw from painful stimuli, such as a pinprick. Skin contact and warmth are the most powerful stimuli in the first few months.

Newborn babies can see to a distance of approximately 22–30 cm and can detect visual patterns; black and white geometric shapes are especially stimulating (Ludington-Hoe, 1983). Their sense of smell is functional and they respond to noxious odours by averting their head (Kenner & MacLaren, 1993). By the time infants are three weeks old, they can imitate the mouth movements of an adult. Because infants have taste buds all over the mouth, they tend to stuff their mouth as full as they can once they start to feed themselves (Pillitteri, 1995).

People often remark on the fact that babies have very large eyes. The eye of a newborn is three-fourths the size of an adult's. During the first 12 months of life, the eyes grow rapidly. This growth gradually slows down until the third year, when the eyes reach anatomical maturity. Visual maturity is reached in the sixth year. Newborns do not shed tears—the tear glands are usually not functional until the infant is two weeks old. Infants are aware of the relationship between sight and sound at a very early age, and by the time children are ready to crawl, they are able to perceive depth.

If the mother was not sedated during the birth process, the baby is likely to be very responsive and alert. If the baby is tired and hungry, however, he or she is capable of shutting out excessive stimulation. During infancy, it is important for the child to have a variety of sensory inputs. A lack of stimulation, as might exist in institutional care, for example, can result in depression and developmental delays. Screening for hearing defects can be done by the time an infant is six to 12 months old.

The major change in sensory perception during the early years of childhood is the maturation of vision. The young child's eye is normally *hyperopic;* that is, a distant image will fall behind the retina. However, because children's eyes have malleable lenses, they accommodate for this easily. Sometimes hyperopia (far-sighted) persists into adulthood. If the eye becomes too long during growth, the child will become *myopic,* that is, nearsighted. Children with myopia do not usually complain of poor vision, since they do not know anything else. With most children, vision usually improves up to the age of five, when most have 20/20 vision. An annual vision screening is done in most school systems from kindergarten through the high school years. Periodic auditory screening is also done in most schools. This is important because a significant hearing loss is one of the most commonly overlooked serious handicaps in children.

By the time the individual reaches adolescence, there is a cessation of growth and a stabilization of sensory powers. As people grow older, their sensory functioning decreases. It takes more stimulation to whet the appetite, for example, because there are fewer taste buds functioning in the mouth.

Vision also deteriorates as people grow older. As people approach middle age, they generally find that they need to wear glasses, even if they have never needed them before. In old age, vision is often impaired by cataracts, glaucoma (increased ocular pressure) or macular degeneration. Most elderly people are farsighted (hyperopia), because the lens of the eye loses elasticity. As a result, it is less responsive to light. Older people usually require much more light to read by than younger people do. They are also more sensitive to glare, and the headlights of oncoming traffic make night driving difficult. Older people are also more at risk for eye injuries because the cornea becomes less sensitive to touch and pressure, heat and cold. A decrease in tearing leads to dry and itchy eyes that are more susceptible to infection. There is also a narrowing of the visual field, with resultant decrease in peripheral vision. The pupils are often small, and there may be white, ringlike deposits of cholesterol just inside the edge of the cornea. Eyeglasses are an important part of the older person's sensory equipment. Nurses should be especially careful to handle them gently and to make sure that the lenses are clean.

Hearing also becomes less acute as a person gets older. Men tend to lose the ability to hear high tones, while women tend to lose the ability to hear low tones. The older person usually needs the radio or television volume set much louder than a younger person does. It is often necessary to speak more loudly and to enunciate words distinctly when talking with an older patient.

[illegible]

sory abilities that deteriorate with age. This makes older people more susceptible to falls for two reasons. First, an increased length of time is required for sensory impulses to travel to the brain and for motor impulses to travel from the brain to the periphery. Hence, reaction time is increased. Second, there are degenerative changes in the sensory organs themselves, which cause decreased vestibular functioning and lessened visual acuity.

Older people are more susceptible to burning themselves. One of the reasons for this is that an older adult's response to temperature is decreased. It is usually the middle ranges of temperature that are not perceived accurately, and the older person can be easily burned by water that is just a little too hot, or a heating pad that has been turned up too high.

Stronger impulses are needed to stimulate the senses as a person gets older. Food loses its flavour as the taste buds atrophy and become less efficient. The sense of smell is often diminished, and the older person may not detect the noxious odour of leaking gas until it is too late. It has been reported, however, that people who have had a keen sense of smell when they were young retain this sensory ability in old age (Ebersole & Hess, 1998). The ability to perceive light touch and vibration is often lost, and even deep pressure sensitivity is diminished. An example of the loss of deep pressure sense is the lessened response to the rectal reflex for evacuation of the bowel. As you will recall from Chapter 22, this reflex is activated by the perception of a feeling of fullness in the rectum.

Until fairly recently, it was assumed that a person's mental functioning gradually deteriorated with age. Studies done in the past few years, however, indicate that intelligence continues to be dynamic over the adult years and that some abilities even improve with age (Ebersole & Hess, 1998). Figure 28.1 depicts the particular strengths of each developmental period from infancy and childhood through to old age. It should be pointed out that "cognitive function among elderly adults is highly individualized based on their health status, experiences and personal resources" (Eliopoulos, 1997, p. 390). Therefore, it is important to have good baseline data on older patients' health status, a personal history and a good assessment of their personal resources.

Common Problems

Problems of cognitive functioning that nurses commonly encounter in patients, both in the community and in-patient facilities, include confusion, delirium, Alzheimer's disease and other dementias. **Confusion** is a clinical term referring to a mental state in which the individual's cognitive functioning is diminished, the person is disoriented as to time and space, may misinterpret sensory stimuli and makes inappropriate statements indicative of loss of memory [illegible]

[illegible] during the day and awake at night, not infrequently wandering about the house or hallways of the hospital in an agitated state. The causes of confusion are numerous, and it is important to investigate all possibilities before labelling a patient mentally incompetent. Some of the more common causes include medications, alcohol, and other toxic substances; anxiety, trauma, stress; infection; malnutrition; disturbances of fluid and electrolyte balance; congestive heart failure and other cardiac and respiratory conditions that interfere with oxygen supply to the brain; and impaired kidney functioning (Eliopoulos, 1997). The older, institutionalized person is particularly likely to become confused. Relocation to a new environment—from home to hospital or extended care facility—may be enough to cause confusion in an older person.

Acute confusional states occur frequently among elderly medical-surgical patients. These are generally transient and self-limiting. The underlying cause should be ascertained and removed (Ebersole & Hess, 1998). **Delirium** is a state of mental confusion and frenzied excitement that is most often the result of physical illness, drug intoxication or overwhelming psychosocial stressors. It develops suddenly and lasts for a short period. It is a common signal of physical illness in the elderly (Ebersole & Hess, 1998). **Dementia** is a broad term used for impaired intellectual functioning severe enough to interfere with a person's normal social and work life. **Alzheimer's disease** is a chronic

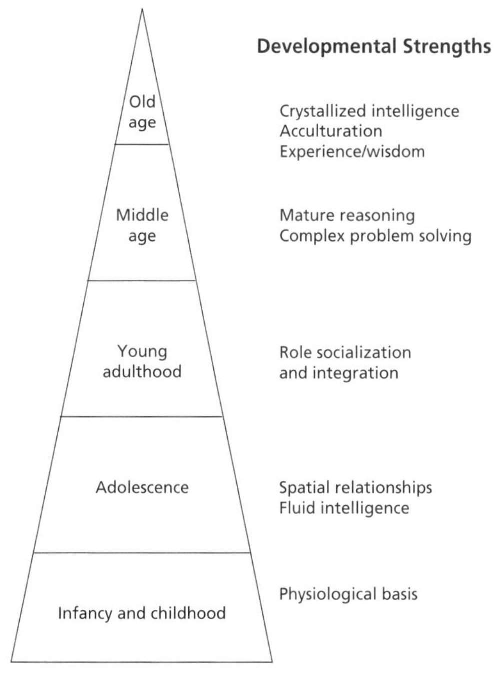

FIGURE 28.1 Lifespan cognitive developmental strengths

SOURCE: Ebersole & Hess, 1998, p. 784.

GERONTOLOGICAL

Changes in Sensory Perception Related to Aging

Factor	Implications for Nursing
In general, compared with younger adults, older adults: • are slower in their ability to process information • have decreased perceptual ability • show decreased reaction time • have more difficulty with tasks that demand concentrated attention	• Allow sufficient time with older people so that neither you nor they feel rushed • Try to relate new situations to familiar ones • See that they have familiar objects around them • Do not demand more of older people than they feel comfortable doing • Ensure consistency in their care (e.g., same staff to look after them whenever possible; consistent approach by all staff)
Vision: • decreased visual field • slowed accommodation to light • increased sensitivity to glare • diminished lacrimal secretions (less tearing) • decreased corneal sensitivity • distorted depth perception	• Ensure adequate nonglare lighting, night lights in bathrooms and hallways • Encourage older persons to wear their glasses at all times if needed; ensure that the glasses are accessible to them, clean and in good condition • Encourage the use of moisturizing eye drops for dry, itchy eyes • Protect the eyes from possible injury (e.g., by using glasses, sunglasses, sun visors, avoidance of rubbing) • Ensure that there are handrails on all stairs and that the stairs are well !it
Hearing: • loss of high-frequency tones • gradual decrease in hearing generally	• Speak clearly, enunciate words carefully
Touch: • lessened ability to sense pressure or pain, differentiate temperatures	• Pay attention to safety precautions regarding hot water bottles and other heating devices • Ensure that bedridden or wheelchair-bound people change position at regular and frequent intervals to prevent pressure sores
Balance and Position Sense: • decreased vestibular functioning, with resultant problems of balance and position sense	• Ensure that pathways and living quarters are clear and uncluttered • Provide handrails in bathrooms and other safety features to prevent falls
Taste: • lessened sense of taste	• Ensure that meals are appetizing and attractively served • Use seasonings judiciously
Smell: • diminished sense of smell	• Ensure that residences where older people live are equipped with smoke and gas detectors

Experience, previous learning and familiarity with the task at hand usually compensate for older adults' sensory deficiencies. They may, however, be more pronounced when the person is in a new situation, or one that is stressful or demanding (Ebersole & Hess, 1998).

dementia that is gradual in onset and progressive in nature. The disease causes atrophy of the brain, and the individual shows signs of progressive deterioriation of mental functioning. It is typically characterized by the four A's: **amnesia** (loss of memory), **agnosia** (loss of comprehension of sensations), **apraxia** (inability to make purposeful movements) and **anomia** (inability to remember names of objects) (Ross & Casey, 1993).

The most common sensory disturbances the nurse will encounter are sensory deprivation, sensory overload and sensory deficit (partial or complete). **Sensory deprivation**

sensory stimuli (Bernstein, Roy, Srull & Wickens, 1988, p. 156). It may result from inadequate or monotonous stimuli, poorly functioning sense receptors, inability to perceive environmental data, physical or social isolation, immobilization or restricted movement, or sensory overload. Humans rely on constant and varied sensory experiences in order to function. A lack of or alterations in sensory input may result in symptoms such as boredom, impaired consciousness, lack of coherent thinking, anxiety, fear, depression and hallucinations (Moore, 1991).

Sensory overload simply means the bombardment of an individual by too many stimuli at the same time. Sensory deprivation and sensory overload are relative terms. What might be sensory deprivation for one person may be peace and tranquillity for another. People who come from large families may enjoy a quiet time by themselves. They may, on the other hand, not find noise as disturbing as those who are used to a quiet household. They may even miss the stimulation of an active, busy home.

Sensory deficit indicates lack or deficiency in one of the sensory abilities. It may be partial, as for example impaired vision, or complete, as in total blindness.

Assessing Cognitive–Perceptual Needs

In order to assess a patient's cognitive-perceptual needs, the nurse obtains a health history and examines the patient for cognitive functioning, sensory deficits and manifestations of sensory deprivation or overload. Tests done on specific sensory abilities, such as a hearing test or an eye examination, will be included in the patient's chart, and the nurse can supplement the nursing data with this information. Similarly, information about the patient's health problems and the plan of therapy for these should also be available to the nurse from the physician's notations and orders on the chart.

Nursing Health History

The health history helps to identify patients' sensory capabilities and to determine the type of assistance they will need. Patients are the most reliable source of information about the condition of their senses. However, the family is a valuable source when the patient cannot communicate adequately. The nurse can add to subjective data by making observations of behaviours that indicate sensory disturbances.

In the health history, the nurse obtains information about the patient's usual and current status with regard to sensory abilities and makes initial observations about his or her cognitive functioning. Basically, the nurse is looking for the four components of cognitive functioning: (a) level of consciousness, (b) orientation to person, place and time, (c)

of the interview, the nurse assesses the patient's alertness and ability to respond to questions (level of consciousness). The nurse notes the patient's orientation to person when asking his or her name. To check orientation to place and time, the nurse may ask if the patient knows where he or she is, what day and time it is and what is the season of the year. The nurse does a cursory check of the patient's memory when asking for address, birth date and place of schooling. During general conversation, the nurse can usually do a preliminary assessment of the patient's recent memory as, for example, whether he or she can remember what the nurse said a few minutes ago. With regard to intellectual ability, the nurse notes the person's educational level, use of vocabulary and ability to answer questions intelligently.

Long-standing sensory deficits or problems the patient has, and any that have occurred recently, are identified. Information about corrective devices that the patient uses, such as eyeglasses or hearing aids, is also obtained. In assessing sensory functioning it is also helpful to gather information about the individual's usual lifestyle and environment to help determine whether these are providing adequate sensory stimulation for health. Through talking with the patient and with the family or friends, the nurse can usually learn something about the patient's basic personality. Is this individual usually quiet or talkative? Is the patient gregarious (does he or she enjoy the company of other people)? What are the person's usual activities during the day? Does the patient live alone or with family? How easily can he or she get out and around? What are some leisure interests?

Physical Assessment

Physical examinations of the sensory organs are outlined in Chapter 16. In this section we will focus on assessments of cognitive impairment, sensory deprivation, sensory overload and sensory deficits.

OBSERVING FOR COGNITIVE IMPAIRMENT

When the nurse observes someone for cognitive impairment it is important to take into consideration the person's age, educational level, cultural background, life experiences and state of health (Eliopoulos, 1997).

Tests for Cognitive Functioning

In addition to the basic information gleaned during the health history, the nurse may wish to employ any of several reliable tests to assess cognitive functioning. Most of these assess:

- orientation to person, place and time
- memory and ability to retain subject matter

- ability to follow directions
- judgement
- ability to do simple arithmetic
- reasoning ability (Eliopoulos, 1997).

Sometimes nurses use a simple test for cognitive functioning when it is not feasible or desirable to have the patient undergo a complete mental status evaluation. One such tool is the Mini Mental State (discussed in Chapter 16), which takes 5–10 minutes to complete (Stuart & Laraia, 1998).

Level of Consciousness

One of the most basic observations that a nurse makes is of the person's level of consciousness. The Glasgow Coma Scale is the most common way of assessing LOC (see Chapter 16). In this assessment, the nurse observes the patient's responses to questions, commands and other stimuli. Descriptions of the different levels into which consciousness is usually categorized are shown in the accompanying box.

Levels of Consciousness

There are four basic levels:

1. Conscious and alert (aware of surroundings)
2. Lethargic (sleepy, needing to be aroused to answer questions)
3. Stuporous or semi-comatose (the person is unconscious but can be aroused and responds to verbal commands)
4. Comatose or unconscious (the person does not respond to verbal commands, nor to painful stimuli; reflexes and respirations are also often abnormal).

SOURCES: Grimes & Burns, 1987; Eliopoulos, 1998

Behavioural Manifestations

Confused individuals may find it difficult to remember what they were saying, or may experience space and time disorientation. They may not know what time of day it is, which meal they have just eaten or where they are. They may make inappropriate responses both in conversation and in action. For example, a person may intend to put on eyeglasses, and instead remove shoes or put on a dressing gown. Thought disorientation may cause distortions in sensory perception and, for instance, cause people to think they are eating fish when in fact they are eating fruit.

The person who is suffering from delirium has lost touch with reality. He or she is disoriented as to place and time, often has auditory, visual or olfactory *hallucinations* (false perceptions unrelated to reality) or **illusions** (false interpretations of environmental stimuli) and engages in continuous, aimless physical activity. The hallucinations and illusions can be very frightening, and the person usually suffers from overwhelming anxiety. For example, the hospital room may become a prison cell and the nurse a sadistic monster. It is as if the person were acting out a play that is running in his or her head. Delirium is usually a transient state that disappears when the underlying cause is removed (Ebersole & Hess, 1998; Eliopoulos, 1997).

People suffering from Alzheimer's disease usually manifest three stages. During the early stage, the person may just seem a little vague and uncertain, loses interest in life and begins to neglect the usual courtesies and rituals of daily living. He or she may have trouble remembering the names of people and objects. As the disease progresses, the changes are more pronounced. The person becomes more forgetful, apt to lose important papers and miss appointments. Health and hygiene are often neglected. Such people have trouble recognizing even familiar faces, places or objects. Their judgement is faulty, and they are unable to follow simple directions. During the latter stages, the person's motor ability is more affected and he or she may have difficulty walking, talking and swallowing (Eliopoulos, 1997; Stuart & Laraia, 1998).

OBSERVING FOR SENSORY DEPRIVATION

It is important for nurses to recognize signs that may indicate possible sensory deprivation in their patients. Once these are recognized, the nurse can take steps to prevent deprivation from occurring or to remedy the situation if it does occur.

Below is a list of the continuum of behaviours manifested by the patient suffering from sensory deprivation:

- boredom
- inactivity
- slowness of thought
- daydreaming
- increased sleeping
- thought disorganization
- anxiety
- panic
- hallucinations (Cameron, Kessler, Kramer & Warren, 1972).

Patients who are *bored* may be overactive, usually doing trivial or inappropriate things. They may annoy other patients or continually push their call button to summon staff members, usually for small requests that they could handle themselves. Often they are irritable. Alternatively, people who are bored may also be *inactive*: they may appear apathetic and just lie or sit in one place without seeming to respond to any form of stimulation.

A person experiencing *slowness of thought* may take considerable time to grasp even simple concepts, and there may be great lapses in conversation as the patient tries to think of what to say. Reaction time will be reduced, and the patient may appear clumsy and awkward.

Daydreaming individuals may sit for seemingly endless periods of time, absorbed in their thoughts and fantasies,

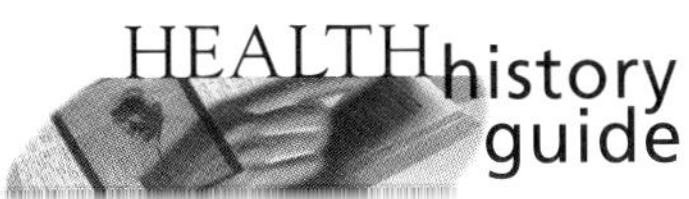

Cognitive–Perceptual Functioning

HEALTH AND ILLNESS PATTERNS

USUAL PATTERNS OF COGNITIVE-PERCEPTUAL FUNCTIONING

- How would you describe your ability to:
  - hear sounds and voices?
  - see near or far objects?
  - differentiate among a variety of tastes?
  - distinguish smells and pick up odours?
  - sense heat, cold and different textures?
  - know where body parts are without looking at them?
  - maintain a sense of body position and balance?
  - react quickly to stimuli, e.g., to a red light?
  - concentrate on an object or activity, such as reading a book?
  - think clearly?
  - remember events, persons, places?
  - solve problems, e.g., a jigsaw or crossword puzzle?
  - communicate your thoughts and feelings?
  - interact with other people?
- Do you use any assistive devices such as a hearing aid or eyeglasses?
- What kind of assistance would you require in caring for these devices?
- Do you live alone or with family? Describe where you live.
- Describe what you do in a typical day.
- What do you usually do for recreation and leisure?
- Do you spend time with other people or do you prefer to do things alone?

RECENT CHANGES IN PATTERN OF COGNITIVE–PERCEPTUAL FUNCTIONING

- Have you noticed any recent changes in your ability to think clearly? In your vision, hearing, sense of smell, taste or touch? If so, describe the changes.
  - Can you identify any recent changes in your life that may be upsetting your functioning, for instance, loss of companionship through death of a spouse, relocating from a quiet environment to one that is noisy?
  - How have these changes affected your daily living?

PRESENTING HEALTH PROBLEM

- Describe the difficulty you are having with your thinking or sensory abilities.
  - Do you have difficulty remembering things?
  - Do you have difficulty concentrating?
  - Do you have difficulty hearing? unusual sensations, such as ringing or humming in the ears? Pain in the ear?
  - Are you having blurred vision, double vision or other visual disturbances, such as sensitivity to light or blind spots?
  - Do you have pain in or around the eyes?
  - Have you noticed an inability to taste foods or distinguish odours?
  - Have you noticed any unusual sensations, such as a bitter or metallic taste in the mouth?
  - Do you have difficulty feeling hot and cold temperatures, or distinguishing different textures?
  - Do you have numbness, tingling or unusual tactile sensations? altered sense of body position? Dizziness or loss of balance? How long have you experienced these disturbances?
- Do you have an acute or chronic condition (such as multiple sclerosis, diabetes, an old head injury or chronic eye or ear infections) that may be causing your sensory disturbance?
- Are you taking any medications or treatments? If, so what are they?
- Do you have a family history of eye disease or deafness?

HEALTH PROMOTION AND PROTECTION PATTERNS

- Do you visit an optometrist or ophthalmologist periodically?
- Do you vary your recreation and leisure activities?
- Do you need rest during the day?
- How would you describe an emotionally stressful situation? How would you handle such a situation?
- Do you use alcohol or other mood-altering drugs?

ignoring whatever is going on in the room. It may be difficult to rouse these people, and they may not know when they have taken a medication or when someone is talking to them. They may confuse reality with fantasy.

The person who *sleeps* for longer than usual periods of time may be bored and consider this an effective way to pass the time. Such a person may find it difficult to stay awake with no stimuli to arouse the nervous system.

Individuals suffering from *thought disorganization* may find it difficult to remember what they were saying, or may experience space and time disorientation. People experiencing *anxiety* may feel that they are losing all faculties one by one or that they have a terrible brain disease affecting sensory perception. These people may become frightened and resort to the use of defence mechanisms (Chapter 9).

Panic, which we discuss in Chapter 36, is a severe state of anxiety. When people reach the stage of panic where sensory functioning is disturbed, they may feel that they will be permanently blind, deaf or paralyzed or that they are going mad.

A person suffering from *hallucinations* has lost all contact with reality. People who have experienced sensory deprivation may also experience hallucinations because:

> *It seems that the brain is always spontaneously active, and that the activity is normally under the control of sensory signals. When these are cut off [as in an isolation chamber] the brain activity can run wild and instead of perception of the world, we become dominated by hallucinations which may be terrifying and dangerous, or merely irritating and amusing.*
>
> (Gregory, 1997)

OBSERVING FOR SENSORY OVERLOAD

The nurse should be alert to factors in the patient's environment that may cause sensory overload and to signs of this in the patient. Ambulatory patients may suffer from an excess of sensory stimulation in their work or home environment, or in the sum of their daily activities. Everyone needs a quiet place in which to relax, to be free from the constant ringing of the telephone and from all the other noises and activities that form a part of the lifestyle of many active, busy people.

The busy parent with a house full of noisy children may show signs and symptoms of stress, as may the harried executive whose phone is constantly ringing, and who goes immediately from one meeting to another. The noise of machines in a factory constitutes a real health hazard to employees, as does the constant noise of planes for people who work in airports. Both the physical and psychological effects of excessive sensory stimulation are significant stress factors contributing to illness.

People who are ill are particularly vulnerable to the effects of excessive stimulation. Rest and quiet are still considered the best therapy for many illnesses. The body will often heal itself if it is not overwhelmed with the exigencies of the usual everyday activities. Indeed, illness is frequently the body's way of telling us that rest is needed.

We have already mentioned some of the sources of excessive sensory stimulation in people who are ill. The nurse should be alert to the factors that have been discussed as well as to excessive noise, interruptions of the patient's rest, too many people attending to the patient or too many visitors, particularly for the patient who is acutely ill.

The primary effect of overstimulation is fatigue. Patients may express weariness verbally but often it is the nurse's responsibility to note if the patient's face looks tired and drawn, if reactions are slowing down and every movement seems an effort, or if the patient is lying quietly in bed, trying to ignore the noise and activity in the surrounding area.

OBSERVING FOR SENSORY DEFICITS

There are a number of basic techniques a nurse can use to assess sensory deficits. These are not usually conducted during the initial patient assessment; however, the techniques are very useful if a sensory deficit is suspected.

Visual

Visual acuity refers to the ability to see objects or persons clearly. The simplest way to test visual acuity is to ask the patient to read printed material. If the patient normally wears glasses, the nurse should also check to see if these are still suitable. Many times, people find that illness affects their sight, and the glasses they used to wear no longer help them. This may be one reason that some ill patients do not read.

Visual acuity may also be measured with a Snellen eye chart (Figure 28.2), which is commonly used as a screening test for vision. The tool measures the ability to read letters or symbols on a chart from a distance of six metres (20 ft). Each eye is tested separately. The patient is asked to read through the chart beginning at the top line and continuing to the smallest line of letters possible. The lines on the chart have standardized numbers representing degrees of visual acuity. Normal visual acuity is 20/20. The first number represents the distance the patient is positioned from the chart. The second number is the visual acuity. It represents the distance at which the normal eye can read a particular line. Thus a reading of 20/20 means the patient can read at 20 feet (6 m) what the normal eye can read at 20 feet. The greater the second number is, the poorer the visual acuity. A score of 20/60 means that a person standing at a distance of 20 feet from the chart can read a line that a normal eye reads from 60 feet (18 m).

The assessment of visual acuity yields information about a person's central vision. Peripheral vision is tested with a visual field test (also called a confrontation test). A **visual field** is the entire area an eye sees when it is fixed on a central point. In a visual field test, the examiner compares the patient's peripheral vision to his or her own, assuming it is normal. To conduct a visual field test, the patient is positioned at eye level about 60 cm away from the examiner. The patient is asked to cover one eye and look directly at the examiner. The examiner also covers the eye opposite to the patient's covered eye and looks at the patient so that their visual fields mirror each other (see Figure 28.3). Holding a pen or other testing object midway between the examiner and the patient, the examiner moves the object from the periphery into the field of vision. The patient is directed to say "Now" as soon as the object comes into view. The object is moved in from several different directions: above, below and laterally. The steps are repeated with the other eye. If the patient is unable to see the object when the examiner does, a peripheral field deficit is suggested.

CONTACT LENSES Contact lenses are small, gas-permeable, saucer-shaped disks worn over the cornea of the eye and are available in both rigid and soft types. They may also be obtained in mono-, bi- and multifocal lenses for correction

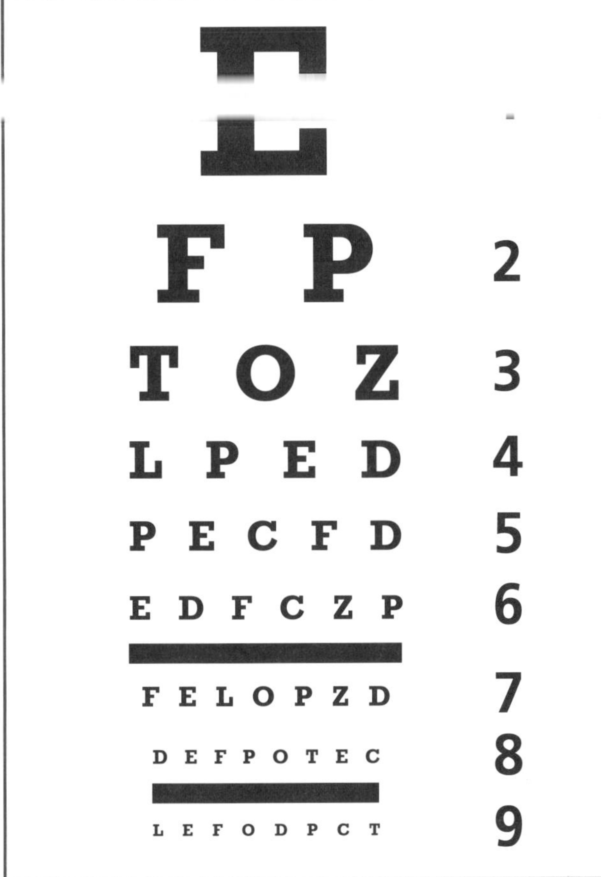

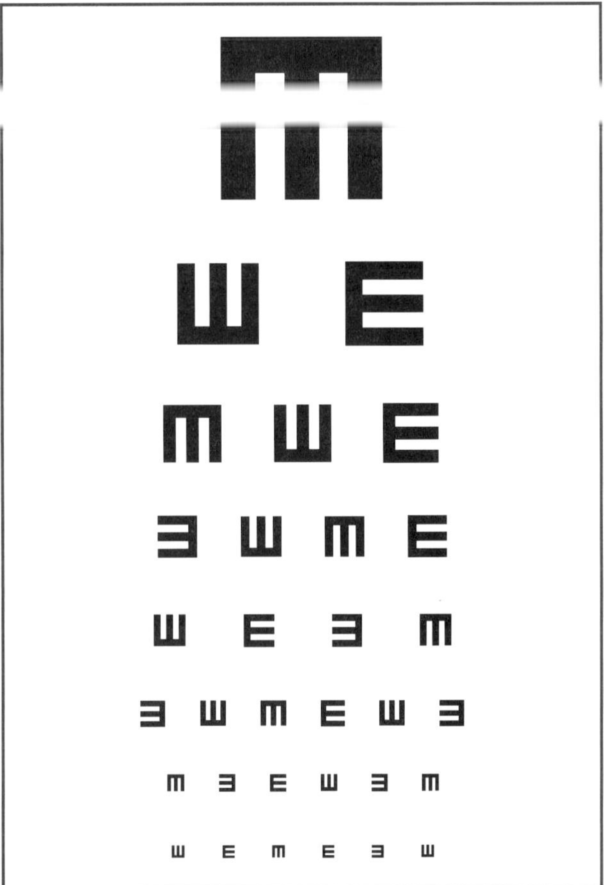

FIGURE 28.2 Snellen charts use letters (A) or symbols (B) to measure visual acuity

SOURCE: Burns & Johnson, 1980, p. 98.

of vision, with UV protection, and may be coloured or tinted for cosmetic purposes. Many types of refractive errors can be corrected: **myopia** (nearsightedness), **hyperopia** (farsightedness), **astigmatism** (unequal corneal curvature), **presbyopia** ("aging eye"; loss of elasticity of the lens of the eye), **anisometropia** (unequal refractive power of the eyes), **aniseikonia** (unequal size and shape of images from one eye), **keratoconus** (conic protrusion of the centre of the cornea) and **aphakia** (absence of lens after cataract removal). As well, contact lenses may be used for treatments such as occlusion therapy in children (for amblyopia), treatment of corneal disorders ("bandage lenses") and as a vehicle for delivering topical medications.

FIGURE 28.3 Position of the examiner and the patient for a visual field test

Soft contact lenses are available as daily wear (removed each night) and extended wear (can be worn continuously for up to seven days). Many are disposable.

Because of the different types of contact lenses available, the manufacturer's instructions for hygiene and handling of them must be strictly observed. The lens care regimen or solutions should not be interchanged or substituted without consulting the eye care professional. (See Procedure 28.1.)

ARTIFICIAL EYES Artificial eyes replace those that have been enucleated due to diseases such as malignancy and severe infection, or because of traumatic injury. The artificial eye is replaced not just for cosmetic purposes; it also prevents remaining soft tissue from collapsing and eyelids and lashes from turning in. It also facilitates proper circulation of tears to continue to lubricate the eye socket and lids (Erickson's Artificial Eyes, 1998).

PROCEDURE 28.1

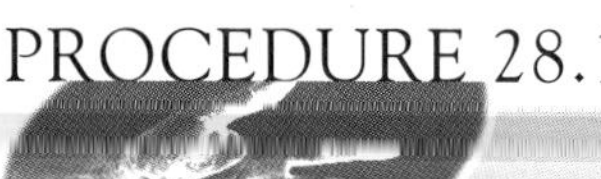

Caring for Contact Lenses

Action	*Rationale*
1. Gather supplies: • lens storage case • gloves (optional) • towel • contact lens solutions: cleaning, wetting, storing, disinfecting, enzyme cleaning and sterile normal saline for rinsing, as required • lens suction cup (optional).	Ensures efficiency and economy of time.
2. Wash hands and maintain medical asepsis.	Reduces transmission of microorganisms and keeps lenses free from bacteria. Poor hygiene may lead to inflammatory conditions and infections of the conjunctiva or cornea, which are hard to reverse and which respond poorly to treatment.
3. Assess patient's knowledge and understanding and elicit additional steps for care.	Determines patient's understanding of the care and level of assistance required; includes and adapts patient's technique and methods of care of contact lens.
4. Position patient in a supine or sitting position. Place towel near the face.	Gives access to the eyes and provides a clean, soft surface if the lens is dropped.
5. Assess eye for redness, excess tearing, corneal irritation, burning or infection.	Enables early identification of problems.
REMOVING CONTACT LENSES	
6. Remove the contact lens from the right eye first: 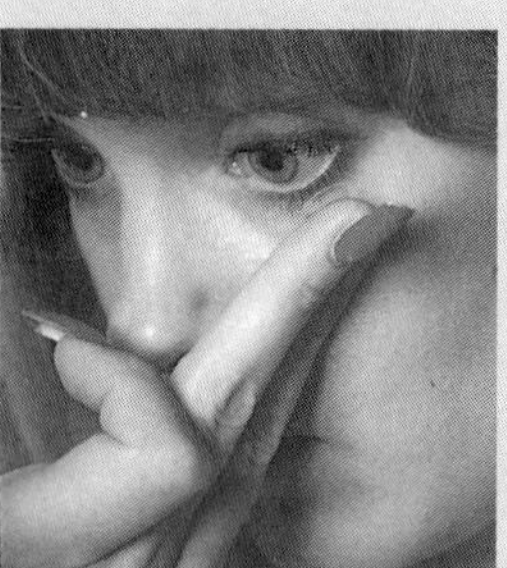	Helps to ensure the correct placement of each lens in the storage container.
Soft lens: Remove by adding a few drops of sterile saline to the eye, and with the patient looking straight ahead or upward, slide the lens off the cornea onto the white of the eye with the pad of the index finger. Then pinch the lens gently between the pads of the index finger and thumb and lift it off the sclera.	Lubricates the lens and eye for easy removal. Reduces the risk of damage to the cornea. Prevents scratching of the eye or lens by the fingernails. Air enters under the lens to break the suction for easy removal.
Rigid lens: Remove by gently pulling on the outer corner of the eye while the lens is centred on the cornea and patient's eye is open; ask the patient to blink, or separate the eyelids to expose the lens, and gently press the lower lid against the lower edge of the lens. The dislodged lens is cupped in the palm or gently picked up.	Dislodges it by catching the lens edge on the eyelid margins to break the suction. Prevents loss.
CLEANING OF LENSES	
7. Clean the lens according to manufacturer's directions, using the solutions recommended.	Prevents infection and ensures longevity of the lenses.
Apply 1–2 drops of cleaning solution on the lens and rub gently between the pads of the thumb and index finger (hard lens), or hold in the palm of the hand and rub with the pad of the index finger on both sides (soft lens), being careful not to scratch the lens with the fingernail.	Cleanses mucous, proteins, lipids and microorganisms from lens surfaces. Soft lenses are up to 80 percent water and can be torn easily.

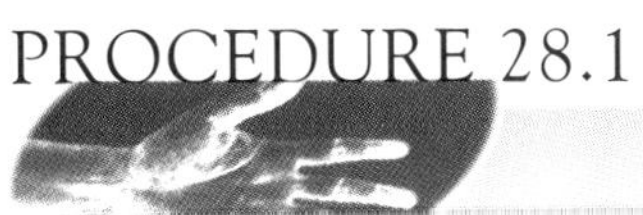

PROCEDURE 28.1 *continued*

Action	Rationale
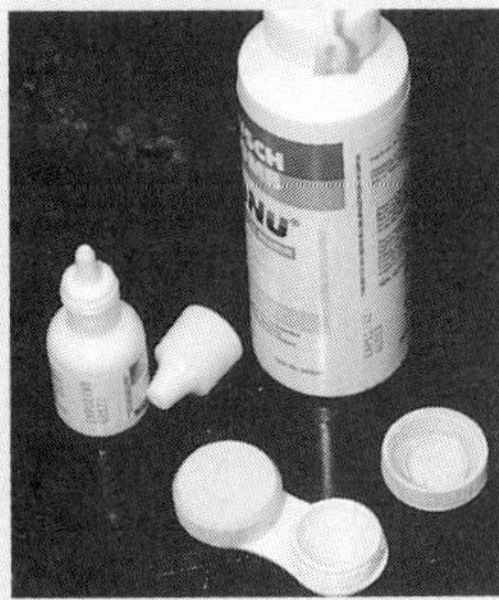	
8. Rinse the soft lens with sterile normal saline, and the hard lens with cool tap water.	Removes the cleaning solution and debris and cleanses the lens for storage.
9. Store the lens in the storage case in the correct compartment (right and left are indicated on the cover), filled with the recommended storage solution.	Prevents mix-up of lenses and ensures proper lens is inserted into the correct eye. Prevents drying and warping of the lenses by keeping them hydrated.
10. Repeat removal, cleaning and storage with the left lens.	Ensures proper care and prevents damage to lenses.
INSERTING LENSES	
11. Proceed after doing steps 1–5.	
12. Open storage case carefully and remove right lens from case without sliding or scratching the lens.	Prevents flipping out of lens and damage by incorrect handling. Always starting with the right lens avoids confusion.
13. Prepare the lens for insertion:	
Soft lens: Inspect for tears, deposits and damage, and rinse with recommended solution.	Prevents eye irritation. Removes storage solution, reduces transmission of microorganisms and prepares lens for insertion.
Rigid lens: Rinse with cool tap water and apply wetting solution to both sides of lens.	Hot water will warp lens. Lubricates lens and promotes adherence of lens to the cornea.
14. Insert the lens on the cornea:	
Soft lens: Place the prepared lens concave side up on the dry index finger and check that the lens is not inverted (an inverted lens causes the edges to point outward or forms a lip). While retracting the upper lid with the nondominant index or middle finger and pulling the lower lid down with the middle finger of the hand holding the lens, place the lens directly on the cornea or on the lower white part of the eye. Slowly release the lower lid first, then the upper lid.	An inside-out lens may feel uncomfortable and may slip off the cornea easily. Soft contact lenses are slightly larger than rigid lenses; this allows room for lens to be placed on the cornea without touching eyelashes or eyelids.
Rigid lens: Place the prepared lens concave side up on the index finger, retract the lower lid and gently place the lens directly on the cornea.	
15. Check that the lens is centred over the iris and pupil; if not, locate the lens in the conjunctival sac and, while using the eyelid to move the lens towards the cornea, have the patient look towards it to slide it onto the cornea.	Vision will be uncorrected if the lens is not centred on the cornea.
16. Tidy supplies; discard solution in the lens storage case. Rinse thoroughly, allow to dry. Wash hands. Store the solution bottles and clean; place dry case in the bedside drawer.	Prevents transmission of microorganisms and cross-contamination. Prevents loss and promotes security of belongings.
17. Record on Kardex that the patient wears contact lenses.	Provides continuity of communication. Alerts personnel to visual impairment when patient is not wearing lenses.

In addition to entire prosthetic eyes that replace an eye after removal, prostheses are available for situations in which the nonfunctional eye, or a remnant of it, is still in place. For example, a thin prosthetic shell fits over the iris and sclera to cover a disfigured eye, or a prosthetic contact lens fits over the cornea when the cornea is disfigured.

Artificial eyes are made of glass or plastic and are removable or permanently implanted. Recent developments in ocular prosthetics include ocular implants that integrate with the tissues of the orbit, deliver lifelike movements to the eye and prevent sagging of the lids due to chronic, unsupported weight on the lower lid by the artificial eye (Cosmetic Optics, 1998).

While most clients with an artificial eye have their own regimen, the nurse may need to provide assistance or care for the prosthetic eye when the patient is unable. It is not necessary to remove the prosthesis on a daily basis. Cleaning regimens vary, and include daily cleaning by application of a warm compress to the front of the prosthesis, rinsing in place (without removal) with saline solution, removal and cleaning with hydrogen peroxide and sterile saline every few weeks and, possibly, professional cleaning and polishing every six to 12 months. (See Procedure 28.2.)

Auditory

Auditory acuity is best tested with an audiometer, which gives a precise quantitative measure of the ability to hear sounds of varying frequencies. This test is conducted by audiologists and other professionals with specialized training in the field. The nurse may conduct a simple voice test to help detect the presence of hearing loss. One ear is tested at a time. While the patient covers one ear, the examiner positions his or her lips 30–60 cm away from the patient's unoccluded ear in such a way that the patient cannot read the examiner's lips. The examiner exhales and, beginning with a low whisper, slowly says two-syllable words that the patient repeats. If necessary the examiner may increase the intensity of the voice to a medium whisper, a loud whisper and then a soft, medium and loud voice (Bates, 1995). The inability to repeat whispered words correctly indicates hearing loss.

HEARING AIDS Hearing aids are available in a variety of sizes and designs, using both analogue and digital technologies; all of them amplify sounds, and many models are programmable for amplifying different frequencies of sound in order to decrease excessive background noise. Digital technology, which is still in development, offers the promise of improved listening. In the future, it may allow more precise adjustments to improve clarity of speech (ASHA, 1998). The different types of hearing aid include those that are worn in the ear, in the ear canal, behind the ear, in eyeglass frames and on the body.

All such devices are delicate and should be kept away from small children and animals, and extremes of temperature such as direct sunlight and hot surfaces. Hearing aids must be handled carefully and protected from breakage by dropping. Dusty and dirty environments, excessive moisture, cosmetics, hair sprays and lotions should be avoided. The hearing aid should be removed when bathing, swimming or showering. (See Procedure 28.3.)

Olfactory

The sense of smell is tested by presenting the patient with familiar and nonirritating odours. Substances such as coffee, vanilla, soap, chocolate or oils of wintergreen, orange or lemon may be used. Patients are asked to close their eyes, occlude one nostril and identify the smell of the substance held under the open nostril.

Gustatory

The taste sensation is tested by applying selected solutions to the tongue with an applicator and asking the patient to discriminate sweet, sour, salty and bitter tastes. A different applicator is used for each substance and the patient takes sips of water between substances to avoid confusing tastes. A simple method is to ask the patient to identify sweet, sour, salty or bitter flavours of foods on the meal tray. While the patient keeps his or her eyes closed, the nurse offers the various foods with a spoon.

Tactile

In testing for touch the patient is asked to discriminate sharp, dull, light and firm touch, as well as heat, cold and pain. The nurse can use a cotton ball for applying light touch and a safety pin or a cracked tongue depressor for inducing pain. The safety pin should be discarded after use to avoid the possibility of transmitting blood-borne pathogens to other patients.

Speech

While interacting with patients the nurse should always observe their formation and perception of speech. Problems in **phonation** (the ability to articulate words), and in the ability to understand and initiate speech, will be evident if there is a deficit.

Diagnosing Cognitive–Perceptual Problems

Altered Thought Processes is the diagnostic label used for people who have alterations in thinking, perceiving, symbolizing, communicating and/or decision making. The definition of *Altered Thought Processes* is "a state in which an individual experiences a disruption in such mental activities as conscious thought, reality orientation, problem-solving, judgement, and comprehension related to coping, personality

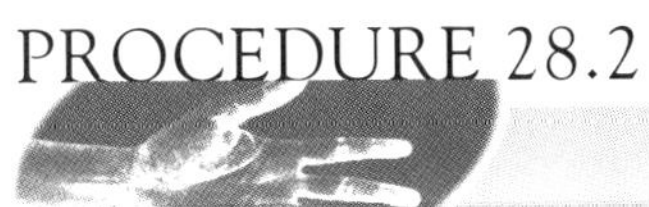

PROCEDURE 28.2 Caring for the Artificial Eye

Action	*Rationale*
1. Gather equipment: • storage case • basin of warm water • soap • soft, dry cloth • hydrogen peroxide and/or saline, per patient's regimen. • clean gloves	Ensures efficiency and economy of time.
2. Wash hands and maintain medical asepsis.	Reduces transmission of microorganisms.
3. Assess patient's knowledge and understanding, and elicit usual regimen for care.	Adapts to patient's method of care of the artificial eye.
4. Don clean gloves and remove the artificial eye by retracting the lower eye lid downward and exerting pressure with the thumb. Gently draw it out of the socket; place in basin.	Exposes the lower margin and releases the suction that holds it in the socket. Prevents loss or damage from dropping it.
5. Assess the lids, socket and surrounding tissue for signs of abrasions, irritation or infection (e.g., redness, inflammation, drainage or crusting).	Enables early identification and intervention for any problems.
CLEANING THE REMOVABLE PROSTHESIS	
6. Expose the eye socket by opening the lids with the thumb and index finger. Clean with normal saline and soft gauze sponges or cotton wipes.	Enables assessment and access to cleansing. Removes debris and prevents spread of microorganisms.
7. Wash the surrounding tissue with mild soap and water or normal saline by wiping from inner to outer canthus and using a fresh wipe each time. Rinse any soap residue completely and dry carefully.	Prevents debris from entering lacrimal ducts if present, and avoids spread of microorganisms to the other eye.
8. Clean the prosthesis with mild soap and water or hydrogen peroxide, according to patient's regimen. Rinse thoroughly with normal saline and dry.	Removes secretions, irritants and microorganisms.
9. Check the prosthesis for cracks, rough edges or need for professional polishing.	Prevents irritation or abrasions to tissues, promotes comfort and identifies any need for professional service.
10. If the eye is not to be reinserted (e.g., removed for surgery), store in a labelled case with sterile saline or water and place in the bedside stand.	Keeps prosthesis moist and prevents damage or loss.
11. To reinsert the eye, retract the upper or lower eyelid, or both, according to patient's regimen, with nondominant thumb and/or index finger. With the dominant index finger and thumb, place the moistened prosthesis into the socket and under the eyelids with the pointed edge towards the nose. Release the eyelids.	Provides access to eye socket. Moisture provides lubrication and easy insertion. Ensures secure fit in the socket and under the eyelids.
12. If the patient uses lubricants, apply as necessary; wipe excess moisture by wiping gently towards the nose.	Keeps eye socket and inner lids moist when lacrimal apparatus is deficient. Prevents dislodgement.
13. Ensure patient comfort. Dispose of used supplies; tidy environment and wash hands.	Reduces spread of microorganisms.
14. Document assessments, if eye has been removed for storage, or any pertinent care information. Document on Kardex that the patient has an eye prosthesis.	Provides continuity of communication. Alerts health professionals to visual impairment.

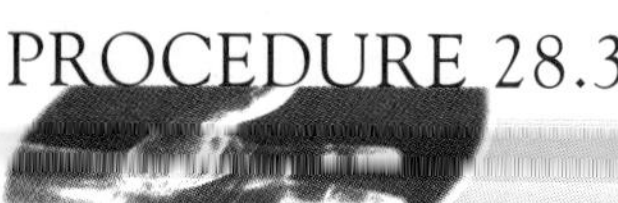

PROCEDURE 28.3 Caring for Hearing Aids

Action	*Rationale*
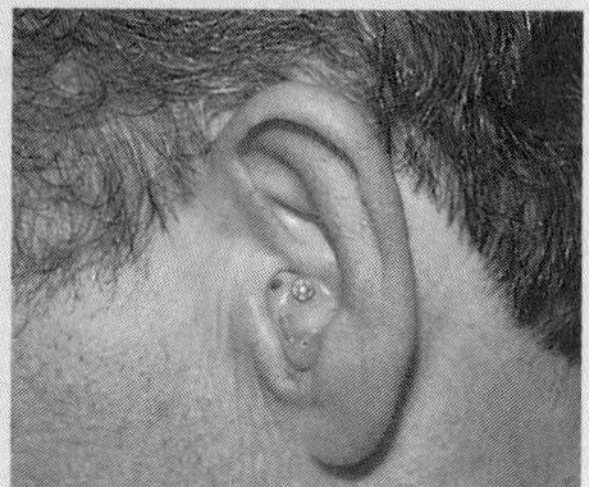	
1. Gather equipment: • kidney basin • soap • warm water • soft, dry cloth • cotton applicators • dry soft toothbrush or tissue.	Ensures efficiency and economy of time.
2. Wash hands and maintain medical asepsis.	Reduces transmission of microoganisms.
3. Assess patient's knowledge and understanding, and elicit additional steps for care.	Determines patient's understanding of the care and adapts to patient's method of care of the hearing aid.
4. Turn the hearing aid off. Assist the patient to remove the hearing aid from the ear by rotating it slightly forward and pulling it outward.	Prevents whistling of device. Follows the natural contours of the ear canal and eases removal.
5. Regardless of the model and size of hearing aid, the casing is usually wiped with a clean, dry cloth and build-up of earwax is removed carefully. The earmould is removed from the receiver in some models (the earmould is the one part that is washed with soap and water and dried daily).	Prevents infection and aids in proper functioning. Prevents wetting or damage to the receiver.
6. Wash and dry the ear canal with soap and warm water; dry carefully. Observe for excess cerumen, redness, sores or exudate from the ears. If necessary, assessment of the ear canal and tympanic membrane may be done with an otoscope.	Prevents infection and enables early identification of any problems.
7. Check the functioning of the device: **Visually:** That it is smooth and uncracked, the battery is not weak or dead; that it is the correct voltage, installed in the right polarity, and that the battery compartment is clean and uncorroded. **Functionally:** Listen for crackling sounds when turned off and on, humming or buzzing noises, and feedback whistle with the earmould occluded (feedback should occur with the earmould unoccluded).	Ensures proper functioning. Identifies problems with the device and possible need to have the hearing-aid dispenser service it.
8. Once the hearing aid is cleaned and checked, insert it into the ear by inserting the canal portion of the earmould first and guiding it snugly into the canal while pulling the outer ear gently up and back.	Ensures proper insertion and functioning. Insecure insertion causes improper function or feedback noise.
9. Check that the device is inserted all the way in, that it is neither too loose nor too tight.	Ensures proper fit.
10. Adjust volume gradually so that conversation at 1 m away is heard at a comfortable level.	Checks that the volume control is set properly, without harsh noise or feedback.
11. If the hearing aid is to be removed and stored, ensure that it is kept in a cool, dry place with battery removed, as recommended with some models.	Ensures continued functioning and longevity of batteries.
12. Document and communicate any communication difficulties and problems that need further servicing. Record on Kardex that the patient uses a hearing aid, and record if stored when not in use.	Provides continuity of communication. Alerts personnel to hearing impairment. Protects from loss when the hearing aid is not being worn.

and/or mental disorder" (Carpenito, 1997, p. 873). The causes or contributing factors associated with *Altered Thought Processes* include cognitive impairment, fear, depression, anxiety, stress

to a patient who is disoriented, has lost his or her memory, is having delusions or illusions, or whose judgement is faulty. Impaired cognitive functioning also gives rise to other problems that may become the focus of the nursing diagnosis, such as *Self-Care Deficit: Dressing, related to impaired cognitive functioning* or *Risk for Injury related to faulty judgement and impaired problem solving due to impaired cognitive functioning*.

Sensory/Perceptual Alterations is a diagnostic label that may be used to describe problems with sensory functioning that are amenable to independent nursing intervention. *Sensory/Perceptual Alterations* is defined as "a state in which the individual/group experiences or is at risk of experiencing a change in the amount, pattern, or interpretation of incoming stimuli" (Carpenito, 1997, p. 803). This may include, for example, the patient who is responding to decreased stimulation from social isolation or excessive stimulation from a noisy environment, or to physiological influences such as pain, immobility or sleep deprivation. Such problems are evidenced by signs and symptoms of sensory deprivation or overload. With respect to sensory deficits (for example, visual loss), nurses independently treat patients' responses to the deficit rather than the deficit itself. In these situations, the nursing diagnosis should describe the response, not the deficit; the sensory deficit becomes the etiology of the problem. Examples of these nursing diagnoses are given in the box below.

Nursing Diagnoses for Sensory Deficits

Visual:

- *Risk for Injury related to blurred vision*
- *Self-Care Deficit related to visual disorder*
- *Diversional Activity Deficit related to impaired vision*

Auditory:

- *Impaired Communication related to hearing loss*
- *Impaired Social Interaction related to hearing deficit*

Kinesthetic:

- *Risk for Injury related to dizziness and loss of balance*
- *Impaired Physical Mobility related to altered balance*

Olfactory:

- *Altered Nutrition related to reduced sense of smell*

Gustatory:

- *Altered Nutrition related to impaired taste buds*

Tactile:

- *Risk for Injury related to inability to perceive heat and cold*
- *Impaired Tissue Integrity related to decreased tactile sensation.*

SOURCE: Carpenito, 1997.

Planning Interventions for People with Cognitive–Perceptual Problems

Once the nursing diagnoses are established, the nurse develops a plan of care to suit the patient's individual needs. The goals or expected outcomes depend on the nature of the problem. For people with a potential problem of cognitive impairment, as, for example, an older person who is being transferred from an acute care hospital to a nursing home, the primary goal is to prevent the problem from developing, insofar as possible. For the person with an actual problem of cognitive impairment, goals would include:

- eliminating the cause whenever possible
- maintaining a stable environment with minimal stimulation
- maintaining the person's orientation to reality insofar as possible
- protecting the individual and others from harm (Eliopoulos, 1997; Stuart & Laraia, 1998; Ebersole & Hess, 1998).

In people with actual or potential problems of sensory deprivation or overload, goals are directed towards preventing the problems or restoring adequate sensory input and normal perception. For people with temporary or permanent sensory deficits, the goals focus on adjusting to the deficit and on maintaining or restoring self-care.

The patient and family should be involved in setting goals and selecting interventions as much as possible. While it is not always possible to involve persons with cognitive impairment in setting goals or planning interventions, the family should always be involved. When a patient is confused, family members are usually very worried and need considerable support to relieve their anxieties. They should be given a realistic explanation of the reason for the confusion, for example, "Your father is not mentally ill. He is very dehydrated and will be much better when he has had the intravenous infusion" (Eliopoulos, 1997). It is important, also, regardless of the person's level of consciousness or degree of impairment, to ensure that you talk to the patient, telling him or her what is being done and explaining procedures and tests (Eliopoulos, 1997). One should never assume that, because a person does not respond to stimuli or appears completely out of touch with reality, he or she does not hear you, or is unaware of what is going on.

It is especially important to involve family in the case of permanent sensory losses, such as those of vision and hearing. In such situations, successful achievement of the goals will depend on the patient's emotional adjustment to the loss and on the support provided by family, health professionals and community organizations. When establishing

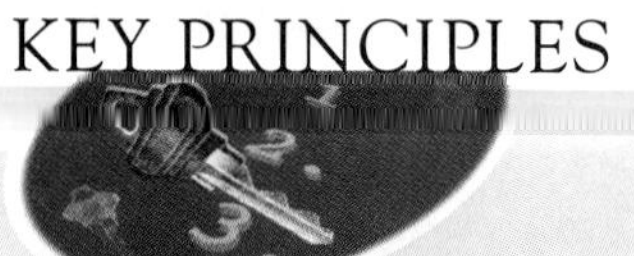

KEY PRINCIPLES

Principles Relevant to Cognitive–Perceptual Functioning

1. Psychosocial equilibrium requires that individuals have adequate sensory stimulation.
2. Stimuli picked up by the sense organs provide the body with information about the external environment.
3. Integrity of the sense organs is essential for sensory perception.
4. Sensory perception can be distorted in persons who are ill.
5. Damage to brain tissues caused by disease processes or by injury can interfere with sensory perception.
6. Communication provides an important means of sensory stimulation.
7. All sensory receptors adapt, either partially or totally, to their various stimuli over a period of time.
8. The brain is active even in the absence of stimuli from the external environment.
9. Sensory perception diminishes as a person ages.
10. The length of time an impulse takes to travel to the brain increases with age.
11. Reaction time to environmental stimuli increases with age.
12. The mechanisms for receiving, interpreting and processing sensations (sensorium) and accessory physiological processes must be intact for optimal cognitive functioning.
13. Cognitive functioning is lessened by anything that clouds the sensorium.
14. Psychosocial factors affect cognitive–perceptual functioning.

the plan of care, the nurse may collaborate with physical, occupational and speech therapists, audiologists and professionals providing specialized services (for example, representatives of the Canadian National Institute for the Blind).

If sensory disturbances are temporary, goals are usually short-term. For instance, the patient with *Diversional Activity Deficit related to impaired vision secondary to eye patches* will need intervention only as long as the eye patches are in place. Adjustment to permanent sensory loss often requires major changes in a patient's life. This may be a long process for some people. It is important to set short-term goals when striving towards long-term accomplishment. Success with short-term goals will help to provide the motivation needed to continue the long-term efforts.

The nurse should ensure that goals are realistic, attainable and measurable for each patient. For example, for a patient who remains in his or her room, sitting in a wheelchair most of the day, the expected outcome might be to increase the number of hours spent outside the room each day. It is helpful to set definite criteria, starting perhaps with two hours, and eventually increasing to eight hours per day. For the patient who takes no initiative in going to arts and crafts or other activities, possible goals might be that the patient will participate in these activities and take

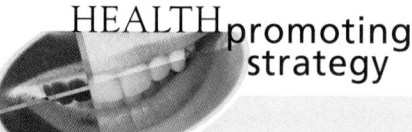

HEALTH promoting strategy

Promoting Healthy Cognitive–Perceptual Functioning

- Have a regular physical examination.
- Participate in a fitness program geared to your capabilities.
- Engage in hobbies that interest you.
- Avoid substances that cloud the senses.
- Avoid situations that cause undue stress.
- See an optometrist or ophthalmologist regularly for eye examinations.
- Watch the ultraviolet index. Wear proper sunglasses or a brimmed hat to avoid direct sunlight.
- Wear protective goggles when handling dangerous chemicals or materials that may fragment.
- Use proper, nonglare lighting for reading, doing close work and in the workplace. Avoid extreme lighting conditions that may be caused by high-intensity light sources.
- Avoid eye strain from excessive use of computers. Rest the eyes about 20 minutes every two hours.
- Avoid persistent loud noise. Wear protective ear covers if exposure is continuous.
- Maintain regular oral hygiene and drink ample fluids to keep the taste buds hydrated. A well-balanced diet with a variety of seasonings and textures will heighten taste perception.
- Keep the environment clean and fresh. Provide pleasant fragrances with deodorizers or flowers.
- Establish a variety of leisure activities to stimulate the senses.
- Balance activities with ample rest.
- Visit with friends and relatives frequently.

increasing responsibility for getting to the arts and crafts room. For the patient who is depressed or apathetic, even the initiation of conversation would be a major achievement.

Implementing Cognitive–Perceptual Interventions

Health-Promoting Strategies

Good physical health is essential for good mental health. As mentioned earlier in the chapter, any injury or disease process affecting the anatomical structures of the sensory organs, brain, nervous system or accessory physiological processes will interfere with cognitive–perceptual functioning. Substances that cloud the sensorium, such as alcohol or drugs, lessen one's ability to think clearly.

The sensory organs enable individuals to relate to and function effectively and safely in their environment. Health practices, lifestyle and occupation can alter sensory functioning and place individuals at risk for sensory loss. Individuals can do much to preserve and promote sensory capabilities in everyday living. Guidelines for promoting optimal cognitive–perceptual functioning are given in the box on page 890.

Health-Protecting Strategies

People who are ill often experience alterations in cognitive-perceptual functioning that may affect psychosocial well-being and interfere with the ability to communicate with others and function safely in their environment. A change in normal environment, exposure to unfamiliar sights and sounds, restricted mobility, medications, treatment measures and lack of diversional activity and meaningful social interactions all contribute to altered sensory patterns. In addition, confusion or cognitive–perceptual impairments such as loss of vision or hearing affect the ability to protect against hazards in the environment and to perform activities of daily living. Measures to promote patient safety and to enable self-protection are outlined in Chapter 30. This section will consider strategies the nurse can use in assisting patients to maintain their cognitive–perceptual functioning, prevent confusion, sensory deprivation or overload, maintain communication and perform activities of daily living.

PREVENTING CONFUSION

Unless the individual's confused state is due to a degenerative disease, such as Alzheimer's, it is usually transient and will disappear when the underlying cause is removed. There are, however, some general guidelines that can help to prevent confusion from increasing to a point where the individual, whether temporarily or permanently confused, becomes agitated and needs to be restrained.

Communicating with the Confused Individual

- Approach the person in a quiet, calm manner.
- Address the person by name and introduce yourself each time you talk to him or her.
- Speak quietly, clearly and calmly.
- Be patient; do not try to rush the person, or appear as if you are in a hurry.
- Try to minimize noise and other distractions in the room.
- Try to limit the number of people interacting with the person.
- Do not "go along" with misinterpretations the person has. Instead, quietly but firmly correct them (e.g., "No, Mr. R., this is not a prison; you are in the hospital").

An important first step is to minimize stimulation. The number of people caring for the person should be limited. Glaring lights and disturbing noises should be eliminated and activity in the room kept to a minimum. Stimuli that might be misinterpreted, such as shadows, or pictures on the television screen, should be removed (Eliopoulos, 1997).

It is also important to maintain stability in the environment. Here it is helpful to have the family involved in planning and carrying out interventions. Insofar as it is possible, all staff and family members should use a consistent approach in their interactions with the individual. Regularity of routines for daily activities such as meals or bathing schedules also contributes to stability. It is helpful, too, if the patient can wear his or her own clothing and have some familiar objects around (Ebersole & Hess, 1998; Matteson, McConnell & Linton, 1997). Suggestions for communicating with cognitively disturbed individuals are given in the box above.

Visits from family and friends can help keep the confused individual oriented to reality. Other contacts that are helpful include radio programs, a calendar and clock in the room and a window from which the individual can see the outside world. It also helps if the person can get out of the room or apartment and participate in activities with others.

People who are confused often neglect their basic physiological needs: they forget to eat, may not drink enough water or other fluids to keep themselves hydrated and may not think of bathing. It is a nursing responsibility to make sure that meals are eaten, fluid intake is maintained and hygiene needs are taken care of when the individual is incapable of looking after these things independently. Documentation of intake and output, bowel functioning and response to meals is important to ensure that other staff are aware of the patient's state of hydration, nutritional status and general physical condition.

Confused patients must be protected from harming themselves or others. Vigilance is essential to guard against hazards such as self-injury or wandering, and all safety precautions should be instituted (see Chapter 30).

PREVENTING SENSORY DEPRIVATION

Sensory deprivation has long been thought to be a problem requiring nursing intervention. Florence Nightingale was evidently concerned about this when she wrote:

> *It is an ever recurring wonder to see educated people who call themselves nurses, acting thus. They vary their own objects, their own employments, many times a day; and while nursing some bedridden sufferer, they let him be there staring at a dead wall, without any change of object to enable him to vary his thoughts; and it never occurs to them at least to move his bed so that he can look out of the window.*
>
> (Nightingale, 1946, p. 35)

The logical approach to nursing action for the patient at risk for sensory deprivation is to ensure that the environment contains adequate meaningful stimuli. This implies a certain amount of environmental management on the nurse's part.

People in the home setting should be encouraged to vary both their physical and their psychosocial environments. The nurse may be able to make some suggestions in this regard, or to involve family and friends or community organizations to assist individuals if they are unable to do this for themselves. Radio and television are great comforts to people who are unable to get out of their everyday environments, and help to keep individuals in touch with the outside world. Active participation in games, crafts and other activities will further promote contact with the environment. For the person who is fond of reading, mobile libraries are available in many communities. A visit by a library staff member not only provides new books and magazines to read, but also the stimulation of a new face and some conversation to relieve the monotony of the day.

Volunteers who deliver Meals-on-Wheels find that their clients often look forward to the social aspects of the service as much as the actual meal. A number of service clubs, lodges and other community groups visit people unable to leave their home, and arrange outings for senior citizens and handicapped persons. The nurse should be familiar with services available in the community. Community centres and organizations also provide activities for those who are ambulatory. Bridge clubs, arts and crafts classes and a variety of courses, including academic subjects as well as gardening, swimming and exercise classes, are among the many activities offered in a number of these centres.

For the person who is ill and in an institutional setting, approaches similar to those in the community setting may be used. Volunteers and community resources can help to provide the individual with sufficient change in both the physical and psychosocial environments to ensure an adequate amount of sensory input. Varying the patient's surroundings, even if this only involves moving the bed near the window, as Florence Nightingale suggested, provides a different perspective.

For the resident in an extended care facility, or one who is low-functioning disabled and confined to home, it is important to maintain contact with reality. It is helpful to provide some devices to enable this contact. The use of clocks, calendars, fixed time schedules, regular television or radio programs, and similar means helps to keep the person oriented to time and place. Newspapers and magazines provide a contact with what is going on in the world outside the agency setting.

The nurse may find brief explanations to the patient of nursing functions and treatments helpful too, even if the activities are routine ones. These explanations help to keep patients aware of where they are and what is being done for and to them. The nurse should not think that just because the patient does not respond means he or she does not hear. It is important to maintain auditory stimuli for the person who is seriously deprived of sensory input.

Therapeutic touch is an effective way of increasing stimulation to the brain and communicating with the patient. The use of touch that is so much a part of nursing has been shown to have definite therapeutic healing properties, from both a physical and a psychological point of view. The nurse's presence also means the patient has someone to talk to, and the different nurses coming on for different shifts help to provide a variety of people, which patients often find stimulating.

The nurse functions both as a source of sensory input to the patient, and as a resource person who can enlist the assistance of family, friends, visitors and volunteers from community organizations to help the patient to receive adequate sensory stimulation. Nurses are frequently called upon to use imagination to think of ways of getting people involved and to provide the type of stimulation needed for particular individuals.

PREVENTING SENSORY OVERLOAD

For the patient at risk for sensory overload, interventions that help to reduce the number of stimuli in the environment are indicated. In the community, the nurse may be able to help the individual plan periods of rest in a busy day or engage in relaxing activities. Physical exercise is often a good antidote for people whose work keeps them in an office, factory or other enclosed surroundings. Some people need assistance in order to be able to rest and relax. Other people enjoy music or reading or a game of bridge. A change of stimuli is often as relaxing as a cessation of stimuli.

Some people need help in learning how to relax and clear their minds of stimuli. Relaxation techniques are discussed in Chapters 27 and 36.

Some of the ways the nurse can help to reduce environmental stimuli for the ill person, at home or in hospital, have already been discussed. In addition, it helps to explain

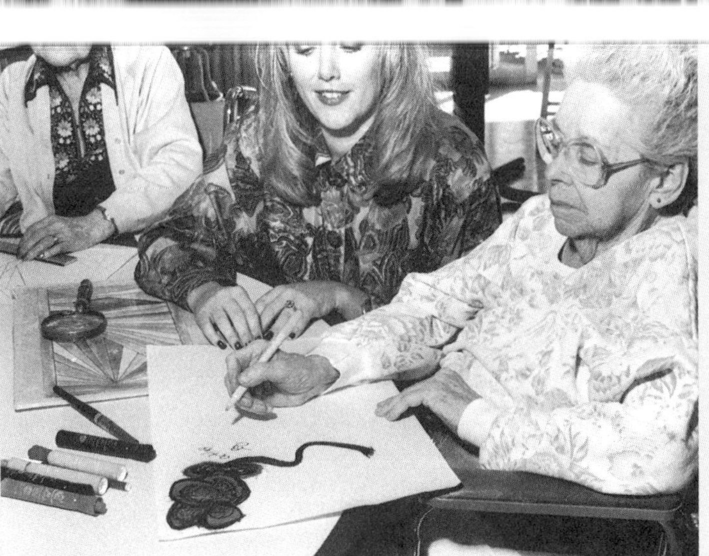

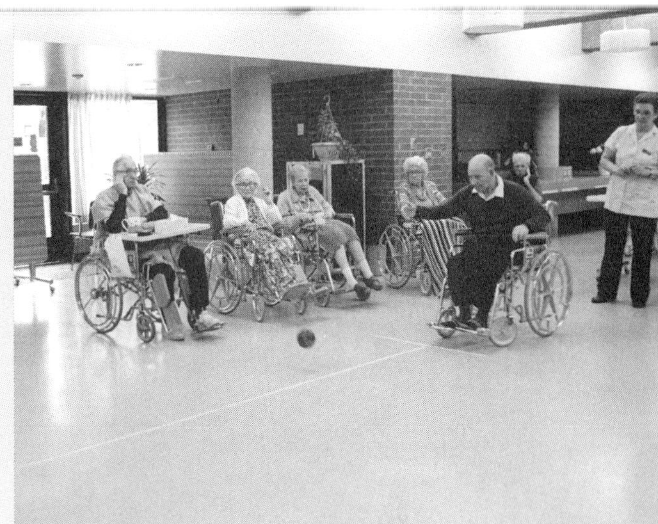

Active participation in games or crafts with other people provides a variety of sensory input and helps to keep an individual in touch with his or her environment.

the reasons for the tubes and machines that are surrounding the patient, the purposes of treatments and the reasons why other personnel come in to visit. Putting a structure to the sensory input helps people to interpret stimuli meaningfully; they are not so apt to feel disoriented, and anxiety is reduced.

MAINTAINING COMMUNICATION

Communicating with the confused or otherwise cognitively disturbed individual can be difficult. It requires patience and a calm, concerned manner on the part of the nurse. Individuals with sensory deficits, such as visual and hearing losses, require alternative methods of communicating with others. People with loss of vision rely on their sense of sound and touch and are very sensitive to spatial perception. Those with hearing loss make maximum use of their sight and may communicate in a number of different ways, such as sign language, lip-reading, hearing aids or note pads. Suggestions for communicating with the confused individual and with people who have vision or hearing loss are shown in the following boxes on page 894.

MAINTAINING ACTIVITIES OF DAILY LIVING

Individuals with cognitive impairment and those with sensory deficits may need assistance in handling their physical environment and maintaining daily activities. The nurse should be sensitive to the patient's needs and offer help before the patient has to ask for it. For example, the nurse can tell the patient who is having problems with vision what foods are on the meal tray and help to locate the food and cutlery. Cutting up food for a patient who has the use of only one hand, anticipating the need for help in putting on a dressing gown or helping a patient to the bathroom are other ways the nurse can assist individuals with sensory impairments to meet daily needs.

The nurse should be aware of tools that have been developed to assist people to maintain physical independence. Many utensils and mechanical devices are now available commercially. It is also possible to adapt ordinary utensils to assist with such activities as eating, reading, getting in and out of bed and moving about. These items eliminate problems for people who are blind, paralyzed or otherwise handicapped in performing both necessary and leisure activities. The nurse can call upon physical and occupational therapists for help in suggesting ways of increasing an individual's independence when one of the sensory abilities has been lost.

Health-Restoring Strategies

As mentioned earlier in the chapter, confusion is often a temporary state. For persons suffering from Alzheimer's disease or other dementia, the confused state may be permanent. In either case, health-restoring strategies are directed towards the same goals and involve the same interventions as those discussed above under health-protecting strategies.

In helping a person to cope with either a temporary or a permanent sensory deficit, the nurse must first of all be aware of the individual's reaction to it. Loss of sensory functioning has both physical and psychosocial ramifications. Some of the psychosocial effects have already been discussed.

Communicating with People with Vision Loss

- Always announce your presence when entering the room.
- Speak in a normal tone of voice.
- Inform the patient when you are going to touch him or her; explain all procedures and explain what will happen next.
- Describe the patient's environment in detail and allow the patient to touch objects in the surroundings.
- Inform the patient when changes have been made in the placement of items in the environment.
- Tell the patient when you are going to leave the room.
- Make sure the call bell is within easy reach.

Communicating with People with Hearing Loss

- Encourage the patient to use a hearing aid. Make sure the aid is in place and working.
- Make your presence known, but avoid startling the patient. Do not approach or do anything unexpectedly from behind.
- Stand where your face can be easily seen and maintain eye contact when speaking. Make sure the lighting is adequate so that the patient can see you.
- Speak clearly and a little more slowly than usual. Do not exaggerate lip movement because this interferes with lip-reading. Refrain from speaking with anything in your mouth. Keep your voice at a normal volume.
- Use visible aids. Speak with your hands, your voice, your face and your eyes.
- If the patient does not understand what you have said, rephrase words or sentences rather than repeat the whole conversation. Use pictures or written information to supplement the spoken word.
- Eliminate background noise; for instance, turn off the radio or television, or close windows to control noise from outside.
- Be sensitive. An ill or fatigued patient may not hear as well as usual.

SOURCE: Chovaz, 1989, pp. 34–36.

If a permanent and total disability of one of the senses has occurred, the patient feels an acute sense of loss and grief. If the nurse is caring for someone who has recently experienced such a loss, it may be helpful at this point to read Chapter 37.

With a partial or a temporary loss of sensory functioning, people may be anxious and worried. Will they regain total functioning? What if they become totally blind or deaf or remain permanently paralyzed? What if their speech never comes back? How are they going to cope with partial impairment? These are some of the spoken and unspoken questions these patients ask.

Often people with sensory losses need the help of specialized health professionals or specialized agencies to enable them to learn to live with a sensory deficit. The nurse supports the work of specialists such as physical, occupational and speech therapists by following through on activities suggested by them. The patient's increased independence is ensured when all nurses are aware of the goals for the patient, and are consistent in their approach to him or her.

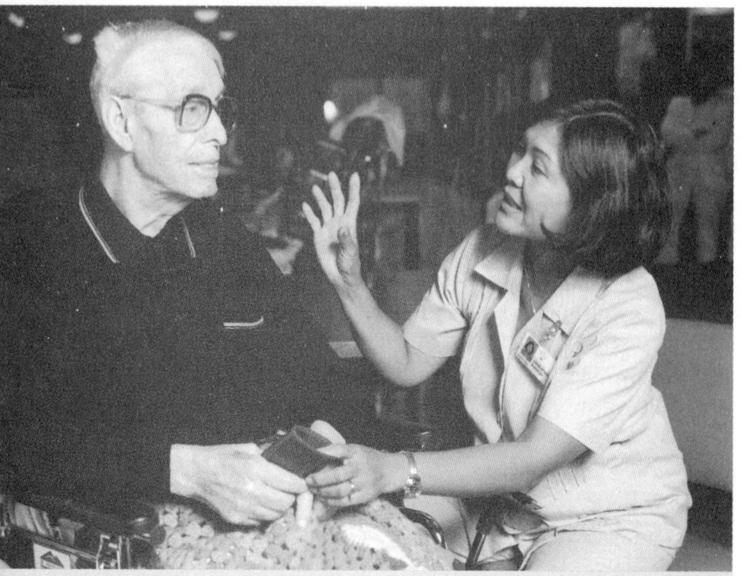

This nurse is speaking with her hands, her face and her eyes.

Rehabilitation centres offer tremendous help for people who are learning to live with a sensory deficit, such as blindness, deafness or paralysis, and also for patients who have lost the ability to speak. The nurse should, if possible, visit one of these centres early in his or her career to become aware of the supports that are available to help individuals with sensory deficits cope with the daily activities of living.

Evaluating Cognitive–Perceptual Interventions

When expected outcomes have been explicitly stated, the nurse is able to evaluate the effectiveness of various interventions or to try alternatives if these have not been successful. It also helps the nurse and the patient to feel a sense of accomplishment when progress towards goal achievement has been made. This aspect of nursing care is important for the nurse as well as for the patient and family.

COMMUNITY health practice: Resources for Alzheimer's Disease

Numerous community agencies have arisen to help people with Alzheimer's disease or sensory deficits and their families to find ways to lead satisfying lives. The Canadian National Institute for the Blind and the Canadian Hard of Hearing Association are both national voluntary agencies with provincial chapters and local branches in most major communities in Canada. Alzheimer's societies have developed provincially and, likewise, are voluntary, nonprofit agencies that have local branches.

The Canadian National Institute for the Blind provides services to individuals across Canada for whom loss of vision is a central problem requiring social adjustment. Core services include:

- counselling and referral to services and resources
- teaching practical skills of daily living (e.g., cooking, banking, personal grooming)
- orientation and mobility training to develop independent travel skills and white-cane techniques
- vision rehabilitation to use remaining sight more effectively
- adaptive technology such as talking watches, Braille playing cards, large-print dictionaries and needle threaders
- career development and employment
- library services—recreational books and magazines in Braille and audiocassette format (in French and English).

The Canadian Hard of Hearing Association is a consumer association of hard of hearing people, dedicated to the assistance of hearing-impaired people across Canada. Programs include:

- education—conferences and workshops
- rehabilitation—managing hearing loss
- information—displays, public speaking
- loan/rental library—videos, books, posters
- advocacy and support.

Alzheimer Canada is a voluntary, nonprofit organization that provides a number of support, information, advocacy and research services. The agency runs information lines through its provincial and local offices. It offers services to people with Alzheimer's disease, their caregivers, health professionals and other concerned individuals. Services include support groups, mainly for caregivers but a few for people with the disease; educational programs; and referrals to other agencies or groups. Alzheimer Canada has a number of publications, including guide books for caring for people with Alzheimer's disease, and lists a number of excellent videotapes in its Video and Kit Title Catalogue, available from its provincial branches.

RESEARCH to practice

Thomas, D.W. (1997). Understanding the wandering patient. A continuity of personality perspective. *Journal of Gerontological Nursing, 23*(1), 16–23.

Much of the literature on wandering patients has focussed primarily on eliminating the contributing factors without considering the reason for the behaviour. Thus, it is not surprising that while many hospitals have adapted their environment to help the wandering patient, some have had positive results, while others have not. The purpose of this study was to explore the relationship between personality and wandering behaviour among patients with dementia.

Subjects for the study were selected from an urban nursing facility and ranged in age from 64 to 94 years. All subjects had a diagnosis of dementia as determined by the Global Deterioration Scale for Assessment of Primary Degenerative Dementia. Subjects were then placed into two groups (wanderers and nonwanderers) following specific criteria developed by the author.

Group A consisted of 20 individuals who wandered. Each wanderer was then matched to a nonwanderer (Group B) based on age, gender and level of dementia. A family member of each of the 40 participants completed the NEO-FFI scale, which measures five personality factors: neuroticism, extroversion, openness, agreeableness and conscientiousness.

The results of the study revealed that wanderers scored significantly higher than nonwanderers on the personality factor of extroversion and agreeableness. In addition, the findings suggested that wanderers have a "continuous active, social-seeking personality where the nonwanderers have a more stand-offish personality" (p. 20).

The author's findings suggest that for individuals who wander, their personality or inherent behaviour may have a greater influence on their wandering then their dementia. With this new information, nurses can critically assess an individual's personality traits to determine whether his or her wandering can be attributed to the disease process or to habits that developed over a lifetime. Perhaps, if nurses viewed wandering as normal behaviour, creative programs could be developed to encourage interaction and thus meet these individuals' needs, rather than current strategies that control or punish.

Owing to the small sample size and the ability for significant others to recall information, the author recommends further study in this area.

IN REVIEW

- Sensory stimulation is:
  - a basic human need
  - necessary for survival.
- Sensory faculties include:
  - sight
  - hearing
  - taste
  - touch
  - smell.
- The sensorium is the appartus for receiving and interpreting sensations. It includes the brain, spinal cord and nervous system.
- Cognition is the act of knowing; it gives meaning to what is perceived.
- Sensory perception:
  - originates in receptors in the five sense organs: eyes, ears, skin, nose and mouth
  - passes information via the nervous system to the brain
  - is modified, refined and interpreted in the light of past experience and data coming in from other sources.
- In addition to the sense organs, the body also has proprioceptive and kinesthetic senses, which enable us to move about smoothly and effectively and to orient ourselves to the environment. Sensory organs for space orientation and balance are believed to be located in the vestibular system in the inner ear.
- Determinants of cognitive–perceptual functioning include:
  - environmental factors (inadequate stimuli leading to sensory deprivation; excessive stimuli leading to sensory overload)
  - biological factors (physiological changes during the life cycle; impairment of any part of the sensorium or accessory systems such as the circulatory and endocrine systems).
- Cognitive development takes place in systematic patterns, reaching its peak at around age 25. It remains dynamic over the adult years and shows improvement (in some abilities) with age.
- Sensory capabilities change from infancy to adulthood:
  - most essential sensory organs are fairly well developed at birth
  - vision matures during the early childhood years
  - all senses are fully developed by the teen years.
- Common problems of cognitive–perceptual functioning include:
  - cognitive (confusion, delirium, Alzheimer's disease and other dementias)
  - sensory (sensory deprivation, sensory overload, sensory deficit).
- Assessment of cognitive–perceptual needs includes:
  - health history
  - examination of the patient for cognitive–perceptual functioning and for manifestation of cognitive impairment, sensory deficits, sensory overload/deprivation
  - tests of cognitive functioning and specific sensory abilities.
- Nursing diagnoses describing cognitive–perceptual problems include:
  - Altered Thought Processes
  - Sensory/Perceptual Alteration
- Cognitive impairment and sensory deficits may be the etiology in other nursing diagnoses in which the focus is on the result of the problem, e.g., Self-Care Deficit/Dressing, due to cognitive impairment.
- Nursing interventions are planned and implemented to meet individual needs. For people with:
  - potential problem of confusion—the goal is prevention
  - actual problem of confusion—goals include: removal of cause, if possible; minimal stimulation; maintenance of stable environment; orientation to reality as far as possible; maintenance of physical health; protection of self and others from harm
  - actual or potential problems of sensory deprivation or overload—goals are directed towards preventing problems and restoring sensory input and perception
  - temporary or permanent sensory deficit—focus is on helping the person to adjust to deficit and to maintain or regain independence. (Collaboration with other health professionals may be required.)

Critical Thinking Activities

1. Mr. Goldman is a 75-year-old retired school principal who had a cerebrovascular accident (stroke) with resultant hemiplegia (left-sided) nine months ago. Following the acute episode, he was admitted to a rehabilitation unit but did not progress as well as expected and was transferred to an extended care facility, where he has been ever since. His mental faculties appear unimpaired and his speech is intact,

but his visual and auditory functioning are decreased. He has some movement in the left leg, but the arm is flaccid. He is helped into a wheelchair daily and can

Mr. Goldman's wife died two years ago; two of his four adult children (a son and a daughter) live in town—the other two sons are at a considerable distance—and both visit frequently, as do their children.

Prior to his disability, Mr. Goldman was active in the local community centre, played golf regularly and liked to travel. However, on the ward, he spends most of his time in his room, staring out the window. He does not go to the TV room and has given up reading newspapers because he says he can see nothing but the headlines. He has his radio on most of the time, but keeps the volume low because other patients were complaining about it. He can never remember if visitors have been in or not.

As his nurse, what can you do to help Mr. Goldman?

2. Visit an agency or rehabilitation centre in your community that offers assistance to people learning to live with sensory deficits such as vision or hearing loss. What types of services do these agencies provide?

3. Miss Ellen Waters is a retired school librarian who lives alone in a one-bedroom apartment in a seniors' complex on a quiet street in Ottawa. Miss Waters is 78 years of age; she is an active volunteer with Meals-on-Wheels, belongs to two book clubs, enjoys long walks in the summer and cross-country skiing in the winter. She likes to take one long trip a year to Europe, the Caribbean or Mexico.

   Miss Waters' eyesight has been deteriorating slowly over the past few years. She had to give up driving two years ago and has now been declared legally blind. She is finding it increasingly difficult to function independently: for example, she has trouble keeping in touch with her friends because she cannot see the numbers on the phone to call them; she can't read the labels on items in the grocery store. She used to love to read, but can no longer do so. Even the images on the television screen are blurred, and she no longer enjoys watching her favourite programs. All this frustrates her. Further, she is becoming increasingly apprehensive about leaving her apartment because she is afraid she may fall or trip over something, which happens frequently at home.

   a. What services are available in your community to help Miss Waters learn to cope with her loss of vision?

   b. What type of health care worker is best suited to help Miss Waters rearrange her apartment to make it easier and safer for her to live there? What kinds of changes can you think of?

   c. What suggestions would you make to help this woman live more independently and make her life more enjoyable (for example, regarding her

   programs, leisure activities)?

KEY TERMS

cognitive functioning p. 873
sensory input p. 873
cognition p. 873
sensorium p. 873
tactile p. 873
olfactory p. 873
gustatory p. 873
perception p. 874
adaptation p. 874
proprioceptors p. 874
kinesthesia p. 874
vestibular system p. 874
aphasia p. 875
hallucination p. 875
receptive aphasia p. 875
expressive aphasia p. 875
confusion p. 877
acute confusional states p. 878
delirium p. 877
dementia p. 877
Alzheimer's disease p. 877
amnesia p. 878
agnosia p. 878
apraxia p. 878
anomia p. 878
sensory deprivation p. 879
sensory overload p. 879
sensory deficit p. 879
illusions p. 880
visual acuity p. 882
visual field p. 882
myopia p. 883
hyperopia p. 883
astigmatism p. 883
presbyopia p. 883
aniseikonia p. 883
keratoconus p. 883
aphakia p. 883
anisometropia p. 883
phonation p. 886

References

AMERICAN SPEECH-LANGUAGE-HEARING ASSOCIATION (ASHA). (1998). Digital technology and hearing aids: The promise and the reality. Healthtouch Online. http://www.healthtouch.com/level/leaflets/aslha/aslha045.htm

BATES, B. (1995). *A guide to physical examination and history taking.* (6th ed.). Philadelphia: Lippincott.

BERNSTEIN, D.A., ROY, E.J., SRULL, T.K., & WICKENS, C.D. (1988). *Psychology.* Boston: Houghton Mifflin.

BURNS, K.R., & JOHNSON, P.J. (1980). *Health assessment in clinical practice* Englewood Cliffs, NJ: Prentice Hall.

CAMERON, C.F. KESSLER, J.C., KRAMER, W., & WARREN, K.E. (1972). When sensory deprivation occurs. *Canadian Nurse, 68*(11), 32–34.

CAPLAN, F., & CAPLAN, T. (1979). *The second twelve months of life.* New York: Grosset & Dunlap.

CARPENITO, L.J. (1997). *Nursing diagnosis: Application to clinical practice.* (7th ed.). Philadelphia: Lippincott.

CHOVAZ, C. (1989). Nursing the hearing impaired patient. *Canadian Nurse, 85*(3), 34–36.

COSMETIC OPTICS. (1998, 28 October). Cosmetic optics: Hydroxyapatite ocular implants raise standards and expectations for the anophthalmic patient. http://www.ioi.com/opt/costmeticopt.html

EBERSOLE, P. & HESS, P. (1998). *Toward healthy aging: Human needs and nursing response.* (5th ed.). St. Louis: Mosby.

EDWARDS, S. (1993). Assessment of the older adult. In A.C. Beckingham & B.W. Du Gas (Eds.), *Promoting healthy aging: A nursing and community perspective* (pp. 185–218). St. Louis: Mosby Year Book.

ELIOPOULOS, C. (1997). *Gerontological nursing.* (4th ed.). Philadelphia: Lippincott.

ERICKSON'S ARTIFICIAL EYES. (1998, 3 March). The prosthetic eye; Caring for your artificial eye; Other kinds of artistic eyes. (Online brochure.) http://www.ericksoneyes.com/brochure/html

GREGORY, R.L. (1997). *Eye and brain: The psychology of seeing.* (5th ed.). Oxford: Oxford University Press.

GRIMES, J., & BURNS, E. (1987). *Health assessment in nursing practice.* (2nd ed.). Boston: Jones & Bartlett.

HALM, M.A., & ALPEN, M.A. (1993). The impact of technology on patients and families. *Nursing Clinics of North America, 28*, 443–457.

KENNER, C.A., & MACLAREN, A. (1993). *Essentials of maternal and neonatal nursing*. Springhouse, PA: Springhouse.

LUDINGTON-HOE, S.M. (1983). What can newborns really see? *American Journal of Nursing, 9*, 1286–1289.

MacKELLAIG, J. (1986). A study of psychological effects of intensive care with particular emphasis on patients in isolation. *Intensive Care Nursing, 2*, 176–185.

MATTESON, M.A., MCCONNELL, E.S., & LINTON, A.D. (1997). *Gerontological nursing: Concepts and practice.* (2nd ed.). Philadelphia: W.B. Saunders.

MOORE, T. (1991). Making sense of... Sensory deprivation. *Nursing Times, 87*(6), 36–38.

MURRAY, R.B., & ZENTNER, J.P. (1997). *Nursing assessment and health promotion: Strategies through the life span.* Norwalk, CT: Appleton & Lange.

NIGHTINGALE, F. (1946). *Notes on nursing: What it is and what it is not.* (rev. ed.). Philadelphia: Lippincott.

PILLITTERI, A. (1995). *Maternal and child health nursing care of the childbearing and childrearing family.* (2nd ed.). Philadelphia: Lippincott.

ROSS, M., & CASEY, A. (1993). Health concerns associated with aging. In A.C. Beckingham & B.W. Du Gas (Eds.), *Promoting healthy aging: A nursing and community perspective.* St. Louis: Mosby Year Book.

STUART, G.W., & LARAIA, M.T. (1998). *Stuart & Sundeen's Principles and practice of psychiatric nursing.* (6th ed.). St. Louis: Mosby.

THOMAS, D.W. (1997). Understanding the wandering patient. A continuity of personality perspective. *Journal of Gerontological Nursing, 23*(1), 16–23.

Additional Readings

BURGENER, S.C., & BARTON, D. (1991). Nursing care of cognitively impaired institutionalized elderly. *Journal of Gerontological Nursing, 17*(4), 37–43.

CANADA NEWSWIRE. (1997, December). Ultravision granted FDA approval to market its soft toric contact lens for astigmatic patients.http://ww2.newswire.ca/releases/December1997/17/c4114.html

CONTACT LENS COUNCIL. (1998). Contact Lens Council answers your general questions about contact lens wear and maintenance. http://www.iglobal.com/CLC.elc-02.htm

CONTACT LENS COUNCIL. (1998). Contact lens wear and care tips: Do's and don'ts. http://www.iglobal.com/CLC.elc-06.htm

CONTACT LENS COUNCIL. (1998). Types of contact lenses. http://www.iglobal.com/CLC.elc-02.htm

CONTACT LENS PRACTICE. (1998). The contact lens practice: Soft lenses for astigmatism. http://www.ctlens.co.uk.astigmat.htm

DAVIDHIZER, R., & GIGER, J.N. (1997). When touch is not the best approach. *Journal of Clinical Nursing, 6*(3), 20–36.

DePAUL, D., & CHAMBERS, S.E. (1995). Environmental noise in the neonatal intensive care unit: Implications for nursing practice. *Journal of Perinatal & Neonatal Nursing, 8*(4), 71–76.

DOOTSON, S. (1990). Sensory imbalance and sleep loss. *Nursing Times, 86*(35), 26–29.

EYE PROSTHETICS OF UTAH, INC. (1998, 27 February). Important information about the wearing and caring of your artificial eye. http://www.citysearchslc.com/EV/SLCUT/0003/88/26/4.html

GERDNER, L. (1997). An individualized music intervention for agitation. *Journal of the American Psychiatric Nurses Association, 3*(6), 177–184.

GILLYON, M., & LAMBERT, T. (1997). Disability: Realm of the senses. *Nursing Times, 93*(9), 32–33.

HAHN, K. (1989). About sensory loss. *Nursing 89*(2), 97–99.

HALFMAN, D., & SCHMEIDLER, E. (1998). Demographics update. Visual impairment among homeless people, prevalence of disability and internet access in school. *Journal of Visual Impairment & Blindness, 92*(1), 90, 92, 94.

HART, B.D., & WELLS, D.L. (1997). The effects of language used by caregivers on agitation in residents with dementia. *Clinical Nurse Specialist, 1*(1), 20–23.

HOROWITZ, A., & REINHARDT, J.P. (1998). Development of the adaptation to age-related vision loss scale. *Journal of Visual Impairment & Blindness, 92*(1), 30–41.

JUPITER, T., & SPIVEY, V. (1997). Perception of hearing loss and hearing handicap on hearing aid use by nursing home residents. *Geriatric Nursing, 18*(5), 201–208, 243.

KEE, C.C. (1990). Sensory impairment: Factor X in providing nursing care to the older adult. *Journal of Community Health Nursing, 7*(1), 45–52.

KELLY, M. (1995). Consequences of visual impairment on leisure activities of the elderly. *Geriatric Nursing, 16*(6), 27–35.

LAMMON, C., FOOTE, A., LELI, P., INGLE, J., & ADAMS, M. (1995). *Clinical nursing skills.* Philadelphia: W.B. Saunders.

LEAHY, J., & KIZILAY, P. (1998). *Foundations of nursing practice: A nursing process approach.* Philadelphia: W.B. Saunders.

LETVAK, S. (1997). Relational experiences of elderly women living alone in rural communities: A phenomenologic inquiry. *Journal of the New York State Nurses Association, 28*(2), 20–25.

LEVINE, M.W., & SHEFNER, J.M. (1991). *Fundamentals of sensation and perception.* (2nd ed.). Pacific Grove, CA: Brooks/Cole.

McCONNELL, E. (1996). Handling your patient's hearing aid: Learn how to manage and clean this in-the-ear device so your patient can hear. *Nursing, 26*(7), 22.

MORGAN, D.G., & STEWART, N.J. (1997). The importance of the social environment in dementia care. *Western Journal of Nursing Research, 19*(6), 740–761.

NEY, D.F. (1993). Cerumen impaction, ear hygiene practices, and hearing acuity. *Geriatric Nursing, 14*(2), 70–73.

OLSEN, D.P. (1997). Development of an instrument to measure the cognitive structure used to understand personhood in patients. *Nursing Research, 46*(2), 78–84.

ROUTASALO, P., & ISOLA, A. (1996). The right to touch and be touched. *Nursing Ethics, 3*(2), 165–176.

SACK, S.Z., & WOLFFE, K.E. (1998). Lifestyles of adolescents with visual impairments: An ethnographic analysis. *Journal of Visual Impairment & Blindness, 92*(1), 7–17.

SCHIFFMAN, H.R. (1990). *Sensation and perception: An integrated approach.* (3rd ed.). New York: Wiley.

SHAW, L. (1997). Protocol for detection and follow-up of hearing loss. *Clinical Nurse Specialist, 11*(6), 240–247.

WILSON, L.D. (1993). Sensory perceptual alteration: Diagnosis, prediction, and intervention in the hospitalized adult. *Nursing Clinics of North America, 28*, 747.

Chapter 2

Movement and Exercise Needs

OUTLINE

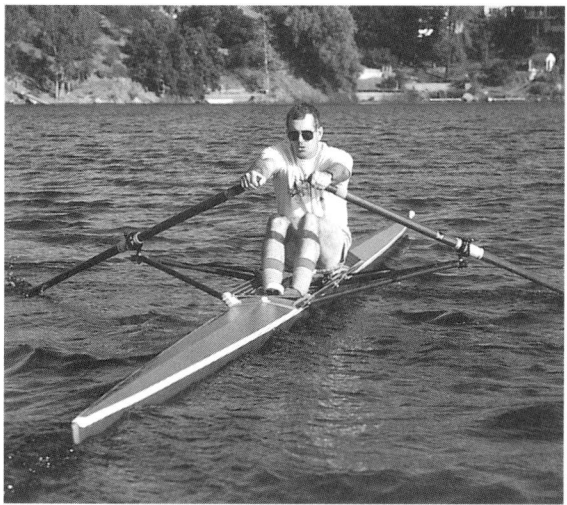

Central Questions

1. How are movement and exercise important to health and well-being?
2. What are the major functions of bones, muscles, joints, nerves and their blood supply in body movement?
3. How does the capacity for coordinated movement and exercise vary throughout the life cycle?
4. What are the main determinants of movement and exercise?
5. What are some common mobility problems?
6. What basic principles does the nurse apply in assisting patients to meet movement and exercise needs?
7. How does the nurse assess movement and exercise needs?
8. What are the common nursing diagnostic statements for patients with movement and exercise problems?
9. How does the nurse develop a plan of care for patients with movement and exercise problems?
10. What strategies does the nurse implement in helping individuals, families or groups promote optimum physical fitness and prevent potential mobility problems?
11. What health-restoring and supportive strategies does the nurse implement in the care of patients with mobility problems?
12. How does the nurse evaluate the patient's response to nursing interventions?

Introduction

Most people take for granted the ability to move around freely. We rely on free movement to carry out activities of daily living (ADL), such as getting out of bed, washing, dressing and eating. We also rely on movement for work, for play, for defending ourselves from danger and for communicating with others. We give little thought to how our skeletal system functions, or how our muscles and joints work, until illness or trauma impairs our capacity to move. Indeed, movement is such a vital part of our lives that we consider permanent loss of the ability to move any part of our body to be one of the major tragedies that can occur.

A loss of mobility lessens self-concept and affects body image. Independence is threatened and, if the immobility affects one or more of the principal locomotor parts of the body, the threat may assume major proportions. Opportunities for communication are also jeopardized if mobility is impaired, and sensory deprivation becomes a real possibility. Communication depends on motor abilities for speaking, writing and using nonverbal "body language" to send messages to other people.

Just as movement is necessary for fulfilling basic human needs, exercise is essential for promoting physical and psychological health. People who exercise regularly not only have higher energy levels; they look better and feel better about themselves. There is growing evidence that exercise, in conjunction with other healthy behaviours, offers some protection against health problems and chronic diseases (Williams, 1993).

When people are ill or become immobilized, the muscles and the nerves that regulate movement become inactive. Disuse of the neuromuscular system quickly leads to degeneration and subsequent loss of functioning. If muscles are immobilized, the process of degeneration begins almost immediately. The restoration of muscle strength and tone, on the other hand, is a very slow process that may take months or years to accomplish. With this in mind, prevention is the better part of care. Nurses caring for patients whose movement is restricted have a responsibility to prevent the degeneration of unused muscles and the development of complications that might limit mobility or prolong the recovery and restoration to health.

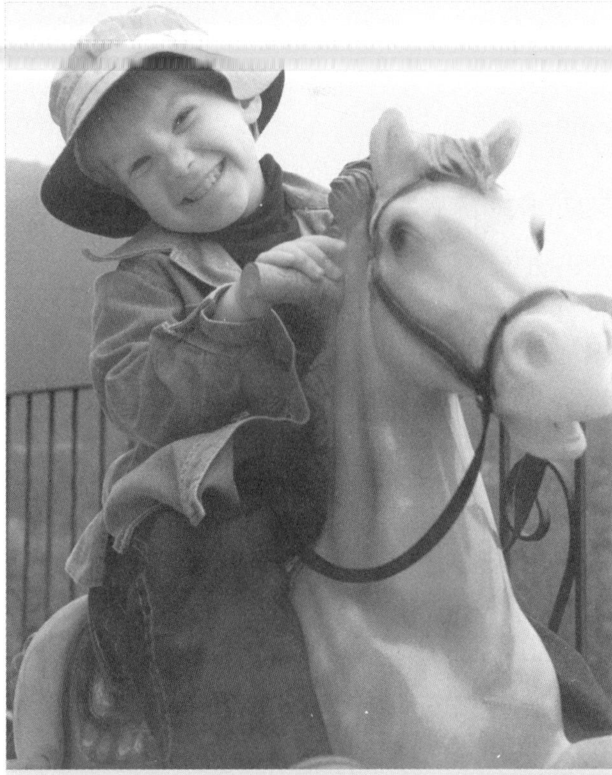

Children will find many ways to exercise.

Physiology Related to Movement

The principal systems involved in body movements are the skeletal system, the muscular system and the nervous system. The circulatory system is also involved in that it provides nourishment to the tissues of these other systems. If circulation to any part of the body is impaired, degeneration of the tissues in the area begins, since body cells cannot live without adequate nourishment. However, it is the bones, the nerves and the muscles, working together, that make movement possible.

Integration of the Bones, Muscles and Nerves in Movement

The bones of the skeletal system have two functions in movement: they provide an attachment for muscles and ligaments, and they act as levers. The *origin* of a muscle is its proximal end; the *insertion* of a muscle is its distal end.

The muscles contract to produce motion. Muscles that are used for movement are always in pairs, one on either side of a bone or joint, and have opposing functions; as one contracts, the other extends (stretches) to cause the bone to move in a certain direction. This action is similar to that involved in the manipulation of a puppet by strings; you shorten one string and lengthen another to make the puppet move in the direction you want it to go.

Muscles tend to work in groups rather than in single pairs. Breathing, for example, requires the coordinated activity of a number of muscles, including the intercostals, the diaphragm, the sternocleidomastoid muscles, the scalenes, the thoracohumeral and the thoracoscapular muscles. Extending the thigh involves the gluteal muscles, hamstrings and lumbar extensor muscles.

The spinal nerves are directly involved in trunk and limb movements. Each spinal nerve has an anterior and a posterior root in the spinal column. The anterior root conducts impulses to the muscles from the central nervous sys- [illegible] peripheral sensory receptors to the central nervous system.

Balance and the progression, coordination and purposefulness of movement require the participation of progressively higher levels of brain function. Motor areas located in the frontal lobes of the cerebral cortex control the voluntary movements of all muscles of the body (Porth, 1998).

Types of Joints

The various types of body movements are made possible by the *joints*, which connect one bone to another. Each movable joint is constructed to make possible a certain type of movement and each has a circumscribed range of motion. These joint movements are defined in Table 29.1 and illustrated in Figure 29.1.

[illegible] such as those connecting the bones in the skull, but the major purpose of joints is to serve as fulcrums to enable the body to move. The body has six types of movable joints (see Table 29.2).

Body Planes and Anatomic Position

Body movements are often described in relation to planes. When the body is in a standing position, as shown in Figure 29.2, the *sagittal plane* divides it into right- and left-side portions; the *frontal plane* into front and back portions; and the *transverse plane* into upper and lower portions.

TABLE 29.1 Types of body movement

Type of Movement	*Explanation*
Abduction	Movement away from the central axis (midline) of the body
Adduction	Movement towards the central axis (midline) of the body
Flexion	The act of bending; the angle between the two moving parts is decreased
Extension	The act of straightening; the angle between the two moving parts is increased
Hyperextension	Extension beyond the normal range of motion, for example, bending the head back towards the spine
Gliding	Movement in one plane, as in sliding
Rotation	Turning in a circular motion around a long axis
Circumduction	Circular motion of a limb or part when the limb or part forms part of a cone, as in swinging the arm in a circular motion. It is a combination of abduction, adduction, flexion and extension
Pronation	A medial rotation of hand or foot down or backwards
Supination	A lateral rotation of hand or foot upward or forward
Inversion	Turning inward towards the midline (foot only)
Eversion	Turning outward away from the midline (foot only)

TABLE 29.2 The six types of movable joints

Type of Joint	*Explanation*
Hinge	This is a uniaxial joint that permits flexion and extension. Examples of a hinge joint include the knee and elbow
Pivot	This is also a uniaxial joint. It permits rotation. An example is the atlantoaxial joint (between the first cervical vertebra and the base of the skull)
Condyloid	This is a biaxial joint. It permits flexion, extension, abduction and adduction. The wrist is a condyloid joint
Saddle	This is another biaxial joint. It permits flexion, extension, abduction, adduction and circumduction. An example is the thumb
Ball and socket	This type of joint is polyaxial. Movements permitted include flexion, extension, abduction, adduction, circumduction, and rotation. The hip joint is a ball and socket joint
Gliding	This is a plane joint and permits gliding movements. Examples include the acromioclavicular joint of the shoulder, wrist and ankle

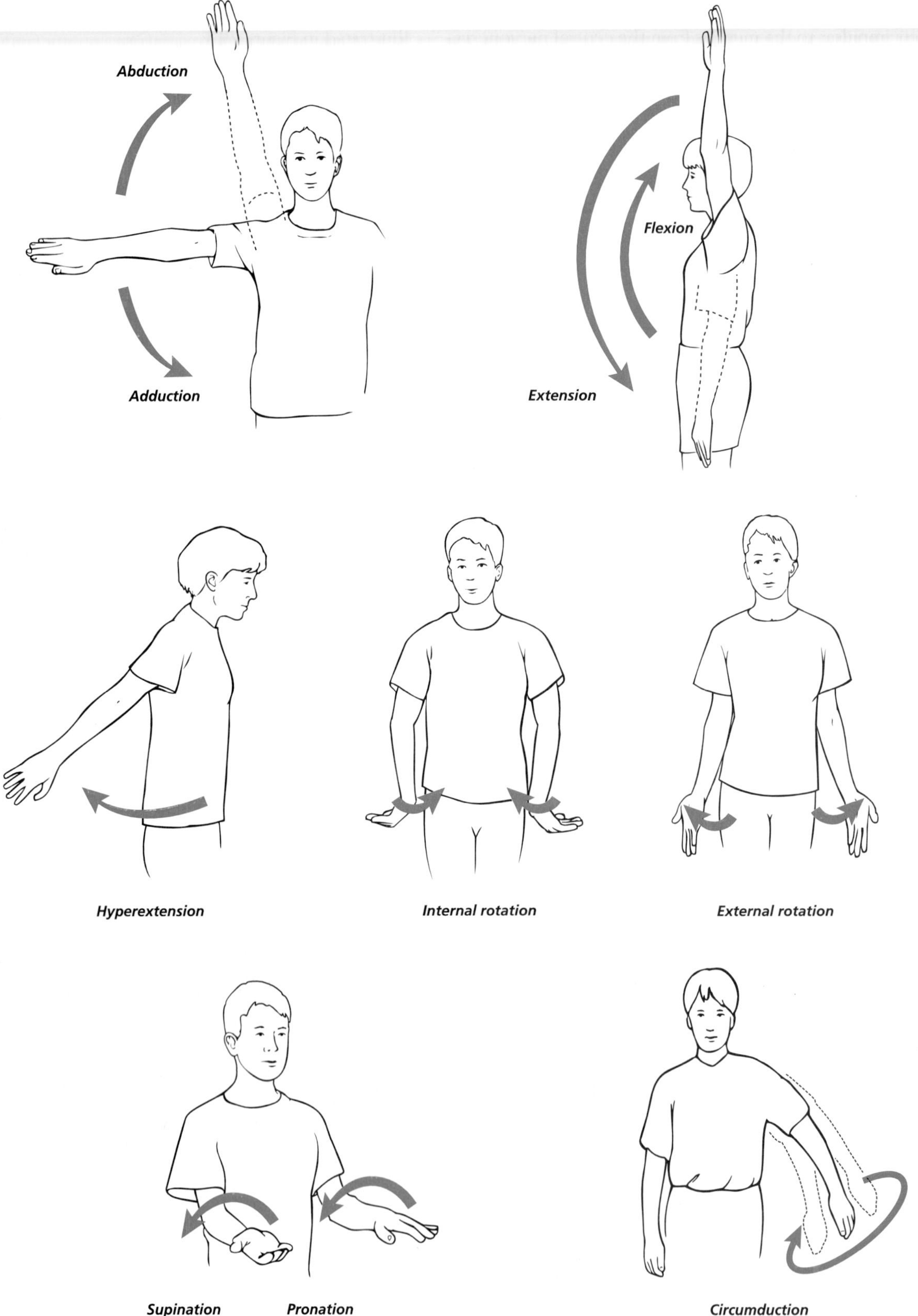

FIGURE 29.1 Types of joint movements

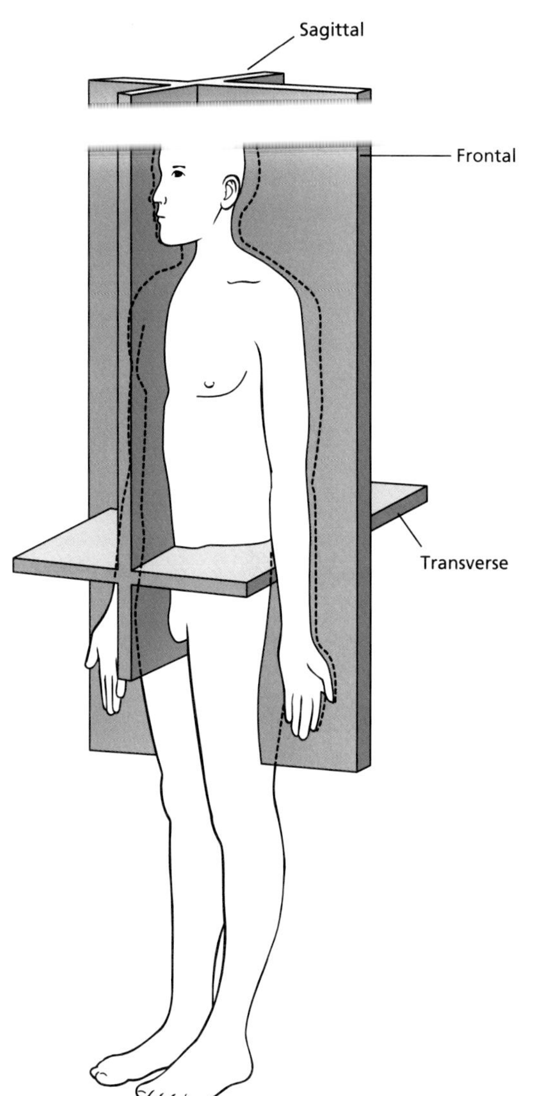

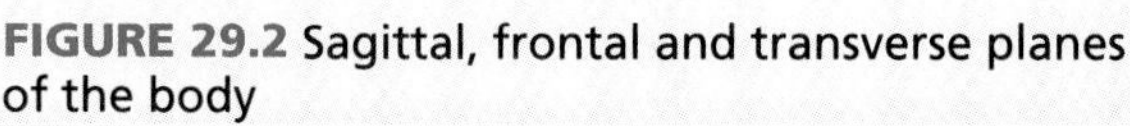
FIGURE 29.2 Sagittal, frontal and transverse planes of the body

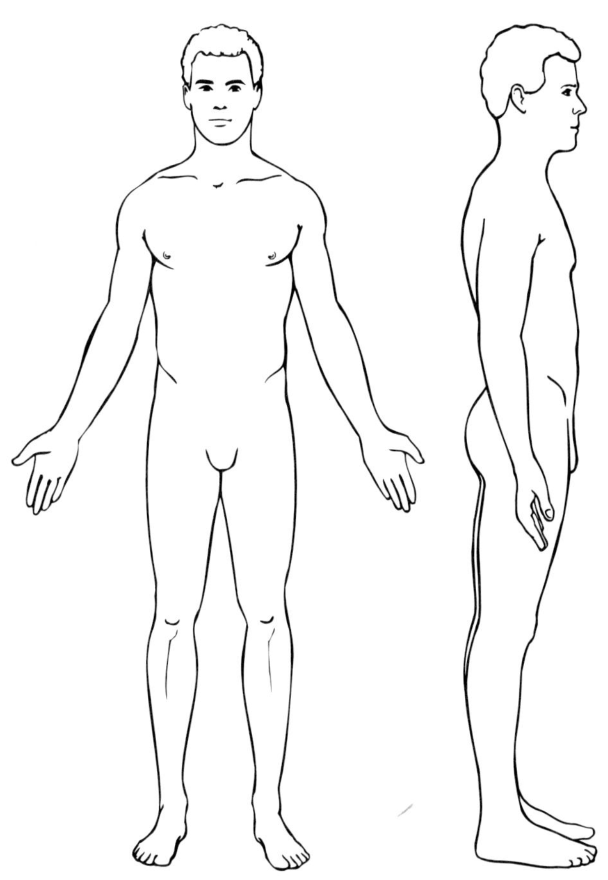

FIGURE 29.3 Normal anatomic position and line of gravity

Anatomic position refers to the **body alignment** or relationship of body parts to the midline of the body. In anatomic position (see Figure 29.3), the body is erect; the head, pelvis, legs and feet are balanced and their weight is evenly distributed. The arms hang down at the sides with the palms facing forward. The feet are slightly apart and pointed forward; the elbows and fingers are slightly flexed.

Movement of the body is much easier when the body parts are well aligned, when the weight of the body is evenly balanced, and when the feet are set a little farther apart (about 30 cm) than in the anatomic position. Setting the feet this far apart provides the body with a wider foundation or **base of support** for its weight than the normal standing posture does.

The **centre of gravity** (also called centre of mass or centre of weight) of the body is located in the pelvis at approximately the level of the second sacral vertebra. The **line of gravity** is an imaginary straight line that passes through its centre of gravity to form a right angle with the ground.

When the body is in anatomic position, the line of gravity falls in the frontal plane downward behind the ear, through the centre of gravity in the pelvis, and slightly in front of the knee and ankle joints, to the middle of the body's base of support, so that the line is perpendicular to the ground, as shown in Figure 29.3. The body is more stable in this position because its line of gravity is in direct line with the gravitational pull of the earth.

The Role of Exercise in Health and Wellness

Exercise increases the efficiency of all body processes. The physiological, psychological and social benefits of exercise have received increasing attention in recent years. The predominantly sedentary way of life of so many North Americans has been a major factor contributing to many illnesses, such as heart disease, stroke, hypertension, diabetes and obesity.

Many studies have been undertaken in the United States, Canada and other countries to determine the exact physiological changes that result from a regular exercise program. Some of the changes indicated by these studies include:

- increased muscle strength, tone and size
- increased efficiency of the heart
- increased pulmonary efficiency
- improved digestion
- increased work tolerance
- better mental alertness
- improved sleep patterns
- increased hemoglobin levels in the blood
- decreased blood pressure
- decreased deposits of fatty tissue
- decreased cholesterol levels in the blood
- increased speed of soft tissue healing
- maintenance of bone density (Greenberg & Dintiman, 1992).

Numerous research studies have also demonstrated that proper exercise can help to slow the aging process. For example, regular exercise has been shown to maintain cardiovascular functioning and pulmonary reserve, glucose tolerance, bone density, physical strength and endurance. It has also been shown to reduce serum lipids, cholesterol and systolic blood pressure (Williams, 1993).

Movement and Exercise Throughout the Life Cycle

Our capacity for movement and exercise is influenced by our age and our current phase of the life cycle. The development of coordinated movement begins in infancy and continues throughout childhood and adolescence. Strength, endurance and motor coordination reach maximum potential in late adolescence and early adulthood, and then gradually decline through middle and late adulthood.

Pregnancy

During late pregnancy, there is a general relaxation of all body ligaments, particularly those involving the pelvic bones and the back. A woman's centre of gravity is moved forward by the enlarging uterus, tending to upset her balance. She usually feels awkward in her movements, being hindered by her increasing bulk as well as her protruding abdomen. A woman needs exercise throughout pregnancy to keep herself in overall good physical condition. Specifically, being in good physical condition aids circulation, strengthens the muscles used in delivery of the baby, and makes it easier to learn relaxation techniques. The relaxation techniques help to make labour and delivery easier. Learning to relax specific muscles used in delivery is essential to ease labour and delivery further.

After delivery, exercises are needed to strengthen the abdominal muscles and the muscles of the pelvic floor, which have been stretched during labour and delivery. Most prenatal programs teach both pre- and postnatal exercises, as well as relaxation techniques.

Expectant parents are usually excited when the mother first feels the baby kick in her womb. This event is called *quickening* and usually occurs during the fourth or fifth month of gestation. The infant continues to move until just before birth, when the head becomes engaged in the birth canal.

Infancy

The newborn's movements are mainly random. Babies have poor motor control at first, because most of their movements are reflex actions. Some infants are much more active than others and some acquire motor skills at an earlier age than others do. It can be very traumatic to a new parent when a one-year-old child is still not walking while the neighbour's child has been running around since nine months of age. It helps if the nurse can reassure parents that their child is just as normal as the neighbour's. A chart of development for the first year of life identifies the *average* age in months when specific achievements are attained by 95 percent of normal infants. The chart is helpful in reassuring parents and is also useful in identifying children who are not developing at a normal rate.

During the first year of life, the major accomplishments in motor skills are learning to walk and learning to use the hands as tools (prehensile skill). These skills depend on physical maturation, although it is generally believed that a stimulating environment can accelerate motor development. A musical mobile, or brightly coloured objects suspended above the crib within the infant's reach, can stimulate a child's interest for movement, grasping and hand–eye coordination.

During infancy, the bones are soft and pliant and the pelvis is usually tilted forward. The back is rounded when the baby is sitting. Because the head is large in comparison with the body, balance is difficult. This is why babies often fall over when first learning to sit and totter in first attempts at walking.

Childhood

During childhood, the extremities grow faster than the trunk of the body; the pelvis straightens and a pronounced spinal curvature develops. The toddler usually "toes out," and the older preschooler may "toe in," when walking. Children delight in activities that use their large muscles, such as running, hopping or jumping. By the time children are six years of age, they have usually acquired rudimentary motor skills that enable them to get about on skates, to ride a two-wheel bicycle and to swim. By the time they are 11, children have gained control of their motor skills to the extent that they appear graceful and coordinated in their movements. The development of fine motor skills usually lags behind that of gross motor skills. Girls as a general rule develop dexterity with their fingers and hands much earlier than boys. Hence, girls' writing is generally better in school, and their drawings are usually neater.

Adolescence

Adolescence is characterized by a rapid growth spurt, and for a while, adolescents look as if they are all arms and legs. Hands and feet grow rapidly in length, pelvic and shoulder diameters increase and head circumference gets larger. Adolescents also attain an adult posture. With all of this growth going on, adolescents often look and feel awkward as they adjust to their new body size. The adolescent usually has a lot of excess energy, which needs to be channelled constructively. This is the time for outdoor sports and active physical exercise. It is during the late teens that strength, endurance and coordination reach their maximum potential.

Adulthood

The maximum potential for movement continues through early adulthood and begins to decline as people approach the middle years. Muscle strength peaks at the age of 30 and begins to decline after that (Timaris, 1988). If the individual continues to put excessive demands on the musculoskeletal system to reach the same levels as before, injury and inflammatory conditions are likely to occur.

During the middle years, bone density and mass progressively decrease. Accidents that previously would have caused only minor injuries may now result in fractures. As people get older, they gradually lose height because dehydration of vertebral discs. The regenerative capacity of articular cartilage is also diminished, and the cumulative effect of injuries to the joints may lead to arthritis. The frequency of joint disease increases with age. Most people do not participate in active sports to the same extent they did in their youth, and this more sedentary lifestyle often leads to "middle-age spread." Functional aerobic capacity also diminishes with age because heart and lung function are not as efficient. Regular exercise is important for several reasons:

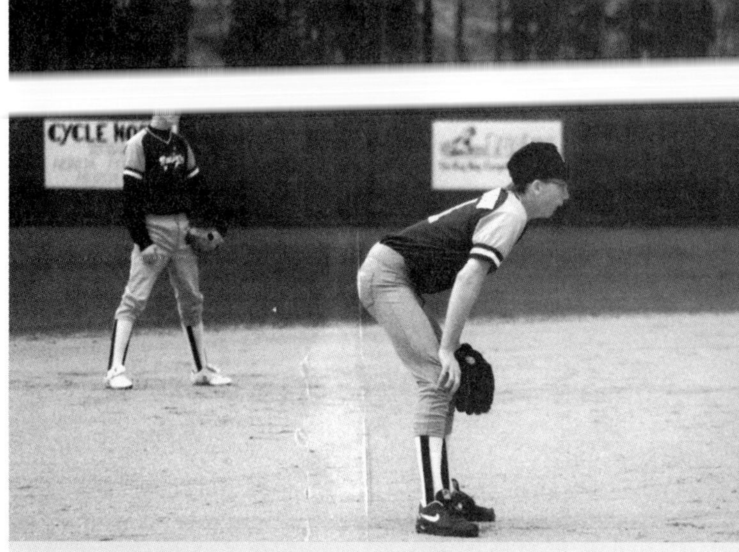

Adolescents enjoy outdoor sports and active physical exercise.

- it improves functional aerobic capacity
- it reduces the risk factors that can lead to coronary artery disease (such as being overweight and developing cholesterol accumulation in the blood stream)
- it maintains joint flexibility and produces a general sense of well-being.

People over the age of 65 are usually about two-and-a-half centimetres shorter than they were in their youth. This is because of the thinning of the intervertebral discs. There is also a loss of cartilage in the large joints and a proliferation of adjacent bone. Women in particular are vulnerable to osteoporosis. The reflexes that minimize sway in the erect posture become sluggish and blunted. There is gradual, progressive loss of muscle bulk and strength. Often, there is limited range of motion in the neck. The changes taking place in the musculoskeletal system and in the nervous system combine to make walking and other coordinated movements more difficult. Exercises that promote joint flexibility and improve circulation are particularly important for the older person.

Determinants of Movement and Exercise

A multitude of factors may affect movement and exercise. Many of these are related to alterations in health status. Others are the result of heredity, immobility and environmental and lifestyle factors.

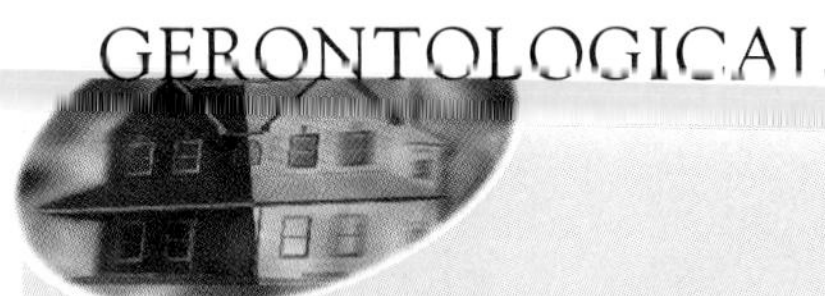

GERONTOLOGICAL

Age-Related Musculoskeletal Changes, Outcomes and Health Prevention, Promotion and Maintenance Approaches

AGE-RELATED CHANGES	OUTCOMES	HEALTH PREVENTION, PROMOTION AND MAINTENANCE
Bones become more porous (osteoporosis)	Dowager's hump (kyphosis)	Have good lighting, dry floors, nonskid rugs
Demineralization of vertebral trabecular bone	Risk of hip fracture	Diet high in calcium
Intervertebral discs dehydrate and narrow	Tremors	Calcium supplements as necessary
Reduced height	Back pain	Do moderate exercise: walking or swimming
Erosion of cartilage through exposure and wearing	Joint swelling	Use assistive devices: cane, walker, if needed
Subchondrial bone becomes hyperemic and fibrotic	Ankylosis	Do range-of-motion activity
Synovial membranes become fibrotic	Crepitation	Seek medical evaluation of back pain
Synovial fluid thickens	Decreased range of motion	Wear shoes with low heels, nonskid soles and good support
Muscle wasting of hand dorsum	Stiffness	Use leg rather than back muscles when lifting
Diminished protein synthesis in muscle cells	Muscle wasting	Rest joints when pain occurs
Glucose mobilizes slowly in response to exercise	Reduced muscle strength	Lose weight when necessary
Diminished muscle mass decreases glucose stores	Night leg cramps	Develop an appropriate exercise program
Bone and muscle weakness changes the centre of gravity	Gait problems	Pace activities
	Smaller steps	Allow for rest periods
	Wider stance base	Break big jobs into small parts
	Poor posture	Adjust activities to high-energy periods of day
		Remove scatter rugs
		Use nonskid rubber mats in tub and shower
		Take stretch breaks
		Eat more potassium- and calcium-rich foods
		Coordinate and balance exercise

SOURCE: Ebersole & Hess, 1998, p. 201.

Alterations in Health Status

The ability of the body to move its various parts and to control these movements and perform them in a coordinated fashion depends on the integrity of the muscles, bones, joints and the nerves innervating these structures, as well as the circulation nourishing them. Injury, disease or congenital problems affecting the bones, muscles, joints or their collateral nerve or blood supply may cause impairment of motor functioning.

Even a minor injury, such as a sprained ankle (which damages muscles and ligaments), will limit the ability to walk until the muscle fibres and ligaments have healed. A bone fracture limits the ability to move the part of the body in which the fracture is located. People injured in car accidents, severe falls or other types of accidents may sustain injury to the spinal cord. Because the spinal cord is essential in the transmission of nerve impulses to and from the area in the brain controlling motor function, all movements below the site of the injury may be cut off. The person may be paralyzed from the waist down (*paraplegic*), if the injury is located at that level, or from the neck down (*quadriplegic*), if the injury is in the cervical region.

A *stroke* is the result of a cerebrovascular accident. This problem frequently impairs the blood supply to motor areas in the frontal lobe of one hemisphere of the brain, with resultant loss of motor functioning on one side of the body (*hemiplegia*). The motor abilities needed for speech may also be impaired if the accident occurs in the speech centre of the brain.

Serious illness of any kind lessens an individual's muscular strength and tone. Ill people may be completely dependent and unable to lift appendages or move around in bed. They may require assistance to do some of these activities. Prolonged inactivity of muscles leads to **contractures**—the abnormal flexion and fixation of joints caused by the shortening and atrophy of muscles fibres. Contractures at the wrist or ankle, for example, will cause limitations in mobility. These contractures frequently result from a hand or foot not being supported in good anatomical position and not being exercised when the patient is immobilized. Correcting contractures requires intensive therapy over a prolonged period of time.

Movement is usually limited in surgical patients because of pain in the operative area. Restrictions are placed [illegible] Limitations may be placed on mobility for therapeutic reasons, even if patients are not confined to bed, for example, in the case of a sprained ankle.

Mobility may also be restricted because of nonmotor-related disabilities that limit the ability to get around without help, for example, vision or hearing loss.

Heredity

Congenital abnormalities are often the cause of hospitalization in infants and small children. Many children whom a nurse will encounter on a pediatric unit are there for correction of congenital malformations that interfere with the ability to walk, for example, club foot or congenital hip dislocation.

Immobility

The dangers of immobility have been well documented in numerous studies, books and articles in both nursing and medical literature over the past 30 or 40 years. Some of the adverse effects of lengthy bed rest include:

- slowing down of the basal metabolic rate
- decrease in muscle strength, tone and size
- postural changes
- constipation
- increased vulnerability to pulmonary and urinary tract infections
- circulatory problems, such as thrombosis (the development of a clot in the blood stream) and embolus (the detachment of a clot that travels through the blood stream until it becomes lodged in a vessel too small for it to pass through)
- decrease in bone density
- decrease in cardiovascular fitness
- decrease in speed of soft tissue healing
- decrease in skin integrity
- increase in risk of skin breakdown.

When the body is in a horizontal position, an extra amount of blood is sent from the legs into the general circulation. When this happens, the pulse rate increases as the heart works harder in an attempt to cope with this extra blood. There is increased excretion of calcium, nitrogen and phosphorus, and the patient may suffer severe depletion of these elements. Patients who are subjected to lengthy bed rest usually develop feelings of anxiety and, frequently, hostility as a result of disturbed functioning of physical and mental activity. Sleep patterns can also be disrupted (Olsen & Johnson, 1990).

Environment

The environment may significantly restrict mobility. People [illegible] nities to move about and may also have physical mobility problems. Mobility is restricted in patients who are isolated because of communicable disease precautions since they cannot leave the immediate surroundings. The movement of some patients may be curtailed by the use of restraints.

Air quality may greatly affect outdoor activity such as walking, jogging or participating in sports. Air pollution can interfere with respiratory function. Weather is another part of the environment that needs to be considered in relation to mobility. Air temperature can be too cold or too hot for many activities, and rain or snow can be a deterrent.

Lifestyle

The growth of technology has contributed to sedentary lifestyles for many people in developed countries. Jobs are often less physically demanding. Computers and electronic information transfer systems (e-mail and fax) have reduced the mobility required for many jobs, while electronic lifts and mechanical devices have eliminated the physical challenge of many others. Highly developed transportation systems and the extensive use of automobiles, coupled with more conveniently placed public services and commercial enterprises, also contribute to reduced physical activity, creating a more sedentary lifestyle. For example, mail is delivered to the door, the bus stop is located nearby, the corner mall contains most of the goods and services necessary for living and, in the extreme, nearly all the essentials of life can be obtained without even leaving the home. In this technological age, individuals must plan for and include physical activity in their daily lives in order to keep fit and healthy.

Overeating, drinking alcohol and smoking are all lifestyle factors that affect the ability to exercise. Financial concerns may also come into play, as some individuals cannot afford to participate in activities that are costly, such as skiing or belonging to a fitness centre.

Common Problems

The ability to make parts of the body move and to control these movements enables us to develop the motor skills (a series of coordinated movements) needed for the functions of daily living. It also permits the development of more highly refined motor skills, such as playing the piano, playing tennis or dancing. Common problems with movement include impaired motor function, limited range of motion, decreased muscle strength, lack of balance and coordination and pain and discomfort.

IMPAIRED MOTOR FUNCTION People whose motor abilities are impaired because of illness or injury often need help to perform the activities of daily living (ADL). Among the common problems for which the nurse's help may be needed is the inability or limited ability to raise the head, grasp objects, move around in bed, turn from side to side, raise the buttocks (necessary for use of the bedpan), sit up, stand, transfer or walk. Such limitations make it difficult to be independent with respect to dressing, grooming, toiletting, bathing, hygiene and feeding. Difficulties in performing these activities of daily living are called self-care deficits (Carpenito, 1997).

LIMITED RANGE OF MOTION (ROM) In expressing how much ROM a person has in all joints, the terms *full*, *partial* and *limited* ROM can be used. Impairment in either the upper or lower extremities or weakness on one side of the body may give patients partial ROM in an affected joint. The patient may need assistance with only some aspects of ADL, such as putting on socks and shoes or fastening snaps or buttons. The patient may have very limited ROM, causing even more difficulty in maintaining ADL without assistance.

DECREASED MUSCLE STRENGTH Immobility associated with illness leads to decreased muscle tone and strength. A common example is the patient who has had a stroke. Patients are usually affected on one side of the body, and are left with weakness or no movement at all. As a result, they are unable to perform the activities of daily living by themselves. Gross motor control may be compromised, denying independence in walking, standing or even sitting in a chair without using assistive devices. A lack of fine motor control may interfere with activities such as handling utensils for eating, combing hair, doing up buttons or holding a pencil.

LACK OF BALANCE AND COORDINATION Falls are common problems that have to do with movement or exercise. They may be due to the type of activity or to a physical impairment, such as one-sided weakness associated with a stroke or abnormal gait related to ataxia (compromised muscle coordination). Neurological disorders will also impair muscle coordination, causing instability when ambulating or when transferring from one place to another (for example, moving from a bed to a chair). All age groups are at some risk of falling, depending upon the developmental stage and the activities in which people participate. Toddlers are prone to falling because they are learning to walk and have unsteady gaits due to balance reactions and undeveloped coordination. Older adults may be at higher risk than other age groups because of slower response time, degenerative disease or disorientation.

PAIN AND DISCOMFORT The ability to move freely may be compromised by pain that occurs with movement. This pain can be related to traumatic injury such as sprains, strains or fractures, or to degenerative disease such as arthritis or osteoporosis. Postsurgical patients may be reluctant to move because of incisional pain.

Assessing Movement and Exercise Needs

In assessing the need for movement and exercise, the nurse uses data from a variety of sources, namely the patient's health history, physical examination and chart, as well as other health team members. The family is a primary source of information when a patient is unable to communicate. The nurse will find the patient's chart a particularly useful source. It contains the medical examination and physician's diagnostic and therapeutic plan for care, along with reports from the physiotherapist, occupational therapist and other allied health team members. Radiology reports and results from laboratory and other diagnostic tests will also be found in the chart. The Kardex is another valuable source: it contains current information about the patient's functional abilities, level of activity, aids to ambulation, ability to transfer and exercise programs.

Nursing Health History

The nursing history provides subjective data about how a patient meets the need for movement and exercise in daily living. This includes information about the patient's usual level of activity and exercise, ease of movement and motor function. Recent changes in mobility, any related health problems and current difficulties with ambulation or activities of daily living are explored. In patients with self-care deficits, the nature of assistance they will need is also determined. The patient's lifestyle, current physical fitness patterns and attitudes and knowledge about the benefits of exercise in health promotion are examined to help identify opportunities for health teaching.

Physical Assessment

Physical assessment is performed to gather objective data about a patient's mobility status. The examination is primarily carried out through the use of inspection and palpation techniques.

GENERAL OBSERVATION By observing the patient as a whole, the nurse can get a sense of the uniformity of the skeletal system, muscle structure, symmetry and posture. Body alignment can be assessed when the patient is standing, sitting and lying. Balance, coordination, weakness, lethargy and fatigue can also be assessed and validated through interviewing. The nurse can then move to more specific areas of the body. It is logical to start at the head and work down systematically to the feet when collecting data. Since there may be great differences in strength, flexibility and ROM in the upper and lower extremities, these areas should be assessed separately.

MUSCLES Muscles are assessed for symmetry, size, tone and strength. Assessment of the strength and equality of the upper extremities can be done using hand grips. The

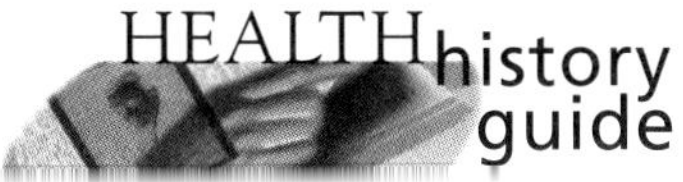

Movement and Exercise

Health and Illness Patterns

USUAL PATTERN OF MOVEMENT AND EXERCISE

- What are the activities you carry out in a typical day (activities of daily living, work-related, home management, cooking, cleaning, gardening, recreation, leisure and social)?
- Do you usually get around by car? By bus? On foot?
- Do you exercise regularly? If so, what type of exercise do you do? How often? For how long?
- Do you use any assistive devices such as a cane, walker or brace?
- What kind of assistance would you require in hospital for ambulating and performing activities of daily living?

RECENT CHANGES IN PATTERN OF MOVEMENT AND EXERCISE

- Have any of your usual activities become difficult or impossible for you? Do you have any problems caring for yourself? Working? Getting around? Exercising? Describe any changes.
- How long have you been experiencing these changes?
- Do you know the cause of these changes? Are the changes due to lifestyle? Environmental factors? Financial resources?
- Have you had a recent illness or health problem that has affected your ability to perform the activities of daily living and to exercise (for example, activity intolerance following a heart attack)?
- Are you taking any medications or treatments that may affect your daily motor activities and exercise?
- Do you think you would be helped by an assistive device such as a cane, walker or brace?

PRESENTING HEALTH PROBLEM

- Describe the symptoms you are experiencing now. Is there any pain? Muscle weakness? Joint stiffness? Swelling?
- Can you point to the area where you feel pain?
- How would you describe the pain? Is it an aching, a burning, a stabbing or a throbbing pain?
- When you have this pain, do you also have pain in another location?
- When did this pain begin? What were you doing at the time?
- What activities seem to decrease or increase the pain?
- Do you have any other unusual sensations, such as tingling, with the pain?
- Describe your weakness. When did you first notice muscle weakness? Did it begin in the same muscles where you notice it now?
- When did you first notice swelling? Did you injure this area?
- When did the stiffness begin? Has the stiffness increased or has it been constant?
- Do you ever hear a grating sound?
- Do weather changes seem to affect the problem? For example, does the pain increase in cold or damp weather?
- What methods have you tried to reduce the stiffness?
- Are you taking any prescription or over-the-counter drugs or using home remedies to treat the problem? If so, which ones, and at what strengths and for how long have you been using them?
- Have you ever had any injury to a bone, muscle, ligament, cartilage, joint or tendon?
- Have you ever had surgery or other treatment involving a bone, muscle, ligament, cartilage, joint or tendon?

HEALTH-PROMOTION AND -PROTECTION PATTERNS

- What are your beliefs about exercise and physical fitness?
- Are you aware of the benefits of a regular fitness program to health and the prevention of illness? If not, would you like to learn about physical fitness and exercise?
- Do you follow a regular fitness schedule? If so, describe it. How has your current problem affected your usual exercise routine?
- Are you experiencing any difficulties with your exercise and fitness activities? Are you experiencing any fatigue? decreased endurance? pain? dyspnea? dizziness?
- Do you supplement your diet with vitamins, calcium, protein or other products?

patient is asked to squeeze both the examiner's hands as firmly as possible. To assess the lower extremities, foot presses can be done. These involve asking the patient to push the foot as hard as possible against the force exerted by the palm of the examiner's hand. This helps to establish whether a weakness exists in one side or the other. Normally, muscle strength should be equal on either side of the body and should fully resist the examiner's opposing force.

BONES AND JOINTS Bones and joints are also assessed through observation and palpation. Contour, prominence and symmetry are observed. Each joint must be examined individually. For the upper extremities, the shoulder, elbow, wrist and finger joints are examined for range of motion. In the lower extremities, the hip, knee, ankle and toes are all assessed separately. Normally, a person should be able to move joints independently through the full range of motion without pain. The nurse notes the degree to which each joint can move, its flexibility or any resistance felt when attempting to move the joint passively. The nurse should never attempt to force a joint if resistance is felt or if the patient expresses pain.

BODY ALIGNMENT It is important to note whether a patient has good body alignment while standing, sitting and lying. In order to assess body alignment, the nurse must be aware of the body's normal anatomic position and know how to determine its centre of gravity (see Figure 29.3).

BODY BALANCE To determine body balance related to gross motor control, the individual is observed in a standing (walking) or sitting position. The patient should be able to maintain balance whether walking independently or with assistive devices, such as a walker or canes. When sitting, a patient should be able to maintain an upright position without leaning to one side or the other. Assessing balance is an important factor in determining risk for injury.

COORDINATION To assess fine motor control, the nurse observes the patient carrying out activities of daily living that involve dexterity, such as handling eating utensils, buttoning buttons, tying shoe laces, combing hair or writing. These activities allow an individual to function independently and are an important part of daily living.

ASSISTIVE DEVICES It is important to note whether patients walk independently or whether they need the help of devices to maintain independence. Do they require the use of a cane, walker, crutches or wheelchair for mobility? How well do they use these devices?

ABILITY TO TRANSFER A person who requires no assistance transferring from bed to chair or from chair to toilet is considered to be independent. It is essential to assess the type of help an individual requires to move from one place to another. Some individuals may require only supervision for safety; others may need the assistance of one or two nurses for a transfer. If the patient is too heavy or too incapacitated, a mechanical lift will be needed.

Diagnostic Tests

The most common diagnostic tests used to assess mobility involve radiographic examination. Fractures, dislocations and other abnormalities can be detected with x-ray. Specific tests that may be done to assess joints, bones and muscles include the arthogram (visualization of a joint), myelogram (visualization of the spinal canal), arthroscopy (examination of a joint through the use of fibreoptic technology), bone scan (evaluation of the presence of inflammation in the joints) and CAT scan (evaluation of the bony and soft tissues of a joint in three dimensions).

Diagnosing Movement and Exercise Problems

Movement and exercise problems pertain not only to difficulties or limitations in physical mobility and motor function but also to the effects of these difficulties on other facets of regular functioning. *Impaired Physical Mobility* is the nursing diagnosis often used for problems in which "the individual experiences or is at risk for experiencing limitation of physical movement but is not immobile" (Carpenito, 1997, p. 565). This can occur in patients with neuromuscular or musculoskeletal conditions such as multiple sclerosis or arthritis; in those who have undergone surgical procedures; or in those undergoing treatment with such measures as casts, traction devices or drainage tubes connected to suction units. Impaired physical mobility may be characterized by the inability to move purposefully within the environment (including bed mobility, transferring and ambulation), limitations in ROM, limited muscle strength and control, impaired coordination and imposed restriction on movement (Carpenito, 1997).

When a patient is unable to endure physical movement and exercise at the usual or desired level, the nursing diagnosis *Activity Intolerance* applies. Many factors can cause activity intolerance. Cardiac, pulmonary, circulatory or chronic diseases, nutritional disorders, treatments such as surgery or chemotherapy, prolonged bed rest, medications and sedentary lifestyle are a few of the possible related factors. Activity intolerance is defined by altered physiological responses to activity, in particular respiratory and cardiovascular function. These may include shortness of breath, dyspnea, change in rhythm, blood pressure and heart rate. Weakness, fatigue, pallor or confusion are other defining characteristics (Carpenito, 1997).

Impairments in motor function that lead to difficulties in performing the self-care activities of daily living are stated as *Self-Care Deficits*. NANDA has identified five categories of self-care deficits:

- feeding
- bathing
- dressing
- toiletting
- instrumental (Carpenito, 1997, pp. 736, 737).

The inability to cut food, open packages or bring food to the mouth defines self-feeding deficits. In the self-bathing deficit, the patient may be unable to wash body parts or attend to personal care. Self-dressing deficits include difficulties with dressing, undressing and grooming. Patients requiring assistance to use the toilet, carry out adequate hygiene, transfer to and from the toilet, handle clothes and flush the toilet have a self-toiletting deficit. Instrumental self-care deficits describe problems in which people experience impaired ability to perform certain activities or use services essential to managing a household, such as dialling a telephone, accessing transportation, shopping or preparing meals (Carpenito, 1997).

functioning, mobility impairments can become the etiology of other nursing diagnoses. For example, a patient with mobility impairment following extensive surgery might experience a self-care deficit. This can lead to a sense of powerlessness if the patient is confined to bed for a prolonged period of time and feels that personal control of the situation has been lost. Mobility impairments may also lead to deficits in diversional activity, alterations in health maintenance, impairments in management at home, fear of falling and difficulties in meeting safety needs. Indeed, when patients cannot move freely, they are at risk for injury because of the limited capacity to protect themselves from harm.

Many people today seek to enhance their level of wellness through lifestyle changes that centre around exercise and fitness. Physical fitness and exercise are key components of health practices that help to improve the quality of life and prevent such health problems as heart disease and stroke. When individuals and families indicate a desire to achieve a higher level of physical fitness and exercise, the diagnostic statement *Potential for enhanced physical fitness and exercise* may be used (Carpenito, 1997).

Following are some examples of nursing diagnoses that may apply to patients with movement and exercise problems.

- *Impaired Physical Mobility related to insufficient knowledge of managing a lower limb prosthesis.*
- *Activity Intolerance related to sedentary lifestyle and inadequate diet.*
- *Diversional Activity Deficit related to prolonged bed rest and inability to perform favourite activities.*
- *Altered Health Maintenance related to decreased flexibility and muscle strength secondary to aging.*
- *Risk for Injury related to unsteady gait secondary to weakness and uncoordinated use of crutches.*

Planning Movement and Exercise Interventions

A plan of care for patients with mobility and exercise problems is based on the nursing diagnoses and is designed to suit each individual's needs. Goals are generally aimed at maintaining, strengthening and restoring mobility and motor function, preventing further deterioration in function and promoting optimal functioning in daily living. The patient and family should be involved in establishing expected outcomes and selecting interventions as much as possible. The nurse works closely with the physiotherapist and the occupational therapist to plan exercises that are consistent with the physician's plan of care for the patient. The prevention of muscle deterioration and the maintenance and improvement of muscle strength and tone in patients whose mobility is limited require the intensive of

The process of recovery for patients who have partially or completely lost one or more of their motor abilities is often a long one. Short-term goals are therefore very important. The achievement of each small step of progress is something to strive for and provides nurse, patient and family with motivation to work towards further goals. In setting goals, the nurse must ensure that the expected outcomes reflect levels of performance that are realistic and attainable in terms of the patient's capabilities.

According to Dr. Sidney Katz (cited in Meissner, 1980), who developed the index of independence in ADL, there is a natural order of progression in regaining independence. Functions such as feeding, continence, transfer, toiletting, dressing and bathing follow a definite hierarchy, beginning with feeding and moving up towards bathing. It is important to note that, in establishing goals, a person who has had a fracture, for instance, will not regain full independence in dressing or toiletting until the ability to transfer has been achieved. Similarly, a patient who has had a stroke will be able to achieve independence in feeding and continence before achieving independence in dressing and bathing (Meissner, 1980).

Examples of expected outcomes include:

- The patient will demonstrate correct body alignment when standing, sitting or lying.
- The patient will show progressive activity tolerance as evidenced by maintaining pulse, respirations and blood pressure within predetermined ranges.
- The patient will feed him- or herself independently using special feeding utensils.
- The patient will walk with crutches, unassisted.
- The patient will demonstrate ways of preventing injury when transferring to, and ambulating, in a wheelchair.

In establishing priorities of care for patients with limited mobility, the nurse considers two sets of problems. For the patient whose mobility is curtailed, the foremost priority is the promotion of optimal strength and tone in unused muscles and the prevention of muscle degeneration and joint contractures. Patients who cannot move by themselves and need the nurse's help in turning and performing the activities of daily living should rank high on the nurse's list of priorities. Patients who cannot feed themselves should be helped while their food is still hot. Patients who need help in turning must be turned at scheduled times or serious skin problems may result. When patients need assistance to use the bedpan or a urinal, the nurse should ensure they receive help immediately. The patient who needs assistance in getting up, getting in or out of bed or getting in or out of the wheelchair likewise should not be left waiting too long.

Potential Benefits of Aerobic Exercise

- Reduces risk of heart attack by:
  - increasing blood serum HDL cholesterol, the "good" cholesterol
  - decreasing blood serum triglyceride levels
  - reducing high blood pressure
  - reducing the desire to smoke
  - improving the efficiency of the heart
- Reduces risk of developing certain forms of cancer
- Reduces risk of developing non–insulin-dependent diabetes
- Reduces excess body weight and helps maintain optimal weight
- Reduces risk of developing osteoporosis
- Increases resistance to stress, anxiety and fatigue; enhances mood and lowers depression
- Increases stamina, strength and working ability
- Improves self-esteem.

SOURCE: Williams, 1993, p. 49.

Priorities of care may change from day to day depending on the patient's status. The nurse must use judgement in scheduling activities to ensure that patients who have problems in meeting basic physiological needs are given assistance at the time they need it. The nurse must also be sufficiently flexible to interrupt other activities that can be deferred in order to assist patients who require immediate assistance. Ignoring or responding slowly to signals for help devalues the patient-centred approach to treatment and is one of the most common complaints patients have when they are in hospital.

Implementing Movement and Exercise Interventions

Health-Promoting Strategies

Since the Lalonde Report (1974) and the fitness revolution that followed, as evidenced by such programs as ParticipAction, *fitness* has become a buzzword. Physical fitness, exercise and other health promotion practices such as proper nutrition, a positive mental outlook and the avoidance of stress enable individuals to increase control over their lives and to function at maximum potential. By definition, physical fitness means "a set of abilities individuals possess in order to perform specific types of physical activity" (Williams, 1993, p. 13). Physical fitness related to health refers to the development of cardiovascular–respiratory vitality, maintenance of an optimal body weight and the development of joint flexibility and muscular strength and endurance. To maintain or improve physical fitness, it is important to participate in some form of regular physical activity and exercise.

TYPES OF PHYSICAL ACTIVITY AND EXERCISE

Physical activity generally involves bodily movement caused by muscular contraction that results in the expenditure of energy. There are two types of physical activity that promote health-related physical fitness—unstructured and structured.

Unstructured Physical Activity

Usual activities of daily living, such as walking, climbing stairs, cycling, gardening and home maintenance, domestic activities (house cleaning, changing bed linen, doing laundry), occupational activities and recreational activities fall into the category of unstructured physical activity. Unstructured activity, because of its low intensity, generally does not improve physical fitness, but it does maintain health and provide some protection against the development of certain chronic diseases, particularly if carried out for long periods of time (Williams, 1993).

Structured Physical Activity

Structured physical activity refers to exercise programs designed to improve physical fitness. These include aerobic, muscle-strengthening and flexibility (stretching) exercises.

AEROBIC EXERCISE Of all the different exercise programs available, those that involve aerobic activity possess the greatest potential for improving health. **Aerobic exercise** refers to sustained physical activity that increases heart rate, blood circulation and metabolic demands for oxygen. Aerobic exercises strengthen cardiopulmonary function and endurance and enhance the capacity of muscle tissues to extract oxygen from the blood and use it to generate energy via the respiratory system (Williams, 1993). Aerobic exercises involve the use of large muscle groups in a rhythmical manner and include speed walking, jogging, stationary bicycling, swimming, cross-country skiing, aerobic dancing and rowing, as well as active games and sports such as basketball, soccer or squash.

MUSCLE-STRENGTHENING EXERCISE Muscular strength and endurance are developed through physical activity in which force is exerted against resistance; thus, the name resistance (weight) training. There are three basic types of exercises in resistance training: isotonic, isometric and isokenetic. **Isotonic exercises** involve muscle contraction used to create a constant force as a joint is moved through its range of motion. The biceps curl with a free weight is an example of an isotonic routine. In **isometric exercise** the tension of the muscles is increased, but there is neither movement of the joint nor change in the length of the muscle. This occurs

adequate to overcome the resistance. Attempting to push or pull against an immovable object is an example of an isometric exercise. **Isokinetic exercise** is defined as an activity in which the speed of limb movement is controlled at a constant velocity. Rehabilitative exercises for knee injuries, for example, use devices to regulate speed through a complete range of motion.

STRETCHING EXERCISE Flexibility is enhanced when muscles and joints are gently moved through their full range of motion. It is necessary to hold stretching exercises for at least 15 seconds in order to increase flexibility or range of motion. Stretching, hatha yoga and calisthenics (systematic exercises for attaining strength and gracefulness) increase range of motion, improve circulation and also promote relaxation.

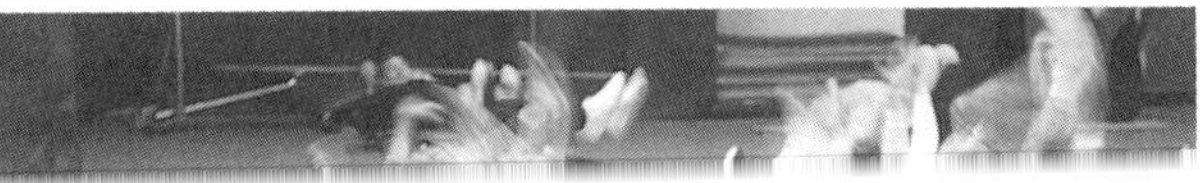

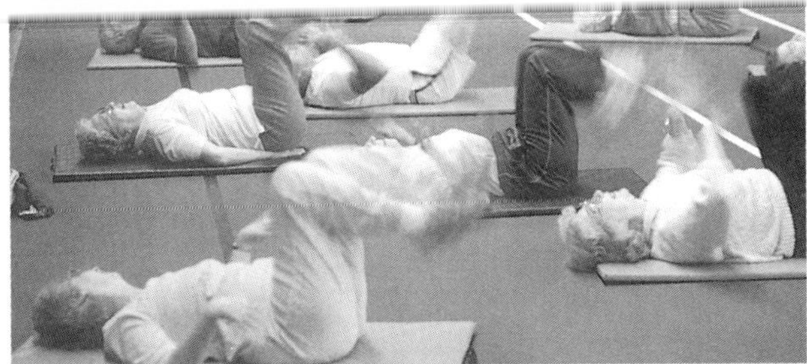

Exercise classes assist people in maintaining physical fitness.

PROMOTING PHYSICAL FITNESS AND EXERCISE

Nurses can help to promote physical fitness by providing education and information to patients. Knowledge of physical fitness and of the benefits and risks of exercise will enable individuals to explore fitness practices and determine exercise needs. Patients may want to know how to go about establishing and maintaining an exercise program, and the nurse should be prepared to provide this information.

Everybody should be encouraged to participate in a regular exercise program, unless health reasons preclude this. Exercises are planned to suit individual needs, interests and motor abilities, taking into consideration age, gender, degree of mobility and limitations imposed by chronic or current health problems and interests. The individual who starts an exercise program should always have a complete physical examination first to make sure there are no contraindications to exercise, and to find out if there are any limitations on the type or amount of exercise planned.

Exercise programs may be carried out at home or outside the home. They can be designed to accommodate all age groups and to cater to virtually all interests, from hiking, swimming and other active sports to simple calisthenics. Many community organizations offer a graded series of exercise classes to assist people in maintaining or regaining optimal physical fitness. Exercises for older people have become a regular feature of many of these programs.

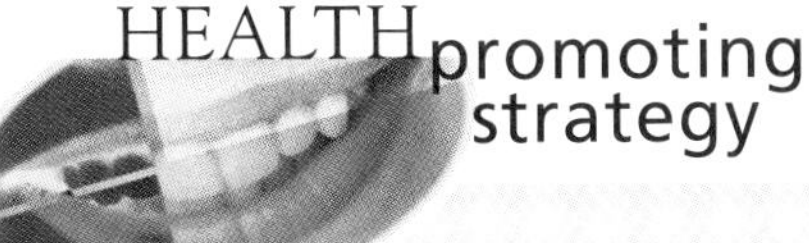

Promoting Fitness and Healthy Exercising

- Make exercise part of your daily routine.
- Use every opportunity for unstructured exercise: for example, take stairs instead of the elevator; walk instead of drive; and walk at a brisk, fast pace.
- Plan a personal fitness program suited to you. If you have any health concerns, consult your physician before planning the program.
- Select activities that are rhythmic, repetitive and that challenge the circulatory system, at an intensity appropriate for you.
- Select a variety of modes of aerobic exercise that you enjoy, that are suited to your needs and that can be done year-round.
- Wear comfortable clothes and shoes with proper support.
- Follow your program regularly, at least three times a week and not more than six, preferably on alternate days.
- Remember to warm up and cool down.
- Begin your sessions with less vigorous activities and gradually build the intensity as your body adapts to the exercise routine and your physical fitness improves.
- Avoid exercising to the point of exhaustion, and never force a joint beyond its range of motion.
- If you experience muscle pain, burning or tingling, stop and rest for a few minutes.
- Stop exercising and consult a physician if you experience:
  - pain in the chest, in the arm or any other unexplained pain
  - irregular pulse rate—too fast or too slow, flutters, rapid rate changes
  - palpitations in the chest or throat
  - dizziness, light-headedness, fainting or confusion.

SOURCES: Williams, 1993; Corbin & Lindsey, 1994.

A regular program of aerobic exercise is recommended. Regular aerobic exercise three to four times weekly, for 30 minutes of continuous activity, has been shown to produce a number of health benefits in all ages (Greenberg & Dintiman, 1992). All exercise sessions should start with a *warm-up* period of exercises that gradually increase respiration, circulation and body temperature and stretch muscles. A proper warm-up helps to prevent excessive strain on the heart as well as muscular soreness and injury. The warm-up is followed by a *stimulus* period of more vigorous activity designed to challenge the cardiovascular system by significantly increasing blood flow to the working muscles over an extended period of time. It is important that the intensity of the activity is moderate, not exhaustive. Exercise tolerance should be built up gradually, through regular sessions of gradually increasing intensity, rather than in intermittent spurts. Exercise levels should be increased only after one level has been performed for three sessions in a row without distress. Sessions should never be carried to the point of exhaustion.

Following the exercise period, a gradual *cooling-down* is advised. This should involve slower movements, such as relaxing exercises or simply walking around for a few minutes, to allow the body time to adjust to lessened physical demand and return the heart rate to near normal. Stretching at this time may help to improve flexibility and prevent muscle stiffness.

Health-Protecting Strategies

Patients who remain in bed for prolonged periods are prone to develop complications as a result of inactivity. Exercise helps to create and maintain good muscle tone and to prevent atrophy. Exercise also helps in the elimination of waste products from the muscles. The contraction of muscles increases circulation and the metabolism of wastes from the body. Increased circulation is particularly important for the person who remains in bed. Stasis of blood is a predisposing factor in the formation of clots, which can lead to serious complications. The increased basal metabolic rate that results from exercise increases the body's need for oxygen. This, in turn, results in an increase in both the rate and depth of respirations, which improves lung aeration and helps to prevent infectious processes that can occur in the lungs as a result of inactive lung areas and stagnant secretions. Improved blood circulation also increases the delivery of oxygen and nutrients to tissues, maintaining their health and preventing deterioration and ulcer formation.

Contractures and stiffening of the joints are other unfortunate side effects of prolonged inactivity. By putting joints through their full range of motion, these complications can often be avoided.

MUSCLE-STRENGTHENING EXERCISE

Patients who are inactive because they are confined to bed or a wheelchair or because they are recuperating from illness can maintain strength and flexibility of muscles and joints and prevent muscle wasting and joint stiffness or contractures through regular exercise. The patient is encouraged to exercise actively those muscles that can be used. Patients can learn how to do isometric exercises while they are otherwise inactive. For example, the patient who is confined to bed can perform isometric exercises of the lower limbs by periodically contracting the quadriceps and gluteal muscles for 10–15 seconds, or by pushing the back of the knee against the bed while the leg is extended. Clenching the fist or squeezing a ball are isometric exercises for increasing hand strength. Isometric contraction, sometimes referred to as *muscle-setting* exercise, can help considerably in maintaining or improving muscle strength and tone. In extended immobility there is a tendency to hunch the shoulders, compromising chest expansion. A useful bed exercise is to pinch the shoulder blades together to squeeze the shoulder retractors. This exercise also reduces the risk of kyphosis.

Isotonic exercise is often prescribed as part of the patient's therapy but it may also be used for preventive care. In isotonic exercise, the muscle actively contracts or shortens,

KEY PRINCIPLES

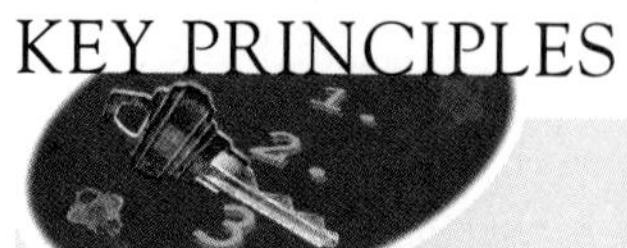

Principles Relevant to Exercise Programs for Patients

1. The process of degeneration starts almost immediately when muscles are unused.
2. The process of degeneration involves bone and skin tissues as well as muscle tissue.
3. All joints have a circumscribed range of motion.
4. Passive exercise of the body's movable parts through their full range of motion prevents the development of contractures that can interfere with joint mobility.
5. Active contraction of muscles is required to maintain and improve their strength and tone.
6. Active contraction of muscles on one side of the body causes the corresponding muscles on the other side of the body to relax.
7. Exercise has beneficial effects on all body systems.

causing the limb to move. Active range-of-motion exercises, which we discuss in the next section, are isotonic activities. This type of exercise is beneficial for preventing joint [illegible] strength and tone. Patients may go to the physiotherapy department for this, or the physiotherapist may come to the nursing unit.

If a program of regular exercise for a patient is not undertaken by another health professional, the nurse institutes one. This is done for all patients for whom active exercise is not contraindicated. Both individual and group exercises are used. Group exercises are helpful from a psychosocial point of view (increasing sensory stimulation) and for their physically therapeutic benefits. There is greater motivation for patients to put forth more effort in a group when everyone is doing the same thing. In many agencies, group classes are organized by the physiotherapy department, but there is no reason why a nurse cannot organize these on a nursing unit. This is frequently done in some obstetrical units to assist patients to regain lost muscle tone resulting from pregnancy and childbirth, or on an extended care unit to reactivate residents.

Occupational therapy also assists people to maintain or regain muscular strength and to prevent loss of joint mobility. The focus of occupational therapy is to assess activities of daily living and to help the patient become as functionally independent as possible.

RANGE-OF-MOTION EXERCISE

Range-of-motion exercises (ROM), in which a body part is moved through a range of motion, are carried out to promote circulation, maintain muscle tone and promote flexibility. In doing this, joint stiffness and debilitating contractures are prevented. **Active ROM** is range of motion carried out by the patient. It is a form of isotonic exercise, and as such it maintains strength, tone and flexibility. In patients unable to move body parts because of paralysis or extreme illness, ROM is performed by someone else. This is called **passive ROM** exercise. Passive exercise helps to maintain joint flexibility and prevent stiffness and contractures. Because this type of exercise involves no active movement on the part of the muscles, it does not contribute to muscle tone or strength.

ROM exercises are planned as a regular part of nursing activities. During a bath, for example, the nurse has an excellent opportunity to move the patient's limbs through their full range of motion. The patient is encouraged to exercise actively those muscles that can be used. However, in certain cases, the nurse may need to assist the patient in performing ROM (active assisted ROM), or to perform passive ROM.

Performing ROM Exercises

The body has six large movable parts: the head, the trunk, two arms and two legs. It also has smaller movable parts, such as the hand, fingers, feet and toes, which form parts of larger parts but may move independently. All these body parts are capable of the various kinds of movements defined previously. You can move your hand without moving [illegible] of any other part of your body.

The degree to which people can tolerate exercise varies considerably. A patient should avoid fatigue and pain while exercising. Joints need to be exercised to the full range of motion. In active assisted and passive exercises, the nurse should not force movement when it is painful to the patient or when resistance is met. When passive range of motion is performed, the joint must be properly supported to prevent muscle strain or injury. The nurse does this by placing the hands directly above or below the joint to be moved. Table 29.3 illustrates, and provides instructions for performing, both active and passive range-of-motion exercises.

When a patient is exercising, the joints should go through their full range of motion. For example, the normal shoulder and upper arm movements are flexion, extension, hyperextension, abduction, adduction, circumduction, inward rotation and outward rotation. The chief muscles involved in these movements are the deltoid (abducts the upper arm), pectoralis major (flexes and adducts the upper arm), trapezius (raises and lowers the shoulders), latissimus dorsi (extends and adducts the upper arm) and serratus anterior (pulls the shoulder forward).

Hand and finger exercises are very important. Flexing, extending, abducting and adducting the hand, as well as flexing and extending the joints of the fingers, are exercises commonly carried out by patients who have some functional impairment as a result of a stroke. It is particularly important to exercise the thumb. The ability to bring the thumb in opposition to the tip and base of the fingers is a key factor in the use of the hands.

The elbows and the knees can be flexed and extended. The biceps, triceps, quadriceps and hamstring muscles are active when these movements are performed. The forearm can be supinated and pronated.

Thigh movement involves the gluteal muscles and the adductor and flexor muscles. The gluteal muscles (gluteus maximus, medius and minimus) extend, rotate and abduct the thigh. The adductor muscles adduct the thigh and adduct and flex the leg. Most hip movements involve movement of the pelvis as well.

Movement of the feet and toes is also important. The ankle is a hinged joint that permits **plantar flexion** (pointing the foot down) and **dorsiflexion** (bending the foot backwards). Inversion and eversion of the feet take place in the gliding joints.

BODY MECHANICS

The practice of good body mechanics is integral to healthy living. In health and in illness, good posture and efficient body movement are essential both therapeutically and aesthetically. The proper use of body mechanics is especially

TABLE 29.3 Assisting with range of motion

	Active		Passive	
Movement	*Illustration*	*Instructions for patient*	*Illustration*	*Description of Nurse's action*
HEAD ***Rotation***	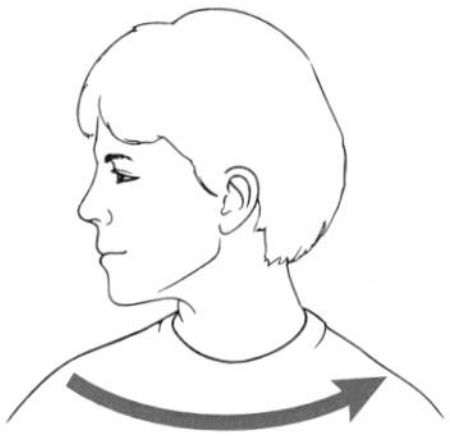	Tell patient to turn head as far as possible to the left, then to the right.	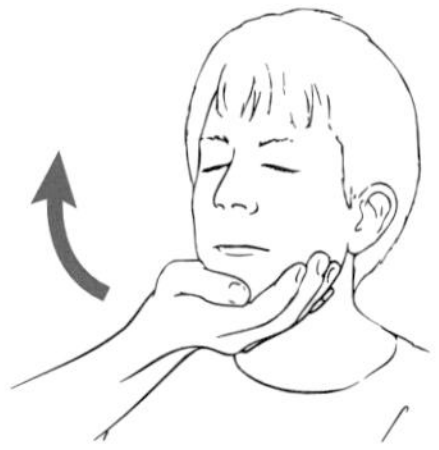	Cup the palm of your hand under the patient's chin. Pull or push chin in an arc towards each shoulder and return. (Note: no pillow)
Forward flexion	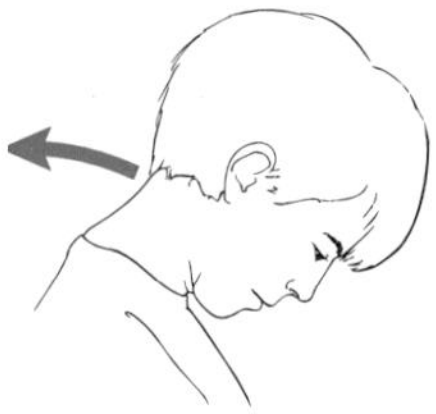	Move head as if to look at feet, then return to resting position.	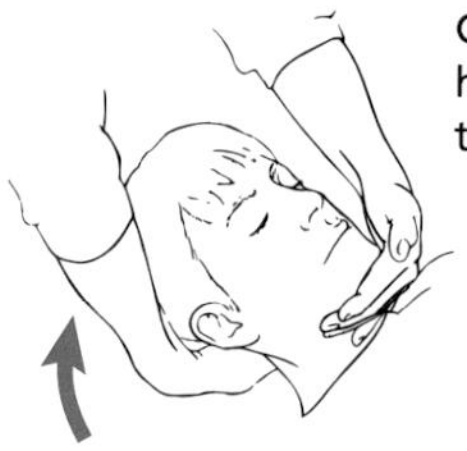	Cup hands behind patient's head, pulling head upward towards chest.
Lateral flexion	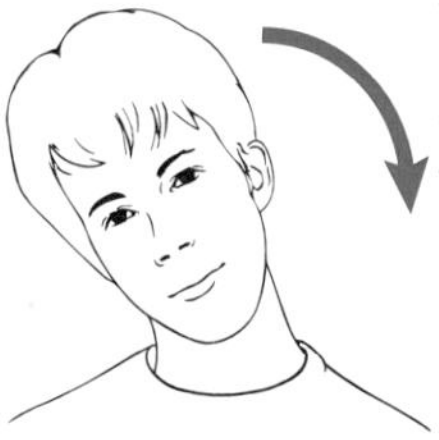	Tilt head so left ear moves towards left shoulder. Repeat for right.	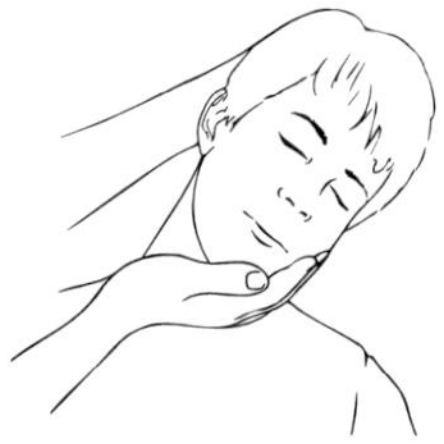	Supporting the head as above, tilt the head so left ear moves towards the left shoulder. Repeat for right.
Hyperextension	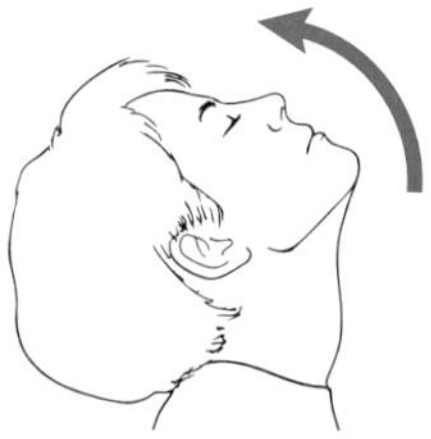	Tip head back as if looking up.	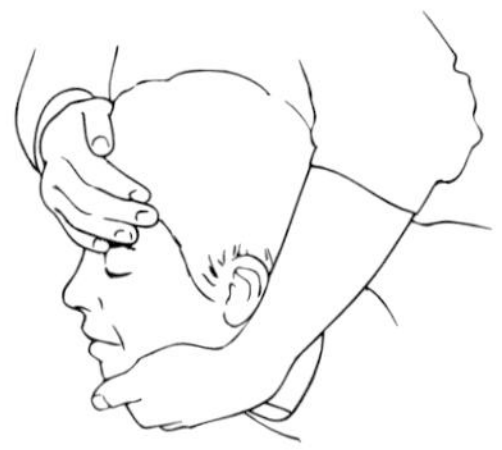	Seated or side-lying—done after all supine exercises. Place one hand on the patient's forehead, the other under chin. Move the head in an arc towards the back (use caution with passive cervical ROM).
Circumduction	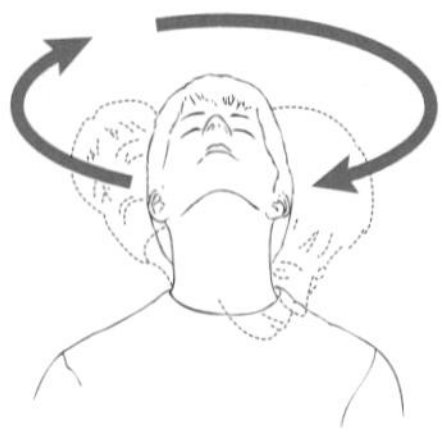	Roll head as if drawing a large circle with the top of the head, left to right, then right to left. Full circumduction of the neck—in particular, bringing it into the extension plane—compromises blood flow to the carotid arteries and therefore to the brain. This ROM is no longer recommended.	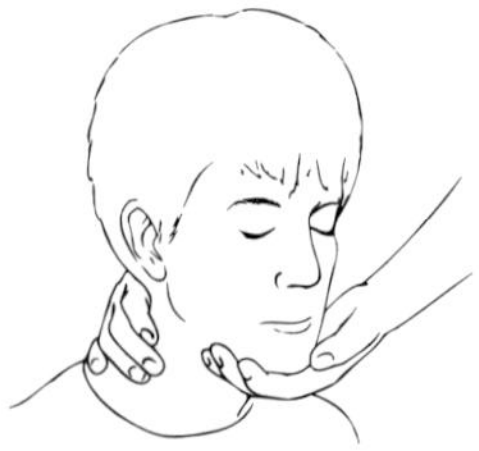	Support chin and occiput (back part of head) with palms of hands when patient is sitting up. Rotate head in circular motion to right, then to left.
UPPER EXTREMITY ***Shoulder flexion***	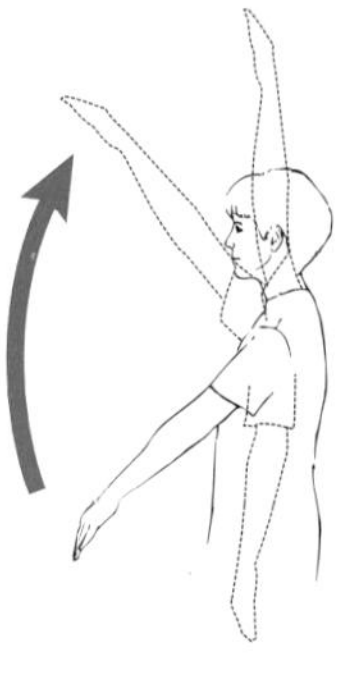	Start with arm at side or flexed so forearm is across chest. Move arm above head in a smooth arc. (Hand or elbow will make a half-circle in movement.)	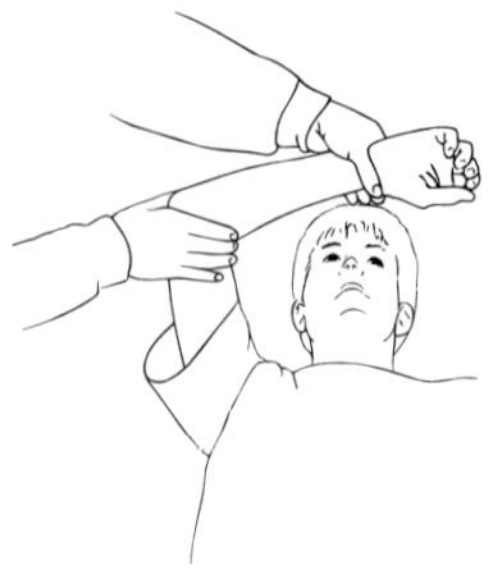	Flex arm across chest. Cup elbow in one hand, grasp wrist joint to support wrist and hand. Move arm above patient's head so elbow makes a 180° arc.

TABLE 29.3 *continued*

Movement	*Illustration*	*Instructions for patient*	*Illustration*	*Description of Nurse's action*
Adduction		Bring arm across chest, moving elbow as close to middle of body as possible.		Bracketed movements are performed together: Grasping elbow and wrist joint as above, move elbow across chest towards midline.
Abduction		After the above, move arm outward, away from the body, then up over head.		Starting in adduction and keeping arm flexed and supported as above, move arm away from the body, then over the head.
Internal rotation		Start with arm straight out to side from shoulder with palm facing front and elbow bent in 90° angle. Move hand downward so fingers point to floor. If lying down, hand should be raised above body. Move hand forward so palm touches bed next to hip. Upper arm remains on the bed.		Move arm straight out from shoulder; flex elbow so hand is raised. Support wrist joint as above and stabilize upper arm. Press gently on shoulder with your other hand. With elbow as fulcrum, move the hand downward so hand makes an arc, touching bed next to patient's hip if possible.
External rotation		After completing internal rotation, move hand so fingers point up. If lying down, keep upper arm on bed and move hand so back of hand touches bed next to head.		After above, move the hand upward so the back of the hand touches the bed next to patient's head.
Circumduction	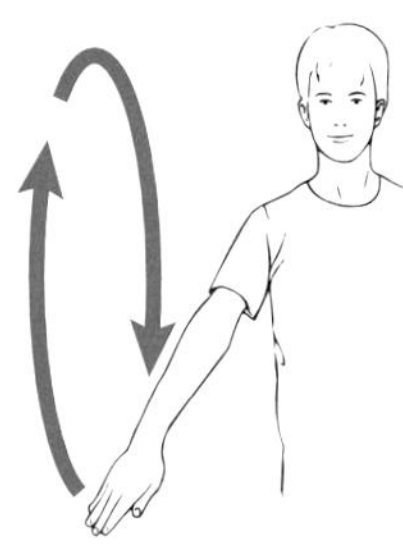	Extend arm straight out from body at shoulder. Move hand as if to draw a circle.	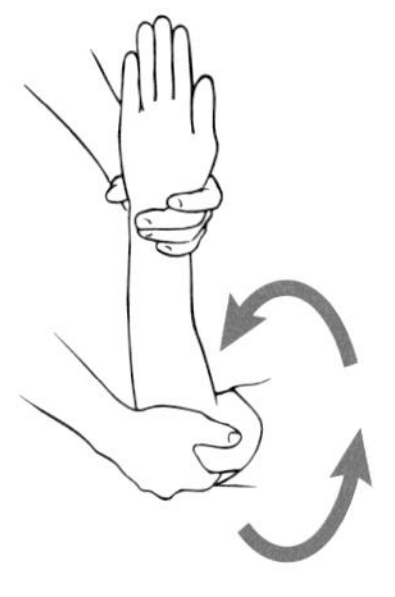	After above, extend the elbow so the arm points out from body. Cupping the elbow and supporting the wrist joint, move the arm in a circular motion.

(continued on next page)

TABLE 29.3 *continued*

	Active		Passive	
Movement	*Illustration*	*Instructions for patient*	*Illustration*	*Description of Nurse's action*
Hyperextension	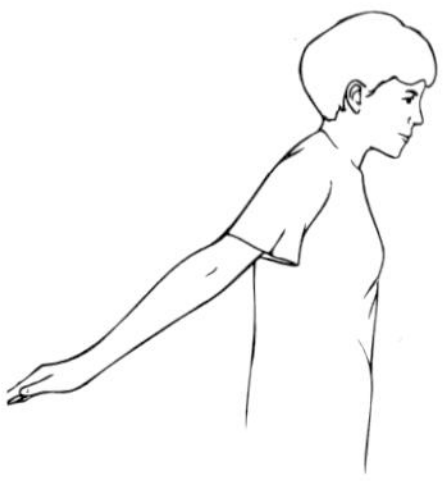	When standing or sitting with arm at side, swing arm backwards as far as possible without turning hand. May also be done lying on side.	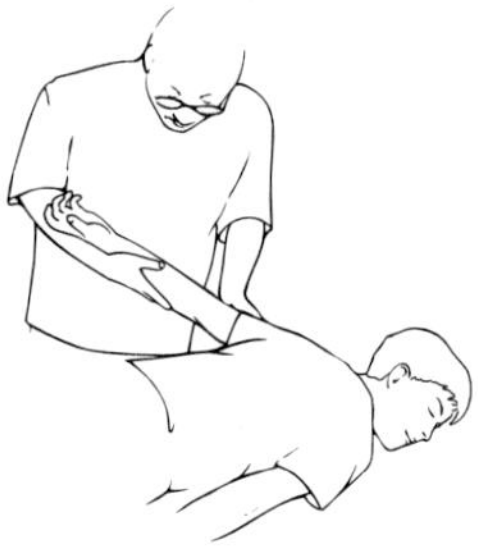	(Done at the completion of all exercises in the supine position.) With patient prone or side-lying, arm at side, cradle arm to support elbow and wrist joint. Move arm towards the back as far as possible, so that hand makes an arc.
Elbow ***Pronation***	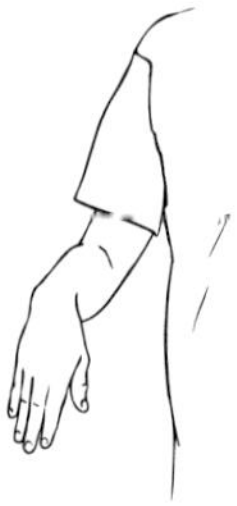	Starting with arms at sides, bend arm with palm facing upward, then turn palm towards floor.	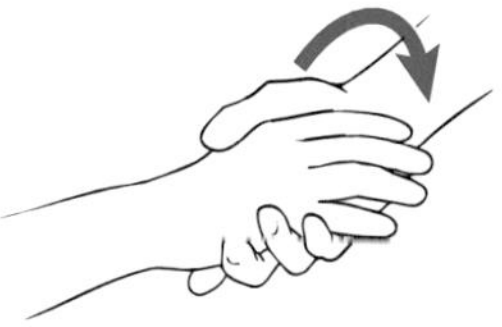	Hold patient's hand as if to shake hands; elbow may rest on bed or be cupped by other hand. Turn your hand so patient's hand faces the floor.
Supination	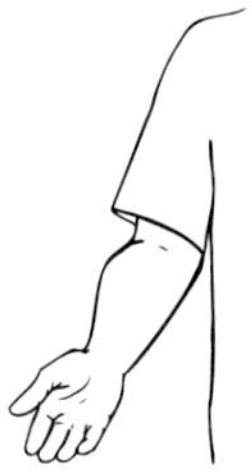	Starting in elbow pronation position, turn palm up towards ceiling.	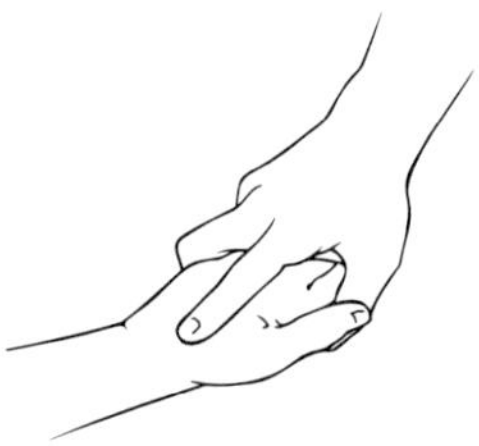	When above is completed, turn palm up towards ceiling.
Flexion	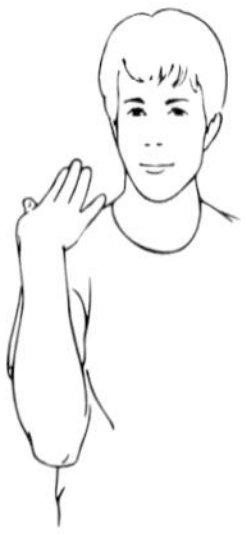	Starting with arm at side, bend elbow, moving hand towards shoulder.		
Extension	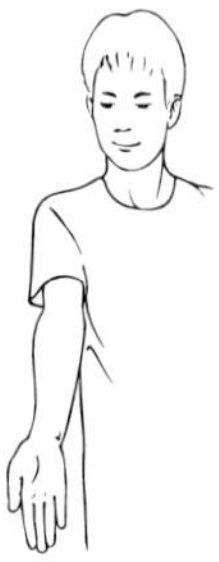	Return to starting position.	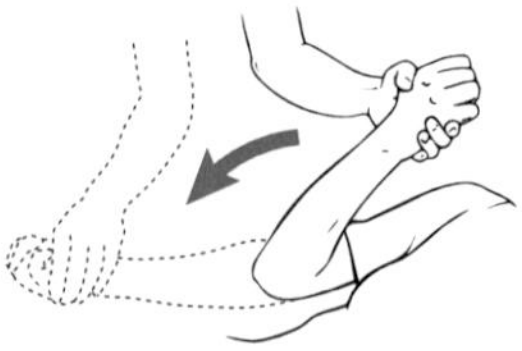	Place patient's arm at the side, palm up or facing thigh. Grasp patient's hand and wrist. With patient's elbow resting on bed, move patient's fingers towards the shoulder and return to straight position.

TABLE 29.3 *continued*

Movement	*Illustration*	*Active Instructions for patient*	*Illustration*	*Description of Nurse's action*
Circumduction	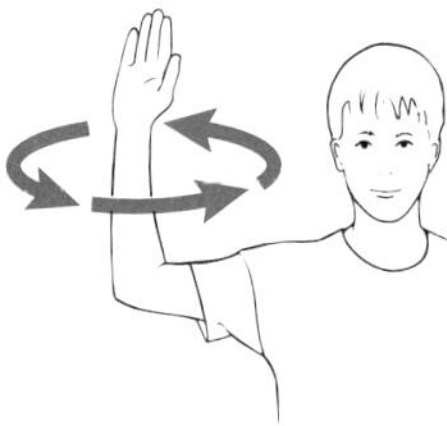	Place elbow out so it is level with shoulder. Move hand in a circle.	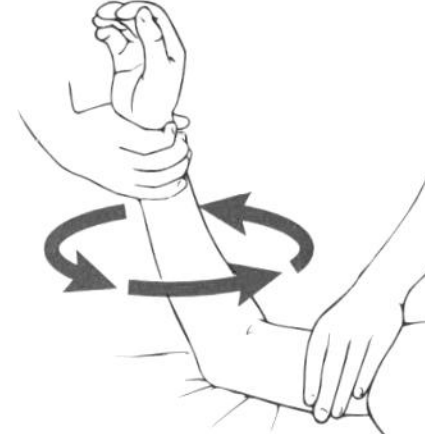	Rest elbow on bed. Grasp wrist and describe circle with hand while stabilizing upper arm with your other hand.
Wrist ***Adduction (ulnar deviation)***	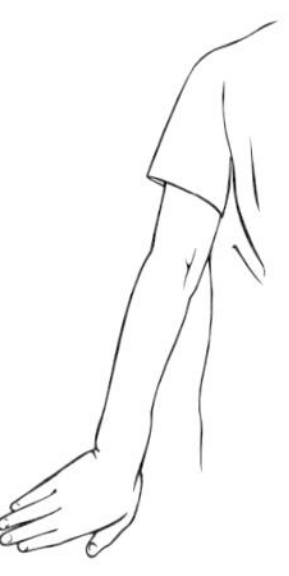	With arm at side, bend wrist as if to touch side of arm with little finger.	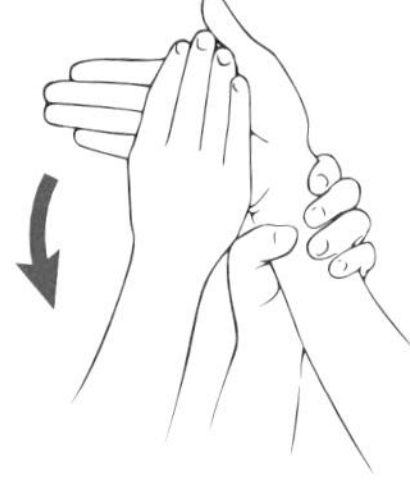	Place patient's palm in yours. Grasp wrist with your other hand. Move patient's hand from side to side as if to touch thumb (abduction) and little finger (adduction) alternately on either side of arm.
Abduction (radial deviation)	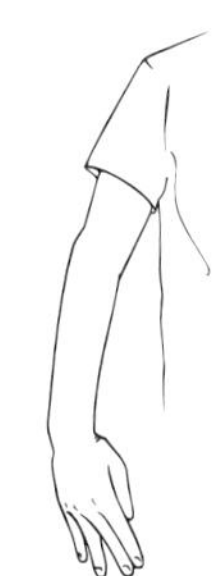	With arm at side, bend wrist as if to touch thumb on side of arm.	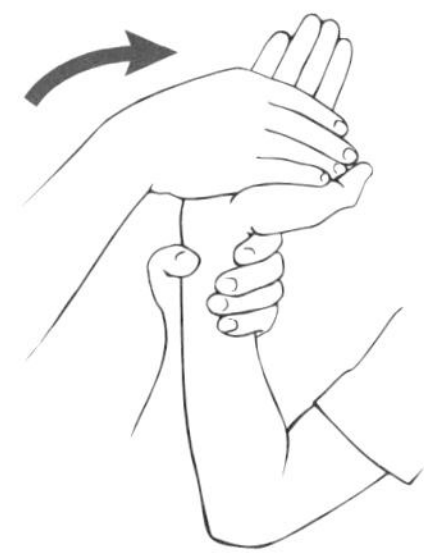	
Flexion	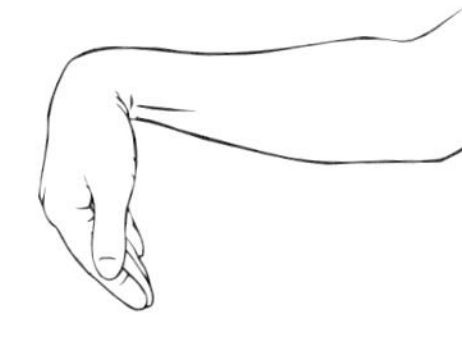	Bend wrist so palm moves towards it.	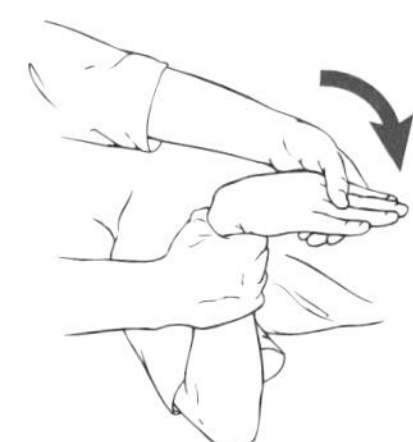	Rest elbow on bed, grasp wrist. Hold patient's hand so yours and patient's fingers are perpendicular. Flex palm towards wrist.
Hyperextension	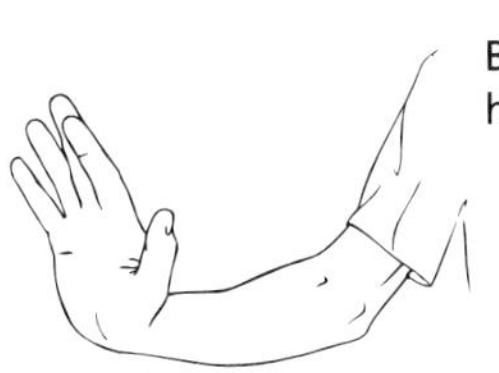	Bend wrist so back of hand moves towards it.	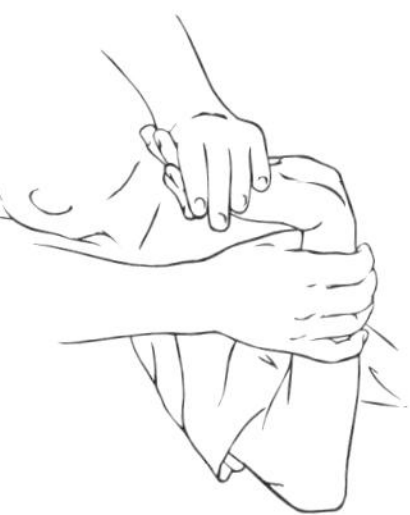	When wrist flexion is completed, extend wrist, then move back of hand towards wrist.

(continued on next page)

TABLE 29.3 continued

Movement	Active: Illustration	Active: Instructions for patient	Passive: Illustration	Passive: Description of Nurse's action
Circumduction	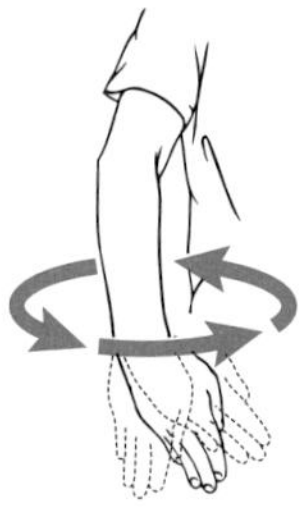	Move hand as if stirring—make a circle with hand.	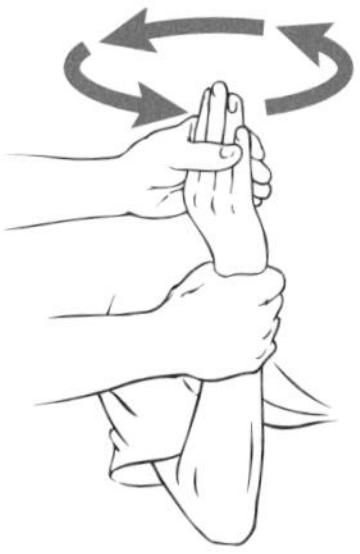	Supporting patient's hand as above, move hand in circular motion.
Fingers ***Adduction/ Abduction***	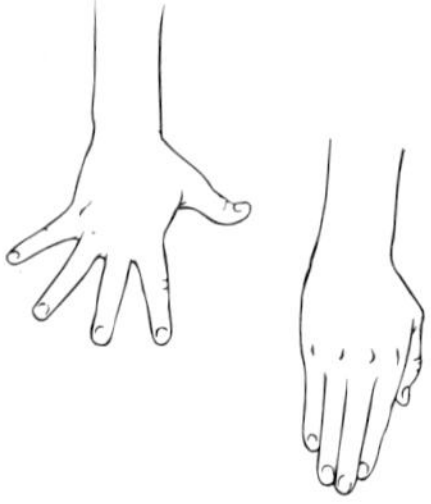	Spread fingers and thumb as far as possible, then bring together.	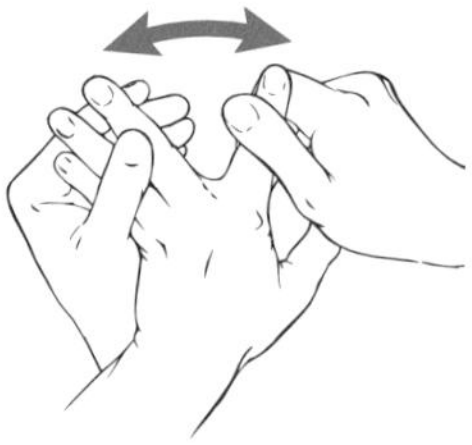	With arm resting on bed or across chest, move the thumb and each finger away from the adjacent finger and return.
Opposition	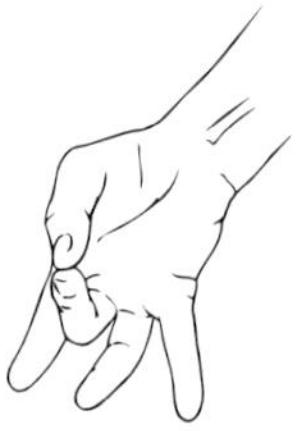	Touch each finger to thumb.	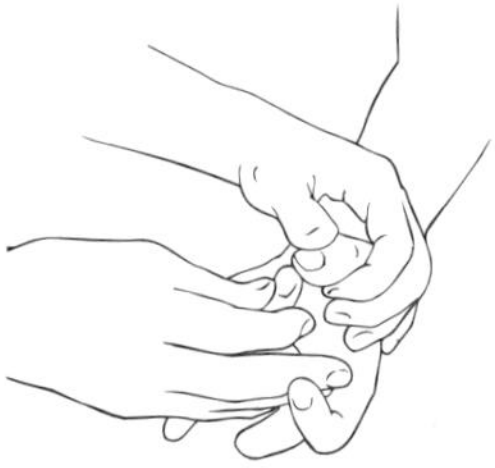	With hand still resting on bed, touch each finger to thumb.
Circumduction	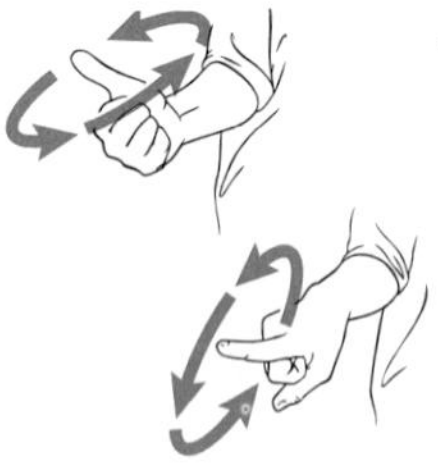	Make a circle with each finger and thumb.	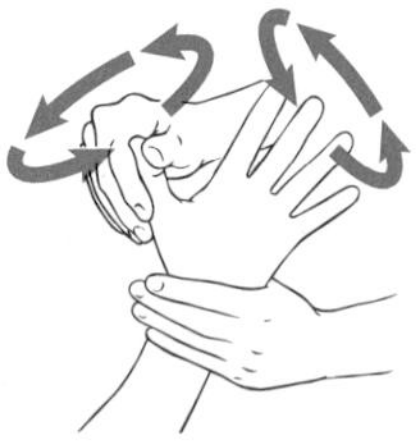	Move each finger and thumb in a circle while supporting wrist.
Flexion/Extension	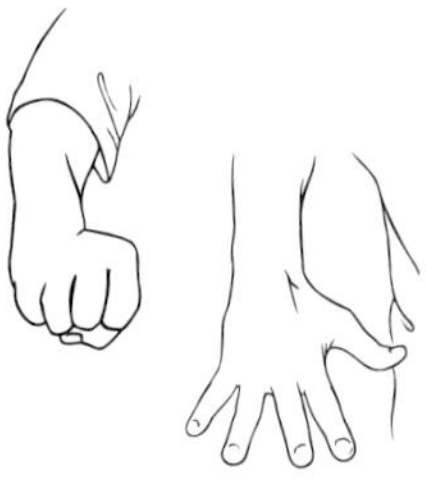	Make a fist, straighten and repeat.	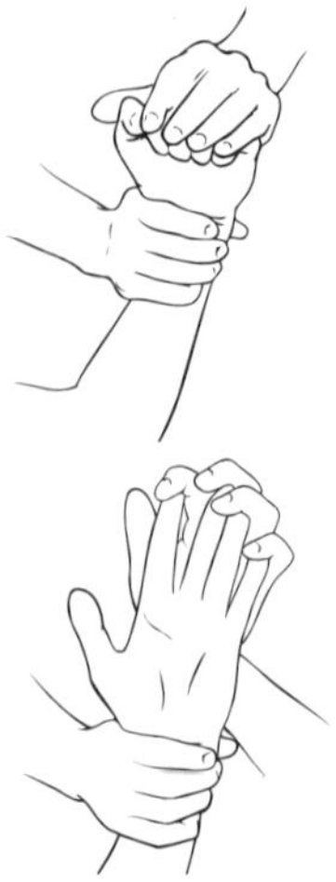	Flex elbow, grasp wrist. Place the palm of your other hand on the back of the patient's hand and flex all fingers and thumb with yours. Hook your fingertips under the patient's flexed fingers and thumb and pull them to extension, or slide your palm under the patient's flexed fingers, extending the

TABLE 29.3 *continued*

Movement	Illustration	Instructions for patient	Illustration	Description of Nurse's action
Hyperextension		Stretch fingers and thumb towards the back of hand.		fingers and thumb as you do. Continue to apply pressure on fingers and thumb to hyperextend them.
LOWER EXTREMITY ***Hip*** ***Internal rotation***		Keeping knee straight and foot perpendicular to leg, turn foot towards centre of body.		With leg resting on bed, rotate leg towards midline.
External rotation		In same position as above, turn foot outward.		With leg resting on bed, rotate leg outward.
Adduction		Bring one leg back to the midline.		Support leg behind ankle and knee. Move leg towards midline.
Abduction		Move leg out to the side as far as possible.		Supporting as above, move leg outward away from midline. Step away from side of bed to fully abduct hip.
Circumduction	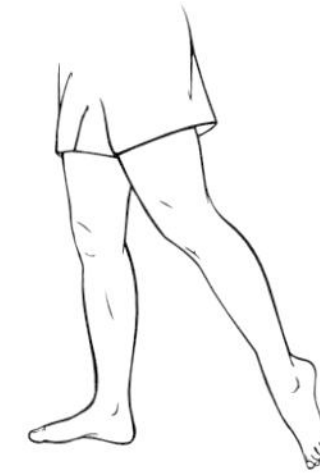	With leg straight, move foot in circular motion.	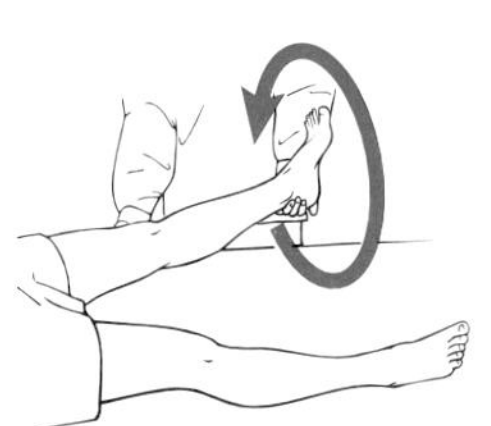	Supporting leg as above, move it in a circular motion, keeping leg straight.

(continued on next page)

TABLE 29.3 *continued*

	Active		Passive	
Movement	***Illustration***	***Instructions for patient***	***Illustration***	***Description of Nurse's action***
Flexion		Bend hip and knee, bringing knee close to chest. Can assist by grasping knee with arms (see knee flexion below).		Support ankle and calf to flex knee and hip, pushing thigh towards abdomen.
Hyperextension		Point toe, move leg backward with knee straight.		(Done after all leg exercises in supine position have been completed.) Place patient on side or prone. Cradle lower leg with arm. Applying counterpressure on buttocks, raise leg off bed. (Move leg backward if lying on side.)
Knee ***Flexion***		Lying on back, bend knee to chest and grasp with arms.		Done with hip flexion.
Circumduction		With knee flexed, move foot in circular motion. (Contraindicated in anyone with knee problems.)		Support back of knee, ankle. With knee flexed, move lower leg in circular motion.
Hyperextension		Sitting with leg extended, push back of knee against surface below. (Contraindicated in anyone with knee problems.)		Cradle knee joint. Apply counterpressure above knee; gently raise lower leg until you feel resistance.
Ankle ***Inversion*** 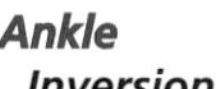	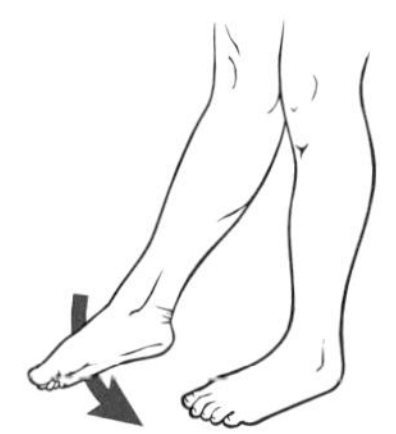	Turn the sole of the foot towards the other leg.	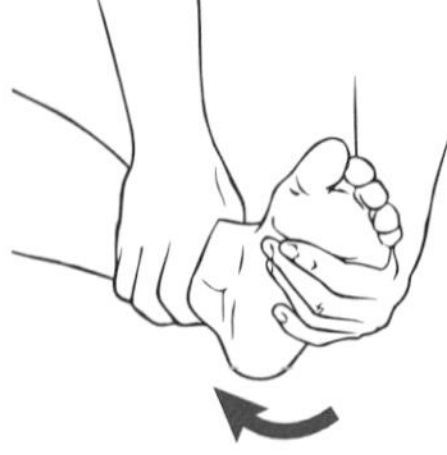	With leg resting on bed, stabilize ankle, grasp forefoot with fingers on sole. Turn sole

TABLE 29.3 *continued*

Movement	*Illustration*	*Instructions for patient*	*Illustration*	*Description of Nurse's action*
Eversion	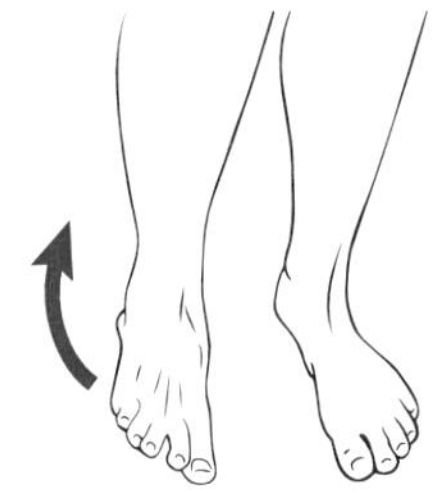	Turn the sole of the foot to the outside.	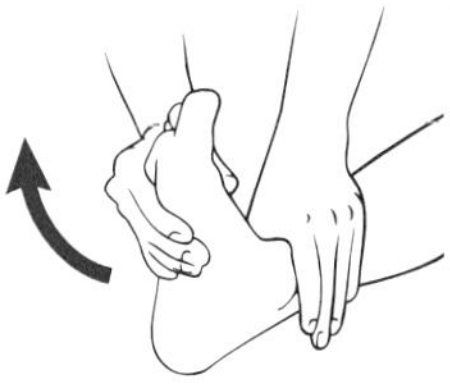	of the foot towards midline. Holding forefoot as above, turn the sole away from the midline.
Dorsiflexion	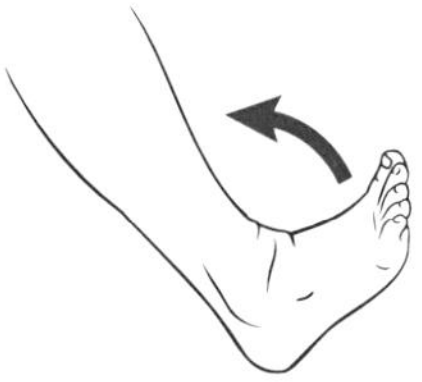	Bend the foot towards the shin.	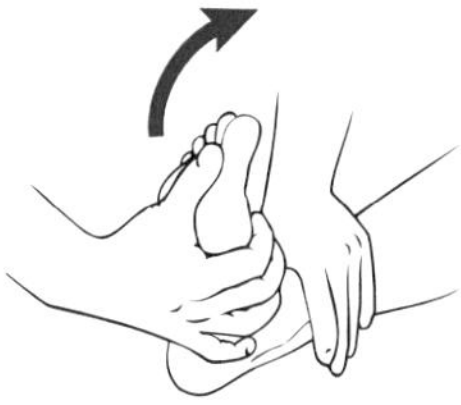	Holding foot as above, flex the foot towards the shin. (May also cup heel with hand and use forearm to flex foot.)
Plantar flexion	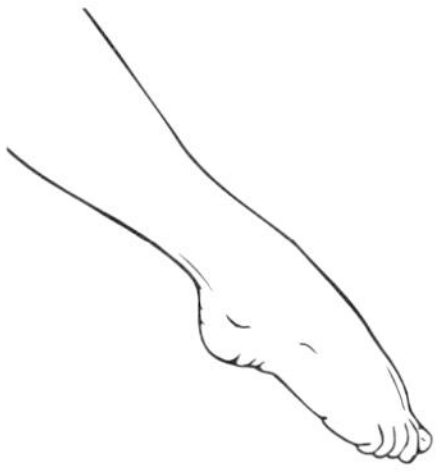	Point the toe.	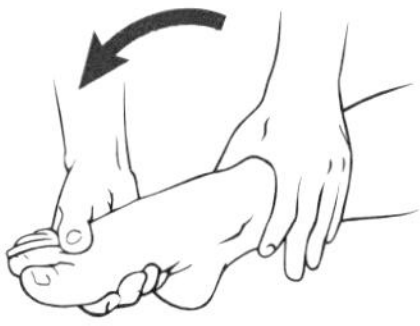	Holding foot as above, straighten foot as if to point toe.
Circumduction	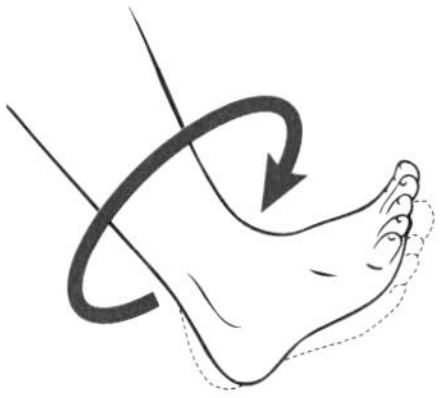	Move foot in circular motion at ankle without moving the knee.	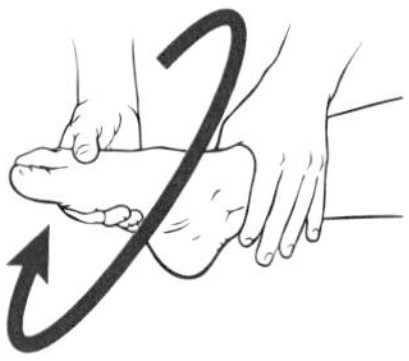	With foot in plantar flexion, rotate forefoot in circular motion.
Toes ***Flexion***	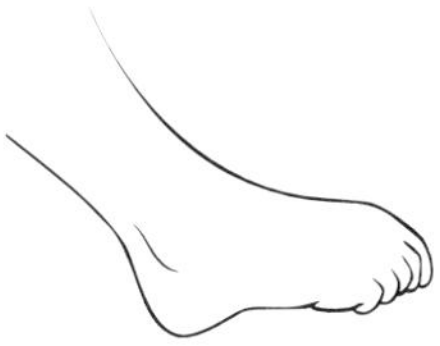	Curl toes.	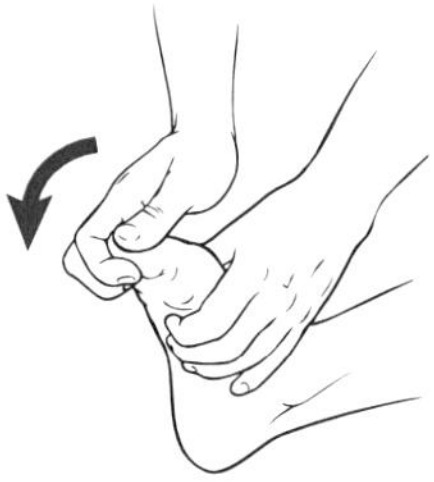	Flex toes towards sole of foot by applying pressure with fingers.
Hyperextension	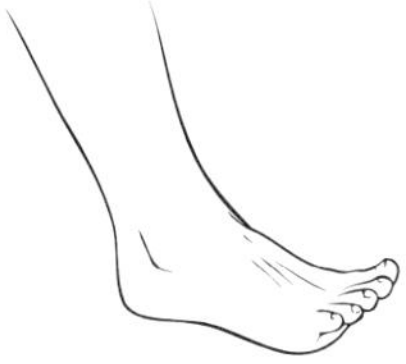	Raise toes off floor without raising foot. Spread toes.	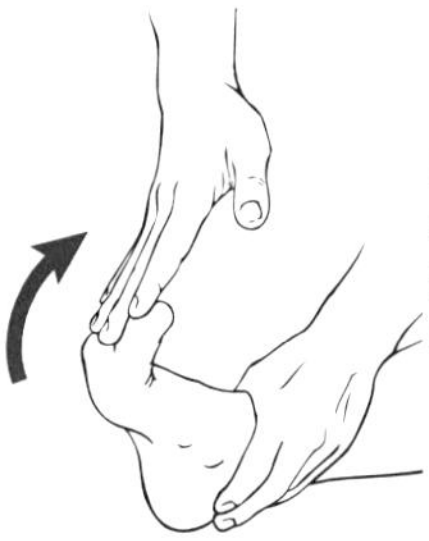	Move one hand behind toes and the other hand to forefoot; apply hand pressure to move toes towards ankle.

(continued on next page)

TABLE 29.3 *continued*

	Active		*Passive*	
Movement	***Illustration***	***Instructions for patient***	***Illustration***	***Description of Nurse's action***
Adduction / Abduction				With leg resting on bed, separate each toe from the one adjacent.
Circumduction				Move each toe in a circular motion.

SOURCE: Berger & Williams, 1998, pp. 1188–1197.

important for nurses, who do a lot of moving and lifting of patients in the course of their work. Improper body mechanics can lead to injury for both the nurse and the patient. Using principles of body mechanics not only prevents injury but also promotes efficient use of energy.

Once people have knowledge of the principles underlying body mechanics, they should put them into practice in order to establish good patterns of body movement. As these patterns are established, movements become smooth and place a minimum of strain upon the muscles. The nurse will find that good patterns of body movement will be beneficial when helping patients to move more easily and be more comfortable.

Understanding the following principles of body movement and their application in the correct use of the nurse's muscular energy and weight will contribute greatly to ease nurse–patient physical interactions and reduce the likelihood of injury to either party.

Large muscles should be used because they are more capable of handling large forces than small muscles. For example, less strain results when a heavy object is raised by bending the knees rather than by bending from the waist. The former movement uses the large gluteal and femoral muscles, whereas the latter utilizes smaller muscles such as the sacrospinal muscle of the back.

Muscles are always in slight contraction. This condition is called *resting muscle tone*. If the nurse prepares the muscles

KEY PRINCIPLES

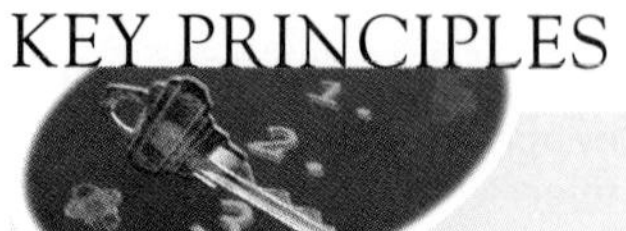

Principles Relevant to Body Mechanics

1. Large muscles generate more force than small muscles.
2. Muscles are always in slight contraction.
3. The stability of an object is always greater when there is a wide base of support and a low centre of gravity, and when the line of gravity is perpendicular to the ground and falls within the base of support.
4. The force required to maintain body balance is greatest when the line of gravity is farthest from the centre of the base of support.
5. Changes in activity and position help to maintain muscle tone and avoid fatigue.
6. The friction between an object and the surface on which the object is moved affects the amount of work needed to move the object.
7. Pulling or sliding an object requires less effort than lifting it, because lifting necessitates moving against the force of gravity.
8. Using one's own weight to counteract patient's weight requires less energy in movement.

Back Programs

"In 1990, Canadian hospitals reported 30 487 time

nurses. Almost half [of the injuries sustained by nurses] were back injuries. Back injury is now recognized as one of the major reasons for ill-health retirement from nursing. Not only is it the most frequent injury sustained by nurses, it is the most debilitating" (Haley, 1994, p. 57). Many programs are available both in the community and in the workplace to deal with the prevention of back problems. Understanding how the back works and developing knowledge of how to use your back correctly are the keys to promoting and maintaining health. Workers' Compensation Boards have developed pamphlets, books and videos to help educate the workforce. Individual hospital programs have developed their own back programs in order to educate staff members about how to use their backs correctly and thereby prevent injury.

for action prior to activity, ligaments and muscles will be protected from strain and injury. For example, the nurse will be better prepared to lift a heavy object if the muscles of the abdomen and pelvis and the gluteal muscles of the buttocks are first contracted. Movement should be smooth and controlled rather than quick and jerky.

The stability of an object is greater when there is a wide base of support and a low centre of gravity, and when the line of gravity is perpendicular to the ground and falls within the base of support. In nursing action movements, the nurse can assume a broad stance and bend the knees rather than bend at the waist. This practice keeps the vertical line of the centre of gravity within the base of support, thus providing greater stability. For example, when standing with feet apart and bending at the knees rather than at the waist, the nurse maintains better balance when helping a patient move.

The force required to maintain body balance is greatest when the line of gravity is farthest from the centre of the base of support. Therefore, the person who holds a weight close to the body uses less effort than the person who holds the weight in extended arms. Thus, when moving a patient from a bed to a stretcher, it is easier for the lifters if they hold the patient's body close to their own.

Changes in activity and position help to maintain muscle tone and avoid fatigue. By changing position even slightly while carrying out a task, and by changing the activity from time to time, better muscle tone will be maintained and undue fatigue will be avoided.

The friction between an object and the surface upon which the object is moved affects the amount of work needed to move the object. Friction is a force that opposes motion. The smoothest surfaces create the least friction; consequently, less energy is needed to move objects on smooth surfaces. When a patient changes position in bed, the nurse can apply this principle by providing a smooth foundation upon which the patient can move.

it, because lifting necessitates moving against the force of gravity. If, for example, the nurse lowers the head of a patient's bed before helping to move the patient up in the bed, less effort is required than when the head of the bed is raised.

Using one's own weight to counteract a patient's weight requires less energy in movement. If nurses use their own weight to move or push a patient, the weight increases the force applied to the movement.

MOVEMENT AND POSITION CHANGE

The goal to safe movement and position change is to promote functional mobility in the dependent or semi-dependent patient while protecting both the patient and the nurse from the risk of injury. The nurse facilitates movement by assisting (as required) the patient to change position using principles of body mechanics and competence in nursing skills. In the following section, various techniques to help patients move and change positions will be outlined. The basic preparation is the same for all the nurse-assisted patient movements.

Preparing the Patient

Inform the patient of the intent to move, in order to avoid startling him or her and to enlist participation. Approach the patient from a direction in which you can be seen and heard. Ensure the patient's freedom of movement by freeing tubes, leads, cords and restraints, and ensure privacy by closing doors or curtains. Enlist help if required, and designate a leader when working as a team to coordinate actions. Remember to use the principles of body mechanics.

Assembling Equipment and Preparing the Work Area

Gather necessary equipment (nonskid shoes, clothing, pillows and transfer aids) prior to movement. Check the equipment for safety. Apply brakes to wheelchairs, beds and stretchers, and clear the work area of obstacles, ensuring freedom of movement.

MOVING A PATIENT TO THE SIDE OF THE BED Procedures 29.1 and 29.2 outline how to help a patient move to the side of the bed using a one-person total and a one-person partial assist. The partial assist procedure is used when a patient has good upper body strength and abdominal muscle tone and can participate in the movement.

MOVING A PATIENT UP IN BED It is easiest to move dependent patients up in bed with two people rather than one; however, it is possible for one nurse to help a patient using a diagonal motion towards the side of the bed. By moving the patient in sections and by using the nurse's own

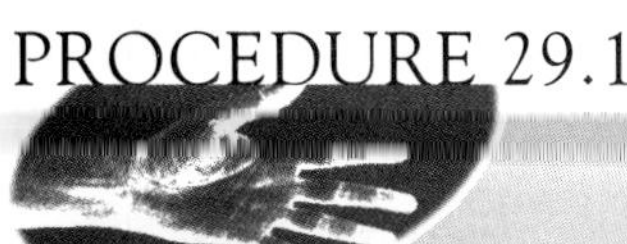

PROCEDURE 29.1 Moving a Patient to the Side of the Bed: Total Assist (One Person)

Action	Rationale
1. Raise the bed to a comfortable working height with the head of the bed flat. Place the patient in a supine position.	Reduces the risk of back strain or injury.
2. Stand facing the patient at the side of the bed towards which the patient is moving.	
3. Assume a broad stance with one leg forward of the other and with knees and hips flexed.	A wide base of support facilitates nurse's stability.
4. Move the patient's body in segments: upper, middle, then lower. Place one arm under the patient's shoulder and neck, and the other arm under the ribcage.	Less energy is expended moving parts instead of whole body.
5. Shift body weight from front foot to back foot, and rock backward and downward with the elbows locked to a crouched position, pulling the patient to the side of the bed.	Large muscles are less easily fatigued.
6. Repeat the procedure for the middle segment, placing the hands under the patient's buttocks and thighs.	

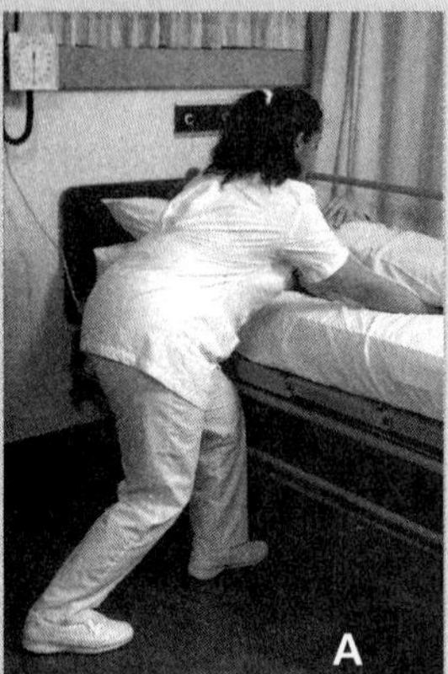

Assume a broad stance.

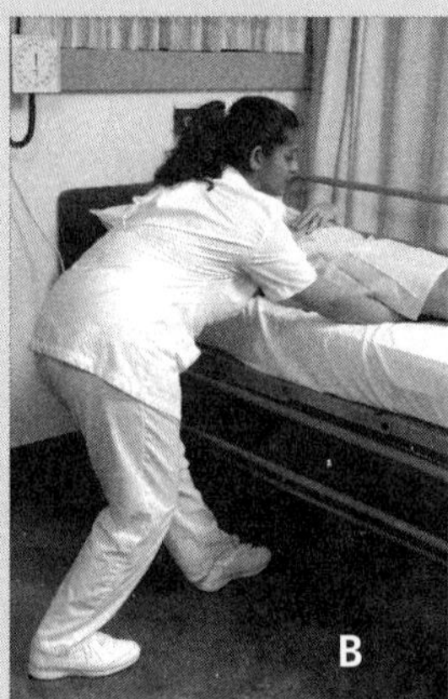

Shift body weight and rock backward and downward, pulling the patient to the side of the bed.

Action	Rationale
7. Align the lower segment by placing arms under knees and ankles.	Maintains body alignment.
8. Avoid excessive friction moving the patient.	Prevents abrasive forces, which cause discomfort and skin breakdown.
9. Assist the patient to a comfortable position. Raise side rails as necessary; lower bed to original height.	

weight to counteract the patient's weight, the nurse can safely move the dependent patient up in bed. This is most easily done if the head of the bed is lowered; this way, the nurse is not working directly against the force of gravity. Procedures 29.3 and 29.4 detail how to move a patient up in bed using a one- and two-person total assist technique.

Patients who have some movement ability may be helped to move up in bed using a partial assist. This movement is facilitated when the patient can assist by flexing the knees and pushing with the legs. In assisting the patient to make this movement, the nurse should take precautions to ensure that the patient's head does not hit the top of the bed. This is done by lowering the head of the bed and putting a pillow there, where it can act as a pad. Helping the patient move up in bed can be done by one or two nurses; in the latter instance one nurse stands on each side of the patient's bed. Procedure 29.5 describes a one-person partial assist.

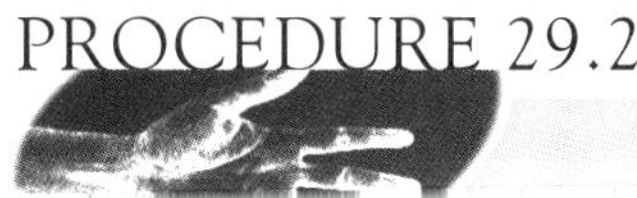

PROCEDURE 29.2 Moving a Patient to the Side of the Bed: Partial Assist (One Person)

Action	*Rationale*
1. Follow steps 1–3 of Procedure 29.1.	
2. Move the middle segment first. Place both arms under the buttock area. Keeping elbows locked and resting on the bed, instruct the patient to bend the knees, push down on the bed with the feet and raise the buttocks. On a count of three, instruct the patient to move over to the edge of the bed, with the aid of the forearms.	Allows the patient to use the femoral muscles for movement.

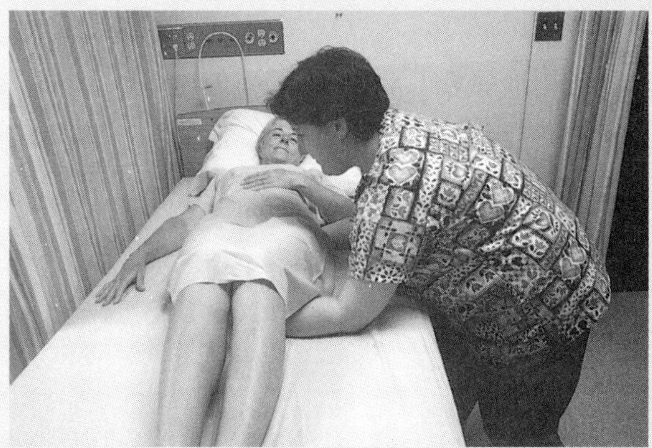

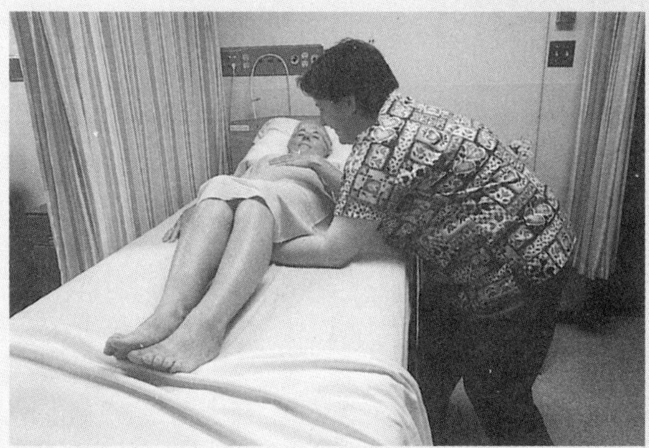

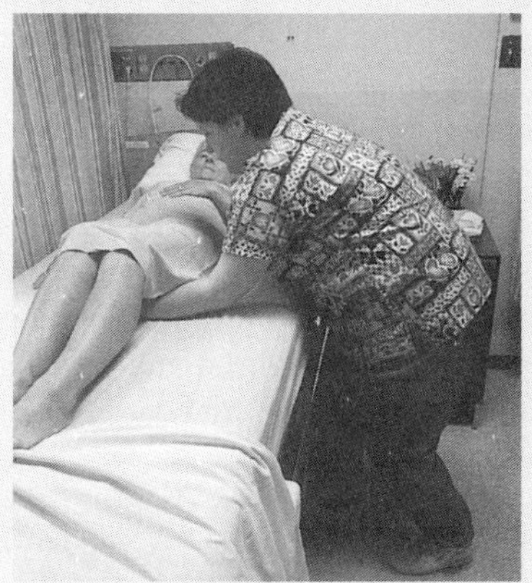

Action	*Rationale*
3. Follow with head and neck, then legs.	Maintains body alignment.
4. Follow step 9 of Procedure 29.1.	

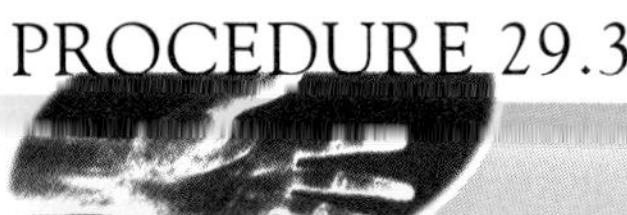

PROCEDURE 29.3 Moving a Patient Up in Bed: Total Assist (One Person)

Action	*Rationale*
1. Follow step 1 of Procedure 29.1.	
2. Remove all pillows; place one pillow at the head of the bed.	Protects the patient's head.
3. Stand at the side of the patient's bed and face the far corner of the foot of the bed. One foot is placed behind the other, assuming a broad stance.	Increases the base of support, which facilitates nurse's stability.
4. Flex the knees so that both forearms are level with the bed. One arm is placed under the patient's head and shoulders, and one arm under the small of the back. 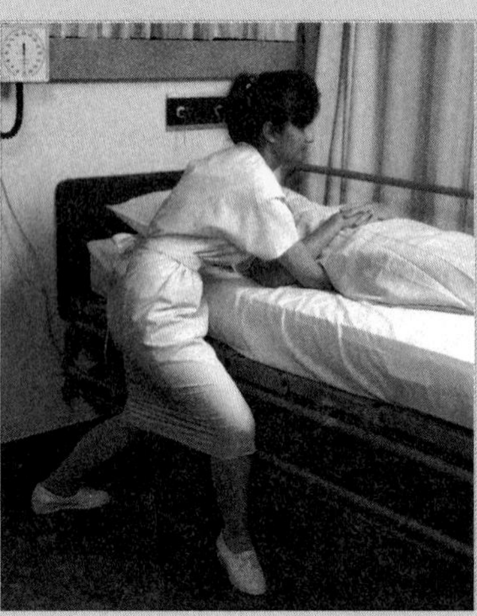	Prevents back injury.
5. Rock forward, then shift weight from the forward foot to the rear foot, hips coming downward. The patient will slide diagonally across the bed towards the head and side of the bed.	Rocking motion develops momentum.
6. Move the patient's trunk and legs as in Procedure 29.1.	Keeps the body in proper alignment.
7. Go to the other side of the bed and repeat the steps. Repeat this process, if required.	
8. Follow step 9 of Procedure 29.1.	

TURNING AND POSITIONING A PATIENT Patients may need assistance turning from side to side or changing position in bed. Procedures 29.6 to 29.8 outline the steps in helping a patient turn from a supine to a side-lying position, from a supine to a semi-prone position, and from a side-lying to a sitting position on the edge of bed.

TRANSFERRING AND LIFTING PATIENTS Movement from one position to another that involves a change in location, position or equipment is referred to as a transfer or a lift. The distinction between the two terms is that transfers are patient-assisted and lifts are not.

Patients may need assistance moving from the bed to a chair, from a chair to the toilet or commode or from the bed to a stretcher. Procedure 29.9 details the steps involved in moving a patient who is able to bear their own weight and take steps from the bed to a chair. The variations in transferring from a chair to the toilet or commode are discussed following the procedure.

To move a patient who must remain in the horizontal position—for example, from a bed to a stretcher—three people are usually needed. The tallest person takes the top third of the patient. This person usually has the longest reach and can most easily support the patient's head and shoulders. The second person supports the middle third of the patient. The shortest person supports the patient's legs. To coordinate movements, the three people must work by counting aloud; the leader, who takes the head of the patient, calls the numbers. The technique of moving a patient from the bed to a stretcher is outlined in Procedure 29.10.

Transferring a patient from a chair to the toilet or commode is the same as transferring from the bed to a chair,

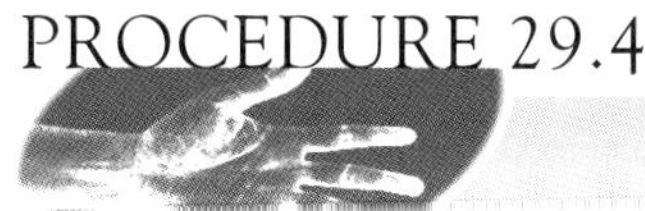

PROCEDURE 29.4

Moving a Patient Up in Bed: Total Assist (Two Persons)

Action	Rationale
1. Follow step 1 of Procedure 29.1.	
2. Remove all pillows; place one pillow at head of bed.	Protects patient's head.
3. Both nurses stand at sides of the bed looking towards the head of the bed.	Movement of the patient is more coordinated.
4. The leader places one arm under the patient's neck and shoulders, supporting the head, and the other arm under shoulder and lower ribs. The second nurse places his or her hands under the patient's buttocks and upper thighs.	Enables equal distribution of body weight.
Drawsheet: Roll the draw sheet close to the patient. Ask the patient to place his or her arms over the chest and flex the knees, if able. It is important to note that with a draw sheet or a lift sheet, the patient is lifted, not dragged.	Acts as a sling to lift the patient upward in bed.

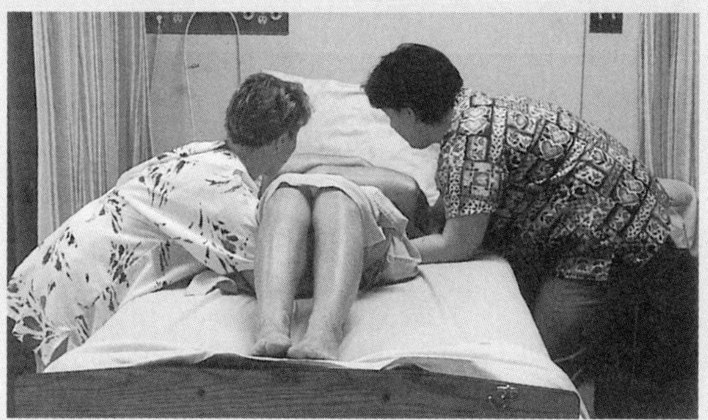

Action	Rationale
5. At leader's direction, the nurses move the patient up in bed by transferring weight to their forward foot.	Promotes smooth, coordinated effort.
6. Follow step 9 of Procedure 29.1.	

with some modification. In moving from a sitting to standing position from a chair, the patient places both feet on the floor, with the legs angled slightly backward behind knees. This provides a base of support, directly below the patient's centre of gravity. The patient then leans forward and, using the arms of the chair, pushes to a standing position. Assistance may be required to help the patient manage clothing. Grab bars and a raised toilet seat facilitate the patient's independence and safety.

TRANSFERRING AND LIFTING DEVICES

There are a number of devices that nurses can use to make the work of lifting, transferring and moving patients easier and safer. These include transfer belts, lift sheets, sliding boards and mechanical devices such as the hydraulic lift.

TRANSFER BELT The main objectives of using a transfer belt are to provide security when moving a patient and to minimize the risks of musculoskeletal injury to both the patient and the health professional. The belt provides a means of guiding a patient's movement from a point close to the patient's centre of gravity while avoiding the use of arms as levers. One of the most important effects of the transfer belt is to extend the reach of the nurse, as the centre of gravity of the patient is the most important factor to control. The belt is positioned securely around the patient's hips; the nurse guides movement by grasping the belt. The nurse should ensure that female patients' breasts are not under the transfer belt. Health professionals who do a lot of patient transfers might consider owning their own transfer belt.

THE LIFT SHEET/DRAW SHEET A lift sheet (catch pad or full sheet folded in half) placed under a dependent patient is a useful aid for changing position in many situations. The lift sheet extends from the patient's arm level to the bottom of the buttocks. At least two nurses are needed to move a patient by this means. The nurses stand on opposite sides of the patient, grasp the lift sheet firmly near the patient and move the patient and lift sheet to the desired position, for example, up in the bed or towards the side (Eustace, 1991). Figure 29.4 illustrates the use of a lift sheet to move a patient up in bed.

To turn a patient to the side, the arms and legs are first positioned safely. The nurse then reaches palms down over

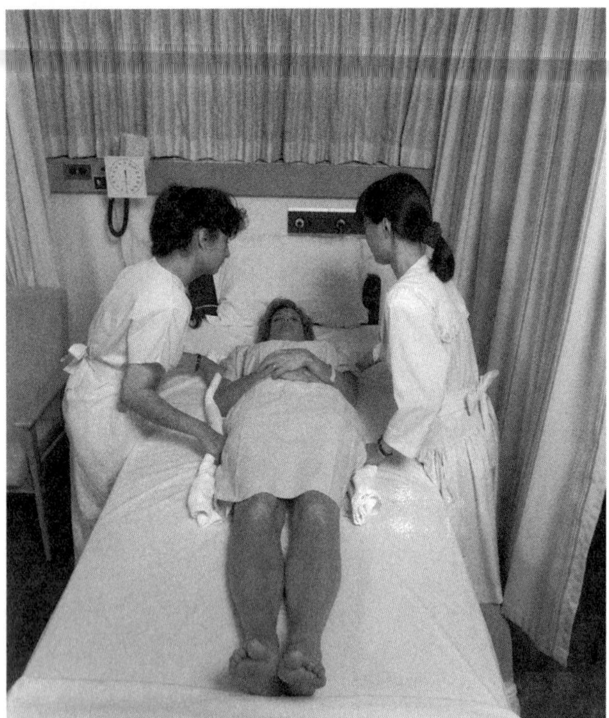

FIGURE 29.4 The use of a lift sheet to move a patient up in bed

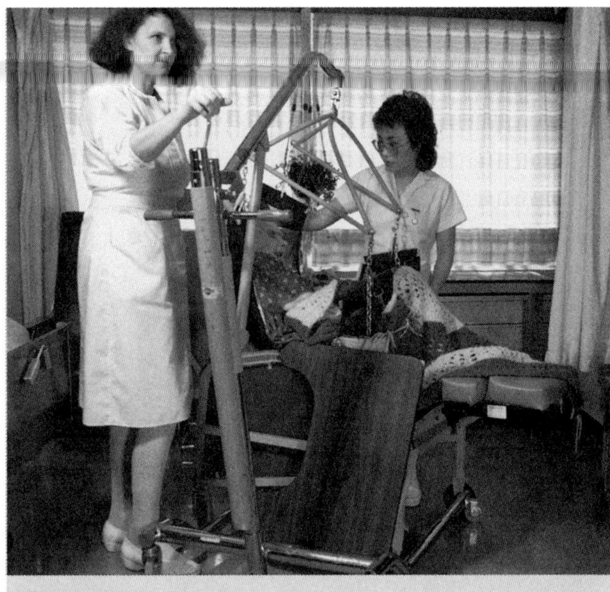

A mechanical lift.

the patient, grasps the lift sheet on the far side, and pulls it forward in such a way that the patient rolls on the side towards the nurse.

SLIDING BOARD A sliding board is a hard plastic board approximately the same length as a hospital bed with cut-out handles. It is placed underneath the patient's drawsheet; the patient is rolled onto the board, and the board is used to slide the patient from the bed to the stretcher. Nurses should receive instruction on the safe use of this equipment.

MECHANICAL DEVICES A wide variety of mechanical devices are available for moving a patient. One is the hydraulic lift, which can raise a person and offers safe, supportive movement. Washable nylon slings fit under the patient's buttocks and back to provide support. These lifts can be used to assist a patient in and out of the bathtub and in and out of bed. The nurse must be taught to use mechanical lifts properly and must have sufficient help to carry out the procedure safely.

Health-Restoring Strategies

Health-restoring strategies involve interventions that help individuals to regain mobility following acute illness or traumatic injury or enable independent movement for people with chronic neurological or musculoskeletal conditions. For instance, mobility interventions may allow a patient with multiple sclerosis to move around with the support of a cane or a walker.

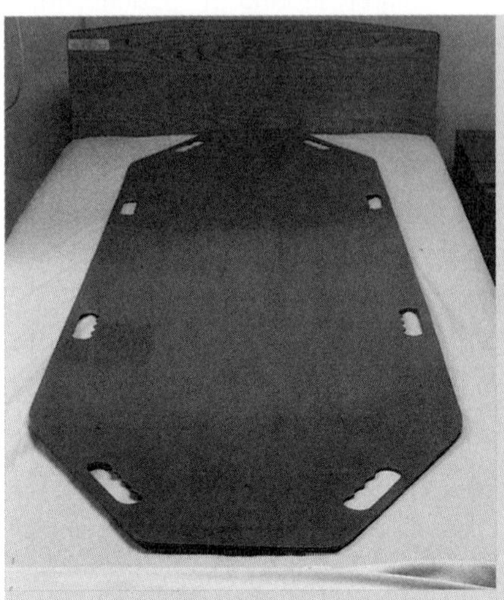

A. An illustration of a sliding board

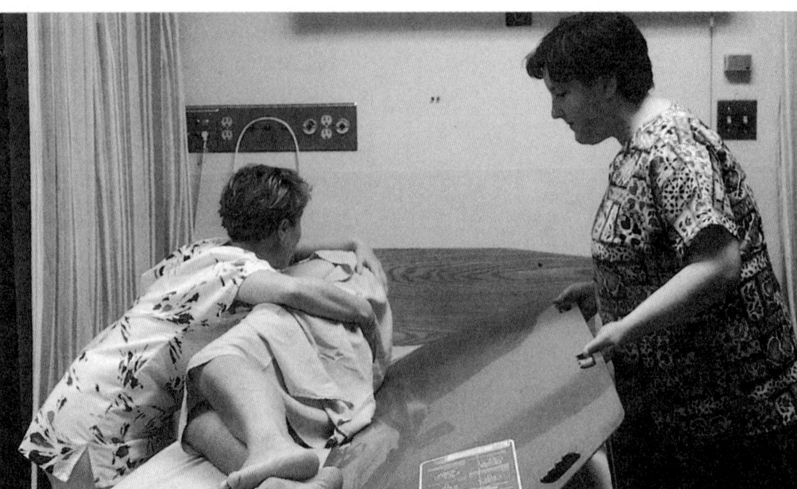

B. Nurses using a sliding board to transfer a patient

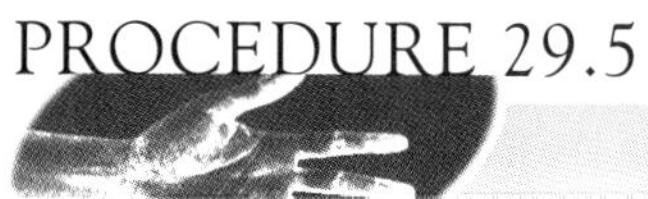

Moving a Patient Up in Bed: Partial Assist (One Person)

Action	*Rationale*
1. Follow step 1 of Procedure 29.1.	
2. Remove all pillows; place one pillow at head of bed.	Protects patient's head.
3. Help the patient get into position with knees flexed and feet flat on the bed, heels near the buttocks.	Permits the patient to use the femoral muscles for movement.

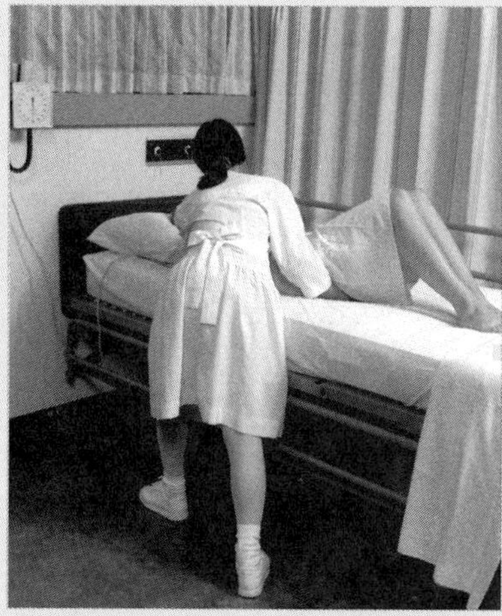

Action	*Rationale*
4. Stand at the side of the bed, facing towards the direction of the movement. One foot is a step in front of the other; the foot that is closer to the bed is positioned to the rear.	Prevents twisting of the nurse's body during the movement.
5. Place one arm under the patient's shoulders and one arm under the upper thighs.	Provides support to heaviest parts of the body.
6. Instruct the patient to place the chin on the chest and push with the feet on count of 3. On the count of 3, shift weight from the rear foot to the forward foot and move the patient up as the patient pushes downward with the feet. The patient may also assist by pulling on an overhead bed bar (trapeze) or by pushing on bent elbows.	Movement is coordinated through a predetermined count of "1-2-3-up." Provides momentum to overcome inertia. Encourages independence.
7. Follow step 9 of Procedure 29.1.	Encourage patient to help in any way they can.

PREPARATION FOR WALKING

Everything possible should be done to help individuals maintain strength and tone in the muscles that are needed for walking, or to regain these if they have deteriorated because of illness. Patients who will require a walker, crutches or a cane need to gain additional strength in their hand, arm and shoulder muscles because much of the weight of the body is supported by these muscles when such aids are used. All patients must strengthen the leg and abdominal muscles in preparation for walking. If active exercises are not contraindicated, the patient should be encouraged to do these while in bed.

Active exercises for patients who require additional strength in the arms and shoulders in preparation for crutch- or walker-assisted ambulation include push-ups and pull-ups.

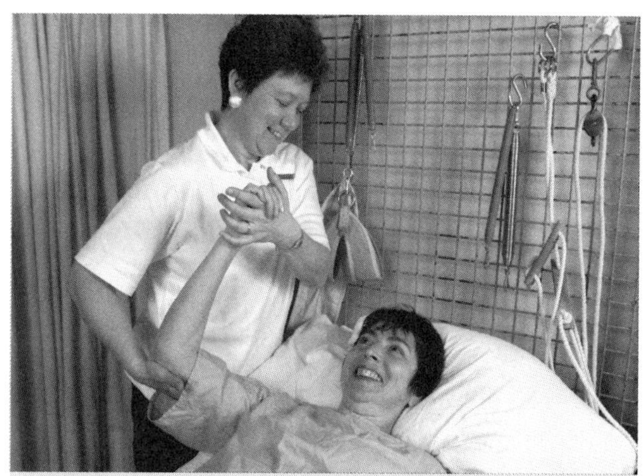

Regaining movement in an injured joint requires gradually increasing exercise.

PROCEDURE 29.6

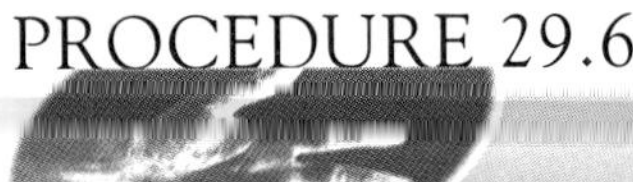

Turning a Patient from a Supine to Side-Lying Position

Action	Rationale
1. Follow step 1 of Procedure 29.1.	
2. Assist the patient to the far side of the bed in supine position.	Keeps the patient away from the edge of the bed when the turn is completed.
3. Stand at the side of the bed towards which the patient is to be turned.	Patient will roll towards the nurse; this allows the nurse to control the amount of turn.
4. Place the patient's far arm across the chest and flex both knees. Check that the patient's near arm is lateral to and away from the body, with palm down.	Uses the patient's weight when rolling. Prevents the patient from rolling on arm during the turn.
5. Stand opposite the patient's waist and face the side of the bed, with one foot a step in front of the other. Slightly flex the knees and put your weight on the leg nearest the bed.	Nurse's body is in the direction of movement, with a wide base of support.

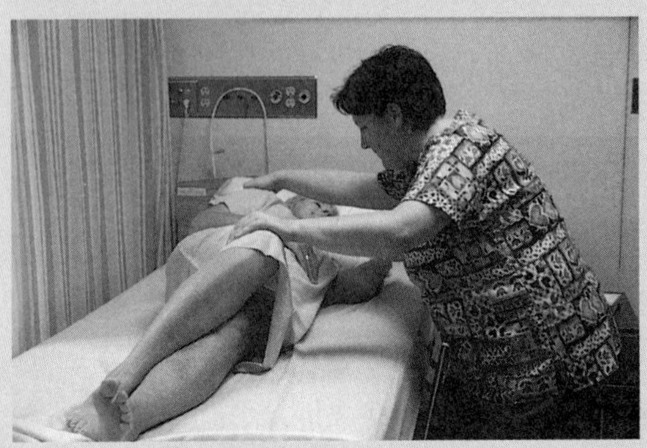

Action	Rationale
6. Place one hand behind the patient's neck over to the patient's far shoulder and the other on both knees. A draw sheet may also be used. The hand position on the draw sheet is the same.	Nurse's weight is used to turn patient.
7. While shifting weight from the forward leg to the rear leg, roll the patient towards you as you move.	Shifting weight provides additional turning force by using large muscle groups.

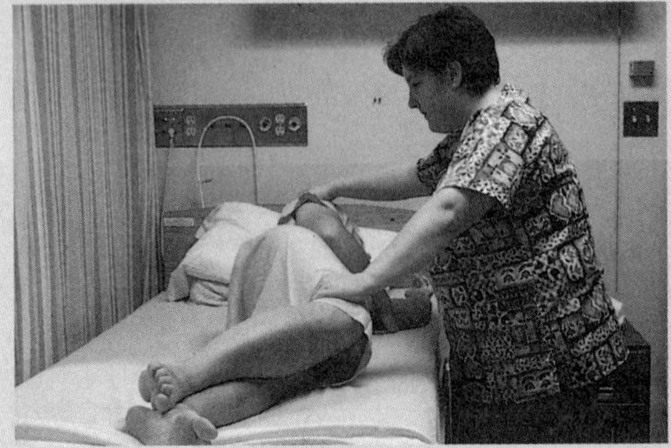

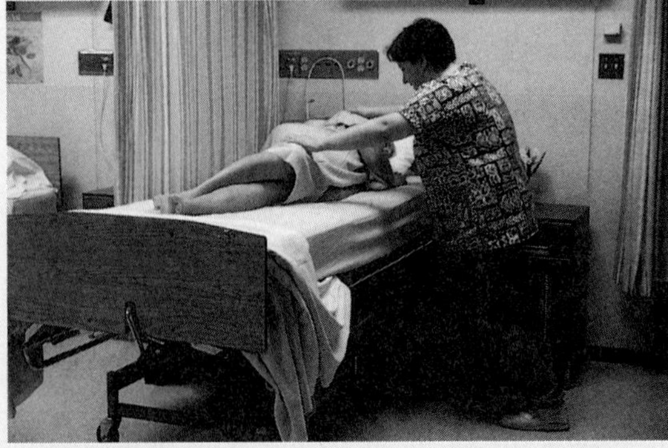

Action	Rationale
8. The patient is stopped by the nurse's elbows, which come to rest on the mattress at the edge of the bed.	Provides security for patient.
9. Place pillows under the head, along the back and between the legs.	Provides support and comfort and maintains body alignment.
10. Check for good body alignment and reposition as necessary.	Prevents muscle strain.
11. Follow step 9 of Procedure 29.1.	

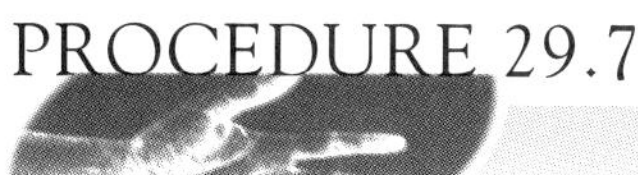

PROCEDURE 29.7 Turning a Patient from a Supine to Semi-Prone (Sims' or Recovery) Position

Action	*Rationale*
1. Follow step 1 of Procedure 29.1.	
2. Move the patient to far side of the bed in supine position.	Ensures the patient will roll to the centre of the bed.
3. Stand on opposite side of bed.	Patient will roll towards the nurse.
4. Tuck the patient's near arm under the buttock. Place a pillow on bed next to the patient's chest. Flex the patient's far leg.	Prepares for the turn. The patient will roll onto the pillow. Uses the patient's weight when turning.
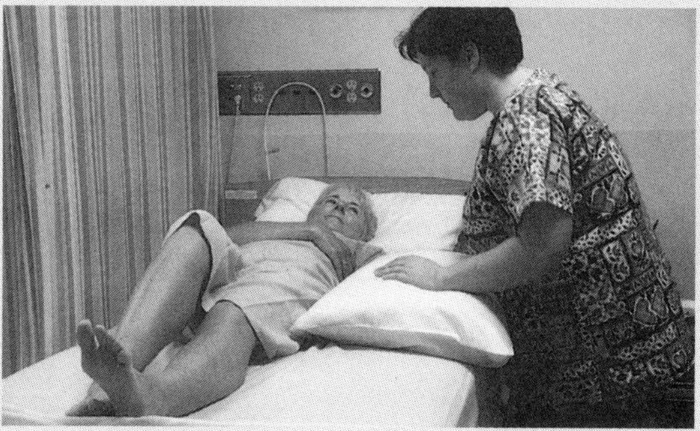	
5. Following steps 5 and 6 of Procedure 29.6, turn the patient, rolling over the bottom shoulder so that the arm is behind the patient.	
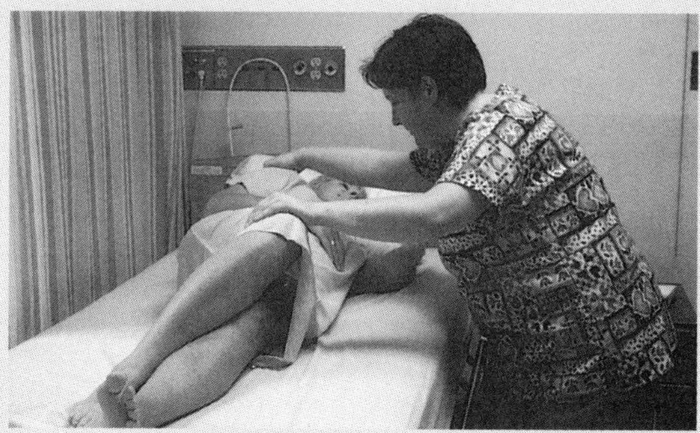	
6. Release the patient's arm from under the buttock.	Maintains patient comfort.
7. Reposition the patient's head.	Maintains an unobstructed airway.
8. Place pillows under head and chest and between legs.	Maintains comfort and body alignment.
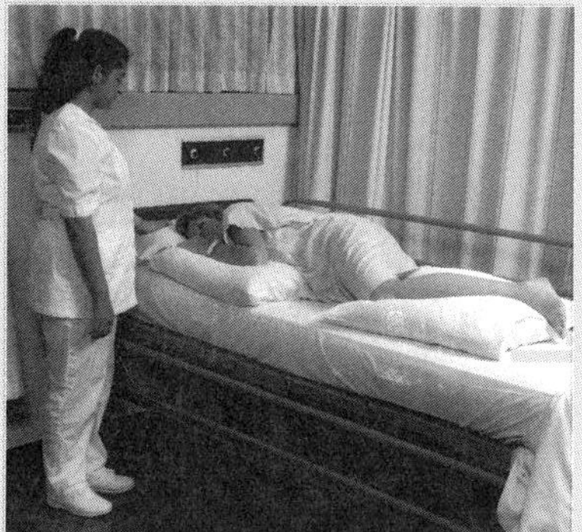	
9. Check for good body alignment and reposition as necessary.	Prevents muscle strain.
10. Follow step 9 of Procedure 29.1.	

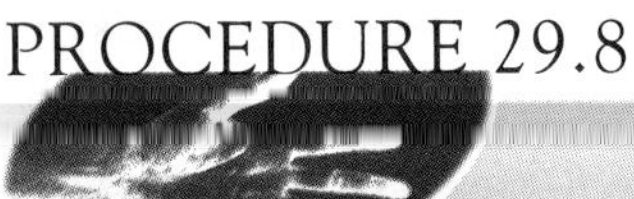

PROCEDURE 29.8 Assisting a Patient to a Sitting Position on the Edge of the Bed (Dangling)

Action	Rationale
1. Assist the patient to a side-lying position, with knees bent and lower legs at edge of bed.	Prepares for the change of position.
2. Raise the head of the bed.	Reduces gravitational force; decreases postural hypotension.
3. Facing the far bottom corner of the bed, support the patient's shoulders with one arm behind the patient's neck, while using the other arm to help the patient extend the lower legs over the side of the bed. Assume a broad stance with the foot that is towards the bottom of the bed positioned to the rear of the other foot.	Nurse's body faces the direction of movement. Provides greater stability and balance, and facilitates use of large muscle groups.
4. While still supporting the patient's shoulders, bring the legs forward close to the edge of the bed. Bring the patient to a natural sitting position on the edge of the bed by pivoting in such a manner that the patient's lower legs are swung downward to the floor. The nurse's weight is shifted from the rear leg to the front leg.	Promotes patient safety. The nurse's weight is used for momentum.

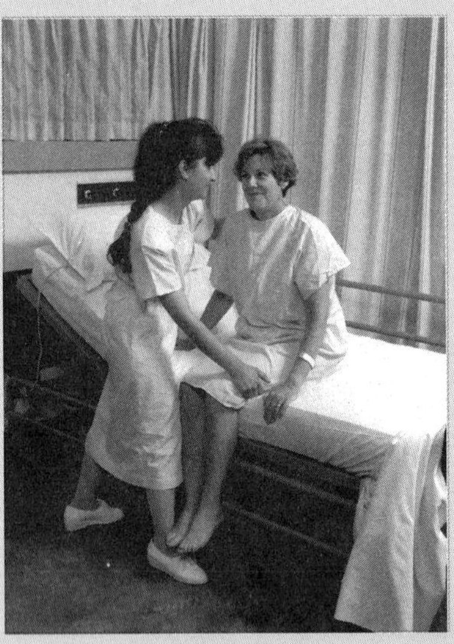

Action	Rationale
5. The patient assists as able by using the elbow to push up from side-lying position.	Promotes independence.

Push-ups are performed while sitting in a chair. The patient raises the buttocks off the chair seat by pushing down on the hands, while keeping the elbows straight. In pull-ups, the patient pulls him- or herself from a lying to a sitting position. A trapeze supported from a Balkan frame is often used to assist patients to pull themselves up to a sitting position if they are unable to manage it unassisted. Another exercise for strengthening hand, arm and shoulder muscles is to have the patient lie flat in bed, reach up to grasp the head of the bed, and pull him- or herself up in the bed.

AMBULATION

It is often necessary for patients to relearn to walk, often with the aid of crutches, walkers or canes. This is usually the responsibility of the rehabilitation department, but it is beneficial for the nurse to be aware of correct use of these aids to ambulation in order to assist the patient.

The patient may be learning to walk again following an extended period of bed rest. Preparing the patient for this task involves both psychological and physical measures. The nurse can help the patient to gain confidence in the ability to walk again. Often encouragement and faith in the patient's ability can bolster self-confidence. If an appropriate exercise program has been maintained throughout illness, the task is easier. Before attempting to stand, the patient must first learn to maintain good trunk balance in a sitting position. Then, he or she must achieve good trunk balance in a standing position before attempting to walk.

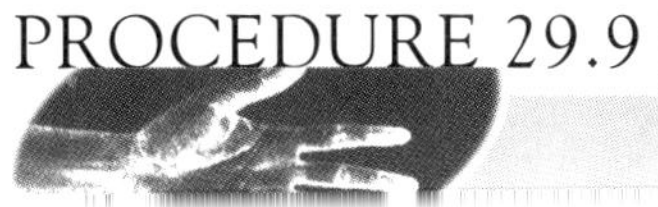

PROCEDURE 29.9 Transferring a Patient from the Bed to a Chair

Action	*Rationale*
1. Lower the bed to a height from which the patient can step naturally to the floor.	Facilitates ease of movement and promotes patient safety.
2. Help the patient assume a sitting position on the edge of the bed and put on the patient's shoes and dressing gown. The patient should wear supportive, nonslip footwear.	Prepares for the transfer. Promotes patient dignity and safety.
3. Place a chair at the side of the bed at a right angle to the bed. Position the chair to the stronger side of the patient. If a wheelchair is being used, secure the brakes and remove the arm and footrest closest to bed.	Enables the patient to use stronger extremities for support. Provides for safety.
4. Stand facing the patient with your feet externally rotated on either side of the patient's feet.	This position prevents the patient's feet from sliding forward as the patient is pulled off the bed.
5. Secure a transfer belt around the patient's waist as described in the section on transfer belts. If one is not available, place your hands over patient's posterior iliac crest. Instruct the patient to place his or her hands lightly around your lower waist.	Promotes patient's sense of security and provides support during the transfer. Allows the nurse to guide movement. Enhances the patient's sense of security and ease of movement.
6. As the patient stands, guide the movement by flexing the knees and positioning the forward knee against the patient's knee.	Prevents the patient's knee from bending involuntarily (buckling).

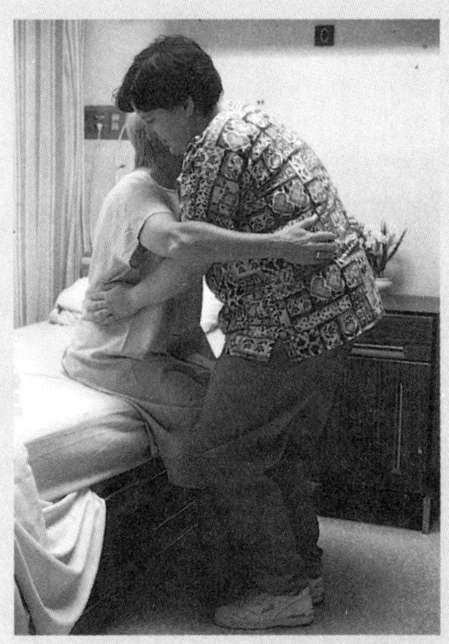

Action	*Rationale*
7. Pivot with the patient while maintaining a wide base of support.	Maintains nurse's balance and stability.
8. Instruct the patient to move backwards until it is possible to feel the back of the chair on the knees and, at the same time, reach for an arm of the chair with an available hand. Ask the patient to bend forward at the waist and squat until he or she is almost in the chair, then to slide the weight towards the back of the chair.	Promotes the patient's sense of space and prevents the patient from sitting down too quickly. Prevents the nurse from having to control the patient as he or she drops down into the chair.

PROCEDURE 29.10 Transferring a Patient from the Bed to a Stretcher

Action	Rationale
1. Move the patient to the side of the bed as in Procedures 29.1 and 29.2.	
2. Position stretcher alongside the bed; raise the bed to the level of the stretcher.	Promotes patient safety.
3. Lock the wheels of the stretcher.	Prevents stretcher from moving during transfer.
4. Have the patient fold his or her arms across the chest.	Makes it easier to move the patient.
5. Two nurses stand on the stretcher side of the bed: one at the head, the other at the trunk. The third nurse positions herself or himself on the bed at the patient's waist level. The nurses grasp the drawsheet at the patient's waist and shoulder.	Decreases risk for injury and maintains body alignment.
6. If a sliding board is available, place it underneath the patient between the bed and the stretcher.	Facilitates easier transfer for nurse and patient.
7. On count of three, the patient is transferred, using a lifting motion.	
8. Raise head of stretcher; raise side rails and cover patient with a blanket.	Provides safety and comfort.

RESEARCH to practice

Goodridge, D., & Laurila, B. (1997). Minimizing transfer injuries. *Canadian Nurse, 93(7)*, 38–41.

Haley and Colgate (1990) identified that, in an eight-hour shift, nurses can lift a cumulative average of two tonnes. Approximately 40 percent of nurses who leave the profession do so because of back pain and injury (Stubbs, Buckle & Hudson, 1983).

The purpose of this retrospective study was to examine injuries sustained by nursing staff during patient handling. The study was carried out at the Riverview Health Centre in Winnipeg, Manitoba.

Data were collected by an interdisciplinary task team that consisted of nurses, physiotherapists and occupational therapists. Data were obtained using secondary sources, for example, incident reports and staff health statistics from 1991 to 1994. Transferring patients (43%) was identified as the highest injury-related task for nurses. The next most common cause of injury was positioning patients in bed (24%), followed by lifting (19%), catching a falling patient (6%), positioning a patient in a chair (4%) and other physical assistance (3%). Data revealed that back injuries were the most reported injury, with shoulder and wrist injuries the next most common complaint.

The team recommended implementation of a transfer assessment program. Two units were used to pilot the program. A number of different transferring aids were evaluated on the designated trial units. Within 24 hours of a patient's admission, nursing staff completed the trial transfer assessment form to identify patient mobility status and appropriate transfer aid. The patient's Kardex, bedside bulletin board, walker and wheelchair were assigned the appropriate pictorial decal that indicated the patient's required level of transfer assistance.

Two years after the end of the pilot program, a significant decline was identified in injuries related to patient transfers. Prior to the initiation of the pilot program, the monthly injury rate was 6.7 percent. Three months after the start of the program, the injury rate had dropped to 3.2 percent.

The program was adopted and continues to be used at this agency. Ongoing audits have demonstrated that compliance with the transfer assessment program has been excellent. For any program to work, it must be simple enough for staff to understand and implement it, and have management support and sufficient resources. However, further comparative research is needed to validate the benefits of this type of transfer assessment program.

When a standing position can be maintained with confidence and balance, a few steps can be tried. Since good balance is essential and the patient must feel steady, it is

pers are worn when standing or walking. The patient should not be allowed to become fatigued and should attempt only short distances at first. The nurse can help to promote the patient's feelings of self-confidence by helping to set small goals for each day's activity and acknowledging the accomplishment of these goals.

Most patients who are learning to walk again require physical support when first starting. There are three ways the nurse can provide this support. The nurse can place the arm that is nearer the patient under the arm at the elbow and grasp the patient's hand. The nurse synchronizes walking steps with the patient's, moving the inside foot forward at the same time as the patient's inside foot. A second method is to grasp the patient's left hand in the nurse's left hand, and encircle the patient's waist with the right hand. Again, the walking is synchronized to provide as wide a base of support as possible. The patient can also be supported during walking by being held at the waist from the rear with the use of a transfer belt. This helps the patient maintain balance. If the patient requires more support than this, it is advisable for the nurse to have a second person to assist in the activity.

In some cases, however, the nurse may have to assist a patient with weakness on one side of the body to walk without the help of a second person. To do this, the nurse stands at the patient's weak side. The nurse puts the arm that is nearest to the patient under the patient's arm and grasps the inside of the upper arm. With his or her far arm, the nurse reaches over and takes hold of the patient's lower arm or hand. In this position, the nurse can also provide support with his or her leg to the patient's weakened one if necessary, providing maximum support for the affected side (see Figure 29.5). Keeping hands on the patient has the advantage of increasing the patient's proprioception to regain balance skills often lost with extended immobility, joint disease or injury.

CRUTCH WALKING

It may be necessary for people to use crutches for a period of time. The patient needs to be measured for crutches and taught how to walk with them.

Measuring a Patient for Crutches

Several methods are used to measure a person for an underarm crutch. One method is to measure the distance from the patient's axilla to the heel of the foot, while the patient is in bed with shoes on. Five centimetres are then subtracted from this distance. A second method is to measure from the anterior fold of the axilla to a point 15 cm lateral to the heel. The top of the crutch should be two to three fingerwidths from the armpit when elbows are flexed approximately 30 degrees. When crutches are the correct length, the hand bar permits slight flexion of the elbow, and the weight is borne by the hand and arms rather than at the axilla. The nerves in the axilla are not protected against pressure except by a layer of fat, which is compressible. If weight is borne on the axilla, the pressure may result in nerve damage and, possibly, paralysis. For this reason the top of the crutch should be five centimetres below the axilla and should not be padded initially.

Safety Measures for Crutch Walking

- Check height of crutches
- Check rubber tips
- Assess environment
- Nonslip footwear should be worn.

Teaching Crutch Walking

Patients should be taught more than one gait. The reason for this is twofold: the patient can use a slow or fast gait as necessary and, since each gait requires a different combination of muscles, gaits can be changed when the patient is fatigued. There are five basic crutch gaits in crutch walking.

1. **Two-point crutch gait:** This gait has the following sequence: right crutch and left foot simultaneously; left crutch and right foot simultaneously.
2. **Three-point crutch gait:** This gait has the following sequence: both crutches and the weaker limb; then the stronger limb.
3. **Four-point crutch gait:** This gait has the following sequence: right crutch, left foot, left crutch, right foot. This is a particularly safe gait because there are always three points of support on the floor at one time.
4. **Tripod gaits:** There are two tripod gaits. A. The patient puts the crutches forward simultaneously and then drags the body forward. B. The patient puts the crutches forward one at a time and then drags the body forward.
5. **Swing gaits:** There are two swing gaits. A. The patient puts the crutches forward and then swings the body up to the crutches. B. The patient swings the body beyond the crutches.

WALKING WITH A WALKER

There are a variety of walkers available to provide support while walking. A safe distance for moving the walker ahead is about 30 cm. The affected leg moves at the same time that the walker is advanced forward. Walker height should be adjusted for maximum efficiency. There should be approximately 15 degrees of flexion of the elbow.

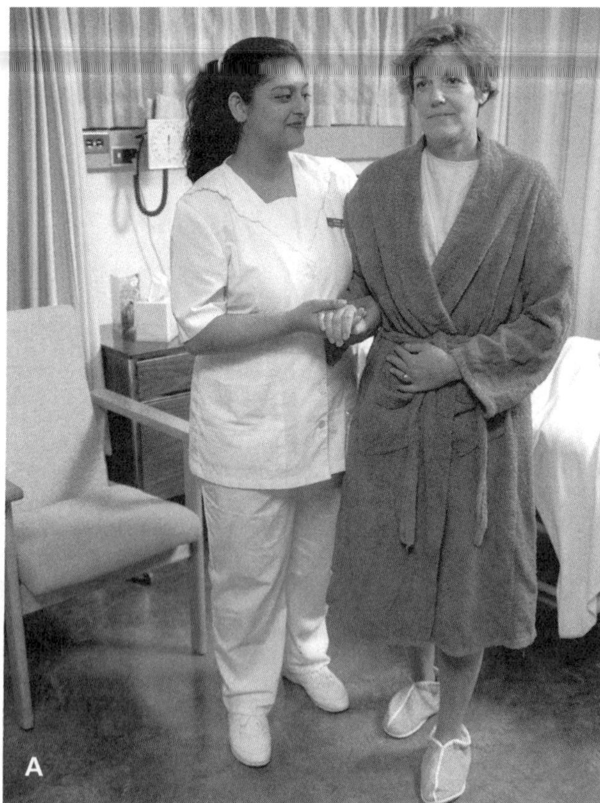

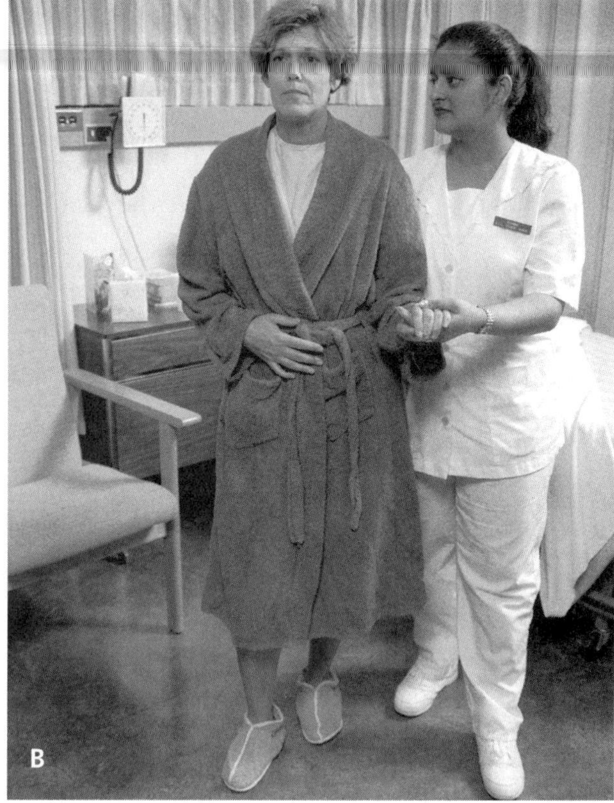

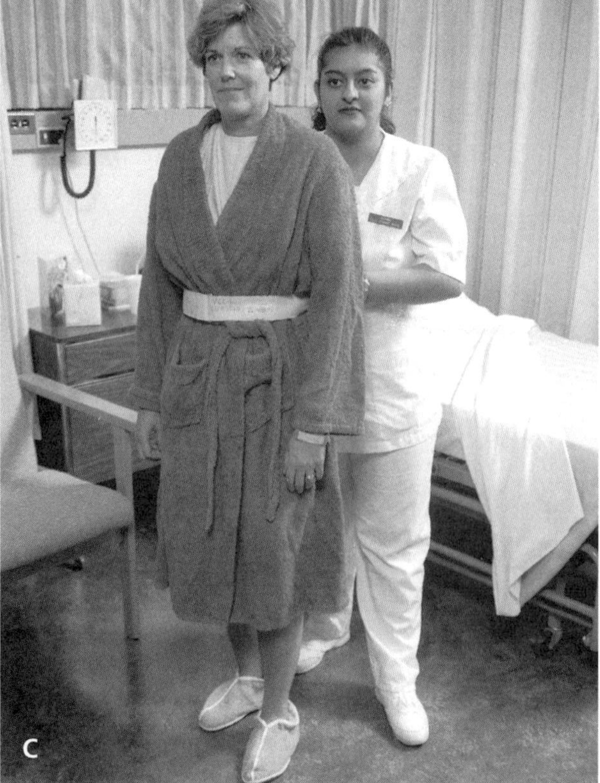

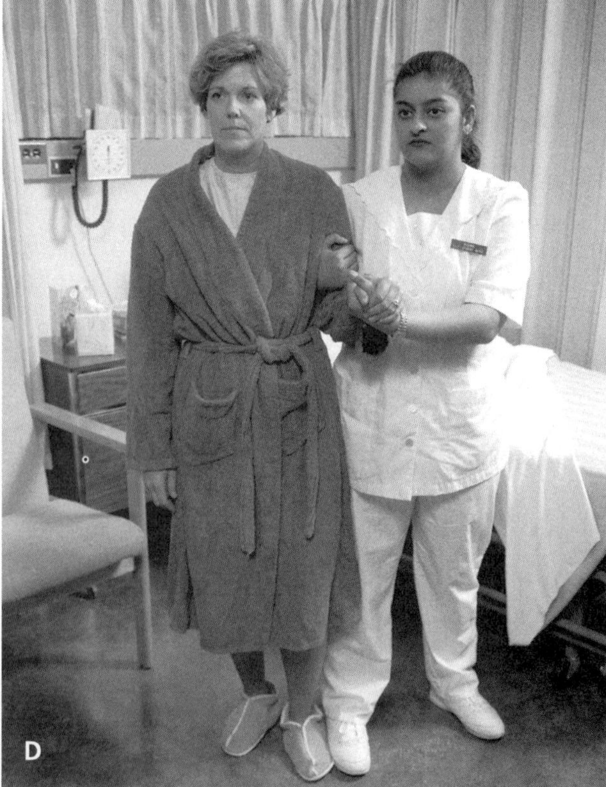

FIGURE 29.5 Supporting the patient while walking. A. The nurse supports the patient under the arm at the elbow and grasps the patient's hand. B. The nurse grasps the patient's left hand in the left hand and encircles the patient's waist with the right hand. C. The nurse supports the patient from the rear with the use of a transfer belt. D. The nurse supports the patient with one-sided weakness

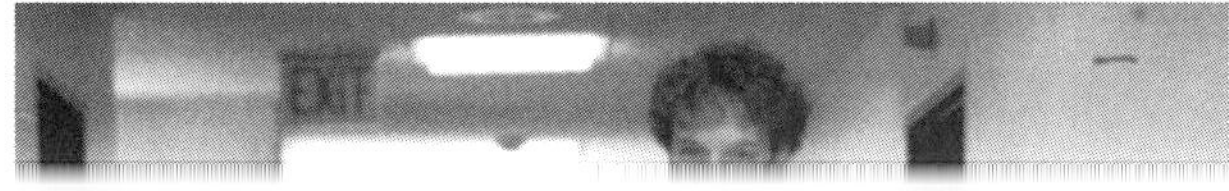

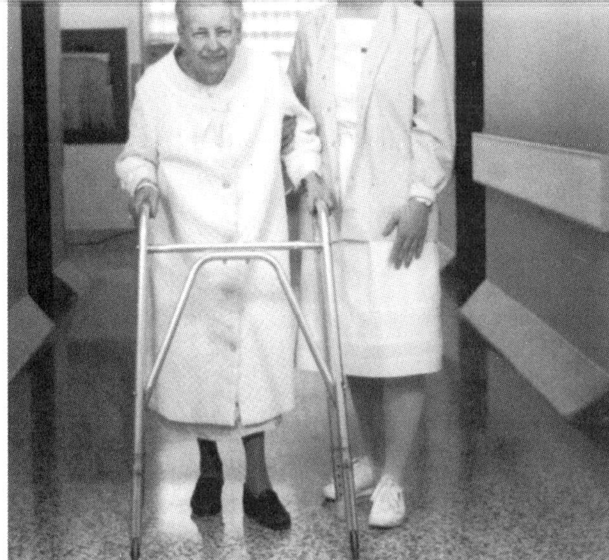

A walker is often used to assist patients who are relearning to walk following illness.

WALKING WITH A CANE

When a patient gradually becomes stronger and has more balance and stability, a cane may be indicated. The patient holds the cane on the strong side of the body. The cane moves forward at the same time that the affected leg moves forward. Stability is increased since there are always two points on the floor as the patient advances (about a 30-cm length at a time). To climb stairs, the patient steps up on the good leg, then follows with the cane and affected leg on the next step. To go down stairs, the procedure is reversed.

ADAPTING TO THE HOME ENVIRONMENT

With the shift in the focus of health care from acute care to community settings, more individuals with mobility problems are returning to home environments. Discharge planning units focus on assisting individuals to be functionally independent by teaching ways to adapt to the environment and to carry out activities of daily living. Occupational therapists assess individual abilities by visiting the home with the patient and seeing what adjustments might have to be made. The occupational therapist may observe the patient cooking a meal or walking up stairs. The therapist will also assess the physical environment in terms of safety and function. The patient may require a homemaker to come in and help with light housekeeping chores, or a community organization such as Meals-on-Wheels to provide the main meal of the day on a daily basis. Many alternatives are available in the community to assist a patient in making the transition from hospital to home. Through a collaborated effort on the part of the patient (and family) and the health team, suitable arrangements may be made.

Evaluating Movement and Exercise Interventions

If the expected outcomes of the nursing interventions have been sufficiently explicit, the process of evaluating the effectiveness of these becomes relatively simple. Have the expected outcomes been achieved? Is the patient's range of motion extended? Can the patient do more of the exercises independently? Does the patient carry out isometric exercises independently, the prescribed number of times as stated in the goals?

The nurse also keeps in mind the long-range goals of nursing action. Have unused muscles for which movement is not contraindicated been maintained in strength and tone? Has the process of degeneration been prevented in these muscles? Have contractures that could interfere with joint mobility been prevented? Has joint mobility been maintained? Have muscular strength and tone been improved? Has the patient regained independence in carrying out activities of daily living or making progress towards this? What progress has been made towards this goal? If the patient requires help in moving to carry out these activities, has help been received when needed, and in such a way as to enable maintenance of other functional abilities? Is there optimal functioning of all other abilities?

IN REVIEW

- Movement and exercise are necessary for fulfilling basic human needs.
- Free movement allows us to:
    - carry out activities of daily living
    - work
    - play
    - protect ourselves
    - communicate.
- Coordinated movement is brought about by the:
    - skeletal system
    - muscular system
    - nervous system
    - circulatory system.
- Movement is easier when the body is in proper alignment. When the weight of the body is evenly distributed, there is a wide base of support and a lower centre of gravity.

- Capacity for movement for exercise is influenced by age and phase of the life cycle.
- The development of coordinated movement begins in infancy and continues throughout childhood and adolescence.
- Strength, endurance and motor coordination reach maximum potential in late adolescence and early adulthood and gradually decline through middle and late adulthood.
- Regular exercise slows the aging process and maintains cardiovascular functioning, pulmonary reserve, bone density and physical strength and endurance.
- Many factors affect movement and exercise. Conditions that interfere with the integrity of muscles, bones, joints and nerves include:
  - bed rest
  - environment
  - lifestyle
  - immobility.
- Common problems associated with movement include:
  - impaired motor function
  - limited range of motion
  - decreased muscle strength
  - lack of balance and coordination
  - pain and discomfort.
- To assess the need for movement and exercise, the nurse uses information from the health history to determine the patient's:
  - usual level of activity and exercise
  - ease of movement and motor function
  - need for assistive devices.
- Physical assessment is performed to determine:
  - integrity of the skeletal system (joints for ROM)
  - muscle structure and symmetry (size, tone, strength, endurance)
  - posture and body alignment
  - balance and coordination.
- Common nursing diagnoses pertaining to mobility status include:
  - *Impaired Physical Mobility*
  - *Activity Intolerance*
  - *Self-Care Deficits*
  - *Risk for Injury*
  - *Powerlessness*
  - *Altered Health Maintenance.*
- Care is planned and implemented to maintain, strengthen and restore mobility and motor function, to prevent further deterioration in function and to promote optimal functioning in daily living.
- To maintain physical fitness, it is important to participate in some form of regular activity and exercise at least three times a week for 30 min.
- Muscle-strengthening exercises and active or passive ROM can be used for patients prescribed bed rest. These exercises:
  - promote circulation
  - maintain muscle tone
  - promote flexibility
  - prevent joint stiffness and contractures.
- Good posture and efficient use of body mechanics are essential for health. Principles of body mechanics are particularly important for nurses when transferring, positioning and moving patients in the course of their practice.
- The nurse can use a number of devices to make the work of moving and transferring easier and safer. These include:
  - transfer belts
  - lift sheets
  - sliding boards
  - mechanical devices.
- Individuals may need help to regain mobility with the aid of assistive devices such as:
  - walkers
  - canes
  - crutches.
- Muscle-strengthening exercises are necessary in preparation for ambulation.
- Shoes with good support, as well as support provided by the nurse, can help the patient maintain balance and feel steady when ambulating.

Critical Thinking Activities

1. **Case Study:** Mr. Guy Francoeur, age 28, had his foot crushed in a logging accident 3 days ago. He works as a scaler for a large forest products company. Following surgery to repair the soft tissue damage, the physician has encased the foot in a cast. He has ordered that Mr. Francoeur remain in bed for an unspecified period of time. He has told Mr. Francoeur that when he is allowed up, he must learn to walk with crutches or use a wheelchair to get around in. Mr. Francoeur is a healthy, active individual and objects strongly to being confined to bed. He says he is not going to use a wheelchair if he can help it. He wants to know if there is anything he can do while in bed that will help him when he is allowed up from bed.

a. What information would you need to help you in planning Mr. Francoeur's care?

b. What sources would you use to obtain this

c. What problems might Mr. Francoeur have in addition to his impaired mobility?

d. What other health professionals might be involved in Mr. Francoeur's care?

e. What factors would you take into consideration in planning Mr. Francoeur's care?

f. What exercises might Mr. Francoeur do on his own to prevent the deterioration of muscular strength and tone? To prepare himself for using crutches?

g. What other help would Mr. Francoeur require in carrying out daily living activities?

2. With the aid of your instructor, arrange to spend a day with a physiotherapist or an occupational therapist in your agency. What types of care does this health care professional provide? In what ways do nurses collaborate with physiotherapists and occupational therapists to provide care in this agency?

KEY TERMS

body alignment p. 903
base of support p. 903
centre of gravity p. 903
line of gravity p. 903
contracture p. 906
aerobic exercise p. 912
isotonic exercises p. 912
isometric exercises p. 913
isokinetic exercises p. 913
range-of-motion exercises p. 915
active ROM p. 915
passive ROM p. 915
plantar flexion p. 915
dorsiflexion p. 915

References

BERGER, K.J., & WILLIAMS, M.B. (1998). *Fundamentals of nursing: Collaborating for optimal health.* (2nd. ed.) Norwalk, CT: Appleton & Lange.

CARPENITO, L.J. (1997). *Nursing diagnosis: Application to clinical practice.* (7th ed.). Philadelphia: Lippincott.

CORBIN, C.B., & LINDSEY, R. (1994). *Concepts of fitness and wellness: With laboratories.* Madison, WI: Brown & Benchmark.

EBERSOLE, P., & HESS, P. (1998). *Towards healthy aging: Human needs and nursing response.* (5th ed.). St. Louis: Mosby.

EUSTACE, C. (1991). Back up and wait. *RN, 54*(6), 49–51.

GOODRIDGE, D., & LAURILA, B. (1997). Minimizing transfer injuries. *Canadian Nurse, 93*(7), 38–41.

GREENBERG, J., & DINTIMAN, G. (1992). *Exploring health: Expanding the boundaries of wellness.* Englewood Cliffs, NJ: Prentice Hall.

HALEY, E. (1994). One approach to patient lifting. *Canadian Nurse, 90*(1), 57–58.

HALEY, E., & COLGATE, W. (1990). Standing up for your back. *Canadian Nurse, 86*(11), 26–27.

LALONDE, M. (1974). *A new perspective on the health of Canadians*

MEISSNER, J.E. (1980). Evaluate your patient's level of independence. *Nursing 80, 10,* 72–73.

OLSEN, E.V., & JOHNSON, B.J. (1990, March). The hazards of immobility. *American Journal of Nursing, 90,* 43–44; 46–48.

PORTH, C.M. (1998). *Pathophysiology: Concepts of altered health states.* (5th ed.). Philadelphia: Lippincott.

STUBBS, D.A., BUCKLE, P.N., & HUDSON, M.P. (1983). Back pain in the nursing profession: The effectiveness of training. *Ergonomics, 26,* 767–779.

TIMARIS, P.S. (1988). Aging of skeleton, joints, and muscle. In P. S. Timaris (Ed.). *Physiological basis of geriatrics.* New York: Macmillan.

WILLIAMS, M. H. (1993). *Lifetime fitness and wellness.* (3rd ed.). Madison, WI: Brown & Benchmark.

Additional Readings

ALEXANDER, R.M. (1992). *The human machine: How the body works.* New York: Columbia University Press.

ALISON, M. (1991). Aging and exercise: Improving the odds. *Harvard Health Letter, 16*(4), 4–6.

ANDERSON, S. (1990). The health club. *Canadian Nurse, 86*(6), 34–35.

CHARNEY, W. (1997). The lifting method for reducing back injuries: A ten-hospital study. *Journal of American Association of Occupational Health Nurses, 45*(6), 300–304.

DAWE, D., & CURRAN-SMITH, J. (1994). Going through the motions. *Canadian Nurse, 90*(1), 31–33.

De VRIES, H.A., & HOUSH, T.J. (1994). *Physiology of exercise.* (5th ed.). Madison, WI: Brown & Benchmark.

EXTON-SMITH, N. (1987). The patient's not for turning. *Nursing Times, 83,* 42–44.

GORDON, M. (1976). Assessing activity intolerance. *American Journal of Nursing, 76*(1), 72–75.

GRAY, J., CASS, J., HARPER, D.W., & O'HARA, P.A. (1996). A controlled evaluation of a lifts and transfers educational program for nurses. *Geriatric Nursing, 17*(2), 81–85.

HEESCHEN, S. (1989). Getting a handle on patient mobility. *Geriatric Nursing, 10,* 146–147.

JAMES, B., & PARKER, A.W. (1989). Active and passive mobility of lower limb joints in elderly men and women. *American Journal of Physical Medicine & Rehabilitation, 68*(4), 162–166.

KANE, M. (1994). Lifting: Why nurses follow bad practice. *Nursing Standard, 8*(5), 34–38.

LAFLIN, K., & AJA, D. (1995). Health care concerns related to lifting: An inside look at intervention strategies. *American Journal of Occupational Therapy, 49*(1), 63–72.

LAMMON, C.B., FOOTE, A.W., LELI, P.G., INGLE, J., & ADAMS, M.H. (1995). *Clinical nursing skills.* Philadelphia: W.B. Saunders.

MASON, D.J., & REDEKER, N. (1993). Measurement of activity. *Nursing Research, 42,* 87–91.

McCONNELL, E. (1990). Placing your patient in the lateral position. *Nursing 90, 20*(7), 65.

MILDE, F.K. (1988). Impaired physical mobility. *Journal of Gerontological Nursing, 14*, 20–24.

NEALE, C. (1997). The assessment of knowledge and application of proper body mechanics in the work place. *Orthopaedic Nursing, 16*(1), 66–69.

ODDY, R., & LODGE, L. (1993). Special support... Scheme to change patient handling practices in a continuing care ward. *Nursing Times, 89*(3), 44–46.

OWEN, B.D., & GARG, A. (1993). Back stress isn't part of the job. *American Journal of Nursing, 93*(2), 48–51.

PAYNE, V.G., & ISAACS, L.D. (1991). *Human motor development: A lifespan approach.* (2nd ed.). Mountain View, CA: Mayfield.

RUBIN, M. (1986). The physiology of bed-rest. *American Journal of Nursing, 86*(3), 8–50.

TARLING, C. (1992). The right equipment. *Nursing Times, 88*(50), 38–40.

WALTON, J. (1993). Lifting techniques for nurse-aiders. *British Journal of Nursing, 2*(7), 385–386; 388.

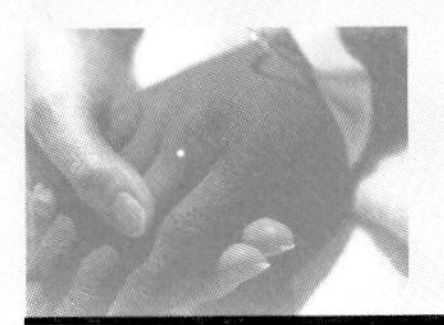

Protection and Safety Needs

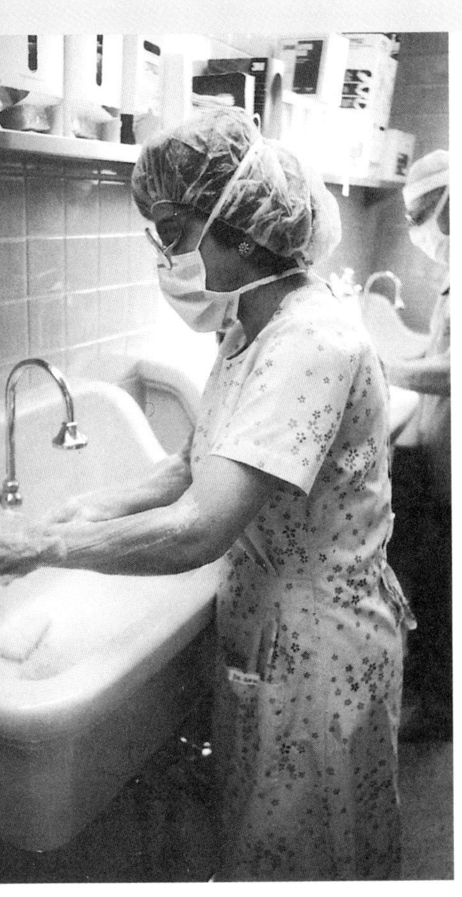

Chapter 30

Safety Needs

OUTLINE

Central Questions

1. What is the nurse's role in protecting against environmental hazards?
2. What are some of the factors affecting a person's capacity for self-protection?
3. How do protection and safety needs vary throughout the life cycle?
4. What are the five principal causes of accidental death in Canada?
5. What are some existing and potential hazards in the home, community, workplace and hospital?
6. How does the nurse assess an individual's safety needs?
7. How does the nurse identify nursing diagnoses pertaining to protection and safety problems?
8. How does the nurse apply relevant principles in selecting, planning and implementing safety interventions?
9. What action does the nurse take to protect the safety of ill persons in case of fire or other disasters?
10. How does the nurse evaluate the effectiveness of nursing interventions?

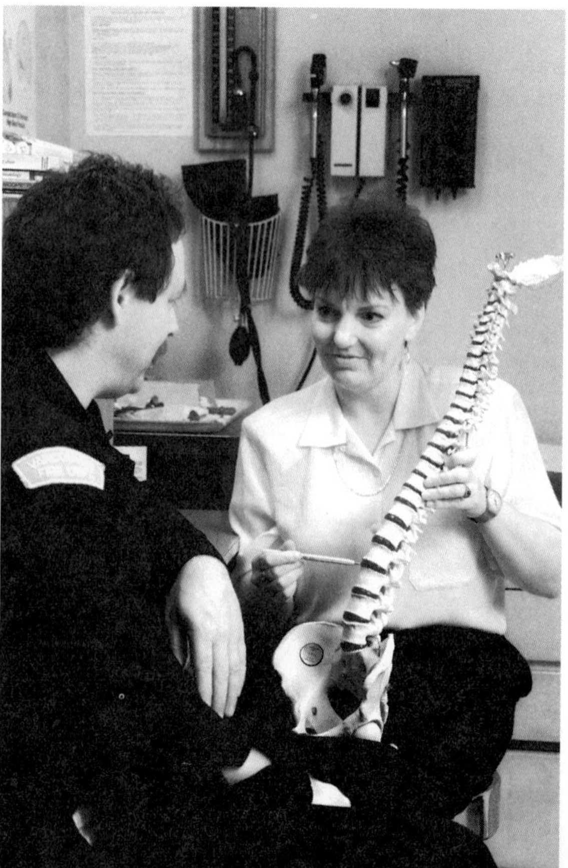

Introduction

A healthy environment is fundamental to life, and attention to the

are to attain the goal of health for all. To achieve concrete results, environmental responsibility must be practised at the individual level, in the workplace and in the home.

As decision makers, caregivers and role models for healthy behaviour, nurses and physicians should encourage and implement measures to achieve environmental responsibility in the settings where they practise, and the health care system in general.

—Joint CNA/CMA Position Statement, 1995

As with so many aspects of the nurse's role today, responsibilities regarding environmental safety are rapidly expanding. Nurses, as informed and knowledgeable health professionals, are not only concerned with health hazards in the communities in which they live and work; they are also taking action and making their voices heard, both individually and collectively, to make the environment more conducive to healthy living. Local, provincial and national nursing associations are expressing concerns about air pollution; the pollution of our rivers, lakes and coastal waters; highway safety; the safety of our water, milk and food supplies; drugs and cosmetics; and the presence of disease-carrying animals, insects and other potential sources

statements and lobbying municipal, provincial and federal authorities to take action to eliminate environmental health hazards, and they are actively participating in community action to detect, minimize or eliminate these hazards.

The International Council of Nurses (ICN) has strongly urged nurses to participate in actions to safeguard the human environment. In 1975, the Council of National Representatives (CNR) of the International Council of Nurses adopted a policy statement that outlines the role that nurses can play in protecting and improving the environment and thereby contribute to better health for all people:

The preservation and improvement of the human environment has become a major goal of man's action for his survival and well-being. The vastness and urgency of the task places on every individual and every professional group the responsibility to participate in the efforts to safeguard man's environment, to conserve the world's resources, to study how their use affects man and how adverse effects can be avoided.

—RNAO, 1976, p. 19.

The Role of Nurses in Protecting and Improving the Environment

The nurse's role is to:

- Help detect ill effects of the environment on the health of humans, and vice versa
- Be informed with the available data and apply knowledge in daily work with individuals, families and/or community groups on potentially harmful chemicals, radioactive waste problems, latest health hazards and ways to prevent and/or reduce them
- Be informed and teach preventive measures about health hazards due to environmental factors as well as about conservation of environmental resources to the individual, families and/or community groups
- Work with health authorities to point out health care concerns and health hazards in existing human settlements and in the planning of new ones
- Assist communities in taking action against environmental health problems
- Participate in research providing data for early warning and prevention of the deleterious effects of the various environmental agents to which we are increasingly exposed. Also, participate in research conducive to discovering ways and means of improving living and working conditions

SOURCE: RNAO, 1976, p. 19.

In Chapter 11, a number of environmental health issues were discussed. The present chapter is concerned with human protection and safety needs, with a focus on injury prevention. Injuries are grouped into two main categories: unintentional and intentional. **Unintentional injuries** are identified as those "due to motor vehicle collisions, drownings, falls, burns and poisonings," while **intentional injuries** include "child abuse, family violence, suicide and homicide" (Government of British Columbia, 1997, p. 1). Factors that influence the capacity for self-protection are described in this chapter, as well as the specific safety and protection needs of individuals throughout the life cycle. Finally, injury prevention and safety in the home, community and workplace, as well as in hospitals and other inpatient facilities, are outlined. Health safety factors that affect nurses and other health professionals are also considered.

Determinants of the Capacity for Self-Protection

Many factors are involved in the ability to protect ourselves from environmental hazards. We must, first of all, be aware of things in the environment that are potentially harmful to health. We must be able to perceive stimuli and to interpret them. We also need to know what action is needed to protect ourselves from hazards we have identified, and we must be capable of carrying out these actions. For example, a small child may see some pretty red berries on a tree and decide to eat them. The child is able to perceive the visual stimulus but does not know that holly berries are poisonous and is therefore not able to interpret the stimulus as dangerous. For self-protection, then, one needs a knowledge of environmental hazards, an intact sensory system, good mental functioning and reasoning ability, a knowledge of the protective measures to take, and adequate motor abilities to take the appropriate action. Age is a factor in all these requirements.

Knowledge

Much of what we know about hazards in the environment and how to protect ourselves from them is gained from personal experience (finding out that the tongue sticks to cold metal if you try to lick a wire fence in the winter) and from learning in the home, the school and the workplace as parents, older siblings, teachers and knowledgeable workers share their accumulated experiences. Books and other media also contribute to our knowledge about the environment, its hazards and how to cope with them. Considerable research is currently being undertaken to increase our knowledge about the effects of pollution and other hazards on our health and to discover ways to make our environments more conducive to health.

Perception and Interpretation of Stimuli

In Chapter 28, we discussed the fact that our sensory receptors provide us with information about our surroundings. It is through our ability to see, hear, smell, taste and feel that we are alerted to dangers in our environment. Impairment of the sensory receptors, of the neural pathways carrying sensory impulses to and through the central nervous system, or of the ability to interpret these impulses results in diminished ability to sense harmful, or potentially harmful, factors.

A person with limited vision may not see obstacles in the path. Someone without the sense of smell may not be aware of the odour of escaping gas from the kitchen stove. The phenomenon of negative adaptation to sensory stimuli can provide hazards. The smell of leaking gas may be so insidious that a person becomes accustomed to it, or is never even consciously aware of it. The sense of smell is one that adapts particularly quickly.

If mental faculties are clouded or impaired for any reason, sensory perception is diminished, as is the ability to interpret stimuli. Being drowsy while driving on the highway is a hazard because sensory abilities are dulled; you may not see cars approaching on your side of the road. Your own car may veer suddenly because your sense of touch is decreased. It may also take longer than usual to realize that you are dangerously close to the edge of the road or in the wrong lane. Alcohol and drugs, which are central nervous system depressants, have the same dulling effect on the senses as drowsiness does.

Any alteration in the state of consciousness will affect the ability to perceive sensory stimuli, to interpret them and to react appropriately. Someone who is roused out of a sound sleep is often confused and disoriented. The confused individual may mistake the door leading to the stairs for the door to the bathroom. Older people may become excited and confused by medications given to help them get to sleep.

Stress, anxiety and other emotions may also affect the perception of harmful stimuli in the environment, the interpretation of these stimuli and the ability to react to them. Mild anxiety increases perceptual awareness, but increased levels of anxiety progressively decrease it. We can attend to only so many stimuli at one time, and if other stimuli are of more importance, we may not be alert to potential dangers. Someone whose thoughts are turned inward or fixed on one object, or who is lost in reverie, may bump into objects because they are not noticed; this person may also step off the curb without looking, or do other things that can endanger life and limb.

Ability to Take Protective Action

The ability to respond to stimuli must also be considered in looking at self-protection. The brain must be functioning sufficiently well to make decisions and to initiate appropriate action in response to sensory stimuli. Some actions are reflexes that are initiated in the spinal cord, such as the withdrawal of the hand from a hot stove. Most actions, however—such as moving out of approaching danger— are initiated and controlled by higher centres of the brain. If the ability to initiate, coordinate and carry out motor actions is impaired for any reason, the ability to protect ourselves from environmental hazards is decreased.

Alcohol is well known for its effect of slowing reactions, thus making people who have been drinking a potential hazard both to themselves and to others. The relationship between alcohol consumption and a substantial proportion of motor vehicle collisions, fires and other types of accidents was mentioned in Chapter 2. Many cities in Canada now set up roadblocks over holiday weekends to check all drivers for the effects of alcohol; police have the power to suspend licences on the spot if drivers are inebriated. The roadblocks have proven to be a good preventive measure.

Injury or illness affecting either the specific areas of the brain that initiate and control movement or the neural pathways that transmit motor impulses will also limit safeguarding abilities. People who have lessened mental faculties because of congenital problems such as cerebral palsy (a motor disorder from nonprogressive brain damage) are hampered in their abilities to protect themselves.

People who have impaired motor functioning of any kind, or who have restrictions (such as a cast) placed on mobility, are at a disadvantage when it comes to protecting themselves from environmental hazards. People in

Determinants of the Capacity for Self-Protection

- age (chronological and developmental)
- knowledge of environmental hazards
- integrity of sensory functioning (vision, hearing, taste, smell, touch)
- level of consciousness
- mental functioning
- emotional state
- knowledge of protective measures
- motor ability
- health status
- medications and other therapies
- ability to communicate.

wheelchairs, for example, may be hampered by having to manoeuvre the chair around obstacles. People who cannot grasp objects or move an arm or leg with normal agility and speed are disadvantaged as far as protective abilities are concerned.

People who are ill are particularly prone to injury. They are often physically weak, and the ability to carry out normal daily activities is impaired. As a result, they may fall while walking, or easily lose their balance on an uneven surface. The protective senses of ill people (for example, sight) may become so impaired that they cannot perceive dangers. Moreover, the anxiety that goes along with illness may interfere with perceptual abilities and with the capacity to concentrate. It may also interfere with the ability to make judgements, and may thus expose ill people to injury. Many people who are ill suffer temporary or prolonged periods of altered states of consciousness. The preoperative patient who is under sedation, the postoperative patient recovering from anesthesia, the person with a severe head injury and the unconscious patient all have decreased sensory perceptual abilities, as well as decreased abilities to respond to environmental stimuli and to make decisions based on good judgement.

In many illnesses, a patient is rendered helpless or semihelpless. Patients who are paralyzed, for example, must depend on others for protection from environmental hazards. In some instances, it is necessary to restrain mobility to afford protection from the patient's own actions that may cause injury, such as pulling out catheters or intravenous tubing. Restraining a confused or disoriented patient is often distressing for both patient and caregivers, especially if the patient fights against the restraints, creating additional safety problems.

Sometimes the therapy that is prescribed makes patients more vulnerable to injuries, or has inherent hazards in itself. Medication therapy carries with it many potential hazards, such as adverse reactions or the possibility that the wrong patient will get the medication. Radiation therapy also has hazards. The very act of penetrating the skin surface for surgery renders a patient more vulnerable to infection and causes physiological stress, which makes the patient more

as fluid and electrolyte imbalance.

Protection and Safety Needs Throughout the Life Cycle

Reproductive Health

The protection of reproductive health concerns the potential not only of both parents, but also of their children, to have healthy offspring (Solomon, 1997; Smith, Hammonds-Ehlers, Clark, Kircher & Fuortes, 1997). Particularly in the workplace, many chemical and physical agents are, or could potentially be, **teratogenic** (causing physical defects), **mutagenic** (causing permanent alterations in the genes) or **carcinogenic** (causing cancer). Agents exist that can affect the male reproductive system, as well as the preconception health of the germ cells of both males and females. A classic example is dichlorobromopropane (DCBP), a chemical used in some pesticides. A study found that male factory workers who were chronically exposed to this chemical became sterile (Tas, Lauwergs & Lison, 1996). Pesticides made with DCBP have now been taken off the market. Exposure to lead compounds has been shown to decrease fertility and cause chromosomal aberrations in males (Roychowdhury, 1990). Organic solvents such as carbon disulfide have been linked with low sperm counts and abnormal genes (Tas, et al., 1996). Radiation is well known for its mutagenic effect on people of both genders. Studies have found an association between anesthetic gas and spontaneous abortions in operating room nurses (Pope, Snyder & Mood, 1995).

Although much is known, more research is needed to investigate reproductive health and to define safe levels of exposure to those chemicals and physical agents that are dangerous to reproductive health. Knowledge of the effects of these substances, and preventing or controlling exposure to them in the workplace, is a key role for the occupational health and safety team.

Pregnant Women

The expectant mother must be protected against potential injury, not only for her own sake but also for the sake of the fetus. The fetus is protected, to the extent that nature is able to do so, by its cushion of amniotic fluid within the uterus. However, trauma to the mother, such as a direct blow to the abdomen, may dislodge the placenta from its attachment to the uterine wall, causing miscarriage or premature labour, depending on the stage of fetal development.

Pregnant women are generally advised not to participate in sports that cause jolting (such as horseback riding), although swimming and most other sports are not contraindicated. As we mentioned in Chapter 29, exercise in moderation is important to the health of both mother and baby.

Maternal exposure to infectious diseases may pose particular risk to the fetus. Protection from exposure to rubella, hepatitis B and human immunodeficiency virus (HIV) is very important, and will be discussed more fully in Chapter 32. The effects of smoking and the consumption of alcohol and caffeine (in large quantities) are detrimental to the health of the developing fetus. Because "safe" limits of alcohol or caffeine consumption on the growing fetus have not been determined, it is best for pregnant women to avoid or eliminate taking these substances during pregnancy. During pregnancy and lactation, drugs should be used only under the supervision of a qualified health professional.

Infants and Children

"Injuries are the leading cause of death for children and youth after the age of one" (Health Canada, 1996, p. 1). Most injuries can be prevented. Newborn infants have very limited abilities to protect themselves and depend on the people who are caring for them to keep them safe. As children grow and develop, they learn—through education and trial and error—to avoid potential hazards in the environment. Injuries often occur because an infant makes a developmental advance for which the parent is not prepared. Although a baby may appear safe in a baby carriage or lying on a bed, six-month-old infants can achieve a sitting position and, because their balance is still not good, may tumble out of the carriage or off the bed.

Infants do not have the ability to push or roll themselves out of water if they fall face down in a pool or bath. Also, the reflex to hold the breath while submerged in water is not fully formed in young children. Therefore, infants and small children need special care around pools and baths. Death rates from drowning are highest in Canada in children from one to four years of age. In 1990, 17 percent of all injury-related deaths in this age group were drownings (Health Canada, 1996).

Very young children have no sense of danger. It is only as the world they know through experience enlarges that they are able to interpret the meaning of potentially harmful stimuli. Children who play with matches are fascinated by the flame. Until they burn themselves or unless their caretaker is sufficiently impressive in terms of correction, they do not perceive matches as dangerous objects. Indeed, the rate of death from fire in children from one to four years of age is higher than in any other age group. In 1990, 15 percent of all injury-related deaths in this age group were from burns (Health Canada, 1996).

Small children cannot read warning labels and may thus ingest poisonous cleaning fluid or other harmful substances. They may ingest chips of lead-based paint from their cribs or from a windowsill and suffer from lead poisoning. Some children suffer from *pica*, the urge to eat unnatural substances. These children must be supervised especially carefully, and potentially harmful substances must be kept from reach.

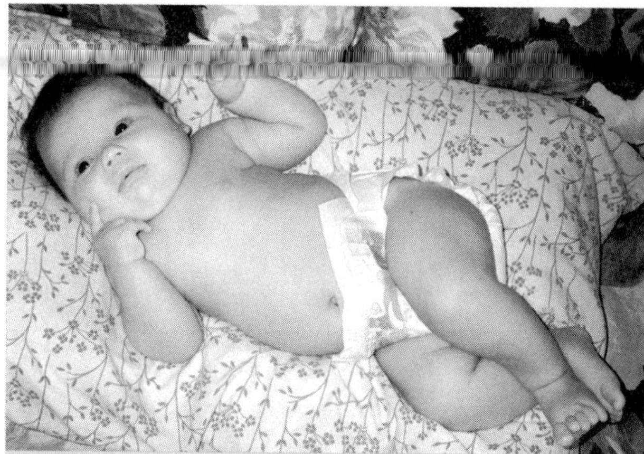

Infants are dependent on others to protect them from harm.

Growing children are most vulnerable to injuries when participating in newly learned activities and when exercising newly won freedom. A four-year-old may be given permission to visit a friend up the block but, during the visit, may dart out into the street to retrieve a ball that has bounced out of reach. The child just learning to ride a bicycle may ride out onto the road and into the pathway of an oncoming car.

Adolescents

By preadolescence, prevention has largely become a matter of self-discipline, but some children are accident-prone, and always seem to suffer from more cuts, bruises and scrapes than their brothers and sisters. This tendency often persists into adulthood. Some people may drive a car for 20 years without an accident, while others have one accident after another. It is believed that emotional disturbances are often the cause of being accident-prone. Tension of any kind is likely to cause increased susceptibility to accidents by impairing critical abilities and exhausting defences.

Young and Middle-aged Adults

Insurance and mortality/morbidity statistics repeatedly point out the disproportionately large number of automobile collisions involving young male drivers (Health Canada, 1996). Risk-taking behaviour is common among young adults (especially among males) because they tend to view their bodies as indestructible. Many, though not all, drive at high speeds, take the steepest trail down the mountain when skiing and generally operate under the philosophy that "it can't happen to me." Many young adults also have unrealistic perceptions about their physical capabilities and will

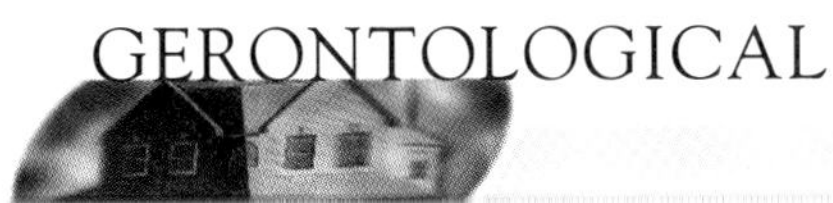

GERONTOLOGICAL

Elder Abuse

Elder abuse has been characterized as a silent assault. The breadth of the problem for Canadians was identified in a national survey of 2000 randomly selected seniors residing in private dwellings. The results indicated that four percent of respondents reported some form of abuse (Podneiks, Pillmer, Nicholson, Shillington & Frizzell, 1990). The offenders were usually people in positions of trust, such as family members or caregivers. Yet, overriding obstacles for the elderly to seek assistance include unwillingness to report the incident and the inability of police to recognize signs of abuse.

Through a collaborative effort between police and health professionals, many communities have developed educational programs, response protocols and interdisciplinary consultation services to help police officers recognize, manage and prevent elder abuse.

push themselves to the limit of endurance. "Shin splints" (periostitis, or inflammation of the periosteum) is a common problem that results from excessive demands on the musculoskeletal system. Much of this trauma is related to sports, although the largest percentage of injuries to young adults still results from car and motorcycle accidents.

In adults, most car accidents are related to the use of alcohol. The trauma resulting from motor vehicle accidents usually gives rise to musculoskeletal problems such as fractures, head injuries and torn ligaments. Repetitive trauma may result in painful inflammatory lesions of the periarticular structures. Because bone mass declines in middle age, injuries to the joints that would affect only ligaments in young adults cause fractures in middle-aged adults.

Stress at any age renders an individual more vulnerable to injuries. People who are troubled—children or adults—are much more likely to stumble and fall, or to act hurriedly without too much thought and injure themselves or others. Stress is said to be the disease of the modern age. Tension related to financial, marital, health, alcohol or drug problems can add to the risk of injury in adulthood. Extra stresses are imposed on the "sandwich generation," who are busy raising children while at the same time helping aging parents with health and housing concerns.

First Nations People

First Nations children have a considerably higher rate of death-related injury than do non–First Nations children. In 1990, First Nations children aged one to four years of age died at a rate over five times higher than the overall Canadian rate. First Nations youth aged 15 to 19 years and infants under the age of one year died at a rate almost four times higher than the Canadian rate (Health Canada, 1996). Disability rates among First Nations adults are greater compared with the total Canadian rate (31% vs. 13% in 1991). Injury was the most cited cause of disability among Canadians of First Nations descent (Ng, 1996).

Older Adults

Falls are the most common type of injury among older people. Those 75 years old and up are more at risk for death or injury from fire than any other age group. The 75-plus age group is also more at risk for death from drowning than any other age group except children aged one to four (Riley & Paddon, 1989).

As people get older, sensory abilities diminish. Vision becomes worse, and hearing may sometimes be considerably decreased. The sensory receptors for smell in the nose are often damaged when people have any kind of head injury and usually diminish with age. Atrophy of the taste buds is one of the aspects of growing older. The receptors for touch also lose acuteness with the changes that occur in aging skin. The older person's skin is less sensitive to heat and cold and is therefore prone to thermal injuries. The older person, like the young child, is very vulnerable to environmental hazards, but for different reasons. The older person's "early warning system" in the sensory receptors is not as efficient, and responses to environmental hazards are slower and not as effective. Vestibular function declines, and there is increased risk of falling. Absent-mindedness is also a major factor in injuries.

Common Accidents

An *accident* is "an unplanned interruption of an orderly process involving the motion of people, objects or substances" (WCB of BC, 1998, ix). An *injury*, a prevalent term in the fields of health and safety and injury prevention, refers to "harm or hurt" to a person (WCB of BC, 1998a, ix). Injuries are among the leading causes of death each year in Canada. They are the principal cause of death among children and young adults and a major cause of hospitalization in people of all ages (Millar, 1995). Injuries are usually caused by hazards in the environment. The hazards that can lead to injuries can be divided into four categories: physical, chemical, biological and psychological hazards. Examples of each are shown in Table 30.1.

TABLE 30.1 Environmental hazards

Physical	*Chemical*	*Biological*	*Psychological*
Noise	Solvents	Bacteria	Shift work
Radiation	Caustics	Viruses	Boredom
Vibration	Fumes	Fungus	Stress
Electricity	Lead	Poisonous plants	Danger
Heat/cold/humidity	Dust	Insects, rodents, reptiles and other disease-carrying animals	
Repetitive motions	Mercury		
Lifting	Gases		
Slips and falls			

Injuries in the Home

Although most injury-related deaths occur on roads and highways, the majority of other injuries take place in the home (Wilkins, 1995; Millar, 1995). Home is a place where children and adults should be safe from harm, but the average home contains many hazards.

FIRE AND BURNS

Fire is probably the most common and the most dreaded accident that can happen in a home. Although no age group is immune to the dangers of fire, the rate of death from fires is higher for the very young and the very old; it is also higher among men than women (Riley & Paddon, 1989). A common cause of fire in the home is an overloaded electrical circuit. About 25 percent of house fires are attributed to heating equipment. Wood stoves and wood-burning fireplaces that are poorly installed and/or poorly maintained cause a large number of these fires. Many homes are not equipped with an adequate escape route or with fire detectors. Many people die in fires because they are trapped or because they are unaware of the fire until it is too late to escape.

Thermal injuries in the home often result from contact with hot water (scalding) or hot pots and pans. Children, in particular, sustain burns while playing with lighters or matches.

FALLS

In Canada, falls are a leading cause of injury-related death in people 65 years of age and up, and are the leading cause of hospitalization for both men and women (Wilkins, 1995).

The Five Most Common Injuries

- motor vehicle collisions
- falls
- drownings
- fires
- poisonings.

Children have their share of falls and sustain injuries from these, but the death rate from falls is not as high as from other types of injuries. Stairs are a principal cause of home injuries. As well, people often fall in slippery bathtubs or showers.

POISONINGS

Deaths due to poisonings appear to be much greater in number for men than for women, with the highest number occurring in the 45–54 age group among Canadian men, and in the 25–34 age group in American men (Riley & Paddon, 1989). Children are also vulnerable to poisoning because of natural curiosity and the tendency to put things into the mouth.

CHOKING AND SUFFOCATION

Choking and suffocation are among the common accidents that occur among infants and small children. Because children like to put many things into the mouth, they may choke on objects that are too big to swallow. In 1990, suffocation accounted for 42 percent of all injury-related deaths of children under the age of one (Health Canada, 1996).

DROWNING AND DIVING INJURIES

Deaths from drowning in Canada are highest among the one to four age group. Many homes and playgrounds have swimming pools, wading pools, whirlpools or hot tubs, to which children are naturally attracted. Drownings unfortunately occur, even with diligent supervision (Health Canada, 1996).

Adolescents and young adults often sustain spinal cord injuries from diving accidents. Diving at night or where visibility is obstructed may cause neck injuries due to hitting the bottom of a lake or pool, or injuries can be sustained by diving into rocks or other submerged objects. Similar to motor vehicle accidents, many drownings are alcohol-related.

Injuries in the Community

Most of the injuries that occur in the community are motor vehicle, bicycle or sport- and recreation-related. Motor vehicle collisions are the number one cause of injury and death among children and young people (Wilkins, 1995). In 1993, motor vehicle collisions accounted for the major cause of death among children aged one to nine years (Wilkins, [illegible]

death and permanent disability in adults. Most of these injuries are preventable.

Bicycling, always a popular sport, has become a common mode of transportation in our country. Many cities in Europe and in other parts of the world have separate lanes for bicycle traffic. In most Canadian cities, however, cars, buses and bicycles all compete for road space on clogged city streets. The risk to the lone rider on a bicycle is much greater than to the occupants of a car, should the two collide. In the community, playgrounds for children, playing fields and sports arenas, as well as schools, are places where accidents can happen. Adult supervision in parks and other recreational areas where children play is essential to identify and remedy potential hazards. Children and adults must be encouraged to wear helmets for cycling, in-line skating and skiing. Indeed, the Canadian Public Health Association (CPHA) recently passed a resolution calling for approved ski helmets to be a part of standard equipment for staff, volunteers and recreational skiers at Canadian ski facilities ("CPHA urges use of ski helmets," 1997).

Injuries in the Workplace

Despite injury prevention programs, millions of occupational injuries and illnesses are still reported in the industrialized world every year. In Canada, over 440 464 time-loss injuries were accepted for Workers' Compensation in 1995 (AWCBC, 1996). The highest number of time-loss injuries occurred in manufacturing, retail trades and health services (AWCBC, 1996). In British Columbia, the highest percentages of claims are found in logging, trucking, sawmills, hospitals and health care, building construction and retail food stores (WCB of BC, 1997).

MUSCULOSKELETAL INJURIES

Musculoskeletal injuries affecting the back, neck and shoulders are common in all types of workplaces. Back injuries due to physical hazards, such as lifting and reaching, are common occupational injuries. Safety improvements have decreased certain types of accidents, but new technology creates new types of problems. A group of disorders called **cumulative trauma disorders** (CTDs), also known as **repetitive strain injuries**, is the silent epidemic of the late 20th century. CTDs are usually caused by sustained, unnatural body postures and repetitive, forceful movements. A common feature of CTDs is overuse of certain joints or muscles groups; therefore, injury is the result of repeated microtrauma leading to chronic injury. Computer operators and assembly-line workers are reporting injuries such as carpal tunnel syndrome, strains, sprains, tendinitis and tenosynovitis. Careful attention to workstation, tool and job task design, training and administrative policies could prevent many CTDs.

COMMON OCCUPATIONAL INJURIES

[illegible] injuries, asphyxiation and thermal injuries. Injuries caused from being trapped by or caught in equipment or other heavy material occur especially in the mining, logging and construction industries. Noise-induced hearing loss can occur in any workplace with excessive noise levels, but hearing conservation programs have now been in place for many years.

OCCUPATION-RELATED DISEASES

Pulmonary diseases can be related to occupational exposure to **hazardous substances**. Environmental dust may be inhaled as a solid, fume or mixture of the two. The type of respiratory injury that could ensue depends on the physical, chemical and toxic properties of the agent involved. Asbestosis (asbestos), coal worker's pneumoconiosis (respirable coal dust), silicosis (silica), meat wrapper's asthma (polyvinylchloride heat process), occupational asthma (various causes), farmer's lung (grain dust) and siderosis (welding fumes, iron oxide) are some of the pulmonary disorders related to occupational exposure.

A number of agents encountered in the workplace have been related to varying types of occupational cancers. These include ethylene oxide, ionizing radiation, coke oven emissions, benzene, radium, asbestos and others (Tas et al., 1997). In addition, skin disorders occur from handling or otherwise being in contact with irritating agents in the workplace. Contact dermatitis and various infections may ensue. Causative agents include latex, solvents, resins, detergents, fibreglass, cutting oils, plastics and infectious agents.

The aging workforce, stress and nonoccupational factors such as arthritis, diabetes, heart disease and lack of fitness all compound occupational injuries, affecting both the severity of injury and length of recovery. Another prevalent occupation-related disease is sick building syndrome (discussed in detail in Chapter 11).

Injuries in the Hospital

A hospital is generally thought of as a place where the sick and injured come for care; it is seldom considered a place where people are injured. Yet the number of injuries that occur in hospitals is high compared with the number that occur in other industries.

Many safety-related problems occur in health agencies. Three groups of people should be considered: patients, who require additional protection because they are ill; staff, who because of the nature of their work are vulnerable to many types of accidental injury (such as back strain from lifting heavy patients); and visitors, who are usually anxious and worried about the person they have come to see.

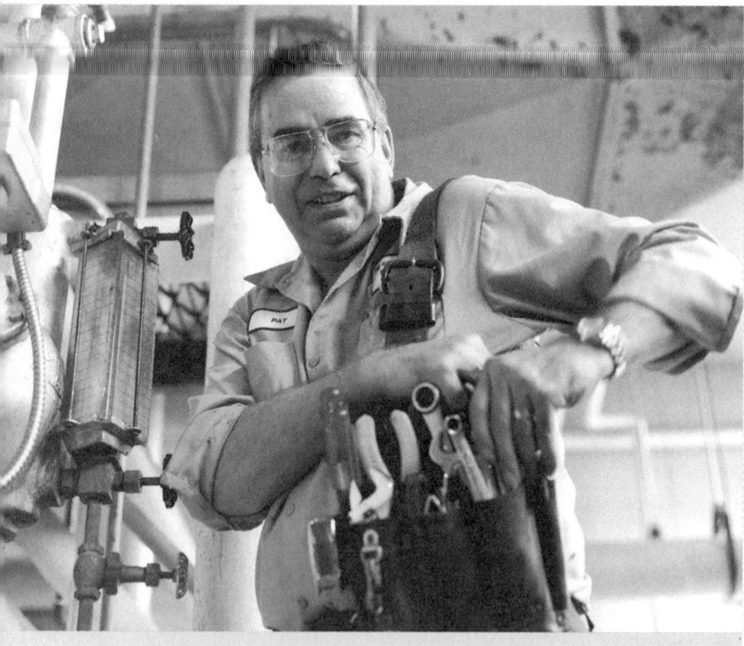

Maintenance personnel ensure a safe mechanical plant.

HAZARDOUS AREAS IN THE HOSPITAL

Many areas of a hospital are particularly dangerous. The nurse should be aware of the dangers of these areas and take extra precautions when working in or around them.

THE MECHANICAL PLANT A hospital usually has a large mechanical plant with heavy equipment, high-voltage areas, hazardous products, boiler rooms, woodworking, machining and paint shops. Potentially dangerous activities such as plumbing, carpentry, welding, electrical work, construction and renovation projects are ongoing.

FOOD AND NUTRITION SERVICES Meal service is part of the daily activities in all inpatient facilities, and safety in food preparation, handling and serving must be considered. Most kitchens have sophisticated food assembly and dish room areas. Many heavy products, raw and prepared, are handled. Cooks and chefs are at risk of sustaining serious cuts. Slips and falls are also common in areas where food and water spills occur.

THE LAUNDRY Laundry functions involve lifting and moving large, heavy loads. There is always the possibility of exposure to sharps inadvertently left in the laundry, thereby posing a risk for infection among laundry workers. Similar to the hospital kitchen, advances in technology have led to computer-controlled mechanical devices and equipment, which in turn have led to decreased injuries in laundry facilities.

DIAGNOSTIC SERVICES Diagnostic and therapeutic procedures are often hazardous because of the potential for chemical and physical injuries to patients and staff, and because of the potential for infection. Staff could be exposed to ionizing and nonionizing radiation, lasers, radioactive isotopes, antineoplastic agents and other hazards.

HAZARDS FOR HEALTH CARE WORKERS

ACCIDENTAL INJURY Back strains accounted for 71 percent of all short-term disability claims in acute care community hospitals between 1991 and 1995 in the province of British Columbia (WCB of BC, 1996b). The cost of these claims was $7 247 579 in 1995 (WCB of BC, 1996a). Most of the back strains were sustained by lifting or transferring patients. Injuries from slips and falls are also common in the hospital, and safe footwear and safe housekeeping signs for wet floors are very important. Cuts, abrasions and contusions can also occur unless proper precautions are taken.

VIOLENCE IN THE WORKPLACE Research shows that "nurses experience high rates of verbal and emotional abuse, physical violence and sexual harassment in the course of their work" (CNA, 1993, p. 1). Over the last decade, society has turned considerable and necessary attention to issues of violence and abuse. While much of this attention has been directed towards child, elder and spousal abuse, interest has been growing in examining abuse within the health care sector. There can be no question that nurses and other health professionals care for individuals and families in a variety of settings and under circumstances where the potential for violence must be recognized and addressed. In recent years, nurses, nursing organizations and health care agencies have worked individually and collectively to identify strategies for preventing violence in the workplace. The position of "zero tolerance" for workplace violence is reflected in the written policies and procedures, reporting systems, advisory committees, education programs and other activities in place in many health care agencies. Recent changes to health and safety legislation in some provinces will also have an impact on how issues related to violence are addressed. In Saskatchewan, for example, health care employers are responsible to satisfy a number of specific requirements with respect to harassment and violence in the workplace (Saskatchewan Labour, 1996). Nurses, and indeed all employees, have the right to be treated with respect and to carry out their duties in a safe work environment.

EXPOSURE TO BLOOD AND BODY FLUIDS Exposure to contaminated blood and body fluids can occur through needle-stick and scalpel injuries, splashes into the eye or mouth or contact with nonintact skin. Housekeeping staff are at a high risk because the source patient is often not known (in the case of a needle-stick from a garbage or sharps container) and therefore cannot be tested for hepatitis B antigen, HIV or other organisms to establish infectiousness. Every health care facility should establish first aid and follow-up treatment for blood and body fluid exposure. Chapter 32 discusses infection control programs and body substance precautions in detail.

STRESS Nurses, as employees within an ever-changing and evolving health care sector, are often pressed by time and budget demands to provide increasingly complex and tech-

many other employers, are recognizing that stress is an occupational hazard and are endeavouring to provide the necessary support services for employees. Most often, services have included an Employee Assistance Program, through which staff can gain access to stress management programs and professional counselling. More recently, hospitals have begun offering special programs for emergency, critical care and other staff who experience the stress associated with unusual, acute, traumatic events. These *critical-incident stress debriefing programs* are "designed to mitigate the impact of the critical incident and to assist personnel in recovering as quickly as possible from the stress associated with the event" (Mitchell & Everly, 1993, p. 7). Indeed, both day-to-day work stressors and acute stress episodes are significant for nurses, and any discussion of hazards for health professionals would be incomplete without considering these important issues.

Safety Needs Assessment Guide

- How old is the patient?

mental faculties? Are there limitations to communication?

- Does the patient require additional safety precautions because of age, physical condition or mental state?
- Is the patient receiving medications that impair the senses?
- Does the patient require restraints of any sort?
- Does the patient smoke?
- Is electrical equipment in use in the patient's room? Does the patient have electrical appliances at the bedside?
- Is heat or cold used as a therapeutic agent in the care of this patient?
- Is the patient receiving oxygen therapy?
- Are there any safety practices or information that can help the patient to avoid injury or accident?
- Is the patient comfortable?
- Can the patient reach everything that is needed?
- Is the call signal within easy reach?
- Is the patient safe from mechanical injuries, such as those resulting from falls?
- Is the patient being protected from burns, for example, those from a heating pad or a hot water bottle?
- What precautions are taken to ensure that medications are given safely?

Assessing Safety Needs

There are two distinct yet related components in the assessment of a patient's safety needs. The first is an appraisal of the factors affecting the patient's (or family's) capacity for self-protection. The second is the identification of potential hazards in the environment that may affect patients, visitors and staff. This appraisal may be conducted in an inpatient facility or in a patient's home.

Assessing the Capacity for Self-Protection

In assessing a patient's capacity for self-protection, the nurse should be aware of both the patient's age and the integrity of the sensory abilities. Does the patient have any sensory deficits, such as loss of sight, hearing, smell, taste or touch? It is necessary to know any restrictions that have been put on the patient's mobility, such as bed rest, position restrictions or immobilization of a body part (as with a cast or traction apparatus). The use of aids for mobility (a cane, walker or wheelchair) may also pose potential hazards for patient safety.

The nurse also needs information about the patient's general state of health, the nature of any health problems, and the physician's plan of diagnostic and therapeutic care. It is important to know if the patient is helpless or semihelpless or whether the nature of the illness may cause loss of strength, impairment of sensory or motor functioning or short or prolonged periods of altered states of consciousness. Is the patient to have surgery, for example, and experience periods when the mental faculties may be lessened by sedation or anesthesia? The nurse should be aware of diagnostic or therapeutic procedures being performed that may involve the use of potentially hazardous equipment, potentially harmful reactions and the possibility of infection. Information about medications that the patient is receiving and the nature of other planned treatments is also essential. Is the patient receiving medications that may cause confusion? Is the patient having treatments, such as oxygen therapy, that require extra safety precautions?

Many patients are anxious, and the nurse should watch for evidence of this. An emotionally upset patient, visitor or staff member may rush blindly into danger. Someone who is worried, preoccupied or emotionally distressed is often less able to make judgements that are in the best interests of physical or mental health. These patients require extra vigilance from nursing staff. The nurse also needs to know if the patient is accident-prone.

Much of the information the nurse requires to assess safety needs may be obtained from the baseline assessment taken at the time of admission. The nursing history and physical assessment will provide data concerning the patient's usual and current patterns of functioning with regard to sensory and motor abilities, state of comfort, rest and sleep and emotional and mental state. The patient's status changes constantly, however, and the nurse must rely on observations and make judgements regarding safety precautions that need to be taken.

The patient's chart is, of course, the most reliable source of information about diagnostic procedures, medications and other therapeutic measures in the overall plan of care. Nurses supplement this information by increasing their own knowledge about medications, tests, examinations and treatments; by consulting other health professionals; and by researching current literature.

To ensure safety at all times, the nurse should conduct a focus assessment during every nurse–patient encounter. This includes a visual scan of the environment for potential hazards and a quick appraisal of patient-related factors. The nurse will find subjective data very helpful. The patient may say that the things on the bedside table are out of reach, for example, or that sitting, standing or trying to walk cause weakness or dizziness. The patient can alert the nurse to factors that are causing pain or discomfort so that appropriate action can be taken. The patient is often aware when mental faculties are impaired and may indicate this by expressing an inability to think clearly or by saying that everything "seems to be fuzzy."

The patient's family or significant others often alert the nurse to dangerous situations. Many agencies permit family members to stay with confused or sedated patients, and this can be of great assistance to the nurse. However, the nurse must ensure that the family member knows what to do when helping the patient and will call for assistance if it is needed. The patient's safety is the nurse's responsibility at all times, and this should not be neglected when a family member is present.

Hospital Hazards Appraisal

- Is all electrical equipment functioning properly? Is it properly grounded (does it have a three-pronged plug)? Are extension cords properly taped to the floor? Look for frayed cords, tangled cords and cords that can be tripped on. Look for loose control knobs, overloaded circuits and placement of appliances near sinks, bathtubs or moisture areas.
- Are "No Smoking" signs clearly displayed in areas where patients are receiving oxygen therapy?
- Could injury be caused by any obstacles present? Equipment? Misplaced footstools? Chairs? Over-bed tables? Bags or suitcases with patients' belongings on the floor?
- Are bathrooms equipped with safety features? Look for hand rails around tubs and toilets, nonslip surfaces, stools or chairs for tubs and showers.
- Is lighting adequate, for instance, can the patient see adequately when getting from bed to bathroom? In the bathroom?
- Are there water spills or wet, slippery areas on the floor? Are "Wet Floor" signs clearly displayed by housekeeping staff when floors are being washed?
- Are hand rails secured properly in bathrooms and hallways?
- Are side rails up for patients who need them?
- Are areas where radiation is in use clearly demarcated?
- Is there a designated smoking area for people who must smoke?

Assessing Hazards in the Environment

In terms of safety, the nurse assesses potential hazards in the environment. In the hospital, these hazards could be a dangling electric cord, a misplaced footstool, a side rail that is down or a slippery floor. In the home, hazards might include inadequate lighting, a stairway with loose steps, slippery surfaces in bathtubs or showers or overloaded electrical outlets. Guidelines for appraising hazards in the hospital and the home are given in the boxes on this page and on the preceding and following pages.

Diagnosing Safety Problems

The patient's safety is an integral component of all facets of the nursing process. Safety needs must be considered when the patient is very young or very old, when perceptual abilities are lessened for any reason, when the ability to react to harmful stimuli is decreased and when potentially harmful equipment is being used in care.

The general diagnostic label for patients with problems meeting safety needs is *Risk for Injury*. Carpenito (1997) defines this as "the state in which an individual is at risk for harm because of a perceptual or physiologic deficit, a lack of awareness of hazards, or maturational age" (p. 509). NANDA has identified four subcategories of potential injury: *Risk for Aspiration, Poisoning, Suffocation* or *Trauma* (Carpenito, 1997). These diagnostic statements identify the nature of the problem more specifically, and thus, facilitate the selection of appropriate interventions.

Examples of nursing diagnoses for patients who are at risk for injury include:

- *Risk for Aspiration related to accumulation of secretions secondary to dorsal positioning.*
- *Risk for Poisoning related to easy accessibility of household cleaners to young children.*
- *Risk for Injury related to insufficient knowledge of accident prevention in the home.*

Planning Safety Interventions

Planning interventions for *Risk for Injury* involves selecting strategies to foster the patient's capacity for self-protection

Home Hazards Appraisal

the treads slip-resistant? If carpeted, is the carpet firm and secure?

2. Are hand rails present on both sides of the stairs? Do they provide a good handhold? Are they strong enough to support an adult's weight?
3. Are stairways well lit?
4. Are balcony and sundeck railings strong enough to resist the impact of a person falling against them? Are they sturdy and secure? Are exterior guard rails at least 1 m high with openings no larger than 10 cm? Can children climb the guard rails without difficulty?
5. Are there decorative decals on glass doors, preventing someone from bumping into or attempting to walk through them?
6. Do floors have nonslip surfaces? Are scatter rugs skidproof?
7. Are walkways and stairways cluttered with objects that are easily tripped over (such as toys, electrical cords, newspapers, garden hoses)?
8. Do bathtubs and showers have nonslip surfaces or rubber mats?

home? Is it tested regularly?

10. Is there at least one readily accessible fire extinguisher in the home? Does every family member know how to use it?
11. Are fireplaces, wood-burning stoves and space heaters properly screened? Are portable heaters away from combustible materials?
12. Are electrical outlets overloaded (having too many items on the same outlet)? Is more than one electrical appliance connected to an extension cord? Are electrical cords worn and frayed?
13. Are all electrical wires placed out of reach of children? Are outlets covered with safety plugs?
14. Are all cleaning products, insecticides, medications and other harmful chemicals placed out of reach of children?
15. Are cigarettes, lighters and matches out of reach of children?
16. Is propane or gasoline stored in the home?
17. Are children's toys in good repair? Do they have sharp edges, loose parts or parts small enough for a child to swallow?

SOURCE: B.C. Ministry of Municipal Affairs, Recreation & Housing, 1991.

or to protect the patient who lacks this capability. Safety is among the most basic of all human needs, especially for those who are ill. The protective aspects of the nurse's role are among the most important of all functions. The nurse must incorporate the patient's safety as the number one priority in all aspects of patient care.

Ensuring patient safety in case of fire or other disasters takes precedence over all other nursing responsibilities. Nurses must know the agency's fire and disaster procedures, understand how to use the equipment for controlling fire and know their responsibilities with regard to patient safety. They must be ever alert to potential hazards and take action to see that dangers are minimized or eliminated, if possible.

Implementing Safety Interventions

The primary goal of nursing action with regard to patient safety is the prevention of accidental injury. A very large aspect of care is educating people to protect themselves from injury in the course of daily living in the home, the workplace and the community. As well, strategies that promote wellness on a personal and occupational level are important because troubled individuals are more prone to accidents. The modelling of safe behaviours is by far the most effective form of teaching safety awareness.

Injury Prevention in the Home

Many injuries such as falls, poisonings, drownings and burns need never happen. A good many of these injuries can be prevented by the careful supervision of children and teenagers and by assessing the home for potential hazards and correcting them. Table 30.2 outlines a number of prevention strategies for protecting children and youth from common accidents.

A report by the B.C. Ministry of Health (Government of British Columbia, 1997) provides a detailed framework for a provincial injury prevention plan for children and youth aged from birth to 24 years. The report outlines how agencies, communities and individuals can reduce the rate of unintentional injuries to children and youth using specific objectives and strategies.

FIRE PREVENTION

The best fire prevention is to practise home fire safety. Every home should have a fire prevention program that includes the installation of smoke detectors, carbon monoxide monitors and sprinklers, fire safety education and an evacuation plan. It should also include other measures such as the use of nonflammable materials wherever possible and care and attention to safety precautions in the use of heat-producing equipment (such as stoves) and all electrical appliances.

TABLE 30.2 Injury prevention strategies for children and youth

Injury Problem	*Intervention*	*Proven Effective*	*Promising*	*More Study Required*
Motor Vehicle Occupants	Air bags	✓		
	Child restraint loaner programs	✓		
	Child restraints/seat belts	✓		
	Education programs for youth		✓	
	Driver training			✓
Pedestrians	Visibility measures	✓		
	Roadway barriers	✓		
	School zone measures	✓		
	Sidewalks	✓		
	Pedestrian education programs		✓	
Motorcyclists	Helmet use	✓		
	Motorcycle rider training		✓	
Bicyclists	Helmet use	✓		
	Visibility measures	✓		
	Bicycle paths		✓	
	Bicycle selection guidelines		✓	
	Bicycle safety education			✓
Home Accidents	Education programs		✓	
Falls	Window guards	✓		
	Parent education		✓	
	Safety gates		✓	
Fire/Burns	Fire-safe cigarettes	✓		
	Flammability standards	✓		
	Reduced tap-water temperature	✓		
	Smoke detectors	✓		
	Sprinkler systems	✓		
	Fire safety education		✓	
Poisoning	Poison control centres	✓		
	Prevention packaging	✓		
	First aid training		✓	
	Prevention education programs		✓	
Suffocation/Choking	Heimlich manoeuvre	✓		
	Product safety regulations	✓		
	Education re: choking risks			✓
Drowning	Barriers for pools	✓		
	Personal flotation devices	✓		
	Supervision	✓		
	CPR instruction			✓
	Parent counselling			✓
	Swimming lessons			✓
Sports and Playground Injuries	Protective equipment	✓		
	Surfacing/equipment standards	✓		
	Education programs		✓	
Occupational Injuries	Education programs		✓	
Injuries in Facilities	Safety standards	✓		
	Training programs for workers		✓	

SOURCE: B.C. Ministry of Health, 1993, p. 18.

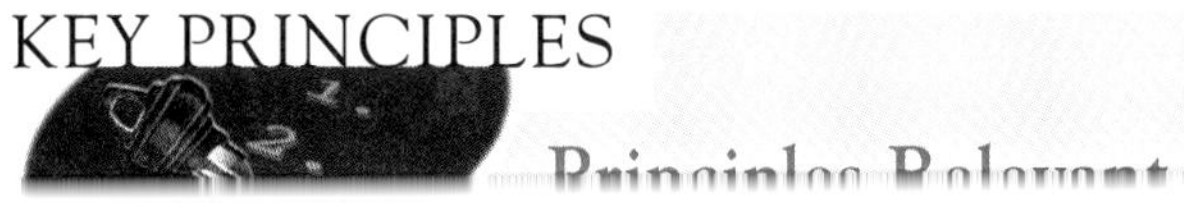

KEY PRINCIPLES

Principles Relevant to Patient Safety

1. Normally functioning body senses inform the individual about potential hazards.
2. Age affects both the ability to perceive and interpret sensory stimuli from the environment and the ability to take effective action to provide protection from harmful stimuli.
3. Familiarity with the environment makes it less hazardous.
4. The ability to provide self-protection is affected by sensory status, mental status, emotional status, mobility status and by the status of comfort, rest and sleep.
5. Illness renders a person more vulnerable to injury.
6. Diagnostic and therapeutic measures have inherent potential for causing a patient harm, even while aiding in the resolution of health problems.

Dwellings should have smoke alarms installed between the bedrooms and the remainder of the house. The batteries should be replaced at least yearly and the alarms tested monthly. A sprinkler system is a good idea for homes, and it is becoming mandatory for apartments under many municipal building codes. If a family member smokes, particular care should be taken to ensure that smouldering cigarettes are not left unattended and that cigarette butts are cold before being put into the garbage. Clothing and upholstery, window drapes and other articles made of cloth must meet flammability standards. People need to be cautioned about the dangers of overloading electrical circuits. Only one appliance should be connected to an extension cord. As mentioned earlier, poorly installed and ill-maintained wood stoves cause a large number of fires in the home. People who have wood stoves or wood-burning fireplaces should ensure that chimneys are cleaned regularly. Wood stoves and fireplaces should always be installed in accordance with local building codes.

Every home should have at least one fire extinguisher, and all family members who are old enough should know how to use it. A 5-lb multipurpose ABC dry chemical extinguisher rated 2A is recommended for homes. A 5-lb container is large enough to put out small fires or contain a fire until the fire department arrives, yet is not so large that it cannot be handled effectively. The ABC type of fire extinguisher is effective against three of the basic classes of fires, described in the following box.

It is dangerous to use water or a fire extinguisher labelled "Class A only" on grease or electrical fires. Class B and C models, however, may be used on Class A fires (National Fire Protection Association, 1997b).

Families are encouraged to prepare an emergency escape plan, which the whole family should periodically review

Three Basic Classes of Fires

- **Class B** Flammable liquids such as grease, gasoline, oil, oil-based paint
- **Class C** Energized electrical equipment including wiring, fuse boxes, circuit breakers, appliances and machinery.

and practise. The local fire department can help families to design this plan. People who live in apartment buildings should make sure that one of the two exit stairs mandatory for apartment buildings under most building codes is always accessible and clear of obstacles. Fire doors should always be kept closed. If the fire alarm rings, people are urged to:

- proceed outdoors as quickly as possible
- take the apartment keys
- walk downstairs, rather than using the elevator.

If a person is trapped in an apartment suite, it is important to let the firefighters know and ensure that the trapped person stays near a window or balcony.

Burns from causes other than fire can be prevented by keeping the temperature of the hot water set at or lower than 54° C (130° F) (B.C. Ministry of Municipal Affairs, Recreation and Housing, 1992). Pots and pans that contain hot foods must be kept out of the reach of small children, as should matches and lighters. Propane and gasoline should be stored outdoors or in a garden shed.

PREVENTING INJURIES FROM FALLS

There are a number of ways to prevent injuries from falls in the home. Stairs should be clear of all objects and should be constructed of slip-resistant material. Hand rails must be strong enough to support an adult's weight and should be shaped to provide a good handhold. Balcony and sundeck railings must be strong, well secured and meet local building code specifications. Bathtubs and showers should be constructed with slip-resistant materials. Window guards and safety gates should be installed where there is a risk of falling. People should never stand on chairs to reach high places, and all carpets and area rugs should be securely fastened.

PREVENTING POISONINGS

People can do much to protect their families from accidental poisonings. Regulated chemical products are required by law to bear appropriate hazard symbols on the labels, and some must be packaged in child-resistant containers. Poisons and medicines should be stored in the original containers and out of reach of children, preferably in a locked cabinet. Parents should never call medicine "candy," nor should they take medicines in front of children. There is a national network of poison control centres in Canada and a poison control centre in every major city in Canada. The phone number of the poison control centre should be posted by each telephone, and baby sitters and relatives should be made aware of it. Every household should have at least one person with first aid training. It is helpful to have ipecac syrup on hand at all times to induce vomiting, although this measure should be taken only after advice from the poison control centre or a physician. For tips on how to poison-proof your home, see the box below.

PREVENTING CHOKING, SUFFOCATION AND DROWNING

Part of home safety is being prepared for possible accidents, such as choking or suffocation. In the home, knowledge of the Heimlich manoeuvre is the most helpful first aid measure. People with swimming pools must take extra precautions to ensure water safety. Rules of conduct, safety barriers, personal flotation devices and adequate supervision protect family and visitors from injuries. Swimming lessons for children and knowledge of cardiopulmonary resuscitation are also essential for safe water activity.

GENERAL SAFETY MEASURES

All home furniture and appliances should meet Canadian Safety Standards specifications. When purchasing clothing, toys, equipment, appliances and furniture, people should give careful consideration to safety features. Parents should be cautious when purchasing or receiving second-hand items such as cribs, playpens, strollers and high chairs, and ensure that these items meet current government safety standard specifications. If parents are uncertain, they should either contact the local health unit, which will have the latest information from Consumer and Corporate Affairs Canada (CCAC), or contact the local office of CCAC directly.

Finally, children must be kept away from construction or carpentry areas, and any work area where dangerous machinery or tools (such as chainsaws or table saws) are being operated.

Injury Prevention in the Community

INFANT AND CHILD RESTRAINT SYSTEMS

Transport Canada publishes regulations governing safety standards for infant and child restraint systems. All provinces require that children be properly restrained when travelling in a motor vehicle. It is imperative that any restraint system meets Canadian Motor Vehicle Safety Standards and is correctly installed according to the manufacturer's instructions. Table 30.3 illustrates the recommended infant and child car restraint systems.

How to Poison-Proof Your Home

The average household contains as many as 250 poisons and, each year in Canada, hundreds of fatalities are caused by poisoning. There are two key steps to poison-proofing your home: identification and storage.

Common Household Poisons

- cleaners and bleaches, including detergents, ammonia, naphtha, oven cleaner and bleach
- solvents, including paint remover, kerosene and turpentine
- polishes and waxes, including paint, car and furniture wax, silver polish
- herbicides, insecticides and insect repellents
- mercury from thermometers
- cosmetics and toiletries, including after-shave, bubble bath, nail polish, hair lotions
- drugs and medicines, including both prescription and nonprescription drugs such as vitamins, ASA, cough medicines and cold medications
- house plants, ornamental plants and flower and vegetable garden plants

How to Store Them

- keep products in clearly labelled original containers
- store prescription drugs out of the reach of children and in containers with safety lids
- store household cleaners on high shelves, not underneath the sink
- return medication and cleaning products to a safe place after using them
- keep all poisonous liquids and solids out of the reach of children; if possible, install child-proof locking cabinets
- never call medicine "candy"; it gives children a distorted idea
- warn children at an early age not to eat household plants or wild plants and berries
- never keep food and household cleaners next to each other
- don't continue to store old products around the house
- don't leave a purse or handbag where a child can reach it, since prescription drugs are often inside
- if poisoning occurs, identify the suspected poison and immediately seek medical help. Many areas have poison information centres. Never attempt to induce vomiting without medical advice.

SOURCE: Colombo, 1992, p. 684.

TABLE 30.3 Recommended infant and child car restraint systems

Type of Restraint	*Weight Limit*	*Description*	*Illustration*
Infant in Rear-facing Restraint in the Centre Back Seat	Birth to 9 kg	• Transport your infant in a rear-facing infant restraint in the back seat. It is safest. Larger restraints prevent snug harnessing and a plastic shield can cause injury if the infant collides with it. Start them in a rear-facing infant seat and when they reach the weight limit of the restraint, switch to a larger rear-facing convertible seat. • Your child is ready to ride the convertible restraint forward-facing when he or she reaches one year of age	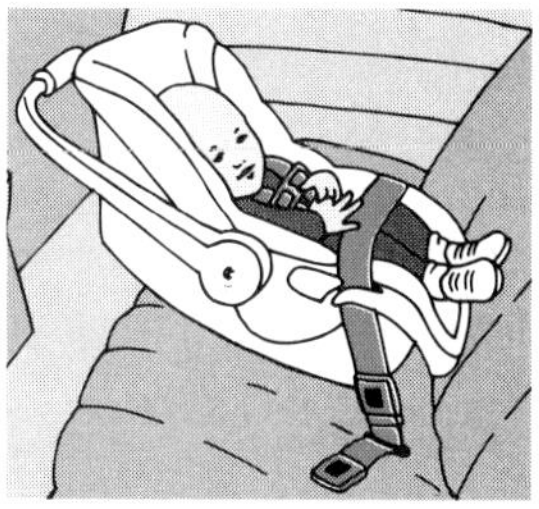
Rear-Facing Convertible Restraints	Birth to 9 kg	• NEVER place a rear-facing restraint in a vehicle seat equipped with an air bag. • Seats faces rear. Place in back seat • Adjust to reclining position • Attach with adult seat belt and, if necessary, use a locking clip. Follow manufacturer's instructions. • Check harness tension each trip.	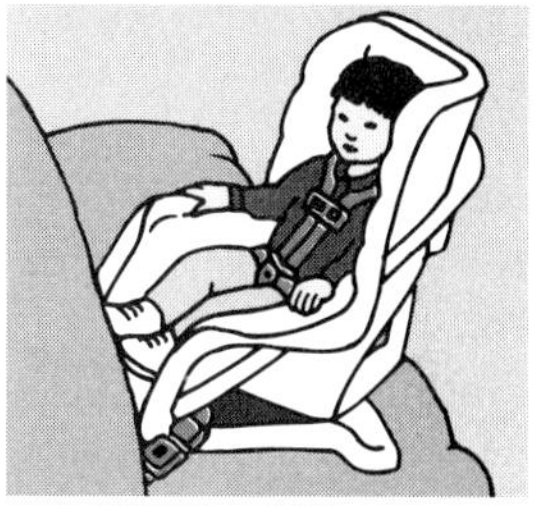
Forward-Facing Child Restraint	9–18 kg	• Seat faces forward. Place in back seat. • Secure tether strap to anchorage hardware in vehicle (check vehicle owner's manual for installation information). • Attach with adult seatbelt and if necessary, use a locking clip. Follow manufacturer's instructions. • Check harness tension each trip.	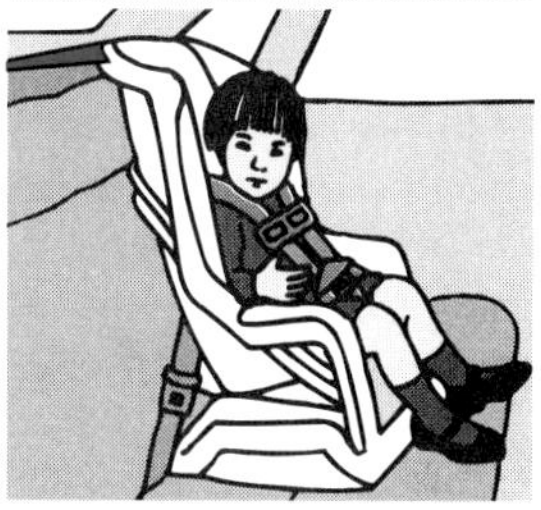
Booster Seat	18–27 kg	• Seat faces forward • Place booster in back seat. • Attach with adult seat belt according to the manufacturer's instructions. • Buckle lap belt low over hips. • Position shoulder belt over shoulders and across chest. • Aftermarket seatbelt adjustment devices are not recommended. • Keep child in booster seat for as long as physically necessary.	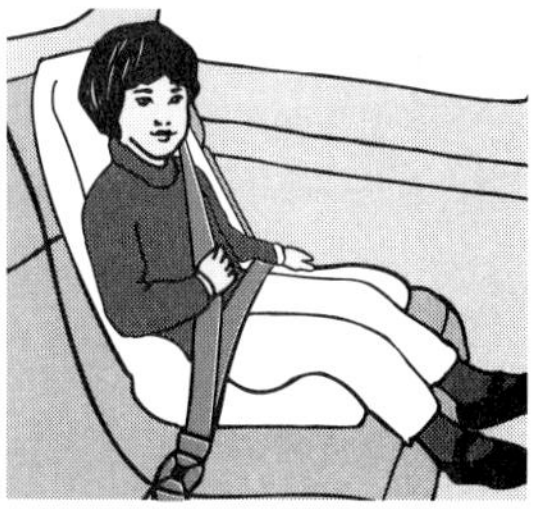
During Pregnancy		• Wear the lap belt snug and low over the pelvic bones and wear the shoulder belt snug against chest. Do not put the belt under your arm.	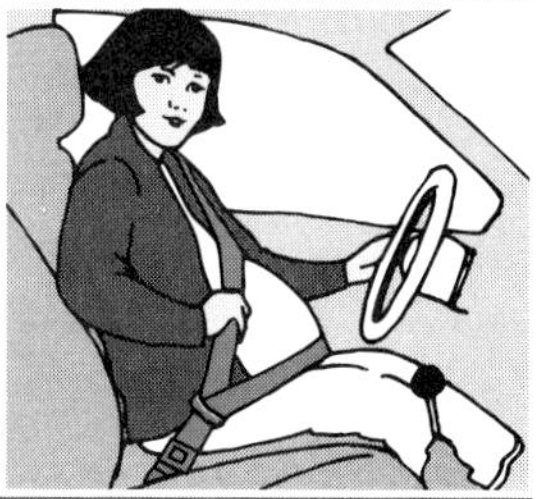

SOURCE: Insurance Corporation of British Columbia, 1997.

The nurse can assist parents by providing information about current legislation and the suggested types of restraint systems. Children should never be allowed to travel in the cargo area of a van, station wagon or truck. Loose, bulky objects in vehicles should be secured. Travel beds and plastic baby seats should never be used in a vehicle, as they are not designed to give crash protection. The infant carrier or seat must be ready for the infant's first ride home from the hospital.

BICYCLE SAFETY

The risk of bicycle-related brain injury can be greatly reduced by the use of bicycle helmets but, as yet, few people actually wear them. Some communities have established mandatory bicycle helmet programs to prevent injuries while cycling.

SCHOOL AND RECREATIONAL SAFETY

In sports arenas and playgrounds, adult supervision is needed to ensure safety for children and youth. Someone skilled in first aid should always be available. Safety is an important area of consideration for school boards, teachers and parents. Both students and teachers need safe working conditions and access to support services (Government of Ontario, 1993).

Injury Prevention in the Workplace

Injury prevention should be part of the overall occupational health and safety program in the workplace. Most large companies and hospitals recognize the importance of promoting health and wellness and preventing injuries, and are hiring staff and allocating funding for occupational health and safety programs.

THE OCCUPATIONAL HEALTH AND SAFETY TEAM

Like any employer, hospitals and other health care agencies are required to adhere to provincial occupational health and safety legislation and regulations. These legally required activities are an essential part of the work of the health and safety team, and serve to support and complement in-house programs and measures. The Occupational Health and Safety team may consist of one or more of the following professionals:

- occupational safety and health manager
- accident prevention/safety officer
- occupational health nurse
- full-time, part-time or occasional occupational health physician
- Workers' Compensation Board claims manager
- clerical support.

In a large corporation, an expanded department might include:

- industrial hygienist
- physiotherapist
- occupational therapist.

Other specialists, such as ergonomists (specialists in environmental hazards in the workplace), toxicologists

Occupational Health and Safety

An occupational health and safety program usually includes, but is not limited to
Education and training of employees about:

- accident prevention and awareness, documentation
- accident investigation and reporting
- workplace inspection and job safety audits
- Workplace Hazardous Materials Information System (WHMIS)
- respirator fit testing, use or any other personal protective equipment
- programs for specific hazards (such as asbestos, noise, lead or mercury)
- back care and lifting education
- Workplace and personal monitoring of physical, chemical, biological or psychological hazards
- Development of safety policies and procedures
- Health assessment and counselling.

Workplace Hazardous Materials Information System (WHMIS)

WHMIS is a system designed to communicate information about hazardous materials in the workplace—from the suppliers of controlled products to employers and to workers through the three key elements: **labelling, material safety data sheets*** and **worker education**. The relationships are shown in the diagram.

*to be completed where the employer produces a controlled product.

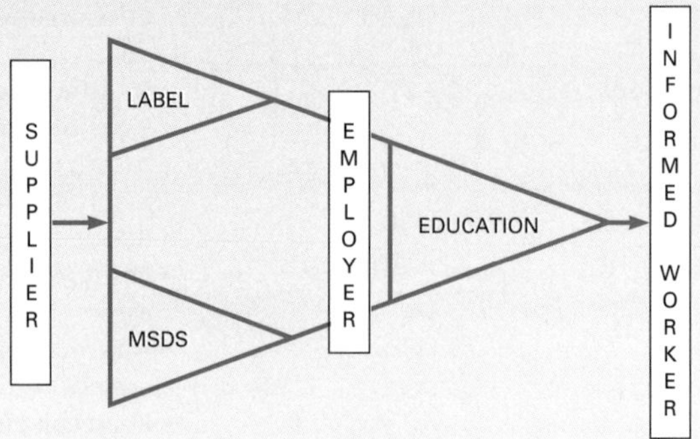

Legislation to implement WHMIS has been enacted at both the federal and the provincial and territorial levels. Federal requirements deal with the importation and sale of controlled products, and provincial legislation covers the storage, handling and use of controlled products in the workplace.

Every province and territory uses a common system of labelling for containers of all controlled products. In addition to this system, WHMIS requires education programs, so that employees will have a thorough understanding of the information on the WHMIS labels (see Figure 30.1) and in the material safety data sheets (MSDS).

SOURCE: Workers' Compensation Board of British Columbia, 1998b, p. 7.

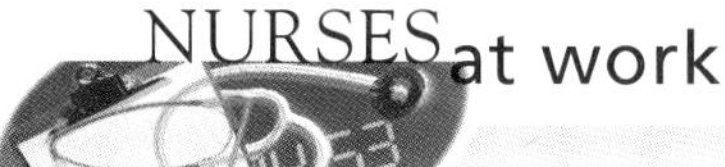

Occupational Health Nurse

Saskatchewan. The 1100 employees in our head offices have direct access to the services and programs offered by the Employee Health Centre. Occupational health nursing is grounded in illness prevention, health promotion and maintenance, health teaching and the control and elimination of workplace hazards. The community of employees that I serve is about 60 percent female and 40 percent male. I have observed that female employees generally request support and assistance from the Employee Health Centre more often than their male colleagues.

Most of the programs that I have contact with have an educational or supportive focus. These programs address such topics as family and women's issues, infant and child care, parenting skills, nutrition, grief/loss, cardiovascular risk factors, migraine headaches, diabetes, workplace stress and conflict management. In addition, employees often come to talk directly to me about their concerns; at other times, employees attend "lunch and learn" sessions or come to borrow videos, books and

to a community agency, when necessary. I believe that part of my role is to ensure that employees and their families have support and assistance to deal with the complexities of the health care system.

I see "walk-ins" in the Clinic Room and, once a nursing assessment is complete, I can provide a variety of direct care services. Frequently, I find that employees come in "to get something for my headache," then stay to talk in confidence about work stress or some personal problem.

Many employees spend all day at a keyboard doing data entry. However, our employees have experienced very few carpal tunnel or other cumulative trauma injuries. Part of this success lies with our aggressive ergonomics program.

Occupational health nursing is an excellent example of nursing within a primary health care model. There is a range of health and wellness programs and services that can be offered to employees. All it takes is knowledge, skill, creativity and self-motivation, and I would not trade it for anything!

—*Lynda Kushnir Pekrul, RN, BScN, MScAdmin*

(specialists in the field of poisons and toxins) and orthopedic specialists (physicians in the field of the prevention and correction of deformities involving locomotor areas of the body, such as muscles, bones and joints) might be brought in on a consulting basis. The type and number of staff required and their responsibilities will depend on the type and size of the business, the type of hazards in the workplace and the activities identified within provincial health and safety regulations. In many agencies, members of the health and safety team also serve as advisors to the Joint Occupational Health and Safety Committee.

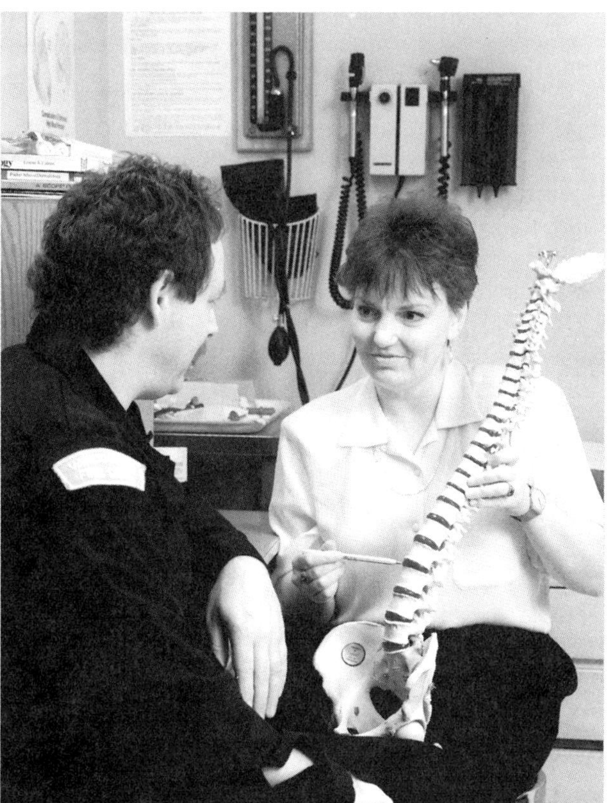

The occupational health team teaches injury awareness and prevention.

Occupational hazards differ greatly from one workplace to another. The types of equipment, chemicals, machinery, work processes and location of work all affect the focus of the safety program. In general, however, the role of the occupational health and safety department includes the identification of occupational hazards, the development and implementation of a safety and accident prevention program and the provision of first aid to injured workers. In addition, the occupational health and safety unit provides health assessment and counselling services for employees of the organization. This is usually one of the responsibilities of the occupational health nurse. The occupational health and safety professional in a health care facility also provides specific expertise regarding infectious diseases.

THE WORKPLACE HAZARDOUS MATERIALS INFORMATION SYSTEM (WHMIS)

The Workplace Hazardous Materials Information System (WHMIS) was developed in response to Canadian workers' request to know—and their right to know—about the hazards of materials used in the workplace to safety and health (WCB of BC, 1998b). A brief summary of the program is given in the box on the previous page. Figure 30.1 illustrates the labels for various WHMIS hazard classes.

A controlled product is a substance or material that meets or exceeds criteria for inclusion in one or more of the following WHMIS hazard classes and divisions:

CLASS A:

COMPRESSED GAS. This class includes compressed gases, dissolved gases and gases liquefied by compression or refrigeration. Examples: gas cylinders for oxyacetylene welding or water disinfection.

CLASS B:

FLAMMABLE AND COMBUSTIBLE MATERIAL. Solids, liquids and gases capable of catching fire or exploding in the presence of a source of ignition. Examples: white phosphorus, acetone and butane. **Flammable** liquids such as acetone are more easily ignited than **combustible** liquids such as kerosene.

CLASS C:

OXIDIZING MATERIAL. Materials that provide oxygen or similar substances and that increase the risk of fire if they come in contact with flammable or combustible materials. Examples: sodium hypochlorite, perchloric acid, inorganic peroxides.

CLASS D: POISONOUS AND INFECTIOUS MATERIALS.

DIVISION 1:

Materials Causing Immediate and Serious Toxic Effects. This division covers materials that can cause the death of a person exposed to small amounts. Examples: sodium cyanide, hydrogen sulfide.

DIVISION 2:

Materials Causing Other Toxic Effects. This division covers materials that cause immediate skin or eye irritation as well as those that can cause long-term effects in a person repeatedly exposed to small amounts. Examples: acetone (irritant), asbestos (cancer-causing), toluene diisocyanate (a sensitizing agent).

DIVISION 3:

Biohazardous Infectious Material. This division applies to materials that contain harmful microorganisms. Examples: cultures or diagnostic specimens containing salmonella bacteria or the hepatitis B virus.

CLASS E:

CORROSIVE MATERIAL. Caustic or acid materials that can destroy the skin or eat through metals. Examples: muriatic acid, lye.

CLASS F:

DANGEROUSLY REACTIVE MATERIAL. Products that can undergo dangerous reaction if subjected to heat, pressure, shock or allowed to contact water. Examples: plastic monomers such as butadiene and some cyanides.

FIGURE 30.1 What is a controlled product?

SOURCE: Workers' Compensation Board of British Columbia, 1998b, pp. 4–5.

WELLNESS PROGRAMS

At one time, it was believed that occupational accidents happened because workers were not "careful enough." More recently, safety experts suggest that lack of management control is an important factor in causing accidents. Safety programs, policies, accident investigation, safety training and providing a safe environment all fall under management's control. However, supervisors and workers both play key roles in developing and maintaining an injury-free workplace. Joint Occupational Health and Safety Committees are mandated by law in each province for most workplaces. Management, unionized and nonunionized staff work together on these joint committees to develop and maintain an effective occupational health and safety program.

Programs such as the Employee and Family Assistance Program (which offers confidential counselling), continuous quality improvement and stress management programs, among others, aim to alleviate or prevent stress-related problems. It has recently been recognized that injuries are often linked to work-related stress and stress from personal, financial or other worries. People take their worries to work; they do not automatically shed them at the company door. A 1984 Canadian study on work and well-being suggests that "troubled employees tend to make more errors, produce poorer quality material and damage equipment" (Thomas, 1993, p. 37).

Corporations have developed wellness programs, realizing that stress is a major factor in absenteeism, work injuries and illnesses, errors of omission or commission and lowered productivity. The wellness program developed in 1986 by Carolyn Mathews and a group of nurses working for Imperial Oil at various sites across the country exemplifies the trend towards wellness in occupational health. Mathews' program was organized in four parts: increasing health awareness in employees, lifestyles examination/risk management, personal prescription (tailoring a program to meet the needs of the individual employee) and behavioural change.

Injury Prevention in the Hospital

In nursing, a knowledge base of safe nursing practices is essential. This involves not only a sound knowledge of the nursing and allied sciences, but also a knowledge of preventive nursing measures. Nurses must recognize circumstances that could result in an injury, and intervene.

ENABLING SELF-PROTECTION

All patients have self-protection learning needs while in the agency. These needs include an orientation to the physical design of the nursing unit and the equipment in the patient's immediate surroundings. Patients must know how to call for assistance if needed (and the call bell must be [illegible] the equipment in and around the bed, and they must be alerted to safety precautions in the use of this equipment. Each nursing measure, diagnostic test or examination and therapeutic measure has important safety precautions that patients need to be aware of to protect themselves from harm. If patients know why the safety measures are being taken, they are more apt to participate.

ENVIRONMENTAL FACTORS

General considerations of environmental factors include arranging everything for the patient's comfort and convenience, as well as that of family members, other visitors and staff. Equipment used in hospitals is generally portable, so that it can be easily moved to a more convenient position or location. Hospitals try to obtain equipment that is also quiet, durable, simple to operate and easily repaired. In many agencies, equipment is built into the patient's unit so that it is easier to use and always convenient. As a result, fewer hazardous objects are in and around the patient's bed. Any electrical equipment being used must be checked and grounded, and must comply with safety standards.

The patient's unit and the nursing unit itself should be kept as free of clutter as possible. When giving care to a patient, nurses should always make sure that there is a clear working space, that they can see what they are doing and that it is possible to practise good body mechanics in any lifting or moving that is involved. It is awkward to work over side rails, for example, or to reach around objects.

REPORTING ACCIDENTS/ INCIDENTS

All accidents—that is, all events that have resulted or could have resulted in injury to a patient, visitor or staff member—are reported so that remedial measures may be instituted. For example, if a patient receives an incorrect medication, notifying the physician and filing a medication incident report help to prevent a recurrence of this error and to remedy the effects of the incorrect medication. Incidents are ordinarily reported on an incident report form (see Figure 30.2). Many hospitals require that employees injured at work complete an employee incident/accident report form (see Figure 30.3) and report to either a designated first aid attendant or the emergency department. Provincial WCB reporting requirements must also be observed when workers are injured.

Reporting accidents also guides the safety committee of an agency in instituting proper preventive measures. The findings of these committees can be used as the bases for changes in medical and nursing practices and as indications of the need for the education of patients and personnel.

PREVENTING FALLS AND SELF-INFLICTED INJURIES

[illegible] falls from beds, from chairs, while walking or while getting into or out of a bathtub. A person who is weakened by illness can lose balance and fall while simply leaning towards a table that is out of reach. Nurses can prevent many injuries of this kind by being alert to potentially dangerous situations and remedying them. For example, adjustable beds can be left in the low position. At this level, the patient will be able to get in and out of bed more safely. Also, patients who have been in bed for several days or who are weakened by illness can be helped to recognize their need for assistance with mobilization.

Slippery floors can be dangerous to people in any situation, not only to patients. To minimize this danger, nonslippery materials are used on the floor surfaces of hospitals. Also, since anything spilled on a floor may make it slippery, spills should be mopped up before an accident occurs. Floors should be washed and polished at a time when there is little traffic, and signs warning that the floor is wet and slippery should be prominently placed.

Untidiness can also contribute to injuries. People can trip over electric cords, footstools and equipment left on the floor. Walkways, such as areas between a patient's bed and the bathroom, can be particularly hazardous when they are not kept clear. Patients have fallen from beds while reaching for articles on bedside tables or while looking for a misplaced call button. The nurse can help the patient to arrange these items so that they are within easy reach.

Other possible causes of falls are movable wheelchairs or stretchers. Often, just as a patient is about to sit in a wheelchair, it moves out of place. Most movable equipment is furnished with locks for the wheels. These locks should be set when the equipment is to be used and released only after the patient is secure.

When a patient first becomes ambulatory after a period of time in bed, some physical support is often required. Many hospitals and other health agencies have rails in the halls to guide and support patients while walking. These and other measures, such as rubber treads on stairs, can help prevent many falls.

Out of concern for a patient's safety, the nurse may employ specific safety devices. There are dangers involved in the use of many of these devices. Disoriented patients may become dangerously entangled in restraints, for example, or a safety device may make a patient unable to move in case of a fire. Many safety devices, therefore, should not be used unless absolutely necessary. In most institutions, devices are used either upon the request of the attending physician, or when, in the judgement of the nurse, they become necessary. Policies vary, however, and the nurse should be familiar with each institution's practices. Students should always check with the primary nurse or with their teacher before using safety devices for patients.

PATIENT/VISITOR INCIDENT REPORT FORM

1. ☐ In-patient 2. ☐ Out-patient 3. ☐ Visitor

A. COMPLETE SECTION A FOR ALL INCIDENTS

Unit/OR #/Dept. reporting incident:
Unit/Dept where incident occurred (if different):

TYPE OF INCIDENT: (Complete appropriate area in Section B)

1. ☐ Fall
2. ☐ Medication/blood/IVs
3. ☐ Operative
4. ☐ Skin Injury/Breakdown
5. ☐ Property Loss, Damage, Theft
6. ☐ Safety/Security/MOAB

Date & Time of Incident: ___/___/___ (YY/MM/DD) ______ (HOURS (00:00))

Person reporting incident: ______________ (Please Print)

BRIEF DESCRIPTION: ______________________________

1. Notified:

	Name	Time
1. ☐ MD		
2. ☐ Charge Nurse/ ☐ Manager		
3. ☐ Family		
4. ☐ Security		
5. ☐ Police: Case #		
6. ☐ Other		

2. Actions taken:

1. ☐ Treatment implemented: ☐ Nurse initiated ☐ Physician initiated
2. ☐ Increased monitoring (NVS, etc)
3. ☐ Additional lab work
4. ☐ X-ray taken : Results ☐ New findings ☐ No new findings
5. ☐ Transferred to ______________
6. ☐ Care plan revised
7. ☐ Other ______________
8. ☐ If equipment related:
   - ☐ Biomed Engineering phoned & equipment set aside for BME
   - ☐ Physical Plant requisition completed & sent
   - ☐ Other

B. COMPLETE APPROPRIATE SECTION ACCORDING TO TYPE OF INCIDENT

1. FALLS

1. Patient's Condition Before Incident: (Check one)

1. ☐ Alert
2. ☐ Oriented
3. ☐ Disoriented: ☐ Time ☐ Place ☐ Person
4. ☐ Restless
5. ☐ Sedated
6. ☐ Unconscious
7. ☐ Anesthetized
8. ☐ Other

2. Contributory Factors:

1. ☐ History of falls: ☐ Identified on admission ☐ Since admission
2. ☐ Unsteady gait
3. ☐ Impaired balance (e.g., dizzy, hypotensive, weak)
4. ☐ Bowel & bladder needs
5. ☐ Visual impairment
6. ☐ Decreased safety awareness
7. ☐ Equipment ______________
8. ☐ Environmental ______________
9. ☐ Faulty footwear
10. ☐ Other ______________

3. Injury

1. ☐ None apparent
2. ☐ Abrasion
3. ☐ Cut
4. ☐ Hematoma
5. ☐ Fracture
6. ☐ Other

2. MEDICATIONS/BLOOD/IV

1. Type (Check one)

1. ☐ Omitted drug
2. ☐ Incorrect drug
3. ☐ Incorrect patient
4. ☐ Incorrect rate
5. ☐ Incorrect dose
6. ☐ Incorrect route
7. ☐ Incorrect time
8. ☐ Extra dose
9. ☐ Unordered drug (given without order)
10. ☐ Incorrect IV solution
11. ☐ Allergy to drug
12. Other ______________

2. Drug (Check any)

1. ☐ Anti-infective
2. ☐ Analgesic
3. ☐ Anticoagulant
4. ☐ Cardiovascular
5. ☐ Insulin
6. ☐ Immunosuppressant
7. ☐ Steroids
8. ☐ Sedatives/anxiolytics
9. ☐ Psychotropic
10. ☐ Large-volume IV solutions
11. ☐ Blood products
12. ☐ Other ______________

Drugs Ordered

____

Drugs Given/# Doses

____

3. Contributing Factors

1. ☐ Allergy sheet overlooked
2. ☐ Unclear order/Order misread
   - ☐ Previous order not D/C
   - ☐ Ambiguous
   - ☐ Illegible handwriting
   - ☐ Look alike/sound alike
   - ☐ Illegible copy of order
3. ☐ Order not processed
4. ☐ Order not received in Pharmacy
5. ☐ Drug incorrectly removed from MAR
6. ☐ Drug not added to MAR
7. ☐ Product/Drug not received on unit
8. ☐ Transcription error
9. ☐ Breach of policy
10. ☐ IV positional
11. ☐ Other ______________

3. O.R.

3. O.R.

1. ☐ No consent/consent incomplete
2. ☐ Incorrect site
3. ☐ Incorrect count/count not done
   - ☐ Sponge/small items
   - ☐ Needles
   - ☐ Instruments
4. ☐ Foreign body left in patient
5. ☐ Equipment malfunction
6. ☐ Supplies not available
7. ☐ Other ______________

4. SKIN INJURIES/BREAKDOWN

1. Type (Check any)

1. ☐ Pressure ulcer
   - ☐ Blisters or abrasions
   - ☐ Exposure of subcutaneous tissue
   - ☐ Exposure of muscle or bone
   - ☐ Dark necrotic tissue (eschar)
2. ☐ Skin tear
3. ☐ Burn: ☐ Chemical ☐ Tape ☐ Thermal ☐ Electrical
4. ☐ Laceration
5. ☐ Hematoma

2. Related Information:

1. ☐ Pressure
2. ☐ Shearing
3. ☐ Prolonged surgery/ Procedure ______________
4. ☐ Hemodynamical IV/unstable/inotropic dependent
5. ☐ Equipment related
6. ☐ Other ______________

5. PROPERTY LOSS, DAMAGE, THEFT

PROPERTY

1. ☐ Loss
2. ☐ Damage
3. ☐ Theft

TYPE:

1. ☐ Dentures
2. ☐ Glasses
3. ☐ Hearing aid
4. ☐ Jewellery
5. ☐ Money
6. ☐ Clothing
7. ☐ Medications
8. ☐ Other ______________

To be completed by manager:

Dentures/Glasses/Hearing aids only:

Recommended reimbursed by hospital:

1. ☐ Yes* 2. ☐ No

*If yes, forward copy to controller

Patient/Family contact person:

Name: ______________

Tel #: ______________

____
Manager's Signature

6. SAFETY/SECURITY/MOAB

1. ☐ Alleged abuse
2. ☐ Missing
3. ☐ Verbal aggressive behaviour
   - ☐ Questioning ☐ Refusal ☐ Release ☐ Intimidation
4. ☐ Physical aggressive behaviour
   - ☐ Self ☐ Other patients/visitors ☐ Staff ☐ Environment
5. ☐ Contributing factors to aggressive behaviour:
   - ☐ Chemical dependency withdrawal ______________
   - ☐ Physiological ______________
   - ☐ Psychological ______________
   - ☐ History of aggression
   - ☐ CAGE score on admission ______________ /4______
   - ☐ Other
6. ☐ Weapons: ☐ Threat ☐ Use
   Description: ______________
7. ☐ Self-inflicted injury
8. ☐ Other ______________

Complete follow-up on reverse side of Canary Copy.
Forward White Copy to Patient Services Administration.

FIGURE 30.2 Patient/visitor incident report form

SOURCE: Vancouver Hospital & Health Sciences Centre, 1996, Vancouver, B.C.

Vancouver Hospital & Health Sciences Centre

EMPLOYEE INCIDENT/ACCIDENT REPORT

SEE REVERSE FOR DIRECTIONS

Surname: ______ Given Names: ______ SIN: ___/___/___ ID #: ______ Date of Birth: ___/___/___ (year / month / day)	Date of Incident: ___/___/___ (year / month / day) Time of Incident: ______ hours Date Reported: ___/___/___ (year / month / day) Time Reported: ______ hours	Department/Unit: ______ Job Title: ______ Immediate Supervisor: ______ Scheduled Working Hours (day of injury): From: ______ h To ______ h
Mailing Address: ______	Home Phone #: ______ Work Phone #: ______	Family Physician: ______
Status: (✓) ☐ Rotating Shifts & Rotating Days Off ☐ Rotating Shifts & Regular Days Off ☐ Full Time ☐ Regular Part-time Days off: M T W T F S S	**Action Taken Following Incident:** ☐ Returned to Work ☐ First Aid ☐ Sent to E.H.U. ☐ Doctor/Emergency **Note:** *If you miss work or see a doctor, contact the Employee Health Unit*	☐ WCB ☐ No Time Loss ☐ Lost Time Injury (missed next shift) ☐ Time off duty ______ h

SECTION B: *DETAILS OF INCIDENT* (EMPLOYEE COMPLETES)

Location of Incident (bldg., floor, room #): ______

Brief Description of Incident: ______

SECTION C: *INJURY DATA* (EMPLOYEE COMPLETES)

Injury Classification:
1. ☐ abrasion
2. ☐ allergic reaction
3. ☐ burn
4. ☐ concussion
5. ☐ contusion
6. ☐ crush injury
7. ☐ dermatitis
8. ☐ dislocation
9. ☐ exposure—BBF
10. ☐ exposure—chemical
11. ☐ foreign body
12. ☐ fracture
13. ☐ hearing loss
14. ☐ infectious disease
15. ☐ laceration—instrument
16. ☐ laceration—other
17. ☐ puncture—needlestick
18. ☐ puncture—other
19. ☐ respiratory condition
20. ☐ sprain
21. ☐ strain—back
22. ☐ strain—repetitive
23. ☐ strain—other
24. ☐ no injury
25. ☐ other ______

Body Part:
1. ☐ head
2. ☐ face
3. ☐ eyes
4. ☐ ears
5. ☐ neck
6. ☐ shoulder/upper arm
7. ☐ upper back
8. ☐ lower back
9. ☐ elbow/forearm
10. ☐ wrist
11. ☐ hands
12. ☐ fingers
13. ☐ chest
14. ☐ abdomen
15. ☐ hips
16. ☐ groin
17. ☐ leg
18. ☐ knees
19. ☐ ankle
20. ☐ foot
21. ☐ multiple
22. ☐ none
23. ☐ other ______

left: ______ right: ______

If strain involving patient, indicate activity:
1. ☐ transfer: Bed to Chair
2. ☐ transfer: Chair to Bed
3. ☐ transfer: Move up Bed/Stretcher
4. ☐ transfer: Rolling side to side
5. ☐ transfer: Sitting up
6. ☐ transfer: Move Bed to Stretcher
7. ☐ transfer: Move from Stretcher
8. ☐ transfer: Reposition pt. in Chair
9. ☐ lift: from Floor
10. ☐ lift: Bed to Chair – Chair to Bed
11. ☐ lift: Mechanical
12. ☐ catch falling patient
13. ☐ bathing patient
14. ☐ prlonged forward flexion
15. ☐ other ______

SECTION D: *ACCIDENT INVESTIGATION* (SUPERVISOR COMPLETES)

IMMEDIATE CAUSES:

Substandard Practice:
1. ☐ communication lacking
2. ☐ equipment/tool use improper
3. ☐ help not obtained
4. ☐ inattentive
5. ☐ insecure grip
6. ☐ lifting improper
7. ☐ load/object not secured
8. ☐ loading/placement improper
9. ☐ lockout procedure not followed
10. ☐ personal protective equipment not worn
11. ☐ repetitive strain/lengthy work in static position
12. ☐ rules/procedures not followed
13. ☐ rushing
14. ☐ unsafe act by another person
15. ☐ workplace conduct
16. ☐ other: ______

Substandard Condition:
1. ☐ aggressive act
2. ☐ awkward position
3. ☐ congestion/limited space
4. ☐ equipment defective/ inadequate/lacking
5. ☐ excessive noise
6. ☐ housekeeping poor
7. ☐ lighting inadequate
8. ☐ maintenance inadequate
9. ☐ personal protective equipment inadequate
10. ☐ surface slippery/uneven
11. ☐ ventilation inadequate
12. ☐ vision obstructed
13. ☐ environmental (heat, cold, etc)
14. ☐ other ______

BASIC CAUSES:

Job Factors:
1. ☐ design, layout inadequate
2. ☐ emergency task
3. ☐ follow-up lacking
4. ☐ hiring procedures
5. ☐ job/skill training inadequate
6. ☐ leadership inadequate
7. ☐ mechanical lift required
8. ☐ orientation inadequate
9. ☐ planning inadequate
10. ☐ poor equipment/tool design
11. ☐ procedure/rules inadequate
12. ☐ signage/labelling inadequate
13. ☐ staffing inadequate
14. ☐ storage/handling problem
15. ☐ unexpected pt behaviour
16. ☐ other: ______

Personal Factors:
1. ☐ fatigue
2. ☐ illness
3. ☐ knowledge/skill/experience lacking
4. ☐ language difficulties
5. ☐ medical condition
6. ☐ personal distraction
7. ☐ physically incapable
8. ☐ pre-existing condition
9. ☐ other: ______

ACTION(S) TAKEN TO PREVENT RECURRENCE:

Corrective Actions: ______ **Date:** ______

	NAME (PLEASE PRINT)	SIGNATURE	LOCAL	DATE
EMPLOYEE				
SUPERVISOR				
DEPT. HEAD				

1. White—Emp. Health Unit within 24 hours 2. Canary—OH&S following completion 3. Pink—Department Head for follow-up

If more space is required, please use additional paper and include with report.

FIGURE 30.3 Employee incident/accident report

SOURCE: Vancouver Hospital & Health Sciences Centre, 1996, Vancouver, B.C.

RESEARCH to practice

Rossy, D., Jourdain-Grand, S., Lamb, G., Armstrong, E., Athrens, S., & Berry, J. (1997). Preventing falls in high-risk patients. *Canadian Nurse, 93*(4), 53–54.

Because patient falls—and the lack of awareness or ability to predict who is at risk—are a major source of injury, the investigators of this study undertook the task of developing and implementing a fall prevention program for high-risk patients in the geriatric assessment unit at Ottawa Civic Hospital. The focus of the study was to facilitate a process to identify high-risk patients, plan appropriate safety interventions, develop a standardized program and educate staff.

The initial phase of the study was intended to define the terms fall and near-fall; to develop a method to calculate the fall rate; to create a fall risk questionnaire, colour-coded identification system and educational tools for patients and families in hospital and in the community; and to develop a standard of nursing care related to safety that included fall prevention strategies. The next phase was to introduce staff of the geriatric assessment unit to the program. The piloting phase began in 1992.

The fall risk questionnaire and colour-coded system identified patients in the geriatric assessment unit who were at high risk for falls. The nurses then implemented the developed standard care for these patients. Fall rates were reviewed on a monthly basis.

Initial findings of this study revealed that the patient who was most at risk for falls was the individual over the age of 75 years with three to four health problems. In addition, once a unit-specific fall-rate standard was identified and it was exceeded, patient monitoring strategies were increased related to the fall rate. A review of the data from 1992 to 1995 indicates that the program proved to be effective, as the number of falls on the unit significantly decreased in the first year of implementation and slightly increased during the second and third years.

Implications for practice that can be drawn from this study include the model, which is expected to prove useful for other units and for all patients, regardless of age. Further, implementation of a fall prevention program increased staff satisfaction, promoted other patient care initiatives and, finally, fostered a collaborative environment.

In recent years, nurses have adopted a least-restraint or no-restraint philosophy and have created policies for hospital settings (Cruz, Abdul-Hamid & Heater, 1997; AARN, 1995; RNANS, 1995; MARN, 1992). The purpose of these policies is to ensure that patients' rights—to live with dignity, to move with freedom and to make individual choices regarding their health—remain intact. Only if individualized assessments determine that the patient's or the staff's safety is at risk, and that the confusion is not attributed to medications, are restraints requested from the physician (Richmond Hospital, 1995). **Restraints** are defined as any mechanical/physical, chemical, environmental or other method used to inhibit, limit or control an individual's behaviour or activity (Richmond Hospital, 1995).

Alternatives to restraints include providing individuals with human company, that is, having friends, family or volunteers sit with them. If family is unavailable, patients can sit in a chair near the nurses' station or in a chair/bed equipped with an electronic device that detects motion. It is commonly known as a chair/bed check. It works when a patient attempts to stand or gets out of bed, an alarm will activate alerting the nurse to investigate. Coat tags are also used, especially with patients who wander. Ensuring that the patient is aware of the day, time and place is also an effective strategy to decrease the use of restraints. Purposeful conversation, calendars, clocks and radio or television can increase patients' cognitive stimulation and help reorient them to reality. Developing routines, such as toiletting and assessing for pain (two major reasons why patients attempt to get out of bed) can help decrease the patient's level of frustration (Stolley, 1995).

Side Rails

Side rails on beds can stop the patient from rolling off the bed. They do not deter the patient from climbing out. Most hospitals have policies regarding the use of side rails. Frequently, side rails are required on the beds of patients who are blind, unconscious or sedated, or who have muscular disabilities or seizures. Some hospitals have adopted a policy of using side rails on the beds of all patients, particularly at night.

It is important when side rails are in use that both rails be up. For example, even when the patient's bed is against the wall both rails should still be used; the wall does not replace the rail. When caring for the patient whose bed has side rails, the nurse should take down the rail on the side at which he or she is working. The nurse should go no farther than an arm's length away from that side of the bed without returning the side rail to its "up" position.

Many patients dislike the use of side rails; they may find them an embarrassing reminder of childhood cribs. Some people are fearful of them, while to others, side rails signify a loss of independence and control. An explanation of the purpose for using side rails often helps patients to accept them. Generally, side rails will not keep patients in bed against their will; if patients need restraining, safety jackets may be used.

Jacket and Belt Restraints

Patients who are confused sometimes try to climb over the side rails of the bed. These patients can often be restrained comfortably in bed by means of a safety jacket or belt (see Figure 30.4). The jacket is a sleeveless garment that has long

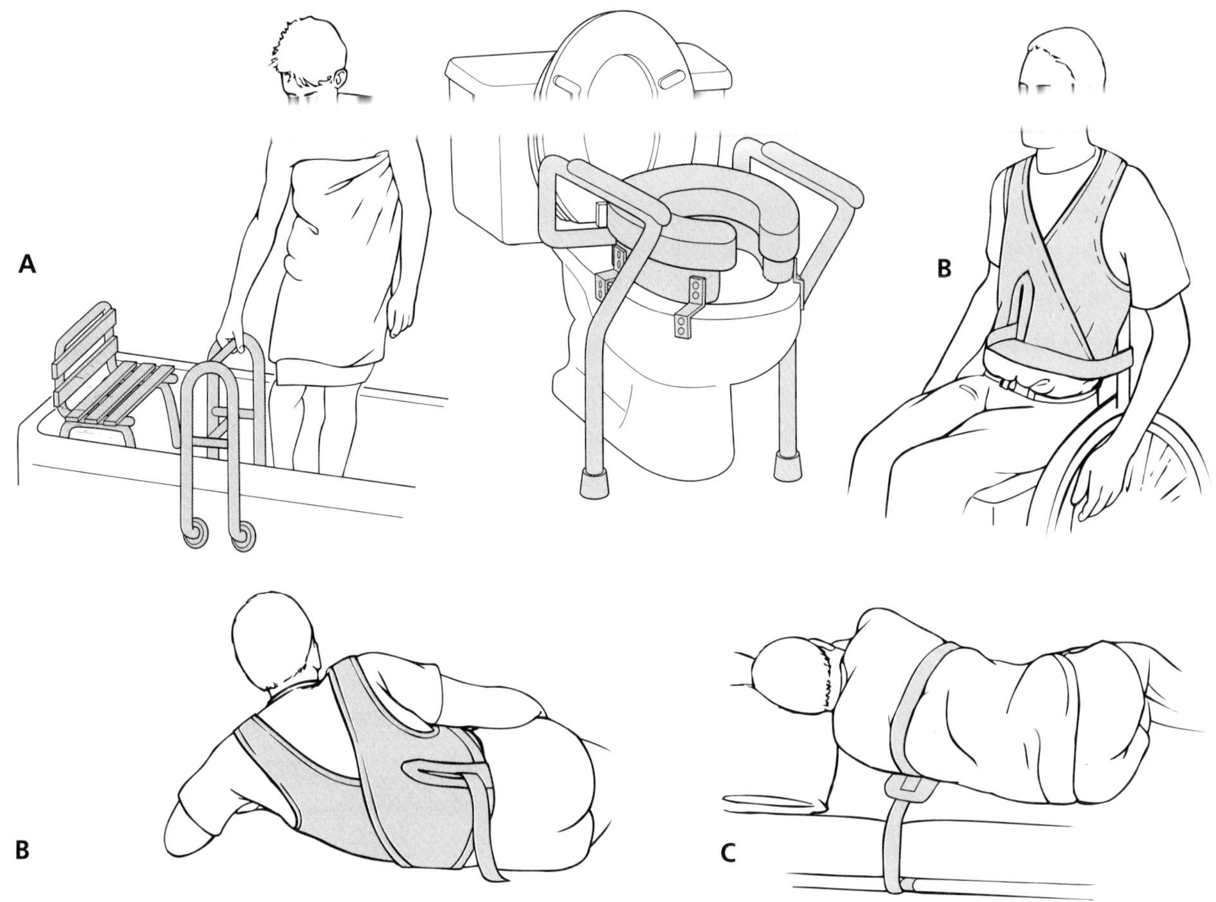

FIGURE 30.4 A. Hand rails. B. Jacket restraint. C. Belt restraint

cross-over ties either in front or in back that can be attached to the frame on either side of the bed but not tied to the side rail. The ties are secured to the frame out of reach of the patient. Some jacket restraints can also be used to hold patients securely upright in wheelchairs. When applying the jacket, ensure that it is not wrapped so tightly that it restricts breathing. Be sure to check the patient regularly to ensure comfort.

The belt restraint performs the same function as the jacket. It is secured around the patient's body, and ties are attached to the bed frame. Both jacket and belt restraints allow patients to move relatively freely in bed, yet restrain them from climbing over the side rails and possibly falling to the floor. When a belt restraint is used, care must be taken to ensure that it is not placed too tightly around the patient's chest or abdomen.

Arm and Leg Restraints

Occasionally it is necessary to apply arm or leg restraints to patients in bed. Generally, this is an undesirable measure because it limits a patient's movements, and this in turn often causes anxiety, increasing restlessness and subsequent fatigue. It is particularly dangerous to restrain only one side of the body because this tends to increase restlessness, and patients may injure themselves as they try to move the restrained side. If only two limbs are restrained, they should be opposite limbs. Few patients like to be tied down, regardless of how irrational they are. The reaction is usually to struggle against whatever is hampering movement, and patients may become quite agitated. Injury to the tissues of the wrists and ankles may result from the friction engendered by rubbing against the restraints. Occasionally, leather restraints may be used. Many agencies will not permit the use of leather restraints except on a doctor's order. There is greater possibility of both adverse patient reaction to leather restraints and injury to the patient as a result of them.

An arm restraint may be prescribed during an intravenous infusion. Its chief purpose in this instance is to remind the patient to keep the arm immobilized during the treatment.

Arms and legs should not be restrained any longer than is absolutely necessary, and at least every two hours the restraints should be loosened and the limbs exercised. A patient's circulation may be restricted if a restraint is tight or if a limb is restrained in an abnormal position. Care must be taken to pad the skin and especially bony prominences before restraints are applied. A washcloth or abdominal pad may be used to protect the skin under the restraint. A knot over the pad serves to keep the restraint from being too tight. Absorbent cotton should never be used because it has a tendency to flatten out and form into lumps. At any sign of blueness, pallor or cold, or if the patient complains of tingling sensations in the extremity, the restraint is loosened and circulation is restored by exercise and massage. A limb is best restrained in a slightly flexed position.

Commercially prepared restraints are available; however, a common restraint used in many agencies is the clove hitch. The clove hitch restraint is made of a piece of cloth or tube gauze, as illustrated in Figure 30.5. The advantage of this restraint is that it does not tighten as the patient pulls on it. To make a clove hitch, first make a "figure eight" with a strip of material. Then pick up the loops and direct the padded extremity through the loops. Adjust the restraint so that it is secure but not too tight on the limb.

Mitt Restraints

Mitt restraints are indicated for patients who are confused or semi-conscious and who may pull at dressings and tubes, for example, a patient with a head injury or one who is confused following a stroke. Mitt restraints have the advantage of not permitting the patient to grasp such objects as dressings, tubing or bed rails, but they do not limit movement. A mitt restraint is like a soft boxing glove that pads the patient's hand. Commercial mitts are available (see Figure 30.6), or mitts may be made using abdominal pads, gauze bandage and adhesive tape. To make a mitt restraint, the nurse first places the patient's hand in a naturally flexed position. This allows unrestricted circulation and places little strain upon muscles. The patient is asked to grasp a soft rolled abdominal pad so that the thumb approximates the fingers. The soft abdominal pad permits flexion of the hand while the mitt is in place. All skin surfaces are separated to avoid irritation. The patient's wrist is padded with an abdominal pad to avoid rubbing bony prominences. Two abdominal pads are then placed over the patient's hand: one medial to lateral, one dorsal to ventral. These are secured by a gauze bandage applied in figure-eight patterns. A stockinette is then fitted over the hand and secured by adhesive tape just beyond the wrist pad. A double fold of stockinette open at one end is sufficient.

The mitts need to be removed regularly. When they are removed, the patient washes the hands and exercises them, or the nurse may do this. Mitt restraints should not be so tight as to impede circulation, but they must be secure and pad the patient's hands well.

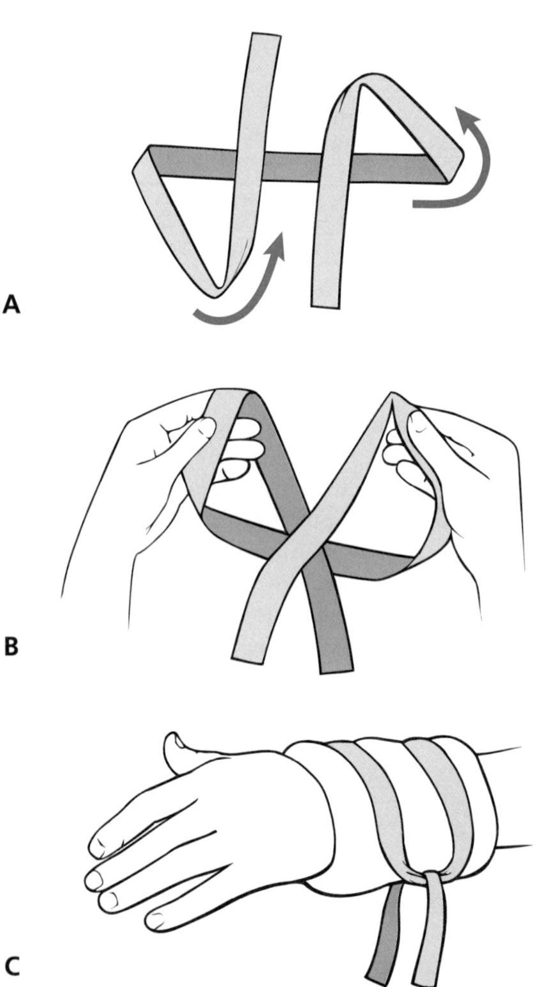

FIGURE 30.5 How to make a clove hitch restraint. A. Make a "figure eight." B. Pick up the loops. C. Put the padded extremity through the loops and adjust the restraint

PREVENTING INJURIES FROM FIRE AND OTHER THERMAL SOURCES

Thermal injuries involve the presence of harmful levels of heat or cold. The most common sources are fire, hot appliances or an improperly functioning electrical circuit. Generally, hospital policy requires electrical appliances to be checked regularly and maintained adequately in order to prevent injury. As an added precaution, patients are often required to have radios, electric razors and other appliances

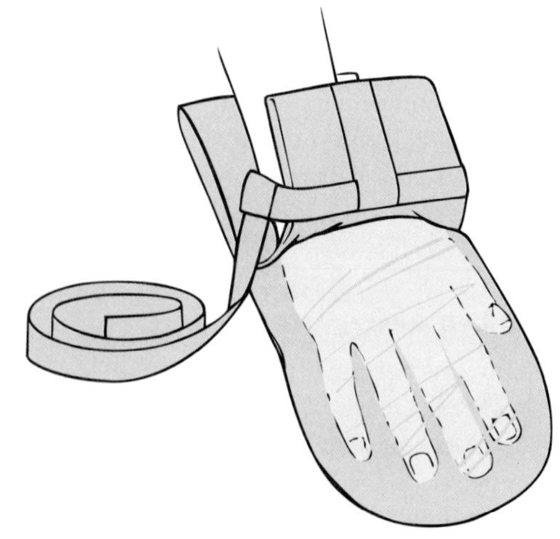

FIGURE 30.6 Mitt restraint

checked by maintenance staff before they use them in hospital. Hot water bottles, heating pads and heat lamps are also possible sources of thermal injury. Heat that is applied

safety limits for that patient.

Fire is a constant threat in institutions. Even though modern construction materials have lessened the danger of building fires, many materials within a hospital are highly combustible, for example, oxygen and ether.

In order for a fire to start, three elements must be present: a combustible material, heat and oxygen. A **combustible material** is anything that will burn, such as paper; textiles (for example, patients' bedding or oily rags); flammable liquids (for example, anesthetics); and electrical equipment. Heat sufficient to ignite the combustible material may come from such sources as a lighted match, a live cigarette, a spark or friction. There is usually enough oxygen in the atmosphere to support combustion if the other two elements are present. Fire prevention is usually directed, therefore, towards controlling combustible materials and heat. Fire-extinguishing measures are geared towards the reduction of heat (as by water cooling) and the exclusion of oxygen.

Fire Prevention

Most hospitals have active programs in fire prevention. These programs are usually designed with input from local fire departments and follow requirements entered in provincial health and safety regulations. Regular education of patients, staff and the public is an essential part of such programs. Some of the areas that are included in the fire control programs of hospitals are discussed in the following paragraphs.

SMOKING REGULATIONS Smoking is prohibited in all public areas of a hospital. Designated smoking areas are well marked and located away from chemical and gas storage areas. Patients who smoke require ashtrays that do not easily tip and that are constructed so that if a cigarette is left burning it will fall into the ashtray. Some patients (those who are confused or under the influence of a sedative or hypnotic drug) should not smoke unattended. Matches and cigarettes may be locked in a cupboard if the patient is confused.

SCRUPULOUS HOUSEKEEPING Thorough housekeeping and adequate maintenance of equipment lessen the likelihood of accidents and fires. Oily rags, paints and solvents are stored carefully in a special area so as to prevent spontaneous combustion.

HAZARDOUS PRODUCTS All hazardous products must be labelled, stored, handled and used according to federal and provincial legislation. Workplace Hazardous Materials Information System (WHMIS) training is usually part of both the orientation program for new staff and the annual in-services for all staff.

Volatile gases and liquids (those that are easily turned into vapour) are distributed to various areas of the agency under strict control, and all necessary fire precautions are observed.

vention program requires that all employees receive regular education in fire prevention and fire extinguishing. All agency personnel should be provided with information about specific policy and practice. Demonstrations in the use of fire equipment, practice in moving patients and knowledge of the established procedure to be followed upon the discovery of a fire are important. It is only through a continuous educational program in fire prevention and extinguishing methods that everyone's safety is ensured.

Types of Fires and Fire Extinguishers

Fires have been categorized into four major classes, based on the type of material that is burning. Class A fires are those involving paper, cloth, wood and similar solid combustible materials; Class B involve flammable liquids and gases; Class C, electrical equipment; and Class D, metals.

Fire extinguishers are simply containers for an agent, such as water or chemicals, that puts out a fire. Many kinds of extinguishers are available for home, institutional and industrial use. They come in dry chemical, carbon dioxide and halogenated types, and some contain pressurized water. The right type of extinguisher must be used to fight a fire. Some are dangerous when used on the wrong type of fire; for example, a water extinguisher (for Class A fires) should not be used on a grease (Class B) or an electrical (Class C) fire. The fire extinguisher should be clearly labelled with picture symbols that identify the type(s) of fire it is intended to extinguish (see Figure 30.7).

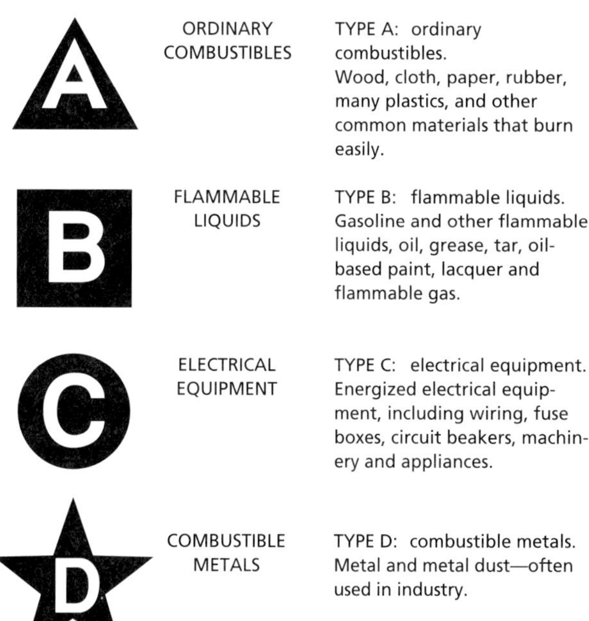

A
ORDINARY COMBUSTIBLES
TYPE A: ordinary combustibles. Wood, cloth, paper, rubber, many plastics, and other common materials that burn easily.
B
FLAMMABLE LIQUIDS
TYPE B: flammable liquids. Gasoline and other flammable liquids, oil, grease, tar, oil-based paint, lacquer and flammable gas.
C
ELECTRICAL EQUIPMENT
TYPE C: electrical equipment. Energized electrical equipment, including wiring, fuse boxes, circuit beakers, machinery and appliances.
D
COMBUSTIBLE METALS
TYPE D: combustible metals. Metal and metal dust—often used in industry.

FIGURE 30.7 Your extinguisher must fit the fire

SOURCE: National Fire Protection Association, 1997a, p. 35B.

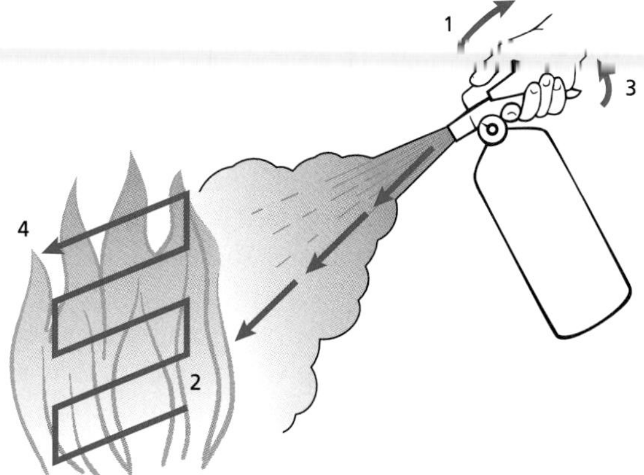

FIGURE 30.8 Most fire extinguishers are operated by the following four steps: 1. Pull the pin. This may involve releasing a puncture lever, inversion or other motion. 2. Aim the nozzle at the base of the fire. 3. Squeeze (or press) the handle. 4. Sweep from side to side at the base of the fire until the contents of the extinguisher are discharged. However, some extinguishers are operated slightly differently. Nurses should be familiar with the extinguishers available in the health agency where they work

Nurses need to know the types of fire extinguishers used in their agency and how to operate them. It is important to read the directions on the extinguisher to check for any variations. The four basic steps for using most types of extinguishers are illustrated in Figure 30.8.

Fire extinguishers must be accessible to personnel. Generally, they are kept in obvious places in all patient and service areas. The kind of extinguisher that is placed in a specific area depends upon the type of fire most likely to occur there. Part of a safety program is the regular inspection and maintenance of fire extinguishers.

In addition to having fire extinguishers, nursing units and other departments of a hospital are usually equipped with fire hoses, and personnel are trained in their use. In the event of a small fire, it may be easier and quicker to use material near at hand, for example, a blanket or a mattress, to smother the fire.

The Nurse's Responsibilities in the Event of Fire

If a fire does occur in a nursing unit, the nurse should make sure that the following steps are carried out:

1. remove patients from the immediate danger area
2. pull the fire alarm and report the location of the fire according to agency protocol
3. shut off the fire area and decrease the ventilation to the area
4. employ available extinguishing equipment.

In some health agencies it is accepted practice to telephone the fire department, directly reporting the exact location of the fire. Other agencies have a fire alarm system that, when activated, causes an alarm to ring in the fire station. A third method of reporting a fire is to telephone the operator at the central hospital exchange, who then notifies the fire department.

THE REMOVAL OF PATIENTS When a fire occurs, the nurse in charge of the unit assumes responsibility for directing the activities of hospital personnel until firefighters arrive. All fire doors and windows should be closed. Patients in immediate danger must be moved to safety quickly. Generally,

Techniques for Carrying Patients

Cradle

This technique is used for people who are not heavy and for children. The nurse lifts the patient by passing one arm beneath the patient's two knees and the other around the back (see Figure 30.9A).

Pack-Strap Carry

With the patient in a sitting position in bed, the nurse faces the patient and grasps his or her wrists: the patient's right wrist in the nurse's left hand, and the left wrist in the nurse's right hand. The nurse then pivots and slips under the patient's arm so that the patient's chest is against the nurse's shoulders and the patient's arms are crossed on the nurse's chest. With one leg forward for balance, the nurse then rolls the patient off the bed and onto the back (see Figure 30.9B).

Piggy-Back Carry

If the patient is conscious and able to give some help, this carry can be used (see Figure 30.9C). The patient sits at the edge of the bed. The nurse stands in front of the patient, back facing the patient. The patient reaches over the nurse's shoulders and clasps hands in front of the nurse. The nurse then grasps the backs of the patient's legs, slightly above the knees. This carry supports the weight of the patient in an easier position for carrying than the pack-strap carry.

Swing Carry by Two Nurses

For a swing carry by two nurses, one nurse stands on each side of the patient. The patient's arms are extended around the nurses' shoulders, and each nurse grasps one of the patient's wrists with the arm that is farthest from the patient. Each nurse then reaches behind the patient's back with the free arm (nearest the patient) and grasps the other nurse's shoulder. The patient's wrists are then released. Each nurse reaches under the patient's knees and grasps the other's wrist. The patient is then in a sitting position between the nurses. This carry is sometimes called a two-handed seat. A variation of this technique is the four-handed seat, which can be used for patients who are able to sit up without support. (See Figure 30.10.)

A

B

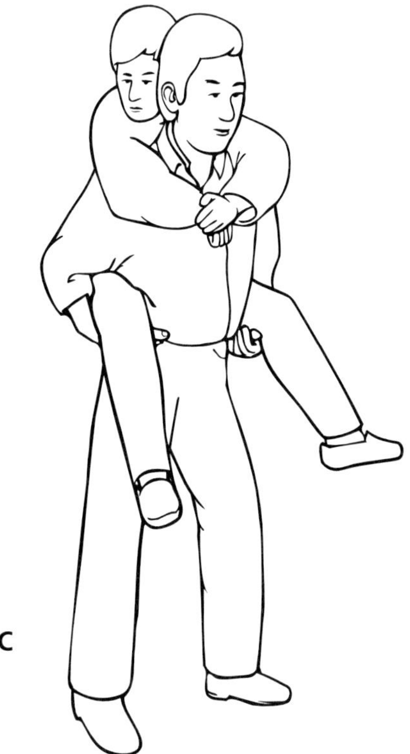

C

FIGURE 30.9 A. Position for cradle carry. B. Position for pack-strap carry. C. Position for piggy-back carry

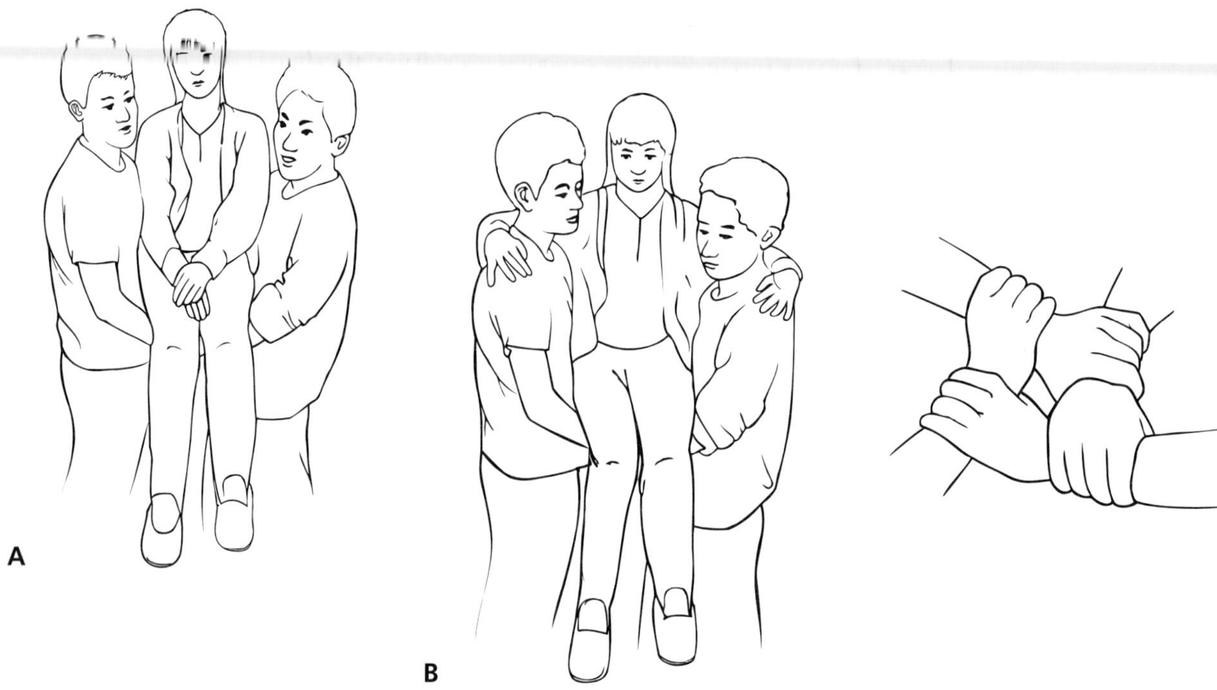

FIGURE 30.10 A. Position for swing carry. B. Position for four-handed seat, with a close view of how the hands are held

ambulatory patients are assisted in walking to safety. In moving immobilized patients, staff wheel the entire bed to a safe area. When it is not feasible to move the entire bed, immobilized patients are moved by stretcher or wheelchair. Occasionally, it is necessary to carry patients in order to remove them from danger. Non-nursing personnel in the agency—for example, housekeeping and maintenance staff—may be called upon to assist with evacuation of patients. Patients may be carried from fire areas using either the cradle technique, the pack-strap carry, the piggy-back carry, or the two-person swing carry (see box on page 971).

HOSPITAL SAFETY PROGRAMS

A safety program is an endeavour to control the physical environment and work procedures in such a manner that injuries can be prevented. In order to be effective, a program must involve all the people who work in the agency. Many hospitals have safety committees whose job it is to plan a safety program for the institution. Nurses are frequently members of these committees.

The safety committee's function is to conduct a continual analysis of the kinds of accidents that occur in the hospital and their causes. On the basis of this analysis, a program is developed. Continual assessment of hospital practices and continual education of employees are important functions of this committee. Another part of a safety program is the regular inspection of agency facilities. To be effective, a safety program must motivate all employees to accomplish the purpose of the program, for it is only through the active cooperation of all people in an agency that accidents can be prevented.

COMMUNITY health practice — Lifeline

Lifeline is a nonprofit, personal emergency response system that connects individuals to a 24-hour emergency help line at the touch of a button. This system can benefit the elderly, the disabled, women with high-risk pregnancies and families with children who have health problems.

The Lifeline communicator is plugged into a phone line. The waterproof help button can be worn around neck or wrist. Once the help button is activated, the Lifeline centre is dialled automatically and will provide assistance from trained professionals who have access to personal health information.

Lifeline personnel can speak directly to the subscriber. If they receive no response, personnel are authorized to follow a prearranged emergency procedure. There is a one-time installation fee and a monthly charge, both of which are tax deductible.

Evaluating Safety Interventions

[illegible] injury almost always results from another problem, such as the nature of the diagnostic or therapeutic plans of care for the patient. The patient's safety may be jeopardized, for example, when under sedation for pain relief. Evaluation of the effectiveness of nursing interventions is based on the degree to which injuries are avoided. The patient's condition is subject to constant change. It is therefore necessary for the nurse regularly both to reassess patients' abilities to protect themselves from environmental hazards and to modify the nursing care plan in accordance with changes in status. The nurse must also be constantly alert to new dangers in the environment that could harm patients, nurses, visitors or staff.

IN REVIEW

- An individual's safety needs include the personal capacity for self-protection and an environment conducive to healthy living. Safety needs vary at different stages of the life cycle.
- Determinants of a person's capacity for self-protection include:
  - age
  - health status
  - sensory and mental functioning
  - motor ability
  - emotional state
  - knowledge of environmental hazards and protective measures.
- Environmental factors may include:
  - physical factors
  - chemical factors
  - biological factors
  - psychological factors.
- Most injuries and injury-related deaths in Canada result from:
  - motor vehicle collisions
  - falls
  - drownings
  - fires/burns
  - poisonings.
- Injuries occurring in the home include:
  - burns
  - falls
  - poisonings
  - chokings and drownings.
- Injuries occurring in the community include:
  - traffic-related injuries
  - recreational and sports injuries.
- Injuries occurring in the workplace include:
  - musculoskeletal injuries
- In hospitals and other health care facilities the most frequent hazards for patients, staff and visitors are injuries, infections and stress.
- Workplace violence has increased in recent years. Nurses, nursing organizations and health care agencies have worked individually and collectively to identify strategies for preventing violence in the workplace.
- The nurse's role in protection and safety includes:
  - determining the person's capacity for self-protection
  - identifying hazards in the environment
  - planning and implementing safety interventions that are specific to the area (home, community and workplace)
  - evaluating the effectiveness of safety interventions
  - joining the safety committee of the practice area
  - reporting and documenting unusual incidents and injuries
  - maintaining a knowledge base related to safety.

Critical Thinking Activities

1. Mrs. R. Ross is a 73-year-old woman in hospital with a fractured femur. The physician has ordered that she sit in a chair for 15 minutes twice a day. Mrs. Ross walks with considerable difficulty and requires support.
   a. What factors should the nurse be aware of in providing a safe environment for Mrs. Ross?
   b. List six specific measures that the nurse should take to prevent mechanical injury to Mrs. Ross.
   c. If there is a fire in this patient's room, what should the nurse do? How should this patient be moved?
   d. By what criteria can the safety of Mrs. Ross's environment be evaluated?

KEY TERMS

intentional injury p. 945
unintentional injury p. 945
teratogenic p. 947
mutagenic p. 947
carcinogenic p. 947
cumulative trauma disorders p. 951
repetitive strain injuries p. 951
hazardous substances p. 951
restraints p. 966
thermal injuries p. 968
combustible material p. 969

References

ALBERTA ASSOCIATION OF REGISTERED NURSES (AARN). (1995). *Position statement on the use of restraints in client care settings.* Edmonton: Author.

ASSOCIATION OF WORKERS' COMPENSATION BOARDS OF CANADA (AWCBC). (1996). *Work injuries and disease: National work injuries statistics program, 1993–1995.* Ottawa: Author.

B.C. MINISTRY OF HEALTH (Office for Injury Prevention, Family Health Division). (1993, September). *Injury prevention strategies for children and youth in British Columbia.* Victoria: Queen's Printer.

B.C. MINISTRY OF MUNICIPAL AFFAIRS, RECREATION, AND HOUSING. (1991). *Home safety: A guide to common hazards around the home.* Victoria: Queen's Printer.

B.C. MINISTRY OF MUNICIPAL AFFAIRS, RECREATION & HOUSING (Office of the Fire Commissioner). (1992). *The British Columbia fire code, 1992.* Victoria: Queen's Printer.

CANADIAN NURSES ASSOCIATION (CNA). (1993). *Policy statement: Violence in the workplace.* Ottawa: Author.

CANADIAN NURSES ASSOCIATION (CNA). (1995, May). *Joint CNA/CMA position statement: Environmentally responsible activity in the health sector.* Ottawa: Author.

CARPENITO, L.J. (1997). *Nursing diagnosis: Application to clinical practice.* (7th ed.). Philadelphia: Lippincott.

COLOMBO, J.R. (Ed). (1992). *The 1993 Canadian global almanac.* Toronto: Macmillan.

CPHA urges use of ski helmets. (1997). *Canadian Nurse, 94*(1), 17.

CRUZ, V., ABDUL-HAMID, M., & HEATER, B. (1997). Research-based practice: Reducing restraints in an acute care setting—Phase I. *Journal of Gerontological Nursing, 23*(2), 31–40, 54–55.

GOVERNMENT OF BRITISH COLUMBIA, MINISTRY OF HEALTH & MINISTRY RESPONSIBLE FOR SENIORS, OFFICE FOR INJURY PREVENTION. (1997). *B.C. injury-free: A framework for action.* Victoria: Author. (Catalogue no. HV675/72/B73-1997)

GOVERNMENT OF ONTARIO (1993). *Nurturing health. Report of the Premier's Council on Health, Well-being and Social Justice (1987–1991).* Toronto: Queen's Printer. (Catalogue 01–93–20M)

HEALTH CANADA. (1996). Fact sheets: All injuries. [Online]. Available at http://www.hc-sc.gc.ca/hppb/cny/factsheets/all_injuries/allinj.htm

INSURANCE CORPORATION OF BRITISH COLUMBIA. (1997). *Doing it up right.* Vancouver: Author. Pamphlet no. TS244A(1097)

MANITOBA ASSOCIATION OF REGISTERED NURSES (MARN). (1992). *Position statement on the use of restraints.* Winnipeg: Author.

MILLAR, W.J. (1995). Accidents in Canada, 1988 and 1993. *Health Reports, 7*(2), 7–16.

MITCHELL, J.T., & EVERLY, G.S. (1993). *Critical incident stress debriefing (CISD): An operations manual for the prevention of traumatic stress among emergency services and disaster workers.* Baltimore: Chevron.

NATIONAL FIRE PROTECTION ASSOCIATION. (1997a). *Fire extinguishers in the workplace.* Quincy, MA: Author. (Pamphlet no. BR–35B)

NATIONAL FIRE PROTECTION ASSOCIATION. (1997b). *Home portable fire extinguishers.* Quincy, MA: Author. (Pamphlet no. BR–3I)

NG, E. (1996). Disability among Canada's aboriginal peoples in 1991. *Health Reports, 8*(1), 25–31.

PODNEIKS, E., PILLEMER, K., NICHOLSON, J., SHILLINGTON, T., & FRIZZELL, A. (1990). *National survey on abuse of the elderly in Canada.* Toronto: Ryerson University.

POPE, A., SNYDER, M., & MOOD, L. (Eds.). (1995). *Nursing, health and the environment.* Washington, DC: National Academy Press.

REGISTERED NURSES' ASSOCIATION OF NOVA SCOTIA (RNANS). (1995). Position statement on the use of physical restraints. Approved by the RNANS board of directors 17 April 1995. *Nurse to Nurse, 6*(3), 19.

REGISTERED NURSES ASSOCIATION OF ONTARIO (RNAO). (1976). ICN Policy Statement. *RNAO News,* 32:19.

RICHMOND HOSPITAL. (1995). *Restraints, least—Adult.* Richmond, BC: Author. (Patient Care Manual PCE4800)

RILEY, R., & PADDON, P. (1989). Accidents in Canada: Mortality and hospitalization. *Health Reports, 1,* 23–49. (Statistics Canada Catalogue no. 82 – 003)

ROSSY, D., JOURDAIN-GRAND, S., LAMB, G., ARMSTRONG, E., ATHRENS, S., & BERRY, J. (1997). Preventing falls in high-risk patients. *Canadian Nurse, 93*(4), 53–54.

ROYCHOWDHURY, M. (1990). Reproductive hazards in the work environment. *Professional Safety, 35*(5), 17–23.

SASKATCHEWAN LABOUR. (1996). *Occupational health and safety regulations.* Regina: Author.

SMITH, E.M., HAMMONDS-EHLERS, M., CLARK, M.K., KIRCHNER, H.L., & FUORTES, L. (1997). Occupational exposures and risk of female infertility. *Journal of Occupational & Environmental Medicine, 39*(2), 138–147.

SOLOMON, G.L. (1997). Reproductive toxins: A growing concern at work and in the community. *Journal of Occupational & Environmental Medicine, 39*(2), 105–107.

STOLLEY, J.M. (1995). Freeing your patients from restraints. *American Journal of Nursing, 2,* 27–31.

TAS, S., LAUWERYS, R., & LISON, D. (1996). Occupational hazards for the male reproductive system. *Critical Reviews in Toxicology, 26*(3), 261–307.

THOMAS, G. (1993). Working can be harmful for your health. *Canadian Nurse, 89*(6), 35–38.

WILKINS, M. (1995). Causes of death: How the sexes differ. *Health Reports, 7*(2), 33–43.

WORKERS' COMPENSATION BOARD OF BRITISH COLUMBIA (WCB of BC). (1996a). *Claims statistics for back strains in the hospital industry.* Richmond, BC: Author.

WORKERS' COMPENSATION BOARD OF BRITISH COLUMBIA (WCB of BC). (1996b). Health and safety now for the workers and employers of BC. *Prevention at Work, 2*(6), 3.

WORKERS' COMPENSATION BOARD OF BRITISH COLUMBIA (WCB of BC). (1997). *Building on common ground: Annual report 1996, Worksafe.* Vancouver: Author.

WORKERS' COMPENSATION BOARD OF BRITISH COLUMBIA (WCB of BC). (1998a). *Industrial health and safety regulations.* Richmond, BC: Author.

WORKERS' COMPENSATION BOARD OF BRITISH COLUMBIA (WCB of BC). (1998b). *What's WHMIS?* Richmond, BC: Author.

Additional Readings

BAIRD, P.A. (1992). Reproductive hazards in the workplace. *Canadian Medical Association Journal, 147,* 157–160.

BECKER, J.H. (1996). The legal side. When you need to use restraints. *American Journal of Nursing, 96*(4), 59.

BRADLEY, L., & DUFTON, B. (1995). Breaking free. *Canadian Nurse, 91*(1), 36–40.

BRAUN, J.V., & LIPSON, S. (1993). *Towards a restraint-free environment: Reducing the use of physical and chemical restraints in long-term and acute care settings.* Baltimore: Health Professions Press.

BREWER-SMYTH, K. (1996). Violence on the job: De-escalating tensions before they explode. *Journal of Christian Nursing, 13*(2), 11–12, 19–22.

CANADIAN NURSES ASSOCIATION. (1991). *Policy statement on human rights.* Ottawa: Author.

CANADIAN NURSES ASSOCIATION. (1992). *Family violence: Clinical guidelines for nurses.* Ottawa: Author.

CANADIAN NURSES ASSOCIATION. (1992). *Position statement on family vi-*

CANADIAN NURSES ASSOCIATION. (1995). *Policy statement: The quality of nurses' worklife.* Ottawa: Author.

CANADIAN NURSES ASSOCIATION. (1996). *Policy statement: Interpersonal violence.* Ottawa: Author.

CANADIAN NURSES ASSOCIATION. (1996) *Policy statement: Necessary support for safe nursing care.* Ottawa: Author.

CHACE, K. (1996). Developing a staff protection program. *Canadian Nurse, 92*(2), 51–52.

CHALIFOUR, R. (1997). Implementing a non-restraint environment. *Canadian Nurse, 93*(6), 47–48.

CONOVER, E.A. (1994). Guarding against fetal toxins. *RN, 57*(7), 28–34.

CONVEY, M.G. (1993). *Fear of falling: The experience of elderly individuals who have previously fallen.* Vancouver: University of British Columbia Press.

COOPER, A., & SAXE-BRAITHWAITE, A.R. (1996). Verbal abuse of hospital staff. *Canadian Nurse, 92*(6), 31–34.

CROKER, K., & CUMMINGS, A.L. (1995). Nurses' reactions to physical assault by their patients. *Canadian Journal of Nursing Research, 27*(2), 81–93.

GARRETT, R.B. (1996). A safer way to move patients. *Occupational Health & Safety, 65*(9), 60–64.

GOODRIDGE, D., & LAURILA, B. (1997). Minimizing transfer injuries. *Canadian Nurse, 3*(7), 38–41.

GUSTAFSON, M.C. (1995). To prevent back injury, change behaviour. *Occupational Health and Safety, 64*(5), 67–69, 80.

HUNTER, E. (1997). Violence prevention in the home health setting. *Home Healthcare Nurse, 15*(6), 403–413.

KUSHNIR-PEKRUL, L. (1992). *Nurse abuse in Saskatchewan.* Unpublished

LANGE, M. (1996). The challenge of fall prevention in home care: A review of the literature. *Home Healthcare Nurse, 14*(3), 198–206.

MAHONEY, D.M. (1995). Analysis of restraint-free nursing homes. *Image, 27*(2), 155–160.

NATIONAL COMMITTEE FOR INJURY PREVENTION AND CONTROL. (1989). *Injury prevention: Meeting the challenge.* New York: Oxford University Press.

OVERMAN, S. (1995). Workplace violence: Threat from within. *Occupational Health & Safety,* 64(7), 24–27.

ROGERS, B. (1994). *Occupational health nursing: Concepts and practice.* Toronto: Saunders.

SHRUGRUE, D.T., & LARACQUE, K.L. (1996). Reducing restraint use in the acute care setting. *Nursing Management, 27*(10), 32H, 32J, 32L, 32O.

SIBBALD, B. (1997). Delegating away patient safety. *Canadian Nurse, 93*(2), 22–26.

SULLIVAN-MARX, E.M. (1994). Delirium and physical restraint in the hospitalized elderly. *Image, 26*(4), 295–300.

SULLIVAN-MARX, E.M. (1996). Restraint-free: How does a nurse decide? *Journal of Gerontological Nursing, 22*(9), 7–14.

THOMAS, G. (1997). Occupational health and safety in Canadian health care facilities. *Canadian Nurse, 93*(5), 36–38.

TURNER, C.J. (1995). Health risk appraisals: The issues surrounding use in the workplace. *Journal of the American Association of Occupational Health Nursing, 43*(7), 357–361.

WHITEHORN, D., & NOWLAN, M. (1997). Towards an aggression-free health care environment. *Canadian Nurse, 93*(3), 24–31.

Chapter 31

Skin Integrity, Wound Healing and Hygiene Needs

OUTLINE

Introduction

Anatomy of the Skin, Mouth, Nails and Teeth

The Process of Wound Healing

Determinants of Skin Integrity and Hygiene Needs

Skin Variations and Hygiene Needs Throughout the Life Cycle

Common Skin and Wound Problems

Assessing Skin and Hygiene Needs

Diagnosing Skin and Hygiene Problems

Planning Skin and Hygiene Interventions

Implementing Skin and Hygiene Interventions

Evaluating Skin Integrity and Hygiene Interventions

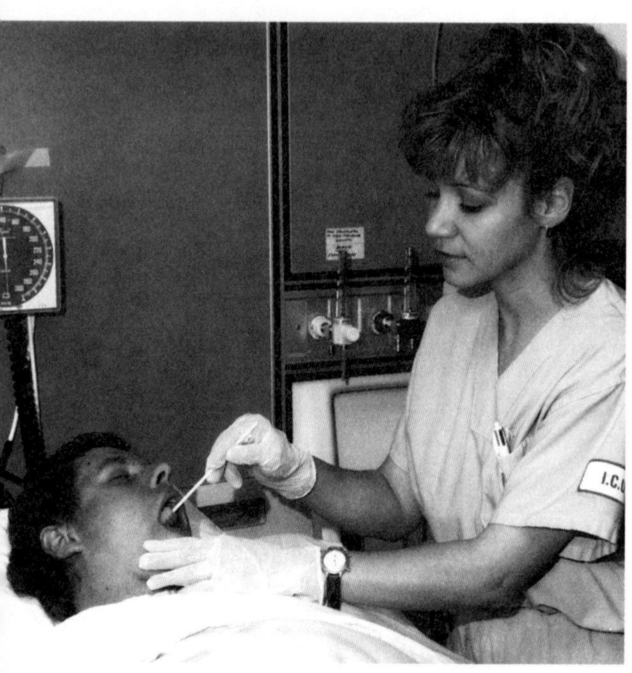

Central Questions

1. Why is good personal hygiene important for health and well-being?
2. What anatomical structures make up the skin, nails, the teeth and the mouth?
3. What are the determinants of skin integrity and hygiene needs?
4. How do skin integrity and hygiene needs vary throughout the life cycle?
5. What are some common problems people have in meeting their hygiene needs?
6. How does the nurse assess skin integrity and hygiene needs?
7. What are the common nursing diagnostic statements for patients with hygiene and skin integrity problems?
8. How does the nurse apply relevant principles in planning and implementing nursing interventions:
   a. to promote good hygiene practices in patients with respect to bathing and the care of the mouth, nails and hair?
   b. to maintain the skin, hair, nails, teeth and soft tissues in the oral cavity in good condition?
   c. to maintain and restore the integrity of the patient's skin?
9. How does the nurse evaluate the effectiveness of nursing interventions?
10. Why is skin integrity important in the prevention of pressure ulcers?
11. What are the physiological functions of the integumentary system?
12. What are some of the common skin problems that people experience?
13. How do wounds heal?
14. Discuss the assessment factors described in various pressure ulcer risk assessment tools.
15. How does the nurse apply relevant principles in planning and implementing nursing interventions in skin and wound care:
    a. to promote healthy skin in everyday living?
    b. to prevent skin breakdown?
    c. to restore wound healing?
16. How does the nurse evaluate the effectiveness of wound care management decisions?

Introduction

Taber's Medical Dictionary (1997) defines hygiene as "the

(p. 67). On a personal level, hygiene usually means those measures a person takes to keep the skin, its appendages (hair, fingernails and toenails) and the teeth and mouth clean and in good condition. Hygiene practices have personal meaning that varies according to cultural and social factors and individual values. Hygiene habits are influenced by family practices and values with respect to cleanliness and by knowledge of hygiene needs in health. Nurses must assess each individual's personal bathing and hygiene practices and incorporate these into the plan of care.

Healthy unbroken skin is the body's first line of defence against infection and injury to underlying tissues (Porth, 1998). The skin is important for the regulation of body temperature and it serves as one means for the excretion of body wastes. It also serves as a sensory organ for touch, pain, pressure and temperature. Healthy teeth and gums are essential for maintaining nutritional status. Decayed teeth and poor condition of the oral cavity are potential sources of infection and discomfort. Thus, proper hygiene is necessary for healthy bodily functions. Altered skin integrity is a potentially serious situation and can be life threatening. As we age or become immunosuppressed, incontinent of urine or stool, malnourished or dehydrated, our skin becomes less efficient in maintaining its integrity or in healing naturally. Individuals who are the most vulnerable to skin breakdown include the elderly, those who are immobile, those with a chronic health condition and those in critical care settings. A fundamental goal of any skin and wound care program should be prevention of skin breakdown (Ferreira & Thorpe-Critten, 1998). The nurse can take a golden opportunity for health promotion by teaching patients about healthy skin care and hygiene practices while assisting with daily hygiene needs.

Attending to personal hygiene and grooming needs is an important independent function both for children (once they have learned to do this themselves) and adults. When ill, people often depend on others for help with their hygiene. The loss of the ability to perform these very personal functions independently often affects self-esteem and contributes to feelings of powerlessness. In addition, having someone else provide very personal aspects of care may be considered demeaning and embarrassing. Both the nurse and the patient feel more comfortable if the nurse can anticipate the patient's needs and provide help in a competent, matter-of-fact manner, and, at the same time, acknowledge the patient's feelings and allow the patient every opportunity for participation in care.

The person who is ill has a lowered resistance to infection. Consequently, the presence of pathogenic bacteria in the environment poses a constant threat. Helping the patient to keep clean by removing dirt, excretory products and secretions eliminates many substances in which these bacteria flourish. In addition to controlling infection, hygienic measures help patients feel more comfortable and

clean, and many who have been unable to rest will sleep soundly after a relaxing bath. Unpleasant odours may be distressing, and attention to hygiene helps eliminate them. Excessive perspiration and the presence of bacteria in the mouth and on the skin are common causes of such odours. Oral hygiene usually eliminates bad breath (halitosis), which is most frequently caused by bacteria and old food particles in the mouth.

In previous chapters, we reviewed health-protecting strategies such as massage, turning and positioning, and the use of therapeutic beds that play a significant role in maintaining skin integrity and preventing skin breakdown. Unfortunately, these measures are sometimes not sufficient. Ferreira and Thorpe-Critten (1998) claim that "with early detection and effective wound management, it is possible to prevent superficial breakdown and tissue damage from becoming a chronic, painful wound that is complicated to treat and costly for the health care system" (p. 31). This chapter will not only discuss oral and hygiene needs but will also deal with pressure ulcers, one of the most common alterations in skin integrity. It will cover the principles of skin and wound assessment and management of wound healing.

Skin and wound care are viewed as collaborative efforts in which the nurse, other health professionals, patient and family are actively involved in prevention of pressure ulcers and promotion of intact skin.

Anatomy of the Skin, Mouth, Nails and Teeth

The Skin

SKIN The skin is composed of two main layers: the outer, thinner layer or **epidermis,** and the inner, thicker layer or **dermis.** Underlying these layers is subcutaneous tissue and adipose tissue. The epidermis itself has four layers on most areas of the body except the palms of the hands and the soles of the feet, where there are five. The outermost, horny layer of epidermis continually flakes off.

NAILS The **nails** protect the distal ends of the fingers and toes from injury. The nails are composed of epidermal cells that have been converted to *keratin*. Epithelial cells lie under the crescent of each nail, and it is from these cells that the epidermal cells of the nails grow.

HAIR **Hair** is composed of a long, cylindrical shaft and a root that is embedded in a depression, called a hair follicle, which penetrates the epidermis to the subcutaneous tissues. The hair receives its nourishment from the blood supply through the root. **Dandruff** is the term used for the dry, scaly material that is shed from the skin of the scalp. While hair does not play a protective role for humans, it is an important factor in individuals' perception of physical beauty and, consequently, their self-image and sense of well-being.

SKIN GLANDS There are three kinds of skin glands in the body. The **sebaceous glands** secrete oil and are present wherever there is hair. The oil (sebum) keeps the hair supple and pliable. The **sweat glands** produce sweat, a mechanism the body uses to cool the skin and reduce body temperature. Waste products are also excreted in sweat. Sweat glands are most numerous in the axilla, on the palms of the hands and the soles of the feet and on the forehead. The action of bacteria on sweat from these glands produces a distinctive odour. The **ceruminous glands,** located in the external ear canal, secrete cerumen (wax). Some people accumulate a large amount of cerumen in their ears, which can impair hearing.

The appearance and condition of the integument (skin, hair and nails) provide valuable information about a person's health status. Thus, a thorough examination of this system is an essential part of the health assessment (Jarvis, 1996). The structures of the integumentary system are illustrated in Figure 31.1.

The Mouth and Teeth

The mouth is the anterior opening of the alimentary canal. It is coated with a mucous membrane and the epithelial tissue layer that lines body cavities and passageways. The mouth contains three important anatomical structures: the tongue, the teeth and the gums. The **tongue**, a movable muscular organ, is an important sensory receptor. It assists in the acts of chewing *(mastication)*, swallowing and sound articulation. Healthy teeth are essential for the chewing of food. Each tooth has a crown and a root or roots. The **tooth** is solid except for the inner soft pulp cavity. The crown is covered with a hard inorganic substance called *enamel*, which protects the soft structures beneath it. The root is protected by *cementum*, which is true bone. The teeth protrude up through the gums **(gingivae),** which are made up of mucous membrane with supporting fibrous tissue. The hard portion of the gum is firm, dense, pink, stippled and tightly attached to the teeth, the periosteum and the bone of the jaws. A soft portion of the gums protrudes upward in the spaces between the teeth (Fuller & Schaller-Ayers, 1994). Figure 31.2 shows the anatomy of the oral mucosa and teeth.

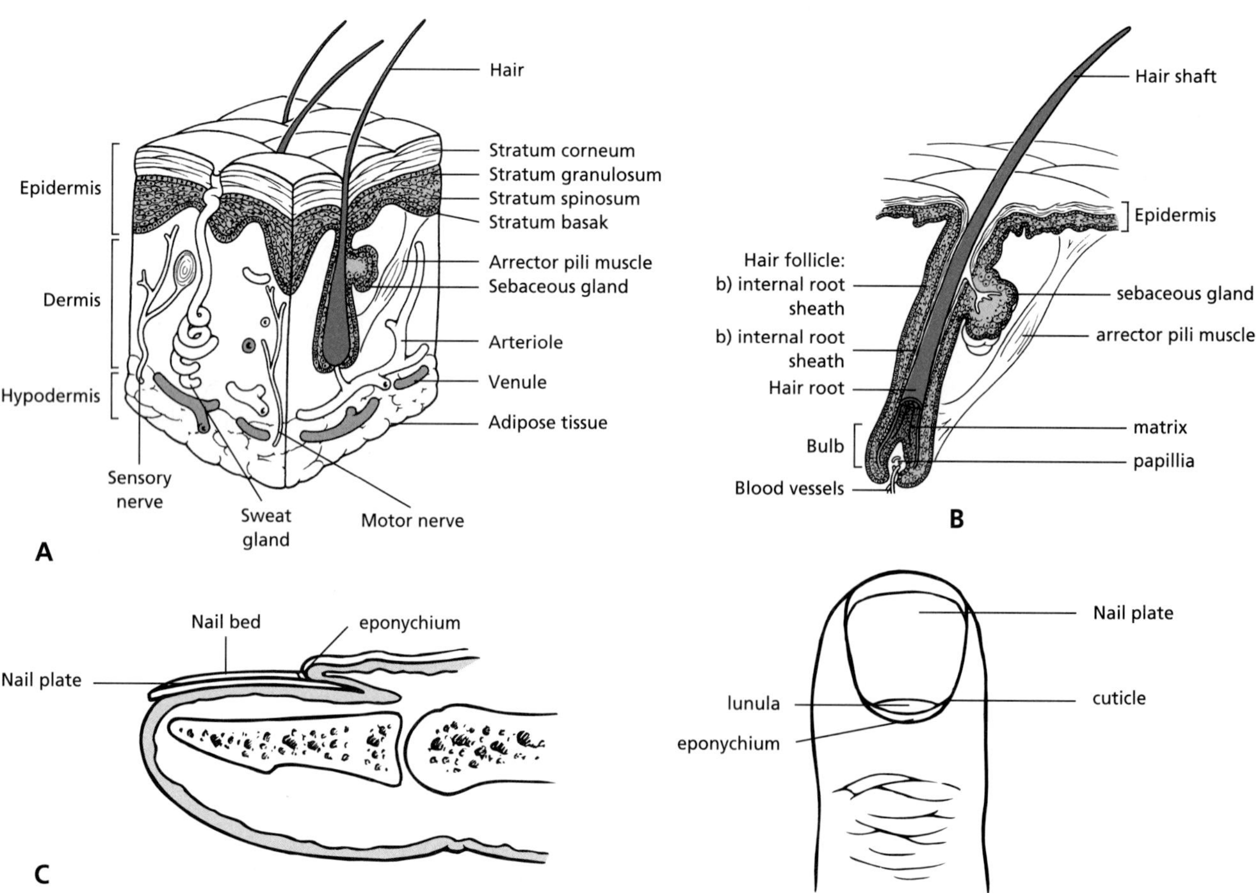

FIGURE 31.1 Anatomy of the skin, hair and nails. A. Skin structure. B. Hair structure. C. Nail structure.

SOURCES: A, B. De Graff & Fox, 1992; C. Thompson & Wilson, 1996.

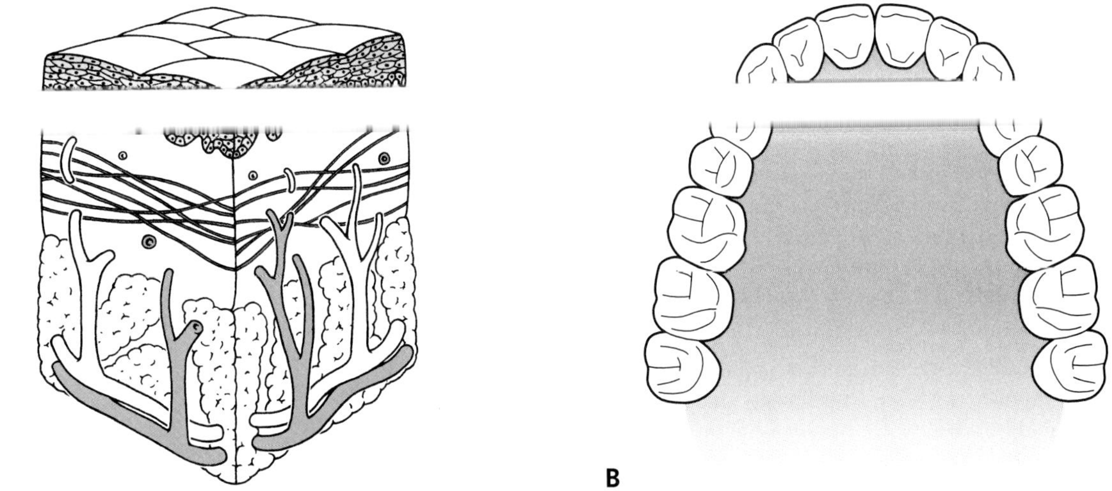

FIGURE 31.2 Anatomy of the oral mucosa and teeth. A. Structure of the oral mucosa. B. Adult's permanent teeth.

SOURCE: Fuller & Schaller-Ayers, 1994, pp. 148–149.

The Process of Wound Healing

Normal healing consists of a series of intricate events that lead to the restoration of tissue continuity. When tissue is damaged, a biochemical process takes place, usually in a sequential and overlapping fashion (Flynn, 1996). There are three phases in the healing process: inflammatory, proliferative and remodelling.

Phase One: Inflammatory Response

This is the first phase of healing. It is the body's initial response to tissue injury. This phase starts immediately after tissue is injured and lasts about three to six days (Flynn, 1996). The functions of this phase are to re-establish homeostasis, produce a local inflammatory response, clear away dead cells and bacteria and initiate a defence. Thromboplastin is released from the injured tissue cells to activate the clotting mechanism, thus re-establishing homeostasis. Histamine is released by the damaged cells and causes dilation of the small blood vessels in the dermal layer. This causes the skin around the injury to appear warm and red. There is also leaking of fluid from these small blood vessels into the surrounding tissue, which causes swelling and pain at the injury site. Neutrophils and lymphocytes rush to the site of injury, engulf bacteria and clear away the debris in the first 24–48 hours of injury. This action creates a creamy yellow exudate. This phase is often confused with signs of infection (Krasner, 1990). Macrophage activity in this phase not only assists in cleansing the wound but stimulates the growth of granulation tissue.

The inflammatory response should last only about three days, but can take weeks or even months. Variables that can inhibit the inflammatory response include medications such as steroids, age, immunosuppressive states and malnutrition (Flynn, 1996). If the injured site has pressure on it, the blood vessels are compressed and the macrophages are unable to reach the wound to clean it. Thus, patients must keep off their wounds, and restrictive dressings should not be used. If the wound is infected or **necrotic** (contains dead tissue cells), or if foreign material such as lint from gauze is present, the macrophages will take longer to cleanse the wound.

Phase Two: Proliferative (Regenerative) Phase

During this second phase of healing, new tissue is being created. It typically begins within 72 hours postinjury and may last for up to 21 days (Flynn, 1996). The functions of this phase include granulation (fibroblasts and collagen activity), re-epithelialization and wound contraction.

Granulation occurs when the body creates new vascular and connective tissue. The developing vascular network brings oxygen and nutrients to the injury site, allowing the fibroblasts to secrete collagen (protein for tissue strengthening). The collagen of a healed wound regains approximately 80 percent of its original strength (Flynn, 1996). The wound will appear pale pink to deep red and moist (shiny). Wound healing occurs from the bottom up as new layers of tissue are created. These new buds of tissue are very fragile, and pressure and caustic agents can destroy them easily.

Epithelialization occurs after the wound is filled with new granulation tissue. The epithelial cells line the wound and begin to multiply and move across the wound surface. These new cells are pale pink and fragile, and can only move across moist tissue. If the wound bed is dry, the epithelial cells must burrow down to the moist layer. If necrotic tissue is present, the epithelial cells cannot move across the wound, and healing will not continue.

Wound contraction occurs at the same time as re-epithelialization. This is the spontaneous decrease in the diameter of the wound. Specialized epithelial cells slowly pull the wound edges towards the middle of the wound (Krasner, 1990). Macerated tissue prevents contraction from occurring.

To promote healing, patients must remain off their wound and should clean it gently using an irrigation procedure (see Chapter 33). Wet-to-dry dressings should be avoided in favour of a wet-to-damp procedure, as dry gauze tears away not only the debris but also the new cells. The wound should be cleaned only with normal saline, as antiseptics will kill the new cells (U.S. Department of Health & Human Services, 1994).

Phase Three: Remodelling

Remodelling occurs after the wound has closed. This phase may begin by day 21 and may last up to two years (Flynn, 1996). Characteristically, maturation of the epidermal and dermal layers takes place. Further, the new tissue is reorganized to create stronger tissue (collagen structure). New granulation tissue is only 10 percent as strong as the previous noninjured tissue, and new tissue will never become more than 70 to 80 percent as strong as the preinjury tissue. A scar is visible to the naked eye.

As mentioned in the introduction to this chapter, there are numerous factors that compromise wound healing, placing the individual at risk for skin breakdown. Chapter 33 explores these factors in greater detail.

Determinants of Skin Integrity and Hygiene Needs

NUTRITION AND HYDRATION The skin is nourished by nutrients delivered by the blood. If food and fluid intake is disrupted, the skin will likely show some effects. If fluid intake is insufficient, a person becomes dehydrated, and the skin appears dry and loose, a condition called *poor tissue turgor*. **Turgor** refers to the elasticity of the skin. Skin heals very slowly when an individual has suffered prolonged nutrient deficiency.

EXERCISE Exercise improves circulation, helping to bring a nourishing supply of blood to the surface tissues. It also aids in the elimination of waste products, both through the skin and other excretory routes.

ENVIRONMENT Weather affects the skin. In cold temperatures, the skin often becomes dry and chapped. Not only is the cold outside a factor, but the indoor environment, which is very dry in many homes with central heating, can also cause problems. Very warm weather can also be hard on the skin. We perspire more in the heat, creating potentially harmful waste buildup on the skin. Frequent bathing will rid the skin surface of bodily wastes excreted via this route. Sunshine was once considered an important factor in healthy skin, but the thinning of the ozone layer now necessitates caution. Exposure to the sun's ultraviolet light has been linked to skin damage, premature aging and skin cancer.

PERSONAL HABITS The health of the skin, hair and nails is affected by hygiene habits. Bathing and grooming rituals vary depending on factors such as culture, access to sanitation facilities, knowledge and personal preference. For example, in some cultures menstruating women believe they should not bathe or wash their hair. In rural Cambodia, salt or lemon is often used for dental care (Richardson, 1990).

SPIRITUALITY Some religions may have cleansings or purification practices as part of their ceremonies. These practices may occur before or during prayers or prior to commencing a meal.

SOCIOECONOMIC FACTORS Maintaining hygiene is more difficult when facilities are not readily available. People who live in poor, crowded or unsanitary conditions often do not have the opportunity to practise good personal hygiene. The person who has to cut a hole in the ice to obtain water in the wintertime or share a bathroom with several other people may not bathe frequently. Teeth may be neglected because an individual cannot afford visits to the dentist.

HEALTH STATUS General health status is very important, both in relation to the ability to maintain hygiene and with respect to the effect of health problems on the skin. Poor health, for whatever reason, is usually reflected by the condition of the skin. The ill person is more susceptible to infection, malnourishment, gastrointestinal problems and other disturbances of body functioning that can affect the condition of the skin. Many types of disorders also specifically affect the skin.

Physical and mental status affects the ability to carry out personal hygiene. Motor abilities, mental capacity and the severity and nature of an illness may have great impact on the level of independence. If a patient is unable to bathe, the nurse's role is to assist as necessary.

Excessive moisture causes the skin to be more susceptible to damage. Fever causes increased perspiration and excretion of wastes through the skin. Irritating drainage seeping onto the skin from wounds can cause problems. Incontinence of urine or feces is a major factor in skin breakdown. Prolonged pressure on any area decreases blood supply and can lead to injury. Friction from rubbing or shearing from being pulled on the bed linen can cause additional trauma. Wrinkled sheets or crumbs in the bed increase the irregularity of the sheet surface and hence increase the friction. A smooth, firm foundation on the bed helps to lessen this friction and aids in preventing tissue breakdown.

MEDICATIONS AND THERAPY Medications and other forms of therapy may cause reactions in the skin. Many medications may cause an allergic skin reaction. Radiation therapy,

destroy malignant cells. The skin and its underlying tissues may also suffer some damage. Mucous membranes, which contain rapidly dividing cells, are frequently affected, leading to sores in the mouth.

Skin Variations and Hygiene Needs Throughout the Life Cycle

Pregnancy

One of the first changes that a pregnant woman notices is increased pigmentation (colouring) of the nipples and areolae of her breasts. *Striae* (stretch marks) and accentuated venous patterns appear over the breasts as they enlarge and prepare to nourish the infant. The tendinous middle line of the abdomen also shows increased pigmentation *(linea nigra)*, and stretch marks usually appear on the abdomen. Darkened brown areas may also appear on the face; these are known as chloasma or the "mask of pregnancy" (Pillitteri, 1995). The changes in skin pigmentation are due to the melanocyte-stimulating hormone secreted by the pituitary gland. As the pregnancy progresses, there is often an increase of vascular spider-like spots, particularly on the legs, and *palmar erythema* (reddened areas on the palms of the hands) is common. These changes are thought to be due to the increased estrogen levels that accompany pregnancy. Sweat gland activity increases during pregnancy, causing increased perspiration. Thus, a daily bath or shower is usually recommended for pregnant women. The gums often become soft and edematous because of increased vascularity. They are sensitive and tend to bleed easily, even with the mild trauma of brushing or flossing.

Infancy

The newborn's skin is usually red, wrinkled and covered with *vernix*, a white waxy coating that has protected the skin in utero. Some newborns are also covered with a downy hair called *lanugo;* premature babies almost always have this additional protective coating. Newborns have many skin variations such as *milia* (white pinpoint papules found on the nose) or *erythema toxicum* (newborn rash), which appear at birth or in the first few days after birth. These require no special care and disappear as the infant's structures mature. Infants need to be handled carefully as their skin is less resistant to injury and infection than an adult's. Mild soaps that are nonirritating to the skin may be used in the infant's bath. Soap should not be used on an infant's face. Daily bathing is not recommended, since frequent washing

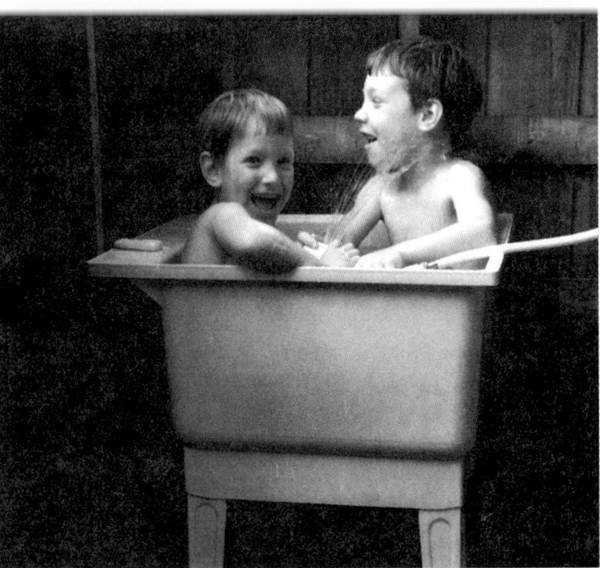

Children can find creative ways to meet their skin integrity and hygiene needs.

removes natural oils and may dry the skin, increasing the risk of infection.

The infant's skin is very sensitive to heat and cold. A warm room for bathing and body temperature, bathwater provide comfort. After bathing, immediately wrapping the infant in a towel reduces heat loss. The hair and the head of an infant should be washed and dried separately, before the rest of the body, because most heat is lost through the head. The nails of infants must be kept short to prevent scratching.

Diaper rash is a common skin problem with infants. "Diapering places a unique set of stressors on the skin. Factors affecting the diaper area include the type of diaper, skin vulnerability, consistency of the stool and diapering practices such as frequency of changing diapers and application of topical preparations and medications" (Wong, Brantly, Clutter, de Simone, Lammert, Nix, Perry, Smith & White, 1992, p. 41). Cleansing the skin before applying a clean diaper is important for removing urine and feces which are irritating to the skin. Getting the infant to take more water will help lessen the effects of skin rash, because water dilutes the urine and makes it less irritating.

Cradle cap is an oily, yellowish crust that develops on the scalp of some infants, particularly in those who are breastfed. It is caused by an excessive amount of secretion from the sebaceous glands of the scalp. Applications of a mild oil (such as mineral oil) or a bland ointment, and frequent shampoos will usually remove the crust within a few days. *Thrush* is a mild fungal infection of the mouth. Having the baby drink approximately 15 mL of sterile water after a milk feeding helps to prevent this problem.

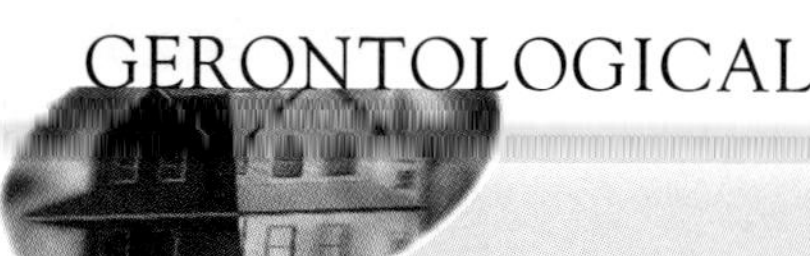

GERONTOLOGICAL

Structural and Functional Changes of the Aging Skin

- Altered cell proliferation
  - Flattened demo-epidermal junction
  - Decreased pigmentation (loss of melanocytes)
  - Cytoarchitectural disarray
- Altered wound healing
- Altered immune responsiveness
  - Reduced Langerhans cells
- Decreased barrier function
- Greater tensile strength (less give of tissue)
- Elastic fibre changes (wrinkles, lax skin)
- Decreased vascularity
- Decreased density
- Altered thermoregulation
- Decreased subcutaneous tissue
- Decreased sweat production
- Nail changes (e.g., brittle)
- Greying of hair (loss of melanocytes)
- Decreased sensory perception

SOURCE: Ebersole & Hess, 1998, p. 244.

Childhood

Usually, school-aged children have learned basic hygienic practices at home. Teachers and the school nurse may need to reinforce the early home teaching.

Owing to vigorous play and still-developing motor skills, children suffer cuts, bruises and scrapes during the preschool and primary school period. The school nurse—and parents—should keep a good supply of mild disinfectant and simple bandage materials on hand to protect childhood wounds from infection. Another common childhood skin problem is allergic eczema, which can be very distressing for both the child and parents. Medical guidance is important in caring for the child with this problem. Children who have a problem with enuresis should have a morning shower or bath, so that they are not sent off to school or to play with the odour of urine on the body, an unpleasant reminder of the problem (Wong, 1995).

Adolescence

The adolescent's skin may be problematic. Acne is a common problem in many teenagers. Hormonal changes occurring at this stage of the life cycle, blockage of the excretions of the sebaceous glands onto the skin surface and bacterial infection are thought to be factors that contribute to teenage acne. Cleanliness, diet and exercise are important factors that help prevent secondary infections. Severe acne requires medical attention.

Adolescents usually demonstrate increased concern over personal appearance and hygiene. This is the time when sweating from the axilla commences, and the teenager is usually very self-conscious about the odour of perspiration.

Adulthood

As a person advances in age, two kinds of skin change take place. First, wrinkling, sagging and increased pigmentation occur due to exposure to sunlight. Secondly, there is a general thinning of the skin accompanied by increased dryness and inelasticity. This aging takes place in the epidermis, dermis and in the subcutaneous fat. The epidermis is generally thinned and flattened, and sometimes there is increased growth of the outer layer of the epidermis. A decrease in oil secretions leads to increased dryness and scaliness. As a result, older people tolerate soap less well than younger adults. If older adults bathe too frequently, the skin will become very dry. Oily liquids and skin creams are often better for the older patient than too much soap and water or alcohol rubs.

The aging process also takes its toll on the hair, the nails, the teeth and other structures in the mouth. Hair often becomes thin and loses its texture. Fingernails and toenails become tougher and more difficult to cut. The mucous membranes lining the mouth become thinner and more fragile with age. After age 20, the teeth are less susceptible to cavities and more susceptible to gum diseases. Half of all Canadians are completely toothless by age 60 (Canadian Dental Association, 1994). Table 31.1 lists the normal and abnormal integumentary variations that occur throughout the life cycle.

Common Skin and Wound Problems

Problems resulting from an inability to maintain skin integrity and hygiene are numerous. The skin, hair, nails and teeth may become dirty, and offensive odours from the body may cause discomfort, both physical and mental. Ingrown nails frequently result from uncut toenails, and may interfere with the ability to walk. If skin care is neglected or carried out inadequately, pressure areas may develop and the skin may break down, causing considerable discomfort and pain and rendering the patient more vulnerable to infection.

TABLE 31.1 Integumentary variations throughout the life cycle

[illegible]	Abnormal Findings
INFANTS	
SKIN	
Pigmentation	
• dark-skinned newborns have a lighter skin tone than their parents because of immature melanocyte function • Mongolian spots (areas of blue-grey pigmentation) are commonly seen over the buttocks and lower back of dark-skinned children; these fade by school age • café au lait spots (irregular, light-brown macules) remain throughout life	• six or more café au lait spots, each greater than 1.5 cm in diameter
Colour	
• pink • transient periods of beefy redness for first 24 hours of life due to vasomotor instability • acrocyanosis (peripheral cyanosis involving the hands, feet and circumoral area) is common during the first 24–48 hours after birth; tends to increase with exposure to a cool environment and chilling; disappears with warming • cutis marmorata (transient mottling; red or blue netlike pattern) occurs when an infant is exposed to a cooler environment • physiologic jaundice occurs on the second or third day of life in about 50% of all newborns due to breakdown of fetal red blood cells	• pallor, generalized cyanosis • jaundice appearing within 24 hours of life
Texture, Moisture and Turgor	
• skin smooth and pliant; visible layer of adipose tissue below • good turgor; superficial peeling after 24 hours • visible veins rare	• thick, leathery skin; cracked; generalized peeling occurs with postmaturity • thin, transparent skin with minimal adipose tissue and many visible veins occurs with prematurity • poor turgor; tenting, generalized edema
Skin Lesions	
• milia (tiny white papules on the cheeks, nose, forehead and chin) are distended sebaceous glands; will resolve in 2–4 weeks as sebaceous glands mature • erythema toxicum (newborn rash; sporadic pinpoint papules on an erythematous base) usually appears during the first to fourth day of life; self-limiting	• skin pustules, vesicles • diaper rash
Vascular Lesions	
• petechiae over presenting part in the newborn; forceps marks on the head • storkbite (flat capillary hemangioma; red or pink patches commonly found at the nape of the neck, also on the eyelids, forehead and upper lip) usually fades during the first year of life	• generalized petechiae • ecchymosis secondary to birth trauma or manipulation during birth of infant • port wine stain (nevus flammeus; macular purple or dark red lesion) frequently appears on the face; remains throughout life • strawberry hemangioma (raised, bright red area 2–3 cm in diameter) may appear at birth or 2–3 weeks after; continues to enlarge during the first year; gradually shrinks in size and usually disappears by 7 years of age • cavernous hemangioma (raised red-blue mass of blood vessels) does not disappear spontaneously but may be removed surgically

continued on next page

TABLE 31.1 *continued*

Normal/Common Findings	*Abnormal Findings*
INFANTS	
NAILS	
Shape and Texture	
• well formed; soft, pliant	• thin and incompletely developed
HAIR	
Distribution and Texture	
• lanugo (fine, downy hair) may be patchy or absent at birth; if present, usually shed by third month • scalp hair silky and soft; may be straight, curly or kinky based on familial traits	• thick lanugo • tuft of hair on spine • fine and woolly; sparse • coarse and brittle
CHILDREN	
SKIN	
Colour, Texture, Vascularity and Lesions	
• may have Mongolian spots, cuts and bruises consistent with play injuries, e.g., on lower legs	• multiple bruising at different stages of healing in unusual areas such as the back, upper arms, buttocks or abdomen may indicate physical abuse • infectious skin disorders such as vesicles of measles, ringworm, impetigo and scabies
HAIR	
• little body or facial hair • scalp hair may darken and thicken	• head lice, nits, scabies, ticks
ADOLESCENTS	
SKIN	
Moisture and Lesions	
• oiliness, acne, comedones (blackheads) • development of axillary perspiration and body odour	
HAIR	
Quantity, Distribution, Texture	
• body hair appearance; progresses towards adult characteristics for gender	• fine, scanty, patchy
OLDER ADULTS	
SKIN	
Colour and Pigmentation	
• senile lentigines (liver spots; tan to brown macules found on surfaces subjected to chronic sun exposure, e.g., forearms, back of hands and face)	
Thickness	
• thin, translucent (parchment-like) appearance; wrinkling and sagging; decreased subcutaneous fat	
Moisture	
• dryness and flaking; decreased perspiration	
Texture	
• acrochordons (skin tags; soft, flesh-coloured overgrowths of skin attached by a stalk) usually found on eyelids, vertical and lateral surfaces of neck and axillae	
Turgor	
• decreased turgor due to loss of elasticity; skin recoils slowly; tenting may occur	• extended tenting

TABLE 31.1 *continued*

	Abnormal Findings
OLDER ADULTS	
Vascularity and Lesions	
• telangiectasis (visible dilated blood vessels) • senile purpura (bruising due to leakage of blood through fragile capillaries into the dermis) • cherry angiomas (papular and round, red or purple; noted on trunk or extremities) • seborrheic keratosis (benign, yellowish to brown, warty lesions with scaly surface) may appear on the trunk and face	• actinic keratosis (pink to reddish, scaly plaques on sun-exposed areas; precursor of squamous cell cancer)
NAILS	
Shape and Texture	
• growth rate slow; may thicken and become yellow; increased brittleness, ridges, longitudinal splitting	
HAIR	
Colour, Distribution, Quantity and Texture	
• greying of hair colour; scalp hair tends to turn grey more rapidly than body hair • thinning of hair on scalp, legs, pubic and axillary regions • eyebrows, nose and ear hair becomes coarser; coarse terminal hairs grow on the chin and upper lip of some women	

SOURCES: Jarvis, 1996; Ebersole & Hess, 1998; Pillitteri, 1995.

Skin Problems

DRY SKIN

Dry skin is one the most common problems that individuals experience, especially the elderly. Diminished amounts of secreted sebum, thinning epidermis and inadequate fluid intake increase the risk of dry skin, as do exposure to environmental elements (sun, dry air), use of harsh soaps and frequent hot showers. **Pruritis** (itching) is aggravated by heat, sweating and many health conditions. Individuals may also experience itching as a result of an allergic reaction (Ebersole & Hess, 1998).

LESIONS

Lesions are defined as "traumatic or pathologic changes in previously normal structures" (Jarvis, 1996, p. 230). There are two basic types of lesions: primary and secondary. *Primary lesions* arise from previously normal skin; *secondary lesions* result from changes in primary lesion (Bates, 1995). *Vascular lesions* originate from arterioles, venules and superficial capillaries in the skin. Primary, secondary and vascular lesions are described and illustrated in Tables 31.2, 31.3 and 31.4, respectively.

BURNS AND SUNBURNS

Burns are among the most common conditions that emergency staff in children's hospitals are called upon to treat. *Thermal burns* are usually the result of fires, playing with matches, scalding and improper handling of firecrackers. *Chemical burns* are the result of ingesting chemical products (Wong, 1995). Individuals may also suffer from sunburns, caused by excessive exposure to sunlight without the proper use of sun protection strategies.

Oral Problems

If the patient has been unable to look after oral hygiene and has not been assisted with it, the teeth and the mucous membranes lining the mouth soon show evidence of this. **Gingivitis,** or inflammation of the gums, is one problem. When oral hygiene is inadequate, a film of mucus and bacteria **(plaque)** and *calculus* (tartar) accumulate on the surface of the teeth and particles of food gather around the teeth and in the crevices of the gums. These substances are removed by brushing the teeth, flossing and regular professional cleaning. Without proper cleaning, the substances accumulate and become a source of mechanical irritation. The tissues of the gums become swollen and inflamed and may separate from the teeth.

Gingivitis not only is uncomfortable for the patient, it also leads to poor nutrition and is a potential source of infection in the parotid glands or the gastrointestinal or respiratory tracts. When oral hygiene is neglected, the teeth and the tongue also suffer. Decay of the teeth **(dental caries)**

TABLE [illegible] Primary skin lesions

Lesions	*Description*	*Examples*
Flat, nonpalpable skin colour change:		
Macule	Circumscribed change in skin colour (may be white, tan, red, purple, brown); less than 1 cm in diameter	Freckles, flat nevi (moles), petechiae, measles, scarlet fever
Patch	Irregular-shaped macule; more than 1 cm in diameter	Mongolian spot, café au lait, port wine stain, chlosma
Elevated, papable solid masses:		
Papule	Firm, circumscribed area less than 0.5 cm in diameter	Elevated mole, verruca (wart), lichen planus
Plaque	Rough, flat surface more than 1 cm wide; may be formed by coalescence of papules	Psoriasis, actinic keratosis
Nodule	Hard or soft circumscribed area; may extend deeper in the dermis than papules; 0.5–2 cm in diameter	Dermatofibroma, intradermal mole
Tumour	Hard or soft area; may or may not be circumscribed; extends deeper into dermis; more than 2 cm in diameter	Lipoma, carcinoma, hemangioma
Wheal	Irregular-shaped, transient, erythematous area of cutaneous edema; diameter varies	Urticaria (hives), insect bites, allergic reactions
Circumscribed, elevated cavities filled with fluid:		
Vesicle	Contains serous fluid; less than 0.5 cm in diameter	Blister, herpes simplex or zoster, contact dermatitis, varicella (chicken pox)
Bulla	Vesicle more than 0.5 cm in diameter	Friction blister, second-degree burn, contact dermatitis
Pustule	Vesicle or bulla containing purulent fluid (pus)	Acne, impetigo

SOURCES: Bates, 1995; Jarvis, 1996; Fuller & Schaller-Ayers, 1994; Morton, 1993; Thompson & Wilson, 1996.

TABLE 31.3 Secondary skin lesions

		Examples
Erosion	Loss of superficial epidermis; shallow depression; moist but does not bleed	Ruptured vesicle, scratch mark
Excoriation	Loss of the epidermis; linear or hollowed-out area; sometimes crusted; often self-inflicted from extreme itching	Abrasion, scratch, scabies, insect bites
Fissure	Linear crack extending into the dermis; may be moist or dry	Athlete's foot, cheilosis (cracks at the corners of the mouth)
Ulcer	Deeper loss of skin surface extending into the dermis; irregular shape; may bleed and form a scar when healed	Decubitus ulcer, stasis ulcer
Atrophy	Thinning of the epidermis; skin level depressed with loss of normal furrows; appears translucent	Aging skin, striae (stretch marks)
Lichenification	Thickened epidermis with accentuated skin markings; results from prolonged rubbing or irritation; resembles the surface of moss (lichen)	Chronic dermatitis
Crust	Dried exudate (serum, pus or blood) on the skin surface, left when vesicles or pustules burst or dry up	Impetigo, scab on abrasion
Scale	Flakes of skin from shedding of exfoliated epidermis; irregular shape; may be thick or thin, dry or oily, silvery or white	Dry skin, flaking following drug reaction, psoriasis
Scar	Fibrotic change in the skin; normal tissue is replaced with connective tissue following injury or laceration to the dermis; young scar often red and purple; mature scar white and glistening	Healed surgical incision or traumatic wound
Keloid	Hypertrophied scar tissue; results from excessive collagen formation during healing; irregular and elevated; extends beyond the borders of the wound	Keloid formation in a surgical incision or traumatic wound

SOURCES: Bates, 1995; Jarvis, 1996; Fuller & Schaller-Ayers, 1994; Morton, 1993; Thompson & Wilson, 1996.

TABLE [illegible] Vascular lesions of the skin

Lesions	*Description*	*Examples*
Vascular changes:		
Cherry angioma	Small, round, slightly raised, bright red dots; appear on the trunk and extremities; increase in size and number with aging	Normally seen in persons over 30 years of age
Spider angioma	Small, fiery red, branching arteriole; capillary branches radiate from a solid centre forming a spider-like shape; blanches with pressure; located on the face, neck, arms and trunk	Associated with pregnancy, liver disease and vitamin B deficiency; normal occurrence in some healthy people
Spider vein (venous star)	Bluish colour from dilation of superficial blood vessels; irregular pattern; may be linear, spider-like or star-shaped; does not blanch with pressure; located most often on legs near veins and also on chest	Associated with increased pressure in superficial veins, as in varicose veins
Purpuric changes:		
Petechiae	Tiny, pinpoint, dark red or purple macules; less than 2 mm; fade away over time; due to bleeding from superficial capillaries; does not blanch with pressure	Associated with bleeding disorders and microembolic formation
Echhymosis	Large, irregular patch; colour changes over time from red-blue or purple at first to green, yellow and then brown before disappearing; size varies; due to capillary bleeding into tissues; does not blanch with pressure	Occurs from trauma; associated with bleeding disorders and liver disease

SOURCES: Bates, 1995; Jarvis, 1996; Fuller & Schaller-Ayers, 1994; Morton, 1993; Thompson & Wilson, 1996.

may result, which requires the assistance of dental health professionals to correct. Lack of oral hygiene also causes the tongue to become coated with a thick, furry substance that is often referred to as **sordes**. This adds to the patient's discomfort and diminishes the ability of the taste buds to receive stimuli, which in turn contributes to nutritional problems such as anorexia and malnourishment.

Hair Problems

One common problem affecting the hair and scalp is excessive dandruff. Normally, dandruff is removed by combing, brushing and washing the hair. These procedures also help to remove the accumulation of excess sebum, the oily secretion of the sebaceous glands that keeps the hair supple and pliable. People whose hair is oily owing to the excessive secretions of sebum need to shampoo frequently to remove the oil. People with an irritation of the scalp should be referred to a physician.

The nurse may encounter patients whose hair and body are infested with lice or other vermin. Head lice is a frequent problem in schools, where the infestation is quickly spread from one child to another.

TABLE 31.5 A comparison of venous, arterial and diabetic ulcers

		[illegible]	Diabetic
Site	gaiter area	any part of the leg, usually below the ankle	any part of the leg, usually below the ankle and on the foot
Size	usually large	usually small	often very small
Edge	shallow, diffuse edges	deep with cliff edge	deep with cliff edge
Floor	exuding	dry	dry
Edema	generalized	localized	localized
Staining	always	never	never
Varicosities	sometimes	never	never
Pulses	normal	reduced/absent	reduced/absent
Pain	some	present, especially at night may be extreme	some neuropathy
Treatment	control edema	increase blood flow—bypass surgery	prevention debride—alert for infection non–weight-bearing

SOURCE: Smith & Nephew, 1992.

Wound Ulcers

TYPES OF WOUND ULCERS

Table 31.5 lists the characteristics of venous, arterial and diabetic ulcers.

VENOUS ULCER A **venous ulcer** usually occurs on the lower leg. It is caused by compromised venous circulation in which leaky venous valves allow fluids to accumulate in the interstitial tissue.

ARTERIAL ULCER An **arterial ulcer** is usually found on the foot or ankle. It is caused by inadequate circulation.

DIABETIC ULCER A **diabetic ulcer** is usually found on the bottom or side of the foot. It is caused by pressure or friction from poorly fitting shoes. The individual may be unaware of the damage, as sensation in the feet is compromised. Poor circulation causes slow healing (Boyton & Paustian, 1996).

MALIGNANT WOUNDS

Occasionally, cancer patients will have a cancerous growth on the outside of the body. **Malignant wounds** can be of any size and are made up of skin and vascular cells. These wounds can sometimes be treated with radiation therapy to shrink them, or they can be surgically removed. Not all malignant wounds can be treated by radiation or surgery. Some wounds have to be treated topically, in which case the goal of care is to prevent bleeding, reduce odour and prevent pain at dressing changes.

PRESSURE ULCERS

Pressure ulcers, also known as decubitus ulcers, bedsores or pressure sores, are areas from which the skin has sloughed. *Decubitus*, which is a Latin word meaning "lying down," is the traditional term for this type of ulcer, because it occurred originally in people who were bedridden. However, pressure ulcers do not only occur in people who are lying down. While decubitus ulcers often develop in people who are ill in bed for a long period of time, especially immobile people, they also occur in people who sit in wheelchairs for hours at a time. Since the primary cause of these ulcers is prolonged pressure on a body part, the term *pressure ulcer* is considered more appropriate, because it "describes both the cause and the condition" (Colburn, 1990, p. 63).

Pressure ulcers are the result of prolonged pressure on one part of the body with resultant loss of circulation to the area and subsequent tissue destruction. Although pressure ulcers may occur in any patient if there is sufficient pressure on one area to cause **ischemia** (decreased supply of oxygenated blood to a body part or organ, often accompanied by pain and dysfunction), they are seen most frequently in individuals with poor nutritional status, especially if there is a negative nitrogen balance. Pressure ulcers are most often seen on the bony prominences of the body such as the sacrum, coccyx, hips, heels, ankles and elbows. Secondary infection may complicate the problem.

Factors that predispose patients to pressure ulcers include continuous pressure on one area, dampness, a break in the skin surface, poor nutrition, dehydration, poor blood circulation and thinness (bony prominences unprotected by adipose tissue). Figure 31.3 shows common sites for pressure ulcers.

Classification of Tissue Damage

All tissue damage is not the same. Wounds can be superficial or deep; they can be clean with granulating tissue, or covered with necrotic debris. Because wounds in different stages are treated differently, nurses must be able to identify what stage the wound is in.

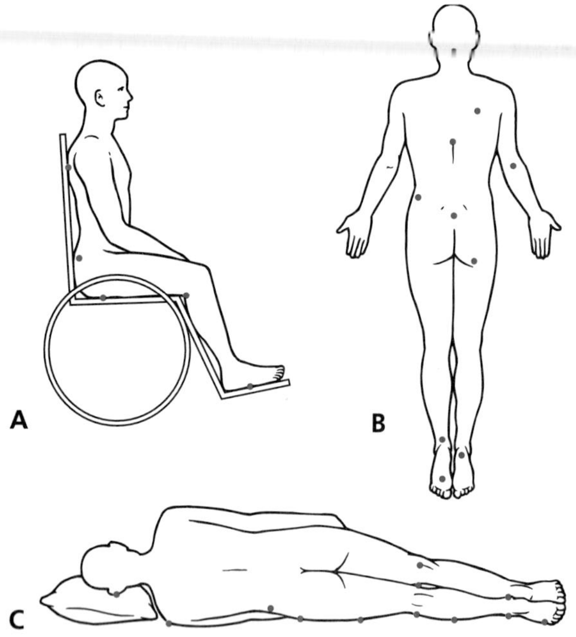

FIGURE 31.3 Common sites for pressure ulcers. Dots show pressure points when sitting (A), when lying on back (B) and when lying on side (C).

SOURCE: U.S. Department of Health and Human Services, 1994, p. 5.

Stage of Pressure Ulcer	*What You See*
A. Stage One: Nonblanchable erythema of intact skin; the heralding lesion of skin ulceration.	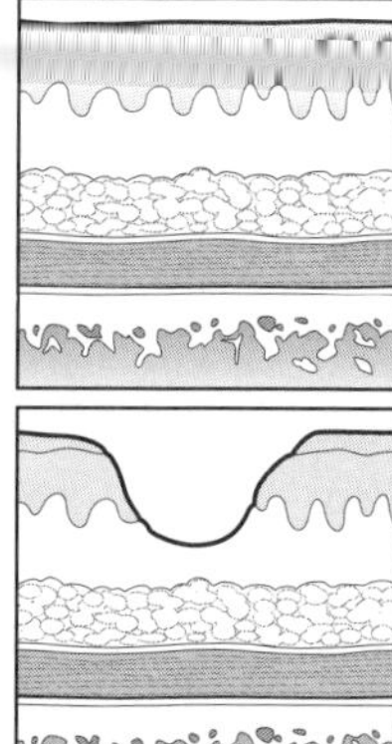
B. Stage Two: Partial-thickness skin loss involving epidermis and/or dermis. The ulcer is superficial and presents clinically as an abrasion, blister or shallow crater.	
C. Stage Three: Full-thickness skin loss involving damage or necrosis of subcutaneous tissue that may extend down to, but not through, underlying fascia. The ulcer presents clinically as a deep crater with or without undermining of adjacent tissue.	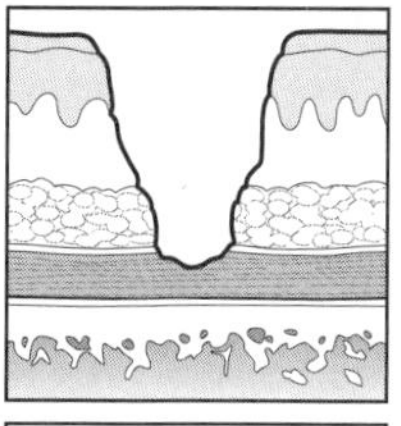
D. Stage Four: Full-thickness skin loss with extensive destruction, tissue necrosis, or damage to muscle, bone or supporting structures (e.g., tendon, joint capsule).	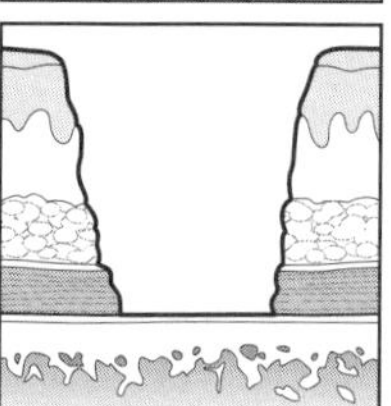

FIGURE 31.4 Stages of pressure ulcers

SOURCE: ConvaTec, 1992.

Pressure ulcers can be classified using various methods. At present, there are two common classification schemes used in health care. It is beneficial to use a consistent method of identifying pressures so that nurses can assess effectively, plan and carry out appropriate nursing interventions, evaluate wound healing and communicate to other health professionals through accurate documentation (Ferreira & Thorpe-Critten, 1998).

THE FOUR-STAGE CLASSIFICATION SYSTEM This system, developed by the National Pressure Ulcer Advisory Panel, enables the nurse to identify the early signs of a pressure ulcer. These signs include redness and tenderness of the particular area. Erythema (redness) lasting more than 30 seconds after pressure is removed is considered Stage One. Unless special measures are taken at this time to relieve pressure and increase local tissue nourishment, a break in the patient's skin usually follows (Stage Two). The ulcer may then continue to increase in size (width, depth, length), and increasing damage ensues to underlying skin layers if the wound is left untreated. Figure 31.4 illustrates the four-stage classification system.

In this classification scheme, however, it is often difficult to distinguish a Stage Three wound from a Stage Four wound, because the wound is usually lined with necrotic tissue and, until this is removed, the precise level of damage often cannot be determined.

THE RED, YELLOW, BLACK CLASSIFICATION SYSTEM This is another system that can be used to assess the condition of a wound and the status of healing (Stotts, 1990). (See box.)

Bacterial Colonization and Infection

Bacterial colonization "stimulates the activity of neutrophils and macrophages" (Flynn, 1996, p. 121). **Colonization** of a wound is considered to have occurred when it contains large numbers of bacteria loosely attached to devitalized tissue cells. **Infection**, on the other hand, is defined as a wound that has organisms that have bonded to tissue, multiplied and then invaded viable tissue (Boyton & Paustian, 1996). All deep wounds (Stages Two through Four) are colonized with bacteria. Cleansing and debridement will usually prevent colonized bacteria from progressing to infection. These procedures are outlined in Chapter 33.

Diagnosing infection can be difficult, as swab cultures will always be positive for bacteria. It is important to look at the bacterial count to differentiate between colonization and infection. Infection is diagnosed if the bacterial count is more that 10^5 organisms per gram of tissue (Boyton & Paustian, 1996). Infected wounds usually have purulent, foul-smelling drainage, are **indurated** (hard or firm) and red at the wound edges; the surrounding skin can be warm to the touch. The best way to diagnose infection is by culture of fluid by needle aspiration or biopsy of ulcer tissue. If these

The Red, Yellow, Black Wound Classification System

Red Stage: Skin Unbroken

[illegible] breakdown, indicated by redness that does not fade. It can be caused by pressure or moisture. The skin at this stage remains intact.

Pressure Damage: This damage is due to circulatory and tissue breakdown. The skin is undergoing an acute inflammatory response in all its layers. The area is irregular in shape, and swelling and pain are present. This stage can be reversed if the pressure is removed in time, though it may take up to 36 hours for the redness to fade. Sometimes the tissue is completely damaged, and a deep wound will eventually open up.

Moisture Damage: This damage occurs when the top layer of skin is red and irritated. It often occurs in skin folds.

Treatment Goal: In either case, the goal is to remove the cause of the redness and to protect the skin while it heals.

Red Stage: Broken Skin

This stage occurs when the wound bed is red or pink in colour. The wound can be superficial or deep.

Superficial Tissue Damage: This is due to pressure, shearing or friction. The damage is localized to the epidermis and dermis. The wound bed appears pink. The wound usually heals in 10–15 days. Drainage is minimal.

Deep Tissue Damage: These wounds extend through all the skin layers to the deep fascia or bone. Usually, they have gone through a necrotic stage. Now the wound is clean and healing and has a red, beefy appearance. These wounds may be crater-like and have a moderate amount of drainage.

Treatment Goal: When the wound is free of **exudate** (fluid from wound) and **necrotic** (dead) tissue, the surface must be protected from trauma so that the wound can continue to heal. The goal is to keep the wound surface moist, clean and warm, and to absorb excess drainage.

[illegible]

This stage is characterized by moderate to large amounts of clear yellow drainage. This can occur in superficial or deep wounds. The wound bed is usually a mix of yellow fragments of necrotic debris and granulating tissue. The drainage is made up of dead cells, bacteria and macrophages. This **autolysis** (disintegration of tissue by the body's own mechanisms) is part of the normal healing process; its goal is to clean the wound so that healing can take place. These wounds are usually not infected.

Treatment Goal: The goal is to clean out the wound bed so that granulation can take place. The wound bed needs to stay moist so that autolysis can occur, and excessive drainage must be absorbed to prevent the wound from becoming macerated.

Black Stage

This is the necrotic stage. The tissue can be yellow-green, grey or black. Yellow-green or grey necrotic (moist) tissue usually occurs in deep wounds. The wound bed is tightly covered with this slough. There are moderate to large amounts of seropurulent drainage. The wound edges may be inflamed, and the wound may be infected. Black, dry necrotic tissue (**eschar**; "thick leather") can be found on the surface. This substance may be dry and hard to the touch; it seals the wound and prevents healing. Eschar on the feet does not need to be removed if the wound edges are free from redness and swelling, and there is no drainage present.

Treatment Goal: Necrotic tissue provides a medium for bacterial growth and slows healing, thus leaving patients at risk for infection. The goal is to remove the dead tissue as quickly as possible. When the necrotic tissue is removed, the wound will appear deeper and wider than before. This is normal and expected.

treatments are unavailable, a swab can be used to identify an infection. Swabbing a wound for culture and sensitivity is described in Chapter 33. If the wound is found to be infected, topical or systemic antibiotics should be initiated.

Assessing Skin and Hygiene Needs

The nurse begins an assessment of skin integrity and hygiene by exploring the patient's usual cleansing and grooming practices, as well as predisposing risk factors to pressure ulcers. The importance and meaning of these rituals should be identified. At the same time, the nurse can assess the patient's knowledge of hygiene. This information is obtained from the nursing history and the use of a risk assessment tool. Following the history, the nurse conducts a physical exam that uses observation and palpation techniques to add information to the data base.

The nurse also takes into consideration factors that affect the patient's ability to carry out hygienic practices. For example, do motor abilities allow the patient to provide for hygiene? Does the physical environment provide the basic necessities for hygiene, such as fresh water? Other health problems may also affect the condition of the skin and need to be considered. Finally, what is the physical appearance of the skin? Are there any lesions, broken skin, allergic reactions? Is there a history of skin cancer?

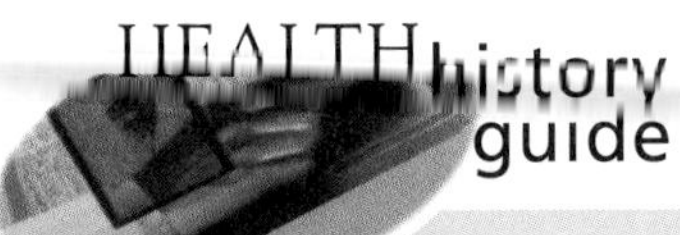

Skin and Hygiene

Health and Illness Patterns

Usual Hygiene Pattern and Practices

- Describe your usual hygiene routine and your usual practices for maintaining hygiene.
- How and when do you bathe and wash hair? How often?
- How do you care for your teeth? What products do you routinely use?
- Do you take any special measures to care for your hair?
- How and when do you clean your ears?
- Do you wash your hands at specific times?
- Do you use any special products for hygiene such as soaps, lotions, creams, deodorants, perfumes?

For women:

- What type of sanitary protection do you use during menstruation?
- Do you have any special hygienic practices during menses?

Overall Appearance of Skin

- Do you have any scars? What injuries caused these scars?
- Have you experienced any difference in skin temperature or sensation anywhere on your body?
- Is your skin normally dry, oily, scaly? If so, where?
- Is this the normal colour of your nail beds?
- Do you have any skin allergies?
- Do you or any member of your family have skin cancer?
- Do you smoke?
- Do you wear sunscreen, a hat and sunglasses when outdoors?
- Do you experience urinary or bowel incontinence?

Recent Changes in Hygiene Pattern and Practices

- Have you had a recent illness or health problem that has affected your hygiene practices?
- Is there anything else that is affecting your ability to keep yourself clean?
- What assistance will you need to meet your hygiene needs?

Recent Changes in Skin Integrity

- Have you noticed any changes in your skin? Any lesions, discoloration, changes in the size of moles, drainage from lesions?
- Has your nutritional status changed recently? Fluid intake?
- Are you more sedentary at present? Do you need assistance with walking?
- Have you noticed any swelling?

Presenting Health Problem

- Do you have any problems with your skin? Any dryness, oiliness, rashes, open areas, changes in pigmentation or moles?
- Where on your body did the skin problem begin?
- When did you first notice the problem?
- How does your skin feel?
- Have you noticed skin changes in other areas?
- Does anything make the problem worse? Better?
- Have you used any home remedies or over-the-counter preparations to try to resolve your problem? What were the results?
- Have you recently had any other illnesses?
- Have you noticed any unusual or patchy hair loss?
- Have you noticed any changes in your nails?
- Have you had any allergic reactions?
- Has anyone in your family had a skin problem?
- What medications or treatments have you been taking recently?
- Do you have any problems with your mouth or teeth?
- Do you experience any unpleasant odours?

Health-Promotion and -Protection Patterns

- How do you try to keep your skin healthy? What things would you like to do for your skin but feel unable to?
- Do you visit the dentist? How often?
- Have you seen a dermatologist? Podiatrist?

Nursing Health History

The nurse may begin a health history by asking a broad, open-ended question such as "What are your usual routines and practices for maintaining hygiene?" More specific questions can be used to elicit more detail, if necessary. For women, the nurse may explore hygienic practices during menstruation. "Feminine hygiene" is a topic infrequently discussed, and many misconceptions exist. Especially with adolescent girls, the nurse may use this opportunity for teaching hygiene practices during menses.

In taking a skin and hygiene health history, the nurse ascertains if the patient has had any changes in usual hygiene practices, nutrition or activity and determines any assistance that may be required to meet hygiene needs. When the patient's presenting health problem relates to the skin or oral cavity, the nurse will then ask specific questions to gather information about it. Finally, as with all needs, the nurse examines the patient's health-promoting behaviours to determine learning needs and opportunities for health teaching. Above is a health history guide to facilitate the gathering of subjective data about skin and hygiene needs.

As part of a nursing health history, nurses can use particular assessment measurement tools to ascertain an individual's degree of risk in relation to pressure ulcers. The first step in preventing pressure ulcers is to identify at-risk individuals and their predisposing factors. Timely and routine risk assessments are essential to preventing skin break- [illegible] 1990). Systematic risk assessments can be done using a risk assessment tool such as the Braden Scale for Predicting Pressure Sore Risk (see Figure 31.5). This tool helps identify the factors that put an individual at risk and can also help the nurse develop a plan of care in order to address and potentially eliminate these factors. Factors included in this scale are mobility, degree of activity, continence, nutrition and level of consciousness. Individuals should be assessed when first seen by members of the health team, such as in hospitals, nursing homes, rehabilitative centres, home care programs and other facilities. Reassessment must be done at predetermined intervals (U.S. Department of Health & Human Services, 1992).

Physical Assessment

The physical assessment for skin integrity and hygiene can be divided into two parts. In the first part, the nurse examines the hair, eyes, ears, mouth, teeth, nails and skin that can be seen without the patient undressing. The second part involves examining areas under clothing. Depending upon the circumstances, this part of the exam may be postponed to a later time, such as during the patient's bath. In any case, a thorough assessment includes an examination of all skin surfaces.

VISIBLE SKIN EXAMINATION

During the first encounter with the patient and during the history-taking, the nurse gains an overall impression of the patient's state of skin integrity. Factors that might affect this impression include general cleanliness, tidiness and any unusual odour. The visible skin is assessed for colour, lesions, moisture (flaking or oiliness) and dirt.

The assessment of hair includes hair on the head (scalp hair), as well as hair on other parts of the body (facial and body hair). Inspect and palpate the hair for distribution, quantity, colour, texture and hygiene. To palpate for texture, rub a few strands of hair between your thumb and forefinger to determine whether it is silky, resilient, dry, brittle or oily.

Normally, coarse terminal hair grows evenly over the scalp. Variations in quantity, texture and colour are influenced by heredity and age. Males, for example, may experience symmetrical hair loss due to a genetic proclivity for baldness, and older adults of both genders experience thinning of the hair. Natural hair colour varies from light blond to dark black, but it can be changed easily with the use of chemical dyes and rinses. Greying of the hair occurs normally with aging; however, premature greying may be associated with underlying disease such as pernicious anemia (Barkauskas, Stoltenberg-Allen, Baumann, & Darling-Fisher, 1994). The texture of scalp hair may be coarse or fine, straight, curly or wavy. It should feel smooth, silky and resilient and be neither excessively dry nor oily. Oiliness, however, is common in both males and females during adolescence because of [illegible] generally be clean, shiny and combed.

Abnormal hair loss (**alopecia**) results from a variety of causes such as radiation or anticancer therapy, overprocessing with chemicals (for example, bleaching) and hypopituitarism. Alopecia may occur as isolated patches, diffuse thinning or total loss of hair. Hair texture may change due to systemic disease. For example, hair becomes very coarse and dry with hypothyroidism, and very fine and silky with hyperthyroidism. Chemical hair products can leave hair dry and brittle. Dirty, uncombed or matted hair indicates poor hygiene practices.

Fine villus hair normally covers the body, while coarse terminal hair grows on the eyebrows and lashes, the axillary and pubic areas and the lower face in males. Hair distribution and quantity varies considerably among individuals and is influenced by race, ethnic origin and gender. For example, people of Mediterranean origin usually have more profuse body hair than do people of Asian descent. Males generally have more noticeable body hair than females. Both males and females develop pubic and axillary hair growth during puberty, but the distribution pattern of pubic hair differs. In males, the pattern is an upright triangle with hair extending midline up the umbilicus, whereas in females, the pattern is an inverted triangle. In both males and females, the quantity of hair gradually increases after puberty and then decreases with age.

When assessing body hair, the nurse should note patterns of distribution and areas of hair loss. **Hirsutism** refers to increased hair growth and may indicate an endocrine disorder. In females, hirsutism assumes the distribution pattern characteristic of males, with an increase of hair on the face and body. The absence of pubic hair or an abnormal distribution pattern of pubic hair in either male or female may signify hormonal abnormalities and should be noted.

The eyes are assessed for redness, swelling, tearing or discharge. The ears are checked for any discharge or wax buildup in the auditory canals. It is important to note any obvious hearing impairment, as it may be related to accumulated cerumen (Ney, 1993). It is helpful to examine hearing aids, if the patient wears them, as they may be plugged with wax. The nurse checks the skin of the external ear and behind the ear.

The nails are inspected and palpated for shape and contour, texture, adhesion to the nail bed, colour and hygiene. At the same time, a blanch test may be performed to determine capillary refill time. See Chapter 24 for details of how to perform this assessment skill.

Normally, the edges of the nails are smooth, rounded and clean, the nail surface is slightly convex and the lateral and posterior nail folds (folds of tissue surrounding the nail) are smooth and rounded. The angle of the nail base (where the skin and nail base meet) is 160 degrees (see Figure 31.6).

Patient's Name ______	Evaluator's Name ______		Date of Assessment		
Sensory perception: Ability to respond meaningfully to pressure-related discomfort	1. Completely limited: Unresponsive (does not moan, flinch, or grasp) to painful stimuli, due to diminished level of consciousness or sedation, or limited ability to feel pain over most of body surface.	2. Very limited: Responds only to painful stimuli. Cannot communicate discomfort except by moaning or restlessness, or has a sensory impairment which limits the ability to feel pain or discomfort over 1/2 of body.	3. Slightly limited: Responds to verbal commands, but cannot always communicate discomfort or need to be turned, or has some sensory impairment which limits ability to feel pain or discomfort in 1 or 2 extremities.	4. No impairment: Responds to verbal commands. Has no sensory deficit which would limit ability to feel or voice pain or discomfort.	
Moisture: Degree to which skin is exposed to moisture	1. Constantly moist: Skin is kept moist almost constantly by perspiration, urine, etc. Dampness is detected every time patient is moved or turned.	2. Very moist: Skin is often, but not always moist. Linen must be changed at least once a shift.	3. Occasionally moist: Skin is occasionally moist, requiring an extra linen change approximately once a day.	4. Rarely moist: Skin is usually dry. Linen only requires changing at routine intervals.	
Activity: Degree of physical activity	1. Bedfast: Confined to bed.	2. Chairfast: Ability to walk severely limited or nonexistent. Cannot bear own weight and/or must be assisted into chair or wheelchair.	3. Walks occasionally: Walks occasionally during day, but for very short distances, with or without assistance. Spends majority of each shift in bed or chair.	4. Walks frequently: Walks outside the room at least twice a day and inside room at least once every 2 hours during waking hours.	
Mobility: Ability to change and control body position	1. Completely immobile: Does not make even slight changes in body or extremity position without assistance.	2. Very limited: Makes occasional slight changes in body or extremity position but unable to make frequent or significant changes independently.	3. Slightly limited: Makes frequent though slight changes in body or extremity position independently.	4. No limitations: Makes major and frequent changes in position without assistance.	
Nutrition: Usual food intake pattern	1. Very poor: Never eats a complete meal. Rarely eats more than 1/3 of any food offered. Eats 2 servings or less of protein (meat or dairy products) per day. Takes fluids poorly. Does not take a liquid dietary supplement, or is NPO and/or maintained on clear liquids or IVs for more than 5 days.	2. Probably inadequate: Rarely eats a complete meal and generally eats only about 1/2 of any food offered. Protein intake includes only 3 servings of meat or dairy products per day. Occasionally will take a dietary supplement, or receives less than optimum amount of liquid diet or tube feeding.	3. Adequate: Eats over half of most meals. Eats a total of 4 servings of protein (meat, dairy products) each day. Occasionally will refuse a meat, but will usually take a supplement if offered, or is on a tube feeding or TPN regimen which probably meets most of nutritional needs.	4. Excellent: Eats most of every meal. Never refuses a meal. Usually eats a total of 4 or more servings of meat and dairy products. Occasionally eats between meals. Does not require supplementation.	
Friction and shear	1. Problem: Requires moderate to maximum assistance in moving. Complete lifting without sliding against sheets is impossible. Frequently slides down in bed or chair, requiring frequent repositioning with maximum assistance. Spasticity, contractures or agitation leads to almost constant friction.	2. Potential problem: Moves feebly or requires minimum assistance. During a move skin probably slides to some extent against sheets, chair, restraints, or other devices. Maintains relatively good position in chair or bed most of the time but occasionally slides down.	3. No apparent problem: Moves in bed and in chair independently and has sufficient muscle strength to lift up completely during move. Maintains good position in bed or chair at all times.		
				Total Score	

FIGURE 31.5 The Braden Scale for predicting pressure sore risk

SOURCE: Bergstrom, Braden, Laguzza & Holman, 1987.

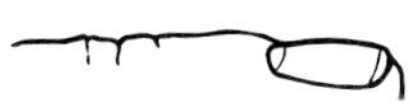

Normal Nail
Nail surface is slightly convex; angle of nail base is 160°.

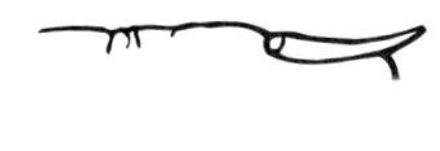

Koilonchia (Spoon Nail)
Thin, depressed nail; lateral edges turn upward. May be congenital; also occurs with anemia and chronic eczema.

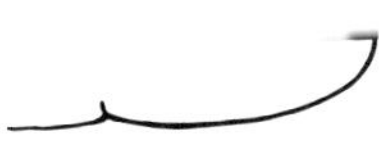

Clubbing
Angle of nail base is 180° or more. Occurs with heart and chronic lung diseases.

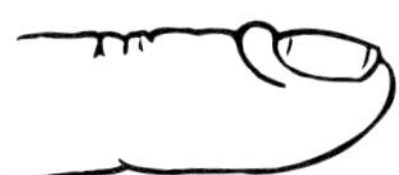

Paronychia
Tender inflammation of the nail folds. Acute infection is usually bacterial; chronic infection usually fungal origin.

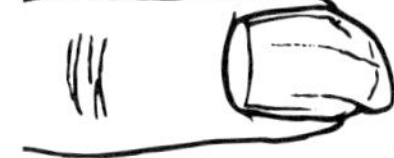

Onychauxis
Thickening or hypertrophy of nail. Occurs with repeated trauma, fungal infection or decreased vascular circulation.

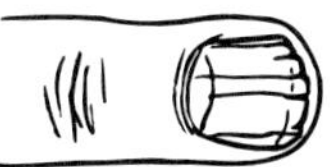

Onychorrhexis
Thinning, fragile, brittle nail with uneven edges. Occurs with malnutrition, chemical trauma and radiation.

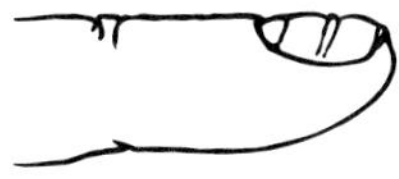

Beau's Lines
Transverse furrow or dent across nail plate. Occurs with acute illness, local trauma, malnutrition.

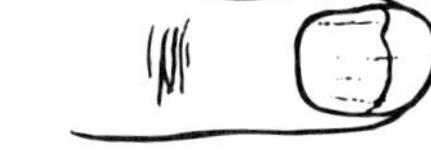

Onycholysis
Loosening of the distal nail occurs at edge from nail bed. May occur with chronic conditions.

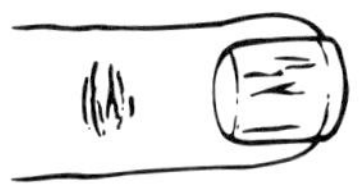

Splinter Hemorrhage
Linear blood streaks occur with trauma and heart disease.

FIGURE 31.6 Normal nails and nail abnormalities

SOURCES: Jarvis, 1996; Thompson & Wilson, 1996; Fuller & Schaller-Ayers, 1994.

The texture of the nail surface is smooth and the thickness uniform. The nail adheres to the nail bed, and the nail base feels firm on palpation. The nail plate is translucent, and the nail bed underneath is pink in colour. In dark-skinned people, brown or black pigment bands or streaks along the nail edges are not unusual. Common nail abnormalities are illustrated in Figure 31.6. These include **koilonychia** (spoon-shaped nail with a concave curve), **clubbing** (increased angle of the nail base), **paronychia** (inflammation of the nail folds), **onychauxis** (excessive thickening or hypertrophy of the nail), **onychorrhexis** (thin, brittle nail with uneven edge), Beau's line (transverse furrow in the nail plate), **onycholysis** (loosening of the distal nail edge from the nail bed) and splinter hemorrhages (Fuller & Schaller-Ayers, 1994).

EXAMINATION OF ALL SKIN SURFACES

The skin surfaces are examined for colour, moisture, temperature, texture and thickness, mobility and turgor, edema, hygiene, vascularity and lesions. Good lighting is necessary for the inspection. Natural light, or artificial light that resembles it, is preferred because artificial light often distorts colours and masks jaundice (Bates, 1995). You may have to correlate your findings with observations of the mucous membranes as diseases may manifest themselves in both areas, and both are necessary for assessing skin colour (Bates, 1995). Techniques for examining mucous membranes are described later in this chapter. You should have a pair of gloves available for palpating any areas that are moist or draining.

Inspect the skin for general colour, pigmentation (skin tone) and colour change. Skin tone varies from person to person, from one part of the body to another and according to genetic make up. These variations may range from ivory or light brown to ruddy or dark pink in lighter-skinned races, or from tan to brown or black in races with darker skin. Some races have yellow-olive overtones to their skin, for example, some Asian people. Dark-skinned individuals usually have areas of lighter pigmentation on the palms, soles of feet, lips and nail beds. In all people, pigmentation is generally darker in areas exposed to the sun, such as the face, neck, arms and hands. Overall, skin tone should be uniform and consistent with genetic background.

Normal alterations in the pattern of pigmentation may also occur as a result of changes in the distribution or function of melanocytes in the epidermis, causing areas of hypo- or hyperpigmentation. An example of hypopigmentation is **vitiligo**, a benign condition consisting of white, patchy areas where melanin pigment is completely absent. While vitiligo can occur in all races, darker-skinned people are more severely affected. Areas of hyperpigmentation, such as freckles (small, flat areas of high melanocyte activity usually stimulated by sunlight), occur in people with white skin. Other hyperpigmented areas, such as nevi (flat or raised areas caused by a proliferation of melanocytes), also known as birthmarks and moles, may occur in all people. Areas of hyperpigmentation, particularly moles, should be examined carefully for signs of skin cancer. The danger signs of pigmented lesions becoming cancerous are outlined in the accompanying box.

Abnormal colour change in the skin may include pallor, cyanosis, erythema and jaundice. **Pallor** is the absence of red-pink colour in the skin due to decreased blood flow to the superficial vessels (for example, fainting) or to decreased amounts of oxygenated hemoglobin in the blood (for example, anemia). Pallor is best assessed in sites with the least pigmentation, particularly the lips and mucous membranes of the mouth, the palpebral conjunctivae (mucosa of the eyelids) and the nail beds. The palms and soles may also be useful in dark-skinned people (Bates, 1995). Pallor appears as a yellowish brown colour in people with brown skin, ashen grey or loss of red tone in those with black skin and whitish-grey in those with light skin.

Cyanosis is a bluish, mottled discoloration in the skin, nail beds and tissues. It is a common finding in people with chronic lung conditions or heart disease. Cyanosis can be central or peripheral in origin. *Central cyanosis* results from insufficient oxygen in the systemic circulation and affects the whole body. It is best detected in the lips, oral mucosa and underside of the tongue (Bates, 1995). *Peripheral cyanosis* pertains to the extremities and is the result of diminished blood flow. The bluish discoloration of the hands, nail beds and sometimes the lips often seen in people exposed to cold temperatures is an example of peripheral cyanosis. The nurse should be careful, however, not to confuse cyanosis with the normal bluish hue on the lips of dark-skinned people of Mediterranean descent, nor the bluish hue to the lips and gums common in black races. The buccal mucosa (inner surfaces of the mouth) or conjunctivae are the most reliable areas for noticing central cyanosis in these individuals. Bluish hands and feet may indicate both central and peripheral cyanosis. The palms and soles may also show cyanosis in people with darker skin.

Erythema refers to redness and is the result of superficial vasodilation. It is seen readily in vascular flush areas such as the cheeks, bridge of the nose, neck, upper chest and genitalia in response to the vasodilation of blushing, excitement, sexual stimulation and fever (Morton, 1993). Erythema may be generalized, as with fever, or localized, as with mild sunburn or inflammation.

Jaundice is a yellow discoloration of the skin and indicates increasing levels of bilirubin in the blood. According to Jarvis (1996), "jaundice is first noted in the junction of the hard and soft palate in the mouth and in the sclera (p. 227). Care must be taken not to confuse scleral jaundice with normal yellow subconjunctival fatty deposits that are common in the outer sclera of darker-skinned people (Jarvis, 1996). As levels of bilirubin rise, jaundice becomes more apparent in the skin.

To assess moisture, use gentle palpation with the dry dorsal surfaces of your fingers so as not to confuse the patient's moisture with your own. Normally, the skin feels dry to the touch without excessive perspiration or oiliness. Increased perspiration may result from warm environmental temperatures, elevated body temperature, muscular activity, anxiety or pain. The skin may be normally drier in winter months, when temperature and humidity are lower. Abnormal dryness may indicate dehydration, in which case the skin remains dry even when the temperature is elevated.

Assess the temperature of the skin using the backs of your fingers or hands because these areas are the most sensitive to temperature perception. Check for generalized warmness or coolness, comparing body parts bilaterally and

Abnormal Characteristics of Pigmented Lesions

The danger signs of cancerous skin lesions are summarized with a simple ABCD mnemonic:

Asymmetry of a pigmented lesion (one that is not regularly round or oval)

Border irregularity (poorly defined margins; edges are notched or ragged)

Colour variation (colour not uniform; variable pigmentation including black, brown, grey, tan, pink, blue)

Diameter greater than 6 mm

In addition, any report of change in mole size, a new pigmented lesion or the development of itching, burning or bleeding in a mole suggests the possibility of skin cancer and should be referred to the physician.

SOURCE: Jarvis, 1996.

noting the temperature of reddened areas. Normally, the skin should feel warm to touch and the temperature should be equal bilaterally. Skin temperature may be affected by [illegible]

become generally warm in a patient with a fever because of vasodilation, or it may feel cool in a patient in shock because of the compensatory vasoconstriction in the skin. Localized temperature changes may also reveal abnormal conditions. For example, warmth around a wound may indicate local inflammation and infection, whereas coolness of the fingers or toes may signify impaired peripheral circulation in a patient with a cast.

Use light palpation with the fingertips to determine the general texture and thickness of the skin and to identify any changes. Normally, the skin feels smooth, soft and supple. Areas of the body exposed to friction and wear, such as the soles, palms, knuckle joints and elbows, may be rough and callused. A **callus** is a thickening of the epidermis in locations subjected to excessive pressure or friction. Skin thickness varies, being thinnest on the eyelids, ears, external genitalia and eardrum, and thickest on the soles of the feet. Skin that is very thin and vulnerable to breakdown must noted.

Mobility is the skin's ease of lifting up (Jarvis, 1996), and *turgor* (elasticity) is the speed with which it recoils (returns to its original shape). To assess turgor, lift a fold of skin under the clavicle or over the sternum, abdomen or inner forearm, then release it and observe how quickly it recoils. The skin should recoil immediately. Turgor is decreased when the pinched skin is slow to recoil. When turgor is poor the skin remains folded and assumes a "tenting" position. Poor skin turgor is a sign of dehydration. Mobility decreases when edema is present in the tissues.

Edema is swelling caused by the accumulation of excessive amounts of fluid in the tissues. It is an abnormal finding that may result from systemic causes, such as congestive heart failure and kidney disease, and from local causes, like obstructed venous or lymphatic drainage (Bates, 1995). The formation of edema may be localized in one area of the body, such as swelling in an ankle, or it may be generalized and spread throughout the whole body. Edematous skin appears puffy, taut and shiny. Edema usually affects the lower or dependent parts of the body first because fluid accumulation relies on gravity drainage. Examine the feet, ankles and legs of ambulatory patients and the sacral area of bedridden patients to detect edema. Press your thumbs firmly but gently into the soft tissues over a body prominence such as the ankle malleolus, the tibia or the dorsum of the foot for at least five seconds and then remove it. Normally, the skin surface remains unchanged when the thumbs are removed (Jarvis, 1996). If pressure of the thumbs leaves an indentation (pit) in the skin, **pitting edema** is present. The extent of pitting is graded on a four-point scale from mild to very deep pitting (see Chapter 16). When edema is present, note its location and whether it is unilateral (confined to one specific area of the body, such as the leg), bilateral (involving areas symmetrically on both sides [illegible]

Along with inspection, olfaction is used to examine hygiene and to detect unusual body odours. Inspect areas carefully, such as those under the breast or in the groin region and the buttocks crease, noting moisture and the presence of secretions or discharge and odour. The collection of moisture and lack of adequate air circulation make these areas particularly vulnerable to skin breakdown. Normally, the skin should be clean and free from body odour. A pungent body odour is normal with perspiration but its presence indicates the need for bathing.

Vascular changes are detected by inspection and palpation. They usually appear as red-pigmented lesions. Some vascular changes, such as cherry angioma, are normal occurrences; others, such as spider angioma, while frequently normal, may be associated with disease (Fuller & Schaller-Ayers, 1994). These vascular changes are described in Table 31.4 on page 988.

Bruising refers to bleeding into surrounding tissues as a result of trauma to underlying blood vessels, and is considered normal if it occurs secondary to the activities of daily living (for example, bumping into a table). However, bruising that is not associated with usual minor injuries should be considered abnormal and investigated further (Thompson & Wilson, 1996). Vascular abnormalities due to bleeding from breaks in the vessels (purpuric lesions), such as petechiae, ecchymosis and purpura, are also described in Table 31.4.

All skin lesions should be examined and described according to their location and distribution, morphology or clinical description (Morton, 1993) and pattern or arrangement. You will need a small ruler to measure the size of lesions and a flashlight for close inspection of their characteristics. Note whether they are generalized over the entire body (diffuse), or region of the body (for example, the trunk), or localized in a specific area (for example, elbows, knees or under rings or watchbands).

Inspect any lesion for size, colour, shape and discharge. Measure the size; in determining the lesion's distinct colour, note also whether it is circumscribed (contained within a well-defined border) or diffuse (spread over a large area). Note whether the lesion looks flat, raised, sunken or pedunculated (connected to the skin by a stem) and whether the edges are regular or irregular. Does the lesion contain any exudate, and if so, what is the colour, amount, consistency and colour? Palpate the lesion, making sure to wear a glove if it is moist and draining. First, apply gentle pressure. Does the lesion feel soft, hard or fluid-filled? Does it blanch (lose colour or fade) with pressure? Next, grasp the lesion between your thumb and forefinger and roll it to assess its depth (Jarvis, 1996). Finally, observe how lesions are patterned, that is, "the arrangement of lesions in relation to each other"

(Morton, 1993, p. 157). For example, the arrangement may be linear (in a line), clustered (grouped together) or annular (arranged in a circle).

WOUND ASSESSMENT

When examining a pressure ulcer the nurse should be able to describe the wound accurately, together with any changes that represent healing or potential infection. Specific components of a pressure ulcer assessment should include location of the wound; its size in centimetres, using a disposable ruler or grid (document width, length and depth); presence and extent of any sinus tracts, **undermining** (tissue destruction underlying intact skin) or tunnelling; stage of the wound; condition of the wound bed and edges (colour, moisture, presence or absence of necrotic/granulating tissue); type, colour and amount of exudate; and presence of edema or odour (Boyton & Paustian, 1996). Many agencies have a flowsheet to document wound care and healing, such as that shown in Figure 31.7.

Diagnosing Skin and Hygiene Problems

When patients have difficulty performing any aspect of hygiene care by themselves, the diagnosis *Bathing/Hygiene Self-Care Deficit* is used. This may include problems in washing, combing the hair, shaving, brushing the teeth, manicuring the nails and applying lotions, creams, deodorants or make-up. The defining characteristics of this diagnosis include situations in which the person is unwilling or unable to wash or to obtain water or regulate the water flow. A hygiene self-care deficit is also indicated by the inability to perceive the need to keep clean (Carpenito, 1997). A multitude of factors, such as severe pain, extreme weakness or paralysis, immobility due to trauma or surgery, and activity intolerance secondary to heart and respiratory problems, can contribute to a bathing/hygiene self-care deficit.

Impaired Skin Integrity identifies "a state in which the patient experiences or is at risk for experiencing damage to the epidermal or dermal tissue" (Carpenito, 1997, p. 676). Patients who are immobilized necessarily have a risk for skin breakdown due to the effects of pressure on body parts and the forces of shearing and friction if the skin sticks to or rubs against bed linen. Moisture, poor nutrition and dehydration also contribute to the problem. Redness and tenderness of an area, particularly over a bony prominence, is the first sign of impaired tissue integrity. A break in the epidermal or dermal tissue is the major defining characteristic of this nursing diagnosis. For example, the nurse in an extended care facility identifies a resident at risk for skin breakdown. The diagnosis might be stated as *Risk for Impaired Skin Integrity related to incontinence and partial immobility*. This nurse has identified a problem for which health-protecting strategies need to be implemented.

KEY PRINCIPLES

Principles Relevant to Hygiene

1. Intact skin and mucous membranes are the body's first line of defence against infection and injury.
2. Individual differences exist in the nature of the skin, hair, teeth and nails.
3. Changes occur throughout the lifespan in the skin, mucous membranes, hair, nails and teeth.
4. The health of the skin and mucous membranes is highly dependent on adequate nourishment, fluid intake and exercise.
5. General health affects both the status of the skin, teeth and mouth, and the ability to maintain proper hygiene.
6. Hygiene practices are learned.
7. Hygiene practices vary with cultural norms, personal idiosyncrasies and values, and the ability to maintain good habits of cleanliness and grooming.
8. The ability to maintain proper hygiene is an important independent function in older children and adults.
9. The skin, hair, nails and teeth may be affected by medication and other forms of therapeutic intervention.

Like the skin, the oral mucous membrane is prone to breakdown if oral hygiene is inadequate or not performed at all. In patients whose oral hygiene is inadequate, the diagnosis *Risk for Altered Oral Mucous Membrane* is used (Carpenito, 1997). Disruptions in the mucous membrane, such as lesions, coated tongue, gingivitis or dry mouth, indicate actual problems.

For patients who engage in poor hygiene practices because of an unhealthy lifestyle or lack of knowledge of how to handle a condition, the diagnosis *Altered Health Maintenance* may be used. Because people are responsible for their own health, this diagnosis indicates a problem that the patient must be motivated to treat, but for which the nurse has a responsibility to raise the patient's awareness that better health is possible (Carpenito, 1997). For example, for a patient with dental caries due to poor oral hygiene practices and lack of dental care, the nurse can provide information about oral hygiene and dental services and encourage the patient to consider changing dental health practices.

The diagnostic label *Knowledge Deficit* may also be used in cases where individuals have a need to learn hygiene self-care. For example, the school nurse may discover an adolescent girl who has just started menstruating and has questions about sanitary products and hygiene practices. A suitable nursing diagnosis might be *Knowledge Deficit of menstrual practices related to change in physical functioning and lack of family discussion of sexuality issues*. This diagnosis illustrates an opportunity for the nurse to practise health promotion.

A bathing or hygiene self-care deficit may become the etiology of other problems. For example, patients unable to

The Richmond Hospital

Wound care

SITE:	MONTH:	DATE / TIME	DATE / TIME	DATE / TIME	DATE / TIME	DATE / TIME	DATE / TIME	DATE / TIME
	YEAR:							
RT/LT:								
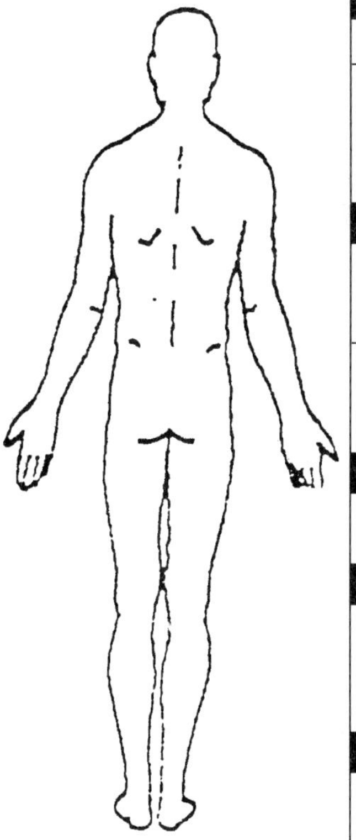	SIZE MEASURE Q WEEK							
	WOUND APPEARANCE							
	D = DRY M = MOIST							
	%R = RED %Y = YELLOW %B = BLACK U = UNDERMINING							
	EXUDATE							
	N = NIL S = SMALL M = MODERATE L = LARGE							
	PUR = PURULENT SER = SEROUS SANG - SANGUINEOUS							
	ODOR							
	N = NONE F = FOUL							
	SURROUNDING TISSUE							
	R = RED IND = INDURATED BL = BLANCHED INT = INTACT							
	DEBRIDEMENT							
	N = NIL S = SMALL M = MOD L = LARGE							
	initial							

TREATMENT:	FREQUENCY:	DIAGRAM OF WOUND

COMMENTS:

FIGURE 31.7 Wound care flow sheet

SOURCE: The Richmond Hospital, Richmond, B.C., 1995.

maintain their preferred pattern of hygiene may experience negative feelings about their body and express embarrassment about how they look. In such cases, the diagnosis *Body Image Disturbance* may be used. Patients may also experience feelings of powerlessness or lack of personal control if they are dependent on others to perform hygiene measures for them. Further, when a break in the integrity of the skin or mucous membrane occurs, the risk of infection increases because the first line of defence against harmful agents is interrupted. These diagnoses may be stated as *Powerlessness* and *Risk for Infection*, respectively.

Planning Skin and Hygiene Interventions

Planning follows naturally from the identification of a problem or nursing diagnosis and involves establishing patient goals or expected outcomes. Hygiene is very personal and goals need to be set individually, taking into account special circumstances and preferences. Goals need to be clearly written, measurable and achievable.

The resident of an extended care facility who is at risk for skin breakdown would have a long-term goal, such as "The resident will show intact skin as evidenced by a lack of redness or open areas." For the adolescent newly experiencing menstruation, one goal might be "The young woman will list two methods for managing menstrual flow." If she has identified that she would like to try using tampons, goals might include "The young woman will list three necessary precautions, when using tampons, that decrease risk of toxic shock syndrome." This goal deals with the prevention of illness as opposed to health promotion.

Assisting patients who need help in carrying out hygiene measures is among the nurse's most important priorities. Serious problems can develop if basic skin care and oral hygiene are not attended to on a regular, planned schedule. As with problems in mobility, *prevention* is the key. Deterioration of a patient's skin or mouth can develop very rapidly, sometimes with little warning. Repair of the damage is a slow process that entails much discomfort and suffering on the patient's part and much work on the nurse's part—work that can be avoided if simple precautionary measures are taken.

Implementing Skin and Hygiene Interventions

Health-Promoting Strategies

Hygiene is a basic requirement for health and well-being. Cleanliness promotes comfort, maintains skin and mucous membrane integrity and reduces the risk of infection from contaminants on the skin. While most people value cleanliness, not everyone engages in healthy hygiene practices. Some do not because they lack knowledge of healthy hygienic measures, whereas others do not because they lack the necessary means. For instance, people living in impoverished or crowded conditions may not be able to perform adequate hygiene care. Strategies for promoting healthy hygiene care involve education and referrals to appropriate resources or to other health professionals. For example, community health and home care nurses may give advice to parents of young children regarding dental health and the need for regular dental visits in this age group. School nurses often teach hygiene care such as washing hands before eating and after using the toilet, brushing the teeth and using dental floss, as well as bathing and shampooing regularly. Skin integrity and hygiene practices for healthy living are given in the accompanying box.

Other health-promoting strategies involve teaching individuals about the risk of excessive exposure to the sun and reviewing sun protection interventions with them. For example, a nurse could review the importance of wearing sunblock or sunscreen with a sun protection factor (SPF) of at least 15, lip balm, sunglasses and a wide-brimmed hat and avoiding the mid-day sun when the ultraviolet rays are the most intense. The nurse could also provide advice to individuals who are at risk for developing a pressure ulcer to eat a well-balanced diet, drink adequate fluids and inspect their skin on a daily basis.

For patients who need help to acquire good hygiene habits, a teaching plan is incorporated into the nursing care plan. Much of the teaching may be done while carrying out specific nursing interventions such as a bed bath. Because hygiene is a very personal matter, tact is needed in this teaching, and care should be taken to protect the patient's self-esteem in the process. Putting the teaching in terms of promoting optimal health and including an explanation of the reasons for the development and maintenance of good hygiene practices help to put the teaching on a more objective and less personal basis.

Health-Protecting Strategies

A very common function of nurses in acute care hospitals, long-term care facilities and in the home is assisting patients who are unable to maintain their own hygiene independently. These individuals may be experiencing an acute illness following traumatic injury or surgery that necessitates temporary assistance. Others may have a chronic or permanent condition such as paralysis following a stroke. This section focusses on procedures nurses employ when helping others with hygiene.

Most inpatient agencies have established routines for providing hygiene care. These include morning care, a daily bath and evening care. The routines are in place to ensure that every patient's need for hygiene is met on a consistent basis. Because these routines take into account staffing patterns, daily baths are usually scheduled in the morning, since there are generally more staff members on the day shift.

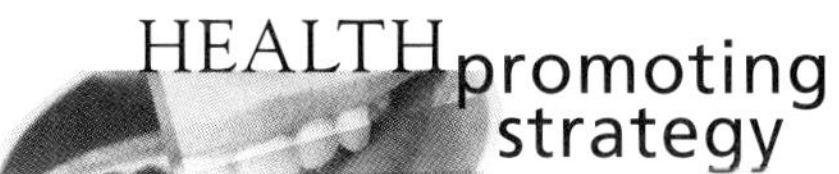

Promoting Healthy Skin Integrity and

HAND-WASHING

- Always wash your hands before starting the day, when visibly dirty, after using the toilet, after blowing your nose, after handling garbage, before eating or drinking, after finishing work and before going to bed at night.
- Use running water to wash your hands. Bacteria can multiply rapidly in standing water, even when a germicidal agent is used.
- Use plain or antimicrobial soap, depending on the purpose.
- Always dry your hands thoroughly. Individual or paper towels are best. Wet dirty towels can spread germs.

ORAL HYGIENE AND DENTAL CARE

- Brush your teeth regularly at least twice a day.
- Use a gentle, circular massaging action to work bristles into the sulcus (the shallow crevice where the tooth and gum meet).
- Brush all other tooth areas—fronts, backs and chewing surfaces.
- Use a soft brush with rounded bristles. A worn brush won't get your teeth clean; if it is worn, replace it.
- Floss your teeth at least once a day. Tartar builds up in 36 hours if plaque (invisible bacterial film) is not removed.
- Work the floss gently between the teeth and then below the gum line. Wrap the floss in "C" shape around each tooth and wipe away from the gum several times.
- If the floss catches and shreds, try waxed floss.
- Visit your dentist and have your teeth professionally cleaned regularly.

PERINEAL CARE

- Wipe area thoroughly if incontinent.

BATHING

- Bathe regularly. If you perspire a lot or have oily skin, daily bathing may be necessary.
- If you are elderly, avoid daily bathing. Frequent washing dries the skin and removes the natural protective oils.
- Showers are best for cleansing because running water washes away contaminants.
- Assess skin (bony prominences) daily.

FOOT CARE

- Keep the feet clean and the toenails cut.
- Cut toenails after the bath or shower; otherwise, soak the feet in a basin of water to soften the nails.
- Cut or file the nail straight across; avoid trimming the lateral corners, as this can cause ingrown toenails. Patients with diabetes should have their nails cut by a podiatrist only.
- Use lotions and moisturizing creams to keep the skin soft and prevent calluses.
- Consult a podiatrist for treatment of corns and calluses.

HAND CARE

- Use lotions and moisturizing creams to keep the skin soft and prevent drying and cracking.
- Regularly trim the nails and push back the cuticles. Keep the cuticle softened with lotion.
- Cut the nails straight across and round the ends with a file.

ENVIRONMENTAL CARE

- Avoid mid-day sun.
- Wear sun protection.
- Eat a well-balanced diet and drink adequate amounts of fluids.
- Choose clothing that is nonabrasive and nonconstrictive.

SOURCES: WHO, 1988; Canadian Dental Association, 1994; Ebersole & Hess, 1998.

GENERAL MORNING CARE

Before breakfast is served, patients who require assistance are offered a bedpan or urinal, or are ambulated to the bathroom if they can get up. Patients who must remain in bed are provided with the necessary materials for washing hands and face and for mouth care, and are assisted with these activities if they require help. Patients are then prepared for the meal—the bed is straightened, they are assisted to the most comfortable position for eating and a place is prepared for the tray.

GENERAL EVENING CARE

The evening care routine is somewhat similar in that the patient who requires assistance is offered a bedpan or urinal or is ambulated to the bathroom, and is given the opportunity to wash the hands and face and clean the teeth. In many agencies, the bed patient's back is washed and a back massage is given as part of the evening routine. The bottom sheet and drawsheet (if one is used) are tightened, and top bedclothes straightened and tucked in. If the patient needs an extra blanket, this is provided. The patient is assisted to a comfortable position; side rails, if needed, are put up on both sides of the bed. The call signal is put within easy reach, and any other items the patient wants near at hand, such as a clock or a jug of water and a glass, are placed within easy reach on the bedside table.

MOUTH CARE

Oral care includes daily cleansing of the teeth as well as regular care by dental professionals. Brushing the teeth removes food particles that provide a likely medium for bacterial growth. Brushing also massages the gums and stimulates circulation. It helps to keep the tongue, the mucous membranes lining the mouth and the lips moist as well as

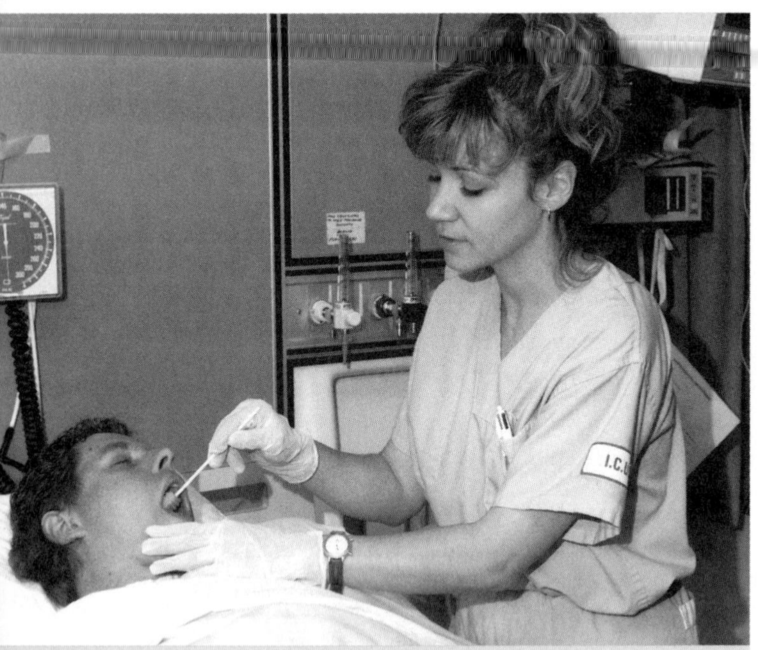

Good oral hygiene is essential for the patient's comfort.

clean. A clean, fresh taste in the mouth is important to the desire for and the enjoyment of food. Thus, good oral hygiene helps to promote good nutritional status.

The Canadian Dental Association recommends brushing the teeth regularly at least twice a day, although many people brush more often. Some people prefer to brush first thing in the morning, while others wait until after eating breakfast. Flossing is equally important in order to clean the spaces between the teeth, which cannot be reached by brushing. Daily flossing is recommended as tartar forms in a minimum of 36 hours.

The nurse helps those patients who cannot brush their teeth unassisted. Patients whose food and fluid intake is restricted or who are unable to eat and drink sufficiently (for example, very weak patients and those who are unconscious) require mouth care at frequent intervals (q4h and as indicated is usually recommended) to keep the tongue, teeth, gums and mucous membranes lining the oral cavity clean, moist and in good condition, and to keep the lips from drying out and cracking. The technique for providing mouth care is outlined in Procedure 31.1.

Preparing the Patient

Assess the patient's needs and preferences for oral hygiene. Explain the procedure and tell the patient how to be of assistance. If patients know what to do, they are better able to participate in the procedure.

Assembling Equipment

Patients usually supply their own toothbrush, dentifrice (toothpaste) or denture cleaner and dental floss. A mouthwash provided by the agency may be used if necessary and depending on the patient's preference. Water or normal saline solution is recommended for oral care. Commercially prepared normal saline swabs are available. Swabsticks can also be made by wrapping soft gauze around one end of a tongue depressor. Nurses traditionally used lemon-glycerine swabs for routine mouth care; however, the use of these kinds of swabs is no longer recommended. Research has shown that lemon-glycerine products may actually harm the patient. Warner (1986) reviewed a number of studies which found that lemon-glycerine dries mucosal membranes, irritates broken tissues and decalcifies the teeth. Petroleum jelly may be used on the lips to prevent drying and cracking. An emesis basin and a towel will also be needed. The nurse should always wear gloves when performing mouth care to prevent exposure to blood and blood-borne pathogens such as HIV and hepatitis B.

When performing mouth care on unconscious patients, a large syringe may be used to rinse the mouth. A catheter connected to a suction unit may be necessary to remove liquid and loosened debris from the patient's mouth to avoid aspiration. The patient should be in a side-lying position for this procedure.

Dentures require special care. Most institutions provide plastic containers for storing dentures that may be removed at night (patient's preference) or taken out for special procedures such as surgery. Lost dentures is not an uncommon occurrence in hospitals. It is important that denture containers are safely stored and clearly labelled with the patient's name.

BATHING

Bathing has several purposes: it cleanses, promotes comfort, stimulates blood circulation and affords an opportunity to exercise. When assisting a patient to bathe, nurses have an excellent opportunity for assessment and health teaching. For example, during the bath the nurse can observe the condition of the patient's skin, note such factors as the presence of edema, the quality of respirations and any difficulty or pain the patient experiences when moving. The nurse can provide teaching such as emphasizing the importance of avoiding pressure over areas of skin breakdown.

Due to the very personal nature of bathing, many patients find it much easier to talk to the nurse during the bath than at other times. It has been suggested that the reason for this is that the act of giving physical attention is perceived by many patients as a sign of caring (Davis, 1970). Thus, the bath provides an excellent opportunity for the nurse to establish rapport with the patient and to facilitate communication.

The type of bath depends on several factors, including the patient's medical condition and restrictions, mobility and mental capacity. A patient with advanced Alzheimer's disease might be physically capable of bathing alone, but for safety reasons should not be left unsupervised.

The three types of baths are the tub bath, the shower and the bed bath. Special aids are available such as pneumatic lifts, as discussed in Chapter 29, for raising immobile

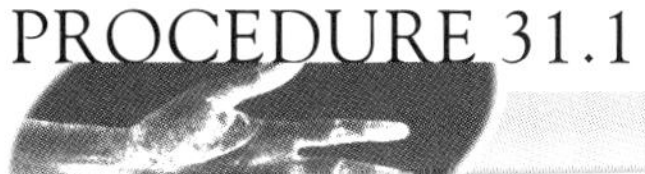

PROCEDURE 31.1 Performing Mouth Care

Action	*Rationale*
1. Assess the patient's needs and preferences for mouth care.	Provides individualized care.
2. Gather equipment: • gloves • toothbrush • toothpaste • warm water or normal saline. **Optional:** • mouthwash • dental floss • petroleum jelly • denture cup • large swabsticks • large syringe • catheter and suction unit.	Ensures efficiency and economy of time.
3. Wash hands.	Reduces risk of transmitting infection to the patient.
4. Explain the procedure to the patient.	Promotes well-being and enables patient participation in care.
5. Assist the patient into an upright or side-lying position. Position the unconscious patient in a side-lying position. Put towel and basin next to the mouth.	Prevents aspiration of fluid.
6. Apply gloves.	Protects both patient and nurse from infection.
7. Clean the teeth: **For dentures:**	
• Remove the upper plate first, using a wiggling motion.	Helps to break suction.
• Hold the dentures over a plastic basin or towel placed in the sink.	Prevents breakage if inadvertently dropped.
• Clean dentures with a toothbrush.	
• Rinse with warm water.	Hot water may damage the dentures.
• Return dentures to the patient. **For teeth:**	
• Place the toothbrush with toothpaste at gum line.	
• Gently vibrate the toothbrush using a circular, massaging action.	Loosens food particles. Minimizes gum irritation.
• Brush front, back and chewing surfaces.	
• If it is the patient's usual routine, wrap dental floss around each tooth and pull away from gum, repeating this several times for each tooth.	Cleans the area between the teeth where the brush cannot reach.
• Have the patient rinse with warm water as needed.	Removes food particles and toothpaste.
8. Clean the mouth.	
• **If patient is able**, have him or her rinse with warm water or half-strength mouthwash.	Removes food particles and debris from the mouth.
• **If patient is unable**, use the large syringe to gently rinse the mouth.	Gentle force reduces the risk of aspiration.
• If necessary, suction out any fluid remaining in the mouth.	Prevents aspiration of remaining fluid.
• Gently wipe the patient's gums and inside of the mouth and tongue with the swab.	Removes any debris. Moistens mucous membranes.
9. Apply petroleum jelly to lips.	Maintains moisture.
10. Examine the mouth for any open areas, redness, secretions or odour.	Provides data for ongoing evaluation of care.
11. Clean and/or dispose of equipment. Wash hands.	Maintains cleanliness and safety in the workplace.
12. Repeat q1–2h (if NPO) and document care given and any pertinent observations.	Facilitates continuity of care.

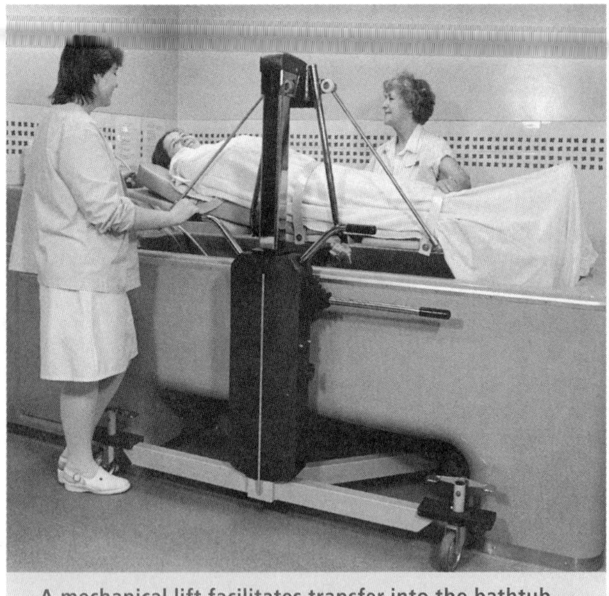

A mechanical lift facilitates transfer into the bathtub.

patients in and out of large bathtubs, and shower chairs for patients who cannot stand. Regular bathtubs are often equipped with railings, nonslip surfaces and special seats to reduce the risk of falls.

Not all patients require a bath every day, nor is it necessary for all patients to receive a bath in the morning. For the patient who tires very easily or who is very ill, the bath may be contraindicated. Because older people's skin will often become overly dry if they bathe too frequently, a partial bath may be indicated. This includes washing the patient's hands, back, axillae and perineal area, as well as providing for oral hygiene and massaging bony prominences. The nurse makes these judgements based on the needs of the patient and the assessment of the situation. In many long-term care facilities, residents receive a tub bath or shower on scheduled days of the week and partial baths on the other days.

The Bed Bath

The steps for giving a complete bed bath are detailed in Procedure 31.2. This basic procedure can be adapted according to patients' abilities to perform some parts of the bath themselves. For instance, some patients may be able to wash the face and hands only, while others may be able to wash most of the body, with the nurse cleansing the back and feet.

PREPARING THE PATIENT Before gathering the equipment, determine the patient's requirements and any personal preferences for bathing. Establish how much of the bath the patient will be able to perform and how much assistance will be needed.

ASSEMBLING EQUIPMENT The equipment required for the bed bath includes bath towels, washcloths, a water basin, soap and moisturising lotions. A bath blanket is also required to cover the patient to avoid embarrassing exposure and to keep the patient warm. The kind of soap used will depend largely on the individual needs of the patient and on the policy of the health agency. In many agencies, patients are permitted, and sometimes even required, to supply their own soap. A moisturizing lotion is supplied by the agency, although many patients may wish to use their own products.

The skin is sometimes irritated by the chemical composition of certain soaps. Soap can be irritating to a patient's skin and particularly to the eyes. Therefore, patients are often advised not to use soap on the face.

The Tub Bath

Tub baths are taken for hygienic and therapeutic reasons. The physician may order a therapeutic bath for some patients—sitz-baths, for example, may be ordered for the patient who has had rectal surgery. Patients with skin diseases often have oatmeal or medicated baths. A tub bath is often a pleasurable experience, but it is important to remember that it can also be very frightening for someone who is weak, unwell or confused.

Bathtubs in hospitals frequently have rails; if they do not, the adjacent wall is often equipped with handles to help the patient climb in and out of the tub. Most tubs also now have safety strips on the bottom which help to prevent slipping. No sick person should lock the bathroom door while unattended; help may be required. The nurse or attendant should know when a patient is bathing, and often it is wise to check on the patient every so often. If a patient is out of bed for the first time after even a few days of bed rest, it is generally unwise to leave him or her unattended in the bath. An attendant can stay just outside the curtains if the patient prefers privacy.

The bathtub is filled one-third full of water. Unless otherwise ordered, the water is drawn at 40.5° C, a comfortable and safe temperature for most people. The length of time that a patient bathes depends upon endurance and strength. A lengthy bath may cause unnecessary fatigue. A very hot bath will cause the blood to be diverted away from the vital centres of the brain to the surface areas of the body. As a result, the patient may feel faint and may even lose consciousness.

Getting into and out of the bathtub is often a difficult manoeuvre, and the patient may need assistance from the nurse. Usually it is easiest if the patient first sits on the edge of the tub with feet inside the tub, then reaches over to grasp the rail on the other side and gradually eases down. In helping the patient out of the tub, it is a good practice to let the water out before the patient attempts to stand up. There are many mechanical devices available today for assisting with tub bath procedures. A mechanical lift, for example, can be used in either hospital or home situations. Shower stools, on which patients can sit while showering, are also available.

A more recent product on the market is called the bag bath (Skewes, 1997). It consists of eight prepackaged, premoistened and disposable cloths that cleanse and hydrate at

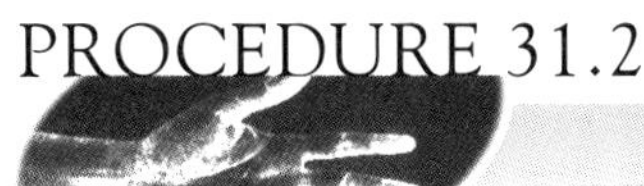

PROCEDURE 31.2 Giving a Complete Bed Bath

Action	Rationale
1. Assess the patient's needs and personal preferences for bathing.	Provides individualized care.
2. Gather equipment: • bath blanket • towels • washcloths • wash basin • soap • gloves • skin lotion • clean hospital gown or patient's own pyjamas.	Ensures efficiency and economy of time.
3. Wash hands.	Reduces the risk of transmitting microorganisms to the patient.
4. Explain procedure to the patient.	Enables patient participation in care.
5. Partially fill the basin with water slightly hotter than desired.	Water cools quickly.
6. Draw the bed curtains, cover the patient with the bath blanket and remove the top bed linen. If a bath blanket is not available, use the top sheet as a cover.	Provides privacy and keeps patient warm during the bath. Prevents the bed linen from getting wet and allows reuse if clean.
7. If the patient or the nurse has any open areas on the skin, wear gloves.	Prevents the spread of infection either to or from the patient.
8. Encourage the patient to do as much as possible.	Promotes independence and provides active ROM.
9. If the patient is unable to do so unassisted, begin by washing the face using clear water. Cleanse each eye from the inner canthus, using a clean area of washcloth for each stroke. Then wash the face, ears and neck.	Prevents soap irritation in the eyes and on sensitive facial skin. Prevents transmission of infection from one eye to the other.
10. Suggested order for bath: • face, ears, neck • arms, hands, axilla • chest, breasts • abdomen • legs, feet • groin and front of perineum • **Turn the patient to the side** • back, buttocks • rectal area • **Change the water** • perineal area	Proceeds generally from clean to soiled areas while minimizing position changes for the patient.
11. Exposing one area at a time, wash, rinse and dry each part well, then cover with the bath blanket or sheet. Place a towel under the extremity or next to the part being washed.	Keeps patient warm and comfortable. Prevents embarrassment from excessive exposure. Protects the bottom sheet(s) from water and facilitates drying.

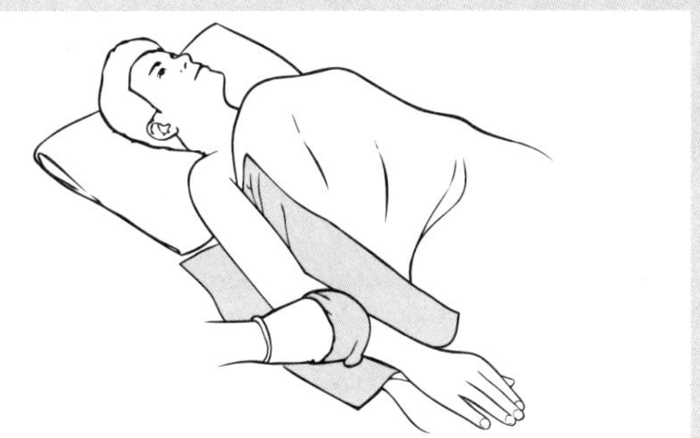

continued on next page

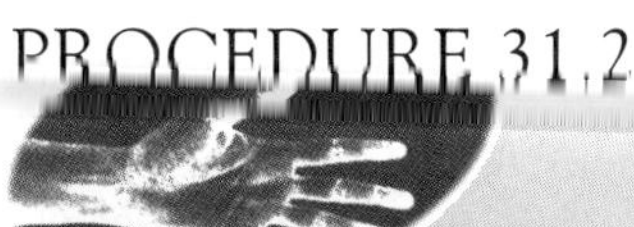

PROCEDURE 31.2 continued

Action	Rationale
12. Use long strokes on the arms and legs directed from the distal to the proximal areas.	Promotes venous return.
13. Change the water as it becomes dirty or cool and as above.	Maintains hygiene and comfort.
14. Apply gloves before perineal and rectal care, if gloves were not used up to this point.	Prevents the spread of infection either to or from patient.
15. Apply lotion to the back, feet and legs as needed.	Promotes comfort and lubricates dry skin.
16. Help the patient put on a clean gown, pyjamas or clothing as appropriate. Replace sheets, remove the bath blanket and assist the patient to a comfortable position. Ensure that the call bell is in reach and that side rails are up.	
17. Clean and/or dispose of equipment. Wash hands.	Maintains cleanliness and safety in the workplace.
18. Document care given and any pertinent observations.	Facilitates continuity of care.

the same time. Each cloth is used to cleanse a separate part of the body, thus reducing cross-contamination. The cleansing solution contains emollients that help maintain the skin's moisture. This solution quickly evaporates, making drying unnecessary. This new product has received support in many health care settings because of its simplicity and health-promotive nature.

PERINEAL CARE

Perineal care involves washing the external genitalia with soap and water or with water alone or in combination with any commercially prepared peri-wash. It may be carried out as part of the patient's bath or as a separate procedure, especially if the patient is experiencing frequent incontinence. It is recommended to clean the area immediately (at time of soiling) to prevent the risk of skin breakdown (Skewes, 1997). Patients who are unable to take care of their own hygiene needs, who are incontinent or who have indwelling or condom catheters require specific perineal care two or three times a day. Perineal hygiene for incontinent patients removes irritating urine and feces which can cause skin breakdown and infection. Patients with condom catheters should have the condom removed, the skin washed and dried and the condom replaced twice daily. The perineal area is inspected regularly for signs of redness or skin breakdown.

Regular and antibacterial soaps and commercially prepared cleaners are commonly used for perineal hygiene. Soap remaining in the genital area can cause damage to the tissues and discomfort for the patient (Lindell & Olsson, 1990; Ravnskov, 1984). Ravnskov (1984) has shown that soap is a major cause of dysuria; it is therefore essential that it be rinsed off thoroughly. If soap cannot be rinsed off completely, warm water alone should be used for perineal cleansing.

Perineal care varies for male and female patients. Procedures 31.3 and 31.4 outline the steps for performing perineal care on female and male patients, respectively.

PREPARING THE PATIENT Providing perineal care can be an embarrassing matter for both the nurse and the patient. When at all possible, patients should do their own perineal care with assistance from the nurse. The nurse will find that if the genital organs are regarded as ordinary body structures and the sexual function (which is often at the root of the nurse's anxiety) is mentally de-emphasized, tasks involving these areas will become less strained (Berger & Williams, 1992). Using a confident, matter-of-fact approach when explaining and performing the procedure will help the nurse and the patient feel more comfortable.

HAIR CARE

Care of the patient's hair is important both to grooming and to the sense of well-being. As a part of daily care, each patient's hair needs to be brushed and combed. Thorough brushing stimulates circulation to the scalp and improves the nourishment of the epithelium. Most patients can attend to this themselves, but the nurse may have to assume this responsibility for the elderly or ill patient.

The nurse, by seeing to daily hair care, can ensure that the patient's hair does not become matted. Long hair may be braided so that it will stay neatly in place. Patients who are in the hospital for long periods will require a shampoo. Permission for a shampoo may have to be obtained from the physician, depending on the patient's medical condition. For example, hair shampooing may be contraindicated for someone with a neck or spinal injury. Commercially prepared "dry" shampoo which absorb oily secretions, may be used as an alternative.

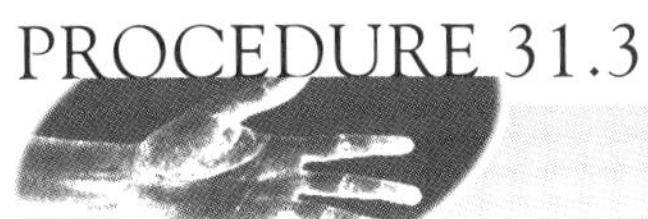

PROCEDURE 31.3 Performing Female Perineal Care

Action	*Rationale*
1. Gather equipment: • towel • washcloth(s) • soap and commercially prepared peri-wash, if available • wash basin • gloves.	Ensures efficiency and economy of time.
2. Prepare the patient.	Enhances the patient's comfort.
3. Prepare a basin of warm water.	
4. Draw bed curtains and assist the patient to a supine or side-lying position. Expose only the perineum.	Promotes privacy, comfort and warmth.
5. Apply gloves.	Prevents transmission of infection.
6. Wash, rinse and dry the groin area and the external labia.	
7. Using the nondominant hand, separate the labia and assess for redness, open areas, swelling, odour or unusual secretions.	Provides data for ongoing evaluation of care.
8. Using a washcloth, cleanse down the centre (over the urethral and vaginal openings) from the mons pubis to the base of the labia.	Prevents bacteria from the rectal area from coming into contact with the vagina and urethra.
9. If an **indwelling catheter** is present, stabilize it with one hand and wash approximately 5 cm of catheter proximal to the patient.	Prevents pulling on the balloon inside the bladder and thus prevents injury to the bladder. Removes mucous that collects on the tube, which can become a medium for bacterial growth and lead to urinary tract infection.
10. Using a clean part of the cloth for each stroke, cleanse each side of the labia minora from front to back.	Prevents transmission of infection from dirtiest to cleanest areas.
11. Gently pat dry.	Prevents injury to the fragile mucosa and prevents patient discomfort.
12. Leave the patient in a comfortable position.	
13. Clean and/or dispose of supplies. Wash hands.	Maintains cleanliness and safety in the workplace.
14. Document care given and any pertinent observations.	Facilitates continuity of care.

Patients prescribed bed rest may have the hair shampooed while in bed or they may be transferred to a stretcher. When a stretcher is used, it is best to move the patient to a sink and support the head on the edge of the sink. If transferring the patient to a stretcher is not possible, the nurse can use a folded plastic sheet or a specially constructed hair washing trough to direct the water from the patient's hair into a pail (see Figure 31.8). The nurse uses pitchers of water to wet and rinse the hair, taking precautions to keep the patient's bed dry. The patient's hair needs to be dried quickly after the shampoo in order to avoid chilling. Today, many large hospitals have hairdressing and barber services for patients.

Shaving

The nurse may sometimes have to shave the male patient who cannot shave himself. If the patient has an electric razor this is often not a problem, but a safety razor requires more skill. Very warm water is needed to give an adequate shave. After the skin has been lathered with shaving soap, it is held taut and the razor is drawn over it in short strokes. The nurse will find that the safest way to shave the patient is to stretch the skin over the bone in a particular area and then to shave in the direction in which the hair grows. Areas around the mouth and nose are particularly sensitive; here the nurse's motions need to be firm but gentle.

NAIL CARE

Care of the nails is another area of grooming that most patients can attend to themselves. For the ill patient or the patient who has difficulty moving, however, nail care may be the nurse's responsibility.

Toenails are cut straight across. Fingernails are also cut straight across; the edges are rounded with a file. For patients who are particularly prone to infection—for example, those with diabetes mellitus or circulatory problems—a referral to a podiatrist (foot specialist) for care is advisable.

To prevent hangnails, it is best to keep the cuticle of the nail pushed well back and lubricated with oil. Some patients

PROCEDURE 31.4 Performing Male Perineal Care

Action	Rationale
1. Gather equipment: • towel • washcloth(s) • soap and commercially prepared peri-wash, if available • wash basin • gloves.	Ensures efficiency and economy of time.
2. Prepare the patient.	
3. Prepare a basin of warm water.	
4. Draw the bed curtains, and assist the patient into a supine or semi-Fowler's position. Expose only the perineal area.	Promotes privacy, comfort and warmth.
5. Apply gloves.	Prevents transmission of infection.
6. Wash, rinse and gently pat dry the groin area and scrotum.	Proceed from cleanest to dirtiest areas.
7. Remove condom catheter, if present.	
8. Using a circular motion, wash around the urinary meatus, rinse and dry well.	The urinary meatus is usually considered to be the dirtiest area due to the presence of secretions.
9. Wash, rinse and dry the shaft of the penis.	
10. If an **indwelling catheter** is present, reverse the order of cleansing, beginning with meatus; also, wash and rinse approximately 5 cm of catheter proximal to the patient. Stabilize the catheter with one hand while washing meatal area and catheter.	When a catheter is present, the meatus is washed first to prevent the introduction of contaminants via the tube, thereby reducing the risk of urinary tract infection. Prevents pulling on the balloon inside the bladder.
11. Reapply a condom catheter.	
12. Leave the patient comfortable.	
13. Clean and/or dispose of supplies. Wash hands.	Maintains cleanliness and safety in the workplace.
14. Document care given and any pertinent observations.	Facilitates continuity of care.

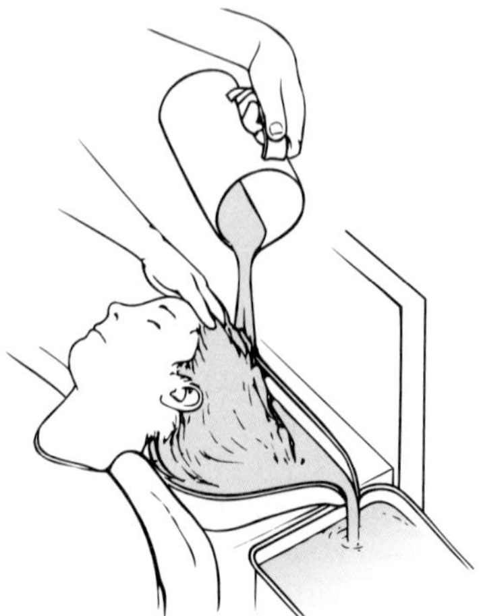

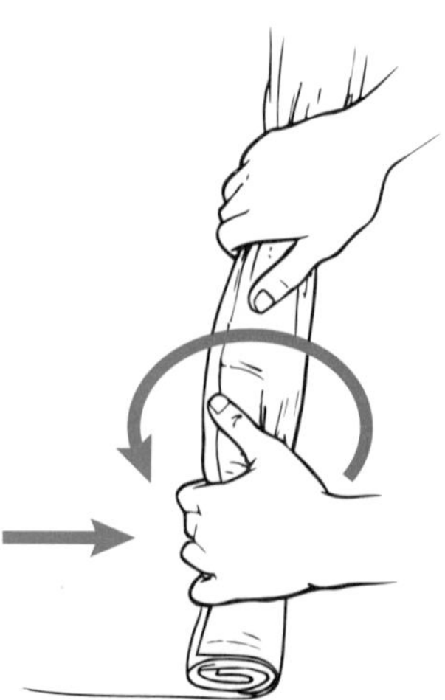

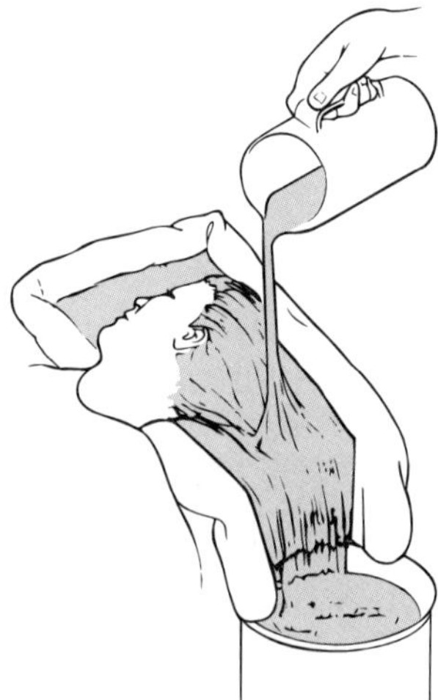

FIGURE 31.8 Shampooing hair while a patient is in bed

SOURCE: Berger & Williams, 1992, p. 1015.

have very hard fingernails and toenails. If the patient soaks the feet for 10–15 minutes in warm water, the nails will soften sufficiently to be cut with nail cutters. Special nail

EYE CARE

Special eye care may be required when the eyes have become irritated or infected. The physician usually orders a special solution to cleanse the eyes. Tap water or normal saline may also be used. With absorbent cotton dipped in the solution, the eye is wiped from the inner canthus to the outer canthus. The nurse uses a clean piece of cotton for each stroke. Water or normal saline will soften crusts so they can be easily removed. The motion from the inner to the outer canthus washes the discharge away from the nasal lacrimal duct, which is located on the inner aspect of the orbit of the eye.

Unconscious patients require special attention to protect the eyes from damage. The upper and lower lids should be kept clean and free from discharge. The lids should be closed when the patient is being turned to prevent scratching of the cornea. Special eye lubricants and "artificial tears" are available to prevent dryness and possible scratches.

Patients' glasses, contact lenses and other prostheses should be looked after carefully, and patients should be assisted with care of these articles if necessary. See Chapter 28 for care of contact lenses and prostheses.

EAR CARE

Hygiene for the ear consists of gentle washing of the external ear. The use of cotton-tipped applicators or other objects to remove earwax (cerumen) is discouraged because the wax may be pushed farther into the ear canal, or the ear canal or tympanic membrane may be damaged (Ney, 1993). Special protocols to remove impacted cerumen involve irrigation of the ear. A physician's order is usually needed to perform this procedure. Care of an individual's hearing aids is described in Chapter 28.

PREVENTIVE CARE FOR PRESSURE ULCERS

There are many preventive measures for pressure ulcers. Frequent changes in position rotate the weight-bearing areas and relieve pressure on any single group of bony prominences. The normal healthy individual shifts body position every few minutes. For the patient who is unable to do this unassisted, it is the nurse's responsibility to ensure that the position is changed. A regular schedule should be set up for turning the patient to keep the skin in good condition. Usual recommendations are to turn the patient every two hours and as needed.

As much as possible, the nurse should encourage patients to maintain their current level of mobility and activity. The effects of **shearing** (trauma caused by layers of tissue sliding against each other) can be minimized by limiting the duration that the head of the bed is elevated, if this does not harm the patient. Pillows and foam wedges should be used to keep bony prominences from direct contact with each other. When repositioning individuals, avoid

the trochanter. If the patient is completely immobilized, it is necessary to relieve total pressure on the heels. This can be accomplished by lifting the heels off the bed with a positioning device, such as a pillow or foam wedge.

When repositioning a patient, lifting devices such as a trapeze or bed linen should be used so that the patient is not dragged along the surface of the bed, causing friction damage. If the individual is at risk for skin breakdown, a pressure-reducing surface for the bed is necessary. See Chapter 28 for further discussion of these devices.

Massage and exercise stimulate circulation and thus improve the nourishment to the skin cells. Avoid massaging over bony prominences. Keeping the skin dry and clean inhibits the growth of disease-producing bacteria and prevents skin from becoming excoriated; body secretions and excreta are particularly irritating to the skin. The nurse should take particular care that a patient's linen and dressings are dry and clean. In areas where secretions cannot be prevented, protective ointments, such as zinc oxide or petroleum jelly, can be used to prevent excessive irritation.

Another preventive measure for pressure ulcers is the use of devices to relieve pressure on specific areas of the patient's body. An over-bed cradle will keep bedclothes off the patient, and other aids such as alternating pressure mattresses, oscillating beds and fluidized air or water mattresses may also be used. The use of sheepskin under pressure areas may be helpful for only short periods of time.

Attention to the patient's nutritional status is essential. Since pressure ulcers occur most frequently in patients with a negative nitrogen balance, the protein intake should be increased. Foods that contain complete proteins, such as eggs, milk and meat, are recommended. Proteins are needed for the regeneration of body tissue. Usually, supplementary amounts of vitamin C are also prescribed because of this vitamin's role in the healing process. Care must also be taken to ensure adequate fluid intake, since dehydration and poor tissue turgor predispose patients to the development of ulcers.

Educating patients, family members and health professionals is also an effective health-protecting strategy. Hospitals and agencies usually have in-services planned so that health professionals can stay abreast of current trends in wound care management. Pamphlets are also available to nurses so that they can provide information to patients and families.

Good skin care and early identification of potential skin breakdown is necessary to prevent pressure ulcers. All individuals at risk should have a systematic inspection of the skin every day to identify any areas that are at risk for breakdown. These areas will appear a pinky-red colour, usually over bony prominences. In individuals with dark skin tone, it is more difficult to identify areas that are at risk. Results of the skin inspection should be documented and a plan of care started to prevent further skin damage.

RESEARCH to practice

Provo, B., Piacentine, L., & Dean-Barr, S. (1997). Practice versus knowledge when it comes to pressure ulcer prevention. *Journal of Wound, Ostomy & Continence Nursing, 24*(5), 265–269.

The purpose of this study was to determine the extent of nurses' current knowledge base and documentation patterns in the prevention and identification of pressure ulcers. Using pre- and postintervention methodology, the authors carried out the study in three phases.

In phase one, they recruited 67 nurses and asked them to complete a modified version of the Bostrom's Patient Skin Integrity Survey on 43 patients (n=43). In phase two, the authors invited all 67 nurses to participate in a 20-minute educational session focussing on identification of pressure ulcers and current trends in pressure ulcer and wound management. Phase three consisted of asking 51 nurses to complete a similar survey as in phase one, but with 49 patients (n=49). Of the 118 nurses who completed phases one or three, 27 completed questionnaires in both phases.

The results revealed no statistically significant difference in nurses' level of knowledge about pressure ulcers before or after the educational in-service, and no significant difference in the identification of patients at risk for pressure sore development. Yet, the number of patients with a comprehensive and documented plan of care for their pressure ulcers increased significantly after the educational in-service.

This study suggests that ongoing educational in-services are essential in helping nurses to maintain their knowledge. More importantly, in-services encourage implementation of current standards in nurses' practice as a way to increase patient comfort and quality of care.

For patients who are wheelchair-bound, repositioning in the chair is also necessary. This will need to be done every hour. If the individual is capable of some movement, small weight shifts in the chair should be done every 15 minutes. Because of the risk for skin breakdown for wheelchair-bound individuals, it is necessary to apply a pressure-reducing surface to the chair.

To prevent venous ulcers, it is necessary to identify patients at risk, that is, individuals with poor venous return. These patients have marked edema of the feet, ankles and lower legs. The valves in the veins are flaccid and can no longer effectively push the fluid up the legs. To improve the flow of venous fluids, support hose (antiemboli stockings) can be used. These stockings increase the pressure on the veins and assist the fluid to move through the venous system, instead of pooling in the feet and ankles. This hosiery is available through local pharmacies and needs to be worn every day to prevent venous congestion. (See Chapter 33 on how to apply antiemboli stockings.) After several months, the stockings lose their elasticity and need to be replaced.

The pumping action of the calf is also necessary for good venous flow; thus, a regular walking program can help keep the calf strong and help to push the venous blood up through the legs. When resting, patients should elevate their legs to decrease the work of venous return. An important aspect of patient teaching is to emphasize that wearing support hosiery is a lifelong change. If the individual wears support stockings only occasionally, rarely walks and forgets to elevate the feet, these interventions will not be effective. People with venous ulcers frequently have them for years, or have recurring ulcers, because the cause of the skin breakdown cannot be corrected. Venous congestion can be improved only by changes in behaviour.

The main intervention for preventing diabetic ulcers is education of persons with diabetes. Good foot care is essential in preventing these ulcers. After bathing, feet must be carefully dried to prevent **maceration** (softening of tissue by soaking in fluid) that can lead to skin breakdown. Good footwear is also critical. Many diabetics develop an abnormal shape to the sole of the foot. Shoes may be custom-made to prevent pressure spots. Because many diabetics have minimal sensation in their feet, they are unable to feel their shoes rubbing. Diabetics should have their toenails trimmed by a podiatrist to prevent small cuts and scratches.

Health-Restoring Strategies

Helping patients to restore their hygiene status involves implementing activities related to specific problems of the skin, hair, nails and oral cavity. Therapeutic care for many of these conditions—for example, skin disorders (such as psoriasis), skin and oral infections or tumours of the skin and mouth—is dealt with in more advanced nursing courses. Problems with a person's gums and teeth, such as gingivitis and dental caries, are referred to a dentist for care.

CARE OF PATIENTS WITH PEDICULOSIS

Occasionally a patient will have **pediculosis** (infestation with lice). Therapy involves killing and removing all the pediculi (lice) and their eggs (nits) that have infested the skin, hair and clothing. There are three main types of pediculosis: *pediculosis capitis* or infestation of the scalp with lice, *pediculosis corporis* or infestation with body lice, and *pediculosis pubis* or infestation of the pubic hair with lice. There are several methods of ridding patients of pediculi. For body lice, the patient's clothing is removed for washing or cleaning, the patient is usually given a cleansing bath and then drugs are applied. In the case of head lice, or if body lice have infected the scalp, medicated shampoo is used. A number of drugs are available that are effective with only one application.

vehicles such as clothing, eating utensils and combs. They are usually found in environments where poor hygienic measures are practised. However, infestation is not necessarily an indication of poor hygiene. For example, in schools pediculi may be acquired even by children who bathe daily. Isolation techniques are discussed in Chapter 32.

CARE OF PATIENTS WITH PRESSURE ULCERS

When a pressure ulcer develops, the nurse faces a challenge in restorative care. The amount of tissue breakdown is often less extensive on the outside area than the inside area of the ulcer. Healing of the ulcer may sometimes be difficult.

Care of the pressure ulcer involves debriding necrotic tissue, cleansing the wound at each dressing change, using a dressing that keeps the ulcer bed continuously moist but the surrounding intact skin dry and preventing contamination from external bacteria (Maklebust, 1996).

Debridement

Debridement refers to the removal of dead tissue from a wound. Tissue observed in the wound should be debrided, as necrotic tissue provides a medium for infection, creates an inflammatory response and slows wound healing. Necrotic tissue is avascular; therefore, systemic antibiotics are of little value. There are several methods of debridement available: sharp, mechanical, enzymatic or autolytic debridement.

Sharp debridement uses a sterile scalpel or scissors to remove necrotic tissue. It can be very painful, as nerves are exposed once the eschar is removed; thus, premedication with analgesia is necessary. Small debridement can be done at the bedside; more extensive debridement is performed in the operating room or special procedure room. A clean, dry dressing should be used for 8–24 hours after sharp debridement to limit bleeding. When there are signs of advancing cellulitis or sepsis, rapid debridement is necessary. Special training is needed to perform this.

Mechanical debridement includes the use of wet-to-dry dressings, hydrotherapy, wound irrigation and dextranomers. A wet-to-dry dressing is one in which a normal saline-soaked gauze pad is applied to an ulcer and, when the pad is dry (usually after four to six hours), it is removed. When the dressing is pulled off, the necrotic tissue that is stuck to the gauze is torn away from the wound bed. The disadvantages of this procedure are that it is painful and that new granulating tissue is also removed when the gauze is pulled off. The debriding function of this type of dressing is minimized if the gauze is moistened prior to removal. Hydrotherapy and irrigation are used to debride wounds and soften eschar. When using this type of debridement, the nurse must ensure that enough pressure is used to clean and debride the wound adequately but also not to destroy granulating tissue (Maklebust, 1996). If the necrotic tissue is firmly adhered to the wound bed, this type of debridement will not

for details on how to irrigate a wound.) Dextranomers are beads that are placed into a wound to absorb exudate, bacteria and debris. One disadvantage is that the beads can be messy to work with as they have to be poured into the wound, and this can be difficult if the patient cannot be positioned correctly.

Enzymatic debridement involves the application of enzyme-containing cream to necrotic tissue. The enzymes effectively break down the dead tissue. There is some concern that they also break down granulating tissue.

Autolytic debridement occurs when fluid from the wound self-digests the eschar. Granulating tissue is not harmed. Wound gels (such as intrasite gel) transfer moisture to the necrotic tissue and help speed up autolysis. The eschar, as a result, is softer and easier for the body to self-digest. A semi-occlusive dressing is needed to cover the wound and to keep wound fluid from drying out.

Enzymatic and autolytic debridement are slow, but both are painless. If the wound becomes infected, a more rapid debridement is needed.

Heel and toe ulcers of dry eschar do not need to be debrided, as it acts as a natural protective layer. If the area is reddened, edematous or draining, debridement will be needed. These wounds should be assessed daily for changes (Maklebust, 1996).

Wound Cleansing

For a wound to heal correctly, it should be cleansed at each dressing change. The purpose is to remove all necrotic tissue, exudate, debris and metabolic waste. Normal saline is the preferred cleansing agent as it is nonirritating and nontoxic. Many of the cleansers on the market today contain harmful chemicals that destroy tissue. Do not use antiseptic agents such as povidone iodine, Dakin's solution, hydrogen peroxide or acetic acid to clean wounds (U.S. Department of Health & Human Services, 1994).

Maintaining a Moist Wound Environment

The goal is to keep the ulcer bed continuously moist while allowing the surrounding skin to remain dry. Moist wound-healing treatments provide faster healing rates than dressings that dry the wound bed. The dressing should control the exudate without desiccating the ulcer bed. Dead space should be filled in, and the dressing should act as a barrier to prevent external bacteria from entering the wound (U.S. Department of Health & Human Services, 1994; Maklebust, 1996).

There are many products on the market that are designed to keep the wound bed moist and the surrounding tissue dry. An advantage that many of these products have is that they do not need to be changed daily, thus decreasing

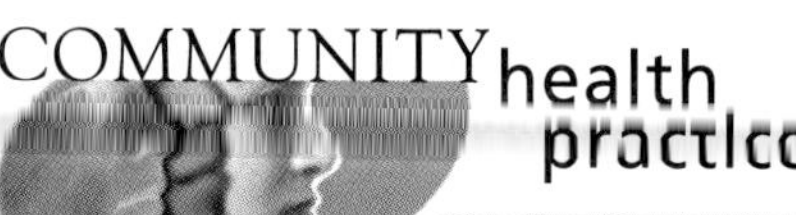

Cast Care

When an individual sustains a fracture of a limb, immobilizing the limb with a cast is often a common medical treatment to help the healing process. Casts can alter skin integrity, and because most individuals will be caring for themselves at home, it is important for the nurse to review essential tips of cast care. Here are some health-restoring teaching tips:

- If plaster was used for the cast, it is important to keep it supported on a firm surface until it is dry. Also, if the cast is to be lifted up, the individual should be instructed to use the palms of the hands. These steps will prevent indentations, which can press inward towards the limb and can potentially rub against the skin, leading to skin breakdown and infection.
- The person may experience edema in the first 24 hours, so it is important to encourage elevation of the casted limb, administration of analgesics/anti-inflammatories and application of ice.
- Occasionally, the skin under the cast will become itchy. Strongly stress to the patient or parent that inserting an object into the cast to relieve the itch could break the fragile skin and lead to infection.
- If the patient detects a foul odour, unusual discomfort or an elevated temperature (after 48 hours), it is important to contact the physician. These signs indicate a developing infection.
- Once the cast is removed, encourage the individual not to scrub off the dead, flaky skin. This action may lead to loss of skin integrity. Encourage the patient to wash gently, pat dry and apply a moisturizing lotion to the affected area.

nurses' workload and increasing patients' recovery and healing time. It is important to remember that every time a wound is cleansed, the wound bed goes into thermal shock from the sudden decrease in temperature. It takes up to three hours for the wound bed to return to its regular temperature; thus, every time the dressing is changed, three hours of healing time is lost. Chapter 33 reviews various dressings and wound management in more detail.

CARE OF VENOUS ULCERS

Venous ulcers can be cared for in the same basic manner as pressure ulcers. Venous ulcers have large amounts of drainage; therefore, effective absorption is needed in the dressings. Patients with venous ulcers are frequently prescribed bed rest and receive diuretics and albumin to correct the edema caused by venous congestion, but these treatments do not cure the underlying etiology. Many people with venous ulcers have them for years; some ulcers may be 20 years old. Topical treatments are not always effective.

A new treatment for healing venous ulcers is a pressure-bandaging system (Profore by Smith & Nephew). This four-layer bandage provides continuous external pressure that improves venous circulation. Improvement in venous ulcers is noticeable in several weeks, and ulcers can be healed in 8–12 weeks. After the ulcer is healed the individual must continue to wear support stockings or the ulcer will return when venous congestion recurs.

CARE OF ARTERIAL ULCERS

Arterial ulcers can be treated in the same ways as pressure ulcers, but because the underlying etiology is poor arterial perfusion, there are unique problems with these types of wounds. Arterial ulcers are usually very dry; thus, it may be necessary to add some moisture to the wound to help maintain a moist wound bed. Gels are useful for this. Some patients may be candidates for vascular surgery that can correct the underlying problem. Unfortunately, many patients are not eligible for this type of surgery.

Because the blood flow to the wound is compromised, arterial wounds are very slow to heal. Frequently, individuals with arterial ulcers have to undergo surgery to remove the necrotic area, and in some cases where infection is present, amputation may be required.

CARE OF DIABETIC ULCERS

Diabetic ulcers are similar to arterial ulcers because diabetics often have poor vascular perfusion to the wound site. This can cause slow healing. Also, because diabetics have limited responses to infection, it may be difficult to identify infection in a diabetic wound. If antibiotics are not effective on an infected wound, amputation may be necessary.

Evaluating Skin Integrity and Hygiene Interventions

Evidence of successful nursing interventions is found in the healthy state of the patient's skin, hair, nails, teeth, mouth and process of wound healing. Continuous reassessment of all of these is required.

More and more criticism is being directed at the ritualistic nature of nursing's hygienic practices. Financial constraints in the health care system also challenge nurses to provide the most efficient and effective care possible. Not only do nurses need to continually evaluate the effectiveness of their care for individual patients, but more evaluation in the form of research studies is also needed.

New advances are being made in wound management. Some of the therapies being tested include electrical stimulation; hyperbaric oxygen; infrared, ultraviolet and low-

growth hormone; and manufactured skin.

IN REVIEW

- Hygiene is the science of health. At a personal level, the term refers to the measures people take to keep their skin, teeth, hair and nails clean and in good condition.
- The body's first line of defence against infection is the skin. It is composed of two layers (epidermis/dermis) and overlies the subcutaneous and adipose tissues.
- Skin integrity is influenced by a number of factors:
  - general state of physical and mental health
  - nutritional and hydration status
  - fitness level
  - personal hygiene practices
  - medications and treatments
  - environment
  - socioeconomic factors
  - religious practices.
- The process of wound healing consists of three phases:
  - inflammatory
  - proliferative
  - remodelling.
- An individual's process of healing may be altered by such factors as:
  - extent of injury
  - patient's age
  - nutritional status
  - weight
  - existing health problems (diabetes, cardiovascular disease)
  - level of mobility/activity
  - immune response system.
- There are variations in skin integrity and hygiene needs throughout the life cycle.
- People commonly experience problems associated with inability to maintain skin integrity and hygiene. These include:
  - gingivitis
  - halitosis
  - dental caries
  - dandruff
  - dry skin
  - burns/sunburns
  - infestations
  - primary, secondary and vascular lesions
  - pressure ulcers
  - wound ulcers (venous, arterial, diabetic).
- In assessing skin and hygiene needs, the nurse uses information from the health history and physical assessment to determine nursing diagnoses

  - *Self-Care Deficits*
  - *Impaired Skin and Tissue Integrity*
  - *Risk for Infection*
  - *Altered Health Maintenance*
  - *Body Image Disturbance*.
- The main focus of nursing intervention is the promotion of healthy and intact skin and the prevention of skin breakdown.
- In promoting healthy skin and hygiene practices, nurses should encourage patient hand-washing and skin care, oral/dental care, bathing, foot care, exercise and eating a well-balanced diet.
- Health-protecting strategies include:
  - assessing skin and bony prominences daily
  - turning/positioning; shifting weight
  - cutting nails
  - identifying individuals at risk for pressure ulcers.
- Restorative care is needed when there is loss of skin integrity or self-care deficit. Strategies include:
  - skin and wound care
  - pressure-reducing devices
  - patient/family education.
- Evidence of effective nursing care is found when an individual has healthy skin, wound/pressure ulcers are healing and the patient participates in health-promoting and health-protecting strategies.

Critical Thinking Activities

1. Mr. Charles Rose was admitted to hospital yesterday for investigative procedures. He is a 32-year-old bachelor who has been working on a trapline in the north woods for the past two years. He lives alone in a remote cabin, coming into town occasionally to replenish his supplies, which consist mainly of canned and dried foods. The cabin does not have electricity or running water; it is heated by a wood stove, and Mr. Rose has to fetch his water from a stream 500 m away.

   He spends several days at a time out in the woods inspecting his lines with only his dog for company. He hit his head two or three weeks ago on a fallen tree trunk when he was straightening up after looking at a trap and he hasn't been feeling too well since. He had headaches of increasing severity, so he went to the doctor in town, who admitted him to hospital.

Mr. Rose is thin, his skin is dry and he has some lesions on his arms and legs, his long hair is matted, his nails are dirty and chipped, and his teeth and fingers are stained with nicotine. The physician has ordered bed rest.

a. What problems can you identify relative to Mr. Rose's hygiene? To the status of his skin, hair, nails and teeth?

b. What factors do you think contributed to these problems?

c. What are the expected outcomes for these problems?

d. What principles can assist you in planning hygiene measures for Mr. Rose?

e. What specific nursing interventions would you implement?

Mr. Rose's condition deteriorates over the next few days; he appears to be very weak and drowsy. The physician and a neurosurgeon who has been called in are contemplating surgery.

f. What additional nursing interventions would you plan for Mr. Rose with regard to hygiene?

g. How would you evaluate the effectiveness of your interventions?

2. Mrs. Santyl is an 87-year-old woman who has history of angina and diabetes. She has been living at home and receives homemaking services twice a week. Recently, she was admitted to the hospital with severe chest pain. Upon admission, the nurse observed a pressure ulcer on Mrs. Santyl's left heel. The wound measures 10 cm x 8 cm x 2.5 cm and presents with a foul odour, necrotic tissue and a slight amount of serous drainage. The doctor has ordered mechanical and sharp debridement.

a. What other data would you collect to document Mrs. Santyl's wound status?

b. What are predisposing factors that put Mrs. Santyl at risk for developing a pressure ulcer? Are there others you would explore with Mrs. Santyl?

c. What principles of wound healing can assist you in devising a care plan for Mrs. Santyl?

d. With whom would you collaborate to develop an effective plan of care for Mrs. Santyl?

e. What specific health-promoting and health-protecting strategies would you explore with Mrs. Santyl in response to her taking responsibility in her healing?

f. How would you prepare Mrs. Santyl for the dressing change?

g. How would you evaluate the effectiveness of your nursing interventions?

KEY TERMS

epidermis p. 977
dermis p. 977
nails p. 977
hair p. 977
dandruff p. 977
sebaceous glands p. 978
sweat glands p. 978
ceruminous glands p. 978
mouth p. 978
tongue p. 978
tooth p. 978
gingivae p. 978
necrotic p. 979
turgor p. 980
pruritis p. 985
lesions p. 985
burns p. 985
gingivitis p. 985
plaque p. 985
dental caries p. 985
sordes p. 988
venous ulcer p. 989
arterial ulcer p. 989
diabetic ulcer p. 989
malignant wound p. 989
pressure ulcer p. 989
ischemia p. 989
colonization p. 990
infection p. 990
induration p. 990
exudate p. 991
autolysis p. 991
eschar p. 991
alopecia p. 993
hirsutism p. 993
koilonychia p. 995
clubbing p. 995
paronychia p. 995
onychauxis p. 995
onychorrhexis p. 995
onycholysis p. 995
vitiligo p. 996
pallor p. 996
cyanosis p. 996
erythema p. 996
jaundice p. 996
callus p. 997
edema p. 997
pitting edema p. 997
bruising p. 997
undermining p. 998
shearing p. 1009
maceration p. 1010
pediculosis p. 1010
debridement p. 1011

References

BARKAUSAS, V.H., STOLTENBERG-ALLEN, K., BAUMANN, L.C., & DARLING-FISHER, C. (1994). *Health and physical assessment.* St. Louis: Mosby.

BATES, B. (1995). *A guide to physical examination and history taking.* (6th ed.). Philadelphia: Lippincott.

BERGER, K.J., & WILLIAMS, M.B. (1992). *Fundamentals of nursing: Collaborating for optimal health.* Norwalk, CT: Appleton & Lange.

BERGSTROM, N., BRADEN, B., LAGUZZA, A., & HOLMAN, V. (1987). The Braden scale for predicting pressure sore risk. *Nursing Research, 36*(4), 205–210.

BOYTON, P.R., & PAUSTIAN, C. (1996). Wound assessment and decision-making options. *Critical Care Nursing Clinics of North America, 8*(2), 115–139.

CANADIAN DENTAL ASSOCIATION. (circa 1994). *Gum disease.* (Pamphlet). Ottawa: Author.

CARPENITO, L.J. (1997). *Nursing diagnosis: Application to clinical practice.* (7th ed.). Philadelphia: Lippincott.

COLBURN, L. (1990). Preventing pressure sores. *Nursing 90, 20*(12), 60–63.

CONVATEC. (1992). *DuoDERM® "S.O.S" wound care: Clinical applications guide.* Princeton, NJ: E.R. Squibb & Sons. (Pamphlet 581–1136).

DAVIS, E.D. (1970). Giving a bath? *American Journal of Nursing, 70,* 2366–2367.

DE GRAFF, K.M., & FOX, S.I. (1992). *Concepts of human anatomy and physiology.* (3rd ed.). Dubuque, IA: W.C. Brown.

EBERSOLE, P., & HESS, P. (1998). *Toward healthy aging. Human needs and nursing response.* (5th ed.). St. Louis: Mosby.

[illegible] care. *Canadian Nurse, 4*(5), 31–35.

FLYNN, M.B. (1996). Wound healing and critical illness. *Critical Care Nursing Clinics of North America, 8*(2), 115–123.

FULLER, J., & SCHALLER-AYERS, J. (1994). *Health assessment: A nursing approach.* (2nd ed.). Philadelphia: Lippincott.

JARVIS, C. (1996). *Physical examination and health assessment.* (2nd ed.). Philadelphia: W.B. Saunders.

KRASNER, D. (1990). *Chronic wound care: A clinical resource for health care professionals.* Philadelphia: Health Management Publications.

LINDELL, M.E., & OLSSON, H.M. (1990). Personal hygiene in external genitalia of healthy and hospitalized elderly women. *Health Care for Women International, 11,* 151–158.

MAKLEBUST, J. (1996). Using wound care products to promote a healing environment. *Critical Care Nursing Clinics of North America, 8*(2), 141–158.

MORTON, P.A. (1993). *Health assessment in nursing.* Springhouse, PA: Springhouse.

NEY, D.F. (1993). Cerumen impaction, ear hygiene practices, and hearing acuity. *Geriatric Nursing, 14*(2), 70–73.

PILLITTERI, A. (1995). *Maternal and child health nursing: Care of the childbearing and childrearing family.* (2nd ed.). Philadelphia: Lippincott.

PORTH, C.M. (1998). *Pathophysiology: Concepts of altered health states.* (5th ed.). Philadelphia: Lippincott.

PROVO, B., PIACENTINE, L., & DEAN-BARR, S. (1997). Practice versus knowledge when it comes to pressure ulcer prevention. *Journal of Wound, Ostomy & Continence Nursing, 24*(5), 265–269.

RAVNSKOV, U. (1984, May). Soap is the major cause of dysuria. *Lancet,* 1027–1028.

RICHARDSON, E. (1990). The Cambodians and Laotians. In N. Waxler-Morrison, J. Anderson & E. Richardson (Eds.), *Cross-cultural caring: A handbook for health professionals in western Canada.* Vancouver, BC: University of British Columbia Press.

SKEWES, S.M. (1997). Bathing: It's a tough job. *Journal of Gerontological Nursing, 23*(5), 45–49.

SMITH & NEPHEW (1992). Differential Diagnosis—Leg Ulcer (pamphlet) #6400153.

STOTTS, N. (1990). Seeing red and yellow and black: Three-colour concept of wound care. *Nursing 90, 20*(2), 59–61.

THOMAS, C.L. (Ed.). (1997). *Taber cyclopedic medical dictionary.* (13th ed.). Philadelphia: F.A. Davis.

THOMPSON, J.M., & WILSON, S.F. (1996). *Health assessment for nursing practice.* St. Louis: Mosby.

U.S. DEPARTMENT OF HEALTH & HUMAN SERVICES, PUBLIC HEALTH SERVICE, AGENCY FOR HEALTH CARE POLICY & RESEARCH. (1992). *Clinical practice guidelines on pressure ulcers in adults: Prediction and prevention.* No. 3. Rockville, MD: Authors. (AHPCPR Publication no. 92-0047)

U.S. DEPARTMENT OF HEALTH & HUMAN SERVICES, PUBLIC HEALTH SERVICE, AGENCY FOR HEALTH CARE POLICY & RESEARCH. (1994). *Clinical practice guidelines on treatment of pressure ulcers.* No. 15. Rockville, MD: Authors. (AHPCPR Publication no. 95-0652)

WARNER, L.A. (1986). Lemon-glycerine swabs should not be used for routine oral care. *Critical Care Nurse, 6*(6), 82–83.

WONG, D.L. (1995). *Whaley and Wong's nursing care of infants and children.* (5th ed.). St. Louis: Mosby.

WONG, D.L., BRANTLY, D., CLUTTER, L., DE SIMONE, D., LAMMERT, D., NIX, K., PERRY, K., SMITH, D., & WHITE, K. (1992). Diapering choices: A critical review of the issues. *Pediatric Nursing, 18*(1), 41–54.

WORLD HEALTH ORGANIZATION (WHO). (1988). *Manual for infection control in health facilities.* New Delhi: WHO Regional Office for South East Asia. (Catalogue SEARO—Regional Health Papers no. 18)

Additional Readings

AYELLO, E.A. (1996). Keeping pressure ulcers in check. *Nursing, 26*(10), 62–63.

[illegible] & MORRIS, J.N. (1995). Pressure ulcers: The minimum data set and the resident assessment protocol. *Advances in Wound Care, 8*(6), 18–25.

DRACUP, K. (1996). Putting clinical practice guidelines to work. *Nursing, 26*(2), 41–47.

DWYER, F.M., & KEELER, D. (1997). Protocols for wound management. *Nursing Management, 28*(7), 45–50.

ENNIS, W.J. & MENESES, P. (1997). Pressure ulcers: A public health problem, an integrated hospital's solution. *Dermatology Nursing, 9*(1), 25–31.

FRANTZ, R.A. (1997). Measuring prevalence and incidence of pressure ulcers. *Advances in Wound Care,* 10(1), 21–24.

GREIFZU, S., RADJESKI, D., & WINNICK, B. (1990). Oral care is part of cancer care. *RN, 53*(6), 42–46.

GROUS, C.A., REILLY, N.J., & GIFT, A.G. (1997). Skin integrity in patients undergoing prolonged operations. *Journal of Wound, Ostomy & Continence Nursing, 24*(2), 86–91.

HANSON, D.S., LANGEMO, D., OLSON, B., HUNTER, S., & BURD, C. (1996). Decreasing the prevalence of pressure ulcers using agency standards. *Home Healthcare Nursing, 14*(7), 525–531.

HARDING, K.G. (1990). Wound care: Putting theory into clinical practice. *Wounds: A Compendium of Clinical Research and Practice, 2*(1), 21–31.

HARRISON, M.B., WELLS, G., FISHER, A., & PRINCE, M. (1996). Practice guidelines for the prediction and prevention of pressure ulcers. Evaluating the evidence. *Applied Nursing Research, 9*(1), 9–17.

HIMES, D. (1997). Nutritional supplements in the treatment of pressure ulcers: Practical perspectives. *Advances in Wound Care, 10*(1), 31–31.

HOFFMAN, R.G., PASE, M.N., & Van LEEUWEN, D.M. (1996). Use and perceived effectiveness of pressure ulcer treatments in extended care facilities. *Advances in Wound Care, 9*(4), 43–47.

KOZIEROWSKI, L. (1996). Treatment of sacral pressure ulcers in an adolescent with Hodgkin's disease. *Journal of Wound, Ostomy & Continence Nursing, 23*(5), 244–247.

LYDER, C.H. (1996). Examining the inclusion of ethnic minorities in pressure ulcer prediction studies. *Journal of Wound, Ostomy & Continence Nursing, 23*(5), 257–260.

MAKLEBUST, J., & SIEGGREEN, M.Y. (1996). How to conquer pressure ulcers. *Nursing, 26*(12), 34–39.

MAKLEBUST, J., & SIEGGREEN, M.Y. (1996). Managing leg ulcers. *Nursing, 26*(12), 41–46.

MURPHY, K.M., & MUSIAK, H. (1997). Options in practice. Patients with occipital pressure ulcer requiring continued cervical collar use. *Journal of Wound, Ostomy & Continence Nursing, 24*(1), 58–60.

OLSON, B., LANGEMO, D., BURD, C., HANSON, S., & CATHCART-SILBERBER, T. (1996). Pressure ulcer incidence in an acute care setting. *Journal of Wound, Ostomy & Continence Nursing, 23*(1), 15–22.

ROBINSON, S.M. (1996). Advancing home care nursing practice with an ET clinical nurse specialist. *Home Healthcare Nurse, 14*(4), 269–274.

STRAUSS, E.A., & MARGOLIS, D.J. (1996). Malnutrition in patients with pressure ulcers: Morbidity, mortality and clinically practical assessments. *Advances in Wound Care, 9*(5, pt 1), 37–40.

VANDEN BOSCH, T., MONTOYE, C., SATWICZ, M., & DURKEE-LEONARD, K. (1996). Predictive validity of the Braden Scale and nurse perception in identifying pressure ulcer risk. *Applied Nursing Research, 9*(2), 80–86.

WHITTLE, H., FLETCHER, C., HOSKING, A., & CAMPBELL, K. (1996). Nursing management of pressure ulcers using a hydrogel dressing protocol: Four case studies. *Rehabilitation Nursing, 21*(5), 239–243, 284.

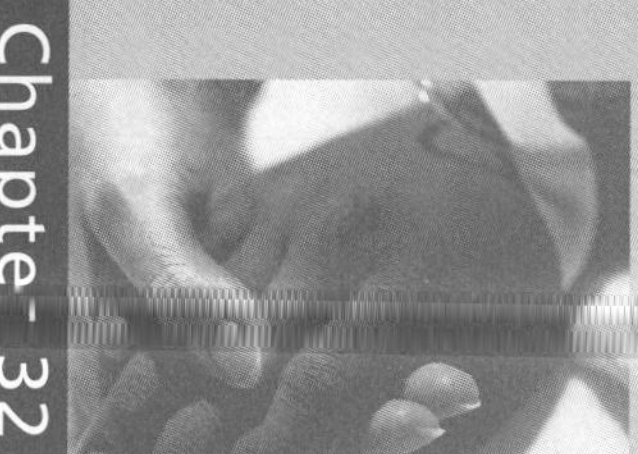

Chapter 32

Prevention and Control of Infection

OUTLINE

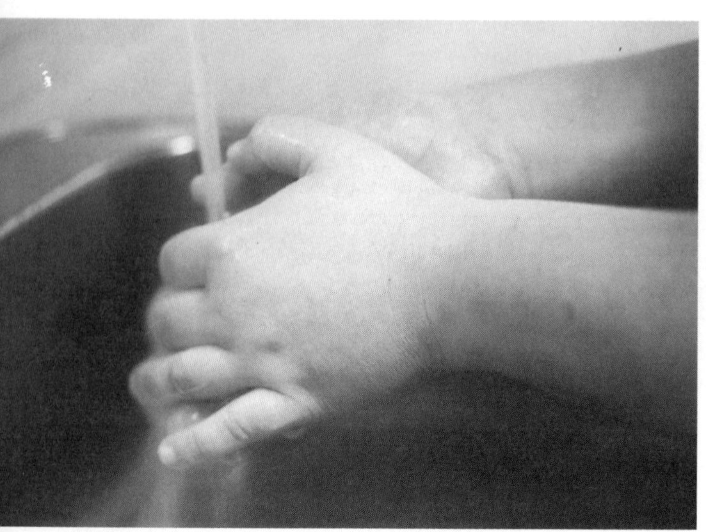

Central Questions

1. Why is the prevention and control of infection important to health?
2. What is the chain of infection, and how does it relate to the infectious process?
3. What are some of the common pathogens that infect people, and how are pathogens spread?
4. What are the major responses of the body to infection?
5. What factors determine the body's response to infectious agents?
6. How do infection prevention and control needs vary throughout the life cycle?
7. What age groups are the most susceptible to infection and why?
8. What are five of the most common infections?
9. What basic principles does the nurse apply in assisting individuals with the control and prevention of infection?
10. How does the nurse assess infection prevention and control needs?
11. What are the common nursing diagnostic statements for patients with infection-related problems?
12. How does the nurse develop a plan of care for patients with infection-related problems?
13. What strategies does the nurse implement in helping individuals, families or groups promote healthy infection control practices?
14. What health-protecting measures does the nurse implement to maintain infection control and to prevent the spread of infection from one person to another?
15. What health-restoring and supportive strategies does the nurse implement in the care of patients with infection-related problems?
16. How does the nurse evaluate the patient's response to nursing interventions?

Introduction

Infectious diseases have plagued humans throughout the

measures to control infection have been developed. One of the principal reasons for the dramatic reduction in infant and child mortality, and the consequent lengthening of the life span in developed countries (and increasingly in developing countries), has been the implementation of infection control programs. The following factors have contributed to this achievement:

- the development and widespread use of specific immunizations against many of the common communicable diseases
- the discovery and widespread use of antimicrobial agents (antibiotics)
- the application of basic sanitary measures to protect the safety of water, milk and food supplies and to ensure the safe disposal of garbage and sewage
- the overall increases in standard of living, with the resulting improvement in the general health of people (from such factors as better nutrition and better housing).

While significant gains have been made in controlling infectious diseases, we have by no means eliminated all illnesses caused by infections. Respiratory infections continue to be a leading cause of death and acute illness throughout the life span. Gastrointestinal infections are one of the most common causes of short-term illness. Sexually transmitted diseases (STDs) have attained epidemic proportions in the past few years, and such diseases as chickenpox and viral hepatitis remain prevalent. AIDS (acquired immune deficiency syndrome), which is caused by the human-immunodeficiency virus (HIV), appeared in the late 1970s and early 1980s. AIDS is a life-threatening disease that suppresses the body's immune system and renders it unable to fight infections. Infection is found worldwide, but sociodemographic factors determine the prevalence of disease in a given population. Institution-acquired infections (called **nosocomial infections**) continue to plague hospitals throughout the world and represent significant concerns regarding morbidity, mortality and cost.

The prevention and control of infection is a primary goal of all health professionals, whether in ambulatory care settings, the community or in inpatient facilities. Infections are caused by microorganisms. Wherever there are sick people, microorganisms that are capable of producing infection pose a constant and serious threat to well-being. Many patients are highly susceptible to infection owing to a number of risk factors, such as underlying disease, altered immune status, the extremes of age, poor nutrition, invasive procedures, drug therapy and irradiation. This is especially true in tertiary care hospitals. It is in fact ironic that medical science is increasingly able to support patients through life-threatening illness or injury that would have been fatal only a few years ago, and yet the risks of infectious complications are rising markedly. The proximity of patients to

infection, as does the intimate contact required when giving care.

Microorganisms are everywhere around us. They are found on our bodies, inside our bodies, in the air, on horizontal surfaces such as floors, table tops and counters, on equipment and furniture and, to a lesser extent, on walls and ceilings. Most microorganisms do not constitute a great threat to a healthy person, but there are a few pathogens that always have the potential to cause infectious disease.

Microorganisms are spread mainly by contact, through the air, by ingesting contaminated food and water and by carriers such as mosquitoes, flies and birds. Health professionals sometimes unknowingly act as carriers of pathogens, creating a potential risk to themselves or to co-workers and an even greater risk to patients. When hand-washing techniques break down, microorganisms are passed on to others. In spite of careful cleaning practices, microorganisms cannot be totally eliminated from the environment. Sometimes an organism highly capable of producing disease may be present and a worker with an open cut or lowered body resistance becomes infected. Workers primarily face the risk of blood-borne diseases such as hepatitis B or C and HIV; patients may be at greater risk for acquiring infections from their own endogenous flora, which gain entrance through an invasive procedure such as the insertion of a urinary catheter, a vascular catheter or surgery. People are increasingly vulnerable to common microorganisms that have developed resistance to previously reliable and usually tolerable antibiotics. The issue of multiple-resistant microorganisms is a growing threat to patients and a sometimes frustrating challenge for infection control. Multiple-drug resistant microorganisms will be one of the more significant infection control issues as we enter the 21st century.

In order to understand the rationale behind nursing measures taken to protect patients and staff from infections, it is important to keep in mind the sources, methods of transfer and modes of spread of microorganisms. Knowledge about the infectious process and the body's responses to it, as well as about specific communicable diseases, will be gained in microbiology, anatomy and physiology courses. Nursing interventions for specific infectious health problems, such as care for persons with AIDS or pneumonia, will be learned in more advanced nursing courses. In this chapter, we will review the history of infectious diseases, briefly describe the infectious process and the body's response to it, and outline common infectious problems in order to provide a framework for understanding the nursing care of individuals with existing or potential problems of infections. Measures to prevent and control the spread of infection, namely immunization, medical and surgical asepsis, as well as the use of universal and body substance precautions, are also outlined.

Historical Perspective

Infectious disease has been cited as the leading cause of morbidity and mortality throughout the world (Hoeprich, 1972). Hospital-acquired infections account for half of all infectious diseases seen in the Western world (Barrett-Connor, 1978). That figure, which is still largely undefined, is even higher in developing countries (Wenzel, 1997). But the people of the Western world were in a similar, perhaps even worse, situation just over a century ago. From earliest times, an aura of mysticism and helplessness pervaded communities when their members were stricken with illness. Faced with what was thought to have been divine anger, witchcraft or the work of demons, early peoples resorted to ritual, incantation and noxious potions as cures. Eventually a rudimentary awareness of the need to isolate infected people developed, but the real causes of disease continued to be elusive. Lepers in biblical times were considered "unclean" and were required to announce their presence when approaching a city or a group of people. Some travellers were kept in huts outside cities for 40 days under observation for evidence of contagion, while sailors entering port were required to remain on board for 40 days. If no one became ill, they could all go ashore. (*Quarantine* comes from the Italian "quaranta giorni" meaning 40 days).

The Black Death, or bubonic plague (caused by the bacterium *Yersinia pestis*), decimated the population of medieval Europe. The plague doctor who went from door to door looking for victims of the dreaded disease wore an outfit that has interesting parallels today. A long hooded gown covered his entire body. On top of the hood he wore a large brimmed hat. A mask that covered his face was equipped with round glass lenses that allowed him to peer out. Attached to the mask was a beak-like projection about 18 cm long. The beak contained pungent herbs and strong-smelling spices. In the 14th century the population of Europe was 105 million. In the four years between 1346 and 1350, 25 million persons died of plague (LaForce, 1997). Remote though it seems now, the Black Death remains the most virulent epidemic in human history.

The Christian church in Europe has a history of caring for the sick and the poor. However, as they believed care of the soul to be of much greater importance than care of the body, washing and general care thereof was opposed. Nevertheless, a 16th-century Italian by the name of Girolamo Fracastora suggested that disease spread from person to person via clothes or other possessions (fomites) or through the air. The scientific knowledge was not available at the time to prove this assumption. However, in 1678, Anton Van Leeuwenhoek, a Dutch merchant, whose hobby was microscopy, took scrapings from his teeth and observed them under the glass lenses he had ground himself by hand. There he observed small creatures believed to be various bacteria and protozoa, which he referred to as his little animalcules. It was Louis Pasteur who in 1855 established the relationship between microorganisms and the occurrence of disease. In 1876 Robert Koch outlined the steps, known as Koch's postulates (shown in the box above), which lead to the production of disease. Koch's postulates are of historical importance. However, as we have acquired more knowledge about disease causation, it has become obvious that these postulates cannot always be realized.

Koch's Postulates

1. The microorganism is found in a high proportion of hosts (human or animal) with disease, but not normally in healthy hosts.
2. The microorganism is isolated and propagated serially in pure culture in the laboratory.
3. The microorganism in pure culture induces a comparable disease in susceptible hosts and can be isolated from these hosts.

SOURCE: McLean & Smith, 1991.

The Hungarian physician, Ignasz Semmelweis, promoted hand-washing as a result of his observations when working at the Allgemeines Krankenhaus (lying-in hospital) in Vienna in 1847. While his findings were recognized far afield, his colleagues in Vienna ridiculed him. Ironically, he died of septicemia in a mental institution in 1865 without the recognition he deserved.

Fairly recently, in 1965, Professor Sydney Selwyn in England uncovered the virtually unknown work of Sir John Pringle who, in the 1740s, was a professor at Edinburgh University and a physician to the British army. He insisted that uncrowded wards and adequate ventilation helped stop the spread of disease. He seems to have been ignored (Selwyn, 1991). Not quite a century later, Florence Nightingale, after observing appalling conditions in the Crimea, returned home to England. Working with William Farr, a noted British health statistician, she prevailed against a hostile military bureaucracy and an indifferent government to show that the mortality rate in British army hospitals could be significantly reduced by improving hygienic practice, avoiding overcrowding and developing a standardized reporting system for army deaths. It has often been pointed out that Nightingale eschewed the germ theory of disease and did not believe the findings of Koch and Pasteur. However, she did appreciate the importance of a clean environment. In her book, *Notes on Hospitals*, she clearly stated that there was a direct relationship between the sanitary conditions of a hospital and postoperative complications due to infectious disease. The type of wards she advocated had high ceilings and adequate space between beds, were well ventilated and were kept clean (Nightingale, 1861).

There were at least three cholera outbreaks in England in the first half of the 19th century. Dr. John Snow observed that all those who became ill obtained drinking water from the same pump. He persuaded authorities to remove the handle, preventing use. It was later discovered that the well was contaminated with raw sewage.

In Glasgow in the 1860s, Joseph Lister (later Lord Lister), who had studied Pasteur's work, decided to try using an antiseptic to dress and pack wounds. He went on to soak [illegible] acid solution prior to surgery. With this approach he demonstrated a dramatic drop in surgical wound infections and became known as the father of antiseptic surgery. Eventually, William Halsted, a U.S. surgeon, introduced the concept of rubber gloves, first to protect the nurse and then to protect the patient. Also around the turn of the century in U.S. hospitals, gowns and masks began to be used for surgery, and the concept of asepsis through sterilization of supplies and equipment was well established by 1910.

However, highly communicable diseases continued to be a source of fear and concern. During the Middle Ages, leprosaria (hospitals for lepers) were common. (We know today, however, that leprosy is *not* a highly contagious disease and requires close prolonged contact for transmission of the pathogen to occur.) Lazarettos were built to confine plague victims, and in the 19th century a large number of infectious disease hospitals were established. Sometimes called fever hospitals, they were used to house those with smallpox and a variety of other communicable diseases. Smallpox had been a dreaded disease for centuries. It decimated populations, sometimes all but wiping out whole communities. Because military personnel became infected very readily due to crowded living conditions, it influenced the outcomes of wars. About 30 percent of children born in 18th-century England died of smallpox before they reached maturity (Parker, 1990). When introduced by Europeans to the native populations of North America, who had never encountered the disease before, smallpox had a devastating effect and was largely responsible for reducing the population to one-tenth of what it had been before contact.

In 1796, Sir Edward Jenner discovered that a person who had had cowpox developed lifelong immunity to smallpox. He observed that the virus causing cowpox was immunologically related to smallpox and that the body could be fooled into producing effective antibodies to smallpox. These observations led Jenner to develop the first vaccine (*vacca* is Latin for cow). He subsequently published his findings, and vaccination was gradually made available to all. Gradually, other vaccines were developed, including pertussis, diphtheria and polio. Today we also have routine immunization for measles, mumps, rubella and *Haemophilus influenzae*, with others being given according to the requirements of the individual. The antibiotic era dawned with the discovery of penicillin in 1928 and the introduction of sulfonamides in 1935. The antibiotic armamentarium is now quite impressive but not without its drawbacks owing to unfortunate side effects, expense and bacterial resistance.

Despite these advances, infectious disease hospitals, leprosaria and tuberculosis (TB) sanatoria continued to be used past the middle of the 20th century. The last surviving Canadian leper who had lived and worked much of his life with his fellows in a leper colony on Bentinck Island off Vancouver Island died in 1956. It was only then that the colony was formally shut down by the [illegible] in places such as Tranquille near Kamloops, British Columbia and Fort San near Fort Qu'Appelle in Saskatchewan. At Vancouver General Hospital, the infectious disease hospital was closed as recently as 1983. Those who practised in the field of infection control had long been advocating the use of decentralized isolation that is done today.

Slowly, over the centuries we have seen the gradual understanding of the role of microorganisms in our environment, how they can cause disease and how disease can be prevented. We now know that certain basic hygienic measures can help ensure a safe community. These include a clean supply of drinking water, clean food and sanitary disposal of sewage. We also know that there are basic measures of hygiene that anyone can practise to help control the spread of infection, such as hand-washing and safe disposal of body secretions and excretions.

Today, we also know enough about our relationship with microorganisms to make informed decisions about our own health and how to care for others so as to prevent the spread of disease. New diseases may arise to challenge us, such as HIV, while old diseases such as tuberculosis or *Staphylococcus aureus* may renew their imperative to survive and multiply by developing resistance to antibiotics that were previously effective. Whatever challenges we meet, it is important to remember the lessons we have learned and to apply that knowledge, understanding and wisdom.

The Infectious Process

Infection is the deposition or invasion and multiplication of microorganisms on surfaces of the body or in body tissues causing adverse or ill effects. Such adverse effects are always assumed in the definition. The disease-producing agent is referred to as a **pathogen**. In certain circumstances, any microorganism may cause disease, even those with which we usually enjoy a **symbiotic** (mutually beneficial) **relationship.** This is especially true of people who are **immunocompromised,** that is, people whose immune system is impaired. Fortunately, only two to three percent of all microorganisms are considered to be true human pathogens. In other circumstances, people may acquire a pathogen, for example, hepatitis B, but never experience any adverse or ill effects. These people become **carriers** of that pathogen and, while they remain symptom-free, they are capable of passing the disease to someone else who can get sick from it. Microorganisms with which we enjoy a symbiotic relationship—which are the vast majority of microorganisms on and in our bodies—are called **commensals**.

The Chain of Infection

An infection does not necessarily begin because a pathogen is present in the environment. Infection is the result of a number of interrelated factors that follow sequentially one after another in a cycle, commonly referred to as the chain of infection. It is best visualized as a chain with its various links (see Figure 32.1). There must first of all be an infectious or *causative agent*. The agent must have a place *(reservoir)* in which it grows and multiplies. It leaves the reservoir, now referred to as a *source*, by an exit route *(portal of exit)* and uses a means of travel (vehicle) or a *mode of transmission*. By using this vehicle, it gains entrance through a *portal of entry* to the body of a susceptible human being, who then becomes its *host* and constitutes a potential reservoir to start the cycle again. It is important to understand the various features of all the links in the chain, as well as other terms used to define infection.

CAUSATIVE AGENTS

The chain of infection begins with an infectious agent capable of causing disease in humans. Causative agents may be bacteria, viruses, fungi, protozoa or helminths (worms) that normally inhabit or have recently entered the body or attached to the skin. **Pathogenic bacteria** are microorganisms capable of invading healthy tissue and causing injury to the body or body part. An example is *Salmonella*, which invades the mucosal surface of the bowel, causing an acute form of gastroenteritis. Other bacteria may invade body tissue when given the opportunity and when present in sufficient numbers. These include, for example, some of the streptococci and staphylococci, which can cause wound and other soft tissue infections. Some bacteria do not invade body tissue but produce toxins that produce disease; *Clostridium* (*C.*) *tetani*, for example, is the causative agent of tetanus, which may cause paralysis and muscle spasm. Some microorganisms, such as *Salmonella*, can cause disease in more than one way, for instance, by inducing local inflammation and producing toxins. Another example is *Staphylococcus* (*S.*) *aureus*, which may invade tissue, spread systemically or produce a toxin in the gastrointestinal tract that in turn acts on the vomiting centre in the brain to cause vomiting, eventual dehydration and, possibly, even cardiac failure.

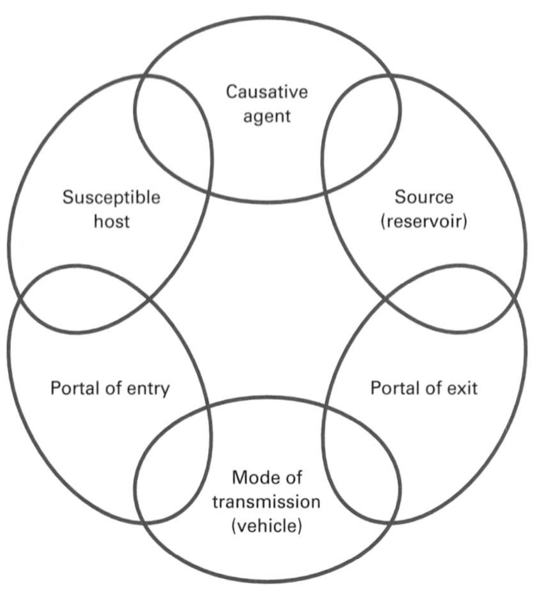

FIGURE 32.1 Chain of infection

Many of the common communicable diseases are viral infections (measles, mumps, chickenpox) that usually occur in children. Diseases in the viral hepatitides group, HIV, influenza and the common cold are all viral infections. Fungal infections include those caused by yeasts and moulds, such as ringworm and athlete's foot. In hospitals, fungal infections most frequently include thrush in newborns (caused by *Candida*) or candidiasis of the esophagus, which is often seen in the immunocompromised patient and may develop into a potentially fatal systemic disease. Another disease seen in the immunocompromised patient is aspergillosis, usually in the form of pneumonia.

Protozoa are single-celled animals that can behave pathogenically. An example is *Entamoeba histolytica*, which causes the intestinal infection of amebiasis, characterized by colicky abdominal pain, frequent bloody stools and, possibly, liver tenderness. Hemorrhage may occur in rare cases. Another example is the protozoan *Giardia lamblia*, which causes an enteric disease called giardiasis, popularly known as beaver fever, since the parasite spends part of its life cycle in water-loving animals such as beavers. Infected people may be asymptomatic, have only mild diarrhea or have watery diarrhea with epigastric tenderness, flatulence, malaise or nausea.

The helminths are common parasites in humans, for example, the pinworms often found in children. In Canada, patients admitted to hospital who have worm infestations most frequently have acquired them from other parts of the world, and since these particular parasites generally do not survive in our temperate climate, there is little risk to others. There is, however, the very rare exception of acquiring *Strongyloides* from skin contact with an infected person who has acquired it in the tropics. Wild meat (game) should always be well cooked to ensure that one does not ingest parasites that the animal has acquired.

It is important to remember that **microbial flora**, which include bacteria, viruses, fungi, protozoa and helminths, are an integral part of our world. They colonize the animate and inanimate environment. They are on and in parts of the body that communicate with the exterior, such as the gastrointestinal tract. The presence of microorganisms in the areas where nature has placed them constitutes a delicate balance that generally sustains us in good health by not leaving room for "foreign" bacteria to gain a foothold. Infections do occur, either when that delicate balance has been upset or when a break in the integument allows invaders to enter. These infections may be either exogenous or endogenous in origin. **Exogenous infections** are those acquired [illegible] are those arising from one's own microbial flora. Colonization may be either transient or permanent, but must always occur before an infection develops (Brachman, 1998).

RESERVOIR OR SOURCE

A reservoir is the agent's natural habitat for growth and multiplication. The most common reservoir for human infectious pathogens is the human body itself. Other reservoirs may include animals, birds, plants, soil and arthropods, such as mosquitoes, fleas, ticks and lice.

PORTAL OF EXIT

The portal of exit is the primary route by which organisms leave their source. Common exit routes in humans include the body systems such as the respiratory, urinary, gastrointestinal and reproductive tracts, as well as breaks in skin and mucous membranes, discharges from wounds and, especially, blood.

MODES OF TRANSMISSION

An infectious agent may be transmitted from its reservoir to a host by a number of routes. Some agents can be transmitted by more than one route or mode.

Contact Transmission

An organism may be transmitted by direct or indirect contact. Direct contact involves physical transfer from the source of infection to the susceptible host. Touching wound drainage from a patient or kissing or engaging in sexual activity with an infected individual are examples of direct contact. Indirect contact involves contact with an intermediate object that has become contaminated from either an animate or inanimate source. For example, infection can be transferred by touching a contaminated bed rail or using a diagnostic instrument that was not properly disinfected after use on a patient. Inanimate objects that carry infectious agents are referred to as **fomites.** Another form of indirect contact is by droplet spread, in which infectious agents are propelled through the air in droplets by coughing, sneezing or even speaking, travelling only a metre before landing on an inanimate surface or on a susceptible host. For example, droplet spread occurs when someone's mucous membrane comes in contact with measles virus or a *Streptococcus* that can cause pharyngitis. Contact spread is by far the most common cause of nosocomial disease transmission and is potentially the easiest to interrupt.

Common Vehicle Transmission

Common vehicle spread is a mode of transmission in which a contaminated inanimate vehicle serves as a source of infection to multiple people. Examples of transmission include *Salmonella* in foods that have become contaminated by an infected food handler or hepatitis A [illegible] contaminated blood. A blood donation from someone with hepatitis C or HIV may be fractionated, resulting in a number of people becoming infected from one person's blood. With blood screening now routine, this is rare but not impossible.

Airborne Transmission

Airborne transmission refers to the spread of microbes through the air. Organisms may be contained within droplet nuclei, dust particles or on skin squames. Droplet nuclei occur when moisture evaporates from droplets. These droplet nuclei, which are five micrometres or less in size, may then become suspended in air, remain there for a long time and travel long distances. Thus, true airborne spread by droplet nuclei is distinguished from spread by indirect contact through droplets that are large and travel only a metre through the air. Two of the most common examples of diseases transmitted by droplet nuclei are tuberculosis and chickenpox.

While dust particles will gravitate to horizontal surfaces, they can be readily resuspended by physical activity and serve as a means of transfer for many microorganisms, although this does not necessarily mean that infection will ensue. All of us shed skin squames on an ongoing basis. These dead epithelial cells carry with them the microbial flora associated with the parts of the body from which they were shed. Outbreaks most commonly associated with shedding skin squames include staphylococcal and streptococcal infections. However, spread of these microorganisms by airborne transmission must be kept in perspective; contact spread is much more likely to occur, as is endogenous acquisition of infection from one's own staphylococci or streptococci. Infectious aerosols are not created easily, and people with rapidly desquamating skin conditions are not admitted to hospital as frequently as in the past.

Vector-Borne Transmission

Vectors include animals, insects and birds that carry infection from a source to a host. For example, flies carry *Salmonella*, the anopheles mosquito carries protozoa that cause malaria and ticks carry *Rickettsia rickettsii*, the organisms responsible for Rocky Mountain spotted fever (tick-borne typhus fever).

PORTALS OF ENTRY

Portals of entry are generally the same as portals of exit. Infectious agents gain access to the body via the respiratory, urinary and gastrointestinal tracts, mucous membranes, nonintact skin and percutaneously (for example, by needlestick or blood transfusion).

HOST

The host is the final link in the chain, and becomes in turn a new reservoir and a potential source of infection. **Susceptibility** refers to the degree of resistance of a host to a pathogen. If people are susceptible to the pathogen—that is, if their resistance is weakened—they are more likely to develop an infection. Susceptibility may also be stated as the degree of vulnerability to a microorganism.

For disease transmission to occur, a potential pathogen must be present in sufficient quantities and with sufficient virulence. **Pathogenicity** is the ability of the organism to cause disease. **Virulence** refers to the power of an organism's ability to cause disease. The pathogen must be able to leave its source, acquire a mode of transmission and gain entry into the tissues of a susceptible host. All these factors must be present simultaneously for disease transmission to occur. The acquisition and multiplication of a microorganism (pathogen or commensal) is referred to as *colonization*. The period leading up to disease manifestation is **incubation**, and infection is the destructive pathological process that ensues.

The Body's Response to Infectious Agents

Humans are equipped with various mechanisms that help to prevent the invasion of body tissues by infectious agents and to control their growth and multiplication in the body if they get past the first lines of defence. However, it should be noted that the quality and quantity of these defences may vary greatly from one person to another. They may be divided into two major categories: nonspecific defence mechanisms and specific defence mechanisms.

NONSPECIFIC DEFENCE MECHANISMS

Nonspecific defence mechanisms include the skin, the mucous membranes and some body secretions. Intact skin and mucous membranes form a barrier that cannot (with very few exceptions) be penetrated by microorganisms. The skin and mucous membranes are considered to be the body's first line of defence. Skin and mucous membrane secretions also have antibacterial activity, sometimes combined with mechanical action. Tears, for example, contain an antibacterial enzyme and, at the same time, mechanically wash away bacteria and other debris. In the nose and upper respiratory tract, mucous serves to entrap infectious agents, while cilia sweep out debris and microorganisms. In the lower respiratory tract, which should remain sterile, tissue macrophages (large phagocytic cells) mobilize to engulf and destroy unwanted invaders. Acid in the gastrointestinal tract acts against enteric organisms, and peristalsis moves ingested products through the gastrointestinal tract, reducing the time that organisms have to multiply and (or invade mucosa). Additionally, acid secretions of the genitourinary tract help to ward off pathogens.

Should a microorganism, through injury or deliberate therapeutic intervention, bypass these outer defences by transecting skin or mucous membrane, a local inflammatory response provides another nonspecific host defence mechanism. The **local inflammatory response** is a readily observable phenomenon with which nurses must become familiar in their day-to-day care of patients. The four classic symptoms of inflammation are *dolor* (pain), *rubor* (redness), *tumour* (swelling) and *calor* (heat). Loss of function may also occur. In all but neutropenic patients the white blood cell **(leukocyte)** count will be elevated. The presence of pus (purulence) confirms the presence of infection. It should be noted that, as neutropenic patients do not have sufficient white blood cells to respond to the microbial invaders, the classic signs and symptoms of infection may be muted or absent.

In **acute inflammation** (which is not always due to infection) the initial response is vasodilation, which causes the redness. Fluid is lost from cells into tissue, causing edema (swelling). Leukocytes, mostly neutrophils, collect in the tissues. Acute inflammation then will be manifested by a cellulitis that diffuses through adjacent tissues. The suffix "itis" is added to a word to indicate inflammation, for example, cellulitis, appendicitis, pharyngitis. The cellulitis may spread via the lymphatic system (lymphangitis) and is seen as red lines extending from the infected area towards the lymph nodes, which become tender and enlarged, causing lymphadenitis.

When pus is evident, the wound is **suppurating**. Pus is the debris that accumulates as a result of the encounter between microbe and neutrophil (granular leukocyte). Tissue necrosis may be present. Should the area become walled off with fibrous connective tissue, an abscess will form. If the abscess consists of pockets or subdivisions, it is referred to as a loculated abscess.

Once someone has been exposed to a significant amount of an infecting agent and the host response does not overpower the invader, the period of *incubation* ensues. This period of time varies from one situation to another. During this interval the host enters the **symptomatic period**, when signs and symptoms of infection are present.

However, in some situations, the infection may be described as inapparent or **asymptomatic**. This happens in the absence of signs or symptoms of infection. In these cases, infection may be demonstrated by laboratory test results, for example, a rise in antibody titre. Inapparent infection also occurs during the carrier state, in which an infectious agent may be present without signs and symptoms of infection. It may be part of the incubation period, or it may follow a recovery from infection. Inapparent infection represents a potential source of infection to others.

SPECIFIC DEFENCE MECHANISMS

A *specific defence mechanism* refers to an immunity that may be either naturally acquired or artificially induced. **Natural immunity** occurs from having had certain diseases such as measles or chickenpox. This contact evokes an antigen–antibody response in which antibodies specific to the disease are formed. These antibodies circulate in the blood and have the ability to recognize the same agent on subsequent encounters. Such immunity [illegible] apparent infection. Some diseases, most notably those in the herpes group of viruses, may manifest themselves again when natural immunity against the retained (and now resident) virus falters. Two of the most frequently seen examples of this phenomenon include the appearance of shingles in a patient who previously has had chickenpox, and the recurrence of herpes virus infections.

Artificial immunity can be active or passive. **Active artificial immunity** is conferred by vaccines. Vaccines may be attenuated during the manufacturing process; that is, the causative agent is weakened to the point of still being able to provoke an antibody response, yet is unable to cause disease. "Killed vaccines" (vaccines prepared from dead microorganisms) are also produced. These are still able to evoke a satisfactory antigen–antibody response. In some instances when the infectious agent produces a toxin that is responsible for disease, a toxoid or antitoxin must be given to ameliorate the effects of the toxin. While active artificial immunity is often lifelong, there are a few diseases for which a booster may be recommended. Pertinent information is readily available through public health agencies.

Passive artificial immunity results from antibodies that are passed from the mother to the fetus through the placenta or to the newborn in the first few weeks of life through ingestion of breast milk. Passive artificial immunity also results from giving immune serum globulin (serum that contains antibodies) to those thought to have been exposed to a specific disease. However, while protection from disease may be conferred with passive artificial immunity, the protection is short-lived, usually no longer than a few weeks to a few months at most.

OTHER RESPONSES OF THE BODY TO INFECTION

The body has both a generalized reaction to stress and a localized reaction that occurs at the site of stress. The early general reaction of the body to the stress of invasion by infectious agents is the same as the "just feeling sick" phenomenon described by Selye (see Chapter 9). This usually includes headache, malaise, a feeling of tiredness, slight elevation in temperature and loss of appetite (sometimes followed by nausea and vomiting). In response to infectious agents, there may be a swelling of the lymph nodes as well.

Determinants of the Body's Response to Infectious Agents

The response of the body (host) to a microbial invader may range from inapparent infection, where there are no observable signs and symptoms, to clinical signs and symptoms of varying degree, to acute fulminating disease [illegible] including agent characteristics and host susceptibility. The inoculum or dose of the infecting organism, its predilection for a particular body site (for instance, hepatitis in the liver or meningococcus in the meninges), its pathogenicity (ability to cause disease) and its virulence (strength), invasiveness and portal of entry, all influence the host response. In the host itself, the quality and quantity of both nonspecific and specific defence mechanisms and the degree of resistance to infection also help determine the onset, spectrum and course of disease. Thus, the same microbial agent may produce a varying degree of illness in different people, in different body sites and at different times of life.

The state of physical, mental and emotional health affects the susceptibility to infection. Proper nutrition, regular exercise, sufficient rest and sleep, emotional well-being, absence of stress and good hygiene practices all contribute to increasing the body's ability to fight off infections. To supplement this general type of resistance, immunization provides acquired immunity against many communicable diseases such as whooping cough, smallpox, measles, tetanus, typhoid fever and poliomyelitis.

Infants and small children are particularly vulnerable to infections, as are older adults. People who are acutely ill and those with chronic conditions are more susceptible to infection because of general debility and, often, altered nutrition patterns. A well-balanced diet with an adequate intake of protein and vitamins is necessary for the production of antibodies and the maintenance and repair of body tissues. When these nutrients are lacking in the diet, healing is impaired and the body's defence mechanisms against infection are lessened.

Poor hygiene practices, unsafe sexual conduct and the sharing of intravenous needles increase vulnerability to infection by providing a portal of entry for microbes. People with lesions or cuts in the skin or wounds of any kind (for example, the surgical patient) have an obvious entry route. Patients who have experienced trauma with excessive blood loss are particularly susceptible owing to inadequate cellular oxygenation and insufficient white blood cells with which to resist infection. Conditions in which the blood supply to a part is lessened, such as peripheral vascular disease, also increase susceptibility.

Any condition that weakens the body's natural defence mechanisms decreases resistance to microbes. Diseases of the immune system, such as leukemia and AIDS, impair the production of white bloods cells and compromise the body's defences. Radiation therapy and medications, such as anticancer drugs, suppress bone marrow function and consequently the production of white blood cells (lymphocytes) needed to fight infection. The use of anti-inflammatory drugs like adrenal corticosteroids increases infection risk by suppressing the immune system and inhibiting inflammatory response.

Stress and poor coping ability can also impair the immune system and increase susceptibility to infectious disease. As part of the body's general response to a stressor, the adrenal cortex secretes cortisone, which increases blood sugar levels and suppresses immune and inflammatory responses. If stress is prolonged, the body's natural immune system is jeopardized, glucose stores are depleted and exhaustion ensues, all of which compromise defences against infection. Additionally, when a person is fatigued or in poor physical condition from lack of exercise, susceptibility to infection is necessarily increased because the efficiency of all bodily processes, including the immune system, is reduced.

Infection Control Needs Throughout the Life Cycle

Pregnancy

Certain infections can be transmitted from the mother to the fetus *in utero* and can seriously affect the health of the fetus and newborn. The most potentially harmful infections are TORCH, HIV and genitourinary infections (Kenner & MacLaren, 1993). TORCH stands for *T*oxoplasmosis, Other infections (chlamydia, group B beta-hemolytic streptococcal, syphilis and varicella zoster), *R*ubella (German measles), *C*ytomegalovirus and *H*erpesvirus type 2 infection. This group of infections can cause congenital abnormalities in the newborn, neonatal infection and death. The human immunodeficiency virus (HIV) readily crosses the placenta and may cause AIDS in the neonate. Genitourinary infections include sexually transmitted diseases and urinary tract infections. Some of these, such as chlamydia, gonorrhea and herpes, can be transmitted to the fetus as it passes through the birth canal during birth. Women are vulnerable to urinary tract infection during pregnancy owing to urinary stasis and asymptomatic bacteriuria. If infection travels up the urinary tract to the kidneys, high fever and a severe systemic reaction may occur. Pyelonephritis has been associated with premature labour, premature rupture of the membranes and fetal loss (Pillitteri, 1995).

Protecting the fetus from infection during pregnancy is complicated because the disease may be asymptomatic in the mother, yet it may injure the fetus. Pregnant women are usually tested for syphilis and immunity to rubella. An HIV-screening test is also offered to women who are at high risk for contracting AIDS. Cervical cultures are taken to identify the presence of specific infections such as gonorrhea and chlamydia, common vaginal infections like candidiasis (yeast infection), as well as group B beta-hemolytic *Streptococcus*. Throughout pregnancy the woman must take precautions to avoid infection. If infection should occur, prompt evaluation and treatment may prevent fetal complications.

Infancy

The first year of life is the period of greatest susceptibility to infection. All newborn infants are to some degree immunologically deficient, their passive immunity being limited to IgG (immunoglobulin G) antibodies received from the mother. (Immunoglobulin G is synthesized in the body in response to bacteria, fungi and viruses that have invaded the body.) Some protection may also be afforded the breast-fed infant by specific immunoglobulin in breast milk and colostrum. Specific IgA (immunoglobulin A) antibodies may be present and become active in the infant's gastrointestinal tract. (Immunoglobulin A is found in body secretions such as saliva, mucus, tears, sweat and bile and provides defence against pathogens on exposed sufaces, especially the intestines and bronchi.) Other protective substances include lysozyme, an enzyme that breaks down bacterial walls, lactoferrin, which can be bacteriostatic for some organisms and macrophages, which can engulf and destroy bacteria. By about two months of age, many of the maternally acquired antibodies are depleted and the infant's body begins to produce its own immunoglobulins. At this point immunization is begun in order to confer artificial immunity against dangerous infections including diphtheria, pertussis, tetanus and poliomyelitis. Mumps, measles and rubella vaccine is administered at 12 months of age, since maternal antibodies for these agents have a longer life span.

Infants are particularly susceptible to infections caused by gram-negative bacteria such as *Haemophilus (H.) influenzae*, gram-positive bacteria such as group B beta-hemolytic *Streptococcus* and *S. aureus* and viruses such as varicella (chickenpox) and cytomegalovirus (Kenner & MacLaren, 1993). They are vulnerable to infections that may be present in health agencies, such as the nosocomial infections caused by *S. aureus* and to infections that may be harboured by staff, as in the case of a person with a herpes simplex eruption (cold sore). Health professionals working in newborn nurseries and pediatric units must be meticulous in their technique and make sure that they are free from infection themselves in order to protect the infants entrusted to their care.

Childhood

There has been a marked decline in the death rate from infections in children since the 1920s. Infection is now the fourth leading cause of death in children aged one to four years (King, Gartrell & Trovato, 1991). Young children succumb very easily to colds, intestinal infections and the common contagious diseases. Smaller children, of course, suffer more quickly from dehydration when they have a fever, are not eating well or are losing fluids from the gastrointestinal tract with vomiting and diarrhea. Children build up their immunity to the common pathogens in their environment upon exposure. Regular immunization boosters are usually given at age 18 months and at four to six years.

Adolescents

Adolescents are susceptible to all types of viral and bacterial

ber of cases of the childhood diseases, so that it is rare for a teenager to come down with measles, mumps or other contagious diseases. One disease that seems to attack adolescents particularly is infectious mononucleosis, a viral infection that has low communicability and is transmitted by droplet infection. A polio booster and an adult type of tetanus and diphtheria toxoid are given at 14 to 16 years of age.

Adulthood

The occurrence of viral hepatitis reaches its peak in the 30- to 39-year-old group, predominantly among males. Among young women, urinary tract and genital chlamydial infections are common (CDC, 1993). Many young adults develop immunological disorders such as allergic rhinitis (hay fever) and sinusitis, which reach their peak incidence in this age group. Eczema and asthma are also common, and arthritis begins to show up as a major problem.

During the middle years, viral infections are common, especially those affecting the respiratory tract. Most people have built up sufficient immunity by this stage of life, however, to ward off the more serious complications of these infections. Bacterial infections are not usually a severe problem, unless the defence mechanisms have been weakened by other stressors. Substance abusers and those who have disorders such as cancer, for example, seem to be much more vulnerable to infections than most middle-aged adults. Allergies causing hay fever or bronchial asthma as well as drug allergies may emerge or become more severe during middle age.

Among older adults, the respiratory tract is the principal site of serious viral infections. Pneumonia is common, and influenza is often fatal, particularly if there are existing cardiopulmonary problems such as heart disease or chronic bronchitis. Older people are also prone to urinary tract infections, which is often related to two factors: most do not drink enough fluids and there is a general slowing of all bodily processes, with more of a tendency towards stasis of urine in the bladder. Diminishing skin integrity increases the risk of infection for the older person. With aging, there is also a decline in the efficiency of immune response to infectious agents. Neoplastic disorders (such as cancer) tend to reduce it further. Treatment of disorders by medications that suppress the immune reaction, for example, chemotherapy, which is often used in treating cancer, may further impair resistance to infection.

Common Problems

People can develop an infection in almost any tissue of the body. Five of the most common infections will be outlined here. These are urinary tract infections, lower respiratory tract infections, surgical site infections, gastroenteritis and bacteremia.

Urinary Tract Infections

Urinary tract infection (UTI) involving only the mucosal surface of the bladder is called cystitis. When the interstitial tissue of the kidney is involved, it is referred to as pyelonephritis. While urine is normally sterile, occasionally an asymptomatic bacteriuria may occur, which is the persistence of bacteria in urine without any symptoms.

COMMON CAUSES AND RISK FACTORS

The bacteria most commonly associated with UTI are for the most part those that colonize the lower gastrointestinal tract such as *Escherichia (E.) coli*, *Klebsiella*, *Proteus*, enterococci, *Enterobacter*, *Serratia* and *Pseudomonas*. In the immunocompromised, *Candida albicans* is occasionally the causative agent.

About 35–45 percent of all nosocomial infections are due to UTI (Stamm, 1998). While 10 percent of hospitalized patients require a catheter, up to 25 percent of these patients may acquire an infection during their stay, usually as a result of the catheter (APIC, 1996). After 7–10 days of indwelling catheterization, fully 50 percent of patients become infected (Stamm, 1998; APIC, 1996). After one month, few escape acquiring an infection. Major risk factors include not only catheterization, especially lengthy catheterization, but also other instrumentation of the urinary tract. Females are at greater risk for infection because of a shorter urethra. Improper catheter care techniques and periurethral colonization with bowel flora further add to the risk. Certain diseases, such as diabetes or multiple sclerosis, may predispose patients to UTI.

Bacteria gain entry to the bladder either by ascending the thin mucous layer between the outer catheter surface and the urethra (periurethrally), or intraluminally within the column of urine inside the catheter. The infecting organism may have colonized the meatus and lower urethra. Bacteria may have originated not only from bowel flora but possibly from the hands of hospital staff manipulating the catheter or touching the perineal area. This can happen whether gloves are worn or not. Good technique is mandatory at all times. Hands must always be washed immediately before and after any catheter manipulation or procedure.

PATHOGENESIS

The microorganism that enters the urinary tract intraluminally most likely enters the catheter collecting system at some point where it can be opened, either the junction between the catheter and tubing or from the emptying spigot when the bag is drained. Organisms ascend the column of urine in the drainage tube. They also may enter the bladder by reflux should the drainage bag be inadvertently lifted above bladder level.

SIGNS AND SYMPTOMS

Signs and symptoms specific to UTI include suprapubic pain and urethral burning. If a catheter is not present, the typical symptoms include urgency, frequency and dysuria. Fever is usually absent. Should a catheter be *in situ*, those symptoms are obscured. However, at least half of all patients with UTI will not have any of the above symptoms, but only a bacteriuria.

About one to two percent of patients with UTI will develop bacteremia (presence of bacteria in the blood), which is manifested by fever, chills, sweats and possible septic shock. Mortality is less than 10 percent if appropriately treated (APIC, 1996). Rare complications include epididymitis and prostatitis with localized and systemic signs and symptoms of infection.

PREVENTION AND CONTROL MEASURES

The risk of acquiring a UTI is much greater in the catheterized patient. Many hospitals follow guidelines published by the Centers for Disease Control (CDC) in the United States and by the Laboratory Centre for Disease Control (LCDC) in Ottawa. If at all possible, catheterization should be avoided altogether. If catheters are necessary, the duration of catheterization should be kept as short as possible or the use of intermittent catheters may be considered, and a condom catheter may be considered for male patients. Insertion of catheters must be done aseptically following hospital procedure. The closed drainage system must be considered sterile, and aseptic precautions must be maintained when entering the system. However, the system must not be entered unless absolutely necessary. Because drainage bags may become colonized (from repeated emptyings) it is important to avoid causing reflux of urine, which can occur if the bag is lifted above bladder level or if the bag is compressed. The perineum is an area that is heavily colonized with microbial flora. Therefore, it is important to ensure that patients are kept clean and at the same time to inspect the catheter site and collecting system for signs of crusting or soreness.

The perineum should be washed with soap and water, rinsed well and dried once a shift. The meatus should be inspected, ensuring that the catheter can rotate freely. Any crusting or other problems must be reported. There is no set time for changing urinary catheters; however, problems such as bypassing or blocking may indicate a need for change.

Very often, then, it is the nurse member of the health care team who can exercise the greatest influence and have the greatest impact on catheter-related infection. In summary, this is done by recommending alternatives or reducing the duration of catheterization, as well as maintaining asepsis in all catheter-related procedures, gravity drainage and good hygiene when caring for the patient.

Lower Respiratory Tract Infections

Pneumonia, the most common expression of lower respiratory infection, may be described as infection of the pulmonary parenchyma (the functional elements of the lung) with consolidation (solidification) and exudation (the escape of fluid from blood cells with deposition in tissues). Once regarded as the "friend of the elderly" because it eased the aged and debilitated to a reasonably quick death, pneumonia remains the most significant cause of death due to infection acquired in inpatient facilities.

COMMON CAUSES AND RISK FACTORS

The bacteria most commonly associated with nosocomial pneumonia include *Klebsiella*, *Enterobacter*, *Proteus*, *Pseudomonas* and *Serratia* among gram-negative microorganisms, while *Streptococcus pneumoniae* and *Staphylococcus aureus* predominate among gram-positive organisms. In immunocompromised patients, pathogens may include *Aspergillus* (a yeast), cytomegalovirus (CMV) or *Pneumocystis carinii* (PCP, which is a protozoan). Opportunist bacteria such as *Acinetobacter* may pose a risk to ventilated patients. Occasionally during a community epidemic of influenza, a viral pneumonia may spread among hospitalized patients, while pneumonia due to respiratory syncytial virus (RSV) may be seen in children.

Nosocomial pneumonia develops in about one-half to one percent of hospital patients, occurring with greater frequency in high-risk patients (APIC, 1996). High-risk patients include those in intensive care units and those who are postoperative, intubated or immunocompromised. The major risk factors for individuals include intubation, intermittent positive pressure breathing apparatus, recent abdominal or thoracic surgery, immunosuppression and decreased level of consciousness, which may lead either to aspiration or to an impaired cough reflex. Other risk factors include pre-existing pulmonary disease or injury and exposure to smoke. In healthy individuals, the respiratory tract is lined with cilia which continuously sweep foreign bodies, including microorganisms, outward and away from the lower respiratory tract. This defence mechanism is bypassed when patients are intubated. Prolonged exposure to smoke will destroy cilia.

PATHOGENESIS

All people are colonized with bacteria, particularly in the oropharynx. Normally, mostly gram-positive cocci reside in the mouth and oropharynx, although a few species of gram-negative rods may be found there. The stomach, owing to its acidity, contains relatively few microorganisms. In ill-hospitalized patients, however, this all changes. The oropharynx becomes colonized heavily with gram-negative bacteria. This predisposition to upper airway colonization increases with the severity of illness, prolonged antibiotic treatment and length of hospitalization. Patients may aspirate these microorganisms into the lower [illegible] growth of these intruders, then nosocomial pneumonia may ensue. Should an endotracheal tube be *in situ*, contaminated aerosols may be delivered directly into the tracheobronchial tree. These aerosols may contain gram-negative rods, as these organisms require moisture. The presence of an endotracheal tube, a tracheostomy or suctioning will facilitate the entry of these organisms to the lower respiratory tract. When patients are intubated and expected to be hospitalized for some time, antacids or histamine$_2$ receptor antagonists may be administered to prevent possible erosion and ulcer formation in the stomach lining. Decreasing the natural acidity provides a more hospitable environment for gram-negative organisms, adding to the risk of nosocomial pneumonia through the aspiration of stomach contents.

SIGNS AND SYMPTOMS

Patients with pneumonia usually have fever, cough and chest pain and produce purulent sputum. On examination, the patient may exhibit signs of pulmonary consolidation, indicated by abnormal breath sounds such as crackles or bronchial breathing. Fever and tachypnea may be noted and may be the only signs present in an immunocompromised patient. When patients are on a ventilator, have just had surgery or have a reduced level of consciousness, it may be difficult to elicit these signs. As well, other clinical syndromes may confuse the picture when presentations are similar to those of nosocomial pneumonia. Such diseases might include congestive heart failure, pulmonary embolus, adult respiratory distress syndrome, atelectasis and aspiration. Radiological findings may help confirm the diagnosis of pneumonia. Findings include a new infiltrate (usually segmental, patchy or lobar), occasionally accompanied by a pleural effusion. A previously present infiltrate may enlarge, suggesting a new superimposed infection, while cavitation of the lung is very suggestive of infection.

PREVENTION AND CONTROL MEASURES

The CDC and LCDC have issued guidelines for the prevention and control of nosocomial pneumonia, and many hospitals use these for guidance. It is important that hospitals have policies and procedures in place to ensure that respiratory therapy equipment is properly managed and reprocessed. Certain patients will require particular attention. For example, those undergoing anesthesia, especially those having abdominal or thoracic surgery, and patients with chronic pulmonary dysfunction or musculoskeletal chest abnormalities are at increased risk. Patients should be brought to an optimum state of health whenever possible before surgery. Preoperative teaching is essential to prepare the patient for coughing, deep breathing and, whenever feasible, early ambulation. To achieve these ends postoperatively it will be necessary to control pain [illegible] effectively.

Hand-washing remains the keystone of infection control practice. Hands must be washed after any contact with respiratory secretions, even after removing gloves. Hands must also be washed after contact with patients who have a tracheostomy or those who are intubated. Emphasis must be placed on good hand-washing after suctioning and any manipulation of respiratory therapy equipment, including care of a tracheostomy.

Fluids being used in nebulizers or humidifiers must be sterile and must be dispensed aseptically. Any unused fluid in dated supply bottles should be discarded after 24 hours and a new bottle used when needed. Multidose vials for respiratory therapy must be stored according to manufacturers' instructions and discarded on expiry. Fluid reservoirs on equipment should be filled immediately before use only and not set up "just in case." Fluid in reservoirs should be discarded first before refilling rather than just "topping up." Water in tubing should be discarded. Newer types of tubing may make opening the system for this purpose unnecessary. Hospital policy regarding the frequency of change for particular pieces of equipment must be observed. All tubing and breathing circuits must be changed between patients and properly reprocessed. Adequate cleaning of all equipment must be done first, whether equipment is to receive high-level disinfection or sterilization. Suctioning should be done only as indicated by the patient's condition, using sterile gloves. Sterile fluid only must be used to rinse the catheter. Suction bottles and tubing must be changed between patients, except for bottles that may be used for more than one patient in short-stay areas such as the recovery room. However, these must be changed at the end of the day. In all instances, this equipment must receive high-level disinfection or sterilization. Room air humidifiers (the sort bought in hardware stores) are not to be used as they become contaminated readily, are difficult to clean and are all but impossible to disinfect.

Surgical Site Infections

Postoperative surgical site infection accounts for approximately 24 percent of all nosocomial infections (Gaynes, 1998). The likelihood of any surgical site's becoming infected varies according to its location, the general condition of the patient and the degree and type of contamination to which a wound is exposed. Surgical site infections may be deep or superficial, and they may involve implants such as artificial joint replacements, cardiac valves or synthetic vascular patches.

COMMON CAUSES

Surgical site infections are almost always bacterial in origin. The specific bacteria likely to cause infection at a given site usually are predictable according to the likely source of contamination. When contamination occurs from an exogenous source, the most likely agents are *Staphylococcus aureus* and group A beta-hemolytic streptococci. Contaminating bacteria from endogenous sources can usually be linked to the flora at the operative site. For example, in bowel surgery, the most common causative organisms include the enteric gram-negative rods found in the gut (*E. coli*, *Klebsiella*, group D streptococci, *Bacteroides fragilis* and *Clostridium*, to name a few). In very clean procedures where only sterile tissue is entered, such as in cardiac bypass surgery, the infecting microorganisms are likely to be skin flora such as *Staphylococcus epidermidis* or *S. aureus*. Many of these endogenous infections are polymicrobial in nature.

RISK FACTORS AND PATHOGENESIS

Risk factors for increased likelihood of infection associated with the host include advanced age, extreme obesity, malnutrition, anemia, chronic obstructive lung disease and diabetes mellitus. Some of these factors may indicate reduced blood supply to the operative site, thus decreased oxygenation and lessened phagocytic activity. Other factors include decreased antibody–antigen response and hypoalbuminemia.

Infection remote from the operative site, for instance, a pressure ulcer, is likely to contain a large amount of bacteria. Similarly, certain skin conditions may contribute to heavier colonization of the operative site. Alternatively, bacteria may travel via the lymphatic system from its source to the operative field. Areas of the body better supplied with blood, such as the head and upper trunk, generally have a lower rate of infection due to better perfusion and greater phagocytic activity. Another important factor in surgical site infection is trauma, in particular when trauma results in heavy contamination of the area, as happens in some motor vehicle or industrial accidents.

The events in the intraoperative period are of prime importance in determining whether or not wound infection will ensue. Much depends on the skill of the surgeon and the particular techniques used, in addition to the factors of host susceptibility and the degree of contamination present.

Good operative technique includes expeditious surgery, gentle handling of tissue, control of bleeding and hematoma formation, eradication of dead space, minimization of the presence of devitalized tissue, removal of foreign materials, choice of suture material and avoidance of drains, especially Penrose drains, where possible. There are, however, specific indications for closed drains, which are preferable to Penrose drains. Drains should not exit through the operative wound, but through an adjacent small incision. Depending on the degree of wound contamination that has occurred, the surgeon may choose to delay closure of the wound until contamination has been reduced, which is usually about five days.

The more people present in an operating theatre, the higher the bacterial air count. Thus, it seems prudent to restrict the number of people in a theatre during surgery, to reduce the flow of traffic in and out of the room and to ensure that operating theatres are constructed so that air changes occur about 25 times per hour. All these considerations will reduce the bacterial air count during an operation.

SIGNS AND SYMPTOMS

The classic signs and symptoms of surgical site infection are pain, redness, induration (hardening), poor healing, dehiscence (separation of all the layers of a surgical wound) and purulent drainage. Systemic manifestations, such as fever, anorexia and malaise, may also be present.

PREVENTION AND CONTROL MEASURES

The prevention of surgical site infections relies largely on the skill of the surgeon. However, there are some host factors, and occasionally environmental factors, in which the nurse can play a role. Whenever elective surgery is planned, the patient should be brought to a state of optimum health. For example, he or she should lose weight and stop smoking; nutrition should be improved; chronic diseases such as diabetes should be brought under control; and remote infections should be treated. Preoperatively, patients must understand the importance of frequent deep breathing and coughing when secretions are present so that nosocomial pneumonia does not develop and interfere with oxygen perfusion. The importance of early ambulation must be stressed. The duration of hospital stay preoperatively must be as short as possible. A preoperative wash with a hospital-approved antiseptic may be desirable, and hair removal must be done by clippers or depilation only as close to the time of surgery as possible and only as much as needed to facilitate surgery. Should prophylactic antibiotics be ordered, timing of the first and subsequent doses is important to ensure that antibiotic levels are highest when surgery takes place. The dose and timing will vary from one antibiotic to another. Personnel must adhere to hospital policy in regard to preoperative scrubbing and operating room attire. Personnel with infections or draining wounds *must not* work in an operating suite. Intraoperatively, the charge nurse in the operating room may be responsible for seeing that traffic is controlled, that the air system has a maintenance schedule, that necessary supplies and equipment are at hand and that the operation proceeds expeditiously.

Postoperatively, the unit (ward) nurse is responsible for ensuring that prophylactic antibiotics are administered until finished, that patients ambulate as soon as they are able, that deep breathing and coughing are done and that the wound is inspected regularly and any signs and symptoms of infection are noted and reported. In addition to the previously described signs and symptoms, nurses should be alert to the presence of fluid collections, such as seromas or hematomas, which may lead to infection. As always, meticulous hand-washing and careful disposal of secretions and excretions are mandatory. [illegible] "No-touch" technique using sterile instruments must be used to maintain asepsis. Alternatively, sterile gloves may be used where direct contact is required.

Gastroenteritis

Gastroenteritis may be defined as increased bowel activity or impaired bowel function caused by an infectious agent. Diarrhea or vomiting may be present with or without associated systemic symptoms. The identity of the infectious agent may or may not be established.

COMMON CAUSES

The most common bacterial agents that cause gastroenteritis seen in patients admitted to hospital in Canada include *Salmonella*, *Shigella*, *Yersinia*, *Campylobacter* and *Aeromonas*. Some bacteria produce toxins in food (for example, *S. aureus*, *C. botulinum* and *E. coli*). Also, pathogenic *E. coli* is a significant cause of diarrhea in newborn nurseries. Viral agents most commonly seen in pediatric facilities include rotavirus, parvovirus, enterovirus and adenovirus, although laboratories in Canada do not always test for these agents. The two parasitic infestations most commonly seen in Canada are *Entamoeba histolytica* and *Giardia lamblia* (beaver fever). Occasionally patients may return from tropical countries with parasitic infestation, for example, *Strongyloides*.

For hospitalized patients, *Clostridium difficile* becomes a significant pathogen, causing pseudomembranous colitis. This particular disease can be attributed to antibiotic usage. With certain antibiotics, normal bowel bacteria may be suppressed, allowing the very small numbers of *C. difficile* present in some people to grow out of proportion in comparison to the usual ratio. When *C. difficile* exists in large quantities, it is capable of behaving pathogenically, causing toxin production leading to severe diarrhea and the formation of a false membrane along the walls of the lower bowel. There have been a number of *C. difficile* diarrhea outbreaks in hospitals involving person-to-person transmission via the fecal–oral route. This happens easily when due care is not taken, as this organism is very hardy and can survive in the environment for long periods of time.

RISK FACTORS

For the most part, enteric pathogens are either food- and water-borne or are transmitted by the fecal–oral route. Some also are transmitted by direct contact such as in oral–anal intercourse. In food- or water-borne illness, the spread of disease may be attributed to fecal contamination through lack of adequate sewage facilities or, in some countries, the use of night soil. Food handlers who lack good hygiene and are carriers of enteric disease may spread it readily to others. In crowded living conditions, the spread of infection is facilitated by the very real difficulties of maintaining both [illegible] tions are exacerbated in times of war or natural disaster and the subsequent displacement of large numbers of people. In developed countries, contamination of well water or of shellfish can occur quite readily if proper precautions or adequate community planning are not undertaken.

Occasionally, food-borne illness or food poisoning can result from a single source. This may typically arise when a number of people become ill who have shared a single meal at a restaurant or social gathering. It is possible to make a relatively accurate assumption about the etiologic agent based on clinical signs and symptoms, the time frame and the likely food vehicle. In some day care centres the parasite *Giardia lamblia* has been found in over 90 percent of the attendees who are not toilet trained, suggesting person-to-person spread (Plorde, 1990). Hepatitis A virus has also been spread under similar circumstances. Several enteric diseases are spread by receptive anal intercourse or oral–anal intercourse. Disease that can be spread in these ways include hepatitis A, *Salmonella*, *Shigella*, *Campylobacter*, *Entamoeba histolytica* and some venereal diseases.

Impaired host defences may predispose a person to acquiring a gastrointestinal infectious disease. Gastric acid in the stomach usually provides protection by reducing or eliminating ingested organisms. A lowering of gastric acidity occurs most often in premature infants or in older adults. Medications designed to reduce stomach acidity may actually provide a favourable environment for potential pathogens, and those with partial gastrectomy or vagotomy are at higher risk. In hospitals, overcrowding and lack of proper hand-washing facilities may contribute to the risk. Another contributing factor in some outbreaks is the ability of some bacteria such as *C. difficile* to survive in the environment or on equipment that is improperly processed after use.

PATHOGENESIS

Microorganisms responsible for enteric illness characterized by frequent fluid intestinal evacuations attack the host in several different ways. Some organisms, for example, *Vibrio parahaemolyticus*, will act directly on the wall of the intestine, stimulating secreting action and producing watery diarrhea. Others, such as *Shigella*, invade the mucosa, producing dysentery (inflammation of the intestine), possibly bloody stools and tenesmus (ineffectual straining at stool), while others, for example *Salmonella typhi* (typhoid fever), may penetrate to local lymphatic tissue and enter the blood stream, possibly producing bacteremia. Some bacteria produce a toxin that, in the case of *S. aureus*, acts on the vomiting centre of the brain. This can quickly create problems with dehydration and cardiac disease in an older adult host. Some microorganisms can cause disease in several ways.

SIGNS AND SYMPTOMS

The frequent fluid intestinal evacuations that occur with gastroenteritis can be characterized in three different ways. The most common form is watery diarrhea. The loss of fluid occurs from the proximal small intestine. The diarrhea may be accompanied by nausea, vomiting, fever and abdominal pain. In most instances, the course is intense but brief, generally lasting from one to three days.

Dysentery (inflamation of the intestine) begins rapidly, but stool may be of smaller volume and contain blood or pus. Fever, abdominal pain, cramps and tenesmus frequently accompany dysentery, but vomiting is not as frequent. The colon is affected by direct invasion or by production of cell toxins. While blood and pus may be present, fluid loss is relatively small as the colon does not absorb or secrete fluid at the same rate as the small bowel. Most cases of dysentery are resolved in two to seven days.

Enteric fever is a systemic infection that originates in the intestinal tract. Diarrhea is usually mild and develops *after* fever and abdominal pain. The causative microorganism spreads through the mucosa of the small bowel to adjacent organs such as the liver and biliary tree. Bacteremia occurs frequently. The most common disease associated with this infection is *Salmonella typhi*, otherwise known as typhoid fever.

PREVENTION AND CONTROL MEASURES

A sanitary sewage disposal system and a safe water supply are fundamental to building a safe community. Additionally, the food supply must be delivered to the end user free of harmful pathogens. People handling food and water for others' consumption must understand and practise good hygiene.

The most important and most common mode of transmission for enteric pathogens is the fecal–oral route via the hands of personnel. Therefore, hand-washing remains the most important activity in preventing the spread of disease. Hands must be washed as necessary, before, during and after patient care, before eating or handling food, after using the toilet and after touching equipment in the patient care environment (where some enteric pathogens can survive for long periods of time). Further, a regular maintenance cleaning schedule and provision for spot cleaning and adequate reprocessing of items such as bedpans are important. Yet, staff should be aware that spores of some microorganisms, notably C. *difficile*, survive exposure to hospital disinfectants. This re-emphasizes the importance of good hygiene and good hand washing. Protective attire must be used when there is likely to be direct contact with stool. Gloves and water-impermeable gowns or aprons should be used; gloves must be changed on completion of each task and hands must be washed. Gloves must not be worn from one patient to another, nor used for subsequent tasks on the same patient. Gowns must be changed between patients and whenever they become soiled. In some instances (in pediatric units, for example), patients must be isolated. Those with the same pathogen may be placed together in the same room (sometimes referred to as "cohorting" patients).

Hand-washing and excretory disposal facilities (bedpan decontaminators) must be adequate, overcrowding must be avoided and the staff–patient ratio must be balanced so as to mitigate risks of cross-infection. These factors are crucial to good infection control in any care setting. Finally, staff should be aware that some people are asymptomatic excreters of certain pathogens, and so care with all secretions and excretions is mandatory to all aspects of patient care.

Therapy for gastrointestinal infections is generally supportive, using fluid replacement and maintaining electrolyte balance. In cases of viral diarrhea, it is the only therapy available and may be necessary also for patients with bacterial diarrhea.

Bacteremia

Bacteremia is the presence of microorganisms (bacteria) in the blood. Terms also used specifically are viremia, fungemia and parisitemia. These organisms are present either as part of an infectious disease (hepatitis B, for example) or reflect a serious and uncontrolled disease process, such as the seeding of microbes into the blood stream from pneumonia or pyelonephritis or direct introduction through a vascular device. Bacteremias may therefore be defined as primary or secondary. Primary bacteremias occur in patients who have no recognized site of infection. However, the two major sources for primary bacteremia are related to intravascular catheters and infusion systems or the gut flora of immunocompromised hosts. Two-thirds of bacteremias are considered secondary as there is a recognizable source of infection such as pneumonia, UTI or a surgical wound (APIC, 1996). Patients are described as septic or having septicemia when the bacteremia is accompanied by oliguria, hypotension, dulling of consciousness and acidosis progressing to septic shock. Occasionally, a transient bacteremia will manifest after manipulation of, or trauma to, a body site that has a population of normal flora. This usually is of no lasting importance, except that it may be a significant factor in the development of infective endocarditis.

COMMON CAUSES AND RISK FACTORS

The most common causes of primary nosocomial bacteremias are *Klebsiella*, *Enterobacter*, *Serratia* and *Pseudomonas*. In secondary bacteremia, the causative organism will be found both in blood and at the site from which the infection spread. Thus, in bacteremias associated with UTI, the agent is likely to be a gram-negative organism such as *E. coli*, while staphylococci would more likely be found in a surgical wound.

In primary bacteremia, the use of an intravascular catheter provides a ready pathway into the blood stream.

The organism may come from the patient's own microbial flora or from the hands of hospital personnel inserting or manipulating the catheter or its dressing. Infusion fluids are [illegible] become contaminated in use by injection of medications, accidental disconnection, monitoring procedures or careless handling of the tubing or ports. Catheter-related sepsis occurs about 10 times as often as infusion-related sepsis (APIC, 1996). In secondary bacteremia, the risk factors are as those for the underlying disease.

PATHOGENESIS

Patients with bacteremia are seriously ill, and require careful observation and immediate treatment. With septicemia, there is increased cardiac output and decreased total peripheral venous resistance. As shock progresses, decreased urinary output occurs, as does acidosis, lactate accumulation, hyponatremia and elevation of serum creatinine. This may be followed by disseminated intravascular coagulation (DIC) resulting in low platelet count, prolonged prothrombin time, low fibrinogen concentration and the presence of fibrin degradation products in the blood.

SIGNS AND SYMPTOMS

Signs and symptoms of bacteremia include fever, chills, perspiration, weakness and myalgia. The signs and symptoms pertinent to disease in the underlying site also will be evidenced in secondary bacteremia. Septic shock, which leads to death in over 50 percent of cases, proceeds to hypotension, oliguria and DIC (APIC, 1996).

PREVENTION AND CONTROL MEASURES

Primary bacteremia can be prevented by taking care when inserting and maintaining vascular lines. First, intravascular lines should be used only as necessary or in anticipation of the need for access. A higher rate of infection is associated with lower extremity use, as in the development of phlebitis. Thus, lines should be inserted in upper extremities. Hands must be washed before insertion or manipulation, and gloves may be needed according to hospital policy for some procedures. The area of insertion should be cleaned with a hospital-approved skin antiseptic first. The catheter should be kept as secure as possible, using a sterile dressing. The intravenous site must be inspected daily and any problems, such as redness or purulence, should be reported immediately. Lines and catheters must be changed according to hospital policy for each particular type of catheter and line as well as after blood products or lipid emulsion. The system must not be entered unnecessarily. Irrigation and blood sampling must also be avoided. Should primary bacteremia occur, it is quite likely that the vascular catheter will be removed if it is considered the source of the microorganism's circulating and being seeded into the blood. Removal of a foreign body also will facilitate antimicrobial therapy.

Secondary bacteremias occur less frequently. Then, prevention is aimed at dealing with the source of infection and eradicating it, for example, by treatment of [illegible] UTI [illegible]

When the source of infection is not known or patients are very ill or immunocompromised, the physician likely will order broad-spectrum antimicrobial coverage empirically.

Multidrug-Resistant Microorganisms

The discovery of anti-infective agents and the subsequent development of immunization programs seemed to signal the possible elimination of illness and death due to infection by the end of the 20th century.

Penicillin, discovered in 1928, came into widespread use during and immediately after World War II. However, after only a few years, strains of *Staphylococcus* had developed resistance to the new wonder drug. By then, medical science had discovered other antibiotics. One was a semi-synthetic penicillin called methicillin. During the 1950s, methicillin was the antibiotic of choice when resistance to penicillin was noted. However, in 1961, the first cases of methicillin resistance were seen in a patient in a U.K. hospital, and shortly thereafter in a European hospital. These reports indicated not that new diseases were emerging and spreading, but rather that bacterial resistance to antibiotics was developing as part of an evolutionary pattern. Bacteria, which like every living organism have the imperative to survive and multiply, were now simply responding to the assault on them by antibiotics. Not only did resistance to semi-synthetic penicillins develop, but other classes of antibiotics were also rendered ineffective—leaving, for the most part, only one antibiotic of value, vancomycin.

The problem of antibiotic resistance continues, and has become a major focus and concern for health professionals. To complicate matters further, development of new antibiotics requires much time and research. Thus far, medical science has failed to find ways to halt the development of resistance to antibiotics. While a number of microorganisms have shown signs of increasing resistance, there are two gram-positive cocci that are problematic in Canadian hospitals.

METHICILLIN-RESISTANT STAPHYLOCOCCUS AUREUS

Staphylococcus aureus is carried on the skin of one-third of the population at any given time. Usually, it causes no harm to healthy people. Yet, it emerged as a significant hospital pathogen in the late 1940s, peaking in the 1950s and early 1960s. Methicillin-resistant *S. aureus* (MRSA) emerged first in 1959 and has evolved throughout the world. By the early 1980s, Canadian hospitals were seeing patients with MRSA, albeit introduced from endemic areas of the world.

By the 1990s, outbreaks of MRSA were becoming much more difficult to control as the number of cases increased. Today, it is generally accepted that MRSA is here to stay. Nevertheless, given the fact that the incidence of this organism in Canadian hospitals remains relatively low, preventive and restorative measures are instituted to contain the organism (Farr, 1997; Sands & Goldman, 1998).

VANCOMYCIN-RESISTANT ENTEROCOCCI (VRE)

The enterococcus is a microorganism of relatively low pathogenicity and virulence that is found in normal flora in the gastrointestinal tract. The first vancomycin-resistant *Enterococcus* was isolated in France in 1988. The incidence of this resistant strain has increased from 0.3 percent of all enterococcal isolates to over 10 percent in both Europe and the United States. In Canada, the number of cases remains relatively low and, like MRSA, it was first introduced by persons returning from endemic areas who were hospitalized. While VRE does not cause disease as readily as *S. aureus*, both organisms pose a threat to the elderly, debilitated and immunocompromised. Unlike MRSA, which can be treated with vancomycin, the only antibiotics that can be used for VRE strains have also produced resistance. At present there are no other effective antibiotics on the horizon. Because of the very limited antibiotic treatment options, it is imperative that preventive measures be established (Farr, 1997; Weinstein & Hayden, 1998).

Assessing Infection Prevention and Control Needs

Every patient in a health agency has the potential for developing infection, as does every health professional. The nurse must always be observant for infections in patients. In the nursing history and physical assessment, information is collected about factors that may influence the development of infection, the general health status of the patient (for example, the current state of functional abilities and of health at the time of admission to the agency), and any existing infectious process. This information is supplemented by data about the patient's past and current health problems, and the physician's diagnostic and therapeutic plans of care as found in the patient's record. Laboratory tests and x-ray reports also provide valuable information.

Nursing Health History

Much of the health history pertaining to infection prevention and control is incorporated into the data collection for each individual need. For instance, information about the usual patterns of hygiene and nutrition, recent changes in these patterns or problems that might suggest infection or place the patient at risk for infection are gathered during the specific need assessment. In addition, information is obtained about general susceptibility to infections, recent exposure to infectious agents, any factors that may place the patient at risk for infection and immunization status.

Physical Assessment

Ultimately, the nurse's observations of the patient are of primary importance in identifying infections. The nurse watches for signs and symptoms of the body's systemic and local responses to invasion. The vital signs—temperature, pulse and respirations—are particularly helpful in early detection of infection. Statements of tiredness, loss of energy, headache, loss of appetite or generally not feeling well are also among the early warning signs of a systemic reaction to infection. If a patient makes any of these statements, it is always wise to check the vital signs to see if they are elevated. Lymph nodes draining the infected area may also be enlarged. Both subjective and objective findings should be reported promptly.

As we discussed earlier, tissue invasion may be manifested by localized signs and symptoms, namely pain or tenderness, redness, swelling, warmth and some loss of function of the affected body part. A foul odour may also be present due either to the by-products of bacterial metabolism or to the death of cells and tissue. These signs and symptoms vary according to the system or body site involved.

Other signs of infection the nurse should observe for include secretions from the nose and throat, coughing, sneezing or the expectoration of sputum. Exudates from wounds or other breaks in the skin, or from any of the body orifices, should also warn the nurse of the possibility of infection, as should any vomiting or diarrhea.

Diagnostic Tests

Blood tests are usually ordered to determine the presence of infection in the body. These include a white blood cell (leukocyte) count, differential white blood count (different types of white blood cells) and erythrocyte sedimentation rate. Generally, increases in the total white blood count, neutrophils, lymphocytes and erythrocyte sedimentation rate are associated with acute and chronic bacterial and viral infections. Specimens of body fluids and wound drainage are also taken to identify the pathogen(s) causing the infection. When collecting specimens for microbiological examination, care must be taken to ensure that the specimens are not contaminated with organisms in the environment.

URINE SPECIMENS In order that patients with urinary tract infections receive the best possible treatment, great care must be taken in the procuring and subsequent handling of urine specimens. Voided specimens must be obtained by the clean-catch (midstream) method while catheter specimens must be obtained aseptically, either on insertion, before the drainage tube is connected, or afterwards by aspirating

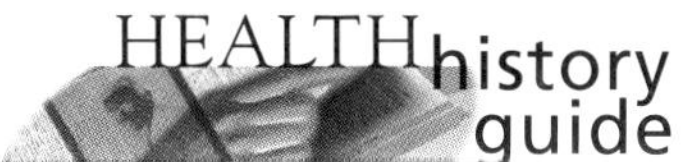
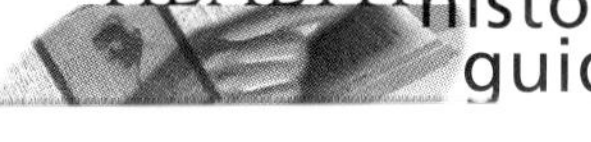

HEALTH history guide **Infection Prevention and Control**

Health and Illness Patterns

- Do you frequently experience infections? If so, how often? What type? Do you know what usually causes these infections? How were they treated?
- When did you last have an infection? How was it treated?
- Have you recently been exposed to any infectious diseases that you know of? If yes, where? How?
- Do you have a history of any acute or chronic illnesses (for example, asthma, diabetes, multiple sclerosis or leukemia) that may place you at risk for infection? Have you had surgery recently?
- Are you taking any medications or treatments (for example, radiation therapy, anticancer drugs or anti-inflammatory drugs) that might increase the risk of infection?

Health-Promotion and Health-Protection Patterns

- What do you ordinarily do to prevent infection?
- Have you been immunized against communicable diseases? If so, what immunizations have you had? When were they done?
- Are you taking any precautionary measures for infection? If so, why? What precautions are being taken?

through the puncture port or the catheter tubing itself. Foley catheter tips are not acceptable for culturing. The techniques for obtaining these specimens are detailed in Chapter 21.

SPUTUM SPECIMENS Obtaining a good sputum sample is a challenge because expectorated sputum will become contaminated with whatever microorganisms are present as it passes through the oropharynx. However, there are a few steps the caregiver can take to help achieve a more accurate result. Because secretions tend to accumulate when one is asleep, an early morning specimen is best. The patient should be instructed to cough deeply since the *lower* respiratory tract is affected. It is advisable to have patients remove dentures first if necessary and to rinse the mouth with plain water. This will help decrease the amount of contamination from the oropharynx. Once a proper specimen has been obtained, it should be sent to the laboratory as quickly as possible. The tests most frequently ordered are for culture and sensitivity and gram stain. However, if a search for tuberculosis, pertussis or *Legionella* is ordered, this must be noted on the requisition. Otherwise, laboratories will not routinely do these tests, nor will they process specimens that appear to be saliva.

WOUND SPECIMENS It is important when obtaining a specimen from surgical wounds that the specimen reflect as accurately as possible the agents that are responsible for the infection. The wound should be cleansed first with normal saline. Fresh pus should be expressed from what appears to be the most affected part of the wound. This is important as fresh pus is most likely to contain live bacteria. Care must be taken to avoid contaminating the specimen with surrounding skin bacteria. The specimen should be sent for processing as soon as possible. The same procedures generally apply to taking a sample from any wound, including pressure or vascular ulcers or traumatic wounds that appear to be infected.

STOOL SPECIMENS Stool specimens ("walnut-sized" or the liquid equivalent) are placed in clean, nonsterile containers for culture and sensitivity and for toxin detection. If other than culture and sensitivity is ordered, it must be specified on the requisition so that laboratory personnel can select the appropriate testing method. With some tests, the specimen must reach the laboratory minutes after it has been obtained, so one should ascertain the proper procedure for each test.

BLOOD SPECIMENS Bacteremia is a serious disease with a 30-percent mortality rate overall and a 50-percent rate in the event of septic shock (APIC, 1996). Expeditious treatment aimed at eradicating the causative organism(s) is imperative. To this end, a sample of the patient's blood is obtained by aseptic venipuncture and sent to the laboratory for culture and sensitivity. Meticulous technique is critical if an accurate result is to be obtained. The skin over the venipuncture site must be cleansed thoroughly with a hospital-approved antiseptic and left to dry. Blood is drawn aseptically through a needle into a syringe or tube. The operator must avoid palpating the site once it has been prepared. The only time that blood can be drawn through a vascular catheter is if it cannot be obtained by venipuncture. Whenever possible, at least 10 mL should be collected from adults, or a correspondingly smaller amount from children. Two to three samples of adequate volume will be collected. Timing of samples will depend on the nature of the bacteremic episodes or underlying disease.

Diagnosing Infection-Related Problems

When patients are at risk for developing an infection, the diagnosis *Risk for Infection* is used. This diagnosis describes people whose host defences are compromised, rendering them susceptible to pathogenic agents from endogenous or exogenous sources. Any number of health problems and conditions may contribute to the risk for infection, including pathophysiological factors such as chronic diseases (respiratory diseases, cancer, diabetes), immunodeficiency, impaired skin and mucous membrane integrity or impaired circulation; treatment-related factors, such as medications (steroids, insulin, immunosuppressants), intravenous therapy or enteral feedings; situational factors, such as a history of recurrent infections, malnutrition, stress or lack of immunizations; and maturational factors, such as age. Treatment measures the nurse may implement focus on minimizing the patient's exposure to microorganisms and increasing the resistance to infection, for example, by improving nutritional status and infection control self-care practices in a person with diabetes. If infection is present in the patient, the diagnosis may be stated as a collaborative problem, for example, *Potential Complication: Septicemia* (Carpenito, 1997). This indicates the nurse's dependent functions in providing care—to implement medical treatments and monitor the patient for related complications.

A known or suspected infection brings additional problems such as controlling the spread of infection to others. In cases where the patient is at risk for transferring opportunistic or pathogenic agents to others, the diagnosis *Risk for Infection Transmission* may be used to direct protective measures towards preventing the spread of infection (Carpenito, 1997). People who are separated or isolated because of airborne communicable disease such as meningitis may experience associated problems. Some may worry and feel anxious about the cause of infection, about spreading it to others and about the seriousness of infection and what it means. These people may experience feelings of hopelessness or powerlessness if they think they have lost control over the situation. They may also feel socially isolated because of limited contact with others, or they may experience sensory deprivation because they are unable to engage in customary leisure and recreational activities. Some common examples of diagnoses for infection-related problems include:

- *Risk for Infection related to malnutrition, skin lesions, and poor hygiene practices.*
- *Risk for Infection related to suppressed immune response secondary to corticosteroid therapy.*
- *Risk for Infection related to the presence of a Foley catheter.*
- *Social Isolation related to airborne isolation precautions.*
- *Risk for Diversional Activity Deficit related to isolation for airborne infection.*

Planning Infection Prevention and Control Interventions

The prevention and control of infection is inherent in the planning and implementation of all nursing activities. The basic goals of nursing action in regard to infection are to prevent infection, to control infection, to promote comfort and lessen or prevent problems associated with infection and to promote infection control self-care practices. The specific plan of care for a patient is based on the nursing diagnoses and must take into account the nature of the infection, the portal of entry of the opportunist or pathogen, its exit routes from the body and its mode of transfer.

Some examples of goals or expected outcomes for patients who are at risk for infectious processes include:

- Patient will describe factors that may cause infection and the precautions that must be taken to prevent it.
- Patient will demonstrate effective hand-washing technique.
- Patient will remain free of nosocomial infection while in hospital.

Implementing Infection Prevention and Control Interventions

During the late 18th and throughout the 19th and 20th centuries, discoveries about the role of microorganisms were made that enabled scientists and other leaders to develop strategies that controlled and prevented the spread of infection. Try to imagine what a hospital or a long-term care facility would be like if concern with the microbial world were unnecessary. There would be no need for protective attire such as gloves, gowns or masks. There would be no need for sterile equipment. Industries devoted to providing hospitals with sterile goods simply would not exist. However, that is not the way the world is. We do have to deal with the unseen microbial world around us and its profound impact on our day-to-day lives.

Health-Promoting Strategies

Not only is the prevention and control of infection important, the promotion of healthy attitudes and practices can enhance the quality of our lives. It is important that the health care provider promote good health in individuals. It is also important to practise what you preach. To practise, teach and exemplify good health, it is necessary to keep informed and up to date on the health care issues of the day. Taking the time to discuss these issues with colleagues will better enable the nurse to deal with patient concerns later. Physical activity in the form of daily exercise and an adequate amount of rest and sleep help the body to maintain its defences against infection. Ensuring good nutrition by eating a balanced diet and also maintaining good dental health will help to maintain defences. Recent research suggests that a positive attitude towards life is beneficial and that humour may boost the immune system (Hall, 1988).

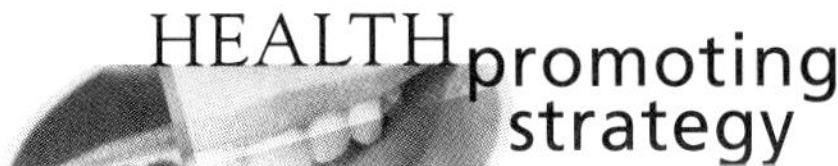

Promoting Healthy Infection Control

- Perform meticulous hand washing:
  - before, during and after patient contact
  - after using the toilet
  - before eating or handling food
  - whenever the hands are soiled
  - after gloves are removed
  - after sneezing or coughing
  - should injury occur.
- Cover the nose or mouth with tissues when coughing or sneezing.
- Keep physically fit and in good condition.
- Obtain adequate rest and avoid fatigue.
- Eat a well-balanced diet and make sure your teeth and gums are in good repair.
- Avoid stress and keep a positive attitude towards life. Humour is said to help maintain resistance against infection.
- If you suffer from a chronic disease, are over 65 years of age or work in an institution such as a day care centre or extended care facility, check with your doctor about getting an annual flu shot. This vaccine can help prevent many cases of influenza.
- Consider a one-time pneumococcal vaccine.
- Keep other immunizations (for example, polio, diphtheria and tetanus) up to date (about every 10 years).
- Health professionals should avail themselves of the hepatitis B vaccine that is available free in most Canadian hospitals.
- Keep informed about health care issues. Infection control programs are found in local community health agencies or hospitals.

SOURCE: Walker, 1991.

Health-Protecting Strategies

The best strategies for dealing with infectious diseases are always preventive. Immunization against infectious diseases, hygiene and aseptic practices are primary forms of health protection.

An understanding of basic asepsis lays the foundation for good infection control practices. While aseptic technique was developed to protect the patient, it also protects the health care provider. **Asepsis** can be defined as an absence of contamination. What that means in practice, according to Sue Crow (1989), a noted U.S. infection control practitioner, is the purposeful prevention of the transfer of infection from one person to another by keeping the microbial count to an irreducible minimum. A hospital environment, both animate and inanimate, including supplies and equipment, must always be kept as clean as is reasonably possible. In some instances, this means that some items must be entirely devoid of microbial life (sterile), and every effort must be made to keep them that way. While it is inevitable in the course of patient care that some items will become soiled, it is essential to know what is dirty, what is clean, what is sterile and how to keep them separate. *Medical asepsis* refers to practices that maintain cleanliness and limit the spread of microorganisms. In this method, also known as "clean technique," objects are described as clean or dirty. Using clean towels for a bed bath, cleaning a bedpan and washing hands before preparing oral medications are examples of medical asepsis. *Surgical asepsis* refers to practices that eliminate microorganisms from objects or areas. This method is known as "sterile technique"; objects are described as sterile or unsterile. Surgical asepsis is the basis of operating room procedure. Nurses practise surgical asepsis at the bedside when they perform such activities as administering injectable medications, inserting urinary catheters or changing sterile dressings.

IMMUNIZATION

The first organized efforts to immunize a segment of the population occurred as a result of Sir Edward Jenner's publication in 1798 citing evidence to support his observations that milkmaids infected by cowpox acquired immunity to the dreaded smallpox (White & Shackelford, 1983). Today in Canada and other countries, federally supported immunization programs ensure that everyone can receive protection from diseases that once were leading causes of morbidity and mortality. Tables 32.1 and 32.2 outline immunization schedules for infants, children and adults as recommended by Health Canada.

The widespread immunization of infants and children has drastically reduced the incidence of diseases such as measles, mumps, rubella, diphtheria and whooping cough (pertussis), and even tetanus and polio, over the past few decades. Many parents today have not experienced the tragic epidemics that used to sweep the country and ended in the deaths of so many infants and children not too many years ago. Many people have, as a result, become unconcerned about the need for immunization. Yet, children are just as vulnerable to these diseases today as they were before the vaccines were developed. The nurse who is counselling young mothers is in an excellent position to give advice on the needed immunizations for children at different ages.

Those who have concerns about immune status or the need for immunization should be encouraged to talk with a physician or other knowledgeable person at the local public health office. Those who work in hospitals must be able to provide, whenever possible, a written record of immunization and may be required to demonstrate immunity to certain specified diseases.

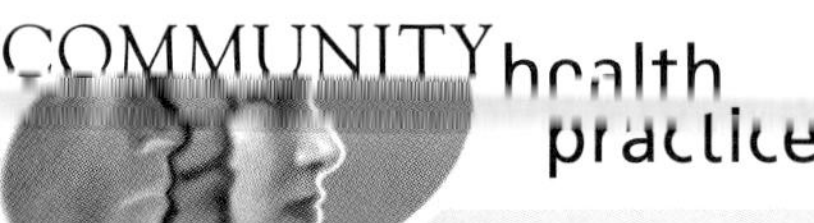

Immunization for World Travel

With more and more people travelling to different parts of the world today, there is no single schedule for immunization agents. Therefore, it is important for travellers to visit their family physician or local health department two to three months prior to their departure. This will allow the nurse or physician time to review the individual's immunization history and to determine the immunizations that are necessary for the countries to be visited, as well as sufficient time to complete appropriate immunizations. One example is hepatitis A vaccine, or serum immune globulin, which is highly recommended for travellers who are visiting developing countries where hepatitis A is endemic.

TABLE 32.1 Recommended immunization schedules for infants and children

Vaccine	*Months*					*Years*		
	2	4	6	12	18	4 TO 6	9 TO 13	14 TO 16
Hepatitis B*	3 doses	3 doses	3 doses	3 doses	3 doses	3 doses	3 doses	
Diphtheria, pertussis and tetanus (DPT)	DPT	DPT	DPT		DPT	DPT		Td**
Haemophilus influenza type b*** (Hib)	Hib	Hib	Hib		Hib			
Polio (inactivated polio vaccine/oral polio vaccine)	Polio	Polio	Polio ****		Polio	Polio		Polio ****
Measles, mumps and rubella***** (MMR)				MMR	MMR *****	MMR *****		

*Adolescents who have not received hepatitis B vaccine (3 doses in total) in infancy (2, 4, 6, 12 or 18 months) should receive it through school programs according to the provincial and territorial policies.

**Td (tetanus and diphtheria toxoids, adult formulation).

***Recommended schedule for both Hib-titre and ActHib.

****If oral polio vaccine is used exclusively, boosters at 6 months and 14 to 16 years of age may be omitted.

*****The second dose of MMR is routinely recommended at either 18 months or at 4 to 6 years of age. It should be given any time before school entry provided that there is at least a one-month interval between receipt of the first and second dose.

SOURCE: Health Canada, 1996, p. 1.

TABLE 32.2 Summary of selected immunization for adults

Vaccine	*Indication*	*Further Doses if Risk Continues*
BCG	High-risk exposure	None
Hepatitis B	Occupational, lifestyle or environmental exposure	None
Japanese encephalitis	Travel to endemic area or other exposure risk	**See page 114***
Meningococcal	High-risk exposure	**See pages 126–28**
Pertussis	Not indicated	
Poliomyelitis	Travel to endemic area or other exposure risk	**See pages 147 and 192**
Rabies pre-exposure use	Occupational or other risk	Every 2 years **See page 155**
Typhoid	High-risk exposure	Every 3–4 years **See pages 170–71**
Yellow fever	Travel to endemic area or if required for foreign travel	Every 10 years **See page 176**

*These page numbers refer to pages in the source

SOURCE: Health Canada, *Canadian Immunization Guide*, 5th edition, 1998.

RESEARCH to practice

Wheelock, S.M., & Lookinland, S. (1997). Effects of surgical hand scrub time on subsequent bacterial growth. *Journal of Association of Operating Room Nurses, 65*(6), 1087–1098.

The purpose of this study was to determine whether a two-minute surgical hand scrub was as effective as a three-minute surgical hand scrub in reducing the number of bacteria on operating room staff hands.

A randomized cross-over design was used whereby 25 surgical staff were recruited from a children's hospital in California. The mean perioperative experience of those in the study groups was 6.7 years. Study participants were randomly assigned to two groups: group A completed a two-minute scrub for seven days. Group B performed a three-minute scrub for the same length of time. After this period, participants were allocated to the alternative scrub time. Existing hand-scrubbing guidelines were followed, and sinks were equipped with timers. Ten participants used 4 percent chlorhexidine gluconate, while 15 participants used 2 percent chlorhexidine gluconate.

Surgical gloves were worn for one hour, and the bacterial count was measured using the "glove juice sampling" procedure. Sample dilutions were then incubated for 48 hours. Study results revealed a higher bacterial count with the two-minute scrub compared with the three-minute scrub. However, these results were not statistically significant. Further research is needed to analyse other factors such as gender, hand size and multiple hospital sites, along with a larger sample size. These considerations will increase the reliability and validity of this study's findings.

CLEANING, DISINFECTION AND STERILIZATION

Cleaning

Cleaning is the removal of any foreign material (soilage or organic matter) from an object. A clean environment provides the background against which all patient care activities are carried out to the required standards of hygiene and asepsis. A clean environment inspires confidence in the hospital's ability to meet these standards. Hospital administrators are responsible for ensuring an adequate routine maintenance cleaning schedule. Those who are involved in direct patient care must ensure that any spillage is cleaned up immediately to remove the potential for microbial contamination as well as to prevent accidents. A good neutral detergent properly diluted is acceptable for basic cleaning. It is essential that nurses and other caregivers develop good work habits that aid in the process of maintaining a clean environment.

On nursing units, there are areas referred to as *clean* or *dirty utility rooms*. The clean area is used for storage of sterile and clean supplies and for set-up of treatment trays. The dirty area is used for dismantling reusable trays and preparing supplies for reprocessing. It also holds garbage containers for disposal of materials and is usually equipped with a "hopper" or clinical sink for the disposal of fluids and excretions (see Figure 32.2).

Supplies to be discarded should be placed securely in appropriate garbage containers according to agency policy. Equipment to be reprocessed should have gross soilage removed prior to its return to the appropriate department. Containers should be rinsed carefully (to avoid splashing) with cold water first, to remove any proteinaceous matter that may coagulate, then with copious amounts of hot water. This will achieve a degree of disinfection as long as gross soilage is removed. These procedures will vary somewhat from one facility to another, depending on which supplies and equipment are reusable and which are disposable. On no account should items such as full urine bags be placed in garbage containers destined for landfill. Neither should a bucket be used for draining urine bags from multiple patients. Bags must be emptied individually. All fluids must be discarded down a hopper or toilet before placing the container in the garbage. An alternative method of disposal such as incineration must be used when it is not possible to open containers safely.

Sanitization

Sanitization is generally used in public health terminology and usually refers to what in hospitals is considered low-level disinfection—the removal of vegetative bacteria, fungi

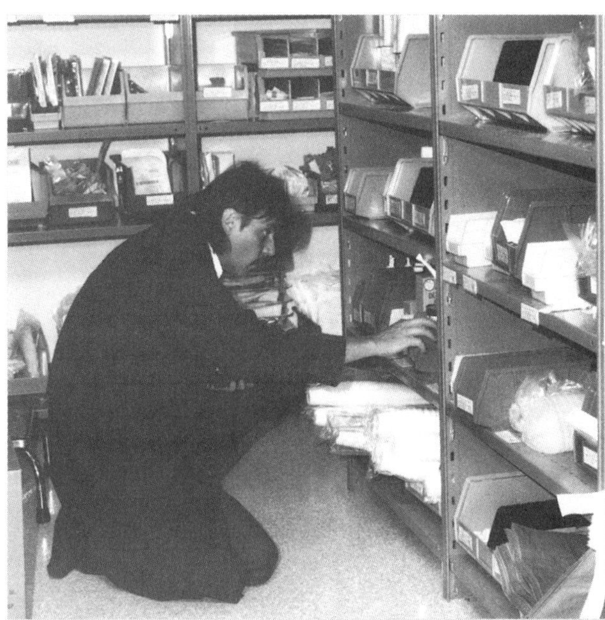

A clean utility room contains clean and sterile supplies.

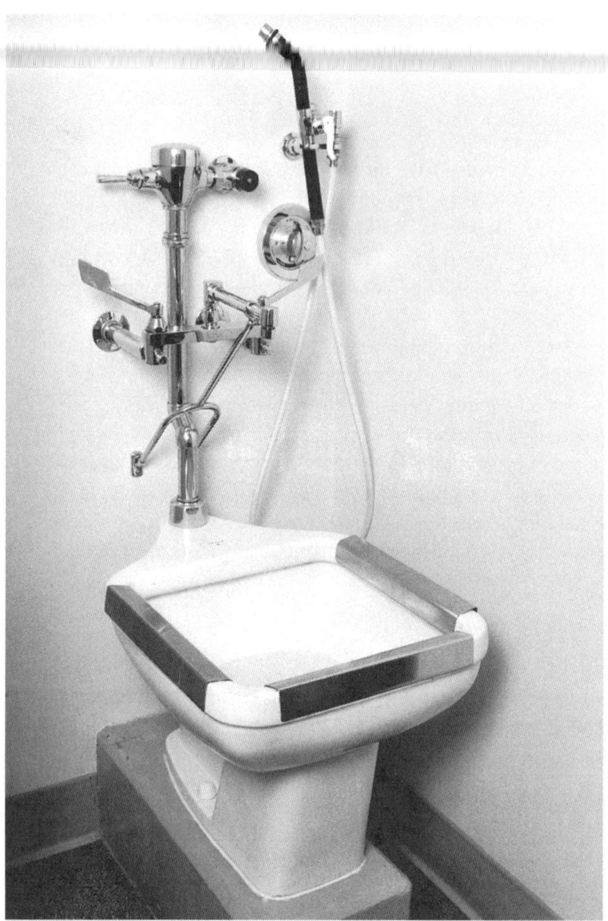

FIGURE 32.2 Hopper or clinical sink

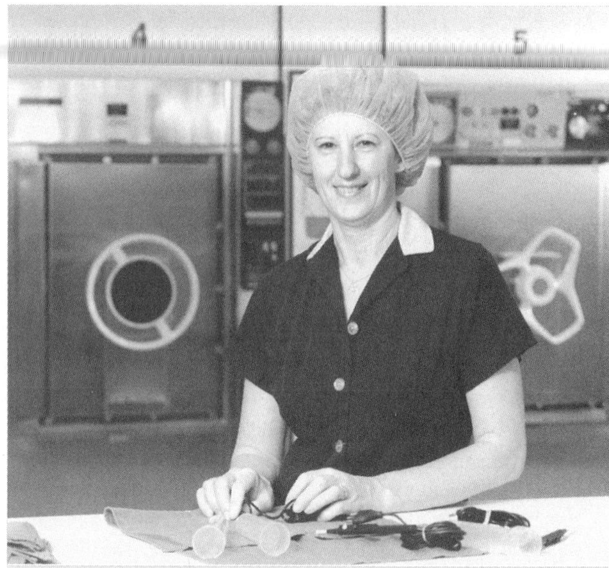

Many health agencies have separate departments in which supplies and equipment are cleaned and sterilized for use.

and some viruses. Sanitization is used, for example, in the reprocessing of bedpans. For many years, bedpan decontaminators functioned by flushing the contents, followed by a steam cycle of one minute or more. In the last few years an improved technology has been introduced. The bedpan and contents (stool, urine, blood, toilet paper) are placed in the decontaminator, which automatically flushes, then washes the utensil with warm water and detergent inside and out, rinses, steams and then allows a cool-down. Stainless steel or plastic utensils can be reprocessed in these machines and returned to circulation once they are dry, as long as the utensil is observed to be clean and the steam cycle lasts for one minute or more at 90°C. In some institutions, hoses have been attached to patient toilets for cleaning of soiled bedpans. This is *not* acceptable because of the difficulty involved in proper cleaning and because there is strong likelihood for aerosolization of stool particles onto the caregiver's clothing or into the environment.

Disinfection

Disinfection is a process wherein all pathogenic microorganisms are removed from an inanimate object with the exception of bacterial spores. Various levels of disinfection (low, intermediate and high) may be used for different items in the hospital, depending on usage. The degree of asepsis required will determine the choice of chemical disinfectant, but proper cleaning *must* be done first. An example of low-level disinfection was described in the sanitization of bedpans. An example of intermediate-level disinfection would be using an approved disinfectant on a hydrotherapy tank. High-level disinfection is applied to respiratory therapy equipment by pasteurization or reprocessing endoscopes with glutaraldehyde.

Sterilization

Sterilization is the complete destruction or elimination of all forms of microbial life. Any item that penetrates skin and mucous membrane must be sterile. This is achieved principally with steam under pressure, dry heat, ethylene oxide gas or chemicals. New technologies are emerging constantly.

MEDICAL ASEPSIS

Medical asepsis is practised to prevent the spread of infection. At a very basic level, medical asepsis is clean technique based on thorough hand-washing and the careful disposal of supplies and equipment. Proper hand-washing before and after giving care to each patient is *the* most important means of preventing the spread of infection from one patient to another. Medical asepsis also involves the use of techniques to protect health care providers, patients and others from known or potential pathogens through what is called universal or body substance precautions and isolation practices.

Body Substance Precautions

Throughout this century, but especially since the 1950s, emphasis has been placed on preventing the spread of disease from patient to patient in hospitals and long-term care

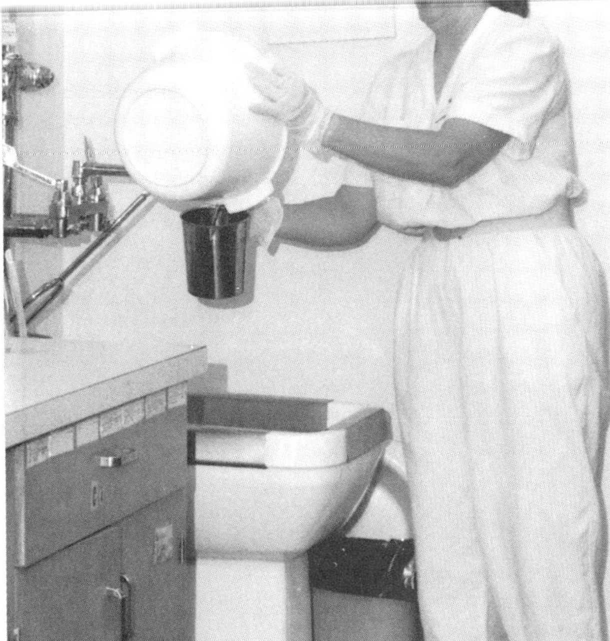

Body substance precautions by all health professionals and agency personnel are necessary to safeguard against infectious disease.

facilities. To this end, agencies established infection control committees to review the problem. The first infection control nurse position was established in England in 1960 because of concerns regarding how infection was transmitted from one end of a big open ward to another. The findings of these infection control pioneers led to renewed emphasis on the importance of simple activities such as hand-washing and the careful handling and disposal of all body secretions and excretions.

Concerns about safety for the health professional had focussed on immunization and ways to protect staff from tuberculosis and polio in the first half of the 20th century. Eventually in the 1970s, risks to health professionals from hepatitis B were recognized, and changes in specimen handling in particular were implemented. It was, however, the advent of HIV (responsible for AIDS) that once again forced another look at safety for the health care provider. Following the report in May 1987 of three health professionals who became infected with HIV in work-related incidents, the Centers for Disease Control (CDC) in Atlanta, Georgia, published their first guideline on **universal precautions** (CDC, 1987). This guideline stated that all blood from all people, as well as all body fluids (including cerebrospinal, pericardial, pleural, peritoneal, amniotic and synovial), should be treated as though potentially infectious. This guideline was supported by the Laboratory Centre for Disease Control (LCDC), Health Canada.

At the same time that this guideline was published (August 1987), infection control practitioners in Seattle and San Diego published their approach to the issue of

as body substance isolation (BSI). Many hospitals in Canada were quick to recognize the simplicity and practicality of this generic system, but chose to call it instead **body substance precautions** or **BSP**. Policies and procedures in infection control manuals and other resources were developed to describe the activities in the system. The guidelines for body substance precautions in the box on the next two pages are consistent with good infection control practice in any hospital. The associated techniques for implementing these guidelines are outlined in Procedures 32.1 and 32.2.

The Centres for Disease Control have published new guidelines for a revised protocol called **standard precautions**, which are a blending together of the major features of universal precautions and body substance precautions. At time of writing, it is unclear whether Canada will adopt these new guidelines.

Isolation Precautions

While the preceding activities are implemented to ensure proper practice of BSP, further precautions are taken to prevent transmission of infectious diseases. These include isolation for airborne and respiratory infection, protective isolation and multiple-drug resistance isolation.

ISOLATION FOR AIRBORNE AND RESPIRATORY INFECTIONS

Isolation precautions are implemented for patients with chickenpox, diphtheria, measles (rubeola, red), meningococcal disease, mumps, pertussis (whooping cough) including parapertussis, rabies and rubella (German measles). Children with respiratory symptoms or those suspected of having influenza, parainfluenza, respiratory syncytial virus (RSV), adenovirus or rhinovirus may be isolated routinely because it is sensible to contain respiratory secretions as much as possible, despite the fact that in some instances (as with RSV) there is little evidence that masks offer any protection. Children with *Haemophilus influenzae* infection also should be isolated until appropriately treated.

The term for this type of isolation may vary from one institution to another. Originally, either *strict* or *respiratory isolation* were used. More recently, the preferred term has been *contact isolation* (a modification). Some hospitals have combined respiratory and strict isolation using a new term, *restrictive isolation*. Others use the term *airborne precautions*. Occasionally, the term *AFB isolation* (acid-fast bacillus) has been used for patients with tuberculosis. The application of isolation precautions differs between adult and pediatric units. Nursing staff, including students, must become acquainted with the infection control and isolation protocols when receiving orientation to any new hospital or any new unit.

PROTECTIVE ISOLATION Patients who are severely immunocompromised may be placed in *protective isolation* to decrease the number of contacts they have with others in order to

Body Substance Precautions

1. Hand-Washing

Hands **MUST** be washed:

- before, during and after patient contact, as necessary
- before eating or handling food
- after using the toilet
- after removing gloves
- whenever the hands appear soiled
- whenever the health care worker's intact skin is penetrated.

NB: Neither jewellery nor nail polish should be worn by caregivers as both may harbour microorganisms, and hand-washing may not be as effective with jewellery in the way.

2. Hand Disinfection

Hands may be disinfected using an antiseptic hand rub made of chlorhexidine, isopropyl alcohol and an emollient. This combination is very effective in reducing the numbers of bacteria on the skin and may be less drying than actual hand-washing. It may be used when circumstances require hand-washing yet the hands appear superficially clean.

Procedure:

a) Apply 3–5 mL of antiseptic hand rub.
b) Massage vigorously all skin surfaces of hand and lower wrist until dry.

3. Gloves

a) Sterile gloves are worn to protect patients from contamination during an aseptic procedure. They also provide protection for the wearer.
b) Clean gloves are worn to protect the wearer from sources of contamination.
c) Gloves **MUST** be worn:
   - when touching body secretions and excretions
   - when touching mucous membrane
   - when touching nonintact skin
   - if the nurse's hands are chapped, cracked or have open lesions.
d) Hands must be washed and wedding band (if allowed by hospital policy) must be removed before donning gloves.
e) If a puncture occurs, remove gloves and wash hands before continuing.
f) Glove use must be task-specific.
g) Gloves must be removed and discarded and hands must be washed after every task is completed.

4. Gowns

a) Hand hygiene must be done before donning gown.
b) Gowns **MUST** be worn:
   - when caring for patients with communicable disease
   - when clothes are likely to be soiled from infective secretions or excretions
   - to prevent visible soilage of clothing
   - for certain procedures when the patient is highly compromised, for example, when changing dressings on severely burned patients (according to hospital policy).
c) Gowns are used only once in patient's room and then discarded in an appropriate receptacle.
d) Hand hygiene must be done when the gown is removed.

5. Masks (also see #6)

a) Masks are worn:
   - by health professionals to protect patient during aseptic procedures (policies may vary from agency to agency; in some instances, they may not be worn)
   - by *susceptible individuals* when entering room of patient in isolation for airborne disease (restrictive isolation)
   - by *personnel* to protect the patient who is immunocompromised (physician's order)
   - by *patients* in isolation when leaving room, as necessary.
b) Masks must be handled by strings (ties) only and removed completely when not needed.
c) Hand hygiene must be done when mask is removed.

6. Masks and Goggles (or face shields)

a) Masks and goggles are worn to protect the mucous membrane and conjunctiva whenever aerosolization of blood or other body fluids is likely.
b) Goggles and face shields may be decontaminated by washing under running water with detergent. After drying, wipe with buffered bleach, alcohol swab or other approved hospital disinfectant and leave to dry.

7. Garbage Handling and Disposal

The principle behind garbage disposal in institutions is that all garbage should be packaged so that it does not:

a) pose a risk to the workers
b) contaminate the environment.

It must remain safely packaged until it reaches its final destination, whether incinerator, autoclave or landfill. Policies will vary from one agency to another and from one jurisdiction to another.

8. Linen Disposal

The principle behind linen handling in institutions is that all linen must be safely packaged so that it does not:

a) pose a risk to the worker
b) contaminate the environment.

Avoid overfilling bags so that they may be secured properly for transport and subsequent handling. Laundry workers must wear protective attire where needed and procedures must ensure adequate processing so that properly disinfected linen is returned to service in all situations.

9. Disinfection—The Environment and Equipment

Maintaining cleanliness is the most important part of the disinfecting process. This is always the first step to be taken. All floors, whether visibly contaminated or simply being routinely cleaned, need only to be cleaned with the agency-supplied neutral cleaner and left to dry. Areas above the floor and all equipment must be cleaned first with the neutral cleaner and, where visibly contaminated, an agency-approved disinfectant must be applied. The

appropriate method, physically remove contaminating matter into garbage.

b) Ensure item or area appears clean, using neutral cleaner as necessary.
c) Apply disinfectant, leaving thin film.
d) Allow to dry.
e) Liquids may be poured down a hopper or toilet and the container then thoroughly rinsed before being returned to the patient or for reprocessing, as appropriate.

A popular disinfectant for general use in all areas is sodium dichloroisocyanurate (NaDCC). This is a buffered bleach solution prepared at approved strength for the appropriate task. Isopropyl alcohol 70% may be used alone in very small items, such as medication vials. Other disinfectants used in institutions may include:

a) chlorhexidine gluconate 0.5% with anti-rust
b) phenolic germicidal 2%
c) glutaraldehyde 2% or glutaraldehyde–phenate solution
d) quaternary ammonia compounds
e) hydrogen peroxide 3%–6%
f) povidone-iodine.

department must have grossly contaminating matter removed.

Disinfectants (for inanimate objects) and antiseptics (for skin) are not interchangeable.

10. Disposable Food Trays

These are not required for any patient. Rather, the standard is that used cutlery, crockery and trays, etc., must be reprocessed so they may be used safely by anyone. Automatic dishwashers are preferred over hand washing.

11. Manual Ventilation Units

These may accompany any patient being transported throughout the hospital if there is thought to be a risk of cardiac or respiratory arrest.

12. Sharps Disposal Containers

Sharps containers that are puncture-resistant must be readily available for disposal of used needles and sharps. Used needles **MUST NOT** be recapped, purposefully bent or broken.

PROCEDURE 32.1

Using Body Substance Precautions: Hand-Washing

Action	*Rationale*
1. Gather equipment: • liquid soap (agency-approved) • warm running water • fingernail stick • paper towel.	Soap and paper towel are usually provided in dispensers at each sink. Fingernail sticks (orangewood or plastic) should be found in the utility room.
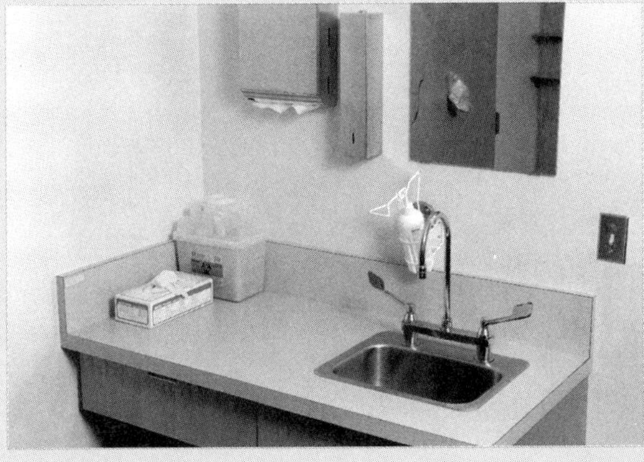	
2. Remove or push watch above the wrist. Long sleeves should be well above the wrists.	Cleanses the wrist area under the band and prevents the watch or the sleeves from becoming wet or contaminated.
3. Stand with clothing clear of sink.	Prevents transfer onto uniform of microorganisms harboured in sink.

continued on next page

PROCEDURE 32.1 *continued*

Action	*Rationale*
4. Turn on the taps and adjust water flow to a comfortable temperature. Avoid splashing; leave water running.	Prevents the spread of contaminants from hands to taps. Hot water depletes natural oils and causes drying of skin. Microorganisms in the sink are transferred onto the nurse's uniform through splashing. Running water washes away microorganisms.
5. Wet hands and wrists, keeping the hands pointing downward and lower than the elbows. 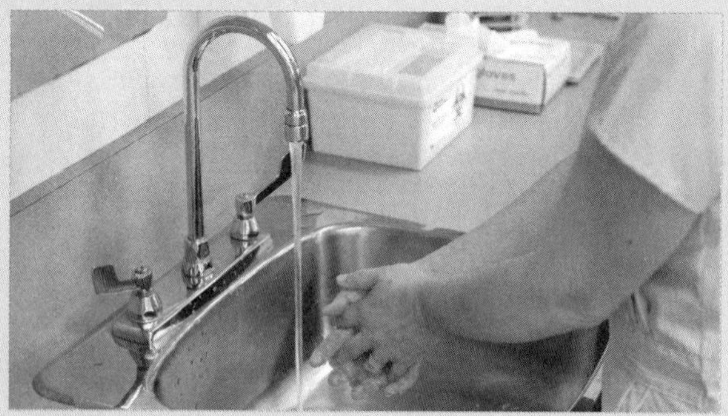	The hands and fingertips are more contaminated than the elbows. Allows water to flow from cleanest to dirtiest area.
6. Apply soap and massage all skin surfaces of hands and lower wrist vigorously for 10–15 seconds.	Dislodges and suspends contaminants in the lather.
7. Clean fingertips and fingernails thoroughly. Use a fingernail stick as necessary. 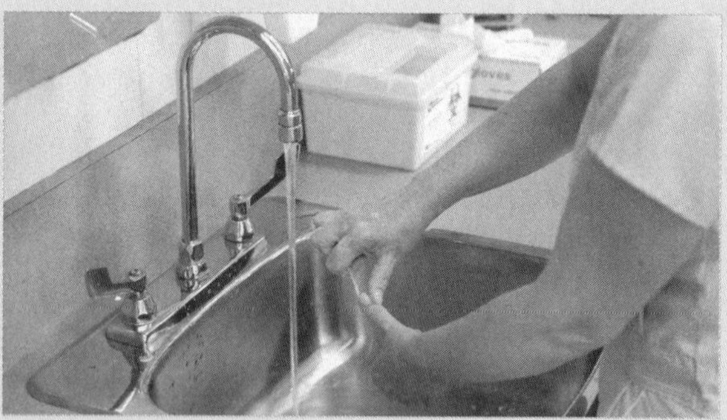	Removes microbes that lodge around and under the nails.
8. Rinse thoroughly and dry hands, holding hands downward. Take care not to abrade the skin. Discard towel. 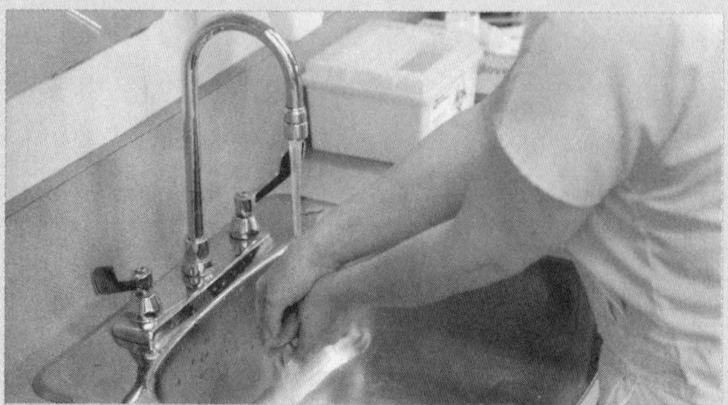	Contaminants and microbes are washed away with flowing water. Drying the hands completely but gently prevents chapping and cracking.
9. Use paper towel to turn off tap.	Prevents contamination of clean hands with microbes harboured on the taps.
10. When not at work, use hand lotion liberally if problems with dry skin develop.	Replaces moisture lost during handwashing and thereby maintains skin integrity.

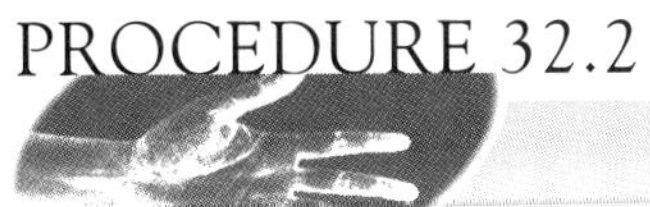

PROCEDURE 32.2 Using Body Substance Precautions: Applying and Removing Mask, Gown and Clean Gloves

Action	*Rationale*
A. Application	
1. Obtain mask, gown and gloves.	Masks are supplied in boxes kept in a central area such as the clean utility room or outside the patient's room. Gowns may be made of reusable waterproof fabric or disposable paper. They open in the back and have ties at the neck and waist. Clean gloves are supplied in boxes kept in the clean or soiled utility room and, in some agencies, in patients' rooms.
2. To apply mask, first bring upper strings above the ears and then tie them at the back of the head. Adjust mask to fit over the nose and under the chin. If nurse is wearing glasses, top edge of mask should fit under them. Tie lower strings at the back of the neck. Wash hands. 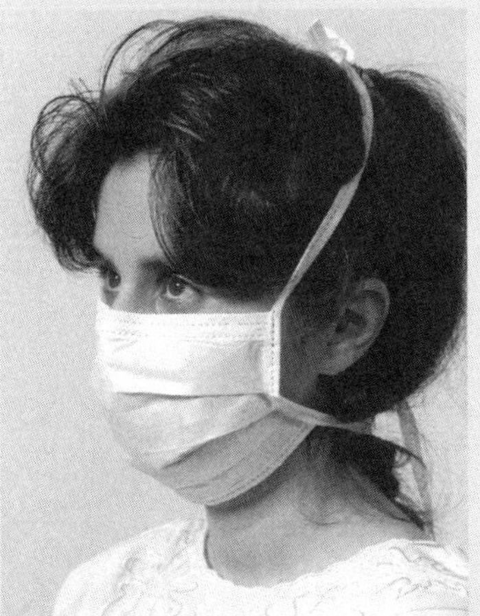	Most masks have a metal strip that helps to secure the mask to the nose. This reduces fogging of glasses.
3. Put on a clean gown and fasten the neck ties. Overlap the gown at the back and tie it together at the waist. 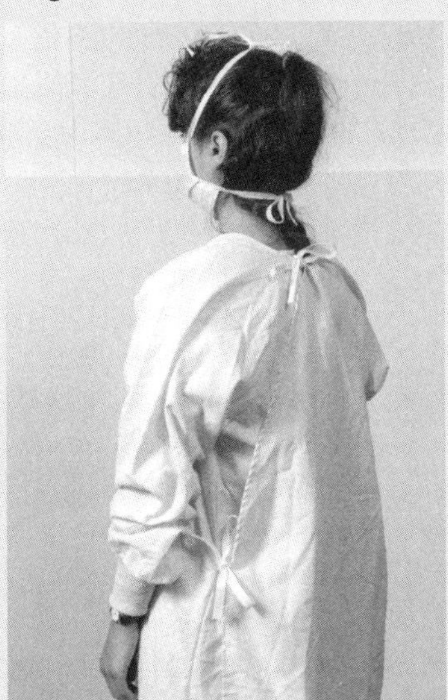	Ensures that clothing is covered to avoid inadvertent contamination.
4. Apply clean gloves in a convenient manner, making sure the cuff covers the wrists and wristwatch.	Prevents contamination of hands, wrists and watch.

continued on next page

PROCEDURE 32.2 *continued*

Action	*Rationale*
B. Removal	
1. Prior to removing gloves, untie the waist ties of the gown. To remove the first glove, grasp the cuff with the other gloved hand and pull the glove over the fingers, turning it inside out. Hold the glove in the fingers of the gloved hand.	Prevents touching the outside of either glove. Allows the first glove to be contained in the second glove when removed.

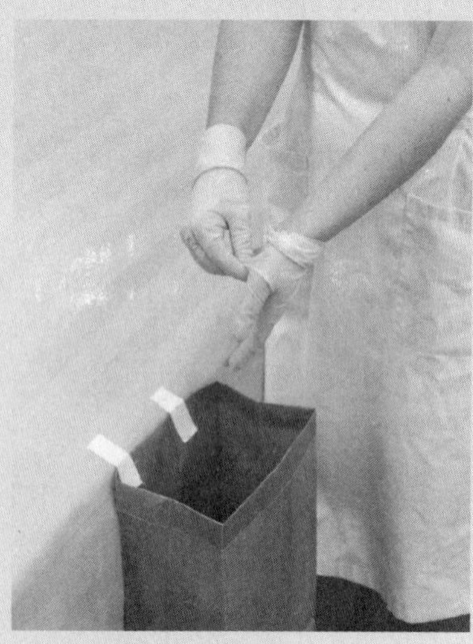

2. To remove the second glove, slide two fingers of the ungloved hand inside the cuff and roll the cuff downward onto the hand. With thumb and fingers, grasp the inside of the glove and peel it off inside out over the first glove. Discard into appropriate container.	Avoids touching the outside of the gloves with bare hands.

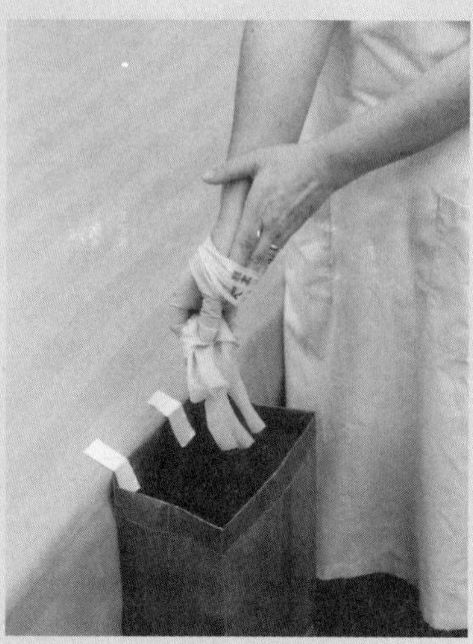

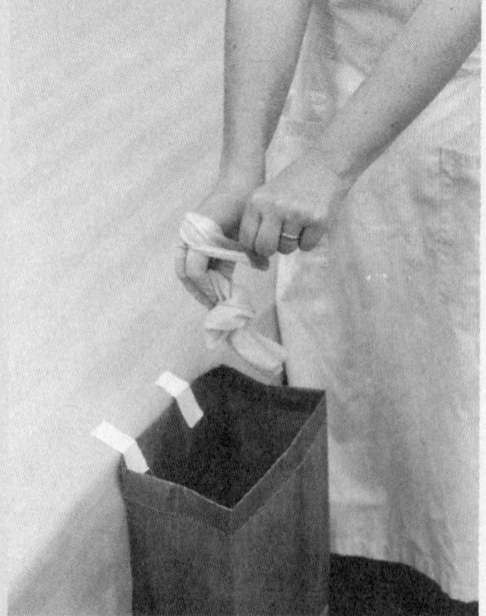

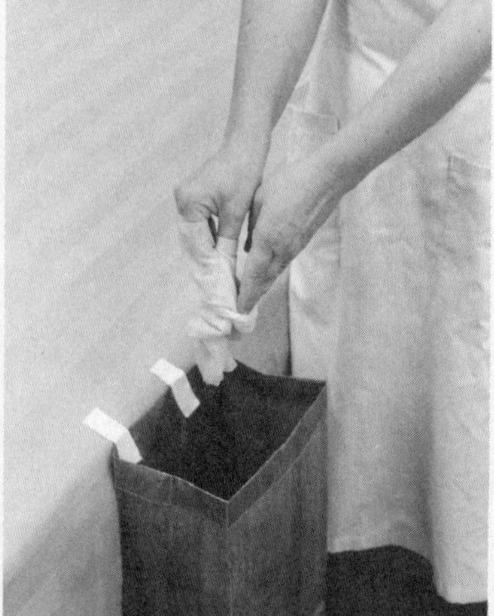

3. Untie neck ties of gown and, without touching the outside of gown, slide your hands into the sleeves, pull the gown off the shoulders and slip out of it.	Prevents transmission of microorganisms from the outside of the gown to the hands.

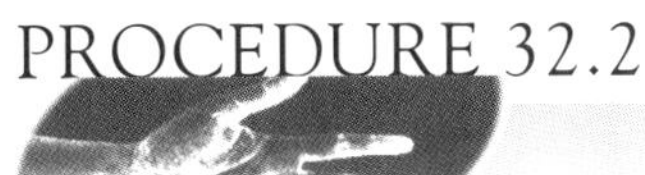

PROCEDURE 32.2 *continued*

Action	Rationale
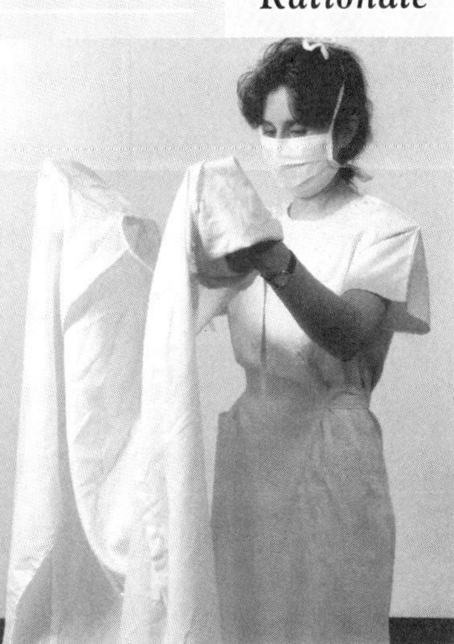 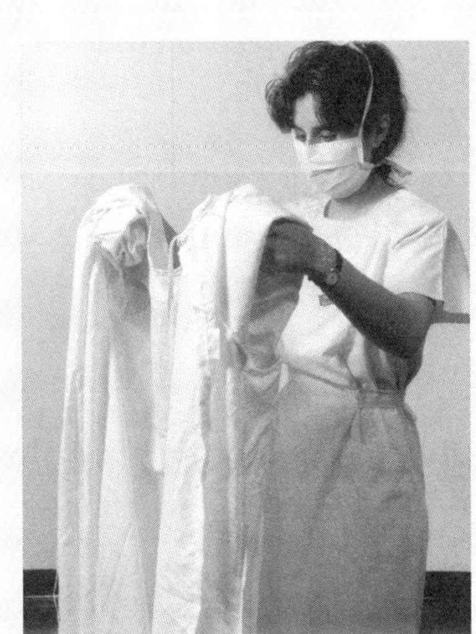	
4. While still holding the gown on the inside, fold the outside surfaces inward and roll it into a ball. Discard into a laundry bag or garbage container.	As above.
5. To remove the mask, handle only the ties/straps. Unfasten them and discard the mask into a garbage container.	The central part of the mask is dirty; the ties are clean.
6. Wash hands thoroughly.	Reduces spread of microorganisms.

reduce the chances of acquiring exogenous infection. However, the value of this practice is in some doubt and it is not done in all hospitals.

MULTIPLE-DRUG RESISTANCE ISOLATION Some bacteria have developed a high degree of resistance to antibiotics that at one time were effective against them. One of the most common of these bacteria is methicillin-resistant *Staphylococcus aureus* (MRSA). Another common drug-resistant bacterium is vancomycin-resistant enterococci (VRE). Many hospitals now are adopting a modified form of strict isolation referred to as *multiple-drug resistance precautions* to prevent these microorganisms from joining the resident microbial flora in the hospital. Following are some common elements of multiple-drug resistance precautions:

- patient is placed in a single room or with cohorts (others with the same resistant organism)
- patient is confined to the room except for diagnostic procedures
- staff are required to don gowns for direct contact
- masks should be considered if the patient has the organism in sputum and is coughing or has a desquamating skin condition
- gloves should be worn for all procedures requiring direct touch (some institutions do not require this, as proper hand-washing at all times obviates their need; in any case, hands must be washed after gloves are removed)
- visitors do not need protective attire, but should be required to wash hands properly on leaving and prohibited from visiting other parts of the hospital
- equipment and supplies in the room must be kept to a minimum, and items such as stethoscopes should be dedicated to the room, if possible
- items removed from the room must be wiped down with disinfectant
- no special precautions are required for garbage, dirty laundry or meal service.

Decolonization may be instituted by having patients whole-body bathed daily with a hospital-approved antiseptic soap. In instances of MRSA, mupirocin ointment may be applied to the anterior nares and around any *in situ* devices.

These precautions may vary from one agency to another; nursing staff should follow the protocols specific to their own facility, as outlined by the infection control department. Figure 32.3 gives an example of a precaution form that is placed outside a patient's door.

As a protective measure, hospitals are now requiring that all inpatient admissions be screened for MRSA and VRE. Figure 32.4 shows one example of a screening tool.

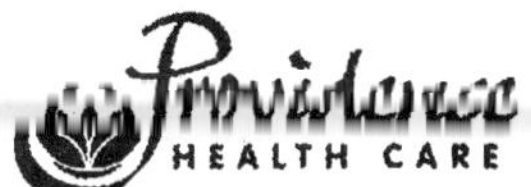

St. Paul's Hospital

MULTIPLE DRUG RESISTANCE PRECAUTIONS

ROOM NO: ________

VISITORS

- **PLEASE SEE CHARGE NURSE ON FIRST VISIT FOR INSTRUCTION**
- Visit patient only. Do not go to other areas of the hospital

PERSONNEL

- **PLEASE SEE CHARGE NURSE ON FIRST VISIT FOR INSTRUCTIONS**
- **INFORM INFECTION CONTROL NURSE WHEN PRECAUTIONS IMPLEMENTED**

ROOM

- DOOR - may remain partially open unless otherwise indicated - refer to page 2 of the protocol.

PRECAUTIONS

- Body Substance Precautions apply in all cases.

PROTECTIVE APPAREL:

1. **MASK** - in specific situations for MRSA only - see Infection Control Manual - Protocol ICM2004 - Page 4.

   Mask Required YES ☐ NO ☐

2. **GOWN** * - is to be worn with all direct patient contact

3. **GLOVES** * - are to be worn when having direct contact with the patient and / or items used by the patient

*** Read specific protocol for additional information as to when gown and gloves are required**

OTHER:

1. **STETHOSCOPE AND TOURNIQUET** - are to be left in the room at all times

2. **DISPOSABLE NON MERCURY THERMOMETER** to be used.

3. **CLEANING AGENT** - Presept (buffered bleach tablet - 2.5 Gram - to one liter of water)

Protocols for multiple drug resistant organisms are located in the Infection Control Manual :

- ICM2004 and ICM2004A - Methicillin (Cloxacillin) Resistant Staphylococcus aureus (MRSA)
- ICM2008 - Vancomycin Resistant Enterococci (VRE)

Form No. NF134 (Rev.07/98)

FIGURE 32.3 Precaution form that is placed outside a patient's door

SOURCE: St. Paul's Hospital, Vancouver, B.C.

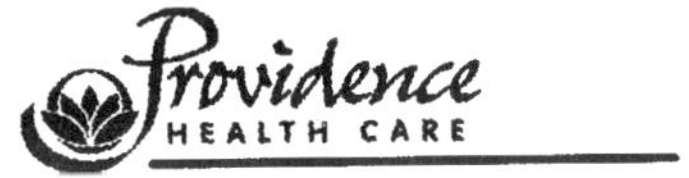

1081 Burrard Street, Vancouver, B.C. V6Z 1Y6
(604) 682-2344

Infection Control

INPATIENT ADMISSION SCREENING FOR ANTIBIOTIC RESISTANT BACTERIA

Directions for form use:

1. Both questions to be asked of all inpatient admissions.
2. Action is required if the response to either or both questions is "Yes" or "Unknown".
3. White copy to remain on the chart.
4. Canary copy, once the is form completed is sent to the Infection Control Nurse c/o Lab.

PART 1: QUESTIONS : for all inpatient admissions:

1. Have you, in the past 3 months been in a hospital (other than St. Paul's) for 48 hours or longer ?

Patient Answer (Circle one)	Action
Yes	Screening required
Unknown *	Screening required
No	No action

2. Have you ever been advised that you were infected or colonized with MRSA and /or VRE ?

Patient Answer (Circle one)	Action
Yes	1. Private room required 2. Multiple Drug Resistant Precautions 3. Screening required
Unknown *	Screening required
No	No action

*** Patient does not understand or does not know. When it is not appropriate to question the patient immediately (eg. in pain or unconscious) send the form to the unit to be completed as soon as possible after admission.**

SCREENING: Nursing staff responsible for obtaining the following swabs for delivery to Lab within 12 hours of the patient's admission.

Organism	Swabs required. Request specific screen for each swab
MRSA	1. Anterior nares (1 swab for both nostrils) 2. Swab of perineum 3. Swab of any open, draining wound, skin lesion or sore
VRE	1. Rectal swab - soiled with faeces

Form completed by: ☐ Admitting Clerk ☐ Nurse Date: ____________

PART 2 - Patients who answer "No" to both questions but who on admission to a Nursing unit are determined to be at increased risk for MRSA - should have swabs obtained for MRSA screen (as outlined above).

Additional information related to individuals at increased risk for MRSA and the protocol in general - refer to the Infection Control Manual - Protocol ICM 2010

Form NF086 (Rev. 11/98) 220079

White Copy : Chart
Canary Copy : Infection Control Nurse

FIGURE 32.4 Antibiotic-resistant bacteria screening tool

SOURCE: St. Paul's Hospital, Vancouver, B.C.

Maintaining Psychosocial Well-Being under Isolation

Patients for whom isolation precautions are being maintained have special needs for emotional support. They are separated from other patients, are frequently in a private room and contact with people is limited. Some patients attach a moral significance to their disease; they feel unworthy and think they are creating extra work for the nurse. Feelings of unworthiness, social isolation and sensory deprivation can seriously affect well-being.

Providing education to patients under isolation precautions is crucial to care. Most people want to participate in their own therapy; moreover, the success of medical asepsis is largely dependent upon the patient's willingness to help. The nurse's explanations are based on the needs of the patient to understand the reason for the various precautionary measures, the possible causes of the infection, how to provide protection from further infection and how to help prevent infection in others. The spread of pathogens from the respiratory tract of patients is thought to be best controlled by teaching safe hygiene practices, which include frequent hand-washing under running water. A patient with a pulmonary infection is taught to use several thicknesses of paper handkerchief to cover the nose and mouth when sneezing or coughing. Also, covered waterproof containers are provided for sputum samples. Facilities are available for the adequate disposal of paper handkerchiefs.

Diversional activities and sensory stimulation are very important in the care of patients under isolation precautions. Such activities should be designed so that they do not interfere with the barrier technique, yet still meet the patient's needs. A television set may help to relieve monotony, and items such as magazines, playing cards or hobby materials can be made safe after they are removed from the contaminated area. However, in some instances they may be discarded. Keeping the room clean and providing space for personal items such as cards and pictures will help create a pleasant environment. Taking time to listen and talk to patients or providing comfort measures such as a back rub will help patients to feel less isolated and better about themselves.

SURGICAL ASEPSIS

Surgical asepsis, or sterile technique, is the method of asepsis carried out to keep an object or area free of microorganisms. In the operating room, a birthing room or a specialized diagnostic area, basic infection control practice specifies that all items transecting the patient's skin (scalpel), or entering a body cavity or tissue (instruments), are sterile.

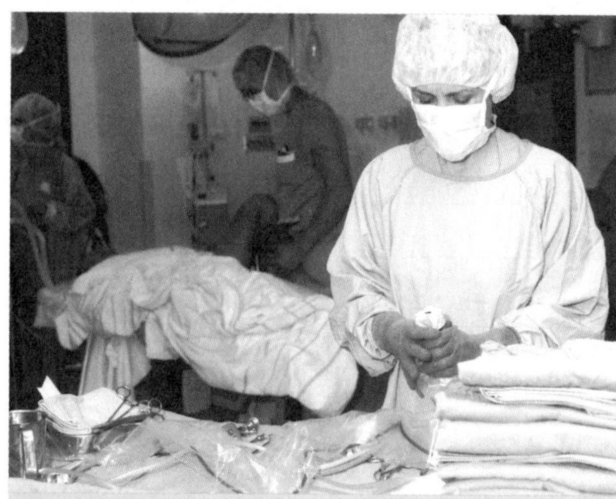

Sterile technique is carried out in the operating room.

Basic Guidelines for Surgical Asepsis

1. A sterile field must be set up only immediately before use to help ensure sterility.
2. Hands and wrists must be washed thoroughly for one minute, preferably with an antiseptic agent such as chlorhexidine gluconate (CHG) or povidone-iodine.
3. The table on which the sterile field is set up must be clean and dry.
4. A sterile package is considered to be unsterile if it passes its expiration date, has been previously opened or is wet. If there is no expiration date, the package must be seen to be intact.
5. The only objects that can touch sterile objects or the sterile field are other sterile objects. If touched by a clean or contaminated object, or by an object of questionable sterility, the sterile object or field must be considered unsterile. If there is any doubt about an object's sterility, it must be considered contaminated.
6. Sterile objects that are out of the range of vision or below waist level are considered to be unsterile. A sterile field must never be left unattended. Edges of a sterile wrapper or towel that hang down over the edge of the table are considered contaminated. The top surface will remain sterile.
7. The outer, approximately 2.5 cm, edge of a sterile field is considered unsterile. This area may be touched with clean hands.
8. Sterile objects are contaminated by transfer of airborne microorganisms. Avoid activities that create air currents such as talking, sneezing, reaching over the sterile field or shaking drapes vigorously.
9. Pour sterile solutions so that they do not splash on the field. When a sterile object or field lying on an unsterile surface becomes wet or damp, it is no longer sterile. Microbes can migrate from the unsterile surface to the sterile field through capillary action.
10. Meticulous aseptic technique must be practised when performing all sterile procedures. A break in technique can lead to infection.

Not only must the set-up procedure ensure that all supplies and equipment used are kept sterile, but the actions of all personnel involved must be such that the sterile field is

ducible minimum during the entire procedure.

Surgical asepsis is also practised at the bedside during procedures that involve entry into a body part or cavity or penetration of skin and mucous membranes. Some of the more common procedures performed by nurses that require sterile technique are administration of injections, insertion of intravenous catheters, urinary catheterization, tracheo-bronchial suctioning and dressing changes. A sterile field is created with sterile equipment, towels and drapes. Sterile gloves or forceps are used to maintain asepsis. In the fol-

sterile technique in performing procedures at the bedside. The student wishing information on surgical asepsis in the operating room should refer to a text on operating room procedure. Basic guidelines for surgical asepsis are listed in the preceding box. The techniques for putting on sterile gloves and setting up a sterile field are outlined in Procedures 32.3 and 32.4.

PROCEDURE 32.3 Donning and Removing Sterile Gloves

Action	Rationale
A. Applying Gloves	
1. Select correct glove size.	
2. Wash and dry hands thoroughly.	Removes transient microorganisms and reduces microbe growth in a dark, moist environment.
3. Carefully open the outer package; remove the inner package and place it on a clean, dry surface.	Prevents the inner package from inadvertently opening and becoming contaminated.

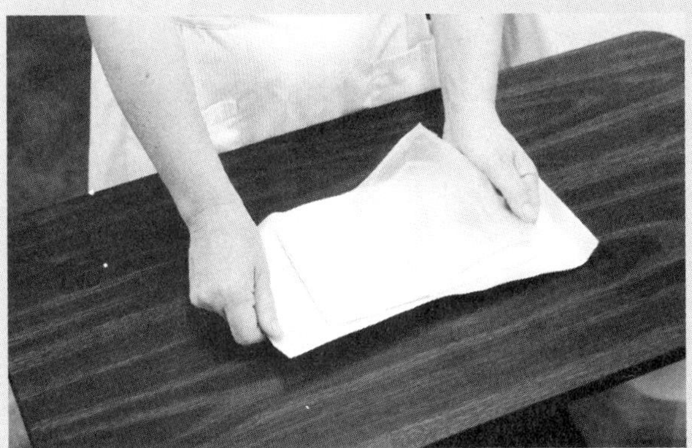

Action	Rationale
4. Open the inner package, touching only the 2.5-cm border. Pull the wrapper gently but firmly to keep it flat. Gloves will be positioned so that the left-hand glove lies on the left and the right-hand glove on the right. Palms will face upward, with thumbs to the outside.	Creates a sterile field for the gloves. If the wrapper falls back to its folded position after being touched, the gloves and inside of wrapper may become contaminated.

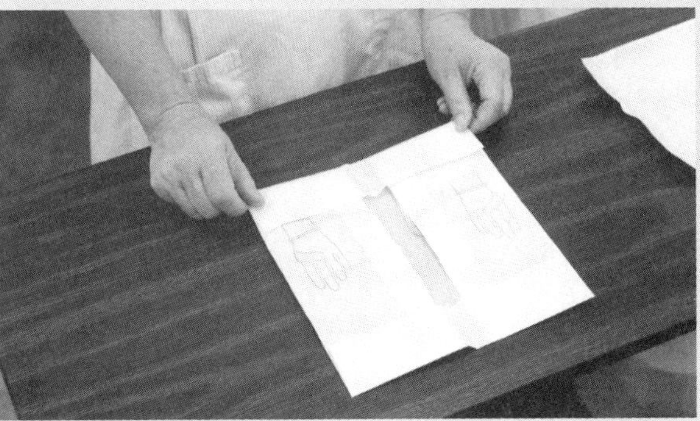

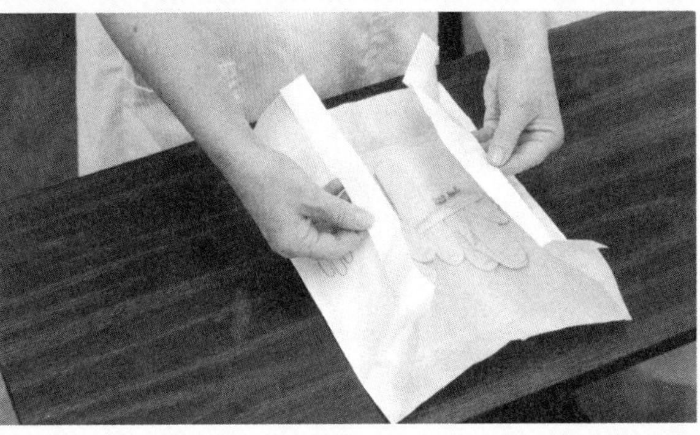

continued on next page

PROCEDURE 32.3 continued

Action	Rationale
5. With the dominant hand* grasp the glove for the nondominant hand by the cuffed edge, lift it from the wrapper and hold it away from your body. 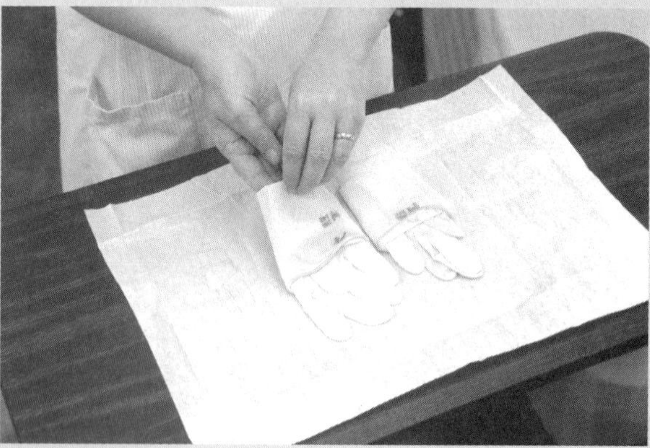	Prevents contamination of the sterile glove by contact with unsterile objects.
6. Slide the nondominant hand into the glove and pull it on. Do not adjust the cuff or placement of fingers inside the glove. 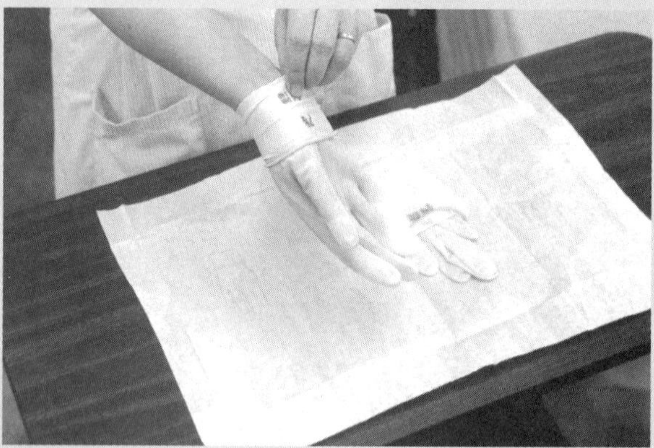	This is accomplished more easily when both gloves are on.
7. Slide the fingers of the gloved hand under the cuff of the remaining glove, and lift it up and away from the wrapper. 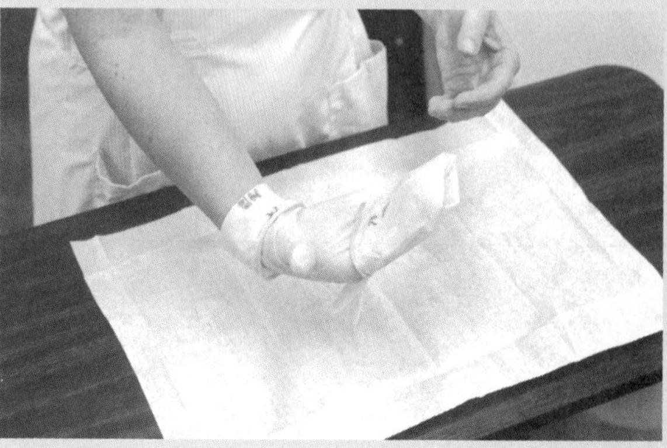	Maintains sterile-to-sterile contact. The cuff protects the gloved fingers.

* If the nurse is right-handed, the left glove is put on first; if left-handed, vice versa.

PROCEDURE 32.3 *continued*

Action	*Rationale*
8. Carefully slide the dominant hand into the glove, keeping the thumb abducted and pulling the cuff up over the wrist with the nondominant (gloved) hand, which is still under the cuff.	Avoids contact with exposed hand.
The cuff of the nondominant glove may then be pulled up over the wrist by slipping the fingers of the now gloved dominant hand under the cuff of the remaining glove and carefully pulling it up over the wrist.	Maintains the technique of sterile surface to sterile surface.
Adjust both gloves, touching only sterile areas.	Smooth fit is necessary for dexterity.

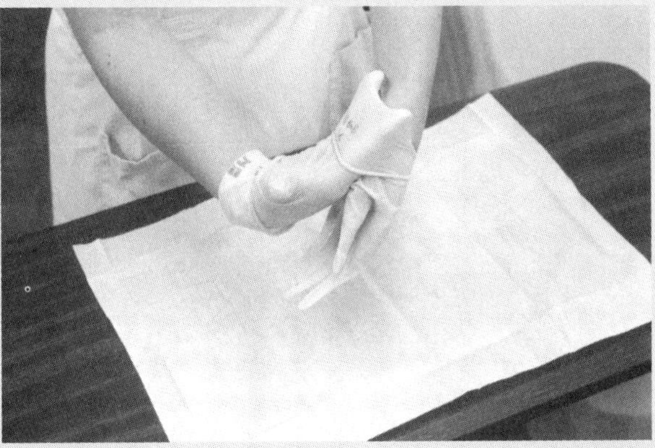

Action	*Rationale*
9. Keep gloved hands in full view and above waist level at all times.	Prevents unintentional contamination.

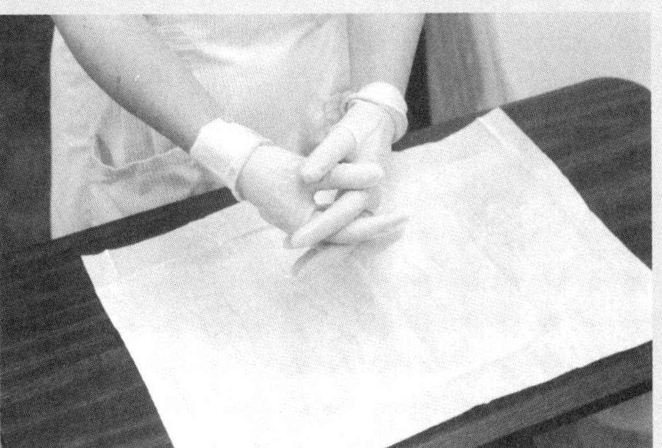

B. Removing Gloves

Action	*Rationale*
1. Grasp the outside of one glove near the wrist and pull it over the hand. The glove will turn inside out.	Prevents transfer of organisms on the gloves (from contact with patient's skin or body substances) to the nurse's hands.
2. Hold on to the glove with the still-gloved hand or discard it with other supplies.	If held, the first glove will be encased in the second glove when removed.
3. Slip the fingers of the ungloved hand inside the remaining glove and pull it off by turning it inside out.	Prevents contamination of the nurse's hands with organisms on the outside of the gloves.
4. Discard gloves and other equipment per agency policy.	Promotes cleanliness and safety in the workplace by limiting the transmission of microorganisms.
5. Wash hands thoroughly.	Removes organisms on the skin.

PROCEDURE 32.4

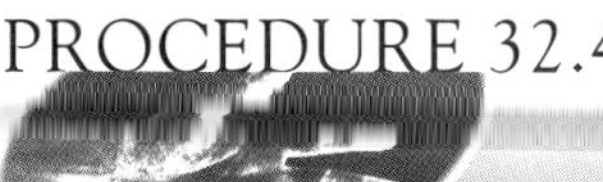

Setting Up a Sterile Field

Action	Rationale
1. Prepare the sterile field immediately before the procedure.	Prevents unnecessary exposure to air and contaminants.
2. Gather necessary supplies and equipment. Check packages for date of expiration, tears, punctures or wetness. Check the solution container for date of expiration.	Promotes efficiency and avoids having to leave the sterile field unattended. Checking packages ensures sterility.
3. Clear a surface area for the sterile field and make sure it is dry. If using an over-bed table, adjust the height to waist level.	Avoids contamination with unsterile objects. Sterile objects held below waist level are considered contaminated.
4. Don a mask if required by agency policy for the procedure.	Reduces the risk of spreading microbes from the nurse's mouth and respiratory tract to the sterile field.
5. Wash hands thoroughly.	Reduces the spread of microorganisms.
6. Create the sterile field.	
Using a sterile drape:	
• Open the outer covering using proper guidelines.	
• Pick up the corner that is folded back, touching only the outer 2.5-cm edge.	The entire 2.5-cm border of a drape is considered unsterile and may be touched with bare hands.
• Lift the drape from the wrapper, hold it away from your body, and let it open without touching any unsterile object. Discard the wrapper with your other hand.	
• Grasp the adjacent corner of the drape with the other hand and lay it on the table. Position the drape on the table, without leaning or reaching over it.	Facilitates positioning the drape on the table. Avoids contamination by air transmission of organisms.
Using a commercially prepared tray:	
• Centre the tray on the work area and open it using the guidelines for an envelope-wrapped package.	Use of these techniques maintains sterility of the field.

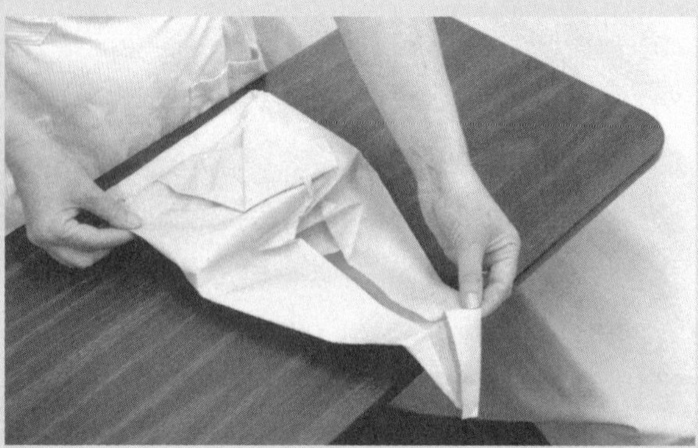

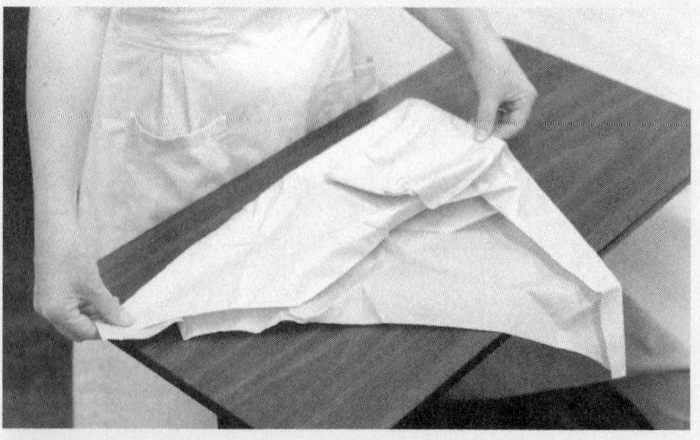

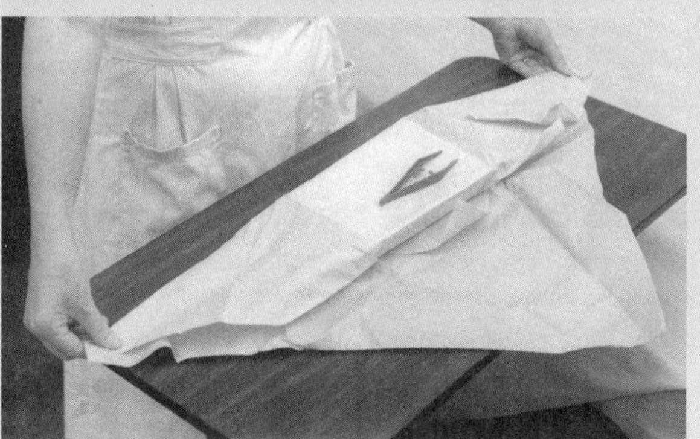

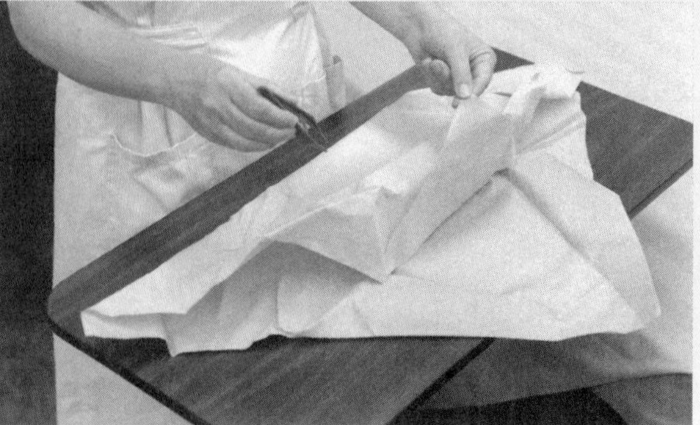

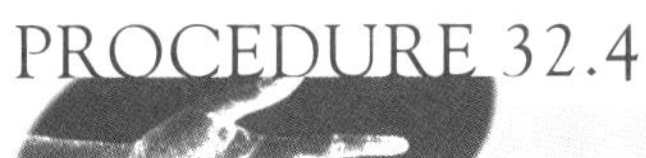

PROCEDURE 32.4 *continued*

Action	*Rationale*
On top of the inner flap, there will be a transfer forcep which must be removed before opening the flap.	Prevents tray from falling on the floor.
• Flatten the wrapper by gently pulling on the sides, touching only the 2.5-cm border.	Prevents corners of the wrapper from falling back on the sterile field and contaminating it.
• Position the wrapper on the table.	
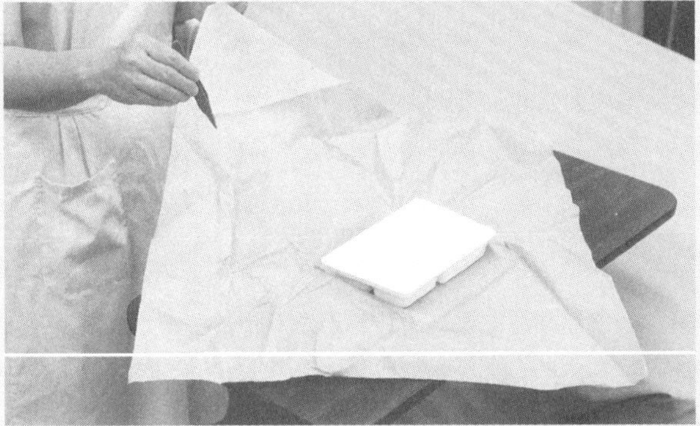	 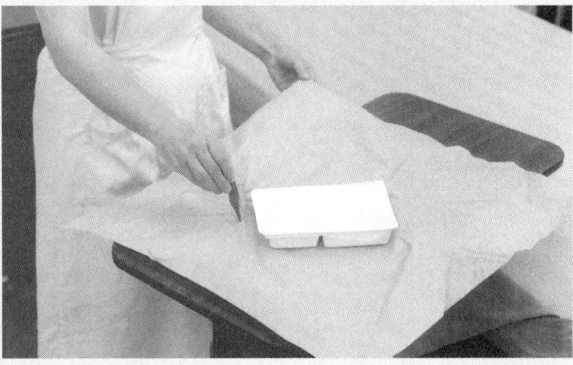
• Arrange items on the tray, placing the handles of the forceps on the 2.5-cm border of the sterile fields.	Prevents contamination of the sterile field when forceps are picked up with bare hands.
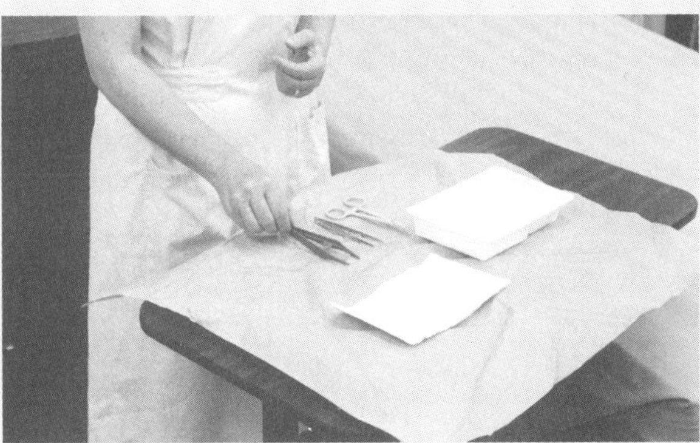	
7. Add supplies to the sterile field as needed.	
• Open packages.	
• Drop small items onto the field from a distance of about 15 cm or use transfer forceps.	Prevents contamination of the sterile field with the outer wrapper.
 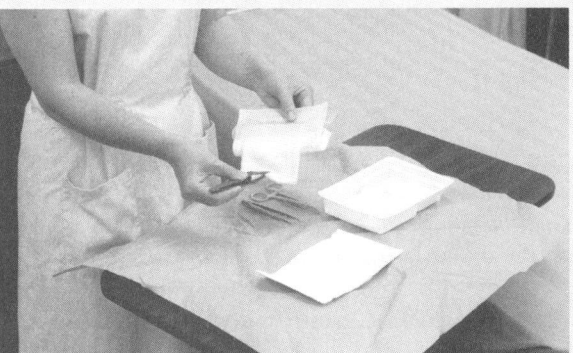	

continued on next page

PROCEDURE 32.4 *continued*

Action	Rationale
• Add heavier items, such as basins or scissors, by holding one edge of the item in its wrapper and covering the hand and wrist with the corners of the wrapper. 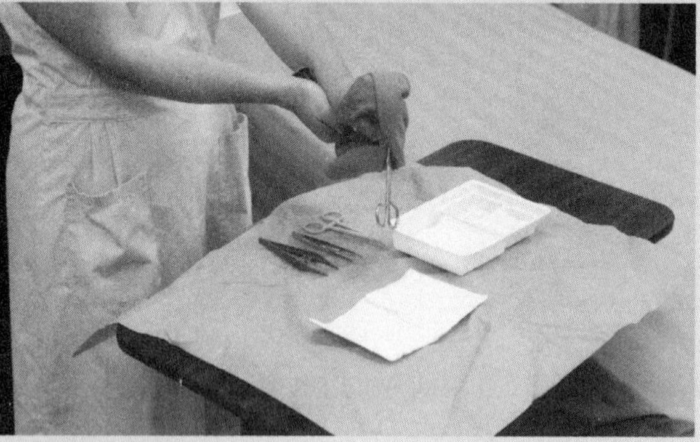	The wrapper provides a barrier between the sterile item and the hand.
• Be sure to place the items within the 2.5-cm border.	Ensures sterility by avoiding contact with an unsterile area.
8. Pour sterile solution.	
• Remove the cap and hold it in the hand or place it on a flat surface, inside up.	Prevents the inside of the cap from becoming contaminated.
• Hold the bottle with the label facing upward.	Avoids wetting and possibly obliterating the label.
• Hold the bottle outside the edge of the sterile field and about 10 cm above the receiving container.	Prevents contamination of the sterile field.
• Pour the solution carefully. Avoid splashing. 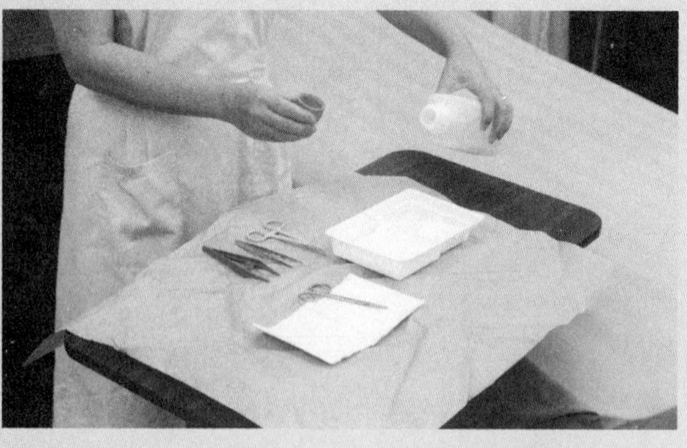	Moisture facilitates the movement of microbes from the unsterile table to the sterile field through capillary action.
• Grasp the outside of the cap and recap the bottle securely.	Maintains sterility of the solution.

Preparing the Patient

In addition to preparing the patient for the specific procedure, the nurse should also explain sterile technique and enlist the patient's participation in ensuring sterility. The patient is asked to avoid touching sterile areas, to avoid sudden movement of body parts covered by the drapes and to refrain from talking, sneezing or coughing over the sterile field. If there is a chance that breathing or coughing may transmit airborne organisms, the patient should be given a mask to wear. If the procedure is anticipated to last a long time, the patient's comfort needs should be attended to first. For instance, the nurse may administer pain medication, assist the patient to the bathroom, or help the patient assume as comfortable a position as possible.

Assembling Equipment and Setting Up a Sterile Field

The nurse begins by gathering all the equipment and supplies that will be needed for the procedure. In most hospitals today, commercially prepared trays or kits are provided that

Guidelines for Opening Sterile Packages

sterile that appear damp or whose wrappers are damaged.

Peel Packs

1. Grasp the tabs above the sealed edge.
2. Peel edges apart to break seal.

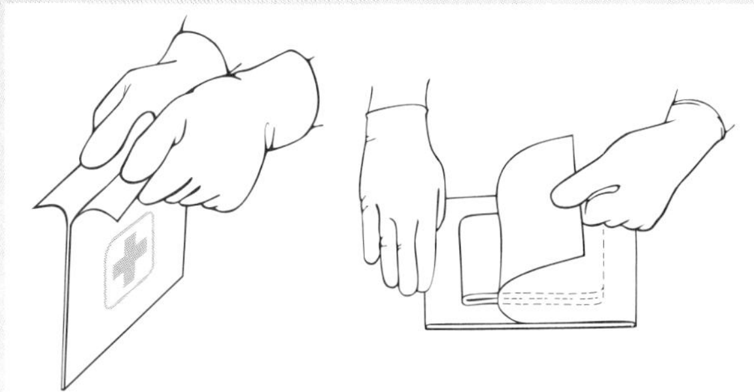

3. Package may be placed on a flat surface and top wrapper removed to expose contents completely, creating a small sterile field for contents of package.
4. Contents may be dropped on another sterile field.

Peelback Containers

1. Hold the bottom of the container with one hand.
2. Grasp corner tab of peelback top; pull to remove top.

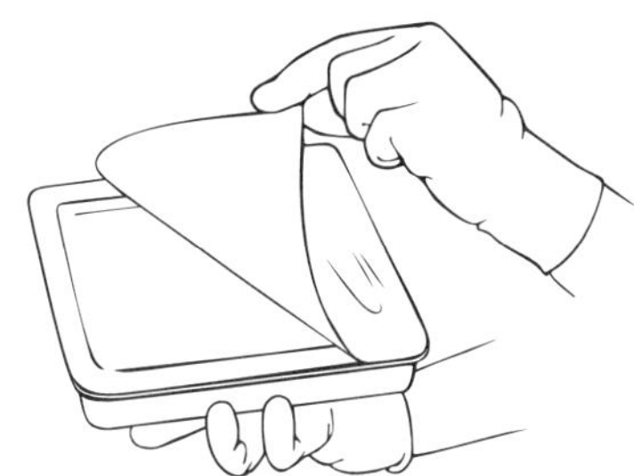

3. Container may be used as self-contained sterile field for contents.
4. Sterile solution may be added if needed, or contents may be placed on another sterile field and container used to hold sterile solution.

Envelope-Wrapped Package on a Surface

1. Centre the package on the work area so the outer flap of the wrapper faces away from you.
2. Reach around, not over, the package and open the flap, pulling it away from you. Touch only the outside of the wrap.
3. Open flaps in sequence, using right hand for right flap and left hand for left flap. Touch outside surface only. Avoid reaching over package.
4. Open inner flap by pulling turned-down corner towards you. If flap is large, step away from the table so wrapper does not contact your uniform. If inner corner is not turned down, touch outside of wrap only, as in step 3.

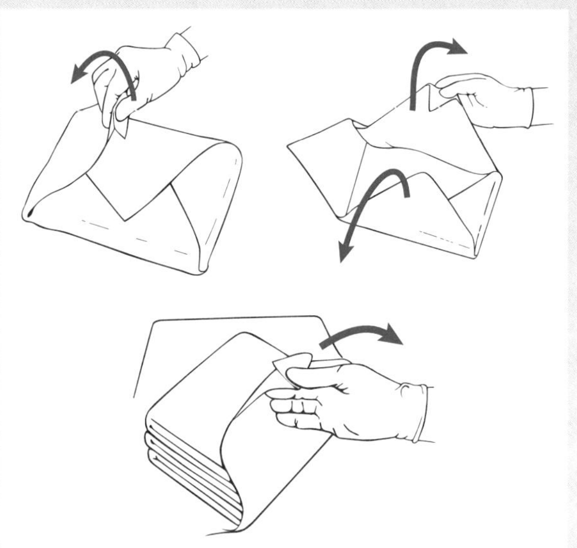

5. Wrapper may be used for sterile field. Additional items may be added as necessary.

Envelope-Wrapped Package Held in Hand

1. Hold the package in one hand so the outer flap of the wrapper faces away from you.

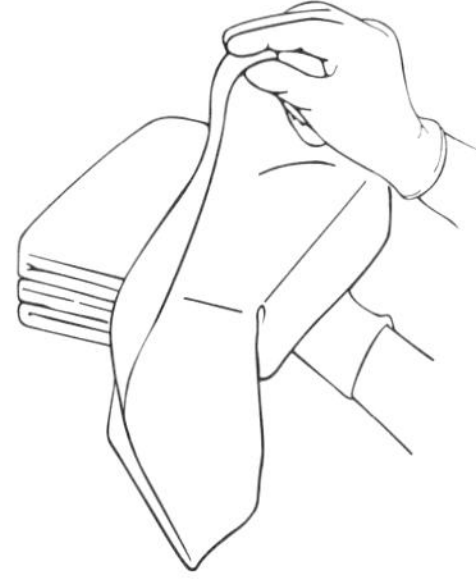

2. Open the package as in steps **2 to 4** above, (envelope-wrapped package on a surface) pulling the flaps back towards you as you open each one.
3. Gather the opened flaps with your free hand and hold them against the opposite arm, as shown. The sterile item can now be placed on a sterile field without risk of contacting the field with the parts of the wrapper that you have touched.

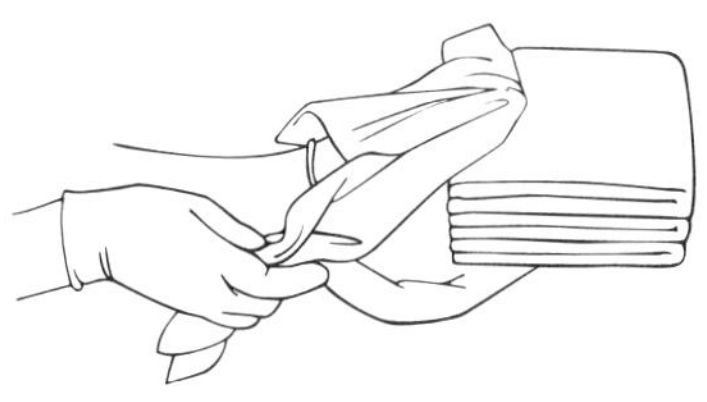

SOURCE: Berger & Williams, 1992, pp. 804–805.

contain the basic supplies for a procedure. For example, a **dressing tray** contains a compartment for cleansing solution, two or three forceps, and some 5 cm x 5 cm and 10 cm x 10 cm gauze sponges. Equipment and supplies are added to the tray depending on the circumstances of each particular situation. The nurse will find it prudent to take a few extra supplies along in case of accidental contamination, because once a tray is opened and a sterile field is established, it must not be left unattended.

ESTABLISHING THE STERILE FIELD A sterile field is set up on a clean, dry surface at about waist level. A bedside table is commonly used for this purpose. The table should be cleared of all items to provide ample surface area and avoid the risk of contamination from unsterile objects. The size of the sterile field depends on the procedure and the amount of equipment needed. In some cases, a sterile field is established by using the inside wrapper of a sterile package; in others it is created with sterile drapes. Supplies are added to the field either directly or with the use of sterile transfer forceps.

OPENING STERILE PACKAGES Sterile items such as catheters, syringes or dressing materials are packaged in plastic or paper packages that are impenetrable by microorganisms as long as they remain dry and intact. Many of these items are wrapped in "peel packs" or "peelback" containers. Reusable equipment such as forceps, towels or drapes is wrapped in paper or cotton (or cotton blend) fabric. An "envelope" method of wrapping is used in which the four corners of the outer wrapper are folded around the object in a uniform manner. The box on page 1053 illustrates how to open the various types of sterile packages.

USING STERILE FORCEPS A variety of forceps are used in sterile procedures (see Figure 32.5). For example, forceps are used for transferring sterile supplies on a sterile field, for handling gauzes and dressings or for anchoring tubes. Forceps are included in prepackaged and reusable trays, but individually wrapped forceps may also be available in some agencies. As with all sterile objects, forceps must always be held above waist level and within full view. The handles are considered contaminated if held with ungloved hands. Dry, sterile forceps that are used with bare hands may be placed on the sterile area so that the tips rest within the sterile field and the handles outside it. Forceps must always be held with the tips downward, especially if they become wet. This prevents contamination from the backflow of moisture from contaminated handles to the sterile tips.

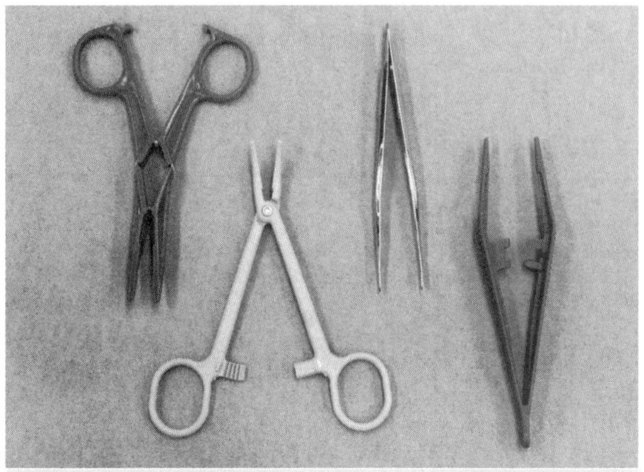

FIGURE 32.5 Forceps used in sterile procedures

POURING STERILE SOLUTIONS Sterile solutions are supplied in glass or plastic bottles. The inside of the bottle and cap are considered to be sterile; the outside surfaces clean. The cap must be removed carefully and held in the hand or placed on a flat surface inside up to prevent the inside from becoming contaminated. The bottle is held with the label facing upward to avoid wetting and possibly obliterating the label. The bottle should also be held outside the edge of the sterile field and about 10 cm above the receiving container to prevent contamination of the sterile field. The lip of the bottle should never touch the receiving container. Solution must be poured carefully to avoid splashing. Only the outside of the cap should be touched when replacing it on the bottle. As with all sterile supplies, check the expiration date on the solution container. Do not use solutions that have expired. After a sterile solution has been opened, the bottle should be labelled with the date and time. Once opened, a solution is considered sterile for 24 hours only.

DONNING STERILE GLOVES Sterile gloves are supplied in a variety of sizes. A proper glove size is necessary for comfort, dexterity and safety. Gloves that fit loosely will make the manipulation of objects difficult, whereas gloves that are too tight may tear and cause contamination.

Health-Restoring Strategies

Nosocomial infections have long been recognized as serious complications of disease or treatment, with significant morbidity, mortality and cost. Even as we continue to find new and more sophisticated ways of supporting people through life-threatening injury or illness, we also expose them to greater risks of infection. Notwithstanding the fact that prevention of illness, coupled with health promotion, is the ideal in a healthy society, in developed countries approximately five to 10 percent of people admitted to hospital develop infection as a result of their stay. This figure remains fairly constant despite best efforts to understand and prevent disease acquisition. Measures must be taken to tip the balance in favour of the infected person. This usually means prescribing antibiotics. The physician doing so will base his or her decision on clinical evidence for disease, possibly with microbiological and radiological support. The decision may be empirical, that is, it may be based on previous experience, at least until culture results are known.

The nurse should have knowledge of the antibiotic agent being administered. The most important aspects include usual dosage and timing, route(s) of administration, potential adverse effects, contraindications and possible drug reactions. In the event of adverse effects or reactions, the nurse must know how to obtain help, especially in a [illegible] [illegible] dertaken to relieve uncomfortable side effects that may not need medical intervention. Ideally, a specimen for culture and sensitivity should be obtained before initiation of antibiotic therapy. Once the specimen is obtained, therapy should be started immediately. The nurse must also monitor and assess whether or not the prescribed treatment appears to be effective. Sometimes a new infection (a **super-infection)** will superimpose itself on the original one, or sometimes the infecting microorganism may have developed resistance to the prescribed antibiotic.

Good nutrition is important to promote good health, and it is vital that someone fighting an infection have proper nutrients. Good nursing care means that the patient will be encouraged to eat and drink and that intake will be monitored. With some patients, especially older adults, it may be necessary to ensure that dentition is in good repair or that their dentures fit properly. The more conscientious the approach to good basic nursing care, the more likely it is that a patient will return to a healthy life.

STAFF EXPOSURE TO INFECTIOUS AGENTS

Health professionals and personnel such as housekeeping staff are at risk for exposure to infectious agents. The greatest concerns expressed are exposure to blood-borne pathogens such as HIV and hepatitis B. The following measures are recommended for health care providers and hospital personnel should they sustain injury from a needle or other sharp instrument that has been used on a patient, or should blood be splashed onto an open lesion or mucous membrane.

1. Wash area thoroughly with soap and water.
2. If stuck with a needle or sharp, squeeze blood from wound.
3. Soak affected area in buffered bleach 1400 ppm (or household bleach 0.5 percent–1 percent) for 10 minutes.
4. Flush eyes and mucous membranes with normal saline at an eyewash station.

Report promptly to the employee health service (or emergency department, depending on agency policy) and to the supervisor for follow-up. If antiretrovival therapy is indicated, it should be started within two hours of injury.

Evaluating Infection Prevention and Control Interventions

Evaluation of the effectiveness of nursing intervention is based on outcome criteria established in the patient's plan of care and by the absence of the infection in other patients, in visitors and in staff. Guidelines the nurse might use in [illegible]

1. Are aseptic practices keeping organisms within defined areas?
2. Are other people in the environment free of the infection?
3. Does the patient (and family) have the knowledge and skills required to prevent the spread of infection and to participate actively in care as much as possible?
4. Does the patient have misconceptions about the infection?
5. Does the patient indicate in any way feelings of isolation? For example, does the patient make verbal statements or show signs of depression?
6. Does the patient have the desired contact with family, hospital personnel and other patients without endangering health?
7. Does the patient get adequate exercise to meet needs?
8. Does the patient demonstrate an active interest in, and is the patient encouraged to participate in, care as much as possible?
9. Does the patient have diversionary materials of interest?

The Role of the Infection Control Service

The vast majority of hospitals in Canada and the United States today have active infection control programs. The basic aim of these programs is to control and prevent the spread of nosocomial infection and to bring its incidence to an irreducible minimum. Three activities form the framework for an effective program. They are surveillance, education and consultation. Surveillance means the "the ongoing, systematic collection, analysis, and interpretation of health data essential to the planning, implementation, and evaluation of public health practice, closely integrated with the timely dissemination of these data to those who need to know" (CDC, cited in Gaynes, 1998, p. 65). This means that data are gathered according to preset criteria, analysed regularly and presented to those persons who can effect appropriate corrective action. Types of surveillance may vary from one agency to another and may be refocussed or retargetted as changing circumstances indicate. Surveillance may also include outbreak investigation and communicable disease reporting to the appropriate authorities.

Educational programs include orientation for all new staff and ongoing inservice sessions as required. Educational needs are identified, programs implemented and evaluation done on a regular basis.

Consultation is an ongoing process, both internally within the facility and externally from the community. Hospital staff at any level are encouraged to bring questions and concerns to the infection control department. Consultation is carried on externally through liaison with other hospitals, health care agencies and facilities, universities, community colleges and other organizations. This is especially true for infection control practitioners in teaching hospitals or in regional referral centres. Infection control practitioners may also sit on a variety of committees and policy-making bodies that deal with issues where infection control aspects must be addressed.

In Canada, the vast majority of people working on a daily basis in infection control are nurses. Usually these nurses have had broad clinical experience and have taken, or are expected to participate in, infection control educational programs. Goals and objectives for such programs have been developed by the Community and Hospital Infection Control Association—Canada (CHICA—Canada). These courses are available through several different educational institutions. Other disciplines active in infection control include laboratory technologists (or others with a science background), infectious disease physicians and medical microbiologists. It is absolutely essential that infection control practitioners have a close working relationship (preferably formalized) with the medical microbiology laboratory. In larger institutions, a multidisciplinary approach is usual and, in fact, desirable. It is contingent on all hospital staff that they support the hospitals' infection control program, and there should be administrative recognition that infection control activities represent continuous quality improvement. In other words, *infection control is everybody's business!*

IN REVIEW

- The prevention and control of infection is a primary goal of all health professionals. It is only in the past 150 years that successful measures to control infection have evolved.
- Infection control measures include:
  - development and widespread use of specific immunizations and antimicrobial agents
  - implementation of basic sanitary measures
  - higher standards of living.
- Important events in the history of infection control include:
  - Leeuwenhoek's invention of the microscope (1678)
  - Jenner's development of the first vaccine for smallpox (1796)
  - Semmelweis's emphasis on hand-washing in lying-in hospitals (1847)
  - Lister's introduction of antiseptics to cleanse the skin prior to surgery ([illegible])
  - Nightingale's demonstration that improved hygiene, reduced overcrowding and standardized reporting of deaths could reduce mortality rates in army hospitals (1861)
  - Koch's postulates on the relationship between microorganisms and disease (1876)
  - the discovery of penicillin (1928)
  - the discovery of sulfonamides (1935).
- The infectious process starts with the invasion and multiplication of microorganisms on or in the body, causing ill or adverse effects.
- A causative agent (pathogen) grows in a reservoir which becomes its source, leaves through a portal of exit via a vehicle (mode of transmission) to a portal of entry in a susceptible host, who becomes the new source.
- Portals of exit and entry may include:
  - the respiratory, urinary, gastrointestinal or reproductive tracts
  - breaks in the skin or mucous membranes
  - wound discharges or blood.
- Modes of infectious transmission include:
  - direct or indirect contact
  - inanimate objects (vehicles)
  - air (droplets) and vectors (animals, insects).
- The host must be susceptible to the pathogen or have a low degree of resistance, and the pathogen must be of sufficient quantity or virulence to cause disease. A period of incubation precedes manifestation of symptoms or the appearance of infection.
- Nonspecific defence mechanisms of the body include:
  - skin
  - mucous membranes
  - some body secretions
  - local inflammatory response
  - generalized stress reaction.
- Specific defence mechanisms of the body include:
  - natural immunity
  - active or passive artificial immunity.
- The host's reaction to an infection may range from no symptoms to acute distress.
- There are a number of factors influencing a host's reaction, including:
  - host's state of physical, mental and emotional health
  - immunization history
  - age (young and old)
  - acute or chronic illness.
- At different stages in the life cycle, people are prone to different types of infection.

- Some of the more common infections affect:
  - the urinary tract
  - the gastrointestinal tract
  - wounds (including surgical sites).
- Multidrug-resistant pathogens are a serious concern for health professionals. The two most common such pathogens are:
  - methicillin-resistant *Staphylococcus aureus* (MRSA)
  - vancomycin-resistant *Enterococci* (VRE)
- Assessing the infection prevention and control needs for each patient starts with the nursing history. The nursing history includes:
  - the patient's health practices
  - the patient's general susceptibility to infections
  - a physical examination.
- The first sign of infection is often an increase in:
  - temperature
  - pulse
  - respirations

  with localized or systemic symptoms.
- Diagnostic tests include laboratory tests on:
  - blood
  - exudates
  - sputum
  - discharges
  - urine or stool.
- Prevention and control of infection are inherent in the planning and implementing of all nursing activities. Basic goals include:
  - prevention of infection
  - control of infection
  - prevention of problems associated with infection
  - promotion of patient comfort
  - promotion of infection control in self-care practices.
- Health-promoting strategies include:
  - good hand-washing technique
  - maintaining good health practices (adequate exercise, nutrition, rest, stress reduction, immunization).
- Communities control infection through ensuring:
  - clean water and food supplies
  - proper sewage disposal
  - a clean environment.
- Health-protecting strategies include:
  - immunization
  - aseptic practices (blood and body substance precautions; universal and isolation precautions)
  - screening for multiresistant organisms.
- Medical asepsis is clean technique involving thorough hand-washing and careful disposal of supplies and equipment to prevent the spread of infection. Proper hand-washing before and after the care of each patient is the most effective method of prevention.
- Surgical asepsis is used to keep an object or area free of microorganisms.
- Health-restoring strategies include:
  - careful technique to prevent nosocomial infections
  - monitoring effects and side effects of antibiotic treatment
  - good nutrition and fluid intake
  - good basic nursing care.

Critical Thinking Activities

1. Mrs. Rose Nakashima is admitted to a hospital for an operation to remove an ulcer on her left leg. Three days after her surgery, Mrs. Nakashima's wound appears reddened and has a purulent discharge. A wound culture has been ordered to identify the infecting organism. Mrs. Nakashima, who is 54 years old, is in a room that has four beds and a shared bathroom.
   a. What specific precautions should be taken?
   b. What factors would you consider prior to explaining these precautions to this patient?
   c. If feasible, what would be the advantages of moving Mrs. Nakashima to a single room?
   d. The infecting organism is found to be *Staphylococcus aureus*. What do you need to know about this organism in order to establish a safe environment?
   e. Mrs. Nakashima's wound is dressed at least twice a day. After this measure, what should be done with the (i) old dressing, (ii) used dressing equipment and supplies, (iii) unused supplies and (iv) unused disinfectant?
2. "The safety of an environment is related to the number of pathogenic organisms in it." What measures in medical asepsis are based on this principle?

KEY TERMS

nosocomial infections p. 1017
infection p. 1019
pathogen p. 1019
symbiotic relationship p. 1019
immunocompromised p. 1019
carriers p. 1019
commensals p. 1019
pathogenic bacteria p. 1020
microbial flora p. 1020
exogenous infection p. 1021
endogenous infection p. 1021
fomites p. 1021
susceptibility p. 1022
pathogenicity p. 1022
virulence p. 1022
incubation p. 1022
local inflammatory response p. 1022
leukocytes p. 1022
acute inflammation p. 1022
suppurating p. 1022
symptomatic period p. 1022
asymptomatic p. 1022
natural immunity p. 1022
active artificial immunity p. 1023
passive artificial immunity p. 1023
asepsis p. 1035
cleaning p. 1037
universal precautions p. 1039
body substance precautions (BSP) p. 1039
standard precautions p. 1039
superinfection p. 1057

References

ASSOCIATION FOR PRACTICE IN INFECTION CONTROL (APIC). (1996). *Curriculum for infection control practice*. Dubuque, IA: Kendall/Hunt.

BARRETT-CONNOR, E. (1978). Nosocomial infection: Definitions and magnitude. In E. Barrett-Connor, S. L. Brandt, H. J. Simon, & D. C. Dechairo (Eds.), *Epidemiology for the infection control nurse*. St. Louis: Mosby.

BERGER, K.J., & WILLIAMS, M.B. (1992). *Fundamentals of nursing: Collaborating for optimal health*. Norwalk, CT: Appleton & Lange.

BRACHMAN, P.S. (1998). Epidemiology of nosocomial infections. In J.V. Bennett & P.S. Brachman (Eds.), *Hospital infections* (chap. 1). (4th ed.). Philadelphia: Lippincott–Raven.

CARPENITO, L.J. (1997). *Nursing diagnosis: Application to clinical practice.* (7th ed.). Philadelphia: Lippincott.

CENTRES FOR DISEASE CONTROL (CDC). (1987). Recommendations for prevention of HIV transmission in health care settings. *Morbidity and Mortality Weekly Report, 36* (Supplement 25), 15.

CENTRES FOR DISEASE CONTROL (CDC). (1993). Recommendations for the prevention and management of *Chlamydia trachomatis infections*. *Morbidity & Mortality Weekly Report, 42* (RR-12), 1–39.

CROW, S. (1989). *Asepsis, the right touch*. Bossier City, LA: Everett Companies Publishing Division.

FARR, B.M. (1997). What to do about a high endemic rate of infection. In R.P. Wenzel (Ed.), *Prevention and control of nosocomial infections* (chap. 11). (3rd ed.). Philadelphia: Williams & Wilkins.

GAYNES, R. (1998). Surveillance of nosocomial infections. In J.V. Bennett and P.S. Brachman (Eds.), *Hospital infections*. (4th ed.). Philadelphia: Lippincott-Raven.

HALL, N. (1988). *Psychoneuroimmunology*. Paper presented at the 15th Annual Educational Conference of APIC, Dallas, TX.

HEALTH CANADA. (1996). *Canadian national report of immunization.* Ottawa: Minister of Supply & Services. Available at http://www.hc-sc.gc.ca/main/lcdc/web/publicat/ccdr/97vol23/imm_sup/imm_e_e.html

HEALTH CANADA. (1998). *Canadian immunization guide.* (5th ed.). Ottawa: Minister of Supply & Services. (Catalogue no. H49–8/1993E)

HOEPRICH, P. D. (Ed.). (1972). *Infectious diseases*. Hagerstown, MD: Harper & Row.

KENNER, C.A., & MACLAREN, A. (1993). *Essentials of maternal and neonatal nursing*. Springhouse, PA: Springhouse.

KING, M., GARTRELL, J., & TROVATO, F. (1991, Summer). Early childhood mortality, 1926–1986. *Canadian Social Trends*. Ottawa: Minister of Supply & Services, 6–10. (Statistics Canada Catalogue no. 11–008E)

LAFORCE, F.M. (1997). The control of infections in hospitals: 1750–1950. In R.P. Wenzel (Ed.), *Prevention and control of nosocomial infections.* (3rd ed.). Baltimore, MD: Williams & Wilkins, 3–17.

McLEAN, D.M., & SMITH, J.A. (1991). *Medical microbiology synopsis.* Philadelphia: Lea & Febiger.

NIGHTINGALE, F. (1861). *Notes on hospitals.* (3rd ed.). London: Longmans.

PARKER, L. (1990). From pestilence to asepsis. *Nursing Times, 86*(49), 63–67.

PILLITTERI, A. (1995). *Maternal and child health nursing: Care of the child bearing and childrearing family.* (2nd ed.). Philadelphia: Lippincott.

PLORDE, J.J. (1990). Flagellates. In J. C. Sherris (Ed.), *Medical microbiology: Introduction to infectious disease.* (2nd ed.) (p. 734). New York: Elsevier Science.

SANDS, K.E.F., & GOLDMAN, D.A. (1998). Epidemiology of *Staphylococcus* and group A *Streptococci*. In J.V. Bennett & P.S. Brachman (Eds.), *Hospital infections* (chap. 41). (4th ed.). Philadelphia: Lippincott-Raven.

SELWYN, S. (1991). Hospital infection: The first 2500 years. *Journal of Hospital Infection, 18* (Supplement A), 5–64.

STAMM, W.E. (1998). Urinary tract infection. In J.V. Bennett & P.S. Brachman (Eds.). *Hospital infections*. (4th ed.). Philadelphia: Lippincott–Raven.

WALKER, M. (1991). What you should know about infection control today—A patient information booklet. *Canadian Journal of Infection Control, 6* (2), 43–45.

WEINSTEIN, R.A., & HAYDEN, M.K. (1998). Mutiple drug-resistant pathogens: Epidemiology and control. In J.V. Bennett & P.S. Brachman (Eds.), *Hospital infections* (chap. 15). (4th ed.). Philadelphia: Lippincott–Raven.

WENZEL, R.P. (Ed.). (1997). *Prevention and control of nosocomial infections.* (3rd ed.). Baltimore, MD: Williams & Wilkins.

WHEELOCK, S.M., & LOOKINLAND, S. (1997). Effects of surgical hand scrub time on subsequent bacterial growth. *Journal of Association of Operating Room Nurses, 65*(6), 1087–1098.

WHITE, P.J. & SHACKELFORD, P.G. (1983). Edward Jenner, MD, and the scourge that was. *American Journal of Diseases in Children, 137*, 846–869.

Additional Readings

BENNETT, J.V., & BRACHMAN, P.S. (Eds.). (1998). *Hospital infections.* (4th ed.). Philadelphia: Lippincott-Raven.

BRAMBILLA, L., MACFARLANE, N., ALFA, M., PLOURDE, P., & HARDING, G. (1997, Winter). *Bacillus cereus* colonization of ventilated patients in two intensive care units. *Canadian Journal of Infection Control,* 136–139.

CANADIAN NOSOCOMIAL INFECTION SURVEILLANCE PROGRAM: Results of the first 18 months of surveillance for methicillin-resistant *Staphylococcus aureus* in Canadian hospitals. (1997). *Canada Communicable Disease Report, 23*, 41–46.

DEDHAR, J., & ENQUIST, G. (1992). Practical guidelines for body substance precautions in long-term care. *Canadian Journal of Infection Control, 7*(3), 77–80.

GARNER, J.S. (1996). Guidelines for isolation precautions in hospital: Part 1. Evolution of isolation practices. *American Journal of Infection Control, 24*, 24–52.

for management of vancomycin-resistant *Enterococci. Canadian Nursing Home, 7*(2), 5–9.

MACDONALD, K.S., MCLEOD, J., & NICOLLE, L. (1993). Clostridium difficile in a Canadian tertiary care hospital. *Canadian Journal of Infection Control, 8*(2), 37–40.

MACKENZIE, D., & EDWARDS, A. (1997). MRSA: The psychological effects. *Nursing Standard, 12*(11), 49–56.

MCGEER, A., ARMSTRONG, M., BLACKLOCK, A., CANN, D., LOW, D.E., & MCARTHUR, M. (1996). VRE: The next epidemic. *Long-Term Care, 6*(2), 10–13.

OLMSTED, R.N., & BARRET, T. (1996). *Infection control and applied epidemiology*. St. Louis: Mosby.

PALMER, S., GIDDENS, J., & PALMER, D. (1996). *Infection control.* El Paso, TX: Skidmore-Roth.

PHILLIP, C. (1998). Fighting back against superbugs. *Nursing BC, 30*(2), 10–13.

PHILLIP, C. (1998). Recognizing and treating a hidden killer. *Nursing BC*

PRESTON, G.C. (1996). HICPAC guidelines for isolation precautions in hospitals: Community hospital perspective. *American Journal of Infection Control, 24*, 207–208.

ROBINSON, K.D.Z., MERCER, J., MARZENA, C., GILL-MORTON, P., & MAIN, S. (1997). Managing vancomycin-resistant *Enterococci.* A winning team approach. *Canadian Nurse, 93*(10), 36–39.

SKIDMORE, A.G. (1993). *Clostridium difficile*—the only important nosocomial pathogen in developed countries. *Canadian Journal of Infection Control, 8*(2), 33.

SOULE, B.M. (1996). The CDC and HICPAC guideline for isolation precautions in hospitals: Commentaries on an evolutionary process. *American Journal of Infection Control, 24,* 199–200.

Chapter 33

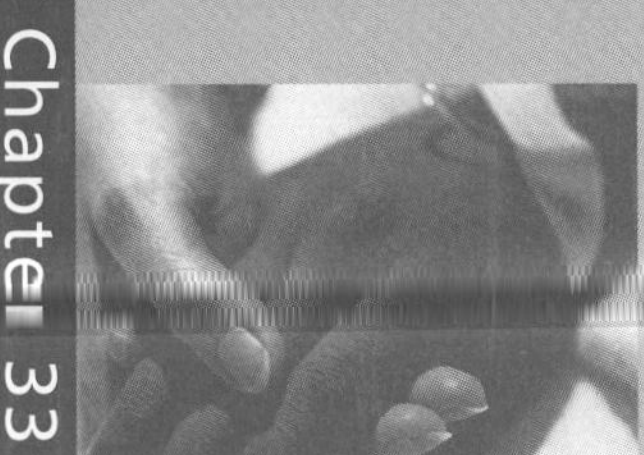

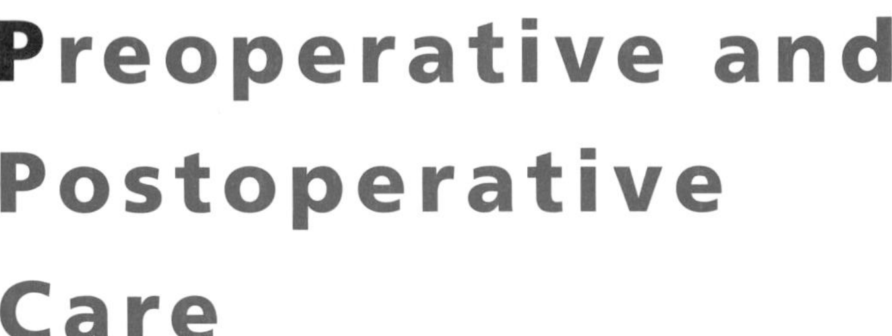

Preoperative and Postoperative Care

OUTLINE

Introduction

Surgery and Health Care

Types of Surgical Intervention

The Preoperative Period

The Postoperative Period

Wound Healing and Restorative Care

Central Questions

1. Why is surgery safer today than in previous times?
2. What are the major goals of nursing care for surgical patients?
3. What are the determinants of a patient's ability to cope with surgery?
4. What is involved in the nurse's preoperative assessment of the surgical patient?
5. What are the common nursing diagnostic statements for patients experiencing surgery?
6. What health-promoting and health-protecting strategies are indicated for preoperative and postoperative patients?
7. What is included in a preoperative teaching program?
8. What are the nursing responsibilities in the immediate and continuing postoperative periods?
9. How do surgical wounds heal, and what determines healing?
10. What restorative strategies promote wound healing and facilitate recovery from surgery?
11. How does the nurse evaluate the effectiveness of nursing interventions?

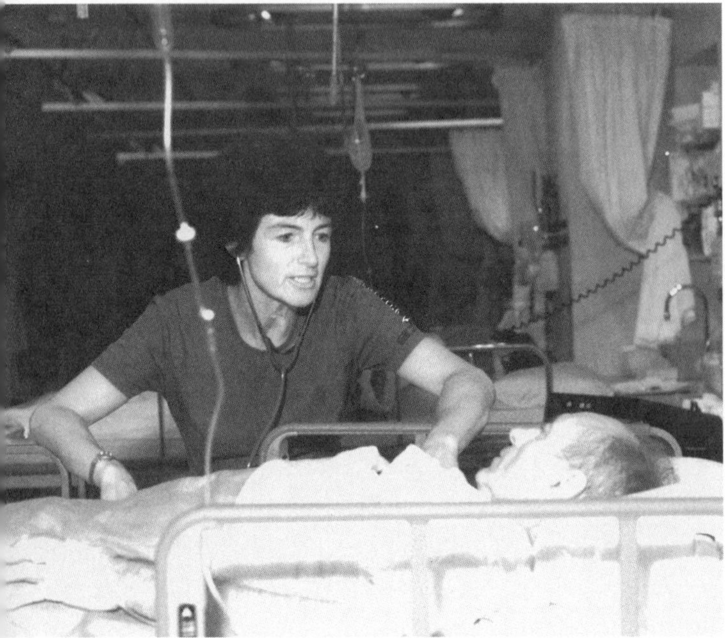

Introduction

Surgery involves the deliberate and planned alteration of

a pathological process, or to repair a traumatic injury. When surgery is recommended, a period of psychological and physiological stress begins; personal control of some aspects of life is surrendered in order to obtain relief from symptoms, to restore normal bodily functions or to retain life itself. In some situations, such as after an accident, there may be no time for the patient to prepare for the surgical experience. In others, there may be ample time to think about and become prepared for surgery.

Nursing care of patients whose illness experience involves surgery is complex and varied. The major goals of nursing practice are to prepare the patient for surgery and to promote a healthy recovery. These goals can be fostered by the nurse who strives to maximize the patient's abilities to cope with the physiological and psychological stressors involved in a surgical experience. Assisting the patient to maintain self-care abilities, ensuring a sense of participation in care, protecting the patient from injury or harm and educating the patient and significant others to manage recovery effectively once home also help to foster these goals.

This chapter outlines the basic knowledge needed to care for patients whose illness experience involves surgery. The developments important to the care of the patient undergoing surgery and the determinants of the ability to cope with it are briefly described. Next, the events of the preoperative phase of the illness experience are discussed, along with the factors that increase physiological and psychological stress, and the nursing intervention of preoperative education. The impact of surgery on basic needs is identified, and potential or actual problems that may be encountered in surgical illnesses are explored within a nursing process framework. The process of wound healing and basic wound care procedures are also described.

Surgery and Health Care

Surgery has been used in the treatment of disease and injury from the beginning of humanity, but it was not until the middle of the 19th century that it began to evolve as a specific type of medical treatment. At that time, surgery was hazardous and was limited either to measures that were essential to save a life, such as amputating a crushed limb, or to minor procedures such as removing a tooth or draining an infected wound. Aseptic techniques were unknown, and surgery was performed by doctors who did not wear gloves or change instruments between successive operations. The rates of infection and mortality were so high that the treatment was not often beneficial.

Today, surgery has become a safe and humane method of treating disease. Advances in surgery have been made possible by the development of knowledge and techniques in the areas of hemostasis, asepsis, anesthesia and technology. The development of critical care units and the increase

the outcomes of the patient undergoing surgery.

Hemostasis is the control of bleeding. Without adequate methods to control bleeding, the patient may die from hemorrhage. The methods used to control bleeding include pressure, cauterization (burning), tying the ends of the blood vessels with some type of material and tissue sealants, which are sprayed on areas to retard or halt blood oozing from capillaries.

Prior to the development of the science of bacteriology, death from infection was common. The modern concept of asepsis is based on the knowledge that microorganisms are capable of causing disease. Factors that need to be controlled in order to prevent microorganisms from gaining access to wounds have been identified, and the application of this knowledge has decreased mortality and morbidity. The development of antibiotics has contributed to the decrease in infection rates after surgery. However, with heavy reliance on antibiotic therapy, the danger always exists that aseptic techniques will be relaxed or that antibiotic-resistant strains of microorganisms will develop, causing massive problems of infection.

The development of anesthesia has made the prevention of pain during surgery possible. The physician can now take time to handle the tissues gently and perform procedures with care. A variety of chemical anesthetic agents are used for inducing unconsciousness, controlling pain and removing sensation in a region of the body or in a small area of the skin or mucous membrane. Chemical agents are delivered by gases, which are inhaled, and by liquids, which are either injected into the skin, veins, sensory nerves or spinal cord or applied directly onto the skin.

Technological advances such as the use of video endoscopes, lasers and microsurgery have improved outcomes for the surgical patient. In video endoscopy, a small telescope-type instrument with a camera is put into a body cavity through a small incision. Another small incision is made for the tiny tools that are used to perform the surgery. The reduction of tissue trauma decreases postoperative pain and diminishes hospitalization time and disability. The removal of a gallbladder by video endoscopy (laparoscopic cholecystectomy) is now a common procedure.

The manner of health care delivery is changing as the cost of prolonged hospital care has become a financial burden to society. Many aspects of care are now delivered safely and effectively in the community. By the year 2000, the majority of patients will be admitted to hospital on the morning of surgery, and 60 percent of them will return home the same evening (Connolly, 1991). At the same time as these advances are taking place, people are exercising their rights and assuming responsibility for their health care. The patient undergoing surgery has the right to informed consent and the responsibility to assume a significant portion of pre- and postsurgical care. The nurse is responsible for the patient education that will allow the patient to fulfill these responsibilities. Much of the education will occur at an outpatient clinic in the hospital or a community centre.

Types of Surgical Intervention

The classification of surgical procedures relates to the seriousness, urgency or purpose of surgery. A surgical procedure may fall into one or more categories. Surgical seriousness is designated as *major* or *minor*, depending on the hazards involved and the physiological effects of the procedures on the body. For example, removal of an ingrown toenail or the incision and drainage of a boil are considered minor surgery, and may not even be done in an operating room. A hysterectomy (removal of the uterus), on the other hand, is considered a major surgical procedure and would be performed in an operating room.

Surgical interventions are also classified by urgency of the problem or time. Surgery for life-threatening problems such as bleeding is termed *immediate* or *emergency* surgery. When intervention is required within 24–48 hours, the surgery is classified as *urgent*, and when a procedure is needed but may be performed within a few weeks, such as in thyroid disorders, it is classified as *required* or *elective*. *Optional* surgery, such as cosmetic surgery, occurs when patient preference determines the time of the surgery.

The purpose of surgery varies. Surgery may be *diagnostic*, such as when a tissue sample is obtained **(biopsy)**, or it may be *curative*, such as when an inflamed appendix is removed. *Reparative* surgery is done, for example, when multiple wounds are repaired. *Palliative* surgery is done to lessen the distressing symptoms of a pathological process, such as when a portion of the intestine is used to bypass an obstruction caused by a cancerous growth. Surgery may also be constructive, reconstructive or cosmetic. *Constructive* surgery involves building or correcting a body part to improve its function or appearance, such as when the upper lip of a child with a congenital cleft is repaired. *Reconstructive* surgery is performed to repair damage to the appearance or functioning caused by trauma or disease in a previously intact anatomical structure. Reconstructive surgery is done, for example, when rebuilding a breast after its removal due to cancer. *Cosmetic* surgery may be done to improve physical appearance and, although it is not necessary for physical health, it is important for self-esteem.

The specific type of surgical procedure performed is described by the use of prefixes and suffixes. Prefixes identify the organ or body part and suffixes explain the procedure. For example, the prefix *gastro-* means stomach; the suffix *-ectomy* means the surgical removal of an organ or gland. Thus, *gastrectomy* refers to the surgical removal of the stomach. Table 33.1 lists some suffixes denoting common surgical procedures.

The Preoperative Period

During the preoperative period, the nature of the illness is determined and a plan of treatment is made. The time before diagnosis may be confusing to the patient who is undergoing a variety of procedures that are time-consuming, embarrassing, strenuous or painful. Once the decision to have surgery is made, the patient will be asked to have more tests done. Frequently, an electrocardiogram is done, a chest x-ray is taken, and blood and urine samples are tested again. The patient must make arrangements to be absent from school or work and to have someone assume responsibilities that cannot be ignored. In addition, patients must cope with fears about the surgery. The illness experience causes changes in

TABLE 33.1 Common surgical procedures

Suffix	*Definition*	*Example of Procedure*
-ectomy	Removal of organ or gland	Nephrectomy (removal of a kidney)
-ostomy	Forming an opening or stoma	Colostomy (an artificial opening from the colon to the surface of the abdomen)
-otomy	Making an incision or cutting into	Laparotomy (a surgical incision through the abdominal wall, often for diagnostic purposes)
-plasty	Repairing or restoring a body part	Mammoplasty (surgical reconstruction of a breast)
-rrhaphy	Suturing an organ or part in place	Osteorrhaphy (surgical fixation of bone fragments with sutures or wires)
-scopy	Visual examination by means of a fibre-optic instrument	Gastroscopy (visual examination of the stomach)

the interactions, roles and relationships between the patient and those involved with the illness. The result is a loss of people's normal way of life (Morse & Johnson, 1991).

mize the patient's psychological and physiological health. The patient who is in physiological homeostasis and is emotionally prepared for surgery has the best chance of tolerating surgery well. Preoperative assessment is done to determine the risk of surgery. Factors such as age, extent of planned surgery and the presence of other health problems may affect the ability to tolerate surgery. If possible, interventions are taken to minimize existing problems. An essential nursing intervention in preparing for surgery is decreasing the patient's psychological stress and enhancing his or her ability to participate in health care.

Determinants of the Ability to Cope with Surgery

Surgery involves an invasion of body tissues. Some people are more vulnerable and at higher risk for developing complications than others. The principal factors affecting surgical risk are discussed below.

EXTENT OF SURGERY

The risk for shock, infection and other complications increases in proportion to the amount of tissue damage, manipulation or removal. The more that tissues are damaged, manipulated or removed, the higher the risk of complications. The patient who undergoes two or more surgical procedures close together in time is more at risk. The body requires time to recover from one surgery before another is imposed upon it.

AGE

The very young and the older patient are more at risk. Before the age of six months, the child's circulatory and renal functions are not fully developed and therefore they do not withstand the stress of surgery as well as older children and adults. Children have small amounts of subcutaneous tissue and fragile thermal regulating mechanisms and are sensitive to chilling and exposure. The child may have adequate heart muscle reserve, but small alterations in fluid and electrolytes may impose significant problems. For example, a small volume of blood loss that would be easily compensated for in an adult may represent a large decrease in the total blood volume of a child.

The physiological changes in older people increase vulnerability to the stresses of surgery. Some of the changes are decreased heart and lung reserves, disturbances in fluid and electrolyte regulation, decreased liver and renal function, decreased gastric and gastrointestinal tract motility, decreased immunological function, decreased sensory abilities, decreased amount of subcutaneous tissue and increased susceptibility to complications from bed rest (Krechel, 1997).

KEY PRINCIPLES

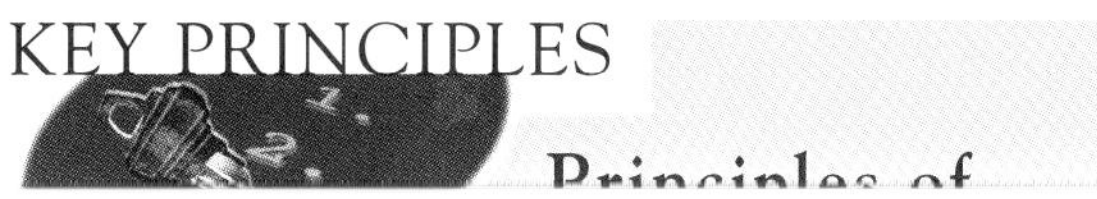

Postoperative Care

1. Surgery evokes a major stress reaction in the body.
2. Surgery is a major assault on the body and lowers the ability to cope with other stressors.
3. Surgery affects the ability to meet basic needs.
4. The skin is the body's first line of defence against harmful agents, and penetration of the skin by surgical incision provides a portal of entry for invading pathogens.
5. The very young and the older patient are vulnerable to the adverse effects of surgery, as are those with respiratory problems, cardiovascular disease, abnormal blood coagulation patterns, diabetes or disorders causing vascular insufficiency.
6. People who are extremely fearful are poor surgical risks.
7. Fear of the unknown is a potent factor in presurgical anxiety, and information may help to alleviate some of this fear.

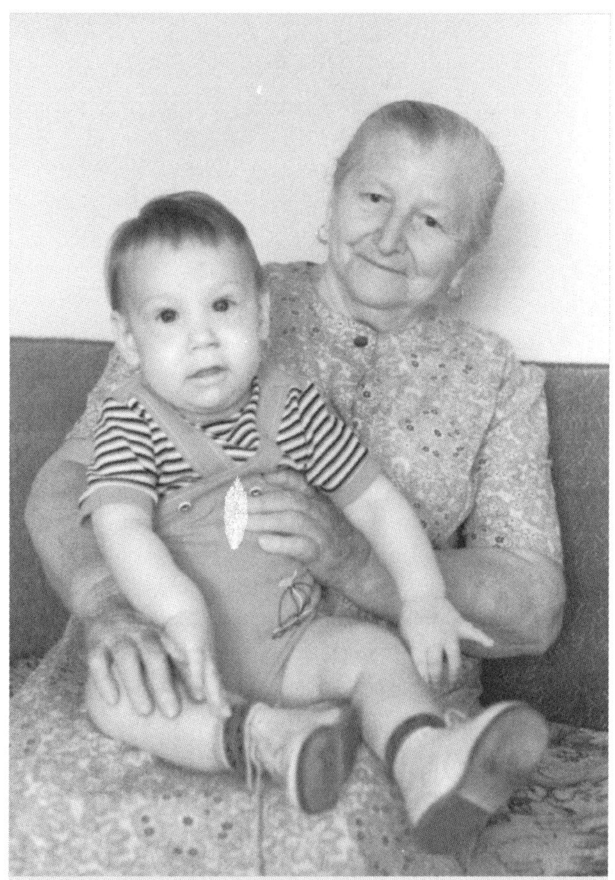

The very young and the older patient are more vulnerable to the stress of surgery.

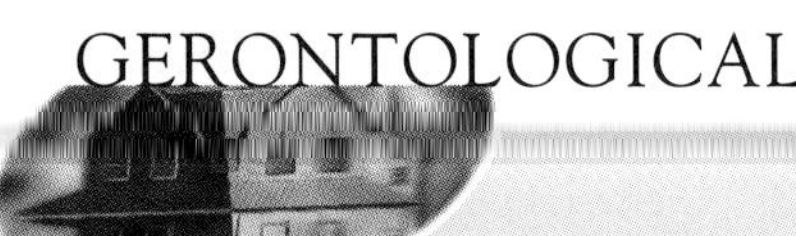

Physical Changes in Older Adults Undergoing Surgery

Physical Change	Nursing Interventions
Cardiovascular	
Decreased cardiac output	Know what anesthesia is used
Moderate increase in blood pressure	Monitor vital signs carefully
Decreased peripheral circulation	Encourage early ambulation and leg exercises
Arrhythmias	Assess for hypo- or hypertension or hypothermia
	Baseline ECG; note any changes
Respiratory	
Decreased vital capacity	Assess for pulmonary aspiration
Reduced oxygenation of blood	Monitor respirations carefully
	Vigorous pulmonary hygiene
	Postoperatively, auscultate lung sounds
	Oxygen saturation monitor
Renal	
Decreased renal blood flow and glomerular filtration rate	Monitor urine output q1–2 h during immediate postoperative period
Decreased ability to excrete waste products	Evaluate intake and output
	Monitor fluid and electrolyte status
Musculoskeletal	
Decrease in lean body mass	Assess level of mobility
Increase in spinal compression	Position on operating table with padding to reduce trauma to bones and joints
Increased incidence of osteoporosis and arthritis	Spine, limbs and pressure points may be padded to prevent fractures
	Early ambulation or exercises to patient's ability
	Provide adequate nutrition
	Provide effective pain management
Sensorimotor	
Decreased reaction time	Orient patient to environment
Decreased visual acuity	Plan individual teaching; allow time to reinforce teaching
Decreased auditory acuity	Provide a safe environment
Thermoregulation	Maintain warmth of patient by use of warm blankets

SOURCE: Black & Matassarin-Jacobs, 1997, p. 454.

The decreased reserves of the heart and the lungs of older people make it difficult for the body to maintain homeostasis in the face of continued strain. The fluid and electrolyte changes include a decline in the ability of the kidney to conserve water and retain sodium, which increases the risk of dehydration. Additionally, there is a decrease in thirst perception, which means that the older patient may not respond to dehydration by independently increasing fluid intake (Krechel, 1997).

The decreased liver function in an older patient may alter or prolong the metabolization of drugs. This, combined with the decline in the ability of the renal tissues to excrete end products, makes the administration of drug therapies difficult. The decrease in intestinal motility prolongs the time of drug absorption and decreases the ability to feel hungry, to take and absorb the nutrients essential for healing and to excrete waste products. A decreased amount of subcutaneous tissue increases the vulnerability to loss of body heat and decreases the resistance to mechanical trauma of the integument. The decrease in immunologic activities increases the susceptibility to infection.

Despite the increased risk, the older patient who has a good outlook, is well nourished and has reasonable cardiac, pulmonary and renal reserves will cope with the stress of a single surgical procedure well.

NUMBER OF OTHER HEALTH PROBLEMS

The patient who has a number of other health problems or is in general poor health is at greater surgical risk than one who is physically fit. Particularly vulnerable to postoperative problems are those with chronic respiratory tract disease such as chronic obstructive pulmonary disease, those with respiratory tract infections or cardiovascular disease, those with blood coagulation problems and those with metabolic disorders such as diabetes.

OBESITY

The patient who is obese is at increased risk for impaired [illegible] tissue on the incision. The obese patient may have shallow breathing or may breathe poorly when lying on the side, causing increased incidence of pulmonary complications. In addition, there is increased incidence of abdominal distention and phlebitis (inflammation of the veins) with increased weight (Flynn, 1996).

PSYCHOLOGICAL STRESS

The patient who is extremely anxious or has multiple life stressors is at increased risk for developing problems during or after surgery. The psychological stressors increase the level of the surgical stress response and may make it difficult for the patient to learn about activities such as deep breathing and coughing, which can improve the outcome of the surgery.

MEDICATION THERAPY

Many prescribed and over-the-counter medications have the potential to affect the physiological functions of the body and may interact with anesthetic agents, causing serious problems. Of particular concern are adrenal corticosteroids, which must be continued to avoid circulatory collapse; diuretics, which can cause electrolyte imbalance; antidepressants, which can increase the hypotensive effects of anesthetics; tranquillizers, which can cause seizures if withdrawn too quickly; insulin, which must be adjusted to account for the rise in blood sugar associated with the stress of surgery; some antibiotics that can interact with anesthetic agents; and, of course, anticoagulants, which alter the normal pattern of blood coagulation. The patient with an addiction to narcotic drugs or alcohol is also at increased risk for developing postoperative complications.

Assessing Preoperatively

A preoperative nursing assessment should begin with the first nurse who is in contact with the patient after surgery is planned. The nurse may work in an outpatient clinic, a preadmission clinic or an inpatient unit of a health care facility. A nursing assessment of each need, as outlined in previous chapters, is done by the nurse, who should have knowledge of the basic nature of the patient's health problem and the purpose of the surgery being planned. The health history is very important in order to establish a data base for future comparisons. Increased attention to oxygen, nutrition, elimination and immune needs is suggested. Each nurse who cares for the patient is responsible for adding to the data base. As the patient will move through several geographical locations in a surgical experience, it is essential to communicate specific information to other nurses and members of the health care team.

SPECIFIC ASSESSMENT OF NEEDS

Oxygen

[illegible] tions are the largest single cause of prolonged hospitalization and death after surgery. Assessment should include information about chronic lung conditions, medications taken for these conditions, smoking history, coughing, wheezing, shortness of breath, orthopnea, ankle edema, cyanosis, clubbing of the fingers, asthma and chest pain on exertion. Signs and symptoms of a cold or other respiratory infection, however minor, are reported, and surgery in non–life-threatening illnesses may be cancelled because of this information. A chest x-ray is done if a respiratory problem is present or suspected. Preoperatively, an improvement in lung reserve may be fostered by encouraging those who are able to walk 1–2 km per day. All patients who smoke are asked to stop prior to elective surgery.

Fluid and Electrolytes

A careful assessment of the circulatory system is essential. Existing problems such as chronic heart conditions, high blood pressure, varicose veins, circulatory disorders causing cold extremities and diabetes are noted. These problems increase the risk of surgery and may contribute to vulnerability to the formation of blood clots in the extremities. The patient should be asked about any medications taken for circulatory health problems. The circulatory system is assessed in relation to the reserve capacity of the heart and blood vessels. Poor exercise tolerance, presence of chest pain, irregularities of the pulse and, in adults, a blood pressure below 90 systolic or above 120 diastolic may indicate a diminished or inadequate ability to tolerate the stress of surgery. Deviations from normal should be reported to the doctor. Surgery may be delayed until treatable problems are corrected. Extremities and the site of planned surgery should be examined for pallor and coldness, which may indicate poor blood supply with decreased ability to heal. An electrocardiogram is taken in all patients over the age of 45 and all patients who report heart problems.

A complete blood count (CBC) test is done preoperatively. A group and screen of the blood type is done in case a transfusion is needed. In situations involving major surgery, a cross-match is done the evening prior to or the morning of surgery. Patients undergoing elective surgery may be able to donate their own blood for use if needed. The availability of the patient's own (autologous) blood should be documented. Prothrombin time (a blood test to assess clotting) is determined to identify potential or actual problems in the blood clotting mechanism. Tests are carried out to assess the electrolyte balance. Of particular importance are the levels of potassium, sodium, chloride and bicarbonate.

Nutrition

Important factors to consider in nutritional assessment are body weight, hemoglobin and recent weight loss. Correction of malnutrition before surgery decreases the risk of surgery. If body weight is 10 percent below the ideal weight for height and if time permits, patients can be referred to a dietitian for dietary counselling, given nutritional supplements, referred to a community resource that delivers meals to the home or helped by family and friends to improve intake (Beckermann & Galloway, 1989). It is important to document information on food and fluid preferences and any food allergies. Cultural or religious practices in relation to food and any special dietary needs, such as a sodium-restricted or diabetic diet, should be noted and the information given to the dietary department. If the patient is overweight and if preoperative time permits, a program of exercise and weight reduction may be advised to reduce the risk of surgery.

Elimination

Kidney function is carefully assessed because the kidneys are involved with the excretion of anesthetic drugs and their end products. Urinary elimination is assessed in relation to the patient's normal voiding pattern and any problems that are currently present. Recent problems in urinary function, such as kidney infections, are noted as they may have to be investigated prior to surgery. A routine urinalysis is usually done. The nurse is responsible for instructing the patient on how to collect the sample, or assisting with the collection if the patient is unable to do so. Results of the urinalysis should be examined for abnormalities. The presence of sugar in the urine is of particular importance and may indicate a diabetic condition. Normal bowel function is assessed, and information about any longstanding or recent problems or aids used for bowel function is gathered.

Immunological Needs

It is important to determine the presence of a history of allergies, including a description of signs and symptoms experienced. Allergies to any medications, blood products or contrast media used in radiological procedures are of special significance. Some medications such as corticosteroids, radiotherapy and chemotherapy produce immunosuppression, and careful assessment of these factors is essential. Body temperature is taken, and the mildest deviation should be reported to the physician.

IMPACT OF SURGERY ON SECURITY AND SELF-ESTEEM

Surgery may be judged as a stressful event that threatens the patient's security and self-esteem. Anxiety is a common problem before surgery. Anxieties may arise if the patient fears death on the operating room table, mutilation or disfigurement, postoperative pain and separation from family and friends. Often the patient is afraid that the surgeon will find evidence of cancer, or worse still a cancer that is too large to remove. The patient may be anxious about how to cope after surgery, both in the hospital and at home. The extent of the surgery, including the discomfort and changes that are anticipated, is often related to the amount of anxiety experienced. The patient who is having surgery for a small hernia may be less anxious than the one who is to have open-heart surgery. Young children may be very anxious prior to any surgery.

During the preoperative period, discharge planning is begun. The patient may express concerns about managing care after hospital discharge. Assistance may be required to plan for care once the patient returns home. The health care system may provide rehabilitative care or professional community nursing care such as that required for wound care. Convalescent care, however, is the responsibility of the patient and significant others. If the patient is unable to make arrangements for help at home, referral to a social worker or a community nurse to assist in this process is beneficial.

The patient may seek information to help control anxiety. The information may be used to formulate a picture of the events to be encountered, to increase the understanding and interpretation of specific elements in the surgical experience and to make plans to minimize the negative aspects of the illness (Johnson & Lauver, 1989). Research studies have shown that nursing interventions related to providing accurate, relevant information, reassurance and attention to individual concerns produce positive outcomes in the postoperative period. These outcomes include improved satisfaction with care, reduced pain, decreased anxiety and minimized postoperative complications (Devine & Cook, 1986; Hathaway, 1986).

Diagnosing Preoperatively

Two major nursing diagnoses of the preoperative period are *Knowledge Deficit regarding the preoperative procedures and protocols and the postoperative expectations* and *Anxiety related to the surgical experience and the outcome of surgery*.

Planning and Implementing Preoperatively

PREOPERATIVE EDUCATION PROGRAMS

A health-promoting strategy that assists the patient and family to prepare for the psychological and physiological stresses of surgery is preoperative education. Preoperative education programs are given prior to hospital admission in preadmission clinics and outpatient clinics or after admission to the hospital. In situations where there is limited time for education, such as before emergency surgery, patients are given small amounts of situational information and psychosocial support. Information about skills training or role expectations is given during the postoperative period.

Preoperative teaching is done in groups or on a one-to-one basis. Whatever the method, it is important to determine the level of understanding of the surgical process and the type of surgery that is to be done. It is important to assess the patient's ability to learn, and to identify any problems that might interfere with learning, such as poor eyesight, hearing

with special learning needs require an alteration in the type and amount of preoperative education. The preoperative assessment and teaching should involve the family or significant others. The family is then able to provide the support and assistance the patient needs in order to review what the nurse has said and to help in the application of the information. Many facilities have excellent teaching aids, but they are not substitutes for education by the nurse who understands about the specific type of surgery, the sensations to expect and the role to be taken by the patient in recovery.

The types of information that are given preoperatively are situational information, sensation and discomfort information, patient role information, psychosocial support and skills training (Schoessler, 1989). Situational information includes descriptions of nursing care activities, equipment and explanation of the sequence and timing of events. Information about sensations and discomfort includes explanation about the sensations the patient may experience and how discomforts can be managed. Role information describes the ways in which the patient will be expected to participate in care so that the treatment goals are met, for example, telling the patient to call a nurse for assistance the first time out of bed after surgery. Psychosocial support refers to the interactions between the nurse and the patient that are aimed at alleviating anxiety or enhancing coping.

Preoperative Education Program

Goals

1. to provide information regarding the surgery and sensations to be expected
2. to assist the patient to manage preoperative anxiety, and thus optimize coping abilities
3. to assist the patient in identifying roles and responsibilities in the preoperative, postoperative and recovery periods.

Expected Outcomes

The patient will be able to:

1. state the nature and purpose of the surgery, and the anticipated course of the surgical illness experience
2. describe the sensations to be expected after surgery and identify strategies to manage the sensations. The patient will postoperatively report pain to the nurse and take analgesics as necessary
3. perform deep-breathing, coughing and leg exercises
4. identify his or her role and responsibilities preoperatively and postoperatively
5. adhere to dietary and smoking restrictions, and any other preoperative instructions.

Skill training is the explanation and guided practice of skills, such as deep breathing and coughing, that aid the patient in protecting or restoring health.

presented beginning at the bottom of this page. This includes the goals, expected outcomes, educational content and evaluation of a teaching program provided at the Scarborough Grace Hospital and Sunnybrook Health Sciences Centre, Toronto, Ontario (Desjardins, Noble, Bubela, McKibbon & Galloway, 1992).

To promote continuity of care, an education checklist is placed on the chart. An example of an education checklist is given in the box below, followed by a description of the information to be given in each category. The content is individualized to reflect the surgical procedure and the circumstances.

1. INFORMATION PROVIDED SPECIFIC TO THE PROCEDURE Document the information provided that is specific to the surgical procedure, such as the nature of the procedure, postoperative nursing care and expected course in hospital.

2. ANESTHETIC Many patients are afraid of being awake or in pain during surgery. Some patients fear not waking up after surgery. Reassure the patient that modern anesthesia is effective and that the anesthetist will monitor the patient carefully. Give general information about how a local or general anesthetic works, and what sensations, such as sore throat, may be experienced afterwards. Ask the patient to write down other questions for the anesthetist. The anesthetist will see the patient the evening before surgery or the morning of surgery. Ask if the patient has had any experience or problem with anesthetics before. Notify the anesthesia department or the on-call anesthetist of the patient's name and unique hospital number if any concerns exist.

Preoperative Education Checklist

Content Given:

1. Information Provided Specific to the Procedure
2. Type of Anesthetic: General, Neuroleptic or Local
3. Dietary Restrictions:
   Pre-OR_______ Post-OR_______
4. Medications:
5. IV Therapy:
6. Dressings and Drainage Tubes:
7. Oxygen Therapy:
8. Sensations Experienced: (Pain)
9. Smoking Restriction:
10. Deep-Breathing and Coughing Exercises:
11. Leg Exercises:
12. Coping:
13. Hospital Policies: Visiting, Smoking, Discharge Time

3. DIETARY RESTRICTIONS All patients are allowed clear fluids until two to three hours before surgery, unless ordered differently by the physician. Postoperatively, diet as tolerated (DAT) is usual. After abdominal surgery, the patient will usually be NPO until he or she has passed gas through the rectum.

4. MEDICATIONS People receiving cardiac medications such as digoxin, antiarrhythmics or antihypertensives (but not diuretics) may be asked by the anesthetist to take medications with a sip of water the morning of surgery. No other medications are to be taken.

5. INTRAVENOUS THERAPY An intravenous (IV) may be inserted preoperatively. The IV is needed to give fluids and medications. It will be removed when the patient is drinking well. Instruct the patient to report pain, swelling or redness at the IV insertion site.

6. DRESSINGS AND DRAINAGE TUBES Ascertain what the surgeon has described to the patient about dressings and drainage tubes and correct any misconceptions.

7. OXYGEN THERAPY The patient may have oxygen given in the post-anesthetic care unit (PACU) or recovery room only. Instruct people who are smokers and those with respiratory disease that they may be required to wear an oxygen mask or nasal prongs for longer.

8. SENSATIONS EXPERIENCED Pain is a major sensation experienced after surgery. Describe the type and severity of pain that the patient can expect. The type of questions asked by patients before surgery (Pogue, 1993) are outlined in the following box. Explain other sensations that the patient can expect pre- or postoperatively, such as nausea, plugged nose or sore throat.

Questions Patients Ask about Pain After Surgery

Being comfortable after surgery is important. You can work with your nurses and doctors to manage your pain after surgery.

What is pain?
People call pain many things. They may say pain is a soreness, a hurt, a pang, an ache, a sting or a cramp. Only the person who has pain knows when it is there, and can describe what it is.

Why is it important to decrease pain after surgery?
With less pain, moving is easier. By moving, you may avoid problems that can delay your recovery. Getting out of bed and walking after surgery keeps your muscles strong and prevents blood clotting. Deep breathing after surgery helps prevent lung problems.

Why will I have pain after surgery?
Pain after surgery may be due to the cutting of skin and tissues, drainage tubes or muscle soreness from the position in which your body was during surgery.

Where will I have pain?
Pain is often in the area of the surgery. Ask your doctor or nurse where you may expect to have pain.

How much pain will I have?
This is a hard question to answer. Two people having the same type of surgery may have different amounts of pain. Medications are available to help decrease your pain.

How will the nurse know how much pain I have?
Tell your nurse how much pain you have. The nurse may ask you how much pain you have on a scale of 0 to 10. No pain is 0. The worst pain you can think of is 10.

When should I tell the nurse about my pain?
Tell your nurse when you start to have pain, if your pain medication does not help or if you have a different type of pain.

When will I get pain medication?
Pain medication will be ordered by your doctor. Ask your nurse for pain medication when you start to have pain. Do not wait until you have severe pain. Ask for pain medication half an hour to an hour before activity.

What medication will I get for my pain?
Medication containing a narcotic is usually given for pain after surgery. This medication may be given by a needle at first. When you can drink, a pain pill is often given. Other ways are used to give pain medication for some patients. If this applies to you, your doctor or nurse will discuss this with you.

Can I become addicted to pain medication?
People seldom become addicted to medication taken for pain after surgery. Unless you have had a problem with drug addiction, this should not worry you. If you have or had a problem with drug addiction, let your doctor know.

Do pain medications have any side effects?
Possible side effects include constipation, nausea or drowsiness. Please ask your nurse or doctor how to manage these symptoms in the hospital and at home.

What can I do to decrease pain?

- Do not wait until you have severe pain before you ask for pain medication.
- Change your position in bed. Ask your nurse if you need help to change your position.
- If you had surgery in the area of your stomach or chest, hold a pillow against your incision while you do breathing and coughing exercises.
- If you have gas pain, walk at least three times per day.
- If you have worries about being in hospital, talk to your nurse.
- Try reading, watching television, listening to music, talking on the telephone, visiting or other quiet activities. These things can help your pain at any time or when you are waiting for pain medication to work.

SOURCE: Pogue, 1993.

9. SMOKING Patients who smoke must stop prior to surgery, as smoking increases mucus production, causing more coughing, and also increases risk for respiratory complications

ing, such as relaxation exercises and discontinuing activities associated with smoking, such as drinking alcohol or coffee.

10. DEEP BREATHING AND COUGHING Review the method for deep breathing and coughing, and have the patient give a repeat demonstration. Explain the rationale for the exercises and give the patient a copy of the instructions, if available.

11. LEG EXERCISES Review leg exercises to be done postoperatively. Instruct the patient to call for assistance the first time ambulating and at any time if feeling unsteady or dizzy.

12. COPING Ask if the patient anticipates any problems coping with the surgery during hospitalization and after hospital discharge. Ascertain if the patient has any recent emotional problems or major losses (for example, loss of a spouse, very ill family member or depression), which may increase the stress response to surgery.

13. HOSPITAL POLICIES Explain visiting hours, the no-smoking policy and the discharge time.

Effectiveness of the preoperative teaching is evaluated by the nurse after surgery using a questionnaire similar to the one depicted in the box below.

IMMEDIATE PREOPERATIVE CARE IN THE HOSPITAL

No matter how well prepared, people are often anxious at the time of hospitalization. They are labelled with an arm band, most of their possessions are taken away and they are given a hospital gown to wear. They may be told when and where they can come and go; they are stabbed with needles and have numerous personal questions asked of them by a variety of health professionals These events happen at a time when they are anxious about the planned surgery.

The nurse is responsible for taking or completing the nursing assessment, and reviewing or giving information in the preoperative period to ease the patient's anxiety. In ad-

is safely prepared for surgery. Vital signs are taken to obtain baseline data and to observe for deviations that indicate the patient is not in good general health. An elevated temperature, irregular heart beat or abnormal blood pressure are vitally important to document and to report. Safe preparation includes nutritional, fluid and integumentary considerations.

Nutrition and Bowel Elimination

Clear fluid may be allowed until two to three hours prior to the administration of an anesthetic. Food and fluids are then withheld so that the stomach will be empty while the patient is under anesthetic. Ensuring that the patient understands and complies with the food and fluid restrictions is vital to prevent the aspiration of regurgitated stomach contents. Such material in the lungs causes irritation and an inflammatory reaction and decreases adequate air exchange (Kaller & Everett, 1993). If the surgery being planned involves the gastrointestinal tract or surrounding area, the intestinal tract is cleared of stool the night prior to surgery. A variety of bowel preparations is used to accomplish the cleaning. These will be ordered by the surgeon and administered according to agency policy.

Skin Preparation

The first line of defence of the body against injury or invading agents is a healthy and intact skin. The objective of preoperative skin preparation is to decrease bacterial sources without injuring the skin. The patient may have a bath or shower using a chemical antimicrobial agent to cleanse the skin. The patient is asked to wash the hair and to clean under the fingernails. The nurse may be responsible for performing certain scrubs or instructing the patient in these procedures.

The skin and the area around the site of the incision are *not* shaved (Cruse & Foord, 1980; Seropian & Reynolds,

Evaluation of Effectiveness of Preoperative Education Questionnaire

Circle the appropriate response.

Rate this patient in relation to:	Poor		Good		Excellent
1. knowledge of the surgical procedure	1	2	3	4	5
2. knowledge of sensations to expect	1	2	3	4	5
3. knowledge of expected hospital course	1	2	3	4	5
4. knowledge of post-op exercises	1	2	3	4	5
5. compliance with post-op exercises	1	2	3	4	5
6. reporting of post-op pain	1	2	3	4	5
7. appropriate taking of analgesics	1	2	3	4	5
8. adherence to NPO and dietary restrictions	1	2	3	4	5

1971), as research has shown that shaving destroys the natural skin defence and can create superficial bacterial growth (Alexander, Fischer, Boyajian, Palmquist & Morris, 1983). If removal of hair at the operative site is necessary, the area is cleaned with a depilatory cream or by electric clippers. Depilatory creams have a chemical base to remove the hair. They result in a clean, smooth and intact skin. The electric clipper with a disposable head is also a safe effective method for hair removal and leaves skin intact (Alexander et al., 1983). If removal of hair by shaving is necessary, it is done 30 minutes or less prior to surgery ("AORN recommended practices," 1992) to minimize the risk of infection.

NURSING INTERVENTIONS ON THE DAY OF SURGERY

There are a number of nursing interventions aimed at safety and at protecting the patient from injury that are performed on the day of surgery. These provisions are instituted prior to the administration of the preoperative medication. Most facilities have a checklist to guide the nurse in completing all the activities before the patient goes to the operating room (see Figure 33.1).

INFORMED CONSENT Determine whether the patient or a legal representative of the patient has given written informed consent. The word "consent" means to agree that something should be done. Physicians have a nontransferable legal duty to obtain a patient's informed consent for any medical or surgical treatment (Curtin, 1993). If the patient has signed a consent form, but the nurse finds that the patient has withdrawn consent, or expresses confusion or uncertainty about the planned surgery, the nurse informs the physician, who is then obligated to explain the matter again to the patient.

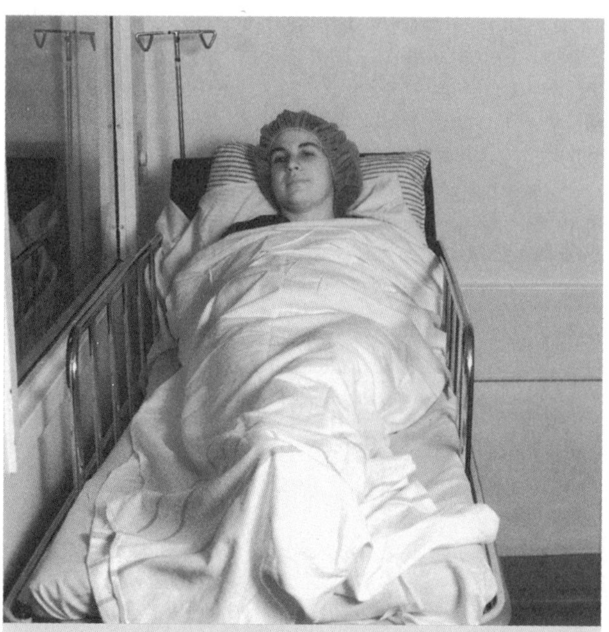

Patient awaiting transfer to the operating room.

THE PATIENT'S RECORD Physician orders are reviewed to ensure that all recommended preparations have been instituted. All pertinent laboratory and preoperative test results are to be present on the chart.

IDENTIFICATION LABEL Ensure that the patient's identification label is correct. The correct spelling of the name and the unique hospital number are carefully checked. The unique hospital number will be used to identify the unconscious patient and to label tissue specimens sent to the laboratory. The patient who has a Medic-Alert bracelet is either to wear it or to have it taped securely to the hospital record.

HYGIENE AND DRESS After bathing, the patient is given a hospital gown to wear. According to hospital policy, all nail polish is removed from fingers and toes to facilitate observation of tissue perfusion in the extremities. All jewellery and hair pins are removed. If the patient does not wish to remove a wedding ring, it is secured with a piece of tape placed around the finger.

DENTURES Check for, remove and store dentures or partial dental appliances. These are removed to decrease the risk of inadvertent aspiration and obstruction of the airway during the surgery. Research has shown that many patients who wear dentures are distressed at having to remove them (Cobley, Dunne & Sanders, 1991). The nurse should not ask the patient to remove dentures until necessary, and if the patient's distress is high, he or she should explore the possibility of the patient's keeping them in place until arrival in the operating room.

HEALTH AIDS AND PROSTHETIC DEVICES Other health aids and prosthetic devices are identified. Contact lenses are removed, as are glasses. If a patient is unable to hear without a hearing aid, it is often left in place. The nurse in the operating room will need to be informed of the hearing aid. Other prosthetic devices such as artificial limbs are labelled, removed and placed in a secure location on the nursing unit.

FAMILY AND SUPPORT PEOPLE The family or support persons are identified by the patient. The patient's wishes are determined about who is to be notified by the physician after the surgery. Family and support people are given guidance about where to wait during surgery, the anticipated length of the surgery and when the physician will speak to them after the procedure.

VITAL SIGNS The patient's pulse, blood pressure, respiratory rate and temperature are taken and documented before administration of preoperative medications or within several hours of the planned surgery if no preoperative medication is ordered. Deviations from the patient's baseline vital signs are reported to the doctor.

URINARY BLADDER The patient is to void so that the bladder is emptied. A distended bladder can obscure the operative area in pelvic and abdominal surgery, increase

ROYAL COLUMBIAN HOSPITAL

OWNED AND OPERATED BY THE FRASER-BURRARD HOSPITAL SOCIETY

PREOPERATIVE CHECKLIST

Signature & Status	Initials	Signature & Status	Initials

MARK EACH ITEM APPROPRIATELY
(✓ = Yes, – = No, N/A Non-Applicable)

				Initials
GENERAL:	1.	Surgical consent complete (signed, witnessed, dated, appropriate procedure(s).		
	2.	Identification band in place?		
	3.	Allergy band in place?		
	4.	Any bruises/bedsores? Specify:		
	5.	Loose or capped teeth; bridge work.		
	6.	Preoperative teaching done?		
	7.	Shave prep done? Location.		
	8.	Hibitane bath/shower? Skin prep?		
	9.	Make-up, nail polish, bobby pins, wigs, contact lenses removed?		
	10.	Jewellery removed or secured: (circle)		
	11.	Prostheses removed: Specify		
		e.g. partials; dentures; glasses; glass eyes; hearing aids)		
	12.	Effects in temporary storage? Specify where.		
SPECIFIC:	1.	Enema given? Type ______ Effect ______		
	2.	Last food or drink at ______ hours.		
	3.	Levine inserted? Time ______ Size ______		
	4.	Catheter inserted + spec. sent? Time ______ Size ______		
	5.	Voided: Time ______ Amount ______ Combistix done?		
	6.	Vital signs operative day: ______ Weight Actual ______ Estimate ______		
	7.	Special pre-op procedures completed? Specify: ______ (e.g., IV, blood gases) ______		
	8.	Pre-med(s) given and charted on Anesthetic Record?		
CHART:	1.	Old chart/thinned charts?		
	2.	Extra consultation forms on chart?		
	3.	Medical history on chart?		
	4.	Electrolytes/hemoglobin report?		
	5.	Cross-match done? Rh factor (if applicable) Pos.______ Neg ______		
	6.	ECG/x-rays? (Circle)		
	7.	Addressograph plate?		
		Patient being transferred to ______ ward following OR? Is Transfer Sheet completed?		

COMMENTS: (e.g., isolation, blind, deaf, positioning restrictions, equipment with patient, physician notified of abnormal results).

______ Date and Time

______ Time

______ Ward Nurse's Signature

______ O.R. Porter

______ Receiving Nurse—O.R.

FIGURE 33.1 Preoperative checklist form

SOURCE: Royal Columbian Hospital, New Westminster, British Columbia.

the risk for inadvertent penetration of the bladder and increase the chance of reflex bladder emptying as muscles relax during anesthesia.

PREOPERATIVE MEDICATION If ordered, the preoperative medication is given. The medication may be ordered to decrease anxiety, make the induction of anesthesia less stressful or decrease secretions in the mouth and throat. Once the medication is given, the patient is asked to remain in bed and, as a safety precaution, the side rails are raised.

FINAL CHECK The nurse makes a final check to ensure that everything has been done for the patient's safety.

When the operating room notifies the nursing unit, the patient is taken to the operating room area on a stretcher. Patients may be transported on a bed if the bed has special attachments, such as traction. The patient's chart is sent to the operating room. A porter may take the patient from the nursing unit to the operating room. The nurse should accompany those individuals who are unable to communicate easily, who are not hemodynamically stable or who are unduly anxious.

PREPARING THE POSTOPERATIVE UNIT The postoperative unit is set up directly after the patient goes to surgery. It involves making a postoperative bed and assembling necessary equipment for postoperative care. The postoperative bed, also called an *anesthetic bed* or *recovery bed,* is a variation of the basic hospital bed. Its purpose is to provide a safe, clean area into which a patient can be easily moved. It is set up so that bed linen can be changed with a minimum of disturbance to the patient.

Making a postoperative bed is similar to making an unoccupied bed (Procedure 26.1). Usually the foundation for an unoccupied bed is completed, and then a cotton drawsheet, flannelette sheet or catch pad is placed over it to protect the bottom sheet. This is done because a short sheet or catch pad can be changed more easily than an entire bottom sheet and therefore causes the least disturbance to the patient. Flannelette sheets are preferred by some because they provide additional warmth. The top covers are applied and then fan-folded to the bottom of the bed in preparation for the patient's transfer into bed upon return to the unit.

Once the bed is made, it is raised to the high position so that it will be at the same level as the stretcher, and a check is made to ensure that the wheels are locked. This will facilitate safe transfer of the patient from the stretcher to the bed. The other furniture and equipment in the room are arranged to make room for the stretcher.

Supplies and equipment needed for postoperative care are gathered and placed for convenient access. The patient's personal belongings are put safely away, and the over-bed table is left clear. Tissues and a kidney basin should be immediately available. An intravenous pole should be either attached to the bed or available in the patient's room.

The Postoperative Period

A patient's postoperative response to surgical intervention can be varied and complex. Any one of the patient's basic needs can be affected, depending on the nature of each situation. The nurse assesses the patient, diagnoses problems and plans, implements and evaluates care by applying knowledge of the impact of the surgery on basic human needs. In this section, we will discuss the immediate postoperative care and initial assessment of the patient upon return to the nursing unit. The impact of surgery on the patient's basic needs and an outline of care organized according to the nursing process will follow. This includes examples of nursing diagnoses and expected outcomes, as well as nursing strategies to achieve patient goals. Evaluation of the effectiveness of care is based on the goal being achieved.

Immediate Postoperative Care

Most patients go to a post-anesthesia care unit (PACU) directly from the operating room. In the PACU, nurses are responsible for the patient's recovery from anesthesia. Nursing care includes assessing the patient's level of consciousness, vital signs and presence or absence of reflexes, as well as drainage from dressings, tubes and collecting bags on arrival and at frequent intervals. Immediate postoperative orders for medications, x-rays, oxygen, intravenous and blood infusions or laboratory work are instituted. Pain control strategies are implemented. These may include setting up and initiating patient-controlled analgesia (PCA) (Maxwell, 1992). The nurse is responsible for coaching patients who are ordered PCA for pain control and providing emotional support and comfort.

The patient is assessed as ready for transfer from the PACU to the nursing unit when vital signs are stable; orientation to person, place and time or the pre-anesthetic

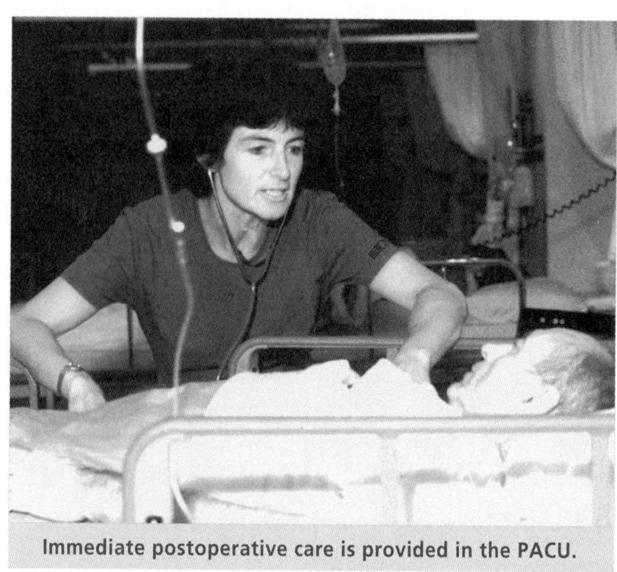

Immediate postoperative care is provided in the PACU.

level of consciousness has returned; airway is satisfactory; no significant bleeding is present; and, if regional anesthesia was used, movement of extremities has returned

who are predicted to need constant monitoring or nursing care are taken to another critical care unit.

Immediate Postoperative Assessment on the Nursing Unit

When the patient is ready for transfer to the nursing unit, the PACU nurse telephones the nurse on the floor to report the patient's condition. The PACU nurse verbally communicates information about the operative procedure, the patient's response during and after the surgery and the nursing management during recovery from anesthesia. The physician's written orders are reviewed. The patient is transferred to the nursing unit on a stretcher and is assisted to transfer to the bed. The nurse who is assuming responsibility for care makes the patient comfortable and assesses the position of the dressing and any tubes, contents of collecting bags and equipment. The assessment is done to ensure that there have been no alterations in the patient's condition during transportation. Safety precautions, such as putting the bed in a low position and positioning the patient so that the airway is patent and secretions can drain easily from the mouth, are implemented.

The nurse immediately assesses the blood pressure, pulse and respirations, and continues to monitor the vital signs every four hours for 24 hours, or more frequently if ordered or if needed. Level of consciousness, colour, temperature and condition of the skin are assessed, as well as the location of any wound or drainage tubes. The dressings, drainage and functioning of the equipment are reassessed every four hours for the first 24 hours, and then as needed.

Ongoing Postoperative Assessment and Intervention

OXYGEN: BREATHING AND AIRWAY

Oxygen needs during and after surgery are of major concern. During general anesthesia, the central nervous system is depressed and the body's muscles are relaxed. Both the anesthetic and the artificial airway inserted to assist in breathing are irritating, and they cause an increase in the secretion of mucous in the throat. The lack of muscle tone means that the patient is unable to keep the tongue from falling back and occluding the airway and is unable to expel the mucous and any other debris that collects. When a patient is recovering from the anesthetic, the nurse must protect the patient's airway by ensuring that it is clear and by assisting the patient to clear the throat and lungs of excess mucous. The patient's body movements may be restricted, and the lack of movement increases the tendency for secretions and other debris to collect in the respiratory tract. The patient is encouraged and assisted to breathe deeply, cough and, if necessary, change positions to prevent the stasis of fluids in the lungs.

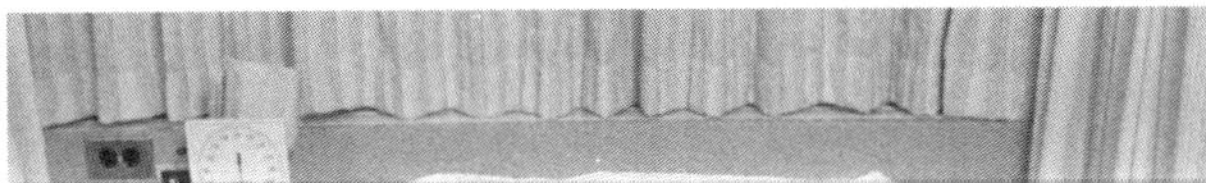

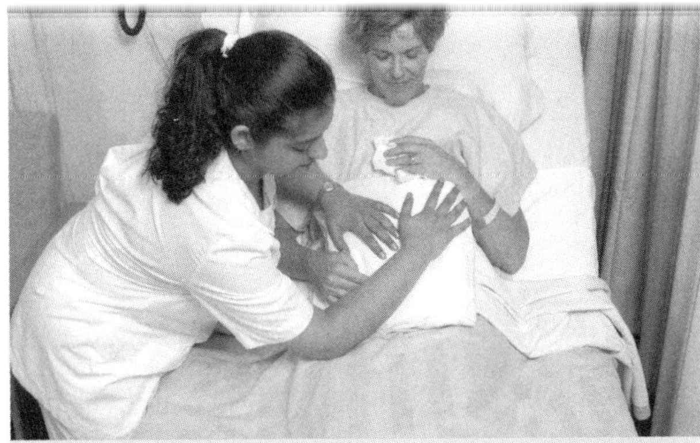

Splinting the incision with a pillow helps the patient cough more effectively.

Diagnosing: Sample Diagnosis

- *Risk for Ineffective Breathing and Airway Clearance related to poor cough effort associated with depressant effects of anesthesia and some medications* (for example, narcotic analgesics, muscle relaxants), *pain, fatigue, tenacious secretions associated with fluid loss and decreased fluid intake.*

Planning: Sample Expected Outcome

- The patient will maintain a clear airway and an effective breathing pattern as evidenced by quiet, easy breathing and normal rate, rhythm and depth of respiration.

Implementing: Health-Promoting Activities

- Promote effective airway clearance by performing actions to decrease pain so that deep breathing and coughing are done with ease. Assist and encourage mobilization as allowed and as tolerated.
- Implement measures to liquefy tenacious secretions by maintaining a fluid intake of at least 2500 mL per day unless contraindicated, and humidify inspired air.
- Instruct and assist with effective deep-breathing techniques every one to two hours unless contraindicated. Monitor the performance of deep-breathing exercises. Assist the patient to cough effectively if secretions are present in the lungs. Encourage the patient to take pain medication if pain is interfering with deep breathing and coughing. Use a small pillow to splint abdominal incisions. Encourage the patient to use an incentive spirometer, if available.

NURSES at work — Staff Nurse, Trauma Unit

I have been nursing for nine and one-half years, and am currently employed as a staff nurse on the trauma unit at the Vancouver General Hospital and Health Sciences Centre. Our patients come from all over the province. The typical patient is young, male and has sustained an injury in a motor vehicle accident. In the past couple of years, we have had more women, more older adults and an increasing number of pedestrians who have been struck by cars. We also have patients who have been injured in industrial or sports-related accidents and falls.

Our unit consists of six beds specializing in trauma care. The nurse–patient ratio is 1:2. We work 12-hour shifts. I work part time, approximately 10 shifts a month.

On my last shift, I was assigned to care for a 46-year-old man and a 62-year-old woman. Mr. J. was a forestry worker who had fallen 7.5 m from a tree, breaking both legs and his sacrum. He was one day postoperative and had a morphine infusion for pain control. An intravenous was *in situ* in his left forearm, and a Foley catheter was in place. Mrs. F. had been in a car accident two weeks ago. Her orthopedic injuries were well healed but she had developed significant postoperative complications. She was very restless and had required restraints.

I started my shift with a head-to-toe assessment. I then prepared the h.s. (bed-time) medications, hung new intravenous bags and settled my patients for the night. I took my supper break at 22:30, then completed some charting and other miscellaneous paperwork. At midnight, I balanced the fluid balance sheets.

At 01:00 hours, we received a new patient from the PACU, which kept us busy for approximately 30 minutes. This included a head-to-toe assessment, vital signs, checking the dressing, drainage, intravenous and other tubes and equipment and transcribing the physician's postoperative orders. Between 02:00 and 05:00, I checked my patients q15 min for any changes in their health status, in particular their comfort level. It is important to continue assessing the patients, because unpredictable events may occur. For example, Mr. J's temperature was elevated at 03:00, and his hemoglobin had dropped from 110 to 90 mg/dL. I immediately phoned the physician on call to notify him of this laboratory result and Mr. J's elevated temperature. When he returned the page, we mutually decided that it would be appropriate to repeat Mr. J's hemoglobin level and administer plain Tylenol to help alleviate his symptoms.

Another busy time on the unit is 06:00 h. I am usually taking another set of vital signs, providing analgesia and turning and positioning my patients. By 07:00, the day staff have arrived and my shift is completed with a verbal patient status report.

At times, the work on the trauma unit can be very hectic, but there are many rewards. The highlight of my work is seeing people recover. I know then that I have made a difference in someone's life.

—*Tina Mettala, RN*

Implementing: Health-Protecting Activities

- Monitor for rapid, shallow respiration, dyspnea and use of accessory respiratory muscles, restlessness, irritability and confusion.
- Monitor for signs of respiratory distress such as the sounds of rasping heard when an airway is partially blocked, wet or noisy breathing and changes in skin colour.
- Monitor for and report signs and symptoms of pneumonia, such as productive coughing of purulent, green or rust-coloured sputum, chills and fever.
- Position the patient on the side so that the tongue does not occlude the airway and any secretions and vomitus can drain from the mouth rather than being aspirated.
- Encourage and assist the patient to change position every two to four hours to prevent the accumulation of secretions and debris in the respiratory tract.
- Perform actions to reduce risk of aspiration, such as withholding food and fluids if gag reflex is absent or if the patient experiences severe nausea and/or vomiting. Place the patient in a semi- to high Fowler's position during eating or drinking and 30 minutes after, unless contraindicated.
- Administer narcotic analgesics, sedatives and tranquillizers judiciously. Withhold medication and consult physician if respiratory rate is less than 10 per minute.

OXYGEN: CIRCULATION AND BLOOD VOLUME

Shock and hemorrhage are always potential problems after surgery. Bleeding may result from the rupture of small surface blood vessels or from trauma to larger, deeper-lying ones. It may be caused by spontaneous rupture of a vessel that is weakened in the process of trauma, by the giving way of sutures that are used to repair damaged vessels, or by problems in the clotting mechanism resulting from a lack of certain clotting factors in the blood.

The presence of bright red blood on dressings from a wound is always a sign of actual or potential hemorrhage, and should be reported promptly. A registered nurse must check a wound when fresh red blood is observed and report to the physician immediately. A bleeding wound is monitored frequently (q15–20 min) to see if the bleeding is increasing. If bleeding becomes excessive, the patient may show signs of shock. Evidence of shock is observed through changes in the vital signs (such as falling blood pressure), rapid weak pulse, pallor, cold and clammy skin, weakness and restlessness. If any of these signs are detected, a registered nurse is alerted immediately and interventions, such as increasing intravenous fluids, are initiated.

Diagnosing: Sample Diagnosis

- *PC: Hypovolemic shock associated with hemorrhage and dehydration.*

Planning: Sample Nursing Goal

- The nurse will manage and minimize postoperative bleeding (Carpenito, 1997).

Implementing: Health-Protecting Activities

- Monitor and report bleeding, gastrointestinal and wound drainage, persistent vomiting and/or difficulty taking fluids orally.
- Monitor for and report signs of hypovolemic shock, such as:
  - restlessness
  - agitation
  - confusion
  - decrease in BP below 90 systolic in a normotensive patient and 30 systolic below baseline in a hypertensive patient
  - decline in BP of 15 with concurrent rise in pulse when patient changes from lying to standing or sitting position
  - resting pulse rate greater than 100 beats/minute
  - rapid or laboured respirations
  - cool, pale or cyanotic skin
  - diminished or absent peripheral pulses
  - urine output less than 30 mL/hour.
- Implement measures to prevent hypovolemic shock, such as administering fluid volume replacement as ordered. Perform actions to prevent nausea and vomiting. When oral intake is allowed, maintain a fluid intake of at least 2500 mL/day unless contraindicated.
- If bleeding occurs, apply firm, prolonged pressure to area, if possible.
- If signs and symptoms of hypovolemic shock occur, notify the physician and continue above measures to control bleeding. Place patient flat in bed with legs elevated 20 degrees unless contraindicated. Monitor vital signs frequently (q10–15 min). Provide emotional support to the patient and significant others.
- Keep the patient warm.

OXYGEN: OTHER CIRCULATORY DISTURBANCES

One potential problem is the development of an embolus.

through the circulatory system until they reach a point at which the vessel is too small to enable them to pass. They then lodge in the vessel, blocking the blood flow to or from the tissues supplied by the artery or drained by the vein. Pulmonary embolism, when the clot travels to the lungs, is a potential hazard for all patients after surgery.

The nurse needs to observe for signs of phlebitis (inflammation of the veins), which predisposes clot formation. A common site for phlebitis is the calf. Characteristic signs are redness, edema, pain and warmth in the area. Postoperatively, one of the best measures to prevent clot formation is to get the patient mobile as quickly as possible.

Diagnosing: Sample Diagnosis

- *PC: Thromboembolism associated with venous stasis resulting from decreased activity and/or trauma to vein walls during surgery.*

Planning: Sample Nursing Goal

- The nurse will manage and minimize complications of phlebitis and pulmonary embolism (Carpenito, 1997).

Implementing: Health-Promoting Activities

- Implement actions to prevent peripheral pooling of blood such as teaching and supervising active leg exercises five minutes every hour when awake, and mobilization at a minimum of three times a day. Maintain a minimum fluid intake of 2500 mL/day unless contraindicated to prevent dehydration and increased blood viscosity, which leads to hypercoagulability.
- Discourage positions that compromise blood flow (for example, pillows under knees, crossing legs, sitting for long periods).
- If ordered, apply antiembolism stockings to decrease pooling of blood in the legs. Remove once a shift and provide skin care (see Figure 33.2 and Procedure 33.1).

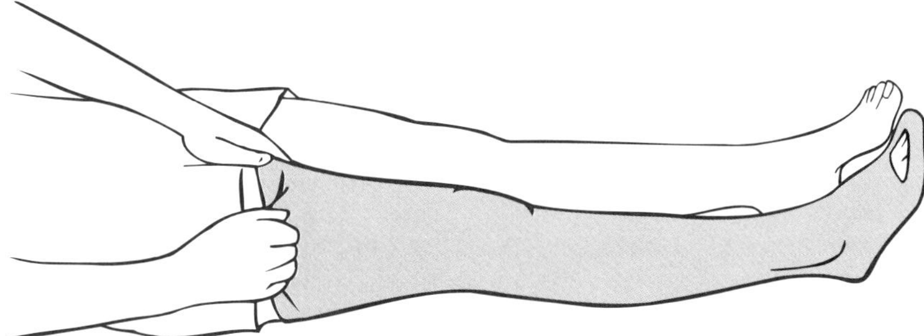

FIGURE 33.2 Antiembolism stockings force blood from smaller vessels into the deep veins and also prevent pooling of blood in the legs. The stockings are removed several times a day to check the colour of skin. To ensure that the stockings are not exerting too much pressure and reducing circulation to the legs, toenail colour can be checked more frequently through the opening in the stocking at the toes

PROCEDURE 33.1

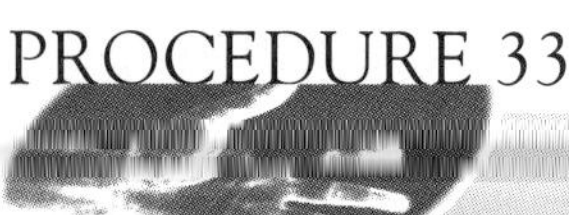

Applying Antiembolism Stocking

Action	*Rationale*
1. Gather equipment: • tape measure • talcum powder • correct size stocking.	Ensures efficiency and economy of time.
2. Wash hands and maintain medical asepsis.	Reduces transmission of microorganisms.
3. Assess patient's understanding of procedure and purpose. Explain procedure and provide privacy.	Allays anxiety and enhances emotional well-being.
4. Measure for correct size of antiembolism stocking according to manufacturer's directions: • **Knee-high:** Measure the circumference of the patient's calf at its widest point (approximately 15 cm below the patella) and length of the leg from the heel to the popliteal space. • **Thigh-high:** Measure the circumference of the patient's calf (as above) and thigh (approximately 15 cm above the patella) and the length of the leg from the heel to the gluteal fold. • **Waist-high:** Measure the calf and thigh as above, and the length of the leg from the heel to the gluteal fold or waist along the lateral aspect of the body.	Ensures that the stocking is not so tight that it impairs circulation by excessive pressure or constriction, nor so large that it does not support the leg.
5. Refer to the manufacturer's size chart and obtain the correct size stocking.	Ensures that the correct size is chosen according to the individual manufacturer's measurements.
6. Apply the stocking before the patient arises in the morning. If the patient has been ambulatory, have him or her elevate the legs for 15–30 minutes.	Facilitates venous return and decreases swelling before applying stocking.
7. Have the patient's legs clean and dry, and apply talc if not contraindicated.	Allows for easy application of stocking
8. Roll the stocking down to the ankle by inserting your hand into the stocking and grasp the heel.	Allows for easier insertion of the foot.
9. Apply the stocking to the leg:	
• Face the patient; slip the stocking over the toes and cover the foot to the heel pocket. Check the fit on the foot.	Ensures that there is no pressure on the toes and no constriction of the foot. Assessment windows or sheer portions of the toes in the stocking allow for assessment.
• Without twisting or leaving wrinkles, pull the stocking up the calf, over the knees or to the thigh (depending on stocking length), and apply adjustable belt if there is one.	Twisted or wrinkled stockings can cause discomfort, pressure on skin and/or impedance of circulation.
10. Make sure the stocking is completely extended, not binding at the top and not rolled or turned down. Teach the patient this.	Rolled or turned-down stockings may constrict circulation and impede venous return.
11. Check the circulation after 1 hour, i.e., colour, temperature, capillary refill and pulses; also skin condition, changes in calf or thigh circumference, patient comfort.	Ensures that circulatory status is satisfactory and that there are no skin allergies or development of thrombophlebitis.
12. Remove stocking once per shift or at least twice a day for up to an hour (unless otherwise ordered) and assess as in #11.	Allows for skin cleansing and assessment for skin redness, lesions, circulatory impairment and tissue edema.
13. Document date and time of application or removal, circulatory and skin assessments before and after application, size and length of stocking, any complications noted and patient comfort.	Communicates patient care given and response to therapy.

Implementing: Health-Protecting Activities

- Monitor for and report signs and symptoms of venous

increase in circumference of calf or thigh (measure at the same place[s] on leg once a shift), unusual warmth and redness in extremity.
- If signs and symptoms of a venous thrombus occur, maintain bed rest until activity orders are received. Prepare the patient for diagnostic studies such as Doppler ultra sonography or duplex scan. Do not rub the affected area, as it may dislodge a formed clot.
- Provide emotional support to the patient and significant others if thromboembolism occurs.
- Administer anticoagulants (blood thinners) as necessary.

WATER, SODIUM, POTASSIUM AND ACID–BASE BALANCE

Surgery always results in a loss of fluids from the body from the blood vessels, from the interstitial spaces and from cells as tissues are cut during the surgical procedure. The body's protective mechanisms are activated and there is increased production of antidiuretic hormone (ADH) and aldosterone. Antidiuretic hormone increases the reabsorption of water by the kidney, protecting the volume of circulating fluid. Aldosterone increases sodium and water retention, enhancing plasma volume and blood pressure. With surgery, there is also a loss of potassium, as large amounts are released from damaged cells and excreted in the urine.

There is usually a disturbance of the body's acid–base balance, with a tendency towards alkalosis. This may be caused by a number of factors. There is a decrease in the ability of the kidneys to excrete sodium bicarbonate, which results in a more acid urine. The retention of sodium and increased loss of potassium appear to reinforce this tendency. Hyperventilation in the early postoperative period also contributes to the acid loss, as carbonic acid (in the form of carbon dioxide and water) is expired from the lungs. If the patient is receiving nasogastric suctioning following surgery, there is a further depletion of acid from the gastric secretions, and this aggravates the tendency towards alkalosis. The nurse should be watchful for disturbances in the acid–base balance as evidenced by physical signs and symptoms and by laboratory findings.

Dehydration and edema are among the common potential postoperative problems. In order to maintain fluid volume and offset the anticipated loss of fluid during surgery, intravenous infusions are given. They are maintained following surgery if the patient is receiving no oral intake. An important set of signs to watch for are those indicating potassium deficit. The patient may experience general malaise, anorexia and gas in the intestinal tract. Muscles become soft, and the patient may have tremors and may become disoriented. It is necessary to be alert for signs of agitation, such as the patient's plucking at the bedclothes, and for signs of disorientation or confusion. If the potassium deficit is severe, muscles in the arms and legs may become flaccid, and there may be paresthesia. A heart block and/or

Diagnosing: Sample Diagnoses

- *Risk for Fluid Volume Deficit related to vomiting, nasogastric tube drainage and profuse wound drainage.*
- *Risk for Fluid Volume Excess related to vigorous preoperative fluid therapy and increased production of antidiuretic hormone (ADH) and aldosterone (output of these hormones is stimulated by trauma, pain, anesthetic agents and narcotic analgesics).*
- *PC: Hypokalemia.*

Planning: Sample Expected Outcome

- The patient will maintain fluid balance as evidenced by normal skin turgor, moist mucous membranes, stable weight, BP and pulse both within the patient's normal range and with position change, urine output greater than 30 mL/hour, balanced intake and output within 48 hours following surgery, clear mental status, quiet, easy breathing and absence of edema.

Planning: Sample Nursing Goal

- The nurse will manage and minimize episodes of potassium deficits (Carpenito, 1997).

Implementing: Health-Protecting Activities

- Monitor for and report signs and symptoms of fluid volume deficit, such as:
  - poor skin turgor
  - dry mucous membranes
  - thirst
  - weight loss greater than 0.5 kg/day
  - low BP and/or decline in BP of 15 mm Hg with concurrent rise in pulse when patient sits up
  - weak, rapid pulse
  - urine output less than 30 mL/hour.
- Implement measures to prevent and treat fluid and electrolyte imbalance, such as performing actions to prevent vomiting and maintaining a fluid intake of at least 2500 mL per day unless contraindicated. When oral intake is ordered and tolerated, assist the patient to select foods/fluids high in potassium (bananas, oranges, tomatoes, fruit juices) and sodium (soups, bouillon).
- Weigh patient daily, if possible.
- Provide mouth care q1-2h if tongue, lips and oral mucous membranes are dry.
- Monitor for and report signs and symptoms of fluid volume excess, such as significant weight gain (greater than 0.5 kg/day), elevated BP and pulse, intake that continues to be greater than output 48 hours postoperatively, change in mental status, dyspnea, peripheral edema.

- Implement measures to prevent and treat fluid volume excess, such as administering fluid replacement therapy judiciously, especially within first 48 hours after surgery.
- Maintain fluid restriction as ordered; restrict sodium intake as ordered.
- Consult physician if signs and symptoms of fluid volume excess persist or worsen.

NUTRITION

All types of injury to the body, including surgery, result in increased metabolic rate. The body mobilizes its forces to repair the damaged tissue, and tissue protein, especially in the skeletal muscles, is metabolized as an energy source. Excess nitrogen is excreted in the urine. There is a breakdown of fat, which becomes a major source of energy in the immediate postoperative period.

At the same time that nutritional needs are increased to keep up with the increased metabolic needs, there is a decrease in food and fluid intake. Most patients having surgery are not allowed any food or fluids for two to three hours prior to surgery. Some are unable to tolerate food and fluids for varying lengths of time postoperatively. Some anesthetic agents may cause nausea and vomiting. The patient's nutritional needs must be met, and intravenous fluids are usually given until the patient is able to tolerate a sufficient amount of nourishment by mouth to meet nutritional needs.

When oral intake is allowed, the patient is started on clear fluids, with the diet modified as tolerance for food and fluids increases. Some patients receive nasogastric feedings postoperatively. Some are maintained on nothing by mouth for a lengthy period of time, in which case total parenteral nutrition may be required.

Diagnosing: Sample Diagnosis

- *Nutrition, Altered: deficit due to food and fluid restrictions preanesthetic, postoperative nausea, vomiting or paralytic ileus (lack of intestinal mobility).*

Planning: Sample Expected Outcome

- The patient will maintain adequate nutrition as evidenced by tolerance of fluids and nutrients, and will maintain weight.

Implementing: Health-Promoting Activities

- The nurse should observe food and fluid intake and encourage the patient to increase intake gradually as tolerance improves.

Implementing: Health-Protecting Activities

- Monitor signs of nausea and vomiting, particularly in a patient who is recovering from anesthetic, is under sedation or has limited mobility.
- Assess patient to determine factors that contribute to nausea and vomiting (for example, abdominal distention, pain, anxiety, certain foods, medications, constipation).
- Implement measures to prevent nausea and vomiting, such as eliminating noxious sights and smells from the environment. Instruct the patient to change positions slowly.
- Provide oral hygiene every two hours or before meals if oral intake is allowed, and after each emesis.
- Keep a careful record of the patient's intake and output.
- When oral intake is allowed, advance the diet slowly (usually beginning with clear liquids and progressing to solid food). Instruct the patient to ingest foods and fluids slowly. Foods/fluids that irritate the gastric mucosa, such as spicy, acidic and/or caffeine-containing items, should be avoided. Encourage dry foods (toast, crackers) and discourage drinking liquids with meals if nauseated. Rest after eating with head of bed elevated to facilitate gastric emptying.
- Consult a clinical nutritionist for help in providing the patient's preferred foods or fluids.
- Monitor for therapeutic and nontherapeutic effects of antiemetic, if administered.
- Consult the physician if the above measures fail to control nausea and vomiting.

ELIMINATION NEEDS

The loss of body fluids during surgery stimulates secretion of the antidiuretic hormone. This directly reduces urinary output, lessening the loss of water from the body. The retention of sodium also helps to hold fluid in body tissues, further contributing to decreased output of urine. A relative oliguria is seen in the postoperative period for the first two to three days. The central nervous system depressant effect of anesthesia and analgesics depress neuromuscular functioning, causing muscle spasm of the sphincter in the bladder and, possibly, inability to void.

Elimination from the gastrointestinal tract is also disturbed by surgery. Lack of solid food intake in preparation for surgery, and usually for a few days postoperatively, means that there is insufficient bulk to stimulate the bowel. The restrictions imposed on activity following surgery also contribute to a sluggish bowel. A paralytic or adynamic ileus (obstruction of the intestines resulting from inhibited motility of the gastrointestinal tract) is also a fairly common occurrence following major surgery, especially if the peritoneum has been entered.

Diagnosing: Sample Diagnoses

- *Urinary Elimination, Altered Pattern due to decreased amount of urine produced (caused by increase in ADH and aldosterone), decreased fluid intake, effect of anesthetic and analgesics in increasing vasoconstriction of bladder sphincter and, possibility, necessity of voiding in a prone position.*
- *Constipation related to decreased physical mobility, decreased motility of gastrointestinal tract and decreased intake of solid food.*

Planning: Sample Expected Outcomes

- The patient will have adequate urinary output as evi- [illegible] every three to four hours with output of [illegible] 30 mL/hour and by emptying bladder when voiding.
- The patient will have adequate bowel elimination as evidenced by a bowel movement at least every three days with easy passage of stool.

Implementing: Health-Promoting Activities

- Establish a regular pattern of urinary elimination by assisting the patient to the bathroom to void every three hours.
- Encourage adequate fluid intake, if permitted, to 2500 mL/day.
- Encourage ambulation as soon as possible.
- Provide privacy in bathroom at time the patient usually evacuates bowel.

Implementing: Health-Protecting Activities

- Monitor the amount and time of first postoperative urination. If the patient has not voided by eight hours after surgery, notify the doctor.
- Monitor amount, frequency, colour and odour of urine.
- Monitor for and report signs and symptoms of urinary tract infection (for instance, cloudy, foul-smelling urine; complaints of frequency, urgency and/or burning on urination; elevated temperature; chills).
- Implement measures to prevent urinary tract infection by acting to prevent urinary retention. Such actions include helping the patient assume a normal position to void (for females, sitting; for males, standing). Instruct females to wipe from front to back after urinating or defecating. Increase activity as tolerated to decrease urinary stasis.
- Request that a stool softener be considered if the patient is taking analgesic medications that contribute to constipation.
- Monitor frequency of bowel movements.

COMFORT, REST AND SLEEP

Pain is usually experienced following surgery because of the tissue damage from mechanical disruption, inflammation and stretching. Pain disturbs comfort and may interfere with rest and sleep. If there has been tissue damage in a part of the body that is involved in mobility, movement is likely to induce and/or increase pain. The intensity of the pain may vary with the extent of surgery, the location of the incision, the degree of intraoperative trauma and the meaning of the surgery to the patient. The intensity of postoperative pain does vary, but it is more severe after intrathoracic, intra-abdominal and renal surgery, and after extensive surgery of the spine, major joints and large bones of the hand and foot (Wasylak, 1992).

The assessment of pain includes the location, the intensity and the quality of pain. The intensity of pain may be assessed by asking the patient how much pain is present on [illegible] worst pain that can be imagined. Pain intensity scales are available for children and adults. Descriptions of the quality of pain, such as "sharp," "shooting" or "dull," are determined. The assessment includes the impact of pain on usual activities and the patient's satisfaction with interventions that are used to control pain.

Diagnosing: Sample Diagnosis

- *Pain related to tissue trauma and reflex muscle spasm associated with surgery.*

Planning: Sample Expected Outcome

- The patient reports satisfaction with pain control and has a relaxed facial expression. Body positioning and activities are not limited by pain.

Implementing: Health-Promoting Activities

- Provide instruction and coaching if the patient is receiving patient-controlled analgesia.
- Provide or assist with nonpharmacological measures for pain management (for example, back rubs, position changes, relaxation techniques, a restful environment).

Implementing: Health-Protecting Activities

- Monitor for nonverbal signs of pain, such as facial grimaces, restlessness.
- Monitor the location, intensity and quality of pain every four hours and following any event that might be expected to cause pain, such as treatments.
- Implement measures to reduce pain, such as administering analgesics as ordered and monitoring for therapeutic and nontherapeutic effects.
- Instruct and assist the patient to support abdominal or chest incisions with a pillow or hands when turning, coughing and deep breathing.
- Consult physician if above measures fail to provide adequate pain relief.

MOVEMENT AND EXERCISE

During World War II, it was observed that the patient who got up and walked around in the early postoperative period recovered sooner and had fewer complications than the patient who remained in bed. Since then, early ambulation has become an important concern for nurses. The patient often needs a great deal of physical and psychological support in order to ambulate. Surgery limits mobility in several ways. If a general anesthetic is given, the patient will be unconscious and unable to move. During surgery, the patient is often maintained in one position for a prolonged period of time. Anesthesia causes muscle paralysis.

When the anesthetized patient is positioned, the muscles cannot contract against the stretching effects of certain positions. The patient may later complain of soreness in the muscles. With a spinal anesthetic, the patient is unable to move parts of the body below the site of the injection of the anesthetic. Even a local anesthetic causes immobility in and around the area being manipulated.

After surgery, pain, the extent and type of tissue damage, weakness and equipment may interfere with mobility. Pain is a major factor limiting mobility. The strain on tissues in the operative area may induce pain when turning in bed or trying to sit up, get out of bed or walk. The patient who has an abdominal incision may not realize the extent to which the abdominal muscles are involved in respiration until asked to breathe deeply or cough after surgery.

With some types of surgery, it may be important to immobilize a limb or other part of the body to allow time for the tissues to heal. The immobility may be achieved by enclosing the part in a cast, or attaching it to various pieces of equipment that severely hamper movement. Often, the patient's freedom of movement is restricted due to intravenous infusion, various tubes or drains that must accompany the patient during ambulation.

Immobility can cause many problems, such as congestion in the lungs and peripheral pooling of blood, as well as loss of muscle tone through disuse. Peripheral pooling of blood makes the patient more vulnerable to clot formation in the blood vessels, with the potential risk of emboli to the lungs and heart. There is also depletion of protein from the muscles and calcium from the bones of immobilized patients, which further interferes with mobility.

The nurse should be observant of the patient's difficulty in carrying out the necessary activities to maintain bodily functions because of limited mobility. Problems with hygiene (for example, because one arm has an intravenous infusion running into it), with feeding, in using a bedpan or in turning over in bed may arise. It is a nursing responsibility to provide the assistance the patient needs.

Antiembolism stockings are often applied in the perioperative period or when there is decreased activity, to promote venous return by maintaining external pressure on the muscles and superficial veins. These stockings prevent circulatory stasis and passive dilation of veins, which contributes to deep vein thrombosis (DVT) of the lower extremities.

Antiembolism stockings come in several types; some apply equal pressure to the entire leg, while others have a graded compression pressure that is greatest over the ankle and is decreased over the length of the leg. Length of stockings also varies, from those that extend from the foot to the knee, mid-thigh or waist. Stockings usually come in small, medium, large and extra-large sizes.

The nurse's assessment of the patient's suitability for wearing these stockings would include adequate arterial blood circulation, pulses, venous return and negative Homans' sign (if the foot is dorsiflexed, the patient will feel a normal stretch and no pain in the calf area. If the patient feels a sharp pain, this can be interpreted as a positive Homan's sign). Contraindications for antiembolism stockings include skin conditions such as open lesions, dermatitis, recent vascular and skin grafts, recent vein ligation, severe arteriosclerosis, gangrene, and pulmonary or massive edema of the extremity.

Diagnosing: Sample Diagnosis

- *Risk for Impaired Physical Mobility related to pain, weakness and fatigue, orthostatic hypotension associated with peripheral pooling of blood and blood loss during surgery, central nervous system depressant effects of some medications, presence of drainage tubing or equipment that must accompany the patient and anxiety over hurting the operative area.*

Planning: Sample Expected Outcome

- The patient will ambulate unless contraindicated three times per day, will perform hygiene in a bathroom and will sit up for all meals.

Implementing: Health-Promoting Activities

- Explain the importance of movement and exercise in promoting healthy recovery from surgery.
- Explain the importance of requesting medication for pain, so that exercises can be done comfortably.
- Keep the bed in low position. Encourage the patient to request assistance whenever needed.
- Assist to a chair for all meals.
- Assist back to bed for frequent rest periods.
- Alternate frequent (every three hours) short walks (for example, one hall length) with periods of rest. Increase length, then frequency, as tolerance improves.
- Give positive acknowledgement of the patient's efforts during and after movement and/or exercise.

Implementing: Health-Protecting Activities

- Determine the existence of conditions predisposing the patient to immobility (weakness, pain, preoperative problems in movement, narcotic analgesics, presence of long tubing and equipment, fear of hurting incision).
- Instruct the patient to wear shoes with nonskid soles and low heels when ambulating. Position tubing and equipment carefully so that they will not interfere with ambulation.
- Accompany the patient during ambulation. Ambulate in well-lit areas and use hand rails if needed. Do not rush; allow adequate time for trips to the bathroom and for ambulation. Increase level of activity as tolerated. Assist in changes of position slowly to reduce dizziness associated with orthostatic drop in BP.
- Consult a physiotherapist if the patient is immobilized or is having difficulty walking.

TEMPERATURE REGULATION

Many general anesthetics cause vasodilation, which results in

of the vasodilation is compounded by surgical exposure. As a result, the immediate postoperative body reaction is shivering. As shivering requires increased metabolism and increased metabolism is also required for tissue repair, body temperature is usually slightly elevated in the early postoperative period. This is generally considered to be a good sign that the body's recuperative mechanisms are functioning. An elevation of temperature should alert the nurse to the possibility of infection, which causes the body's metabolism to be greatly speeded up in efforts to combat the invading pathogens.

INFECTION CONTROL

One of the most important needs for all patients undergoing surgery is protection from infection. Cutting through the skin penetrates the body's first line of defence and provides ready access to deeper tissues for infectious agents. The trauma of surgery, the stress of the illness which necessitated it, the pain and decreased nutrients all are stressors that increase vulnerability to infection. The nurse should also be alert to the possibility of generalized infection following surgery. Observations the nurse should make in regard to both generalized and localized infectious processes were discussed in Chapter 32. They include signs of redness, pain, swelling, unusual discharge, elevated temperature and increased white blood cell count.

Diagnosing: Sample Diagnoses

- *Impaired Tissue Integrity related to surgical trauma.*
- *Risk for infection related to surgical incision.*

Planning: Sample Expected Outcome

- The patient will show normal healing of the surgical wound as evidenced by gradual reduction of redness and swelling at the wound site and the presence of granulation tissue or intact, approximated wound edges.

Implementing: Health-Promoting Activities

- Perform actions to maintain optimal nutritional status and adequate circulation to the wound area (for instance, do not apply dressings tightly unless ordered, as excessive pressure impairs circulation to the area).

Implementing: Health-Protecting Activities

- Monitor and report signs and symptoms of impaired wound healing (such as increasing redness and swelling at wound site and separation of wound edges).
- Inspect dressings, wounds and skin areas in contact with wound drainage (drains or puncture sites) and tape for signs of irritation and breakdown.
- Use aseptic techniques in all wound contacts.
- Decrease stress on wound by instructing and assisting the patient to support the involved area when moving and to splint abdominal and chest wounds when coughing.

that dressings are secure enough to keep them from rubbing and irritating the wound.
- Cleanse the skin and change dressings, if appropriate.
- To prevent skin irritation due to drainage, maintain the patency of drainage tubes to decrease the risk of leakage around them. Apply a collection pouch over drains, or paste to skin areas likely to be in contact with drainage. Caution the patient against lying on drainage tubes. Secure all tubing to prevent excessive movement, which can irritate mucous membranes or skin.
- To minimize skin irritation resulting from tape, use necessary amounts of tape only, and use hypoallergenic tape whenever possible to secure tubing and dressings (see Figure 33.4). Use elastic netting or Montgomery ties to avoid repeated tape application and removal. Apply skin sealants or barriers such as Stomadhesive before application of tape, if necessary. Remove tape by pulling in the direction of hair growth and using adhesive solvents, if necessary.
- If skin irritation or breakdown occurs, notify the physician. To prevent further irritation and breakdown, monitor closely and report signs and symptoms of infection (such as elevated temperature; redness, warmth and edema around incision or area of breakdown; unusual drainage from site).

SENSORY FUNCTIONING

General anesthetics depress all sensation, and the patient is maintained in an unconscious state for the length of time the surgery takes. After surgery, sensory perception may be dulled by the administration of sedatives and analgesics. These drugs may result in confusion, poor defence responses and postural imbalance. If surgery was performed on the nose or mouth, vision, smell or taste may be affected. Neural pathways may have been disturbed, by accident or by design, during the course of surgery, and any deviations from the initial baseline data in regard to sensory functioning must be observed. If deviations occur, adequate precautions are taken to assure safety, and the doctor is notified.

PROTECTION AND SAFETY

After surgery, mental function may be affected by a number of factors, including medication, anesthesia and disturbances in physiological processes. The patient will have experienced varying levels of consciousness during induction and recovery from anesthesia. Some people have untoward reactions to sedation and to anesthetic agents. Older people are particularly sensitive to drug reactions. All these factors may interfere with the patient's capacity for self-protection. Protective strategies for confused and disoriented patients and those with altered levels of consciousness were discussed in Chapter 30.

SELF-ESTEEM, SECURITY AND HEALTH MAINTENANCE

After surgery, anxiety may arise concerning pain, dependency on health care providers, equipment and the outcome of surgery itself. The nurse assists in decreasing anxiety by attending to the need for comfort, by providing competent technical care, by providing clear explanations about what is expected in the patient role and by encouraging the expression of emotions related to the surgical illness experience.

The patient may express many emotions after surgery. There may be uncertainty related to the future outcome of illness or relief that the surgery has been successful. If the surgery has altered a body part, the patient may express grief over the alteration in body image. The predischarge and early postdischarge periods may be times that are particularly distressful for the patient. The distress may be associated with the recognition that recovery will now be a personal responsibility, and the patient may be concerned about how to manage at home. Nursing research has shown that at hospital discharge, people feel it is important to know what complications may occur and if a complication occurs, what actions to take, how to manage symptoms such as pain and fatigue, what diet and activity guidelines to follow and how to take medications (Bubela, Galloway, McCay, McKibbon, Nagle, Pringle, Ross & Shamian, 1990; Galloway, Bubela, McKibbon, McCay & Ross, 1993).

Diagnosing: Sample Diagnosis

- *Knowledge Deficit related to safe management at home after hospital discharge.*

Planning: Sample Expected Outcome

- The patient will be able to manage recovery at home, as evidenced by verbalizing what complications to monitor for, what activity and dietary guidelines to follow, how to care for the incision and how to take medications as directed.

Implementing: Health-Promoting Activities

- Refer to community support groups specific to the health problem if the patient is agreeable.
- Encourage patient to remain a nonsmoker if he or she smoked preoperatively.
- Provide information about adequate nutritional intake to promote wound healing.
- Explain that frequent rest periods during the day may be needed, but that energy level will begin to return in several weeks.
- Encourage exercise. Unless contraindicated, the best exercise is walking.

Implementing: Health-Protecting Activities

- Provide teaching about complications specific to surgical procedure. For example, after bowel surgery, instruct about what action to take if diarrhea or constipation occurs.
- Provide teaching about wound care. Instruct the patient to keep the wound clean and to notify the doctor if signs of infection develop (for example, if the wound becomes red, swollen or warm to the touch or discharge becomes green or yellow).
- Explain that a shower may be taken, but that perfumes, creams or powder should not be put on wounds.
- Provide information about prescribed medications to take and how to take them.

Wound Healing and Restorative Care

A physical wound is an injury caused by anything that disrupts the normal continuity of the body's structure. Wounds are classified as open or closed. An **open wound** refers to tissue injury with a break in the skin or mucous membrane. A surgical incision is one example of an open wound. Injury to the skin and underlying tissues without a break in the skin is called a **closed wound**. A contusion is a closed wound. The names of wounds correspond to the manner in which they are acquired and to the extent of injury to the skin. Table 33.2 presents a description of the common types of wounds. The major goals of restorative wound care are to promote wound healing, prevent damage to surrounding tissues and to prevent infection (Timby, 1996).

The Process of Healing

As we discussed in greater detail in Chapter 31, normal healing is a series of complex events that lead to the restoration of tissue continuity. The localized response of the body to tissue injury begins at the time of injury and occurs in three major phases: the inflammatory phase, the proliferative phase and the remodelling phase (Byers, 1996; Flynn, 1996).

TABLE 33.2 Types of wounds

Type	*Cause*	*Characteristics*
Open:		
Incision	Surgical or traumatic cut with a sharp instrument (scalpel or knife)	A clean cut; straight, smooth edges. A surgical incision is more likely to heal well, with less chance of infection, because it is made under controlled, aseptic conditions.
Abrasion	Surgical or traumatic scraping off of the outer layer of the skin	Superficial wound of the skin only. Often painful because nerve endings are exposed. Prone to infection.
Puncture	Surgical or traumatic stab with a penetrating object or instrument	Well-defined penetration of skin and underlying tissues. May damage nerves and arteries. Traumatic wounds may have concealed blood loss and foreign objects.
Laceration	Traumatic tearing apart of skin and underlying tissues	Opening of the skin with ragged, irregular edges. Not likely to heal well.
Ulceration	Tissue injury caused by excessive pressure with a lack of blood circulation to underlying tissues	A crater in which skin or mucous membrane is missing.
Closed:		
Contusion	Direct blow from a blunt object	Damage to tissues and blood vessels under the skin; a bruise. Edema and tenderness are often present.

SOURCES: Earnest, 1993; Timby, 1996.

Determinants of Wound Healing

The factors that affect the speed and character of the healing process may be either systemic or local (Byers, 1996). Systemic factors refer to conditions within the body, while local factors are conditions in the area near the wound that may impair healing. Some systemic and local factors are described below.

SYSTEMIC FACTORS

EXTENT OF THE INJURY The process of repair and regeneration depends upon the extent of the tissue damage. Wounds with minimal tissue damage or loss, for example, clean surgical incisions or simple lacerations, heal very quickly by what is termed *primary intention*. On the other hand, wounds in which tissue loss is extensive, for example, burns or ulcerated areas, heal by *secondary intention*.

Primary intention healing occurs when there is little or no tissue loss. The wound edges are approximated (brought together) and secured with sutures, staples or tapes. This enhances the migration of epithelial cells from the wound edges. Because epithelialization is rapid, the risk of infection is decreased. Some inflammation may occur. Granulation tissue is not noticeable and scar formation is minimal (Flynn, 1996).

Secondary intention healing occurs when damage and loss of tissue are extensive. In secondary intention healing, wounds cannot be approximated and secured with sutures or staples. The wound edges remain open until scar tissue fills the wound site. The phases of healing are prolonged because drainage, necrotic tissue and debris in the wound space must be removed. Granulation tissue replaces the tissue that has been destroyed, providing a connective tissue base for the growth of epithelial (skin) cells. Inflammation persists, and infection is a high risk. Scar formation is sometimes excessive and may result in permanent loss of function (Flynn, 1996).

AGE Healing is more rapid in children than in adults. It is slowed in older patients owing to the lessened efficiency of circulation, which can result in inadequate delivery of nutrients, blood cells and oxygen to the wound. Older patients often have other underlying chronic illnesses that make wound healing difficult. With aging there is decreased thickness in the dermis and subcutaneous tissue, as well as decreased sensation. Wound healing is also compromised by poor eating habits and malnutrition, which is often found in the elderly (Resnick, 1993).

NUTRITION Nutrients are essential for normal healing, as they provide the ingredients for cellular repair and regeneration. Specific nutrients needed for healing include protein, carbohydrates, fats, vitamins, minerals and oxygen. Protein is needed for revascularization, lymphatic formation, fibroplastic proliferation, collagen synthesis and wound remodelling. Carbohydrates and fats are needed for cellular energy. Vitamin C is needed for the formation of new capillaries and is involved in the maturation of collagen fibres during the later stages of healing. Vitamin K deficiencies may cause bleeding and result in anemias or hematomas, which may interfere with wound healing. Although injury increases the use of specific B vitamins, the mechanism by which they influence protein, fat and carbohydrate metabolism is not well understood (Flynn, 1996; Telfer & Moy, 1993).

OBESITY Patients who are obese may have poorer wound healing. Adipose tissue has poor vascularization; this, combined with the increased tension of the excess tissue, increases the incidence of incisional hernias, infections and dehiscence (the breaking open of a wound) (Weingarten, 1993).

DIABETES Diabetes, one of the most common metabolic disorders, causes disturbances in carbohydrate, protein and fat metabolism, and makes the patient more vulnerable to impaired or prolonged wound healing. Wound infections are more common in patients with diabetes, as the leukocytes malfunction with hyperglycemia. It is also possible that there is poor oxygenation to the healing tissue owing to thickened capillaries, which are related to diabetes (Flynn, 1996).

IMMUNOSUPPRESSION The immune system of the body is important for the regeneration and repair of wounds and for other functions, such as promoting phagocytosis during the inflammatory phase. The normal immune response may be artificially prevented or diminished by radiotherapy or by the administration of steroids, antimetabolites, antilymphocyte serum or specific antibodies. The nurse must be aware of the effects of immunosuppression and protect the surgical wound from pathogenic organisms. The normal signs and symptoms of infection may not all be present, although fever is often seen (Wahoff-Stice, 1995).

RADIATION Healing is slowed after radiotherapy owing to the systemic effects of immunosuppression and the local effects of decreased blood supply and increased fibrotic (scar) tissue. If an area is to be radiated before surgery, the best operative time is considered to be four to six weeks after the therapy is completed. This is because the tissues are in the proliferative stage of healing before fibrosis and vascular narrowing occur. Complications that are common with patients who have received radiotherapy include delayed healing, dehiscence and fistula formation. The tissues of the irradiated area are more friable than normal and require very gentle handling (Mosiello, Tufaro & Kerstein, 1994).

LOCAL FACTORS

CHEMICAL, MECHANICAL OR THERMAL The disinfectants and medications used to cleanse and treat a wound and the surrounding tissue should be strong enough to be effective but should not irritate healthy tissue. Protective ointments such as sterile petrolatum can be used to protect the skin when it is necessary to use irritating disinfectants on open wounds. Mechanical stress, such as friction over a new wound, may strip the new epithelial cells and delay healing. To avoid mechanical injury, all wounds should be handled gently. Adhesive tape near the wound must be removed carefully. Special solvents may be used to loosen the adhesive. Thermal injury can be avoided by the use of solutions at a temperature that is not dangerous to tissue. Room temperature is generally considered to be safe for most tissues.

SUTURE MATERIAL Some people have an allergic response to sutures, staples or wound care supplies. Each patient is asked about prior allergies; in patients with no known allergies, the wound should be observed for localized reactions.

INFECTION The major complication in surgical wounds is infection. Infectious processes result in tissue destruction, delay the healing process and contribute to increasing the size of surgical scars. All solutions, dressings and equipment that come into contact with an open wound should be sterile. There are several organisms that are commonly found in wound infections. Of the gram-positive group, *Staphylococcus (S.) aureus* and *S. epidermidis* are found most commonly. These spherical, asymmetric bacteria are normally found in the nose, skin and feces. The alpha- and beta-hemolytic streptococci also cause many infectious processes. An estimated eight percent of all people carry these bacteria in the nasopharynx.

Of the gram-negative bacteria, *Escherichia coli* and species of *Aerobacter* and *Alcaligenes* are frequently found in wounds. These, together with *Proteus* and *Pseudomonas*, are the principal inhabitants of the intestine. They can also often be isolated in the anogenital area, and are frequent causes of urinary tract infections.

BLOOD SUPPLY Blood supply is necessary for healing as it brings the nutrients, blood cells and oxygen to the wound.

strictive bandages or casts, restraints and gross edema, will interfere with wound healing and render the area more vulnerable to infection. Healing is also slowed in patients with anemia or blood disorders that cause vascular insufficiency, such as atherosclerosis, in which there is a build-up of fatty deposits in the walls of large and medium-size arteries (Flynn, 1996).

Assessing Wounds

A wound is assessed every eight hours for signs of healing, infection and discharge. Approximation of skin edges is observed. The skin edges may be held together by metal skin clips (staples) or sutures. After five to seven days the clips or sutures are removed. The incision and surrounding area are assessed. Normally, there is slight redness along an incision for 48 hours. Redness extending 2 cm or more away from incision, edema and tissue heat are signs of infection, which are reported to the doctor. The physician may now ask you to obtain a wound culture of the incision site. A wound culture and sensitivity test will indicate the presence of a pathogenic organism causing the suspected infection. Collect a sterile wound culture swab, sterile gloves, and normal saline. To obtain the culture, don the sterile gloves and cleanse the area with normal saline. This will remove any surface microorganisms that may interfere with the results. With the tip of the sterile-cotton swab, gently rotate it at the site then place it in the accompanying culture tube, label the specimen and send it to the laboratory. Surgical wound infections are not uncommon. The incidence is markedly reduced by shortening preoperative stays (Cavanillas, Rodriguez-Contreras, Rodriguez, Abril, Gigosos, Solvas & Vargas, 1991), avoiding preoperative shaving of hair, flawless aseptic technique and elimination of drains in clean wounds. If infection is suspected, the patient's temperature is taken, and an assessment is done for pain in the area, headache and malaise. The latter are indicators of systemic infection.

The colour, type and amount of discharge are observed. **Serous discharge**, from the clear portion of blood, is amber in colour. **Sanguineous discharge** is blood, which may be bright red (indicative of fresh blood) or dark red (old blood). A combination of blood and serum is called **serosanguineous drainage. Purulent drainage** contains pus and may be white, yellow, green or pink. The colour is associated with the type of organism that is growing. The drainage is thick and may have an unpleasant odour.

The amount of discharge from a wound is monitored. The nurse first determines what amount of discharge is usual. For example, an abdominal incision is not expected to have more than a few drops of drainage after 24 hours. An incision in the perineum, however, may have 20–30 mL of drainage every 12 hours for several days. The amount of drainage is given in millilitres (mL) whenever possible.

Wounds are assessed for the presence of complications such as hematoma, dehiscence or evisceration. A **hematoma** occurs when there has been bleeding and a clot forms beneath the skin. The old clot (hematoma) may be absorbed, or may have to be removed. Removal is accomplished by a doctor who opens a small area of incision, allowing the hematoma to drain out. **Dehiscence** occurs when there is a splitting open of wound edges, whereas **evisceration** is the protrusion of body organs through a wound.

KEY PRINCIPLES

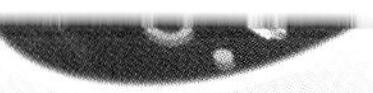

to Wound Care

1. Skin and mucous membranes normally harbour microorganisms.
2. Microorganisms are present in the air.
3. Moisture facilitates the growth of microorganisms. Dressings that are wet with drainage are more likely to foster the growth of organisms than are dry dressings. Dressings should be changed when they become wet.
4. Moisture facilitates the movement of microorganisms. When a dressing becomes soaked, movement of microorganisms towards the wound is facilitated as the moisture provides a vehicle for their transport. Because the outside of a dressing is generally highly contaminated, the movement of organisms from the outside inward must be prevented. Maintaining dry dressings inhibits the multiplication and the transfer of organisms.
5. Fluids move through materials by capillary action. Loosely woven fabrics such as gauze provide a good surface for capillary action. The fluid is absorbed through the material as each thread in the material conducts the fluid away from the wound by the action of the surface tension of the fluid and the forces of adhesion and cohesion. (Adhesion and cohesion are forces that draw two things together.)
6. Fluids flow downward as a result of gravitational pull. In a draining wound, the area of greatest contamination is likely the lowest part, where the drainage collects.
7. The respiratory tract often harbours microorganisms.
8. Blood transports the materials that nourish and repair body tissues. When dressing and bandaging a wound, exercise care to ensure that circulation to the area is not restricted. Dressings are never made restrictively tight, and they are applied starting at the distal portion of the body and proceeding to the proximal portion as a means of promoting venous flow.

Implementing Restorative Strategies

Operative wounds may be sutured with a wide variety of nonabsorbable sutures, including those made of polyester, polypropylene or silk, or with absorbable sutures made from surgical gut or a synthetic fibre or metal clips (staples). A wound is covered with a sterile dressing to provide a proper environment for healing, to absorb drainage, to protect the new epithelial tissue from mechanical injury, to promote hemostasis in a pressure dressing and, at times, to reduce anxiety in patients who are distressed by an incision in their body. Some wounds are clean, dry wounds, others are draining wounds.

CLEAN, DRY WOUNDS

The initial dressing that is applied to a clean, dry incision is left in place until the wound edges are sealed. Wound edge sealing usually occurs in 24–48 hours. Then, the dressing is removed and the area is gently cleaned and left uncovered (Maklebust, 1996). The absence of a dressing is beneficial as it allows easy observation of the area, eliminates conditions of warmth, moisture and darkness that promote microorganism growth, and avoids reactions from tape. **Occlusive dressings** allow insulation of a wound and have been shown to reduce the rate of wound infection when compared with nonocclusive dressings such as gauze (Maklebust, 1996). Occlusive dressings that are impermeable to bacteria, that are transparent and that are gas- and vapour-permeable are preferred for some wounds such as intravenous insertion sites. The occlusive dressings are changed when dirty or damaged, or according to the guidelines of the specific product.

DRAINING WOUNDS

Wounds heal more quickly if accumulated blood clots, body fluids, pus or debris are adequately drained. The accumulated materials provide a rich medium for microorganism growth; thus, soiled dressings need to be changed several times a day. If a wound is draining, the skin is not completely closed and a pathway exists for the entry of microorganisms. Dressings are therefore placed by sterile technique. If a wound is expected to drain excessively, a drain or packing is inserted by the physician to facilitate this process. Soft and firm rubber drains, as well as plastic drains, are used for this purpose. Packing is usually made of a long strip of gauze, often impregnated with an antiseptic or antibiotic.

When dressings on draining wounds are wet, they need to be changed. The drainage is irritating to the skin and increases the risk of infection. The dressing procedure is called a *dry dressing change* because the wound is cleansed and dry dressings are then applied.

CHANGING A DRY DRESSING

Dry dressings are usually applied to wounds that heal by primary intention. A dressing is changed to cleanse the wound, to remove excessive drainage and to apply a clean covering. It also provides an opportunity for careful assessment of wound healing. The technique for changing a dry dressing is detailed in Procedure 33.2.

Preparing the Patient

Prior to the dressing of a wound, the patient is given information about the procedure. If the patient will be seeing the wound for the first time, information is given about its appearance and what will happen during the dressing change. Often a wound has meaning for the patient, and concerns may be discussed. The nurse should be careful that words such as "contaminated" and "dirty" are not used, since they may make a patient feel uncomfortable and not acceptable. A wound infection is, however, a legitimate cause for concern, and the patient needs to know if it is present. The patient may ask whether changing a dressing is painful and may worry about coping with the pain. Most dressing procedures have some discomfort but the pain is usually mild. If the procedure is going to be uncomfortable, the patient should be offered a pain medication beforehand. Dressings that stick to the skin because of dried discharges can be removed with little discomfort by soaking them with sterile normal saline or sterile water. Another possible source of discomfort is the use of a cleansing solution with an alcohol base. These agents may feel cold and may sting when in contact with an open wound. The use of a cleansing solution without an alcohol base is often advisable. The most common cleansing solution is normal saline. The patient can participate in the procedure by lying still and keeping hands away from the wound area so that the wound and the equipment do not accidentally become contaminated.

Before assembling equipment for the dressing change, the nurse inspects the patient's dressing to determine the supplies and equipment that will be needed. Once a dressing tray is opened and set up, the nurse cannot leave the sterile field to obtain additional supplies, since doing so would constitute a break in sterile technique. Because of this, the nurse needs to make a quick check to determine the type of dressings, the presence of drainage tubes and the type of tape used to anchor the dressing. At the same time, the nurse should clear space on the patient's bedside or over-bed table for the dressing equipment and supplies.

Assembling Equipment

Changing a dry dressing is a sterile procedure. Supplies and equipment are needed for removing the old dressing and for cleansing and redressing the wound. The specific cleansing solution and the dressings that will be needed depend upon the kind of wound, the physician's order and the agency policy.

The safest aseptic technique in wound care is carried out by using individual trays containing only materials and equipment that can be discarded or sterilized after the wound is dressed. In most agencies, it is standard practice to use a disposable tray, referred to as a *dressing set.* While variations may exist from one manufacturer to another, the dressing set consists of a tray with a compartment for the cleansing solution, some 5 cm × 5 cm gauze sponges, some 10 cm × 10 cm gauze sponges, a metal thumb forceps, a plastic thumb forceps, a plastic locking forceps (Kelly forceps) and a sterile drape (see Figure 33.3). Separately packaged dressing materials are added to the set according to the specific needs of the patient. Sterile scissors may also be needed to shape the dressings and tape. Many agencies no longer require masks to be worn for sterile dressing changes, but the nurse should consult agency policy.

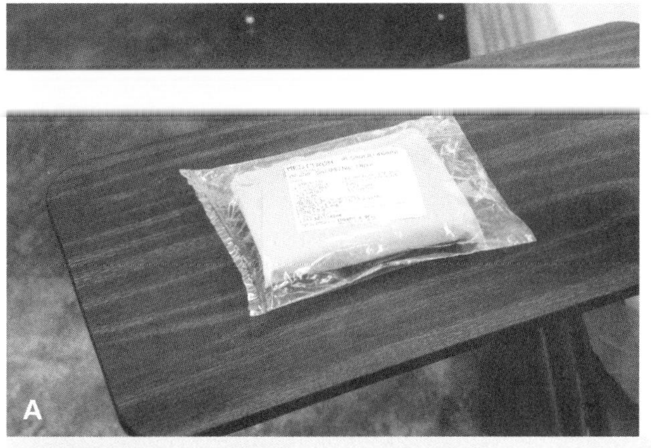

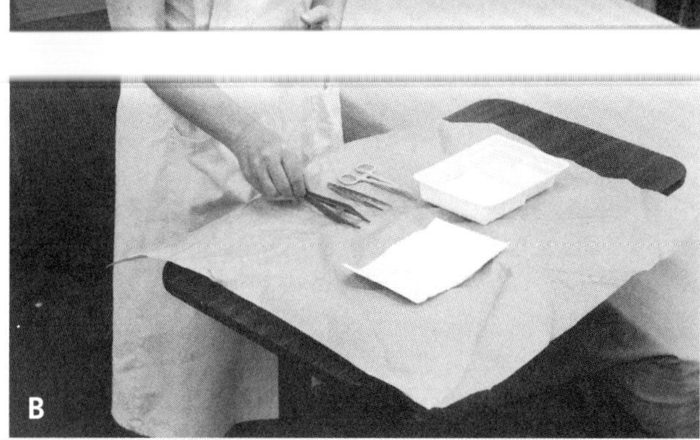

FIGURE 33.3 Dressing set. A. Unopened set. B. Set-up tray

SUPPLIES FOR REMOVING OLD DRESSING A large moisture-proof bag is needed to contain the old dressing materials. Clean gloves are required for removing the outer dressing. The inner dressings may be removed using transfer forceps (from the dressing set). Because sterile gloves are costly, their use should be reserved for special circumstances only. In some cases, the adhesive surface of the tape anchoring the dressing adheres to the patient's skin after the tape is removed. When this happens, an adhesive remover such as acetone may be used to loosen the adhesive. It is applied with clean 10 cm × 10 cm gauze sponges and the area is then washed with soap and water.

CLEANSING SOLUTIONS AND SUPPLIES Normal saline is commonly used to cleanse wounds; however, other topical solutions may be ordered by the physician. Incisions are cleansed with sterile 5 cm × 5 cm gauze pads. Sterile supplies are handled with sterile forceps.

DRESSINGS The most commonly used dressings are fine mesh gauze pads made of cotton or rayon fabric or synthetic materials, such as viscose polyester. Gauze is beneficial in wound care because it is highly absorbent and draws drainage away from the wound. In addition, the inert nature of gauze minimizes wound irritation. Gauze dressings come in a variety of sizes and textures, including 5 cm × 5 cm and 10 cm × 10 cm squares, 10 cm × 20 cm rectangles and gauze bandage rolls. The gauze dressings are placed directly over the wound to form the inner dressing. In some cases, a dressing with a nonadherent surface is first applied to the wound. This is done to prevent further injury to the delicate healing surface when the dressing is removed. There are many nonadherent dressings on the market. These include dressings made of silicone and silk, gauze pads with a nonadherent surface (for example, Telfa) and gauze rolls permeated with petroleum jelly. The external or outer dressing is usually a large, thick cotton pad, commonly called an abdominal or combination pad. Its purpose is to absorb drainage and protect the wound from external contaminants. An abdominal pad is more absorbent on one side than on the other. The more absorbent side is placed against the inner gauze dressings; the less absorbent side faces outward. Some manufacturers mark the outward side with a blue line running through the centre.

Dressings are secured by adhesive tape, elasticized tape, waterproof tape, adhesive ties, binders, bandages or plastic tape. The type of tape used and the method by which it is applied depend upon the site of the wound and the specific needs of the patient. For the patient who is allergic to adhesive tape, some other type of commercially prepared bandage can be used. Adhesive ties or Montgomery straps, illustrated in Figure 33.4, are selected when frequent dressing changes are necessary, since only the ties are undone

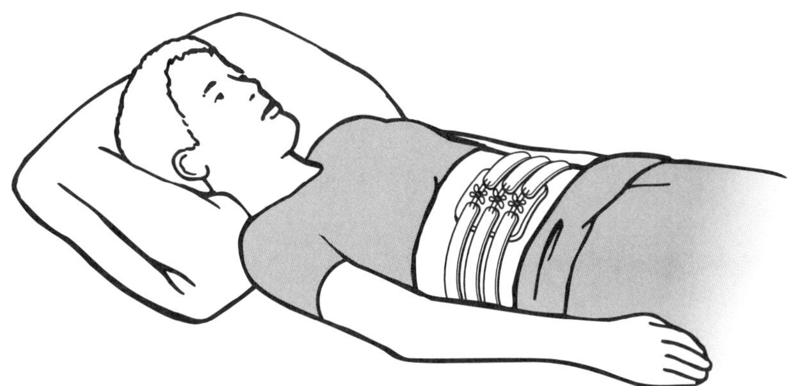

FIGURE 33.4 Montgomery straps

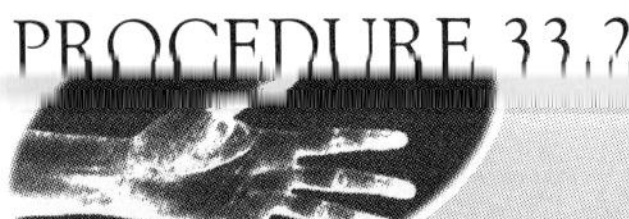

PROCEDURE 33.2 Changing the Dry Dressing

Action	Rationale
1. Check the physician's order for specific instructions.	Promotes accuracy and avoids error.
2. Prepare the patient and check the existing dressing.	Promotes the patient's well-being and participation in care. Indicates the supplies and equipment that will be needed.
3. Wash hands thoroughly.	Maintains aseptic technique.
4. Gather equipment: • dressing set • cleansing solution • moisture-proof bag • clean gloves • gauze squares • gauze dressings and abdominal pad(s), as necessary • tape, bandage or binder • sterile scissors (optional) • sterile gloves (optional) • mask (optional) • acetone and clean 10 cm × 10 cm gauze squares (optional).	Facilitates efficiency and economy of time.
5. Help the patient into a comfortable position. Expose the wound area; drape the patient with a sheet or bath blanket.	Provides privacy and avoids unnecessary exposure of the patient.
6. Fold down the top of the moisture-proof bag to make a cuff. Place the bag within easy reach and in an area away from the sterile field such that soiled dressings and sponges are not passed over the wound and sterile field.	Prevents contamination of the outside of the bag, protecting the nurse from contact with contaminants. Placing the bag within reach and away from the sterile field facilitates the nurse's work and reduces the risk of contaminating sterile areas.
7. Apply a mask, if required.	Some agencies require masks to be worn to prevent droplet contamination of the wound from the nurse's respiratory tract.
8. Apply clean gloves and remove tape, ties or bandages. To loosen tape, apply gentle pressure to the skin and pull the tape in the direction of hair growth and towards the wound.	Protects the nurse from contaminants on the outer dressing. Prevents stress on the wound and lessens patient discomfort.

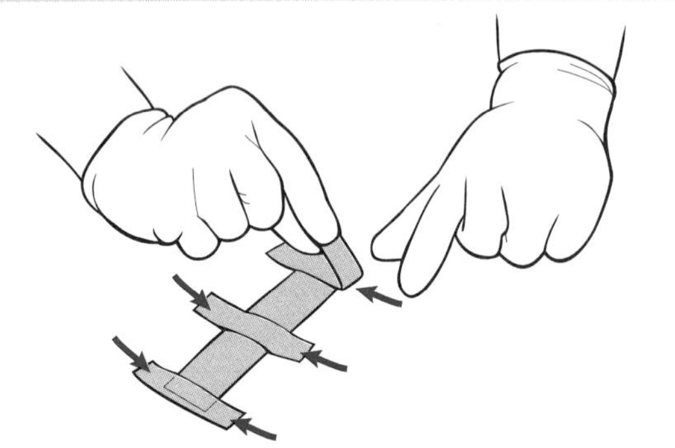

Action	Rationale
9. Remove the external dressing. Note the amount and character of drainage. Fold the dressing inward and discard it into the moisture-proof bag. Avoid touching the outside of the bag. Remove and discard gloves.	Provides data for ongoing evaluation of wound healing. Prevents the transmission of microorganisms.
10. Open the sterile dressing tray on the over-bed table. Add solution. Open packages and add supplies, ensuring aseptic technique.	Readies the equipment for the dressing change.

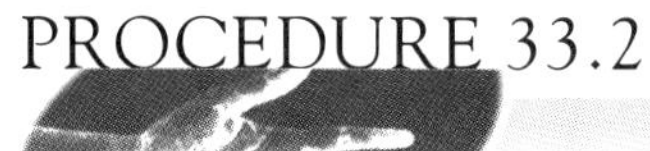

PROCEDURE 33.2 *continued*

Action	*Rationale*
11. Using sterile transfer forcep, remove the inner dressings, taking care not to dislodge any drains. If the gauze sticks to the drain, use another forceps to anchor the drain while taking off the dressings.	Prevents contamination of the nurse's hands from wound drainage.
12. Observe the dressings for amount and character of drainage and discard. Place the transfer forcep aside (on the sterile area but away from the supplies) or discard.	Provides data for ongoing evaluation of wound healing. Reserves the forceps if needed for anchoring a drain during the cleansing procedure.
13. Using sterile forceps and sponges moistened with solution, cleanse the wound:	
• Use one gauze pad for each stroke.	Prevents the spread of microorganisms from dirty to clean areas.
• Work from clean to dirty (see Figure 33.5). Discard the gauze sponge.	
• After cleaning the wound itself, work away from the wound to a distance of about 5 cm.	
• If a drain is present, clean it after the incision is cleaned.	The drain is dirtier than the incision, since moisture harbours microorganisms.
• Keep the tips of the forceps lower than the handle.	Prevents contamination of the tips with backflow of solution.
• Do not carry contaminated sponges over sterile areas.	Prevents contamination from solution dropping on sterile equipment.
• Do not reach over a sterile field.	Prevents contamination from the nurse's arms or uniform.
14. Dry the wound with gauze as necessary, using the same sequence as for cleansing.	
15. Inspect the wound for appearance, integrity and drainage.	Provides data for ongoing evaluation of healing and effectiveness of care.
16. Using sterile forceps, place the new dressing over the wound. It should be dropped in place rather than moved over the skin. The outer dressing should extend at least 5 cm beyond an open wound.	Avoids transfer of microorganisms from the skin to the centre of the wound and prevents mechanical injury to the wound.
17. Secure the dressing as appropriate with tape, ties, bandages or binders.	Prevents contamination of the wound should the edges be accidentally turned back.
18. Using acetone, remove tape surfaces that have adhered to the skin and are outside the dressing. Wash the area with soap and water.	Prevents skin irritation.
19. Assist the patient into a comfortable position.	Promotes patient well-being.
20. Discard supplies and wash hands.	Maintains cleanliness and safety in the workplace.
21. Document the procedure, the condition of the wound, the cleansing solution and the type of dressing applied.	Fulfills requirement for nurse accountability. Promotes continuity of care.

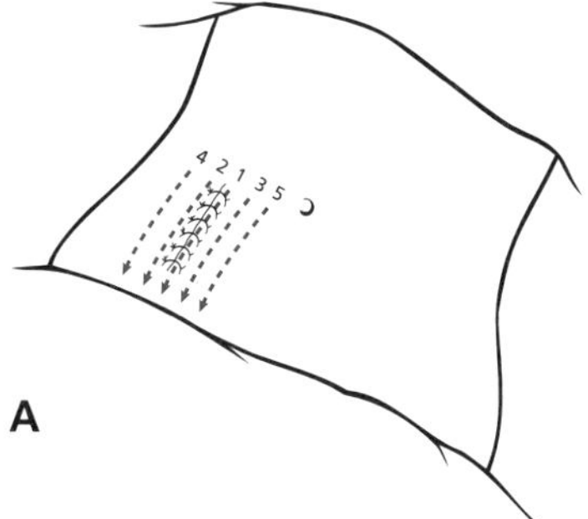

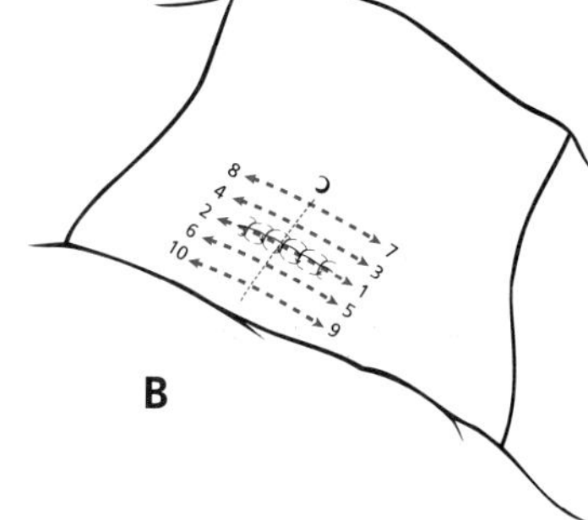

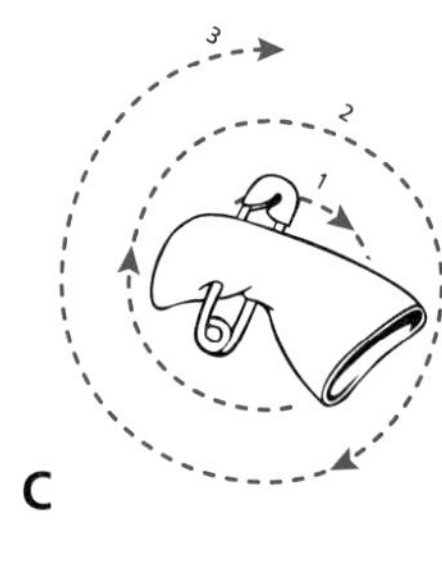

FIGURE 33.5 Cleansing wounds. A. A vertical wound is cleaned from the top, where there is the least amount of drainage, to the bottom, where drainage is the greatest. B. A horizontal wound is cleaned from the centre of the incision outward. C. A drain or stab wound is cleaned in a circular fashion, working from the centre outward.

RESEARCH to practice

Stotts, N.A., Barbour, S., Griggs, K., Bouvier, B., Buhlman, L., Wipke-Tevis, D., & Williams, D.F. (1997). Sterile versus clean technique in postoperative wound care in patients with open surgical wounds: A pilot study. *Journal of Wound, Ostomy & Continence Nursing, 24*(1), 10-18.

The purpose of this study was to identify whether there were differences in the rate of wound healing and supply costs when using sterile versus clean dressing technique for open surgical wounds. The study included a two-group random design. The sample consisted of 30 multiethnic participants—15 men and 15 women—who were undergoing elective gastrointestinal surgery.

Participants were recruited from five surgical units in two urban hospitals. Patients were randomly assigned after informed consent was obtained to have their dressing changed by a clean or a sterile procedure. Dressings were changed on postoperative day 1 and repeated three times daily until discharge. Healing time was analysed using the Mann-Whitney U Test. A T-test was used to analyse supply costs. Data were collected over a period of three to nine days.

The results revealed that there was no difference in the rate of wound healing between the clean and sterile groups. However, the mean cost was significantly less for the clean group versus the sterile group. The authors suggest that due to the small sample size, further investigation is required, in particular into the rate of wound complications.

when the dressing is changed. The adhesive portion is not removed from the skin unless the tape becomes soiled. Use of Montgomery straps prevents skin irritation and breakdown caused by frequent removal and application of tape.

CHANGING A WET-TO-DRY (-DAMP) DRESSING

Wet-to-dry (-damp) dressings are ordered as a means of removing drainage and debriding (removing necrotic tissue and debris) wounds that heal by secondary intention. Moistened dressings are placed over the wound and are then covered with a dry dressing. The moist dressing traps drainage and necrotic tissue as it slowly dries. Wound debris is removed with the dressing when it is changed. This may be painful and can harm healthy granulation tissue. Moist dressings must be placed within the wound bed only and not on the surrounding skin. Constant contact of the surrounding tissue with a moist dressing will cause the skin to macerate. To prevent this, a thin layer of petroleum jelly or a hydrocolloid may be placed around the wound edges as a skin barrier (Maklebust & Sieggreen, 1996). The moist-to-damp saline dressing should not dry out completely, nor should it be moistened if stuck to the wound bed (Leahy & Kizilay, 1998).

At time of writing there is controversy within the wound care literature with regard to wet-to-dry dressings. Research has demonstrated that a moist environment promotes faster wound healing than a dry environment. Therefore, use of the term *wet-to-damp* appears more current.

Dressings are changed every four to six hours. A method for applying a wet-to-dry (-damp) dressing is given in Procedure 33.3.

Preparing the Patient

The wet-to-dry dressing can be painful. Therefore, the nurse should discuss the need for analgesia with the patient prior to the procedure. If needed, pain medication is given about 30 minutes before the dressing change.

Assembling Equipment

The equipment for a wet-to-dry dressing change is similar to that for a dry dressing. Additional 10 cm × 10 cm gauze squares or ribbon gauze will be needed. If the wound is large, sterile gloves are recommended to expedite the wound-packing procedure. Sterile forceps are sufficient if wounds are small. Normal saline is commonly used to cleanse and debride wounds; however, other solutions may be ordered.

CHANGING AN OCCLUSIVE DRESSING

Occlusive dressings are used on ulcerated areas, pressure sores, minor burns, abrasions, lacerations and postoperative wounds. They might also be used to protect skin areas from irritation and breakdown. The transparent occlusive dressing is commonly used to anchor venipuncture devices in intravenous therapy. Occlusive dressings are self-adhesive. They adhere to the skin around the wound, not the wound itself. The advantage of these dressings is that they keep wounds moist, thereby speeding the healing process (Maklebust, 1996). Moreover, the dressings are left in place until healing has occurred or until they have loosened away from the skin (up to a week or more). This protects the healing basin (the migration of epithelial cells across the open area) from damage caused by the shearing effect of frequent removal and reapplication of dressings. The technique for changing an occlusive dressing is outlined in Procedure 33.4.

Assembling Equipment

There are two types of occlusive dressings: transparent and hydrocolloid (see Figure 33.6). These dressings come in a variety of sizes. The nurse should choose a size that will extend about 5 cm beyond the wound edge.

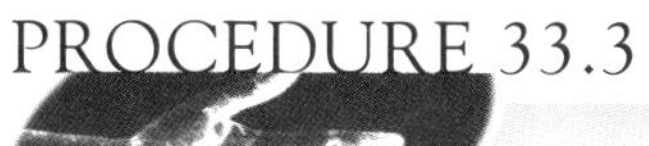

PROCEDURE 33.3 Changing the Wet-to-Dry (-Damp) Dressing

Action	Rationale
1. Follow steps 1 to 10 of Procedure 33.2. In addition to equipment necessary for changing a dry dressing, gather: • extra 10 cm × 10 cm sterile gauze pads • normal saline or solution as ordered.	
2. Using a sterile transfer forcep, remove the contact dressing. If it adheres, warn the patient of discomfort. Do not moisten it to ease removal. Discard dressings and forcep into the moisture-proof bag.	Moistening the dressing would counteract the effectiveness of debridement. Moisten only if absolutely necessary, as it preserves new tissue and prevents the disruption of new granulation tissue, which would retard wound healing.
3. Observe the dressings for amount and character of drainage and discard. Inspect the wound for appearance, necrotic tissue and drainage.	Provides data for ongoing evaluation of healing.
4. Put on sterile gloves.	Maintains sterile technique.
5. Saturate ribbon, packing-strip gauze or 10 cm × 10 cm gauze pads with normal saline. Wring out excess solution so that pads are damp but not dripping.	Creates an optimal environment for absorbing and trapping exudate. Use of noncytotoxic solutions prevents damage to new granulation tissue.
6. Lightly pack the wound with the moistened gauze pads, making sure that all surfaces are covered. Sterile forceps may be used to tuck the gauze into deep areas.	Effective debridement requires complete contact between the wound surface and the dressing.
7. Place dry, sterile 10 cm × 10 cm gauze pads over the moist dressings and cover the wound with an abdominal pad.	
8. Complete the procedure as for a dry dressing change (steps 17–21, Procedure 33.2).	

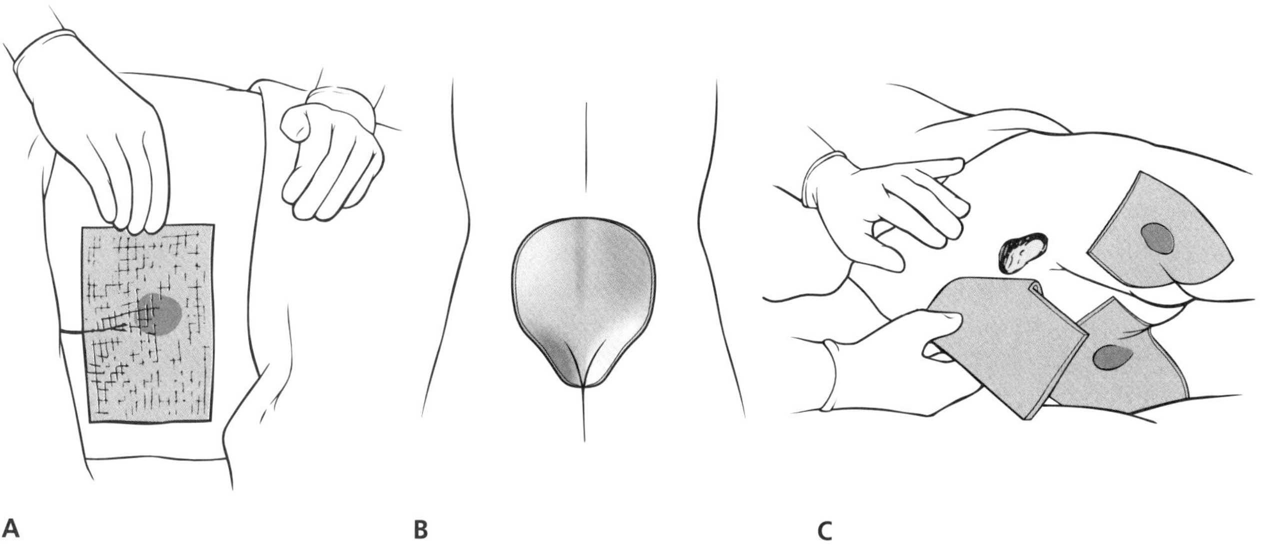

FIGURE 33.6 Occlusive dressings. A. Transparent dressing: OpSite™ Flexigrid*. B. Hydrocolloid dressing: DuoDerm CGF Border Tri-Angle. C. Hydrocolloid dressing: DuoDerm CGF Control Gel Formula dressing

SOURCES: A. Smith & Nephew Inc., Lachine, QC. B & C. E.R. Squibb & Sons, Inc., Princeton, NJ. *Trademark of Smith & Nephew.

PROCEDURE 33.4 Changing an Occlusive Dressing

Action	Rationale
1. Follow steps 1 to 7 of Procedure 33.2, but gather the following only: • dressing set • cleansing solution and supplies • occlusive dressing • clean gloves • moisture-proof bag • mask (optional) • soap and water.	
2. Don clean gloves.	Protects the nurse from contact with contaminants and secretions.
3. Gently press down on the skin at the edge of the dressing with one hand and, with the other, peel the dressing away from the wound. Work from the edges towards the centre of the dressing.	Avoids tearing the newly healed surface that could be pulled away with the dressing.
4. Discard dressing and gloves into the moisture-proof bag.	Reduces spread of contaminants.
5. Cleanse the wound in an appropriate manner, making sure to remove loose necrotic tissue and debris. If a solution other than normal saline is used to clean the wound, rinse with normal saline.	The wound must be clean and free of necrotic tissue and debris for effective healing to occur.
6. Wash the skin around the wound with soap and water. Dry it well.	Removes secretions and dried exudates.
7. Inspect the wound for appearance, integrity and drainage.	Provides data for ongoing evaluation of healing and effectiveness of care.
8. Remove the paper backing from the dressing. Centre the dressing over the wound and gently press it in place. Working from the centre outward, smooth out wrinkles and mould the dressing to the contour of the skin surface.	Avoids air bubbles being trapped beneath the dressing.
9. If necessary, secure the dressing edges with paper tape.	
10. Assist the patient into a comfortable position.	Promotes patient well-being.
11. Discard supplies and wash hands.	Maintains cleanliness and safety in the workplace.
12. Document the procedure, the condition of the wound and the type of dressing applied.	Fulfills requirement for nurse accountability. Promotes continuity of care.

TRANSPARENT DRESSING The *transparent dressing*, such as Op-Site™ or Tegaderm, is a thin, selectively permeable membrane that is applied to a wound. It permits moisture vapour and oxygen to move towards the wound while providing a barrier against bacteria and fluids. Because it is pliable, this dressing conforms easily to irregular skin surfaces and can be placed over joints without disrupting the patient's mobility. The dressings are commercially prepared to facilitate ease of application. Wounds are assessed through the dressing since it is transparent. In addition, some dressings (for example, Op-Site™) have a grid incorporated into the film that permits accurate measurement of the healing process. Transparent dressings, however, are not absorbable. Wound drainage can accumulate and cause the dressing to separate from the skin. A transparent pouch dressing is now available for containing wound drainage. With a pouch dressing, some of the drainage is eliminated through evaporation, extending the dressing's integrity (Maklebust, 1996).

HYDROCOLLOID DRESSINGS *Hydrocolloid dressings* (for example, DuoDerm) are used for covering wounds that yield a lot of drainage and for those that heal by secondary intention. The underside of the dressing contains a preparation that absorbs moisture and wound secretions to form a gelatinous substance, hence the label "hydrocolloid." The moist environment promotes healing and protects the newly formed epithelial tissue from damage and contamination. The dressing may remain in place for up to three days unless it becomes loosened.

Hydrocolloid dressings can be used as a skin protector with Montgomery straps. The hydrocolloid is placed on the skin along the incision line. The Montgomery straps are

dermis is not removed each time the dressing is changed (Maklebust, 1996).

MANAGING WOUND DRAINS AND DRAINAGE SYSTEMS

Wound healing is hastened if blood clots, body fluids, pus and debris are adequately drained. This process is facilitated by the insertion of a drain or packing at the time of wound closure in the operating room. A rubber or plastic drain may be inserted through the incision line or, more commonly, through a stab wound situated a few centimetres away from the incision. This allows the fluid to drain from the wound without excessive moisture accumulating on the incision line. Some drains are sutured in place, whereas others are freely movable.

Soft rubber drains (Penrose drains) have a suture or sterile safety pin attached to the distal portion of the drain to prevent them from slipping completely inside the wound (see Figure 33.7). These drains are open drains because liquid secretions flow by gravity from the wound into the dressings. Similarly, microorganisms can migrate upward to the wound through contaminated dressings. A closed drain, on the other hand, is a perforated plastic tube connected to a drainage receptacle that draws secretions from the wound by vacuum action. The Hemovac or Davol units are examples of portable wound suction devices (see Figure 33.8). A closed drain may also be connected to a wall suction unit or a suction machine set at low pressure. Because the system is closed, the possibility of microorganisms entering the wound through the drain is reduced. Packing is usually made of a long strip of gauze, often impregnated with an antiseptic or antibiotic. Open drains and packing are sometimes withdrawn a little each day to encourage healing from the base or depth of the wound. Closed drainage systems are left in

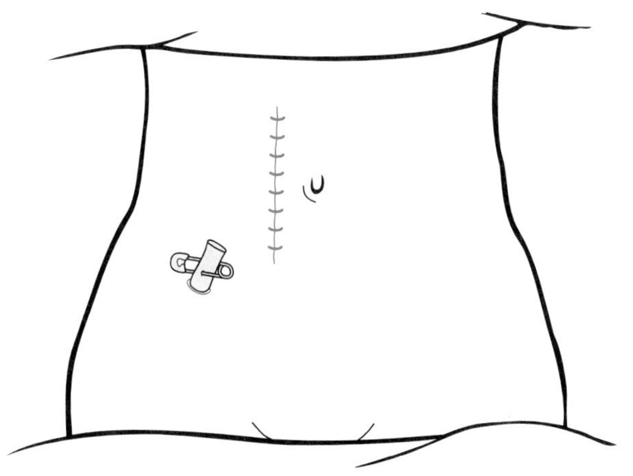

FIGURE 33.7 Penrose drain exiting from a stab wound

Choosing the Appropriate

Superficial Wounds—Minimal Drainage
Wounds that are superficial (only in the epidermis) have minimal amounts of drainage. A dressing is needed that will maintain a moist environment for the wound and allow the surrounding skin to stay dry. Transparent film dressings are useful in this situation (e.g., Op-Site). This dressing is semi-occlusive, allowing oxygen to flow through while water vapour can pass out. In addition, a film dressing will protect the wound from external contamination while keeping the wound bed moist. It needs to be changed every seven days, or when it leaks.

Superficial Wounds—Minimal to Moderate Drainage
These wounds need a dressing that can absorb some drainage to prevent the wound from becoming macerated. A hydrocolloid (e.g., DuoDerm, Replicare) can be used. This type of dressing is an adhesive, mouldable wafer that forms a gel when in contact with exudate. It will provide an occlusive environment, maintain a moist wound bed and absorb small amounts of drainage. These dressings need to be changed every three to five days.

Deep Wounds—Moderate to Large Drainage
These wounds need a dressing that can absorb large amounts of drainage. Gauze pads can be used, but they quickly become saturated and provide an easy path for bacteria to be drawn into the wound bed, causing contamination and possibly infection. Foam dressings are able to absorb large amounts of drainage and need to be changed only every three days or when saturated. Hydrogels (e.g., Intrasite gel) can also be used with deep wounds, but only with light exudate. Hydrogels facilitate debridement and maintain a moist environment. They can also be used in the presence of infection. A highlight of hydrogel is that it cools the wound and thus increases comfort for patients with painful wounds. Alginate, a seaweed derivative, can be used in the management of deep wounds with moderate to large drainage. It is usually placed within the wound and conforms to eliminate dead space while promoting a moist environment.

Barrier Products
There are some products available that provide a barrier on the skin that prevents surrounding tissue from becoming macerated. These barriers can be sprayed or wiped on and will provide a protective layer for intact skin. They are especially useful for skin surrounding large draining wounds.

Filling in Dead Space
Wound cavities and fistulas need to be filled so that the area does not grow over and become abscessed. These areas should be loosely filled with a packing material. If the wound is overpacked, the pressure on the tissue in the wound bed could be enough to cause additional damage, thus delaying healing.

SOURCES: Maklebust, 1996; Thomas-Hess, 1995; Bryant, 1992.

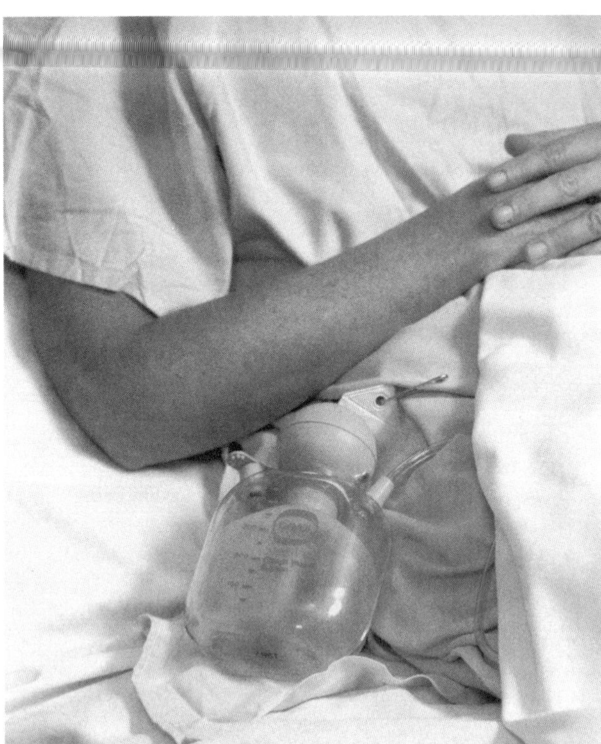

FIGURE 33.8 Closed drainage system

place until the wound is free of drainage (three to seven days). The drainage receptacle is emptied once per shift and the amount of drainage is measured. Procedures 33.5 and 33.6 outline how to shorten a drain and how to empty a closed drainage receptacle.

Preparing the Patient

Drain shortening should be a relatively comfortable procedure. The patient may experience a pulling sensation when the drain is withdrawn.

Assembling Equipment

A sterile safety pin, sterile scissors and sterile gloves are needed in addition to the equipment for a dry dressing change. Suture scissors are added for the first drain shortening if the drain is anchored with a suture. Clean gloves and a calibrated pitcher are required for emptying a closed wound drainage receptacle.

IRRIGATING WOUNDS

A **wound irrigation** is "the introduction of a solution called an irrigant into the wound to wash out exudate, drainage and debris so that the wound can heal" (Earnest, 1993, p. 920). Wounds are often irrigated to cleanse deep cavities or to debride large open areas. A wound may also be irrigated to apply warmth to an area or to administer medication. Because wounds constitute a break in skin integrity, wound irrigations are performed using sterile technique. Procedure 33.7 outlines the steps for executing a wound irrigation.

Preparing the Patient

Wound irrigations may be painful. Therefore, the nurse should ascertain the patient's need for pain medication. If necessary, the analgesic should be administered at least 30 minutes before performing the procedure.

Assembling Equipment

A wound irrigation is usually done in conjunction with a dressing change. The irrigation procedure itself will require a syringe, an irrigant and a collecting basin. The wound needs to be irrigated with enough force to clean it but not to damage the wound bed. Four to 15 pounds of force per square inch (psi) is needed to irrigate a wound effectively. A bulb syringe administers too little pressure; a WaterPic administers too much. A 35-mL catheter with an 18- or 19-gauge over-the-needle catheter delivers sufficient irrigation pressure (Longmire, Broom & Burch, 1987).

Sometimes, deep wound cavities have small surface openings. In such cases, a soft, straight catheter is necessary to reach the base of the wound. Normal saline is a common irrigant; however, other solutions, such as Dakin's solution or hydrogen peroxide, may also be prescribed. Approximately 200 mL of solution may be required to cleanse the wound; a large sterile basin is needed to hold the irrigant. The irrigant should be warmed to 32.2°–35°C. This can be done by placing the solution container in a basin of warm water. The collecting basin for irrigant return does not have to be sterile since it will not come in direct contact with the wound. A large, clean kidney basin is sufficient for this purpose. If an irritating irrigant such as Dakin's solution will be used, a skin protectant, such as zinc oxide or petroleum jelly, will also be necessary.

REMOVING SUTURES AND STAPLES

Sutures and staples hold the skin and underlying tissues together in wounds that heal by primary intention. Some sutures are made of absorbable materials that slowly dissolve as the wound heals. These require no care. Nonabsorbable sutures are made of natural fibres, such as silk, or synthetic materials, such as polyester or polypropylene. Some are made of wire. Staples are wide metal clips made of wire or silver. They resemble ordinary paper staples. Staples do not fully encircle the wound edges. They simply form a trough that keeps the wound edges together (see Figure 33.9C). Sutures and staples remain in place until the wound has healed sufficiently. This can be as soon as three days or as long as 14 days postoperatively. A physician's order is required for removal of both sutures and staples. The order may be to remove one half of the sutures and staples one day, and the other half the next day.

There are many different types of suturing methods the surgeon may use for skin closure. You will learn more about these as you advance through your course of study. Here, we will discuss two methods of suturing skin: intermittent and continuous suturing. With intermittent suturing, separate sutures are placed in the skin and tied in a knot

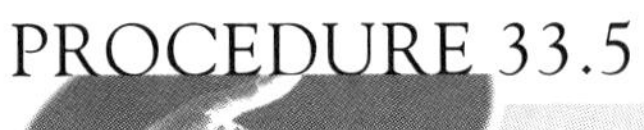

PROCEDURE 33.5 Shortening a Wound Drain

Action	*Rationale*
1. Follow steps 1 to 12 of Procedure 33.2. In addition to the equipment necessary for changing a dry dressing, gather: • sterile safety pin • sterile scissors • sterile gloves • sterile suture scissors (for first drain shortening).	
2. Cleanse and dress the incision as in Procedure 33.2.	
3. Cleanse the drain wound.	
4. Put on sterile gloves.	Maintains sterile technique and expedites the procedure.
5. If necessary, clip and remove the suture securing the drain, as in step 6, Procedure 33.8.	Provides a measurement marker for shortening the drain.
6. Open a 10 cm × 10 cm gauze and wrap it around the drain adjacent to the skin. Place another piece of gauze on the skin beside the drain site.	Facilitates application of countertraction needed for drain withdrawal.
7. With the nondominant hand, withdraw the drain as required. Then, with the dominant hand, insert the sterile pin about 1.5 cm away from the skin.	Allows space for placing dressings between the drain and the skin. The pin prevents the drain from slipping back into the incision.
8. Using sterile scissors, cut the drain between the pins. Discard the piece of drain and the gloves.	Reduces the spread of microorganisms.
9. Using forceps, cleanse the wound again.	Removes secretions that may have accumulated when the drain was withdrawn.
10. Dress the drain site. Use precut 10 cm × 10 cm gauze pads around the drain site. Layer the gauze snugly under the drain. Encircle the drain with the dressings and make sure the edges overlap. Apply gauze dressings over the drain.	Provides a surface for absorption of drainage and protects the skin.

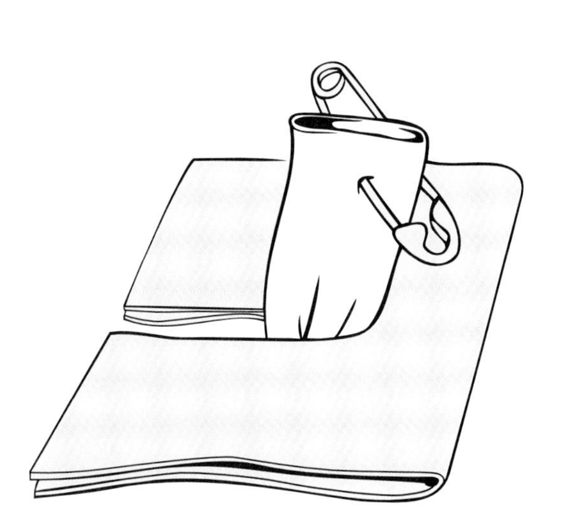

11. Cover the incision and the drain area with an abdominal pad.
12. Complete steps 17 to 20 of Procedure 33.2.

PROCEDURE 33.6 Emptying a Closed Wound Drainage Receptacle

Action	*Rationale*
1. Gather equipment: • measuring pitcher • clean gloves • waterproof protective pad.	
2. Lay a protective pad on a flat surface and place the measuring pitcher on it.	Catches spills that might occur when the receptacle is emptied.
3. Apply gloves and maintain aseptic technique when emptying the receptacle.	Prevents the introduction of contaminants into the system.
4. Open the receptacle cap, invert the receptacle and empty the contents into the measuring pitcher.	
5. Re-establish suction mechanism according to the manufacturer's directions.	Suction mechanisms vary according to the manufacturer.
6. Measure the amount of drainage and note the colour, odour and consistency.	Provides data for ongoing evaluation of care.
7. Record the procedure and the characteristics of drainage in the patient's record. Enter the amount of drainage on the intake and output record.	Fulfills requirements for nurse accountability and communicates assessment information to members of the health care team.

PROCEDURE 33.7 Irrigating a Wound

Action	*Rationale*
1. Check the physician's order for type of irrigant and specific instructions.	Promotes accuracy and avoids error.
2. Prepare the patient and check the existing dressing. If necessary, administer pain medication 30 minutes prior to the procedure.	Promotes the patient's well-being and participation in care. Indicates the supplies and equipment that will be needed.
3. Wash hands thoroughly.	Maintains aseptic technique.
4. Gather equipment: • dressing set and dressing materials as necessary • 35-mL syringe with 18- or 19-gauge over-the-needle catheter • soft, straight catheter (optional) • irrigant as ordered • sterile basin • clean kidney basin • sterile gloves • clean gloves • moisture-proof bag • waterproof protective pad • skin protectant (for example, petroleum jelly) • sterile tongue blade • mask (optional).	Facilitates efficiency and economy of time.
5. Help the patient into a position in which the wound is accessible and drains downward. Make sure the patient is comfortable. Expose the wound and drape the patient with a sheet or bath blanket.	The force of gravity is used to flush and drain the wound.
Put a protective pad under the wound area. Position the clean kidney basin below the wound.	Protects the bed linen from drainage.

PROCEDURE 33.7 *continued*

Action	*Rationale*
6. Prepare the sterile equipment for the irrigation and subsequent dressing application.	Promotes efficiency and ease of performing procedure.
7. Remove the dressing and discard it as in Procedure 33.2.	
8. If necessary, apply a skin protectant to healthy skin around the wound and especially between the wound and the collecting basin.	Provides a barrier against the irritating solution.
9. Don sterile gloves and fill the syringe with irrigant; attach the angiocatheter to the syringe.	
10. **Syringe:** Gently flush the entire wound surface, beginning at the top and working downward, using slow, continuous pressure.	Flow of solution with gentle force loosens debris and washes it downward, without damaging the fragile healing surface of the wound.
Catheter: Insert the catheter into the wound until resistance is felt and then pull back about one to two centimetres. Gently flush the wound using slow, continuous pressure.	Ensures that catheter tip is off the fragile surface of the wound.
11. Continue irrigation until all irrigant is used up or the returning solution is clear.	
12. Using sterile forceps or gloves, dry the wound edges with gauze.	
13. Inspect the wound for appearance, integrity and drainage.	Provides data for ongoing evaluation of healing and effectiveness of care.
14. Dress the wound as required.	
15. Assist the patient into a comfortable position.	Promotes patient well-being.
16. Discard supplies and wash hands.	Maintains cleanliness and safety in the workplace.
17. Document the procedure, the irrigant used, the appearance of the returning fluid and the condition of the wound.	Fulfills requirement for nurse accountability. Promotes continuity of care.

(see Figure 33.9A). In continuous suturing, one suture is woven through the tissues just below the surface of the skin (see Figure 33.9B). A knot is tied at either end. Often, a piece of tubing is placed between the skin surface and the knot to prevent the knot from entering the incision. Sometimes, if incisions are long, the surgeon brings one or more loops of suture over the surface of the skin to facilitate removal. Sutures are removed by clipping the side next to the skin surface and then pulling them out with forceps. The most important principle to remember in removing sutures is *never* to pull loops of suture from the surface of the skin through underlying tissue. Doing so can cause infection. The techniques for removing sutures and staples are detailed in Procedure 33.8.

Preparing the Patient

The removal of sutures and staples may be uncomfortable. As with all procedures, knowing what to expect eases some of the patient's discomfort. A stinging sensation and a feeling

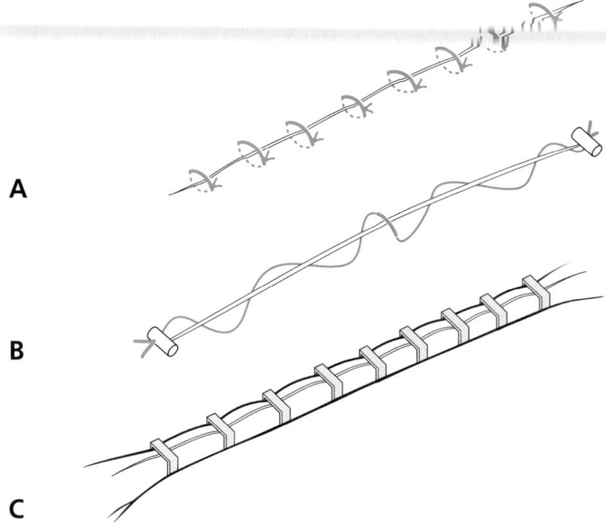

FIGURE 33.9 Examples of suturing methods and staples. A. Intermittent sutures. B. Plain continuous sutures. C. Staples

of pressure is commonly experienced as a continuous suture is being pulled out. Patients often express the most discomfort when an intermittent suture is being lifted away from the skin so that it can be cut with the suture scissors. Removal of intermittent sutures and staples cause a pinching or "mosquito bite" sensation. Tension can worsen the discomfort. The patient will find that use of relaxation and distraction techniques (described in Chapter 27) will significantly help cope with the discomfort accompanying suture and staple removal. The nurse should also assess the patient's pain level and administer analgesia prior to the procedure, if necessary.

Assembling Equipment

Suture and staple removal are sterile techniques. The incision is cleansed first; a dressing set and cleansing solution are required. Sutures are clipped with special suture scissors having a short, curved cutting tip that slides easily under the suture. Staples are taken out with a special surgical staple remover (see Figure 33.10). In some cases, a bit of

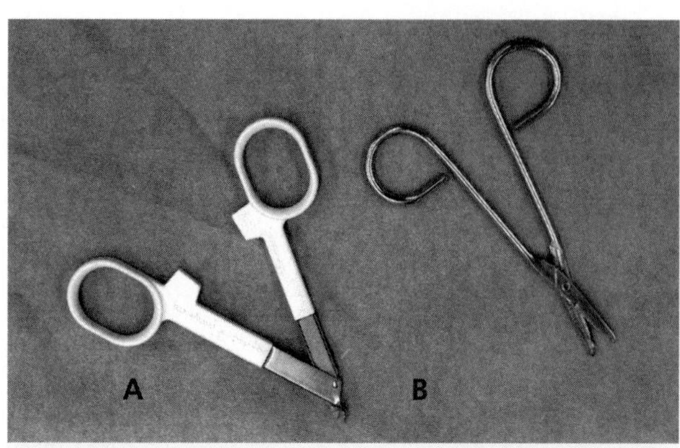

FIGURE 33.10 A. Staple remover. B. Suture scissors

wound dehiscence may occur when the sutures and staples are removed. When this happens, the separated edges are brought and held together with tape strips, such as butterfly tape or Steri-Strips. The wound may be left exposed, or covered with a light dressing such as a 10 cm × 20 cm gauze rectangle, or an adhesive wound dressing (such as Hypafix or Mepore plaster) may be applied following the procedure.

APPLYING BANDAGES

A bandage is a piece of material that is used to wrap a part of the body. The purposes of applying a bandage are:

1. to limit movement
2. to apply warmth (for example, to a rheumatoid joint)
3. to secure a dressing
4. to keep splints in position
5. to provide support (for example, to the legs to aid venous blood flow)
6. to apply pressure in order to control bleeding, promote the absorption of tissue fluids or prevent the loss of tissue fluids
7. to shape or mould a stump.

Materials Used in Bandaging

GAUZE Gauze is one of the most frequently used materials for bandaging. It is a soft, woven cotton that is porous but not bulky, light in weight and readily moulded to any contour. Gauze is sometimes impregnated with various ointments such as petrolatum. Cotton gauze is not commonly used anymore because of its cost. It is the safest bandage material, however, when there is concern about pressure on the wound.

KLING GAUZE OR KERLIX GAUZE Kling gauze and Kerlix gauze are woven to allow the gauze to stretch, moulding to body contours. The gauze has a crepe-like texture and tends to cling to itself, an attribute that helps keep it in place after it has been applied.

STOCKINET Stockinet is a stretchable material in the shape of a tube. It comes in various widths and can be applied to many parts of the body, such as the head, chest, arms, legs or fingers. It is easy to use, moulds well to the body and provides uniform pressure.

FLANNEL Flannel makes a soft and pliable bandage. It is heavy and keeps in the heat of the body; it can be used to apply warmth to body joints.

MUSLIN Muslin (factory cotton) is a strong, heavy cotton that is not pliable. It is used to provide support, as for splints, or to limit movement.

ELASTICIZED BANDAGES Elasticized bandages made of cotton with an elastic webbing (Ace bandages) are often used as tensor bandages to apply pressure. They are expensive but can be washed and reused.

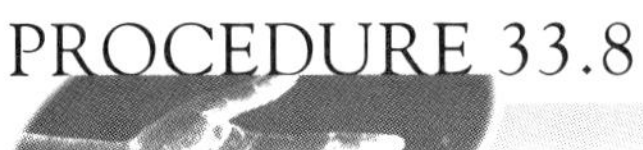

PROCEDURE 33.8 Removing Skin Sutures or Staples

Action	*Rationale*
1. Validate the physician's order.	Promotes safety; avoids error.
2. Prepare the patient. Determine the need for analgesia and administer medication, if necessary.	Promotes the patient's well-being and participation in care.
3. Wash hands thoroughly.	Maintains aseptic technique.
4. Gather equipment: • dressing set • cleansing solution • sterile suture scissors or staple remover • Steri-Strips or butterfly tape • light wound dressing (optional) • moisture-proof bag • clean gloves.	Facilitates efficiency and economy of time.
5. Remove the dressing and cleanse the incision as outlined in Procedure 33.2.	Removes surface microorganisms and moistens sutures, which may ease removal.
6. Removing Intermittent Sutures	
• Using forceps, grasp and lift the knot. Slide the scissors under the suture, away from the knot.	Facilitates insertion of the scissors underneath the suture.
• Cut the suture as close to the skin as possible.	Prevents surface suture material from being pulled through underlying tissue.
• Gently pull the freed stitch up and out.	
• Remove alternate sutures. If there is no evidence of dehiscence, remove the remaining sutures. Should a large dehiscence occur, cover the wound with sterile gauze and notify the physician immediately.	Provides support to the incision should dehiscence occur.

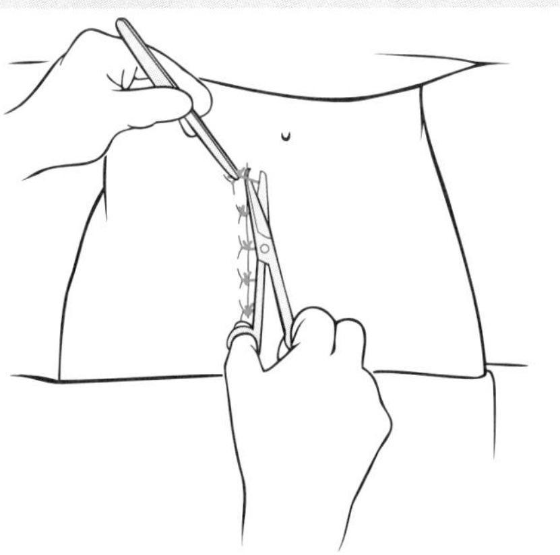

Action	*Rationale*
Removing Plain Continuous Sutures	
• Grasp the first loop of suture with forceps. Lift it gently and cut it at the end opposite to the knot. Then cut the same end of the adjacent suture.	As above.
• Grasp the knot of the freed suture and pull the suture out, pulling parallel to the body.	Reduces patient's discomfort.
• Next, grasp the freed end of the suture and cut it off close to the skin.	
• Grasp the next loop, pull out the underlying suture and cut it off. Repeat this sequence until all loops have been removed.	
• Grasp the remaining knot and pull out the suture.	

continued on next page

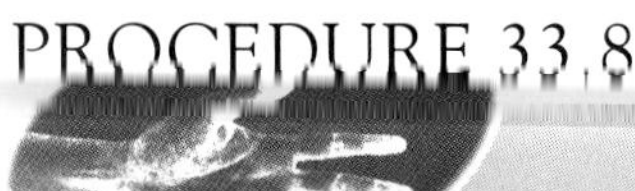

PROCEDURE 33.8 *continued*

Action	*Rationale*
Removing Staples	
• Slide the lower tips of the staple remover under the middle of the staple. Squeeze the handle and when both edges of the staple are visible, lift it from the skin. Remove staples in the same alternate fashion as for intermittent sutures.	Bends the centre of the staple and straightens the embedded ends.

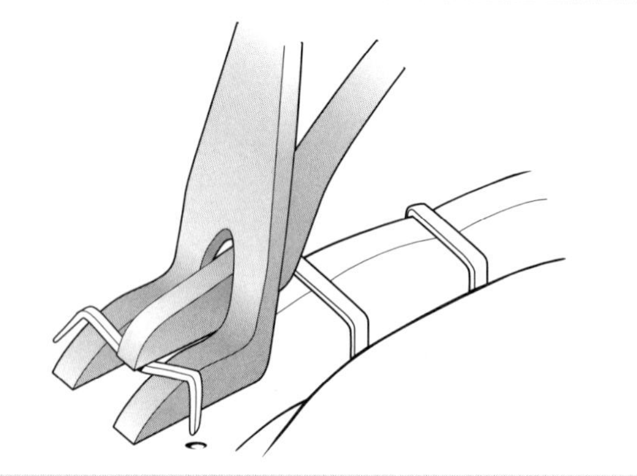

Action	*Rationale*
7. If necessary, clean the incision again.	Sometimes, bleeding may occur.
8. If small areas of wound separation are present, bring the wound edges together with butterfly tape or Steri-Strips. These tapes may be placed intermittently along the entire length of the wound.	Holds the wound edges together and provides support to the wound.
9. Cover the incision with a light dressing, if necessary.	Protects the wound from external contaminants.
10. Assist the patient into a comfortable position.	Promotes patient well-being.
11. Discard supplies and wash hands.	Maintains cleanliness and safety in the workplace.
12. Document the procedure, the condition of the incision, any wound separation and whether tape strips or a dry dressing were applied.	Fulfills requirement for nurse accountability.

ELASTIC ADHESIVE Elastic adhesive (Elastoplast) is a woven bandage with an adhesive side. It is applied to give support, for example, when dressings are being secured.

PLASTIC ADHESIVE Plastic adhesive is a waterproof bandage with an adhesive side. It is somewhat elastic and can be used to apply pressure and at the same time keep an area dry.

Fundamental Turns in Bandaging

There are five fundamental turns in bandaging (see Figure 33.11). These turns are used to make up the variety of bandages applied to the various parts of the body.

The **circular turn** is used to bandage a cylindrical part of the body or to secure a bandage at its initial and terminal ends. In a circular turn, the bandage is wrapped about the part in such a way that each turn exactly covers the previous one. Two circular turns are usually used to initiate and to terminate a bandage. For comfort, the initial and terminal ends are not situated directly over the wound.

The **spiral turn** is used to bandage a part of the body that is of uniform circumference. The bandage is carried upward at a slight angle so that it spirals around the part. Each turn is parallel to the preceding one and overlaps it by two-thirds of the width of the bandage. A spiral turn is used on parts of the body such as the fingers, arms and legs.

The **spiral reverse turn** is used to bandage cylindrical parts of the body that are of varying circumference, such as the lower leg. To make a spiral reverse turn, the thumb of the free hand is placed on the upper edge of the initial turn; the bandage is held firmly. The roll is unwound about 15 cm and then the hand is pronated so that the bandage is directed downward and parallel to the lower edge of the previous turn, overlapping it by two-thirds of the width. The roll is then carried around the limb and another reverse is made at the same place so that the turns are in line and uniform.

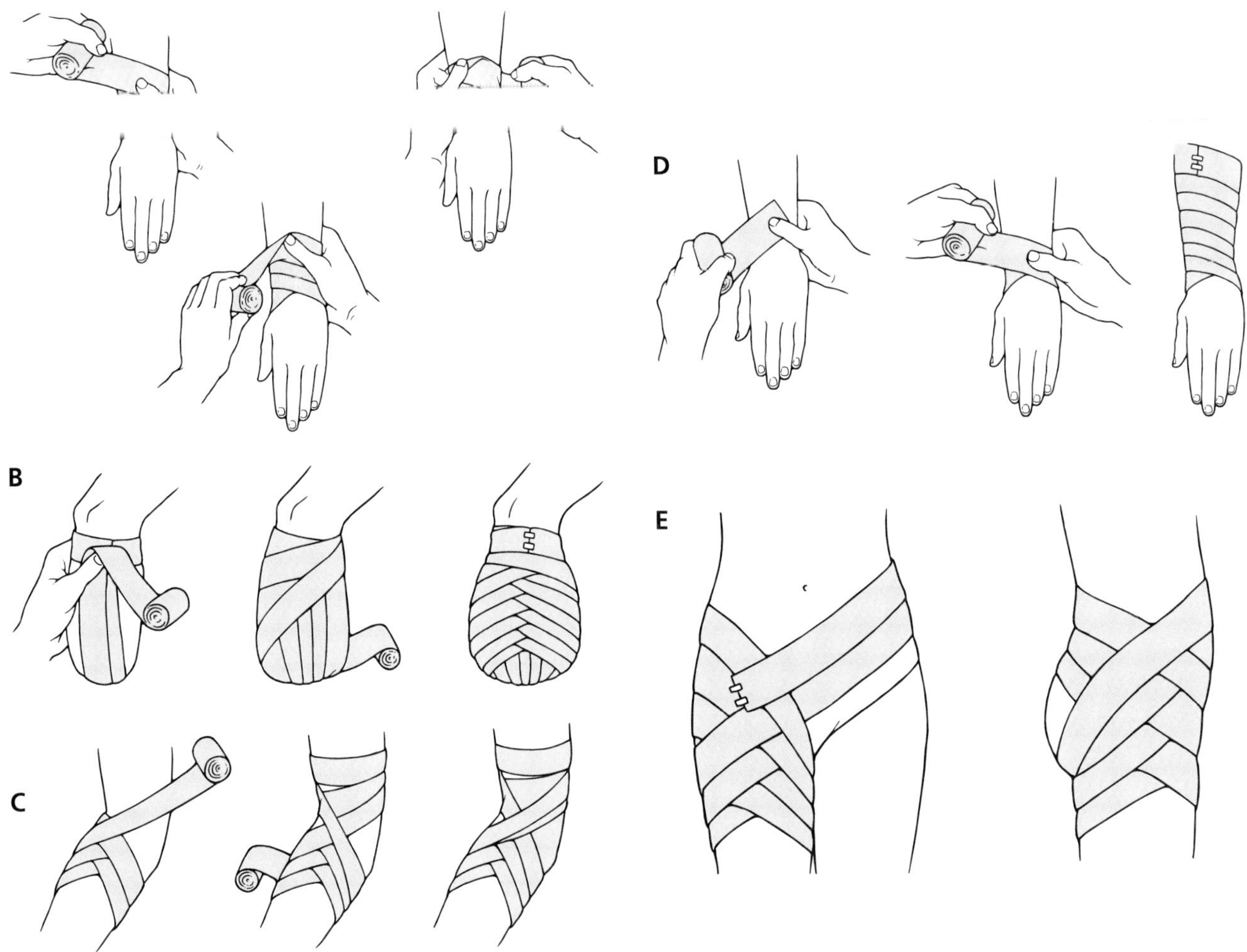

FIGURE 33.11 Types of bandages. A. Spiral reverse turn. B. Spiral turn. C. Recurrent turn. D. Circular turn. E. Figure-eight turn

SOURCE: Timby, 1996, pp. 577, 580.

The **figure-eight turn** is usually used on joints but may also be used for the entire length of an arm or leg bandage. It consists of repeated oblique turns that are made alternately above and below a joint in the form of a figure eight. After the initial circular turns are made over the centre of the joint, the next turn is superior to the joint and the next is inferior to the joint. Thus the turns are worked upward and downward, with each turn overlapping the previous turn by two-thirds of the width of the bandage.

The **recurrent turn** is used to cover distal portions of the body, such as the tip of a finger or the toes. After the bandage is anchored with a circular turn, the roll is turned and brought directly over the centre of the tip to be covered. It is then anchored inferiorly, and alternate turns are made, first to the right and then to the left, over the original turn covering the tip so that each turn is held above and below. Each turn overlaps the preceding one by two-thirds of its width. The bandage is secured by circular turns that gather in the ends.

Generally speaking, bandages for the hands, arms and feet are made with circular, spiral and spiral reverse turns. Bandages for the joints are made with figure eights, and bandages for the distal portions of the body are done with recurrent turns. In addition, there are many special bandages, such as the thumb spica, ear and eye bandages and skull bandages. It is suggested that the nurse consult a bandaging text for more detailed information.

APPLYING BINDERS

Binders can be used to retain dressings, to apply pressure, to support an area of the body and to provide comfort. They are generally made of a heavy cotton material that is strong and durable. Scultetus binders are occasionally lined with flannel, which absorbs moisture and provides additional comfort. When the purpose of the binder is to provide support to abdominal muscles, a two-way stretch type of binder, similar to a girdle, is sometimes used.

Types of Binders

There are five basic types of binders: T-binder, straight abdominal binder, scultetus (many-tailed) binder, breast binder and triangular binder (see Figure 33.12).

KEY PRINCIPLES

Principles Relevant to Bandaging

1. *Microorganisms flourish in warm, damp and soiled areas.* A bandage is applied only over a clean area; if it is to be placed over an open wound, the wound is dressed aseptically beforehand. Skin surfaces are dry and clean and are not pressed together when bandaging. Adjacent skin surfaces may be kept separated by inserting a 5 cm × 5 cm piece of gauze between them. Bandages are removed at regular intervals and the skin surfaces are washed and dried. Soiled bandages are never reused.
2. *Pressure exerted upon the body tissues can affect the circulation of blood.* A bandage is applied from the distal to the proximal part of the body to aid the return of the venous blood to the heart. Bandages are always applied evenly so that they do not restrict circulation. They should be checked frequently to make certain that there is no interference with blood supply to the part.
3. *Friction can cause mechanical trauma to the epithelium.* A bony prominence of the body is padded before it is bandaged, so that the bandage does not rub the area and cause an abraded wound. Skin surfaces are separated to prevent friction and maceration.
4. *The body is maintained in the natural anatomical position with slight flexion of the joints to avoid muscle strain.* Bandages are applied with the body in good alignment to avoid muscle extension, which is fatiguing and produces strain. In particular, adduction of the shoulder and hip joint is avoided.
5. *Excessive or uneven pressure upon body surfaces can interfere with blood circulation and therefore with the nourishment of the cells in the area.* Bandage evenly and, if possible, leave the distal portion of the bandaged limb exposed so that any restriction in circulation can be detected. Signs and symptoms of restricted circulation are pallor, erythema, cyanosis, tingling sensations, numbness or pain, swelling and cold.

   When a bandage is applied over a wet dressing, allowances are made for shrinkage as the bandage becomes wet and subsequently dries.

Guides to Bandaging

1. Face the patient being bandaged.
2. Start a roller bandage by holding the roll of the bandage upward in one hand, the initial end in the other hand.
3. Bandage from the distal to the proximal and from the medial to the lateral.
4. Do not initiate or terminate a bandage directly over a wound or an area where the patient is likely to exert pressure.
5. Bandage evenly and firmly, overlapping the preceding turn by two-thirds of the width of the bandage.
6. Use the bandage material that best serves the purpose of the bandage.
7. Cover a dressing with a bandage that extends past each side of the dressing.
8. Separate the skin surfaces and pad bony prominences and hollows to prevent friction and to apply even pressure.
9. Check the bandage and look for any signs of restricted circulation.
10. A bandage should be safe, durable, neat, therapeutically effective and economical.

The **T-binder** is made of two strips of cotton attached in the shape of a T. The top of the T serves as a band that is then placed around the patient's waist. The stem of the T is passed between the patient's legs and is then attached to the waistband in front. In some T-binders, the cotton strip that goes between the patient's legs is split into two tails about 22.5 cm from the end. These tails provide wider support to the perineal area and add to the comfort of the male patient particularly. T-binders are used chiefly to retain perineal dressings. Because of the profuse drainage that often occurs from this area, they are usually changed frequently.

The **straight abdominal binder** is a rectangular piece of cotton from 15 cm to 30 cm wide, and long enough to encircle the patient's abdomen and overlap at least 5 cm in front. This type of binder is used to retain abdominal dressings or to apply pressure and support to the abdomen.

The **scultetus binder,** which is also known as the many-tailed binder, is a rectangular piece of cotton, usually 22.5 cm to 30 cm wide and 37.5 cm long, with six to 12 tails attached to each side. It is usually used to provide support to the abdomen, but it can also be used to retain dressings. It can be applied to the chest as well. The advantage of the scultetus binder is that it fits the contours of the body closely.

The **breast binder** is a rectangular piece of cotton shaped roughly to the contours of the female chest. It usually has straps that fit over the shoulders and pin to the binder in front.

Guides for the Applying of Binders

1. Binders are applied in such a manner as to provide even pressure over an area of the body.
2. Binders should support body parts in their normal anatomical position, with slight joint flexion.
3. Binders are secured firmly so that they do not cause friction and irritate the skin or mucous membrane.

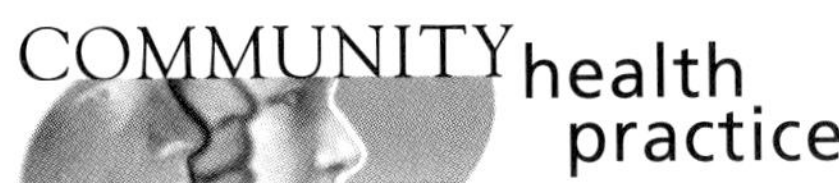

Same-Day Surgery

Health care reform has meant that an increasing number of surgical procedures are being performed on an outpatient basis. Some of the benefits of same-day surgery include improved patient care, decreased anxiety and fear, improved cost-effectiveness, decreased risk of nosocomial infections and increased support of individual and family preferences. The literature supports that individuals have a better recovery in their home environment.

Many hospitals have developed preoperative preparation programs that include a night-before-surgery routine, a nursing physical assessment the morning of surgery, follow-up postoperative care and discharge planning. These programs appear to be successful in preparing and supporting patients and their families before, during and after hospitalization.

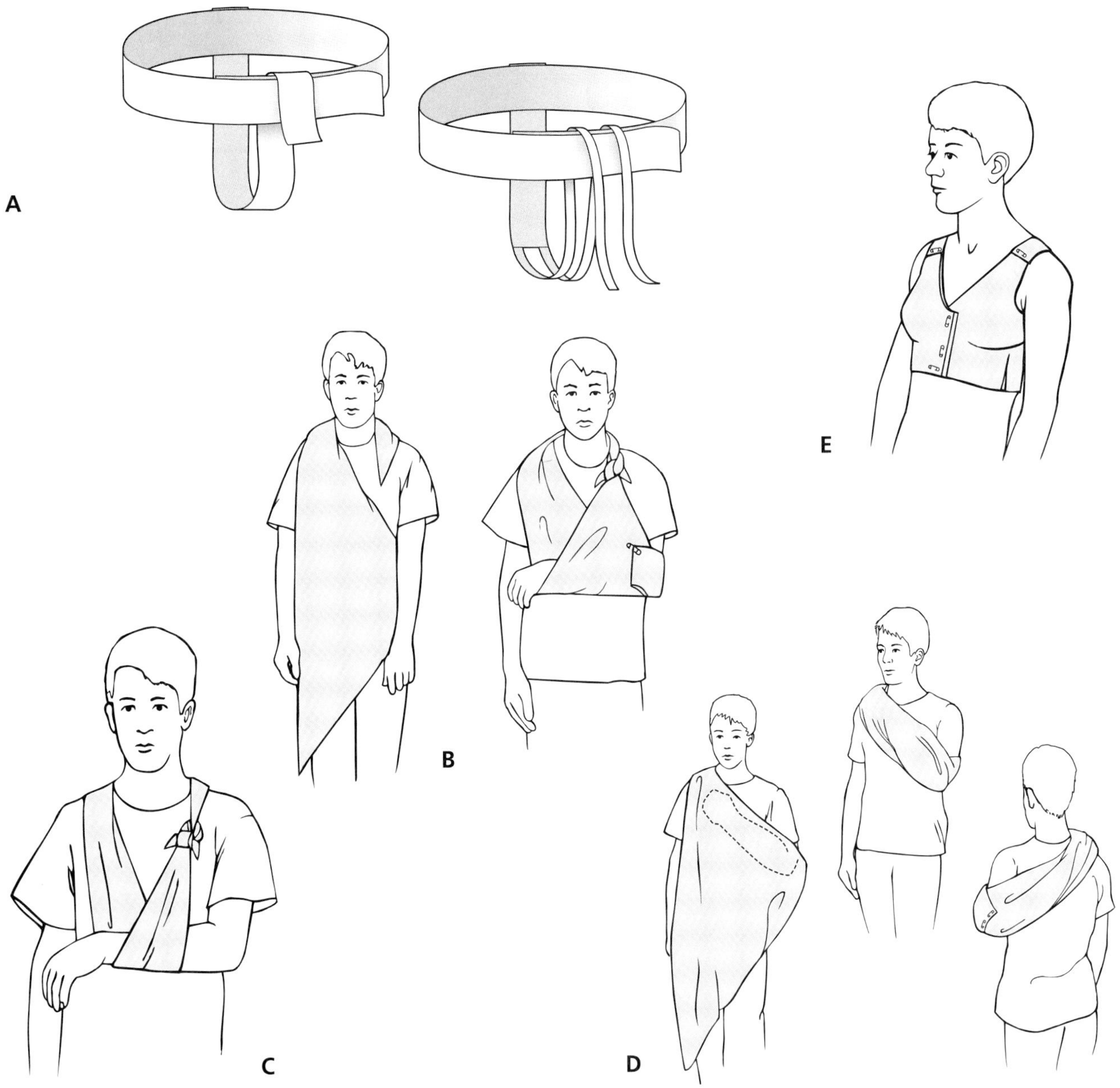

A

E

B

C

D

FIGURE 33.12 Types of binders. A. The T-binder is used for women and the double T-binder is used for men. B. A large arm sling. C. A small arm sling. D. A triangular sling. E. Breast binder.

Various forms of the **triangular binder** (sling) are used to support a limb, to secure a splint (as a first aid measure) and to secure dressings. The triangular binder is made of heavy cotton, is triangular in shape and has two sides approximately 1 m in length. It can be applied as a full triangle or folded for a variety of applications.

As a full triangle, the binder is used frequently to make a large arm sling. Folded into a broad bandage, it can be used as a small sling to support the patient's wrist and hand. A triangular binder can also support a patient's arm in such a manner as to elevate the hand. This is called a triangular sling.

Problems Related to the Use of Binders

Binders are most often used for large areas of the body, and since they are not secured to skin surfaces, they have a tendency to slip out of position. A binder should be changed or reapplied as often as necessary to maintain its intended function of support, comfort or application of pressure. Soiling is also a problem with binders. Because a dirty binder can be a source of both irritation and infection, it is essential to see that soiled binders are changed promptly.

When a binder is applied, it should be secured firmly, but the nurse should be careful that there is no interference with normal body functioning. An abdominal or breast binder that is too tight, for example, can restrict movements of the chest wall and interfere with respiration. In postoperative patients this could lead to serious complications. The nurse should be alert for signs of impaired respiration, such as shallow breathing, which could indicate that a binder is too tight and should be loosened.

IN REVIEW

- Surgery involves the deliberate and planned alteration of anatomical structures to arrest, alleviate or eradicate a pathological process or to repair a traumatic injury. Major nursing goals are to prepare individuals for and promote healthy recovery from surgery.
- Surgery may be:
  - major
  - minor.
- Depending on the severity of existing pathology, surgeries are classified as:
  - immediate
  - urgent
  - elective
  - optional.
- The purpose of surgery may be:
  - diagnostic
  - curative
  - constructive
  - reparative
  - palliative.
- The determinants of an individual's ability to cope with surgery include:
  - extent of surgery
  - patient's age
  - physiological and psychological health
  - overall coping abilities
  - ability to assist in postoperative planning
  - support received from family and significant others.
- A nurse's preoperative assessment includes:
  - health history
  - assessment of basic needs.
- In the preoperative patient, attention is paid to various needs, including:
  - oxygen
  - nutrition
  - fluid and electrolyte balance
  - elimination
  - immunological status
  - security
  - self-esteem.
- Preoperative teaching is an important health-promoting and health-protecting strategy. Teaching may be accomplished:
  - singly or in groups
  - before or after admission to a health facility.
- Preoperative teaching includes:
  - situational information
  - sensation/discomfort information
  - patient role information
  - psychological support
  - skills training.
- Most agencies have specific protocols for pre- and postoperative care that are essential for the health and safety of the patient on the nursing unit, in the post-anesthesia care unit and after transfer back to the nursing unit.
- Following surgery, the patient goes to the post-anesthesia care unit where he or she is monitored frequently. When conscious and stable, the patient is transferred back to the nursing unit.
- Postoperative complications include:
  - ineffective breathing and airway clearance
  - shock
  - development of thrombosis or embolism
  - electrolyte and acid–base imbalance
  - altered nutritional status
  - altered urinary elimination
  - altered bowel elimination
  - pain and anxiety
  - increased risk for infection.

- Healing occurs from a surgical wound by:
  - primary intention (little or no tissue loss)

extensive).

- The healing process for a surgical wound has three phases:
  - inflammatory
  - proliferative (granulation)
  - remodelling.
- Systemic and local factors may impede wound healing. Systemic factors include:
  - extent of injury
  - patient's nutritional status
  - obesity
  - diabetes
  - immunosuppression
  - use of radiation treatment.

  Local factors may be:
  - chemical
  - mechanical
  - thermal
  - caused by suture material
  - caused by infection
  - caused by lack of blood supply to the affected area.
- Restorative strategies include the use of aseptic technique:
  - for cleaning the wound and changing dressings
  - for management of wound drains and drainage systems.
- Specific techniques are used for:
  - changing dressings
  - shortening drains
  - irrigating wounds
  - removing sutures and staples.
- Bandages may be used to:
  - secure a dressing
  - apply warmth
  - keep splints in place
  - provide support
  - apply pressure
  - limit movement.
- Binders are used to:
  - retain dressings
  - apply pressure
  - provide comfort.
- Common binders include:
  - T-binders

  - breast binders
  - triangular binders.

Critical Thinking Activities

1. Mr. John Eberhardt is a 30-year-old law enforcement officer who is married, has four children and is in excellent physical condition. He was admitted to hospital three days ago with a bullet wound to his right shoulder. The bullet has been removed, but since there may still be particles of foreign matter present, the physician has not sutured the wound. The physician's orders for Mr. Eberhardt include: change dressings b.i.d. and as necessary; flush wound with normal saline; fluids to diet as tolerated.

   When you arrive to change his dressing, Mr. Eberhardt complains of headache and a burning sensation in the region of his wound. You notice a yellow discharge seeping through the previous dressing. Mr. Eberhardt also remarks that he feels hot, although a fresh breeze is blowing through the open window beside his bed.

   Mr. Eberhardt has been worried that he may not regain full use of his right arm, and since he is right-handed, he fears he may have to resign from active duty.

   a. What would you do first when faced with this situation?

   b. What might be causing the yellowish discharge from the wound?

   c. What other observations might you expect to note in the area of Mr. Eberhardt's wound?

   d. What other observations might you note about his general condition?

   e. How would you record your observations concerning Mr. Eberhardt?

   f. What could you do to assist in relieving his anxiety?

KEY TERMS

biopsy p. 1064

open wound p. 1084

closed wound p. 1084

primary intention healing p. 1085

secondary intention healing p. 1085

serous discharge p. 1087

sanguineous discharge p. 1087

KEY TERMS

serosanguineous drainage p. 1087
purulent drainage p. 1087
hematoma p. 1087
dehiscence p. 1087
evisceration p. 1087
occlusive dressings p. 1088
wound irrigation p. 1096
circular turn p. 1102
spiral turn p. 1102
spiral reverse turn p. 1102
figure-eight turn p. 1103
recurrent turn p. 1103
T-binder p. 1104
straight abdominal binder p. 1104
scultetus (many-tailed) binder p. 1104
breast binder p. 1104
triangular binder p. 1106

References

ALEXANDER, J.W., FISCHER, J.E., BOYAIJIAN, M., PALMQUIST, J., & MORRIS, M.J. (1983). The influence of hair-removal methods on wound infections. *Archives of Surgery, 118*, 347–352.

AORN RECOMMENDED PRACTICES (1992). Proposed recommended practices skin preparation of patients. *Journal of the Association of Operating Room Nurses, 55*(2), 555–562.

BECKERMANN, S., & GALLOWAY, S. (1989). Elective resection of the liver: Nursing care. *Critical Care Nurse, 9*(10), 40–48.

BLACK, J.M., & MATASSARIN-JACOBS, E. (1997). *Medical–surgical nursing: Clinical management for continuity of care.* (5th ed.). Philadelphia: W.B. Saunders.

BRYANT, D. (1992). *Acute and chronic wounds.* St. Louis: Mosby Year Book.

BUBELA, N., GALLOWAY, S., McCAY, E., McKIBBON, A., NAGLE, L., PRINGLE, D., ROSS, E., & SHAMIAN, J. (1990). Factors influencing patients' informational needs at time of hospital discharge. *Patient Education & Counselling, 16*, 21–28.

BYERS, J.F. (1996). Local and systemic effect of major traumatic wounds. *Critical Care Nursing Clinics of North America, 8*(2), 107–113.

CARPENITO, L.J. (1997). *Nursing diagnosis: Application to clinical practice.* (7th ed.). Philadelphia: Lippincott.

CAVANILLAS, A.B., RODRIGUEZ-CONTRERAS, R., RODRIGUEZ, M.D., ABRIL, O.M., GIGOSOS, R.L., SOLVAS, J.G., & VARGAS, R.G. (1991). Preoperative stay as a risk factor for nosocomial infection. *European Journal of Epidemiology, 7*(6), 670–676.

COBLEY, M., DUNNE, J.A., & SANDERS, L.D. (1991). Stressful pre-operative preparation procedures. *Anaesthesia, 46*, 1019–1022.

CONNOLLY, M.L. (1991). Ambulatory surgery and prepared discharge. *Nursing Clinics of North America, 26*(1), 105–112.

CRUSE, P., & FOORD, R. (1980). The epidemiology of wound infection: A 10-year prospective study of 62,939 wounds. *Surgical Clinics of North America, 60*, 27–40.

CURTIN, L.L. (1993). Informed consent: Cautious, calculated candor. *Nursing Management, 24*(4), 18–20.

DESJARDINS, L., NOBLE, J., BUBELA, N., MCKIBBON, A., & GALLOWAY, S.C. (1992). *Preoperative Education Program, Scarborough Grace Hospital/Sunnybrook Health Science Centre.* Toronto, Ontario.

DEVINE, C., & COOK, T. (1986). Clinical and cost-savings effects of psycho-educational intervention with surgical patients. A meta-analysis. *Research in Nursing and Health, 9*(2), 89–105.

EARNEST, V.V. (1993). *Clinical skills in nursing practice.* (2nd ed.). Philadelphia: Lippincott.

FLYNN, M.B. (1996). Wound healing and critical illness. *Critical Care Nursing Clinics of North America, 8*(2), 115–123.

FRAULEIN, K.E. (1987). After anesthesia: *A guide for PACU, ICU, and medical–surgical nurses.* Norwalk, CT: Appleton & Lange.

GALLOWAY, S.C., BUBELA, N., McKIBBON, A., McCAY, E., & ROSS, E. (1993). Perceived information needs and effect of symptoms on activities after surgery for lung cancer. *Canadian Oncology Nursing Journal, 3*(3), 116–119.

HATHAWAY, D. (1986). Effect of pre-operative instruction on post-operative outcomes: A meta-analysis. *Nursing Research, 35*(5), 269–275.

JOHNSON, J.E., & LAUVER, D.R. (1989). Alternative explanations of coping with stressful experiences associated with physical illness. *Advances in Nursing Science, 11*(2), 39–52.

KALLER, S.K., & EVERETT, L.L. (1993). Potential risks and preventive measures for pulmonary aspiration: New concepts in preoperative fasting guidelines. *Anesthesia & Analgesia, 77*, 171–182.

KRECHEL, S. (1997). Special considerations in the geriatric population. In M. Brown & E.M. Brown (Eds.), *Comprehensive postanesthesia care.* Philadelphia: Williams & Wilkins.

LEAHY, J., & KIZILAY, P. (1998). *Foundations of nursing practice: A nursing process approach.* Philadelphia: W.B. Saunders.

LONGMIRE, A.W., BROOM, L.A., & BURCH, J. (1987). Wound infection following high-pressure syringe and needle irrigation. *American Journal of Emergency Medicine, 5*, 179–181.

MAKLEBUST, J. (1996). Using wound care products to promote a healing environment. *Critical Care Nursing Clinics of North America, 8*(2), 141–158.

MAKLEBUST, J., & SIEGGREEN, M. (1996). *Pressure ulcers: Guidelines for prevention and nursing management.* (2nd ed.). Springhouse, PA: Springhouse.

MAXWELL, L. (1992). Acute pain management: IV patient-controlled analgesia places the patient in control. *Canadian Operating Room Nursing Journal, 10*(3), 12–15.

MORSE, J.M., & JOHNSON, J.L. (Eds.). (1991). *The illness experience: Dimensions of suffering.* Newbury Park, CA: Sage.

MOSIELLO, G., TUFARO, A., & KERSTEIN, M. (1994). Wound healing and complications in the immunosuppressed patient. *Wounds, 6*, 83.

POGUE, P. (1993). *Questions patients ask about pain after surgery.* Sunnybrook Health Science Centre: Toronto, Ontario.

RESNICK, B. (1993). Wound care for the elderly. *Geriatric Nursing, 14*, 26.

SCHOESSLER, M. (1989). Perceptions of pre-operative education in patients admitted the morning of surgery. *Patient Education & Counselling, 14*, 127–136.

SEROPIAN, R., & REYNOLDS, B.M. (1971). Wound infections after preoperative depilatory versus razor preparation. *American Surgeon, 121*, 251–254.

STOTTS, N.A., BARBOUR, S., GRIGGS, K., BOUVIER, B., BUHLMAN, L., WIPKE-TEVIS, D., & WILLIAMS, D.F. (1997). Sterile versus clean technique in postoperative wound care in patients with open surgical wounds: A pilot study. *Journal of Wound, Ostomy & Continence Nursing, 24*(1), 10–18.

TELFER, N., & MOY, R. (1993). Drug and nutrient aspects of wound healing. *Dermatology Clinics, 11*, 729.

THOMAS-HESS, C. (1995). *Wound care: Nurse's clinical guide.* Springhouse, PA: Springhouse.

TIMBY, B.K. (1996). *Fundamental skills and concepts in patient care* (6th ed.). Philadelphia: Lippincott.

WAHOFF-STICE, D. (1995). Surgical wound management. In R.A. Roth (Ed.), *Perioperative nursing core curriculum.* Philadelphia: W.B. Saunders.

WASYLAK, T.J. (1992). Surgical pain management. In J. Watt-Watson and M. Donovan (Eds.). *Pain management: A nursing perspective.* St. Louis: Mosby.

WEINGARTEN, M. (1993). Obstacles to wound healing. *Wounds, 5*, 238.

Additional Readings

BALL, K.R. (1997). Treating the whole person: One women's surgical experience. *Today's Surgical Nurse, 19*(6), 25–30.

[illegible] (1997). Preparation of children for surgery and invasive procedures: Milestones on the way to success. *Journal of Pediatric Nursing, 12*(4), 252–255.

CLEMENT, S.B. (1997). Postoperative considerations: Geriatric surgical patients and cardiovascular function. *Today's Surgical Nurse, 19*(5), 19–22.

DALEY, M.D. (1997). Positioning and the geriatric surgical patient. *Today's Surgical Nurse, 19*(5), 13–18.

DOUGHERY, J. (1996). Same-day surgery: The nurse's role. *Orthopedic Nursing, 15*(4), 15–18.

GALLACHER, B.P. (1997). Anesthesia for the older ophthalmic patient. *Today's Surgical Nurse, 19*(5), 23–27.

GALLAGHER, T.J. (1995). *Postoperative care of the critically ill patient.* Baltimore: Williams & Wilkins.

GARRETT, J.M. (1997). Hypothermia—Is it cold in here? *Today's Surgical Nurse, 19*(6), 17–24.

GERMAINE, E., ISMAN, C., PRICE, J., & ROSS, E. (1996). Surgical preadmission clinics in Canada: The expanding need with changing technologies. *Seminars in Perioperative Nursing, 5*(4), 199–202.

GIGER, J.N., & DAVIDHIZAR, R. (1996). When the operating room has a multicultural team. *Today's Surgical Nurse, 18*(5), 26–32.

HEISER, R.M., CHILES, K., FUDGE, M., GRAY, S.E. (1997). The use of music during the immediate postoperative recovery period. *Journal of the Association of Operating Room Nurses, 65*(4), 777–778, 781–785.

JACOBSEN, A.F. (1997). Research for practice. Preop fluid bolus reduces adverse surgical effects. *American Journal of Nursing, 97*(3), 62.

JANIKOWSKI, D.L. & ROCKEFELLER, C.A. (1998). Awake and talking: Ambulatory surgery and conscious sedation. *Nursing economics, 16*(1), 37–43.

KAEMPF, G., & GORALSKI, V.J. (1996). Monitoring postop patients. *RN, 59*(7), 30–35.

KELLY, M. (1997). Postoperative delirium in the elderly. *Today's Surgical Nurse, 19*(5), 10–12.

KEOUGH, V., & LETIZIA, M. (1996). Elder care: Perioperative care of elderly trauma patients. *Journal of the Association of Operating Room Nurses, 63*(5), 932–937.

[illegible] oxygen therapy protocol on use of pulse oximetry and oxygen therapy. *Respiratory Care, 40*(11), 1125–1129.

KRASNER, D. (1992). The 12 commandments of wound care. *Nursing, 22*(12), 34–41.

KRISTENSSON-HALLSTROM, I., & ELANDER, G. (1997). Patients' experience of hospitalization: Different strategies for feeling. *Pediatric Nursing, 23*(4), 361–367, 376–377.

LAMMON, C.B., FOOTE, A.W., LELI, P.G., INGLE, J., & ADAMS, M.H. (1995). *Clinical nursing skills.* Philadelphia: W.B. Saunders.

LANCASTER, K.A. (1997). Patient teaching in ambulatory surgery. *Nursing Clinics of North America, 32*(2), 417–427.

LUSIS, S.A. (1996). The challenges of nursing elderly surgical patients. *Journal of the Association of Operating Room Nurses, 64*(6), 954–955, 957–962.

MAZIARSKI, F.T., & PETTY, W.C. (1997). RNs: Conscious sedation providers? *Today's Surgical Nurse, 19*(1), 38–40.

McCONNELL, E. (1990). Applying antiembolism stockings. *Nursing, 20*(10), 92.

McEWEN, D.R. (1996). Home study program. Intraoperative positioning of surgical patients. *Journal of the Association of Operating Room Nurses, 63*(6), 1058–1063, 1066–1075, 1077–1082, 1084–1086.

NEAL, L.J. (1996). Outpatient ACL surgery: The role of the home health nurse. *Orthopedic Nursing, 15*(4), 9–13.

NELSON, S. (1996). Surgical nurse. Pre-admission education for patients undergoing cardiac surgery. *British Journal of Nursing, 5*(6), 335–340.

NORMAN, E.M. (1997). Critical care extra positioning patients to promote oxygenation. *American Journal of Nursing, 97*(8), 16C.

PALMERINI, J. (1996). Practical innovations: Developing a comprehensive perioperative nursing documentation form. *Journal of the Association of Operating Room Nurses, 63*(1), 239–242, 245, 247.

SUTHERLAND, M., & BRUCE, B. (1998). Same day pediatric surgery. *Canadian Nurse, 94*(4), 36–39.

ZALON, M.L. (1997). Pain in frail elderly women after surgery. *Image, 29*(1), 21–26.

Chapter 34

Administering Medications Safely

OUTLINE

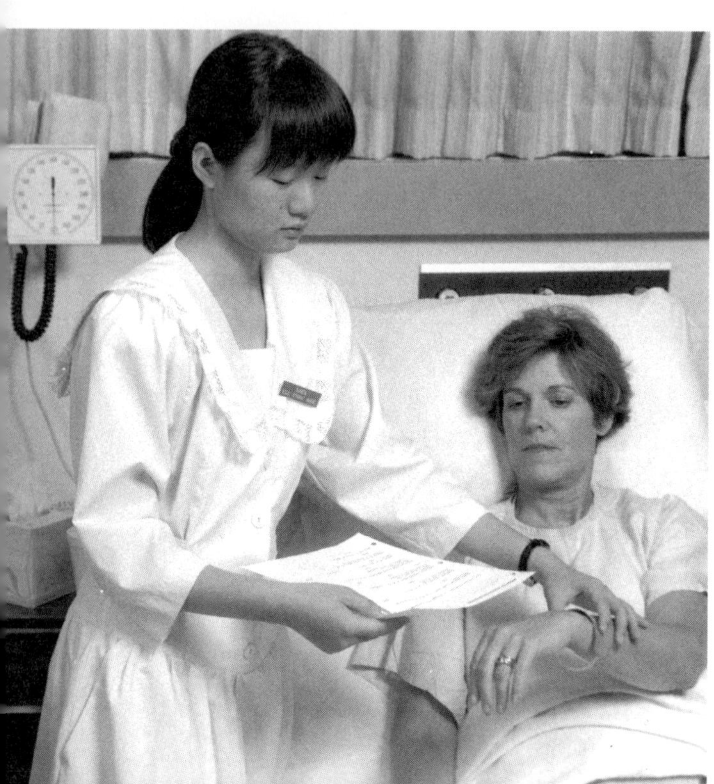

Central Questions

1. Why do some drugs have several different names?
2. How do drugs produce their effects in the body? What is pharmacokinetics? What is pharmacodynamics?
3. What determines the action and effects of drugs on different people?
4. What controls exist on drugs in Canada?
5. How are standards for drugs determined?
6. What information is required for medication orders to be valid?
7. What are the nurse's responsibilities in administering drugs safely?
8. How does the nurse assess the medication needs of patients?
9. What are some problems associated with drug therapy?
10. In order to promote healthy medication use, what advice should nurses give patients?
11. What is involved in teaching the self-administration of drugs?
12. What are the five rights of drug administration?
13. What methods are used for administering drugs? How are these carried out?
14. How does the nurse record the administration of medications?
15. How does the nurse evaluate the effectiveness of medications?

Introduction

By definition, a **medication** is a substance taken to treat a [illegible] agents (also referred to as drugs) and other "medicines" such as Therapeutic touch, laughter or hugging. In this chapter we will deal only with the administration of pharmaceutical agents.

Medications have been used throughout history to promote, maintain and restore health. In recent years, however, the number of different medicines manufactured commercially for distribution has increased exponentially. We take drugs to go to sleep, to reduce pain, to settle our nerves, to reduce ulcers, to provide vitamins and minerals—the list goes on. Health professionals have the enormous task of keeping up to date with the new drug products that are introduced each year, so that they may safely prepare and administer these drugs and provide patients with adequate information for self-administration. Medications can offer huge benefits for our health, but they are not without potential hazards. We must always be aware of these.

The administration of medications is a therapeutic nursing function that chiefly depends upon the orders of the physician. Some medication orders state the exact time of administration; others leave this to the nurse's judgement. For example, ferrous sulfate is usually prescribed three times a day after meals; morphine sulfate, on the other hand, is often ordered so that it can be given when the patient *requires* medication for pain. While the administration of medications is a delegated task, the responsibility for safe and effective administration rests with the nurse. Legally, nurses are responsible for any medications they administer. Safe, effective administration of medications begins with a basic understanding of pharmacology and the legal implications of drug administration. It requires knowledge and skill in preparing, administering and recording the administering of medications. It also requires knowledge and skill in assessing the patient's health status, in identifying problems and in implementing nursing interventions to enhance the effectiveness of drug therapy, minimize adverse reactions and promote patient safety and well-being.

Basic Pharmacology

The term **pharmacology** comes from the Greek *pharmakon*, which means "drugs," and *logos*, which means "science." By definition, pharmacology means the study of drugs, their actions and their effects on living organisms (Pinnell, 1996). An understanding of the basic concepts of pharmacology is fundamental to the safe administration of drugs.

Names of Drugs

A drug usually has at least three names: its trade name, a chemical name and a generic name. The beginning nurse often finds it difficult to decipher these names when first learning to administer drugs, because the same drug may be referred to by three [illegible]

[illegible] name, is the name of a drug chosen and copyrighted by the manufacturer. An example of a trade name is Valium. Manufacturers market drugs under the trade name. One drug may therefore have several trade names, since the same drug may be manufactured by several drug companies, each one giving it a different trade name. The **chemical** name of the drug is a description of its chemical constituents. For instance, the chemical name for Valium is 7-chloro-1,3-dihydro-1-methyl-5-phenyl-2H-1,4-benzodiazepin-2-one. A **generic** name is the original name assigned by the individual or company that develops the drug. It is usually a simpler representation of the drug's chemical name. The generic name for Valium is diazepam (Pinnell, 1996).

An increasing number of health agencies are promoting the use of generic names of drugs for writing prescriptions. This practice eliminates confusion about the nature of the drug prescribed. It also means that products from different drug companies can be used alternatively, except in cases where the physician requests a specific product. In addition, if the drug is ordered in its generic form, the patient can often save money, since brand-name products are frequently more expensive.

Mechanisms of Drug Action

Drugs act on the body in a number of different ways. The study of the mechanisms of drug action and the effects on cellular function is called **pharmacodynamics** (Pinnell, 1996). Drugs act by replacing missing or deficient substances, by altering the environment of the cell or by affecting the rate of cellular functions. Replacement therapy consists of administering an essential component of the body, such as insulin in diabetes mellitus or iron in iron-deficiency anemia. Drugs may alter the environment of cells through physical and chemical processes. For example, some drugs act by the mechanism of lubrication. Mineral oil given orally acts as a lubricant on the surface of the bowel, facilitating the passage of feces. Other drugs act by altering the chemistry of body fluids. Administering intravenous fluids and electrolytes will change the serum levels of the individual ions and may also influence the pH level of body fluids. Drugs that affect the rate of cell functions do so by acting on *receptors* found on cell membranes to stimulate (activate) or depress (block) a tissue response. Mechanisms of stimulation "increase the rate of cellular activity or increase the secretion from a gland" (Kee & Hayes, 1993, p. 14). Mechanisms of depression decrease or block cellular activity and reduce organ function. Drugs that stimulate or produce a response are called **agonists**. For example, epinephrine, which acts on alpha- and beta-adrenergic receptors to stimulate an adrenergic response, is an agonist. Drugs that block a cellular response are called **antagonists**. For example, cimetidine is an antagonist because it blocks the histamine$_2$ (H_2) receptors of the parietal cells of the stomach, thereby reducing gastric acid secretion.

A drug's action in the body is related to the amount of drug that reaches its target sites, or sites of action. Drug action is influenced by the dose of the medication (the quantity or concentration of the drug in a unit of volume or weight) and four basic processes: absorption, distribution, metabolism and excretion. The study of these four processes is called **pharmacokinetics** (Pinnell, 1996). *Absorption* is the process by which a drug moves from its site of entry to circulating body fluids, the blood stream and the lymphatic system. Absorption occurs in the mouth when medication is placed under the tongue (sublingual), in the gastrointestinal tract, in subcutaneous tissue, in muscle tissue and in the skin. Drugs given intravenously are injected directly into the blood stream and thus do not have to be absorbed. Once the drug molecules are absorbed, they are transported throughout the body to their sites of action (*distribution*). Drug molecules are also delivered to sites in the body, where they are chemically changed into active or inactive compounds. This process is called biotransformation or *metabolism* and takes place primarily in the liver. Most drugs are deactivated by this process and converted into water-soluble compounds for excretion from the body. However, some drugs are modified into active forms that can produce new pharmacological effects. *Excretion* is the process that eliminates drugs from the body. Excretion occurs primarily through the kidneys. Other routes of excretion include bile, feces, lungs, saliva, sweat and breast milk.

There is an ever-changing balance between the processes that increase active drug levels in the blood (absorption and distribution) and those that reduce active drug levels (metabolism and excretion). This balance "determines how soon the drug's actions will appear, how intense and widespread they will be, and how long they will last" (Shlafer, 1993, p. 46). The **onset of action** is the time it takes for a drug to enter the blood stream and begin its action on the body (or reach its minimum effective concentration). The point at which a drug reaches its highest blood level (concentration) and maximum effect is called **peak action** or **peak effect**. Once the peak effect and concentration are reached, levels begin to fall as a result of metabolism and excretion (Pinnell, 1996).

The term **half-life** is generally used to indicate the time it takes for 50 percent of the plasma concentration of a drug to be eliminated from the body. For instance, if a person takes 325 mg of acetaminophen and the half-life is three hours, the plasma concentration would drop to 162 mg in three hours, 81 mg in six hours, 40 mg in nine hours, and so on. **Duration of action** refers to the length of time a drug produces a pharmacological effect. This may be hours, days or months, depending on the half-life of the drug. Most drugs have a half-life of only a few hours. Therefore, dosages must be repeated regularly to maintain the concentration of the drug in the blood at a relatively constant level (the **plateau**). The object of drug therapy is to keep the plateau in a safe therapeutic range. This is accomplished by spacing repeated doses according to known influences on the absorption, distribution, metabolism and excretion, as well as the half-life of drugs. Drugs with a short half-life, such as ASA or penicillin, are given several times a day. Those with a long half-life, for instance digoxin, are given every one or two days (Pinnell, 1996).

Drug Action and Effects

Drugs are administered to produce desired or intended effects on the body. The desired response of drug action is called the **therapeutic effect.** Generally, drugs are administered for one of two therapeutic effects: systemic or local. A **systemic effect** refers to the action of a drug on the whole body after it is absorbed and distributed to the tissues. In a **local effect,** drug action is confined to the specific area of application. Eye drops, ear drops or ointments are examples of preparations administered for their local effects. Drugs that are administered locally, however, can produce systemic effects if they are absorbed into the blood stream. For example, an anticholinergic agent instilled into the eyes may cause systemic effects such as flushing of the skin, dry mouth or rapid pulse.

No drug exerts a single effect on the body. All drugs have the potential to affect more than one body system and to produce physiological responses that are unrelated to the therapeutic effect. These responses are called **adverse reactions** or **side effects.** An adverse reaction "is an unwanted, undesired and possibly harmful side effect of a drug" (Pinnell, 1996, p.47). The reaction can happen right away or may take days or weeks to occur. Some adverse reactions are predictable with normal doses, for example, CNS depression with barbiturates. However, some patients respond unpredictably with CNS stimulation. Most side effects are undesirable; however, some may be desirable. For example, diphenhydramine (Benadryl), which may be used as an antihistamine to counteract allergic itching, also causes drowsiness. This sedative effect may be helpful to patients who are feeling distressed by the itchiness and cannot relax. Side effects may be harmless or they may cause mild to severe injury. Some side effects may even be lethal; for example, a severe allergic reaction can cause death.

An **allergic reaction** is a hypersensitive (antigen–antibody) reaction to a drug in a person who was previously exposed to the drug or a related chemical and has developed antibodies to it. Reactions may vary from mild to severe itching, skin rashes and urticaria (hives); to exfoliative dermatitis and fever, rhinitis or bronchospasm; or to life-threatening respiratory distress and cardiovascular collapse, known as **anaphylactic reaction**. Although patients with a history of allergies are more likely to develop hypersensitive drug reactions, all patients must be carefully monitored for allergic responses to medications. A mild allergic reaction should be regarded as a warning that if the drug is continued, a more serious reaction will likely occur. The drug should not be administered again, and the physician should be notified.

(Shlafer, 1993, p. 115). **Drug toxicity** refers to the effects produced by an overdosage, an accumulation of a drug in the body or an abnormal sensitivity. Drug accumulation is a common cause of toxicity, which often results when a drug is metabolized or excreted more slowly than it is being administered. Older adults or people with hepatic and renal impairment are prone to drug accumulation. However, toxicity is not always the result of drug overdosage or accumulation. It can also occur as an abnormal reaction to a drug taken in therapeutic doses (Shlafer, 1993). Toxic effects may appear as exaggerated therapeutic or side effects. For example, a drug used for sedation may cause coma. Careful monitoring of the serum levels of drugs can avoid toxicity.

Drug tolerance describes the circumstance in which a therapeutic response to a dosage lessens after days or weeks of continued administration. A larger dose of the drug is often required to maintain the desired effect. Patients commonly develop tolerance to opiate analgesics and sedative drugs.

Effects resulting from the combined actions of two or more drugs are called **drug interactions**. The interaction of two or more drugs can modify the mechanisms of action and alter the way in which any of the drugs are absorbed, distributed, metabolized and excreted from the body, all of which ultimately influence the therapeutic effects. Two drugs that are administered simultaneously may have an additive, potentiating or antagonistic effect. An **additive effect** is the result of administering two drugs with similar actions. For example, if nitroglycerin (for angina) is taken with an alpha-adrenergic blocker such as prazosin, the blood pressure will drop significantly, causing syncope or faintness. A **potentiating** or **synergistic effect** is one in which the combined effect of two drugs is greater than the intended effect of the single drug. For example, alcohol, when combined with a hypnotic drug, has an enhanced hypnotic effect. An **antagonistic effect** occurs when two drugs in opposing categories cancel out the effects of both drugs. For instance, if a beta-adrenergic stimulant such as isoproterenol (Isuprel) were given with an adrenergic beta-blocker such as popranolol (Inderal), the actions of each drug would nullify the other. There would be no therapeutic effect in this case (Kee & Hayes, 1993).

Determinants of Drug Action and Effects

A number of factors determine the action and effects of any medication, and the nurse must be aware of them all. These factors can alter the effects of medication to varying degrees within and among patients. One patient may respond differently to repeated doses of a medication after a period of time. Similarly, the same dose of a drug may cause different effects in different patients.

AGE The age groups at opposite ends of the life cycle are most predisposed to alterations in the effectiveness of medications. Very young people and older adults are particularly affected—children because of the immaturity of the entire system and older adults because of changes associated with aging. Both these age groups are discussed more fully later in this chapter.

BODY SIZE, WEIGHT AND GENDER The actions, and therefore the effectiveness of a medication, are greatly influenced by body size, weight and gender. Generally, the greater the body weight, the higher the dosage required to produce a therapeutic effect. Children, for example, usually require smaller dosages of a medication, as do severely emaciated patients. Conversely, obese people may require larger doses in order to obtain an effective action from a medication.

Males and females respond differently to certain drugs because of differences in body size and weight, as well as differences in the distribution of adipose tissue, water, muscle mass, hormones and metabolic levels.

Typically, men have more muscle mass and less adipose tissue, and therefore a greater basal metabolic rate (BMR), than women. During pregnancy, a woman's BMR may increase by 20 percent owing to the metabolic rate of the fetus. An increased BMR produces faster drug biotransformation (Pinnell, 1996). Further, because males have more body water than women and women have more adipose tissue than men, drugs that are soluble in water are more readily absorbed in men, whereas those soluble in fat are better absorbed in women.

ENVIRONMENT The physical, mental and spiritual environments have an impact on the effectiveness of a medication. Environments that are disruptive may provoke anxiety in some patients, reducing the maximum effect of an analgesic. Similarly, a patient who is completely isolated and feels shut out and uncared for, in spite of the nurse's best intentions, often experiences less pain relief from analgesics. Environmental temperature also affects the action of medications. For example, topical medications are absorbed more quickly in a warm environment because warm temperatures cause peripheral vasodilation. Conversely, topical preparations are absorbed more slowly in cold temperatures because the peripheral blood vessels constrict. For the most part, the patient's environment is an aspect of preference, and the nurse should attempt to create an environment in which the patient can feel comfortable. Finally, smoking and high altitudes also affect drug response.

GENETIC MAKEUP Genetic variations cause some individuals to react differently to certain medications. Frequently, these differences are hereditary, with family members experiencing similar drug sensitivities or reactions.

When taking a medication history, the nurse should ask the patient if other family members have particular sensitivities.

DISEASE AND ILLNESS The actions and effects of many medications depend on the proper functioning of body organs and processes within the individual, particularly gastrointestinal absorption and circulatory, hepatic and renal function. Thus, in addition to the problem being treated, the nurse must explore other health problems the patient may have, such as chronic illnesses or secondary problems.

PATIENTS' EXPERIENCES WITH MEDICATIONS Many patients have had past experience with medications and carry beliefs about the effectiveness of these drugs. Often, the medication that the patient believes will work has a much greater effect than one in which the patient has no faith. On the other hand, if a patient has been using a medication, such as an analgesic, for a long period of time, the dosage may need to be altered since the degree of tolerance developed will decrease its effectiveness.

PSYCHOLOGICAL FACTORS Lack of trust in health professionals and negative emotions such as anger, sadness and high anxiety will inhibit the action of medications; on the other hand, positive emotions and beliefs will enhance the effects. It is therefore crucial that the nurse develop a trusting relationship with the patient and acknowledge and assist him or her to cope with negative emotions.

TIME OF ADMINISTRATION The time that oral medications are administered can affect the action of drugs and cause unpleasant side effects. The existence of food in the stomach generally slows the absorption of medications; thus, oral medications should be given on an empty stomach. Notwithstanding, some medication must be administered with food or milk to prevent gastric irritation.

ETHNIC DIFFERENCES Some variations in drug response can be attributed to ethnic differences. For example, studies have shown that some ethnic groups respond differently to antihypertensive drugs. Chinese patients are especially sensitive to the hypotensive actions of propranolol (Inderal), and thus require less medication than patients from other ethnic groups. Further research is needed regarding the differences in drug response among diverse ethnic populations (Pinnell, 1996).

Drug Action and Effects Throughout the Life Cycle

While the nurse must be prudent about administering medications to any age group, there are certain stages of the life cycle that have special needs and warrant further attention. These include pregnant women, infants, children and older adults.

Pregnant Women

As a general rule, pregnant women are advised to avoid all medications except acetaminophen, since most drugs will cross the placental barrier and affect the fetus. The fetus is most susceptible to the effects of drugs during early pregnancy (the first three months), when the brain and other organs are developing. Drugs administered during this time may cause *teratogenesis*, the creation of physical defects in the fetus during development. Some drugs—such as alcohol, nicotine (to a lesser degree) and opiates—may cause mental deficiencies and growth retardation in the developing fetus. If fetal growth has been retarded by medications, there is usually no major "catch-up" growth after birth.

Smoking has been linked to both low birth weight babies and prematurity (Naeye, 1981; Shiono, Klebanoff & Rhoads, 1986). Alcohol, in any amount, affects fetal development and birth weight. Excessive alcohol taken in early pregnancy can affect the development of the fetal facial features and central nervous system (CNS) or cause full-blown fetal alcohol syndrome, characterized by craniofacial abnormalities, growth retardation, CNS dysfunction (hypotonia, irritability), mental retardation, hyperactivity, poor coordination and fine motor dysfunction. It is also associated with congenital defects of the cardiovascular, genitourinary and musculoskeletal systems (Butters & Howie, 1990). There is some evidence, although not conclusive, to suggest that caffeine in ordinary tea, coffee and cola, if consumed in large quantities, may harm the fetus (Aaronson & MacNee, 1989; McKim, 1991). The narcotic addiction of a pregnant woman can cause neonatal dependency and withdrawal trauma (neonatal abstinence syndrome) during the first few days or weeks of life. Drugs that are given to a woman during labour also cross the placenta and affect the newborn. Women who have been given opiate analgesics and sedatives during labour usually find that their babies are drowsy for the first two to three days after birth.

Women who use cocaine during pregnancy have increased risk for abruptio placenta, prematurity and growth retardation of the fetus. Infants exposed to this drug are smaller at birth and, in the first few weeks of life, show poor sucking and feeding, irritability, tremulousness, hypertonia, regurgitation, yawning and sneezing (Butters & Howie, 1990; Aaronson & MacNee, 1989).

Infants

Infants require a smaller amount of medication than adults do. The dosage of medications for infants is usually ordered according to body weight. Infants are often more sensitive to the pharmacologic effects of drugs because of smaller body size and rapidly developing tissues. They are also more prone to drug accumulation and side effects due to immature functioning of the liver and kidneys. Because they are unable to swallow tablets or pills, infants are usually given oral medications in liquid form. These may be administered by

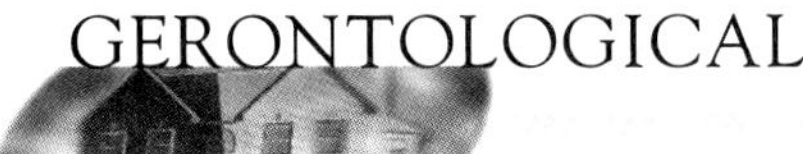

GERONTOLOGICAL Safe Drug Administration for Older Adults

- Always follow your prescription.
- Read all labels carefully.
- Take medications as scheduled.
- Understand the reason for taking a medication.
- Advise your physician or pharmacist of over-the-counter medication use.
- Keep medications in labelled containers.
- Never take medications in a dimly lit room.
- Throw away old or expired medications.
- Keep medications out of reach of grandchildren.
- Never take medication prescribed for others.
- Inform your physician and pharmacist of previous medication complications.
- Keep a daily log of all prescribed medications and their effects.
- Ask your pharmacist for easy-to-access containers, if required.
- If your vision is impaired, ask your pharmacist to provide larger print on medication labels.
- Avoid mixing alcohol with medications.
- Alert your physician or pharmacist to any unusual drug reactions you may experience.
- If travelling, ensure you have a sufficient supply for the duration of your vacation.
- If your doctor's verbal instructions were unclear, ask the pharmacist to repeat them and/or provide written instructions for taking your medications.
- Do not discontinue any medication without your physician's guidance.
- Inform significant others of your medication regime.
- Ask your pharmacist what to do if you miss a dose of medication.

SOURCE: Ebersole & Hess, 1998.

dropper, on a spoon or with a medicine dispenser that is specially designed for children.

Children

With older children, drug dosage is usually calculated in relation to height and weight, with weight being considered the more important factor. When an exact dosage for size is necessary, surface area (SA) may be used. Surface area is estimated from both height and weight measurements.

Adolescents and Young and Middle-Aged Adults

Allergies to drugs often begin to develop in adolescence and young and middle adulthood. The nurse should be particularly alert for allergic reactions in patients in these age groups. The problem of drug abuse, which is discussed at the end of this chapter, is also most prevalent among people of these ages.

Older Adults

Drug overdoses in older patients have become fairly common. They may result from a number of factors related to dosages, multiple prescriptions, drug interactions, the aging process and intentional overdose.

Kidney and liver function decline with age, and often older people simply cannot process and excrete drugs as efficiently as before. Drug concentrations increase, resulting in cumulative effects and the potential for toxicity (Matteson & McConnell, 1988; Blair, 1990). The nurse must be aware that a dosage may be too large for an older individual to process.

With the increase in life expectancy and the concomitant increase in the incidence of chronic illness, older adults often take many medications, once or more daily or every other day; the frequency of dosages can vary tremendously. This can be confusing for the older individual, who may have difficulty reading the label on a prescription bottle because of failing vision. The patient may not understand what medications to take or when to take them. The nurse often has to help the older adult set up a simple, orderly system for ensuring that the right dosage of the right drug is taken at the right time. Dispensing a week's supply of pills into small envelopes for daily consumption or distributing them in egg cartons are two possible methods.

Drug interactions are a potential problem for older adults on multiple drug regimens. This frequently happens when a patient is being treated by more than one physician for different conditions. The patient's general practitioner may prescribe medications for a heart problem and other long-standing conditions, but the urologist who is treating a urinary tract obstruction may order other drugs. The two sets of drugs are not always compatible. The nurse should encourage the patient to keep a current list of medications readily available for different members of the health care team to consult. It is also wise to give a copy of this list to a family member in case of emergency.

Idiosyncratic reactions to drugs because of the age factor are also possible. Older people often react poorly to certain drugs. Barbiturates and tranquillizers are two groups of drugs that many older people do not tolerate well. Barbiturates often cause excitement in older patients instead of sedation, while tranquillizers may cause mental disturbances such as delusions.

Malnourishment is a factor that contributes to adverse drug reactions in older adults. Malnourished patients have less plasma protein to bind with highly protein-bound drugs. Consequently, plasma concentrations of these drugs is greater, and there is more free drug to enter cells. Dehydration also contributes to altered drug distribution, since it leads to increased plasma concentrations of drugs. The results are more intense drug effects. Factors influencing nutrition and hydration in the older patient include finances, physical ability, disease, condition of teeth or dentures, mental status, decreased thirst drive and decreased ability to concentrate urine (Pinnell, 1996).

Intentional overdose is the final factor that must be considered. Suicide rates are high among older people. Because sedatives and tranquillizers are so commonly prescribed, they are readily available, and drug overdose is a common method of committing suicide. The nurse must be aware of older patients who appear depressed, lonely or despondent, as they are at a greater risk for intentional overdose.

Nurses are often in the best position to assist older adults with safe medication administration. The nurse can frequently both identify and intervene in problems that the older person is experiencing in taking medications. The nurse's responsibilities include explaining the actions of various medications, reviewing the administration schedule and helping the patient to set up a simple medication regimen that is physically manageable. The nurse is also frequently the first person to observe untoward reactions to drugs in patients. Therefore, he or she must be alert to side effects and possible interactions with other drugs the patient is taking. Often the nurse takes the position of patient advocate, who can discuss the patient's difficulties with taking certain medications with the physician.

Legal Aspects of Medication Administration

Nurses are not only responsible for knowing the pharmacological aspects of drug therapy; they must also be knowledgeable about the legal implications of drug administration and abide by established laws and regulations.

Drug Legislation

All aspects of drug production, distribution, advertising and sale are governed by laws. In Canada, the drug laws include the *Food and Drugs Act* of 1953 (with yearly amendments) and the *Narcotic Control Act* of 1961 (with periodic amendments). Table 34.1 outlines the provisions of these laws. Both laws are administered under the Health Protection Branch of Health Canada. Enforcement of the *Narcotic Control Act* is delegated to the Royal Canadian Mounted Police. In the United States, the *Food, Drug and Cosmetics Act* (1938) and the *Controlled Substances Act* (1970), both with amendments, provide the governing laws.

TABLE 34.1 Canadian federal drug legislation

Legislation	*Provisions*
Food and Drugs Act (1953)	• Provides for regulation of the manufacture, distribution, advertising and sale of drugs. • Prohibits the sale of drugs that are contaminated, adulterated or unsafe. • Prohibits the sale of drugs whose labels are false, misleading or deceptive. • Prohibits the advertising and sale of food, drugs, cosmetics or devices for diseases listed in Schedule A of the act (such as alcoholism, arteriosclerosis and cancer). • Classifies drugs into groups with varying degrees of control over distribution and sale. • Stipulates that drugs must comply with the professed standards of the manufacturer or the standards set out in recognized pharmacopeiae or formularies.
Narcotic Control Act (1961)	• Restricts the manufacture, sale, possession and distribution of narcotics. • Allows authorized professionals to prescribe and dispense narcotics to those patients for whom the drug is prescribed. • Requires the maintenance of complete records of the disposition of the narcotic drugs.

Drug laws regulate the availability and use of drugs in a country, the purpose being to ensure that all drugs available for use are safe, effective and wisely administered. [illegible]

[illegible] group of substances, including nonprescription preparations that may be purchased in any retail outlet or in a pharmacy; prescription preparations that are available for medical management by a physician or dentist; and restricted preparations, obtainable only by a research institution that has received authorization from Health Canada. Many of the regulations pertaining to the availability of drugs are based on federal law, but provincial laws may further restrict the distribution of a drug. For example, ephedrine is a nonprescription drug at the federal level; in British Columbia, however, ephedrine, as the single active ingredient for internal use, is ruled to be a prescription drug. Provincial laws may be more, but not less, restrictive than federal law. Drugs placed on the list of prescription drugs by federal law may not be removed by provincial regulation (Health & Welfare Canada, 1991). Table 34.2 outlines the categories of drug control and availability of drugs for public use in Canada.

Drug Standards and Control

Drugs are derived from natural sources (plants, animals or inorganic substances such as minerals) or produced from synthetic chemicals. For example, digitalis is extracted from a plant called purple foxglove; some insulins are obtained from the pancreases of cattle and pigs; and biosynthetic insulin is synthesized in the laboratory. Natural sources of drugs are not uniform in their pharmacological quality or strength, and synthetic processes may not always be consistent. Therefore, drugs can vary in strength and purity and thereby produce unpredictable effects. Drug standards ensure that drugs meet requirements for purity, that dosages are uniform and that effects are predictable. Many countries have official or recognized formularies or pharmacopeiae that prescribe standards for drugs and drug use.

In Canada, drugs are evaluated according to the manufacturer's own standards and those of the *United States Pharmacopeia* and the *British Pharmacopeia*. The manufacturer's standards for a drug must be equal to or more stringent than the standards of the recognized pharmacopeiae. Once drugs are approved they can be entered into the *Compendium of Pharmaceuticals and Specialties* (CPS). The CPS is a drug reference book compiled and revised annually by the Canadian Pharmaceutical Association for the use of all health professionals. The World Health Organization (WHO) also publishes a guide entitled *Specifications for the Quality Control of Pharmaceutical Preparations*. This is an international pharmacopoeia listing important drugs used in many countries. The WHO publication has been a major step towards establishing international standards for drugs.

The Nurse's Legal Responsibility

As members of a profession and as individuals who admin-

under the laws regulating drug administration. Nursing legislation in every province further outlines the nurse's legal responsibility for conduct. It is illegal for a nurse to practise in a manner that is beyond, or does not adhere to, the defined limits of the law. The nurse must know the legal specifications in his or her region, because practices vary among provinces. For example, nurses employed in the Yukon and Northwest Territories prescribe a range of drugs according to standard protocols; in other provinces, this practice would be illegal.

As professionals, nurses are responsible and accountable for all their actions, including the administration of medications. It is important for nurses to maintain an adequate knowledge base, clarify orders when necessary and refuse to administer a prescribed medication if a potential problem is indicated. For example, a nurse may refuse to administer a dosage that is beyond recommended safe limits or if the patient's condition is in jeopardy.

Unfortunately, even the most careful nurse may make a medication error. When this happens, it is important to confront the error in an honest and professional manner so that patient safety can be maintained and the occurrence can be documented swiftly and accurately. A medication error is reported immediately to the physician and the nurse in charge so that immediate steps can be taken to protect the patient from injury. The error is also analysed to determine the exact cause as a safeguard against making the same mistake again. Most agencies have incident report forms that the nurse fills out, describing the details of the error. Mistakes do happen, and it is important for the nurse to acknowledge them, learn from them and seek appropriate support. Finally, no nurse ever *plans* to make a medication error and so must forgive him- or herself once the incident is over.

Basic Foundations for Administering Medications

The safe administration of medications is based on knowledge and skill, and requires collaboration with other health professionals. The physician, pharmacy department and agency administrators are also responsible for safe drug therapy. To this end, health care agencies have established policies and systems for ordering, processing, communicating, storing and dispensing medications. Medications are not always supplied in the exact dosages ordered. Therefore, mathematical skills are needed for the computation of individual drug dosages.

TABLE 34.2 Categories of drug control and availability

Category	*Description*	*Availability and Identification*
Nonprescription Drugs		
• *Proprietary medicines*	For treatment of minor, self-limiting illness that does not require advice of a health professional; for example, cough drops, medicated shampoos, fluoride toothpastes.	Any retail outlet. Have letters **GP** (General Public) on labels.
• *Over-the-counter drugs*	For treatment of minor, self-limiting illness but may require the advice of a health professional for proper use; for example, decongestants, laxatives, many vitamins, mild analgesics.	Any pharmacy. Have letters **DIN** (Drug Identification Number) followed by an eight-digit number.
• *Limited public access*	For use only after consultation with and upon recommendation of physician; for example, muscle relaxants, insulin, nitroglycerin, analgesic preparations containing low doses of codeine (not more than 8 mg per tablet or 20 mg per 30 mL oral solution).	Dispensed by pharmacist. Not on open shelves.
Prescription Drugs		
• *Vitamins A, D, K and folic acid*	When recommended daily dose of vitamin A and D exceeds 10 000 IU and 1000 IU, respectively; when recommended daily dose for folic acid is greater than 1 mg; and all vitamin K preparations.	By prescription.
• *Schedule F Drugs*	Diversity of drug classes ordered by a physician or dentist to treat diagnosed conditions; for example, antibiotics, diuretics.	By prescription. Have the symbol Pr on the label.
• *Controlled Drugs (Schedule G)*	Stimulants and sedatives that have mood-modifying effects, are habit-forming and may be abused; for example, amphetamines and barbiturates.	By prescription. Have the symbol ◇C on the label.
• *Narcotic Drugs*	Drugs that are controlled by the *Narcotic Control Act* and Regulations; for example, cocaine, opium derivatives (codeine, morphine), phencyclidine, and *cannabis sativa* (marijuana).	By prescription. Have the letter **N** on the label.
• *Restricted Drugs (Schedule H)*	Drugs that have no recognized medicinal use but cause dangerous physiological and psychological effects; for example, LSD (lysergic acid diethylamide).	Available only to authorized institutions involved in highly specialized research.

SOURCE: Health & Welfare Canada, 1991.

Knowledge About Medications

It is never acceptable to administer a medication without [illegible] and its effects helps to safeguard against the administration of a medication that could harm a patient. For example, if a patient has very slow respirations (say, 10 per minute), morphine may be contraindicated, because it can depress respiration even further. This knowledge helps the nurse to make intelligent observations that assist in the assessment of the effectiveness of both the medication and the nursing care.

In an ideal world, the nurse would be able to take the time to review the overall classification of each drug to be given and to stay abreast of research on specific drugs in that category. The information the nurse should gather includes indications for use (the diagnoses and conditions that are treated with the drug); actions, therapeutic effects and adverse reactions; food and drug interactions; dosage; contraindications (problems or conditions in the patient in which giving the drug may be harmful); and nursing implications (specific concerns related to administration of a drug).

On the other hand, the realities of daily practice must also be recognized. Nurses are at times faced with the situation of administering an unfamiliar medication with little time to research it. However, the nurse can still gain a safe level of knowledge and administer the medication within minutes. While shortcuts are possible, it is never acceptable to administer a medication without knowing the following basics: classification and main action, key adverse effects, safe dosage and nursing considerations. A quick search will often only take one to two minutes, and the nurse can pursue a more complete review later.

There are a number of sources of drug information available in the agency for the nurse's use. These may include the *CPS*, the agency pharmacy department, physicians, professional nursing and medical journals, nursing drug guides, and information supplied by commercial drug companies. In many health agencies, the pharmacy department maintains an up-to-date *formulary*, which lists and describes drugs currently used in the agency. Copies of the formulary are usually distributed to all nursing units, where they are readily available for reference. In addition, many unit managers like to keep a drug file on their unit containing information about new drugs. The pharmacist is, of course, an excellent reference source, and the nurse should not hesitate to request information from this health professional. Physicians, too, are usually very willing to explain the nature and purpose of new drugs they have prescribed for patients.

Medication Orders

Medications are, in most instances, ordered or prescribed by a physician. In an ambulatory care setting, the physician usually writes the prescription on a form that the patient later gives to the pharmacist. The prescription should tell the pharmacist what medication(s) the patient is to have, the dosage required, the amount to be supplied, how to prepare it and the instructions the patient is to be given. In many [illegible] on the label of the medication the patient receives.

In an inpatient facility, the prescription is usually in the form of a written order that is dated and signed by the physician, although in some health agencies, physicians are permitted to issue orders to the nursing staff by telephone. In such cases, the physician is often required to countersign the order within a defined period of time, usually 24 hours. In an emergency, medications are often prescribed via verbal orders that are later written and countersigned. Generally speaking, written orders are considered to be the safest practice.

TYPES OF MEDICATION ORDERS

There are two types of written orders: the self-terminating order and the standing order.

Self-Terminating Orders

Self-terminating orders have a time limit on them. A **stat order** is a type of self-terminating order that is to be carried out immediately and only once; for example, *meperidine hydrochloride (Demerol) 100 mg IM (intramuscularly) stat*. The order is not repeated unless there are specific instructions to do so. Another type of self-terminating order is one in which the time limit is actually specified; for example, the physician orders *acetaminophen (Tylenol) 650 mg for six doses*, or *digitalis 0.25 mg June 12th and 14th*. Sometimes a self-terminating order is dependent upon the condition of the patient, such as when an order is written *acetylsalicylic acid 325 mg q4h until temperature remains below 37.8°C for 24 hours*. Some agencies have policies that place a time limit on orders regardless of how they are worded. For example, a narcotic order often remains in effect for 72 hours, after which time it is automatically discontinued unless the physician writes another order.

Standing Orders

Orders that are carried out indefinitely are called standing orders (for example, *vitamin C 1000 mg PO o.d.*). Some standing orders contain the direction "prn" (*pro re nata*) which means the medication is to be given as necessary. The administration of a drug under a **prn order** is left to the nurse's judgement and the patient's need. These orders, however, often specify minimum time intervals between doses, for example, *dimenhydrinate (gravol) 25–50 mg IM, sc, PO, IV, q4h prn*.

COMPONENTS OF A MEDICATION ORDER

There are a number of essential components to a medication order. An order should *always* include the patient's name, the date of the order, the name of the drug, the dosage, the route of administration, the time and frequency of administration and the prescriber's signature.

PATIENT'S NAME The patient's full name should appear on the drug order form to avoid confusion among patients of the same surname. Most agencies require an imprint of the patient's name and identification number on the physician's order form.

DATE OF THE ORDER The date of the order must include the day, month and year. Many agencies also require that the prescriber specify the time the order is written. Specifying the time is essential for orders that are automatically terminated because it indicates precisely when the order should end.

NAME OF THE DRUG The name of the drug should be clearly written and correctly spelled. Many agencies require the use of generic names in the drug order; however, a large number of agencies still use common trade names.

DOSAGE The order must specify the exact strength and amount of drug to be administered. Sometimes a range of amount may also be given. For example: *acetaminophen 325 mg* (strength) *1 or 2 tabs* (range of amount).

ROUTE OF ADMINISTRATION A medication may be administered by a number of different routes. Thus, it is necessary to specify the route in the drug order. The route of administration is often indicated through the use of common abbreviations, such as PO (oral route) or IV (intravenous route).

TIME AND FREQUENCY OF ADMINISTRATION The time and frequency of giving medications must be indicated. Again, common abbreviations may be used, for example, *ferrous gluconate 300 mg b.i.d.* Many inpatient facilities have standard times for administering medications. For example, b.i.d. or twice-daily medications may have standard times of 10:00 h and 22:00 h. If the physician wishes a medication to be given at a time other than the standard time, this should also be specified. Thus, the order *ferrous gluconate 300 mg b.i.d. with meals* would be written.

SIGNATURE The signature of the prescriber is a legal requirement on all medication orders. An order that is not signed is not valid in a court of law. When a medication order is obtained over the telephone, the nurse must indicate that it is a telephone order, identify from whom the order was taken, and sign it. In most agencies, the physician who gave the telephone order will then countersign it at a later date.

If any one of the components is omitted in a medication order, it is appropriate for the nurse to contact the physician and seek clarification. The nurse has an obligation to question any order that is ambiguous or seems to be unsafe for a patient. It is not acceptable to administer a medication merely because it was ordered by the doctor. It never hurts to clarify orders, and if the dosage exceeds the limits defined by the medication manuals, it is unwise to administer it. In health agencies, it is customary practice for all of a patient's orders to be written on a doctor's order sheet, which is kept in the patient's chart. Hospitals use a variety of methods of flagging charts to indicate that a patient has new orders.

PROCESSING AND COMMUNICATING MEDICATION ORDERS

Once an order has been written, it is then processed. A nurse or a unit clerk may process the order by transcribing it onto appropriate forms and notifying the pharmacy department. In some agencies, the order is copied onto the medication record in the patient's chart and the nursing unit Kardex or nursing care plan. In addition, a medication card is filled out. In other agencies, the new order is entered on the patient's medication administration record, called the MAR.

Medication cards are still used in some agencies, although this system is not as widespread as it once was. With this system, each medication is recorded on a separate card that includes the patient's name, the medication, dosage, route and times to be administered (see Figure 34.1A). Often these cards are filed on a central shelving system that is divided into each hour of the day. The nurse then searches through all the medication cards at the specific time, pulls the cards and prepares those medications. Once the medication has been administered, the card is advanced to the next time slot when the medication is to be given. The nurse must be especially careful when using the card system because cards may get lost or put into the wrong time slot, or they may go home in the nurse's pocket.

The MAR set-up is a computerized system that is being used with increasing frequency in hospitals. Once a day, the pharmacy department prints out the medications that have been ordered for a patient and sends the computer printouts to the nursing units (see Figure 34.1B). These printouts are often stored in binders so that nurses have

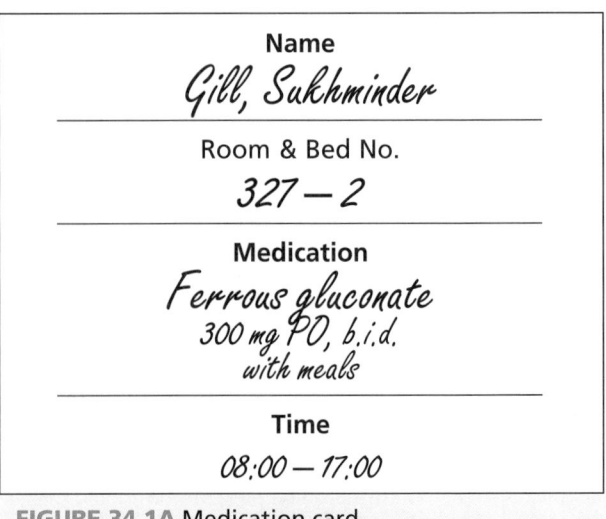

Name

Gill, Sukhminder

Room & Bed No.

327 — 2

Medication

Ferrous gluconate
300 mg PO, b.i.d.
with meals

Time

08:00 — 17:00

FIGURE 34.1A Medication card

Medication Administration Record

Time and Date: 24 h from 08:00 18 Apr 98 through 07:00 19 Apr 98

Name: Giardino, John Location: 6 6DUM 604 1

Patient ID: 12345678 Physican: Elaine Rosenthal, MD

08 09 10 11 12 13 14 15 16 17 18 19 20 21 22 23 24 01 02 03 04 05 06 07

Solutions

Order #1 Aminophylline 500 mg *1st*
Dextrose 5% in Water 50 mL
Infuse 50 mg (50 mL)/h

08 09 10 11 12 13 14 15 16 17 18 19 20 21 22 23 24 01 02 03 04 05 06 07

Order #2 Ampicillin 500 mg *1st*
0.9% sodium chloride 50 mL
Infuse over 30 min q 8h

14 22 06

Medications

Order #3 Digoxin tab 0.125 mg Lanoxin *1st*
0.125 mg (1 tab) PO daily

08

PRN Medications

Order #4 Meperidine 100 mg/mL (1 mL) Demerol *1st*
50–100 mg (0.5) IM q3–4-h prn

Allergies: Sulfa* Checked by: Jean Singer, RN

FIGURE 34.1B Sample medication administration record (MAR)

easy access to them. When new orders are written or when medications are terminated, notations are made on the existing MAR. The changes are then displayed on the next day's computer printouts. The MAR printout often groups medications according to solutions, oral medications and prn and/or stat dosages. The time of administration is printed beneath each regular medication, to cue the nurse. The nurse simply looks through the patients' MARs and notes the times that the medications are to be prepared and administered. The MAR system has at least two advantages over the card system: it offers a more complete picture of the medications that each patient is taking, and it avoids the problem of losing medication cards.

Although different methods of posting medication orders are used in various agencies, the nurse should remember that the original written order is the primary source of information. Whenever orders are copied, whether onto a Kardex file, a nursing care plan, a medicine card or an MAR, the possibility of error is always present. The nurse who administers the medication should always check the original order to ensure accuracy.

Agencies have different methods of indicating that a medication has been discontinued. In hospitals, it is common practice for "discontinued" to be imprinted across the physician's order once it is no longer valid. In agencies that use the MAR system, the discontinued medication is often highlighted in yellow. If the card system is used, the medication card is destroyed and an appropriate notation is made on the medication record. In a public health agency, the notation "discontinued" and the date are entered on the nursing care record.

Medication Distribution and Storage

Every agency has a system for the distribution and storage of medications. Some medications are considered stock, while others are specifically obtained for the individual patient (private drugs). Additionally, some agencies use a unit dose system. Each of these systems is designed to minimize error and maximize efficiency.

STOCK DRUGS Stock drugs are the more commonly used medicines, and a supply is kept on the unit at all times. Stock drugs are sometimes grouped according to action; for example, all vitamin preparations are kept together. Another method of grouping stock drugs is to arrange them alphabetically according to generic or trade names. Either method facilitates finding a specific preparation quickly.

PRIVATE DRUGS Private or personal drugs are specially prepared for a patient, and a small supply is obtained from the pharmacy department with the patient's name on it. The drug is then stored either in a common drawer with all the other personal drugs, or in the individual's medication drawer if a medication cart system is used.

UNIT DOSE SYSTEM The unit dose system is the safest method of distributing medications. In this system, each dose of the patient's prescribed medication is individually packaged. The nurse simply double-checks the order and takes the entire packet supplied by pharmacy. Normally, the pharmacy department sends enough doses for a 24-hour period. This method is advantageous to the nurse because it saves nursing time and decreases the opportunity for error.

STORAGE OF CONTROLLED DRUGS

Narcotics, barbiturates and other controlled drugs are under strict governmental control. In hospitals, narcotics and other controlled drugs are kept in locked cupboards, and distribution is closely managed. The administration of these drugs is recorded not only on the patient's chart but also in a special book commonly referred to as the narcotics book. The information recorded in the narcotics book includes the name of the patient to whom the narcotic will be administered, the name of the physician who ordered the drug, the drug, dosage, date and time, and the signature of the nurse administering the drug. Any narcotics that are wasted are also recorded, along with the quantity of drug wasted. In addition, wastages must be co-signed by another nurse, who validates the wastage.

The narcotics book is usually kept near the narcotics cupboard. Narcotics, barbiturates and other controlled drugs are counted at specific times, and totals are recorded in the narcotics book. For example, narcotics and controlled substances are often counted at the end of each shift, and the number distributed plus the number remaining on hand must equal the number assigned to the nursing unit or agency. The count is usually done by two nurses, a nurse going off duty and one coming on duty. This practice helps to protect the nurses on both shifts. Any discrepancies in the count must be reported immediately and the appropriate paperwork filed.

CALCULATIONS OF DRUG DOSAGES

In order to prepare and administer medications safely, the nurse must be adept at converting measurements from one system to another and calculating dosages (see Table 34.3).

Systems of Measurement

There are three systems of measurement used to prescribe drugs: the apothecary, the household and the SI metric systems.

APOTHECARY SYSTEM The apothecary system is based on the "troy pound" with 5760 grains as a standard pound. The pound is divided into 12 ounces; the ounce is divided into eight drams; the dram is divided into 60 grains. Fluid measures use the quart (32 oz), which is divided into two pints. The pint is divided into 16 ounces; the (fluid) ounce into

TABLE 34.3 Approximate equivalents, household, apothecary and metric measures

Household	Apothecary	Metric
60 drops (gtt)	1 teaspoon (tsp)	5 mL (or cc)*
1 drop (gtt)	minim 1 (m)	0.065 g
	minims 15 or 16	1 mL
1 teaspoon (tsp)	1 fluidram (ʒ)	5 mL
1 tablespoon (tbsp)	4 fluidrams	15 mL
2 tablespoons (tbsp)	8 fluidrams = 1 ounce (℥)	30 mL
1 measuring cup	8 ounces	240 mL
1 pint	1 pint or 16 ounces	500 mL
1 quart	1 quart or 32 ounces	1000 mL

*The abbreviations mL and cc are used interchangeably; however, mL should be used for liquids, cc for solids and gases, and g for solids.

SOURCE: Brown & Mulholland, 1996.

eight fluid drams; the fluid dram into 60 minims. Roman numerals are used to express numbers (grains X), and quantities less than one are written as fractions. This system is seldom used anymore, as it is inconvenient and not as accurate as the metric system (Brown & Mulholland, 1996; Norville, 1994).

HOUSEHOLD MEASUREMENTS The household system is widely used in the home environment. Most people are likely to be familiar with the basis of the household system, as it is frequently used in cookbooks. The teaspoon, tablespoon, teacup and glass are commonly used household measures. As this system is the least accurate of the three, it is rarely used in professional health care settings (Norville, 1994).

METRIC SYSTEM The metric system (or *Système international*, SI) is the most accurate and convenient system of measurement. It is based on multiples of 10, with the basic units being the metre (linear), the litre (volume) and the gram (weight). The nurse should become familiar with the metric units outlined in Table 34.4.

Computing Drug Dosages

It is not uncommon for the nurse to have to calculate drug dosages. While calculations may be done in the pharmacy department, this is not always possible, nor do all nurses work directly with a pharmacy. Further, it is prudent for the nurse to double-check all calculations. Given all this, the nurse must be familiar with formulas for computing drug dosages. Several methods can be used, but the dosages to be calculated must always be in the same unit of measurement. One common method uses a formula based on simple algebra:

$$\frac{\text{Dose available}}{\text{Quantity available}} = \frac{\text{Dose desired}}{\text{X (Quantity desired)}}$$

EXAMPLE 1

Order: Morphine sulfate 100 mg PO q4h is ordered for a patient with cancer pain. The morphine is supplied as a solution 5 mg/1 mL.

1. Set up proportions: $\frac{5\text{ mg}}{1\text{ mL}} = \frac{100\text{ mg}}{X\text{ mL}}$
2. Cross-multiply: $5X = 100$
3. Compute X: $100 \div 5 = 20$ mL to be administered

EXAMPLE 2

Order: Digoxin 0.125 mg PO once a day. Supplied: Digoxin 0.25 mg pills.

1. Set up proportions: $\frac{0.25\text{ mg}}{1\text{ tablet}} = \frac{0.125\text{ mg}}{X\text{ tablet}}$
2. Cross-multiply: $0.25X = 0.125$
3. Compute X: $0.125 \div 0.25 = 1/2$ tablet to be administered

TABLE 34.4 Conversion of metric calculations

Linear			Volume			Weight		
10 millimetres	=	1 centimetre	1000 millilitres	=	1 litre	1000 micrograms	=	1 milligram
100 centimetres	=	1 metre				1000 milligrams	=	1 gram
1000 metres	=	1 kilometre				1000 grams	=	1 kilogram

RESEARCH to practice

Ashby, D.A. (1997). Medication calculation skills of the medical–surgical nurse. *Medical–Surgical Nursing, 6*(2), 90–94.

The purpose of this exploratory research was to assess the medication calculation skills of practising medical–surgical nurses. A convenience sample was taken from a large midwestern hospital of 62 practising medical–surgical nurses. The Bayne-Bindler Medication Calculation Test was used to measure medication calculation skills.

This study found that 56.4 percent of nurses who took the Bayne-Bindler Medication Calculation Test were unable to calculate medications correctly in 90 percent of the problems posed. Medical–surgical nurses made the highest errors in calculating intravenous medications. Scores on the Bayne-Bindler Medication Calculation Test were not significantly influenced by educational preparation or the number of years of clinical practice.

Today, medication errors are a problem in many hospitals. Such errors incur significant costs to the health care system and contribute to detrimental patient outcomes. Thus, medication calculation skills of nurses should be regularly tested. To help improve nurses' performance, continuing education is mandatory.

Calculating Pediatric Dosages

The administration of medications to infants and children requires extra caution. Because of the smaller size of children, the administration of adult doses could be lethal. Special methods have been developed to convert adult dosages to safe dosages for children. The method most often used is based on body surface area (BSA) and uses a nomogram to estimate the BSA according to the child's height and weight. As shown in Figure 34.2, a child's BSA is obtained by drawing a straight line on the nomogram from the child's height on the left side to his or her weight on the right side. The point on the surface area (SA) column indicates the body surface area (m^2). The BSA is then used in a formula for calculating the safe dosage for the child. This formula is a ratio of the child's BSA to the body surface area of an average adult (that is, 1.7) three times the normal adult dose. Thus:

$$\text{Child's dose} = \frac{\text{Child's BSA (m}^2\text{)}}{\text{Average adult's BSA (1.73 m}^2\text{)}} \times \text{adult dose}$$

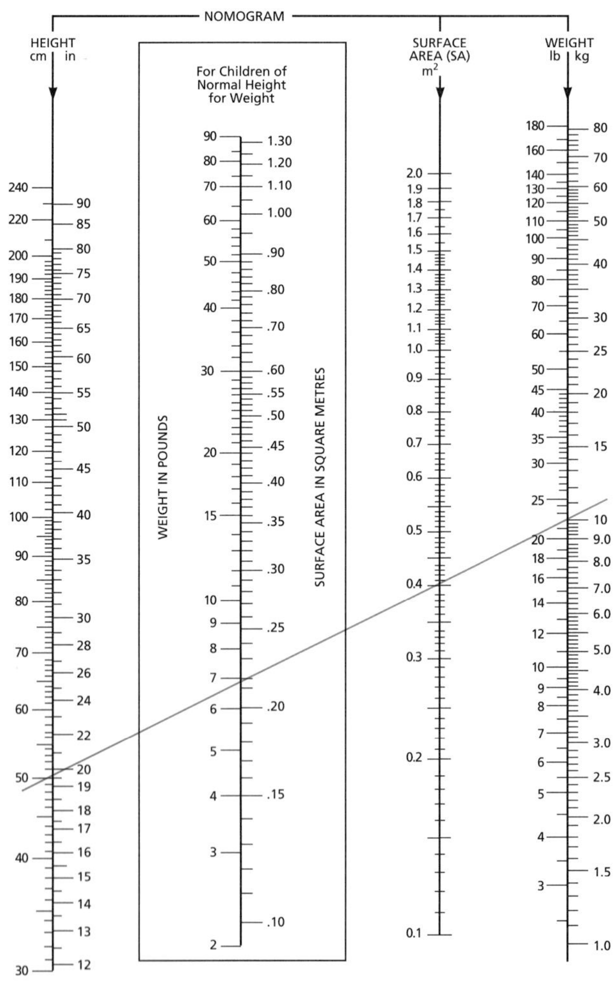

FIGURE 34.2 Nomogram of body surface area for infants and children. To find the BSA, draw a straight line from the child's height (in the left column) to the child's weight (in the right column). The point at which the line intersects the SA column is the estimated BSA.

SOURCE: Behrman, Kleigman, Arvin & Nelson, 1996, p. 670.

Assessing Medication-Related Needs

Nothing in the human body happens in a completely isolated fashion; the nurse must consider the entire person when assessing medication-related needs of patients. This involves an appraisal of factors in the patient's health history pertaining to the use of medications that would contribute to health or place the patient at risk for complications. The nurse should be aware of disease or illness states, such as chronic conditions or secondary problems, that may influence the effectiveness of medications or cause adverse effects. Physical and psychological assessments may indicate actual and potential problems that may influence if, when or how a drug is given and provide a baseline for evaluating the patient's response to medication. In addition, an understanding of the patient's medical plan of care and the desired therapeutic effect of the prescribed medications is essen- [illegible] known. Personal concerns, cultural values and religious beliefs that may cause the patient difficulty in accepting medication therapy or maintaining a regimen must also be examined. Throughout all aspects of assessment, the nurse must be aware of the special needs of patients throughout the life cycle and those with specific health challenges.

The patient's medical history should provide the nurse with information about physical and emotional conditions that may affect the overall response to a new medication or contraindicate its administration. For example, patients with congestive heart failure may be at risk for altered drug responses owing to the generalized slowing of drug distribution throughout the body. Similarly, the potential for cumulative effects is common in patients with renal and hepatic diseases because of impaired biotransformation and excretory functions. The medical history may also provide information about a patient's physical capabilities to self-administer medications at home, for example, physical deficits such as poor eyesight, impaired mobility or inability to remember dosages and times for medications.

Nursing Health History

The patient's medication history is one facet of the nursing health history. In the medication history, the nurse focusses on the patient's patterns of drug use, both current and in the recent past, responses to the medications and any related problems. Health promotion and protection patterns pertaining to medication use are also explored. These include the patient's understanding about the medication's action, purpose, administration and adverse effects, as well as any associated expectations and concerns. The patient's ability to self-administer and adhere to a medication regimen must also be determined. This information is necessary in order to identify actual and potential problems with the use of drugs and find opportunities for assisting and teaching people how to use, or not to use, medications that will promote optimum health for themselves or their family members.

In the event the patient is admitted in an unconscious state, the nurse should attempt to contact a member of the family or close friend for a medication history. Many medications interact with one another; therefore, it is necessary to know about all types of drugs the patient uses, including prescription and nonprescription drugs, recreational/illicit drugs (for example, marijuana, tobacco) and alcoholic beverages. It is important to note that patients may not openly admit to using illegal drugs or alcohol. Nevertheless, the nurse should attempt to explore the patient's use of these substances. This information might also be found in the physician's history. Knowledge of medications used in the past few months is important because such medications can have an effect on newly prescribed preparations. It is wise to encourage patients to carry with them a current list of medications they take. The patient's food and eating pattern is [illegible] patible with certain drugs, for example, foods high in active amines (aged cheese, beer, yeast, chocolate) can provoke a dangerously high blood pressure if consumed by a person taking monoamine oxidase (MAO) inhibitors such as tranylcypromine (Parnate). The patient's age, weight and any allergies are also noted.

Measurements and Diagnostic Tests

Vital signs and laboratory tests are necessary for assessing the effectiveness of many medications and for monitoring adverse effects. For example, blood pressure readings are taken to assess the therapeutic effectiveness of antihypertensive medications. Serum potassium levels are monitored for the development of hyperkalemia, a potentially dangerous side effect when patients are given a daily potassium supplement in conjunction with a potassium-sparing diuretic such as triamterene (Dyrenium). Dosages of some medications are based on serum levels of certain substances. For instance, insulin dosage is ordered according to blood glucose levels, and prothrombin times determine dosage adjustments for the anticoagulant, warfarin (Coumadin). The plasma levels of drugs that have a very narrow therapeutic index (margin of safety), such as digoxin (lanoxin) or anticonvulsants, must be monitored frequently because they pose a high risk for the development of toxic effects. In collecting data for determining medication-related problems and needs, the nurse must examine vital signs and review laboratory results as required.

Physical Assessment

During physical assessment, the nurse examines the patient for indications of therapeutic and adverse effects of the specific medications the patient is taking. For instance, if a patient is prescribed a heart pill and a diuretic for congestive heart failure, the physical examination would focus on such things as colour, shortness of breath, ease of breathing, coughing, activity tolerance and edema to determine therapeutic effectiveness. When the prescribed diuretic is a potassium-wasting agent, the physical assessment would include observations for signs of hypokalemia and digitalis toxicity, since the most common cause of digitalis toxicity is hypokalemia secondary to associated use of potassium-wasting diuretics.

The physical assessment also includes an appraisal of the patient's ability to take medications and any indicators that may contraindicate the administration of a particular medication. For example, nausea and vomiting may contraindicate the use of an oral medication. The nurse observes the patient for wakefulness, alertness, ability to swallow and ability to participate in the administration procedure. For example, can the patient assume the necessary position for

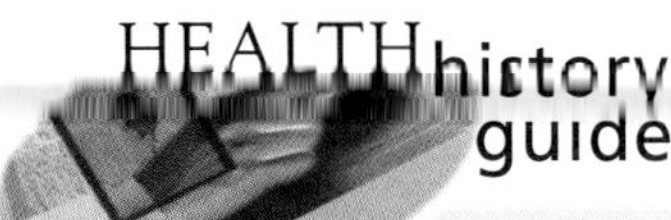

Medication

Health and Illness Patterns

Current Medication Pattern

- What medications are you presently taking that have been prescribed by your doctor? What are the medications for? What dosage are you taking? How frequently? By what route are you taking them?
- Describe the response to these medications. What are the therapeutic effects? Adverse effects? Do you have problems taking these medications?
- What nonprescription medications do you use, for example, vitamins, laxatives, sleep aides, analgesics, decongestants or antihistamines? What for? How often do you take them? How much do you take? By what route do you take them? What is your response to these medications?
- Do you smoke or use recreational or street drugs? If so, what kind? How often do you take them? How much do you take? By what route do you take them? What is the response when habitual use of these substances is interrupted?

Past Medication Patterns

- What medications have you taken during the past few months? What for? How frequently? What dosage? What route?
- Describe your response to these medications. What are the therapeutic effects? Adverse effects? Allergic reactions? What problems have occurred while taking these medications?
- Do you have medications saved from past use? How are they stored? What is the expiration date?

Health Promotion and Protection Patterns

- What do you know about the medications you are currently taking? How much do you want to know? Do you want to know the reasons for the medications? The expected therapeutic effects? Side effects? What to do if side effects occur? When medications should be taken? Any special precautions? Whether there is a need for follow-up?
- What do you expect from the current drug therapy as prescribed by the doctor? As self-prescribed? (For example, a patient may be taking self-prescribed garlic pills in conjunction with a prescribed antihypertensive drug to control blood pressure problems.)
- What are your personal views about the use of medications?
- Do you have any concerns about taking medications? Any fear of medications? Fear of side effects? Any religious or cultural influences?
- What things help or prevent you from taking your medications as prescribed?
- How do you usually take oral medications at home? With water? Milk? Juice? Food?
- Do you usually take your medications with meals? Before meals? At bedtime?
- If taking multiple medications, how do you keep track of the medications you take?
- Do you have any problems self-administering medications? Reading and understanding labels? Knowing or remembering when to take the medication? Using special techniques, for example, eye drops, injecting insulin? If so, do you have a relative or a friend who can help you take your medications as prescribed?
- Where do you store your medications? Are they kept out of reach of small children?
- Do you have any concerns about the cost of the medications? Would you require help with financing the medication?

administering ear drops? If the patient is going home while still on the medication, the nurse must also observe the patient's self-administering capabilities. This includes the patient's visual acuity, mobility, mental processes and manual dexterity. For instance, someone with arthritis may have difficulty opening and closing containers or self-administering insulin.

Diagnosing Medication-Related Problems

Problems pertaining to safe medication administration may relate to the medication therapy itself or to the distinctive circumstances of patients taking the drugs. Potential problems caused by the side effects of medications that may be prevented independently by the nurse are labelled *Risk for Injury*. For instance, if the side effect of a drug is dizziness and orthostatic hypotension, the nursing diagnosis would be *Risk for Injury related to dizziness and fainting secondary to medication*. However, adverse effects of medications may cause potentially serious reactions that require medical intervention for treatment or prevention. These are collaborative problems and, in drug therapy, they are identified as *Potential Complications: medication therapy adverse effects*. For example, for a patient taking anticancer drugs, the diagnosis would be *PC: antineoplastic adverse effects* (Carpenito, 1997).

A wide range of problems may apply to the distinctive circumstances of patients receiving medication therapy. When a new medication is prescribed to a patient th

apeutic and side effects and self-administration. Lack of knowledge about the use of nonprescription and recreational drugs may lead to unhealthy lifestyles and problems with health maintenance. In addition, personal concerns, cultural values and religious beliefs may cause difficulties for patients in accepting drug therapy or maintaining a medication regimen. Sensory/perceptual impairments, such as poor vision, inability to read, forgetfulness or drowsiness, may interfere with the ability to self-administer and maintain a medication schedule. Likewise, physical problems such as difficulty swallowing or difficulty handling medication supplies and equipment may affect the ability to take medications. Examples of nursing diagnoses are listed below.

- *Knowledge Deficit about drug action, therapeutic and adverse effects, and administration.*
- *Altered Health Maintenance related to unhealthy lifestyle and lack of knowledge about over-the-counter drugs and substance abuse.*
- *Altered Health Maintenance related to personal concerns, cultural values and religious beliefs about the prescribed medication.*
- *Ineffective Management of Therapeutic Regimen related to sensory/perceptual or physical impairments affecting correct self-administration of medication.*
- *Risk for Injury related to lack of knowledge or sensory/perceptual or physical impairments affecting correct self-administration of medication.*

Planning Medication Administration

As with all needs, a plan for the safe administration of medications is based on goals or expected outcomes that are derived from the nursing diagnoses. Planning must be done jointly with the patient and/or family and must consider individual beliefs and values, lifestyle practices, preferences and socioeconomic factors. Emphasis is placed on strategies to enable the optimal use of medications for therapeutic interventions and health maintenance. These include health teaching about drug actions, effects and safe use, as well as safe self-administration. The patient may need help developing a dosage schedule and arranging for follow-up evaluation and care.

Some examples of goals or expected outcomes pertaining to safe medication administration are listed below.

- Patient will explain the reasons for and expected effects of the medication, describe the route and method of administration, state the times for self-administration and describe interventions for common side effects.
- Patient will correctly and independently administer the prescribed dose of insulin.

Implementing Medication Administration

Health-Promoting Strategies

We are in an age of empowerment; people want to participate actively in health care and have some control over their situation. In medication therapy, this means having the right to give an informed consent, having the right to refuse medication and taking responsibility for self-administration. Patient education, teaching and supportive care are key nursing strategies for helping patients to promote optimal health through the use of medications.

INFORMED CONSENT

Patients have the right and want to make informed decisions about care and their prescribed medications. Informed consent requires adequate knowledge on which to make a decision. The patient needs to know the reasons for drug therapy, the effects and the resulting alterations in habits and lifestyle. Simple explanations given in terms the patient can understand are not only reassuring but also help to provide conditions of acceptance that can enhance the effectiveness of a drug. In the rare occurrence when a physician does not want the patient to receive information about a medicine from the nurse, it can be suggested that the patient confer with the physician.

RIGHT TO REFUSE MEDICATION

Sometimes a patient may refuse to take a medication. With rare exceptions, it is *not* the nurse's duty to administer the medication no matter what. The patient has the right to refuse treatment. It is the nurse's responsibility to determine, if possible, why the patient is refusing the medication and to take reasonable action to gain the patient's consent. There are a myriad of reasons why patients refuse medications, and it is imperative that the nurse explore these. Often, the problem can be remedied and the medication administered. Some of the common reasons for refusal, along with suggested interventions, are outlined in Table 34.5. If the patient refuses to take a medication, the nurse must inform the physician and document the event immediately.

PATIENT EDUCATION AND TEACHING

All people taking medications should be aware of the nature of the drugs they are taking, along with the reasons for the drug, the dosage, possible side effects, the route and method

TABLE 34.5 Refusal to take medications

Reason for Refusal	*Nursing Intervention*
• Finds the medication to be nauseating and causes vomiting.	• Administer antiemetic as ordered 30–60 min prior or administer with food.
• Is allergic to the medication. A record of the patient's allergies should be noted on admission; however, this is not always possible. For example, the patient may have been unconscious upon admission.	• Notify the pharmacy department and initiate appropriate references on the patient's chart, Kardex and wristband and at the bedside.
• Believes the medication does not help.	• Explain medication effects to the patient in terms that he or she can understand.
• Thinks it is the wrong medication.	• When this occurs, always double-check the order and the medication. If it is the correct medication, spend time discussing the issue with the patient. It may be a different brand than the patient is used to taking and will appear different.
• Believes the physician has changed the order.	• Check the physician's orders. The doctor may have changed the order and it may not be processed yet, or the physician may have intended to change the order, but has not written it yet.
• Finds injections painful.	• Use techniques to minimize the pain of injections. Give the patient as much choice as possible.
• Finds the medication has an unpleasant taste.	• Administer the medication with a pleasant-tasting juice or food. Give with a cold fluid to decrease the sensitivity of the taste buds.
• Does not want medication because of religious or cultural beliefs. A Hindu patient may refuse a hormonal preparation that contains extracts from cattle. A patient who belongs to the Jehovah's Witness faith may refuse a blood transfusion. Many people who believe in naturopathic remedies will refuse any medicine prepared from inorganic chemicals.	• Respect the patient's beliefs and collaborate with the physician and the patient to determine alternatives.
• Does not understand the purpose of the medication and is afraid it will be harmful.	• Provide information and pamphlets in terms the patient can understand.
• Thinks the medication is given at an inconvenient time, such as when visitors are present.	• If possible, collaborate with the patient to find a more convenient time. If this is not possible, minimize time nurse spends in the room.
• Is afraid of becoming addicted to the medication.	• Explain that addiction is a remote possibility when medications are used for short periods of time.

of administration and any specific things that should or should not be done when taking the medication. They should also be alerted to adverse signs and symptoms to watch for and the dangers of altering the dosage or neglecting to take medications. Unfortunately, some people mistakenly believe "If one tablet is good for me, two tablets are twice as good." Some people also need help to understand why they should take a prescribed dose and require realistic explanations of the action and anticipated effects of the drug. Not only is this a need for hospitalized patients; it is also crucial for people who take medications at home. People experience various reactions to specific drugs. The patient's reaction to any single medication is important and should be recorded. Thus, patients require information about what reactions to report to the nurse or the physician. This is particularly true for the person who is taking medication at home and does not have constant contact with a health professional.

A checklist for patient teaching in medication therapy is given in the box on the next page. Many agencies provide written information about medications for patient use; some agencies print this information in a variety of languages so that non–English-speaking people can benefit as well. If a patient is unable to self-administer medications, a family member or friend should be given the necessary instruction.

Checklist of Teaching in Medication Therapy

- [illegible] medication history
- reason for medication therapy
- expected results
- side effects and other adverse reactions
- when to notify physician, pharmacist or health care provider
- drug–drug and drug–food interactions
- required changes in activities of daily living (ADL)
- demonstration of learning; may take several forms, such as listening, discussing or return demonstration of psychomotor skills (for example, insulin injection)
- medication schedule, associated with ADL as appropriate
- recording system
- discussion and monitoring of access to financial resources, medication and associated equipment
- community resources

SOURCE: Kee & Hayes, 1993, p. 22.

Patient teaching is an ongoing process. It is wise to review medications periodically, even if the patient has been taking the same drugs for some time. The nurse will often be surprised at the gaps in knowledge. In addition to learning about specific medications, there are a number of general things people can do to facilitate the effectiveness of medication use and promote optimum health.

Health-Protecting Strategies

Safe administration of medications is imperative, as mistakes can lead to dangerous effects. Because the possibility of error is always present, special precautions are taken to avoid mistakes. Nursing has adopted the practice of checking medications using the "five rights" when preparing and administering medications as a means of avoiding error. The five rights include the right drug, the right dose, the right time, the right route and the right patient. If the nurse consistently practises the five rights for each medication, the potential for error is reduced dramatically.

RIGHT DRUG

The nurse uses the MAR or medication card to choose the appropriate medication. When using the MAR, if a number of medication orders are present on the same page, it is wise to cover up the other orders while pouring a particular medication. This practice will help to prevent errors. To ensure the right drug is obtained, the nurse uses a three-check system when pouring the medication. The first check occurs when the nurse obtains the medication from the drawer or cupboard. He or she then compares the MAR or medication card with the label on the medication container, making sure the drug name is the same on both. The second check is done when the nurse plans to pour the medication into the [illegible] medication in the drawer or cupboard. If the unit dose is used, the package will be empty, but the nurse will compare the information on the package.

RIGHT DOSE

The dose of a drug is ordered by the physician in consideration of the patient's weight, age, gender, physical condition and level of drug tolerance. Therefore, a medication must be administered in the exact dose that is ordered by the physician. When calculating the right dose, the nurse will check the MAR or medication card and compare the information with the supplied medication. It is important to calculate the dosage considering what the pharmacy supplies and what is ordered, since there may be a difference. Again, it is prudent to use the three-check system described above. Frequently, the pharmacy department calculates the ordered dose, particularly when small doses are required (for example, for children) and includes the information on the MAR or personal medication package. It is still important for the nurse to calculate the dosage as well, since errors can occur anywhere and the nurse administering the medication is ultimately responsible. In situations requiring dose calculation, the safest practice is for a second nurse to check the calculations made by the first nurse.

The nurse should *never* "guestimate" a dosage. It is not safe practice to break an unscored tablet to obtain a dosage, since the amount of drug in an unscored tablet is not evenly distributed. When pouring liquid medications, the nurse should place the receptacle on a flat surface and keep it at eye level in order to obtain an accurate dosage.

RIGHT TIME

Many agencies have standard times for administering medications, and the nurse should become familiar with these. Many oral medications that are ordered for more than once per day are given during waking hours, while intravenous medications are given around the clock. Thus, if an intravenous antibiotic is ordered three times per day, the nurse would administer it at regular eight-hour intervals, such as 06:00, 14:00 and 22:00. Also, if patients have been taking medications at home, their usual schedule should be considered. Wherever possible, medication times should be similar to the patient's usual schedule.

Finally, the realities of nursing are such that it is rarely possible to give every medication at the exact moment of the exact hour that it is ordered. Thus, the rule of 30 minutes is used. This gives the nurse 30 minutes on either side of the time the medication is due in which to administer it. However, the nurse must consider all the medications to be administered and assign certain ones a higher priority than others. Insulin, for example, must be administered before meals and not 30 minutes after the meal has been consumed.

HEALTH promoting strategy — Promoting Healthy Medication Use

- Take all the medication as prescribed by your physician. Do not stop taking the medication just because you feel better.
- Consult your physician if you are experiencing undesirable side effects.
- Keep the medication in its original container. Make sure the label remains clear.
- Keep all medications in a cupboard *well out of reach of children*. Remind visitors to keep any medications they bring with them safely out of children's reach.
- When taking prescribed medications, check with your physician or the pharmacist about using over-the-counter drugs such as cold remedies, decongestants, ASA, acetaminophen, antihistamines or laxatives.
- Take all medications with you when you visit your physician.
- Know why you are taking each medication and the reactions you should immediately report to your physician or health care provider.
- Avoid using alcoholic beverages because these alter the action of medications. Abstain from alcohol when it is absolutely contraindicated.
- Nicotine affects the actions of some drugs. If you are a smoker, check with your physician or the pharmacist for specific information.

SOURCE: Kee & Hayes, 1993, p. 21.

RIGHT ROUTE

It is important to verify that the medication supplied coincides with the prescribed route. The nurse can administer the medication only by the ordered route; the route cannot be arbitrarily changed. If the nurse believes the ordered route is not appropriate, he or she must contact the physician. Sometimes, the physician will provide some variance with the route order. For example, the physician may order dimenhydrinate (Gravol) 25–50 mg PO, IM or IV q6h and the route can be decided by the nurse and patient together.

RIGHT PATIENT

One of the most important factors in the administration of a medication is the identification of the patient. Any method that accurately identifies a patient is satisfactory. Some agencies provide each patient with an identification band. Many protocols suggest asking the patient his or her name before administering a medication. If this is the case, the nurse should not say, "Are you Mr. Smith?" nor should the nurse rely on the patient to answer to the name he or she uses. In both situations, the patient may give an automatic affirmative answer. It is better to say, "What is your name?" or "Please state your full name." The habit of relying on bed numbers and even room numbers in order to identify patients is also dangerous. Patients' rooms often change, and patients also move to other units. Situations in which patients are continually reassigned to new rooms make identification especially difficult. Further, it is not entirely unheard of for patients to lie down in the wrong bed. Therefore, it is prudent to check the patient's identification band prior to the administration of *every* group of medications.

The beginning nurse often feels foolish pursuing this suggestion, since this person often administers medications to only one or two patients. The nurse who administers a number of medications to a multitude of patients knows only too well that lack of time, not knowing what each patient looks like and being constantly distracted all carry huge potential for error. The measure of checking wristbands is the final stopgap to prevent the wrong medication from being given to the wrong patient. Good habits formed early in a career save errors later.

OTHER STRATEGIES FOR PREVENTING MEDICATION ERRORS

If a nurse is ever in doubt about whether or not to give a medication, he or she should consult a reliable source before

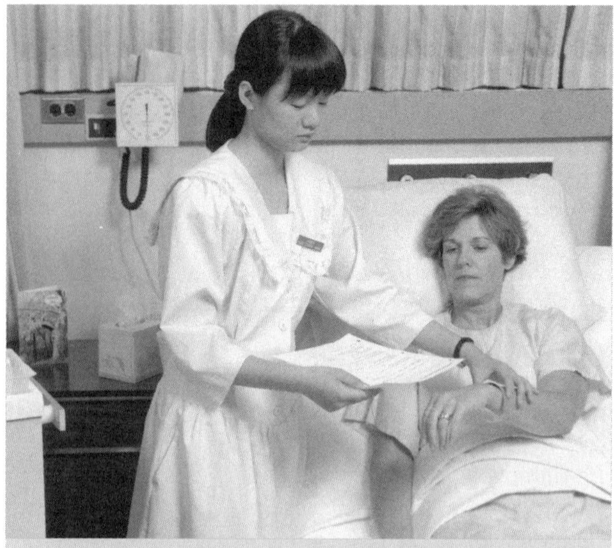

The safest method of ensuring the "right patient" is to check the patient's identification band.

going ahead. As mentioned earlier, most agencies have literature to which the nurse can refer. If the agency possesses no resources and the nurse is routinely unable to contact a [illegible] a current drug book.

The pharmacist should be the only one to label a container of medication. Therefore, when the nurse finds an unlabelled container or a label that has been partially obscured, the entire container is returned to the pharmacy for clarification. It is also considered safe practice not to return medications to a container once they have been removed; instead, they should be disposed of by flushing down a toilet or hopper. Most agencies require a witness to be present when narcotics and controlled substances are discarded. Finally, medications should not be transferred from one container to another, even when two containers with the same medication are in use.

In order to avoid error, the nurse who prepares a medication should administer it immediately after it has been prepared and should observe the patient take it. If prepared medications are left unattended, the chances of the drug's being misplaced or taken by another patient are increased. Moreover, the nurse is legally responsible for the medications to be administered and only if the nurse has prepared a medication can he or she testify to the actual drugs in the medication container. The identification of medication by its appearance alone is dangerous practice, since many drugs have similar appearances. If it happens that medications are distributed when a patient is unavailable to take the medication (for example, if the patient is having a test done in another department), that medication can be returned to the nursing unit and locked in the cupboard with the identifying medication card.

Health-Restoring Strategies

The administration of medications is a therapeutic nursing function, often implemented on the order of the physician to treat a specific illness or disease. The nurse requires not only knowledge but also psychomotor skills in preparing and giving medications. In this section we will focus on the skills required to administer medications by the various methods and routes.

METHODS OF ADMINISTERING MEDICATIONS

Medications can be administered using a variety of methods and routes.

ORAL The most common method of administering medications is by mouth (orally). Not only is this route simple, it is also the most economical way. Capsules, liquids, lozenges, tablets and powders are all administered by mouth. A *capsule* contains a powder, oil or liquid within a gelatinous covering. A *lozenge* or *troche* contains a drug in a flavoured base and releases the drug as it dissolves in the mouth. *Tablets* are solid dosages of medication that are often coloured. Some tablets are *enteric coated*. These tablets are coated with a substance that is insoluble in gastric acids, thereby reducing [illegible] mixture of finely ground drugs.

SUBLINGUAL Sublingual administration involves placing the drug (for example, nitroglycerin) under the patient's tongue, where it is dissolved and absorbed.

PARENTERAL Parenteral administration refers to the giving of drugs by needle. Intramuscular, intradermal, subcutaneous and intravenous injections are common methods of parenteral therapy. Intracardiac, intrapericardial, intrathecal (intraspinal) and intraosseous (into bone) injections are less common methods that may be used by physicians. All parenteral therapy involves the use of sterile equipment and sterile, readily soluble solutions.

INHALATION Inhalation is the administration of a drug into the respiratory tract, where it is almost immediately absorbed. Volatile and nonvolatile drugs can be inhaled, the latter by means of a vehicle such as oxygen.

INSTILLATION Instillation is a method of putting a drug in liquid form into a body cavity or orifice, for example, the ears, the eyes, the urinary bladder or the rectum. Liquid medications can be instilled with a dropper (into the ear) or with a syringe (into the urinary bladder).

TOPICAL Medications are also applied to the skin and mucous membranes; this process is called topical application. Antiseptics, astringents and emollients can be applied as liquids or ointments. An *ointment* is a semi-solid mixture that is applied topically to mucous membranes or skin. Some medications are available in the form of *transdermal patches*, which are applied directly to the skin.

SUPPOSITORY A *suppository* is moulded into a firm base and is most commonly used for insertion into a body cavity or orifice, such as the rectum or vagina. As the suppository gradually dissolves at body temperature, the drug is released and is absorbed through the mucous membrane. Although a suppository is sometimes used to administer medications when a systemic action is desired (for example, an antipyretic), it is not considered as efficient as a medication administered by other routes. Suppositories are therefore used principally for local action. They may be used, for instance, to administer an analgesic to the rectal area, or to stimulate peristalsis and bring about a bowel movement.

PREPARING MEDICATIONS

There are two common places for preparing medications: a medication room and a medication cart (see Figure 34.3A). A medication room is usually in or near the nursing unit, yet separate from it so that medications can be prepared with minimal disturbance. If the nurse prepares the medication in a medication room, the medication is placed on a tray for transport to the patient's room. The trays often have

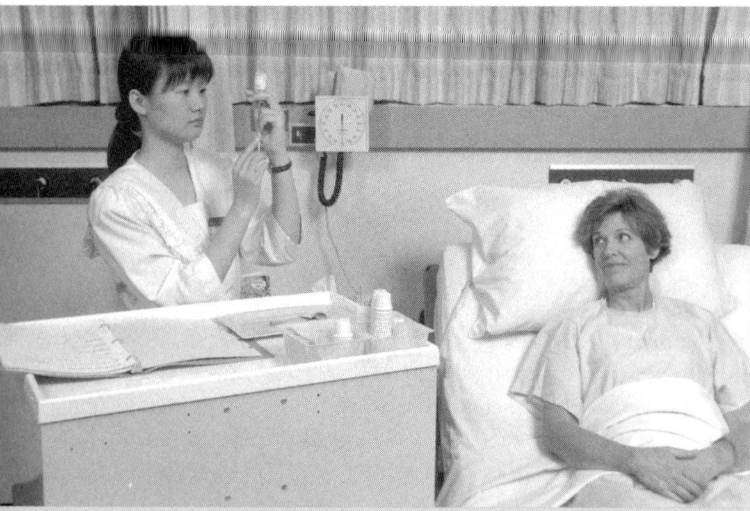

Medications may be prepared at the bedside table from the medication cart.

special slots so that the medicine card stands upright and can be read easily (see Figure 34B).

Medication carts are similar to medication rooms, except that they are portable. They are designed to save the nurse time by allowing preparation and administration of the medication directly from the cart. Trays for medications are not needed. The cart can be positioned close to the area where the medications will actually be administered. Nurses should take time to familiarize themselves with the cart, as it is often possible to prepare all medications without leaving it. Medication carts may be locked (check the hospital policy).

A hospital medication cupboard is sometimes locked, the key being kept by a nurse responsible for administering medications (if this system is used). Adjacent to the medication cupboard are usually a locked narcotics cupboard and a refrigerator. Medications that lose their potency unless kept cold are stored in the refrigerator.

The first step in preparing medications is to obtain the medication card or MAR and verify the order. This is done by checking the MAR or medication card against the original doctor's order. Errors in transcription occur, especially with medication cards and less often with the MAR. In some agencies, all medication orders are checked with the doctor's orders during the night shift. Any discrepancies are communicated to the pharmacy department, who contact the physician.

The second step in the preparation of any medication is to get the complete order and make sure it is understood. Sometimes agency policy or the medication order governs the administration of a specific drug or the special nursing measures that accompany its administration. For example, an order might read "withhold drug if apex is below 60 beats per minute." Specific directives in the order may influence how the medication is poured, as we will discuss later. Occasionally, medications are inadvertently ordered to which the patient has an allergy. Because allergies can cause severe and sometimes life-threatening reactions, the nurse must always check for allergies. The presence of allergies is noted at the top of the physician's order form. Additionally, in many agencies, patients with allergies are given a red identification band, and the label on the chart is also red.

The medication is obtained from the patient's personal medication package, from the stock drug section in the cart or medication room or from the refrigerator. Often the MAR will distinguish whether the medication is a personal or a stock drug. The techniques for preparing medications vary according to the route of administration. These are outlined in the specific procedures that follow.

When a nurse is preparing a variety of medications for a group of patients, the medications for one patient are

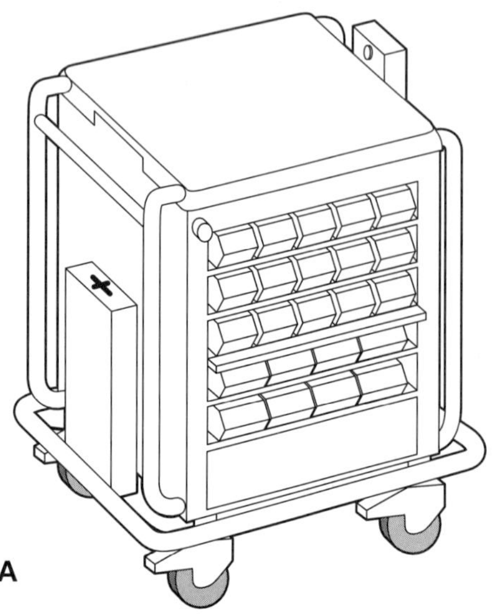

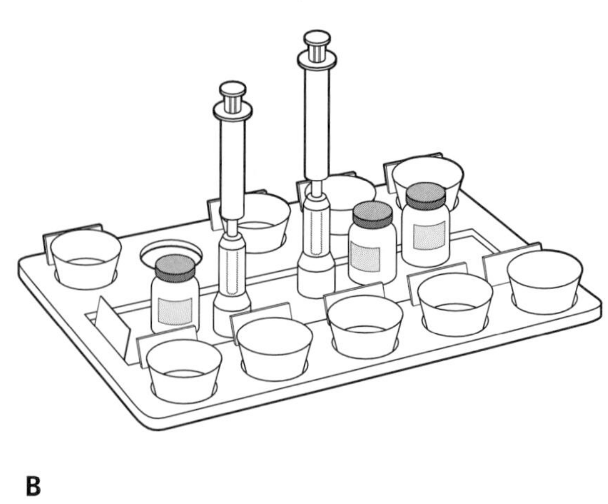

FIGURE 34.3 A. Medication cart. B. Medication tray

separated from those for another. Generally, all medicines that are administered by the same route for one patient can be placed in the [illegible] upon some specified criterion. For example, if digoxin (Lanoxin) 0.125 mg is to be withheld when the patient's pulse is below 60 beats per minute or as stated in the hospital policy, this drug is put in a separate container from the other oral medications for that particular patient.

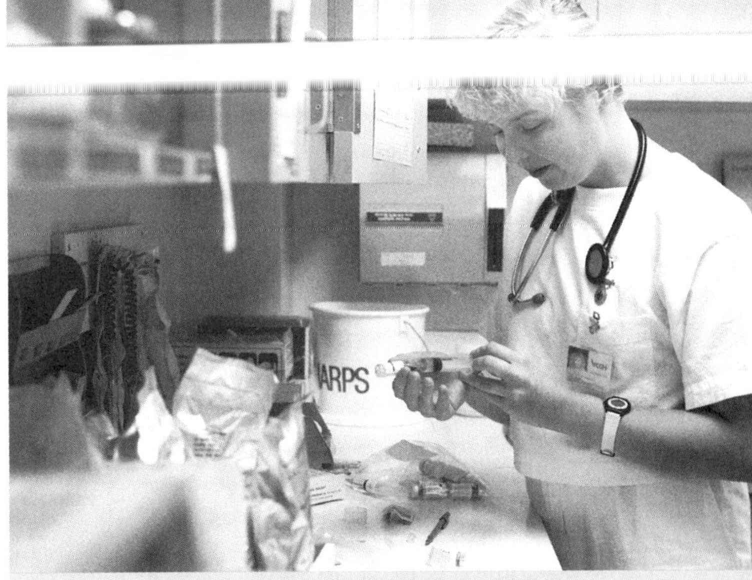

This nurse prepares medications in a medication room.

ADMINISTERING MEDICATIONS

Procedure 34.1 lists the steps involved in general preparation of medications.

Preparing the Patient

Medications are given to individuals, and the nurse will find that each individual is different. Some people want to know about medications; others prefer not to know. The amount of knowledge that a patient desires is highly dependent upon individual circumstances. The seriously ill patient in a hospital may be too ill to learn about the drug. The information that each patient should have depends on intelligence, age, education, illness and emotional needs. The nurse is guided by the patient and the physician as to the amount of information provided. When a patient does express a desire to learn about the medication, the patient should be informed, in an understandable manner, of the basic action of a medication, the main adverse effects, dosage and how to take the medication. It is always wise to ask the patient about allergies, even if these are not indicated in the chart. Sometimes, people do not recall allergies when first asked. It is also possible that the physician unintentionally orders a medication to which the patient has known allergies.

Giving the Medication

Any technician can safely administer medications, but the nurse who views the patient in a holistic way will be better able to assist. Complementary to the administration of many medications is the provision of nursing care measures that serve to supplement the action of a drug. For example, giving the patient a back rub and straightening the bed might increase the effectiveness of a sedative, while teaching a patient to drink fluids properly can help prevent the crystallization of sulfonamides in the kidneys. Similarly, spending a few extra moments to ensure the patient has the preferred type of juice, or gets the pills in the preferred order, lets patients know they matter as individuals. It is *how* the medications are administered that makes the difference.

Sometimes the administration of a medication is contingent upon some factor, such as the patient's apical rate or blood pressure, and this is assessed first. With few exceptions the nurse stays with a patient until the medication has been taken. The exceptions are medications that have been ordered to be left with a patient, for example, a drug that the patient has for immediate use (such as nitroglycerin for

PROCEDURE 34.1 General Steps in Preparing a Medication

Action	*Rationale*
1. Obtain MAR or medication card and verify order.	Protects the patient from injury and promotes accuracy.
2. Check for allergies.	Ensures safety and economy of time.
3. Clear working surface on medication cart or in medication room.	Allows nurse to focus and prevents errors.
4. Wash hands.	Prevents spread of microorganisms.
5. Gather equipment.	Facilitates efficiency and economy of time.
6. Maintain cleanliness and aseptic technique as necessary.	Prevents contamination and the spread of microorganisms.
7. Prepare medications using the "five rights."	Ensures safety and accuracy.

cardiac pain) or a drug that is contained in an intravenous infusion for gradual administration. If medications are left at the patient's bedside, it is the nurse's responsibility to check at frequent intervals to ascertain the dosage that has been consumed. Such intervals vary depending upon the drug; the nurse is referred to the agency policy manual for these.

Some circumstances call for a number of different forms of oral medications to be administered at the same time. In these cases, tablets and capsules should be administered before liquid forms, particularly syrups and antacids. This will ensure that the benefits of syrups and antacids on the oropharynx, esophagus and stomach are not washed away with the water consumed with the tablets or capsules.

When administering medications to children, the nurse should attempt to incorporate play into the session. Generally, it takes longer to administer medications to children than to adults. At all times, be honest, and negotiate with the child. Give medications in as small amounts of food or fluid as possible, since large quantities often cause difficulties. Abstain from bribing the child with a favourite food as a mixing agent—this may turn the child against the favourite food.

Assessing for Adverse Effects

An important part of administering a medication is assessing the patient afterward for drug effectiveness, side effects or allergic reactions. The patient should be observed for adverse reactions within an hour of taking the medication. If the reaction is severe (such as difficulty breathing), notify the doctor immediately and prepare to administer interventions as ordered.

RECORDING MEDICATION ADMINISTRATION

As for all nursing procedures, medications must be recorded to provide legal documentation that they have been administered. The record also keeps other members of the health care team informed. It is important to note the exact time and dosage (if a range is provided) with prn or stat medications. Medications are recorded immediately after they have been administered. The recording should include the name of the drug, the time it was administered, the exact dosage, the method of administration and the signature of the nurse. Some agencies also require that the status of the person administering the drug be designated, for example RN or SN.

When the card system is used, the nurse enters the time of administration and his or her name on the medication record in the patient's chart. The MAR system often requires the nurse to take the MAR to the bedside to provide a final check for the correct patient. Once the medication has been administered, the nurse then signs the MAR. In some agencies, prn and stat medications are recorded in the nurses' notes, along with the assessment of the patient's condition and the reason the medication was given. In other agencies, these are recorded on the MAR. In both systems, a notation should be made later in the nurses' notes or on the MAR describing the patient's response to a prn or a stat medication. Additionally, many agencies require that the nurse indicate on the doctor's order sheet that stat dosages have been administered.

ORAL MEDICATIONS

Oral medications are taken by mouth. They are chiefly absorbed in the small intestine, although they can also be absorbed in the mouth and the stomach. Medications in liquid form, either upon administration or upon dissolution within the stomach, are absorbed through the gastric mucosa. Absorption of a drug is slowed by the presence of food in the stomach as well as by its administration in concentrated form. Dilution, an alcoholic base and an empty stomach facilitate absorption. Table 34.6 outlines the advantages and disadvantages of oral medications.

TABLE 34.6 Advantages and disadvantages of oral medications

Advantages	*Disadvantages*
• convenient: simple method of administration • economic: cost less to manufacture • safe: do not invade body defences	• taste: can stimulate nausea and vomiting • gastric irritation • destroyed by gastric secretions • harmful to the teeth: can damage enamel and discolour teeth • inaccurate measure of absorption: some drugs are destroyed to a variable extent by gastrointestinal secretions • limited use: patient must be able to swallow or have a feeding tube • patient must be able to retain medication

Nursing measures can often minimize the disadvantages of oral medications. For example, medications that are administered in liquid or partially dissolved form tend to

form. Unpleasant-tasting liquids can be given with cold fluids or with ice, since cold is less stimulating than warmth and helps to desensitize taste buds.

Irritation of the gastric mucosa, caused by some medications, can be minimized by administering the drug after a meal, while food is still in the stomach. Also, the more diluted the medication is, the less irritating it will be to the mucosa. A medication that is particularly irritating can sometimes be given with another drug or with food, such as bread, in order to modify its undesirable effect.

Medications that are destroyed by gastric secretions can still be administered by the oral route if they are manufactured with an enteric coating so that they do not dissolve in the stomach. Otherwise, these drugs may be ordered to be given via parenteral administration.

Medications such as hydrochloric acid and liquid iron preparations are harmful to the teeth. These undesirable effects can be avoided by giving highly diluted forms and by using a straw in order that the teeth do not come in contact with the liquid. It is also wise to have the patient rinse the mouth with water or a mouthwash after taking these medications.

Another disadvantage of the oral administration of medications is the relative inability to measure absorption accurately in the gastrointestinal tract. Certain disorders affect absorption; for example, accelerated peristalsis will decrease absorption because of the drug's speedy propulsion through the gastrointestinal tract. Moreover, some medications are destroyed to a variable extent by gastrointestinal secretions. In addition, the adequacy of the circulation of the blood to the tract affects the rate of absorption. If a patient vomits after ingesting a medication, the amount of drug retained in the body is questionable. Generally, when this happens the physician is consulted in order to assess the patient's need for a repeated dose of the medication.

Considering the list of disadvantages, it quickly becomes evident that the use of oral medications is limited to patients who are able to swallow and retain them. The unconscious patient, the patient who is unable to swallow and the vomiting patient cannot take oral medications. Patients who are restricted to taking nothing by mouth are occasionally allowed oral medications. Some patients cannot take oral medications because of gastric suction, and some find swallowing difficult because of surgery or paralysis. Frequently, it is the nurse who first becomes aware that a patient has difficulty swallowing a medication. The nurse needs to inform the physician so that a change to a more easily consumed drug can be made. Tablets can be crushed and a scored tablet can be broken for easier administration, but the protective coverings of capsules or enteric-coated pills should not be removed to facilitate administration. The techniques for preparing and administering oral medications are outlined in Procedure 34.2.

Dry medications are generally distributed in disposable paper cups. Liquid medications are given in plastic or waxed paper containers. The advantages of using disposable containers are obvious: cleanliness is assured and washing and sterilizing are eliminated. It is difficult to pour the exact amount of tablets into a medication cup. This poses a problem when a number of tablets are being poured into the same container. Therefore, pills should first be dropped onto the bottle cap or into an empty medicine container and then transferred to the medication cup. Medications should not be handled indiscriminately. Pouring pills into the hands increases the transmission of microorganisms. If there is any doubt about administering a specific drug, it is kept separately from the other tablets for a specific patient. For example, digoxin is poured into a separate container, since the nurse cannot administer the medication until the patient's apical beat has been determined to be above the specified rate.

In order to obtain an accurate measurement when pouring liquids, the dose is measured from the bottom of the concave meniscus. It is important to view the container at eye level with the container on a flat surface (see Figure 34.4). Excess amounts are sometimes poured into the cup. These should not be returned to the medication container but should be discarded instead. Some liquids separate after standing in a bottle and need to be shaken before they are used. The medication container should be held so that the medication flows from the side opposite to the label. This prevents medication from staining and obstructing the label. Drips from the lip of the bottle can be wiped with a clean, damp paper towel before the lid is replaced. Minims (0.06 mL) and drops are not interchangeable measures. Special droppers or glasses and, in some agencies, syringes, are used for measuring small amounts of liquid medications.

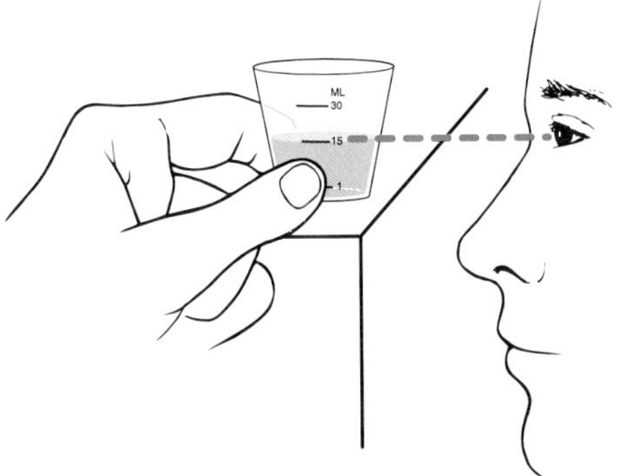

FIGURE 34.4 When pouring a liquid solution, the dose is measured from the bottom of the meniscus. A meniscus is the result of the surface tension of the solution against the wall of the container, which causes a concave curvature on the surface of the solution.

PROCEDURE 34.2

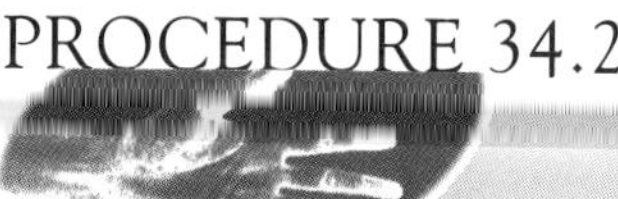

Administering Oral Medications

Action	*Rationale*
1. Follow steps in Procedure 34.1.	Facilitates efficiency and economy of time.
2. Gather equipment: • MAR or medication card • medication container • prescribed medication • food or fluid • drinking straw (optional) • mortar and pestle (optional).	
3. Pour medications:	
Tablets or capsules: Pour into lid of container and then transfer to medication cup. If using unit dose system, remove tablet or capsule from self contained pocket directly into medication cup.	Ensures safety and accuracy.
Liquids: Set plastic container on flat surface and bend (using correct body mechanics) so that eyes are at the level of the cup. Place lid of medication container top down on table. Pour medication into container until meniscus reaches desired level.	Prevents contamination of lid. Ensures accuracy of measurement.
Separate drugs that require special consideration.	
4. Place medication cup in medication tray with appropriate medication cards or notation on MAR.	Allows correct identification of medications.
5. Return medication to appropriate storage place (such as a drawer or refrigerator) and tidy area.	Promotes cleanliness and safety.
6. Take medication, medication card or MAR and selected fluid (water, juice) to patient's room. Identify the patient.	Ensures the correct patient is receiving the medication.
7. Explain the medication(s) to the patient and encourage questions.	Facilitates the patient's well-being and participation in care.
8. Ask the patient to sit upright, if possible, or roll the head of bed up unless contraindicated.	Assists patient to swallow and prevents choking.
9. Give the medication cup to the patient and offer selected fluids.	Gives patient control and individualizes care.
10. Ensure the patient has swallowed oral medications.	Ensures effective administration. Some people may require more fluids. Patients with paralysis may not feel whether medications have been swallowed. Rarely, patients will collect medications inside mouth and remove later.
11. Position the patient for comfort and offer any further explanation regarding medications.	Promotes patient well-being.
12. Record administration of medication on appropriate form.	Provides legal record of medication administration.
13. Assess the patient for therapeutic effects, side effects or allergic reactions.	Provides evaluation of care and promotes patient safety.

Occasionally, patients require tablets to be crushed. In this instance, it is more palatable to administer crushed medications with food such as jam, pudding or ice cream to enhance the taste. The choice will depend upon the type of medication and the patient's preference. It is not wise to try to "hide" the medication in these foods and administer them without the patient's knowlege. This may threaten the patient's trust in the nurse and may turn the individual against that particular food. A mortar (small ceramic bowl) and pestle (little hammer with a rounded end) are used to crush tablets. Fluid, such as water, juice or milk, will also be required for swallowing tablets and capsules and following liquid medications. A drinking straw will be needed for any liquid medication that stains the teeth.

ADMINISTERING ORAL MEDICATIONS THROUGH A TUBE

Some patients cannot tolerate oral medications because of the presence of a nasogastric (NG) tube. Fortunately, it is

TABLE 34.7 Oral medications that cannot be given by tube

Medication	Rationale
Buccal or sublingual tablets	These medications are intended to be absorbed by veins under the tongue, or in the cheek.
Enteric-coated tablets	The enteric coating prevents release of active drug until the drug passes through the stomach. Administration without coating would cause premature release of medication.
Uncoated gastric irritants	May cause adverse gastrointestinal reactions.
Sustained-release tablets and capsules	Since they are designed to release medication slowly and contain two to three doses, crushing them could cause overdose.

still possible to administer some oral medications. Ideally, it is best if the medication is in a liquid form, but some tablets and capsules can also be administered. For example, some tablets can be crushed and administered with water, and some capsules can be punctured or opened and the contents removed. Table 34.7 outlines the tablets and capsules that should not be given via nasogastric tube.

The administration of medications by nasogastric tube is a relatively simple procedure, but because clogging of the tube is a common problem, care must be taken to flush it properly. Procedure 34.3 outlines the steps for administering oral medications via tube.

SUBLINGUAL MEDICATIONS

Sublingual medications are basically prepared and administered like oral medications. The difference is that the patient places the medication under the tongue rather than swallowing it. Absorption occurs swiftly through the epithelial layer under the tongue. Sublingual medications bypass the liver and do not come into contact with contents of the gastrointestinal tract, resulting in a higher concentration of the drug in the blood (Pinnell, 1996).

PARENTERAL MEDICATIONS

It is becoming more common to administer medications by the parenteral route. In fact, next to oral administration, parenteral administration is the most common route. Parenteral medications are delivered through a needle into the dermal layer of the skin (intradermal injection), into subcutaneous tissue (subcutaneous injection), into designated muscle tissue (intramuscular injection) and into veins (intravenous injection). Drugs administered by parenteral routes are absorbed more quickly than by oral routes, and because of this, have a more rapid effect. Additionally, once administered, parenteral medications are not retrievable. Therefore, caution and precision are essential when preparing and administering them. Considerable skill and dexterity are needed to perform the procedures safely and accurately. Furthermore, because parenteral injections penetrate the skin barrier, the risk of infection is always present. Solutions and equipment must be sterile, and aseptic technique must be used throughout the procedure. The techniques for administering medications by each of the parenteral routes will be outlined separately. All parenteral medications are prepared in the same basic way.

Assembling Equipment

The basic equipment for administering parenteral medications consists of syringes, needles and medication containers, namely vials and ampoules.

SYRINGES A syringe consists of the barrel, the plunger and the tip, which attaches to a needle. The parts of a syringe are shown in Figure 34.5A. Syringes are made of glass or plastic material. Plastic syringes are usually disposable and are commonly used in hospitals, offices and clinics. Syringes are supplied in sizes ranging from 0.5-cc to 50-cc capacities ("cc" stands for cubic centimetre). The *standard* 3-mL syringe is commonly used for subcutaneous and intramuscular injections. The standard syringe is calibrated in millilitres (1 mL = 1 cc) and minims (M), as shown in Figure 34.5B. A larger syringe may be needed for preparing intravenous medications. An *insulin syringe* is used specifically for administering insulin. The units of measurement on the syringe are equated to the concentration of insulin in units per millilitre. Since most insulins are manufactured in concentrations of 100 U/mL, the most common insulin syringe is the U-100, which is calibrated in 100 U/cc (Figure 34.6). A low-dose insulin syringe is also available for patients requiring 50 U or less of U-100 insulin. The *tuberculin syringe*, originally designed to administer tuberculin, is now used to enable accurate measurement of small volumes of solution. A tuberculin syringe is calibrated in tenths and hundredths of a millilitre and in 0.5 and 1 minim scales (16 minims equals 1 cc), as shown in Figure 34.7.

NEEDLES A needle consists of the hub, the shaft or cannula and the bevel (see Figure 34.8). The hub is the larger section that connects to the barrel of the syringe; the shaft is the long narrow part. The weakest point in a needle is where the cannula joins the hub. The bevel is the sharp slanted tip at the end of the cannula. Bevels vary in slant or length.

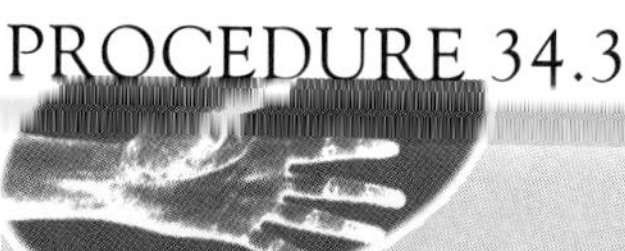

PROCEDURE 34.3 Administering Oral Medication by Nasogastric Tube

Action	*Rationale*
1. Follow steps in Procedure 34.1.	
2. Gather equipment: • MAR or medication card • prescribed medication • 2 paper medication cups (if pills to be crushed) or plastic medication cup (if liquid suspension) • mortar and pestle • 50-mL syringe • water • clean gloves.	Facilitates efficiency and economy of time.
3. Pour medications using the "five rights." Prepare medication according to type: **Tablets:** Crush between 2 paper cups. **Capsules:** Open and pour into plastic medication cup. Some capsules may need to be pierced with a needle.	Ensures safety and accuracy.
4. Continue as in steps 4 to 7 of Procedure 34.2.	
5. Put on clean gloves.	Prevents transmission of microorganisms.
6. Aspirate fluid from the NG tube and test for acidity with a pH test strip (see Procedure 20.1).	Checks placement of the tube.
7. Flush NG tube with 30–50 mL water.	Ensures patency of the tube.
8. Administer each medication separately with at least 5–10 mL of water.	Dilutes medication in order to prevent clogging of the tube.
9. Repeat step 8 for each medication.	
10. When all medications have been administered, flush the NG tube with 15–30 mL water.	Maintains patency and prevents clogging of the tube.
11. If the NG tube is attached to suction, keep the suction off for 30 minutes after administration.	Allows absorption of medications.
12. Rinse large syringe with water and keep at patient's bedside. Label and date all equipment.	Economizes use of supplies.
13. Follow steps 11 to 13 of Procedure 34.2.	

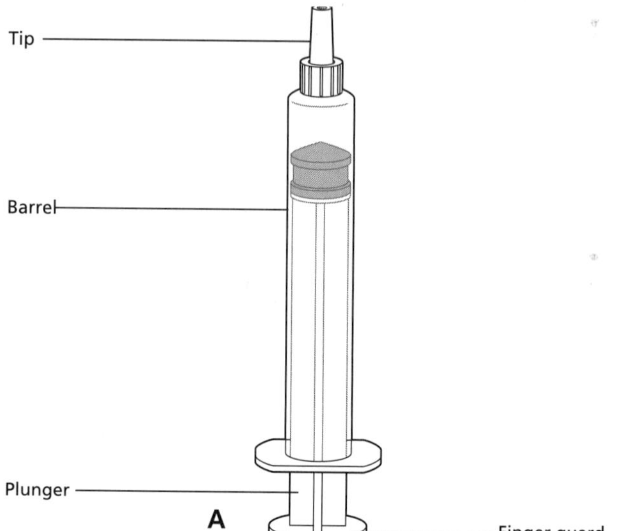

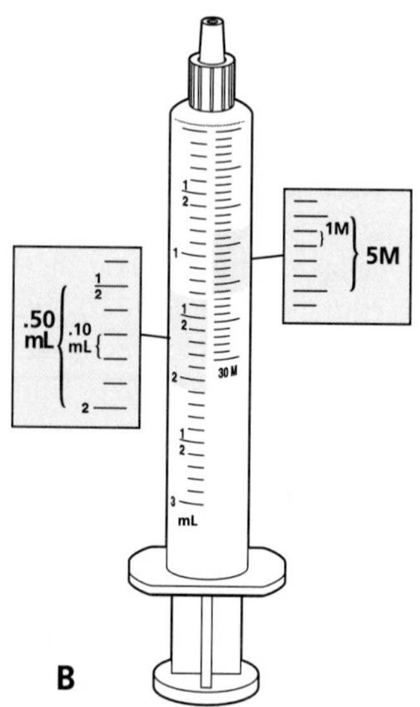

FIGURE 34.5 A. Parts of a syringe. B. Calibrations of a 3-mL syringe

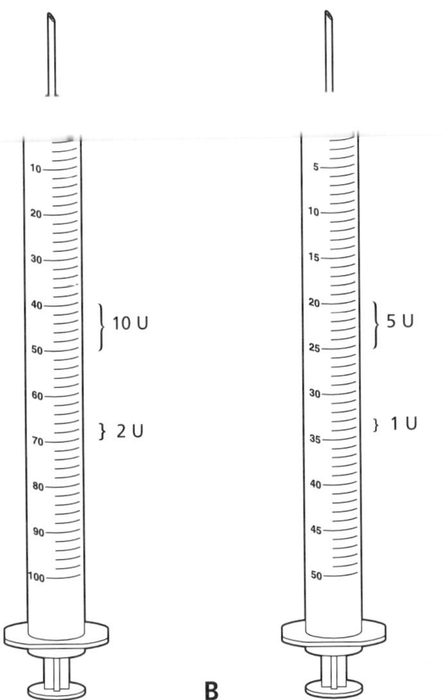

FIGURE 34.6 A. U-100 insulin syringe. B. Low-dose insulin syringe

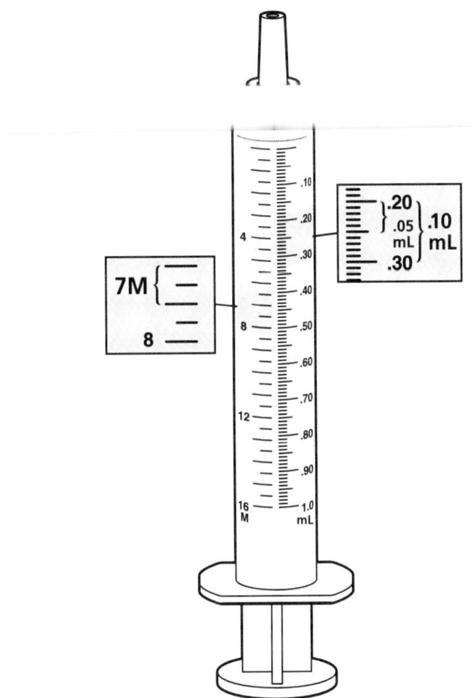

FIGURE 34.7 Calibrations of a tuberculin syringe

A longer bevel means a sharper needle, which minimizes discomfort when it penetrates the tissues. It is used for subcutaneous and intramuscular injections. A needle used for any injection should be straight and sharp. A short or small bevel is used when the risk of occlusion in a larger bevel is high, as in intravenous injections in which the bevel could rest against the side of the vein.

Needles vary in the length and diameter of the shaft. The length may range from about one to five centimetres. The diameter of the needle shaft is expressed as the *gauge*. The higher the gauge, the smaller the needle diameter. For example, an 18-gauge needle is larger than a 26-gauge needle. Needles used for parenteral administration range from 18 to 26 gauge. Figure 34.9 shows the various needle lengths and sizes.

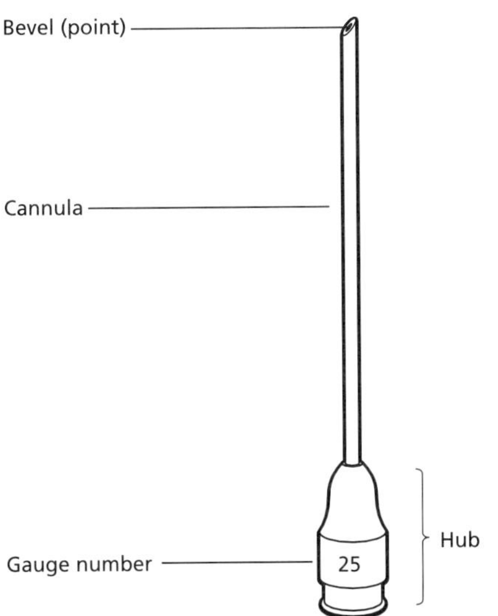

FIGURE 34.8 Parts of the needle

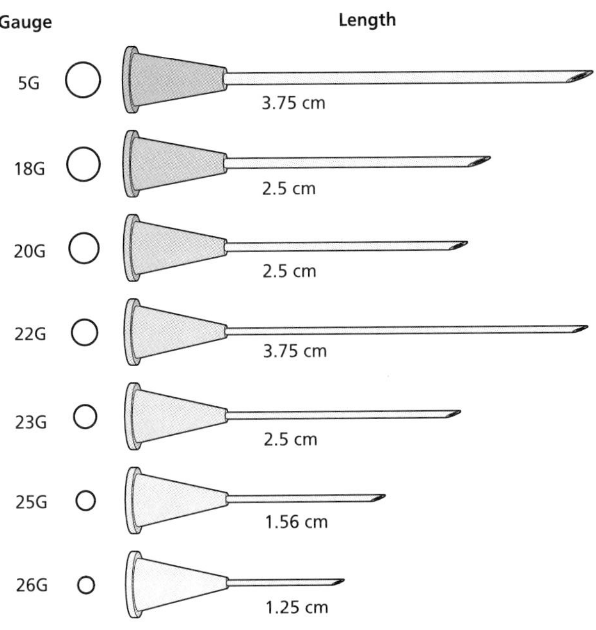

FIGURE 34.9 Needle lengths and gauges

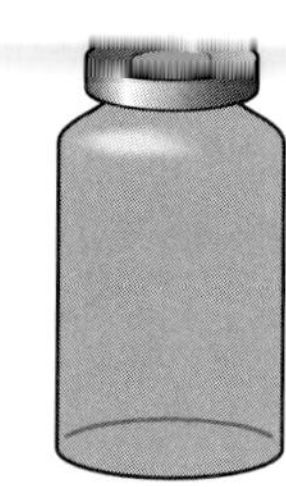

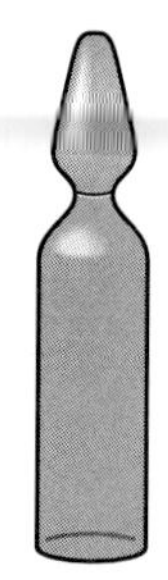

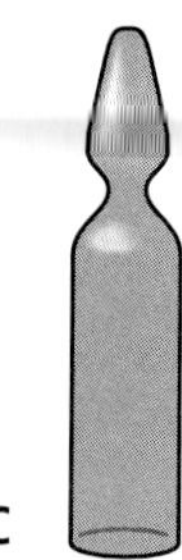

FIGURE 34.10 A. Vial. B. Prescored ampoule. C. Unscored ampoule

MEDICATION CONTAINERS Parenteral medications are usually prepared from vials and ampoules containing sterile powdered or liquid medication. A *vial* is a glass container with a self-sealing rubber stopper that may contain one or more doses of medication. An *ampoule* is a sealed glass container that contains a single dose of medication (see Figure 34.10). Vials contain liquid or dry powdered medication. Medications that are unstable in solution are packaged as powders, which have to be reconstituted before use. A vial is a closed system and, as such, requires the creation of positive pressure inside the container in order to withdraw medication from it. This is accomplished by injecting air equal to the amount of medication to be removed. The neck of an ampoule must be broken in order to withdraw the medication. Many ampoules are prescored to facilitate opening; scoring is depicted with a coloured ring around the neck. Those that are not prescored should be scored with a file to facilitate opening.

Preparing Injections

Parenteral medications are supplied in liquid or powder form. Both forms must be kept sterile during preparation and administration. The techniques for preparing injections depend on the form of the drug and on the container (ampoule, single-dose vial, multidose vial or a two-compartment vial). Sometimes two drugs are ordered by the same route. Providing the drugs are compatible, they can be mixed together in one syringe, saving the patient the unnecessary discomfort of another injection. Nursing units have a compatibility chart that identifies which drugs are compatible. Medications may be mixed from two ampoules, from two vials or from a vial and an ampoule. The various techniques for preparing drugs for parenteral administration are outlined in the following Procedures 34.4–34.8.

PROCEDURE 34.4 Preparing a Medication from an Ampoule

Action	*Rationale*
1. Follow the steps in Procedure 34.1.	Facilitates efficiency and economy of time.
2. Gather equipment: • medication card or MAR • prescribed medication • syringe and needle • alcohol swab.	
3. Hold the top of the ampoule between the thumb and forefinger and flick the wrist. Hold the body of the ampoule and tap the top sharply with your finger. 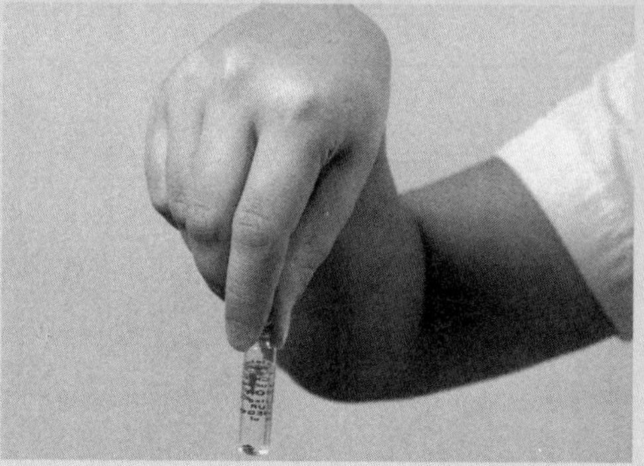	Transfers solution from the top of the ampoule into the bottom from which it is withdrawn.

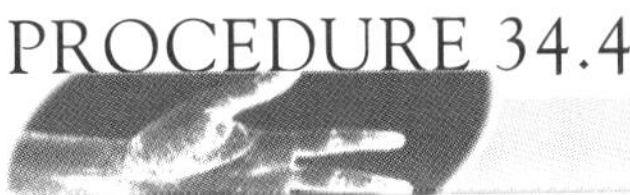

PROCEDURE 34.4 *continued*

Action	Rationale
4. Wrap the neck of the ampoule with an alcohol swab.	Prevents cuts when opening.
5. Grasp the ampoule with one hand and with the thumb of the other hand on the neck; apply pressure to the neck while bending it backward away from the face.	Prevents injury from splinters.

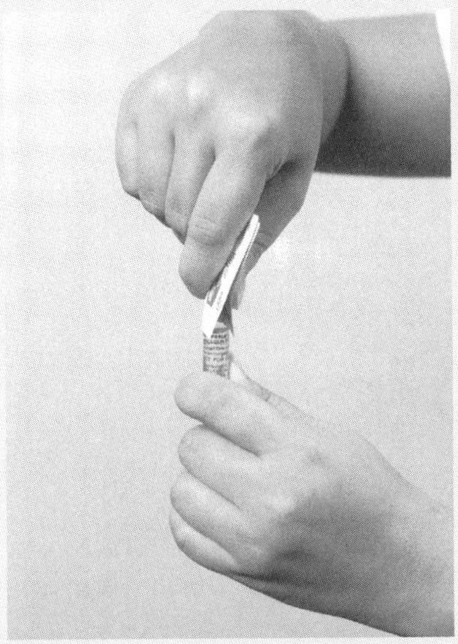

Action	Rationale
6. Deposit the top directly into the sharps container.	Swift disposal prevents injury and keeps working area clean.
7. Twist the needle onto the syringe, and remove the needle cap. Leave the cap on a flat, accessible surface.	Prepackaged syringes and needles are not always tightly fastened.
8. Insert the needle into the ampoule without touching the neck of the ampoule.	Maintains sterility of needle.
9. Withdraw the desired amount of solution:	
A. Hold the inverted ampoule and syringe in one hand and gently pull on the plunger with the other hand until the desired amount of solution is withdrawn. Ensure that the ampoule is directly upright and that the tip of the needle is below the level of solution.	Pulling on the plunger creates a negative pressure in the syringe, drawing fluid from the ampoule into the syringe. Air will also be drawn into the syringe if the needle tip is not in solution. Solution will not drip out of ampoule because of surface tension. *DO NOT push solution or air into an ampoule while it is inverted or medication will drip out.*

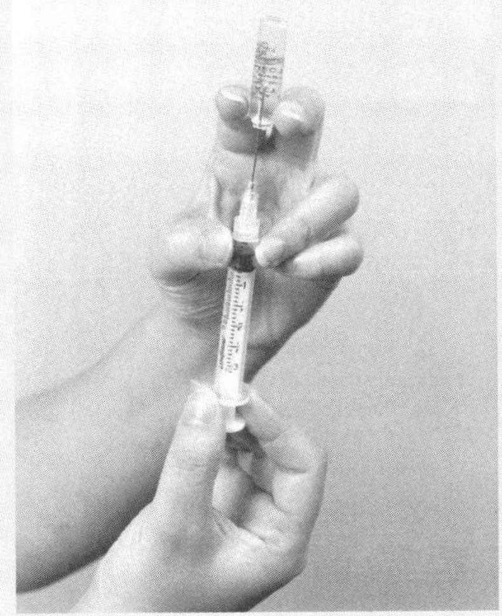

continued on next page

PROCEDURE 34.4 *continued*

Action	*Rationale*
B. Place the ampoule on a flat surface and gently pull on the plunger until the desired amount of solution is withdrawn. Make sure the tip of the needle is below the level of solution and does not scrape the bottom. 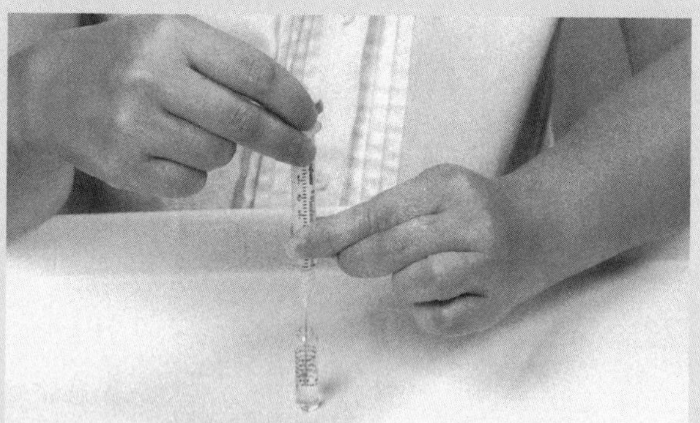	
10. Place the ampoule on a flat surface and remove the syringe.	Facilitates manual dexterity.
11. Hold the syringe upright and tap the barrel using the heel of a hand (or fingertips). 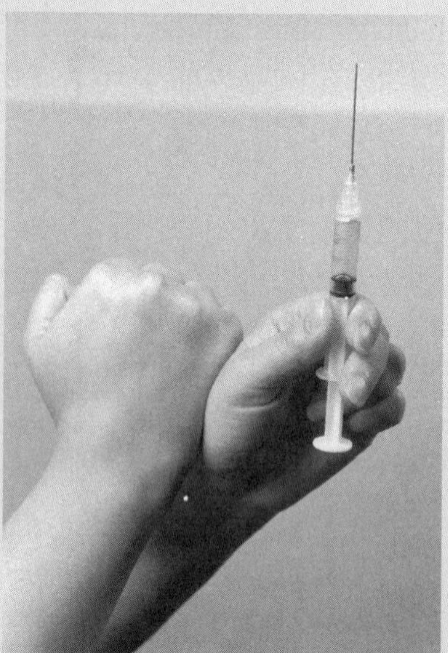	Causes air bubbles to rise to the hub of the syringe.
12. Aspirate approximately 0.25 mL.	Any time the syringe is tapped, small amounts of solution escape into the needle. Aspirating draws this solution back into the syringe and prevents spurting when dosage adjustments are made.
13. With the syringe in a vertical position, eject any air remaining in the syringe.	Syringe must be exactly vertical, as even a slight tilt causes air bubbles to sequester in the syringe.
14. Check the dosage in the syringe against the MAR. Expel excess solution into a paper towel or container.	Ensures accuracy of dosage.
15. Recap the needle by sliding it into the needle cap.	Ensures safety for nurse and others.
16. Discard the ampoule into a sharps container.	Correct disposal ensures workplace safety.

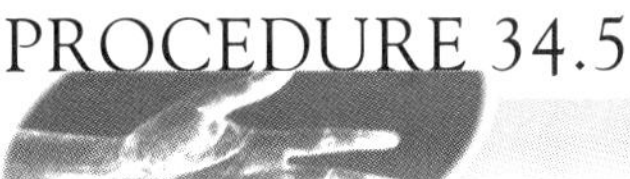

PROCEDURE 34.5 Preparing a Medication from a Vial

Action	Rationale
1. Follow the steps in Procedure 34.1.	
2. Gather equipment: • medication card or MAR • prescribed medication • syringe and needle • alcohol swab.	Facilitates efficiency and economy of time.
3. Remove the metal or plastic cap from the top of an unopened vial. 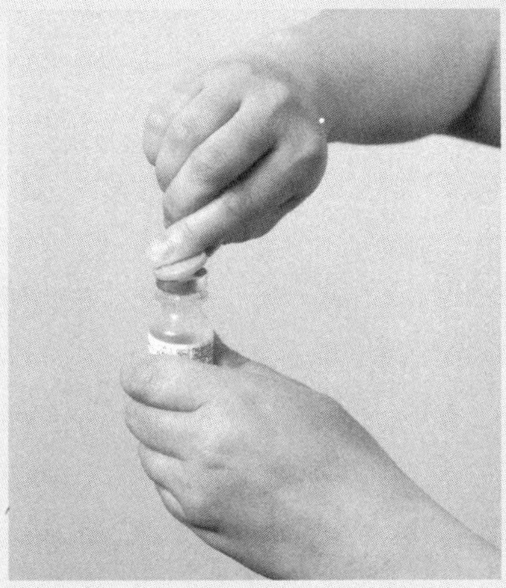	
4. Cleanse the rubber top of a previously opened multidose vial with an alcohol swab. If the surface of a newly opened vial has not been touched, this step is unnecessary.	Removes surface microorganisms.
5. Twist the needle onto the syringe and remove the needle cap. Leave the cap on a flat accessible surface.	Prepackaged syringes and needles are not always tightly attached.
6. Draw back on the plunger to fill the syringe with an amount of air equal to the amount of solution to be withdrawn.	Because a vial is a closed container, the amount of fluid withdrawn must be replaced with air to keep the pressure inside the vial equalized. This prevents the formation of a vacuum, which would make the withdrawal of medication difficult.
7. With the vial placed firmly on a flat surface, insert the needle into the vial and inject the air into the space above the solution. 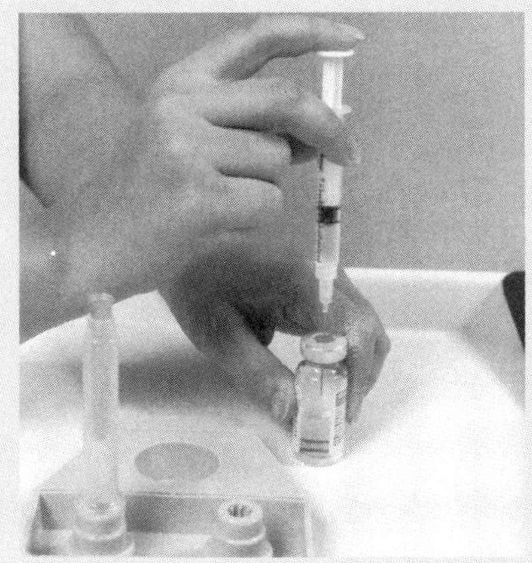	Prevents the formation of air bubbles, which could cause difficulty in withdrawing the correct amount of medication.

continued on next page

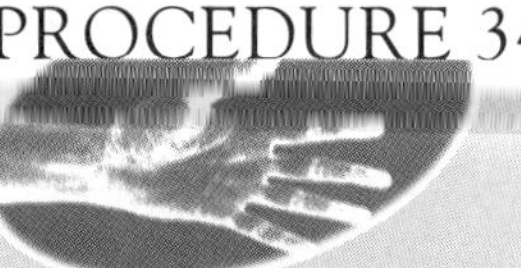

PROCEDURE 34.5 continued

Action	Rationale
8. Invert the vial and syringe unit, ensuring that the needle tip is below the level of fluid in the vial. 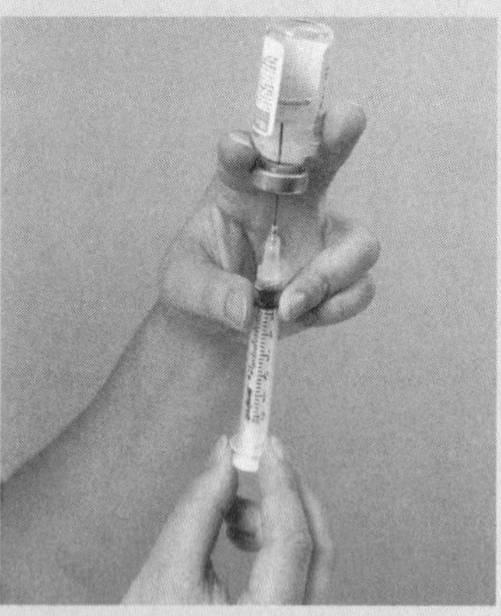	Prevents air from being drawn into the syringe.
9. Holding the syringe at eye level, pull down on the plunger to withdraw the required amount of solution. 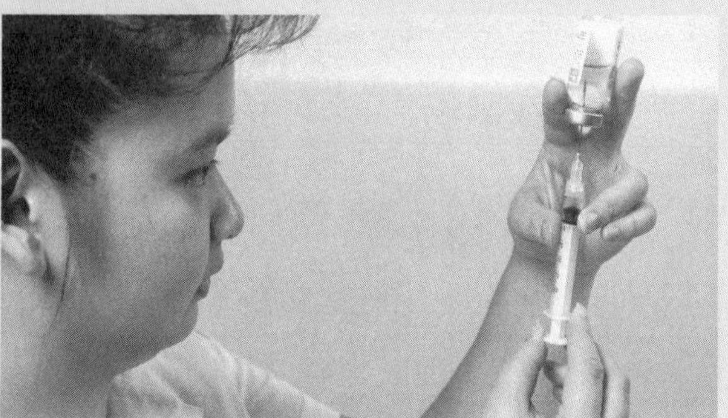	
10. With the needle still in the vial, and holding the syringe upright, tap on the barrel. 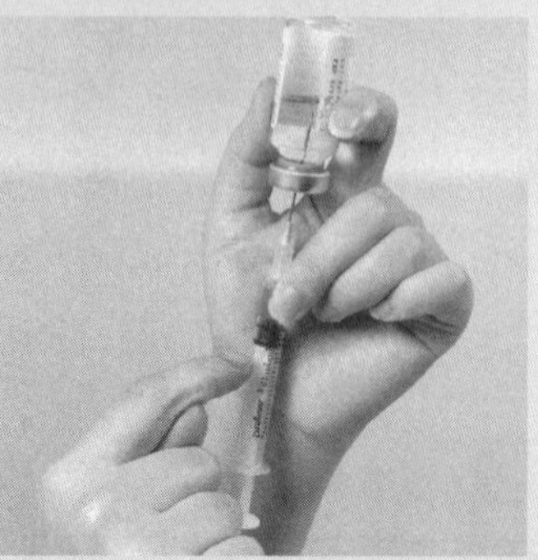	Dislodges air bubbles and displaces any air to the top of the syringe.
11. Inject air at the top of the syringe into the vial.	
12. Check the amount of solution in the syringe. Return excess or withdraw more solution as necessary.	Ensures accuracy of measurement.
13. Place the vial in an upright position on a flat surface. Remove the needle.	Removing the syringe with the vial inverted may cause spraying of medication.
14. Recap the needle by sliding it into needle cap.	Ensures safety for nurse and others.
15. Return a multidose vial to storage. Discard empty vial and used supplies.	Promotes cleanliness and safety in the workplace.

PROCEDURE 34.6 Preparing a Medication from a Powder

Action	Rationale
1. Follow the steps in Procedure 34.1.	Facilitates efficiency and economy of time.
2. Gather equipment: • medication card or MAR • prescribed medication • diluent (as specified on label) • syringe and needle • alcohol swab.	
3. Read the instructions on the package insert.	Provides specific instructions regarding reconstitution.
4. Withdraw air from the vial equal to the amount of diluent to be added.	Prepares the vial for the diluent, to balance the pressure in the vial.
5. Draw the required amount of diluent into the syringe and inject it into the upright medication vial.	Mixes with powder to reconstitute the medication.
6. Remove the syringe and without using a second hand, replace the needle by sliding it into the needle cap. Set it aside.	Promotes safe habits and prevents needle-stick injuries.
7. Roll the medication vial between the palms of the hands. *Do not shake!*	Rolling promotes mixing, whereas shaking often causes multiple bubbles or foaming to occur. This wastes time and can impede accuracy of measurement.
8. Withdraw the desired amount of medication as in Procedure 34.5.	
9. Label the vial indicating the date, time, type, amount of diluent and amount of drug per mL if it is to be reused. Store the vial as directed.	Ensures safe reuse. Many reconstituted drugs are effective for a limited period of time.

PROCEDURE 34.7 Mixing Medications in One Syringe Using Two Vials

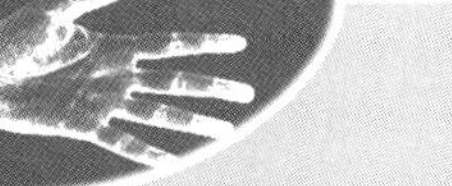

Action	Rationale
1. Follow the steps in Procedure 34.1.	
2. Gather equipment: • medication card or MAR • prescribed medications • syringe and needle • alcohol swab.	Facilitates efficiency and economy of time.
3. Check a compatibility chart.	Protects the patient by ensuring that two medications can be mixed in the same syringe.
4. Determine which medication will be withdrawn first (vial 1) and which will be withdrawn last (vial 2).	
5. Prepare vials as in Procedure 34.5.	
6. Inject an amount of air equal to the volume to be withdrawn into vial 2 and remove the syringe.	Creates a positive pressure in the vial.
7. Repeat step 6 for vial 1 but do not remove the needle. Invert the vial and withdraw the correct dose. Ensure that this amount is accurate and that no air bubbles are present.	Since two medications are being mixed in the same syringe, accuracy is essential for correct dosage.
8. Insert the needle into vial 2, taking care not to depress the plunger. Withdraw the exact dose. Check the dosage.	Prevents contamination of medication in vial 2 and ensures accurate dosage. Excess medication cannot be returned to the vial because the syringe now contains a mixture of the two medications.
9. Recap the needle by sliding it into the needle cap.	Ensures safety for nurse and others.

PROCEDURE 34.8 Preparing Medication from an Ampoule and a Vial

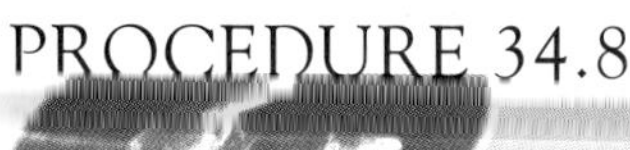

Action	*Rationale*
1. Follow the steps in Procedure 34.1.	
2. Gather equipment: • medication card or MAR • prescribed medications • medication ampoule • syringe and needle • alcohol swab.	Facilitates efficiency and economy of time.
3. Check a compatibility chart.	Protects the patient by ensuring that two medications can be mixed in the same syringe.
4. Prepare the ampoule as outlined in Procedure 34.4.	
5. Withdraw the correct dose from the vial as outlined in Procedure 34.5.	Prevents contaminating a multidose vial with medication from the ampoule.
6. Ensure that the dosage from the vial is accurate and that no air bubbles are present.	Since two medications are to be mixed, accuracy is essential for correct dosage.
7. Withdraw the exact dose from the ampoule as in Procedure 34.4.	
8. Recap the needle by sliding it into the needle cap.	Ensures safety for nurse and others.

Body Substance Precautions

The disposal of syringes and needles requires a special word of caution. Nurses must be meticulous in discarding needles and syringes. This is an area where short cuts are not acceptable, as carelessness can lead to disastrous results. One of the problems that can occur relates to people who may be looking for needles and syringes to assist their habit of illicit drug use. Nurses can prevent these opportunities from occurring by swiftly disposing of needles and syringes into sharps containers. In many hospitals and clinics sharps containers are placed in every room. Needles and syringes should *never* be put in the garbage can after use. Uncapped needles can easily prick an unsuspecting housekeeping worker and cause injury. Furthermore, the nurse should *never* recap syringes once an injection has been administered. Current literature indicates that most needle-stick injuries occur when the nurse recaps the needle following an injection (Ford, 1990). Needle-stick injuries carry the risk of transmitting hepatitis B and HIV. Therefore, the safest method is to deposit the syringe into a sharps container directly after giving the injection.

It is permissible to recap a needle before it is used on a patient. Once the medication has been prepared the needle is covered to keep it sterile and to protect others from needle-stick injury. The needle may be recapped by sliding it into the protective cover (cap). *Do not* use the other hand. This prevents needle-stick injury and fosters safe habits.

Common Problems in Preparing Medications from a Vial

There are several problems commonly associated with drawing fluid from a vial into a syringe. One problem occurs when the nurse begins to draw the fluid into the syringe only to find that large air bubbles form in it. There are two reasons for this. First, if the needle has not been tightly secured to the syringe, air from the outside is drawn into the syringe. Second, the needle may be above the level of the fluid inside the vial, in which case air will be drawn into the syringe instead of fluid. Another problem occurs when the nurse forgets to put air into the vial prior to withdrawing solution. When this step has been forgotten, the solution will flow sluggishly into the syringe because of the resulting negative air pressure inside the vial. The air pressure inside the vial must be positive (greater than atmospheric) for fluid to flow freely.

Using Two-Compartment Vials

Some drugs are commercially prepared in two-compartment vials. One compartment contains the powdered medication and the second contains the sterile liquid for dissolving the drug. The insertion of a sterile needle or pressure exerted upon a rubber diaphragm releases the liquid to mix with the powder, which is then ready for injection. Some drugs are packaged this way because they are more stable in a dry state and can be kept for a longer period of time in this form.

SUBCUTANEOUS INJECTIONS

Injections into subcutaneous tissues entail the delivery of medication into the loose connective tissues between the dermis and muscle layer. This route has been used since the 1860s and has been traditionally called the hypodermic injection. It has a relatively slow rate of absorption—about one to two millilitres per hour per injection site. The result is a lower concentration of drug in the body but with longer-lasting effects. The [illegible] The duration of action is from hours to weeks. As outlined in Table 34.8, the maximum volume of solution that can be given comfortably by this route is thought to be less than 1.0 mL. Certainly anything greater than 1.5 mL will cause pressure on surrounding tissues and will therefore be painful. The advantages and disadvantages of subcutaneous injections are presented in Table 34.9.

The nurse can minimize the risk of infection by using strict aseptic technique for all injections. Unfortunately, it is not possible to prevent entirely the development of lipomas or leathery skin in patients who require repeated injections over a long period of time, such as with insulin-dependent diabetics. However, it is possible to minimize the potential by rotating sites appropriately and allowing sites to rest for at least a month between injections. The variability in the rate of absorption can be reduced with consistent exercise and by remaining in the same position following injection for about 15 minutes. In addition, if the patient's temperature is elevated, every effort should be made by the nurse to reduce it to a normal range. The technique for administering a sub- [illegible]

TABLE 34.8 Recommended quantity of solution for route

Route	*Amount of Solution*
Subcutaneous	0.1–1.0 mL
Intramuscular	
Adults:	
deltoid	0.1–2.0 mL
ventrogluteal	0.1–5.0 mL
dorsogluteal	0.1–5.0 mL
vastus lateralis	0.1–5.0 mL
Children:	
vastus lateralis	0.1–1.0 mL
Intravenous	
Adults and Children	0.1–1000 mL/h (children are at the lower end)
Infants	0.1–10 mL/h

Preparing the Patient

As with many procedures, patients are concerned about the impending discomfort an injection may cause. The nurse should explain to the patient that the subcutaneous tissue is just below the cutaneous tissue or skin. It has fewer sensory receptors than the skin itself; therefore, once a needle is through the skin, an injection is relatively painless. Some drugs sting upon injection, but an isotonic solution can usually be administered painlessly. (The term *isotonic* refers to a concentration that is the same as the saline composition of body fluids.)

Assembling Equipment

The MAR or medication card, a syringe, a needle, the medication and an alcohol swab are collected. The standard 3-mL or the 1-mL tuberculin syringe with a 24-, 25- or 26-gauge needle is commonly used for subcutaneous injections. An insulin syringe is required for administering insulin. The length of the needle may vary from 1 cm to 2.5 cm, depending on the amount of subcutaneous fat and the degree of hydration of the patient. A longer needle is needed for the obese patient, a shorter needle for the dehydrated or emaciated person. Generally, a 25-gauge, 1.6-cm needle is used for the average adult.

There are two variations to the traditional method of administering subcutaneous injections. These are the injection syringe and the jet injector. The *injection syringe* is equipped with a spring that releases the needle for rapid insertion. The *jet injector* introduces the medication into the subcutaneous tissue by means of high pressure rather than through a needle. Although these methods are preferred in some instances, they have not replaced the usual subcutaneous injection by hypodermic syringe.

Choosing Subcutaneous Injection Sites

The exact site for a subcutaneous injection depends on the need of the specific patient, on the medication and, to some extent, on the policy of the institution. There are, however,

TABLE 34.9 Advantages and disadvantages of subcutaneous injections

Advantages	*Disadvantages*
• virtually complete absorption, as long as patient's circulation is adequate	• invasive; breaks natural barrier (skin) against infection
• accurate measure of the amount of drug absorption as a result of complete absorption and no disruption in absorption from gastric secretions	• skin changes with repeated injections can lead to development of lipomas or leathery skin
• not dependent upon consciousness or rationality of the patient	• absorption rate varies with the patient's exercise, temperature and position following injection

PROCEDURE 34.9 Administering Subcutaneous Injections

Action	Rationale
1. Explain the procedure and the medication(s) to the patient. Encourage questions.	Facilitates patient well-being and participation in care.
2. Follow the steps in Procedure 34.1.	
3. Gather equipment: • MAR or medication card • prepared medication with appropriate needle attached • alcohol swab • clean gloves.	Facilitates efficiency and economy of time.
4. Don clean glove or gloves per hospital policy.	Follows body substance precautions to prevent contact with blood.
5. Identify the patient.	Ensures the right patient.
6. Select the appropriate injection site.	Facilitates consistent absorption of medication.
Assess the area for redness, birthmarks, scars, swelling and lesions. Ask the patient if the area is tender, itchy or burning. If any of these conditions are present, choose another site.	Ensures a clean site which promotes absorption and prevents discomfort and inflammation.
7. Open the alcohol swab, loosen the needle cap from the syringe and move close to the selected area.	Readies supplies for injection. Maintains safe body mechanics.
8. Cleanse the injection site with the alcohol swab using a circular motion, starting at the site and moving outward. Allow the area to dry completely.	Removes surface contaminants and bacteria. A circular motion pushes microorganisms away from the selected site.
9. **Patients with ample subcutaneous tissue:** With the thumb and forefinger of the nondominant hand, spread a fold of skin surrounding the site.	Assists in penetration of needle and causes less discomfort.
Patients with minimal subcutaneous tissue: With the nondominant hand, pinch a fold of skin around the site.	Pinching the skin elevates it from muscle tissue.

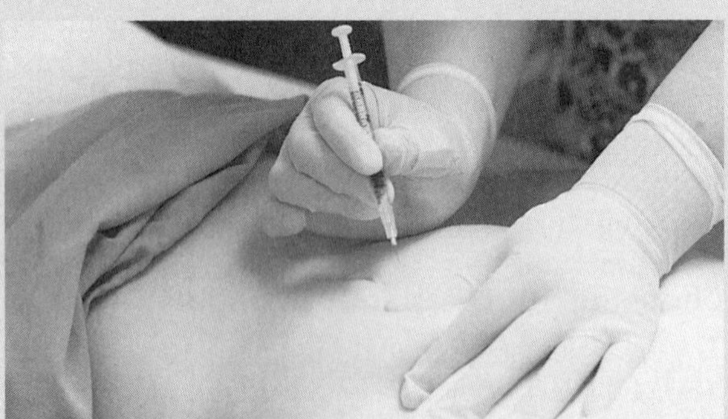

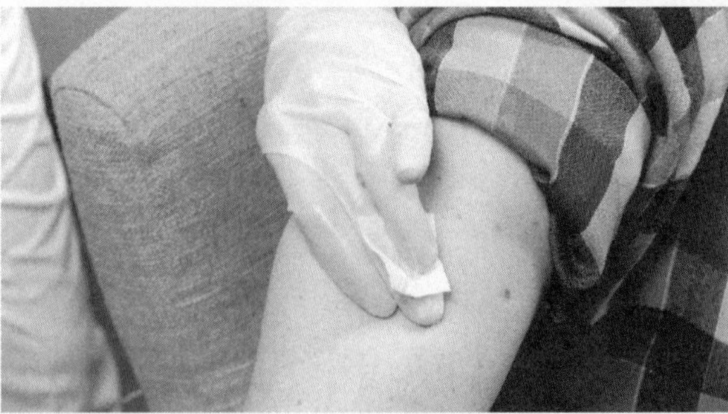

Action	Rationale
10. Hold the syringe, bevel upward, between the thumb and four fingers or the thumb and forefinger of the dominant hand and swiftly insert the needle using a 45°–90° angle.	Most patients have enough subcutaneous tissue to warrant a 90° angle; very thin patients may require a 45° angle to prevent injection into the muscle and artery.

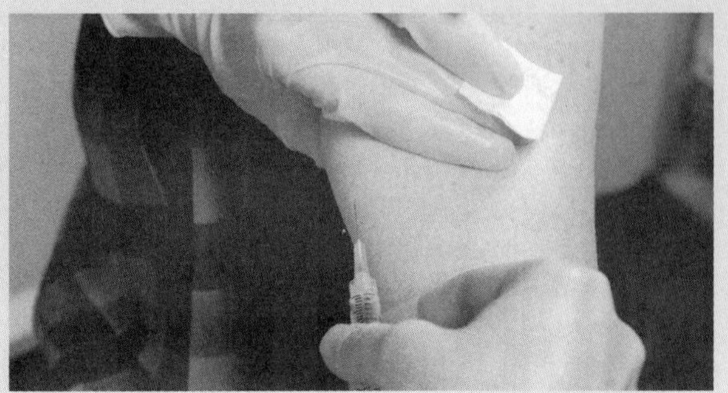

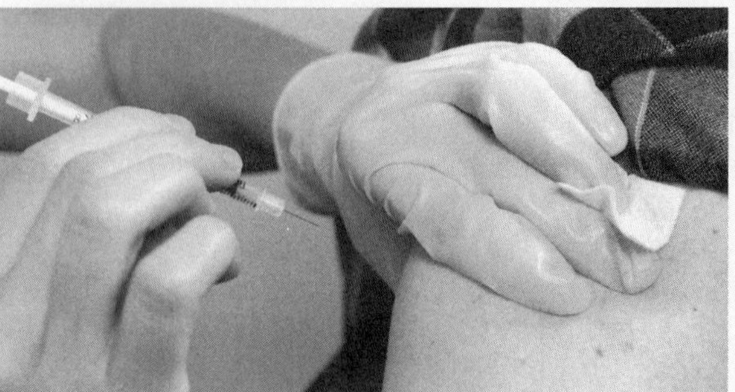

PROCEDURE 34.9 *continued*

Action	*Rationale*
11. Release the nondominant hand and move it to the plunger end of the syringe. 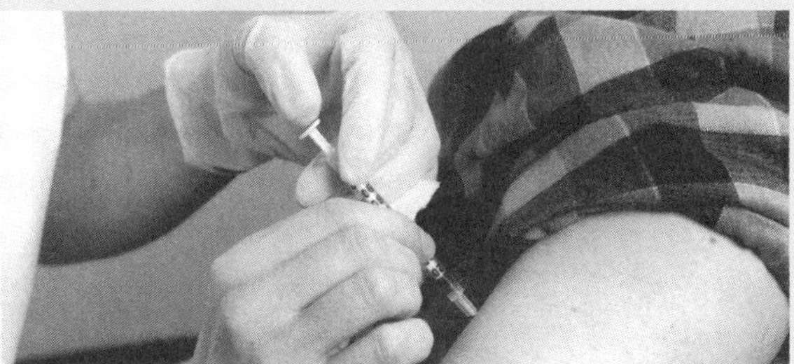	Once the syringe is in the patient, it is no longer necessary to stretch or pinch the skin. *Never leave a syringe unattended while in a patient's body!*
12. Aspirate by pulling back slightly on the plunger and inspect the syringe for the presence of blood. If blood appears, prepare a new syringe. **Do not aspirate for insulin or heparin.**	Blood in the syringe indicates the needle is in a blood vessel and should be removed.
13. If no blood present, slowly inject the solution.	Prevents rapid tissue distention and discomfort.
14. Swiftly remove the needle and massage the site with an alcohol swab unless contraindicated for the specific drug. If blood appears on site, cover the alcohol swab with the swab package.	Swift removal decreases discomfort. Massaging the site decreases bleeding and facilitates distribution of the medication. If bleeding does occur, the package from the swab will act as a barrier between the nurse and the patient if gloves are not used.
15. Do not recap the needle. Discard directly into the nearest sharps container.	Prevents needle-stick injury.
16. Ensure patient comfort, wash hands and record medication.	Promotes patient well-being, prevents the spread of micro-organisms and fulfills requirements for nurse accountability.

exceptions to this rule, such as with insulin and heparin, and these will be discussed separately. Generally, areas of the anterior and lateral aspects of the thigh, lower ventral abdominal wall, and the fat pads on the lower back and posterior aspect of the arms are recommended as usable sites (see Figure 34.11). To avoid the umbilical veins, do not use a one-inch area around the umbilicus. In the past, the anterior aspect of the upper arms and the back of the thighs have been portrayed as potential injection sites, but these are no longer advocated (Drass, 1992). The skin and subcutaneous tissue should be free of irritation, such as itching, and any signs of inflammation, such as redness, heat, edema, tenderness or pain. Areas in which scar tissue is present should be avoided.

ROTATING INJECTION SITES If a patient is receiving a series of repeated injections, the sites are rotated to minimize trauma and to allow unused areas the chance to heal completely between uses. An anatomic region is selected, for example, the lower ventral abdominal wall, and injections are made into that region until all sites have been used. This is called intrasite rotation. The sites progress in clockwise direction, and each injection should be 2.5 cm away from the previous one. A region should not be reused for a month (Drass, 1992). It is important to chart the site every time it is used so that two consecutive doses are not given in the exact same area. Sometimes a map is made indicating the sites to be used for rotating injections, or a chart may be attached to the nursing care plan for the patient. Another method for keeping track of used sites is to put a spot bandage on the first site used in a region. The nurse can then rotate the sites as described above.

Subcutaneous Injection of Insulin

The subcutaneous injection of insulin is virtually the same as other subcutaneous injections, but with a few variations. The nurse must be especially aware of the types of insulins that can be mixed in the same syringe. Only insulins of the same brand should be mixed together. Similarly, there should never be cross-mixing of insulins with different bases, such as pork-based insulins and humulin insulins. Regular insulin can be mixed with most other types, that is, Lente and NPH (neutral protamine hagedorn) insulin. However, care must be taken to ensure that the vial containing the regular (short-acting) insulin is not contaminated with longer-acting insulins. The accidental instillation, on repeated occasions, of a drop of longer-acting insulin into a vial of short-acting insulin can appreciably decrease the insulin's onset, peak and duration of action. Short-acting insulin should always be drawn up first, followed by the longer-acting insulin (Drass, 1992; Pinnell, 1996).

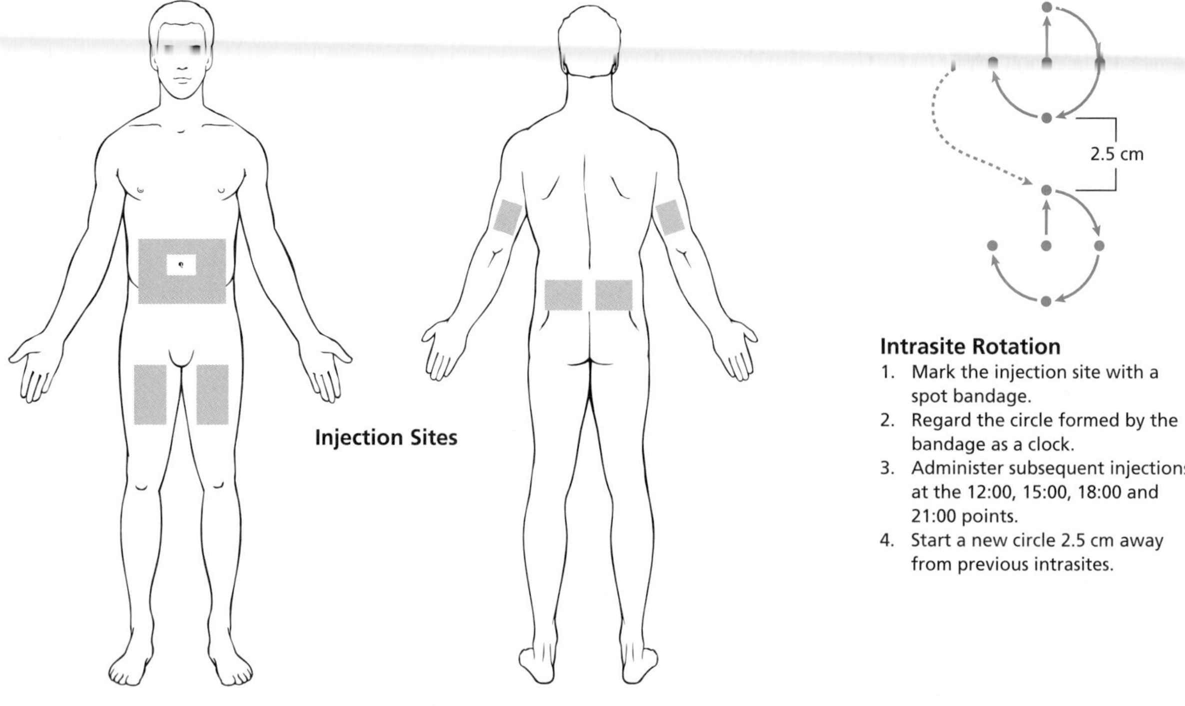

FIGURE 34.11 Subcutaneous injection sites and intrasite rotation

SOURCE: Drass, 1992.

When administering insulin, the nurse does not need to pull back on the plunger before injecting the solution. The potential for entering a blood vessel is minimal and tissue disruption is at risk. However, Drass (1992) recommends that the nurse should consider aspiration "for children, thin adults, or any patient who has many superficial blood vessels at the injection site or well-developed underlying muscle (common among diabetic athletes)" (p. 42). The insulin is slowly injected into tissues. The syringe is then withdrawn, and firm pressure is applied with an alcohol swab. The area must not be massaged because this will cause inconsistent absorption.

Subcutaneous Injection of Heparin

Heparin is frequently administered via the subcutaneous route at 90 degrees and requires several deviations from routine procedure. After the correct dose of heparin is drawn up, the needle is changed. A clean needle will be free of any heparin that may cause tissue damage. A second difference pertains to site selection. The abdomen is the site of preference for subcutaneous heparin injection. However, using the thigh or arm does not alter the drug's effectiveness. Research has shown that there is no increase in bruising with the use of alternative sites (Fahs & Kinney, 1991). As with insulin administration, the plunger is not aspirated prior to injection. The medication is injected slowly; the syringe is removed, and firm pressure is applied with an alcohol swab. Massaging is not recommended, as it can cause greater tissue damage.

INTRAMUSCULAR INJECTIONS

Intramuscular injections are administered under the muscle fascia below the subcutaneous layer. This route is often the choice for administering some medications, particularly those that are viscous and irritating, since the scarcity of sensitive nerve endings in deep muscle tissue results in less pain. Because muscles have a good vascular supply, medications are absorbed more quickly than when they are administered subcutaneously. However, there is danger of damaging nerves and injecting drugs into blood vessels. Medications administered by this route begin to work in less than an hour; the duration may last from hours to weeks, depending on the medication. Table 34.10 outlines some advantages and disadvantages of intramuscular injections.

While there are disadvantages to the intramuscular route, it is possible to minimize them. Nurses who consistently use proper techniques in locating injection sites (landmarking) will minimize damage to blood vessels and nerves. In addition, as with any injection, it is important to maintain aseptic technique in order to decrease the chance of infection. Many people shy away from intramuscular injections because they are uncomfortable. Although injections are not as easy to take as an oral medication, the nurse can often minimize discomfort. A number of suggestions are given in the box on the next page. The technique for administering intramuscular injections is detailed in Procedure 34.10.

TABLE 34.10 Advantages and disadvantages of intramuscular injections

Advantages	*Disadvantages*
• provides a less painful route for medications • muscles can absorb larger amounts of fluid than can subcutaneous tissue • absorption is more rapid than by the subcutaneous route • can be used for potent drugs that are not cytotoxic • can be used for aqueous suspensions and solutions in vegetable oil that may cause emboli if given intravenously	• greater danger of damaging nerves and blood vessels • invasive; breaks skin, thus potentiates infection • many patients fear intramuscular injections

Reducing the Pain of Intramuscular Injections

1. Involve the patient in the choice of site. Any patient who has had more than a few injections may have a preference.
2. Choose the smallest gauge of needle possible, giving consideration to the site and solution to be administered.
3. Assist the patient to relax the muscle to be used. If the gluteal muscle is to be used, have the patient lie prone, or stand with toes pointed inward, or lie on the side with knees flexed. If the vastus lateralis muscle is to be used, ask the patient to point the toes inward so the hips rotate internally. If the deltoid muscle is to be used, flex the elbow and support the lower arm.
4. Avoid sensitive areas. Roll the selected muscle mass with thumb and forefinger to assess for twitching.
5. Numb the site with ice if the patient is very apprehensive.
6. Make sure that the antiseptic used to wipe the site is dry. Wet antiseptic can cling to the needle and cause discomfort during insertion.
7. Change the needle if it was used to puncture a rubber stopper during preparation. This will also obliterate any medication on the needle, which can be another cause for discomfort.
8. Insert and remove the needle quickly and smoothly. If possible, distract the patient by asking him or her to wiggle the toes, take a deep breath and exhale, or participate in discussion.
9. Inject the medication slowly to minimize the creation of high pressure in the muscle.
10. Never leave the needle unattended while it is in the patient. Instead, hold it steady.
11. Use all possible sites.
12. Massage the muscle following injection, unless contraindicated.
13. Administer only the recommended amount of fluid into a muscle.

Assembling Equipment

The MAR or medication card and the prescribed medication are gathered. If the medication is in a powdered form, a diluent will also be necessary. Most intramuscular injections require a 3-mL or 5-mL syringe. The standard prepackaged 3-mL syringe with a 21- or 22-gauge, 3.8-cm needle is commonly used for adults. If more than 5 mL of solution is ordered, the amount is given in two injections. Viscous fluids require a larger needle—19 gauge, for example. The length of the needle depends on the injection site, the size of the patient's muscle and the amount of adipose tissue that is present. A person with a large amount of adipose tissue will need a longer needle in order to reach the muscle tissue; a thin person will need a shorter needle. Smaller, shorter needles are required for infants and small children.

Locating Intramuscular Injection Sites

Regardless of the site chosen, the area must be exposed adequately so that the nurse can clearly see it. The selection of an area for an intramuscular injection depends on a number of factors: the size of the patient and the amount of muscle tissue available for injection; the proximity of nerves and blood vessels; the condition of the skin around the area; the nature of the drug to be administered; and the patient's preference. There are four recommended sites for administering intramuscular injections, all of which are anatomically safe. Each area has little potential of hitting a nerve or large blood vessel. When choosing a particular site, the nurse must inspect the tissue in the area to make sure it is free from bruises or soreness. There should be no abrasions on the skin, and areas with hardened tissue (such as scar tissue) should be avoided.

It can sometimes be difficult to locate a suitable site on a patient who has had repeated injections. The patient should be involved in picking the general area of safe sites where he or she would feel comfortable getting the injection. If a patient has been receiving intramuscular injections over a long period of time, the nurse should collaborate with the physician to evaluate the effectiveness of this route and to consider alternatives.

PROCEDURE 34.10 Administering Intramuscular Injections

Action	*Rationale*
1. Explain the procedure and the medication(s) to the patient. Encourage questions.	Facilitates patient well-being and participation in care.
2. Follow the steps in Procedure 34.1.	
3. Gather equipment: • MAR or medication card • prepared medication with appropriate needle attached • alcohol swab • clean gloves.	Facilitates efficiency and economy of time.
4. Follow steps 5 and 6 of Procedure 34.9.	
5. Once the general site has been selected, position patient and provide privacy.	Promotes physical comfort and emotional well-being.
6. Place the syringe and alcohol swab close to selected site.	Maintains safe body mechanics.
7. Locate the injection site by identifying the correct landmarks. Cleanse it as in Procedure 34.9. It is often possible to mark the site with the corner of the alcohol swab.	Essential for a safe injection. Positioning the alcohol swab pointing towards the selected area allows the nurse to obtain the syringe without losing the site.
8. With the dominant hand, take the syringe and slide the needle cap off the needle.	
9. Using the thumb and forefinger of the nondominant hand, pull the skin taut within 5 cm of the selected site. If the patient is emaciated, it may be necessary to pinch the skin.	Facilitates needle insertion and lessens pain when the injection is given.

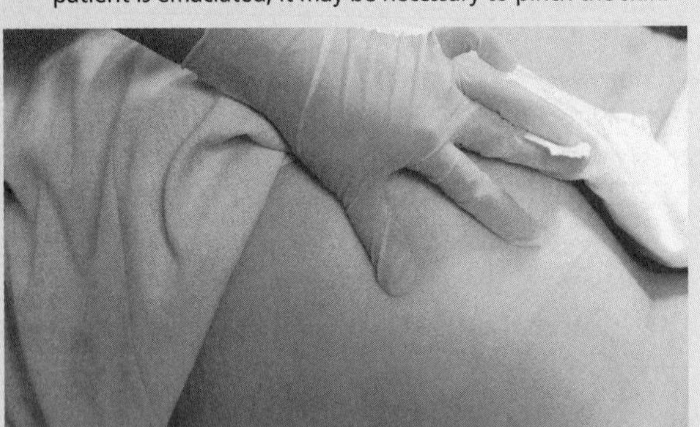

10. Ask a question, or instruct the patient to take a deep breath or wiggle the toes.	Distracts the patient and decreases the discomfort of the injection.
11. Hold the syringe between thumb and forefinger of the dominant hand and, with a swift, smooth motion, insert the needle at a 90° angle, completely into the muscle.	A quick motion decreases the patient's discomfort.

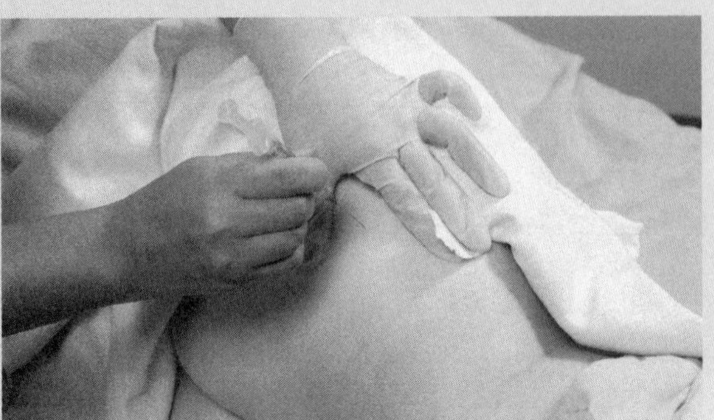

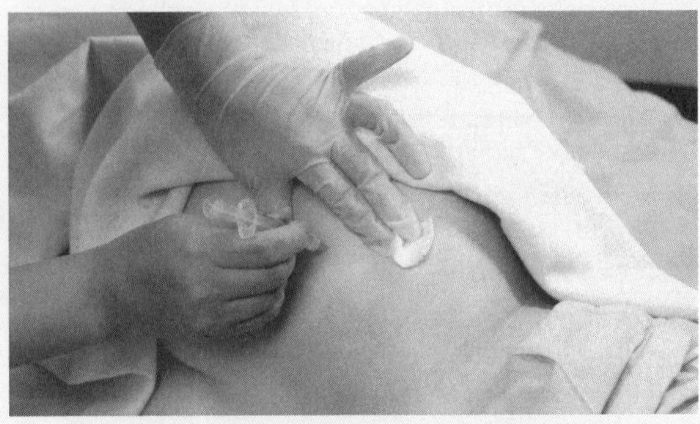

12. Follow steps 11 to 15 of Procedure 34.9.

Three areas of the body are commonly used for intramuscular injections: the gluteus muscles in two areas of the buttocks, the quadriceps muscles [illegible] tate the areas when a series of injections is given. The gluteal muscles are thick and permit the injection of larger quantities of fluid. The use of these muscles in many normal daily activities also aids in the absorption of drugs.

THE DORSOGLUTEAL MUSCLE The dorsogluteal site uses the gluteus maximus muscle. This site should not be used in patients younger than three years, as muscle is not sufficiently developed. The site may be located by drawing an imaginary line from the posterior superior iliac spine to the greater trochanter of the femur. This line runs lateral and parallel to the sciatic nerve; consequently, an injection lateral and superior to it is in a safe area (see Figure 34.12).

To position a patient for an intramuscular injection in the gluteal muscle, ask the patient to lie in a prone position with his or her toes internally rotated in plantar flexion. In this position the gluteal muscles are relaxed and there is good visualization of the injection site. If the patient is unable to lie prone, ask the patient to lie on the side with knees flexed.

THE VENTROGLUTEAL MUSCLE The ventrogluteal site is the primary site for individuals over seven months old because there are no large nerves or blood vessels in the area (Beyea & Nicoll, 1996). In addition, the ventrogluteal area is usually less fatty than the buttocks, meaning that more medication is administered directly to the muscle.

When the ventrogluteal site is used, the injection is made into the gluteus minimus and the gluteus medius muscles. The site is situated in a triangle within three palpable bony landmarks: the iliac crest, the anterior superior iliac crest and the greater trochanter of the femur (Figure 34.13A). [illegible] part of the greater trochanter with the index finger on the anterior superior iliac spine. Then the middle fingers are stretched dorsally as far along the iliac crest as possible (Figure 34.13B). An alternative method of locating the ventrogluteal site has been developed by Rhoda Brooke through her nursing experiences with adults and children. With this method it is not necessary to lay the nurse's hands on the body. Rather, the individual's anatomy is relied on more specifically. In Brooke's method, an imaginary line is drawn from the top of the iliac crest down to the trocanter. Then another line, parallel to the waistline, is drawn from the anterior superior iliac spine (hip bone) to join the first line. The point of intersection is the ventrogluteal site (Figure 34.13C). It is important to palpate the injection site; it should feel soft and fleshy. If it feels hard, the site is likely too close to the bone and will have to be adjusted accordingly.

An injection may be given into the ventrogluteal site with the patient in a prone, supine or side-lying position. The beginning student may find it easier to locate the site when the patient is side-lying. If the patient's gluteal muscles are tense, flexing the knees will promote relaxation (Beyea & Nicoll, 1996).

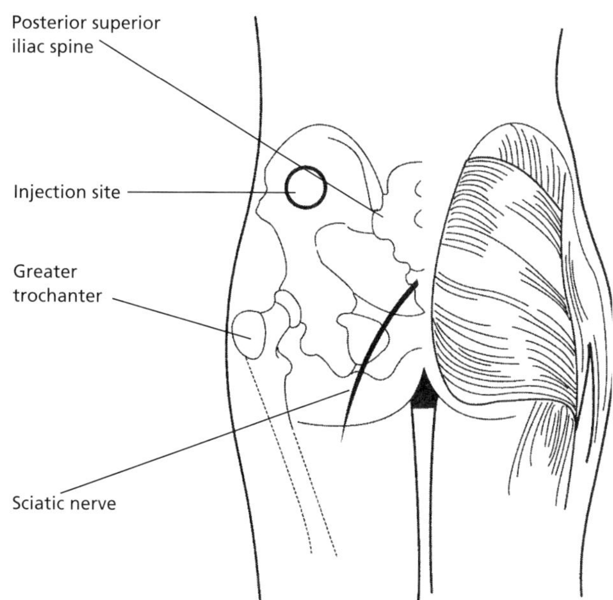

FIGURE 34.12 Locating the dorsogluteal injection site

SOURCE: Nursing Department, Langara College, Vancouver, BC.

THE VASTUS LATERALIS The vastus lateralis muscle on the lateral aspect of the thigh is also being used more frequently for intramuscular injections. This is the site of choice for infants and young children. It can also be used for debilitated patients whose gluteal muscles are poorly developed. The area is free of major blood vessels and nerve trunks. By virtue of its length, the vastus lateralis muscle provides a long area, which is useful when numerous injections have to be given. The muscle extends the full length of the thigh from mid-anterior to mid-lateral and is approximately 7.5 cm wide. The injection may be given anywhere from approximately 10 cm above the knee to approximately 10 cm below the hip joint (see Figure 34.14). While this muscle is excellent to use because it lacks major nerves or vessels, the injection can be painful for individuals with large musculature on the upper leg.

THE DELTOID MUSCLE The deltoid muscle of the arm is also used for intramuscular injections. This site is two to three finger-breadths down from the acromion process on the outer aspect of the arm (see Figure 34.15). In most people this is a smaller muscle than the gluteal muscle and therefore is not capable of absorbing a large volume of medicine comfortably. The danger of administering an injection in this area is that harming the radial nerve, as well as the humoral circumflex artery, is a possibility.

With careful technique, complications from intramuscular injections can be avoided. Abscesses, nerve injuries, cysts and necrosis of tissue do occur as a result of intramuscular injections. Aseptic technique, the correct use of landmarks in determining injection sites and alternating sites help to avoid these complications.

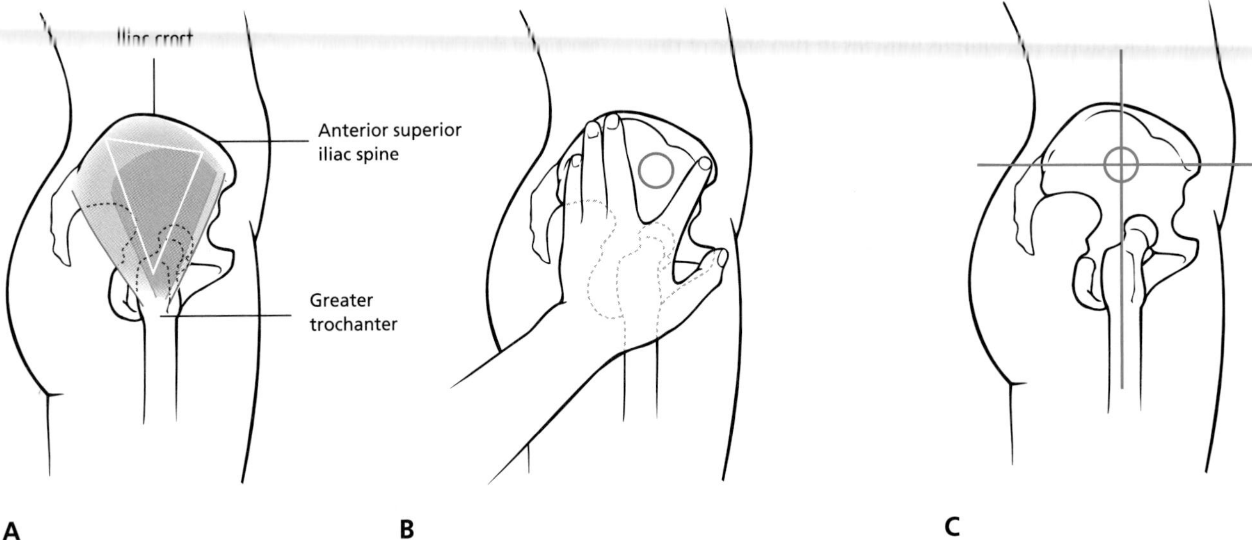

FIGURE 34.13 Locating the ventrogluteal injection site: A. Ventrogluteal site. B. Standard method. C. Brooke method

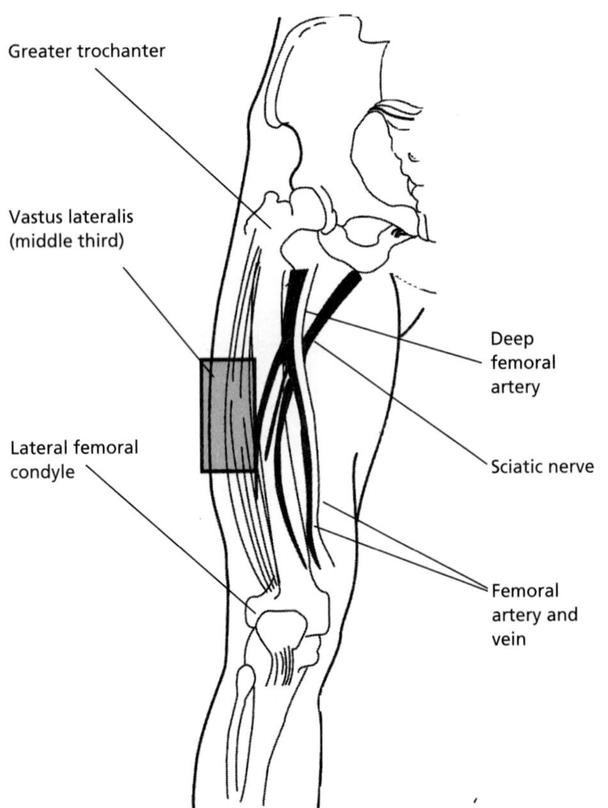

FIGURE 34.14 Locating the vastus lateralis injection site

SOURCE: Nursing Department, Langara College, Vancouver, BC.

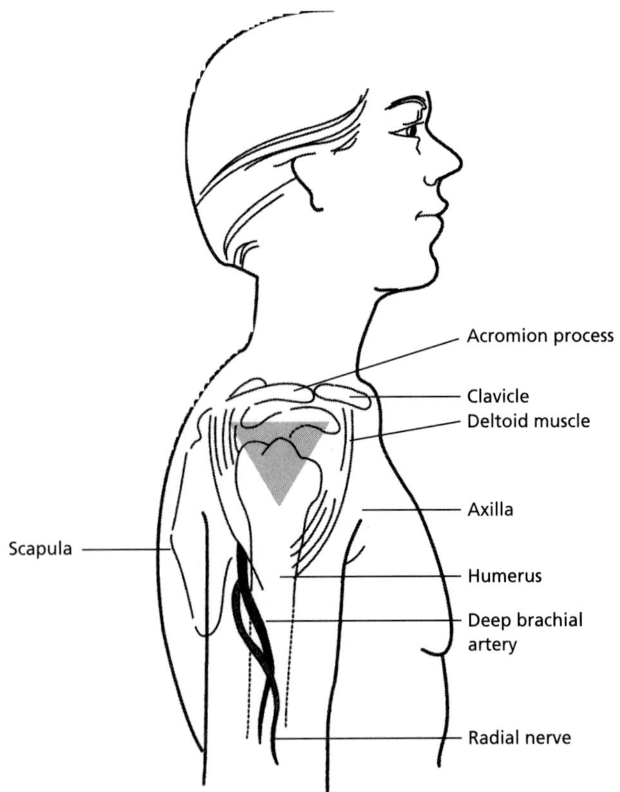

FIGURE 34.15 Locating the deltoid injection site

SOURCE: Nursing Department, Langara College, Vancouver, BC.

Z-TRACK INJECTIONS

Some medications are best given by the Z-track method, [illegible]

of those which discolour tissues. It is also used for people who have had multiple intramuscular injections and consequent reflux leaking. The Z-track injection is prepared and administered in the same way as a routine intramuscular injection, with the following exceptions. The needle is always changed after the medication has been drawn up. This ensures that there is no medication on the needle that could cause irritation to the tissues. In the Z-track method the skin and subcutaneous tissues are laterally displaced, and traction is maintained while the medication is injected. Release of the tissues after injection seals the medication in the muscle and creates a leak-proof zigzag path (see Figure 34.16). With the nondominant hand, the skin and subcutaneous tissue are displaced about 2 cm over the target muscle. The needle is inserted at a 90° angle, and the medication is injected while lateral traction is being maintained. Once the medication has been administered, the needle is quickly removed and then the traction is released. An alcohol swab is held firmly over the site but the site, is not massaged. Massage may cause seepage of medication into delicate tissue, resulting in discomfort or staining.

INTRADERMAL INJECTIONS

An intradermal injection is the administration of a small amount of fluid (0.1 or 0.2 mL) into the dermal layer of the skin. It is frequently done as a diagnostic measure, as in tuberculin and allergy testing. Since the blood supply to the dermis is decreased, medications absorb very slowly, and the effects are generally localized. It is important to reassess the area for the next few days, as this is generally when reactions appear.

Assembling Equipment

A tuberculin syringe with a very fine 26- or 27-gauge, 1-cm

Choosing Intradermal Sites

The areas of the body commonly used for intradermal injections are the fat pads over the medial aspect of the forearms, the upper arms, the scapula and the upper chest (see Figure 34.17). The area should be free of hair, veins and discoloration. Procedure 34.11 outlines the steps involved in administering an intradermal injection.

INTRAVENOUS ADMINISTRATION

Use of the intravenous route to administer medications is increasing. Intravenous medications begin to work immediately, and that can be both an advantage and a disadvantage. Although IV medications are very beneficial when a rapid effect is needed, adverse reactions or errors can cause serious, life-threatening complications. Intravenous medications can be delivered through a variety of methods: by adding a medication to a primary IV container (continuous infusion); by using a separate container connected to the primary line with secondary tubing (secondary line or piggyback set-up); or by the direct push method (small amount of solution is injected directly into an existing IV line). These same methods can also be used for the patient who has an intermittent infusion device, commonly referred to as a saline or heparin lock. The duration of action of a medication administered intravenously varies from a few seconds to hours. Table 34.11 outlines some of the advantages and disadvantages of using the intravenous route for administering medications.

The most effective way to deal with the disadvantages of intravenous medications is to prevent their occurrence.

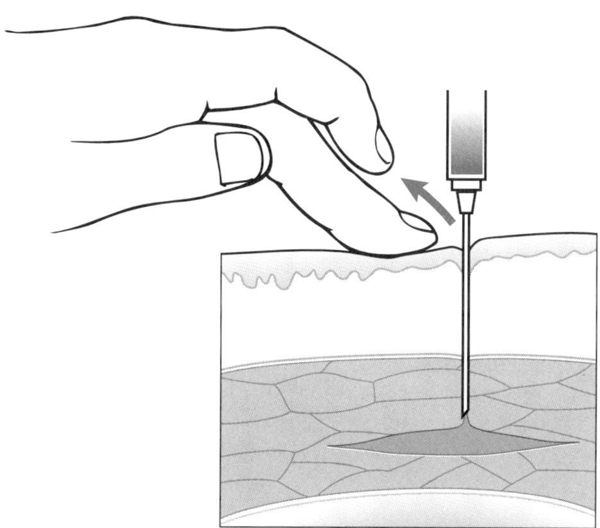

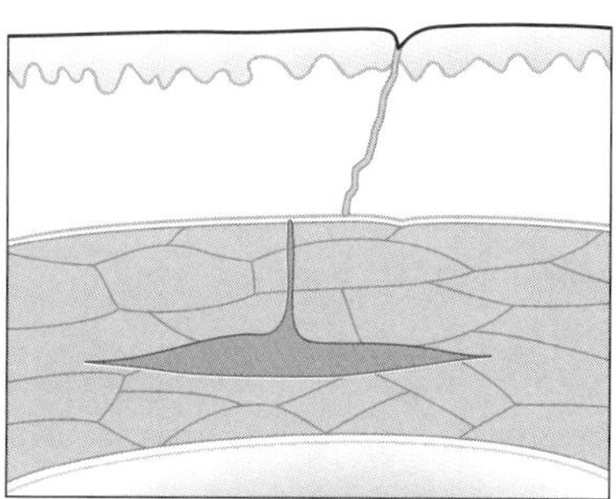

FIGURE 34.16 Z-Track method. This technique converts the needle track into a zigzag, which prevents leakage of solution into tissues

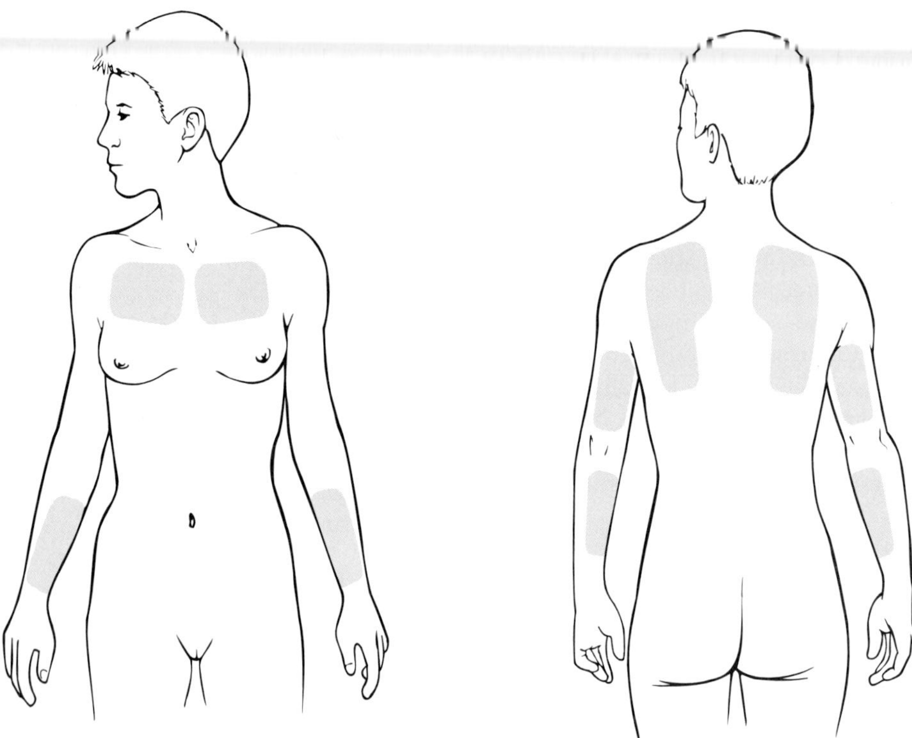

FIGURE 34.17 Intradermal injection sites

Drug incompatibilities can largely be prevented by scrupulous checking of the compatibility of the solution, the medication and the diluent. Most agencies have current compatibility charts available, and the nurse can always contact the pharmacist to double-check. Effective vascular access is sometimes beyond the nurse's control; however, the insertion of intravenous needles can be performed with excellent technique, thus avoiding repeated attempts that serve only to cause discomfort and injure the patient. When irritating drugs are to be infused, the nurse must follow recommendations for solution quantities and times. Adverse reactions can occur either immediately or following an infusion and the nurse must be alert to this possibility. While the nurse cannot necessarily prevent adverse reactions, he or she can check carefully for known allergies or drug sensitivities prior to administering a medication.

ADDING MEDICATION TO A PRIMARY IV CONTAINER

Some drugs are best administered by continuous infusion in a large volume (500 mL or 1000 mL) of compatible solution. Multiple vitamins and potassium chloride are two

TABLE 34.11 Advantages and disadvantages of intravenous medications

Advantages	*Disadvantages*
• no absorption problems; medication is administered directly into the patient's circulation, thus rapidly achieves therapeutic levels • accurate titration due to accurate absorption • less discomfort; the pain associated with IM and SC routes is generally avoided since the veins have a much higher pain threshold • alternative to the oral route when patient is unconscious, uncooperative or NPO • immediate discontinuation (if an adverse drug reaction does occur, the infusion can be stopped)	• potential incompatibility when any two drugs are mixed in a syringe or solution • poor vascular access (in emergencies with venipunctures, or with infusions of extended irritating drugs, normally accessible veins may collapse or develop scarring) • severe adverse reactions may occur quickly due to high blood levels

PROCEDURE 34.11 Administering an Intradermal Injection

Action	Rationale
1. Explain the procedure and the medication(s) to the patient. Encourage questions.	Facilitates patient well-being and participation in care.
2. Follow the steps in Procedure 34.1.	
3. Gather equipment: • MAR or medication card • prepared medication with appropriate needle attached • alcohol swab • clean gloves.	Facilitates efficiency and economy of time.
4. Follow steps 5 to 8 of Procedure 34.9.	
5. With the nondominant hand, pull the skin taut between thumb and forefinger with selected site in the centre.	Taut skin is easier to pierce and less painful for the patient.
6. Using the dominant hand, allow loosened needle cap to slide off. Position the needle with bevel facing up and fingers below the syringe, almost parallel to the skin.	Hand position provides stability.
7. Using a 15° angle, insert the needle gently but firmly through the epidermis into dermis.	Using a greater angle will ultimately inject solution into the subcutaneous tissue, instead of the dermal tissue.
8. Without aspirating, slowly inject the fluid into the dermis to produce a small bleb (blister) under the skin.	Intradermal tissue contains no large blood vessels; thus, aspiration is not necessary. Slow injection causes gradual distention and is less painful for the patient.
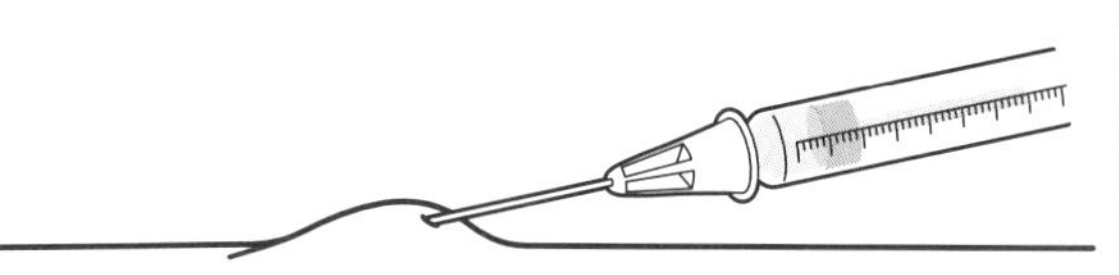	
9. Remove the needle swiftly and at the same angle as insertion.	Maintains patient comfort.
10. Do not recap needle. Discard directly into the nearest sharps container.	Prevents needle-stick injury.
11. Ensure patient comfort; wash hands and record medication.	Promotes patient well-being; prevents the spread of microorganisms and fulfills requirements for nurse accountability.

examples of medications administered in this way. Procedure 34.12 outlines the steps for adding medication to a primary IV container.

Assembling Equipment

The procedures for establishing and maintaining a primary IV line are described in Chapter 23. It is recommended that medication be added to a new solution container rather than an existing one. In some agencies the medication is prepared in the pharmacy department, while in others this is done by the nurse in the unit. The supplies and equipment the nurse will need include the IV solution (as ordered by the physician), the prescribed medication, a diluent if the medication is to be first reconstituted, a syringe with a 3.8-cm needle, alcohol swabs and a medication label. The IV container must be clearly labelled with the name of the

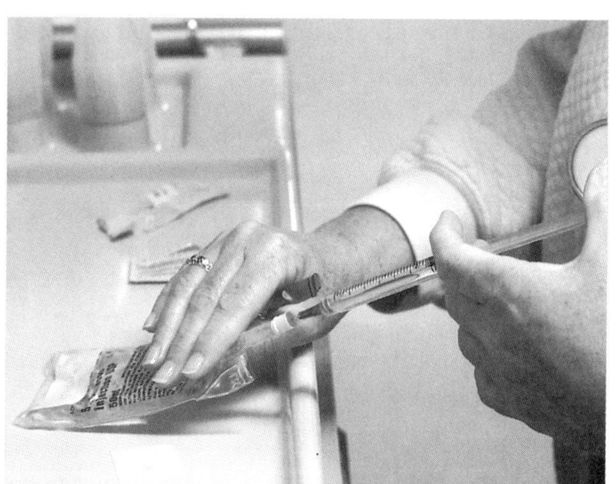

A nurse adds medication to an IV minibag.

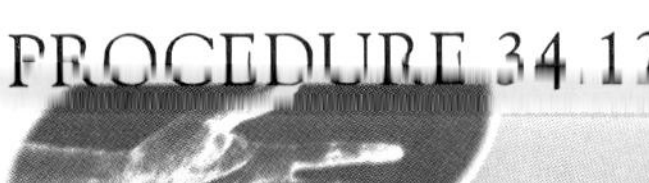

PROCEDURE 34.12 Adding Medication to a Primary IV Container

Action	*Rationale*
1. Explain the procedure and the medication(s) to the patient. Encourage questions.	Facilitates patient well-being and participation in care.
2. Follow the steps in Procedure 34.1.	
3. Check compatibility of diluent, medication and IV solution.	Prevents adverse reactions.
4. Gather equipment: • MAR or medication card • IV solution as ordered • prescribed medication • diluent • syringe with 3.8-cm needle • alcohol swabs • medication label.	Facilitates efficiency and economy of time.
5. Prepare the medication as in Procedure 34.4 or 34.5.	
6. Lay the solution container on a flat surface.	Facilitates ease of injecting medication.
7. Clean the resealable injection port.	Removes surface microorganisms.
8. Hold the injection port with thumb and forefinger of the nondominant hand, keeping the container horizontal on the flat surface.	Acts as a guide to insert the needle. If the bag is kept in a vertical position, the needle can easily travel through the side and poke the nurse. The nondominant hand will feel if the needle is coming through the side and it can easily be repositioned.
9. With the syringe in the dominant hand, slowly insert the needle into the centre of the port up to the hub. Inject the medication.	The needle must be inserted to the hub to ensure that the medication is injected into the container, not the port.

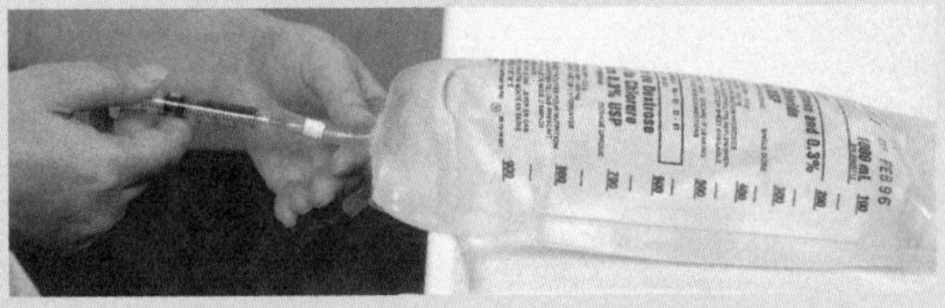

Action	*Rationale*
10. Remove the needle and dispose of syringe in the nearest sharps container.	Prevents needle-stick injury.
11. Prepare the medication label with the patient's name, medication, dosage, date and time and infusion rate of flow. Apply the label right side up on the solution container.	Provides identification. When the nurse is preparing numerous medications, an added safety measure is to put the label halfway on during preparation and remove the backing completely once the medication is in the bag.

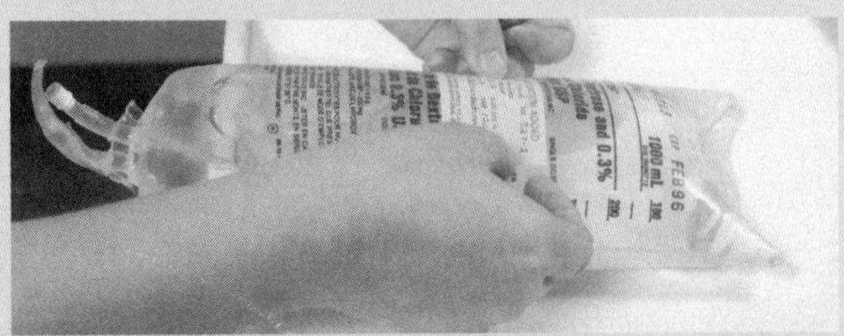

Action	*Rationale*
12. Gently agitate the solution container 4–5 times.	Distributes medication evenly and prevents a bolus of medication from forming.
13. Identify the patient.	Ensures the right patient.
14. Change the solution container, using principles of IV therapy outlined in Chapter 23.	
15. Ensure patient comfort; wash hands. Record medication and enter the solution in the fluid balance record according to agency policy.	Promotes patient well-being; prevents the spread of microorganisms. Fulfills requirements for nurse accountability and promotes continuity of care.
16. Carefully monitor the IV infusion and the patient for therapeutic and adverse effects of the medication.	Promotes safety and establishes need for care.

medication, the dose, the duration of infusion and the infusion rate of flow in order to avoid inadvertent error in administration.

ADMINISTERING MEDICATION THROUGH A SECONDARY IV LINE

Many intravenous medications are administered intermittently through the use of a separate, small-volume container that is connected to the patient's primary IV line. The medication is delivered over a short period of time, usually 30–60 minutes. This method permits the infusion of medications that are not compatible with the solution in the primary line or those that are stable in solution for only short periods of time (for example, antibiotics). Diluting the drug in a small amount of solution also decreases the risk of immediate drug reactions or local vein irritation. The steps in administering medication via a secondary IV line are outlined in Procedure 34.13.

Assembling Equipment

A secondary IV line is made up of a small solution bag, usually of 50-mL or 100-mL capacity (but may be more), that is connected to the highest injection port of the primary IV line by a short section of tubing, called a secondary medication set. This system is often called a *piggyback set-up* because the secondary unit "borrows the use of the primary line and equipment" (Earnest, 1993, p. 885). The secondary line is connected to the primary infusion by an 18-gauge needle, equipped with a protective needle lock which protects the nurse from needle-stick injury. If your agency is using a needleless IV access system, the secondary line is connected to the primary line via a lever lock or a threaded lock. The highest injection port is used because it has a backcheck valve that stops the infusion from the primary container when solution flows from the secondary container. Since IV flow is assisted by gravity, the secondary container is held higher by lowering the primary container on an extension hook. When the secondary infusion is finished and the level of fluid in the secondary tubing is lower than the fluid in the drip chamber of the primary line, the backcheck valve opens and the primary infusion begins to flow again. An extension hook is included in each secondary medication set. Figure 34.18 illustrates a secondary IV (piggyback) line. If medications are different or incompatible, a secondary line can be flushed. To clear the line of medication, open the secondary clamp and lower the bag below the primary line. This allows the primary solution to flow into the secondary line, and flushes the tubing.

When patients receive intermittent IV medications, for example q6 h, the secondary tubing is not changed every time a dose is given. The IV bag is left hanging after the medication has infused to maintain a closed system and reduce the risk of contamination. The secondary IV line is changed every 72 hours or per agency policy.

ADMINISTERING MEDICATION BY IV PUSH

circulation by direct injection (push) through an existing intravenous line. This route is selected when a rapid response is necessary and therefore is used frequently in emergencies. It is also used to deliver drugs that cannot be diluted, such as dilantin. Extreme caution must be used, since the complete dose of a medication is delivered in a short period of time and the drug is irretrievable. Many agencies have policies that specify the nurses permitted to administer drugs by this route, as well as the drugs they can administer. Some IV push drugs may be given only by the physician. All nurses, including students and graduates, must check agency policies before giving a medication by direct push. The steps in delivering medications by push through an existing IV line are outlined in Procedure 34.14.

Assembling Equipment

The size of the syringe will depend upon the amount of solution to be delivered. A larger needle is required to draw up the medication and a smaller one to administer it. Usually a 22-gauge, 2.5-cm needle is used for giving the medication in order to minimize the puncture holes created in the injection port with repeated instillations. In agencies employing a needleless IV administration (access) system, a blunt syringe cannula will be used instead of the needle. A watch with a second hand is also needed, because the medication must be administered carefully over a specified period of time.

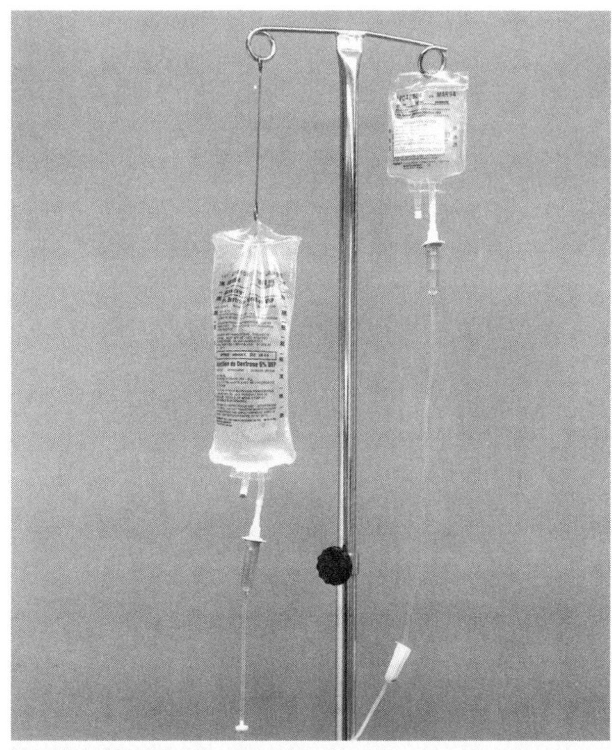

FIGURE 34.18 Secondary IV line (piggyback set-up)

PROCEDURE 34.13 Administering Medication Through a Secondary IV Line

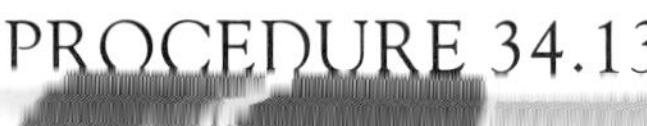

Action	Rationale
1. Explain the procedure and the medication(s) to the patient. Encourage questions.	Facilitates patient well-being and participation in care.
2. Follow the steps in Procedure 34.1.	
3. Check compatibility of diluent, medication and IV solution.	Prevents adverse reactions.
4. Gather equipment: • MAR or medication card • 50- or 100-mL solution bag • prescribed medication • diluent • syringe with 3.8-cm needle • alcohol swabs • medication label • secondary medication set with needle or secondary medication set with lever lock (needleless IV access system).	Facilitates efficiency and economy of time.
5. Add the medication to the solution bag and label it as in Procedure 34.12.	
6. Calculate the infusion rate of flow based on the amount of solution, the time in which it is to be administered and the drop factor of the tubing.	Promotes efficiency and economy of time at the bedside.
7. Assemble the secondary medication set. Close the roller clamp.	Prevents solution from leaking out while tubing is being primed.
8. Remove the protective cover from the tubing port on the secondary bag. Uncap the spike and, while holding the port with one hand, insert the spike with the other hand, using a firm, twisting motion.	Pulling downward quickly removes the cover and maintains sterility of the port. A twisting motion is needed to puncture the seal on the bag.
9. Prime the tubing by slowly opening the roller clamp. Close the roller clamp when the tubing is primed.	The tubing is short and will prime quickly. To decrease the risk of wasting medication, a secondary tube can be primed by backflushing the secondary tubing with primary solution.
10. At the bedside, hang the secondary bag on the IV pole.	Facilitates manual dexterity.
11. Identify the patient. *Note:* If a secondary line is already set up, the medication bag is changed using principles of IV therapy outlined in Chapter 23, and then steps 14 to 21 are implemented.	Ensures the right patient.
12. Clean the highest injection port on the primary tubing with alcohol.	Removes contaminants from port.
13. Remove the protective cap from the needle or lever lock on the secondary tubing and insert it into the injection port of the primary line.	Connects the secondary set to the primary line.
14. Lower the primary bag, using the extension hook.	Force of gravity assists the flow of solution from the secondary bag.
15. Completely open the clamp on the secondary set.	Establishes flow of the secondary infusion.
16. Regulate the rate of flow by adjusting the roller clamp on the primary tubing.	Solution ultimately flows into primary tubing; thus, it will regulate rate of flow.
17. Monitor the patient and the infusion.	Ensures safety.
18. When the secondary infusion is finished, clamp the secondary tubing, raise the primary bag to its original position and regulate the flow rate.	Re-establishes primary infusion at the required flow rate.
19. If the secondary line is to be reused, leave the empty bag attached to the system.	Decreases risk of contamination by minimizing disruption of the closed system.

PROCEDURE 34.13 *continued*

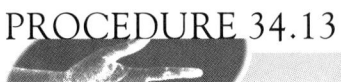

Action	*Rationale*
20. If the secondary line is not to be reused, remove it and discard. Make sure the needle is disposed of in a sharps container. The lever lock can be disposed of in a garbage container.	Promotes safety of nurse and others.
21. Record the medication and enter the solution and amount absorbed onto the fluid balance record per agency policy.	Fulfills requirements for nurse accountability and promotes continuity of care.

PROCEDURE 34.14 Administering a Medication by IV Push Through a Primary Line

Action	*Rationale*
1. Explain the procedure and the medication(s) to the patient. Encourage questions.	Facilitates patient well-being and participation in care.
2. Follow the steps in Procedure 34.1.	
3. Check the type and amount of diluent and the recommended administration time.	Ensures safety. The length of time required for injection varies with each medication. It is usually between one and five minutes.
4. Gather equipment: • MAR or medication card • prescribed medication • syringe • 22-gauge, 2.5-cm needle or syringe cannula, if using a needleless IV access system • diluent • alcohol swabs • watch with second hand.	Facilitates efficiency and economy of time.
5. Prepare the medication as in Procedures 34.4 and 34.5.	
6. Identify the patient.	Ensures the right patient.
7. Inspect the IV site for redness, swelling or discharge, and ask if the patient feels discomfort.	Ensures a patent site.
8. Sit on a chair or on the patient's bed and bring the tubing close.	IV push medications take several minutes, and sitting will allow the nurse to use proper body mechanics and talk to the patient.
9. Cleanse the port closest to the IV insertion site with an alcohol swab.	Removes surface particles.
10. Turn off the primary IV, if indicated.	
11. Insert the needle or syringe cannula completely into the port.	Inserting the needle only partway into the port will sequester the medication in the port, and it will not be delivered to the patient.
12. Administer the medication over the recommended period of time while monitoring the injection rate with a watch.	Permits the medication to disperse, thus decreasing irritation to the vein wall and promoting patient comfort. A bolus of medication delivered too fast may cause shock or embolism.
13. Reopen the primary IV and infuse slowly for 2–5 minutes.	Some of the medication will remain in the primary tubing.
14. Re-establish the prescribed rate.	Resuming the original primary rate will permit ample dispersion and prevent the problems mentioned above.
15. Observe the patient closely for reactions.	IV medications begin to work immediately.
16. Do not recap needle. Discard directly into nearest sharps container.	Prevents needle-stick injury.
17. Ensure patient comfort; wash hands and record medication.	Promotes patient well-being; prevents the spread of microorganisms and fulfills requirements for nurse accountability.

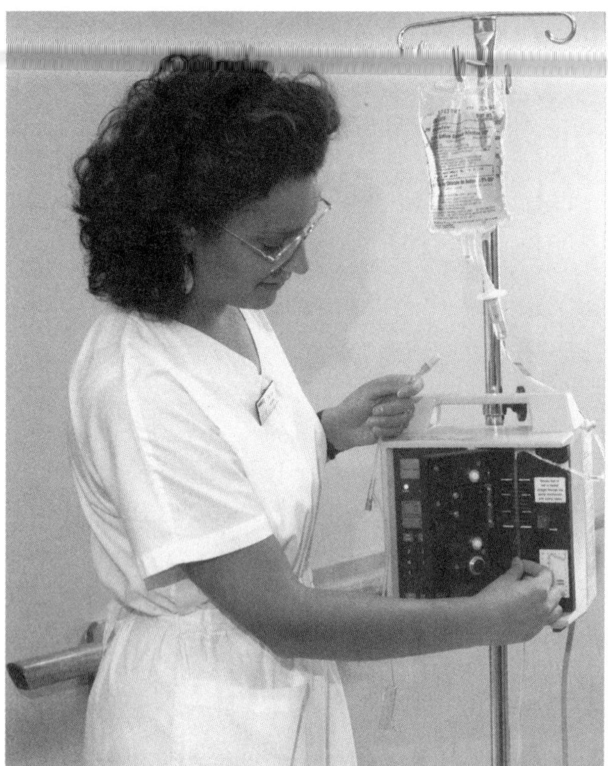

The use of an infusion pump facilitates accurate infusion of medications administered by continuous infusion.

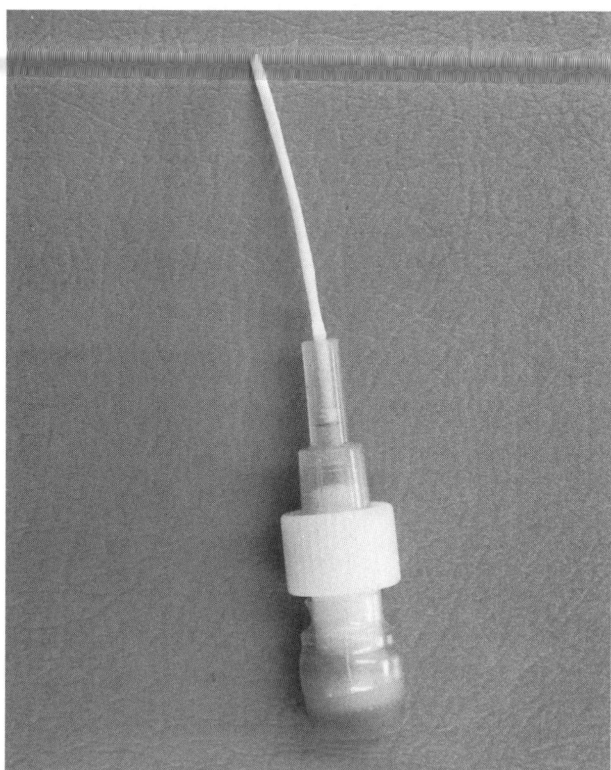

FIGURE 34.19 Intermittent infusion device connected to an angiocatheter

ADMINISTERING MEDICATION THROUGH AN INTERMITTENT INFUSION DEVICE

An intermittent infusion device is a reusable membrane or injection site connected to either a winged-tip needle with tubing or an angiocatheter placed in the patient's vein and maintained for regular, intermittent use (see Figure 34.19). Medications are administered either through a secondary IV line piggybacked to a primary IV line that is attached to the infusion device or by the direct push method. Between use, the infusion device is kept patent with normal saline or a dilute solution of heparin, thus the name *saline* or *heparin lock*. The advantage of a saline or heparin lock is that it allows intermittent access for intravenous medications while affording the patient freedom of movement when it is not being used.

An intermittent infusion device may be inserted specifically for administering medications, or an existing IV line may be converted to a heparin or saline lock when the patient no longer requires continuous infusion of fluids. The technique for inserting an intermittent infusion device is the same as for inserting a peripheral venipuncture device (see Procedure 23.2). However, instead of attaching a primary IV administration set to the venipuncture device, a male adapter plug is inserted into the needle or cannula hub. The infusion device is flushed after each use and according to agency policy with normal saline or dilute heparin solution to keep it patent. The care for the venipuncture device and site is the same as for peripheral intravenous infusion, outlined in Chapter 23. In this section we will describe the technique for converting an existing IV line to a saline or heparin lock (see Procedure 34.15). We will also detail how to administer medications through an intermittent infusion device using an IV line (see Procedure 34.16) and by IV push (see Procedure 34.17).

Assembling Equipment

An intermittent infusion device consists of an injection site or cap at one end and one of two basic types of adapter plugs at the other. The two types are the long male adapter plug (slip lock), which slides into the needle or cannula hub by friction, and the short male adapter plug (Luer lock), which twists into place. The injection site is a membrane made of a resealable rubber material similar to the injection ports on IV administration sets. The sites are usually accessed with a 22-gauge, 2.5-cm needle. In agencies using the needleless IV access system, a needleless syringe cannula is used for piercing the injection site.

As mentioned in the previous section, intermittent infusion devices must be flushed regularly to maintain patency. Agencies vary with regard to the type and amounts of solution used for flushing these devices. Heparin lock flush procedures call for 0.5–1 mL of dilute heparin solution, either 100 U/mL or 10 U/mL. Saline lock flushes require from 1–2 mL of normal saline.

PROCEDURE 34.15 Converting an IV Line to an Intermittent Infusion Device

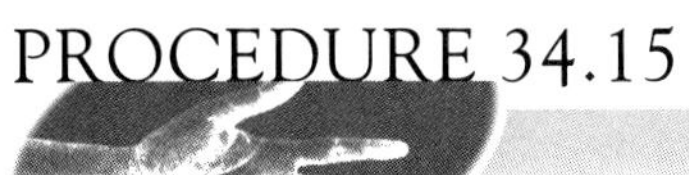

Action	*Rationale*
1. Check physician's order.	Ensures safety and avoids error.
2. Gather equipment: • intermittent infusion device per agency policy • dilute heparin or normal saline in a syringe with a 22-gauge, 2.5-cm needle or a syringe cannula, if using needleless IV access system • sterile gauze sponges • sterile protective cover • alcohol swab • clean gloves.	Facilitates efficiency and economy of time.
3. Identify the patient and explain the procedure.	Avoids error and promotes patient well-being.
4. Wash hands and maintain sterile technique throughout the procedure.	Prevents the spread of microorganisms.
5. Ready the equipment. Remove the tape anchoring the IV tubing and place a gauze sponge under the connector site. Open the sterile packages containing the intermittent infusion device and the protective cover. Place them within easy reach.	Facilitates efficiency. The gauze sponge absorbs moisture.
6. Turn off the IV.	
7. Apply gloves.	Protects the nurse from backflow of blood during the conversion.
8. Grasp the hub of the venipuncture device firmly with the nondominant hand and, at the same time, apply pressure to the distal end of the catheter tip with the little finger. With the dominant hand, disconnect the IV tubing from the venipuncture device and quickly insert the male adapter plug, keeping all ends sterile.	Stabilizes the venipuncture device and prevents it from becoming displaced during the procedure. Prevents backflow from the venipuncture device.
9. Apply the sterile protective cover over the connecter end of the tubing.	Maintains sterility of the connector end between uses.
10. Clean the injection cap with alcohol.	Avoids possible contamination.
11. Slowly inject the normal saline or heparin flush solution. Use positive pressure technique: remove needle from device at the same time the last 0.5 mL is being injected.	Prevents trauma to the vein wall and avoids a burning sensation. Prevents reflux of blood into the catheter as the needle is being withdrawn.
12. Do not recap needle. Discard directly into the nearest sharps container.	Prevents needle-stick injury.
13. Ensure patient comfort; discard supplies, wash hands.	Promotes patient well-being; ensures cleanliness and a safe work environment.
14. Document the procedure, noting the time, type of intermittent infusion device inserted, amount and type of flush solution.	Fulfills requirements for nurse accountability and promotes continuity of care.

When a medication is administered via an intermittent infusion device using an IV line, the procedure is similar to that for administering medication through a secondary line (see Procedure 34.13). A primary line is set up and a secondary administration set is usually piggybacked to it. A solution of 5 percent dextrose in water (D5W) is usually used in the primary line because it is the solution with which most medications are compatible. The exception to this rule is the diabetic patient for whom sugar is contraindicated; normal saline is used for these patients instead.

TOPICAL APPLICATIONS

Medications may be applied to the skin or mucous membranes in the form of aerosol sprays and foams, creams, gels and jellies, liniments, lotions, ointments, pastes, powders and transdermal patches.

PROCEDURE 34.16

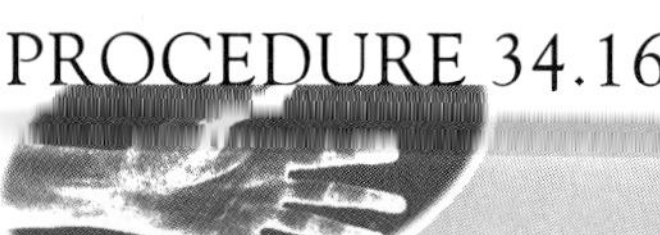

Administering Medication Through an Intermittent Infusion Device Using an IV Line

Action	Rationale
1. If one has not been established, prepare a primary IV line as outlined in Procedure 23.1.	Provides the IV line for the secondary medication set.
Place a protective covering over the connector end of the tubing.	Prepares for connection to the intermittent infusion device.
2. Prepare medication and secondary medication set as in Procedure 34.13. In addition, gather, per agency protocol: • 1-mL or 2-mL normal saline solution in a syringe with a 22-gauge, 2.5-cm needle or needleless syringe cannula • alcohol swabs.	Promotes efficiency and economy of time.
3. Connect the secondary medication set to the primary IV line as in Procedure 34.13. (This is done at the bedside if there is an existing primary IV line.)	
4. At the bedside, identify the patient.	Avoids error.
5. Cleanse the injection cap with alcohol and flush the device with normal saline.	Determines patency and placement of the venipuncture device. Checks patient comfort at the site.
6. Cleanse the injection cap with alcohol and connect the primary IV line.	Prevents entry of surface contaminants into the system.
Note: If using an existing primary line, first attach a sterile 22-gauge, 2.5-cm needle or a needleless lever lock to the connector end of the tubing.	Ensures sterility of connector.
7. Establish the primary line infusion, then lower the primary container and open the roller clamp on the secondary tubing. Regulate the rate of flow.	Establishes flow of medication.
8. Monitor the patient and the infusion.	Ensures patient safety.
9. When the medication infusion is finished, prepare dilute heparin or normal saline solution per agency policy.	Prepares for disconnection of primary IV line and flush procedure.
10. Close the roller clamp and disconnect the primary line. Remove and discard the needle into a sharps container. Place a sterile protective cover over the connector end of the tubing.	Maintains sterility of connector end between uses.
11. Cleanse the injection cap with alcohol and slowly inject heparin or normal saline solution. Use positive pressure techniques: remove needle from device at the same time the last 0.5 mL is being injected.	Maintains patency of the venipuncture device and vein. Prevents reflux of blood into the catheter as the needle is being withdrawn.
12. Do not recap needles. Discard directly into the nearest sharps container.	Prevents needle-stick injury.
13. Ensure patient comfort; discard supplies, wash hands and record medication.	Promotes patient well-being; prevents the spread of microorganisms and fulfills requirements for nurse accountability.

Aerosol sprays provide a thin layer of medication on a designated area. They are generally used when large areas of the skin are to be treated or when manual application would be uncomfortable for the patient.

Aerosol foams provide a layer of medicated foam and are generally used in hairy areas such as the rectum or vagina.

Creams are semi-solid, nongreasy, water-soluble preparations that are usually applied on an area where esthetics is a consideration or on moist areas.

Gels and *jellies* are semi-solid preparations that are often clear or translucent. These preparations contain water or alcohol. They liquefy when applied to the skin and are especially useful for lubrication.

Liniments are liquids that are applied to the skin by rubbing. They are frequently used to warm an affected area through the superficial dilation of blood vessels. This also helps to relax tight muscles. The application of lotions or liniments is often a clean rather than a sterile procedure in

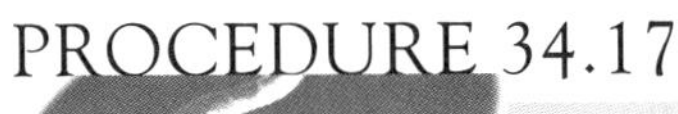

PROCEDURE 34.17 Administering an IV Push Medication Through an

Action	Rationale
1. Prepare medication as in Procedure 34.14. In addition, gather, per agency policy: • syringe with 1–2 mL normal saline • syringe with 2–3 mL normal saline • syringe with dilute heparin or normal saline solution • 3 22-gauge, 2.5-cm needles or needleless syringe cannulas (one for each syringe) • alcohol swabs.	
2. At the bedside, identify the patient.	Ensures the right patient.
3. Inspect the IV site for redness, swelling or discharge, and ask if the patient is experiencing discomfort.	Assesses for inflammation and patency of site.
4. Sit on a chair or on the patient's bed and bring the extremity with the infusion device close.	IV push medications take several minutes; sitting will allow the nurse to use proper body mechanics and talk to the patient.
5. Cleanse the injection cap with an alcohol swab each time a needle or needleless cannula is inserted.	Removes surface particles and prevents entry of contaminants into system.
6. Attach the syringe with 1-mL or 2-mL normal saline and flush the intermittent infusion device.	Determines patency and placement of the venipuncture device. Checks patient comfort of the site.
7. Administer the medication over the recommended period of time while monitoring the injection rate with a watch.	Permits the medication to disperse, decreasing irritation to the vein wall and promoting patient comfort. A bolus of medication delivered too fast may cause shock or embolism.
8. Attach the syringe with 2–3 mL normal saline and slowly instill the solution into the infusion device.	Flushes medication out of the venipuncture device, ensures medication is dispersed into the system and prevents a bolus effect.
9. Attach the syringe with dilute heparin or normal saline and slowly instill the solution. Use positive pressure technique: remove the needle from the device at the same time the last 0.5 mL is being injected.	Maintains patency of the venipuncture device and vein. Prevents reflux of blood into the catheter as the needle is being withdrawn.
10. Do not recap needles. Discard directly into the nearest sharps container.	Prevents needle-stick injury.
11. Ensure patient comfort; discard supplies, wash hands and record medication.	Promotes patient well-being; prevents the spread of microorganisms and fulfills requirements for nurse accountability.

a home situation. In a hospital or other inpatient facility, however, it is advisable to use sterile cotton balls or gauze to apply the liquid. More commonly, clean disposable gloves are worn on the hand being used for the application, unless the skin is broken, which would require the use of sterile gloves.

Lotions are liquid preparations that are usually applied to protect, soothe or soften surface areas, to relieve itching or to prevent the growth of microorganisms.

Ointments are preparations with a fatty base, such as lard, petroleum jelly or oils. They may be applied to the skin or mucous membranes, where they are melted by the heat of the body and absorbed. Ointments are frequently used for antiseptic or antimicrobial purposes. As with lotions and liniments, it is advisable in an institutional setting to use sterile equipment for applying them. Sterile gloves are not needed, since the ointment is applied with a sterile tongue depressor.

Pastes are similar to ointments, but they do not penetrate the skin; they contain more powder and are stiff in consistency. They may absorb moisture and provide protection from secretions such as urine and feces.

Powders are nonabsorbable, finely ground preparations that are applied as protection to reduce friction on dry areas. However, they cause clumping on wet areas and must be used selectively.

Transdermal patches are an effective means to administer drugs for local or systemic effect. This method of drug therapy utilizes a multilayered adhesive patch consisting of an occlusive (often skin-coloured) backing film, a film that contains a drug reservoir, a microporous semi-permeable membrane that controls the rate of drug delivery, an adhesive layer and a protective strip that is peeled off before application. The drug is made lipid-soluble; once it penetrates the epidermis by passive diffusion, it is then absorbed into the systemic circulation at a constant rate. The advantages of this route include noninvasiveness, ability to maintain a consistent serum drug level and suitability for people who are unable to take oral medications. It is also a good means of delivering drugs that are not well absorbed in the gastrointestinal tract or metabolized by the liver. Finally, the convenience of transdermal patches encourages compliance, as some are effective for up to seven days. The disadvantages of patches include the possibility of dislodgement from active patients, slow onset of action (up to 72 hours for peak serum levels) and difficulty in making dosage adjustments or reversing toxic effects (up to 12 hours). Transdermal patches may also cause skin redness, irritation or hypersensitivity. Some examples of drugs administered transdermally are nitroglycerin (Nitro-Dur), fentanyl (Duragesic), scopolamine (Transderm-V), hormones (estrogen and testosterone) and nicotine prescribed for smoking cessation (Nicoderm).

Procedure 34.18 describes the steps in applying topical medications, while Procedure 34.19 deals with application and removal of a transdermal patch.

INSTILLATIONS INTO THE EAR

Instillation means introducing small amounts (drops) of a medication into a body opening. Common sites for instillations are the ear, eye, nose, throat, vagina and rectum.

Liquid medications are instilled into the ear cavity usually for one of two purposes: to insert a softening agent so that earwax can be removed easily, or to introduce an antibiotic suspension in cases where the ear canal or the eardrum is infected. The technique of instilling medication into the ear is presented in Procedure 34.20.

Assembling Equipment

A medicine tray, a sterile medicine dropper, the bottle of medication and some sterile cotton balls will be needed.

PROCEDURE 34.18 Application of Topical Medication

Action	*Rationale*
1. Follow the steps in Procedure 34.1.	
2. Gather equipment: • MAR or medication card • container of prescribed medication • sterile 5 cm × 5 cm gauze or cotton balls • tongue depressor • clean gloves • sterile gloves and dressing tray (optional, if the area is covered).	Facilitates efficiency and economy of time.
3. At the bedside, identify the patient.	Ensures the right patient.
4. Explain the procedure and purpose of medication.	Promotes patient well-being and enables participation in care.
5. Ensure that the area to be treated is clean.	Removes drainage, reduces microorganisms and enhances effectiveness of application.
6. Observe the area for discharge, redness, swelling, bleeding or odour, and ask if the patient is experiencing discomfort, itchiness, burning.	Provides information that is necessary for ongoing evaluation of treatment.
7. Apply gloves, if necessary.	Gloves reduce transmission of microorganisms and accord with body substance precautions. Also, it is often easier to apply some medications wearing gloves rather than by using tongue depressors.
8. Place a small amount of medication on a sterile gauze or a tongue depressor. If a tongue depressor or gauze is used, do not return it to the container.	Prevents the transmission of microorganisms.
9. Apply the medication to the desired area according to package directions (for example, liniments should be rubbed in long, smooth strokes).	Each preparation is different. Some require massage, others should be put on skin with minimal disruption of tissue.
10. Remove gloves: peel from the wrist downward, and collect one glove inside the other.	Prevents transmission of microorganisms.
11. Wash hands and apply a sterile dressing, if necessary.	Keeps medication from soiling bed linen and patient's gown.
12. Wash hands and record procedure.	Prevents the spread of microorganisms and meets requirements for nurse accountability.

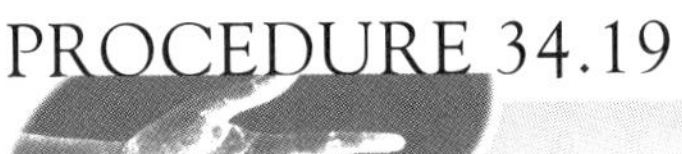

PROCEDURE 34.19 Applying and Removing a Transdermal Patch

Action	*Rationale*
A. APPLICATION	
1. Prepare patient; explain procedure.	Reduces anxiety and fear, and enables patient participation.
2. Assess the patient's status.	Provides baseline data for medication effect.
3. Wash hands and gather equipment and supplies: • clean gloves • wash basin • water • towel • scissors or clippers, if necessary.	Reduces transfer of microorganisms and facilitates efficiency and economy of time.
4. Draw bed curtains.	Promotes privacy.
5. Consult manufacturer's directions and assess the patient's skin to locate a suitable area for application. Generally, locations are nonhairy, flat, clean, dry, intact areas—behind the ear; on the front or the back of the torso, chest or shoulders, side, lower back or buttock; or the inner or outer aspect of the upper arm.	Promotes good adhesion and absorption of medication and even distribution through areas of smooth, permeable skin.
Areas to be avoided include: • skin folds (trunk or lower abdomen, breasts)	Wrinkles interfere with patch adhesion.
• areas distal to the knee or elbow	Excessive movements may dislodge patch or speed absorption owing to dilated capillaries and increased circulation from exercise.
• areas of irritation, rashes, burns, or abrasions	Increased absorption may occur from inflamed areas.
• scarred areas.	Decreased drug absorption may occur owing to skin changes.
6. Wash the chosen skin area with water; dry thoroughly. Unless otherwise indicated in package directions, do not use soap, oils, lotions, alcohol or other products. If hair must be removed, clip with scissors or clippers but do not shave the skin.	Washing removes debris from skin; drying promotes good adherence of patch. These products alter the absorption of drug. Shaving irritates the skin or may alter the skin's integrity, letting the drug penetrate too quickly.
7. Put on clean gloves; remove the patch from the pouch and avoid cutting or tearing the patch.	Protects nurse's skin from medication. Preserves integrity of the medication reservoir.
8. Remove the protective liner from the adhesive and avoid touching the adhesive surface.	Ensures that the patch will adhere.
9. Stick the adhesive surface onto the skin and press firmly with the palm of the hand for about 10 seconds. Run a finger around the edge. Write the date and time on the patch.	Ensures secure adhesion to the skin, especially around the edges. Provides visual reminder and ensures correct administration times.
10. Remove gloves and wash hands thoroughly.	Prevents nurse from absorbing any medications that may have been left on hands.
11. Record medication administration information on MAR: drug, dose, site, time; assessment of skin before application of patch.	Documents treatment, teaching and response to therapy; provides baseline for future assessments.
B. REMOVAL	
1. Wash hands thoroughly; don clean gloves.	Prevents the spread of microorganisms; projects nurse's hands from medication.
2. The old patch is removed and a new one applied, according to the schedule prescribed by the physician and recommended by the manufacturer. Generally, with a daily schedule, the patch is changed at the same time each day. The sites are rotated; a different area of skin is used for each patch.	Ensures medication is administered as prescribed. Ensures a continuous effect. Avoids skin irritation.

continued on next page

PROCEDURE 34.19 continued

Action	Rationale
3. To remove the patch, press down on the centre of the patch, then grasp the edge or tab if present. Gently and slowly peel the patch from the skin.	Raises the outer edge away from the skin and aids in loosening the edge for removal.
4. Fold the used patch in half with the adhesive sides together; place in the pouch from the new patch (if available) and discard safely away from children and pets.	Avoids exposure to residual medication. Prevents inadvertent absorption of residual medication; may also be toxic if ingested.
5. Wash the area and dry thoroughly.	Removes residual medication.
6. Assess the skin for irritation, excess redness or itching.	Some medications result in mild redness, itching or contact dermatitis and should disappear in a few hours.
7. Remove gloves; wash hands thoroughly.	Prevents inadvertent absorption of medication.
8. Record time of removal, assessment of skin and therapeutic effects.	Provides communication and documents care.

PROCEDURE 34.20 Instilling Medication into the Ear

Action	Rationale
1. Follow the steps in Procedure 34.1.	Facilitates efficiency and economy of time.
2. Gather equipment: • MAR or medication card • container of prescribed medication • medicine tray • sterile medicine dropper • sterile cotton balls • cotton-tipped applicators • clean gloves.	
3. At the bedside, identify the patient.	Ensures the right patient.
4. Explain the procedure and the purpose of the medication to the patient.	Promotes patient well-being and enables participation in care.
5. Ask the patient to lie on the side with the ear to be treated facing upward.	Facilitates instillation and absorption of medication.
6. Put on gloves.	Gloves should be worn when there is potential contact with body secretions.
7. Observe the auditory meatus for discharge, redness, swelling, bleeding or odour, and ask if the patient experiences discomfort, itchiness or burning.	Provides information that is necessary for ongoing evaluation of treatment.
8. Clean the auditory meatus with a cotton-tipped applicator.	Removes any drainage.
9. Draw medication into applicator.	Facilitates instillation and absorption.
10. With nondominant hand, straighten the auditory canal. **Adult:** Gently pull the pinna upward and back.	The anatomy of the ear canal of adults and children is quite different and must be taken into account.

PROCEDURE 34.20 *continued*

Action	*Rationale*
Children under 3 years: Gently pull the pinna down and back.	
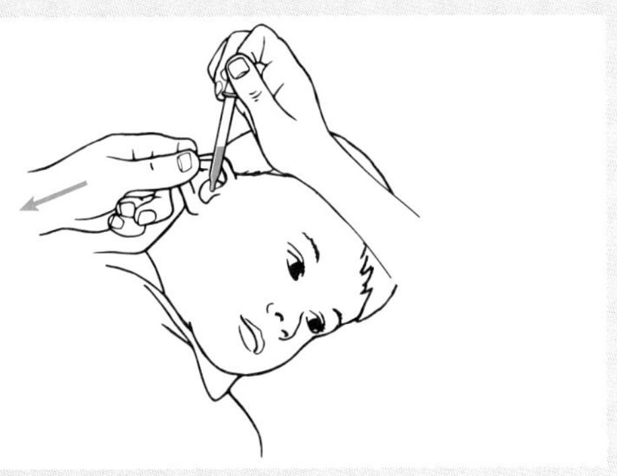	
11. With dominant hand, instill the medication along the side of the ear canal, counting the correct number of drops.	Facilitates distribution of medication into the ear canal.
12. Gently massage tragus (cartilaginous protrusion at the entrance to the ear canal).	Prevents medication from escaping out of the ear canal.
13. Loosely place a cotton ball at the meatus of the auditory canal and leave there for 20 minutes. Encourage the patient to remain on the side for five minutes following treatment.	
14. Wash hands and record the procedure.	Prevents the transfer of microorganisms and meets requirements for nurse accountability.

Many preparations are packaged for individual use and come with an attached dropper.

The medication should always be warmed before being inserted into the ear. A temperature of 40.6° C is recommended. Cool solutions are not comfortable and may cause dizziness or nausea because the equilibrium sense receptors in the semi-circular canals are stimulated. The bottle of ear drops may be placed in a small open container of warm water for a few minutes before it is to be used. The temperature of the solution may be tested by dropping a small amount on the inner aspect of the wrist. If it feels comfortable (neither hot nor cool), the solution should be comfortable for the patient.

INSTILLATIONS INTO THE EYE

Liquid medications in the form of eye drops or ointments are instilled into the eye for several reasons: to soothe the irritated eye, to dilate the pupil for an eye examination, to apply an anesthetic or to combat infection. It is best to use aseptic technique, since the eye is vulnerable to infection. Eye medications should *never* be shared between patients. The technique for instilling medications into the eye is outlined in Procedure 34.21.

Assembling Equipment

Most eye medications come in bottles with their own dropper or in tubes of ointment. A soft cloth or cotton balls

PROCEDURE 34.21 Instilling Medications into the Eye

Action	*Rationale*
1. Follow the steps in Procedure 34.1.	Facilitates efficiency and economy of time.
2. Gather equipment: • MAR or medication card • prescribed eye drops or ointment • medicine tray • soft cloth or cotton balls • warm water • sterile eye pad, if needed • clean gloves.	
3. At the bedside, identify the patient.	Ensures the right patient.
4. Explain the procedure and the purpose of the medication to the patient.	Promotes patient well-being and enables participation in care.
5. Put on gloves.	Gloves should be worn when there is potential contact with body secretions.
6. Cleanse secretions or crusts on the eyelid and lashes with a soft cloth or with cotton balls dipped in warm water.	Cleaning the eye will give the medication the opportunity to work and is more esthetically pleasing for the patient.
7. Give the patient a cotton ball or tissue to use after the instillation.	With some medications, it is necessary to block the nasolacrimal duct after liquid applications to prevent systemic effects. The cotton ball or tissue can also be used to catch excess medication and prevent it from running down the cheek.
8. If possible, have the patient sit or lie supine with the head tilted back.	Permits absorption of the medication into the canthus or cornea.
9. Observe the eye for redness, discharge or swelling. Ask if the patient experiences burning, itching, blurring, diplopia or photophobia.	Provides information that is necessary for ongoing evaluation of treatment.
10. Open the medication container and, if there is a dropper, fill it with the prescribed amount of medication.	
11. Ask the patient to look toward the ceiling.	Lessens the urge to blink by partially protecting the cornea.
12. While resting the nondominant hand on the cheek and using the thumb and forefinger, gently pull downward on skin below the eye.	Exposes the conjunctiva and provides stability. Prevents fingers from poking cornea; does not put pressure on eyeball, and prevents the patient from blinking.

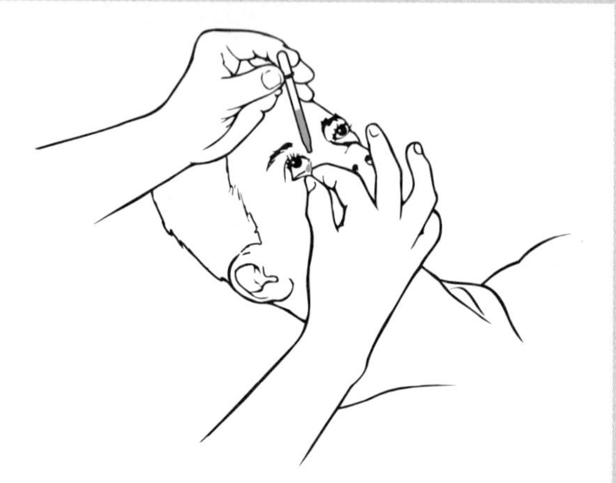

13. Hold the medication in the dominant hand and rest the hand on patient's forehead.	Provides stability and prevents poking the cornea.

PROCEDURE 34.21 *continued*

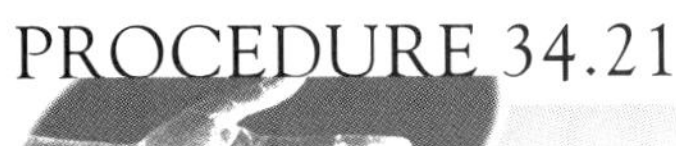

Action	Rationale
14. **Eye drops:** Squeeze the bulb of the dropper gently, being careful to dispense only the required amount of drops. **Ointment:** Gently squeeze the tube to fill the length of the conjunctival sac, moving from inner to outer canthus.	
15. Ask the patient to close the eye for 2–3 minutes, but avoid tightly squeezing the eye shut.	Allows absorption and dispersal of medication. Squeezing the eye will force the medication out of the eye.
16. Instruct the patient to block the nasolacrimal duct for 30 seconds.	Prevents medication from running out of eye and into duct.
17. Gently wipe the eyes from inner to outer canthus.	Collects excess medication.
18. If necessary, apply a sterile eye pad.	
19. Wash hands and record procedure.	Prevents transmission of microorganisms and meets requirements for nurse accountability.

and warm water may be necessary to remove secretions and crusting on the eyelids.

INSTILLATIONS INTO THE NOSE

The usual purpose of instilling medication into the nose is either to heal infection or to shrink swollen membranes. The instillation of medication into the nose is not usually a sterile procedure. The technique is presented in Procedure 34.22.

Assembling Equipment

Nasal instillations may be in the form of drops, administered with a dropper that is attached to the medication bottle. They may also come in the form of an inhaler or an atomizer.

PROCEDURE 34.22 Instilling Medications into the Nose

Action	Rationale
1. Follow the steps in Procedure 34.1.	
2. Gather equipment: • MAR or medication card • prescribed medication with dropper • medicine tray • towel or tissues.	Facilitates efficiency and economy of time.
3. At the bedside, identify the patient.	Ensures the right patient.
4. Explain the procedure and the purpose of the medication to the patient.	Promotes patient well-being and enables participation in care.
5. Ask the patient to blow the nose and assess the discharge noting colour, consistency and odour. Ask the patient to describe any congestion or difficulty breathing, and note facial discomfort and any discharge from the nares.	Provides information that is necessary for ongoing evaluation of treatment.
6. Position the patient according to the area to be used.	
Eustachian tube: Back-lying position. The drops will flow into the nasopharynx.	Eustachian tube opens into the nasopharynx.
Ethmoid and sphenoid sinuses: Proetz position. That is, back-lying with the head over the edge of the bed, or place a pillow under the shoulders to tip the head backwards.	Allows drainage into ethmoid and sphenoid sinuses.

continued on next page

PROCEDURE 34.22 *continued*

Action	*Rationale*
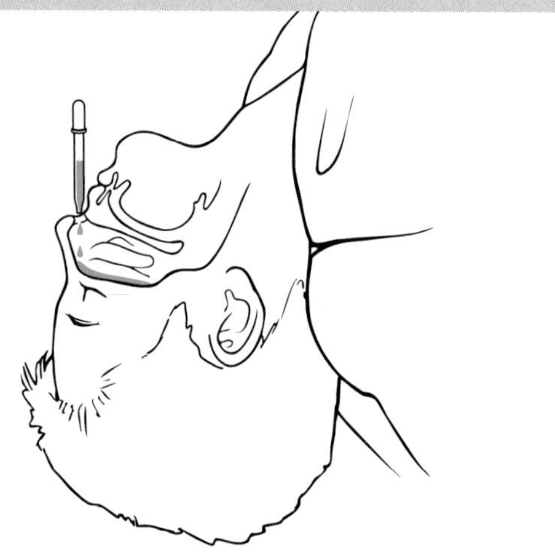	
Maxillary and frontal sinuses: Parkinson position. That is, the same as Proetz position except that the head is turned to the side to be treated. Ensure patient comfort by supporting the head.	Allows drainage into maxillary and frontal sinuses.
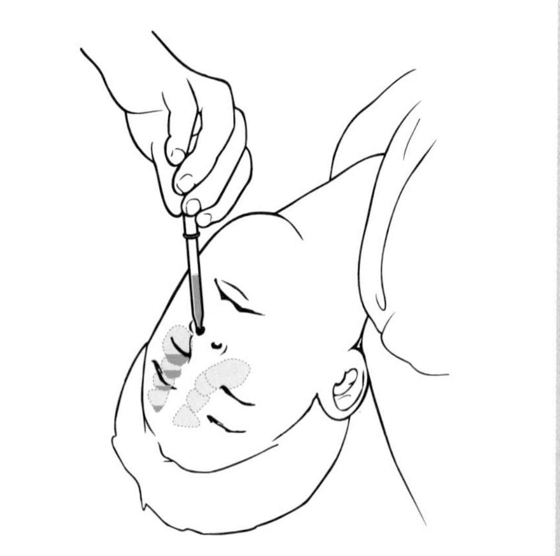	
7. Draw up prescribed amount of solution into dropper.	
8. With the dropper slightly above the nostril, instill the medication towards the midline. Do not touch the mucous membranes of the nares with dropper.	Allows maximum solution to be absorbed. Touching mucous membranes with dropper would contaminate it and cause potential cross-contamination of the medication.
9. Ask the patient to remain in the position for 5–10 minutes.	Allows the solution to disperse into the entire area.
10. Reassess the patient immediately and when medication is expected to be effective.	Provides information for evaluation of care.
11. Leave the patient comfortable.	
12. Wash hands and record procedure.	Prevents transmission of microorganisms and meets requirements for nurse accountability.

INSTILLATIONS INTO THE THROAT

The throat may be either sprayed or painted as means of [illegible] are outlined in Procedure 34.23.

Assembling Equipment

Cotton-tipped applicators are used to paint medications onto tissues of the throat. A tongue depressor is needed to keep the tongue out of the way. A flashlight will help to visualize the area.

INSTILLATIONS INTO THE VAGINA

Medications are usually instilled into the vagina to combat infection or to relieve discomfort. They may be applied in the form of a suppository or an ointment. Suppositories are inserted with the index finger of the nurse's gloved hand. Ointments for use in the vagina usually come in a narrow tube with an attached plunger. Procedure 34.24 outlines the steps for administering vaginal instillations.

Assembling Equipment

In addition to the medications, the nurse will need clean [illegible] suppositories that do not come prelubricated. A perineal pad may be used to absorb any leakage.

INSTILLATIONS INTO THE RECTUM

Medications are inserted into the rectum to provide local or systemic effects. Rectal suppositories are commonly used to stimulate bowel function. The steps in administering a rectal instillation are given in Procedure 34.25.

Assembling Equipment

The medication, clean gloves, water-soluble lubricant and a disposable incontinence pad will be needed. If the suppository is used to stimulate defecation in a patient, a commode or toilet should be nearby.

PROCEDURE 34.23 Administering a Medication into the Throat

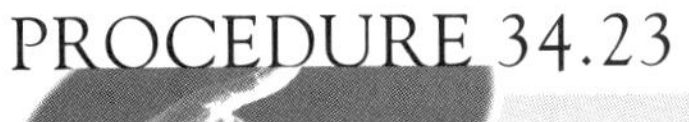

Action	*Rationale*
1. Follow the steps in Procedure 34.1.	Facilitates efficiency and economy of time.
2. Gather equipment: • MAR or medication card • prescribed medication • medicine tray • cotton-tipped applicators • tongue depressor • flashlight.	
3. At the bedside, identify the patient.	Ensures the right patient.
4. Explain the procedure and the purpose of the medication to the patient.	Promotes patient well-being and enables participation in care.
5. Ask the patient to sit upright. Stand directly in front of the patient and look down into the throat. A good light is essential for this procedure.	Provides the best position to visualize throat and instill the medication.
6. Ask the patient to tilt the head backward (or help him or her to do this) and to open the mouth. Using the nondominant hand, hold down the tongue with a tongue depressor.	Permits the nurse to view the throat.
7. Apply the spray or medication, using either an atomizer for spraying or cotton-tipped applicators for painting the tissues.	Ensures the prescribed dose has been delivered.
8. Inspect the throat and ensure that the entire area has been covered.	
9. Leave the patient comfortable.	Promotes patient well-being.
10. Wash hands and record procedure.	Prevents transmission of microorganisms and meets requirements for nurse accountability.

PROCEDURE 34.24

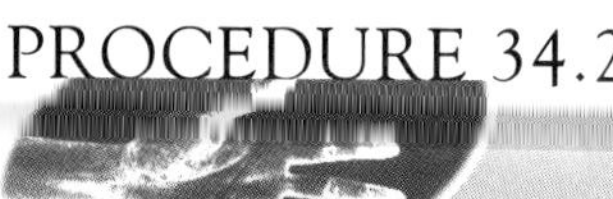

Administering a Medication into the Vagina

Action	Rationale
1. Follow the steps in Procedure 34.1.	
2. Gather equipment: • MAR or medication card • prescribed vaginal cream or suppository • lubricant, if necessary • clean gloves • perineal pad, if necessary.	Facilitates efficiency and economy of time.
3. At the bedside, identify the patient.	Ensures the right patient.
4. Explain the procedure and the purpose of the medication to the patient.	Promotes patient well-being and enables participation in care.
5. Ask the patient to void prior to the procedure and, if possible, to wash the perineum.	An empty bladder will promote patient comfort. A clean perineum facilitates accurate assessment. A clean surface promotes absorption.
6. Ensure privacy.	Promotes patient well-being and decreases embarrassment.
7. Don gloves.	Prevents the spread of microorganisms and accords with body substance precautions.
8. Ask the patient to lie on her back with knees flexed and hips rotated laterally. If the patient can tolerate it, place a pillow under the hips. Drape the patient so that only the perineum is exposed.	A pillow will help to prevent the medication from leaking out. Ensures comfort and warmth and decreases embarrassment.
9. Observe the vagina and perineum for redness, lesions, discharge or odours. Ask if patient experiences discomfort, itchiness, burning or other symptoms.	Provides information that is necessary for ongoing evaluation of treatment.
10. **Vaginal suppository:** Remove the suppository from the package; lubricate it if necessary.	Facilitates insertion and decreases discomfort.
Using the nondominant hand, separate the labia majora and minora. With the middle and forefinger of the dominant hand, insert the suppository approximately 8–10 cm along the posterior wall of the vagina.	Exposes the vaginal orifice. The posterior aspect of the vagina is longer than the anterior wall, because of the protrusion of the cervix into the anterior wall.
Vaginal cream, jelly, foam: Using manufacturer's directions, instill the required amount of medication into the applicator. Insert the applicator approximately 5 cm and slowly inject the plunger until medication has been distributed. Remove the applicator and place it on a paper towel or directly into garbage.	
11. Remove gloves: peel from the wrist down and collect one glove inside the other.	Turning the gloves inside out will minimize spread of the vaginal discharge and microorganisms.
12. Assist the patient to straighten her legs, and instruct her to remain supine for 10 minutes following treatment.	Returns the patient to a position of comfort and ensures the medication will be absorbed into the posterior fornix once it has melted.
13. Apply a clean perineal pad.	
14. Wash hands and record procedure.	Prevents the spread of microorganisms and meets requirements for nurse accountability.

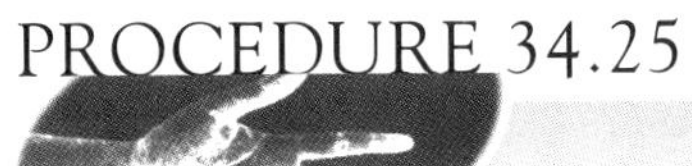

PROCEDURE 34.25 Administering a Medication into the Rectum

Action	*Rationale*
1. Follow the steps in Procedure 34.1.	Facilitates efficiency and economy of time.
2. Gather equipment: • MAR or medication card • prescribed suppository • lubricant, if necessary • clean gloves • incontinence pad.	
3. At the bedside, identify the patient.	Ensures the right patient.
4. Explain the procedure and the purpose of the medication to the patient.	Promotes patient well-being and enables participation in care.
5. Provide privacy and ask the patient to lie on the left side with knees flexed.	In this position, the sigmoid is in the lowest position and decreases the potential for feces to be expelled.
6. Drape the patient so that only the buttocks are exposed.	Ensures comfort and warmth and decreases embarrassment.
7. Apply gloves.	Prevents the spread of microorganisms.
8. Assess the anal area for redness, swelling, lesions, hemorrhoids, discharge and odour and ask if patient experiences any burning, itchiness or discomfort.	Provides information that is necessary for ongoing evaluation of treatment.
9. Remove the suppository from the wrapper and, if necessary, lubricate it. Lubricate the middle finger of the dominant hand.	Facilitates insertion.
10. Ask the patient to breathe through the mouth. Touch the anal sphincter with middle finger.	Facilitates relaxation of anal sphincter.
11. Using the middle finger, insert the suppository into the anal sphincter (small pointed end first) as far as possible along the wall of the rectum. This will be approximately 10 cm for an adult and 5 cm for a child.	The middle finger is the longest and will be able to insert the farthest. The pointed end will facilitate insertion and decrease discomfort. The suppository will be absorbed by the mucosa of the wall of the rectum.
12. Remove the finger and peel off the glove by pulling down from the wrist and turning it inside out.	Reduces possibility for transmission of microorganisms.
13. Cover the patient and advise him or her to lie in this position for up to 30 minutes (if possible).	Facilitates absorption of the medication.
14. Wash hands and record procedure.	Prevents transmission of microorganisms and meets requirements for nurse accountability.

SPECIAL CHALLENGES IN ADMINISTERING MEDICATIONS

Alterations in Consciousness or Orientation

It is important for the nurse to assess for and report *any* difficulties that are encountered when administering a medication, as these can lead to further problems for the patient. For example, a patient with a decreased level of consciousness may not have a gag reflex and is at risk for aspirating an oral medication. The nurse may request that another route be ordered or that a feeding tube be inserted. Similarly, the disoriented patient may simply refuse to swallow an oral medication. The nurse must consider other routes and also, whenever possible, give medications when the patient is most alert and oriented.

Illness

Some illnesses do not affect the patient's ability to take and retain medications; others do. The nauseated patient may not be able to retain oral medications. In this instance, an antiemetic may be administered one hour prior to the administration of other oral medications, or another route may be considered. On the other hand, some patients are so fatigued that it is overwhelming to attempt to swallow numerous oral medications. The nurse can often work around this by offering medications at spaced intervals throughout the day, giving the medications when the patient has the most energy, or considering another route.

Other Potential Challenges

Another area of nursing practice is concerned with idiosyncratic reactions to medications, overdoses of drugs and the ingestion of poisonous materials. Many medical centres provide immediate information to people about the antidotes and emergency measures for common poisons. Poison control centres are located in many large cities. A list of poison control centres in Canada is contained in the *Compendium of Pharmaceuticals and Specialties of Canada* (CPS).

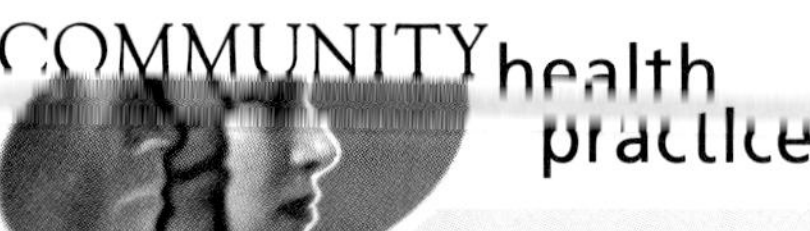

Computerized Pharmacy Data Bases

As our population ages, Canadians are seeing an increase in chronic illnesses, many of which require treatment with multiple medications (polypharmacy). In order to decrease the potential for adverse drug interactions, the Government of British Columbia has instituted a policy whereby all pharmacies are required to link up with Pharmanet, the province's computerized pharmacy data base. This system permits monitoring of use or abuse of prescription medications.

Shoppers Drug Mart has developed the Health Watch System, which is unique to this retail chain. This system maintains updated records of individual medication histories and can identify potential problems, such as allergic reactions or adverse drug interactions. This information allows the pharmacist to alert the prescribing physician of actual or potential concerns. When a new prescription is entered into the Health Watch System, the computer prints out an information sheet ("Health Watch Reminder") that provides the customer with details about the dosage, side effects, adverse effects and safe administration of the medication purchased.

Evaluating Medication Administration

After the administration of any therapeutic agent, the nurse should observe the patient for effectiveness and reaction. The criteria by which the nurse judges the effectiveness of a medication depends upon the purpose for which it was administered: the alleviation of pain, the reduction of fever, a decrease in swelling or even the appearance of orange-coloured urine. These are anticipated results, and they reflect the effectiveness of the particular medication. The observations are recorded in detail on the patient's chart. Adverse reactions to the medication are always reported to the charge nurse and the physician. If a reaction is severe, that is, if the patient is acutely uncomfortable or essential body functions are impaired, the physician is notified immediately so that measures to stop the reaction can begin. In severe allergic reactions, the tissues of the throat may become so edematous that breathing is difficult. Prompt intervention at the earliest sign of an allergic reaction is required. These reactions are also recorded in detail on the patient's chart.

Quick Guide to Evaluating the Effectiveness of Medications

1. Is the patient taking the medicines that have been prescribed?
2. Have the medications been administered safely?
3. Does the patient show signs or symptoms indicating that the medications are effective (or ineffective)?
4. Has the administration of the medications been accurately reported on the patient's record? Have pertinent observations been recorded and reported to appropriate personnel?

Quick Guide to Safe Medication Administration

1. Does the patient have any allergies?
2. How old is the patient?
3. What medications have been prescribed for the patient?
4. Why is the patient receiving these medications?
5. What observations should the nurse make relative to the effect of these medications on the patient?
6. Are specific nursing measures indicated because of the action of drugs contained in these medications?
7. How are the patient's medications to be administered?
8. What precautions should be taken in administering these medications? Are there special precautions that should be taken because of the patient's age, physical condition or mental state?
9. Do any of the medications require special precautionary measures for administration?
10. Does the patient have learning needs relative to medicinal therapy?
11. Does the patient or family require specific skills or knowledge in order to continue medicinal therapy at home?

Illegal Use of Drugs

While drug abuse can result from the use of drugs for therapeutic purposes, it is a more widespread problem among those who use drugs illegally. Experimentation with drugs such as marijuana, hashish, cocaine and alcohol is common among young people under the influence of peer groups. It may constitute both a new experience and an escape from reality for the user.

There is considerable lack of public understanding about the effects of drug abuse. Professional controversy exists regarding the consequences of the use of "soft" drugs and [illegible] and the question of whether their use leads to use of "hard" drugs. Attempts are under way by several groups to decriminalize the possession and use of marijuana. However, it is clear that marijuana, like alcohol, can severely impair the user's ability to drive and can lead to automobile accidents.

Health professionals are in contact with drug users in all types of settings. However, the effects of "hard" drugs such as cocaine, heroin and LSD (lysergic acid diethylamide) are usually seen and dealt with in emergency departments. These drugs are mind-altering and mood-changing. The sense of being "high" on these drugs is usually followed by a "low" or hangover of some type, which may be difficult for the patient to cope with alone. Someone may be needed to "guide" or "talk down" the person on an LSD "trip" who is hallucinating badly and experiencing a distorted sense of reality.

As we mentioned earlier in this text, drug overdose has become a leading cause of death among teenagers. Drug overdoses often seen in emergency departments include both accidental overdoses of illegal drugs and deliberate attempts at suicide, which may involve the use of either illegal drugs or prescribed sedatives. The combination of sedatives with alcohol is particularly dangerous.

On the other hand, several drugs that are widely used illegally may also have uses in medical therapy. Cocaine and morphine are used as anesthetics, and it has been proposed by some people that heroin, which like morphine is derived from opium, should be used to alleviate pain in terminally ill patients. Marijuana—in the form of nabilone (Cesamet)—is currently administered to some cancer patients to lessen the nausea and vomiting that often accompany radiation and chemotherapy. Marijuana has also been proposed as a treatment for the eye disease glaucoma.

IN REVIEW

- Throughout history, medications prepared from pharmaceutical agents have been used to promote, maintain and restore health.
- Medications are often referred to as "drugs" or "medicines" and are usually ordered by physicians. The administration of medications is a therapeutic nursing function, and the nurse has a legal responsibility to dispense medications safely.
- The nurse must have:
  - knowledge and understanding of pharmacology
  - knowledge and skill in assessing patients' health status
  - skill in preparing, administering and recording medications
  - skill in monitoring the effectiveness of medications' actions.
- The nurse must implement nursing interventions:
  - to enhance drug therapy
  - to promote patient safety and well-being.
- Each drug has three names:
  - trade name
  - chemical name
  - generic name.
- Drugs act by:
  - replacing missing or deficient substances
  - altering the cellular environment
  - affecting the rate of cellular functions.
- Drug reaction is influenced by:
  - dose of the drug reaching its target site
  - pharmacokinetics (absorption, distribution, metabolism and excretion of the drug).
- Determinants of drug action and effects include:
  - age
  - gender
  - body weight and size
  - genetic makeup
  - presence of disease or illness
  - medication history
  - psychological factors
  - time of administration
  - environmental conditions.
- Because drugs can cause adverse effects, all patients should be monitored. Special monitoring is necessary for:
  - pregnant women
  - infants
  - children
  - older adults.
- Older adults are particularly prone to problems with medication because of:
  - failing vision
  - lessened efficiency of excretion
  - possibility of malnourishment and dehydration
  - multiple medications for multiple health problems
  - widespread use of over-the-counter medications
  - confusion about dosages and administration times
  - idiosyncratic reactions
  - intentional overdose.
- In Canada, all aspects of drug production, distribution, advertising and sale are governed by the federal *Food and Drugs Act* and the federal *Narcotic Act*, with some provinces having additional drug legislation.

- Provincial nursing legislation outlines the nurse's legal responsibility regarding medications.
- Drugs are derived from either:
  - natural substances (plants, animals or inorganic matter)
  - synthetic chemicals.
- Once approved for use in Canada, drugs can be listed in the *Compendium of Pharmaceuticals and Specialties (CPS)*, a drug reference book compiled and revised annually by the Canadian Pharmaceutical Association.
- All health care agencies have their own policies and procedures regarding medications, including:
  - ordering
  - processing
  - communicating
  - storing
  - dispensing.
- Before administering a drug, the nurse should know its:
  - classification
  - main action
  - key adverse effects
  - safe dosage limits
  - nursing considerations.
- Medication orders may be:
  - standing orders
  - self-terminating orders.
- Nursing responsibilities include:
  - questioning any order that is unclear or unsafe
  - checking the original order with the MAR to confirm accuracy of transcription
  - following the "five rights" of drug administration (right drug, right dose, right route, right patient, right time)
  - reporting medication errors to the appropriate person, using a medication error form.
- Controlled drugs are stored in a locked cupboard and their distribution is closely monitored. Controlled drugs are recorded in the:
  - patient's record
  - narcotics book.

  At designated times in a 24-hour period, a narcotics count is done by two nurses, and any discrepancy is reported immediately.
- When the dosage ordered for a drug is different from the dosage supplied, the nurse needs mathematical skills to compute the exact dosage.
- Calculating drug dosage can be done by the:
  - apothecary system
  - SI metric system
  - household system.
- The nurse must be able to convert from one system to another, as well as calculate the dosages. This is particularly true with pediatric drug orders, which are usually calculated according to body surface area (BSA).
- A nursing history includes:
  - assessment of the medication-related needs of the patient (including medication and medical history)
  - actual or potential problems that might influence the effectiveness of the drug
  - monitoring of lab values.
- Many problems associated with drug therapy are collaborative problems that require accurate observation of the patient to assess effectiveness of the therapy as well as any adverse effects.
- Patient education and supportive care are key nursing strategies to promote optimal health.
- Medications are administered:
  - orally
  - sublingually
  - parenterally
  - topically
  - by inhalation, instillation or suppository.
- For parenteral administration, sterile equipment, supplies and aseptic technique are maintained. All needles are disposed of in a sharps container.
- Intramuscular injections can be given in the:
  - dorsogluteal site
  - ventrogluteal site
  - vastus lateralis site
  - deltoid site.
- Intravenous medications may be delivered by adding a medication to a:
  - primary line
  - secondary line
  - IV push.
- An intermittent infusion device may be used for a patient who no longer requires continuous intravenous infusions or medications.
- After the administration of any medication, the nurse observes the patient for effectiveness and reactions, and documents any changes.

Critical Thinking Activities

1. You are a home care nurse assigned to an 86-year-old woman whose memory is failing and who has difficulty reading because of poor eyesight. She tells you

she has to take medications for a heart ailment, for high blood pressure, for joint pain and for indiges- [illegible]

2. In the health agency in which you are having clinical practice, find out the following information:
   a. The method of ordering medications for patients.
   b. The methods of processing and communicating medication orders.
   c. The location of medications on a nursing unit, storage facilities and system for arranging medications.
   d. The equipment used for preparing and administering medications.
   e. Safety precautions taken in the preparation and administration of medications.
   f. The approved method of recording medications by various administration routes, including narcotic and controlled drugs.
   g. The location of resources and reference material on drugs.
   h. Pertinent agency policies regarding the administration of medications.

KEY TERMS

medication p. 1111
pharmacology p. 1111
trade (brand/proprietary) name p. 1111
chemical name p. 1111
generic name p. 1111
pharmacodynamics p. 1111
agonists p. 1111
antagonists p. 1111
pharmacokinetics p. 1112
onset of action p. 1112
peak action (peak effect) p. 1112
half-life p. 1112
duration of action p. 1112
plateau p. 1112
therapeutic effect p. 1112
systemic effect p. 1112
local effect p. 1112
adverse reactions (side effects) p. 1112
allergic reaction p. 1112
anaphylactic reaction p. 1112
drug toxicity p. 1113
drug tolerance p. 1113
drug interactions p. 1113
additive effect p. 1113
synergistic (potentiating) effect p. 1113
antagonistic effect p. 1113
stat order p. 1119
prn order p. 1119

References

AARONSON, L.S., & MACNEE, C.L. (1989). Tobacco, alcohol, and caffeine use during pregnancy. *Journal of Obstetric, Gynecologic and Neonatal Nursing, 18*(4), 279–287.

ASHBY, D.A. (1997). Medication calculation skills of the medical–surgical nurse. *Medical–Surgical Nursing, 6*(2), 90–94.

BEHRMAN, R.E., KLIEGMAN, R.M, ARVIN, A.M., & NELSON, W.E. (1996). *Nelson textbook of pediatrics.* (16th ed.). Philadelphia: W.B. Saunders.

[illegible]

BLAIR, K.A. (1990). Aging: Physiological aspects and clinical implications. *Nurse Practitioner, 15*(2), 14–28.

BROWN, M., & MULHOLLAND, J.L. (1996). *Drug calculations: Process and problems for clinical practice.* (5th ed.). St. Louis: Mosby.

BUTTERS, L., & HOWIE, C. (1990). Awareness among pregnant women of the effect on the fetus of commonly used drugs. *Midwifery, 6*(3), 146–154.

CARPENITO, L.J. (1997). *Nursing diagnosis: Application to clinical practice.* (7th ed.). Philadelphia: Lippincott.

DRASS, J. (1992). What you need to know about insulin injections. *Nursing 92, 22*(11), 40–43.

EARNEST, V.V. (1993). *Clinical skills in nursing practice.* (2nd ed.). Philadelphia: Lippincott.

EBERSOLE, P., & HESS, P. (1998). *Towards healthy aging: Human needs and nursing response.* (5th ed.). St. Louis: Mosby.

FAHS, P.S.S., & KINNEY, M.R. (1991). The abdomen, thigh, and arm as sites for subcutaneous sodium heparin injections. *Nursing Research, 40*(4), 204–207.

FORD, C. (1990). Disposal of sharps. *Journal of Intravenous Nursing, 13*(1), 42–47.

HEALTH AND WELFARE CANADA. (1991). *Health protection and drug laws.* Ottawa: Minister Supply & Services Canada. (Health & Welfare Canada Catalogue no. H49-5/1991E)

KEE, J.L., & HAYES, E.R. (1993). *Pharmacology: A nursing process approach.* Philadelphia: W.B. Saunders.

MATTESON, M., & McCONNELL, E. (1988). *Gerontological nursing—concepts and practice.* Philadelphia: W.B. Saunders.

McKIM, E.M. (1991). Caffeine and its effects on pregnancy and the neonate. *Journal of Nurse Midwifery, 36,* 229–231.

NAEYE, R. (1981). Influence of maternal cigarette smoking during pregnancy on fetal and childhood growth. *Obstetrics & Gynecology, 57*(1), 18–21.

NORVILLE, M.A.F. (1994). *Drug dosages and solutions.* (3rd ed.). Norwalk, CT: Appleton & Lange.

PINNELL, N.L. (1996). *Nursing pharmacology.* Philadelphia: W.B. Saunders.

SHIONO, P., KLEBANOFF, M., & RHOADS, G. (1986). Smoking and drinking during pregnancy: Their effects on preterm birth. *Journal of the American Medical Association, 255*(1), 82–84.

SHLAFER, M. (1993). *The nurse, pharmacology, and drug therapy: A prototype approach.* (2nd ed.). Redwood City, CA: Addison-Wesley.

Additional Readings

ABRAMS, A.C. (1998). *Clinical drug therapy rationales for nursing practice.* (5th ed.). Philadelphia: Lippincott.

AHRMEDZAI, S., & BROOKS, D. (1997). Transdermal fentanyl versus sustained-release oral morphine in cancer pain: Preference, efficacy, and quality of life. *Journal of Pain & Symptom Management, 12,* 254–261.

BUTTARO, M. (1994). Staying on top of transdermal drug patches. *Nursing 94, 26*(11), 41–45.

CLAYTON, B.D., STOCK, Y.N., & SQUIRE, J.E. (1997). *Basic pharmacology for nurses.* (11th ed.). St. Louis: Mosby.

DERIVAN, M.C., & FERRANTE, C. (1993). How to apply a transdermal drug patch. *Nursing 93, 23*(8), 32C–32F.

DICKERSON, R. (1992). 10 tips for easing the pain of intramuscular injections. *Nursing 92, 22*(8), 55.

HACKEL, R., BUTT, L., & BANISTER, G. (1996). How nurses perceive medication errors. *Nursing Management, 27*(1), 33–34.

HUNT, J.R., MAX, L., & RAPP, R.P. (1996). Intravenous medication errors. *Journal of Intravenous Nursing, 19*(3S)(suppl.), S9–S15.

KALSO, E., HELSKANEN, T., TANTIO, M., RESENBERG, P., & VAINIO, A. (1997). Epidural and subcutaneous morphine in the management of cancer pain. *Pain, 67*, 443–449.

KENNEDY, D. (1996). Medication "safety checks" in pediatric acute care. *Journal of Intravenous Nursing, 19*(6), 295–302.

KONICK-McMAHON, J. (1996). Full speed ahead—with caution: Pushing intravenous medications. *Nursing 96, 26*(6), 26–32.

LESTER, R.M. (1995). *Intravenous medications of critical care.* (2nd ed.). Philadelphia: W.B. Saunders.

MATTINSON, K., & HAWTHORNE, J. (1996). Harm reduction: A realistic approach toward injection drug users. *Canadian Nurse, 92*(2), 22–26.

McCONNELL, E. (1997). Using transdermal medical patches. *Nursing 97, 27*(7), 18.

McCURDY, D.E., & ARNOLD, M.T. (1995). Development and implementation of a pediatric/neonatal IV syringe pump delivery system. *Neonatal Network, 14*(3), 9–18.

MORRISON, R. (1993). Medication non-compliance. *Canadian Nurse, 89*(4), 15–18.

RIPAMONTI, C., ZECCA, E., & BRUERA, E. (1997). An update on the clinical use of methadone for cancer pain. *Pain, 70*, 109–115.

ROSE, K., & SIMMS, D.P. (1996). Focus on quality: Drug administration made safer. *Canadian Nurse, 92*(6), 53–54.

SPRINGHOUSE CORPORATION. (1996). *New nursing photobooks: Giving medications.* Springhouse, PA: Author.

VALLERAND, A.H. (1996). *Davis's guide to IV medications.* (3rd ed.). Philadelphia: F.A. Davis.

VARELLA, L., JONES, E., & MEGUID, M.M. (1997). Drug–nutrient interactions in enteral feeding: A primary care focus. *Nurse Practitioner, 22*(6), 98–104.

WEINSTEIN, S.M. (1997). *Plumer's principles and practice of intravenous therapy.* (6th ed.). Philadelphia: Lippincott.

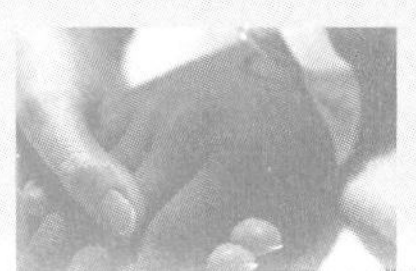

Psychosocial Needs

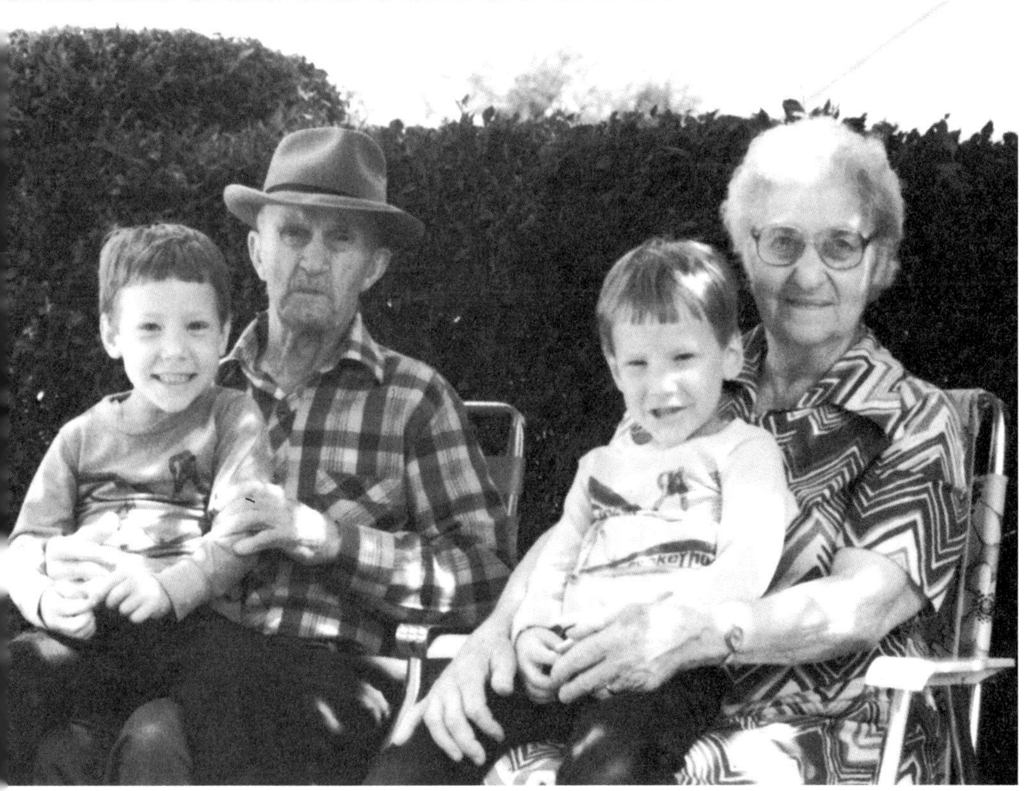

Chapter 35

Sexuality Needs

OUTLINE

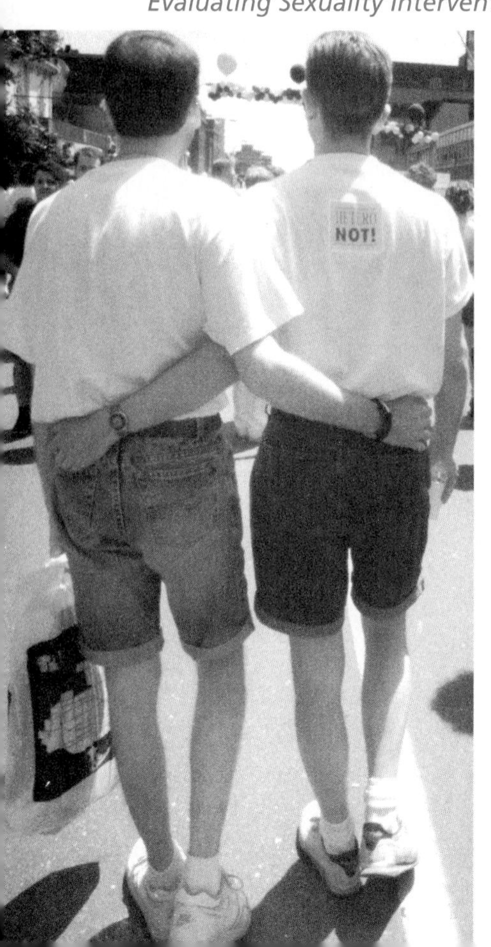

Central Questions

1. What is sexuality?
2. Is there a difference between sex and sexuality?
3. What are the structures and functions of the female and the male reproductive systems?
4. What are the four phases of the human sexual response cycle?
5. What are the major determinants of sexual functioning?
6. How do sexuality needs vary throughout the life cycle?
7. What are some sexual behaviours, orientations and variations?
8. What are some common sexual concerns and problems?
9. What basic principles does the nurse apply in assisting individuals to meet sexuality needs?
10. How does the nurse assess an individual's sexuality needs?
11. What are the common nursing diagnostic statements for patients with sexuality problems?
12. How does the nurse develop a plan of care for individuals with sexuality problems?
13. What strategies might the nurse implement in helping individuals, families or groups promote and protect sexual health?
14. How does the nurse assist in providing restorative and supportive care for individuals with sexuality problems?
15. How does the nurse evaluate the patient's response to nursing interventions?

Introduction

The recognition and acceptance [illegible] relatively new. Prior to the 20th century, sexual intercourse was believed to be for procreation and not for pleasure, especially for women. Sexual mores were dictated by religious and cultural doctrines, and it was considered inappropriate for a woman to initiate or to enjoy sexual activity. As the disciplines of psychiatry and psychology developed, beginning with the work of Freud and others, an interest in sexuality as a separate concept emerged, evolving into the science of sexology. The Kinsey Reports (1948 and 1953) and the works of researchers such as Masters, Johnson and Kolodny in the 1960s did much to provide a clearer understanding of sexual attitudes and practices and to encourage open discussion of sexuality. The development of sexology was dominated at this stage by a biomedical model, which did not deal with the psychosocial aspects of sexuality. It was a commonly held belief that female sexuality should be a "mirror image" of male sexuality, without consideration of the vast differences in male and female sexual needs. For example, from a male perspective, "normal" sexual behaviour was believed to be coital activity that resulted in orgasm. Today, most countries view sexual needs of women as distinctly different from those of men. Safety, trust, intimacy and sensuality are often more important to women than the physical aspects of sex alone. Unfortunately, in some areas of the world, women are not yet allowed sexual rights and are still legally considered the property of their husbands.

In 1975, the World Health Organization recognized sexuality as a health entity. It defined sexual health as "the integration of the somatic, emotional, intellectual, and social aspects in ways that are positively enriching and that will enhance personality, communication, and love" (WHO, 1975, p. 2). WHO recommended that health care professionals become involved in the education, counselling and treatment of sexual health problems (WHO, 1975).

Social developments in the latter half of the 20th century have increased public awareness of sexuality and the sexual needs of people. Television, music videos and movies provide a source of education about sexuality for many people, particularly children and adolescents. Whether these sources are positive or negative depends upon their content and the context in which they are viewed. Political and social pressures from groups opposed to sexuality education and reproductive choice have resulted in limited access to safe, effective birth control measures and to safe, legal abortions in many areas of the world. HIV infection (which leads to AIDS) and hepatitis B viral infections, the results of which can be fatal, have emerged as major health and social problems, along with other sexually transmitted diseases. There has been an increase in the incidence of child sexual abuse and sexual assault—crimes that have devastating effects on the emotional and physical health of victims unless effective intervention is available.

[illegible] providers of sexual health education and services. There is a need to counteract negative influences and inaccurate information while empowering people to care for their own sexual and reproductive health. The challenge for nurses when promoting sexual and reproductive health or when providing restorative care after sexual problems occur is in being a helpful, accurate and culturally sensitive resource. Comfort, competence, confidence and a nonjudgemental attitude enables nurses to address sexuality issues in an appropriate and professional manner. Talking to someone about sex and sexuality is not easy. To deal competently with the sexuality needs of patients, nurses must first feel comfortable discussing sexuality. A solid base of knowledge and understanding of sexuality and sexual health problems will help to reduce a nurse's discomfort in this area. Nurses must also examine their own values and beliefs about sexuality and be able to recognize situations where personal biases could interfere with meeting the needs of patients. An awareness of changing sexual needs throughout the life cycle and a sensitivity to variations in values, beliefs and behaviours will enhance the nurse's effectiveness in providing care.

Human Sexuality

"Where do babies come from?"

"I'm 13 and my period hasn't started yet. All my friends have theirs. What's wrong with me?"

"Is it harmful for a man to get all excited and then nothing happens?"

"I'm a virgin. Is intercourse always painful at first for the woman?"

"I'm 70 now and I guess sex shouldn't even be on my mind anymore."

"I feel inadequate, less than a woman, because I can't conceive a baby."

"I look like a man, but inside I feel like a woman."

Questions and statements such as these reflect the variety of concerns individuals have regarding sexuality. Human sexuality is a multifaceted phenomenon which "encompasses the biological, psychological, social, cultural, and ethical aspects of sexual behaviour" (Knowlton, 1988, p. 420). It involves two related concepts—sex and sexuality. **Sex** refers to the biological distinctions that identify a person as male or female, based on the characteristics of the sex organs. This is called **biological sexual identity**. Sex also refers to the

KEY PRINCIPLES

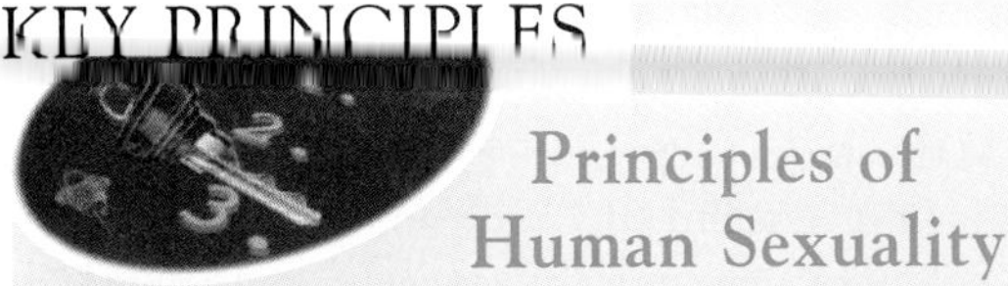

Principles of Human Sexuality

1. Sexuality is an integral aspect of the human personality.
2. Sexuality is a life-long component of the personality.
3. The components of sexuality include physical, biological, psychological, social and cultural aspects.
4. Everyone has the right to be recognized as a sexual being, regardless of age, physical, emotional or cognitive status, or sexual orientation.
5. Sexuality may be expressed in many physical and emotional ways, only one of which is sexual intercourse.
6. Everyone has the right to consent to activity related to sexuality or reproduction.
7. Everyone has the right to possess personal values.
8. No one has the right to impose sexual values on another person.

sexual functions for reproduction and pleasure, namely sexual intercourse. **Sexuality** is a broad concept that brings together the expression of self and the totality of feelings, attitudes, beliefs and behaviours related to being male or female. Sexuality is expressed in how people relate to others, how they dress and look, how they behave and how they express feelings of intimacy, tenderness and love. It includes the need for emotional attachment with another human being, for tenderness, intimacy and affection, for sensuality and for procreation (Knowlton, 1988).

The concept of sexuality includes a number of components. **Gender definition** or **identity** is the perception of the self as a male or female. This definition may or may not coincide with one's biological sexual identity, as in the case of the man who said, "I look like a man but inside I feel like a woman." **Gender role identity** refers to behaviours identified by one's culture as appropriate to each gender, or how a person behaves as a male or female. Gender role identity includes all of the learned behaviours of masculinity or femininity, sexual behaviours and orientations (how sexuality is expressed) and sexual relationships (how sexuality is shared).

Sexuality also includes attitudes and values, feelings and judgements about sexual behaviour. It includes choices people make about reproduction (whether or not to become a parent) and about sexual pleasure (whether or not to engage in a physical relationship with a sexual partner).

Human sexuality exists in two dimensions: private and public. The private dimension includes feelings, values and beliefs that are very personal. The public dimension manifests itself through behaviours that are influenced by values and beliefs, and may disclose how the person is feeling. Illness, chronic disease or disability can have an impact on both dimensions. For example, someone who holds the belief that sexuality is limited to the domain of healthy, able-bodied, young people may be devastated by the onset of a debilitating disease or disability. In the public dimension, this same person may also develop poor personal hygiene and grooming, as well as a "what's the use?" attitude.

Sexuality pervades virtually every aspect of life, from birth to death. It is an integral part of the human personality and a significant factor in a person's self-identity. Successful gender identification in early childhood is important for health and well-being throughout life. Sexual fulfillment is a very basic need. Actual or potential damage to the integrity of an individual's sex organs can pose a considerable threat to self-esteem and self-identity.

Sexual Anatomy and Physiology

Embryology

All cells in the human body, with the exception of the *gametes* (germ cells), contain 23 pairs of *chromosomes*. Twenty-two of these are homologous pairs; they are like each other and bear genes for the same traits. The twenty-third pair are the sex chromosomes. Females have two similar sex chromosomes, designated as *X chromosomes*. Males have two dissimilar sex chromosomes: one is an X chromosome, and the other is a *Y chromosome*.

During the process of maturation, the gametes (the male sperm and the female ovum) divide, and the number of chromosomes each carries is reduced by half to 23. The mature ovum always contains an X chromosome, while the sperm cell may contain either an X or a Y chromosome. If the ovum is fertilized by a sperm carrying an X chromosome, the resultant embryo will be a female (XX) who will develop a female reproductive system. If the sperm carries a Y chromosome, a male (XY) embryo will result and the *gonads* (sex organs) will develop into testes. Under the influence of the Y chromosome, the embryonic testes secrete the hormone *testosterone*, stimulating the formation of the male external genitalia, duct system and accessory sex organs. In the absence of the Y chromosome and without the influence of testosterone, female reproductive organs develop. Testosterone is also responsible for sex differentiation in the brain.

Hormonal Control of the Reproductive System

The gland controlling the sex hormones in both genders is the *hypothalamus*. This gland, located in the brain, secretes *gonadotropin-releasing hormone* (GnRH), which stimulates the pituitary gland to secrete the gonadotropic hormones *follicle-stimulating hormone* (FSH) and *luteinizing hormone* (LH). FSH stimulates maturation of germ cells in the ovary and testes, while LH stimulates production of estrogen (female) and testosterone (male).

The hypothalamus is sensitive to external stimuli such [illegible] tion can affect the pituitary gland, resulting in changes in ovarian or testicular function. For example, a woman who is undergoing intensive training for a competitive sport may stop menstruating because of stress or a lowered body-fat content. Men who have a severe systemic illness will likely have a temporary lowering of the sperm count.

The principal female hormones are the *estrogens* and *progesterone*. The estrogens are secreted by the ovarian follicle, by the corpus luteum and, during pregnancy, by the placenta. The functions of these hormones include:

1. stimulating the growth of the reproductive organs and the development of secondary sex characteristics at puberty
2. inducing regeneration of the endometrium following menstruation
3. promoting growth of the duct system of the mammary glands
4. maintaining matrix formation in the bones
5. increasing the motility of the uterus and its sensitivity to oxytocin during labour and delivery.

Progesterone is also secreted by the corpus luteum and during pregnancy by the placenta. Its primary functions include:

1. causing the vascular and glandular structure of the endometrium to assume its mature form during the luteal (post-ovulatory) phase of the cycle, making it ready to supply glucose to the blastocyst (embryonic stage) and creating an environment hospitable to implantation. If pregnancy does not occur, corpus luteum function declines, estrogen and progesterone levels fall and endometrial shedding (menstruation) occurs
2. promoting growth of the mammary gland alveoli
3. decreasing motility of the uterine muscle.

Female hormone levels are cyclic from the onset of puberty until the onset of menopause. During childhood and after menopause, the levels of estrogen and progesterone are consistently lower than during the reproductive years.

The male hormones are collectively known as *androgens*. The principal male hormone is testosterone, the functions of which include:

1. inducing sexual differentiation during embryonic development
2. stimulating growth and development of the genitalia and secondary sex characteristics
3. initiating and maintaining the process of spermatogenesis
4. promoting body growth through protein anabolism
5. stimulating the sex drive.

Hormone production in the male is not cyclic as it is in the female, although minor fluctuations of testosterone lev- [illegible] testosterone levels and sperm counts are as much as 17 percent higher in the winter (Levine, 1993). This finding may account for the higher birth rates in summer and early fall. The production of male hormones declines with aging, but because the change is gradual, it should not cause concern.

The Female Reproductive System

The female reproductive system includes organs that produce and transport the female germ cells, receive the sperm, support conception and furnish an environment that promotes growth and development of a fetus (see Figures 35.1 and 35.2). The system includes a birth canal for the passage of the mature fetus and a mechanism for suckling the infant after it is born.

Ovaries

The ovaries are small, ovoid organs located in the pelvic region of the abdominal cavity. They are suspended from the lateral pelvic wall by a section of the broad ligament. At birth, the ovaries contain approximately 10 million *primordial follicles* (primitive ova), of which about 350 to 500 will mature to become *graafian follicles* during the woman's reproductive years.

A few years before puberty, the ovaries begin to secrete increased amounts of the hormones estrogen, progesterone and some androgens (male hormones). Puberty starts when the production of female hormones becomes cyclic and continues in a regular pattern. Approximately every 28 days, the pituitary hormone FSH stimulates the maturation of a small number of oocytes within their follicles. The follicles secrete ever-increasing amounts of estrogen. One or two mature ova are extruded from the surface of the ovary in a process called *ovulation*. An ovum is capable of being fertilized for about 24 to 36 hours, after which it disintegrates. The cyst-like structure left on the surface of the ovary then begins to secrete progesterone.

Fallopian Tubes (Oviducts)

The fallopian tubes or oviducts are two small, tube-like structures approximately 10 cm long that extend from the uterus to the ovaries. They are attached to the broad ligaments and open into the lateral aspects of the uterus about one-third of the way down. The distal end of each tube has a fringe of finger-like projections, called *fimbria*, which lie in close proximity to the ovaries. They help to direct the ovum into the outer (distal) portion of the fallopian tube, where fertilization usually takes place. During the three or four days following conception, the fertilized ovum is transported to the uterus for implantation. The ovum is propelled through the tubes by a series of peristaltic contractions and the wave-like motion of *cilia*, which line the fallopian tubes.

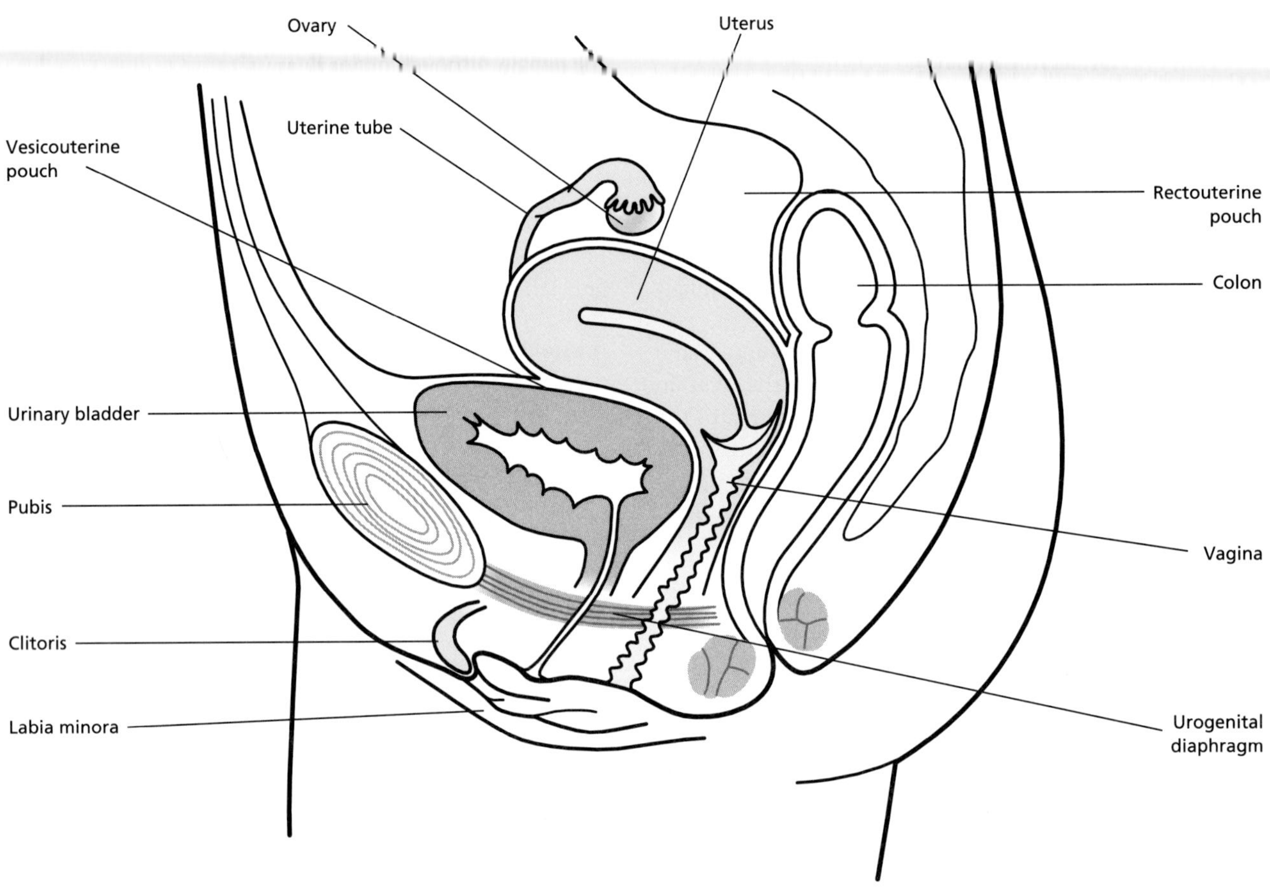

FIGURE 35.1 Female reproductive organs

Uterus (Womb)

The uterus is a hollow muscular organ about the size of a fist, located in the pelvic portion of the abdominal cavity between the rectum and the bladder. The lining of the uterus consists of a specialized layer of tissue, the *endometrium*, which is the primary site for implantation of the fertilized ovum. If conception does not occur, the hormone levels decrease, and about 14 days following ovulation, the endometrium is shed in a process called *menstruation*.

Cervix

The cervix is the muscular, conical neck of the uterus. It is firm to the touch and protrudes into the posterior vault of the vagina. It has a narrow opening in its centre, the cervical os. The cervical os leads to the cervical canal, which forms the passageway from the vagina to the uterine cavity. During pregnancy, the muscle in the cervix helps to keep the developing pregnancy within the uterus by keeping the cervix tightly closed. A mucus plug, present in the cervical canal during pregnancy, helps to prevent entry of substances from the vagina.

Vagina

The vagina is an elastic tube lying, with its walls against each other, between the bladder and the rectum. It is approximately 10 cm long and 4 cm wide in its resting state, but expands during sexual arousal. The vagina functions as the birth canal and is capable of expanding to allow passage of a full-term fetus. During coitus (sexual intercourse), the erect penis is inserted into the vagina. When ejaculation occurs, sperm are deposited at the cervical os to make their way through the uterus to the fallopian tubes.

Vulva

The external female genitals are collectively known as the vulva (Figure 35.2). The *mons pubis* is a soft pad of adipose tissue located over the symphysis pubis and is covered with pubic hair. The *labia majora*, which are somewhat similar to the scrotum in the male, are longitudinal folds of skin that cover and protect the opening of the vagina, the urethral meatus and the labia minora. The *labia minora* are small folds of erectile tissue that extend from the *clitoris* to the *fourchette*.

The clitoris is a short, erectile organ located just below the mons pubis and just above the urinary meatus. It is similar to the glans penis of the male, but contains a relatively greater concentration of sensory nerve endings. The clitoris is highly sensitive to tactile stimuli.

The vestibule is the ovoid area between the labia minora that contains the vaginal introitus (opening), the urethral meatus, the hymen and the openings of several glandular ducts. The vaginal opening is the site of the Bartholin's glands; the urethral opening is the site of the Skene's glands.

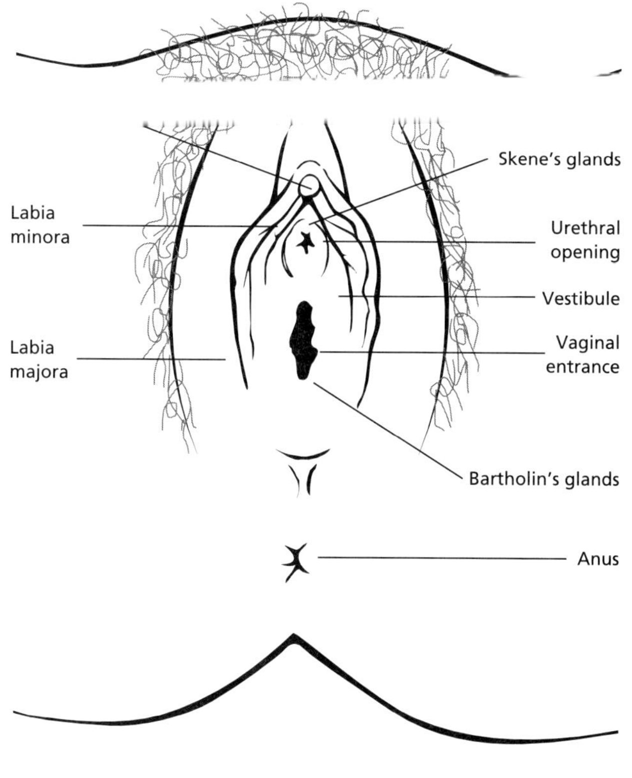

FIGURE 35.2 External female genitalia

Both glands have a lubricating function. The *hymen* is an elastic fibrous membrane that may or may not be visible at the introitus. Th [illegible] of whether or not a woman has had sexual intercourse, although the presence of a very thick membrane (imperforate hymen) would likely be an impediment to vaginal intercourse.

Mammary Glands (Breasts)

The mammary glands are accessory sexual structures in the female. Their purpose is to secrete milk to nourish an infant. Each breast contains lobes separated by adipose tissue and is made up of lobules. The lobules contain grape-like clusters of milk-secreting cells called *alveoli*. The milk is conveyed to storage areas (ampullae), and then to the lactiferous ducts that lead to the nipple. During pregnancy, increased levels of estrogens and progesterone begin to prepare the breasts for milk production. After childbirth, the hormone prolactin stimulates this function (see Figure 35.3).

THE MENSTRUAL CYCLE

The average length of the menstrual cycle is 28 days, counting the first day of menstrual flow as day 1 of that cycle. Ovulation occurs an average of 14 days before the onset of menstrual flow. The length of cycles may vary from woman to woman, and also in the same woman from cycle to cycle,

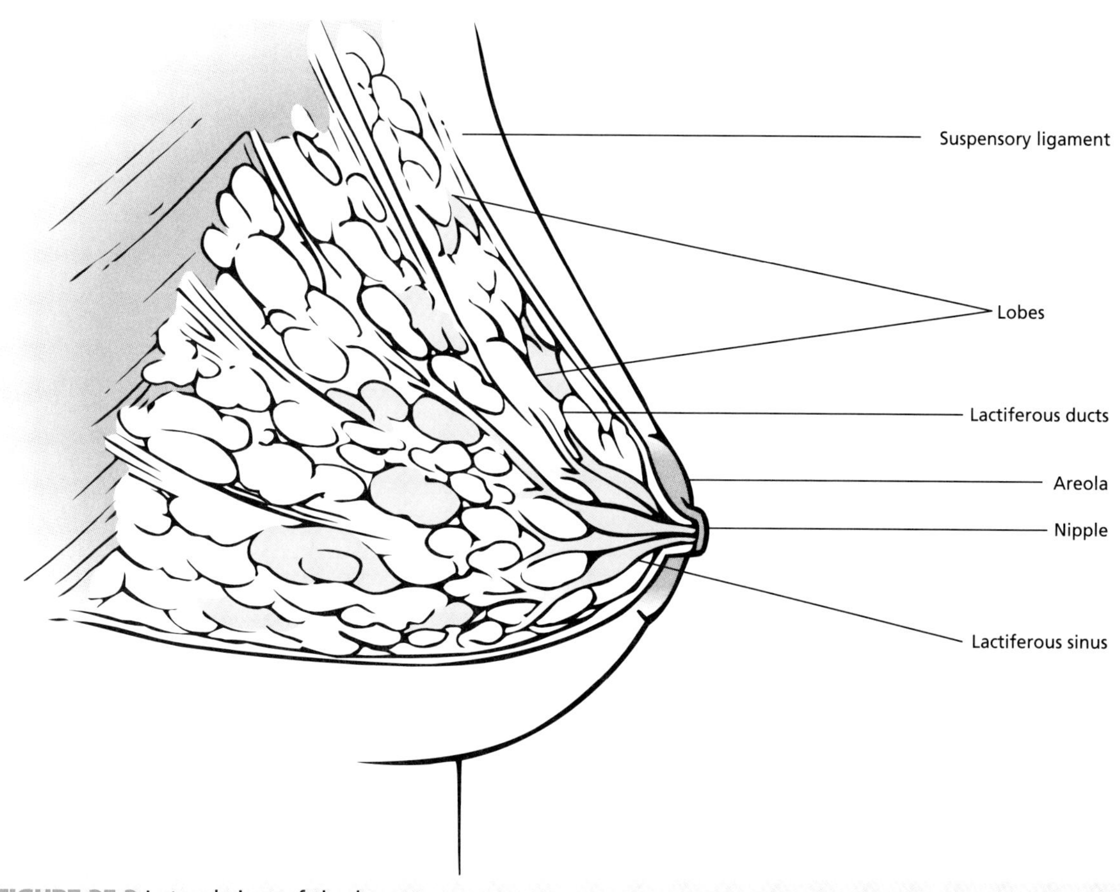

FIGURE 35.3 Lateral view of the breast

reflecting variations in the follicular phase. The duration of menstrual flow can also vary, ranging from two to seven days on average, with about 40 mL to 50 mL of blood loss. The menstrual cycle consists of three phases: the menstrual phase, the proliferative or follicular phase and the secretory or luteal phase.

The Menstrual Phase

The menstrual phase occurs about 14 days after ovulation, when the hormone secretion of the corpus luteum decreases and the endometrium disintegrates. Separation between the innermost basal layer of the endometrium takes place, with shedding of the two outer layers lining the uterus.

The Proliferative (Follicular) Phase

Under the influence of FSH, the ovarian follicle begins to develop and secrete increasing levels of estrogen. This initiates glycogen storage and regeneration of the endometrium.

The Secretory (Luteal) Phase

As the ovum matures, the hypothalamus and pituitary glands respond to increased estrogen levels by lowering production of FSH and sharply increasing production of LH (luteinizing hormone). The mature ovum ruptures the surface of the ovarian follicle and is released into the pelvic cavity during ovulation. Ovulation occurs 10 to 12 hours after the peak level of LH. The ruptured follicle forms the *corpus luteum*, which secretes progesterone. Under the influence of progesterone, the vascular and glandular structure of the endometrium assumes its mature form as a hospitable environment for implantation. If conception occurs, *human chorionic gonadotropin* (HCG) is produced and supports the continued function of the corpus luteum until the placenta is able to provide these hormones at six to eight weeks gestation. If conception does not occur, the corpus luteum degenerates, estrogen and progesterone levels fall, and a new menstrual cycle begins.

Menarche and Menopause

The onset of the first menstrual period is called **menarche**. In North America, the average age of menarche is 12 years, with a range extending from age 9 to age 16.

Menopause is considered to have occurred when a woman has not experienced menstrual flow for one to one-and-a-half years. The average age of menopause is 51 years, and ranges from age 45 to 55 (Uphold & Graham, 1994). Approximately 1 percent of women experience the onset of menopause as early as age 35.

Menopause is a normal physiological event that results from the lowered response of the ovaries to hormone stimulation. "Surgical menopause" can occur at any age if the ovaries are removed or rendered nonfunctional in the treatment of life-threatening diseases within the reproductive system.

In addition to marking the end of a woman's reproductive years, lowered estrogen levels can produce a variety of effects on the body. Ongoing research is being conducted into the short- and long-term effects of menopause on women's health. These effects are more acute in women who have had a surgical menopause. Some women experience few, if any, problems with menopause. Others have a difficult time with physical symptoms and/or emotional reactions to this significant life event and may require support and counselling from a health care professional. These women may also benefit from hormone replacement therapy.

The Male Reproductive System

The male reproductive system (see Figure 35.4) includes the organs that produce both the male hormone and germ cells, a duct system to transport the germ cells outside of the body, various internal structures which aid in the process, and the penis that, during sexual intercourse, allows the deposit of the germ cells into the reproductive tract of the female. A successful outcome—achieving a pregnancy—depends upon a complex interplay of physical and emotional factors.

Testes

The testes are a pair of ovoid organs that produce testosterone and spermatozoa (germ cells) in the mature male. They develop within the abdominal cavity and descend into the scrotal sac during fetal development. Human sperm production and viability require a narrow range of temperatures just below normal body temperature. The *scrotum* acts as a thermostat, relaxing with warmth to keep the testes away from the body, contracting when cold to bring the testes up towards the perineum.

Each testicle consists of about 250 wedge-shaped lobes. Each lobe contains a few narrow, coiled tubes known as the *seminiferous tubules*, which produce spermatozoa. Also located in the testes are *Sertoli's cells*, which supply nutrients to the sperm, and *Leydig's cells*, which produce testosterone.

Duct System

The process of spermatogenesis takes about 60 days in the seminiferous tubules. After another 14 days in the *epididymis*, the sperm are usually motile (able to move) and capable of fertilizing an ovum.

The sperm then move through the *vas deferens* towards the *urethra*. Several glands in this area contribute secretions that ensure the survival of the sperm. The first of these are the *seminal vesicles*, which lie behind the bladder and secrete a thick nutrient-containing fluid. The *prostate gland* surrounds the urethra at the neck of the bladder. It secretes a thin, milky, alkaline fluid essential for maintaining viability of the sperm. The *bulbourethral (Cowper's) glands* are a pair of pea-shaped structures that lie along the lower portion of

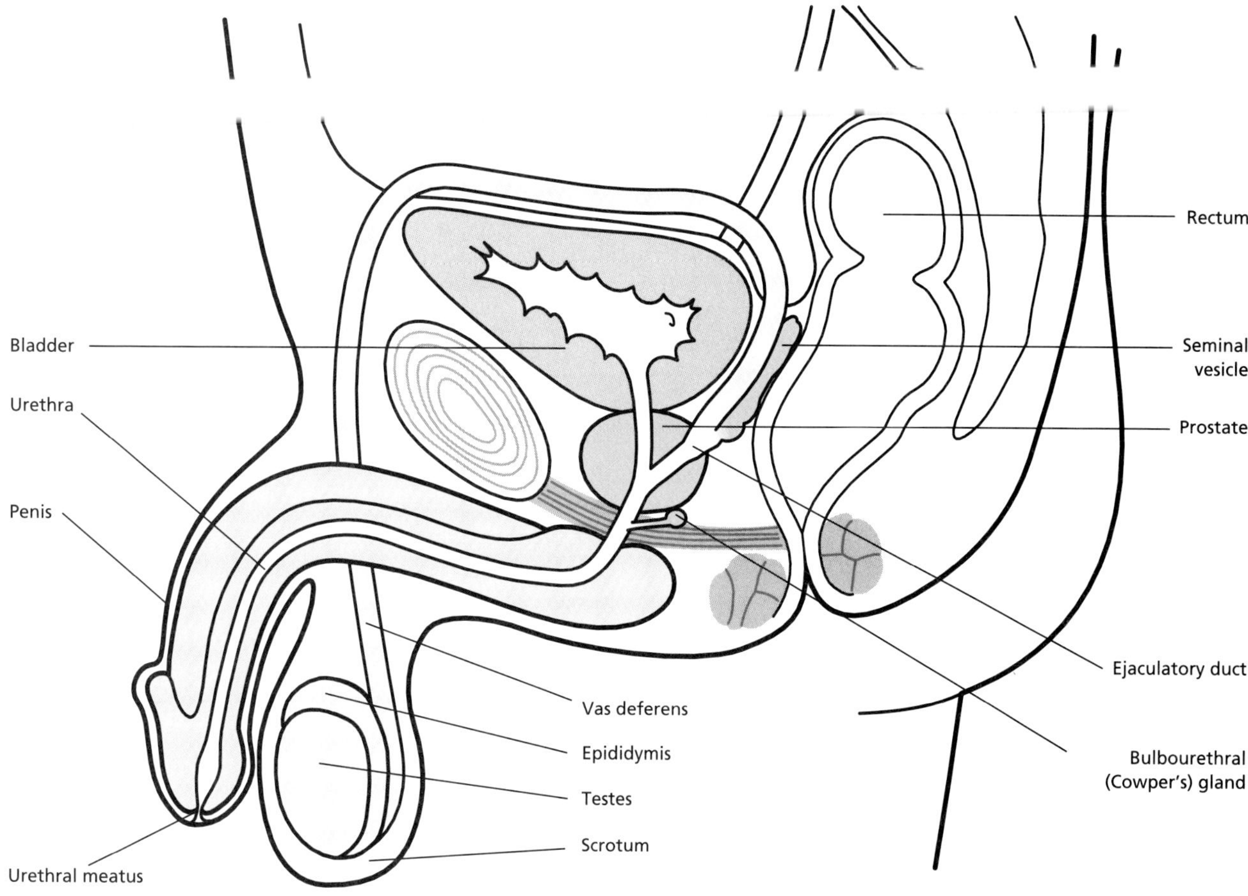

FIGURE 35.4 Male reproductive organs

the urethra. They secrete a mucous substance during sexual stimulation, called pre-ejaculatory fluid. This fluid is slightly alkaline and protects the sperm from residual acidity of urine in the urethra. It may also contain significant numbers of sperm.

The combination of spermatozoa and fluids from the various glands is known as *semen* or *seminal fluid*. During the process of ejaculation, about 2 mL to 6 mL of seminal fluid containing several hundred million sperm are discharged by a healthy male. The average normal sperm count is about 120 million per mL, of which an average of 60 percent to 80 percent will be motile. Semen is thick and milky when first ejaculated, but rapidly becomes watery due to the action of hydrolytic enzymes from the prostate gland.

Penis

The penis is the male organ of copulation. In the flaccid or nonerect state there is some degree of difference in size among individuals. In the erect state, however, size variations are less marked (the average size is 15 cm by 2.5 cm). The penis consists of three cylindrical structures (cavernous bodies) of erectile tissue bound together by fibrous bands. They extend into the pelvis where they are attached to the anterior and lateral walls of the pubic arch by muscle fibres. Two of these structures located in the dorsal portion of the penis are called the *corpus cavernosa*. The third structure, located more ventrally, is called the *corpus spongiosum*. The corpus spongiosum also forms the *glans penis*, the enlarged conical structure at the end of the penis. The urethra is contained within the corpus spongiosum and the opening in the glans penis is called the *urethral meatus*. The glans is covered by a fold of retractable skin, the *foreskin* or *prepuce*, which may be removed by circumcision for cultural, religious or health reasons.

During sexual arousal or in situations where nerve reflexes are activated, blood flow increases to the pelvic area and the cavernous bodies, causing the penis to become erect. Vascular pressure increases, slowing blood flow out of the penis and allowing the erection to be maintained. Erection of the penis is essential for vaginal intercourse to take place.

The Sexual Response Cycle

The human sexual response can be triggered by a variety of stimuli. These may be mental, such as sexual fantasies or thoughts; or sensory, involving vision, smell, taste, hearing or touch. Responsiveness to any particular stimulus is highly individual and can vary in the same person from time to time. Sexual responsiveness and function also depend upon the emotional status of the individual. Some "turn-offs" are anxiety, pain, lack of privacy or lack of trust in one's partner.

Physiologists divide the human sexual response cycle into four phases: excitement, plateau, orgasm and resolution. This commonly used definition of the human sexual response cycle evolved from laboratory situations in which researchers Masters and Johnson (1966) used male and female volunteers who were chosen because of a history of sexual responsiveness. The conclusions were reached after measuring physiological changes in a laboratory setting and so probably do not reflect the great variation in sexual responses of people in general. Because of this same fact, the definition does not reflect the variations that happen within each person on different occasions either. The human sexual response cycle definition is best used as a guideline, but not as a standard against which all sexual experiences should be evaluated.

Generally, two main physiological changes take place during sexual response: vasocongestion and myotonia. Vasocongestion occurs when the sexual response is triggered. There is a rise in heart rate and blood pressure. The blood vessels (chiefly the venous system) in the lower pelvic area and the genitals become engorged with blood. Myotonia is the increase in muscle tension, which in turn enhances the response to sensory stimuli. The awareness of these physical changes also contributes to the arousal process.

EXCITEMENT PHASE

Touching and caressing various body parts can promote arousal. These are called the "erogenous zones," after Eros, the Greek god of love. The most sensitive areas in many women are the breasts and the genitals, particularly the clitoris. As a woman becomes sexually aroused, vaginal lubrication begins, the inner two-thirds of the vagina expands, the outer lips of the vulva open and the clitoris enlarges. The vaginal walls become a dark purplish colour due to vasocongestion. As the excitement phase continues, the breasts swell, the nipples become erect and the areolae become engorged. A redness or maculopapular rash appears on the skin of the epigastric region and breasts, known as a "sex flush."

In men, the response to sexual stimuli may appear to be more rapid than in females, although the physiological changes are the same. The most obvious sign of male sexual arousal is erection of the penis. At the same time, the scrotal sac is pulled up towards the body and the scrotal skin becomes thick and rigid.

As the stimulation continues, the blood pressure and heart rate in both sexes increases. Rising sexual tension causes involuntary tensing of the intercostal and abdominal muscles.

PLATEAU PHASE

During the plateau phase in women, the uterus is elevated within the pelvis and the vaginal barrel elongates. Vasocongestion causes swelling of the labia minora and the outer third of the vagina. The colour of the labia minora changes from bright red to dark purple. The Bartholin's glands secrete a small amount of mucoid material and the clitoris retracts against the symphysis pubis. The muscles of the pelvic floor retract, allowing for comfortable insertion of the penis.

In the male, the plateau phase includes a further increase in size of the head of the penis and the testicles. The glans may also darken in colour, and clear fluid (pre-ejaculatory fluid from Cowper's glands) may appear at the urethral meatus. As muscle tension increases, the blood pressure becomes markedly elevated. Just prior to ejaculation, a valve located in the urethra at the bladder neck closes to prevent discharge of urine and to create a path through the penile urethra for the semen.

ORGASM

In both men and women, orgasm is characterized by a series of involuntary muscle contractions. In the female, there may be 5 to 12 contractions at 0.8-second intervals. They involve the uterus, the muscles of the lower abdomen and the pelvic floor. Contractions of the anal sphincter also occur.

In the male, clonic contractions along the length of the urethra transport the semen and expel it from the urethral meatus. The epididymis, vas deferens, seminal vesicles and prostate gland also contract at 0.8-second intervals. The contractions become less frequent as the ejaculatory process is completed (within a few seconds). Separate, but closely related, reflex centres in the spinal cord govern erection, ejaculation and orgasm. These three events are thus interrelated, but can occur independently.

Sexual response can occur regardless of the type of sexual activity that is taking place. It may occur during a fantasy or a dream, during sexual activity with a partner or during self-stimulation. The experience of orgasms is highly individual and subjective. It can be different each time, depending on how it is achieved (for instance, fantasy, vaginal intercourse, anal intercourse, partner or self-masturbation, or use of sexual aids). Following orgasm, a woman may be able to become sexually aroused again almost immediately and experience second, third or more orgasms. In males, however, a period of 10 to 45 minutes (or more depending upon the age and health status of the man) is required before the arousal cycle can recur. This is called the *refractory period*.

RESOLUTION

In the resolution phase the heart rate, respiration and blood pressure return to normal. In women, nipple erection subsides, breast size decreases and the skin flush disappears.

Resolution occurs within 10 to 15 minutes or, if no orgasm occurs, it may last a day. In men, the penis, testes and scro- [illegible]

[illegible]

Determinants of Sexual Functioning

There is probably no other area of human functioning that is affected by as many factors as sexuality. Successful sexual functioning combines a range of sensory and motor responses that are mediated by cognitive, emotional, social and biological influences. These determinants are listed in the box below. A disturbance in any area can interfere with sexual functioning. In a way, the experience of healthy sexuality depends on the absence of negative factors almost as much as it depends on the presence of positive ones.

Psychosocial Factors

Cognitive

As a child grows towards maturity, the development of cognitive skills provides the ability to seek out and maintain relationships, to understand the concept of consent, to evaluate possible risks and benefits and to recognize and adopt rewarding behaviours. With regard to sexual functioning, the stage of cognitive development is as important as chronological age. For example, someone who has well-developed cognitive skills may prefer to seek sexual gratification through masturbation rather than through more risky involvement with a partner.

Emotional

Mental health professionals have long been aware that depressive illnesses have a dampening effect on sexual function. The primary effect is a decrease in desire and a subsequent loss of sexual interest. Emotional well-being is integral to a positive self-image, which in turn contributes to a healthy interest in all aspects of life, including sexuality.

Factors Influencing Sexual Function

Psychosocial Factors	Biological Factors
Cognitive	Age
Emotional	Genetics
Educational	Health related:
Personal	Acute illness
Societal	Chronic illness
Situational	Disability
	Treatment related:
	Medications
	Other treatments
	Recreational substance use

[illegible]

Myths and misinformation about human sexuality abound, often causing individuals to make decisions that have unfortunate results. For example, a young woman who thinks that pregnancy cannot occur the first time she has intercourse may not even consider using a condom for birth control, or for protection from sexually transmitted diseases. Studies have shown that access to accurate, relevant information, such as that provided through comprehensive health education programs in schools, promotes healthy sexual decision making (Orton & Rosenblatt, 1986).

Personal and Societal

Every society in history has attempted to control sexual behaviour to some degree through societal norms. Children learn very early what constitutes acceptable sexual behaviour within their culture. These early lessons are very powerful and can have a lifelong influence on personal values. For example, a person raised in an atmosphere of strict sexual repression may have difficulty learning to be sexually responsive even in a marital situation where sexual behaviour is sanctioned.

Although there may be some variation from one culture to another, certain sexual taboos are nearly universal. One of these is prohibition of incest, which is sexual intercourse between members of the same family (father with daughter, mother with son, or between siblings). Sexual taboos are frequently enforced by legal controls. Sexual assault (the violent sexual assault on one person by another), sexual activity between an adult and a child, and indecent exposure (inappropriate exposure of the body) are all illegal acts described in the Canadian *Criminal Code*. In addition to major impacts on emotional health in general, sexual abuse or assault during or after childhood can have a damaging influence on subsequent sexual function. Although many survivors of childhood sexual abuse and trauma are able to develop into sexually healthy adults, therapists note that a high percentage of people who seek help for sexual problems have a history of sexual abuse (Maltz, 1992; Beitchman, Zucker, Hood, DaCosta, Akman & Cassavia, 1990).

Some religions exert important influences on the sexual behaviour of followers and, in a general way, on society at large. For example, the Judeo–Christian and Islamic faiths have strict codes allowing sexual contact only within marriage and teach that the principal objective of marriage is to have children. Although not strictly adhered to, these codes of behaviour influence general attitudes in subtle ways.

Personal factors also have a significant bearing on sexual functioning. Restrictive attitudes, ignorance and fear shroud with feelings of guilt, repression and anxiety what is a normal biological function. During the latter part of this century, societal attitudes have changed, with more general acceptance of consensual sexual activity regardless of marital status, with a recognition of the right of women to sexual satisfaction in relationships and with a tolerance of pregnancy and parenthood for unmarried women. The availability and widespread use of contraception has provided women with reproductive choices that were not possible even 50 years ago. With the ability to postpone childbearing, women have been able to exercise other life choices in career, relationships and lifestyle.

Other issues related to sexuality remain controversial. One such area is homosexuality, which is still considered abnormal and deviant by many religious and cultural groups. The scientific community, however, now recognizes that sexual preference is inherent. Homosexuality is not a perversion, but a reflection of one facet of the large spectrum of human sexual preference.

Situational

A number of situational factors may influence sexual functioning. These include the availability of a compatible partner, the capacity to sustain an intimate relationship with a sexual partner and opportunities for sexual expression. For instance, a young couple, both of whom are pursuing successful careers while raising a family, may find little time or energy for intimacy and sexual expression. Freedom from anxiety about sexual performance, pregnancy and sexually transmitted diseases are other factors that affect sexual functioning.

Biological Factors

Age

Age and physical development are very important factors in determining sexual function. Neurological pathways for sensory input and for certain reflex responses are intact and functioning prior to birth. For example, erection of the penis may be observed on ultrasound scans of the fetus, and small children are known to be capable of experiencing orgasm. The anatomical structures required for reproduction are present at birth, but do not become capable of this function until puberty.

The sexual response cycle, from arousal to orgasm, can occur, if conditions allow it, in either sex throughout the life cycle. Women are capable of bearing children from the onset of puberty until menopause and can fulfill this function even if the sexual response cycle is absent. After puberty, the male produces sperm on a more or less continuous basis and is capable of biological fatherhood even in old age. For reproductive purposes, an erection response is necessary to insert the penis into the vagina. The only other requirement is for ejaculation to occur within the vagina. For most males, orgasm and ejaculation occur simultaneously or within seconds of each other. Although increasing age can have a negative effect on general health, which in turn can affect sexual function, sexual response patterns change with age, but do not disappear.

Genetics

The primary biological agents controlling reproductive and sexual function are the genes and the hormones. Initial differentiation of the sexual organs *in utero* is determined by the XX or XY chromosome combination in the newly formed embryo. Further development of the sexual organs is controlled by hormones produced under the influence of these chromosomes. Defects in the sex chromosomes or disturbances of the hormone balance can give rise to problems in growth, development, future sexual function and fertility. One example is *Klinefelter's syndrome*, which occurs in males. It is caused by the presence of an extra X chromosome and can result in low testosterone levels, small testicles, a nonmasculine stature and no sperm production. *Turner's syndrome* is a genetic defect that affects females. This syndrome results from the absence of one of the X chromosomes. The ovaries and breasts fail to develop adequately, menarche does not appear and stature may remain short. Women with Turner's syndrome are no less feminine than other women. If treated with female hormones, they can develop an adult female body type, however, pregnancy is not possible.

Health-Related Factors

Sexual function can be altered by a disease or disability if sensory loss, motor disability, loss of reflexes or muscle weakness occur as part of the disease process. Some of the effects of illnesses, such as pain, fatigue, depression, anxiety, grief reaction, altered self-image or changed sex roles, can also impact on sexual function, as can some medications and other treatments. Therapeutic medications and recreational drugs can affect sexual function by causing a decrease in the sex drive or by interfering with the vascular or neuromuscular systems. Table 35.1 outlines the effects of treatments and recreational drugs on sexual functioning.

Sexuality Needs Throughout the Life Cycle

The biological purpose of the sex drive is to ensure continuation of a species. In most other species, coital activity is mostly limited to episodes when the female is fertile and biologically programmed to be receptive. In human beings, however, sexual needs include more than the physical need to propagate the race. The cognitive abilities of human beings allow recognition that sexual activity is inherently rewarding. The pleasure obtained from physical contact with another person and from positive sensory stimulation is reinforced by the pleasurable experience of orgasm. The "reward" of orgasm is probably a factor in the desire for sexual contact, whether or not procreation is intended. Human sexuality involves a complex set of relationships between

TABLE 35.1 Effect of surgery, medications and recreational drugs on sexual function

Alcohol	Small amounts: decreased inhibitions, increased libido Chronic use: lowered testosterone, erectile and ejaculatory dysfunction, infertility
Tobacco	Long-term use: *Men:* erectile dysfunction, infertility *Women:* infertility
Cocaine	Short-term use: said to enhance sexual pleasure Long-term use: decreased libido, impaired erectile, ejaculatory and orgasmic responses
Marijuana	Long-term use: Same as cocaine, infertility
Anabolic steroids	*Women:* menstrual disturbances, infertility *Men:* testicular atrophy, lowered testosterone, low sperm production, possibly permanent sterility
Tricyclic antidepressants ***Monoamine oxidase inhibitors*** ***Anticholinergic drugs*** ***Antihypertensives*** ***Antihistamines*** ***Antispasmodics*** ***Beta blockers*** ***Radiation therapy***	All of these commonly used medications can affect sexual function, depending on dosage and individual response. The most common effects in men are problems with erection, orgasm or ejaculation. In women, libido and orgasmic response may be affected. May have a negative effect on general health as well as on the reproductive glands and organs
Surgery	Includes structural and functional changes in the body, altered body image and grief in reaction to perceived loss.

people. These include the need to develop and express the self as a male or female within society, the need to engage in close, reciprocal relationships with others and the need to mate and reproduce children.

INFANCY

As has been mentioned, sex differentiation begins *in utero*, and sexual and reproductive organs are intact but immature at the time of birth. The first "sexual" experiences of an infant are related to gratification of basic needs for nourishment, warmth and touch. If these early experiences are positive, the infant's feelings of love, trust and self-worth are engendered. These form a solid basis for a personality that allows people to take risks and extend themselves to others in future relationships.

CHILDHOOD

One of the most important developmental tasks of childhood is the establishment of gender identity and gender (sex) role identity. The child learns his or her gender, that he is a "boy" or she is a "girl," and incorporates the appropriate gender role at the same time. Gender role behaviours include mannerisms, deportment, demeanour, preferences for play or recreational activities, daydreams and fantasies, life goals and performance on projective tests. Overemphasizing the importance of gender roles can have the unfortunate consequence of gender role stereotyping. In the absence of rigid gender role behaviour guidelines, children are able to learn more complete life skills and enjoy the expression of creativity.

Gender identity and role are imprinted during the first three years of life, by which time the child's self-concept includes the gender-appropriate label. Some children may briefly experiment with the opposite gender identity by role-playing behaviours specific to that gender.

Although a same-gender role model is helpful in early childhood, children need role models of both genders to develop a sexual identity and later to establish comfortable relationships with others. A safe, loving and nurturing environment is now considered to be a much more important factor than the gender of a parent. In addition, during the preschool years, children need clear, honest answers to questions about sexuality. They need to know the correct names for reproductive anatomy and should have a basic understanding of the male and female roles in reproduction.

Gender roles are firmly entrenched during the early school years. By age nine or 10, segregation of the sexes is reflected in different interests and play activities. Boys may prefer sports such as soccer, baseball and football, while girls seem to enjoy such activities as skipping rope, dancing and skating. As barriers based on gender are lowered, the differences in activity preferences are becoming less marked.

Children explore and derive pleasure from their own bodies, including the genital area. **Masturbation**, the stroking and stimulation of one's own genital area, is quite common throughout childhood. School-aged children are usually very curious about sexual matters as they develop the ability to understand abstract concepts, such as relationships and consequences of behaviours. They need to know about the physical and emotional changes that occur during puberty before they are experienced, about sexuality and reproductive function, about sexual assault and about sexually transmitted diseases. Decision-making and communication skills are also important for a healthy sexuality to develop.

PUBERTY

Puberty is defined as the process by which the body gains the physical ability to reproduce. In girls, estrogen levels begin to rise at about age eight or nine. There may be a marked increase in height, and breast development begins with the growth of "breast buds." Axillary and pubic hair appears, hips broaden and further breast development is followed by menarche.

The first few menstrual cycles may be anovulatory; that is, the ovaries do not release an ovum. However, ovulation does take place in some early cycles as pregnancies have occurred in young women who have not yet had a menstrual period. Adolescent women may experience difficulties with menstruation, including irregular cycles, amenorrhea (absence of menstruation) or dysmenorrhea (painful menstruation). The fluctuations of hormones can produce uncomfortable premenstrual symptoms and strong emotional reactions. Dysmenorrhea can be treated successfully in most cases by medications such as nonsteroidal anti-inflammatory drugs that have an antiprostaglandin (antispasmodic) effect on smooth muscle.

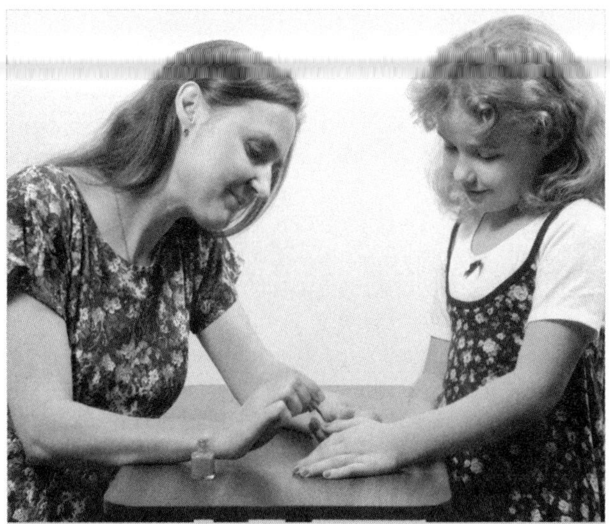

In developing gender role identity, a girl often imitates her mother.

Societal or cultural attitudes tend to be very negative towards menstruation, as reflected by commercial advertising of sanitary products where the need for deodorants and for internal, unseen protection (tampons) is emphasized. Positive attitudes towards menstruation can be fostered in young women by female relatives, by peer groups and by health professionals, particularly nurses and health educators.

In boys, levels of testosterone are low until about eight years of age. The early physical changes of puberty are not as obvious as they are in girls. Nonetheless, they include enlargement and an increase in pressure sensitivity of the testes, reddening and stippling of the scrotal skin, an increase in penis size, the appearance of axillary, pubic and facial hair, activation of axillary sweat glands, voice change, nocturnal emissions ("wet dreams"), an increase in height and a broadening of the shoulders. These changes can begin as early as age eight or nine years old but may not be completed for several years. The age range for puberty in boys is between nine and 17, with the average age of first ejaculation of semen at about age 12.

ADOLESCENCE

Adolescence encompasses the physical changes of puberty, and includes the psychological, cognitive and social transition from childhood into adulthood. Adolescence is a process involving coming to terms with a new physical appearance, as well as with an emerging self-identity.

Up until the early part of the 20th century, puberty was generally followed closely by marriage, with childbearing occurring as a natural consequence. Adolescents now seem to reach puberty about three years earlier than is thought to have been the average 100 years ago. The need to attain greater levels of education and to "grow up" before seeking a spouse causes a delay between the onset of biological maturity and the time when sexual behaviours are officially sanctioned.

Adolescents frequently find themselves caught between their own biological urges and desires, the need to conform to peer pressure, the "pro-sex" messages in advertising and the

ents, religious groups and well-meaning health educators. In the book *The Dynamics of Psychological Development*, Thomas and Chess (1980) outline the developmental tasks involved in attaining sexual adulthood, expressed in terms of cultural norms. There is no end-point to these tasks, some of which require lifelong effort. These developmental tasks include:

1. establishing basic identity as a male or female (usually by age three or four)
2. adopting appropriate gender role behaviours as dictated by the particular cultural milieu (an ongoing process)
3. developing sexual attraction to the opposite gender
4. knowing how to give and receive sexual pleasure
5. having ability to establish intimacy in a relationship
6. establishing sufficient self-control over pleasure-seeking to control reproduction (and to practise safer sex).

Achievement of these developmental tasks requires that the adolescent learn behaviours involved in giving and receiving sexual pleasure. Skills required for establishing intimate relationships must also be gained. The challenge for our society is to allow adolescents sufficient opportunity to learn these behaviours and skills while ensuring that there will be few if any undesired consequences. Society must also learn to tolerate and accept the fact that a percentage of people are unable to conform to the expectation that they will develop heterosexual attraction. As a result of the strong need for social and peer-group conformity, any uncertainty about sexual preference can be devastating to an adolescent. Mental health professionals have observed a higher suicide rate among homosexual youth (*Suicide among gay and lesbian youth*, 1993). Other problems associated with adolescence and sexuality are high rates of unplanned pregnancy, sexual assault and abuse and very high rates of sexually transmitted infections. For example, chlamydia is the most often reported of all communicable diseases in North America (CDC, 1996).

To become sexually healthy adults, adolescents need comprehensive health education with curricula that include all topics relevant to sexuality. Whether they are gay or straight, adolescents need access to health care and other resources that will allow them to make responsible decisions about managing sexuality safely. When they make mistakes, special support services are needed to help diminish any negative effects.

YOUNG ADULTHOOD

Young adulthood marks the period of life when pair-bonding takes place and families begin. Although the traditional concept of the family as a basis for bearing and raising children is still strong, the definition of family can be expanded to include any group of two or more people who

"blended"; with higher rates of divorce and remarriage, new families are often formed with children from two or more previous relationships.

In addition to reproductive functions, sexual behaviour during young adulthood may foster closeness and intimacy, give pleasure and bolster self-esteem. Although there is a widespread belief that young adults are at their "sexual peak," the demands involved in raising and supporting a family and establishing an acceptable standard of living can be detrimental to relationships and sexual function. Fatigue, stress and unrealistic expectations about sexual performance can lead to dissatisfaction and distress. Approximately 15 percent to 20 percent of the population will experience infertility, which contributes to stress and sexual problems (Canadian Research Institute for the Advancement of Women, 1989). The incidence of both cancer of the cervix and infertility is associated with increased rates of sexually transmitted diseases within the general population. The rates of unplanned pregnancies and sexually transmitted diseases are also very high in men and women between the ages of 20 to 30. Taking the example of chlamydia genital infections, the prevalence rate is as high as 5–10 percent in women aged 15–24 (CDC, 1993). The incidence of testicular cancer is also highest in this age group, affecting, for example, 4 of every 100 000 white males per year (Reinisch, 1990). Based on 1996 statistics, an estimated 770 new cases were reported (Statistics Canada, 1998).

Young adults need ongoing access to reliable information about sexual function, contraception and safe sex practices. Some of the sexual difficulties in this age group can be addressed through health-promoting education and lifestyle changes.

MIDDLE ADULTHOOD

During the years commonly referred to as "middle age," ongoing changes in sexual and reproductive anatomy and function become more noticeable. Some women experience an increase in sexual drive while others note a decline in sexual interest and activity. The lowering of female hormone levels with menopause can cause vasomotor disturbances such as hot flushes, dizziness or headaches and disturbed sleep patterns. Lowered estrogen levels can also cause atrophy of the vaginal mucosa, leading to dryness, painful intercourse and increased susceptibility to vaginal infections. Prior to menopause, pregnancy is possible. The risk of sexually transmitted diseases does not disappear with menopause. Because the risks of cancer in the reproductive system increase with age, women in the middle years need information on how to promote sexual health and need access to regular health screening including mammography and gynecological examinations.

GERONTOLOGICAL

Physical Changes in Sexual Response in Old Age

	Female	**Male**
Excitation phase	Diminished or delayed lubrication (1 to 3 min may be required for adequate amounts to appear) Diminished flattening and separation of labia majora Disappearance of elevation of labia majora Decreased vasocongestion of labia minora Decreased elastic expansion of vagina (depth and breadth) Breasts not as engorged Sex flush absent	Less intense and slower erection (but can be maintained longer without ejaculation) Increased difficulty regaining an erection if lost Less vasocongestion of scrotal sac Less pronounced elevation and congestion of testicles
Plateau phase	Slower and less prominent uterine elevation or tenting Decreased muscle tension Decreased capacity for vasocongestion Decreased areolar engorgement Less evident labial colour change Less intense swelling of orgasmic platform Less sexual flush Decreased secretions of Bartholin glands	Decreased muscle tension Nipple erection and sexual flush less often No colour change at coronal edge of penis Slower penile erection pattern Delayed or diminished erectal and testicular elevation
Orgasmic phase	Fewer and less intense orgasmic contractions Rectal sphincter contractions with severe tension only	Decreased or absent secretory activity (lubrication) by Cowper gland before ejaculation Fewer penile contractions Fewer rectal sphincter contractions Decreased force of ejaculation (approximately 50%) with decreased amount of semen (if ejaculation is long, seepage of semen occurs)
Resolution phase	Observably slower loss of nipple erection Vasocongestion of clitoris and orgasmic platform quickly subsides	Vasocongestion of nipples and scrotum slowly subsides Very rapid loss of erection and descent of testicles shortly after ejaculation Refractory time extended (time required before another erection ranges from several to 24 hours, occasionally longer)

SOURCE: Ebersole & Hess, 1998, p. 591.

Although there is no such phenomenon as "male menopause," many men are distressed by changes in sexual function and may become concerned about sexual performance. These changes may include a slower erectile response, a decrease in the degree of erection or a decrease in the intensity of orgasm and/or force of ejaculation (or, occasionally, a loss of ejaculation). Many men require more direct manual stimulation to become aroused and have a longer refractory period following orgasm. In some men, the interval between arousal and orgasm is prolonged, which could have the beneficial effect of allowing more time for a partner to achieve orgasm. Male fertility declines gradually with the lowering of testosterone levels, but healthy men have been known to father children even in older adulthood.

Men in their middle years are at increased risk for benign or malignant overgrowth of the prostate gland. In addition to reassuring information about the normal and gradual changes in sexual function, men need regular health examinations that include a rectal examination of the prostate gland.

OLDER ADULTHOOD

During the later years, the changes that occurred in the middle years may become more pronounced. The myth that older adults are not interested in sex was shattered by a Canadian study on sexuality by Judith Stryckman. She found that "seven out of ten couples who do not have major health problems were sexually active, sometimes into their late eighties" (Government of Canada, 1990, p. 2). "Age, it seems, has less of an effect on interest in sexual activity than previous patterns of sexual activity. Those with a strong interest in sex in their younger days continue to have it as they grow older" (DuGas, 1993, p. 148).

An older adult who has access to a willing and capable partner can enjoy a full range of sexual activities. A loving sexual relationship, even one that does not include sexual

Respecting the Sexuality of Older Adults

- Support and encourage interest in appearance and individuality.
- Encourage children to accept their parents' sexuality and their need for intimate contact.
- Recognize that sexuality may be expressed in many physical and emotional ways, only one of which is sexual intercourse.
- Ensure that older adults have the opportunity to meet members of the opposite gender.
- Do not deprive older adults of the privacy they need to develop an intimate relationship.
- Encourage older adults to speak up for themselves and make others aware of their right to make decisions about their own sexuality.

SOURCE: Du Gas, 1993, p. 152.

intercourse, contributes significantly to the health and well-being of an older person. Because women in general have a longer life span than men, older women are more likely to lack a partner and may suffer from loneliness or even touch deprivation. Some suggestions for respecting the sexuality of older people are highlighted in the box above.

The incidence of cancer and degenerative diseases is higher in older people and these diseases can have a negative impact on sexual function. If sexuality is recognized and validated, older people are more likely to seek assistance with sexual difficulties, especially if these are associated with a health concern.

Sexual Behaviours, Orientations and Variations

There are many possible sexual behaviours known to most sexually active adults. Some other behaviours are not so familiar, or may be viewed as strange, risky or uninteresting. Generally, an activity can be considered within the range of "normal" if it is mutually desired and enjoyed when shared, if it provides sensual pleasure and if it causes no mental or physical harm.

Some sexual behaviours such as fantasies and dreams require little or no physical effort. These behaviours are **autosexual activities**, referring to self-involvement only. Masturbation is also an autosexual behaviour, and often takes the form of rhythmic stroking of the genital area. As recently as 50 years ago, masturbation was considered to be unhealthy and a probable cause of mental illness and other ailments that commonly afflicted young people. It is now being accepted more and more as a natural and healthy manner of sexual expression for people of all ages and as a safe way for young women and men to learn about their own sexual responses.

Heterosexual behaviours include activities that are

Many people who are unable for one reason or another to have intercourse discover, to their delight, that the activities usually called foreplay can be just as satisfying as intercourse. Stimulation of a woman's genitals by a partner's mouth or tongue is called *cunnilingus*, and the same activity performed on a man's genitals is called *fellatio*. Both activities are called "oral sex" and may or may not be a prelude to intercourse. Couples may also engage in *outercourse*, or the rubbing of the penis between the thighs or breasts. This is often done as a form of contraception.

Although anal intercourse has been generally considered a homosexual form of activity, in two recent surveys, between 9 and 13 percent of women reported that they engaged in anal intercourse regularly. Another survey indicates that up to 43 percent of heterosexual couples engage in anal intercourse at least occasionally (Reinisch, 1990).

Homosexual behaviours can include any possible combinations of the previously mentioned activities, but take place between partners of the same gender. **Homosexuality** is a sexual orientation, defined as the romantic and sexual attraction to a same-gender partner. There is no clear explanation for homosexuality, but it existed in ancient cultures, and is considered to be an inherent aspect of a person's identity. **Bisexuality** refers to the preference and attraction to either gender.

There are four stages of homosexual and bisexual identity formation: (1) *sensitization*, the time when the child may feel different and recognize some attraction to persons of the same gender; (2) *sexual identity confusion*, often occurring in adolescence, when the young person attempts to understand internal feelings while attending to negative societal pressures against homosexuality or bisexuality; (3) *sexual identity assumption*, in which the individual explores homosexual or bisexual practices and lifestyles; and (4) *integration and commitment* to his or her sexual orientation. One study indicates that the average time between recognition of homosexual or bisexual orientation and disclosure to others is more than four years. Some individuals never disclose their orientation to others (Mattox, 1998).

There are a number of other variations in human sexual identity and sexual behaviour. Gender dysphoria, commonly known as **transsexualism**, occurs when an individual's gender identity does not match their biological gender. In this situation, a man may feel like a woman trapped in a male body or a woman may view herself as a man in a woman's body. **Transvestism**, or cross-dressing, refers to the activity of dressing like the opposite gender for sexual pleasure or psychological comfort. Another variation in sexual behaviour is **paraphilia**. In Greek, "para" means beyond or outside of the usual and "philia" means love. Paraphilias range from sexual preferences not considered very unusual—for example, a desire to see one's partner dressed in seductive underwear, to more extreme or possibly dangerous activities such as bondage or asphyxiation. A more thorough discussion of these variant sexual preferences and behaviours is beyond the scope of this book.

Common Sexual Concerns

A large number of factors can influence sexual function. Problems may arise when people feel that patterns of sexual interest or response that are normal for them have been impaired. For instance, fear of the effect of sexual activity on the heart following a heart attack may inhibit sexual desire for both partners. Sometimes sexual problems are actually culturally based differences in expectations. For example, a male partner may view his female partner's sexual arousal and orgasm as a direct reflection of his masculinity. His partner, however, may not be easily aroused or may not need frequent orgasm. The pressure of his expectations can generate feelings of inadequacy and stress, which can further suppress sexual desire. Table 35.2 presents an outline of some common sexual concerns.

Persons with Disabilities/Chronic Illnesses

There is a prevalent belief that persons with physical and mental disabilities are asexual. In most instances, sexual desire is not affected by physical or mental limitations. When working with individuals who have a disability, the nurse must include sexuality in her assessment, just as she would for any client in her care. Many clients with disabilities are sexually active. This means that information about safe sex, contraceptive methods and special approaches to the expression of sexuality will be required. Couples may have to experiment with a variety of techniques and positions to find those that result in comfort and pleasure. For example, individuals with rheumatoid arthritis, multiple sclerosis, spinal cord injury or any other mobility-limiting disease may benefit from suggestions about the following: use of baths and massage to relax muscles prior to engaging in sexual activity; use of analgesic medication to reduce pain; use of pillows under joints after determining which positions will be most comfortable; and timing to avoid excessive fatigue. Aromatherapy and music might also assist with relaxation. For those people lacking sensation due to spinal cord injury, stimulation of erogenous zones above the level of injury can result in something called paraorgasm. **Paraorgasm** results from a buildup of sexual tension and goes through similar phases (but with less intensity) as the sexual response outlined earlier in this chapter. Advice on how to manage possible bladder and bowel responses to sexual stimulation will be helpful to those with spinal cord lesions.

Individuals with developmental delay also experience sexual feelings, thoughts and desires. Because understanding these feelings and knowing how to respond to them appropriately may be problematic for persons with mental disabilities, special educational programs have been developed that assist both parents and professionals in presenting information in a way that will be helpful and understandable.

Persons with disabilities need to know how their functional abilities influence their sexual practices, but sexual response is influenced by more than functional ability. The broader aspects of sexuality must be appreciated for all individuals. Some couples choose to become parents and may need special assistance with the demands of the childbearing cycle.

Female Circumcision

Female circumcision is widely practised in some areas of Africa, the Middle East and southeast Asia. Nurses need to be aware of this practice, as some of their clients may present with symptoms such as dysmenorrhea, nonconsummation, urinary tract infection or psychosexual problems occurring as a consequence of the particular form of genital surgery. The term *circumcision* is used to describe the removal of the hood of the clitoris. *Excision* is the amputation of the clitoris, sometimes with the removal of the labia minora. *Infibulation* involves the removal of the clitoris, the labia minora and much of the labia majora. The procedure is carried out before the girl is 16 years of age. A culturally sensitive approach by the nurse is critical when working with clients who have undergone this procedure (Andrews, 1997).

Treatment of Sexual Concerns

Treatment of sexual problems may involve both psychological and physical treatment and will depend upon the cause of the dysfunction and the context in which it occurs. Sexual therapy begins with a detailed assessment that includes the time of onset of the problem (whether it has existed since the onset of sexual experiences or whether it began after a period of satisfactory sexual experiences); the extent of the problem (whether it is present in all situations or only in particular situations or with certain partners); and an exploration of the effects of the problem on the person and his or her partner. An educational component is often required. If problems are evident within the relationship in general, couple therapy may be required before sexual issues can be addressed. In most cases, and especially in those in which the sexual problem has had an impact on both partners and the relationship, therapy is most effective if both partners participate.

SEXUALLY TRANSMITTED DISEASES

There are a number of diseases caused by bacterial or bacteria-related organisms that are spread by infected people through intimate or sexual contact. These diseases are called sexually transmitted diseases or STDs. The human immunodeficiency

TABLE 35.2 Common sexual concerns

Problem	Women	Men
Impaired sexual desire	Also called *low libido*. Most frequent problem in women. May be associated with relationship problems, depression or organic causes.	In both primary and secondary cases, organic causes (for example, hypogonadism) may be a factor. In secondary cases, relationship with partner or depression may be a factor.
Impaired sexual arousal	Lack of sensations associated with sexual excitement. Absence of vaginal lubrication and engorgement. May occur secondary to impaired sexual interest following childbirth or menopause and in women with strong sexual inhibitions.	Manifested as erectile dysfunction. Most common problem in men who seek help.
Orgasmic problems	Absent or very infrequent orgasm in both men and women. If orgasm can occur with masturbation but not with the partner, this may be associated with relationship problems.	Same as for women.
Ejaculatory problems		*Premature ejaculation*: Ejaculations occur consistently before or very soon after vaginal penetration. Common in first sexual encounters and in stressful situations. *Retarded (delayed) ejaculation*: Relatively uncommon. Can affect both ejaculation and orgasm. *Retrograde ejaculation*: Usually due to physical causes (surgery to bladder, neck; spinal cord injury). Orgasm may be experienced, but ejaculation is directed into the bladder.
Other problems	*Dyspareunia* (Pain during intercourse): May be localized at introitus or deeper. Causes include lack of arousal or lubrication, vaginal or pelvic infection, endometriosis or constipation. *Vaginismus*: Involuntary muscle spasm at introitus, which occurs with attempted penetration. May be a primary problem or secondary to vaginal trauma or infection. Most women with vaginismus are otherwise sexually responsive.	

virus (HIV) and the hepatitis B virus are STDs that may be contracted through sexual contact with body fluids such as blood, semen, urine, or contact with feces.

STDs may also be found in areas of the body other than the sexual organs. For example, gonorrhea and chlamydia can infect other warm, moist areas such as the throat, the nasopharynx or the eyes. A person may be infected by more than one STD at a time. In addition, many STDs have similar or overlapping symptoms. In Table 35.3, the more common and serious STDs are listed as syndromes, or groups of symptoms that result from one or more infective agents.

Treatment of Sexually Transmitted Diseases

STDs are usually treated successfully with antibiotics. Unfortunately, reinfection can occur. Bacteria (such as gonococcus) may form resistance to antibiotics, which necessitates the development of ever more potent medications.

The virus that causes herpes simplex usually can only be treated symptomatically. Once the infection subsides, the virus is then harboured within the nerve pathways and becomes symptomatic and infectious when the body's natural defences are weakened through stress or illness.

TABLE 35.3 Common sexually transmitted diseases

Syndrome and Causative Agent	*Symptoms*
Urethritis • Gonococcus • Chlamydia and others	Penile pain or itching Dysuria Urethral discharge (30% to 50% asymptomatic)
Vaginitis • Candida albicans • Bacterial vaginosis: Gardnerella Trichomonas	Vulval, vaginal itching Abnormal vaginal discharge Redness, edema of vulva Dyspareunia Dysuria Unpleasant odour
Cervicitis • Chlamydia • Gonorrhea • Herpes simplex 2	Often asymptomatic Abnormal vaginal discharge Systemic symptoms (herpes) Dyspareunia Menstrual spotting Postcoital bleeding
Pelvic Inflammatory Disease • Chlamydia • Gonorrhea • Other non-STDs • HIV in women	Lower abdominal or back pain Menstrual spotting Abnormal vaginal discharge Fever, general malaise Dyspareunia
Ulcerative Skin Lesions • Syphilis (Treponema Pallidum)	Painless ulcer at area of contact Skin rash, fevers, general malaise **Late stage**: deterioration of neurological and cardiovascular systems, death
• Herpes simplex virus	**Primary infection**: malaise, fever, itching, pain in genital area, blister-like genital lesions lasting for three to six weeks **Recurrences**: same as primary but without malaise
Nonulcerative Skin Lesions • Condyloma acuminata (human papilloma virus) • Certain sub-types of HPV are implicated in some types of genital cancers, for example, cervix, vulva, penis, rectum	Cauliflower-like growths on genitals, in oral cavity, vagina or rectum; may be difficult to see
Other Viral Infections • HIV: causative agent of acquired immunodeficiency syndrome (AIDS)	**Early infection**: usually no symptoms **Later stages**: symptoms are related to loss of immune defences. Opportunistic infections and cancers develop in the majority of cases, leading to death. AIDS-related symptoms vary widely from person to person and for men and women. Tests for antibodies, indicating infection with HIV, may be negative for up to six months following exposure, but the person may infect others during that time.
• Hepatitis B Virus	**Acute hepatitis:** • malaise • fever • jaundice **Late complications:** • cirrhosis of the liver • cancer of the liver
• Hepatitis C Virus	Acute phase is usually asymptomatic and without jaundice; abnormal liver function tests and mild to severe symptoms for months or years

Viruses such as hepatitis B (HBV) and HIV are capable of surviving within the body for many years without symptoms, but they may be transmitted through unpro-

ing street drugs. Treatment for both HBV and HIV/AIDS is aimed at treating opportunistic infections and diseases and supporting the body's natural defences as much as possible. A vaccine is available for the prevention of hepatitis B but a vaccine preventing HIV infection has not yet been developed. Neither disease is yet curable, which leads to an emphasis on prevention. Health Canada recently pubished the 1998 edition of *Canadian STD Guidelines* for health professionals working for the prevention/management of STD.

Assessing Sexuality Needs

An assessment of a patient's sexual health status is an essential part of the general health assessment. This includes an appraisal of physical or functional status and an exploration of the psychosocial aspects of sexual health. Reproductive health issues will be briefly discussed here because the reproductive system is involved in both sexual function and childbearing.

Nursing Health History

When taking a health history, a thorough exploration of the patient's sexual practices and patterns of sexual functioning is neither appropriate nor necessary in the majority of cases. For instance, when a patient comes into the hospital for the removal of a gallbladder, it is not necessary to inquire about sexual practices, but when admitted for an investigation of genitourinary symptoms, a sexual health history becomes necessary. It is important to discover any effects the current illness or treatment measures may have on sexual functioning and on sexual self-image. For example, how has gallbladder disease and the need for surgery affected a woman's ability to function as a mother and as a wife? When taking a sexual health history, the nurse begins with questions about the effects of the current illness on sexual functioning. If it is known that sexuality is likely to be affected by a specific illness, treatment regimen or surgery, more specific information about sexual functioning may be gathered. Should significant sexual needs and concerns become evident, a more thorough examination may then ensue. A guide for obtaining a brief sexual health history is given in the box that follows. The beginning student who does not feel ready to pursue this level of examination should seek the help of an instructor or experienced nurse.

Many people view sexuality as very private and are often reticent to discuss their sexual health. As a result, they may be reluctant to talk openly about sexual matters. In some cultures, discussing female and male physiologic functions and problems is taboo. It is therefore necessary to first obtain the patient's permission before asking sex-related questions. Patients may be more willing to discuss sexual functioning if they know why the information is needed and that the information will be kept strictly confidential. If the patient

cept this decision, stressing that they will be available to talk about any concerns the patient may have in the future.

To generate a level of trust that will allow for open discussion of personal issues, nurses must arrange for privacy and they must be sensitive to the patient's concerns in this regard. Because confidentiality is a critical point when information about sexual matters is being shared, nurses must emphasize that what is said in the interview will remain confidential. Taking the history when the patient is dressed and using terms they understand will enhance comfort. Terminology and anatomical language may pose barriers to obtaining accurate data about body functions. The use of slang terms may be necessary to impart meaning. Only those areas that are pertinent to the needs of the patient should be discussed.

Physical Assessment

Physical assessment begins with a general inspection of appearance. This includes body shape and stature (Is it appropriate for the gender?), hair distribution, skin texture and growth patterns. These aspects vary according to the age and developmental stage of the individual. Inspection and palpation techniques are used to assess the genital structures of both men and women. Just as many people do not like talking about sexual matters, they also do not like others looking at their genitals. Nurses must exercise the same consideration and sensitivity to patient privacy during physical assessment as they do during the history-taking. A confident, thoughtful and reassuring approach, along with proper draping will do much to enhance patient ease and reduce embarrassment. In addition, unless the patient is admitted with a sexual health problem, conducting the physical assessment while performing routine measures may alleviate embarrassment. For instance, the nurse might wait to carry out an external genital appraisal on an older adult until administering perineal hygiene care.

FEMALE PATIENTS

Female physical appraisal involves examination of the breasts, the external genitalia and an internal (pelvic) examination. Breast examination provides a good opportunity for teaching breast self-examination. The breasts are examined for age-appropriate contour, symmetry of structures, areas of skin pigmentation, the presence of redness, rashes, lesions and edema, as well as discharge from the nipple. It is not unusual for breasts to be slightly asymmetrical and unequal in size, particularly in growing women. The breasts, nipples and axillary and clavicular nodes are palpated for consistency of tissues, masses and tenderness.

The external genitalia are examined for the size, shape and colour of structures and the presence of lesions, inflammation

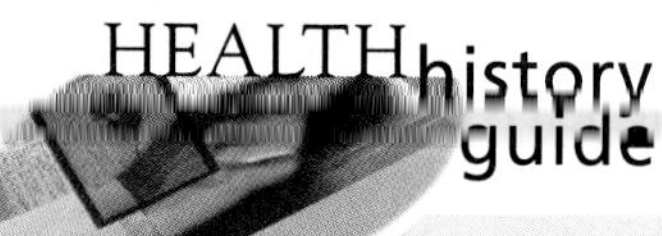

Sexuality

Health and Illness Patterns

- Are you sexually active?
- Has your illness or anything else affected your sexual function? If so, how?
- How has your illness or anything else affected your ability to function in your role as a spouse or sexual partner or parent?
- How has your illness or anything else affected the way you feel about yourself? As a man/woman?
- Do you have any concerns about your sexuality and sexual function?
- What do you expect from health care professionals in promoting your sexual health?

Health Promotion and Protection Patterns

For Females:

- Do you have a regular health checkup? Pap smear? Mammography?
- Do you examine your breasts on a monthly basis?

For Males:

- Do you examine your testes regularly?

For Both Sexes:

- Do you practise safe sex?
- Would you like some information on sexual self-care and on safe sex practices?

SOURCES: Carpenito, 1997; Woods, 1984.

and discharge. A mirror can be used to teach women about their own anatomy, showing them the mons pubis, the clitoris, the labia majora and minora, the urethral and vaginal openings and the openings of the ducts of Bartholin's and Skene's glands. Normally, the vulva is darker in colour than other skin areas, and the mucous membranes are dark, pink and moist. Abnormalities that should be noted include tenderness, irritations or lesions of the skin, discolouration, lumps or swelling in any area, abnormal size or adhesions of the clitoris and unusual discharge from the vagina. A small amount of clear or whitish discharge is normal.

The vaginal and internal pelvic examinations are ordinarily performed by physicians, midwives and nurses specializing in sexual health care. However, nurses may be called upon to assist with the procedure and certainly to prepare the patient and answer questions. The vaginal examination involves the use of a speculum and light source to examine the vagina and the cervix. The examiner looks for lesions, discolouration or unusual discharge from either the vaginal walls or the cervix, abnormalities in size or position of the cervix, and signs of infection, damage or growths in either area. If the speculum is metal, it should be warmed prior to use. The speculum should also be lubricated with a water-base jelly or warm water. While the speculum is in place, specimens may be obtained for laboratory examination, which will be discussed later. During the internal pelvic examination, the examiner inserts two gloved fingers into the vagina and exerts pressure to move the uterus and other organs towards the front of the abdominal wall, allowing palpation with the other hand. Any pain or abnormality in the size or consistency of the internal organs are noted.

In preparation for a vaginal or internal pelvic examination, the woman is asked to void immediately prior to the procedure. This facilitates ease of examination, since a full bladder distorts the position of the pelvic organs. A full bladder also makes the procedure more uncomfortable for the patient. The patient is usually placed in a lithotomy position to permit full visualization of the genital area. A lateral Sim's position may be used for patients who are unable to assume a lithotomy position, for example, women with arthritis or musculoskeletal deformity.

MALE PATIENTS

The genital examination includes visual inspection of the size and shape of the organs, the condition of the skin and the presence of lesions, edema, inflammation or discharge. The inguinal region is observed for hernias. Using a gloved hand, the penis is palpated for masses or tenderness. The tip of the glans is compressed to determine the presence of penile discharge (an abnormal finding). The scrotal contents are examined by holding the scrotum in the palm of one hand and gently palpating the structures with the thumb and first two fingers of the other hand. The testes are examined for size, shape, consistency and mobility and the epididymis and spermatic cord are examined for masses, tenderness and swelling. Normally, the testes are asymmetrical, the left usually being slightly lower than the right. Their size varies: approximately two centimetres in diameter at the larger end is average. The testes feel firm on palpation and move around easily. Because testicular cancer is common in young adult men, men should learn how to perform testicular self-examinations on a periodic basis. Again, a good time for patient teaching is during the physical assessment.

Diagnostic Tests

A number of laboratory tests are performed on a regular basis on any woman who is sexually active, regardless of age, and on every woman beyond the age of 20. The *Papanicalaou (Pap) test* is done to screen for cervical cell dysplasia (abnormal changes that can lead to cancer). The presence of trichomonas, herpes simplex and human papilloma virus. A small amount of tissue for laboratory examination is scraped from the cervix during a pelvic examination. Culture samples are taken to identify infectious diseases, caused mainly by *Candida albicans* (yeast), *Gardnerella vaginalis* (bacterial vaginosis), *Trichomonas vaginalis, Chlamydia trachomatis* and *N. gonorrhoeae*. At the same time, the vaginal walls and cervix are carefully scrutinized for herpes or HPV lesions. Reproductive hormone level assays are also done. Abnormal hormone levels may be a factor in disrupted sexual function or reproductive (fertility) problems. Reproductive hormone level changes can also confirm that menopause has occurred. The levels of male reproductive hormones may also be tested to confirm or rule out hormonal factors in sexual or fertility problems. Males who have ever had sexual intercourse should have routine cultures taken for chlamydia and gonorrhea. Cultures should also be obtained if any suspicious skin lesions are present.

Prostate-specific antigen is a serum blood test that can assist in the identification, classification and localization of a prostate tumour. This test can be administered pre- and postoperatively. It can also be used to monitor ongoing disease and assessment of treatment protocols (Chernecky & Berger, 1997).

Diagnosing Sexuality Problems

Sexuality problems that fall under the domain of nursing therapy are labelled *Altered Sexuality Patterns*. This diagnostic statement represents problems in which the patient is experiencing or is at risk for experiencing a change in sexual health (Carpenito, 1997). The diagnosis is used primarily when patients express concern about sexuality. For example, a diagnosis of *Altered Sexuality Pattern* applies to a woman who worries about her femininity and ability as a sexual partner following a radical mastectomy; or the middle-aged male who expresses concern about altered sexual function as a result of antihypertensive medications. Patients may experience a range of responses to conditions affecting sexuality. In these cases, nursing diagnoses reflecting these responses should be used. For instance, in an adolescent who is sexually active, but lacks knowledge of contraception and safe sex practices, the more appropriate diagnosis would be *Knowledge Deficit*. Similarly, the diagnosis for a patient who is anxious about the effects of treatment on body image would be stated as *Anxiety related to altered body image*.

Planning Sexuality Interventions

As with all nursing needs, the nurse formulates a plan of care based on the established nursing diagnoses. In many cases, patients' problems fall outside the domain of independent nursing intervention. A nursing plan of care might centre on examining feelings, providing information and making referrals to appropriate health care professionals. For instance, impaired sexual function due to physical problems may be referred to gynecologists or urologists or, if available, physicians or mental health professionals with training in sexual therapy. Marital difficulties and relationship problems might be referred to mental health professionals or to sex therapists. Collaboration with the patient and, if appropriate, the sex partner is essential in identifying patient goals and in formulating the plan of care. Effective achievement of goals or expected outcomes is more likely if the patient is involved in setting goals and has a desire to achieve them. Some examples of expected outcomes are listed below.

- Patient will identify limitations on sexual activity caused by health problem.
- Patient will express positive statements about body image and desirability as a sexual partner.
- Patient will report increase in sexual desire and arousal.
- Patient will verbalize proper use of contraceptive methods.
- Patient will verbalize safe sex practices.

Implementing Sexuality Interventions

There are three principal goals of nursing action regarding human sexual health and sexuality:

1. to provide the knowledge and skills that will enable people to promote and protect their sexual health
2. to assist in the detection of illnesses, abnormalities or other disorders that can have a damaging impact on sexual health
3. to assist with or carry out therapeutic measures and to provide support that may improve or restore sexual health.

The PLISSIT Model

Many nurses and health care providers are reluctant to address sexual issues, often because of their own discomfort or lack of special training. They may also be concerned about invading the privacy of patients. One model that is used frequently in sexual counselling is the PLISSIT Model,

The PLISSIT Model

P
(PERMISSION)
LI
(LIMITED INFORMATION)
SS
(SPECIFIC SUGGESTIONS)
IT
(INTENSIVE THERAPY)

developed by Annon in 1976. Annon's PLISSIT model identifies four levels of intervention and provides a guideline based on the skills and training of the health professional. The first, permission, would always be included in any intervention because it is important to promote questions and communication about concerns at every level.

PERMISSION

The primary element of the permission level of intervention is the encouragement of discussion about sexual matters. The message is given that "sex is spoken here." The role of the nurse at this level is to be sensitive to verbal or behavioural cues about sexual concerns (questions, inappropriate comments or sexual acting out). The nurse then acknowledges that any changes in a patient's sexual life can be of great concern, that many people have questions but are reluctant or unable to ask them. The other aspect of permission is listening respectfully to patients' concerns, and, if knowledge and training are appropriate, providing the next level of intervention. If not, the nurse can assist in locating an appropriate resource.

Mr. G. is a 68-year-old man who is in a rehabilitation facility and starting his recovery from a cerebral vascular accident (stroke). Whenever a female staff member enters his room, he greets her flirtatiously, invites her into his bed "for a good time," and requests back rubs for his "lower back pain."

The permission level of intervention in this situation could involve a gentle, but firm, setting of behavioural limits for Mr. G., pointing out that his behaviour causes the staff discomfort, making them feel reluctant to enter his room and provide the care that he needs. The nurse could then state that many people who have had Mr. G.'s type of illness also have concerns about what changes may have occurred sexually and that arrangements could be made for him to talk to someone who is knowledgeable in that area.

Many people will not express questions or concerns unless directly encouraged to do so. The nurse can anticipate this and, once rapport is established with the patient, the topic of sexuality may be introduced. One method that promotes comfort is the making of a "ubiquity" statement—a statement that validates the "normality" of such concerns. For example, the nurse might say, "Many people who have had a spinal cord injury have concerns about what their sexual function might be like when they go home from hospital. Is this something you have thought about?"

LIMITED INFORMATION

The next level of the PLISSIT model is limited information. The patient is provided with information that pertains to the specific situation. For example, myths or misinformation may be clarified, the basic sexual response cycle may be explained, contraception or safer sex practices may be discussed or the possible effects of certain medications on sexual function may be outlined.

Sally is a 16-year-old secondary school student who has been visiting the health office at school frequently, with a number of minor concerns. The nurse's time in the school is limited, with only one session per year in each classroom. The session in Sally's class dealt with making healthy decisions. It was enthusiastically received because of the nurse's creative approaches to the topic and nonjudgemental manner. Later, Sally comes to the nurse's office complaining of a sore throat. While the nurse is checking Sally's throat, she asks, "You can't get pregnant the first time you have sex, can you?"

The nurse, who has had training in counselling and adolescent health, encourages Sally to talk about her concerns. The permission level is applied here (and was implicitly applied in the classroom). The nurse can provide information about the possibility of pregnancy in that situation (limited information) and then assist Sally in finding appropriate resources.

SPECIFIC SUGGESTIONS

The use of specific suggestions usually requires a level of specialized expertise achieved through training and experience. This level may be viewed as the "problem-solving" level, where the health care provider's knowledge and skills can assist the patient in improving the quality of sexual experiences.

Mrs. H. is a 31-year-old woman whose first baby is now six weeks old. During a visit to the well-baby clinic, the nurse inquires about how things are going at home, sleeping habits, breast-feeding and concerns about contraception. Mrs. H. states, "Sex is pretty well a nonevent at our house these days. Not only am I too tired most of the time, but it also hurts when we try to have intercourse."

The nurse is aware that in the postpartum period and during the time the mother is breast feeding her baby, there can be a decline in sexual desire. In addition, hormonal changes involved in lactation can decrease the amount of vaginal lubrication, in turn causing dyspareunia. The nurse could discuss some strategies (specific suggestions) with Mrs. H. to promote positive sexual functioning, for example, finding some time to herself, and getting some extra rest by having her partner bottle-feed the baby once during the night with breast milk that has been expressed. The use of water-soluble vaginal lubricants for intercourse can relieve the discomfort when Mrs. H.'s interest in sex returns. In the meantime, Mrs. H. and her partner might explore some mutually acceptable alternative approaches.

INTENSIVE THERAPY

Intensive therapy is the final level of intervention and is usually provided by specialized health care professionals. In- [illegible] selling, sexual therapy or other specialized techniques. The use of intensive therapy requires very careful assessment of all aspects of sexual function and consideration of the impact that such treatment may have on the person and, if appropriate, on the partner.

Mrs. T. is a 24-year-old woman whose marriage was arranged by her family. Shortly after the wedding, the couple moved to Canada and Mrs. T. learned to speak English. She was referred for sexual therapy because all attempts to have sexual intercourse had been extremely painful and unsuccessful.

In this situation, the sexual therapist, who could be a nurse with special training, would conduct a sexual health assessment from a physical perspective and within a psychosocial and cultural context. The diagnosis of vaginismus, confirmed by a careful examination, would provide a basis for a comprehensive therapeutic approach. This approach would include sexual and relationship counselling and sexuality education for both partners, the use of vaginal introducers to relieve spasm of the vaginal muscles, and referral to community agencies that provide social contact for women from other cultures who are also isolated from customary support systems. The nurse is aware that the use of vaginal introducers alone, without the other interventions, would likely be unsuccessful.

Nurse–Patient Relationships

One of the most difficult challenges of nursing practice is the setting of boundaries between professional and personal relationships. Situations involved in nurse–patient interactions, particularly where personal care or sexuality issues are involved, can engender a form of intimacy that could then "spill over" into other interactions between the nurse and patient. A patient may become sexually attracted to or infatuated with a nurse. This attraction could become mutual.

Many institutions and nursing organizations have developed guidelines or regulations regarding relationships between patients and staff, but some have not. In any case, the onus is on the nurse to behave in a responsible manner that also recognizes and respects the patient's needs. Listed below are some approaches the nurse may find helpful in such situations.

1. Recognize and accept that sexual attraction can and does occur between people. Recognize that there is no need to act on this attraction just because it is there.
2. Recognize that the physical closeness and dependency inherent in a health care setting is different from the usual mutuality and independence found in healthy relationships.
3. Whether or not the feelings of attraction are mutual, address this in a calm, professional manner that recognizes and affirms the patient's sexuality and [illegible] to remain asexual and professional.
4. Recognize that many people are embarrassed and sensitive about sexual matters and have a strong need for privacy. Nurses may become so accustomed to nudity or exposed genitalia that the patient's discomfort may not be acknowledged. Providing suitable coverings during a complete physical examination can help preserve a sense of dignity.
5. Before asking about sexual matters, alleviate patient discomfort by asking permission. For example, "Would it be all right if I asked you a few questions about what your sex life has been like since your illness?" Respect the right of the person to decline this discussion. Respond with a statement such as, "I understand that this is a very private matter for you. If you have any questions later on, I would be happy to try to find you some answers."
6. Avoid making assumptions and avoid expressing them in your terminology. For instance, ask, "Are you currently in a relationship?" rather than, "Are you married?" And refer to a "partner" rather than "wife" or "husband." Use phrases such as "people who have a spinal cord injury" or "people with disabilities" rather than "the spinal cord injured" or "the disabled." A balance between a professional manner and the warmth of genuine caring is beneficial in the nurse–patient relationship.

Health-Promoting Strategies

Sexuality is a fundamental aspect of life that is influenced by a complex system of physiological, psychological, developmental and social factors. To assist patients in achieving an optimum level of sexual health, the nurse must understand these influences and recognize differences in sexual orientation and experience. Nurses can help patients, and if appropriate their partners, to maintain optimum sexual health in two basic ways. First, nurses can encourage people to explore lifestyle factors, cultural and personal values and health practices that might have an impact on sexual health. Second, nurses can provide information that will enable patients to make informed decisions and take responsibility for sexual health. Sexuality education and supportive care are the chief nursing strategies that help to promote optimal sexual health.

SEXUAL DECISION MAKING

An underlying element in the promotion of healthy and responsible sexual decision making is the concept of empowerment and ownership of the sexual self. People who lack a sense of control over a situation may have difficulty

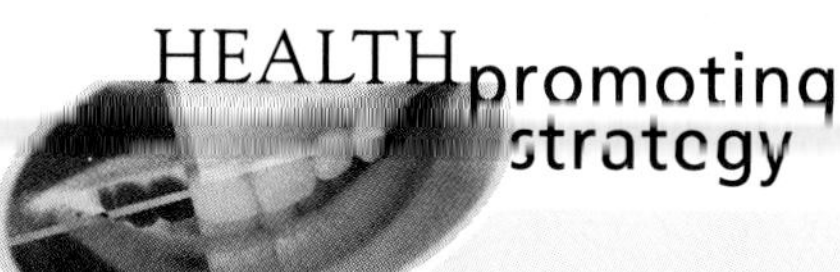

Promoting Healthy Sexuality

- Develop a sense of control over your sexual life. Learn about sexual health and sexual functioning so that you can make the best decisions for your needs. Information may be obtained from school health nurses, occupational health nurses or community clinics.
- Develop a reproductive life plan so that you can make choices about your sexual health.
- If appropriate, learn about contraception or birth control and make an informed decision. Information and counselling may be obtained from community clinics, such as Planned Parenthood, community health agencies and women's health clinics.
- If single, become involved in activities where you can meet people of the opposite gender (or of the same gender if you are homosexual), such as church groups, sports and health clubs, special interest groups.
- Maintain physical fitness. This helps you feel good about yourself and enhances relationships with others.
- Remember that sexuality is expressed in many physical and emotional ways, not only in sexual intercourse. Enjoy close relationships with others you care about and who love you; share feelings, give hugs; and accept touch as an expression of warmth, caring and love.

making decisions about sexual health. For example, someone whose low self-esteem is the result of sexual or other forms of abuse may be unable to make decisions about the use or care of his or her own body and may continue to be victimized. Many people who have not been victimized also lack this ability. With proper support, a sense of self-ownership and an ability to exercise control over one's sexual life can be gained.

In addition to a sense of control, people need sufficient information to allow informed decision making. Very often, health-promoting measures are not followed because of a lack of information or because the information is incorrect. An example might be a woman who not only believes that oral contraceptives cause heart attacks and cancer, but also rejects condoms "because men don't like to use them." Access to appropriate health-screening services and safe, effective contraceptive methods also facilitates decisions that need to be made about sexual health. People who know where to go and how to find the available services are much more likely to act responsibly.

SEXUALITY EDUCATION

Just as sexuality is a lifelong issue, the need for education and counselling continues throughout the life span. Three common areas of sexuality education in which nurses play a key role include reproductive health, contraceptive education and the prevention of sexually transmitted diseases (STDs). Teaching about preventive measures for STDs is a health-protecting strategy. The role of the nurse in providing sexuality education or counselling depends on the nurse's level of training and expertise and on the policies of the health care agency.

Reproductive Health

One way of assisting people to promote optimal sexual health is the concept of a reproductive life plan. A reproductive life plan allows individuals to consider sexuality from a long-term perspective. This plan would include an exploration of hopes and dreams for future relationships, career plans, and whether or not to have children. The impact of sexually transmitted diseases on health and fertility would be discussed, as would possible options if an unplanned pregnancy were to occur. The management of sexuality from a long-term perspective offers the opportunity to make choices. In so doing, it provides a sense of control over life. People who choose safe sex practices and protection from unwanted pregnancy will be likely to have a positive attitude towards these practices.

Contraceptive Education

The use of contraception or birth control is a personal choice. The nurse's primary role in contraceptive teaching and counselling is to provide accurate, unbiased information to enable the patient to make an informed decision. The selection of a contraceptive method is a collaborative endeavour between the health care provider and the patient. There are several factors that must be considered when selecting a contraceptive method:

1. the effectiveness of the method in preventing pregnancy
2. the safety and possible side effects
3. the cost
4. the long-term effects on future fertility
5. the effectiveness of the method in preventing STDs.

Table 35.4 gives a description of common birth control methods along with typical failure rates and contraindications for use. The typical failure rates are expressed as a percentage of couples who initiate use of a method, experience accidental pregnancy during the first year, and do not stop use of the method for any other reason. If left to chance, 85 percent of women will become pregnant within one year.

TABLE 35.4 Birth control methods

Method and Description	Failure Rate	Contraindications
Coitus Interruptus Removal of the penis from the vagina prior to ejaculation.	16%–23%	Any situation in which pregnancy is absolutely contraindicated.
Fertility Awareness Methods (Rhythm Methods) Methods of determining probable fertile period during a menstrual cycle (Calendar Method, Sympto-Thermal or Billings).	2%–25%	Women who have irregular menstrual cycles or where pregnancy is absolutely contraindicated.
Lactation Amenorrhea Method (LAM)	2%	Baby is more than six months old or is being supplemented with formula; woman has had vaginal bleeding after the 56th day postpartum.
Vaginal Spermicides Foams, suppositories, tablets or jellies inserted intravaginally prior to intercourse.	10%–21%	Sensitivity to chemicals or perfumes in the product; physical or mental disability.
Vaginal Contraceptive Sponge Small, pillow-shaped polyurethane sponge, containing 1 gm nonoxynol 9, inserted intravaginally prior to intercourse, effective for 24 hours.	18%–28%	History of toxic shock syndrome, vaginal infection, including *S. Aureus*; allergy to polyurethane or nonoxynol 9; anatomic abnormalities of the pelvis or vagina; physical or mental disability.
Female Condom A polyurethane pouch that is held in the vagina by an inner flexible ring; an outer ring holds the condom in place, covering the entire area of the labia; provides better protection from STDs for the female than does the male condom. Can be inserted up to 8 hours prior to intercourse.	21% typical user 5% perfect user	Allergy to condom material; physical or mental disability.
Male Condom Latex sheath worn over the penis during genital contact; the latex forms a barrier to the transmission of semen or organisms that cause STDs.	12%	Allergy to latex or spermicidal agent; mental or physical disability; some men cannot maintain erections if condoms are used.
Diaphragm, Cervical Cap Vaginal barrier methods used in combination with spermicidal creams or jellies.	18%–23%	History of toxic shock syndrome, vaginal infections, including *S. Aureus*; repeated urinary tract infections, pelvic inflammatory disease; allergies to rubber or spermicides; anatomic abnormalities; cervical biopsy or cryosurgery in past six weeks (cervical cap); full-term delivery in past six to 12 weeks; requires refit a few weeks after first sexual experiences, after each pregnancy regardless of whether the pregnancy ended in abortion or a full-term baby, and after a weight loss of between 10 and 20 pounds.

TABLE 35-4 *continued*

Method and Description	*Failure Rate*	*Contraindications*
Intrauterine Device Plastic device usually wrapped with copper, or may have hormone added; inserted into the cavity of the uterus where it prevents passage of sperm to fallopian tubes; may also prevent implantation if fertilization occurs.	1.5%–5%	Risk factors present for sexually transmitted diseases, acute pelvic infection, history of ectopic pregnancy, known or suspected pregnancy; anatomic abnormalities or malignancy of the reproductive system; valvular heart disease, bleeding disorders, anemia; concern for future fertility.
Oral Contraceptives		
a. **Combined**: tablets containing estrogen and progesterone taken in a series; suppress ovulation, diminish growth of endometrium, increase viscosity of cervical mucous.	0.5%–3%	Personal or family history of cardiovascular disorders, risk factors for thrombosis, known or suspected estrogen-dependent neoplasms; pregnancy; liver disease; over age 35 combined with any other risk factor; smoking, (15 or more cigarettes per day), classic migraine headaches (with aura), hypertension, inability to take pills consistently or correctly.
b. **Progestin-Only:** The "mini-pill" has fewer estrogen-related health risks than combined pill; 40% to 60% of women on mini-pill have ovulatory cycles; possible method once lactation is well established in breast-feeding mothers.	1%–3%	A history of functional ovarian cysts or ectopic pregnancy, unexplained abnormal or irregular vaginal bleeding during previous three months; inability to take pills consistently and correctly.
Long-Acting Progestin Provides long-term contraception; most common side effects are irregular bleeding and some weight gain; may be a delay of six to 12 months in return of fertility following use.		
a. **Norplant (levonorgestrel)**: Progestin is contained in small silastic capsules that are inserted subcutaneously; provides contraception for up to five years.	0.04%	Acute liver disease; jaundice; unexplained vaginal bleeding; history of blood clots in legs (thrombophlebitis), lungs (pulmonary embolism) or eyes; pregnancy, within six weeks postpartum in lactating women; smoking; the presence of other medical conditions such as diabetes, epilepsy, hypertension; elevated cholesterol or triglycerides should be carefully reviewed prior to administering Norplant.
b. **DepoProvera (medroxyprogesterone acetate)**: Progestin is given by injection every three months.	0.3%	Same absolute contraindications as in combined oral contraceptives, (except DepoProvera does not appear to increase the risk of thromboembolic disease); unexplained irregular vaginal bleeding; where a rapid return to fertility will be desired.

TABLE 35.4 *continued*

Method and Description	*Failure Rate*	*Contraindications*
Postcoital Methods		
a. **Hormonal**: Can prevent pregnancy if taken within 72 hours of unprotected intercourse; must be only episode of unprotected intercourse in that cycle; consists of two tablets of 50 μg ethinyl estradiol, 0.5 mg D1-norgestrel (Ovral-Wyeth), and two tablets 12 hours later.	less than 1%	Same as for combined oral contraceptives but, because postcoital use is short term, the advantages of using may outweigh possible risks.
b. **Intrauterine Device**: A copper-bearing IUD can be inserted within five days of unprotected intercourse. Left in place, it can then provide ongoing contraception.	1%–3%	Same as for IUD.
c. **Menstrual Extraction**: Insertion of a sterile cannula into the uterine cavity and removal of uterine contents by suction, if menstrual period more than two weeks late.	Not well documented	Any situation where risks of hemorrhage or infection outweigh other considerations.
Sterilization A permanent method which involves surgical procedures.		Where informed consent cannot be obtained, where future pregnancy might be desired, or where surgical risks outweigh other considerations.
Female: Tubal ligation, in which the fallopian tubes are ligated or sealed by cautery.	0.4%	
Male: Vasectomy, in which the vas deferens is cut and either ligated or cauterized through an incision made into the scrotal skin.	0.15%	

Unreliable Methods

A. Attempting to calculate ovulation using only a calendar.

B. Douching or washing out the vagina following intercourse. This cannot prevent sperm from entering the uterus immediately after ejaculation. Douching should only be used if a special solution is prescribed for treatment of vaginal infection. The use of strongly acidic solutions can cause severe damage to the vaginal mucosa.

C. Coitus interruptus or withdrawal is not effective because of the difficulty of interrupting sexual intercourse at the peak of sexual feelings and because the pre-ejaculatory fluid may contain a significant number of sperm.

D. The insertion of spermicidal products into the vagina following intercourse is unlikely to be effective (see item B).

E. Lactation decreases fertility in some women, particularly if the breast-feeding is constant and the infant has no other source for suckling. However, lactating women may ovulate without warning as their menstrual cycles resume. Conception can occur at this first postpartum ovulation.

SOURCES: Hatcher, *et al.*, 1992; *Population Reports*, 1996.

RESEARCH to practice

Richardson, R.L., Beazeky, R.P., Delaney, M.E., & Langille, D.B. (1997). Factors influencing condom use among students attending high school in Nova Scotia. *Canadian Journal of Human Sexuality, 6*(3), 185–195.

Many Canadian adolescents have had intercourse by the time they have completed high school. Because teens feel invulnerable, they may engage in behaviour that puts them at risk of pregnancy and sexually transmitted disease. The purpose of this study was to examine levels of sexual activity and condom use in a high-school population and to examine the ability of the theory of planned behaviour to predict condom use. Some 796 students (of 830 enrolled in the school) participated in the survey. The following measures were used: attitudes towards condom scale (modified), social normative beliefs regarding condom use scale, attitudes towards difficulty of using condoms scale and the intentions to use condoms scale. The results indicate inconsistent condom use in a population of adolescents of whom more than 50 percent have had sexual intercourse. Overall, 58 percent of these students did not use condoms for each of their last three episodes of vaginal intercourse, even though 75 percent indicated they would always use condoms with all sexual partners. Females were less likely to use condoms despite having strong intentions to do so. The implications for sexuality education are numerous.

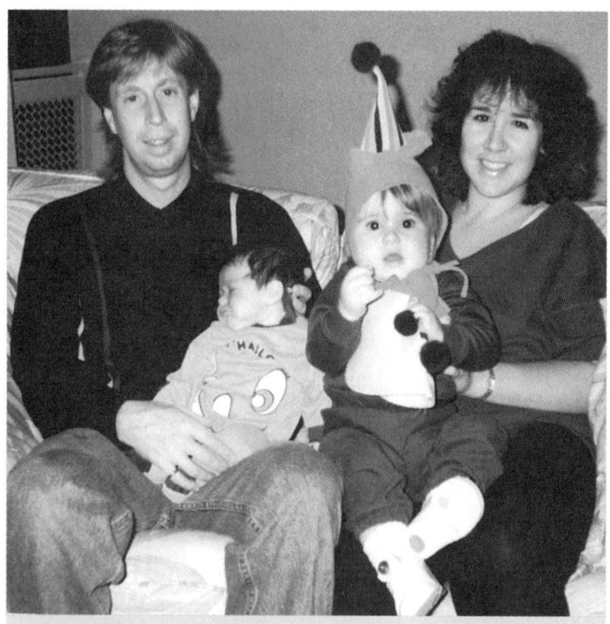

Contraceptive methods permit couples to regulate the number and timing of children.

Health-Protecting Strategies

Many aspects of reproductive health screening, such as breast and testicular examinations and the teaching of self-examination, are performed by nurses. In some agencies, Pap tests and tests for STDs may also be performed by nurses. This offers a unique opportunity to discuss sexual anatomy and sexual function in a nonthreatening setting. Another major element of health protection is the teaching of safe sex practices and prevention of sexually transmitted diseases. Guidelines for safe sex practices and the prevention of STDs are presented in the box below. Figures 35.5 and 35.6 outline methods for breast and testicular self-examination. Nurses can also assist individuals in maintaining safe sexual health by promoting public education and access to resources that encourage healthy sexual behaviours and awareness of possible risks.

In addition, there are a number of strategies that health care providers can implement to prevent the transmission of STDs. Because many STDs, including HIV/AIDS and hepatitis B, are infectious even when asymptomatic, body substance precautions must *always* be exercised by health

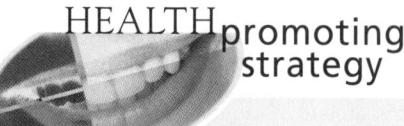

HEALTH promoting strategy — Protective Strategies

Promoting Safe Sex Practices

- Take some time to get to know your sex partner. Share your sexual health histories with one another.
- Avoid anal intercourse.
- Use latex condoms for vaginal intercourse.
- Use latex condoms or dental dams for oral sex.
- Minimize the number of sexual partners.
- Avoid sharing sex toys or devices.

Preventing Sexually Transmitted Diseases

- Do not share needles used for injecting drugs.
- Practice safe sex and
  - avoid any sexual behaviour that involves exchange of or contact with body fluids
  - limit sexual activity to one partner who is guaranteed not to be infected.

Before a Mirror

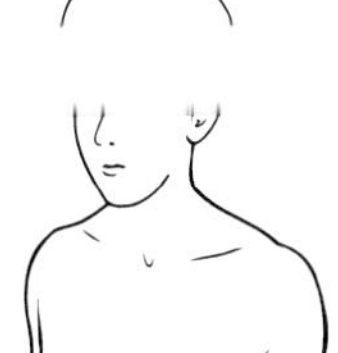

1
With your arms relaxed at

breasts carefully for any changes in size or shape. Look for any rashes, puckered or dimpled skin, and for any discharge or change in the nipples.

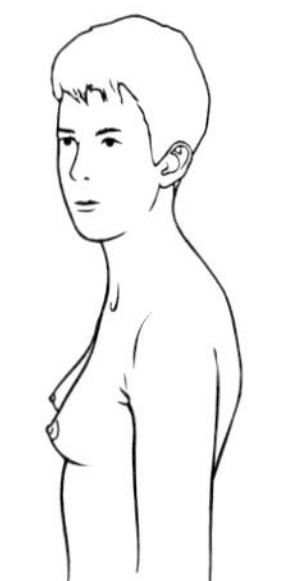

Turn and inspect each side view of the breast. Observe for any flattening in side view. When turned, inspect back and bra line areas for moles and skin irritations.

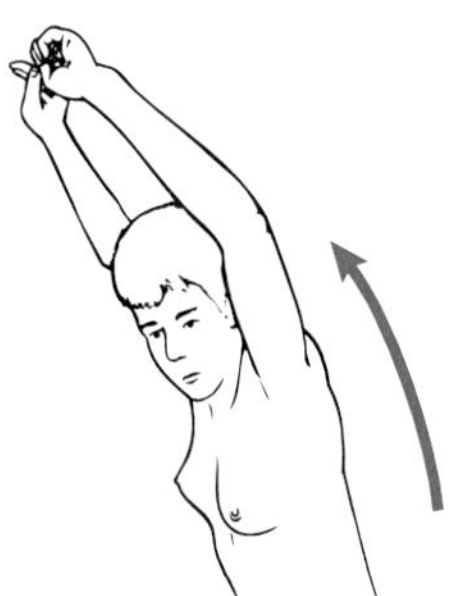

2
Raise your arms over your head and bend forward from your waist inspecting both breasts for any changes.

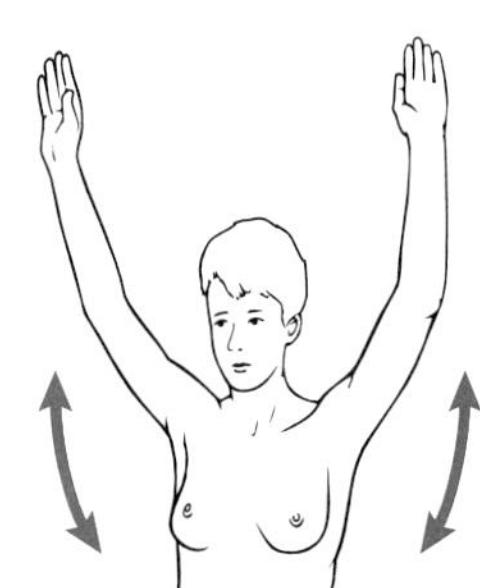

3
Standing straight, raise your arms over your head and move them *slowly* up and down (3 times), observing that the breasts move freely over the chest wall. TURN left and right, observing sides of breasts in same manner.

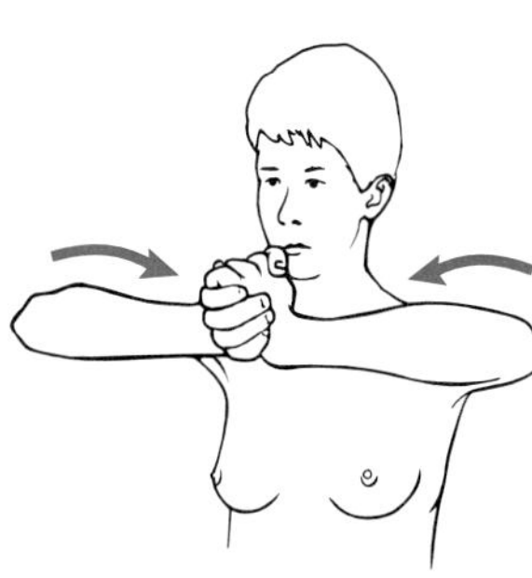

4
Press hands together at chin level and push firmly (3 times) to flex your chest muscles. Turn left and right, observing sides of breasts and underarm breast tissue in the same manner.
5
Regular inspection shows what is normal for you and will give you confidence in your examination.

Lying Down

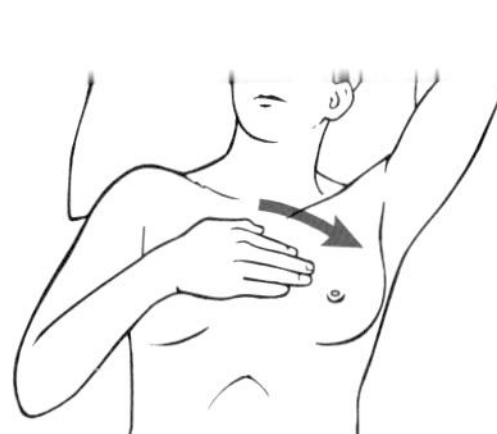

1
To examine your left breast

hand on your forehead. This spreads breast tissue more evenly on the chest. With the fingers of your right hand held together flat, press gently but firmly with small circular motions around an imaginary clock face, feeling the breast tissue between your fingers and your chest wall.

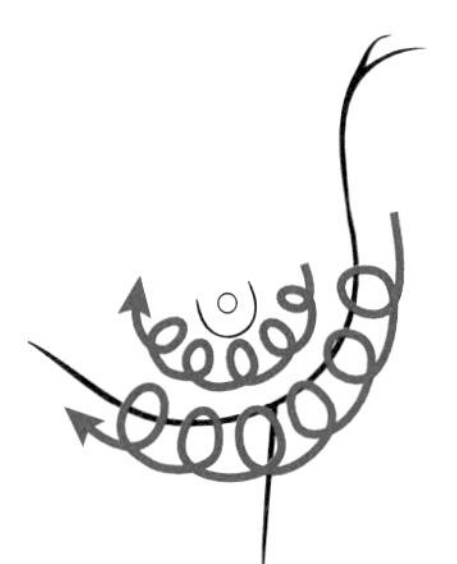

2
Begin at the outermost top of your left breast for 12 o'clock, and without lifting your fingers from your breast feel slowly and carefully with small circular motions all the way around the rim of your breast back to 12. A ridge of firm tissue in the lower curve of each breast is normal. Now move your fingers in toward the nipple about 2 cms and feel all the way around again. Repeat this action as many times as necessary to be sure you have covered the entire breast, finishing over the nipple.

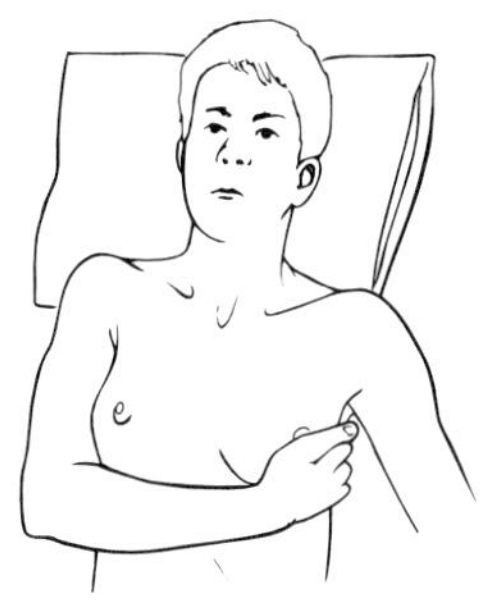

3
Bring your left arm down to your side and, still using the flat part of your fingers, feel under your armpit, since breast tissue is found there as well.

Sitting

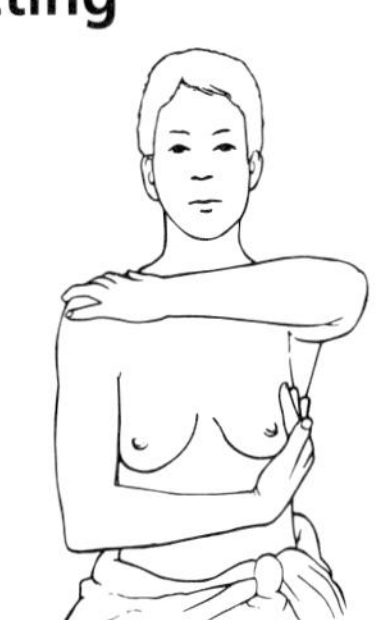

1
With left hand on right shoulder lift elbow to expose left or right hand, still using flat part start at upper edge of left breast with a circular motion to bottom of armpit.

To examine right breast repeat the procedure using your left hand.

Examine your breasts *regularly* once a month, 7 to 10 days after each menstrual cycle begins, when breasts are usually not tender or swollen. If you are not menstruating, pick a special day, the first day of the month or your birth date, to practise BSE. Doing BSE will protect your health.

When you practise BSE you quickly learn what is usual for you, so if anything unusual develops you'll discover it at a very early stage. If a lump, thickening, or *any change* is discovered during BSE, it is important to see your doctor right away. Don't be frightened. Most breast lumps or changes are *not* cancer, but only your doctor can make that diagnosis.

FIGURE 35.5 Breast self-examination

SOURCE: Canadian Cancer Society, 1993.

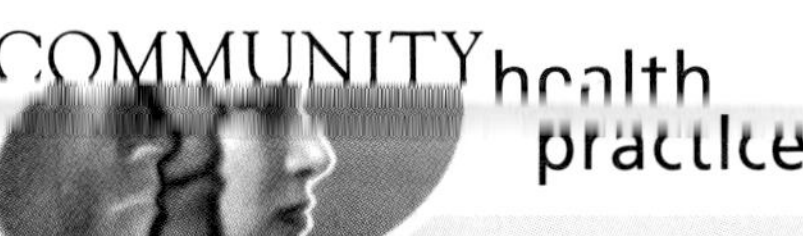

COMMUNITY health practice — Sex Education for Children

A common question parents may ask nurses is "What books are available to explore sex education with my children?" *Speaking of Sex: Are you ready to answer the questions kids will ask?* is a book written by Meg Hickling, a Canadian author, which is available in libraries and bookstores. Recently, this book was reviewed in detail by Ann Barrett, in *Canadian Journal of Sexuality*. This is a humorous book that has as its main theme that parents are an important source of information for their children. Hickling makes effective use of children's questions and comments, in their own handwriting and spelling throughout the book, and suggests that parents have to deal with these topics directly, even if their children are embarrassed. She talks about dealing with sexuality questions from children of all ages. Hickling's examples of how to present content are very interesting. For example, "The vagina constantly makes moisture, just like your eyes do ... sometimes it dries to a yellowish or whitish colour on your underpants. This is a good sign that your vagina is clean and healthy." This book is extremely comprehensive; most adults will learn new information from it as well.

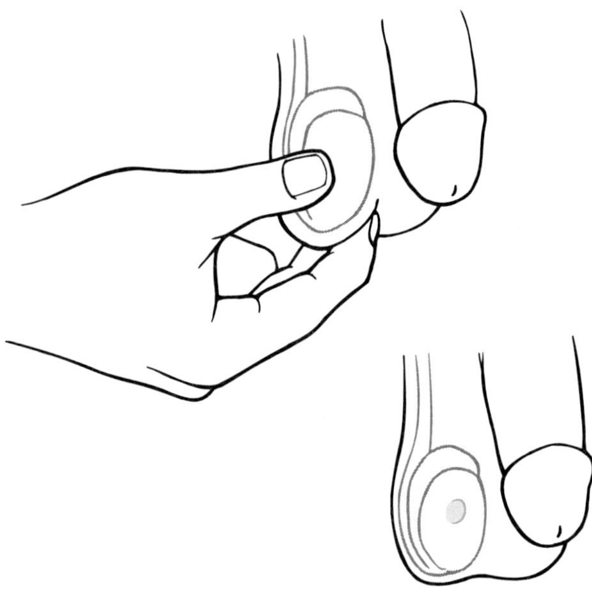

1. The best time to examine your testicles is right after a hot bath or shower because the scrotal skin is more relaxed and the contents can be felt more easily.
2. Place your index and middle fingers on the underside of the testicle and your thumbs on the top. Gently roll your testicle betwen your thumb and fingers. The normal testicle feels slightly soft with an even consistency and a smooth surface. The epididymis can be felt at the back of the testicle and feels slightly different in consistency. Examine both testicles.
3. Any thickening or lump, however small (even pea size), should be reported to your physician.

FIGURE 35.6 Testicular self-examination

SOURCE: Canadian Cancer Society, 1989.

care providers when in contact with any body substances, just as safer sex practices must always be used by all sexually active people. Blood, tissues, organs and sperm that will be used for transplant or donation must be carefully screened as well as blood that will be used for transfusion.

RESEARCH to practice

Lierman, L.M., Young, H.M., Cope, G.P., Georgiadou, F. and Benoliel, J.Q. (1994). Effects of education and support on breast self-examination in older women. *Nursing Research, 43*, 158–163.

The purpose of this study was to determine how an educational program and structural support affect the frequency of breast self-examination (BSE) by middle-aged and older women, their proficiency in doing the examination and their perceptions of their skill in BSE. The study population consisted of 175 women 50 years of age or older from a prescreened group of health maintenance organization (HMO) subscribers who volunteered to participate. The women were divided into three groups. One received only the basic teaching program with no support. The second group was paired with peer partners assigned by the researcher. The third group brought partners of choice to the instructional sessions. Women in both partner groups contracted to work together for six months after instruction, using self-determined strategies of support.

The educational program consisted of a sound and slide presentation about BSE, and a discussion of the risk factors for breast cancer and factors influencing the performance of BSE. This was followed by individualized, one-on-one instruction and supervised practice with a registered nurse. An initial interview was held with each participant and data was gathered in two subsequent interviews (six and 12 months after the educational program).

Data analysis based on the differences between initial interviews and the follow-up interviews indicated that the educational program was very successful in increasing the frequency of breast self-examination, the women's proficiency in carrying it out and their perceived skill in doing it. There was no significant difference in the scores of women in the three groups, which the authors feel may have been due to the high level of motivation of all participants. The study shows that older women are willing and able to change their behaviour, given the necessary instruction, skills and support.

Health-Restoring Strategies

Sex therapy is a specialized area for nurses as well as for [illegible] chologists and mental health counsellors. A discussion of restorative care for sexual health challenges is beyond the scope of this book. However, this topic will be covered in more advanced courses.

Evaluating Sexuality Interventions

Evaluation of the effectiveness of sexual health care follows implementation and is based on the patient goals and the plan for care. The criteria listed below represent the range of nursing interventions that a general staff nurse or student may implement in meeting patients' sexuality needs.

1. Has the patient gained the knowledge and skills that will enable the promotion of sexual health? Exercise of informed consent in areas of sexual behaviour? The prevention of unwanted pregnancy? Protection against sexually transmitted diseases? Identification of the presence of disorders of sexual or reproductive function? The ability to seek and obtain appropriate treatment?
2. Are you, the nurse, aware of your personal values and beliefs, and sufficiently comfortable with them to be able to deal with patients' sexuality issues in a matter-of-fact manner? Does your patient show embarrassment or distress when sexual issues are discussed? If so, what steps have you taken to alleviate the distress? What could you have done differently or in addition that might have been more effective?
3. Have female patients learned and demonstrated skills in breast self-examination? Are they aware of the importance of Pap testing and infection screening? Are male patients able to practise regular testicular self-examination? Are they able to discuss and use condoms appropriately?

IN REVIEW

- Sexuality is a broad concept that brings together not only reproduction and sexual pleasure, but also the need for love, personal fulfillment and self-expression and the totality of feelings, attitudes, beliefs and behaviours related to being male or female.
- Sex refers to the biological distinctions that identify a person as male or female and to the sexual functions for reproduction and pleasure.
- Sexual functioning combines a range of sensory and motor responses that are mediated by:
    - emotional
    - social and
    - biological influences.
- Sexual needs change throughout the life cycle.
- Infants develop feelings of trust and self-worth through the gratification of three basic needs:
    - nourishment
    - warmth and
    - touch.
- In childhood, gender identity and gender (sex) role identity develop.
- Puberty is the age of hormonal changes affecting growth and secondary sex characteristics.
- Adolescence encompasses the physical changes of puberty and includes the psychological, cognitive and social transition from childhood to adulthood.
- Young adulthood is a period when marriage and families are often begun.
- Middle years of adulthood produce changes in sexual and reproductive anatomy and function. Women may experience an increase or decrease in sexual interest. Men may experience a change in sexual function that may cause distress and concern.
- Older adults do remain sexually active, providing a capable partner is available.
- Through the teen and adult years, there may be problems with:
    - sexually transmitted diseases
    - pregnancy into the menopausal years
    - cancer of the reproductive organs (breast and cervix in women and prostate in men)
- Common sexual concerns may require physical and psychological treatment for both partners.
- Sexually transmitted diseases (STDs) are spread through intimate or sexual contact, or contact with any body fluid.
- A nursing health history should include sexual health questions that are relevant to the patient's condition or expressed concern. The patient's permission is necessary before asking sex-related questions.
- *Altered sexuality patterns* is a nursing diagnostic label that may be used for problems in which patients are experiencing changes in sexual health or expressing concern about their sexuality.

- The PLISSIT model, often used in sexual counselling, provides a guideline based on the skills and [illegible] of the health care provider. The letters stand for:
  - permission
  - limited information
  - specific suggestions and
  - intensive therapy.
- Correct information is needed in:
  - reproductive health
  - safe sex practices
  - contraceptives
  - prevention of STDs.
- Reproductive health screening includes:
  - breast exam
  - testicular exam
  - teaching of self-examination.

Critical Thinking Activities

1. Mr. Ivanovitch is a divorced 70-year-old patient in extended care with a leg injury. He likes to play cribbage, and he frequently tells you that he is lonely. According to Sarah, another nurse on the unit, he requests her attention often. Over the past week, he has started to make overtures and then direct passes at her, saying "I just want a woman." Apparently, it is fairly typical of his cultural background to be direct.
   a. How should Sarah deal with his behaviour?
   b. What are some of the ways to redirect his attention?
   c. What community resource groups can be called upon to help this gentleman?
2. Candy Lane, 18, is a very unkempt girl who shows up repeatedly in the women's health clinic for treatment of an STD. Her records indicate she is slightly mentally deficient and has a ninth-grade education. She lives with her family. Her five brothers and sisters have various learning disabilities. Her father is an occasional labourer; her mother stays at home. Both parents are alcoholics. Apparently she engages in prostitution.
   a. How can you assist Candy in improving her situation?
   b. Which resource people can be contacted?
   c. What are some of the factors affecting her situation?
   d. Should Candy be sterilized?
   e. Should prostitution be legalized? Why or why not?

KEY TERMS

sex p. 1183
biological sexual identity p. 1183
sexuality p. 1184
gender definition (gender identity) p. 1184
gender role identity p. 1184
menarche p. 1188
menopause p. 1188
masturbation p. 1194
puberty p. 1194
autosexual activities p. 1197
homosexuality p. 1197
bisexuality p. 1197
transsexualism p. 1197
transvestism p. 1197
paraphilia p. 1197
paraorgasm p. 1198

References

ANDREWS, G. (Ed.). (1997). *Women's sexual health.* London: Bailliere Tindall.

ANNON, J.S. (1976). The PLISSIT model: A proposed conceptual scheme for the behavioural treatment of sexual problems. *Journal of Sex Education and Therapy, 2,* 211–215.

BEITCHMAN, J., ZUCKER, K., HOOD, J., DACOSTA, G., AKMAN, D., & CASSAVIA, E. (1990). *A review of the long-term effects of child sexual abuse.* (Revised version of a final report submitted to Health and Welfare Canada.)

CANADIAN CANCER SOCIETY. (1989). *TSE: The most important minute in a man's life.* (Pamphlet). Vancouver: Author.

CANADIAN CANCER SOCIETY. (1993). *BSE: Breast self-examination.* (Pamphlet). Vancouver: Author.

THE CANADIAN RESEARCH INSTITUTE FOR THE ADVANCEMENT OF WOMEN. (1989). *What you should know about infertility and sterility.* Ottawa: Author.

CARPENITO, J.B. (1997). *Nursing diagnosis: Application to clinical practice.* (7th ed.). Philadelphia: Lippincott.

CENTERS FOR DISEASE CONTROL. (1993). Recommendations for the prevention and management of chlamydia trachomatis infections. *1993 Morbidity and Mortality Weekly Report, 42*(RR-12), 1–39.

CENTERS FOR DISEASE CONTROL. (1996). Ten leading nationally notifiable infectious diseases—United States. *1995 Morbidity and Mortality Weekly Report, 45,* 883–884.

CHERNECKY, C.C., & BERGER, B.J. (1997). *Laboratory tests and diagnostic procedures.* (2nd ed.). Philadelphia: Saunders.

DUGAS B. W. (1993). Healthy life-styles. In A. C. Beckingham and B. W. DuGas (Eds.). *Promoting healthy aging.* St. Louis: Mosby.

EBERSOLE, P., & HESS, P. (1998). *Towards healthy aging: A human needs and nursing response.* (5th ed.). St. Louis: Mosby.

GOVERNMENT OF CANADA. (1990–91). Sexuality: A lifelong issue. *Seniors' Info Exchange,* Winter, 1990, 2, 3.

HATCHER, R.A., STEWART, F., TRUSSELL, J., LOWAL, D., GUEST, F., STEWART, G., & CATES, W. (1992). *Contraceptive technology, 1990–1992.* New York: Irvington Publishers.

HEALTH CANADA. (1998). *Canadian STD Guidelines.* Ottawa: Author.

HICKLING, M. (1996). *Speaking of sex: Are you ready to answer the questions kids will ask?* Kelowna, BC: Northstone.

KINSEY, A.C., POMEROY, W.B. and MARTIN C.E. (1948). *Sexual behaviour in the human male.* Philadelphia: Saunders.

KINSEY, A. C. et al. (1953). *Sexual behaviour in the human female.* Philadelphia: Saunders.

KNOWLTON, C. N. (1988). Human sexuality. In J.M. Flynn and P.B. Heffron (Eds.). *Nursing: From concept to practice* (2nd ed.). Norwalk, CT: Appleton & Lange.

LIERMAN, L.M., YOUNG, H.M., COPE, G.P., GEORGIADOU, F., & BENOLIEL, J.Q. (1994). Effects of education and support on breast self-examination in older women. *Nursing Research, 43*, 158-163.

MALTZ, W. (1992). *The sexual healing journey*. New York: Harper Perennial.

MASTERS, W.H., & JOHNSON, V.E. (1966). *Human sexual response*. Boston: Little, Brown.

MATTOX, J. (1998). *Obstetrics and gynecology*. St. Louis: Mosby.

ORTON, M. J., & ROSENBLATT, E. (1986). *Adolescent pregnancy in Ontario: Progress in prevention*. Toronto: Planned Parenthood Association of Ontario.

POPULATION REPORTS. (1996). *Lactational amenorrhea method*; Maryland: Population Information Program, Center for Communication Programs, The Johns Hopkins School of Public Health, XXIV(2).

REINISCH, J. (1990). *The Kinsey Institute new report on sex: What you must know to be sexually literate*. New York: St. Martin's.

RICHARDSON, R.L., BEAZEKY, R.P., DELANEY, M.E., & LANGILLE, D.B. (1997). Factors influencing condom use among students attending high school in Nova Scotia. *The Canadian Journal of Human Sexuality, 6*(3), 185–195.

STATISTICS CANADA. (1998). *Cancer Statistics, 1996.* Major releases available: http://www.statcan.ca/Daily/English/960213/d960213.htm/ART1.

SUICIDE AMONG GAY AND LESBIAN YOUTH. (1993). Anecdotal Report. Annual AIDS Conference, Vancouver.

THOMAS, A., & CHESS, S. (1980). *The dynamics of psychological development*. New York: Brunner/Mazel.

UPHOLD, C., & GRAHAM, M. (1994). *Clinical guidelines in family practice*. (2nd ed.). Gainesville, FL: Barmarrare Books.

WOODS, N. (1984). *Human sexuality in health and illness* (3rd ed.). St. Louis: Mosby.

WORLD HEALTH ORGANIZATION. (1975). *Education and treatment in human sexuality: The training of health professionals*. (Technical Report Series No. 572.) Geneva: Author.

Additional Readings

BALLARD, J.D. (1997). Treatment of erectile dysfunction: Can pelvic muscle exercises improve sexual function? *Journal of Wound, Ostomy and Continence Nursing, 24*(5), 255–264.

CLARKE, H.F., JOESPH, R., DESCHAMPS, M., HISLOP, G., BAND, P.R., & ATLEO, R. (1998). Reducing cervical cancer among First Nations women. *Canadian Nurse, 94*(3), 36–41.

BC, 30(2), 10–19.

EKLAND, M., & McBRIDE, K. (1997). Sexual health care: The role of the nurse. *Canadian Nurse, 93*(7), 34–37.

FRALEU, A.M. (1992). *Nursing and the disabled*. Boston: Jones and Bartlett.

MacLAREN, A. (1995). Primary care of women: comprehensive sexual health assessment. *Journal of Nurse Midwifery, 40*(2), 59–64, 104–119.

MATICKA-TYNDALE, E. (1997). Reducing the incidence of sexually transmitted disease through behavioural and social change. *Canadian Journal of Human Sexuality, 6*, 89–104.

McLAREN, P., MALLESON, R., & KLEIN, M. (1998). Teenage pregnancy and adolescent sexuality: Present status, practice issues, effective strategies. *BC Medical Journal, 40*(2), 64–67.

MEADUS, R.J. (1995). Testicular self-examination (TSE). *Canadian Nurse, 91*(8), 41–44.

MURRAY, R.B., & ZENTNER, J.P. (1997). *Health assessment and promotion strategies through the life span*. Stamford, CT: Appleton & Lange.

SHARESKI, D. (1996). Integrating traditional beliefs with western practice. *Nursing BC, 28*(5), 27–29.

SHORTEN, A. (1995). Female circumcision: Understanding special needs. *Holistic Nursing Practice, 9*(2), 66–73.

SOKOLSKI, E.H. (1995). Canadian First Nations women's beliefs about pregnancy and prenatal care. *Canadian Journal of Nursing Research*, 27(19), 89–100.

STATISTICS CANADA. *Reproductive Health: Pregnancies and Rates in Canada, 1974–1993.* (Statistics Canada Catalogue no. 82/568).

STEBEN, M. & SACKS, S.L. (1997). Genital herpes: Epidemiology and control of a common sexually transmitted disease. *Canadian Journal of Human Sexuality, 6*, 127–134.

STUART, G.W., & LARAIA, M.T. (1998). *Stuart and Sundeen's principles and practice of psychiatric nursing*. (6th ed.). St. Louis: Mosby.

SULPIZI, L.K. (1996). Issues in sexuality and gynecologic care of women with developmental disabilities. *Journal of Obstetric, Gynecologic and Neonatal Nursing, 25*(7), 609–614.

TEPPER, M.L., & GULLY, P.R. (1997). Lovers and livers: Hepatitis B as an STD. *Canadian Journal of Human Sexuality, 6*, 135–142.

VARNEY, H. (1997). *Varney's midwifery*. Boston: Jones & Bartlett.

Chapter 36

Self-Esteem Needs

OUTLINE

Central Questions

1. Why is self-esteem important to well-being?
2. What are the main determinants of self-esteem?
3. How is the sense of self-esteem developed and nurtured throughout the life span?
4. What sorts of problems stem from a lack of self-esteem?
5. How does the nurse assess self-concept?
6. What are some problems related to low self-esteem?
7. What specific nursing diagnoses might apply to patients with problems related to low self-esteem?
8. What basic principles are applicable in planning care to promote, protect and restore self-esteem?
9. What strategies might be used for promoting self-esteem? for protecting self-esteem? for helping to restore self-esteem?
10. How does the nurse evaluate the individual's or the group's response to nursing interventions?

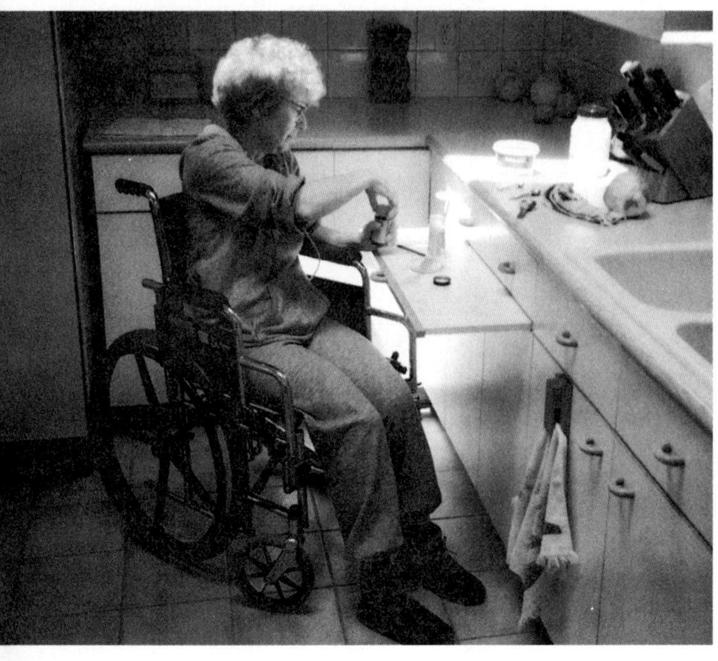

Introduction

Self-esteem is to the mind as food is to the body: and all human [illegible] being.

— Simmermacher, 1989

Self is the most complex attribute that an individual possesses. The concept of self is not clearly defined. "The self is the most real aspect of one's experience, however, and it is the frame of reference through which a person perceives, conceives and evaluates ones' world" (Stuart & Sundeen, 1995, p. 376).

Self-concept "develops over a lifetime and represents the total beliefs about the self" (Boyd & Nihart, 1998, p. 281). "The self-concept reflects the individual's integration of self-body, mind, spirit" (Haber *et al.*, 1997, p. 145). Theorists agree that self-concept does not exist at birth, but evolves or is learned by interaction with the self, with others and with the environment (Stuart & Laraia, 1998). Self-concept has three interrelated dimensions: body image, personal identity and self-esteem. **Body image** "represents an individual's beliefs and attitudes about his or her body and include such dimensions as size (large or small), attractiveness (pretty or ugly), perfection ..." (Boyd & Nihart, 1998, p. 281). **Personal identity** is "knowing 'whom I am' and is formed through the numerous biological, psychological, and social challenges and demands throughout the stages of life" (p. 282).

Self-esteem, it has been said, is the key to a person's behaviour. It influences thinking processes, emotions, desires, values and goals. It affects virtually all aspects of our lives: how we function in school, at work, in love and as parents, and how successful we are in life (Simmermacher, 1989). Maslow (1970) contends that attainment of self-esteem is only possible when lower-level needs have been fulfilled. A healthy self-esteem can only develop when we feel secure. Our sense of security depends on having basic physiological needs met, feeling safe from harmful elements in the environment and feeling safe and secure in our relationships with other people.

Self-esteem involves a critical self-evaluation: How do I measure up physically, socially, psychologically and behaviourally to the standards and values I have chosen for myself? Although they may not be aware of their self-evaluation on a conscious, verbalized level, people experience it as a feeling about themselves. People feel "good" about themselves if, in their opinion, they have done something well, or they feel small and miserable because they believe they can never do things right.

The way we see ourselves, and the way we feel and think about ourselves, is learned through our interaction with others and through their responses to us. It is not something we are endowed with at birth (Boyd & Nihart, 1998). If the way we see ourselves is learned, it follows that positive self-esteem can be promoted and negative self-esteem can be transformed through successful learning experiences.

Poor self-esteem has been linked as a causative factor to [illegible] matic disorders and to numerous social problems, such as delinquency, child abuse, prejudice, alcoholism and drug addiction (Boyd & Nihart, 1998; Stuart & Laraia, 1998). Poor self-esteem is a common factor among the groups of people in Canadian society who are most vulnerable to poor health—those in poor socioeconomic situations, the unemployed, older adults, single mothers, new immigrants and First Nations people (Epp, 1986).

Today, we are hearing a lot about the need to "empower" people so that they can assert control over factors that affect their health. **Empowerment** is a key concept in the socioeconomic model of health. Empowerment has been defined as "the promotion of continuing growth and development of strength, power and personal excellence" (Boyd & Nihart, 1998, p. 1054). If health is viewed as "the ability [of people] to realize their aspirations and satisfy needs and, on the other hand, to change or cope with the environment" as defined by the World Health Organization (WHO) (1980), then empowerment is a vital component in helping people realize their health potential (Epp, 1986).

In this chapter, we will look at the determinants of self-esteem, its development throughout the life cycle, and some of the common problems experienced by people when these needs are unfulfilled. We will also discuss the nurse's role in helping to promote self-esteem, in protecting feelings of self-worth and in helping people to overcome feelings of low self-esteem.

Determinants of Self-Esteem

Basic Needs

Self-esteem is derived from a number of different elements, including the fulfillment of basic physiological and security needs. Physiological needs must be met first. People need food, clothing and protection from the elements for themselves and their families. They do not feel very secure if their stomachs are empty and they do not know where the next meal is coming from, if they are constantly worrying about paying the rent, or, if they are among the growing number of homeless in this country, where they are going to sleep at night. People also need freedom from pain. In addition to having physiological needs met, people have to feel that they can go about their daily activities without fear, that they are safe in their home at night and that their children are safe. These very basic components of feeling safe are essential for a sense of security.

Adequate finances are important to provide the basic essentials of security—food for the table, housing, clothing and the other necessities of life. An economic recession puts strains on individuals and families, especially when there is not enough money to pay all the bills and still buy necessary items. The uncertainty of not knowing whether there will be a job tomorrow is devastating to anyone's security and self-esteem.

Money is also the way our society rewards people for the work they do. The higher the income, the more valuable the position is considered to be. Although we would like to think otherwise, in this materialistic world of ours success is to a large extent judged by the amount of income earned.

Love and a Sense of Belonging

Meeting basic physical needs is not enough. People also need a sense of belonging and a feeling that they are part of a particular segment of the population. They also need the love and companionship of other people, although sometimes a pet will provide its owner with the needed affection. People also need attention and recognition from others—an acknowledgement that they are accepted members of society.

Social Support

Of primary importance in both the development and nurturing of self-esteem are the significant people who inhabit our social world. These people include family members; peers and teachers at school; colleagues and supervisors in the workplace; and friends and neighbours in the community.

HOME The importance of the family in helping people grow up comfortable and secure with themselves and their environment cannot be stressed too much. It is the family or significant others who provide people with the support they need to make their way in the outside world.

SCHOOL People also need attention and recognition from others outside the family. The school is usually the first place where the outside world is confronted. The way children are accepted and the way that their development is nourished in classrooms and on playing fields is crucial to the formation of the feelings of security and self-esteem that are carried throughout life (Government of Ontario, 1993). Level of education is probably more important now than ever before in helping people to meet security needs and in contributing to self-esteem. Today, a minimum of a high-school education is required to even begin to compete in the job market. To enter most professions and occupations requires post-secondary education at a community college, technical institute or a university. A high-school diploma provides a sense of achievement and a certain amount of security when obtaining employment; a college certificate or diploma or a university degree provides even more security and increased feelings of self-worth (Oderkirk, 1993; Gilbert & Orok, 1993).

WORKPLACE Work, how people feel about it, the pleasure they receive from it, and the companionship and respect they obtain from co-workers and supervisors all contribute to feeling comfortable and secure in daily living. A warm, supportive atmosphere at home can help nullify the damaging effects of a work environment filled with stress. More and more, however, employers are finding it advantageous to make the workplace more conducive to developing employees' self-esteem. Employers are fostering a cooperative team spirit that gives people the feeling of being an important part of the organization.

COMMUNITY Social networks in the community are also important contributors to feelings of self-worth. These social networks include friends, people in our neighbourhood, clubs and other organizations and communities of worship. These networks provide emotional, material and companionship support. People who lack this support are much more likely to experience feelings of low self-esteem, anxiety, depression, self-blame and helplessness than those with strong social support systems (RNABC, 1992; Government of Ontario, 1993). The supportive (nurturing) community fosters social contacts by providing places where people can meet and interact, such as libraries, schools, churches, parks and playgrounds and community centres. A supportive community also provides services that people need to feel secure, such as health and social services and law enforcement services.

Cultural Customs and Mores

The traditional customs and mores of a community also play a part in self-esteem. They help maintain a sense of the continuity of life and give people a sense of identity. There is an order that is reassuring, for example, in the fact that Thanksgiving comes in fall every year. The ceremonies that mark life events—starting, for example, with circumcision of the male Jewish child a few days after birth, the baptism of the Roman Catholic infant, the marriage ceremony and the death service—are all important in that they help family members to develop a sense of continuity. The ceremonies also contribute to the self-esteem of participants and their families, since the event is being marked in the approved manner. "Healing" and "talking" circles are used by people of the First Nations as a means of remaining connected to their traditions and culture (Clarke, 1997). It has been government policy in Canada to help ethnic groups to maintain their own cultural identity, and many of the traditional customs have been passed down from generation to generation. Vancouver is noted for its Chinese New Year celebrations, Edmonton for its celebrations of the Ukrainian Christmas, Toronto for Caribana and Kitchener-Waterloo for Oktoberfest. These events all help people whose roots are outside Canada to maintain their identity.

Religion–Spirituality

Many ceremonies and traditional events are religious in nature. Religion has always provided many people with a refuge from the uncertainties of life. It can be reassuring for

Determinants of Self-Esteem

- fulfillment of basic physiological needs
- [illegible]
- an adequate income to purchase the necessities of life
- a supportive, nurturing family, school and work environment
- a nurturing community
- cultural customs and mores
- a sense of purpose in life
- good health
- successful transitions through developmental stages in the life cycle
- religion–spirituality.

people to feel that there is an order to the universe and that a supreme being is in charge to whom they can go for comfort, support and guidance. The stress of living in today's fast-paced world, with all the uncertainties brought about by rapid change, has no doubt contributed to the growth of many churches in recent years. People seem to be looking for a semblance of order and a meaning to life to renew their faith and security in the world (see Chapter 12 for more details).

A Purpose in Life

Rapid changes in institutions and in the economic situation have an effect on our sense of security and the way in which we view ourselves. According to Toffler (1981), we derive our sense of purpose, our feeling that our lives "count," from our relationships with family, our place of work, our community of worship and our political involvement. We also need to be able to see ourselves as part of the cosmic scheme of things.

Health-Related Factors

Self-esteem is threatened by illness—sometimes very much so—particularly in the case of sudden illness or accident that requires hospitalization. Sometimes in agencies, health professionals are so busy taking care of the technical aspects of health care that they forget that people are attached to all the tubes and equipment. An important responsibility of the nurse is to look after people—to help them to feel secure and to support both self-confidence and self-respect. This responsibility is part of the *caring* aspect of the nurse's role, which is the core of nursing.

The loss, or potential loss, of independence, for example, poses a very real threat to people with health problems. It can cause them to lose self-esteem and to think that other people will not respect them. It is important, therefore, to make sure that nothing the nurse does or says causes patients to think that they are any less themselves because of the health problem.

Illness can interfere with people's careers, or with the fulfillment of their potential. The loss or threatened loss of the ability to use the hands, for instance, would be a [illegible]

[illegible] outdoor ones, such as skiing or riding, would be anxious if a health problem threatened the loss of motor function.

Developmental Crises

At certain times in the life span, major changes, often referred to as **developmental crises,** take place during transitions from one developmental stage to another. These transitions were discussed extensively in Chapter 8. These crises cause a considerable threat to self-esteem, as people wonder if they can cope with the demands that will be made upon them in the next stage of development.

Self-Esteem Needs Throughout the Life Cycle

PREGNANCY

Building self-esteem is probably our most important developmental task (Simmermacher, 1989). It begins in infancy—some say even before, when the fetus is still in the womb.

During pregnancy, many women say that they have never looked or felt better, and they feel a sense of satisfaction and completion that they have not known before. The woman begins planning more and more for the coming birth. During this period, some men feel excluded. Both men and women need reassurance at this time. Women have to deal

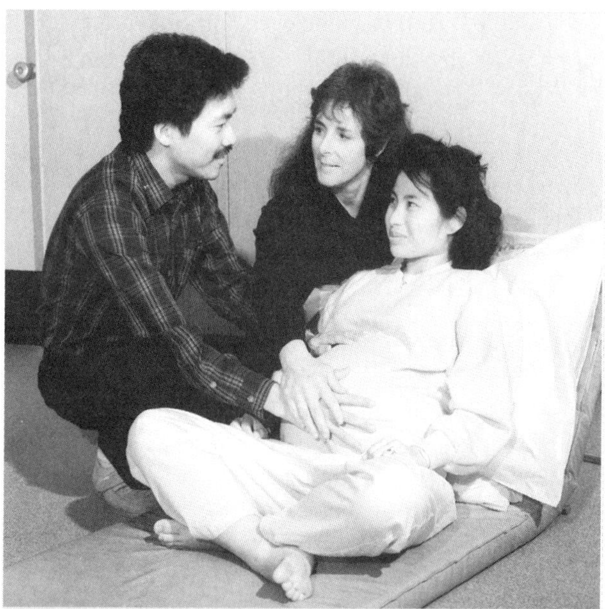

Prospective fathers need to feel they are an important part of the birthing process.

with clumsiness and ungainly proportions and a sense that their earlier self-image has been distorted and their equilibrium disturbed. Pregnant women need to know that they are still attractive and that the changes in appearance are normal. They should be encouraged to see the beauty of the body during pregnancy, exemplified by the many paintings and sculptures focussing on motherhood. A woman can invest her emotions in the care of the fetus better when she feels secure. There is a desire for deeper intimacy during this period, and a new sense of family develops.

Single pregnant women need a supportive environment such as a nuclear family, a cooperative housing arrangement or an extended family environment.

Prenatal classes are invaluable for both the mother and her partner; the latter needs to be an important part of this process and needs reassurance and peer support. The birth of a child causes a major change in the lives of a man and woman. After birth, the family must be reorganized to accommodate the new member. Feelings of security and a sense of self-esteem develop from the moment of birth. Considerable emphasis is now put on the importance of parental bonding during the first few hours after birth and throughout the first week to give the infant a sense of security. At one time, the mother's partner was barred from the delivery room in most Canadian hospitals. Now, if there is no "birthing room," a separate room is usually set aside where the mother, her partner and baby can get to know each other immediately after birth. The quality of the contact—with an emphasis on touching and caressing—is considered more important than the quantity of interaction. The voice of the mother is very important, as it gives positive reassurance of her presence to the infant.

INFANCY

Erikson (1963) feels that one of the major developmental tasks of infancy is the development of trust—of oneself, of the environment and of other people. At first, infants do not distinguish between themselves and their environment. They can, however, sense and respond to feelings of approval or disapproval on the part of a mother or a nurse. Approval leads to a sense of well-being and disapproval causes discomfort. At three months of age, children begin to explore their sense of self. They watch their hands and their feet with great interest and examine other areas of their body. At four months, children are aware of themselves as distinct from the rest of the world. They begin to explore this world, using the mother as a security base. Infants who have developed security in their attachment to their mothers are more likely to actively explore the world around them, although they will cry if she leaves them, showing happiness only when she returns.

Anxious infants may be more passive, showing less curiosity and less interest in exploring their environment than secure ones. "Stranger anxiety" is a common trait at six to 10 months, the time when infants begin to distinguish between mother and others.

An infant's emotional security rests to a considerable extent on the relationship that develops with the mother. If the relationship is a positive one, a rapport is established that permits interaction on a nonverbal basis, with the mother responding empathetically to her infant's needs. If the mother–infant relationship is cold, inconsistent or rejecting, mistrust and insecurity are built into the personality of the infant. Parents who respond promptly to their infant's cries have happier, calmer and more outgoing children as a general rule. Inconsistency or lack of response to the infant's needs can lead to infant anxiety, which is manifested by crying and clinging behaviour.

Body-image—the way we perceive our physical being—begins to develop in infancy from sensory input. Infants begin to notice the parts of their body that they can see, and to explore both their own body and that of their mother, using touch, smell, taste, sight and hearing. As children become a little older, they begin to associate the reflections they see in the mirror with themselves and they hear other people complimenting them on their appearance. Because the bony prominences of the body (such as the knees and the elbows) and the body openings are what come into contact most often with other objects, they serve as the most immediate points of reference for orienting children to their environment and are particularly important in developing body image. People's attitudes towards their body and its parts and functions are largely a product of their early socialization. Children absorb without question the attitudes of their parents regarding "clean" and "unclean" parts of their body, the appropriate state of cleanliness of the body and whether it is good to be fat or lean.

CHILDHOOD

During the toddler stage, children gain new motor skills, learn to walk, and extend their range of activities to investigate different aspects of their surroundings. Verbal and

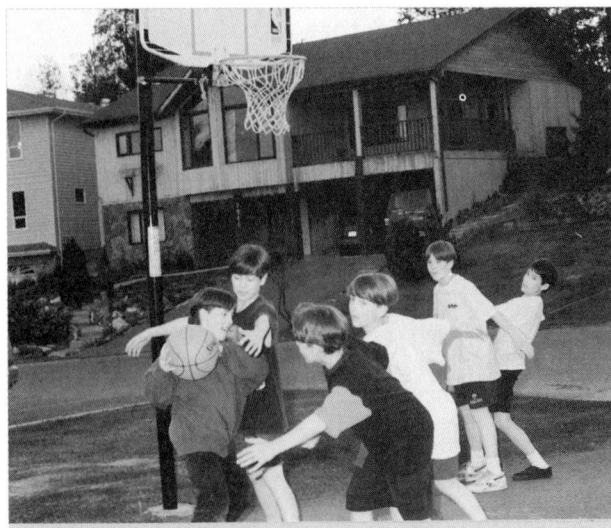

Through sports, school-age children learn to interact and cooperate with others their same age.

intellectual abilities develop at a rapid rate. They begin to comprehend and test out the meaning of the word "no." For the first time, children learn that there are restrictions

needs to be childproofed, so that the restrictions and limitations can be kept to the minimum needed for the child's safety. During the toddler stage and until about age four, the principal developmental task is to gain a sense of autonomy, without developing doubt or a sense of shame. Thus, the child needs to learn to negotiate the stairs (under watchful eyes) when they are ready to do so, without too many admonishments about being careful. Positive reinforcement will greatly enhance the situation. Toddlers' expanding communication skills enhance the development of self. Their first and most deeply learned perception of themselves is a composite reflection of how significant persons around them—their parents (or others taking a parental role), siblings and grandparents—perceive them.

The preschooler needs to learn initiative and to develop skills that build self-confidence. It is important for preschoolers to be given the opportunity to try new things and to receive the support of their parents while doing so. The self-confidence that is gained is reflected in the children's sense of eagerness, their spontaneity and the "bounce" in their steps. The development of routine times for meals, bedtime and outings helps to provide security for the child by developing the sense of expectation with reinforcement. During the preschool stage, the child is beginning to develop a conscience. Until approximately age seven, however, children are still very egocentric.

When children enter school, they are suddenly confronted with an expanding circle of people and new activities. They must learn how to interact and cooperate with others. In school, children also have a wider range of roles to emulate as teachers and older students provide appropriate role models. They learn how others (teachers, students and principals) evaluate their strengths and how others care for them as people. They learn the difference between work and play and they learn to enjoy work for the rewards it brings. If children feel a sense of inferiority or mediocrity, they may tend to withdraw and be discouraged. The school may provide reinforcement for a child's self-esteem through recognition of achievements, which can often offset an adverse atmosphere at home. On the other hand, problems at school may counteract the benefits of a supportive home environment. The chief task of this age group is to develop a sense of industry rather than inferiority to others.

ADOLESCENCE

The adolescent stage begins at approximately 12 years of age and lasts until about age 19. During puberty, when adolescents tend to be very self-conscious, a sense of identity and belonging is gradually achieved, usually through the stabilizing influence of peer groups. Adolescence is a period of great ambivalence, with the desire to be free of authority,

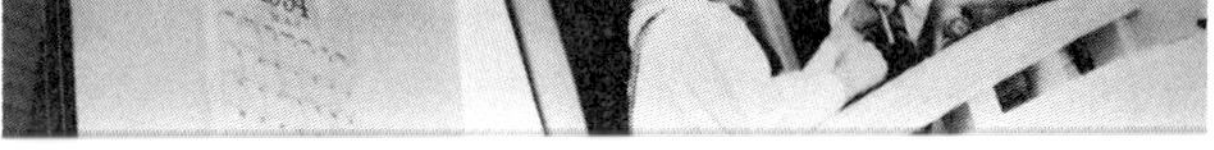

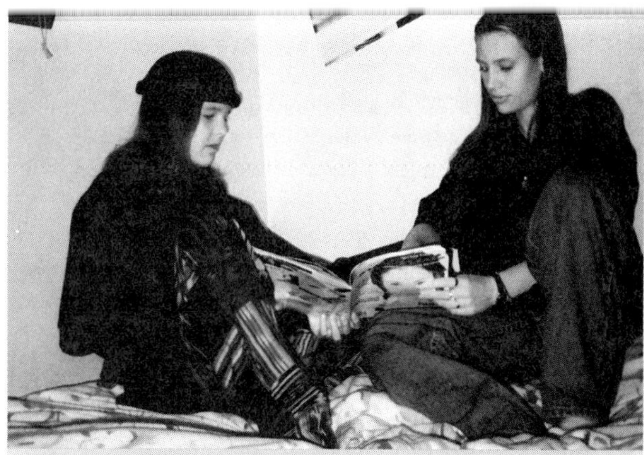

Adolescents need their own space to help them develop a sense of their own identity.

most importantly parents and school, conflicting with the dependence on them for emotional and financial support. Adolescents are dealing with who they are, what they want to work at and what they want to do with their lives. The major task at this stage is to gain a sense of identity. Failure to resolve this may lead to confusion, depression or an identification with a group or cult that supplies an identity. It may also lead people to seize the first job that arises or the first mate who offers a sense of identity, or else to "opt out," through the use of alcohol and drugs, of the difficult transition from adolescence to adulthood.

Positive reinforcement is vital during this period. One goal of education is to reinforce adolescents' identity through teamwork and the development of skills that can support them throughout their lifetime. To achieve a secure identity, adolescents need a sense of community in which they can exchange learning skills and support each other, especially since a vast number of adolescents are now being raised in single-parent homes. The establishment of sexual identity is a major developmental task of adolescence. Issues surrounding sexual identity are discussed in Chapter 35.

YOUNG ADULTHOOD

The young adult is mainly concerned with developing more intimate relationships with others. Without these relationships, they can experience a feeling of isolation. Intimacy has traditionally centred on marriage, although an increasing number of people are postponing marriage and devoting the early part of the adult years to establishing careers. It is necessary for the young adult to have a firm sense of identity at this point, although in today's society, people often experience a sense of isolation and insecurity. Young women in particular appear to have a difficult time at this stage because of conflicting societal expectations to marry and have children on the one hand, and to have a career on the other.

RESEARCH to practice

Marottoli, R.A., Mendes de Leon, C.F., Glass, T.A., Williams, C.S., Cooney, L.M. Jnr., Berkman, L.F. & Tinetti, M.E. (1997). Driving cessation and increased depressive symptoms: Prospective evidence from the New Haven EPESE. *Journal of the American Geriatric Society, 45*, 202–206.

The purpose of this cohort study was to identify whether there was a relationship between depressive symptoms among older adults and giving up driving. The urban setting of New Haven, Connecticut, was the site of the study. Participants were drawn from the established population for epidemiological studies of the elderly program, and included 1316 noninstitutionalized men and women over 65 years of age who completed all seven annual interviews. During the 1989 interview, participants were asked if they were still driving or had ever driven and had stopped. If participants had stopped driving they were asked when this had taken place. Other factors that could affect the outcome were assessed, for example, age, gender, educational level, marital status, sensory problems, cognitive status and difficulty performing activities of daily living.

Depressive symptoms were measured using the Center for Epidemiologic Studies depression (CES-D) scale during home interviews in 1982, 1985 and 1988. Of the study participants, 38 percent were still driving, 7 percent had given up driving between 1982 and 1987, and 55 percent had never driven or gave up driving before 1982. An increase in depressive symptoms was seen in each group over the six-year period. The group who were active drivers had the lowest CES-D scores at all three interviews. The group that had given up driving had intermediate scores at the baseline interview with higher depressive scores at the end of the six-year period.

The results indicate a substantial increase in depressive symptoms in noninstitutionalized seniors who give up driving.

There is a tendency to view oneself during young adulthood as being "indestructible" and able to "burn the candle at both ends." This attitude often leads to accidents and to the physical and mental state known as "burn out." This in turn may alter the self and adversely affect self-esteem. Damaged self-esteem and feelings of helplessness contribute to many of the suicides and homicides committed by people in this age group. Stable young adults, however, who are married or in an intimate relationship with another and have careers under way tend to see their lives as more secure, productive and self-actualized.

MIDDLE ADULTHOOD

Erikson (1963) feels that during middle age, there is a need to focus on a sense of "generativity" as opposed to stagnation in one's life, socially, at work and in the community. He feels that emphasis should be placed on the ability to impart wisdom to the young, and on innovation, rather than on simply going through life in a mechanical routine. Many men often become more concerned with feelings and are less aggressive in the middle years. Parents feel more free as their children become less dependent. A person's sense of security comes from the home one has created and the abilities one has developed. Somatic disorders frequently develop in response to psychic stress and anxiety. Diarrhea, colitis, bronchial asthma, hyperventilation and diabetes insipidus are among the health problems that are thought to have a strong psychosomatic component. Essentially, middle age is a time for stock-taking and re-evaluation. A sense of order in this world and a sense of one's life as an aspect of history has been developed.

OLDER ADULTHOOD

During the older years, there is increased attention to the maintenance of dignity to preserve the sense of self-esteem. Older people value their independence. Home care services are now making it possible for seniors to stay in their own homes when they become ill. An increasing number of people are choosing to die at home, surrounded by friends, relatives and belongings.

During the older adult years, security is ensured partially through financial means such as pensions, savings and retirement plans and partially through the ability to adapt, often to the situation of being dependent upon others. The main task during this period of the life cycle, according to Erikson (1963), is the maintenance of integrity as opposed to despair: accepting what has been, feeling useful and receiving respect. The older years are a time for looking back; the self-concept is related to past experience.

The problem of dependency on others for support and assistance may weigh heavily on older adults' sense of integrity. Depression may follow the loss of a spouse, friends, home, health and income, coupled with a feeling of rejection by society. Help in dealing with daily situations is usually welcome, along with visits from friends and relatives. The problem of decreased mobility may deepen the sense of isolation, although many communities have transportation systems geared to serving older adults. A large number of older people live alone and many are lonely. The alienation of the elderly is reflected in the high percentage of suicides among the older population. Older people need a social support network within their own communities, such as seniors' clubs, which can help to provide them with a sense of belonging. A network of friends helps to fulfill the need for love and affection that is vitally important to security and self-esteem.

Common Problems

[illegible] unsure of themselves, unhappy and afraid to take the chance of doing something for fear of failing. People with low self-esteem often blame themselves for their problems: they believe that it is their fault they are inadequate, that they did not try hard enough or that they did something wrong. Often there is an associated feeling of guilt and a need for punishment. People with low self-esteem may punish themselves with self-destructive behaviour to atone for wrongdoing. Alternatively, they may blame others for their problems and become hostile and angry. They are prone to illnesses that originate in the body's reaction to real or imagined threats. People in low income brackets, such as some single mothers living in low rental housing complexes, older adults who have insufficient income to live comfortably, First Nations people, chronically ill, disabled and some unemployed people often experience a pervasive feeling of powerlessness—they feel that there is nothing they can do to make their situation better (Epp, 1986).

Disturbances of self-concept and many of the problems related to negative self-esteem, such as anxiety, depression, negative body image, ineffective individual and family coping, and powerlessness are addressed in depth in psychiatric and mental health nursing courses and texts. The effects of low self-esteem are so pervasive, however, affecting so many aspects of a person's well-being, that it is important to develop early in your course of study some skills in assessing self-concept and identifying some of the common problems.

In this chapter, we will focus on three of the most common problems related to lack of self-esteem: feelings of powerlessness (hopelessness/helplessness), anxiety and depression. These problems often cluster together with other problems such as negative body image, social isolation and ineffective individual or family coping; one problem is often related to another. For example, a patient may develop a poor body image because of the loss of a leg in an accident; the patient may become depressed and may withdraw from contact with friends.

Powerlessness

Powerlessness has been defined as "The state in which an individual or group perceives a loss of personal control over certain events or situations which affects outlook, goals and lifestyle" (Carpenito, 1997, p. 658). It is probably the most devastating problem related to self-esteem—the feeling that nothing you can do is going to make any difference. It is unpleasant when people believe that it is impossible to obtain the things they want or need to protect themselves or their family, and it leaves people feeling very vulnerable and insecure. The future looks bleak and people become anxious, uneasy and constantly worried.

People often react to feelings of powerlessness with anger and hostility towards the government, employers, the school system—whatever is seen as the power that is controlling their lives. Violent behaviour, such as the vandal- [illegible] mentioned in Chapter 3 that the social unrest, the strikes and the riots during the 1930s were due to feelings of powerlessness on the part of unemployed workers who were unable to do anything to remedy the situation. If a patient is ill and the prognosis is poor, there is often anger towards the physician, the hospital and the nurses (Staples, Baruth, Jefferies & Warder, 1994). Sometimes friends and family bear the brunt of this anger as the patient fights against his or her fate. The anger may fade into apathy or turn into depression as the patient becomes resigned to the situation.

Anxiety

Anxiety is defined as "...an unpleasant feeling of tension and apprehension, accompanied by physiological, psychological and behavioural symptoms, that serves as an early warning signal that alerts people to impending real or symbolic threat to self, significant others or a way of life" (Haber *et al.*, 1992, p. 794). There are varying degrees of anxiety, ranging from mild apprehension to overwhelming panic. Unresolved anxiety, or anxiety to a more-than-mild degree, can be incapacitating. In Chapter 9, in the section on stress, we discussed the individual's reaction to perceived threats. The material in Chapter 9 provides a theoretical background for our discussions about anxiety in this chapter.

Threats to the individual cause certain physiological reactions to take place within the body. These reactions vary to a certain extent depending on physical makeup. Anxiety also brings about changes in a person's behaviour. Again, these changes vary, depending on the individual's basic personality structure and the ways in which he or she has coped with anxieties in the past. There are also changes in *feeling tone (affect)* and in the person's *mental functioning (cognitive ability)*. Physical condition affects the ability to tolerate anxiety. Something that may constitute only a minor worry when a person is healthy may create an overwhelming anxiety when the body's defences are lowered.

Physiological Manifestations

The principal physiological mechanism operating in anxiety is the fundamental stress reaction as the body attempts to protect itself from harm. The most easily observable physical signs of anxiety in an individual are the circulatory changes that take place. The action of the heart is strengthened and accelerated. Blood pressure may be elevated. Pulse rate may be as much as 30 percent above normal and respiratory pattern is often disturbed as well—there may be increases in rate and depth, or there may be irregularities. There may be a marked pallor of the skin or sometimes a flushing of the face, and often the skin surfaces are cold.

Muscular tension is almost invariably present with anxiety. In some people this tension may be observed in a taut expression of the face or in a clenching of the fists. Some people assume a very rigid posture. At times, muscular tension is revealed by a tremor of the hands, in a facial, arm or shoulder tic, or in a generalized shivering or trembling of the body. The tightening of the abdominal muscles and the "butterflies" in the stomach that are commonly experienced with anxiety are the result of muscular tension. The tension headache is another common symptom of anxiety.

Many people perspire excessively in anxiety-provoking situations. The palms of the hands or the soles of the feet may be the most affected. This increased perspiration combined with a coldness and pallor of the skin (due to lessened peripheral circulation) results in the typical cold and damp hands of very anxious people.

Gastrointestinal symptoms often accompany anxiety. The "knot" or "butterflies" in the stomach may progress to nausea and vomiting. Often people say they cannot face the thought of food when they are going to take an exam or undergo an important interview and, some people vomit. Diarrhea is also a common symptom of anxiety, and people often have urinary frequency as well.

Feeling Tone (Affect)

People react to threatening situations in a variety of ways. Behaviour usually reflects the ways in which people have learned to cope with life's dangers. While some people can talk easily about their fears and openly express them to the nurse, others may be expressing fear in less easily recognizable forms. Some people attempt to deny the existence of anxiety. These people ask no questions and frequently make a point of keeping conversation off the subject of themselves. In our culture, many men still feel that it is "unmanly" to express fear, particularly to women. Men (and sometimes women) frequently cover up feelings of anxiety with loud assurances that they are not frightened, and may joke and laugh in an attempt to minimize the seriousness of the condition.

Some people react to the threat of danger with anger and hostility. They may criticize the care they are receiving and be loud and insistent in demanding special treatment. People who react in this way often engender hostility on the part of nurses and other staff, who label them consciously or unconsciously as "difficult" patients. If nurses can accept this type of behaviour as being indicative of the patient's anxiety and not take it as a personal attack, they will be in a better position to take positive measures to help the patient.

Severe anxiety may become **panic,** in which the patient is unable to say or do anything meaningful. Behaviour may be completely out of context—people may laugh when they should be crying—and thoughts and speech become incoherent. People who have "panicked" need someone calm to stay with them, to take charge of the situation and to tell them what to do. People cannot think for themselves at this point.

Common Manifestations of Anxiety

Physiological

- increased pulse and blood pressure rates
- altered respirations; increased or irregular
- pale skin (sometimes flushed)
- increased perspiration
- muscular tension (clenched fists, rigid posture, nervous tics, trembling or shivering, headache)
- lack of interest in food
- diarrhea
- frequency of urination

Affective

- feelings of tension
- uneasiness
- a sense of dread; a feeling that something bad is about to happen
- anger and hostility

Cognitive

- heightened mental activity
- insomnia, nightmares, early morning wakening
- inability to focus on any topic other than the one that is the centre of attention
- short attention span

Behavioural

- rapid speech in a loud, high-pitched or quavery voice; sometimes hesitancy of speech with stammering and stuttering
- restlessness, may become agitated as tension mounts
- rapid movements, hurried gait
- verbal or physical hostility towards others
- inappropriate behaviour (for example, laughing when they should be crying)
- crying
- use of defence mechanisms

We said in Chapter 9 that a little anxiety is a good thing because it stimulates us to put forth the effort needed to accomplish things. However, when the anxiety persists too long, or is too overpowering, the body's defences break down and illness results.

Mental Functioning (Cognitive Ability)

In patients experiencing anxiety, mental activity is usually increased. When anxiety is mild, increased mental activity may mean that the individual is simply more alert and better able to think clearly. As anxiety mounts, however, perceptual awareness decreases. People become unaware of their immediate surroundings, except possibly the one thing on which their attention is focussed. Anxious people often have difficulty concentrating on anything other than that one thing. Attention span is usually short and people may be unable to answer even simple questions. Worried parents [illegible] so distraught that they cannot remember their own address.

With increasing anxiety, heightened mental activity may hinder rest, and insomnia frequently results. If anxious people do manage to get to sleep, they are often troubled by nightmares. They may awaken early in the morning and be unable to get back to sleep.

Behavioural Manifestations

People seek relief from muscular tension in a number of ways: by biting nails, drumming fingers on the table or pacing. Restlessness and overactivity are usually fairly reliable indications of anxiety.

Changes in the patient's voice and speech patterns are also possible indications of anxiety. Some people talk very rapidly or constantly when anxious, and sometimes the voice becomes very loud or high-pitched, or may quaver. In others, there may be a hesitancy of speech; people may appear to be having difficulty finding the right words. Stammering and stuttering are not uncommon in people experiencing anxiety.

Some people react to anxiety by crying. Many nurses are embarrassed to discover a patient in tears and find it difficult to know what to say or do. Attempts to reassure patients that "everything is going to be all right" are not usually effective in helping them to cope with their feelings. Crying often denotes a feeling of helplessness and an inability to handle certain problems. Tears serve to relieve tension, and the nurse can perhaps be most helpful by staying with the patient and being ready to listen when the crying is over.

Depression

Depression has been defined as "a feeling of profound sadness, low self-esteem and hopelessness about one's life" (Haber *et al.*, 1992, p. 797). It may range from being minor and transitory (the "blues" that everyone has once in a while) to a severe feeling of sadness that is pervasive and persistent. Someone whose security is threatened and who feels helpless in a situation may react with depression rather than anxiety. Often the same stressors that cause anxiety in some people give rise to sadness and melancholy in others. Depression may also be created by a situation or an event that would normally cause a person to be sad, such as the death of a spouse or a good friend; this is called **reactive** or **situational depression.** A change in the weather may precipitate a period of depression. This is called Seasonal Affective Disorder (SAD).

Depression is said to be the single most common problem that nurses and other health professionals encounter (Haber *et al.*, 1997). Social surveys undertaken in recent decades in Canada indicate that people in lower socioeconomic groups are "on the average, more unhappy, more worried, and [tend to be] less hopeful about the future" (Stolzman, 1988). We noted in Chapter 12 the high rate of suicide among First Nations people and the high incidence [illegible]

Depression is a common problem among people of all age groups. Although it was once more common among adults in the 25–44 age bracket, it appears to be becoming more prevalent among 18–24-year-olds; the age when depression is prevalent is decreasing with each generation (Haber *et al.*, 1997; Statistics Canada, 1995). In Canada, suicide and motor vehicle accidents are the leading causes of death in young adults from age 15 upward. Generally speaking, depression affects women more than it does men, except in the older age group when more men than women suffer from depression (Ebersole & Hess, 1998).

Depression is so prevalent among the population that it is said to be the "common cold" of mental illness. It is often hidden by people who may wear a mask of joviality to cover sadness, or it may masquerade as physical illness. Nurses encounter depression among people living in the community and in patients in all units of an inpatient facility. Nurses should be particularly watchful for depression in teens and young adults who are having difficulty "finding themselves," in people who are going through middle-age turmoil and in older people, particularly those living alone.

Depression and anxiety both cause certain physiological reactions to occur within the body. They also both give rise to specific behavioural manifestations, although the two sets of responses are quite different. The observant nurse should be able to distinguish between these two problems in most cases. Sometimes, however, a person will show manifestations of both anxiety and depression, a state which is called **agitated depression.**

Physiological Manifestations

Gastrointestinal functioning slows down, and depressed patients tend to become constipated. They usually have no appetite and will say that they no longer enjoy food. As a result, depressed people will probably lose weight. A loss of anywhere from five to 20 pounds is not unusual. On the other hand, some people overeat when they are depressed. Men and women tend to lose their sex drive when they are depressed, and women may have a cessation of menses.

Sleep disturbances are associated with depression. Research finds that REM sleep often begins too early in the night and lasts longer than normal. This finding may explain why depressed individuals often complain of feeling tired after a night's sleep. Other sleep disturbances associated with depression include decreased overall sleep time, increased number of dreams, trouble falling asleep and increased natural awakenings (Stuart & Laraia, 1998).

Feeling Tone (Flat Affect)

Three basic feelings are experienced as part of depression and these feelings are evident in the behaviour of depressed

Common Manifestations of Depression

Physiological

- loss of appetite leading to loss of weight
- weight gain
- constipation; may have retention of urine in severe cases
- slow movements
- lessened response to stimulation
- lessened sex drive
- amenorrhea
- psychomotor retardation

Affective

- feeling of sadness, melancholy; loss of enjoyment of usual activities
- feelings of worthlessness and low self-esteem
- anger towards self
- feelings of hopelessness
- guilt

Cognitive

- poor concentration
- difficulty remembering things
- may become obsessed with one topic
- difficulty making decisions
- disturbed sleep patterns; often waking in the night; may sleep excessively

Behavioural

- stooped posture, slouching gait
- lack of interest in clothes, grooming
- withdraw from social contacts
- reluctant to talk, speech slow
- may use drugs or alcohol in seeking temporary relief
- difficulty finishing tasks

people. They often do not want to socialize, often do not want to do anything at all. They have feelings of worthlessness and experience a loss of self-esteem. They also may want to hurt or even destroy themselves because they feel they are not worthy of life.

Even if people have accomplished a great deal in life, when depressed, they often speak of their achievements as meaningless. Sometimes people turn to alcohol or drugs to find temporary relief from depression.

Depressed people may describe their feelings in terms such as "blue," "down," "low," "sad" or even "depressed." Others may complain of being irritable. Often, people say they feel "hopeless," "guilty" or "worthless."

Mental Functioning (Cognitive Ability)

Depressed people usually find it difficult to concentrate and to remember things. They may forget appointments or feel that it is too much effort to go. Often, activities are started but not completed. People either lose interest or just do not have the energy to finish.

Behavioural Manifestations

In most types of depression, people claim to feel as if everything is happening in slow motion. They feel less active, and their movements and reaction time are slow. They are less responsive to any form of stimulation, they talk less and their speech is slower than normal. Severely depressed people may be totally unresponsive and may have thoughts of suicide (Boyd & Nihart, 1998).

Depressed people usually walk with a stooped, slouching gait, the head down near the chest, often shuffling along. They seem to want to make themselves as small as possible. They are also unconcerned about what they wear. It is an effort just to get out of bed in the morning. Depressed people begin to neglect their appearance, by not bathing or shaving. Most depressed people find that the worst time of the day is when they are waking up (Haber *et al.*, 1997; Morales-Mann, 1990).

Many different theories, such as cognitive, biological, social and family role theories, as well as a "learned helplessness" theory, have been proposed to account for the phenomenon of depression. There is no single theory, however, that accounts for all types of depression. Rather, it is important to look at all the factors in an individual's life to understand the reasons for depression (Haber *et al.*, 1997).

Other Problems

NEGATIVE BODY IMAGE

Body image is the mental picture we have of our bodies (Haber *et al.*, 1997). It reflects the perceptual image we have of our physical being and our attitudes towards our body and its various parts and functions. This mental picture is derived from sensory input over the years, from our social interactions with other people and from our responses to them. How we see our bodies is very much a cultural matter. Children whose appearance is different from other children in the prevailing culture, for instance, soon become aware of the fact that they are different. If they are teased by the other children, they begin to feel that they are not as good as the others.

Whether a child develops a positive or a negative body image is a product of the early social environment. Children's body image reflects the image parents project of them and it is subsequently modified by others in the home, school and playground. Our body image changes over the years as our bodies change. People are always disturbed by changes in their body—adolescents wonder how to cope with the physical signs and inward changes in their maturing body. Pregnant women may be disturbed by changing body shape. With the emphasis in our society on a lean and physically fit body, people who do not fit this image tend to think poorly of themselves. People in their middle years often regret the loss of physical prowess and view the sight of the first grey hairs with dismay. Older adults often perceive

will make deprecating remarks about themselves.

Any alteration in body image can seriously upset a person's equilibrium. Alterations may be caused by illness or accident as well as by developmental changes in body structure and functioning. For example, a scar on the face may result from a motor vehicle accident; a person with diabetes may lose a limb from complications of the disease; a loss of hair commonly happens with chemotherapy. The loss of hair with chemotherapy is usually temporary, ending when the treatment does—but it is nonetheless traumatic. Almost all illnesses cause temporary or permanent changes in the body; even the common cold makes the eyes water, the nose run and the body function less efficiently. People can be disturbed by even the slightest change in the body's appearance or its functioning. Major changes can be devastating.

People who are worried about body image may feel ashamed or embarrassed about the defect they see in their body. They may also feel guilty if they think the perceived defect is the result of some wrongdoing on their part. It is not uncommon for people who have had a mastectomy or a colostomy to show revulsion towards their body. Some people are able to express their feelings openly. For others, the disturbance in self-image may be inferred from a reluctance to look at or touch the offending part. These people may try to hide the disturbance in self-image, although some say, "Let the world see me for what I am." Often, people with self-image problems are preoccupied with the change or loss; they may express feelings of depression and they may engage in self-destructive behaviour. They will often limit contact with other people, and some may use denial, refusing to believe what has happened or trying to convince themselves that the affected part of their body does not belong to them (Carpenito, 1997).

SOCIAL ISOLATION

People who have low opinions of themselves are usually hesitant about making social contacts. Social support is one of the most important factors in the development and maintenance of self-esteem, but people with low self-esteem are often unable to make the contact with others that is necessary to gain this support. Being alone should not be confused with loneliness. Some people are "loners" and quite content with solitary pursuits; these people make the choice to be alone. It is important to verify that the reason for not having many social contacts is a matter of personal choice, not one of difficulty in making friends, or fear of reaching out to other people. We all need the company of other human beings, some more than others. People who have difficulty meeting and interacting with other people are often lonely.

INEFFECTIVE INDIVIDUAL OR FAMILY COPING

with life's stresses. They may have difficulty making decisions, solving problems and resolving conflicts. Often angry at themselves as the cause of their failures, they may become self-destructive or hostile and aggressive in their behaviour towards others. Playground bullies, for example, are frequently the children who receive more punishment than love and affection at home and consequently grow up with strong negative feelings about themselves. People who have been abused as children are likely to abuse their own children in a vicious cycle that may persist for generations. People often turn to alcohol or drugs that give them temporary respite from feelings of inadequacy. Some join cults, which provide them with the security of a supportive group and give them a sense of identity (Morales-Mann, 1990; Haber *et al.*, 1997).

An Ontario study found that more people with a low income, and with a low level of education, reported living in dysfunctional families than those with higher incomes and higher educational attainment. According to the report, "...people with lower incomes and less education report poorer personal and social well-being..." (Government of Ontario, 1992, p. 13).

Assessing Self-Esteem Needs

Low self-esteem may have a number of causes and it may be manifested in many ways, making it difficult to identify. The assessment process is ongoing. It begins with the nursing health history and continues as the nurse and the patient interact during the process of nursing care.

Nursing Health History

The amount of information disclosed during the health history depends on the relationship that is established between interviewer and interviewee. Trust is essential in this relationship, and as patients develop security in the relationship with the nurse, they are more open when talking about feelings, thoughts and perceptions. Most people will talk quite freely if the nurse has established a climate in which the patient feels free to communicate, and if the nurse takes the time to be an attentive listener.

To assess self-concept and identify actual or potential problems related to negative self-esteem, the nurse needs to know something about the patient as a person, the present stage of physical and psychosocial development, and about lifestyle, health status and immediate concerns.

The nurse needs to know the patient's personality characteristics and value systems. What are the most important things in the patient's life? The patient's interests, especially those that can be enjoyed in spite of the health problem(s), should also be determined.

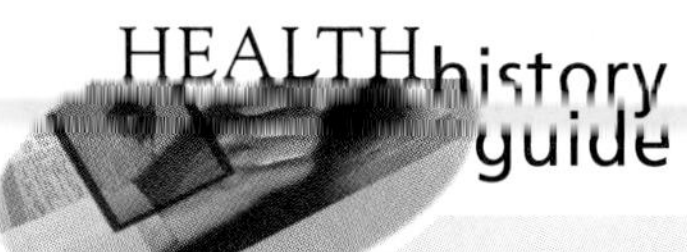

Assessing Self-Concept

1. How old are you?
2. What is your marital and family status?
3. Do you live with someone other than a family member?
4. Do you have many friends? Do you feel lonely?
5. What is your occupation?
6. Have you experienced major changes in your life recently? If so, what were they? What kind of adjustments to your life did they require?
7. What are some of your immediate concerns? Do you have any fears or worries?
8. What is your health problem? Are you worried about pain, surgery, disfigurement or death related to this problem? Are you afraid that this problem will prevent you from pursuing your normal lifestyle?
9. What are some sources of stress in your life?
10. How do you usually handle stress? What gets you through tough times?
11. Briefly describe your personality. Are you happy? sad? optimistic? pessimistic? outgoing? self-sufficient? an idealist? a realist? a perfectionist?
12. Do you usually feel better in the morning or at night?
13. What things are important to you?
14. Do you have any hobbies? What leisure activities do you enjoy?
15. Are you a member of any religious or cultural groups? If so, would you like to meet with representatives of these groups?
16. Can you think of any resource people on our staff whom you would like to see?
17. What helps you cope?

The nurse considers age and the current stage of physical and psychosocial development. Is there a possibility that the patient is going through a developmental crisis? The nurse should also be aware of marital and family status, and how the patient fits in to the family structure. The patient's friends and significant others can also influence self-esteem.

Behaviours Associated with Low Self-Esteem

Criticism of self or others
Decreased productivity
Destructiveness
Disruptions in relatedness
Exaggerated sense of self-importance
Feelings of inadequacy
Guilt
Irritability or excessive anger
Negative feelings about one's body
Perceived role strain
Pessimistic view of life
Physical complaints
Polarizing view of life
Rejection of personal capabilities
Self-destructiveness
Self-diminution
Social withdrawal
Substance abuse
Withdrawal from reality
Worrying

SOURCE: Stuart & Laraia, 1998, p. 324.

The patient's occupation and socioeconomic status may be sources of insecurity, leading to self-esteem problems. Where does the patient stand in relation to the fulfillment of basic needs? Is self-actualization important at this point in life, or is the patient struggling to make enough money to provide the basic essentials of food, shelter and security?

Another matter to consider is whether there have been any major changes in the patient's life recently. If so, what sort of changes were they? Did they necessitate major readjustments in the patient's life?

In regard to health status, the nurse considers the patient's main concerns at the present time. What brought the patient to the health agency? Verbalizations of feelings, and statements made in regard to physical or mental symptoms being experienced, also help the nurse to identify low self-esteem or problems associated with it. The patient's attitude towards the illness and the hospital staff—lightheartedness, joking, hostility or crying—may also reflect self-esteem needs. Even the patient's willingness or reluctance to talk about their social, emotional or health problems may indicate self-esteem needs.

Some questions that are helpful in assessing the self-concept of individuals and identifying problems related to low self-esteem are listed in the Health History Guide above.

Physical Assessment

During both the nursing health history and the physical assessment of the patient, the nurse looks for behavioural manifestations of negative self-esteem. For example, is the patient angry and irritable? In Chapter 17, we discussed nonverbal behaviour as a means of communicating attitudes and feelings.

During the physical assessment, the nurse notes general appearance. Is the patient well-groomed or untidy in appearance? With the exception of the very ill, most people [illegible] health centre or when the nurse or physician is visiting them.

The nurse also looks for physical signs of anxiety or depression, such as altered heart rate, constipation or diarrhea, change in appetite, poor posture or altered rates of speech and movements. Does the patient speak in monotone or in a high-pitched voice? Does the patient show signs of muscular tension?

Diagnosing Self-Esteem Problems

The effects of low self-esteem are pervasive and related to numerous problems that are in the domain of nursing practice. Carpenito (1997) lists body image disturbance, personal identity disturbance, self-esteem disturbance, chronic low self-esteem and situational low self-esteem in one broad category that she calls self-concept disturbance. The person who has had a debilitating health problem may have a *Disturbance of the self-concept* related to the health problem. For the woman who has had a mastectomy, the diagnosis would be written as *Body Image Disturbance related to surgery.* For a young man who has never done well in school and drops out in grade 10, the nursing diagnosis might be written as *Self-Esteem Disturbance due to repeated failures.* In other problems where low self-esteem is a major factor, the nursing diagnosis would be written as PROBLEM *related to* CAUSE, for example, *Anxiety related to low self-esteem* or *Anxiety related to actual or perceived threat to self-concept.* "Depression" is not on the NANDA list of nursing diagnoses. Any of the following nursing diagnoses may be related to depression: *Powerlessness*, any of the *self-care deficit* family of diagnoses, such as *Self-Care Deficit in dressing and grooming, Risk for self-harm, self-mutilation or suicide* and *Social Isolation* (Carpenito, 1997).

Planning Self-Esteem Interventions

Nursing care is based on planning to meet the nursing needs of individuals and groups. As we noted in discussing the determinants of security and self-esteem, self-esteem is the product of many factors including home life, school environment, workplace and social networks. To nurture self-esteem, then, requires a multisectoral approach involving collaboration with people in numerous fields. In planning nursing care to promote, protect, support and restore self-esteem, the nurse works in collaboration with members of many disciplines.

KEY PRINCIPLES

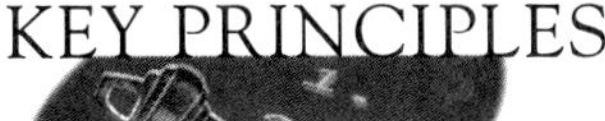

[illegible] Self-Esteem

- self-esteem is an internal evaluation of the sum total of people's perceptions, feelings and beliefs about themselves
- self-esteem exists in relation to the individual's total psychological environment
- fulfillment of the basic physiological, security, love and belonging needs is necessary for the development of positive self-esteem
- self-esteem is acquired through the process of growth and development
- negative (or low) self-esteem has been linked to numerous physical and social ills
- negative self-esteem can be transformed through successful learning experiences.

Basic principles regarding self-esteem that are relevant to planning nursing measures are shown in the box above.

The nurse's responsibilities are:

- to work with parents and families to foster the development of self-esteem in children
- to work with others at the community level and in the public forum to promote conditions that will nurture feelings of self-worth
- to protect the self-esteem of individuals and families
- to plan and implement nursing care for individuals and families to meet the needs of people with specific nursing diagnoses.

It is essential that the individual or family participate in identifying goals and in planning strategies to meet these goals. It is important that the goals become the patient's own, with the nurse acting as a facilitator instead of as an authority.

Some examples of outcome criteria for nursing diagnoses related to low self-esteem and to specific problems are given in Table 36.1.

Implementing Self-Esteem Interventions

The specific goals of nursing care related to the need for self-esteem are:

- to promote the fostering of self-esteem in individuals, families and communities
- to protect the individual's or family's feelings of self-worth

TABLE 38.1 Examples of outcome criteria for nursing diagnoses related to low self esteem

Nursing Diagnoses Related to Low Self-Esteem	*Sample Outcome Criteria*
Low self-esteem	• The person will identify ways of exerting control and influencing outcomes. • The person will verbalize and demonstrate acceptance of appearance (grooming, dress, posture, eating patterns, presentation of self). • The person will describe strategies to promote effective socialization.
Powerlessness	• The person will identify and explore how she or he can update employable skills. • The person will make decisions regarding his or her care, treatment, and future when possible.
Anxiety	• The person will describe his or her own anxiety and coping patterns.
Depression	• The person will state the desire to live.

- to enhance the individual's power to improve his or her life situation
- to facilitate the acquisition of knowledge and the development of skills that will enable people to take control of their lives, make decisions about choices and improve their life situation.

Health-Promoting Strategies

Nursing interventions to promote self-esteem include individual counselling, teaching, working with groups, and working with people in other sectors, such as school teachers and employers, to foster environments in which self-esteem is nurtured. Nursing interventions to promote self-esteem also involve political action at times, such as forming coalitions and lobbying.

The Epp framework for health promotion suggests three mechanisms for health promotion: self-care, mutual aid and healthy environments. Nurses use all three in fostering self-esteem.

SELF-CARE

"Simply put, encouraging self-care means encouraging healthy choices" (Epp, 1986, p. 6). In this context, **self-care** refers to the decisions people make and the practices they adopt to promote and protect their own health. To make healthy choices, people need access to information and they need motivation and a supportive environment to adopt healthy practices. Nurturing self-esteem is a lifelong process that begins before a child is born. To nurture self-esteem, the nurse works with:

- prospective parents to provide them with access to the information they need to become nurturing parents

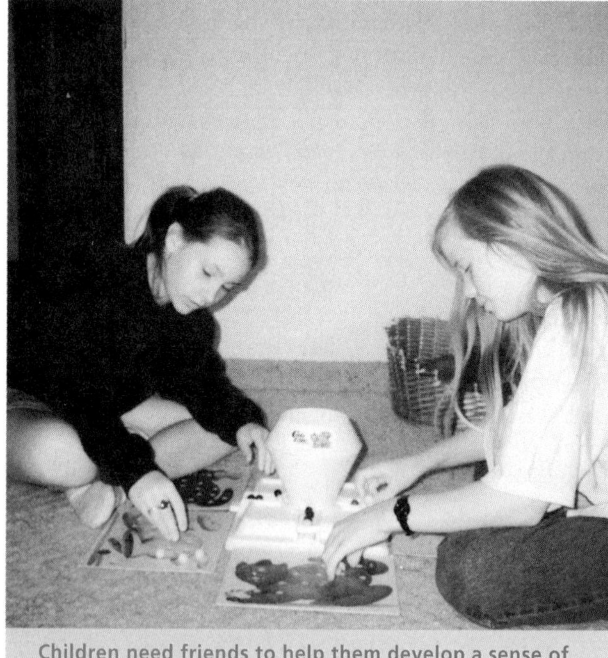

Children need friends to help them develop a sense of belonging.

- mothers and partners during labour and delivery to foster "bonding" between parents and child
- new mothers to encourage breast-feeding and with both parents to help them gain the knowledge and skills needed to care for their infant and develop a good relationship with the child
- parents of young and school-age children to assist them in learning how to help their children grow up with positive feelings of self-worth.

Children reflect the image their parents have of them. If parents communicate to their children that each one is loved, wanted and an important being, those children are [illegible] themselves than children who are constantly criticized. The different ways we have of communicating are summarized in the box opposite.

MUTUAL AID

Mutual aid refers to the concept of people helping other people. Much of the nurse's work with parents is done with groups such as prospective parent's classes, or with young parents, helping them to learn to foster self-esteem in their children. It is reassuring for young parents to learn that their child's behaviour is not so different from that of other children the same age, and to share with other parents ways to help their children grow up confident and sure of their worth. We talked in Chapter 4 about self-help groups, and

Different Ways of Communicating

- verbally—through spoken or written words
- nonverbally—nonverbal sounds (for example, groans, laughter, facial expressions, body positions and movements)
- behaviourally—our actions communicate our thoughts, feelings and desires very clearly. For example, if someone says, "I really want to lose weight" but continues to overeat, it looks as if eating is more important than losing weight.
- silently—silence can mean "I do not want to communicate with you" or "I am afraid to communicate with you" or "I am too angry to communicate with you."

SOURCE: Holloway, 1991.

Qualities of the Healthy Personality

Characteristic	Definition	Description
Positive and accurate body image	Body image is the sum of the conscious and unconscious attitudes one has toward one's body, function, appearance and potential.	A healthy body awareness is based on self-observation and appropriate concern for one's physical well-being.
Realistic self-ideal	Self-ideal is one's perception of how one should behave or the standard by which behaviour is appraised.	A person with a realistic self-ideal has attainable life goals that are valuable and worth striving for.
Positive self-concept	Self-concept consists of all the aspects of the person of which one is aware. It includes all self-perceptions that direct and influence behaviour.	A positive self-concept implies that the person expects to be successful in life. It includes acceptance of the negative aspects of the self as part of one's personality. Such a person faces life openly and realistically.
High self-esteem	Self-esteem is one's personal judgement of one's own worth, which is obtained by analyzing how well one matches up to one's own standards and how well one's performance compares with others. It evolves through a comparison of the self-ideal and self-concept.	A person with high self-esteem feels worthy of respect and dignity, believes in his or her own self-worth, and approaches life with assertiveness and zest. The person with a healthy personality feels very similar to the person he or she wants to be.
Satisfying role performance	Roles are sets of socially expected behaviour patterns associated with functioning in various social groups.	The healthy person can relate to others intimately, receive gratification from social and personal roles, trust others, and enter into mutual and interdependent relationships.
Clear sense of identity	Identity is the integration of inner and outer demands in one's discovery of who one is and what one can become. It is the realization of personal consistency.	The person with a clear sense of identity experiences a unity of personality and perceives herself or himself to be a unique person. This sense of self gives life direction and purpose.

SOURCE: Stuart & Laraia, 1998, p. 323.

in Chapter 18, the enterostomal therapist talked about working with the Ostomy Association, a self-help group for people with colostomies or ileostomies. Associations such as these help people and their families to feel comfortable with their illness by sharing experiences, feelings and ways of coping with the stresses of their everyday lives. In so doing, feelings of self-worth are nurtured; people are part of a group with similar problems.

In working with all of these groups, it is important for nurses to remember that their role is that of *resource* for the group—a source of information and professional expertise when it is needed, a teacher of skills and sometimes an advocate for the group with official governmental and other agencies. The nurse's task is to *facilitate* the work of the group.

HEALTHY ENVIRONMENTS

Self-esteem requires fostering in the home, school, workplace and community. The nurse works with parents and other family members, with teachers and school principals, with employers and with other people in the community to foster environments that will nurture people's self-esteem. Nurses are also involved in promoting the fostering of self-esteem as citizens and through professional associations by developing healthy public policies to provide a supportive environment for everyone.

Characteristics of a healthy school environment and a healthy workplace taken from the Ontario document *Nurturing Health* (1993) are shown in the boxes. The information in these boxes emphasizes the importance of nurturing self-concept in the promotion of health and suggests strategies for doing so.

A Healthy School Environment

- involves students, staff and parents in decisions affecting the school and community
- ensures that students and teachers have safe working conditions and access to support services
- builds students' and teachers' self-esteem and fosters values such as mutual responsibility, caring and personal power
- provides instruction in health matters and gives opportunities to practise decision-making skills
- prepares students for productive employment, positive social relationships and full participation in the community

SOURCE: Government of Ontario, 1993.

A Healthy Workplace Environment

- provides a healthy and safe physical environment
- invests in employees by offering ongoing training and by rewarding good work
- recognizes that fairness, job security, recognition, good management, teamwork and personal wellness are important to employees
- involves employees in making decisions, and in defining and responding to workplace needs
- offers flexible work hours that alleviate the stress of balancing home and workplace responsibilities
- offers workplace health promotion programs and opportunities for positive interactions with co-workers.

SOURCE: Government of Ontario, 1993.

Health-Protecting Strategies

In Chapter 13 we discussed the writings of some of the "human care" theorists in nursing, including Leininger, Watson, Orem and Roach. That material is particularly pertinent to our discussion here on protecting self-esteem. Watson, for example, has stated that "the end [goal of nursing] is protection, enhancement and preservation of human dignity" (Watson, 1988, p. 35). The treatment of people in health care agencies has become increasingly impersonal as our predominantly "cure-oriented" care has become more technological and the institutions more bureaucratized (Watson, 1988). The reforms that are taking place in health care across the country are attempting to make the system more humane by de-emphasizing institutional care and bringing health care closer to home, and by encouraging people to be partners in the health care process rather than simply the recipients of services.

Still, there are many agencies where the patient feels like a cog in a machine. To cite one example, an individual phones to make an appointment with her physician, who is in a busy family practice clinic. The office nurse who answers the phone tells the woman she does not need her name, just her clinic number. One cannot blame the woman for changing her family physician to one in a smaller practice where she will be treated as a person instead of a number.

Hospitals have been especially criticized for the impersonal manner in which admission procedures are carried out, and the depersonalization that results from the routines many hospitals consider necessary. First, patients are asked a lot of personal questions; they are expected to give answers to a stranger. They are then given a number and "tagged" with an armband. They are taken to a nursing unit that is usually also designated with a number, not a name, and assigned to a room or bed, likewise numbered. Once there, patients are stripped of all their clothes and most of the valuables that help to identify them as people. A procession of strangers then begins to arrive at their bedside, to ask more personal questions and perform various examinations. Sometimes, these strangers do not even introduce themselves, and the patient is left to guess who they are by the uniform they are wearing. If patients are assigned to a room where there are other patients, they often have to make introductions themselves.

Ways of Conveying Respect for Personhood

Verbally

- addressing patients by the name they wish to be called
- using "active listening" skills
- telling patients what the nurse or others are going to do to them, or for them, and asking permission
- giving praise for each accomplishment

Nonverbally

- using nonverbal sounds like "Mmmm" to convey interest in what is being said
- being conscious of facial expressions and careful not to show negative feelings such as hostility, anger, disinterest or disgust
- looking at the patient's face when talking and using frequent eye contact (in some cultures, eye contact is considered disrespectful)
- avoiding quick movements that give the impression of being in a hurry

Behaviourally

- carrying out requests that have been made, such as phoning a patient's child and reporting back on the conversation
- seeing that members of the patient's family feel welcome
- ensuring the privacy of the patient's family when discussing personal matters
- getting an interpreter to help patients to communicate if they do not speak English
- adapting care so that the individual can maintain traditional religious and ethnic customs
- respecting the patient's modesty

Silently

- being there when the patient needs support, for example, during a painful procedure
- holding patient's hands, touching the arm or putting an arm around the shoulder

Many agencies have changed admission procedures to make them less impersonal. Pre-admission clinics make the procedure of admission more "people-oriented." The introduction of primary nursing on nursing units has also been helpful because it gives patients one person to whom they can relate throughout their stay in hospital—one person they feel really cares about them. Regardless of whether primary nursing is in operation or not, nurses can do a great deal to dispel the impression of agency impersonality and to minimize patients' feelings of depersonalization.

Nurses protect the self-esteem of the people they care for by conveying feelings of respect for the personhood of the individual. This is done in the same way other feelings are communicated. Some of the ways the nurse conveys to the individual or group respect for their personhood are listed in

Health-Restoring Strategies

STRATEGIES FOR POWERLESSNESS

The most pervasive problem related to low self-esteem is the feeling of powerlessness (helplessness/ hopelessness) it engenders. Strategies used to restore self-esteem so that people are able to meet their own needs, solve their own problems and mobilize resources so that they can take control of their lives are referred to as "empowering" strategies.

The overall goals of empowering strategies are twofold: (1) "...to transform internal feelings of powerlessness (hopelessness/helplessness); and (2) to initiate changes in the physical and social living conditions that create or reinforce inequalities in power" (Rappaport; Labonte. Both cited in RNABC, 1992, p. 9).

These goals imply that there needs to be a continuum of empowering strategies, beginning with the individual through personal empowerment, and including small group development, community organization, coalition advocacy and political action. This continuum of empowering strategies is shown in Figure 36.1.

Nurses work at the individual and group-development level and, increasingly, in community development; they work through their professional organizations, in coalition advocacy and in political action to improve physical and social conditions. You will learn more about working with groups and community development in more senior courses on community nursing, and more about coalition advocacy and political action in courses on issues in nursing. We will focus here on personal empowerment strategies. The following assumptions suggested by Gibson (1991) are pertinent to our discussion:

- individuals are primarily responsible for their own health
- the individual has the right and the capacity for self-determination
- individuals empower themselves, but nurses provide the resources that foster empowerment
- individuals' input into decisions must be valued, and their opinions must be the bottom line
- mutual respect must exist between the individual and the nurse
- trust is a necessary part of empowerment.

Some *personal empowerment strategies* are listed below.

- Provide people with the information they need to change their behaviour or their environment, for example, information about courses in assertiveness training; courses to upgrade skills; services that are available such as a

X	X	X	X	X
Personal Empowerment	**Small Group Development**	**Community Organization**	**Coalition Advocacy**	**Political Action**

PERSONAL EMPOWERMENT:	• Developmental casework • Enhancing personal perceptions of control and power
SMALL GROUP DEVELOPMENT:	• Improving social support • Promoting personal behaviour change • Providing support for lifestyle choices
COMMUNITY ORGANIZATION:	• Developing local actions on community-defined health issues • Critical community/professional dialogue • Raising conflict to the conscious level
COALITION ADVOCACY:	• Lobbying for healthier public policies • Achieving strategic consensus • Collaboration and conflict resolution
POLITICAL ACTION:	• Support for broad-based social movements • Creating vision of sustainable, preferred future • Enhancing participatory democracy

FIGURE 36.1 A continuum of empowering strategies

SOURCE: Registered Nurses Association of British Columbia (RNABC), 1992, p. 10.

rent ombudsperson, health services, shelters for battered wives; government grant programs such as New Horizons, which provides funds for senior citizen projects.

- Encourage participation in decisions regarding the person's own actions—to take a course, to go to the Family Services Bureau, and to make decisions regarding the small things in everyday life. For people in an inpatient facility, it means giving them the opportunity to make as many decisions on their own as possible, such as when they are going to take their bath, what they want to eat for breakfast, lunch and dinner, what they are going to wear for the day and what services they want to have.
- Help people to develop positive coping skills.
- Help people to derive power from other sources, such as prayer, or stress-reduction techniques; help people to maintain religious or cultural rituals; offer to call the patient's religious leader or leader in their ethnic community (Carpenito, 1997).
- Support and encourage existing positive coping skills.
- Understand patient's perspective.
- Work with what patients do well.
- Encourage the patient to participate in groups, such as self-help and support groups (Carpenito, 1997).
- Help people to form a group with other people in similar situations. Quarrington (1992) discusses starting a patient self-help group on a psychiatric unit and helping the patients to overcome feelings of powerlessness and low self-esteem by letting them have a say in their care and the services they receive, and by encouraging them to share successful coping strategies with each other.

We discussed in Chapter 11 numerous other examples of ways to help people form groups to tackle problems that they feel powerless to address on their own. Forming these groups is part of the nurse's role in community development, and is a role which is shared with other professionals in the field, such as social workers and health educators.

STRATEGIES FOR ANXIETY

In the course of daily practice, nurses meet many people who are anxious. Most people are at least a little nervous when they visit a health agency for the first time. Even if they are going for a routine checkup, there is always the nagging worry that something may be wrong. Anxiety almost invariably accompanies the person who is being admitted to a hospital or coming into the emergency department. When

into account the fact that the plan of care has to be individualized. No two people are alike in regard to the nature of anxieties, reactions to these, or the type of help needed to overcome them. The nurse also considers whether this patient needs the help of another member of the health team. There is, therefore, no easy set of rules for the nurse to follow. The assumptions about anxiety listed below can be used to guide your selection of strategies that may be helpful with a particular individual:

- it is easier to allay a known fear than to ease anxiety from an unknown source
- people generally feel less anxious when they know what is going to happen to them
- anxiety is lessened when people feel they have some control over their situation
- loneliness aggravates anxiety
- a feeling of depersonalization contributes to anxiety
- physical activity helps to relieve muscular tension
- anxiety can often be relieved by diversional activity.

The following nursing interventions are based on the assumptions listed above and might be considered in the care of specific individuals.

Identify the cause of the anxiety, if possible We have already discussed some of the ways the nurse can gather information to help identify the sources of a patient's potential or actual anxiety. The nurse always verifies with the patient that the interpretation of the source of the anxieties is consistent with the patient's perceptions. The nurse may think that the patient is very worried about the treatment when in actual fact the patient may be anxious about a family member who has not come in to visit.

Help the patient to explore the problem It is important to remember that talking with the patient can also be therapeutic. Talking gives the patient an opportunity to explore the causes of anxiety, to discuss them with someone and to work out solutions to some of the things that are worrisome.

Refer the individual to specialized counselling services Beginning nurses should not feel that they are skilled counsellors at this stage in their career. If you do not feel comfortable dealing with a patient's anxiety, or feel the patient needs more highly skilled counselling than you are able to provide, you should not hesitate to call in someone else. Nor should you feel guilty in doing so. The clinical instructor, or the charge nurse on the unit (case manager in home care), may be able to help the patient. If a clinical nurse specialist in psychiatric/mental health nursing is available, this person is often able to help patients with their anxiety more effectively than someone else. A psychiatric/mental health nurse may also be able to provide the beginning nurse with help in the approach to caring for the patient. Some patients need the counselling services of a psychologist or psychiatrist, and they should be referred

Providing information is important both in preventing and in allaying anxiety. If patients know what is going to be done during a laboratory test, they are usually less apprehensive about it. Similarly, the patient who has been told that a certain procedure may hurt a little is better able to face the pain. Teaching plans that identify patient information needs should form a part of every nursing care plan.

Encourage the person to take some control of the situation Enlisting patient cooperation and having the patient participate in care whenever possible helps to give them a feeling of control over the situation. The use of self-administration techniques for pain-relieving medications has been helpful in this regard. Giving patients a voice in the scheduling of their activities or in the way some interventions are carried out is one way of helping them to feel some control over events.

Promote social contacts People need the company of other people and a group with whom they can identify. We have mentioned the importance of social support in nurturing self-esteem. Family, friends and a group identity help to provide individuals with the security and support needed to overcome threats to self-concept. Many groups, such as churches, have visitor committees to visit the sick and people who are confined to their homes. Senior citizens' centres, in connection with community centres, help to fill the need for socialization and the provision of a group identity. Among inpatients, the nurse needs to be alert to those who have no visitors, to encourage family to visit, or if the patient has no family close by, to arrange for visits from the patient's church, lodge or other organization.

Show respect for the patient as an individual When patients feel that they have lost their identity, that they are just a health agency number or an interesting "case," their confidence in the care they are receiving diminishes. It is important to help patients to retain the feeling that they are respected.

Provide opportunities for exercise or relaxation techniques Exercise to a patient's limits of tolerance is a good way of relieving the muscular tension that accompanies anxiety. Relaxation exercises and techniques can also help. A physical therapist is often helpful for teaching people relaxation exercises or for suggesting other measures to reduce muscular tension.

STRATEGIES FOR DEPRESSION

The subject of depression will be treated in more detail in psychiatric nursing courses. The beginning student, however, should be alert to the possibility that depressed people may try to injure themselves, and they may attempt to commit suicide. Most of the time, someone who is contemplating suicide will signal their intentions. They may say, "I wish I

GERONTOLOGICAL

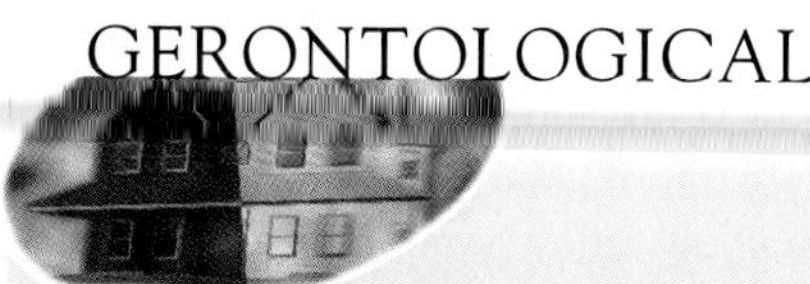

Medications that Can Cause Depression in the Elderly

Antihypertensives and cardiac medications
Hormones
Central nervous system depressants
Alcohol
Anti-anxiety agents
Benzodiazepines
Anti-psychotic
Antiulcer (histamine H2 antagonist)
Antiparkinsonian (dopamine agonist)
Antineoplastic (estrogen blocker)

SOURCE: Eliopoulos, 1997.

could do away with myself" or "I'd like to kill myself," and may even discuss ways of doing so. The nurse should always be watchful of any patient who seems to be getting more depressed. The nurse may notice that the physiological and behavioural manifestations are becoming more pronounced. It is important to remember that depressed patients are not always on a psychiatric unit in a hospital; they may be on a surgical or a medical unit or at home. The patient's physician should be alerted if the nurse suspects that the patient is becoming more depressed, so that psychiatric counselling and appropriate therapy can be instituted promptly. Often, mood-elevating medications are administered.

In selecting specific strategies to help depressed people, the nurse may find the following assumptions helpful:

- a person who is depressed will show changes in physiological functioning, in feeling state, in cognitive functioning and in behaviour
- prolonged or deep depression may cause general metabolic retardation, mental confusion and/or dullness
- emotions are influenced by physiological state
- depressed people usually have very low self-esteem
- depressed people may not want to live because they feel unworthy.

Nursing interventions for the depressed patient are directed towards three principal goals: preventing patients from injuring themselves or taking their own lives; supporting and maintaining the patient's basic physiological processes, such as nutrition and elimination; and helping the patient to overcome the depression.

Protect the patient from self-injury Constant vigilance is needed to protect severely depressed patients from injuring themselves or committing suicide. Patients who are seriously depressed are usually placed on a psychiatric nursing unit so that the specialized care they require is available. If they are on a general ward, often a private duty nurse or one staff nurse is assigned to care for the patient. The nurse who has a depressed individual among the regular patient load should be particularly careful to make sure that he or she takes all medications. There should be no opportunity for the person to collect a large number of sleeping pills or other medications. When visiting a patient in the home, the nurse should also make sure the patient who shows signs of depression is not collecting too many tranquilizers or other medications. Sharp instruments should not be accessible. The medication cart on the unit should be kept locked at all times, unless a nurse is actually in the process of dispensing medications. This is a good general rule: Nurses should be direct with patients about their concerns.

If the patient is known to be suicidal, all potential sources of self-injury, such as belts and shoe laces, are removed. There should also be a check on the patient at irregular but frequent intervals. Depressed patients who wake up in the early morning hours (when a person's body processes are at their lowest ebb) often need someone to talk to, and the nurse should take time to stop and chat for a few minutes. Occasionally, patients will need to be physically restrained to keep them from injuring themselves.

Maintain physiological processes Because depressed people are inactive, nutritional status may suffer. Depressed people often have no appetite and must be encouraged to eat. Appetite often improves in mildly depressed people if they have company during meals. Some community organizations have potluck suppers on a regular basis so that people who live by themselves do not have to eat dinner alone.

The nurse should be alert to the problem of constipation in depressed people because of the slowing down of gastrointestinal functioning and inactivity. These people need to be encouraged to take a sufficient amount of fluids. The slowing down of physiological functioning also causes a tendency for urine to be retained in the bladder and infections can result. Because depressed people tend to sit a lot, they may develop edema in the dependent limbs, or in the sacral area.

Help with hygiene and grooming Depressed people often need help with hygiene and grooming, since it requires too much effort for them to do it themselves. Often, assisting a person to improve their personal appearance will help to lift a mild depression. A new article of clothing may also stimulate an individual, helping with mild depression.

Promote socialization People who are lonely often get depressed. Everyone needs the stimulation of other people (or a pet) to stay alert and responsive. One of the things the nurse can do for lonely people is to encourage them to participate in group activities. Loneliness is a common companion to old age. Community centres have a wide

Examples of Evaluative Observations

- Does the person (or group) identify factors that he or she can control?
- Has the person verbalized acceptance of his or her appearance?
- Has the person demonstrated acceptance of his or her appearance, for example, by taking more care with grooming and dress, standing tall and presenting themselves better and eating better?
- Does the person describe strategies to promote effective socialization? Does the person demonstrate use of these strategies?
- Has the person identified and explored ways to update employable skills, e.g., obtained calendars or brochures about educational programs or sought the advice of an employment counsellor?

For powerlessness:

- Does the person have the information needed to make decisions about his or her care or situation?
- Does the person appear more confident in making decisions about his or her care, treatment and future?
- Does the person verbalize feelings of greater control of situations?

For anxiety:

- Is the person able to express his or her own anxiety and coping patterns?
- Have the physical and behavioural manifestations of anxiety lessened or disappeared? For example, is the person's facial expression more calm and relaxed? Is muscle tension reduced? Are speech and voice patterns more normal? Have distressing symptoms such as diarrhea, urinary frequency, or headache disappeared?
- Can the person describe techniques for stress reduction? Does the person use these techniques?
- Does the person state that he or she is feeling better?

For depression:

- Does the person state that he or she wants to live?
- Have the physical and behavioural manifestations of depression been lessened? For example, are movements faster? Is posture improved? Is the person more animated? Does the person sleep well at night? less in the daytime?
- Does the person socialize more with other people?
- Is the person eating well? Maintaining proper weight?

variety of activities for seniors and have become the drop-in centres for older people in many places. Many long-term care facilities employ recreational therapists who help stimulate residents' interests. There are also transportation aides, so that people who are not mobile can be taken by wheelchair to activities or special programs.

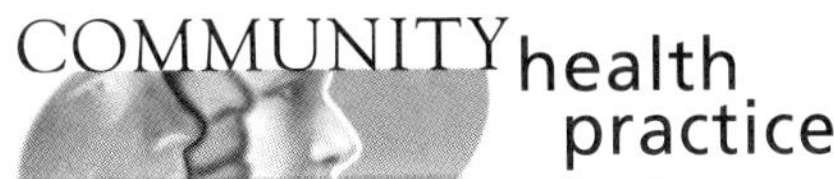

COMMUNITY health practice

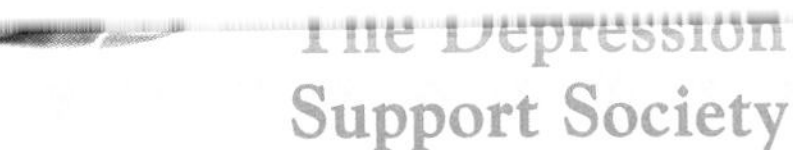

The Depression Support Society

The Depression Support Society (DSS) is a nonprofit organization that was founded in 1996. The DSS provides education and support for the entire family. Its approach is to assist the patient and family to:

- accept that the patient has a medical disorder
- identify symptoms
- examine changes to care-taking roles
- understand the current preventive measures to control symptoms
- distinguish between medication side effects and the medical disorder
- improve coping skills

Resources available include current journals, videos and books. All facilitators are well trained and have many years of experience. Services are available within the lower mainland of British Columbia.

In long-term care agencies, a resident's depression will often lift when a companion with shared interests can be found. It is good to discover patients' interests, and to try to match them with someone else who is interested in the same things.

Use nonverbal communication Unlike the anxious patient, the person who is depressed may not like to talk with the nurse—or with anyone—because talking really does not help. Still, the presence of the nurse, with a touch on the arm or an arm around the shoulder, often goes a long way towards making a depressed person feel that someone still cares.

Try music therapy Music is being used quite extensively now to assist in overcoming depression. Happy lively music will often lift spirits. Many people come out of depressed moods when they start to play a tune on a musical instrument.

However, it is important not to try to force severely depressed patients into activities to "cheer them up." Sitting beside the person and giving quiet companionship is often helpful in gradually drawing a response. Very often the patient needs to work through a problem, as in the case of a woman who has had a mastectomy and must adjust to her altered figure. Many people need the help of a psychiatric nursing specialist or a psychiatrist to assist them to overcome depression.

Encourage good nutrition and regular exercise One should not forget the vital role of good nutrition and regular exercise both in helping to prevent depression and in helping people overcome it. Some of the most enthusiastic marathon runners took up the sport to overcome the effects of depression. All report that they feel a "high" when they are reaching their maximum potential in running.

Vigorous exercise also helps to promote sleep and better quality rest. It encourages good nutrition and promotes a more regular daily schedule. There is much truth in the old adage, "healthy mind, healthy body."

Administer antidepressant medication Many people who experience periods of depression control their symptoms with antidepressant medications. It is important for the nurse to ensure that medications are taken as prescribed, monitor side effects and provide ongoing education. Education is a significant role for the nurse, as many antidepressants may take up to 10 days to show a therapeutic response.

Evaluating Self-Esteem Interventions

In evaluating the effectiveness of interventions for self-esteem, the nurse observes the patient for changes in affect, behavioural patterns, cognitive functioning and physiological status indicating progress towards resolution of the individual's specific problem(s). The nurse observes whether the outcome criteria established in planning care for patients have been met.

IN REVIEW

- Self-esteem is said to be the key to our behaviour, affecting virtually all aspects of our lives—our thinking, emotions, desires, values and goals.
- The determinants of self-esteem include the following:
  - fulfillment of basic physiological needs
  - freedom from pain and fear
  - a sense of belonging
  - the love and companionship of others
  - social support in:
    - home
    - school
    - workplace
    - community
    - cultural customs and mores
    - religion
    - having a purpose in life.
- The building of self-esteem is probably our most important developmental task. The successful accomplishment of other developmental tasks at each stage of the life cycle builds self-confidence and is important in fostering self-esteem.
- Lack of accomplishment in developmental tasks fosters:
  - feelings of worthlessness
  - inferiority
  - low self-esteem.
- People with low self-esteem:
  - feel anxious
  - feel unsure of themselves
  - are often unhappy
  - are afraid of failing
  - feel responsible for their own problems and feel guilty because of it
  - blame others for their failures.
- Three common problems related to lack of fulfillment of self-esteem needs are:
  - powerlessness (hopelessness/helplessness)
  - anxiety
  - depression.
- People experiencing powerlessness:
  - feel unable to control their own destiny
  - react with anger and hostility towards whatever is seen as the power controlling their lives
  - become resigned to the situation
  - feel anger and hostility, which may fade into apathy and depression.
- The unpleasant feeling of anxiety alerts people to a real or symbolic threat to themselves, their significant others or their way of life. Ranging from mild anxiety to overwhelming panic, it is manifested in changes in feeling tone (affect), physiological reactions, behavioural changes and changes in cognitive ability.
- Feelings expressed with anxiety include:
  - tension
  - uneasiness
  - a sense of dread or anger
  - hostility.
- Physiologic changes with anxiety may include:
  - increased blood pressure, pulse and respirations
  - pallor or flushing
  - cold skin
  - loss of appetite
  - increased frequency of voiding
  - muscular tension
  - headaches
  - perspiration
  - nausea and vomiting or diarrhea.
- Behavioural changes with anxiety include:
  - biting nails
  - drumming fingers
  - pacing

- restlessness and overactivity
- talking loudly or constantly
- [illegible]
- stammering or crying
- rapid movements
- inappropriate behaviour
- increased mental activity
- inability to rest.

■ Depression is a common problem among all segments of the population but is particularly prevalent in young and older adults, immigrants (especially refugees) and people in low socioeconomic groups.

■ Feelings expressed with depression include:
  - sadness
  - lack of enjoyment
  - low self-esteem
  - anger directed towards the self
  - feelings of hopelessness.

■ Physiological changes with depression include:
  - lack of appetite with resultant weight loss
  - slow movements
  - constipation
  - amenorrhea
  - lessened response to stimulation
  - lessened sex drive.

■ Behavioural changes with depression include:
  - stooped posture
  - slouching gait
  - lack of interest in clothes and grooming
  - withdrawal from social contacts
  - reluctance to talk
  - slow speech
  - difficulty finishing tasks.

■ Cognitive changes with depression include:
  - poor concentration
  - obsession with one topic
  - disturbed sleep patterns
  - inability to make decisions
  - use of drug or alcohol for temporary relief.

■ Other problems resulting from unfulfilled self-esteem needs include negative body image, social isolation and ineffective individual and family coping.

■ Assessment is ongoing, but starts with the nursing health history and physical examination. The nurse learns about:
  - personality
  - present stage of physical and psychological development
  - [illegible]
  - health status
  - immediate concerns.

■ Nursing diagnoses related to low self-esteem are usually written as specific problems related to causes, for example, *Anxiety related to pending surgery*.

■ Common nursing concerns for depression are:
  - powerlessness
  - self-care deficits
  - risk for self-harm
  - self-mutilation
  - suicide
  - social isolation.

■ The nurturance of self-esteem requires a multidisciplinary approach, and the nurse works in collaboration with people in many different disciplines in planning nursing care.

■ Nursing intervention for health promotion include:
  - counselling
  - teaching
  - working with groups
  - working with people in other sectors, for example, school teachers and employers
  - conveying respect for the personhood of the individual.

■ Personal empowering strategies nurses can use include:
  - providing people with information
  - encouraging them to participate in making decisions about their own actions
  - helping them develop positive coping skills
  - teaching them to derive power from sources such as prayer or stress-reduction techniques
  - helping them form and participate in groups with people in similar situations.

■ Nursing interventions for anxiety include:
  - identifying the cause of the anxiety where possible
  - helping the individual explore the problem
  - providing necessary information
  - encouraging the individual to take some control of the situation
  - showing respect for the person as an individual
  - promoting social contacts
  - providing opportunities for exercise and relaxation techniques
  - referring to specialized counselling services as needed.

- Nursing interventions for people who are depressed include:
  - protecting the patients from self-injury
  - maintaining physiological processes
  - helping with hygiene and grooming
  - encouraging good nutrition and regular exercise
  - promoting socialization
  - music therapy
  - using nonverbal communication to convey care.
- In evaluating self-esteem interventions, the nurse looks at changes in the patient's feeling tone, behaviour, cognitive ability and physiological status that indicate progress towards resolution of the problem(s); for example, the patient may be better able to take control of his or her situation, may have less anxiety or may be less depressed.

KEY TERMS

self p. 1217
self-concept p. 1217
body image p. 1217
personal identity p. 1217
self-esteem p. 1217
empowerment p. 1217
developmental crises p. 1219
powerlessness p. 1223
anxiety p. 1223
panic p. 1224
depression p. 1225
reactive (situational) depression p. 1225
agitated depression p. 1225
self-care p. 1230
mutual aid p. 1231

Critical Thinking Activities

Delcina Arias is a 38-year-old single mother of two boys, aged nine and 12. Recently divorced, she returned to teaching after a refresher course and is now in her first full-time position at a local elementary school as a grade 4 teacher. During the Easter vacation period, she noticed a small lump in her right breast. Her family doctor referred her to the cancer clinic where she underwent a number of diagnostic tests and examinations before being admitted to hospital for a mastectomy.

1. What threats does the impending surgery pose for Delcina's self-esteem?
2. How would you assess Delcina's self-esteem?
3. What emotional, physiological, behavioural or cognitive manifestations might you observe in Delcina that would indicate that she:
   a. was anxious about the surgery?
   b. depressed when told she had to have radiation therapy after the surgery?
   c. felt that she no longer had any control over her life?
4. What nursing diagnoses might be applicable in Delcina's care?
5. What nursing interventions might you use to promote and protect Delcina's self-esteem? to relieve her anxiety? to help her overcome depression if this occurs? to regain feelings of control over her situation?
6. How would you evaluate the effectiveness of your interventions?

References

BOYD, M.A., & NIHART, M.A. (1998). *Psychiatric nursing: Contemporary practice*. Philadelphia: Lippincott.

CARPENITO, L.J. (1997). *Nursing diagnosis: Application to clinical practice*. (7th ed.). Philadelphia: Lipincott.

CLARKE, H.F. (1997). Research in nursing and cultural diversity: Working with First Nations peoples. *Canadian Journal of Nursing Research, 29*(2), 11–25.

EBERSOLE, P. and HESS, P. (1998). *Toward healthy aging: Human needs and nursing response*. (5th ed.). St. Louis: Mosby.

ELIOPOULOS, C. (1997). *Gerontological nursing*. (4th ed.). Philadelphia: Lippincott.

EPP, J. (1986). *Achieving health for all: A framework for health promotion*. Ottawa: Minister of Supply & Services.

ERIKSON, E. (1963). *Childhood and society*. New York: Norton.

GIBSON, C.H. (1991). A concept analysis of empowerment. *Journal of Advanced Nursing, 16,* 354–361.

GILBERT, S. and OROK, B., (1993, Autumn). School leavers. *Canadian Social Trends, 30,* 2–7.

GOVERNMENT OF ONTARIO. (1992). *Ontario health survey 1990 highlights*. Toronto: Ontario Minister of Health.

GOVERNMENT OF ONTARIO. (1993). *Nurturing health*. Report of the Premier's Council on Health, Well-being and Social Justice (1987–1991). Toronto: Ontario Minister of Health.

HABER, J., KRAINOVICH-MILLER, B., McMAHON, A.L., & PRICE-HOSKINS, P. (1997). *Comprehensive psychiatric nursing*. (5th ed.). St. Louis: Mosby.

HABER, J., LEACH, McMAHON, A., PRICE-HOSKINS, P., & SIDELEAU, B.F. (1992). *Psychiatric nursing*. (4th ed.). St. Louis: Mosby.

HOLLOWAY, S. (1991). *Critical skills for communicating in conflict*. Vancouver: Justice Institute of British Columbia.

MAROTTOLI, R.A., MENDES de LEON, C.F., GLASS, T.A., WILLIAMS, C.S., COONEY, L.M. Jnr., BERKMAN, L.F., & TINETTE, M.E. (1997). Driving cessation and increased depressive symptoms: Prospective evidence from the New Haven EPESE. *Journal of American Geriatric Society, 45,* 202–206.

MASLOW, A. (1970). *Motivation and personality*. (2nd ed.). New York: Harper & Row.

MORALES-MANN, E.T. (1990). Child with depression. In A. Baumann, N.E. Johnston and Antai-Otong, D. (1990). *Decision in psychiatric and psychosocial nursing*. Toronto: B.C. Decker Inc., 58–59.

ODERKIRK, J. (1993, Autumn). Educational achievement. An international comparison. *Canadian Social Trends, 30,* 8–12.

QUARRINGTON, D. (1992). The power of self help. *The Canadian Nurse, 88*(2), 26–28.

REGISTERED NURSES ASSOCIATION OF BRITISH COLUMBIA (RNABC). (1992).

SIMMERMACHER, D. (1989). *Self-image modification.* (Revised ed.). Dunfield Beach, Florida: Health Communications Inc.

STAPLES, P., BARUTH, P., JEFFERIES, M., & WARDER, L. (1994). Empowering the angry patient. *The Canadian Nurse, 90*(4), 28–30.

STATISTICS CANADA. (1995). Prevalence of depression by age and sex. *National Population Health Survey.* Ottawa: Author.

STOLZMAN, J.D. (1988). The distribution and treatment of mental disorders by social class: A review of the research and theoretical implications. In B.S. Bolaria and H.D. Dickinson. (1988). *Sociology of health care in Canada.* Toronto: Harcourt Brace Jovanovich.

STUART, G.W., & LARAIA, M.T. (1998). *Stuart and Sundeen's principles and practice of psychiatric nursing.* (6th ed.). St. Louis: Mosby.

STUART, G.W. & SUNDEEN, S.J. (1995). *Principles and practice of psychiatric nursing.* St. Louis: Mosby.

TOFFLER, A. (1981). *The third wave.* New York: Bantam.

WATSON, J. (1988) *Nursing: Human science and human care.* New York: National League for Nursing.

WORLD HEALTH ORGANIZATION. (1980). *Health for all by the year 2000.* (Pan-American Health Organization). Washington, DC.: Regional Office for the Pan American Sanitary Bureau.

Additional Readings

BOHLANDER, J.R. (1995). Differentiation of self: An examination of the concept. *Issues in Mental Health Nursing 16*, 164–184.

BUFFUM, M.D., & BUFFAM, J.C. (1997). *The psychopharmacologic treatment of depression in elders, 18*(4), 144–149.

CLEELAND, E.A. & DAVIS, L.L. (1997). Depression in dementia with implications for home healthcare practice. *Home Healthcare Nurse, 15*(11), 780–787.

CONSTANTINO, R.E., SUTTON, L.B., & ROYAH, J. (1997). Assessing abuse in female suicide survivors. *Holistic Nursing Practice, 11*(2), 60–68.

ERMALINSKI, R., HANSON, P.G., LUBIN, B., THORNBY, J.I., & NANORMEK, P.A. (1997). Impact of a body-mind treatment component on alcoholic inpatients. *Journal of Psychosocial Nursing and Mental Health Services, 35*(7), 39–45.

HAGGERTY, B.M., & PATUSKY, K. (1995). Developing a measure of sense of belonging. *Nursing Research, 44*(1), 9–13.

HALL, P. (1996). Providing psychosocial support. *American Journal of Nursing, 96*(10), 16N–16P.

HASSELL, J.S. (1996). Improved management of depression through nursing model application and critical thinking. *Journal of the American Academy of Nurse Practitioners, 8*(4), 161–166.

growth. (4th ed.). Philadelphia: Lippincott-Raven.

LEIBERMAN, M., & FISHER, L. (1995). The impact of chronic illness on the health and well-being of family members. *The Gerontologist, 35*, 94–102.

LOVEJOY, N., & MATTEIS, M. (1997). Cognitive–behavioural interventions to manage depression in patients with cancer: Research and theoretical initiatives. *Cancer Nursing, 20*(3), 155–168.

MILLER, C.A. (1997). Drug consult. Keeping up with new developments in antidepressants. *Geriatric Nursing, 18*(4,) 180–181.

PARIS, B., MEIER, D., GOLDSTEIN, T., WEISS, M., & FEIN, E. (1995). Elder abuse and neglect: How to recognize the warning signs and intervene. *Geriatrics, 50*, 47–51.

PASACRETA, J.V. (1997). Depressive phenomena, physical symptom distress, and functional status among women with breast cancer. *Nursing Research, 46*(4), 214–221.

REICHMAN, W., & COYNE, A. (1995). Depressive symptoms in Alzheimer's disease and multi-infarct dementia. *Journal of Geriatric Psychiatry and Neurology, 8*, 96–99.

SIBBALD, B. (1997). Beating the odds: Helping problem gamblers. *The Canadian Nurse, 93*(5), 22–23.

TIEDEMAN, M.E. (1997). Anxiety responses in parents during and after the hospitalization of their 5–11-year-old children. *Journal of Pediatric Nursing, 12*(2), 110–119.

VALENTE, S.M., & SAUNDERS, J.M. (1997). Diagnosis and treatment of major depression among people with cancer. *Cancer Nursing, 20*(3), 168–178.

VALENTE, S.M., & SAUNDERS, J.M. (1997). Managing depression among people with HIV disease. *Journal of the Association of Nurses in AIDS Care, 8*(1), 61–67.

WADE, B. (1994). Depression in older people: A study. *Nursing Standard, 8*(40), 29–35.

WASSON D., & ANDERSON, M.A. Chemical dependency and adolescent self-esteem. *Clinical Nursing Research*, 4(34), 174–289.

WILLIAMS, S.A. (1997). Caring in patient-focused care: The relationship of patients' perception of holistic caring to their levels of anxiety. *Holistic Nursing Practice, 11*(3), 61–68.

WILLOUGHBY, C., KING, G., & POLATAJKI, G. (1996). A therapist's guide to children's self-esteem. *American Journal of Occupational Therapy, 50*(2), 124–132.

Chapter 37

Death, Loss and Grief

OUTLINE

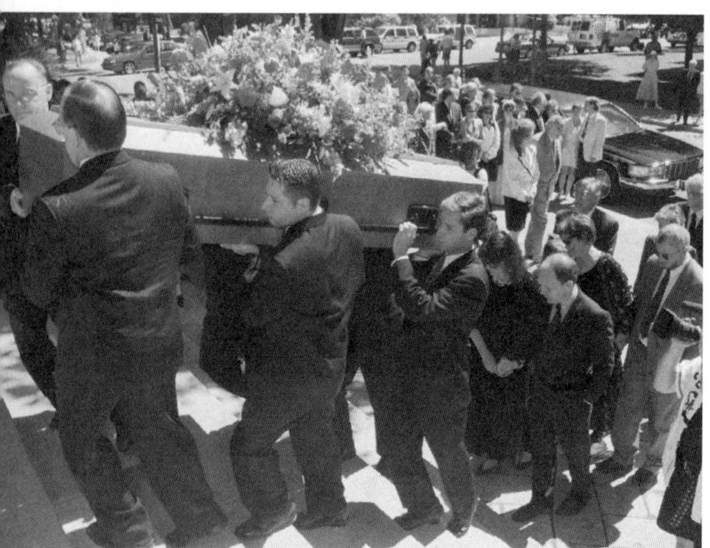

Central Questions

1. What are the meanings of loss, death, bereavement, grief and mourning?
2. What are some different types of loss?
3. What are some common manifestations of the grief response?
4. What are the most common causes of death?
5. What physical changes occur in the body as death approaches?
6. How do the Victoria Hospice Society's phases of grief and the dimensions of the fading-away model explain the psychological responses to death and dying?
7. How does a bereaved person work through the process of grieving?
8. What are the determinants of bereavement and grief?
9. How do the concept and understanding of death and grief vary throughout the life cycle?
10. How does the nurse assess the needs of dying patients and their families?
11. What are some common nursing diagnoses related to death, dying and grieving?
12. How does the nurse plan and implement appropriate interventions to assist dying patients and their families to meet their needs?
13. How does the nurse evaluate the effectiveness of care?

Introduction

Inextricably involved in nursing is the preservation of life

Our society celebrates health, life and youth. Death is a subject that generally is avoided; even when death is imminent, it is frequently denied. Yet death is not an uncommon occurrence on hospital wards, in nursing homes or among the sick in the community. By the very nature of their work, nurses and physicians encounter death more often than do most people.

Encountering death as part of their job does not make it easy for nurses to deal with. Regardless of whether death is sudden or follows a lengthy illness, the care of the terminally ill patient, and the comforting and consoling of the patient's family, presents one of the most demanding and stressful situations in nursing practice. Yet, caring for the dying can also be one of the more satisfying nursing responsibilities.

The difficulty that nurses and other health professionals have in caring for the dying stems in part from membership in the larger North American society which does not openly deal with death very well. As members of a society focussed on youth, productivity and activity, we are not prepared to accommodate into our lives what is seen as a process of deterioration, nor are we prepared to allow for expression of the intense responses that accompany death. When a person becomes terminally ill, others are reminded of their own mortality. Death is an unfamiliar experience that provokes many feelings—fear, futility, uncertainty, joy, grief, loneliness, hope, anger, a longing for death and a longing to avoid it. These feelings are as much present in nurses as they are in patients and families. To provide comprehensive and compassionate care to dying people and their families, however, is to learn to cope with strong emotions and to learn that death really is a part of life.

Coping with the prospect of one's own death and with the loss of loved ones through death is perhaps the greatest challenge humans must face in the course of living. Death brings about disruptive changes in individuals and families that threaten the ability to satisfy needs and to change and cope with the environment. How people are able to meet these challenges—to die peacefully and with dignity, or to restore emotional, social and spiritual health and harmony after the death of a loved one—depends on a number of influences. These may include the coping strategies that individuals and families have learned in dealing with past losses, as well as their support systems, cultural, religious and spiritual beliefs and age. We will discuss these determinants later in this chapter.

To cope with death in a healthy way, people need sensitive, caring support from health professionals. In this chapter we will describe basic concepts of loss, death, grief and grieving. This knowledge will enable nurses to:

- assess the needs of dying patients and their families
- provide comprehensive and compassionate care for
- promote healthy grieving in individuals and families.

Loss and Death

All of us have experienced loss at some time in our lives. Perhaps our first encounter with loss came when we were weaned from our mother's breast or from the bottle and taught how to drink milk from a cup. As we grew and moved through the developmental stages of life, we weathered other losses—our first day at kindergarten, taking the school bus by ourselves, graduating from high school or moving away from home to attend college or university. All these experiences meant leaving behind both a degree of dependence on our parents and the security of a familiar environment. Some of us may also have lost someone or something very significant, such as a husband, wife or partner through separation or divorce; a dear friend who has moved away; a job or a valuable piece of jewellery. Some of us may have lost a part of our body or its function from illness or trauma, or experienced the death of someone close to us. All these losses have one thing in common: the individual who loses something is separated from and deprived of the lost person, object, status or relationship (Corr, Nabe & Corr, 1994).

Loss refers to any life event in which one is deprived of something that is valued. This may include loss of external objects, developmental loss, loss of a part of the self, secondary losses, symbolic losses, loss of a significant other or impending loss of self through death (Shapiro, 1993). The experience of loss through death is called **bereavement** (Corr et al., 1994). The term *bereaved* is used as an adjective ("the bereaved family") or as a noun ("the bereaved") to refer to those who have experienced the loss of a loved one through death. The different types of losses are defined in Table 37.1.

Loss brings about a variety of feelings, from shock and disbelief, to resentment, sadness, despair and even relief. For example, we may feel very saddened when a close friend dies from cancer, but at the same time we may feel relief that this friend is no longer suffering. The degree of loss one feels depends on the magnitude of attachment to that which has been lost and on the availability of its replacement. For instance, the loss that might be felt when a perfect new car sustains its first scratch or dent may cause minor distress requiring minimal emotional adjustment and a trip to the automotive repair shop to re-establish a sense of well-being. On the other hand, the loss of something or someone very important and irreplaceable will cause profound distress and place heavy demands on adaptive resources and on the capacity for coping with adversity and change. Such losses might include the loss of a body part or function, a highly esteemed occupation or role in society, or a significant

TABLE [illegible] Types of losses

Type	*Definition*	*Example*
Loss of external objects	Loss of valued material things	Family residences and possessions are lost in a hurricane. A child's teddy bear wears to shreds.
Developmental loss	Maturational loss resulting from normal life transitions	Adolescents lose their childhood identity as they assume their own self-image. Elderly people lose their physical endurance as a result of aging.
Loss of a part of self	Loss of one's sense of identity, body image or physical functioning	A person is disfigured owing to burns sustained in a house fire. A patient loses a limb due to injury or illness. An employee loses self-esteem owing to job restructuring.
Secondary losses	Losses associated with other losses	Patients in hospital lose the comforts of home, their sense of autonomy and control. A family loses financial security when one parent loses a job. A person recuperating from a prolonged illness experiences financial loss.
Symbolic losses	Perceived losses associated with the psychological aspects of a physical loss	Women who lose a breast to cancer perceive a loss of sexual attractiveness and femininity. Men who develop sexual impotence feel "less than a man."
Loss of a significant other	Loss of significant other through death, separation or divorce	A family loses a child through a drowing accident. Children lose a parent through divorce. A beloved pet must be euthanized owing to illness or old age.
Impending loss of self	Personal losses experienced as one approaches death	A dying patient grieves the loss of relationships, status or roles. An elderly client broods over missed experiences and opportunities in life.

SOURCE: Shapiro, 1993.

other through separation or death. In addition, one's own impending death is a major loss that must be resolved (Kübler-Ross, 1969).

Although death is a biological process, it is accompanied by a multitude of social, emotional and spiritual experiences both for dying people and for their survivors. Death can have many meanings for the dying person. Some may view death as a punishment for past wrongdoings; others may see it as a loss of self and self-identity and missed future goals, opportunities, pleasures and relationships. For others, death may mean relief of prolonged suffering from a terminal illness or a reunion with loved ones in an afterlife. What death means for the survivors will depend upon the value of the lost person and on the ways in which they interpret that loss (Corr *et al.*, 1994). For instance, the death of a spouse may mean the end of sharing life experiences with a partner, loneliness and perhaps loss of economic and domestic security. For parents, the death of a child may mean never seeing the child grow to be an adult or enjoying the gratification of watching his or her accomplishments in life. Bereavement is painful because death is final (Corr *et al.*, 1994). No two individuals will cope with death in the same way because people are different. Each person will approach the experience of loss using available resources and coping strategies learned in dealing with other stressful events in life. Our goal as health professionals is to try to understand others' ways of coping with death and to support their coping abilities. We will discuss this aspect further on in the chapter.

Grief and Grieving

Grief refers to the total response to loss. When individu-

and painful state that involves strong emotions and affects how one thinks, feels, behaves and continues the functions of daily living. Grief is manifested in a number of ways, including the physical, psychological, behavioural, social and spiritual realms (Corr *et al.*, 1994). Examples of these manifestations are given in the accompanying box.

Mourning is associated with grief and grieving. **Mourning** refers to "the process of incorporating the experience of loss into our everyday lives" (DeSpelder & Strickland, 1992, p. 234). Also referred to as *grieving* or *grief work* (Lindeman, cited in Corr *et al.*, 1994), mourning denotes the long-term process of moving forward and working through the grief towards the resumption of a satisfying life. It involves an internal process in which individuals struggle with the grief response and an outward process in which they acknowledge the loss to others (Corr *et al.*, 1994). The outward display of loss is influenced by culture. Culture defines certain behaviours as socially appropriate for disclosing the fact that a person or family is mourning. For example, in some cultures, families who are in mourning often wear dark colours and abstain from social functions for a period of time after the death of a loved one. In others, such as the Hindu or Sikh religions, mourning attire is traditionally white.

Manifestations of the Grief P

Feelings
- Profound sadness, emptiness, loneliness, sorrow, helplessness, anger, numbness or relief.

Physical Sensations
- Hollowness in the stomach; dry mouth; tightness in the throat or chest; a frequent need for sighing; fatigue or muscle weakness.

Cognitions (Thoughts)
- Distress, confusion; events perceived as unreal; absentmindedness, difficulty concentrating; preoccupation with thoughts of the lost person or object; a sense of presence or hallucinations of the deceased person or object.

Behaviours
- Sleep pattern disturbances; loss of appetite; general restlessness or hyperactivity; searching for the deceased, talking incessantly about the deceased or visiting places and cherishing objects or pictures reminiscent of the deceased person.

Social Dimension
- Difficulties in interpersonal relationships; problems in functioning at home and at work.

Spiritual Dimension
- Search for a sense of meaning or recognition that one's value framework is inadequate to cope with this particular loss.

SOURCES: Worden, 1991; DeSpelder & Strickland, 1992; Corr, *et al.*, 1994.

Death and Dying

Causes of Death

When people consider death, a question often asked is "What did the patient actually die from?" When death is not sudden (as from a myocardial infarction), its actual cause is most often cancer-related, since cancer is the second leading cause of death, next to cardiovascular problems. The most common causes of death in advanced cancer are infection, organ failure, infarction and hemorrhage.

Infection results in death in almost half of terminal cancer patients. There are various types and locations of infections:

- septicemia and/or septic shock
- major visceral infection including pneumonia, peritonitis and pyelonephritis
- gram-negative bacteria, including *Escherichia coli*, *Klebsiella* and *Pseudomonas aeruginosa.*

Organ failure is due to the consequence of tumour invasion, except for the heart. Failure leading to death occurs more often in some organs. In decreasing frequency, organ failure occurs in the lungs, heart, liver, central nervous system and kidneys.

Death attributable to infarction in cancer patients is uncommon. Pulmonary infarction is more frequent than myocardial infarction. Pulmonary emboli derive in equal frequency from distal venous thrombosis and tumour cell emboli.

Death directly related to persistent or massive bleeding is rare. In descending order, hemorrhage is more common in the gastrointestinal system, the brain, the cardiovascular system and the lungs. The bleeding may be related to direct tumour invasion and erosion, thrombocytopenia or coagulopathy.

Physical Changes at the End of Life

Unless death occurs suddenly, there is usually a progressive failure of the body's homeostatic mechanisms as the individual becomes weaker. Changes are noted in every major body system. Table 37.2 gives a summary of the changes in body systems as death approaches.

The Psychological Response to Dying

No two people react to dying or death in exactly the same way. Yet, most people experience characteristic responses as

TABLE 37.2 Physical changes approaching death

System	*Areas to Discuss*	*Outcome*
Respiratory	Breathing patterns	Will decrease to death
	Respiratory congestion	Will be relieved if death occurs
	Hemoptysis	Very rare
Neurological	Level of consciousness	Will decrease to death
	Predeath restlessness	Treat if a problem
	Twitching	Treat if moderate
	Convulsions	Rare unless prior history
Cardiovascular	Blood pressure	Will fall
	Heart rate	Often rapid and weak
	Heart failure	Part of dying process
	Pulmonary edema	Uncommon; treat if occurs
	Arrhythmias	Part of dying process
Integumentary	Temperature	Skin often cool; may be febrile
	Colour	Often pale, blue, blotchy
	Skin breakdown	Minor at end is common and acceptable
Excretory	Rectal incontinence	May occur
	Bladder incontinence	Common
Gastrointestinal	Food	Intake will become zero
	Fluid	Intake will become zero
	Medications	
	• which to keep	Analgesics, antiemetics
	• which to stop	
	• which routes	
	Mouth care	Important
Prognosis	How long	
	When to call family	

SOURCE: Victoria Hospice Society, 1993.

they face significant losses, such as the loss of physical ability, the loss of a loved one or the loss of one's own life from a terminal illness. Both the patient and the family experience grief. The concept and theories of grief are tools for the nurse to use in anticipating the needs of patients and families and in planning interventions to help them understand and cope with grief.

PHASES OF COPING WITH DYING

Individuals

Weisman (cited in Gonda & Ruark, 1984) describes the common reactions during the process of dying as phases that are connected to the course of terminal illness. The phases are existential plight, mitigation and accommodation, decline and deterioration, and preterminality and terminality. The phases tend to occur in a particular order; however, they may persist or recur throughout illness and dying.

The first phase, *existential plight*, refers to the initial shock people experience when faced with the irrefutable evidence of their own vulnerability and mortality. During this phase patients and families may exhibit numbness, shock and bewilderment. Weisman's second phase, *mitigation and accommodation*, often follows initial treatment of the disease. During this time, patients and families focus on achieving a balance among their new roles as potentially dying patients, their old identities and their related coping capacities. In this process, the acute threat of death is allayed or mitigated. An accommodation is made between the reality of the prognosis and the customary requirements for daily living. For example, a patient with ovarian cancer may state, "I know I have cancer. I will get sicker in time. But for now, I will carry on life as usual."

The third phase of coping with dying is *decline and deterioration*. This phase occurs when the patient's disease advances, when he or she has minimal energy for daily functions and when treatment brings shorter periods of freedom from symptoms. This period of a terminal illness may be the most difficult for patients and families. The signs of advancing illness are unavoidable, and the prospect of death becomes real. While patients may continue the struggle to maintain their functioning, the ability to maintain hope and a positive attitude may begin to fade. The support of [illegible] omy and control of their life.

The fourth of Weisman's phases is *preterminality and terminality*. In this phase, response to treatment is minimal and the focus shifts to palliative care of symptoms and management of discomfort. Both the patient and family may come to the realization that they have limited time together. Thus, they may alter their goals to much narrower outcomes. For example, the goal might be living to see the birth of a grandchild, the graduation of a son or daughter, or the marriage of a favourite niece (Gonda & Ruark, 1984).

Families

The entire family unit is affected when one of its members is terminally ill. Anything that affects one member affects the family system, just as anything that affects the family unit affects each individual member. Therefore, to provide optimal care in palliative situations, nursing actions must focus not just on the patients, but on the family as well. Findings from one nursing research study offer some insight into understanding the family's experience. Based on interviews with dying patients, their spouses and adult children, the researchers described the transition of "fading away" (Davies, Chekryn-Reimer, Brown & Martens, 1995). The following theoretical scheme serves as a foundation for nursing approaches for helping families engaged in the transition of fading away (Chekryn-Reimer, Davies & Martens, 1991).

Even though families may have been told about the patient's poor prognosis, they describe a moment when they "suddenly" realize that the patient's death is inevitable. Unrecoverable weakness, inability to get around, loss of independence in personal care and loss of mental clarity are visible signs of the patient's demise. Though difficult, the acknowledgment that the patient will not recover enables the patient and other family members to face the challenges that lie ahead.

The transition of fading away incorporates several components that are not discrete entities, nor do they occur in sequence. They are interrelated and intertwined. *Redefining* is the central component that influences how families adjust to the change in the patient's status. Through redefining, patients and family members identify and acknowledge the losses they have incurred, are incurring and are anticipating. *Dealing with burden* is the second component. Patients confront the possibility of being a burden to others, and family members grapple with being burdened by the extra responsibilities inherent in caring for a dying loved one.

The central struggle for all family members rests in the paradox of living and dying at the same time. The patient's increased dependency requires many changes in roles and responsibilities, socializing patterns, values and health status. Family members seek answers that help them come to terms with their situation through a search for meaning. [illegible] is a common way of finding meaning. The search for meaning appears to form a bridge between the struggle and a new perspective. When people can find some meaning and can put the situation into perspective, they experience less turmoil. They see more clearly the need to live day to day and to make the most of the time they have left. They are able to engage in preparing for death by making concrete plans for the practical aspects of dying.

How patients and family members face the transition of fading away is related to their own styles of coping and their past experience. In particular, experience with loss and death within the family plays an influential role in how families face the current transition.

PHASES OF COPING WITH DYING AND GRIEF

Kübler-Ross's (1969) description of coping with dying and grief is considered pioneering work in the field of thanatology (the study of death and dying). After considerable experience in counselling terminally ill patients, Kübler-Ross developed a theoretical model consisting of five stages in the process of death and dying. The stages include denial, anger, bargaining, depression and acceptance. According to Kübler-Ross, these stages are defence mechanisms that "will last for different periods of time and will replace each other or exist at times side by side" (1969, p. 138). These stages do not necessarily proceed in an orderly fashion. They may occur in varying order, and any one stage may recur a number of times during the course of a terminal illness. Further, any one of the stages may be totally absent in some individuals.

Since Kübler-Ross's research, health professionals have come to see grief as a series of phases rather than stages. A phase-oriented approach depicts grief as a process rather than a sequential series of steps. One phase blends into another, and there is movement back and forth between phases.

Individual reactions to grief vary and cover a wide range of behaviours and responses. Some responses may be perceived by others as peculiar, though the responses may be normal within the context of the individual's grief. For example, after her mother's death, Jane did not want to be around people who were happy and having fun. She was irritated by their happiness, and either avoided them or interacted angrily. Some people might criticize Jane's behaviour as antisocial or rude, but her response is one normal manifestation of grief.

In another example, Mr. Zeller's wife wanted to sit with her husband's body after his death on an acute care hospital ward. Some nurses considered this behaviour abnormal, and wanted to encourage Mrs. Zeller to leave the room. Other nurses understood that some families need this time to say their final good-byes. Similarly, a mother in a maternity ward whose baby was stillborn asked that her other children come to see and hold their deceased sibling. Some people might perceive this request as morbid. However, such behaviour helps the family to say good-bye and is conducive to the children's learning about death.

The Victoria Hospice Society (1993) describes grief as a healthy, normal process in response to loss. Its model, derived from the work of Rando (1984) and Worden (1991), is based on the idea that grief is work and, as such, requires time and energy. Knowing this can be empowering for some people. By acknowledging the process of grief, nurses can help people perceive their experience as constructive personal growth, rather than hopelessness or harmful self-indulgence. The Victoria Hospice Society model describes three phases of grief: the occurrence of death, confronting the pain and re-establishing connections. These phases are outlined, and the tasks associated with each phase are identified, in Tables 37.3, 37.4 and 37.5.

Bereavement and Grieving

Bereaved people grieve the loss of a loved one in much the same manner as those anticipating their own death. The process includes periods of shock, disbelief and somatic distress; feelings of guilt, anger and hostility; disruption in the daily functions of living; preoccupation with thoughts of the deceased; and finally, working through to a healthy

TABLE 37.3 Phase I—when a death occurs

Griever Responses	Nurse Contacts
Immediately following a death, there is a sense of shock, numbness and disbelief that can last minutes or weeks. The bereaved may feel panicked and overwhelmed, and may experience strong physical reactions. When there has been a lengthy illness, grievers may experience a sense of relief for the person who died and for themselves now that the stresses of caregiving are over. This period allows individuals to take in information at a slower rate and to prepare for the adjustments that lie ahead.	The nurse will have contact with a griever at the time of death, when attending the funeral or when checking in with the family to acknowledge the death, offer condolences or provide follow-up bereavement support.
Healthy Responses of Grief	**What Helps**
Social • Withdrawal from others • Dependence on others • Fear of being alone	**Social** • Establish a relationship; be comfortable and present • Make sure support is available
Physical • Palpitations • Shortness of breath, crying • Diarrhea, constipation, vomiting • Physical symptoms of shock • Change in appetite and sleep patterns	**Physical** • Acknowledge griever's physical reactions and respond in practical ways, e.g., if person is having trouble eating, suggest some high-calorie/high-protein snacks
Emotional • Numb, empty, flat expression • Indifference to daily activities • Withdrawal or explosive emotions • Need to review death	**Emotional** • Listen; acknowledge and encourage repeated review of the loss • Allow expression of emotions
Cognitive • Confusion, sense of unreality • Poor concentration, forgetfulness, daydreaming • Denial, disbelief • Constant thoughts about the deceased	**Cognitive** • Accept denial without supporting false hopes • Offer practical suggestions for enhancing organization or memory, e.g., making lists of tasks to do
Spiritual • Blaming God • Lack of meaning or direction • Wanting to die/to join the dead person	**Spiritual** • Begin to understand what this loss means to the bereaved, e.g., possible difficulties, other losses • Acknowledge person's feelings

SOURCE: Victoria Hospice Society, 1993, p. 477.

TABLE 37.4 Phase II—confronting the pain

[illegible] Responses	Nurse Contacts
As the numbness wears off, the bereaved will begin to feel the emotional pain of grieving. The intensity of feelings may surprise and frighten them, but the pain is healthy and can be affected by the quality of support, other losses, preparation for the death, the nature of the lost relationship and general approach to life.	The nurse may schedule checkups with grievers who are at risk for health problems or who are experiencing overwhelming emotional reactions, trouble with eating or sleeping or panic attacks. A family member may consult the nurse about a griever when the support network is at the end of its patience. Some grievers attend bereavement follow-up programs; alternatively, some return to the place where the death occurred or seek to talk with the nurse or other health professional who cared for their loved one.
Healthy Responses of Grief	**What Helps**
Social • Continued withdrawal, lack of interest • Need for company but inability to ask • Rushing into new relationships • Self-consciousness	**Social** • Help bereaved identify how loss affects them, e.g., changes, self-esteem, finances • Assess person's support system and consider whether a support group would be beneficial
Physical • Tight chest, shortness of breath, sharp pangs • Diarrhea, constipation • Restlessness, aimless activity, gnawing emptiness • Nightmares, vivid dreams, hallucinations • Symptoms of illness	**Physical** • Acknowledge bereaved's physical reactions and respond in practical ways • Encourage people to remember that these physical reactions are normal, healthy responses to grief
Emotional • Acute, conflicting, extreme feelings • Anger, sadness, guilt, depression • Feelings of loss, overwhelmed, general anxiety • Unrealistic fears about others or self	**Emotional** • Listen; acknowledge and be comfortable with expressions of feelings and pain • Refer particular concerns to a counsellor
Cognitive • Forgetfulness, daydreaming, confusion • Continuing denial • Inability to concentrate or understand • Sense of going crazy, losing touch with reality	**Cognitive** • Give information about grief • Continue to normalize reactions • Encourage personal timetable for grief
Spiritual • Continued blaming • Lack of meaning or purpose in life • Attempts to contact the dead person	**Spiritual** • Help people find ways to maintain positive connections with the deceased, e.g., compiling a memory book, developing rituals around anniversaries

SOURCE: Victoria Hospice Society, 1993, p. 478.

resolution and an integration of the loss into life. The desired outcomes of grieving are to remember the loved one without major emotional pain and to preserve the capacity to love. Successful achievement of these outcomes requires that bereaved individuals face the pain by recognizing that what is happening is a normal part of life and by acknowledging and expressing the full range of feelings associated with grief (Martocchio, 1985).

Martocchio (1985) identified four elements in grieving: breaking the emotional bond to the deceased, readjusting to an altered environment, developing new or renewed relationships, and learning to live comfortably with memories of the deceased. In breaking the emotional bond to the deceased, the survivor must work through unfinished business. "The content of unfinished business, how it is handled, and how the survivor is affected by it all have an impact on the experience of grief" (DeSpelder & Strickland, 1992, p. 255). An unresolved conflict, words that were unspoken or deathbed promises, for example, constitute unfinished business that must be resolved before normal grieving can continue. Suffering is heightened when survivors feel unable to resolve conflicts left by unfinished business. Such individuals may need the help of health professionals to work through these aspects. "Perhaps the key to

TABLE [illegible] Phase III—Re-establishing connections

Griever Responses	Nurse Contacts
Over time, the bereaved will have increased energy and desire to reconnect with the world.	At this time the nurse may be consulted for concerns that are not directly grief-related. It remains important to ask the bereaved about their grief. Some people may come with concerns about a new relationship. Nurses who counsel clients in bereavement may have continued contact with grievers. Others may encounter grieving persons in other realms of practice.
Healthy Responses of Grief	**What Helps**
Social • More interest in others' daily affairs • Ability to reach out • Energy for social relationships • Renewed desire for independence	**Social** • Give gentle "push" as appropriate • Encourage new social connections • Refer to community resources
Physical • Decrease in dreams and hallucinations • Decrease in physical symptoms • Return of normal appetite • Gut-wrenching emptiness comes and goes • More settled sleep	**Physical** • Acknowledge that continuing physical responses are normal and may be long-lasting • Be alert to ongoing symptoms that may indicate medical conditions
Emotional • More settled, less extreme emotions • Feeling of coming "out of the fog" • More peace and happiness • Some guilt about how life goes on	**Emotional** • Review person's grief process • Acknowledge strengths and abilities • Listen, knowing that the grieving person's need to tell the story may continue
Cognitive • Fewer thoughts of being crazy • Increased perspective about death • Ability to remember with less pain • Improved concentration	**Cognitive** • Encourage the person to take on responsibilities, make choices, learn skills • Remind people that grief reactions will surface with major transitions
Spiritual • Reconnection with religious beliefs • New direction; sense that life has meaning • Acceptance that death is part of life	**Spiritual** • Ensure that the person is not moving into this phase prematurely • Suggest that the spiritual journey is often long and time-consuming and may be an ongoing process

SOURCE: Victoria Hospice Society, 1993, p. 479.

unfinished business is forgiveness; accepting the situation as it is" (DeSpelder & Strickland, 1992, p. 256). Breaking bonds with the deceased also includes establishing a new or renewed identity. This includes learning new skills and re-establishing roles. For example, a widow who has been staying at home with young children may have to re-enter the workforce, take on the role of single parent and manage the household and family on her own. Readjustment to an altered environment means learning to live without the presence of the loved one and becoming comfortable with symbols of the deceased in everyday life. For example, an elderly widow now eats and sleeps alone and finds ways to replace the time and activities shared with her husband. She may take a trip with a friend and develop new interests to fill the void in her life.

In developing new or renewed relationships, the survivor re-enters social life and invests emotional energy in other people. Sometimes this takes the form of joining mutual-aid support groups and helping others who are experiencing crises or losses in life. This element of grieving may also include the renewal of the spiritual dimension in the survivor's life and the integration of the loss into his or her religious beliefs.

The last element, learning to live comfortably with memories of the deceased, requires that the survivor say good-bye to his or her loved one. The survivor achieves a level of resolution in which he or she can treasure memories of the deceased with a sense of peace and personal equilibrium. The process of grief is highly variable among indi

works to integrate the loss and re-establish a "normal" life. Time is also variable. It often takes two to five years for most people to work through grief and to feel fully integrated into a new and satisfying life.

Grief work may not always be successful. Sometimes grief is complicated with unfinished business, personality variables or ineffective coping abilities. Grief may become prolonged or chronic, in which case the survivors experience a sense of hopelessness and resist moving forward. Anger, self-blame and depression may be intensified. Grief can also be delayed. In delayed grief, survivors refuse to acknowledge grief and carry on with life as though nothing has happened. While people may appear to be doing well on the surface, they do so at great cost to themselves. Some people may never begin the normal process of grieving and may eventually require professional intervention (Martocchio, 1985).

Attig (1995) has criticized the limitations of much of the literature on grief and bereavement. He suggests that standard stage–phase and medical models of bereavement are based on the belief that grieving is experienced passively. Common to nearly all standard concepts is the view of grieving as yet another event that happens to bereaved persons, a process into which they are thrust against their will, that they undergo or endure and that they must somehow survive.

In contrast, Attig (1995) distinguishes between the specific emotion of grief and the far more complex coping process that is grieving. The emotion, says Attig, renders bereaved individuals passive in the face of their losses. The choicelessness of death and bereavement prompts feelings that the work is out of control and that survivors are powerless to influence major events in their lives. Heightened anxiety, depression and immobilization ensue. The grieving process, on the other hand, presents challenges and opportunities: it requires that energy be invested, tasks undertaken and choices made. As such, grieving is an active process that involves relearning one's physical and social worlds, one's relationship to oneself and to the deceased. This position acknowledges the innate strengths and resilient nature of grieving persons. It also recognizes people's abilities to make sound decisions about matters of importance to them, even in the face of adversity and grief. Respecting others when they grieve involves respecting individual ways of flourishing and individual vulnerabilities.

Recent work in the field has challenged another commonly held assumption about grief: that the goal is to break emotional ties with the one who has died. Instead of assisting grieving individuals to become emotionally detached from their loved ones, health professionals now believe that it is important to help grieving persons find ways of maintaining connections to their loved ones. Relationships do not die with the death of a person; they are changed, and are kept alive in memories, rituals, dreams, thoughts and ongoing influences (Attig, 1995; Klass, Silverman & Nickman, 1996).

Determinants of Bereavement and Grief

Several factors can influence how people experience loss and determine the ability to grieve and the capacity to cope. Principal among these are:

1. the degree of prior attachment to the deceased
2. the type of death
3. the age of the deceased
4. the personality and coping strategies of the bereaved individual
5. the social support upon which the bereaved individual is able to draw.

Knowledge of these factors will help the nurse understand the nature of grief and facilitate the assessment of needs, strengths and coping abilities of bereaved persons and families.

PRIOR ATTACHMENT TO THE DEAD PERSON Bereavement and grief are greatly influenced by the prior attachment to (or the perceived value of the relationship with) the deceased person. How important was the deceased person in the survivor's life? How will the survivor's life change because of the loss? Generally speaking, feelings of loss and grief are more intense when the deceased and the survivor shared a strong relationship and when the death causes significant changes in the survivor's life. Thus, the loss of a spouse, partner, parent, child or close friend or relative has a far greater impact on the survivor than the loss of an acquaintance or co-worker. The quality of the relationship may also affect bereavement and grief. For example, a woman who was ambivalent about her relationship with an abusive husband may not find his death to be so devastating; she may even inwardly feel glad that he is gone. However, this very ambivalence may bring about feelings of guilt, which will affect her grieving and coping capacity.

TYPE OF DEATH The way in which death takes place, whether expected or unexpected, affects one's bereavement and grief. Sudden, unexpected, traumatic deaths—for example, accidental death, homicide or suicide—are overwhelming and very difficult to cope with. Furthermore, suicide is accompanied by guilt, self-reproach and blame on the part of the survivor. "Why didn't I see it coming?" "If I had done something better, this would not have happened!" As well, survivors may see suicide as a personal affront or "final insult" and consequently "direct strong feelings of anger and blame toward the person who committed suicide" (DeSpelder & Strickland, 1992, p. 252). Such feelings compound grief and grieving.

Knowledge of an impending death as a result of a terminal illness is believed to alter bereavement and the experience of grief. The "response to prior knowledge of an impending death, with the result that the survivor has time to contemplate its effect before it actually occurs" is called **anticipatory grief** (DeSpelder & Strickland, 1992, p. 251). Some believe that anticipatory grief facilitates mourning by lessening the intensity of feelings following the actual loss. However, anticipatory grief does not significantly diminish the grief experienced when the loss becomes an objective fact (DeSpelder & Strickland, 1992). Nevertheless, knowledge of an impending death does temper the element of shock that accompanies the news that a loved one has died.

AGE OF THE DECEASED Humans hold an intrinsic belief that people should live to an old age and enjoy a multitude of successes and opportunities before they die. Therefore, premature death, whether sudden or expected, is among the most difficult to cope with. The death of a child causes the most profound and intense grief in survivors (Rando, 1986). Corr *et al.* (1994) cite Sanders, saying that research has shown that "adult bereavement is usually impacted most significantly by the death of a child, a spouse, and a parent—in that order" (p. 302). In addition, they quote a familiar saying that "the death of my parent is the death of my past; the death of my spouse is the death of my present; the death of my child is the death of my future" (Corr *et al.*, 1994, p. 302).

PERSONALITY AND COPING STRATEGIES We noted earlier that people cope with bereavement using strengths and skills they have acquired in dealing with past losses or crises in their lives. "Developing new and more effective coping skills requires more time and energy than are usually available in the immediate aftermath of a death or other significant loss" (Corr *et al.*, 1994, p. 174). Personality influences how a person relates to life events in general. A person with a healthy personality and a positive self-concept is likely to grieve in a more effective manner than someone with a dependent and emotionally immature personality (DeSpelder & Strickland, 1992).

SOCIAL SUPPORT Social support is a crucial determinant in the ability to grieve and to cope with death. In the period immediately after the death of a loved one, survivors experience profound feelings of grief and isolation. They devote all energy to the loss, and have little left to reach out to others or even feed and care for themselves. People cannot cope successfully with the challenges of mourning if they do not obtain adequate nutrition, hydration, rest and exercise (Corr *et al.*, 1994). The presence of caring people is paramount during this time. Having someone present who can give emotional support and ensure that the bereaved person eats, drinks and gets some rest and exercise is essential for effective coping. In many communities and societies, relatives, friends and neighbours function in this capacity. Similarly, social support is necessary as bereaved individuals progress through the grieving process. This may take the form of continued support from a close friend or relative, a health professional or a community mutual-aid group.

Death and Grief Throughout the Life Cycle

A person's concept and understanding of death develop maturationally in accordance with cognitive and emotional readiness and past experiences with death. As with other developmental processes, children who have had "firsthand encounters with death may arrive at an understanding of death beyond that which is characteristic of children of the same age group" (DeSpelder & Strickland, 1992, p. 90). However, there are certain characteristic responses to and levels of understanding of death at different ages and developmental stages.

CHILDREN BELOW THE AGE OF FIVE Generally, children below the age of five see death as a reversible state or a temporary departure; the deceased are still somewhere eating, sleeping and doing the things they usually do. This is evident in questions and statements such as: "Will Grandpa come back for Christmas?" "Who will cook for Grandpa in heaven?" "Can we take some birthday cake to Grandpa in his grave?" Although children under the age of five may use the word "death," they do not fully understand its meaning and have difficulty understanding abstract explanations of it. Because children at this age think in concrete terms, telling a four-year-old that his mother is in heaven and at the same time buried in her grave will cause confusion. "How can Mom be up in heaven when she is in a grave?" "Can we go to heaven to see Mom?" Because young children lack understanding of the finality of death, they may not show severe emotional response when told of someone's death. For example, they may want to go out and play shortly after hearing of a loved one's death and then come back later and ask when that person is coming back (Dyregrov, 1991).

CHILDREN AGED FIVE TO NINE Children between the ages of five and nine develop the understanding of death as a finality. They accept death as irreversible; however, they resist thinking that death is a possibility for themselves. They personify death as an external force—a "death man" or bogeyman who takes people away. In this way, children view death as avoidable and not inevitable. They believe that "those whom the external force catches, do die; those who escape or get away from the clutches of that force do not die" (Corr *et al.*, 1994, p. 244). Children in this age group are still concrete in their thinking. Therefore, they need concrete expressions such as rituals, pictures and tombstones to support them in their grief work. In addition, because children in this age span are less self-focussed, they are able to comprehend the perspective of others' loss and [illegible] towards others who are grieving a loss (Dyregrov, 1991).

CHILDREN AGED 10 THROUGH ADOLESCENCE After the age of nine, children recognize death as universal, inevitable and no longer avoidable. It is seen as something that "can happen to me" even though this thought is kept at a distance. Adolescents fear lingering death and view death in philosophical or religious terms (Murray & Zentner, 1997). Like all human beings, adolescents respond to death by grieving. However, their mourning processes may not correspond to those of adults; rather, the processes may reflect characteristics of their developmental stage (Corr et al., 1994). Adolescents may not outwardly display grief for a loved one because they may fear a loss of emotional control and worry how others will perceive them. Instead, they will often occupy themselves with usual activities, for example, playing games, listening to music, studying or playing a musical instrument. At the same time, they will manifest distress in behaviours such as withdrawal, disturbances in eating and sleeping, fatigue or ambivalence in other relationships (Murray & Zentner, 1997; Corr *et al.*, 1994).

ADULTS Adult attitudes, understandings and expressions of death and grief are influenced by personal, cultural and religious beliefs. These aspects differ among individuals and, furthermore, change within individuals over the course of a lifetime. In a study on attitudes towards death across the life span, Gesser, Wong and Reker (1988) found that fear of death and dying was relatively high among young adults; it peaked during the middle years and fell to the lowest level among the elderly. Corr *et al.* (1994) maintain that the worries or concerns of young adults about death are likely in relation to the deaths of others, perhaps grandparents or parents. As they encounter the illness and deaths of others (peers, spouses or parents, for example) and learn from life's experiences, people in the middle years develop a new sense of mortality and the realization that they, too, will die someday. The developmental tasks of older adults (Erikson's *integrity versus despair*) relate directly to death and dying because they denote the end of our given course of life. As a developmental task, death "can be viewed as a goal and as fulfillment" (Murray & Zentner, 1997, p. 776). People who have lived happy, rich and productive lives and have achieved the developmental task of ego identity are able to accept the realization that life is limited and that the self will cease to be. They begin preparing for this eventuality, physically, emotionally, philosophically and spiritually, long before death actually takes place (Murray & Zentner, 1997).

Assessing the Needs of Dying Patients and their Families

Assessment of loss, death and grief involves the patient who is dying and the family or significant others who are responding to the death. Effective care for dying patients and their families is based on an assessment of everyone's needs—physical, psychological, social and spiritual. The methods of data collection are the same as for standard assessments. The nurse uses communication and interviewing techniques, observation and physical assessment skills, as well as interaction with other health professionals. However, data collection is an ongoing process rather than a one-time health history or physical examination, and is oriented towards understanding the strengths as well as the vulnerabilities of the dying patient and members of the family (Benoliel, 1985).

Nursing Health History

The initial interview is an important tool for obtaining information about the patient and family, the understanding of the terminal illness, problems being encountered and coping capacities. During this time, the nurse will focus on patient and family goals and expectations; concerns about the challenges being faced; knowledge and understanding of the disease and medical treatment; knowledge about the patient's health status and prognosis; perceptions of relationships with physician and other health professionals; effect of illness and treatment on the patient's activities of daily living; environmental supports and barriers in the home; and availability of support systems (Benoliel, 1985).

As we discussed in a previous section, the needs and coping capacities of dying patients and their families are complex and very personal. The nurse has to take into account social, cultural and religious and spiritual factors, as well as personal experiences, family beliefs and practices that are influencing individual and family responses at the time. This requires open communication with and active listening to those who are coping with dying and loss in order to identify, with them, their own needs.

Because the ability to cope with challenges in life is variable and rooted in previous experience, asking patients and families how they usually cope with loss and crises will give a good indication of how they will cope with this terminal illness and the eventual death and bereavement.

AWARENESS OF IMPENDING DEATH

In order to talk openly and freely with patients and families, the nurse must first identify the state of awareness of the impending death. Glaser and Strauss (1965) described four states of awareness of impending death: closed awareness, suspected awareness, mutual pretence and open awareness.

CLOSED AWARENESS Closed awareness is the state in which the dying person does not realize the impending death. The family may or may not be aware. The physician, and perhaps the family, determine that it may not be in the patient's best interest to disclose the diagnosis or prognosis. While the intention is to protect the patient, difficulties result for the family and the nurse. Families and patients are cheated of the opportunity to communicate openly, to express feelings, to share the burden of grief, to plan realistically for the family's future and to close life with the proper rituals. Likewise, nurses caring for the patient find it difficult because they are unable to communicate openly and freely (Murray & Zentner, 1997).

SUSPECTED AWARENESS Dying patients do not remain unaware for long. The deteriorating state of health, changes in physical appearance and altered behaviours of family members and health professionals lead to suspected awareness. The patient begins to suspect that things are not as they are said to be. Because patients may feel that trust has been undermined, they may not voice suspicions to others, which further complicates communication.

MUTUAL PRETENCE In mutual pretence the patient, family and health professional all know that death is pending but continue to pretend otherwise. Patients may avoid talking about their death to protect the family from distress, and nurses may not bring up the subject because they think they are preserving the patient's privacy. Mutual pretence is very demanding for everyone involved and interferes with a healthy response to death.

OPEN AWARENESS In open awareness, the dying person, the family and the health professional realize and are willing to discuss the impending death. While it is not easy, open awareness allows the patient and family to share grief, to support one another, to finish important business and to make appropriate future plans. "The anguish is not reduced but can be faced together" (Murray & Zentner, 1997, p. 789).

Physical Assessment

The physical assessment of a dying patient follows the format for assessing all needs. The patient will exhibit signs and symptoms related to the disease process and responses to it. In addition, certain signs indicate the imminence of death. These are outlined later in the chapter in the section dealing with care of the dying patient.

Diagnosing Problems Related to Death, Dying and Grieving

Patients who are in the terminal phase of illness and are facing the ending of life can experience the total range of nursing diagnoses, depending on individual circumstances. Dying people will have concerns about challenges being encountered, and their usual coping abilities may not always be effective. In a study on the concerns (fears and anxieties) about death among those coping with dying, Davidson (cited in Corr *et al.*, 1994) found that the majority of terminally ill patients were concerned firstly about abandonment and rejection by significant others; secondly about losing control or ability to manage their lives; and thirdly about intractable pain. This study revealed that people who are dying have a mixture of physical, psychological, social and spiritual concerns and suggested that coping with dying "may be closely linked to what is involved in coping with living" (Corr *et al.*, 1994, p. 106). Thus, three diagnoses that may apply specifically to dying patients are *Fear*, *Anxiety* and *Ineffective Individual Coping*. The diagnoses of *Fear* and *Anxiety* can take many forms, as they are related to a number of different attitudes and beliefs that individuals and societies hold about death and dying. The same is true for *Ineffective Individual Coping*, since people cope in ways that are vastly different.

People who are coping with the impending death of a loved one may also experience a range of problems, including physical responses to the stresses being experienced. They may have concerns related to the suffering of a loved one, as well as fears and anxieties related to the consequences of the death. For example, there may be fear of loneliness and of the anticipated changes the loss will bring. In fact, people may already be experiencing losses—for example, the loss experienced by a husband whose wife becomes too weak to participate in the activities of daily living. How effectively people will be able to cope with the impending death depends on personality and on coping abilities.

Grieving is the diagnosis used for individuals and families who have experienced a loss, including bereavement (Carpenito, 1997). As we discussed earlier, people experience and manifest grief in many different ways. Normal grief and mourning may cause a variety of problems for individuals or families that nurses may independently treat. For example, a widow may experience *Sleep Pattern Disturbance*, *Social Isolation* or *Altered Role Performance*; a family may experience *Decisional Conflict* or *Ineffective Family Coping*. When grief is unresolved or when it is unusually long, the diagnosis of *Dysfunctional Grieving* is used (Carpenito, 1997). *Dysfunctional Grieving* constitutes an abnormality in the normal process of grief and mourning that is beyond the realm of this introductory work. The beginning nurse will learn about dysfunctional grieving in more advanced courses.

Planning Interventions for Death, Dying and Grieving

The goals for care of patients facing impending death are highly individual and age-dependent, reflecting patients' fears, anxieties, concerns and desires, as well as the physical needs brought about by the illness and the process of death. In general, expected outcomes of dying patients that may be

- Patient will achieve a peaceful, dignified death.
- Patient will maintain physical comfort, primarily control of pain.
- Patient will verbalize fears, anxieties, concerns.
- Patient will maintain control over aspects of care.
- Patient will express positive feelings, optimism and hope about the present and future.
- Patient will share reflections of his or her life in a positive manner.
- Patient will share reflections of his or her values and the personal meanings of life and death.
- Patient will die with the support of loving family members and individuals who care.

As we discussed earlier, the general goals or expected outcomes of grieving for a bereaved person are "to remember the loved one without major emotional pain and to reinvest emotional energy in life so that the capacity to love is not lost" (Martocchio, 1985, p. 331). Understandably, these are long-term goals, the achievement of which will be determined by the multiplicity of factors that affect grief and mourning. Care for bereaved persons and families may be better guided by setting short-term goals based on their individual responses and perceived needs. Some examples of short-term expected outcomes include:

- Survivor will verbalize the reality of the loss.
- Survivor will express the pain of the loss.
- Survivor will express feelings of hope about the future.
- Survivor will express regained interest in life.
- Survivor will establish new roles.

Again, it is important to keep in mind that these goals are individual. Not achieving them should not be viewed as a failure on the part of the patient, survivor or health care provider, since every person is different and will cope in different ways.

Implementing Interventions for Death, Dying and Grieving

Principles of Palliative Care

In recent years, the development of the hospice movement has fostered special programs to care for the dying. Hospices or programs of care for the dying began in Britain in the 1960s. In the 1970s, the first program in Canada was started in Montreal. The term "palliative care" was adopted to

Suggested Principles of Palliative Care

1. Care is directed towards meeting the physical, psychological, social and spiritual expectations and needs of the patient and family with sensitivity to their personal, cultural and religious values, beliefs and practices.
2. Patients and families have timely access to information and services when they need and are prepared to accept them. Information and services are provided in language that can be understood. Essential palliative care services are available 24 hours per day, seven days per week.
3. Palliative care services are equally available regardless of the patient's and family's age, gender, national or ethnic origin, geographical location, race, colour, language, creed, religion, sexual orientation, diagnosis, disability, availability of primary caregiver, ability to pay, criminal convictions or family status.
4. The ethical principles of autonomy, beneficence, nonmaleficence, justice, truth-telling and confidentiality are integrated into the provision of care.
5. It is the patient's right to be informed about his or her disease, potential treatments and outcomes, appropriate resources and options. It is the family's right to be informed about the disease, potential treatments and outcomes, appropriate resources and options, respecting the patient's right to confidentiality.
6. Decisions are made by the patient and family in collaboration with the caregivers and service providers, respecting the level of participation desired by the patient and family. The patient's and family's choices for care, settings of care and information sharing are respected.
7. The unit of care is the patient and family.
8. Care is provided by an interdisciplinary team of caregivers and service providers working collaboratively with the patient and family.
9. A coordinated, continuous plan of care that minimizes duplication is maintained across all settings of care, from admission of the patient through bereavement support for the family.
10. The palliative care needs of a community can be met only through the collaborative efforts of available services in partnership at the patient care and programmatic levels.
11. Care is delivered by all service providers within professionally accepted standards of conduct and practice.

SOURCE: Canadian Palliative Care Association, 1995, pp. 16, 17.

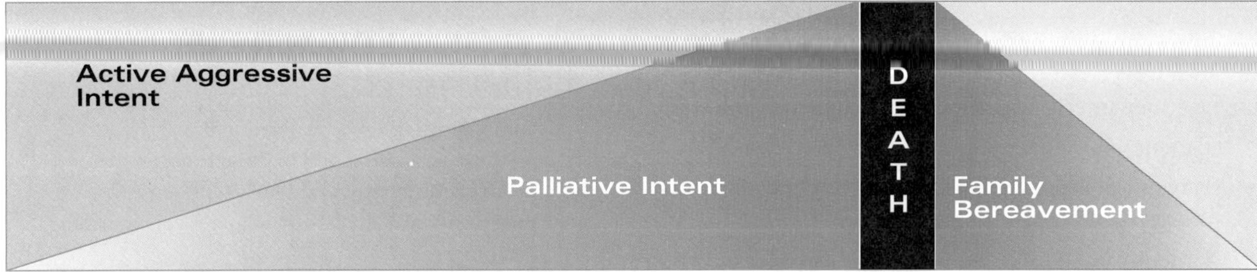

FIGURE 37.1 Hospice view of medical treatment

SOURCE: Health & Welfare Canada, 1989, p. 2.

describe this program, and has become the term used more frequently than "hospice" in Canada. **Palliative care** is active, compassionate care of the terminally ill at a time when goals of cure or prolongation of life are no longer paramount and when the emphasis of care is on the comfort and quality of life until death. Care encompasses the terminal phase, death and period of grieving after death (see Figure 37.1) (Canadian Palliative Care Association, 1995).

Palliative care programs may be located within special units of hospitals or within freestanding agencies, or they may operate through a variety of home care programs. Palliative care programs are rapidly increasing in number and exist in every province. Not every patient who dies, however, does so within the context of a palliative care program. Many deaths occur in critical care units and in nursing homes. Regardless of location of care at the time of death, the philosophy and principles of palliative care should guide the care of the terminally ill.

In 1995, the Canadian Palliative Care Association suggested a set of principles that can be used to guide the care of the terminally ill (see box on preceding page).

The Health Care Team

Roles and relationships among health professionals also affect the care of terminally ill and dying patients. Clearly, they greatly determine the emotional climate of any care setting. Traditional authoritarian relationships, which have in the past characterized physician–nurse relationships in particular, have no place in the care of the terminally ill. For professionals interested in providing optimal care to the dying, collaboration and cooperation are essential.

Needs of the Dying Patient

Dying patients have many needs involving physical, psychological, social and spiritual dimensions. A summary of these needs appears in Table 37.6.

Perhaps the need that can best guide the nurse is the patient's need to die gracefully, or with dignity. To treat another with dignity is to acknowledge that each dying person is to be seen as a unique individual, one whose life history is solely his or her own. Further, it means acknowledging that this person is just as important as anyone else in the health

COMMUNITY health practice — May's Place

The May Gutteridge Hospice, commonly called May's Place, was the first freestanding hospice facility for the terminally ill in British Columbia. The hospice is named after May Gutteridge, who received the Order of Canada for her 30 years of service with the St. James Social Services Society. The hospice has been in operation since 1990 and is a member of the St. James Social Services Society. May's Place is situated in the downtown east side of Vancouver and gives priority admission to those living in this area.

The philosophy of the hospice emphasizes the individuality and autonomy of the resident. Therefore, each resident has the right to remain active in treatment decisions. The emphasis of care is on the patient, family and friends, and is provided by specially trained staff in a comfortable, unstructured, home-like setting. Each patient is treated as an individual with respect for his or her autonomy and dignity.

The hospice is open to terminally ill residents of British Columbia who are over the age of 20 and have a life expectancy of a few months. Residents must be eligible for provincial long-term care benefits. A small, affordable *per diem* rate is charged to each resident, which covers the cost of rent and food.

The hospice has six private, fully furnished rooms with cable television and phone access. Each resident is encouraged to bring personal belongings to decorate his or her room. There is 24-hour nursing care from trained palliative care nurses and nurses' aides. Residents may receive primary care from their family physician or from the hospice's medical director. The caregiving team is complemented by a dedicated group of volunteers. At time of writing, the St. James Social Services Society Cottage Hospice Campaign has begun. This campaign is to acquire funds to establish a Cottage Hospice which would be the second freestanding hospice in Vancouver, B.C.

TABLE 37.6 Needs of dying patients

[illegible]	Need
Physiological	Good symptom control
Safety	A feeling of security
Belonging	The need to be needed
	The need not to be a burden
Love	Expressions of affection, human contact (touch)
Understanding	Explanation about the disease and its symptoms
	Opportunity to discuss process of dying
Acceptance	Regardless of mood and sociability
Self-esteem	Involvement in decision making, especially as physical dependency on others increases
	Opportunity to give as well as receive

SOURCE: Victoria Hospice Society, 1993.

care system and is entitled to the same rights and privileges. The dying person's bill of rights (see box on following page) assures comprehensive and compassionate care.

Care of the Dying Patient

Nursing interventions for death and dying involve strategies that support the needs and goals of dying patients. Care focusses on maintaining physiological functioning as well as psychological, social and spiritual well-being. Ethical dilemmas may arise when serious decisions have to be made concerning death and dying. Throughout all aspects of care, the nurse implements activities that enable patient participation, foster a sense of control and promote a peaceful death with grace and dignity.

Many religions and cultures have specific rituals associated with the process of dying. For example, most Christians receive the sacrament of the sick; Buddhists may wish a quiet place for meditation, and prayers may be offered by a Buddhist monk. Muslims may prefer to sit or lie facing Mecca. Nurses need to be aware of the cultural and religious preferences of the patients they care for (see Chapter 12). Consultation with patient, family and pastoral counsellor will allow the nurse to provide culturally specific nursing care.

MAINTAINING PHYSIOLOGICAL FUNCTIONING

The physical needs of people who are dying are similar to the needs of all seriously ill patients. In addition, one of the most crucial needs is to control pain. Assisting patients and families through this period requires art and compassion. Knowledge of the process of dying is basic to supporting patients and families.

Sensory–Perceptual Needs

Changes in the level of consciousness may be the first symptom, occurring over a period of weeks or days in patients with cancer. In other diseases, such as with stroke or cardiac arrest, change in the level of consciousness may be an event, not a process.

Consciousness is an integral component of being human, of relating to the environment and to others and an indication of the extent of influence or control an individual has. Although patients may have intellectually accepted that they are dying and will lose consciousness, most have great difficulty in letting go of the conscious awareness of life. Some will be so fatigued from the disease and its limitations that "just going to sleep" becomes the wish; such patients often die very quickly once they "let go." For other patients, however, the inner drive to survive continues. Any impairment of consciousness creates a turbulent, restless phase during which they continually seem to struggle. The box on page 1259 summarizes the states of consciousness in dying patients. The information is based on the work of Plum and Posner (1980) as adapted by the Victoria Hospice Society.

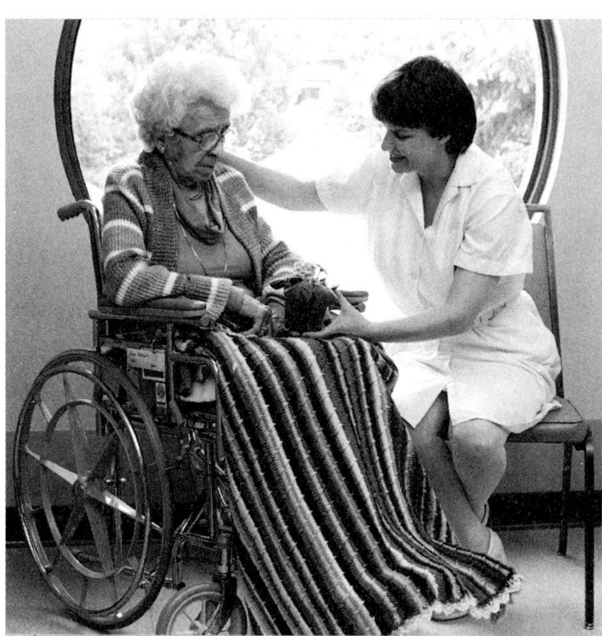

Listening to patients warmly and affectionately is important in palliative care.

The Dying Person's Bill of Rights

I have the right to be treated as a living human being until I die.

I have the right to maintain a sense of hopefulness, however changing its focus may be.

I have the right to be cared for by those who can maintain a sense of hopefulness, however changing this might be.

I have the right to express my feelings and emotions about my approaching death in my own way.

I have the right not be deceived.

I have the right to have help from and for my family in accepting my death.

I have the right to die in peace and dignity.

I have the right to retain my individuality and not be judged for my decisions which may be contrary to beliefs of others.

I have the right to participate in decisions concerning my care.

I have the right to expect continuing medical and nursing attention even though "cure" goals must be changed to "comfort" goals.

I have the right not to die alone.

I have the right to be free from pain.

I have the right to have my questions answered honestly.

I have the right to discuss and enlarge my religious and/or spiritual experiences, whatever these may mean to others.

I have the right to expect that the sanctity of the human body will be respected after death.

I have the right to be cared for by caring, sensitive, knowledgeable people who will attempt to understand my needs and will be able to gain some satisfaction in helping me face my death.

SOURCE: Barbus, 1975.

Breathing Needs

Respiratory difficulty is one of the most distressing symptoms for patients, and it is agonizing for families to witness. As the patient's condition deteriorates, he or she may experience changes in breathing patterns. There are three common breathing patterns that may occur close to death. *Cheyne-Stokes respirations* (CSR) are commonly seen, characterized by:

- regular alternation of hyperpnea and apnea
- smooth crescendo and smooth decrescendo
- hyperpneic usually greater than apneic period.

CSR appears to be due to a combination of abnormal increased response to carbon dioxide, causing hyperpnea, and abnormal decreased forebrain ventricle stimulus, thereby allowing posthyperventilation apnea and bilateral cerebral dysfunction in the deep cerebrum or diencephalon. This breathing pattern may occur in conscious, frail patients, such as those in mild congestive heart failure or with chronic obstructive pulmonary disease, during sleep and may disappear upon awakening. CSR occurs very commonly in the terminally ill who are receiving moderate to high doses of narcotic agents and who are very weak. It must be pointed out that the narcotic dose should not be reduced if patients are receiving a stable dose and require this amount. If the dose is being titrated upward and the patient is now pain-free, the doses should be either continued at the present level or reduced slightly. However, it is exceedingly rare that CSR alone is a sign of drug toxicity. Finally, CSR also occurs in comatose patients who are imminently dying.

Cluster breathing is also commonly seen prior to death and is often confused with CSR. Here the nurse will see short patterns of sudden deep breathing of three to five breaths in decreasing volume. The depth of breathing will gradually decrease several hours prior to death; periods of apnea are prolonged (10–60 seconds) and variable in duration. Some families may refer to this as "gasping" for breath, since after the period of apnea there are sudden and deep breaths. Finally, *ataxic breathing* is generally seen within minutes or hours of death. This pattern is characterized by complete irregularity in breathing that varies in depth, rate and periods of apnea.

Respiratory congestion is another common problem observed prior to death. It has also been referred to as the "death rattle," "suffocation" or "drowning in sputum." However, such language is often inaccurate and inappropriate, leading to emotional reactions that bring fear and anxiety for everyone involved. Respiratory congestion is a more appropriate and accurate term. There are several contributing factors. For example, as patients become weakened, they lose the energy required to raise sputum so that the sputum may sit in the minor or major bronchi and cause the characteristic noise. As well, bronchial infection, pneumonia or blood in the airways create excess exudate and give rise to a congested sound. Whether the congestion is mild or severe, it should be treated, since it can be very distressing to the family.

It is important to raise the possibility of respiratory congestion and the reasons for it beforehand, so that family members are prepared in the event that it occurs. While it seems obvious to family members (and many nurses) that suctioning would help, in most cases suctioning is an inappropriate intervention, as secretions are often below the trachea and inaccessible to suction. On occasion, massive pulmonary edema or copious amounts of mucous and saliva in the mouth and throat may warrant suctioning, but this is not the norm. A more humane and dignified approach would be to use medications to relieve respiratory congestion. The goal is to prevent these symptoms from occurring. Therefore, regularly scheduled medication to prevent and control respiratory congestion is advised.

States of Consciousness in Dying Patients

self and the surrounding environment. There are two aspects:

1. *Content.* The sum of mental processes, including the ability to discriminate among both the sensory inputs and the internal cognitive aspects.
2. *Arousal.* A state of wakefulness or alertness to external and internal processes.

B. Clouding of Consciousness: Defined as a reducing state of wakefulness or through any or all of these as death approaches.

1. *Mild clouding.* For the terminal patient, fatigue and periods of drowsiness are common. After a period of rest, the patient remains fully conscious. Several other features may occur intermittently, and may be attributed to anxiety. They may not be observed or appreciated by caregivers in the early part of this phase. These are:
   - excitability and irritability, which alternate with drowsiness
   - tendency to be startled by minor stimuli
   - distractibility
   - misjudging sensory perceptions, especially visual
   - inability to think clearly or quickly.
2. *Advanced or subacute confusional state.* In this phase, the intensity and persistence of the symptoms is increased. The patient is "confused." Symptoms include:
   - consistent misinterpretation of stimuli
   - shortened attention span
   - bewilderment, including difficulty following commands

   [illegible] and familiarities to place and person
   - faulty memory
   - drowsiness (which may alternate with nighttime agitation).
3. *Semi-consciousness.* This phase is frequently seen in toxic and metabolic states including poisoning, alcohol withdrawal, uremia, acute hepatic failure and severe systemic infections. Symptoms at this level include:
   - intensified disorientation, fear or irritability
   - misinterpretation of stimuli; often visual hallucinations
   - lucid periods that often alternate with delirium (while lucid, the patient may be afraid of mental failure)
   - delusions
   - loud, talkative, offensive, suspicious or agitated behaviour.
4. *Stupor.* This state is reached when the patient is unresponsive but briefly arousable only during vigorous and repeated stimuli, and then immediately drifts back to unresponsiveness. In this phase, the patient may moan or be briefly restless when being turned or when given skin care. The nurse needs to ascertain whether this moaning is due to insufficient pain control or simply being partially aroused from a deeper level.
5. *Coma.* The true comatose state is defined as complete unresponsiveness or the absence of any psychologically understandable response to external stimuli or inner need. The patient is breathing on his or her own, but is totally unarousable by any stimulus.

SOURCE: Victoria Hospice Society, 1993.

Cardiovascular Needs (Tissue Perfusion)

Decreasing blood pressure, lessening heart rate and arrhythmias are part of the dying process. As blood circulation slows, the patient's extremities appear cyanosed or mottled and feel cool and clammy to the touch, even though the patient may perceive warmth and the body temperature is above normal. When circulation is considerably decreased, the effectiveness of analgesics administered intramuscularly or subcutaneously is decreased. As a consequence, the patient may require intravenous analgesia.

Elimination Needs

Dying patients experience inability to control urination and defecation. This is usually due to loss of muscle tone. The sphincter muscles of the rectum and bladder relax and, as a result, there is involuntary micturition and defecation. A retention catheter may be required; absorbent pads can be used to help keep the patient dry and comfortable. Since patients are often embarrassed about the inability to control these functions, it is important that the nurse be discreet and understanding. Deodorants are frequently used to keep the air in the patient's room fresh and free from unpleasant odours.

Involuntary micturition and defecation predispose the patient to pressure ulcers. By helping patients to keep dry and clean and to change position regularly, the nurse can usually prevent these complications.

Movement and Activity Needs

Because of the progressive loss of muscle tone, dying patients find it increasingly difficult to maintain position in bed without support. If patients are conscious, Fowler's position is usually indicated in order to increase the depth of ventilation of the lungs. If they are unconscious, a semi-prone position promotes the drainage of mucous from the mouth. Family members may become anxious when they see the patient positioned in this manner, and it is wise to explain the reasons for it. Ultimately, however, each patient is different, and if able, should be allowed to choose how he or she wishes to be positioned. Patients are the best judge of their comfort. Regardless of the patient's position, supportive measures, such as pillows, can add comfort. If possible, the various parts of the body should be kept out of dependent positions to prevent the pooling of blood.

Nutritional Needs

There is progressive diminution in peristalsis of the gastrointestinal tract of dying patients. Desire for food is usually minimal, but they may want frequent sips of water. The mouth may be dry, owing to dehydration and perhaps to a slight fever, which sometimes precedes death. Good oral hygiene is essential. Because of reduced peristalsis, flatus accumulates in the stomach and intestines, often distending the patient's abdomen and causing nausea. More than a few sips of water at a time, consequently, can cause vomiting. Dying patients are often given nourishment and fluids parenterally, but rarely are sips of fluid contraindicated.

Pain Management

One of the greatest fears of terminally ill patients is that they will have unbearable pain during their final days. In fact, research suggests that 50 percent of cancer patients experience pain (Anderson, 1982; Fainsinger, Miller & Bruera, 1991). Pain control is important because pain alters sleep, appetite, mobility, energy levels and psychological functioning. Yet, pain in both cancer and noncancer patients is often poorly controlled. The many reasons for this include lack of understanding of the differences between acute and chronic pain; inappropriate beliefs, attitudes and fears held by patients, families and health professionals; and lack of knowledge about current techniques in pain control.

Most nurses are educated in the observation and assessment of acute pain. Outward manifestations of severe acute pain are dramatic and demand immediate attention. In contrast, patients with chronic pain often display few outward indications or may appear drowsy and depressed. However, when questioned, such patients will often state that they are in a great deal of pain. Thus, lack of expression of pain does not mean lack of pain. Nurses, therefore, need to be aware of the differences between the acute and chronic signs of pain.

Owing to the subjective nature of pain, the first strategy in its management is an individualized pain assessment. This will provide valuable baseline information for making treatment decisions. Treatment of chronic pain is an essential element in promoting comfort for the terminally ill and in helping them to maintain activities of daily living.

Analgesics are often used to treat chronic pain. Generally, these medications are most effective if administered regularly rather than on a prn basis. Frequently, when patients are receiving a regular dosage of analgesia, pain may "break through," necessitating additional doses of medication to keep it under control. Medications for pain management are not limited to analgesics and can also include corticosteroids, antidepressants, anticonvulsants and anxiolytics. Determining which kind of medication to use is based on the pain assessment. As well as medications, other strategies can greatly enhance comfort for those who are dying. Relaxation, guided imagery, distraction and peripheral nerve stimulators can also provide relief for patients. These interventions and others are described in detail in Chapter 27.

MAINTAINING WELL-BEING

Psychological Well-Being

Denial and feelings of anger, fear, anxiety and sadness are common during terminal illness and the period of dying. Throughout the denial state, the nurse must accept the fact that patients vary in their ability to acknowledge the seriousness of the illness. Most patients seem to experience these denial responses fairly often during terminal illness. Some maintain denial up to the point of impending death, and continue to talk optimistically of future plans. Many patients, however, are aware of the prognosis, even though they have never been told in words; yet, they may pretend not to know. Often, patients maintain a facade of cheerfulness for the benefit of families, in whom they sense discomfort talking about death, or because they believe that they are expected by hospital staff to behave in this manner. For these patients, it is frequently a relief to drop the facade in the presence of someone who understands what they are going through.

Expressions of anger, hostility, fear, anxiety or sadness are feelings nurses often have the most difficulty responding to because nurses innately want to find answers that will make the patient's pain and distress go away. Anger is especially hard to deal with, particularly because it is often projected onto the caregiver. The important element in providing psychological support is to realize that these feelings must be identified, acknowledged and expressed. Careful listening to the patient is the key. Giving patients "permission" to share feelings, to talk about what they feel and why they feel as they do may be the most helpful intervention (Corr *et al.*, 1994). The nurse can also use touch in some cases as a healing activity. Because not all people are comfortable with physical touching, the nurse must pay attention to the patient's verbal and nonverbal responses when touch is used.

People lose their sense of dignity, self-esteem and self-worth when they lose control over their lives and their environment and become dependent on others for their care. The nurse can do much to maintain a dying patient's psychological well-being by continually involving him or her in decisions, asking for preferences and offering choices in regard to care.

Social Well-Being

Dying people need ongoing interaction with loved ones to maintain a sense of security and social well-being. Within the security of a loving relationship, one is able to talk about concerns, find meaning in experiences and work through problems. Sometimes all that is needed is the presence of a

that nurses be aware of and feel comfortable with their own spiritual beliefs and values before offering support to patients, so that the nurse's own needs do not

support to family members and significant others in coping with their own grief so that they, in turn, are able to maintain meaningful relationships with the patient. When these individuals are not present, the nurse can facilitate the patient's well-being by showing an interest and encouraging him or her to talk about family members and significant others.

People who are coping with impending death also have concerns about changes in social roles and about family circumstances that will be left behind. For example, patients may worry about a work project not completed, the economic security of their family and how their partner will cope as a single parent. Nurses can help by allowing patients to talk about such concerns and by enabling them to act for themselves. This is done by listening and helping patients explore problems, consider options and find resources to fulfill needs. Nurses may also become advocates for dying patients by finding needed resources, such as social workers, counsellors or lawyers.

Spiritual Well-Being and Hope

Hope is characterized by a confident yet uncertain expectation of achieving a future goal (Dufault & Martocchio, 1985). Hope is not a single entity, but rather a combination of thoughts, feelings and actions that change frequently. Even when there is not a shadow of doubt in the nurse's mind that the present illness will result in death for the patient, it still proves possible to maintain hope in a realistic sense. The key is that the object of the hope is shifted to a shorter range. Patients shift from hoping for a cure to hoping for longer periods of remission. As illness progresses, the focus of hope changes to even more immediate objects: hope for survival until a special occasion has passed, for example, or hope for symptom-free days. Finally, patients may hope for a relatively peaceful and dignified death. If given the opportunity and the encouragement, patients will remain hopeful, often right until the moment of death.

As death approaches, patients often seek comfort by analysing values and beliefs related to life and death. If they have had questions about their life, these also emerge when they are dying. A dying patient seeks to find purpose and meaning in life before surrendering to death (Conrad, 1985).

Providing a patient with spiritual comfort implies much more than arranging for clergy to visit. The nurse must support patients in the expression of a philosophy of life. The nurse or family can assist the patient with spiritual matters through careful listening, expressing empathy, reading scriptures and praying, if that is in line with the patient's desires, or by arranging for clergy to visit if the patient so wishes.

Attentive listening encourages patients to express feelings, clarify them and accept death. However, it is crucial

ETHICAL ASPECTS OF CARE

There are many decisions to be made surrounding patients whose life is slipping away. Can the medical condition be reversed? Should present treatments be continued or stopped? If so, when?

Ethics and the decision-making process is a vast area that is rapidly increasing in importance in the health care system. Decisions concerning dying and death are at the very roots of medicine, since one of its main goals is the reverse—to sustain and improve life. When the possibility of death enters, a host of reactions and decisions are necessary. The professional mandate of nurses is to promote health, to care for those who are ill and, in cases where cure is not possible, to provide comfort to those who are dying. Discrepant views about sustaining life and accepting an inevitable death are at the root of the ethical dilemmas that many nurses face.

Ethical issues arise in all facets of health care when serious decisions have to be made. Preferences are expressed or not expressed by patients about their care or future; differing futures are envisioned for the patient by others. From time to time, the goals of care must be revised. As well, patients, family members and health professionals need to adjust to partial achievement of goals. What is possible and what is desirable must be considered. Several factors must be taken into account, including the nature of the disease; the patient's status and preference; the values of the patient, his or her family and health care providers; and social, cultural, political and financial realities.

In recent years the concept of **advance directives** has developed as a mechanism for dealing with some of the decisions that arise when caring for the terminally ill. Advance directives apply when there is no hope of recovery. Their purpose is to speak for an incapacitated patient who cannot speak for himself or herself by outlining the patient's medical treatment wishes. Advance directives incorporate the concepts of the **living will**, the patient's right to refuse unwanted life support. Every state in the United States has passed some legislation authorizing the use of advance directives. Several Canadian provinces have adopted the concept, and the Canadian Medical Association has issued a policy statement supporting the use of living wills (Keatings & Smith, 1995). The University of Toronto Centre for Bioethics will provide copies of their living will upon request (Singer, 1993). Figure 37.2 illustrates an advance directive form; a living will prepared by the organization Choice in Dying Inc. is presented in the box that follows.

Some patients will talk about and seriously consider euthanasia. They may feel that their lives are without meaning, or they have completed the life they enjoyed. Or, they may feel a burden to themselves, their families or the

Advance Directive

Physician Order for: Degree of Intervention and Resuscitation

A. Resuscitation In the event of witnessed cardiac and/or respiratory arrest (indicate one):

- ❑ Do not resuscitate.
- ❑ Initiate basic and advanced cardiopulmonary resuscitation.
- ❑ No decision about resuscitation is made at this time.

B. Degree of Intervention In the event of life-threatening illness (indicate one):

- ❑ **Degree One:** Supportive care only (i.e., nursing care, pain and other symptom relief, oral nutrition and hydration).
- ❑ **Degree Two:** Therapeutic measures without transfer to acute care hospital (includes supportive care as outlined in Degree One and medications such as antibiotics, if indicated).
- ❑ **Degree Three:** Transfer to an acute care hospital if necessary but excluding admission to intensive care unit.
- ❑ **Degree Four:** Transfer to an acute care hospital with maximum therapeutic effort and, if necessary, admission to intensive care unit.
- ❑ No decision about Degree of Intervention made at this time.

C. Other Specific Recommendations:

____

____

____

____

D. Physician Statement I have satisfied myself that the above identified person (indicate one):

- ❑ is competent to make treatment decisions and these orders reflect his/her wishes; or
- ❑ is not competent to make treatment decisions, but has previously given advance directive to me or a family member or representative that is consistent with these orders; or
- ❑ is not competent to make treatment decisions and these orders are consistent with the preferences expressed by (family member or representative); or other (specify).

Attending Physician's Signature:________________________ Date: ____________________

E. Authorization by Patient or Representative

I have discussed with Dr. ____________________ the above options and understand the implications. This order shall remain in effect unless rescinded and should be reviewed in one year. This form will accompany the above identified patient if transferred to another health care facility.

Patient's or representative's signature Relationship Date

F. Annual Review (If revised, destroy this form and complete another; if review only, date and sign below).

Physician's Signature: Date: Physician's Signature: Date:

FIGURE 37.2 Advance directive form

SOURCE: Capital Health Region. (1996). Victoria, B.C.

The Living Will Prepared by Choice in Dying Inc.

In addition to the basic form of the will, Choice in Dying Inc. notes the following:

"Declarants may wish to add specific statements to the Living Will to be inserted in the space provided for that purpose above the signature. Possible additional provisions are suggested below:

1. a) I appoint ______________________ to make binding decisions concerning my medical treatment.

OR

b) I have discussed my views as to life-sustaining measures with the following, who understand my wishes:

____

____

____

2. Measures of artificial life support in the face of impending death that are especially abhorrent to me are:

   a) electrical or mechanical resuscitation of my heart when it has stopped beating

   b) nasogastric tube feedings when I am paralyzed and no longer able to swallow

   c) mechanical respiration by machine when my brain can no longer sustain my own breathing

   d) ______________________________________.

3. If it does not jeopardize the chance of my recovery to a meaningful and sentient life or impose an undue burden on my family, I would like to live out my last days at home rather than in a hospital.

4. If any of my tissues are sound and would be of value as transplants to help other people, I freely give my permission for such donation."

SOURCE: Choice in Dying Inc., New York, NY.

community. **Euthanasia** means an easy or painless death, the word being derived from the Greek words meaning "good death." The term is often used synonymously with "mercy killing," a concept that has caused considerable controversy over the years. There are two forms of euthanasia. *Passive* or *negative euthanasia* means the withholding of life-preserving techniques. It involves an omission (or failure to do something). *Active* or *positive euthanasia* is the initiation of life-shortening measures, and involves taking deliberate action to end life.

The issue is an ethical one that has not been fully resolved. It revolves around two fundamental beliefs: the right of individuals to decide their own time and means of dying and the equally strong argument that all measures must be tried before death is accepted as inevitable. Often, it becomes a matter of "to treat or not to treat." Passive euthanasia is much more widely accepted than active life-shortening measures. Often, in hospitals and long-term facilities, directions will be left for ways that prolong life-

family wish it. Some patients and families may request that the terminally ill person not be subjected to resuscitation attempts in the event of death, in which case the physician should enter a "do not resuscitate" (DNR) order in the patient's chart.

Traditionally, hospice programs have acted as an alternative to the euthanasia movement by pointing out that patients often request euthanasia because they are in physical distress. As the symptoms are relieved, most patients regain a sense of life and wish to live until they die, but in comfort.

Care When Death is Imminent

SIGNS OF IMMINENT DEATH

Patients' reflexes gradually disappear as they approach death and are unable to move. Sensation and power of motion, as well as reflexes are lost first in the legs and then gradually in the arms. Because pressure on the legs is especially uncomfortable, sheets should not be snug and special attention should be paid to the positioning of the legs. Respirations become increasingly difficult; Cheyne-Stokes respirations, cluster breathing or ataxic breathing may occur.

Typically, a faint cyanotic pattern becomes discernible in the face. As peripheral circulation fails, there may be a drenching sweat, and the body surface cools. Although the patient's skin feels cold and clammy, he or she may display restlessness that, paradoxically, is caused by the sensation of heat, and may actually throw off the bedclothes. At this point, patients need lighter covering and fresh circulating air. The nurse may have to explain to family members that even though the patient feels cold to the touch, he or she is not aware of being cold, because the internal temperature is quite high.

The pulse accelerates and becomes weaker. With increasing anoxia, the pupils become dilated and fixed. Low blood pressure, elevated temperature, and a rapid respiration rate are common.

For the comfort of dying patients and their families, the room must be kept clean and tidy. In hospital, dying patients may be given a private room on the nursing unit so that they may have privacy. Staff must ensure frequent visits into the room so that the patient and family do not feel forgotten. As sight and hearing fail, the patient frequently sees only what is near and hears only what is spoken directly to him or her. Indirect lighting should be provided, and family members should be encouraged to sit near the patient's head. Nurses and family members should not draw the shades in the room, talk in whispers in a corner or fail to answer honestly any of the patient's questions. There may be an interval of peace just before death occurs.

RESEARCH to practice

Patterson, C., Molloy, D.W., Guyatt, G.H., Bedard, M., North, J., Hassard, J., Willison, K., Jubelius, R., & Darzins, P. (1997). Systematic implementation of an advance health care directive in the community. *Canadian Journal of Nursing Administration, 10*, 96–108.

This study examined chronically ill elderly who were receiving home care and were willing to complete an advance directive. Study exploration included psychosocial factors associated with directive completion, treatment choices and satisfaction with care.

Two hundred and two elderly individuals were recruited from a Canadian urban area using a randomized control design. The experimental group consisted of 114 participants with 49 individuals in the control group. All participants in the experimental group were assessed for competency using the Specific Instrument to Assess Competency Tool (SIACAD).

Home care nurses attended a one-day workshop on advance directives and were provided practice time before a follow-up educational session. The nurse then made an appointment with study participants to educate them about the purpose of an advance directive. In a follow-up visit, nurses reviewed the directive with those individuals wishing to participate in the study.

Study results indicate that, of the experimental group, 70 percent completed an advance directive. Interaction with the study nurse was a strong predictor of directive completion. A proxy was chosen by all study participants: 45 percent chose either a daughter or son, while 25 percent chose a spouse. With respect to life-threatening illness, 84 percent of participants requested surgical or intensive care if their condition was reversible, compared with 7.5 percent if the condition was deemed irreversible. In the event of an irreversible condition, 92 percent did not want cardiopulmonary resuscitation (CPR), whereas 24 percent did request it. Completion of the directive was not influenced by mood, depression or uncertainty. Furthermore, satisfaction with decision making was not influenced by participation in this study.

The authors suggest that it is reasonable to expect elderly individuals in a community setting to complete an advance directive when provided with continuing education. This is consistent with other research. Workload, time, scope of practice and policy development are all issues that require further examination.

SIGNS OF DEATH

Death is considered to have occurred when the patient's respirations and heart have ceased to function for several minutes. Usually, breathing stops first; the heart stops beating a few minutes later.

For the purpose of human transplants, it has become necessary to have a more precise definition than the cessation of breathing and heartbeat as the absolute signs of death. The absence of brain wave activity as measured by an electroencephalogram is usually used to confirm that death has occurred.

Care After Death

In caring for the body of the patient after death, whatever procedures are carried out are performed with dignity and respect. In some religious faiths, only family members are permitted to care for the body of the deceased. However, this is generally a nursing responsibility. Although each agency usually has its own specific procedures, there are some general guidelines for the care of the body after death which are fairly universal.

The body is generally placed in a supine position in bed with one pillow under the head. The head is slightly elevated to prevent postmortem hypostasis of blood, which could discolour the face. The body is positioned immediately after death and before rigor mortis sets in.

Rigor mortis, a stiffening of the body after death, is a result of a chemical action within the muscles in which glycogen is coagulated and lactic acid is produced. It generally occurs shortly after death, progressing from the jaw down the trunk to the extremities. Once rigor mortis has set in, the body remains rigid for one to six days. When relatives wish to see the body, the nurse first tidies the room and removes extraneous equipment. The body should appear clean, comfortable and peaceful. A slightly shaded room affords a comforting effect.

In some hospitals, it is the policy to insert dentures immediately after death; other institutions send the dentures with the body to the morgue, where they are inserted later by the mortician. In most institutions, rings are removed; if a ring cannot be removed, it is taped in place, and a notation is made on the patient's chart and on the form that goes with the body to the morgue.

The preparation of the body by the nurse involves the application of pads to the perineal area or the insertion of packing into the rectum and vagina. Rarely is it necessary to bathe the body; this procedure is carried out by the mortician. It is, however, necessary to cleanse the body of any blood or drainage that may have accumulated after death.

After the family has left, the nurse places identification tags on the body. At most hospitals, bodies are labelled twice: one label is attached to the ankles, the other to the shroud in which the body is wrapped. If a patient had a transmissible disease, this information also needs to be noted for the protection of others who will be handling the body. When agency protocol requires the ankles and wrists to be tied together, they should be well padded in order to prevent bruising. In some agencies, it is the practice to treat the body as if the patient were still living, and no shroud is used. When the preparation of the body is complete, it is

a morgue, the mortician should be notified to come for the body.

The patient's valuables and clothes should, whenever possible, be sent home with the relatives. If there is no one present who can assume responsibility for these, valuables should be placed in the hospital safe and the clothes labelled and stored until such time as the family collects them.

The laws of each province may vary with regard to the requirements of certifying death. This is usually the responsibility of a physician. For the medical record, nurses should note the time that respirations cease and the heart stops beating. In many agencies, it is the nurse's responsibility to inform families who are not present at the time of the death.

The physician often asks families about organ or tissue donation when the patient is a suitable donor. The nurse, however, may have to answer questions asked by the family and to support them in their decision. In some provinces, it is common for individuals to indicate whether they want their eyes donated for corneal transplantation. Enucleation of the eyes for corneal transplant must follow a rigid procedure as developed by the Canadian National Institute for the Blind (CNIB) and as carried out by a physician. Nurses must be aware of the patient's choice and may assist with this procedure.

The decision to conduct an autopsy (postmortem examination) usually rests with the family. The physician discusses with the family the need or the desire for an autopsy

order to provide appropriate follow-up should the family ask additional questions or express concerns about the procedure. Procedure 37.1 lists the steps in caring for a patient's body after death.

Support for the Grieving Family

Family members must be supported through the patient's dying and death and, at the same time, be encouraged to provide support to the patient. In the hospital setting, particularly outside palliative care units, the family has greater difficulty in providing support. The nurse must recognize family members as potential resources in providing optimal care to the patient.

The family is more involved when the patient is being cared for at home. Most families prefer to have their loved one at home, but to do so four factors must be present: a caregiver is able and available, support from health care providers is readily available, the patient's symptoms are under control, and the physical environment of the home is conducive to the patient's mobility (Brown, Davies, Reimer & Martens, 1990). Regardless of location of care, however, families sometimes have great difficulty coping with terminal illness. Benoliel (1985) describes circumstances that make it difficult to cope with the demands of terminal illness.

PROCEDURE 37.1 Caring for the Body After Death

Action	*Rationale*
1. Prepare the patient for family viewing:	
• Place in supine position with the head on a small pillow, arms by the sides, palms down, or with hands folded on abdomen. Do not place hands one on top of the other.	Raising the head prevents face discolouration from blood pooling. Provides comfortable appearance. Prevents the discolouration of underlying hand.
• Close the eyes by gently holding the eyelids closed for a few moments. Place dentures in the mouth according to agency policy; close the mouth and, if necessary, prop it closed with a roll under the chin. Comb the hair.	Provides an appearance of resting peacefully. Provides natural appearance.
• Determine whether there will be tissue/organ donation, autopsy or inquest. Remove and/or document equipment. Remove, cut or secure tubes, catheters, dressings and other attachments according to agency policy.	
• Remove jewellery according to family's wishes and/or agency policy. Gather personal effects and place in a bag.	Provides for return of items to the family.
• Place clean absorbent pads where necessary for containing any drainage.	
• Change the bed linens and gown as needed.	

continued on next page

PROCEDURE 37.1

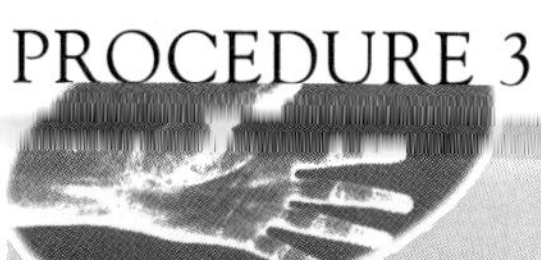

Action	*Rationale*
2. Close the door and pull curtains around the bed.	Provides privacy for the family.
3. Allow the family to spend time with the patient. Stay with the family to provide support or, if they wish, leave them alone with the patient. Involve the family in after-death care according to cultural needs.	Meets family's needs.
4. If possible, have all personal articles and valuables signed for and taken home by the family.	Prevents loss of personal effects.
5. After the family leaves, bring in equipment: shroud pack with body tags; dressings, absorbent pads; clean gloves; disposal bag; basin, water and towels.	Ensures efficiency and economy of time.
6. Don gloves.	Prevents transmission of microorganisms.
7. Remove the gown; wash body of any soiled areas or drainage. Assess appearance of skin and any marks.	Helps to identify any marks present and those that may occur after death and after preparation.
8. Place body on shroud. Check identification carefully and attach identification tags on toe, wrist or ankle, according to agency policy. Agency identification bracelets are generally not removed.	Ensures correct identification. Clothing or bed linen conceals any marks from ties.
9. Change or place absorbent pads at orifices and drainage sites.	Contains leakage after sphincter muscles relax upon death.
10. According to policy, use ties on the wrists and ankles to keep them together, otherwise place hands on abdomen. If necessary, tie a bandage under the jaw and up onto the head; pad all ties.	Maintains body alignment. Prevents jaw from dropping open. Prevent marks on skin from ties.
11. Wrap the body in the shroud according to package instructions or agency procedure. Use tape or ties to secure the shroud, if necessary. Some hospitals use zippered shroud bags.	
12. Place identification tag on the outside of the shroud.	
13. Gently transfer the body to the morgue stretcher. Use side rails or stretcher straps.	Prevents injury, as the body bruises easily.
14. Remove gloves, wash hands, tidy room.	Maintains medical asepsis.
15. Transport the body to the morgue as inconspicuously as possible. Close other doors; have elevator waiting.	Avoids upsetting other patients and visitors.
16. Take the body to the morgue and sign the log book according to agency policy.	Identifies location.
17. Record and report, as appropriate:	Documents care; ensures accurate legal records.
• vital signs, and time of absence of same	
• events leading up to the death	
• time the physician pronounced death	
• any marks, wounds, bruises on the body before death or made during care of the body	Enables differentiating marks that may occur after this time.
• removal or securing of drains and tubes	Documents care of tubing and drains according to agency policies.
• time of notification of family	
• removal of jewellery or securing of items left on, and removal or replacement of dentures	Prevents loss of items.
• consent forms, release forms signed	Meets legal requirements.
• belongings as taken and signed for by family	
• time body was taken to the morgue.	

NURSES at work Pediatric Hospice Nurse

I am a nurse at Canuck Place, North America's first freestanding pediatric hospice. The program is designed to care for children who have progressive, life-threatening illnesses and for their families. Referrals come from across the province, frequently through British Columbia's Children's Hospital, and also from community social workers, nurses, physicians and families themselves. Some of these children are in the early stages of degenerative neuromuscular, neurological or metabolic disorders. They may participate initially in the respite aspects of the program, which emphasize social and recreational activities, monitoring of changing needs and provision of anticipatory grief support. Other children may require immediate palliative care, which includes pain and symptom management as well as intense holistic care for the dying child and grieving family.

Canuck Place is a facility with eight inpatient beds and family accommodation in a beautiful old mansion surrounded by gardens. It is also a philosophy of family-centred, comprehensive care that reaches beyond the walls of the house into the community and the province. Nursing in this environment requires many skills and a flexible approach to life. Let me describe my work in terms of one child's story.

Mark was a toddler referred to us by the oncology department at the local children's hospital. He suffered from a rare brain tumour and had already received extensive chemotherapy and radiation. No further curative treatment was possible. His parents were new immigrants from Hong Kong and spoke very little English. Devastated by the diagnosis and bewildered by the health care system, they came to Canuck Place with great trepidation. One of our first actions was to obtain the services of a reliable translator who attended family meetings, first at the hospital and then at Canuck Place. With the translator's help, we learned of the family's background, including *feng shui* (the Chinese system of holistic design), folk medicine and beliefs about health and illness. An appropriate room was found for Mark, and his mother grew comfortable preparing his favourite dishes in our kitchen. His older sister at times attended classes in our school and became a favourite around the house.

As Mark's primary nurse, I worked with community services to enable him to spend brief periods at home. As his condition worsened, however, religious and cultural restrictions made it impossible for the family to care for him there. As Mark's disease process was relatively slow, he stayed at Canuck Place for several months. We worked with the family to create a comfortable, accepting and joyful environment for Mark to spend his last months, and we supported the family in their grief and in decision making about his care.

Mark died peacefully in his mother's arms, surrounded by loving family and caring staff. His parents kept a place of honour for his nurses at the funeral service. They have stayed in touch with us through our bereavement program. Mark's sister and parents attend grief support groups every two weeks, and I will follow them—by phone and mail—over the next two years.

Being a nurse at Canuck Place is a challenge, especially in our culturally diverse province. But it is one of the most rewarding things I have ever done.

—*Anne Compton, RN*

These include a lengthy period of dying, symptoms that are difficult to control, unpleasant sights and smells, limited coping resources, poor relationships with caregivers and a dying child.

It is important that the family feels the patient is receiving the best care possible. Helping the patient to die in a dignified and peaceful manner is perhaps one of the most valuable contributions the nurse can make to the comfort of both the patient and family.

The nurse must first determine the degree to which family members want to be involved in the patient's care. Giving family members an active role in the care of their loved one can help them feel useful and help preserve the relationship with the patient. Though relieved of some nursing chores, the nurse must still supervise the care given to the patient and support the family in the care they provide. Explanations of treatments, procedures and changes in the patient's condition, in particular, are crucial to helping the family cope with the impending death.

At times, it is up to the nurse to tell the family that a patient has died. Breaking such news requires a delicate and sensitive transaction. It is best to tell the family group in privacy. The nurse should anticipate that they will be upset and will look to him or her for supportive understanding. Care does not stop with the event of death. Dying with dignity means, in part, respect for the body and for those who remain. Suggestions for discussion with family members include the following:

1. Reassure family members about the normalcy of grief reactions. Allow them to sit with the body, if they so choose.
2. Reassure them that tears are natural for some; they are not abnormal or an indication that the person is "falling apart." For others, tears do not come easily, or the person may not feel any need to cry. This is also normal, and it doesn't mean that the loss is any easier to bear.
3. Allow families to stay with the body and to decide for themselves when they wish to leave. Some families may want to stay with the body for a long time after death; others may want to leave immediately. Neither decision is callous or morbid. On rare occasions, excess preoccupation or rejection of the dead may signal abnormality, but on the whole there is great variance in people within a normal range.

Children require special attention. Allow them to touch the body. They may ask many questions, which should be answered accurately at their level of understanding.

4. Provide families with an opportunity for prayer. Some families appreciate this opportunity; others do not feel it is necessary. The nurse can support a family's wishes to say their own prayer, offer to call the chaplain or the family's own minister or, in some cases, offer a universal prayer such as the following:

   "Oh God, in whose presence we came into life, in whose care we live and die, we come at this moment of death to remember with one another the life of ——, who has lived with us. Our love goes with him/her as we now in silence commend him/her to your care."

5. Allow families to engage in other rituals specific to their faith or cultural beliefs. Some ethnic groups expect that members of the immediate family will be vocal in their outpouring of grief. With others, more stoical behaviour is expected.

Nurses should be prepared to provide support to the bereaved regardless of the mode in which their grief is expressed. Grief is the normal, natural response to loss, and it is a very individualized process. Nurses, therefore, should avoid instructing the family on how to respond. Nurses need to listen and provide small acts of kindness that will make families feel cared for. Nurses can offer support even by making a cup of coffee, allowing adequate time to pack up the deceased's belongings (or helping with this painful task) or walking with the family to the front door of the agency. The gentle actions of the nurse at the time of death can greatly assist the family by starting them on a positive bereavement course.

Evaluating Interventions for Death, Dying and Grieving

It is especially important to evaluate nursing interventions for effectiveness in the care of dying patients because their needs and goals change as death approaches. Outcome criteria should be evaluated and the plan of care revised on a regular basis to meet the changing needs of patients and their families.

IN REVIEW

- People experience loss throughout their lifetime. When loss involves death, it is called bereavement. Grief refers to an individual's total response to loss.
- Grief affects many dimensions of a person's life, including the:
  - physical
  - psychological
  - behavioural
  - social
  - spiritual.
- Mourning is the process of incorporating the experience of loss into everyday life.
- Davies, Chekryn-Reimer, Brown and Martens (1995) have offered the concept of "fading away" as a means of conceptualizing a family's phases of coping with dying. They have explained this concept as a transition that incorporates several interrelated and intertwined components.
- There are three phases of grief:
  - the occurrence of death
  - confronting the pain
  - re-establishing connections.
- While grief has been viewed as essentially a passive process, Attig (1995) has suggested that, in actuality, it is an active process involving relearning one's physical and social worlds.
- Weisman (1980) has described four phases in the process of dying:
  - existential plight
  - mitigation and accommodation
  - decline and deterioration
  - preterminality and terminality.
- Bereaved people need:
  - to express feelings associated with the loss
  - to establish a new relationship with the deceased that enables them to cherish memories without suffering undue pain
  - to adjust to a new environment and new roles
  - to develop new or renewed relationships.
- Factors that influence how people experience, grieve and cope with loss include:
  - degree of attachment to the deceased
  - type of death
  - age of the deceased
  - survivor's personality
  - usual coping strategies
  - survivor's social support system.
- Assessment of the dying patient and the grieving family is based on a holistic approach in which the nurse uses:
  - communication
  - interviewing techniques
  - observation
  - physical examination
  - collaboration with other health professionals.
- People who are in the terminal phase of illness and who are coping with impending death can experience the total range of nursing diagnoses.

- Palliative care includes:
  - active, compassionate care of the terminally ill
  - emphasis on patient comfort and quality of life until death
  - aftercare of the bereaved.
- Ethical dilemmas often revolve around sustaining life or accepting inevitable death.
- Advance directives and living wills provide a mechanism for dealing with some of the decisions that arise when patients are no longer capable of speaking for themselves.
- Care of the body after death is performed with dignity and respect.
- Nurses should provide support to grieving families, regardless of how grief is expressed. Supportive interventions include:
  - listening
  - providing warmth and kindness
  - making the family feel cared for.

Critical Thinking Activities

Mr. Edward Chang is in hospital with a malignancy that his doctors consider terminal. He is 93 years old and has three sons and seven grandchildren. Mr. Chang has been in a stuporous state and, upon waking, he experiences pain.

1. What are some of the nursing needs of this patient?
2. What is stupor?
3. What needs of the family could be met by the nurse?
4. Which other members of the health team might be able to assist Mr. Chang and his family?

KEY TERMS

loss p. 1243	*palliative care p. 1256*
bereavement p. 1243	*advance directives p. 1261*
grief p. 1245	*living will p. 1261*
mourning p. 1245	*euthanasia p. 1262*
anticipatory grief p. 1252	*rigor mortis p. 1264*

References

ANDERSON, J. (1982). Nursing management of the cancer patient in pain: A review of the literature. *Cancer Nursing, 5*, 33.

ATTIG, T. (1995). *How we grieve: Relearning the world*. New York: Oxford University Press.

BARBUS, A.J. (1975). The dying person's bill of rights. *America Journal of Nursing, 75*, 99.

BENOLIEL, J. (1985). Loss and terminal illness. *Nursing Clinics of North America, 20*, 439.

BROWN, P., DAVIES, B., REIMER, J., & MARTENS, N. (1990). Families in supportive care (Part II): Palliative care at home—a viable care setting. *Journal of Palliative Care, 6*(3), 21–27.

CANADIAN PALLIATIVE CARE ASSOCIATION. (1995). *Palliative care: Towards a consensus in standardized principles of practice.* Ottawa: Author.

CAPITAL HEALTH REGION. (1996). *Capital Health Region advance directive.* Victoria, BC: Author.

CARPENITO, L.J. (1997). *Nursing diagnosis: Application to clinical practice.* (7th ed.). Philadelphia: Lippincott.

CHEKRYN-REIMER, J., DAVIES, B., & MARTENS, N. (1991). Palliative care: The nurse's role in helping families through the transition of "fading away." *Cancer Nursing, 14*(6), 321–327.

CHOICE IN DYING INC. (n.d.). *The Living Will.* New York, N.Y.: Author.

CONRAD, N.L. (1985). Spiritual support for the dying. *Nursing Clinics of North America, 20*, 415.

CORR, C.A., NABE, C.M., & CORR, D.M. (1994). *Death and dying, life and living.* Pacific Grove, CA: Brooks/Cole.

DAVIES, B., CHEKRYN-REIMER, J., BROWN, P., & MARTENS, N. (1995). Fading away: *The experience of transition in families with terminal illness.* Amityville, NY: Baywood.

DESPELDER, L.A., & STRICKLAND, A.L. (1992). *The last dance.* (3rd ed.). Mountain View, CA: Mayfield.

DUFAULT, K., & MARTOCCHIO, B.C. (1985). Hope: Its spheres and dimensions. *Nursing Clinics of North America, 20*, 379.

DYREGROV, A. (1991). *Grief in children: A handbook for adults.* London: Jessica Kingsley.

FAINSINGER, R., MILLER, M., & BRUERA, E. (1991). *Journal of Palliative Care, 7*(1), 9–15.

GESSER, G., WONG, P.T.P., & REKER, G.T. (1988). Death attitudes across the life span: The development and validation of the death attitude profile (DAP). *Omega: Journal of Death and Dying, 18*, 113–128.

GLASER, B., & STRAUSS, A. (1965). *Awareness of dying*. Chicago: Aldine.

GONDA, T.A., & RUARK, J.E. (1984). *Dying dignified: The health professional's guide to care.* Menlo Park, CA: Addison-Wesley.

HEALTH & WELFARE CANADA. (1989). *Guidelines for establishing palliative care services.* Ottawa: Department of National Health & Welfare.

KEATINGS, M., & SMITH, O. (1995). *Ethical and legal issues in Canadian nursing.* Toronto: W.B. Saunders.

KLASS, D., SILVERMAN, P.R., & NICKMAN, S.L. (Eds.). (1996). *Continuing bonds: New understandings of grief.* Washington, DC: Taylor & Francis.

KÜBLER-ROSS, E. (1969). *On death and dying.* New York: Macmillan.

MARTOCCHIO, C.B. (1985). Grief and bereavement. *Nursing Clinics of North America, 20*, 327–341.

MURRAY, R.B., & ZENTNER, J.P. (1997). *Nursing assessment and health promotion: Strategies through the life span*. Norwalk, CT: Appleton & Lange.

PATTERSON, C., MOLLOY, D.W., GUYATT, G.H., BEDARD, M., NORTH, J., HASSARD, J., WILLISON, K., JUBELIUS, R., & DARZINS, P. (1997). Systematic implementation of an advance health care directive in the community. *Canadian Journal of Nursing Administration, 10*, 96–108.

PLUM, F., & POSNER, J. (1980) *The diagnosis of stupor and coma.* (3rd ed.). Philadelphia: F. A. Davis.

RANDO, T.A. (1984). *Grief, dying, and death.* Champaign, IL: Research Press.

RANDO, T.A. (1986). *Loss and anticipatory grief.* Lexington, MA: Lexington Books.

SHAPIRO, C. H. (1993). *When part of the self is lost.* San Francisco: Jossey-Bass.

SINGER, P.A. (1993). *Centre for Bioethics living will.* Toronto: Centre for Bioethics, University of Toronto. (Individuals interested in obtaining copies may send requests to the Centre for Bioethics, University of Toronto, 88 College Street, Toronto, Ontario M5G 1L4; tel. 416 978-2709, fax 416 978-1911)

VICTORIA HOSPICE SOCIETY. (1993). *Hospice resource manual. Volume 1: Medical care of the dying.* (2nd ed.). Victoria, BC: Author.

WORDEN, J.W. (1991). *Grief counselling and grief therapy: A handbook for the mental health practitioner.* New York: Springer.

Additional Readings

BROWN, M.A., & POWELL-COPE, G. (1993). Themes of loss and dying in caring for a family member with AIDS. *Research in Nursing & Health, 16*(3), 179–191.

CAVANAUGH, T. (1996). The ethics of death-hastening or death-causing palliative analgesia administration of the terminally ill. *Journal of Pain & Symptom Management, 12*, 248–254.

COWLEY, L.T., YOUNG, E., & RAFFIN, T.A. (1992). Care of the dying: An ethical and historical perspective. *Critical Care Medicine, 20*(10), 1473–1482.

CZERWIEC, M. (1996). When a loved one is dying: Families talk about nursing care. *American Journal of Nursing, 96*(5), 32–36.

DAVIES, B., & OBERLE, K. (1990). Dimensions of the supportive role of the nurse in palliative care. *Oncology Nursing Forum, 17*(1), 87–94.

ERICKSEN, J., RODNEY, P., & STARZOMSKI, R. (1995). When is it right to die? *Canadian Nurse, 91*(8), 29–33.

GAUTHIER, P.A. (1997). Living with dignity to the end. *Canadian Nurse, 93*(3), 38–40, 42.

GOETSCHIUS, S.K. (1997). Families and end-of-life care: How do we meet their needs? *Journal of Gerontological Nursing, 23*(3), 43–50, 55–56.

GRANDE, G.E., TODD, C.J., & BARCLAY, S.I.G. (1997). Support needs in the last year of life: Patient and career dilemmas. *Palliative Medicine, 11*(3), 202–208.

KAZANOWSKI, M. (1997). A commitment to palliative care: Could it impact assisted suicide? *Journal of Gerontological Nursing, 23*(3), 35–42, 50, 54, 56.

LINDLEY-DAVIS, B. (1991). Process of dying: Defining characteristics. *Cancer Nursing, 14*(6), 328–333.

McCLAIN, M.E., & SHAFER, S.M. (1996). Supporting families after sudden infant death. *Journal of Psychosocial Nursing & Mental Health Services, 43*(4), 30–34.

McINTYRE, M. (1997). Understanding living with dying. *Canadian Nurse, 93*(1), 19–25.

McWHAN, K. (1991). Caring for dying patients in acute hospital wards: A review. *Nursing Practice, 5*(1), 25–28.

MOLLOY, D.W., & MAPHAM, V. (1996). *Let me decide.* (3rd ed.). Toronto: Penguin.

MOODY, R. (1976). *Life after life.* Harrisburg, PA: Stackpole Books.

RANDO, T.A. (1988). *Grieving.* Lexington, MA: Lexington Books.

RANDO, T. (1993). *Treatment of complicated mourning.* Champaign, IL: Research Press.

ROACH, S.S., & NIETO, B.C. (1997). *Healing and the grief process.* Albany, NY: Delmar.

ROSS, M.M. (1998). Palliative care: an integral part of life's end. *Canadian Nurse, 94*(3), 28–31.

ROSS, M.M., & McDONALD, B. (1994). Providing palliative care to older adults: Context and challenges. *Journal of Palliative Care, 10*(4), 5–10.

RUTMAN, D., & PARKE, B. (1992). Palliative care needs of residents, families, and staff in long-term care facilities. *Journal of Palliative Care, 8*(2), 23–29.

SMITH, A.A. (1995). Patient-induced dehydration: Can it ever be therapeutic? *Oncology Nursing Forum, 22*(1), 1487–1492.

SMITH, N., & REGNARD, C. (1993). Managing family problems in advanced disease—a flow diagram. *Palliative Medicine, 7*(1), 47–58.

SMITH, S.A. (1997). Controversies in hydrating the terminally ill patient. *Journal of Intravenous Nursing, 20*(4), 193–200.

STANHOPE-GOODMAN, S. (1997). Loss as a part of aging. *Canadian Nurse, 93*(2), 55–56.

STILES, M.K. (1990). The shining stranger: Nurse–family spiritual relationships. *Cancer Nursing, 13*(4), 235–245.

TIPTON, K.D. (1997). How to discuss death with patients and families. *Nursing 97, 27*(9), 32hn10–32hn12.

VAN WEEL, H. (1995). Euthanasia: Mercy, morals and medicine. *Canadian Nurse, 91*(8), 35–40.

WHEELER, S.R. (1996). Helping families cope with death and dying. *Nursing 96, 26*(7), 25–30.

Appendix A

Code of Ethics for Registered Nurses

PREAMBLE

The *Code of Ethics for Registered Nurses* gives guidance for decision-making concerning ethical matters, serves as a means for self-evaluation and reflection regarding ethical nursing practice, and provides a basis for peer review initiatives. The code not only educates nurses* about their ethical responsibilities, but also informs other health care professionals and members of the public about the moral commitments expected of nurses.

The Canadian Nurses Association (CNA) periodically revises its code to address changing societal needs, values, and conditions that challenge the ability of nurses to practise ethically. Examples of such factors are: the consequences of economic constraints; increasing use of technology in health care; and, changing ways of delivering nursing services, such as the move to care outside the institutional setting. This revised *Code of Ethics for Registered Nurses* provides nurses with direction for ethical decision-making and practice in everyday situations as they are influenced by current trends and conditions. It applies to nurses in all practice settings, whatever their position and area of responsibility.

Ethical problems and concerns, as well as ethical distress at the individual level, can be the result of decisions made at the institutional, regional, provincial and federal levels. Differing responsibilities, capabilities and ways of working toward change also exist at the client,[1] institutional and societal levels. For all contexts the code offers guidance on providing care that conforms with ethical practice, and on actively influencing and participating in policy development, review and revision.

The complex issues in nursing practice have both legal and ethical dimensions. The laws and ethics of health care overlap, as both are concerned that the conduct of health professionals show respect for the well-being, dignity and liberty of clients. An ideal system of law would be compatible with ethics, in that adherence to the law ought never require the violation of ethics. Still, the domains of law and ethics remain distinct, and the code addresses ethical responsibilities only.

ELEMENTS OF THE CODE

A value is something that is prized or held dear; something that is deeply cared about. This code is organized around seven primary values that are central to ethical nursing practice:

- Health and well-being
- Choice
- Dignity
- Confidentiality
- Fairness
- Accountability
- Practice environments that are conducive to safe, competent and ethical care.

Each value is articulated by responsibility statements that clarify its application and provide more direct guidance. Where it is clear that an action or inaction would involve an **ethical violation** (i.e, the neglect of a moral obligation) the level of guidance is prescriptive. The statement is intended to tell the nurse and others what is ethically acceptable and what is not. Where the situation involves an **ethical problem**[2] or dilemma, guidance is advisory. No ready-made answers can be offered and thoughtful consideration is required to increase the quality of decision-making. Where the situation provokes feelings of guilt, concern, or distaste, it is a situation of ethical distress. In instances of **ethical distress** the level of guidance is more limited but there remains a responsibility for the nurse to examine the situation in light of the provisions of the code. Decisions will be influenced by the particular circumstances of the situation. Ethical reflection and judgement are required to determine how a particular value or responsibility applies in a particular nursing context.

There is room within the profession for disagreement among nurses about the relative weight of different ethical values and principles. More than one proposed intervention may be ethical and reflective of good practice. Discussion is extremely helpful in the resolution of ethical issues. As appropriate, clients, colleagues in nursing and other disciplines, professional nurses' associations and other experts are included in discussions about ethical problems. In addition to this code, legislation, and the standards of practice, policies, and guidelines of professional nurses associations may also assist in problem-solving.[3]

The values articulated in this code are grounded in the professional nursing relationship with clients and indicate what nurses care about in that relationship. For example, to identify health and well-being as a value is to say that nurses care for and about the health and well-being of their

* In this document *nurse* means *Registered Nurse*.

[1] In this document *client* means the individual persons, and groups of persons such as families and communities, with whom the nurse is engaged in a professional relationship.

[2] Ethical problems arise when ethical reasons both for and against one or more courses of action are present and choices must be made. Disagreement about the type and amount of information needed to reach an ethically acceptable decision may further complicate efforts to reach agreement on the appropriate course(s) of action.

[3] The CNA and its member associations publish policy statements and guidelines on a variety of issues, e.g., advance directives, resuscitative interventions, boundary violations, the use of technology in health care, quality of nurses' worklife, support for safe nursing care, etc.

clients. The nurse–client relationship presupposes a certain measure of trust on the part of the client. Care and trust complement one another in professional nursing relationships. Both hinge on the values identified in the code. By upholding these values in practice, nurses earn and maintain the trust of those in their care. For each of the values, the scope of responsibilities identified extends beyond individuals to include families, communities and society.

VALUES

HEALTH AND WELL-BEING Nurses value health and well-being and assist persons to achieve their optimum level of health in situations of normal health, illness, injury, or ill the process of dying.

CHOICE Nurses respect and promote the autonomy of clients and help them to express their health needs and values, and to obtain appropriate information and services.

DIGNITY Nurses value and advocate the dignity and self-respect of human beings.

CONFIDENTIALITY Nurses safeguard the trust of clients that information learned in the context of a professional relationship is shared outside the health care team only with the client's permission or as legally required.

FAIRNESS Nurses apply and promote principles of equity and fairness to assist clients in receiving unbiased treatment and a share of health services and resources proportionate to their needs.

ACCOUNTABILITY Nurses act in a manner consistent with their professional responsibilities and standards of practice.

PRACTICE ENVIRONMENTS CONDUCIVE TO SAFE, COMPETENT AND ETHICAL CARE Nurses advocate practice environments that have the organizational and human support systems, and the resource allocations necessary for safe, competent and ethical nursing care.

HEALTH AND WELL-BEING

Nurses value health and well-being and assist persons to achieve their optimum level of health in situations of normal health, illness, injury, or in the process of dying.

1. Nurses provide care directed first and foremost toward the health and well-being of the client.
2. Nurses recognize that health is more than the absence of disease or infirmity and assist clients to achieve the maximum level of health and well-being possible.
3. Nurses recognize that health status is influenced by a variety of factors. In ways that are consistent with their professional role and responsibilities, nurses are accountable for addressing institutional, social, and political factors influencing health and health care.
4. Nurses support and advocate a full continuum of health services including health promotion and disease prevention initiatives, as well as diagnostic, restorative, rehabilitative and palliative care services.
5. Nurses respect and value the knowledge and skills other health care providers bring to the health care team and actively seek to support and collaborate with others so that maximum benefits to clients can be realized.
6. Nurses foster well-being when life can no longer be sustained, by alleviating suffering and supporting a dignified and peaceful death.
7. Nurses provide the best care circumstances permit even when the need arises in an emergency outside an employment situation.
8. Nurses participate, to the best of their abilities, in research and other activities that contribute to the ongoing development of nursing knowledge. Nurses participating in research observe the nursing profession's guidelines, as well as other guidelines, for ethical research.

CHOICE

Nurses respect and promote the autonomy of clients and help them to express their health needs and values, and to obtain appropriate information and services.

1. Nurses seek to involve clients in health planning and health care decision-making.
2. Nurses provide the information and support required so that clients, to the best of their ability, are able to act on their own behalf in meeting their health and health care needs. Information given is complete, accurate, truthful, and understandable. When they are unable to provide the required information, nurses assist clients in obtaining it from other appropriate sources.
3. Nurses demonstrate sensitivity to the willingness/readiness of clients to receive information about their health condition and care options. Nurses respect the wishes of those who refuse, or are not ready, to receive information about their health condition.
4. Nurses practise within relevant legislation governing consent or choice. Nurses seek to ensure that nursing care is authorized by informed choice, and are guided by this ideal when participating in the consent process in cooperation with other members of the health team.
5. Nurses respect the informed decisions of competent persons to refuse treatment and to choose to live at risk. However, nurses are not obliged to comply with clients' wishes when doing so would require action contrary to the law. If the care requested is contrary to the nurse's moral beliefs, appropriate care is provided until alternative care arrangements are in place to meet the client's needs.

6. Nurses are sensitive to their position of relative power in professional relationships with clients and take care to foster self-determination on the part of their clients. Nurses are sufficiently clear about personal values to recognize and deal appropriately with potential value conflicts.
7. Nurses respect decisions and lawful directives, written or verbal, about present and future health care choices affirmed by a client prior to becoming incompetent.
8. Nurses seek to involve clients of diminished competence in decision-making to the extent that those clients are capable. Nurses continue to value autonomy when illness or other factors reduce the capacity for self-determination, such as by providing opportunities for clients to make choices about aspects of their lives for which they maintain the capacity to make decisions.
9. Nurses seek to obtain consent for nursing care from a substitute decision-maker when clients lack the capacity to make decisions about their care, did not make their wishes known prior to becoming incompetent, or for any reason it is unclear what the client would have wanted in a particular circumstance. When prior wishes of an incompetent client are not known or are unclear, care decisions must be in the best interest of the client and based on what the client would want, as far as is known.

DIGNITY

Nurses value and advocate the dignity and self-respect of human beings.

1. Nurses relate to all persons receiving care as persons worthy of respect and endeavour in all their actions to preserve and demonstrate respect for each individual.
2. Nurses exhibit sensitivity to the client's individual needs, values, and choices. Nursing care is designed to accommodate the biological, psychological, social, cultural, and spiritual needs of clients. Nurses do not exploit clients' vulnerabilities for their own interests or gain, whether this be sexual, emotional, social, political, or financial.
3. Nurses respect the privacy of clients when care is given.
4. Nurses treat human life as precious and worthy of respect. Respect includes seeking out and honouring clients' wishes regarding quality of life. Decision-making about life-sustaining treatment carefully balances these considerations.
5. Nurses intervene if others fail to respect the dignity of clients.
6. Nurses advocate the dignity of clients ill the use of technology in the health care setting.
7. Nurses advocate health and social conditions that allow persons to live with dignity throughout their lives and in the process of dying. They do so in ways that are consistent with their professional role and responsibilities.

CONFIDENTIALITY

Nurses safeguard the trust of clients that information learned in the context of a professional relationship is shared outside the health care team only with the client's permission or as legally required.

1. Nurses observe practices that protect the confidentiality of each client's health and health care information.
2. Nurses intervene if other participants in the health care delivery system fail to respect client confidentiality.
3. Nurses disclose confidential information only as authorized by the client, unless there is substantial risk of serious harm to the client or other persons, or a legal obligation to disclose. Where disclosure is warranted, both the amount of information disclosed and the number of people informed is restricted to the minimum necessary.
4. Nurses, whenever possible, inform their clients about the boundaries of professional confidentiality at the onset of care, including the circumstances under which confidential information might be disclosed without consent. If feasible, when disclosure becomes necessary, nurses inform clients what information will be disclosed, to whom, and for what reasons.
5. Nurses advocate policies and safeguards to protect and preserve client confidentiality and intervene if the security of confidential information is jeopardized because of a weakness in the provisions of the system, e.g., inadequate safeguarding guidelines and procedures for the use of computer databases.

FAIRNESS

Nurses apply and promote principles of equity and fairness to assist clients in receiving unbiased treatment and a share of health services and resources proportionate to their needs.

1. Nurses provide care in response to need regardless of such factors as race, ethnicity, culture, spiritual beliefs, social or marital status, gender, sexual orientation, age, health status, lifestyle or the physical attributes of the client.
2. Nurses are justified in using reasonable means to protect against violence when they anticipate acts of violence toward themselves, others or property with good reason.
3. Nurses strive to be fair in making decisions about the allocation of services and goods that they provide, when the distribution of these is within their control.

4. Nurses put forward, and advocate, the interests of all persons in their care. This includes helping individuals and groups gain access to appropriate health care that is of their choosing.
5. Nurses promote appropriate and ethical care at the institutional/agency and community levels by participating, to the extent possible, in the development, implementation, and ongoing review of policies and procedures designed to make the best use of available resources and of current knowledge and research.
6. Nurses advocate, in ways that are consistent with their role and responsibilities, health policies and decision-making procedures that are fair and comprehensive, and that promote fairness and inclusiveness in health resource allocation.

ACCOUNTABILITY

Nurses act in a manner consistent with their professional responsibilities and standards of practice.

1. Nurses comply with the values and responsibilities in this *Code of Ethics for Registered Nurses* as well as with the professional standards and laws pertaining to their practice.
2. Nurses conduct themselves with honesty and integrity.
3. Nurses, whether they are engaged in clinical, administrative, research, or educational endeavours, have professional responsibilities and accountabilities toward safeguarding the quality of nursing care clients receive. These responsibilities vary but are all oriented to the expected outcome of safe, competent and ethical nursing practice.
4. Nurses, individually or in partnership with others, take preventive as well as corrective action to protect clients from unsafe, incompetent or unethical care.
5. Nurses base their practice on relevant knowledge, and acquire new skills and knowledge in their area of practice on a continuing basis, as necessary for the provision of safe, competent and ethical nursing care.
6. Nurses, whether engaged in clinical practice, administration, research or education, provide timely and accurate feedback to other nurses about their practice, so as to support safe and competent care and contribute to ongoing learning. By so doing, they also acknowledge excellence in practice.
7. Nurses practise within their own level of competence. They seek additional information or knowledge; seek the help, and/or supervision and help, of a competent practitioner; and/or request a different work assignment, when aspects of the care required are beyond their level of competence. In the meantime, nurses provide care within the level of their skill and experience.
8. Nurses give primary consideration to the welfare of clients and any possibility of harm in future care situations when they suspect unethical conduct or incompetent or unsafe care. When nurses have reasonable grounds for concern about the behaviour of colleagues in this regard, or about the safety of conditions in the care setting, they carefully review the situation and take steps, individually or in partnership with others, to resolve the problem.
9. Nurses support other nurses who act in good faith to protect clients from incompetent, unethical or unsafe care, and advocate work environments in which nurses are treated with respect when they intervene.
10. Nurses speaking on nursing and health-related matters in a public forum or a court provide accurate and relevant information.

PRACTICE ENVIRONMENTS CONDUCIVE TO SAFE, COMPETENT AND ETHICAL CARE

Nurses advocate practice environments that have the organizational and human support systems, and the resource allocations necessary for safe, competent and ethical nursing care.

1. Nurses collaborate with nursing colleagues and other members of the health team to advocate health care environments that are conducive to ethical practice and to the health and well-being of clients and others in the setting. They do this in ways that are consistent with their professional role and responsibilities.
2. Nurses share their nursing knowledge with other members of the health team for the benefit of clients. To the best of their abilities, nurses provide mentorship and guidance for the professional development of students of nursing and other nurses.
3. Nurses seeking professional employment accurately state their area(s) of competence and seek reasonable assurance that employment conditions will permit care consistent with the values and responsibilities of the code, as well as with their personal ethical beliefs.
4. Nurses practise ethically by striving for the best care achievable in the circumstances. They also make the effort, individually or in partnership with others, to improve practice environments by advocating on behalf of their clients as possible.
5. Nurses planning to participate in job action, or who practise in environments where job action occurs, take steps to safeguard the health and safety of clients during the course of the action.

SOME SUGGESTIONS FOR APPLICATION OF THE CODE IN SELECTED CIRCUMSTANCES

Steps to Address Incompetent, Unsafe and Unethical Care

- Gather the facts about the situation and ascertain the risks;
- Review relevant legislation and policies, guidelines and procedures for reporting incidents or suspected incompetent or unethical care and report, as required, any legally reportable offence;
- Seek relevant information directly from the colleague whose behaviour or practice has raised concerns, when this is feasible;
- Consult as appropriate with colleagues, other members of the team, professional nurses' associations, or others able to assist in resolving the problem;
- Undertake to resolve the problem as directly as possible consistent with the good of all parties;
- Advise the appropriate parties regarding unresolved concerns and, when feasible, inform the colleague in question of the reasons for your action;
- Refuse to participate in efforts to deceive or mislead clients about the cause of alleged harm or injury resulting from unethical or incompetent conduct.

Nurse Managers, Professional Associations and Client Safety

- Nurse managers seek to ensure that available resources and competencies of personnel are used efficiently;
- Nurse managers intervene to minimize the present danger and to prevent future harm when client safety is threatened due to inadequate resources or for some other reason;
- Professional nurses' associations support individual nurses and groups of nurses in promoting fairness and inclusiveness in health resource allocation. They do so in ways that are consistent with their role and functions.

Considerations in Student–Teacher–Client Relationships

- Student–teacher and student–client encounters are essential elements of nursing education and are conducted in accordance with ethical nursing practices;
- Clients are informed of the student status of the care giver and consent for care is obtained in compliance with accepted standards;
- Students of nursing are treated with respect and honesty by nurses and are given appropriate guidance for the development of nursing competencies;
- Students are acquainted with and comply with the provisions of the code.

Considerations in Taking Job Action

- Job action by nurses is often directed toward securing conditions of employment that enable safe and ethical care of current and future clients. However, action directed toward such improvements could work to the detriment of clients in the short term;
- Individual nurses and groups of nurses safeguard clients in planning and implementing any job action;
- Individuals and groups of nurses participating in job actions, or affected by job actions, share the ethical commitment to client safety. Their particular responsibilities may lead them to express this commitment in different but equally appropriate ways;
- Clients whose safety requires ongoing or emergency nursing care are entitled to have those needs satisfied throughout any job action;
- Members of the public are entitled to information about the steps taken to ensure the safety of clients during any job action.

A Code of Ethics History

1954 CNA adopts the ICN Code as its first Code of Ethics

1980 CNA moves to adopt its own code, entitled *CNA Code of Ethics: An Ethical Basis for Nursing in Canada*

1985 CNA adopts new code, called *Code of Ethics for Nursing*

1991 *Code of Ethics for Nursing* revised

1997 *Code of Ethics for Registered Nurses* adopted as updated code for CNA

References

1. Canadian Health Care Association/Canadian Medical Association/Canadian Nurses Association/Catholic Health Association of Canada/in association with the Canadian Bar Association. (1995). *Joint statement on resuscitative interventions*. Ottawa: Authors.
2. Canadian Home Care Association/Canadian Hospital Association/Canadian Long Term Care Association/Canadian Nurses Association/Canadian Public Health Association/Home Support Canada. (1994). *Joint statement on advance directives*. Ottawa: Authors.
3. Canadian Nurses Association. (1992). *The role of the nurse in the use of health care technology*. Ottawa: Author.
4. Canadian Nurses Association (1994). *A question of respect: Nurses and end of life treatment dilemmas*. Ottawa: Author.

5. Canadian Nurses Association. (1994). *Ethical guidelines for nurses in research involving human participants*. (2nd rev. ed.) Ottawa: Author.
6. Canadian Nurses Association. (1996). *Necessary support for safe nursing care*. Ottawa: Author.
7. Canadian Nurses Protective Society. (1993, September). *Confidentiality of health information: Your clients' rights*. *Info Law*, **1**(2). Ottawa: Author.
8. Canadian Nurses Protective Society. (1994, December). *Consent to treatment: The role of the nurse*. *Info Law*, **3**(2). Ottawa: Author.

Appendix B

CNA Nurse Registration/ Licensure Examinations[1]

NATURE AND PURPOSE OF THE EXAM

The CNA Examination (subsequently referred to as the RN Examination), like registration/licensure examinations in general, has a well-defined purpose: to protect the public by ensuring that those who are licensed possess sufficient knowledge and skills to perform important occupational activities safely and effectively (Canadian Psychological Association, 1987).[2] In the case of the RN Examination, the purpose is to determine whether or not examinees are prepared to practise nursing, without risk to their clients.

The examination content is based on nursing competencies—that is, the knowledge, abilities, skills, attitudes and judgement expected of a beginning practitioner are expressed within the examination, according to explicit guidelines and specifications, such that accurate decisions can be made on the ability of examinees to practise safely and effectively.

USE BY ALL PROVINCES

Since August 1980, passing the Canadian Nurses Association Registration/Licensure Examination has been one of the requirements for registration/licensure in all provinces and territories.[3] (From 1970 to this date, candidates from Quebec who wrote in French took an examination developed by the Order of Nurses of Quebec).

The registering/licensing authorities (see the list at the end of this appendix) impose eligibility criteria (e.g., completion of an approved program of nursing education) that provide additional guidelines for determining an individual's readiness to practise nursing.

ENGLISH AND FRENCH VERSIONS

Both English and French examinations are developed from a common document, entitled *The Blueprint for the Criterion-Referenced Nurse Registration/Licensure Examination (1993)*. Therefore, the content domain (i.e., the list of competencies) is common, as are the specifications for structural and contextual variables. The examinations are developed in each official language; that is, items are written by nurses in French or English for the respective examinations. To facilitate equivalency between different versions of the examination (i.e., English/French, or from one year to the next), a psychometrically sound test equating method is employed.

MINIMUM PASSING GRADE

The pass mark (standard) to be met on the RN Examination is established prior to the administration of the exam. The procedure involves extensive input from a panel of content experts who are familiar with the roles and responsibilities, scope of practice and expectations of a beginning practitioner. In addition to the expert input, other relevant data are carefully considered to ensure that the standard that examinees are required to achieve is fair and valid.

WHO IS ELIGIBLE TO WRITE?

All graduates of diploma and baccalaureate nursing programs from Canadian schools are eligible to write the RN Examination. Nurses trained outside Canada must apply through one of the provincial/territorial registering/licensing authorities to determine if they are eligible to write the examination.

WHERE ARE THE EXAMS WRITTEN?

The RN Examination is offered in all provinces and territories. The registering/licensing authorities are responsible for administering the examination in their province or territory. They determine the number and location of the examination writing centres in their jurisdiction. Writing centres are usually established in proximity to the nursing schools in each province.

HOW LONG ARE THE EXAMS?

There are 240-260 operational questions on the RN Examination, represented in two books. As well as the operational questions (i.e., those on which the exams are scored), there are a number of experimental questions which are included in order to assess their suitability for use on future examinations. Examinees are not scored on these experimental questions.

HOW OFTEN ARE THEY WRITTEN?

Since August 1995, the RN Examination will be offered in a one-day administration. The RN Examination is administered four times a year: in January, June, August and October. However, the number of times the RN Examination is offered in a particular jurisdiction is at the discretion of each registering/licensing authority.

EXPLANATION OF CONTENT

The content domain for the RN Examination is a list of 238 competencies[4] required for the safe and effective practice

---

[1] The information in this section was provided by Assessment Strategies Inc., the testing agency that develops the RN Examination for the Canadian Nurses Association.

[2] Canadian Psychological Association. (1987). *Guidelines for educational and psychological testing*. Old Chelsea, QC: Author.

[3] The following information deals with the examination that is in use until January 2000. Future versions may be different, as the exam is revised periodically.

[4] The list of competencies is currently under revision. The revised list of competencies will be used to develop the examinations to be introduced in the summer of 2000.

of beginning nurses in Canada. The content domain was developed from a nursing focus. This means that the metaparadigm nursing—namely, the concepts of person (client), health, environment and nursing—was accepted as a basic tenet.

A number of assumptions were made in developing the list of competencies for nurses beginning to practise. Specifically, the competencies are assumed to:

- include knowledge, abilities, skills, attitudes and judgement
- focus on the individual client, who is a member of a family, group or community
- focus on the client's responses to common predictable health situations throughout the life cycle
- include health promotion, illness prevention, restoration and maintenance of health, and care of the dying
- recognize that nurses beginning to practise are generalists prepared to practise collaboratively, in structured, supervised environments
- be directed towards the practice of the beginning nurse on entry into practice, regardless of education preparation.

The list of competencies is classified into seven categories, the first five representing the nursing process and the last two representing more general and ongoing aspects of nursing:

- Data Collection
- Analysis and Interpretation of Data
- Planning Care
- Implementation
- Evaluation
- Collaboration and Coordination
- Professional Practice

CRITERION-REFERENCED BASIS

The RN Examination is criterion-referenced. This means that the exam measures an individual's command of a specified content/skills domain. As well, scores on a criterion-referenced examination are interpreted in comparison with a predetermined performance standard, independent of the results obtained by other examinees.

TYPES OF QUESTIONS AND EXAMPLES

Questions on the RN Examination are of the objective type and are presented in one of two formats: case-based (i.e., a brief introductory text accompanied by approximately five related questions) or independent items (i.e., stand-alone questions that are not specifically connected with any other text or questions).

Sample Questions: Case-Based

Case 1

Mr. Robert Lowry, an 82-year-old married man, collapses at home. Mr. Lowry is rushed to the community hospital where it is determined that he has suffered a cerebrovascular accident (CVA). Mrs. Lowry tells the nurse that, prior to this incident, her husband had been taking hydrochlorothiazide (HydroDiuril) to control his hypertension.

Questions 1 to 5 refer to this case. (*indicates correct answer)

1. Which one of the following initial nursing assessments would determine Mr. Lowry's level of consciousness?

  1. Visual fields
  2. Auditory acuity
  3. Reaction to cold
  *4. Responses to painful stimuli

2. Mr. Lowry regains consciousness and is found to have loss of movement on his left side and hemianopsia. Which one of the following responses by the nurse would be appropriate to give Mrs. Lowry when she asks questions regarding her husband's potential for recovery?

  1. "It sounds as though you may be somewhat anxious to resume your former lifestyle."
  2. "It's difficult to know, but most people take at least a year to recover completely."
  *3. "Concern about recovery is common. Rehabilitation takes time and progress is often slow."
  4. "To be anxious is normal. Unfortunately, there is no way of estimating your husband's recovery potential."

3. Mr. Lowry is receiving a thiazide diuretic. Which one of the following manifestations would indicate mild hypokalemia?

  *1. Anorexia; irregular and weak pulse
  2. Agitation; redness and dryness of skin
  3. Hyperrefliexia; numbness and tingling of fingers
  4. Abdominal cramps; anxiety and changes in personality

4. Which one of the following interventions should the nurse implement to encourage Mr. Lowry to feed himself?

  1. Assist him to position the cutlery in his hands
  2. Suggest that Mrs. Lowry take him to the cafeteria
  3. Allow sufficient time for him to cut up his own food.
  *4. Arrange food items on his tray so that he can see them

5. Which one of the following nursing observations of Mrs. Lowry's behaviour would best indicate her readiness to participate in her husband's care at home?
   1. She selects his daily menus
   2. She visits her husband every day
   3. She brings his shaving kit and pajamas from home
   *4. She asks if she is correctly positioned to help him walk

Sample Questions: Independent

1. Which of the following nursing measures would most likely facilitate a client's acceptance of an altered body image following a total laryngectomy and tracheostomy?
   1. Emphasize what the client can do within the limitations resulting from the treatment
   2. Encourage the client's family to refrain from discussing the tracheostomy while visiting
   3. Demonstrate a sympathetic approach when providing the client's tracheostomy care
   *4. Reassure the client that following discharge there can be a complete return to pre-hospitalization activities
2. What should the nurse do if, in the nurse's opinion, the physician's order for a postoperative analgesic seems excessive?
   1. Assess the client closely for side effects after giving the drug
   *2. Seek clarification from the physician before giving the medication
   3. Give the medication and document the concern in the nursing notes
   4. Withhold the medication and document the reason in the nursing notes

To obtain information on writing the Nurse Registration/Licensure Examination, contact any of the provincial/territorial registering/licensing authorities:

Alberta Association of Registered Nurses
11620- 168th Street
Edmonton, Alberta T5M 4A6
(403) 451-0043
Fax: (403) 452-3276

Association of Nurses of Prince Edward Island
17 Pownal Street, Box 1838
Charlottetown, Prince Edward Island C1A 3V7
(902) 368-3764
Fax: (902) 628-1430

Association of Registered Nurses of Newfoundland
55 Military Road
P.O. Box 6116
St. John's, Newfoundland A1C 5X8
(709) 753-6040
Fax: (709) 753-4940

College of Nurses of Ontario
101 Davenport Road
Toronto, Ontario M5R 3P1
(416) 928-0900, ext. 860
Fax: (416) 928-6507
Toll Free: 1-800-387-5526

Manitoba Association of Registered Nurses
647 Broadway Avenue
Winnipeg, Manitoba R3C 0X2
(204) 774-3477
Fax: (204) 775-6052

Northwest Territories Registered Nurses Association
P.O. Box 2757
Yellowknife, Northwest Territories
X1A 2R1
(403) 873-2745
Fax: (403) 873-2336

Nurses Association of New Brunswick
165 Regent Street
Fredericton, New Brunswick
E3B 3W5
(506) 458-8731
Fax: (506) 459-2857

Ordre des infirmières et infirmiers du Québec
4200 ouest boulevard Dorchester
Montréal, Québec H3Z 1V4
(514) 935-2501
Fax: (514) 935-1799
Toll Free: 1-800-363-6048

Registered Nurses Association of British Columbia
2855 Arbutus Street
Vancouver, British Columbia
V6J 3Y8
(604) 736-7331
Fax: (604) 738-2272

Registered Nurses Association of Nova Scotia
Suite 104, 120 Eileen Stubbs Ave.
Darmouth, Nova Scotia
B3B 1Y1
(902) 468-9744
Fax: (902) 468-9510

Saskatchewan Registered Nurses Association
2066 Retallack Street
Regina, Saskatchewan
S4T 2K2
(306) 757-4643
Fax: (306) 525-0849

Yukon Registered Nurses Association
Suite 14, 1114-1st Avenue
Whitehorse, Yukon
Y1A 1A3
(403) 667-4062
Fax: (403) 668-5123

Appendix C

The Internet, Nursing Research and Continuing Education

FRANK J. KNOR

Today we are in the throes of the *Information Age*. This means, in part, that mankind's knowledge, as a whole, will double in approximately seven years. This rate of change is even greater in some disciplines—including those in nursing and general health—where some experts state that doubling time may be as brief as two years. The dynamics of these rapid changes mean that in order to remain current in our chosen fields and avoid becoming functional "dinosaurs," we must continue to be students and researchers throughout our working lives.

Many of us will employ textbooks, such as this one, to bring us tried and tested information. We must recognize, however, that the information in textbooks is not as current as the material one can find in periodical publications (the journals, magazines, newspapers, etc. that are published every year, month, week, or day). Since the growth of computer usage, finding information on reports or articles in these publications is no longer limited to use of print-based indexes or abstracts. Today, a rapidly increasing number of sources to which we look for both historical and current documents are electronic tools and databases presented in digital formats. We can access these documents using special search strategies, moving from documents, to indexes, to graphics, to pictures, all found in a network of computers located in over 150 countries around the world. The network referred to, of course, is *the Internet*, and the use of this network to move from resource to resource has been called *surfing the Internet*. Let's have a look at what recent Internet developments mean to nursing students and other healthcare researchers.

An Overview of the Internet

Please note that the inclusion or exclusion of companies, services, or sites referred to or cited does in no way constitute specific recommendations or lack thereof.

Information on the Internet is practically inescapable today. All forms of media, be they television or radio programs, magazines, newspapers, or books, now advertise their locations on the growing network of millions of computer sites that can be found on the Internet. The Internet addresses for these locations are known as URLs (meaning Universal Resource Locators). These URLs consist of letters and/or symbols separated by periods, and when activated, will lead you to a coded page of information on a computer site somewhere in the world. The URLs usually appear in the following form:

http://name_of_site.computer_name.country

In North America, a three-letter code is sometimes used instead of a country suffix, to indicate the type of organization hosting the site, e.g.:

.com	(for commercial organizations)
.gov	(for government organizations)
.edu	(for educational institutions)

A URL example: http://www.hc-sc.gc.ca.

(The Internet address for *Health Canada Online)*, where:

http:	= hypertext telnet protocol 'transmission code type'
www	= the World Wide Web (WWW)
hc-sc.gc	= the name of computer site (or "domain name"), i.e. Health Canada, Government of Canada
.ca	= country where the site is located (in this case, Canada)

URL names actually represent an equivalent number, which in this example is 198.103.237.8. You can enter this number (rather than the URL) on your browser and it will find *Health Canada Online*.

As an example of the wealth of information on just this *Health Canada Online* Web site, there is information on and links to: The Minister of Health, AIDS, cancer, children, consumer products, disease info, drugs, First Nations, funding, healthy living, heart health, hepatitis, home care, media literacy, men's health issues, news releases, nutrition, pharmacare, pregnancy, provincial links, safety, schools, seniors, sexuality/STDs, smoking, warnings, women's health, etc.

Due to the huge growth of information and the numbers of computers connecting to the Internet, there is a rapid change in domain names and URLs. In some cases the URLs are changing because there simply are not enough numbers to cover the demand for domain names and URL addresses. Unfortunately there are no "change of address" forms as we have with regular mail address changes. Currently, URLs are in a great state of change, so you may encounter errors when trying to connect to Web sites. When an Internet URL changes, you will have to search to find the new URL. You may be able to find the site if it has moved, but do not be surprised if the information simply has been dropped and no longer exists online.

One can find the addresses for and information from companies, businesses, educational institutions, government resources, research publications, commercial publications, training materials, professional and special interest news and information groups covering just about any topic imaginable. Growth and change on the Internet is abundant, with hundreds of thousands of new pages of information in a variety of forms being developed daily. But don't let these numbers daunt you: the search process is relatively simple, and will be dealt with briefly in a following section.

Technically, *the Internet* means more than just the World Wide Web (WWW) and finding pages on computers as directed by their URL addresses. There is the very popular form of communication called *e-mail*, whereby electronic "mail" messages can be sent between computer mailboxes. Other forms of communication can be used between computer sites; however, these are rapidly being replaced by the more common Internet communication protocols. There is also an increased emergence of digital radio and digital video imaging and transmission, animated graphics, and a multitude of interactive options due to the use of special applets and programming languages such as CGI, and Java. Some of these formats require specialized microcomputer equipment and software for effective use. These variable requirements mean that a new microcomputer probably has a functional life of about two to three years. Remember that the Internet itself is the best teacher of technical developments, as it provides a variety of sites with detailed, and very often up-to-the minute explanations. You can quickly learn the skills necessary to find information on the Internet by following the tips presented in this guide.

How To Use The Internet—Self Study

The Internet is so easy to use that, even with limited exposure, most of us experience an early feeling of confidence. Unfortunately, this feeling is often misleading. You may discover that you are jumping from page to page to image to picture, and surfing up a storm, but you may be wasting a lot of time and missing some of the most valuable information the Internet has to offer. It is well worth your time to visit one or more of the following self-study sites, which can help you to use your time on the Internet most effectively.

NETSCAPE: WHAT IS IT AND HOW TO USE IT

http://www.lib.berkeley.edu/TeachingLib/Guides/Internet/NetscapeBasics.html#what

This excellent tutorial gives written and illustrative explanations on how to use the Netscape browser.

LEARN HOW TO USE NETSCAPE: A TUTORIAL

http://home.netscape.com/eng/mozilla/2.02/handbook/docs/learn.html#C0

A tutorial presented by the creators of Netscape to help you understand the basics of the popular Netscape program. Other infomation options are also available.

FINDING INFORMATION ON THE INTERNET

http://www.lib.berkeley.edu/TeachingLib/Guides/Internet/FindInfo.html

This excellent program gives you an extensive set of tutorials—including the Netscape tutorial mentioned above—that help you learn from a variety of programs. Everything from Internet basics, to advanced user techniques, to examples for use with specific search engines are available.

INTERNET SEARCH TOOLS & TECHNIQUES

http://www.ouc.bc.ca/libr/connect96/search.htm

A second tutorial choice designed to help you learn basic functions of the WWW search engines and search results by using some of the specialized search engines that have been mentioned.

USING AND UNDERSTANDING THE INTERNET

http://www.pbs.org/uti/

This self-study site from PBS includes tips for the beginner as well as details for the more advanced user. This site also supplies links to a variety of software choices you can download to add onto Netscape and Microsoft Explorer.

How To Access The Internet

The Internet is a network of computers connected to each other by a variety of telecommunication systems. These systems include high-speed telephone lines, cable or fibre-optic lines, microwave transmission links, and even wireless radio wave connections including satellite up- and down-links. In order to access the Internet, you must connect your microcomputer (or terminal) to this network, just like a lamp must be connected to an electrical outlet, whereby electrical wires provide it with electricity. An Internet connection differs from an electrical connection in that the Internet connection requires another gateway computer link between your microcomputer and the network. This gateway computer functions to interpret and direct your user messages and commands. A computer that functions in this manner is called an *Internet Service Provider* (ISP). Connections to ISPs are usually provided in two general ways: via networks provided by institutions or via home connections through your computer modem or cable television.

You can connect to an ISP and the Internet in many major modern institutions. In these cases, your microcomputer plugs into a specially designed internal wiring system called a computer network, usually an "Ethernet" or "Token Ring" network. Plugging into this network and operating appropriate software connects your single microcomputer station to other single stations and to another larger computer within the institution called *a server*. In most instances, these institutional networks provide a special host computer. This host computer will likely operate as your ISP, providing a gateway from your microcomputer to the Internet at large. If the institution does not provide an ISP computer, then it will at least direct you to an outside service agency which offers this service. Your ISP computer may also provide you with the home address for your e-mail. In such a cases, your e-mail address may be something like the following:

Your_name@Your_institution.Province.Country, such as "fknor@bcit.bc.ca," (where the institution's Internet URL is http://www.bcit.bc.ca)

As a home microcomputer user, you also must connect to an ISP before you can access the Internet. Currently, the most common method is to purchase a modem for your microcomputer that will permit you to make a telephone connection to an ISP company. An increasingly popular option is to connect to an ISP and the Internet via your cable television. New equipment is being developed for cable that can offer subscribers a small "black box" with built-in software. You may have heard or seen advertisements for these under the name of *WebTV*. You simply connect this black box to your television set and cable, register as a user, and you are set. You then use the black box with a remote mouse/keyboard to surf and control Internet access, which you view on your television set. Depending upon the method of connection and ISP company you choose, your monthly fee will probably fall into the range of $20-60 for Internet access. This fee will also include use of a personal e-mail account. This address will enable you to use Internet software to send and receive electronic messages via the ISP's computers. In order to use/surf the Internet, send e-mail and be able to employ other Internet user options, you must be running Internet software. The following are references to some Internet Service Providers where you can obtain further details:

Internet Gateway Service
http://www.intergate.bc.ca

An example of a service provider with competitive rates.

National Capital Region ISPs
http://home.on.rogers.wave.ca/mreid/ottisp/index.html

A Web site that gives details of major service providers in the Ottawa area and those with outlets across Canada.

Rogers' Wave—Cable Internet Access
http://home.on.rogers.wave.ca/mreid/rogwave/index.html

A good explanation of cable access to the Internet available from Rogers.

Sympatico Internet Service Provider
http://www.mb.sympatico.ca/Sympatico_Help/About/

Sympatico is a Canadian national Internet service. Sympatico membership gives you free Internet software, reliable connections, friendly toll-free support, and a Web site made by and for Canadians.

Internet Software

When you select your ISP, part of the fee you are charged pays for special Internet software, collectively known as *Web browser software*. This software has been developed to allow you to use the Internet, receive text pages, images, sounds, and much more. For all but the most sophisticated computer users, it is safe to say that this software must be operational on your microcomputer before you can access the Internet. Once your browser software is operational and your ISP connects you to the Internet, you can become an Internet user. The vast majority of Internet Web users run one of two software packages: *Netscape Communicator*, or *Microsoft Internet Explorer*. This software provides your microcomputer station with the ability to use all of the features available on the Internet, mainly, the ability to view pages of text and images. In many cases, the text or the images you view are active links. You will recognize these because the text is underlined, the images are surrounded with a line, or they may cause a change in your mouse cursor arrow when they are pointed to. These are active (or "hot") links you use to move from one page or image to another. To do this, you simply use your computer's mouse. Place the mouse cursor arrow on active text reference or image reference link to where you want to go, click the mouse button, and the software will take you to the page indicated by the link. In this manner you can move within a Web site or change from one Web site to another. In addition, the software will let you print pages, save text and images, and open up windows that allow you to reply to interactive Internet pages or send e-mail. You are even able to download copies of the most recent versions of Web browser software, free of charge. Downloading software to your own computer is easily accomplished; however, large programs and files can take a long time to be transferred.

Speed of file transfer and Internet performance depends, to some degree, upon the quality and features of your local microcomputer; however, it primarily depends upon the speed of your Internet connection. Modem connection over telephone lines is the slowest, followed by cable, with fibre-optic connections being the fastest. The faster your personal computer and the faster your Internet connection, the faster your Internet performance will be. Remember, in computers and in telecommunications, the faster the speed the greater the costs. Your needs as well as budget will help you decide on your options. Details on the two most popular software packages may are available from the following company Web sites:

Netscape Netcenter
http://home.netscape.com

The front door to the Netscape Corporation, with numerous links to company and general Internet options, including search engines. This site allows you to download the *Netscape Communicator* Web browser.

Microsoft Corporation
http://microsoft.com/default.htm

The main corporate page of the giant Microsoft Corporation. This page is filled with general information and software on the Internet including free software from Microsoft—featuring their Internet browser *Internet Explorer*.

In summary, to use the Internet, you simply need a microcomputer (or a special television "black box"), Internet software, and a telecommunication connection to an Internet Service Provider (ISP). With these pieces in place, you are ready to join approximately 50 million other Internet users.

Tips on Using the Internet

Perhaps the easiest way to visualize the information on the Internet is to consider it as existing in two forms. The most common form for information is Web pages. The second form is for information to appear as databases. Let's deal with the pages first.

Web pages can be likened to millions of newspaper or magazine pages that exist in millions of filing cabinets around the world. To find these pages, you must use search strategies to direct you to the filing cabinet (i.e. computer site) and then to the actual page or series of linked pages (i.e. the Internet Web pages) that you want. Fortunately, a number of companies have developed search software and huge digital indexes that help us find these pages according to the contents and topics the pages cover. Using a search engine is similar to searching in a library computer catalogue for a book. Likewise, Internet search strategies are also similar to those you use to search for topics in a book by using the book's index. So, at the basic level, searching is really not rocket science. Let's expand and explain searching further.

Keyword or Word Basic Searching

In this method, you simply identify the word, words, or phrases that you want to find on Internet pages. These words may represent topics, names (of people, companies, places or things), or other significant words that identify what you seek.

e.g.: Enter words such as: *herbs*, *"herbal remedy"*, *homeopathy*, *carcinogen*, *myotome*, *"Jean Chretien"* ,*"Health Canada"*, *Vancouver*.

TIP: The more specific and unique the words you use, the more precise your search response will be. The use of common words such as "computer," and "nurse," will result in thousands of vague references that will be of low precision and of limited value to you. Some of the search engines will deal with phases if you indicate that they are phases by using quotation marks, as in the examples shown. If this phrase connection is not used, each word will be searched separately, resulting in an imprecise search with a large number of references you do not want or need, called garbage output or *false drops*.

Subject Heading Basic Searching

As you will recall from your experience using library catalogues and book indexes, you can often find information by searching for subject headings. The advantage of using subject headings is that when they are properly employed, they will group and list together a number of items—in this case Web pages—that are of the same or similar topics. Thus, one-well chosen subject heading can lead you to a wealth of related pages. Subject heading searching can only be performed using Web search engines where the pages have been arranged according to these headings (as opposed to the random keyword arrangements).

e.g.: Enter your subject heading terms: *Psychiatric nursing*, *critical patient care*, *hospice*, *etc*.

TIP: The more specific the subject heading, the more precise the response. For example, the subject term *psychiatric nursing* will give a more focussed response than *nursing*. The problem, however, is that the index you are searching uses only a limited vocabulary and number of subject terms. The index may not use some of the subject headings you enter. It is always better to start with more general headings, such as *nursing*, and then browse the index to see if more specific headings are employed. Remember, all possible subject headings are not necessarily used. Thus, if you cannot find one subject heading, then try entering synonyms for the subject heading.

e.g.: If you can't find *cars*, then try searching for *automobiles*.

References

The following sites provide excellent examples of health-related subject searching:

Medsite: Your online source for medical information.
http://www.medsite.com

Provides medical subject heading groupings and information on a wide range of health- and medical-related topics. Current medical news is provided. For those of you who like to get into Internet chat forums, their Medical Community forum might be just what you are looking for. This impressive and well-supported medical ISP provides an opportunity for users to establish a free e-mail address.

Sympatico Health Link Reviews
http://www.mb.sympatico.ca/healthyway/health.html

This Canadian service provider allows subject searching including a vast array of Canadian-focussed health-related information. Topical areas as diverse as active living and health food recipes to sex and sexuality are covered.

Yahoo Canada - Health Sources
http://www.yahoo.ca/Health

An excellent subject heading approach to health resources and topics. You may limit your searches to Canadian only resources or make your search "world-wide".

Advanced Boolean Logic Searching

The Internet contains millions of references. One of the most frustrating situations that new users often experience is the inability to find what they seek. Searchers are often either overwhelmed with incorrect (false drop) results, or they can't find anything at all. If you are going to become an effective Internet researcher, you will have to learn how to do advanced searching using Boolean logic. Simply stated, Boolean logic is the combination of sets of keywords; constructed by joining the terms with the words "and," "or," and "not". It works something like this:

"Or" Boolean Searches

Enter: *children or infants*

This finds and combines a search set for children and a set for infants.

This is useful for broadening your search because you are including synonyms.

"And" Boolean Searches

Enter: *children and nutrition*

This finds and combines sets that include *only both* of the terms.

This is useful for narrowing your search—by ensuring that *all concepts* are present.

Caution: When you do an "and" search and when one of the sets you are combining contains nothing, the total result will be nothing. It is always best to first start with broad terms and then narrow your search by using "and."

Combining "Or" and "And" Boolean Searches

It is easy to see the efficiency that can be gained by performing either of the preceeding examples, but you can achieve even greater efficiency by combining these searches. You simply enter the search sets using brackets to group search activities, as shown by the following:

Enter: *(children or infants) and (diet or nutrition)*

This one search statement finds and combines all of the preceding searches. The results will contain either of the words *children* or *infants*, and either *diet* or *nutrition.*

Using Truncation to Expand Search Options

Most of the search engines also permit you to search for prefixes (stems) of words. You do this by truncating your search words using an asterisk (*). This is especially useful for finding singular and plural forms of words, as *infant* and *infants*. Notice the results of the following search using truncation.

Enter: *child**

Will find: *child's, childbirth, childhood, childish, childless, childlike, and children.*

Putting it All Together

Now that you have become familiar with all of the individual Boolean logic options, you are able to put together some very sophisticated searches. Remember that if any of the search words have zero results, your final search results will be zero when the "and" combination function is used. The following example shows how to do both Boolean and truncation in a detailed search statement designed to find information on the all of the examples cited earlier, using one search statement.

Enter: *(child* or infant*) and (nutrition or diet*)*

TIP: Remember that the Internet itself is the best teacher of online information. In addition to the general training references provided in this section, do check the help pages with all the search engines. These help pages give excellent guidance for using the features of their specific search engines.

Search Engine References

Some of the Internet search companies that provide word searching also provide excellent subject searching. The best known and largest company that specializes in providing subject headings is Yahoo. Most of these search engines offer basic keyword searching as well as advanced searching options which permit Boolean searching and the use of truncation. Keep in mind that there is currently a tremendous amount of activity in this very competitive market, with a number of recent sales that may impact some functions of the Internet search companies. *Remember also that the major library catalogues from around the world are now on the Internet.* You can locate these libraries by searching for the name of the institutions with which they are associated. You can try the same searches on a number of search engines and decide on your favourite—there are major differences among the services. Also be certain to check under subject headings in those engines that offer this feature. Some subject areas are excellent sources.

Alta Vista Canada
http://www.altavistacanada.com

Offers a large database with both simple and advanced Boolean and phrase search options. Also includes a full-text index of newsgroups updated in real-time. A great choice for Canadian information which may not appear in the U.S. Alta Vista search site.

Excite Netsearch
http://www.excite.com

One of the largest widely-used sites offering basic and advanced search engine options plus the ability to browse/search by subject categories. Excite allows you to search using keywords and concepts. You can also search and browse a collection of Web site reviews, and set up your own version of the Excite home page.

Hotbot
http://www.hotbot.com

A highly-rated, good all-around search engine. In addition to regular and advanced searching, it offers a number of specialty databases which are useful for searching special Internet resources, such as images, pictures, sounds, telephone numbers and stocks.

InfoSeek Net Search
http://www2.infoseek.com

Claims to be one of the fastest and most comprehensive search engines with the largest databases on the Internet. Offers a basic word plus advanced searching. You can also browse/search by subject categories. Search results are ranked according to relative accuracy.

Lycos, Inc.
http://www.lycos.com

Uses a keyword search and permits Boolean as well as phrase searching. It has the added feature of providing subject-oriented search/browse options as well as a directory and critical reviews of the top five percent of popular Web sites.

Magellan
http://www.mckinley.com

This site offers basic searching plus search/browse by subject. As a special features, it permits you to locate reviewed Web sites by subject. You can also restrict your search to their recommended "green light" sites.

Metacrawler
http://www.metacrawler.com/index.html

One of the more popular meta (multiple site) search programs. This engine displays your search results simultaneously from a number of major search engines. In effect, this unified Web search engine queries the Web's most popular engines for you at the same time, collates and verifies the results. Keep in mind that each Web engine site is not fully searched and the *levels* of searches on these other sites are not as complete as searching each site individually. This meta search is particularly useful when you are having problems locating anything from individual search sites. Search results can be overwhelming and imprecise for regular searches.

WhoWhatWhere
http://www.whowhere.com

One of the best people search locations. Includes other special advanced search options that help you locate people with special interests, from certain organizations and companies.

WebCrawler Searching
http://Webcrawler.com

A WWW search site that also includes subject/browse search capability. It searches Web page titles and contents, and returns a sorted list of links. WebCrawler is easy to use and now capable of simple Boolean searching.

Yahoo
http://www.yahoo.ca (the Canadian database site)
http://www.yahoo.com (the U.S.A. site)

One of the first successful search sites to use a subject/browse approach to organizing WWW information. Keyword search options are offered, plus special features including a weekly selected listing of new sites. The relatively new Canadian site is an excellent choice for Canadian companies, organizations, and associations.

Researching Using Internet Indexes and Databases

The other form of research technique that exists is the searching of databases and indexes of published information. Librarians and researchers have long been using this information in printed form, and most of these printed indexes for the health areas still exist in this form. Fortunately for us, most of the important health indexes also exist in digital form that can be searched on the Internet using our browser software. This means that you can use the Boolean and sophisticated search strategies that have been discussed. Thanks to computers and Boolean searches, you can look up complicated search concept results in minutes, whereas a similar search without the computer using only printed indexes could take hours. Since health-care is subsidized by governments, we now can find some of these major indexes available for our use without charge. Unfortunately, some of the other significant database indexes are available as *pay-for-use*, and require subscription and sometimes user charges.

In these pay-for-use cases, most of us turn to our academic libraries or large institutions where database subscription and user fees are usually paid for by the libraries. Members of these institutions can access these valuable resources free or for little cost. Certainly this is an option that should be explored—visit your local libraries to check them out.

Following is a listing of some major professional indexes that you should be aware of and employ if you plan on doing serious nursing and medical research:

CINAHL®
http://www.cinahl.com/

The CINAHL® database, published by Cinahl Information Systems, provides access to nursing and allied health literature and information from 1982 to the present. Coverage of virtually every nursing journal published, this database also features physical therapy, occupational therapy, emergency services, consumer health, alternative therapies, and health sciences librarianship. You can test this pay-as-you-search Internet database from this location, the CINAHL® home page.

EBSCO Host Online
http://www.epnet.com/

Ebsco Publishing provides this pay-for-use online Internet database service as part of their company offerings. Active subscribers may connect from the Internet and search for articles written in periodicals and, in many cases, view and print the full text of the article from their microcomputer Internet station. Of particular interest to the health and medical areas is the *Health Source Plus* database—a database providing abstracts and indexing for nearly 500 consumer health, nutrition and professional periodicals. Over 200 periodicals and 1000 health pamphlets are covered in full text. Unfortunately, few graphic images are yet available in this service.

MEDLINE: PubMed and Internet Grateful Med
http://www.nlm.nih.gov/databases/freemedl.html

Every health researcher should know about Medline, the online version of *Index Medicus*, produced by the National Library of Medicine. *PubMed* provides free access to the Medline database of more than nine million references to articles published in 3800 biomedical journals. Also accessible free of charge on the World Wide Web is *Internet Grateful Med,* which provides free access to Medline, Aidsline, HealthSTAR, Aidsdrubs, Aidstrials, Dirline, Histline, HSRproj, and Oldmedline databases.

MEDLINE via HealthGate: Free MEDLINE Access
http://www.healthgate.com/HealthGate/MEDLINE/search-advanced.shtml

Another link to a wonderful service that provides free database searching access. This site also offers an index of recent articles in Medline, as well as the following: *aidsdrugs; aidsline; aidstrials; bioethicsline; cancerlit; healthstar;* free pages for publications and services including *Doodys Review Service, Diagnostic Procedures, Healthy Living, Healthy Eating, Healthy Parenting, Healthy Sexuality, Healthy Woman,* and much more.

UMI and ProQuest Direct Service
http://www.umi.com

The UMI is a company that also provides pay-for-use information. Their library includes materials in subjects from Asian studies to zoology. Of particular importance for Internet users, UMI offers a service called *ProQuest Direct*. This service provides immediate online access to UMI's extensive collection of newspapers, journals, periodicals, magazines, and other information sources. Abstracts and indexing to articles from over 3000 publications are represented. You can obtain many of these publications in full text, meaning you can print or download the complete article to your computer site. Full graphs, charts and photo images are also available as part of these articles and are fully searchable. Of particular interest for health is *ProQuest's* Medical Library. It combines MEDLINE indexing with full text and images for more than 100 key medical titles. You can even test drive examples from their home page.

UnCover Reveal
http://uncWeb.carl.org/reveal/index.html

This pay-for-use service offers tremendous potential for the researcher. In addition to viewing the tables of contents of over 16 000 periodicals, you can set up a free automated alerting service. Your service is based upon your choice of periodical titles and search strategies. The printed periodical tables of contents are sent directly to your e-mail box as each new issue appears. Should you want copies of an article, you can order and pay for individual articles from UnCover online and interactively. UnCover will also rapidly fax copies of articles you order.

Cautionary Advice About The Internet

The preceeding references provide you with some excellent resources that you can find and use on the Internet largely without cost. I am sure you have heard the adage: *if something is free that's exactly what it is worth.* Unfortunately, for some of the information on the Internet, this statement is very true. Even worse, some of the information you may encounter is incorrect. This may be accidental and relatively harmless, or may in fact be maliciously misleading, with possible unpleasant consequences.

A recent, highly publicized example of erroneous information provides us with an apt anecdote: a U.S. Senator went into the U.S. Senate and reported that the world famous comedian Bob Hope had died. You can imagine how surprised the alive and well Bob Hope was when he heard news reports about this, and you can envision the scramble to correct this error by the Senator and by the news media. Fortunately, this piece of bad Internet information did not have any lasting or fatal results. The message from this example is that you must ensure, as much as possible, that the information you receive and use is, in fact, correct and accurate, free from bias and can withstand scrutiny, including the verification of credible references.

Sometimes a little information can be dangerous, especially if the information is taken out of context. As a further example, consider the following cautionary notice given by Medsite, the major health information provider:

> *The information on Medsite.com is for educational purposes only. Medsite.com is not engaged in rendering medical advice or professional services. The information provided throughout medsite.com should not be used for diagnosing or treating a health problem or disease. It is not a substitute for professional care.*

Also consider the message from the Canadian Red Cross Web site, which may seem especially cautious, perhaps due to the multi-million dollar legal suits they are facing in other arenas. This notice also points out the fact that information on the Internet is often covered by copyright, with ownership and use in accordance to Canadian and international copyright laws.

> *Authorized Use: The materials available from this Web site may be viewed and copied subject to the following conditions:*
>
> 1) *use must be for private, informational, and non-commercial purposes only;*
> 2) *graphics or photos available from this Web site may not be reproduced without the accompanying text and written permission from Canadian Red Cross and any other individual or group identified as having rights in the photo or graphic;*
> 3) *documentation, text, photos, or other information from this Web site may not be modified or altered in any way; and*
> 4) *all proprietary rights notices must be reproduced with any copy of any material reproduced in any form.*
>
> *You represent and warrant that it is legal to view this Web site in the jurisdiction to which you are subject and confirm that you are responsible for compliance with all laws of that jurisdiction, in viewing or using the information on this Web site.*

Considering these examples, you now are warned that use of information from the Internet should be tempered with common sense and with good judgement on behalf of the researcher.

An Annotated List Of Sites

The following list of URLs have been randomly selected as representing areas in which nursing students and health-care workers may be interested. While there is definitely a Canadian bias to this listing, most of the major nursing, health, and medical information sources are located outside of Canada.

Canadian and International Health Resource Associations and Organizations

The following represents a selected list of Web sites giving a cross-section of the thousands of health-related associations, societies, and special interest groups that can be found in Canada and on the Internet. Wherever possible, sites have been provided that offer indexes which point to more of these organizations.

About Face International
http://www.interlog.com/~abtface/

AboutFace is an international organization that provides information and emotional support for individuals and families with individuals who have facial differences.

Aboriginal Nurses Association of Canada (ANAC)
http://www.anac.on.ca/

ANAC is a non-governmental, non-profit organization whose membership works mainly in First Nations Communities. An affiliate group of the Canadian Nurses Association, it is the only Aboriginal professional nursing organization in Canada.

Al-Anon Family Groups
http://www.ycn.library.ns.ca/alanon/al-anon.html

The Al-Anon Family Groups are a fellowship of relatives and friends of alcoholics who share their experience, strength and hope in order to solve their common problems. Al-Anon believes alcoholism is a family illness and that changed attitudes can aid recovery.

Alcoholics Anonymous World Services, Inc.
http://www.alcoholics-anonymous.org/

This Web site is created and maintained by Alcoholics Anonymous World Services, Inc. ("The General Service Office" of U.S./Canada). The General Service Office is the national office serving AA in the U.S./Canada.

Alzheimer Society of Canada
http://www.iaw.on.ca/~asnr/alz_can.htm

This is a new site from the Alzheimer Society of Niagara Region. The site is dedicated to ensure quality services for individuals with Alzheimer disease and related dementias. They support and advocate for individuals, families, caregivers and community through counselling, education, and the promotion of research to compassionately respond to the very special needs of those experiencing dementia.

Anorexia Nervosa and Bulimia Association (ANAB)
http://www.ams.queensu.ca/anab/moreinfo.htm

An excellent resource for information on eating disorders.

Aplastic Anemia Foundation of America, Inc.
http://www.aplastic.org/

Provides information on and links to sites dealing with fighting Aplastic Anemia, Myelodysplastic Syndromes, and other bone marrow failure.

Arthritis Canada
http://www.arthritis.ca./new.html

This site provides links and resources to support Arthritis Canada's mission statement: *to search for the underlying causes and subsequent cures for arthritis, and to promote the best possible care and treatment for people with arthritis.*

Associations on the World Wide Web
http://www.knowres.on.ca/associations/

A useful listing of many Canadian family and general health-related associations, sponsored by the commercial company Knowledge Resources.

Asthma Society of Canada
http://www.asthmasociety.com/

A national volunteer-based organization devoted to enhancing the quality of life of people living with asthma and to eliminating the disorder.

Autism Society Manitoba (ASM)
http://www.enable.aroundmanitoba.com/orgs/asm/index.html

ASM has provided this guide for parents to offer information on their child's disorder and on services available in Manitoba. General links to other sites are included.

Big Brothers and Sisters of Canada
http://www.clo.com/~bbsc

Provides information on this organization stated as being dedicated to helping in the development of children growing up in primarily lone-parent families. There are over 950 000 boys and girls in Canada who live with one parent. These are the children served by 180 agencies across Canada.

Canada's Physical Activity Guide To Healthy Active Living
http://www.csep.ca/Canada's_Physical_Activity.html

The Fitness and Active Living Unit of Health Canada and the Canadian Society for Exercise Physiology (CSEP), have announced that they are working jointly on a project to develop Canada's Physical Activity Guide for use by the Canadian public.

Canadian AIDS Society (CAS)
http://www.cdnaids.ca/index_e.html

CAS is a national coalition of over 100 community-based AIDS organizations across Canada. They are dedicated to strengthening a positive response to HIV/AIDS across all sectors of society and to enriching the lives of people and communities living with HIV/AIDS. This site provides Canadian community contacts, general information resources, listing of events, general advocacy information and more.

Canadian Association on Gerontology (CAG)
http://www.cagacg.ca/

CAG is a professional organization which provides leadership in the area of aging in Canada. Through its many activities, CAG helps to foster research, education, and policy aimed at improving the quality of life of the elderly in Canada.

Canadian Association of Occupational Therapists (CAOT)
http://www.caot.ca/pages/About.html

This organization provides services, products, events and networking opportunities to assist occupational therapists achieve excellence in their professional practice. Also, CAOT provides national leadership to actively develop and promote the client-centred professions of occupational therapy in Canada and internationally.

Canadian Association of Optometrists
http://opto.ca

This site represents the profession of optometry and the association's 2800 members. In addition, it provides public information, member information, a link to the Eye Health Council of Canada, and general eye-care links.

Canadian Association of Social Workers
http://www.wlu.ca/~wwwcassw/english/index.html

States itself as being "a national non-governmental membership organization of educational institutions and associated individuals whose purpose is to advance the standards, effectiveness and relevance of social work education and scholarship in Canada." This site has sections dealing with the organization, board of accreditation, editorial board, Canadian social work review, publications, a directory of accredited schools, forthcoming conference lists, and general member information.

Canadian Association of Speech Pathologists and Audiologists (CASLPA)
http://www.caslpa.ca/

CASLPA is the single national body that supports the needs, interests and development of speech-language pathologists and audiologists across Canada. This site provides support for members, the membership exam and general information about the disciplines.

Canadian Association of the Deaf (CAD)
http://www.cad.ca/English/Introduction/WIS.htm

CAD is the national consumer organization of the deaf people of Canada. This site helps further the purposes of the association, which are to act as a research and information centre, an advisory council, a representative body, a self-help society, and a community action organization.

Canadian Cancer Society and the National Cancer Institute
http://www.cancer.ca/EnglishPages/mission.html

A national, community-based organization of volunteers, whose mission is the eradication of cancer and the enhancement of the quality of life of people living with cancer. This site provides resources and links to cancer-related sites.

Canadian Centre on Disability Studies
http://www.escape.ca/~ccds

The Canadian Centre on Disability Studies is a consumer-directed, university-affiliated centre involved in research and education on disability issues. This site offers a wide variety of resources and links for field workers as well as for people with disabilities.

Canadian Chiropractic Association
http://Home.InfoRamp.Net/~ccachiro/

An Internet source for information about chiropractic services in Canada, this page contains links to public and professional sites, each of which is designed to meet the unique needs of their audience.

Canadian Cultural Society of the Deaf (CCSD)
http://www.connect.ab.ca/~ccsd/

The CCSD is comprised of deaf people working together for deaf people. This site provides access to significant papers, general information of interest and links to further resources.

Canadian Diabetes Association (CDA)
http://www.diabetes.ca

This site was posted in the fall of 1995 as another way for the CDA to reach its members, persons with diabetes or anyone interested in furthering their knowledge on the subject.

Canadian Health Promotion Research Centres
http://duke.usask.ca/~sproat/CENTRES.htm

Web page links are supplied for those Canadian centres who have Web pages up and running.

Canadian Nurses Association/Association des Infirmièrs du Canada (CNA)
http://www.cna-nurses.ca

The Association's mission is to advance the quality of nursing. Included in this site are a calendar of events, publications, inside CNA and number of nursing profession related site links and lists. The Web site of this major nursing federation of 11 provincial and territorial nursing associations represents more than 110 000 registered nurses.

Canadian Red Cross
http://www.redcross.ca/index1.htm

This site provides publications, details and resources related to the services and focus areas of this important organization.

Canadian Society of Allergy and Clinical Immunology (CSACI)
http://csaci.medical.org/index.html

CSACI is one of the oldest specialty societies in Canada, founded in 1945. A wide range of information is presented.

Canadian Sport
http://www.canadiansport.com/

Lists the major Canadian sports-related links including: Canadian national and provincial organizations; Canadian sports facilities, clubs & associations; individual sports; team sports; sport for athletes with a disability; multisports organizations; major games organizations; and Sport Canada.

Chatelaine Partners in Health Resource Guide
http://www.chatelaine.com/chatelaine/sources/health/partners.html

This excellent guide and index contains descriptions and phone numbers of various Canadian health-related agencies and organizations to help you find necessary information quickly and easily.

Dying with Dignity: A Canadian Society Concerned With The Quality of Dying
http://www.Web.apc.org/dwd/

Dying With Dignity is a registered charitable society whose mission is to improve the quality of dying for all Canadians in accordance with their own wishes, values and beliefs. The site helps them to inform and educate Canadians about their rights to determine and choose health-care options at the end of life.

Epilepsy Canada
http://www.epilepsy.ca

Resources and links provided by Epilepsy Canada, the only national nonprofit organization whose mission is to promote and support research into all aspects of epilepsy, and to create awareness and understanding about epilepsy through educational programs. There are 65 provincial and regional epilepsy associations across Canada.

Family Living: General Resources
http://www1.nb.sympatico.ca/healthyway/LISTS/B9-C00_res1.html

Provided by the Sympatico service provider, this location lists a number of unreviewed Canadian family and social health-related sites.

Family Services Canada
http://www.cfc-efc.ca/fsc/

Founded in 1982, Family Services Canada is a national, nonprofit, voluntary organization representing the concerns of families and family-serving agencies across Canada.

Health and Nutrition Organizations Links
http://www.freespace.net/~lsmedmor/p10.htm

This site offers links to Canadian and American non-government organizations. These organizations are often nonprofit and employ health professionals of various types. The links usually contain information about the goals and objectives of the organization and information for nutrition educators and consumers.

Heath Promotion Online (HPO), Health Canada
http://www.hc-sc.gc.ca/hppb/

HPO is your door to Health Canada's health promotion information on the Internet. Developed by Health Canada's Health Promotion and Programs Branch (HPPB), HPO gives health promoters the resources they need in an easy-to-use, bilingual Web site.

Health Related Internet Resources
http://www.hlth.gov.bc.ca/exsites/exlinks.html

Established by the B.C. Ministry of Health, this page provides Canadian links to other health-related Internet sites and resources. These information resources have been selected to serve the information needs of Ministry of Health staff and stakeholders.

Heart and Stroke Foundation of Canada
http://www.hsf.ca

This Web site helps to further the mission of the Heart and Stroke Foundation of Canada which is stated as being: "to further the study, prevention and reduction of disability and death from heart disease and stroke through research, education and the promotion of healthy lifestyles."

Learning Disabilities Association of Canada
http://edu-ss10.educ.queensu.ca/~lda

This page presents information on the association itself; as well as resources related to learning disabilities in general.

Multiple Sclerosis Society of Canada
http://www.mssoc.ca

A wide range of information, resources and links to sites that deal with multiple sclerosis.

Muscular Dystrophy Association of Canada
http://www.mdacbc.org

The purpose of the Client Services program of the Muscular Dystrophy Association of Canada is to work in partnership with persons affected by neuromuscular disorders to contribute to their quality of life.

Ontario Interdisciplinary Council for Aging and Health (OICAH)
http://www.ahs.uwo.ca/orcn/academic/Gerontology/

Includes information on the Council as well as links to Canadian Association of Gerontology and other significant links.

St. John Ambulance Canada
http://www.sja.ca

This site includes information on training, products, First Aid, CPR, health promotion, and community service.

United Way of Canada
http://www.uwc-cc.ca

This agency supports a multitude of volunteer and care organizations. Details on local organizations, history, and resources are provided.

World Federation of Neurology Amyotrophic Lateral Sclerosis (WFN/ALS)
http://www.wfnals.org

This Web site is sponsored by the World Federation of Neurology to link researchers and clinicians world-wide, with the goal of finding effective treatment and a cure for ALS.

Computer, Internet and Software

Following are a few sites that will lead you to important sites on computing, use and growth of the Internet, and a site to use for finding software.

Canarie
http://www.canarie.ca/

This is the spot to check for Canadian Internet developments. As stated on their Web site: "CANARIE Inc. is a not-for-profit, industry-led and managed consortium which was created as an innovative way for the federal government, the research community and the private sector to collaborate in stimulating the development of the Information Highway in Canada."

HotWired!
http://www.hotwired.com

The most popular and fun major reference magazine on and for the Internet. It is also available in regular magazine form.

Internet Encyclopedia
http://clever.net/cam/encyclopedia.html

This is an encyclopedia composed of information available on the Internet. There are two main divisions. The MacroReference contains references to large areas of knowledge, frequently asked questions where available, and pointers to relevant areas of the MicroReference. The MicroReference contains information and references to specific subjects, sometimes with instructions on finding the specific subject inside a general reference. Each specific subject will reference its general subject in the MacroReference if one is present.

The National Center for Supercomputing Applications (NCSA)
http://www.ncsa.uiuc.edu

NCSA is the home of Internet research and development. It is one of the major sites to check in order to keep up-to-date on Internet developments.

Tucows: The Ultimate Collection of Winsock Software
http://www.tucows.com

Don't let the silly name fool you—Tucows is one of the largest and best collections and sources for software available on the Internet. There are mirror sites available around the world that you can use to discover and download software.

Employment, Career and Job Search Links

As students, you are likely looking forward to the day you will be finished your education and working in your new career. The following sites provide excellent career and job search assistance:

BC WorkInfoNet: Labour Market Information for Career Practitioners and Job Seekers
http://workinfonet.bc.ca/

This B.C. site is a career development site providing links to information on future job prospects as well as postings for presently available positions.

Bridges CX98
http://cdn.cx.bridges.com

A Canadian, subscription-based employment information service offering free trials of its services.

British Columbia Job Postings
http://www.postings.gov.bc.ca/index.htm

Find out about current job offerings from the B.C. government.

Canadian Job Search
http://www.truro.nscc.ns.ca/hrdc/canjobs.htm

This page contains Canadian job search sites, which are designed to specifically search for employment opportunities that are currently available throughout Canada. They can also be useful for those who are in secondary or post secondary education. By viewing these job sites, you will see what potential employers are looking for in today's rapidly changing and challenging job market.

CanWorkNet
http://www.workinfonet.ca/cwn/english/main.html

CanWorkNet is a gateway site to career and job activities and vacancy information across Canada.

FAQ: Canada to US Immigration for Businesses and Professionals
http://www.grasmick.com/canimfaq.htm

From the law offices of Joseph C. Grasmick comes this site containing useful information regarding requirements for Canadians interested in working in the U.S.A.

Health Care Source
http://www.healthcaresource.com/

One of the most established sites for information on the American job market and health careers.

Human Resources Development Canada—National Job Bank®
http://www.hrdc-drhc.gc.ca/common/home.shtml

Home page of Human Resources Development Canada, including the National Job Bank. The Job Bank provides links to postings for specific job openings throughout Canada.

Resume Writing Tips: 40 Free Online Workshops by Regina Pontow
http://www.provenresumes.com

A great site for job seekers and students to learn how to identify and market their top skills to match the jobs and salaries they want.

CareerPath
http://www.careerpath.com/res/owa/rb_applicant.display_rblogin?

Job advertisements from six major U.S. cities.

The Monster Board Canada
http://english.monster.ca/welcome.htm

This is the Canadian version of the Monster Board job list. Post resumés, get help on composing resumés, and search for jobs.

WorkWeb
http://www.cacee.com

Designed to help students and recent graduates use the Internet in their search for work.

General Health, Nursing and Medicine References

The following references should be of general use to nursing and health-care workers. Keep in mind that the URLs cited are in a constant state of change, and may become invalid.

Academic Journal Directory
http://www.son.utmb.edu/catalog/catalog.htm

Online directory from the University of Texas School of Nursing at Galveston, Texas. This document contains listings for approximately 400 professional academic journals in clinical nursing, nursing education, nursing research and related health-care fields. A typical entry includes journal name, publisher, frequency, readership and statement of purpose.

Alternative Medicine
http://www.pitt.edu/~cbw/altm.html

This page is a great source for sites that have information on unconventional, unorthodox, unproven, or alternative, complementary, innovative, or integrative therapies.

American Association of Neuroscience Nurses (AANA)
http://www.aann.org

The AANA is a specialty organization serving nurses throughout the world with more than 4000 members. The AANA home page provides news, continuing education, a bulletin board, membership information, special focus groups, core curriculum for neurosurgical nursing as well as partial contents of their journal, *The Journal of Neuroscience*, and other relevant links.

American Medical Association (AMA)
http://www.ama-assn.org

This site helps the AMA serve physicians and their patients by establishing and promoting ethical, educational, and clinical standards for the medical profession and by advocating for the highest principle of all—the integrity of the physician/patient relationship.

American Red Cross
http://www.crossnet.org

An interesting and informative home page for this worldwide organization.

Association of Operating Room Nurses, Inc. (AORN)
http://www.aorn.org

The home page of AORN provides information about the association, clinical practice, education, AORN products and services and online perioperative employment opportunities.

Atlas of Pathology
http://www.med.uiuc.edu/PathAtlasf/titlePage.html

This atlas provides a series of images in clinical pathology of systemic and diseases.

Canadian Network of Toxicology Centres (CNTC)
http://www.uoguelph.ca/cntc

Provides information about the organization, online newsletters and documents and links to other toxicology-related sites.

Cardiology Resources on the Web
http://www.fis.utoronto.ca/~burns/

This Web site was created to serve as a communication tool and as a vehicle for information exchange among the Canadian Association of Interventional Cardiology members. It offers an array of didactic and research instruments as well as an overview of products available from their sponsors, with particular emphasis on new developments.

Center for Education and Drug Abuse Research
http://www.pitt.edu/~mmv/cedar.html

Provides information and links to publications designed to educate in order to help reduce drug abuse.

Centers for Disease Control (CDC)
http://www.cdc.gov

The CDC, located in Atlanta, Georgia, U.S.A, is an agency of the Department of Health and Human Services. The CDC's mission is to promote health and quality of life by preventing and controlling disease, injury, and disability. Includes such publications as the *Weekly Morbidity and Mortality Reports*.

CHORUS: Radiology Encyclopedia
http://chorus.rad.mcw.edu/chorus.html

Offers a series of medical radiology images with corresponding case information. Provides an excellent quick reference for physicians and medical students. More than 1200 documents describe diseases, radiological findings, differential-diagnosis lists ("gamuts"), pertinent anatomy, pathology, and physiology.

Chemical Industry Institute of Toxicology (CIIT)
http://www.ciit.org

Founded in 1974 and supported by 36 industrial organizations, CIIT is a non-profit toxicology research institute dedicated to providing an improved scientific basis for understanding and assessing the potential adverse effects of chemicals, pharmaceuticals, and consumer products on human health.

Custom Medical Images
http://www.cmsp.com

Custom Medical brings a view of its library of medical, scientific, sonographic and other images.

Emergency Medicine at the Crossroads
http://x-roads.com/directory.html

Offers download files (FTP), relevant electronic journals, emergency medicine organizations mailing lists, marketplace information, medical information resources relevant to emergency medicine and other medical information resource links.

Ethics and Genetics
http://www.med.upenn.edu/~bioethic/genetics.html

An imaginative home page site concept that leads you to ponder questions such as "What do you think about genetic testing, genetic enhancement, gene therapy, genetic engineering?" This "electric conversation" lets you post your comments instantly and engage in live conversations with any of the hundreds of people who visit this site every week.

The Global Health Network (GHNet)
http://www.pitt.edu/HOME/GHNet/GHNet.html

GHNet is a multilingual site alliance of experts in health and telecommunications who are actively developing the architecture for a health information structure for the prevention of disease in the 21st century.

Go Ask Alice!
http://www.goaskalice.columbia.edu

Go Ask Alice! is an imaginative and useful interactive health question/answer database located at Columbia University Health Science Library, N.Y. You enter your medical and health question and Alice gives you responses. The site also includes additional search options plus the online *Healthwise Highlights* newsletter.

Health Canada/Santé Canada
http://www.hc-sc.gc.ca

From the Canadian government, this site provides a variety of health-related sources, as outlined earlier in the examples cited.

Health-Economics.com
http://www.healtheconomics.com/

Established as a guide to searching health economics, as well as medical and pharmacy resources by subject category on the Internet.

HealthSeek
http://www.healthseek.com

A well-established database that offers a wide range of health-care industry news, information and resources, as well as links galore on a multitude of health-related topics.

Hospital Web
http://neuro-www.mgh.harvard.edu/hospitalWeb.shtml

Scroll down the page past the useful career links to find listings and links to hospitals around the world. The hospital index is divided into two sections: U.S. hospitals and global hospitals. Many of these hospitals include a nursing department home page.

HyperDOC: The Visible Human Project
http://www.nlm.nih.gov/research/visible/visible_human.html

The Visible Human Project is an outgrowth of the NLM's 1986 Long-Range Plan. It is creating a complete, anatomically detailed, three-dimensional representations of the male and female human body. The current phase of the project is collecting transverse CT, MRI and cryosection images of representative male and female cadavers at one millimetre intervals.

Injury Control Resource Information Network (ICRIN)
http://www.injurycontrol.com/icrin/

An annotated list of key Internet-accessible resources related to the field of injury research and control. New users may want to look at the online ICRIN slide show (also available in a Microsoft PowerPoint format) that presents an overview of ICRIN's structure, content and benefits.

Interactive Patient
http://medicus.marshall.edu/medicus.htm

The Interactive Patient at Marshall University School of Medicine is a truly unique Interactive World Wide Web program that allows the user to simulate an actual patient encounter. This teaching tool for physicians, residents and medical students offers a case with a chief complaint to the user who then has to interact with the patient-requesting additional history, performing a physical exam, and reviewing laboratory data and x-rays.

Infomedial
http://home.ipoline.com/~guoli/home/index.htm

This useful site provides links to medical dictionaries, professional information, articles, links to medical sites, links to search engines, and more.

Med Help International
http://medhlp.netusa.net/index.htm

Med Help International, a nonprofit organization, is dedicated to helping all those who are in need find qualified medical information and support. You are free to search their medical libraries, which they state as being the largest and most comprehensive medical library on the Internet.

Medical i-Way
http://www.largnet.uwo.ca/med/i-way.html

A Canadian database of medical cases and diagnosis. You can retrieve the cases according to anatomical areas. Classic and typical cases available give the patient case history, various CT and other medical images, and the medical diagnosis.

Medical Library Association (MLANET)
http://www.mlanet.org/

The Medical Library Association is a professional organization of more than 1200 institutions and 3000 professional institutions in the health information field.

Medical Online
http://www.medicalonline.com.au

Medical Online is an Internet site designed to put both health care professionals and the general public in contact with medical information.

Medical Radiography
http://Web.wn.net/ricter/Web/medradhome.html

This site is designed to be a gateway to learning through exploration for technologists, students, educators and others interested in the radiologic sciences. Your exploration of the many resources available can be as structured or as unstructured as you want it to be.

Medical Research Council of Canada (MRC)
http://www.mrc.gc.ca/title.html

MRC is the major federal agency responsible for funding health research in Canada. While not specific to medical radiography, this supporting site includes information on grants, jobs, research and other medical information.

Medinet: Directory of BC Health Providers
http://Web20.mindlink.net/medinet/medlinks.htm

An excellent B.C. and Canadian index of health provider Web links.

MedWeb: Electronic Newsletters and Journals
http://www.gen.emory.edu/MEDWEB/medWeb.html

Offers a searchable database of medical sites and databases.

MEDwire: Medical Products on the Web
http://www.callamer.com/itc/medwire

MEDwire is a medical products news service that gives desktop access to medical press releases.

Medscape®
http://www.medscape.com

Medscape®, for health professionals and interested consumers, features the Web's largest collection of free full-text, peer-reviewed articles, medical news, MEDLINE, interactive quizzes, and is updated daily.

The Merck Manual: Merck & Co., Inc.
http://www.merck.com/!!r_7n50cwSr_7n50cwS/

This Merck company site includes a computer-accessible copy of the *The Merck Manual of Diagnosis and Therapy*, 16th Edition, Copyright © 1992 by Merck & Co., Inc. This is one of the most widely-used medical reference books.

MIR Nuclear Medicine
http://gamma.wustl.edu/home.html

This site provides a number of nuclear medicine cases by study type and diagnosis or of an unknown diagnosis. Also included are links to other related Web sites.

Morbidity & Mortality Weekly Report
http://www.cdc.gov/epo/mmwr/mmwr.html

Prepared by the Centers for Disease Control and Prevention (CDC), this series reports health-related statistics provided by U.S. health agencies.

National Centre for Training & Education in Prosthetics & Orthotics
http://www.strath.ac.uk/Departments/NatCentre/index.htm

This is the home page of the National Centre at the University of Strathclyde, U.K. It provides information on postgraduate courses, research interests, distance learning courses, recent publications, and the soon-to-be implemented Recall Online (the abstracting database in the field of prosthetics & orthotics).

U.S. National Health Information Center (NHIC)
http://nhic-nt.health.org

The NHIC is a health information referral service. NHIC puts health professionals and consumers who have health questions in touch with those organizations that are best able to provide answers.

National Institutes of Health (NIH)
http://www.nih.gov

The NIH mission is to uncover new knowledge that will lead to better health for everyone. This site reflects this mission by publishing NIH research and general health information.

National League of Nursing (NLN)
http://www.nln.org

This site includes support for the Center for Nursing Education and Interdisciplinary Education, Nursing Practice & Interdisciplinary Health Care, Research in Nursing as well as the products, services and meetings of the NLN in New York City.

The U.S. National Library of Medicine
http://www.nlm.nih.gov

One of the most comprehensive libraries of medical resources in the world, located on the NIH Campus in Bethesda, MD.

New England Journal of Medicine Online
http://www.nejm.org/content/index.asp

The New England Journal of Medicine Online, a weekly journal reporting the results of important medical research worldwide. The journal is owned and published by the Massachusetts Medical Society.

Nurse: From the University of Warwick, UK
http://www.csv.warwick.ac.uk

This is one of the first specialized Internet nursing sites. Includes a journal called *Nursing Online*, and a variety of information sources, links and info on jobs in the U.K., and more.

Nurseweek
http://www.nurseweek.com

Nurseweek is a California-based resource for nurses which lists nursing job opportunities, continuing education, event guides, company information and hot links to over 200 sites on the World Wide Web.

Nursing HealthWeb
http://www.lib.umich.edu/hw/nursing.html

Cites international sources for nursing sites, resources, and related information.

Nursing Web Server, University of Maryland
http://www.nursing.ab.umd.edu/

This University of Maryland, Baltimore nursing site provides a listing of some nursing Web sites from around the world. Also included with local information are nursing publications links, as well as information on general nursing education.

Nursing World of the American Nurses Association (ANA)
http://www.nursingworld.org

The ANA Home Page, Nursing World includes information about the Association, American Nurses Credentialing Center, and ANA NET. Links to other Web sites are included.

NPWeb: Nursing Practitioner
http://www.npWeb.org/

Offers professional news and information, conference info, The Harding Files, NH government sites, clinical resources, health-related sites, reference tools, other nursing sites, and more.

PharmInfoNet
http://pharminfo.com/pin_hp.html

Pharmaceutical Information Network leads the way on the Internet with up-to-date, free and accurate drug information and serves as the primary entry point into the World Wide Web for health professionals and patients who are seeking high-quality information about drug therapies and medical information.

Radiology Webserver, University of Washington
http://www.rad.washington.edu

This site includes a variety of education, training and information sources.

Radiopharmaceuticals (ICP)
http://www.icppet.org/radio.html

A discussion of position emission tomography (PET) radiopharmaceuticals.

University of British Columbia Division of Nuclear Medicine
http://www.triumf.ca/ubcnucmed/default.html

This home page includes some interesting cases online as well as the Nuclear Medicine Grand Rounds dating from September 1996 to the present. Five teaching hospitals are affiliated with the division, and the site includes links to the UBC Radiology and Faculty of Medicine.

Ultrasound Scans
http://home.hkstar.com/~joewoo/joewoo2.html

A highly regarded site with extensive text and graphical treatment of use of ultrasound in obstetrics.

University of Washington School of Nursing
http://www.son.washington.edu

An excellent site with special education and health links, as well as local information on the school and its activities such as nurse midwifery, continuing education and Center for Women's Health Research.

The Virtual Hospital (VH)
http://vh.radiology.uiowa.edu

The VH may be used to answer patient care questions, thus putting the latest medical information at physicians' fingertips. This same information may be used for Continuing Medical Education (CME), delivering CME to physicians' offices and homes at their convenience. The VH is a project of the Electric Differential Multimedia Laboratory, Department of Radiology, at the University of Iowa College of Medicine. It is a continuously updated digital health sciences library and is available over high-speed networks.

Virtual Nursing Center
http://www-sci.lib.uci.edu/HSG/Nursing.html

This is a very comprehensive nursing site. Included within are world-wide news reports, travel warnings and immunization international services, language dictionaries, medical dictionaries and glossaries, primary technical support metabolic pathways and genetic maps, interactive anatomy browsers, online nursing journals, courses and tutorials, clinical examinations, protocols and procedures, interactive nurse case studies and patient browsers, codes, calculators and laboratory diagnostics, and much more.

Visible Human Project
http://www.crd.ge.com/esl/cgsp/projects/vm/

This project at the National Library of Medicine, called the "Visible Man," has already produced computed tomography, magnetic resonance imaging and physical cross-sections of a human male cadaver.

The World Health Organization (WHO), Geneva, Switzerland
http://www.who.ch

This home page opens the door to major world health databases and information sources including WHO publications and its library.

Whole Brain Atlas
http://www.med.harvard.edu/AANLIB/home.html

Roentgen-ray computed tomography (CT), magnetic resonance imaging (MRI), and single photon/positron emission computed tomography (SPECT/PET) images and descriptions can be found on this rather impressive site.

General Science References

The following are some general science references that relate to subject areas often studied by students in the health professions. These include some Canadian and U.S. government sources and databases which provide useful tools.

ATSDR - HazDat Database
http://atsdr1.atsdr.cdc.gov:8080/hazdat.html

The hazardous materials database compiled by the United States Government.

Biodidac Biological Images
http://biodidac.bio.uottawa.ca

A bank of digital images and resources useful for teaching or studying biology. Anyone can use this site to find images relating to biology. The search feature allows you to search this databank using scientific nomenclature or common language keywords.

Biology: Dictionaries, Glossaries, and other Reference Materials
http://www.library.wisc.edu/guides/Biology/refer.htm#science

Dictionaries, lists of all kinds, encyclopedias and more are available here. The material covers many aspects of biology, including botany, zoology, life sciences, chemistry, molecular biology, and more.

The Biology Project
http://www.biology.arizona.edu

Online tutorials on such topics as biochemistry, cell biology, developmental biology, human biology, Mendelian genetics, immunology and molecular biology. The site is similar in concept to the introductory chapters of first-year general biology textbooks.

Commission for Environmental Cooperation (CCE/ CCA/ CEC)
http://www.cec.org

Commission for Environmental Cooperation of NAFTA based in Montreal is a site which contains full-text documents related to Canada, United States and Mexico, including legal aspects.

Chemfinder
http://chemfinder.camsoft.com/

Chemfinder is a wonderful tool that lets you find lots of data on specific chemicals. There are several search options including chemical name or formula, and there is a good set of instructions. Chemfinder Webserver indexes over 150 chemical information sites.

Chemistry Helper
http://www.gc.cc.va.us/~gcsteid/chem/chemhelp.htm

Ye Olde Professor provides links to online textbooks, encyclopedias, tutorials, and more. A site with hard data in addition to the more commonly found set of further links.

ENVIRO-NET Material Safety Data Sheets (MSDS) Index
http://www.enviro-net.com/technical/msds

This MSDS database has a searchable index in which you may type the chemical name or find it manually in the alphabet. This site, ENVIRO-NET MSDS is also mirrored at the University of Utah MSDS database.

Environmental Health Perspectives
http://ehis.niehs.nih.gov/

The online source for Environmental Health Perspectives and other publications of the National Institute of Environmental Health Sciences.

Hazardous Chemical Database
http://ull.chemistry.uakron.edu/erd/

This database, maintained by the University of Akron in Ohio, will allow the user to retreive information for any of over 1300 hazardous chemicals based on a keyword search.

Health and Safety Related Internet Resources
http://www.ccohs.ca/resources/wwwo.html

An outstanding collection of related Internet resources and links.

The International Labour Office (ILO) - CIS International Occupational Safety & Health Information Centre
http://turva.me.tut.fi/cis/home.html

The Geneva-based ILO provides a wealth of occupational health and safety data including ILO publications, Directories of institutions, chemical safety databases, ILO Code of Practice and further names and addresses of collaborating centers.

National Institute of Environmental Health Sciences (NIEHS)
http://www.niehs.nih.gov

The NIEHS site contains a number of online databases, including toxicological data, MSDS and reports from the NTP (National Toxicology Program) Divison, which may be searched via a search engine.

National Pollutant Release Inventory (NPRI)
http://www.ec.gc.ca/pdb/npri.html

NPRI provides information on the on-site releases to air, water and land, as well as transfers off-site in wastes, of 178 substances. The NPRI is the only legislated, nation-wide, publicly accessible inventory of pollutant releases and transfers in Canada. NPRI reports and information about Accelerated Reduction/ Elimination of Toxics (ARET), and a list of proposed substances for reduction/elimination are also provided.

North Atlantic Treaty Organization (NATO) Environmental Clearinghouse System (ECHS)
http://www.nato.int/ccms/

The NATO-ECHS Web site is a tool for the multiple CCMS pilot studies and participating nations to acquire, organize, retrieve, and disseminate environmental information of common interest. The NATO-ECHS Web site provides access to environmental data, reports, and studies. The NATO-ECHS Web site does not provide access to nor support for classified, restricted, or otherwise sensitive data.

National Institute for Occupational Safty and Health (NIOSH)
http://www.cdc.gov/niosh/homepage.html

Being one of the leading government agencies in this field, NIOSH covers a wide information spectrum on occupational health and safety issues.

Physical Reference Data
http://physics.nist.gov/PhysRefData/contents.html

From the National Institute of Standards and Technology, this site links to physical constants, units, conversion factors, spectroscopic data, and much more.

Science Council of British Columbia
http://www.scbc.org/home.asp

A good source of B.C. and Canadian scientific and technological information.

Selected Internet Resources for Chemistry
http://www.indiana.edu/~cheminfo/cisindex.html

An excellent site for finding information on many aspects of chemistry. The approach here uses a back-of-the-book type of indexing system.

Units of Measurement Conversion Tables
http://eardc.swt.edu/cgi-bin/ucon/ucon.pl

An interactive weights and measures conversion source. You type in the unit and the system gives the conversions.

Libraries as Major Sources of Information

Don't forget libraries as being very valuable sources of information. The majority of these are now available and searchable on the Web.

The Canadian Library Index
http://www.lights.com/canlib

Remember, libraries are one of the best sources leading you to books and reports or other resources. This site provides a province-by-province index and links to the major Canadian libraries, which enable you to search their resources from the Internet.

Libraries on the Web
http://sunsite.Berkeley.EDU/LibWeb/

This University of Berkeley digital library database, called LibWeb, currently lists over 2300 home pages from libraries in over 70 countries around the world.

In Conclusion

For futher health and Internet information, you may also want to check Prentice Hall Canada's Web site (http://www.phcanada.com) for the 1997 publication by Jim Carroll and Rick Broadhead, titled *Good Health Online: A Wellness Guide for Every Canadian*.

It my hope that this information will be especially valuable to Canadian students, health workers and the community at large. Should you care to send me an e-mail message, you may contact me at: fknor@bcit.bc.ca, or you can have a virtual visit with me at my home page at: **http://www.lib.bcit.bc.ca/fknor.htm**

May your Internet searches be great ones.

Frank Knor

July, 1998.

Glossary

abduction movement away from the central axis (midline) of the body.

absorption process whereby soluble nutrients pass through the intestinal wall into the blood or lymphatic circulation.

abstract a brief summary of a study.

accessibility one of the five principles on which the Canadian health insurance plan is based; health services are available to all insured persons on uniform terms and conditions with no impediments to services, by charges or other means.

accessible population a population that is a feasible source of sample members.

accountability a person is answerable (or accepts responsibility) for his or her own actions.

accreditation/approval (of basic nursing education programs) (1) a process to ensure that schools of nursing meet certain minimum standards established by the registering body in a province (2) the process of certifying that an educational program has not only met minimum standards, but is considered "good" by national standards.

acculturation process whereby individuals learn the beliefs, values and lifeways of a culture other than the one into which they were born and accept these as their own.

accupressure use of massage (light to moderate pressure) to stimulate energy flow through the body.

accupuncture to correct energy imbalance, fine needles are inserted on the body meridians.

acid a compound that releases hydrogen ions when dissociated in solution.

acidosis a condition in which there is an excessive proportion of acid (H^+ concentration) in the blood or a depletion of base (bicarbonate) reserves.

action potential a change in electrical charge on the cell membrane that activates nerves to transmit impulses to muscles.

active artificial immunity immunity conferred by vaccines.

active ROM range of motion exercises carried out by the individual.

active transport the movement of solute particles from an area of lower concentration to an area of higher concentration with the use of a carrier molecule.

actual diagnosis represents a problem that has been validated by the presence of major defining characteristics.

actual problem situation in which data in the cluster are similar to the defining characteristics for a hypothesized problem.

acupressure massage technique which uses manual pressure to stimulate energy points on the body.

acute pertaining to a condition with a sudden, severe onset and a relatively short course.

acute confusional states occur most frequently among the elderly medical-surgical patients. These states are transient and self-limiting once the underlying cause is ascertained and removed.

acute illness is one which the onset is rapid and the symptoms are severe and the patient usually recovers fairly quickly.

acute pain is a protective mechanism that warns of potential or actual tissue damage.

adaptation a condition in which the brain no longer perceives the available stimuli because the receptors are not picking up enough stimuli or are picking up too much of the same stimulus.

addiction refers to the psychological need to use drugs for other than medical reasons.

additive effect the result of administering two drugs with similar actions.

adduction movement toward the central axis (midline) of the body.

advanced directives statements by people specifying the type of care they wish to receive when they are terminally ill in the event that they are incapable of expressing their wishes at that time.

adverse (side) effects physiological responses to a drug other than the therapeutic effect.

advocate to see that the patients rights and interests are protected.

aerobic exercise sustained physical activity that uses the oxygen system to strengthen cardio-respiratory function and endurance.

affective domain the domain of learning tasks involving the changing of attitudes.

agitated depression a state in which a person may experience anxiety and depression at the same time.

agnosia loss of comprehension of sensations.

agonists drugs that stimulate or produce cellular response.

air embolism the presence of a large amount of air in the circulatory system.

airway passageway for air in the body.

alarm reaction where the bodies defense mechanisms are mobilized.

alkalosis a condition in which there is a reduced proportion of acid (H^+) in the blood or an excess of base (bicarbonate) reserves.

allah Muslim name for God.

allergic reaction a hypersensitive reaction to a drug in a person who was previously exposed to the drug or a related chemical and has developed antibodies to it.

allophone a Canadian whose mother tongue is neither English or French.

alopecia abnormal hair loss.

alternative/complementary medicine any approach to solving a health problem that is different from that used by conventional Western practitioners.

Alzheimer's disease Is a chronic dementia that is gradual in onset and progressive in nature. The disease causes atrophy of the brain and the individual shows signs of progressive deterioration of mental functioning.

amino acid the structural unit of protein.

amnesia loss of memory.

amniotic sac the protective membrane filled with fluid that surrounds the developing embryo, providing warmth, moisture and relative freedom of movement.

anabolism the building process of metabolism in which simple substances are converted to more complex compounds; synthesis of enzymes and proteins needed by the body cells.

anal canal forms the last 2.5 cm of the rectum.

analgesic relieving pain; a pain relieving agent.

analogic usual nonverbal communication such as body posture, facial expression and tone, as well as creative expression such as music, poetry and painting.

analytic study investigates data obtained from descriptive studies and attempts to determine relationships with other factors.

anaphylactic reaction life-threatening respiratory distress and cardiovascular collapse as a result of an allergic reaction to a drug.

anion ion that carries a negative charge.

aniseikonia unequal size and shape of images from one eye.

anisometropia unequal refractive power of the eyes.

anointing of the sick a sacrament in the Roman Catholic Church interpreted as an aid to healing and a source of strength.

anomia inability to remember names of objects.

anorexia loss of appetite or lack of desire for food; it involves the subjective perception of a distaste for food.

antagonistic effect two drugs whose effects cancel each other out.

antagonists drugs that block cellular response.

anthropometric measurement measurements of the size and proportions of the body: height, weight and skinfold (fatfold) thickness.

anticipatory grief the response to prior knowledge of an impending death.

antidiarrheal agents agents which counteract diarrhea.

anxiety an unpleasant feeling of tension and apprehension. It is often accompanied by physiological, psychological and behavioural symptoms that alerts people to an impending real or symbolic threat to self.

aphakia absence of lens after cataract removal.

aphasia the state of being unable to speak at all.

apical pulse the beat of the heart auscultated at its apex.

apnea the absence of breathing.

appetite the desire for food.

apraxia inability to make purposeful movements.

aquathermia pad a type of heating pad, consisting of channels through which heated water circulates and transmits dry heat of a constant temperature.

aromatherapy makes use of aromatic essences extracted from wild or cultivated plants for beauty treatments and for therapies similar to those used in herbal medicine.

arterial blood gas (ABG) the test measures the partial pressure of oxygen and carbon dioxide dissolved in the arterial blood.

arterial ulcer located on the foot or ankle. It is caused by inadequate circulation.

artificial airway a tube inserted into a person's airway by way of the mouth or nose, or through a tracheostomy.

asepsis the absence of contamination.

assault a threat to do physical harm to another and an apparent ability to carry out that threat.

assessment the first step in the nursing process; the collection and interpretation of clinical information.

assumption an idea or concept that we take for granted; provisional suppositions.

astigmatism unequal corneal curvature. Vision is blurred and eye use causes discomfort. Accomadation does not correct the problem.

asymptomatic a condition without signs or symptoms.

audibility the adequacy of information about the researchers decisions, choices and insights that directed each step of the research.

auscultation listening to body sounds produced by the heart, lungs and abdomen.

authenticity genuineness; often manifested by spontaneity, self-disclosure and a lack of defensiveness.

authority the status attributed to individuals or groups giving them the power and right to command and be obeyed.

autocratic a teaching style in which the teacher makes all decisions about learning.

autologous transfusion blood is collected from a person, stored and then transfused back into the same person at a later time.

autolysis disintegration of tissue by the body's own mechanisms.

autolytic debridement the removal of dead tissue from a wound by using dressings that allow enzymes in the wound fluid to dissolve the dead tissues.

autonomous thinking thinking for oneself.

autonomy the right to self-determination.

autosexual activities sexual behaviours which involve the self only.

ayurvedic medicine based on natural phenomena as the cause of illness, rather than spirits, with treatment based on a belief in the body's innate ability to heal itself.

Baha'i a religion based on the belief that mankind is one human race; it teaches the unity of religions and the unity of mankind.

Balkan frame a metal frame that extends lengthwise above the bed supported at either end by a pole attached to the bed frame.

baptism a Christian ritual in which the individual is immersed in or sprinkled with water as a sign of purification and admission to the church.

basal metabolic rate (BMR) the minimum energy requirements of the body when the individual is awake and at digestive, physical and emotional rest.

base a compound that combines with acids to form salts; neutralizes the effects of acids.

base of support foundation that gives an object stability.

battery touching without consent.

bed cradle a device used to keep the weight of the top bed covers off the patient.

behaviour modification substituting desired behaviour for undesired behaviour using reinforcement.

behavioural model an approach to health based on the premise that there are four principal factors affecting both individual and group health; namely, heredity, environment, lifestyle, and health care organization. (Also known as the *health fields approach* or *lifestyles model*).

behaviourist school a theory that believes learning is observable and can be controlled by manipulating the environment.

beneficence an ethical principle that requires that we do good and prevent harm.

bereavement the experience of loss through death.

binuclear family families in which children are members of two households as a result of joint-custody arrangements following divorce.

biofeedback ability to control body systems by self -monitoring.

biological sexual identity the biological distinctions that identify a person as male or female based on the characteristics of the sex organs.

biomedical model an empirical approach to health, based on scientific research and training, that focusses on the physiological determinants of health and disease.

biopsy surgery to obtain a tissue sample from the body.

bisexuality romantic and sexual attraction to partners of either sex.

blended or reconstituted family a husband and wife, at least one of whom has been married before. The blended family can include one or more children from a former marriage as well as offspring from the new union.

blood group the type of blood classification.

blood pressure the pressure of the blood within arteries.

body alignment relationship of body parts to the midline of the body.

body image represents an individual's beliefs and attitudes about his or her body.

body substance precautions (BSP) a more generic version of CDC's universal precautions.

body temperature the balance between heat production and heat loss.

bonding attachment that occurs between parent and newborn.

boundaries filters which permit varying degrees of exchange between the system and the environment; in family systems theory, physical demarcations such as the family's property line or a member's bedroom, or abstract entities like rules, norms, attitudes and values which separate families and subsystems from their environments, and which require human interaction inside and outside the family.

brachial pulse the pulse located on the anterior surface of the arm just below the elbow where the brachial artery passes over the ulna.

bradycardia a very low pulse rate (less than 60 beats per minute).

bradypnea an abnormal decrease in respiratory rate.

brainstorming the spontaneous consideration of ideas or solutions.

braxton-hicks contractions a tightening of the uterine muscles in preparation for labour.

breast binder a rectangular piece of cotton shaped roughly to the contours of the female chest with straps that pin to the binder in front.

bronchoscopy an examination of the larynx, trachea and bronchi with the use of a fiberoptic bronchoscope, a tubular instrument with an attached light source.

bruising refers to bleeding into surrounding tissues as a result of trauma to underlying blood vessels.

Buddhism a world-wide religion with no gods but encompassing various philosophical beliefs and ethical systems. A central belief is that the ultimate state is one of self-enlightenment.

buffering is the immediate chemical response to changes in the hydrogen ion concentration of body fluids.

burn an injury to the body's tissue cause by heat, electricity, chemicals or gases. .

calcium mineral important for the proper formation of teeth and bones, for muscle tone and nerve transmission and blood coagulation.

callus is a thickening of the epidermis in a location subjected to excessive pressure or friction.

calorie a unit of heat; the amount of heat required to raise the temperature of one gram of water by one degree Celsius.

Canada Pension Plan (CPP) a pension plan that is compulsory for all employed persons in Canada, except in the Province of Quebec which has its own Quebec Pension Plan (QPP).

cancer pain is the pain attributed to advancing disease or clinical treatment.

capillary refill nail bed occluded becomes pale; when nail bed released oxygenated blood returns to it.

carbohydrate an organic compound composed of carbon, hydrogen and oxygen found in most plants, fruit sugars and natural starches; the primary source of energy for the body.

carcinogenic pertaining to influences causing cancer.

cardiac output the amount of blood ejected from the heart with the force of each ventricular contraction.

care is the basis for ethical decision making in health care; action towards assisting, supporting or enabling another individual (or group) with evident or anticipated needs to ameliorate or improve a human condition or lifeway.

carotid pulse the pulse found over the carotid artery.

carriers individuals who acquire a pathogen but do not experience any adverse effects; however, these individuals may transmit the pathogen to others.

case management responsible for coordinating multidisciplinary services to assist the patient to achieve standardized expectation.

case mix groups (CMGs) diagnosis-related groups of patients.

case study a teaching strategy that uses an imaginary situation as the basis for questions and discussion.

catabolism a complex metabolic process in which compounds are broken down or oxidized for energy.

cathartic a substance that promotes the passage of watery soft stool accompanied by some cramping.

cation an ion that carries a positive charge.

causality relating of causes to the effect they produce; determination that one variable causes another.

cecum receives unabsorbed chyme from the small intestine.

central pain syndrome usually arise from injury to sensory nerves, neural pathways or areas in the brain concerned with pain perception.

centre of gravity also called centre of mass or centre of weight of the body. It is located in the pelvis at approximately the level of the second sacral vertebra.

certification a legal document from an official body attesting that an individual or an institution has met certain standards or an individual has successfully completed a course of training.

ceruminous glands skin glands located in the external ear canal that secrete cerumen (wax).

change agent outside consultant who is called in to assist with the dissemination of information about new ideas and/or practices in an organization (or in a social system) and their adoption in practice.

channel the means of conveying a message.

charting by exception (CBE) documents only significant findings or exceptions to the norm.

chelation therapy removal of poisons and toxic metals from the body with a chemical agent.

chemical name the description of a drug's chemical components.

Chi the finite amount of energy we are endowed with at birth.

chill involuntary contractions of the voluntary muscles with shivering and shaking.

Chinese/Oriental medicine a doctrine revolving around theories of energy and elements, with 3 basic types of intervention: (1) herbal remedies, (2) acupuncture, and (3) exercise.

chiropractic medicine a branch of medicine primarily concerned with the examination and treatment of the spine.

cholesterol a fat-like substance (an alcohol) found in all animal fats and oils; an essential component of some body tissues and compounds.

Christianity the doctrine of Christ and his apostles, based on the belief that Jesus is the Christ and the Son of God.

chronic pertaining to a condition which develops slowly and persists for a long duration, often throughout the remainder of a person's lifetime.

chronic illness an illness of long duration, usually progresses slowly often with little change over time.

chronic pain pain lasting longer than six months, that may or may not be connected to a pathological process.

circadian (diurnal) rhythm a regular pattern which recurrs in cycles of about twenty-four hours; the biological clock which regulates many body processes including the daily sleep-wake cycle.

circular turn is used to bandage a cylindrical part of the body or to secure a bandage as its initial and terminal ends. .

circumduction circular movement, as of a limb or eye.

cleaning the removal of any foreign material from an object.

cleansing enema given to remove feces from the colon.

client education is the use of the educational process for individuals who are partners in the health-education effort.

client system term Neuman's model uses to refer to an individual or a group.

climate of trust a situation in which the patient feels able to trust the nurse as a person concerned first and foremost with the patient's welfare.

clinical laboratory technologist a member of the health team who collects specimens for laboratory tests, treats and analyzes these specimens and advises physicians and nurses on the results of these tests.

clinical nurse specialist a registered nurse who holds a master's degree in nursing and has expertise in a clinical nursing specialty.

clinical significance the usefulness of the findings of a study in clinical practice.

closed systems systems that limit interaction with their environment.

closed wound injury to the skin and underlying tissue without a break in the skin.

clubbing is an increase in the angle between the base of the nail and fingernail.

cluster categories or groups of data.

cluster sampling taking progressively larger random samples from different units within a population.

code of ethics describes the values and obligations considered important in nursing practise.

coenzyme an essential element needed for the activation or control of enzyme activity in the body.

cognition the mental process characterized by knowing, thinking, learning and judging.

cognitive appraisal a person's perception of a situation as harmful and an assessment of his or her ability to cope with it.

cognitive coping skills the mental processes used to regulate the emotional and physiological responses to stress by attempting to see at least some part of a stressful situation in a positive way.

cognitive domain the domain of learning tasks involving the acquisition of knowledge.

cognitive functioning a broad term used to encompass competencies of perceiving, thinking, solving problems and communicating thoughts and feelings.

cognitive school a theory that believes learning is an intellectual process similar to information processing.

cohabiting family a man and a woman living together without the sanctity of marriage. Also known as a common-law relationship.

collaborative relationship that develops between the nurse and the patient.

collaborative problem complications that occur or may occur in association with specific pathology and treatment.

collaborative research studies done in collaborative teams with colleagues, people in other agencies, people in other provinces or countries, or with members of other disciplines.

colonization the acquisition and multiplication of a microorganism.

colostomy a surgically created opening from the large intestine to the abdominal wall.

colostrum a thin yellowish substance rich in maternal antibodies produced by the breasts.

combustible material a substance capable of burning.

comfort a subjective experience indicating a sense of physical, psychological, social, spiritual and environmental ease.

commensals microorganisms with which people enjoy a symbiotic relationship.

commitment a complex, affective response characterized by convergence between one's desires and one's obligations and by a deliberate choice to act in accordance with them.

communal family an intimate network of unrelated adults and their children who make a commitment to live together as one large family unit.

communication the process by which people transmit information to one another through verbal and nonverbal messages or cues.

communion (or eucharist) a Christian sacrament in which the person partakes of bread and wine. The bread represents the body of Christ; the wine his blood.

community (1) a group of people living in a given geographical area (which may not necessarily be defined by legislation) who interact with one another and work collectively on matters of common concern. (2) Any group of people with a common bond.

community health centre a health agency that provides primary health care services in an ambulatory setting.

commuter family spouses live in separate cities or countries on a voluntary basis.

compassion a sensitivity to the pain and brokenness of another; a quality of presence which allows one to share with and make room for another.

compensation over-achieving in the same sphere or one different from that in which we feel inferior.

competence having the knowledge, judgement, skills, energy, experience and motivation required to respond adequately to the demands of one's professional responsibilities.

complete protein food that contains all of the essential amino acids in amounts and proportions for proper use in the body.

compliance the ease with which the lungs and the chest wall can expand to fill with air and contract to empty the air.

comportment bearing, demeanour, dress and language.

comprehensiveness one of the five principles on which the Canadian health insurance program is based. The term is used to mean the provision of all insured services provided by hospitals, medical practitioners, or dentist, and, where permitted, by other health care practitioners.

concept a complex mental formulation of an object, a property (characteristic) or an event that is derived from an individual's perceptual experience.

conceptual model (conceptual framework) the diagrammatic representation of a theory.

confidence the quality which fosters trusting relationships.

confirmability is achieved when other criteria are met.

confirmatory data analysis involves the use of various techniques in order to (1) test proposed relationships between variables, (2) ascertain (infer) that the findings from a sample are representative of the total population, (3) examine causality (that a specific change in 'a' caused reaction 'b'), (4) predict that under similar circumstances, 'a' will probably cause 'b' again, and (5) infer from the sample to a theoretical model.

confounding variables variables that cannot be controlled or are not recognized until the study is in progress.

confusion is a clinical term referring to a mental state in which the individual's cognitive functioning is diminished.

congenital problems encountered by the unborn infant *in utero*.

conscience a state of moral awareness which grows with experience.

constipation infrequent, hard, dry bowel movements.

consumers' bills of rights statements developed in both the United States and Canada that have sought to clarify an individual's basic rights as these are applicable to health care.

continent urostomy a urinary diversion procedure consisting of an internal pouch, a stoma and two nipple valves which prevent urine from draining out of the stoma; urine is stored in the pouch until it is emptied with a catheter passed through the stoma.

continuum of care where each phase of care merges into another.

contracture a shortening or distortion of muscle tissue.

control group one that can be compared with the experimental group.

controlled drugs drugs whose use is controlled by federal legislation (in Canada, the Narcotic Control Act and Regulations). Included are the narcotics and certain other drugs such as barbiturates.

convenience sampling (accidental sampling) allows the entry of any available (convenient) subject into the study until the desired sample size is reached.

core temperature temperature of the internal, deep structures of the body as compared to temperature of peripheral tissues.

correction implies the return of all acid-base components to normal.

correlation the extent to which values of one variable are related to values of another variable.

crackles abnormal breath sounds described as discontinuous crackling sounds produced by air passing through fluid in the small airways.

credibility degree to which the researcher has captured, accurately interpreted and faithfully described, human experiences.

crime a wrong committed against the public and punishable by the crown.

critical path an outline of care for an individual patient.

critical thinking purposeful thinking that takes into consideration focus, language, frame of reference, attitudes, assumptions, evidence, reasoning, conclusions, implications and context when they matter in deciding what to believe or do.

critique a critical assessment of a piece of research involving a systematic appraisal according to specified criteria.

cross match procedure that is performed to establish compatibility between donor and recipient blood.

crowning when the head of the baby becomes visible.

cue a piece of information that one perceives from the environment.

cultural mosaic ethically plural society in which people retain a distinct sense of cultural identity.

cultural relativism endeavor to see people within the context of his or her culture.

cultural sensitivity (cross-cultural competence/intercultural effectiveness/ethnic competence) the ability to work effectively with people of different cultures in a way that people of these cultures find acceptable.

culture the basic beliefs, values and lifeways of groups of people.

cumulative trauma disorders a group of disorders caused by sustained, unnatural body postures and repetitive, forceful movements.

cyanosis bluish tinge in the skin and mucous membranes frequently associated with respiratory distress.

cybernetics the science of systems of control and communications in animals and machines.

cystitis inflammation of the urinary bladder.

cytoscopy an examination of a patient's bladder with a lighted instrument inserted up the urethra.

daily hassles the irritating, distressing and frustrating demands of everyday life.

daily uplifts things in a person's daily life that help to balance stressors such as relating well to one's spouse or lover, relating well to friends, completing a task or feeling healthy.

dandruff dry, scaly material shed from the scalp.

data information the researcher (investigator) collects from subjects or participants in the research study, or about objects in a non-human study.

data base a component of the POMR including the physician history and physical exam and the nursing history and functional health assessment.

data base assessment an evaluation of the patient, conducted on admission to a health care agency or upon initial contact with the patient.

debridement removal of dead tissue from a wound.

deductive working from existing theory to hypothesize relationships that can then be tested.

deductive reasoning involves the development of specific predictions or the generation of certain details from a major theory, generalization, fact or assumption.

defamation of character damage to a person's reputation by written or spoken words that tend to lower his or her esteem in the eyes of other people.

defecation the evacuation of feces.

defence mechanisms strategies that people commonly use in day-to-day life to buffer the emotional component of a stressful situation.

defining characteristic lists or categories of signs and symptoms or risk factors that depict hypothesized problems.

dehiscence the disruption of a surgical wound.

dehydration loss of water from body tissues.

delayed gratification the ability to put off immediate rewards in order to achieve long-term goals.

delirium A state of temporary and reversible mental confusion and frenzied excitement. It is characterized by disorientation, restlessness, clouding of the consciousness and fear. It may result from metabolic disorders, postpartum or postoperative stress, ingestion of toxic substances or shock.

dementia a broad term used for impaired intellectual functioning severe enough to interfere with a person's normal social and work life.

democratic a teaching style advocated by the humanists where the students participate in decisions about learning but are not the sole decision makers.

demonstration method of teaching by exhibition and explanation of a procedure.

demonstration project involves studying a new method of delivering health care in the community.

denial refusal to acknowledge a threat.

dental caries decay of the teeth.

dependence is the state in which the individual experiences symptoms of withdrawal, which occur when the drug is abruptly discontinued.

dependent variable (outcome variable) the characteristic that is being measured to show results in a research study.

depression profound feeling of sadness, low self-esteem and hopelessness.

dermis the inner, thicker layer of skin.

descriptive study measure the amount and distribution of a health concern within a given population.

descriptive theory classify or describe phenomena of concern to a discipline.

developmental crises at certain times in an individual's life, major changes occur.

Dewali Festival of Lights.

diabetic ulcer located on the bottom or side of the foot. It is caused by pressure or friction.

diagnosis a deliberate, systematic process of data analysis and synthesis that ends with a clinical judgement, the nursing diagnosis.

diagnostic cue one that gives strong, valid information for making inferences.

diagnostic reasoning the process of critical thinking in which the nurse uses his or her clinical knowledge and experience to collect information, interpret the information collected, and form a conclusion about the patient's health or illness status (the nursing diagnosis).

diaphoresis sweating or perspiration.

diarrhea the frequent discharge of loose, watery stools.

diastolic pressure the force exerted against the arterial wall during ventricular relaxation.

dietary thermogenesis where food is ingested and the body uses energy to digest, absorb, transport and further process the nutrients.

dietitian a member of the health team usually responsible for planning meal service for patients and staff, supervising other workers in the preparation of food and counselling patients about their nutritional problems.

diffusion the process whereby dissolved particles (ions and molecules) distribute themselves equally within a given space; the particles move from an area of higher concentration to an area of lower concentration until equilibrium is reached.

digestion the process by which complex food forms are changed into simpler, soluble chemical parts so that they can be absorbed into the circulation for use by the body.

digital verbal communication.

dilation cervical opening.

discharge summary concludes the POMR which includes a discussion of each problem and its outcome.

disciplinary bodies monitor the practice of nurses to whom they have granted registration/licensure.

discussion involves participation on the part of the patient, facilitates the retention of learning.

disease an interruption in the continuous process of health, manifested by abnormalities or disturbances in the structure and function of body parts, organs or systems.

displacement type of behaviour in which one transfers anger at one person to another person or object.

distal farther from a point of reference or point of attachment.

distress detrimental, harmful, unpleasant or damaging stress.

diuresis excretion of an increased amount of urine.

diuretic a drug given to increase the secretion of urine in the kidneys.

documentation the communication in writing of essential facts in order to maintain a continuous history of events over a period of time.

donor blood taken from an individual.

dorsal recumbent position lying on the back with the head and shoulders slightly elevated on a pillow.

dorsalis pedis pulse the pulse located on the dorsum of the foot in a line between the first and second toes, just above the longitudinal arch.

dorsiflexion flexion of a body part toward the back, such as upward bending of the fingers, hand, foot or toes.

drug addiction the psychological need to use drugs for other than medical reasons, such as pain relief.

drug dependence symptoms of withdrawal which occur when a drug is abruptly discontinued.

drug interactions the effects of two or more drugs on the body.

drug tolerance the circumstance in which a therapeutic response to a drug dosage lessens after continuous exposure to it.

drug toxicity the effects of a drug produced by an overdose, accumulation of the drug in the body or an abnormal sensitivity to the drug.

dual-career family a family in which both heads of the household pursue careers and at the same time maintain a family life together.

duodenum is the primary site in the small bowel for iron and calcium absorption.

duration of action the length of time a drug produces a pharmacological effect.

dyspnea difficult or laboured breathing.

dyssomnias conditions characterized by difficulties with the quantity and quality of sleep; insomnia, hypersomnia and narcolepsy.

dysuria difficulty or pain on voiding.

ecological (environmental) equilibrium the balance maintained by human organisms in their interactions with the physical environment.

ecology the study of organisms and how they relate to their environment.

ecomap depiction of the family members' contact with their outside world.

ectoderm outer layer of the uterine wall.

edema the accumulation of excessive amounts of fluid in the tissues.

effacement the cervix shortens and becomes thinner.

elastic recoil when the inspiratory muscles relax, these elastic components are able to contract, returning the ribcage and the lungs to their normal position.

electroacupuncture uses electrical charges to pulse the needles rather than manual rotation.

electrolyte a substance which, when dissolved in solution, splits into electrically charged ions of individual atoms or molecules that conduct an electrical current.

emancipated minor a teenager who no longer lives at home and is self-supporting.

emergency medical technician a member of the health team who has had training in advanced life support skills, can do basic and advanced first aid and CPR and can start intravenous infusions.

emesis stomach contents expelled during vomiting.

empathy the ability to recognize and understand another person's feelings.

empirical concrete, based on observation, experiment or experience, not on theory.

empirical abstract meaning inferred from examples of direct or indirect evidence in the real world.

empowerment the social process of recognizing, promoting and enhancing people's abilities to meet their own needs, solve their own problems, and mobilize necessary resources to take control of their own lives.

endoderm inner layer of the uterine wall.

endogenous infection infection originating from a person's own microbial flora.

endorphins large polypeptides with an opioid-like pharmacological action.

enema the instillation of fluid into the rectum to stimulate peristalsis and remove feces or flatus from the colon.

entrepreneurial health care model one in which health care services are provided by private agencies and paid for by the consumer of these services.

enuresis bedwetting.

environment includes physical, psychosocial and related variables that can effect teaching and learning.

environmental illness is one manifestation of hypersensitivity to the environment.

enzyme a compound, almost always a protein, that speeds the rate of a chemical process but is not altered by the process.

epidemiological model basic components are (1) the systematic collection of health data through epidemiological surveys and (2) the search for causes of various states of health.

epidemiology the study of the distribution and determinants of various health-related states or events in specified populations and the application of this study in the control of health problems.

epidermis the outer, thinner layer of skin.

epidural analgesia a method of pain relief by injecting analgesic medication into the epidural space of the spinal column.

erythema refers to redness and is the result of superficial vasodilation–flushing, blushing.

eschar black, dry, "thick, leather-like" necrotic tissue.

esteem needs need to feel that you are worthwhile as a human being.

ethical dilemma a problem with two or more moral claims.

ethics a branch of philosophy that focuses critical reflection upon action and events from the standpoint of right or wrong.

ethnicity the ethnic or cultural group(s) to which an individual's ancestors belonged; it pertains to the ancestral roots or origins of the population and not to place of birth, citizenship, nationality or language.

ethnocentricity viewing people from other cultures from our own cultural perspective.

ethnography the scientific description of human races (ethnic groups).

ethnomethodological a descriptive analysis of a culture or sub-culture which can be used as a basis to develop theories about that culture.

etiology the search for the causes of disease and other health states.

eupnea normal breathing (effortless, regular and noiseless).

eustress "good" stress.

euthanasia easy or painless death; often synonymous with "mercy killing.".

evaluation planned, ongoing deliberate activity in which the nurse, client, significant others and other health care professionals determine the extent of client outcome achievement and the effectiveness of the nursing care plan; a comparison against accepted standards.

eversion turning outward away from the body.

evisceration the protrusion of body organs through a wound.

examination an objective, systematic assessment of the patient's physical status.

excretion a substance discharged by the body.

exhalation the phase of breathing when air is passed out of the lungs; expiration.

exogenous infection an infection acquired from the local animate or inanimate environment.

expected outcome the behaviour the patient is expected to achieve.

experimental studies the researcher intervenes and changes one variable, then observes what happens.

expiration breathing out.

explanatory theory specify relationships among phenomena.

exploratory or descriptive data analysis involves tabulating, depicting and describing collections of data.

expressive aphasia individuals know what to say but cannot verbalize their thoughts.

extended care health services required by persons with long- term illness or disability and provided in nursing homes, intermediate care facilities, adult residential care, home care and ambulatory care.

extended family network of two or more related nuclear families, known in everyday language as relatives or kinsfolk. This family unit consists of grandparents, aunts, uncles and cousins, who may live near by or far away from one another.

extension the act of straightening.

external respiration breathing.

external validity things that happen in a study that make it difficult to apply study findings to other samples.

extracellular fluid fluids situated outside the cells of the body.

extraneous variables factors that might influence the measurement of study variables and the relationships between them.

exudate an inflammatory fluid discharged from an infected area of the body.

fair mindedness the ability to recognize bias and narrow thinking in themselves and in others.

faith healing based on the belief a person has in the healing power of an object or the healing ability of an individual.

false imprisonment individuals who are unjustifiably detained, or confined against their will and without a legal warrant for detention.

family two or more people, who may or may not be related by blood, marriage, or adoption, bound by strong emotional ties, a sense of belonging, and a commitment to live with and care for one another over time.

Family Allowance a universal social program in Canada through which every family with children receives an allowance, based on a certain amount per child.

family crisis state of disorganization in the family unit.

family dynamics interrelationships among members of a family, namely their roles, relationships and communication patterns.

family functions those activities a family performs in order to meet the needs of both individual family members and society as a whole.

family health is a dynamic process in which family members create adaptive patterns of interaction with one another and with an ever changing physical and social environment.

family stress a state of imbalance in the family.

family stressors life events or demands that impact on the family, producing stress or having the potential of producing stress, and ultimately require change.

family structure the way a family is organized.

family systems theory views the whole family as a unit of care, such that the family is the patient or client.

family therapy a branch of psychotherapy concerned with the use of family process to treat psychopathological conditions or other dysfunctions in families.

fantasy day-dreaming.

fat an organic water-insoluble compound found naturally in animals and plant seeds; also called lipid.

fatty acid a unit of fat consisting of a chain of carbon atoms linked to hydrogen ions and an acid group attached; may be saturated, monounsaturated and polyunsaturated.

fecal impaction a large, hardened mass of stool that cannot be expelled.

fecal incontinence a lack of control over bowel evacuation.

feces waste products excreted from the intestines.

feedback a process created by the output of a system which permits the system to maintain stability of its internal function; in family systems theory, a continuous process of input and output exchanges between families and the community that surrounds them.

femoral pulse the pulse located in the middle of the groin where the femoral artery passes over the pelvic bone.

fever an elevated temperature.

fidelity is based on trust and generates rules for promise-keeping based on respect for autonomy.

fight or flight mobilization of the bodies physiological defense mechanism as the body prepares for action.

figure-eight turn is used to bandage joints but also the entire length of an arm or leg.

filtration the process whereby water and dissolved substances are forced across a membrane from an area of high pressure to an area of low pressure by hydrostatic or fluid pressure.

First Nations the earliest settlers in Canada; the term includes native North American Indians and the Inuit.

fittingness is the criterion against which the applicability of qualitative findings be evaluated.

flexion the act of bending.

flowsheet graphic recording of interventions or observations that occur within a designated period of time.

fluid volume deficit used to designate a condition in which the body or tissues are deprived of water.

focus assessment information collected on an ongoing basis to determine changes in the patient's health status and the need for change in the nursing plan for care.

focus charting a type of charting in which the nurse identifies client concerns rather than problems and focusses on a behaviour, change, event or a nursing diagnosis.

fomites inanimate objects that carry infectious agents.

footboard a device made of plastic or wood that is placed at the foot of the patient's bed to serve as a support for the feet.

Fowler's position a sitting position in which the person's head and trunk are raised 45° to 90°.

fracture board a board made of wood or plexiglass that is placed under the patient's mattress to increase support.

frail elderly people who require nursing care or supervision.

fremitus a vibration that can be felt on the exterior chest wall when a person speaks.

frequency distribution analysis method that involves determining how often scores or values appear in a data set.

function the dynamic interaction among component parts of a system.

gay or lesbian family form of cohabitation in which individuals of the same gender live together, with or without children, and share a sexual relationship.

gender definition (gender identity) the perception of self as male or female.

gender role identity the behaviour identified by one's culture as appropriate to that gender; how a person behaves as male or female.

general adaptation syndrome (GAS) the response of the body to physiological stress.

generic name a drug's original name assigned by the individual or company that originally marketed the drug.

genogram diagram of the family constellation. It shows the structure of the intergenerational relationships of a family.

gestation term used to describe the development of new life that takes place in the womb between conception and birth.

gingivae the gums.

gingivitis inflammation of the gums.

gliding movement in one plane, as in sliding.

glomerulus each nephron consists of a glomerulus(cluster of capillaries).

gluconeogenesis the formation of glucose from proteins and fatty acids when carbohydrate stores are depleted.

glycogen a polysaccharide stored in the cells after the breakdown of carbohydrate.

glycogenolysis the conversion of glycogen to glucose in the liver.

good samaritan laws legislation designed to protect the professional practitioner from malpractice suits arising from care given to the injured at the scene of an accident or other emergency.

grand theory/mega theory a global statement that identifies phenomena (concepts or ideas) that are of interest to the discipline.

graph shows how many times each score has occurred, displaying the frequency of each score and illustrating the distribution of scores.

grief the total response to loss.

grounded theory a theory that has been grounded in reality derived from data systematically obtained from social research.

gurgles abnormal breath sounds described as a coarse, continuous sound produced by air flowing through large passages narrowed by secretions, mucosal swelling or obstruction.

gustatory pertaining to the sense of taste.

hair a filament of keratin, composed of a long, cylindrical shaft and a root. .

halal the lawful meat of Muslims.

half-life (of a drug) the time it takes for 50 percent of the plasma concentration of a drug to be eliminated from the body.

hallucinations false perceptions unrelated to reality.

hardiness a particular constellation of personality characteristics that helps people stay healthy despite facing stressful life events. It includes (1) commitment, (2) the ability to view change as a challenge, (3) a sense of personal control over life.

hazardous substance substance capable of causing injury upon exposure.

healing means to make whole.

health (1) a positive state of being that includes physical fitness, mental (or emotional) stability, and social and spiritual ease. (2) the extent to which an individual or group is able, on the one hand, to realize aspirations and satisfy needs; and, on the other hand, to change or cope with the environment.

health education a planned process aimed at helping individuals and communities achieve and maintain a level of health which is appropriate for them.

health educator a member of the health team who is responsible for the development of health education programs in a community.

health maintenance organization a form of prepaid group practice. They provide a comprehensive range of services on a fixed contract basis, which is paid for in advance by people enrolling in the organization.

health promotion the process of enabling people to increase control over, and to improve, their health.

health within illness an event that can expand human potential, not an enemy that the patient is expected to fight against. This is an opportunity for personal growth and transformation.

healthy communities process a means to identify and resolve local health issues.

healthy public policy public policy that is concerned with health and equity and with accountability for the health impact of the legislation.

hematest test that is used to determine occult blood in the stool.

hematoma a clot formed beneath the skin as a result of bleeding.

hematuria indicates blood in the urine.

hemiplegic a person with loss of function on one side of the body.

hemodialysis a procedure in which waste products and excess water are removed from the body by circulating blood from an artery through an external dialyser (sometimes referred to as the artificial kidney).

hemoccult slide commercial test that can be used to determine occult blood in the stool.

hemoptysis the coughing up of sputum containing varying amounts of blood.

hemorrhoids swollen veins of the anus or rectum.

herbal medicine plants or parts of plants that may be used for their medicinal effect.

herbalist a person who treats people with potions, salves and brews made from various plants.

hesitancy difficulty initiating urination.

high-risk diagnosis describes a potential problem.

Hinduism a religion, a social system and a way of life for most of population of India with a belief in numerous gods and in reincarnation.

hirsutism increased hair growth.

histogram a graphic display of a frequency table using rectangular bars with heights equal to the frequency in a particular class.

holistic focussing on the total person, the reaction to stress and the factors influencing the person's ability to cope with stress and restore equilibrium.

holistic health an approach to wellness that recognizes the interaction between the whole person and his or her environment, and emphasizes harmony within oneself, with nature and the world.

homeopathy is a holistic system of therapeutics in that it takes a broad view of illness and how individuals express illness.

homeostasis the process by which the body brings into play certain mechanisms to maintain stability in its internal environment.

homeothermic warm-blooded.

homologogous or indirect transfusion carries the potential for incompatibility between the donor's blood and the recipient's blood and for exposure to blood borne disease.

homosexuality the romantic and sexual attraction to the same-gender partner; a sexual orientation.

hospice/palliative care refers to both a philosophy of care and an agency for inpatient and outpatient services for the dying person.

hospital postgraduate course an educational program in a clinical nursing specialty given in a hospital.

hot compress applications of either sterile or unsterile gauze sponges moistened with heated normal saline or antiseptic solution.

humanist school a theory that believes learning must involve the whole person (intellect and emotions).

humidifier a device that adds moisture to inspired air.

hunger an uncomfortable sensation that indicates a physiological need for nourishment.

hydrolysis a process of chemical digestion whereby nutrients are split into simpler elements by the addition of water to molecules.

hydrotherapy water treatments which include tubs, tanks and whirlpool baths.

hypercalcemia an excessive amount of calcium in the blood.

hyperextension straightening beyond the normal range of motion.

hyperkalemia an excessive amount of potassium in the blood.

hypermagnesemia an excessive amount of magnesium in the blood.

hypernatremia an excessive amount of sodium in the blood.

hyperopia farsightedness, a condition resulting from an error of refraction. It occurs behind the retina.

hyperphosphatmia an excessive amount of phosphate in the blood.

hypersomnia excessive sleeping, especially during the day.

hyperthermia an abnormally high body temperature; fever.

hypertonic having more solute concentration than another solution, thus exerting greater osmotic pressure than the other solution.

hyperventilation increase in rate and depth of respirations; a condition in which the amount of air in the alveoli exceeds metabolic demands.

hypervolemia an abnormal increase in blood volume.

hypnosis employs an artificially induced state that characterized by greater receptivity to suggestion.

hypnotic a drug that acts to induce sleep.

hypocalcemia a decrease in the amount of serum calcium.

hypochloremia a reduced concentration of chlorides in the blood.

hypokalemia a reduction in the amount of potassium in the blood.

hypomagnesemia a reduction in the amount of magnesium in the blood.

hyponatremia a decrease in the amount of sodium in the blood.

hypophosphatemia a reduction in the amount of phosphate in the blood.

hypothermia excessively low body temperature.

hypothesis suggests solutions or answers by translating the problem into a precise prediction of expected outcomes.

hypotonic having less solute concentration than another solution, thus exerting less osmotic pressure than the other solution.

hypoventilation an irregular slow, shallow pattern of alveolar ventilation which does not meet metabolic demands.

hypoxemia a decrease in the oxygen content of the blood.

hypoxia an insufficient supply of oxygen to the tissues.

identification modelling oneself on a successful person.

ileal conduit a urinary diversion procedure consisting of a reservoir constructed from a portion of the ileum and a stoma.

ileostomy a surgically created opening from the ileum of the small intestine to the abdominal wall.

ileum primary site in the small bowel for vitamin and bile salt absorption.

illness the personal experience of feeling unhealthy.

illusions false interpretations of environmental stimuli.

immunocompromised having an immune system that is impaired.

implementation step in the nursing process in which nurses use their knowledge and skills to carry out planned interventions.

incentive spirometer used to increase lung functioning and improve pulmonary ventilation.

incidence the number of instances of illness commencing, or of people falling ill, during a given period in a specific population.

incomplete proteins deficient in one or more essential amino acids.

incubation the period leading up to a disease.

independent variable (experimental/ intervention variable) a variable that the researcher establishes independently, e.g. treating Group A differently from Group B, or variations in population under study, e.g. age, gender.

inductive working from data collected to identify variables in order to generate theory.

inductive reasoning begins with specific details and facts and uses them to arrive at conclusions and generalizations.

induration hardening or firming of tissue.

industrial hygienist a member of the health team whose main concern is the detection and control of hazards in the work environment.

infection the deposition or invasion and multiplication of microorganisms on surfaces of the body or in body tissues causing adverse or ill effects.

inference the subjective interpretation of cues.

inflammation the protective response of body tissues to injury.

informed consent the consent must be consensual, freely given, informed, and specific to both the treatment and the caregiver.

inhalation the phase of breathing when air is taken into the lungs; inspiration.

input energy, information and resources that the system receives from the environment and then processes.

insensible water loss losses of fluid from the lungs and the skin through respiration and perspiration.

insomnia difficulty falling asleep or staying asleep, or excessive wakefulness.

inspection using the senses to assist in making judgements, comparisons and decisions.

inspiration breathing in.

instrument device used to record the data obtained from subjects.

intellectual humility that they (nurses) do not know everything.

intellectual integrity requires nurses to be consistent in the standards that they apply.

intentional injury are injuries caused with intent such as child abuse, family violence, suicide and homicide.

intermittent pain exacerbations and remissions of acute episodes of pain.

internal validity factors within a study design that may have influenced the findings.

interstitial fluid the fluid in the spaces between the cells.

intracellular fluid fluids situated within the cells of the body.

intrathecal analgesia a method of pain relief by injecting analgesic medication into the subarachnoid space for dispersion throughout the spinal fluid.

intravascular fluid the fluid in the blood and lymph vessels; plasma.

intuition experienced nurse's ability to assess a situation quickly, make decisions and act.

Inuit a separate group of the First Nations occupying small communities north of the treeline in Canada's Far North, stretching from the Mackenzie River Delta, through the Arctic Islands and Baffin Island, along the coast of Hudson Bay and Ungava Bay in Quebec, to the east coast of Labrador.

inversion turning inward towards the body.

iron important for building hemoglobin in red blood cells and preventing nutritional anemia.

ischemia decreased supply of oxygenated blood to a body part or organ.

Islam the religion of the Muslims, based on the revelations of the god Allah through his prophet Mohammed.

isokinetic exercise exercise in which the speed of muscle shortening is controlled by a machine or electronic device.

isometric exercise exercise in which muscle tension is increased with little movement of the joint or change in muscle length.

isotonic having the same solute concentration as another solution, thus exerting the same osmotic pressure as the other solution.

isotonic exercise exercise in which the tension of a muscle remains constant while its length changes to move the resistance (weight) through a range of motion.

isotonic fluid deficit occurs when water and electrolytes are both lost in approximately the same proportions and the osmolality of the remaining fluids is normal.

jargon technical terms common to a particular field but not common outside of that field.

jaundice is a yellowish discoloration of the skin and indicates increasing levels of bilirubin in the blood.

jejunum primary site in the small bowel for fat and carbohydrate absorption.

Judaism a religion of the Jewish people with a belief in one God and based on mosaic and rabbinical teaching.

kaccha in Sikhism, special undershorts worn by members of both genders, as a reminder of modesty and sexual morality for women.

kanga a comb worn in the hair by Sikhs.

kara a steel bangle, worn on the right wrist by Sikhs.

karma the law of cause and effect.

kegel exercises pelvic floor strengthening exercises.

ketosis abnormal accumulation of ketones in the body resulting from a deficiency or inadequate utilization of carbohydrates.

kilocalorie a thousand calories; the amount of heat needed to raise the temperature of one kilogram of water by one degree Celsius.

kinesiologist a member of the health team who specializes in human movement and human performance.

kinesthesia the sense that tells the person where body parts are in relation to one another.

Kirpan a symbolic dagger, worn under the clothes by Sikhs as a symbol of readiness to fight.

knee-chest position a person kneels with the buttocks upward. The upper body part is support by flexed elbows.

knowledge deficit not a nursing diagnosis; refers to the lack of knowledge a patient has about his or her condition or about aspects of his or her care.

koilonychia spoonshaped nail with a concave curve.

Koran the Holy Scriptures of the Islamic religion.

kosh uncut hair maintained by Sikhs.

kusti a woven cord worn around the waist.

labour the process by which the baby is expelled from the uterus.

laissez-faire a teaching style in which the students make all decisions about learning.

lanugo fine downy hair covering the body of the fetus.

large intestine primary function is to absorb water, electrolytes and remaining nutrients, the synthesis of vitamins, and the storage and elimination of feces.

lateral position lying on the side.

laxative a substance that promotes the passage of a soft stool.

laying on of hands the use of touch to promote healing, for example, the anointing of the sick.

learned resourcefulness learned repertoire of skills that people use to regulate their lives and overcome the stresses of life.

learning a change in the individual caused by the person's interaction with the environment.

lecture uninterrupted talk that presents information.

lesion traumatic or pathologic change in previously normal structures.

leukocytes white blood cells.

libel term used for defamation of character through written words, as in a letter to a third party, or depicted in a cartoon that causes the person to be the subject of ridicule or contempt.

licence a permit granted by a government agency to an individual to engage in the practice of a profession and to use a particular title.

licensed practical nurse (LPN) (Registered Nursing Assistant (RNA) in Ontario and Certified Nursing Assistant (CNA) in Alberta). A person trained in basic nursing techniques and direct patient care who practises under the supervision of a registered nurse or a physician in hospitals and other health care settings.

line of gravity is an imaginary straight line that passess through its centre of gravity to form a right angle with the ground.

linea nigra a vertical line of dark pigment which appears between the pubic area and the naval.

listen attentively hear a person speaking.

lithotomy position a position in which the patient lies on the back with the hips flexed and slightly abducted and the knees flexed.

living will an advance directive in which an individual writes down preferences for treatment in the event that he/she cannot decide for him/herself.

local adaptation syndrome (LAS) localized reactions which occur when a specific part or organ of the body is affected by a stress.

local effect drug action which is confined to a specific area of application.

local inflammatory response during injury, the body activates a visible protective response. It begins with four classic signs, redness, heat, swelling and pain. Loss of function may also occur.

long-term goals goals that will be achieved over a long period of time, sometimes weeks or months.

loss any life event in which one is deprived of something that is valued.

love and belonging need the need for love and affection and for a supportive network of friends, family and/or significant others.

maceration softening of tissue by soaking in fluid.

macrosystems the whole individual is viewed as a part of larger systems.

magnesium mineral important in the regulation of body temperature, nerve conduction and muscle contractions.

malignant wound a cancerous growth on the outside of the body. It is made up of skin and vascular cells.

malnutrition a state of poor health resulting from a long-standing dietary intake that either fails to meet or greatly exceeds nutritional needs.

malpractice negligent or incorrect treatment of a patient by a health professional; may include other claims such as breach of contract.

massage therapy the systematic use of friction, stroking and kneading to improve circulation and mobility, drain lymph and release tension.

masturbation the stroking and stimulation of one's own genital area.

material justice equal share according to need, effort or merit.

mature minor one who has demonstrated that he/she has the intelligence, understanding, and independence to make his/her own decisions in regard to the acceptance or rejection of medical treatment.

mean (average) a measure of central tendency derived by dividing the sum of the values in a data set by the total number of values, scores, or subjects in it; represented by the symbol $\bar{x}$, read as x bar.

measures of central tendency a statistic that summarizes the data into one representative value.

meatus an opening.

meconium the first bowel movement of the newborn infant; a greenish black, tarry substance.

median measure of central tendency that corresponds to the middle score.

meditation used to treat stress and manage pain.

Medicaid a federal government program in the US that provides personal health care services for the poor.

Medicare in Canada, a national medical insurance program that covers the total population. In the United States, a national government program that provides personal health care services for older people.

medication a substance taken to treat a disease or condition.

melena black tarry-like stools.

melting pot the blending of various nationalities who have come as immigrants into a homogenous identity.

menarche the onset of the first menstrual period.

menopause the cessation of the menstrual cycle, occurring when a woman has not experienced menstrual flow for one to one-and-a-half years.

mensa the mind.

meridian the path of energy channels in the body.

mesoderm middle layer of the uterine wall.

message the thought, feeling or idea being conveyed in communication.

metabolism the physical and chemical changes that nutrients undergo after their absorption from the gastrointestinal tract; the use of simple sugars, amino acids, and glycerol by the body cells.

microbial flora microorganisms that live on or within the body and provide a natural immunity against certain infections.

micturition the act of emptying the bladder; urination, voiding.

midwifery the care of women and their families throughout the maternity cycle. Its mandate is to provide care for normal versus high-risk pregnancies and for normal newborns.

minimal justice equals must be treated equally.

minimal responders small reactions, such as a nod or single word, that signify a person is listening to a speaker.

mode category or class that has the highest frequency. It is the simplest measure of central tendency.

modular nursing in this method, the nurse is assigned a group of patients, usually eight to twelve, whose beds or rooms are close together in one geographic area of the nursing unit.

moral distress term used when a person knows the right thing to do but is unable to do so because of agency constraints.

morbidity the incidence of illness.

mortality rate the number of deaths relative to the population.

mosque house of worship.

motivation the stimulus of interest in carrying out a task.

mourning the process of incorporating the experience of loss into our everyday lives.

mouth is the anterior opening of the alimentary canal. .

mucosal folds small folds within the mucosal surface of the small intestine.

Muezzin a crier in the Muslim religion who calls the faithful to prayer five times a day.

multi-service agency the single entry point for people needing long-term care services at home or in the community, or who require care in a nursing home, or a charitable or municipal residential facility for older people. The range of services to be delivered includes visiting nurses, supporting housing, homemaking, friendly visiting, security programs, physiotherapy, nutrition counselling, meal programs and transportation as well as palliative care either at home or in the community.

multisectoral involving collaboration between different sectors, for example, actions that involve collaboration between the health care sector and the business, education, justice and law enforcement sectors, such as the passage of mandatory seatbelt legislation.

multi-skilling the consolidation of responsibilities for diverse work assignments within a single job description.

music therapy used to reduce anxiety and increase relaxation.

Muslim one who practises Islam.

mutagenic pertaining to influences causing permanent alterations in the genes.

mutual-aid a concept that refers to people helping other people.

myopia nearsightedness caused by the elongation of the eyeball. Refraction occurs in front of the retina.

nail a flattened, epidermal structure at the end of a finger or a toe. .

narcolepsy sudden, irresistible sleep attacks.

narcotics drugs that depress the central nervous system, relieving pain and producing sleep when taken in moderate doses, producing unconsciousness, stupor, coma and possibly death in excessive doses.

narrative charting progress notes are written in simple paragraph form and in chronological order as patient issues are presented; also known as source-oriented medical recording.

national health insurance model (public insurance model) one in which the government is the insuring agency. People pay a predictable sum to government, or a quasi-governmental agency, either through a premium or through taxes, to cover their health care costs.

national health services model model in which health services are provided and organized by the national government of a country.

natural immunity immunity acquired from having had certain diseases.

naturopath practitioner of natural medicine.

naturopathy a health doctrine based on drugless therapy and natural therapeutic and healing techniques.

nausea gastric distress accompanied by an urge to vomit.

nebulizer a device that generates a fine spray (aerosol) that is inhaled deeply into the respiratory tract.

necrotic contains dead tissue cells.

necrotic tissue dead tissue.

negative copers ineffective coping strategies.

negligence the omission to do something which a reasonable person, guided by those considerations which ordinarily regulate the conduct of human affairs, would do, or doing something which a prudent and reasonable person would not do.

nephron the functional unit of the kidney.

neuropathic pain can occur from injury to peripheral nerves that have been cut or exposed to chemotherapeutic agents or viruses.

neutral thermal environment the relatively narrow range of environmental temperature in which an infant can maintain normal body temperature with the least amount of oxygen consumption.

neutropenia abnormal decrease in neutrophils in the blood.

neutrophil granular leukocyte necessary for phagocytosis and the removal of bacteria and cellular debris.

night terrors often occur during stage 4 sleep.

nightmare frightening dream causing the individual to wake up; occurs during REM sleep.

nociceptor free sensory nerve ending responsible for pain reception.

nocturia the need to get up during the night to void.

nonmaleficence an ethical principle that requires that we do no harm.

nonproductive cough a cough without the production of mucous.

normothermic for humans, this means a temperature ranging from 36.6 to 37.5.

nosocomial infections institution-acquired infections.

noxious causing harm or injury.

nuclear family a husband and wife with their own or adopted children, who share a residence, divide their labour, and cooperate economically.

nuclear-dyad family comprised of a couple without children.

nuisances factors in the environment that may endanger health (such as excessive noise, offensive odours, and the like).

null hypothesis a hypothesis which, if rejected, indicates that the reverse is true and the relationship is considered to exist.

nurse manager charge nurse of a nursing unit.

nurse's aides also called nursing attendants, personal care attendants or health care aides, workers in this category are frequently trained on the job, or in a formal course of a few weeks' duration. The nature of the tasks varies from one agency to another.

nursing the actions taken by the nurse on behalf of, or in conjunction with the patient.

nursing audit method of evaluating nursing care through a review of patient records which document the care given.

nursing diagnosis a clinical judgement about individual, family, or community responses to actual or potential health problems/life processes.

nursing health history a primary tool for collecting baseline data which relies on skilful interviewing techniques.

nursing informatics a combination of computer science, information science and nursing science designed to assist in the management and processing of nursing data, information and knowledge to support or enhance the practice of nursing and the delivery of nursing care.

nursing practice act laws that govern the practice of nursing.

nursing problems patients' problems, which can be helped by nursing action.

nursing process a systematic and logical approach to practice which embodies a series of interrelated steps the nurse takes in planning and giving nursing care.

nutrient a chemical substance found in foods that provides energy for human metabolism and is needed for growth and repair of tissues, synthesis of enzymes and hormones and regulation of body processes.

nutritionist a member of the health team who advises people about good dietary habits, counsels them about nutrition problems and undertakes nutrition education programs for people in the community.

objective data information that can be observed, perceived, or measured through the use of the sense organs or through the use of instruments.

observation the collection of information through the use of the physical senses (sight, sound, touch, smell, and taste).

occlusive dressings self-adhesive dressings used on ulcerated areas, pressure sores, minor burns, abrasions, lacerations and post-operative wounds.

occult blood blood in stool that is only seen by a microscope.

occupational health a field of health concerned with the physical, mental and social well-being of people in relation to work and working environment and people's adjustment to work and the adjustment of work to people.

occupational therapist a member of the health team who is primarily concerned with the restoration of bodily functions through specific tasks or skills, rather than exercises and treatments.

Old Age Security a universal pension program in Canada that provides income security for older people.

olfactory pertaining to the sense of smell.

oliguria decreased production of urine; less than 30 ml per hour.

one-on-one discussion nurse directly relays content and engages the patient in informal discussion.

onset of action the time it takes for a drug to enter the bloodstream and begin its action on the body.

onychauxis excessive thickening of the nail.

onycholysis loosening of the distal nail edge from the nail bed.

onychorrhexis thin, brittle nail with an uneven edge.

open system a system that exchanges energy, resources and information with its environment.

open wound tissue injury with a break in the skin or mucous membrane.

operational definition definition of a concept such that someone else will measure it in the same way.

ophthalmoscope an instrument used to examine the eyes.

oral airway a curved, plastic device which slides over the tongue to hold it down and forward.

orderlies nursing attendants who assist with the care of patients in hospitals, extended-care facilities, nursing homes and similar establishments.

orientation phase the time it takes for a nurse and patient to get to know each other and begin to trust each other.

orthopnea the inability to breathe except when in a sitting or standing position.

orthostatic hypotension abnormally low blood pressure occurs when an individual stands too quickly from a lying position.

osmolality a measure of the number of osmotically active particles per kilogram of water (mmol/kg).

osmolarity the quantity (concentration) of dissolved substances in a solution.

osmosis the movement of a solvent, such as water, across a selectively permeable membrane from a solution that has a lower solute concentration to one that has a higher solute concentration.

osmotic pressure the force exerted by the nondiffusible particles in a solution which tends to draw water toward it; the amount of pressure required to prevent osmotic movement across a membrane.

otoscope an instrument used to examine the ears.

output energy, information and resources that are released back to the environment.

oxygenation the supply of oxygen to body cells.

pain a subjective experience; an unpleasant sensation resulting from the noxious stimulation of sensory nerve endings.

pain threshold the point at which a stimulus has reached sufficient intensity to activate pain receptors and produce a sensation of pain; the point at which the pain is first felt.

pain tolerance the amount of pain an individual is willing to endure.

palliative care active, compassionate care of the terminally ill at a time when goals of cure or prolongation of life are no longer paramount and when the emphasis of care is on the comfort and quality of life until death.

pallor is the absence of red-pink colour of the skin due to a decrease blood flow to the superficial vessels or to a decrease in hemoglobin.

palpation using touch to detect characteristics of the body.

pancha karma many means to cleanse the body of wastes.

panic severe form of anxiety.

paralysis loss or impairment of motor or sensory function due to neural or muscular disease.

paraorgasm stimulation of erogenous zones above the level of spinal injury.

paraphilia sexual preferences beyond or outside the usual.

paraplegic a person who is paralysed from the waist down.

parasomnias conditions characterized by disruptions of the sleep cycle; somnambulism, enuresis and night terrors.

parasympathetic nervous system a division of the autonomic nervous system.

paronychia inflammation of the nail folds.

partial pressure the pressure exerted by a single gas in a mixture, with the pressure directly related to its relative amount to the total pressure of the mixture.

participant observation researcher-involvement in the activities of the group.

passive artificial immunity immunity conferred by antibodies passed from the mother to the fetus through the placenta and/or breast milk.

passages turning points or changes taking place in adulthood.

passive ROM range of motion exercise performed by someone else.

pastoral care is the ministry of compassionate individuals who offer emotional and spiritual support to patients, family and staff.

pathogen the disease-producing agent of an infection.

pathogenic bacteria microorganisms capable of invading healthy tissue and causing injury to the body.

pathogenicity ability of an organism to cause disease.

pathos and machos bond that exists between the suffering and its meaning.

patient recipient of care can be an individual, family or a community.

patient contract a systematic agreement between the patient and the nurse that grants reinforcement to the patient for performing a specific desirable behaviour.

patient education is the use of the educational process for individuals, their families and other significant persons when dependent upon the health-care system for diagnosis, treatment or rehabilitation.

patient record an account of the patient's history, present health status, treatment and response to treatment; a means of communication among health care providers.

patient-centered care where decision-making is decentralized and put into the hands of those closest to the patient.

patient-controlled analgesia a drug delivery system that permits patients to self-administer small amounts of predetermined doses of narcotic analgesics as they need them.

PCIS (Patient Care Information System) a computerized system that documents patient care; in hospitals known as HIS (Hospital Information System).

peak action (peak effect) the point at which a drug reaches its highest blood level and maximum effect.

peak flow measurement of peak expiratory flow rates.

pediculosis an infestation of lice.

peer review a method of assessing the quality of care provided by a practitioner through a review of his/her work by a group of peers.

perception the conscious recognition and interpretation of a sensory stimulus.

percussion striking or tapping the body surface to produce sounds that correlate with the type of underlying tissue density.

peripheral vascular resistance the resistance to blood flow primarily caused by friction within the vascular walls.

peristalsis the rhythmic wave-like muscular contractions that move food down the gastrointestinal tract.

peritoneal dialysis a procedure in which waste products and excess water are removed from the body by instilling and later removing a dialyzing fluid into the peritoneal cavity.

person the individual, family, group or community that is the recipient of nursing care.

personal identity knowing who you are; formed through numerous biological, psychological and social challenges and demands throughout life.

personal space the amount of room a person prefers to keep between him- or herself and others.

pH the abbreviation for potential hydrogen, a measure of the hydrogen ion concentration in solution.

phagocytosis a process by which certain body cells engulf and destroy microorganisms and cellular debris.

phantom pain pain experienced after the cause of the pain has been removed, as pain in amputated limbs.

pharmacist a member of the health team whose primary area of responsibility is the preparation and dispensing of drugs and other chemical substances used in the detection, prevention and treatment of illness.

pharmacodynamics the study of the mechanisms of drug action and the effects on cellular function.

pharmacokinetics the study of a drug's four basic processes (absorption, distribution, metabolism and excretion).

pharmacology the study of drugs, their actions and their effects on living organisms.

phenomenological research concerned with how people perceive experiences.

phonation the ability to articulate words.

phospholipids act as structural lipids found in cell membranes and myelin sheath.

phosphorous mineral which aids in the formation and strengthening of bones and is necessary for energy production, calcium metabolism and muscle function.

physician's assistant (US) member of the health team usually employed by a physician who performs, under the supervision of the physician, many tasks traditionally considered a part of medical practice.

physiological needs include the need for water, for food, for air, for elimination, for rest and sleep, for temperature maintenance, and for the avoidance of pain.

physiotherapist a member of the health team who assists in assessing the patient's functional ability, strength and mobility; carries out therapeutic treatments, particularly those dealing with the musculoskeletal system; and teaches families and individuals exercises and other measures that can contribute to the patient's recovery and rehabilitation.

PIE charting acronym for Problem, Intervention and Evaluation (of nursing care); a problem-oriented approach to charting that eliminates the Care Plan and incorporates it into the daily documentation.

pitting edema small, indentation in the skin when pressure is applied to an edematous area.

placenta organ that attaches itself to the uterine wall and to the fetus by means of the umbilical cord.

plan of care the written plan of nursing action (interventions) for a patient.

plantar flexion extension of the foot away from the body.

plaque a film of mucous and bacteria on the teeth.

plateau a relatively constant level of a drug in the blood.

pleural friction rub where the lining of the pleura (visceral and parietal) rub together.

pneuma the spirit.

point of maximal impulse (PMI) the place in the fifth intercostal space of the thorax, 7–9 cm to the left midclavicular line. Below the left nipple.

policy a decision or an action taken in an organization by which other specific proposals are judged for their acceptability.

polyuria excretion of an excessive amount of urine.

popliteal pulse the pulse located on the inner aspect of the back of the knee.

population participants in a study.

populations at risk a group of people who, because of certain factors, are more likely to develop a disease or condition.

portability one of the five principles on which the Canadian health insurance plan is based. The term is used to mean that residents moving to another province continue to be covered by their home province until eligible for insured services in their new province (maximum 3 months), and that people absent from their home province temporarily will have insured services paid for (a) in another province at the rate set in the province of temporary residence (b) out-of-country at the rate normally paid in the home province.

possible problem identifies that a problem may exist but more information is needed in order to validate that a problem actually exists.

post-basic education formal educational programs offered by educational institutions for graduate nurses.

posterior tibialis pulse the pulse located on the inner aspect of the ankle.

postural drainage a form of chest physiotherapy that uses positioning to aid in drainage of secretions by the flow of gravity and deep breathing.

potential problem presence of risk factors in a data base without the accompanying defining characteristics of a hypothesized problem.

power hierarchy the actual or potential ability of individual family members to control, influence or change the behaviour of other family members.

powerlessness state in which an individual or group perceives a loss of personal control over certain events.

praxis is a reciprocal process of reflection and action that produces opportunities for transformation and emancipation.

predictive theory moves beyond explaining relationships, to predicting precise relationships among certain characteristics of a phenomenon or specific differences among groups.

presbyopia farsightedness resulting from a loss of elasticity of the lens. More commonly known as the aging eye.

pressure ulcers areas from which the skin has sloughed; also known as decubitus ulcers, bedsores or pressure sores. They occur from prolonged pressure on one part of the body with resultant loss of circulation to the area and subsequent tissue damage.

prevalence the number of instances of a given disease or other condition in a given population at a designated time.

primary health care the first level of service in a comprehensive health care system.

primary intention healing the process of repair to a wound where there is little or no tissue loss.

primary nursing a system of delivering nursing services where the nurse is responsible for planning complete 24-hour care for each patient.

primary source data collected from the patient.

Priory Model a philosophy of restorative care for older people.

prn order a type of standing order that is to be carried out as necessary, as determined by the nurse's judgement and the patient's need.

probability sampling/random sampling measure to ensure that each element in the study population has an equal and independent chance of being selected.

problem describes the state (e.g., health concern) that exists as specifically as possible.

problem list multidisciplinary and generated from the data base.

problem statement/research question outlines the stated purpose and identifies the general problem under study.

Problem-Oriented Medical Record (POMR) a patient record organized by the patient's problems in which members of the health care team document issues relevant to their discipline.

problem-solving teaching strategy using problems the student might encounter in practice.

problem-solving (discovery) nurse helps the patient identify the problem and work through possible solutions.

professional conduct review is the process (or processes) used by a regulating authority to respond to a complaint about a registrant or licensee.

program management new approach to the delivery of clinical services to specific patient groups in the hospital or the community.

progress notes documentation of patient issues as these are presented.

projection ascribing one's own unacceptable feelings to others.

pronation turning down toward the ground.

prone position lying on the abdomen with the head turned to one side.

proprietary hospital a small hospital, providing specialized mental health or addiction-related services.

proprioceptors sensory nerve endings that provide information about movement and the position of the body in space.

prostate gland located below the bladder neck, surrounding the urethra in the male.

protein a complex organic compound containing carbon, hydrogen, oxygen and nitrogen found in animals and plants.

proximal closer to the point of reference or the point of attachment.

pruritis the symptom of itching.

psychogenic pain arises from an emotional or psychological origin.

psychomotor domain the domain of learning tasks involving the development of skills.

psychosocial equilibrium a balance in a person's relationships with other people.

puberty the period of sexual maturation in humans when they become functionally capable of reproduction; marked by menarche in females and the production of sperm in males.

public general hospital a non-profit general hospital.

public health inspector (US: "sanitarian") a member of the health team concerned with the elimination or control of "nuisances," ensuring the safety of water, milk, and food supplies; ensuring that garbage and sewage disposal is properly carried out; enforcing public health laws with regard to sanitation; and assisting in control of communicable diseases.

public health nurse nurse whose role is health promotion and illness prevention throughout the life span.

public policy a policy that has been established and legislated by a public body, duly constituted to make policy in the area of concern.

pulmonary function tests a number of tests performed to assess lung function and identify the presence and severity of respiratory disease.

pulse a wave of blood caused by the contracting of the left ventricle of the heart.

pulse oximetry non-invasive method of measuring a patient's arterial blood oxygen saturation.

pulse pressure the difference between the systolic and diastolic pressure.

pulse rate the number of ventricle contractions per minute.

pulse rhythm the pattern of heart beats.

pulse tension the compressibility of the arterial wall.

pulse volume the size of the pulse wave.

purposive sampling selection of subjects based on the investigator's knowledge of the population under study and the elements of the study.

purulent drainage thick discharge which contains pus; white, yellow, green or pink in colour.

pyelogram a radiological procedure which outlines the renal pelvis, calices, ureters, and urinary bladder by means of a contrast medium.

pyrexia (fever) condition in which the body temperature is above normal.

quadraplegic a person who is paralysed from the neck down.

qualitative studies, usually descriptive in nature, in which knowledge is developed inductively from the data.

quality assurance a program designed to try to ensure that health care provided to patients is consistently of good quality.

quantitative includes experimental and non-experimental studies in which knowledge is derived deductively.

quasi-governmental agency one that is closely related to government and is responsible to it, although it operates autonomously, as, for example, in Canada, a Crown Corporation.

Qui Gong the healing art of building up a person's energy.

quota sampling selecting participants by proportional representation of different groups or strata within the total population.

rabbi the spiritual leader in Judaism (a teacher—not a priest).

radial pulse the pulse located in the inner aspect of the wrist on the thumb side where the radial artery passes over the radius.

radiology technologist a member of the health team who carries out diagnostic and therapeutic measures involving the use of radiant energy.

range of motion exercises exercises in which a body part is moved through a range of motion.

rapid eye movement (REM) stage of sleep where dreaming occurs.

rationalization giving socially acceptable reasons to defend one's actions.

reaction formation protesting too much against something for which someone secretly yearns.

reactive (situational) depression depression occurs as a result of a situation or an event in a person's life that would cause sadness.

reasonable prudence an individual acting with the care that any reasonable person with his or her knowledge, education and experience would take.

receiver the recipient of a message.

receptive aphasia individuals cannot understand what is being said.

receptivity the willingness to enter into the perspective of another.

recipient the receiver of donated blood.

recreation specialist a member of the health team concerned with promoting health and physical fitness. Responsibilities include the development of recreation, sports, and physical fitness programs in the community.

rectum peristaltic movements force stool into the rectum for defecation.

recurrent turn is used to bandage distal portions of the body, such as a finger.

refereed journal journal in which articles have been reviewed, assessed for accuracy, scholarliness and scientific merit and accepted for publication by an editorial board of experts.

referred pain pain that may be felt in one region of the body from a stimulus in another.

reflection is a mental exercise used to review and reconsider ideas and situations, and is very important to the development and use of critical thinking skills.

reflective practice enables the students to access, understand and learn through their lived experiences.

reflexes automatic responses to stimuli.

reflexology also known as "zone therapy," the study of the reflexes of the foot, which are believed to correspond to specific parts of the body.

registration the listing of an individual's name on the official roster of a governmental or non-governmental agency.

reframing ability to redefine a situation in order to consider it from many perspectives.

regionalization decentralizing the health care system by giving local authorities the power to make decisions about health care.

regression reverting to a form of behaviour that was acceptable at one stage of our development but is no longer considered appropriate.

regulating authorities purpose is the protection of the public from risk or harm.

rehabilitation the restoration of an individual who has been ill to the most complete level of social, physical and mental functioning possible.

reliability the extent to which a measuring device yields the same results wherever the same quantity is measured.

religion adherence to a belief system(doctrine).

remedial gymnast a member of the health team who specializes in rehabilitation through exercise.

renal anuria the cessation of urine production; urine output of less than 100 ml per day.

repetitive strain injuries a group of disorders caused by sustained, unnatural body postures and repetitive, forceful movements.

reporting the communication of information to another individual or a group of individuals; may be written or oral.

repression unconsciously forgetting that which we do not want to remember.

research concepts elements that are abstract and only measurable indirectly.

research design structure of an investigation, through which answers to research questions are sought.

research-based practice practice which includes three components: (1) the conduct of studies, (2) the dissemination of research findings, and (3) the utilization of research in practice.

respect the recognition of a person's worth and dignity.

respiration the exchange of oxygen and carbon dioxide between the atmosphere and the cells of the body.

respiratory character digressions from normal, effortless breathing.

respiratory depth the amount of air inhaled and exhaled with each breath movement.

respiratory rate the number of breath cycles per minute.

respiratory rhythm the regularity of the inhalation and exhalation cycles.

respiratory technologist a member of the health team who is an expert in diagnostic procedures and therapeutic measures used in the care of patients with respiratory problems.

rest repose or relaxation; implies freedom from emotional tension and physical discomfort.

restraints are any mechanical, physical, chemical, environmental or other method used to inhibit, limit or control an individual's behaviour or activity.

return demonstration a demonstration performed by the patient in order to learn a skill previously demonstrated by the nurse.

Rh factor inherited antigen on the surface of red blood cells.

rigor mortis a stiffening of the body after death.

risk the probability that an event will occur, e.g., that an individual will become ill within a stated period of time, or age.

risk diagnosis describes a potential problem.

role structure behaviours expected of members in designated positions.

role-play a teaching strategy in which students participate in a situation (real or imaginary) to learn appropriate actions or responses.

rotation turning in a circular motion around a fixed axis.

safety and security needs such fundamental components as adequate shelter from the elements and protection from harmful factors in the environment; includes feeling secure and protected from both real and imagined dangers.

safety to practise confirmation that beginning practitioners have the knowledge and skills necessary to practise their profession competently and without harming the people to whom they render care.

salwar kameze a traditional garment worn by Hindu and Sikh women consisting of a blouse or long tunic over loose trousers.

sample a small portion of a total population which serves to give information about the characteristics of the population sampled.

sanguineous discharge discharge of blood from a wound.

sanitarian term used for public health inspectors in the USA.

sari a traditional garment worn by Hindu and Sikh women consisting of a length of cotton or silk draped around the body as a skirt.

saturated fatty acid a form of fatty acid in which all carbon atoms are linked to hydrogen ions; it cannot take up any more hydrogen atoms.

scapegoating hostility directed at one particular person or group of people.

scope of practice defined and exclusive domain of practice for designated health professional.

screening a preliminary examination or testing to determine whether or not a person might have a particular condition and whether further diagnostic testing is indicated.

scultetus (many-tailed) binder a rectangular piece of cotton with 6 to 12 tails attached to each side; used to provide support to the abdomen or to retain dressings.

seasonal affective disorder (SAD) a depression that affects people at certain seasons of the year, particularly in winter.

sebaceous glands skin glands that secrete oil; located with hair.

secondary intention healing the process of repair to a wound where there is extensive tissue loss.

secondary source data collected from "significant other".

secretion a product produced by a gland.

selectively permeable membrane a type of membrane that allows some substances to pass through it but not others.

self is the most real aspect of one's experience. It is a frame of reference through which a person perceives, conceives and evaluates one's world.

self-actualization the need to attain one's highest potential and achieve one's ambitions in life.

self-care encouraging people to make healthy choices.

self-concept represents the total beliefs about the self. It is the individual's integration of self—body, mind and spirit.

self-disclosure a willingness to disclose opinions and feelings.

self-efficacy a belief in personal responsibility for one's own behaviour and in one's ability to influence events.

self-esteem the key to a person's behaviour. It influences thinking processes, emotions, desires, values and goals.

sensorium the part of the consciousness that includes the special sensory-perceptive abilities and the mental awareness of time, place and person.

sensory deficit a lack of or a deficiency in one of the senses.

sensory deprivation a prolonged reduction in exposure to sensory stimuli that may result from inadequate or monotonous stimuli, poorly functioning sense receptors, an inability to perceive environmental data, physical or social isolation, immobilization or restricted movement, or sensory overload.

sensory input receiving and accurately interpreting stimuli from the external environment.

sensory overload an overabundance of sensory stimulation.

serosanguineous drainage discharge of a combination of serous and sanguineous matter from a wound.

serous discharge discharge of the clear portion of blood, amber in colour, from a wound.

serum electrolyte electrolyte concentrations are measured on serum, the portion of plasma remaining after clotted blood is removed.

sex biological sexual identity or sexual intercourse.

sexuality the expression of self and the totality of feeling, attitudes, beliefs and behaviours related to being male or female.

shaman medicine man who deals with the spirit world.

shared governance the organization of hospital patient services in which staff nurses have more autonomy and decision-making authority than in the traditional structure. Also called "participatory management.".

shearing trauma caused by layers of tissue sliding against each other .

shiatzu Japanese form of acupressure in which pressure is applied to the body along the meridians (energy lines).

short-term goal expected outcomes that can be met in a relatively short period of time (a week or less).

sick building syndrome (SBS) an increase in the frequency of building-occupant-reported complaints associated with acute, non-specific symptoms in non-industrial environments that improve while away from the building.

sickness a status defined by the social actions or roles that an individual assumes when he or she experiences illness or is diagnosed with a disease.

Sikhism an offshoot of Hinduism with a belief in one God and in reincarnation.

simple random sampling selecting a sample using a table of random numbers.

Sims' position a lateral position in which the patient is semi-prone (sometimes called 3/4-prone).

single-parent family a mother or father living with one or more dependent children.

situation-based interpretive approach to grasp a principle and to learn it at a functional level requires many practical experiences in which the principle is embedded.

situational constraints aspects of our structural and interpersonal work environments that impede our implementation of the standards of our practice and thus jeopardize the quality of patient and family care.

sitz bath a special bath used to cleanse and to provide comfort and warmth to the perineal area.

skill mix each team member's knowledge, skills and judgement are maximized, duplication of effort is reduced and quality of care is enhanced.

skin turgour elasticity of skin, provides an indication of hydration.

slander defamation of character through spoken words.

sleep a period of decreased mental alertness and physical activity which is part of the normal daily pattern of living and is necessary for life.

sleep apnea a sleep disorder characterized by repetitive pauses in breathing lasting from 10 seconds to 2 minutes.

sleep deprivation a decrease in the amount, quality, or consistency of sleep.

small intestine is a narrow muscular tube 2.5 cm in diameter and 7 m in length which accepts food from the stomach.

SOAPIE format method of charting information in which information is organized on a POMR; SOAPIE is an acronym for Subjective data, Objective data, Assessment, Plan, Interventions and Evaluation.

social climate atmosphere created by interpersonal relationships between people in a group.

social safety net a network of programs to protect people from the crippling effects of unexpected financial, social or health problems as, for example, by ensuring income security for those in need and universal health care.

social worker a member of the health (and social services) team who assists in evaluating the psychosocial situation of the patient and helps people with social problems.

socialization the process by which people learn the beliefs, values and lifeways of a culture.

socioeconomic model an approach to health that recognizes the importance of the relationship between health and the economic and social dimensions of a community.

solo research study conducted by a researcher working independently.

solute a substance that dissolves in a solution.

solvent the fluid (water) in which substances are either dissolved or suspended.

soma physical body.

somatic pain pain which originates from the skin, muscles, or joints; it may be superficial or deep.

somatization expression of emotional and psychosocial discomfort through physical symptoms or body language.

somnambulism sleepwalking.

sordes a thick, furry substance which coats the tongue; caused by lack of oral hygiene.

source the sender of a message.

speciality a specifically defined area of clinical and functional nursing with a narrowed, in-depth focus, necessary for the safe delivery of the full range of services required in that area of nursing.

specificity clarification of the nature of a patient's problems.

speech language pathologists carry out diagnostic and therapeutic measures with individuals who have language and speech difficulties.

sphygmomanometer an instrument used to measure blood pressure consisting of an inflatable cuff, an inflation bulb with a release valve and a mercury manometer or an aneroid pressure gauge.

spiral reverse turn is used to bandage cylindrical parts of the body that are of varying circumference.

spiral turn is used to bandage a part of the body that is of uniform circumference.

spirit comes from the Latin word for breath.

spirituality that part of ourselves that gives us power, energy and motivating force.

splinting a method that provides support to the incision during coughing; involves applying external pressure to wound site.

sputum mucous secretion from the lungs, bronchi and trachea; not saliva.

stage of exhaustion occurs if the stressor is severe enough and persists over a period of time. Depletes the body's resources for adaptation.

stage of resistance when the battle for equilibrium is most active.

standard deviation the average distance of the deviations from the mean.

standard precautions a revised set of guidelines published by the Center for Disease Control. They blend the major features of the universal s and body substance precautions.

stat order a type of self-terminating order that is to be carried out immediately and only once.

statistics the systematic collection, organization, analysis and interpretation of numerical data.

stertor a snoring sound made when secretions are present in the trachea or large bronchi.

stethoscope an instrument used to amplify body sounds.

stoma an opening.

storytelling method of teaching using stories that present information, usually to children.

straight abdominal binder a rectangular piece of cotton long enough to encircle the abdomen and overlap at least 5 cm; used to retain abdominal dressings or to apply pressure and support the abdomen.

stratified sampling a random selection made from different sub-groups within the population.

street clinics storefront or free clinics developed in the 1960s and 1970s in both Canada and the United States. Set up in poor neighbourhoods, they provide services for people who are reluctant to use the traditional agencies. The clinics offer readily accessible care, usually on a 24-hour free basis in a setting that is as devoid of "red tape" as possible.

strengths physical and psychosocial capabilities, the cultural and religious values and beliefs, and the spiritual dimensions of persons or families which enable them to cope with the challenges of daily living.

stress the body's response to any demand made upon it.

stress incontinence the excretion of small amounts of urine involuntarily with exertions such as coughing or laughing.

stress response physiological response to stress which is modulated by the emotion a person attaches to the stressor.

stressor any factor that disturbs the organism's equilibrium.

stretch marks reddish streaks that develop on the breast and abdomen during pregnancy.

stridor a harsh high-pitched "crowing" sound heard on inspiration caused by a narrowing of the larynx or trachea.

structure the arrangement of the specific parts of a system.

structured interview an interview controlled and directed by the interviewer for the purpose of gathering specific information.

subject in research, a participant in a study.

subjective data in nursing, information reported primarily by the patient or the patient's family or significant other.

sublimation channelling socially unacceptable motives into acceptable forms of behaviour.

subsystems hierarchies in family systems theory; two or more interrelating family members can form subsystems, such as the spousal subsystem, the parent-child subsystem, or the sibling subsystem.

sudreh a white muslin vest.

suffering is a state of distress induced by the threat of the loss of intactness or the disintegration of a person from whatever cause.

superinfection a new infection superimposed upon a previous infection.

supination turning upward (the opposite of pronation).

supine position lying on the back without a pillow under the head and shoulders.

support/mutual aid groups assist people with a variety of specific problems and illnesses.

supporting cue information used to assure the certainty of the patient state when combined with other cues.

suppression deliberately putting something unpleasant out of one's mind.

suppuration the production and exudation of purulent matter or pus.

suprasystem in family systems theory, the physical, social and cultural environment with which the family interacts in order to sustain its life, continuity and growth.

susceptibility the degree of resistance of a host to a pathogen.

sweat glands skin glands that produce sweat.

symbiotic relationship a mutually beneficial relationship.

sympathetic nervous system a division of the autonomic nervous system, "fight or flight response".

symptomatic period the stage of infection when signs and symptoms of the infection are present.

synagogue the Hebrew place of worship.

syndrome diagnosis cluster of actual or high-risk nursing diagnoses that are predicted to be present because of a certain event or situation.

synergistic (potentiating) effect the combined action of two drugs which is greater than the intended effect of a single drug.

system two or more connected elements or parts which mutually interact to form an organized whole.

systematic sampling taking every *n*th member of the population, e.g. every 10th name on a list.

systemic effect the action of a drug on the whole body after it is absorbed and distributed to the tissues.

systems theory is a science of wholeness. It examines the interconnection of two or more parts that form an organized whole and that interact with each other. The whole is greater than the sum of its parts.

systolic pressure the force exerted against the arterial wall as the left ventricle contracts.

T-binder two strips of cotton attached in the shape of a *T*; used to retain perineal dressings.

tachycardia a very high pulse rate (over 100 beats per minute).

tachypnea an abnormal increase in respiratory rate; also called polypnea.

tactile pertaining to the sense of touch.

Tai Chi a form of medication in motion, used both as part of a spiritual quest and as a lifestyle health practice.

teaching is an interactive process that facilitates learning.

teaching plan includes content to be taught and strategies to be implemented.

temporal pulse the pulse located anterior to the ear at the mandibular joint, where the temporal artery passes over the temporal bone.

tenesmus painful straining in unproductive attempts at defecation.

TENS a small machine that can be operated by the patient to relieve pain and promote wound healing.

teratogenic pertaining to influences during pregnancy that result in physical defects to the fetus.

termination phase the stage when the nurse ceases to care for the patient.

testator the individual making a will.

theoretical pluralism in the case of an educational program, the teaching of several nursing models.

theoretical sampling used in grounded theory as a process for generating theory.

theory a supposition, or system of ideas that has been proposed to explain a given happening in the world.

therapeutic effect the desired response of drug action.

therapeutic relationship the relationship between the nurse and a patient that enables the nurse to administer care.

therapeutic touch a non-invasive type of therapy involving the laying on of hands.

thermal injury tissue injury caused by exposure to extreme heat.

thermoregulation the physiological control of body temperature (heat production and heat loss).

thoracentesis the insertion of a needle through the chest wall and into the pleural space for the aspiration of fluid or air.

tolerance occurs when there is a need to increase the dose of the drug in order to achieve the same initial effect.

tooth a dental structure of the jaw used to cut, grind and chew food for the process of ingestion.

tort legal wrong committed by one person against the person or property of another.

total pain describes the multidimensional (physical, psychological, social and spiritual) suffering experienced by cancer patients.

trade (brand/proprietary) name the manufacturer's copyrighted name for a drug.

traditional Chinese medicine a preventive rather that curative approach revolving around theories of energy flow and elements.

transcendence an experience that is outside normal sensory phenomenon.

transformation the changing of input into meaningful forms that can be used for an organism's survival.

transsexualism also known as gender dysphoria; occurs when gender identity does not match biological gender.

transvestism cross-dressing; dressing like the opposite gender for sexual pleasure or psychological comfort.

triangular binder a triangular piece of cotton with two sides approximately one metre in length; used as a full triangle or folded for a variety of applications; often called a sling.

triglyceride a lipid compound made up of three fatty acids to one glycerol base.

trochanter roll used to prevent external hip rotation.

turgor refers to the elasticity of the skin.

type A personalities (workaholics) people who tend to drive themselves to the brink of exhaustion while ignoring the need for rest and relaxation.

typing blood test that is done to confirm a person's blood group.

ulnar pulse the pulse located on the opposite side of the wrist to the radial.

umbilical cord cord through which the fetus receives nourishment and oxygenated blood and disposes of wastes.

undermining tissue destruction underlying intact skin.

unintentional injuries are injuries caused for the most part, without purpose, such as motor vehicle collisions, drownings, falls, burns and poisonings.

universal precautions guidelines published by the Center for Disease Control that state that all blood and body fluids should be treated as though they are potentially infectious.

universality one of the five principles on which the Canadian health insurance plan is based—all insured persons of a province must be entitled to the services provided by the plan on uniform terms and conditions.

unsaturated fatty acid a form of fatty acid which is capable of absorbing more hydrogen ions.

uremia an excessive amount of urea and other non-protein waste products of metabolism in the blood.

ureter the tube that carries urine from the kidney to the urinary bladder.

urethra a short, muscular tube which carries the urine from the bladder to its exit point from the body.

urgency the need to void in a hurry.

urinalysis an examination of urine.

urinary bladder a distensible muscular sac which serves as a reservoir for urine.

urinary frequency voiding more often than usual.

urinary incontinence the inability to control urination.

urinary retention the inability to pass urine despite bladder distention.

urostomy an artificial opening or stoma made to divert urine from the kidneys to the abdominal wall.

vaccine a preparation of attenuated or dead microorganisms administered to induce active immunity against infectious diseases.

validate the knowledge base explore how a study relates to and builds on previous research and theory in the field.

validity the extent to which tests measure what they are intended to measure.

values the ideas, attitudes and beliefs about the worth of any entity that bind together the members of a common culture.

variable in research, a quality, characteristic or property of an object, a person, or a situation that can and does change in different circumstances.

vector carrier of disease.

venipuncture insertion of a needle or catheter for intravenous therapy.

venous ulcer located in the lower leg area and comprised venous circulation in which leaky valves allow fluid to accumulate in the interstitial tissue.

vernix a creamy white substance which protects the baby's skin in the womb and eases its passage through the birth canal.

vestibular system a proprioceptive sense, located in the inner ear that conveys information about the position of the body in space; the sense of balance.

villi tiny finger-like projections within the folds of the mucosal surface of the small intestine which serve as sites of absorption of fluids and nutrients.

virulence an organism's ability to cause disease.

visceral pain pain which arises from sources in the abdominal cavity.

visual acuity the ability to see objects or persons clearly.

visual field the entire area an eye sees when it is fixed on a central point.

vital signs temperature, pulse and respirations; also known as cardinal signs.

vitiligo a benign condition consisting of white, patchy areas of the skin where the melanin pigment is completely absent.

vomiting the forceful ejection of the stomach's contents.

warmth implies a genuine liking for people.

welfare society a society characterized by a multisectoral approach to the promotion of health; consumer participation in the formulation of health and social policies; and partnerships in research and training between business, government, educational institutions and health agencies.

welfare state one which provides a wide range of health and support services for its people, as, for example, unemployment insurance, universal old age pensions, national health insurance.

well-being the personal experience of a feeling of ability, harmony and vitality.

wellness a state of optimal health or optimal functioning.

wellness diagnosis clinical judgement about an individual, family, or community in transition from a specific level of wellness to a higher level of wellness.

wheeze a high pitched "whistling" sound often made on inspiration when the airway is partially obstructed.

will a declaration of an individual's wishes regarding what is to be done with his/her property after death.

working phase the time when the nurse and patient determine and implement a plan of care.

wound irrigation the introduction of a solution called an irrigant into the wound to wash out exudate, drainage and debris so the wound can heal.

yarmulke a skull cap.

YinYang flow two opposing but complementary forces which Chinese philosophers believe balance everything in the universe.

yoga the use of postures, breathing and visualization exercises to improve mobility, circulation, digestion and energy level.

Zoroastrianism the oldest monotheistic religion practised today with a highly moral belief system that salvation is the reward for those who follow "good thoughts, good words and good deeds.".

zygote fertilized ovum.

Index

A

I

N

O

Q

R

S

X

Y

Z

Photo Credits

Al Harvey: 33, 321, 393, 407, 479, 534 (right), 543, 544, 627, 670 (right), 672 (E, F, G, and H), 674, 675, 679 (left), 681 (both), 706 (both), 747 (both), 927 (all), 929, 930 (bottom left, bottom right), 932 (all), 933 (top and middle), 935, 1016, 1157

Augustine Medical, Inc. Reproduced with permission: 773, 791

Beverly Du Gas/Emily Knor: 10, 66, 158, 166 (bottom), 168, 171(both), 175, 193, 216, 217, 484, 900, 905, 948, 981, 1065, 1210, 1216, 1220, 1221, 1230

Bill Wittman: 213, 219

Bill & Peggy Wittman: 166 (top)

Canada Wide: 1182

Canapress/Paul Chiasson: 1242

Canapress/Ryan Remiorz: 243

Cindy Goodman, North Shore News, Courtesy of Lion's Gate Hospital, North Vancouver:, BC: 155, 707

Courtesy of Appleton & Lange from their title *Clinical Nursing Skills: Basic to Advanced Skills: Fourth Edition* (1996) by Smith and Duell: 578, 674 (bottom left, bottom right)

Courtesy of Appleton & Lange from their title *Fundamentals of Nursing: Collaboration for Optimal Health* (1992) by Berger and Williams: 123, 592, 672 (A, B, C, and D), 673 (top), 723

Courtesy of Lion's Gate Hospital, North Vancouver BC: 325, 801, 807, 819, 831, 843 (both), 860, 875, 893 (right), 930 (top right), 976, 1002, 1004, 1037, 1038 (right), 1039, 1048, 1062, 1072, 1074, 1162, 1181, 1257

Courtesy of Registered Nurses Association of British Columbia: 201, 202, 1133

Courtesy of Respiratory Services, St. Paul's Hospital, Vancouver, BC: 53, 739

Courtesy of the IVAC Corporation, San Diego CA: 392 (both)

Courtesy of the Vancouver General Hospital Nurses Alumnae Association Archives: 36

Courtesy of Vancouver Hospital and Health Sciences Centre: 677 (bottom), 678 (middle left, middle right, bottom left, bottom right)

Dick Hemingway: 173, 179, 185, 776

First Light/Bob Gomel: 177

FPG International LLC/Artic Rawls: 438

Image Network: Inc.: 98

Image Network/Chris Minerva: 406

Image Network Inc./Gary Hofheimer: 299

Image Network Inc./Ken Glaser: 805

Image Network Inc./Matthew Borkoski: 351

Image Network Inc./Patricia Levy: 466

Image Network Inc./Tom Campbell: 286

Image Network Inc./Tomas Del Amo: 72

Image Network Inc./Willie Hill Jr.: 285

Kate Williams, Courtesy of The Richmond Hospital, Richmond, BC: 408, 416, 871 (top right), 894, 931, 939, 952

Lakehead University, Native Nurses Entry Program: 268

Langara College, Nursing Department, Vancouver, BC: 483, 683

Lauchlin McKenzie: 205, 382, 385, 396 (both), 405, 433, 534 (left), 552, 562 (both), 583 (both), 608, 670 (left), 673 (bottom left, bottom right), 678 (top left, top right), 680 (all), 685, 720, 750, 758 (all), 799 (right), 817 (all), 818 (all), 871 (bottom left), 883, 926 (both), 928, 930 (top left), 931, 933 (bottom), 934, 938 (all), 1038 (left), 1041, 1042 (all), 1043 (both), 1044 (all), 1045 (all), 1049 (all), 1050 (all), 1051 (all), 1052 (all), 1053 (all), 1054 (both), 1056, 1075, 1089 (both), 1096, 1100, 1110, 1130, 1132, 1140, 1141, 1142, 1143, 1144, 1148 (all), 1149, 1152, 1158 (both), 1159, 1162, 1194

Marta Tomins: 872

Memorial Nurse Portrait Collection of the BC History of Nursing Groups. Dolls designed by Sheila Rankin Zerr: 81

Multicultural Health Education Program of The Vancouver Heath Department:: 6, 43, 71, 87, 131, 172, 254, 269, 364, 499, 944, 961, 1219

National Archives of Canada: 3

North Shore News/Courtesy of Lion's Gate Hospital, North Vancouver, B.C.: 893 (left)

Photo Researchers, Inc.: 778

Prentice Hall Archives: 485

Prentice Hall Inc.: 677 (top), 679 (right)

Prentice Hall Inc./George Dobson: 441, 526

Prentice Hall Merrill Publishing/Tom Watson: 446

Scott Cunningham: 13

Simon & Schuster/Prentice Hall College Inc.: 77

Simon & Schuster/Prentice Hall College Inc./ Michael Heron: 464

Stock Boston/David J. Sams/Texas Imprint: 342

Stock Boston/Miro Vintoniv: 300

The Slide Farm/Al Harvey: 58, 156, 178, 252, 899, 913

The Vancouver Hospital and Health Sciences Centre, the British Columbia Children's Hospital, and the Canadian Liver Foundation. Reprinted with Permission: 455

Tony Stone Images/Bruce Ayres: 184

Unicorn Stock Photos/A. Ramey: 1, 456

Unicorn Stock Photos/Aneal Vohra: 2

Unicorn Stock Photos/Greg Greer: 884

Unicorn Stock Photos/Jeff Greenberg: 731

Unicorn Stock Photos/Jim Shippee: 888

Unicorn Stock Photos/MacDonald Photography: 943

Unicorn Stock Photos/Paul A. Hein: 885

Victoria General Hospital,Winnipeg: 799 (left)

Procedures and Special Features

Procedures

Continued from previous page

Health History Guide

Key Principles

Health-Promoting Strategy

Community Health Practice

Gerontological